BLACKWELL'S FIVE-MINUTE VETERINARY CONSULT: RUMINANT

SECOND EDITION

BLACKWELL'S FIVE-MINUTE VETERINARY CONSULT

RUMINANT

SECOND EDITION

Edited by

Christopher C.L. Chase, DVM, PhD
Diplomate ACVM (Immunology and Virology)
Professor, Department of Veterinary and Biomedical Sciences
College of Agriculture and Biological Sciences
South Dakota State University, Brookings, South Dakota, USA

Kaitlyn A. Lutz, VMD
Diplomate ABVP (Food Animal)
Consultant in Production Animal Agriculture – International
Pennsylvania, USA;
Private Practitioner – Dairy, Ashburton, New Zealand

Erica C. McKenzie, BSc, BVMS, PhD
Diplomate ACVIM
Professor, Large Animal Internal Medicine
Department of Clinical Sciences
College of Veterinary Medicine
Oregon State University, Corvallis, Oregon, USA

Ahmed Tibary, DMV, MS, DSc, PhD
Diplomate ACT
Professor, Department of Veterinary Clinical Sciences
College of Veterinary Medicine
Washington State University, Pullman, Washington, USA

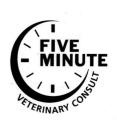

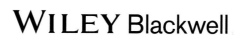

This second edition first published 2017 © 2017 by John Wiley & Sons, Inc.

Edition History
John Wiley & Sons, Inc. (1e, 2009)

The right of Christopher C.L. Chase, Kaitlyn A. Lutz, Erica C. McKenzie, and Ahmed Tibary to be identified as the authors of the editorial material in this work has been asserted in accordance with law.

Registered Office
John Wiley & Sons, Inc., 111 River Street, Hoboken, NJ 07030, USA

Editorial Office
111 River Street, Hoboken, NJ 07030, USA

For details of our global editorial offices, customer services, and more information about Wiley products visit us at www.wiley.com.

Wiley also publishes its books in a variety of electronic formats and by print-on-demand. Some content that appears in standard print versions of this book may not be available in other formats.

Library of Congress Cataloging-in-Publication Data

Names: Chase, Christopher C.L. (Christopher Civilian Louis), 1956- editor. | Lutz, Kaitlyn A. (Kaitlyn Ann), 1985- editor. | McKenzie, Erica C. (Erica Claire), 1974- editor. | Tibary, A. (Ahmed) editor.
Title: Blackwell's five-minute veterinary consult. Ruminant / edited by Christopher C.L. Chase, Kaitlyn A. Lutz, Erica C. McKenzie, Ahmed Tibary.
Other titles: Five-minute veterinary consult. Ruminant | Ruminant
Description: Second edition. | Hoboken, NJ, USA : Wiley, 2017. | Includes bibliographical references and index. |
Identifiers: LCCN 2017028666 (print) | LCCN 2017029572 (ebook) | ISBN 9781119064695 (pdf) | ISBN 9781119064701 (epub) | ISBN 9781119064688 (cloth)
Subjects: | MESH: Ruminants | Animal Diseases | Veterinary Medicine–methods | Handbooks
Classification: LCC SF997.5.R86 (ebook) | LCC SF997.5.R86 (print) | NLM SF 997.5.R86 | DDC 636.2089–dc23
LC record available at https://lccn.loc.gov/2017028666

Cover design by Wiley

Set in 9/10pt GaramondPro by Aptara Inc., New Delhi, India
Printed in Singapore by C.O.S. Printers Pte Ltd

10 9 8 7 6 5 4 3 2 1

To Mary Chase, my wife and best friend, whose support and patience was essential for the completion of this project. Thank you for always being there.

Christopher C.L. Chase

To Drs Michaela Kristula, Billy Smith, and Rob Callan whose tireless attention to detail rubbed off and gave me the tools to complete this project, Dr Tim Holt whose passion is contagious, and to my very encouraging friends and family.

Kaitlyn A. Lutz

Dedicated with gratitude to my husband, David, for his endless love and patience, and his understanding of the demands of academic life.

Erica C. McKenzie

To my families in Morocco and Minnesota, my wife Brigitte for her support, and to all who share their clinical knowledge through books.

Ahmed Tibary

PREFACE

With production animal agriculture changing at an alarming rate, the individuals who service these animals, producers, and businesses are called upon to remain current in a myriad of areas. Every farm visit confirms the necessity of possessing knowledge beyond traditional medical and surgical techniques. Veterinarians are challenged to advise producers in areas such as advanced reproductive techniques, precision-feeding, farm economics, facility design, governmental regulations, and biosecurity, to name a few. This second edition of *Wiley-Blackwell's Five-Minute Veterinary Consult: Ruminant* is designed to build upon the first edition by providing food animal practitioners, veterinary students, animal scientists, extension specialists, and researchers with concise and timely chapters relevant to these new challenges. The Five-Minute format allows busy practitioners to access up-to-date information in an easy-to-use format when time does not allow for sifting through the literature. The companion website for the second edition also allows for easier access to information in the field and use of full-color illustrations for improved information transfer.

As we see the consolidation of animal agriculture in many parts of the world, we are also seeing a resurgence of smallholder farming in other areas. To this point, food animal practitioners must be well versed in individual animal care as well as herd management recommendations and production parameters. This textbook, like the first edition, comprehensively covers information useful across a variety of production systems and species and strives for global relevance. Although this text focuses on cattle, sheep, and goats, a significant effort has been made to include key information on other ruminant species including bison, water buffalo, yak, and cervidae as well as pseudoruminants, camelids.

The book editors, along with the hundreds of veterinary specialists who contributed to this second edition of *Wiley-Blackwell's Five-Minute Veterinary Consult: Ruminant*, are delighted to provide this updated text. Our sincere hope is that the reader finds this textbook to be a useful reference guide. Many thanks are also due to Scott R.R. Haskell for his dedication to bringing the first edition of this book to fruition.

Kaitlyn A. Lutz
Christopher C.L. Chase
Erica C. McKenzie
Ahmed Tibary

ACKNOWLEDGMENTS

Immense gratitude is owed to the contributing authors, who dedicated much time and energy towards updating and rewriting chapters for this edition. Their combined knowledge and expertise spanning a multitude of ruminant topics has resulted in a greatly improved reference for practitioners of ruminant and camelid medicine.

It was through the vision and perseverance of Dr. Scott R.R. Haskell that this series was originally born. Many thanks for the efforts of Scott and his team who worked on the first edition.

The perseverance of Mirjana Misina was integral in seeing this project to completion. The editors extend their fervent gratitude to Mirjana for unwavering professionalism and patience. We would also like to thank Heather Addison, copy editor, for her attention to detail and ability to "catch" the little things. Thank you also to the team of editors at Wiley Blackwell who ensured that this project ran smoothly: Purvi Patel, Nancy Turner, Melissa Wahl Hammer, Susan Engelken, and Erica Judisch.

CONSULTING EDITORS

CHRISTOPHER C.L. CHASE, DVM, PhD
Diplomate ACVM (Immunology and Virology)
Professor
Department of Veterinary and Biomedical
Sciences
College of Agriculture and Biological
Sciences
South Dakota State University
Brookings, South Dakota
USA

KAITLYN A. LUTZ, VMD
Diplomate ABVP (Food Animal)
Consultant in Production Animal Agriculture –
International
Pennsylvania, USA
Private Practitioner – Dairy
Ashburton
New Zealand

ERICA C. MCKENZIE, BSc, BVMS, PhD
Diplomate ACVIM
Professor, Large Animal Internal Medicine
Department of Clinical Sciences
College of Veterinary Medicine
Oregon State University
Corvallis, Oregon
USA

AHMED TIBARY, DMV, MS, DSc, PhD
Diplomate ACT
Professor
Department of Veterinary Clinical Sciences
College of Veterinary Medicine
Washington State University
Pullman, Washington
USA

CONTRIBUTORS

SAMEEH M. ABUTARBUSH, DVM, MVetSc
Diplomate ABVP, Diplomate ACVIM
Associate Professor
Department of Veterinary Clinical Sciences
Faculty of Veterinary Medicine
Jordan University of Science and Technology
Irbid
Jordan

AMBER L. ADAMS-PROGAR, PhD
Assistant Professor
Dairy Management Specialist
Department of Animal Sciences
Washington State University
Pullman, WA
USA

ARN A. ANDERSON, DVM DipL ABUP
(Beef Cattle)
Cross Timbers Veterinary Hospital
Bowie, TX
USA

KEVIN L. ANDERSON, DVM, PhD
Diplomate ABVP (Dairy Specialty)
Professor
Department of Population Health &
Pathobiology
College of Veterinary Medicine
North Carolina State University
Raleigh, NC
USA

CHANCE L. ARMSTRONG, DVM, MS
Diplomate ACT
Assistant Professor
Department of Clinical Sciences
School of Veterinary Medicine
Louisiana State University
Baton Rouge, LA
USA

LORA R. BALLWEBER, DVM, MS
Diplomate ACVM (Parasitology)
Professor
Department of Microbiology, Immunology &
Pathology
College of Veterinary Medicine and
Biomedical Sciences
Colorado State University
Fort Collins, CO
USA

GEORGE M. BARRINGTON, DVM, PhD
Diplomate ACVIM
Professor
Department of Veterinary Clinical Sciences
College of Veterinary Medicine
Washington State University
Pullman, WA
USA

JULIÁN A. BARTOLOMÉ, MV, FRVCS, MSc,
PhD
Diplomate ACT
Professor, Animal Reproduction
Facultad de Ciencias Veterinarias
Universidad Nacional de La Pampa
La Pampa
Argentina

MICHELLE HENRY BARTON, DVM, PhD
Diplomate ACVIM (Large Animal)
Fuller E. Callaway Endowed Professor
Department of Large Animal Medicine
College of Veterinary Medicine
University of Georgia
Athens, GA
USA

ADRIENNE C. BAUTISTA, DVM, PhD
Diplomate ABVT
Veterinarian
Banfield Pet Hospital
Roseville, CA
USA

SANDRA BAXENDELL, PSM, BVSc(Hons),
PhD MANZCVS, GCertAppSC(RurExt),
GCertPSectMgt, PGDAppSc, MRurSysMan
Goat Veterinary Consultancies – goatvetoz
Brisbane
Queensland
Australia

RONALD E. BAYNES, BSc, MS, PhD
Professor of Pharmacology
Director, Center for Chemical Toxicology
Research and Pharmacokinetics
College of Veterinary Medicine
North Carolina State University
Raleigh, NC
USA

DANIELA BEDENICE, DrMedVet
Diplomate ACVIM (Large Animal)
Diplomate ACVECC (Equine)
Associate Professor
Department of Clinical Sciences
Cummings School of Veterinary Medicine at
Tufts University
North Grafton, MA
USA

DANELLE BICKETT-WEDDLE, DVM, MPH,
PhD, Diplomate ACVPM
Associate Director
Center for Food Security and Public Health
Iowa State University
Ames, IA
USA

NORA M. BIERMANN, MagVetMed
Resident Large Animal Surgery
Department of Health Management
Atlantic Veterinary College
University of Prince Edward Island
Charlottetown
Prince Edward Island
Canada

JENNIFER L. BORNKAMP, DVM, MS
Clinician, Anesthesiology
Veterinary Clinical Sciences
Lloyd Veterinary Medical Center
College of Veterinary Medicine
Iowa State University
Ames, IA
USA

MARGARET M. BROSNAHAN, DVM, PhD
Diplomate ACVIM, Large Animal Internal
Medicine
Research Associate
Baker Institute for Animal Health
Cornell University College of
Veterinary Medicine
Ithaca, NY
USA

DAVID R. BROWN, PhD
Professor of Pharmacology and Vice Chair
Department of Veterinary Biomedical
Sciences
College of Veterinary Medicine
University of Minnesota
Saint Paul, MN
USA

BARBARA A. BYRNE, DVM, PhD
Diplomate ACVIM (Large Animal)
Diplomate ACVM (Bacteriology and Mycology)
Professor of Clinical Veterinary Microbiology
Department of Pathology, Microbiology, & Immunology
School of Veterinary Medicine
University of California, Davis
Davis, CA
USA

ALEXIS J. CAMPBELL, DVM, MS
Diplomate ACT
Clinical Instructor of Comparative Theriogenology
Department of Veterinary Clinical Sciences
College of Veterinary Medicine
Washington State University
Pullman, WA
USA

FRANCISCO R. CARVALLO, DVM, DSc
Diplomate ACVP (Anatomic Pathology)
Assistant Professor
California Animal Health and Food Safety Laboratory
San Bernardino Branch
School of Veterinary Medicine
University of California, Davis
San Bernardino, CA
USA

ALEJANDRO CEBALLOS-MÁRQUEZ, DVM, MSc, PhD
Associate Professor
Research Group on Milk Quality and Veterinary Epidemiology
Faculty of Agricultural Sciences
Universidad de Caldas
Manizales
Colombia

CLEMENCE Z. CHAKO, BVSc, MPH, PhD
Diplomate ACVIM
Assistant Professor
College of Veterinary Medicine
Midwestern University
Glendale, AZ
USA

MANUEL F. CHAMORRO, DVM, MS, PhD
Diplomate ACVIM (Large Animal)
Clinical Assistant Professor
Department of Clinical Sciences
College of Veterinary Medicine
Kansas State University
Manhattan, KS
USA

CHRISTOPHER C.L. CHASE, DVM, PhD
Diplomate ACVM (Immunology and Virology)
Professor
Department of Veterinary and Biomedical Sciences

College of Agriculture and Biological Sciences
South Dakota State University
Brookings, SD
USA

CELINA CHECURA, DVM, MS, PhD
Diplomate ACT
Clinical Assistant Professor
Department of Medical Sciences
School of Veterinary Medicine
University of Wisconsin-Madison
Madison, WI
USA

MUNASHE CHIGERWE, BVSc, MPH, PhD
Diplomate ACVIM (Large Animal)
Associate Professor
Department of Veterinary Medicine and Epidemiology
School of Veterinary Medicine
University of California, Davis
Davis, CA
USA

MICHELA CICCARELLI, DVM
Comparative Theriogenology Resident
College of Veterinary Medicine
Washington State University
Pullman, WA
USA

THOMAS M. CRAIG, DVM, PhD
Diplomate ACVM (Parasitology)
Professor
Department Veterinary Pathobiology
Texas A&M University
College Station, TX
USA

BRENT C. CREDILLE, DVM, PhD
Diplomate, ACVIM (Large Animal)
Assistant Professor
Food Animal Health and Management Program
Department of Population Health
College of Veterinary Medicine
University of Georgia
Athens, GA
USA

MAISIE E. DAWES, DVM, PhD
Diplomate ACVIM (Large Animal)
Assistant Professor
Immunology & Large Animal Internal Medicine
College of Veterinary Medicine
Western University of Health Sciences
Pomona, CA
USA

ANDRÉS DE LA CONCHA-BERMEJILLO, DVM, MS, PhD
Veterinary Pathologist
Regents Fellow
Texas A&M Veterinary Medical

Diagnostic Laboratory
Texas A&M University System
College Station, TX
USA

SARAH DEPENBROCK, DVM, MS
Diplomate ACVIM (Large Animal Internal Medicine)
Clinical Instructor
Department of Production Animal Health
University of Calgary
Faculty of Veterinary Medicine
Calgary, Alberta
Canada

ALFREDO DICONSTANZO, PhD
Professor
Department of Animal Science
University of Minnesota
St Paul, MN
USA

DOUGLAS C. DONOVAN, BVetMed, PhD, MRCVS, PAS
PhD Dairy Nutritionist
Standard Dairy Consultants
Omaha, NE
USA

SIAN A. DURWARD-AKHURST, BVMS, MS
Diplomate ACVIM (Large Animal)
PhD Student
Equine Genetics and Genomics Laboratory
University of Minnesota
Department of Veterinary Population Medicine
Saint Paul, MN
USA

RICHARD EHRHARDT, PhD
Small Ruminant Extension Specialist
Departments of Animal Science and Large Animal Clinical Science
Michigan State University
East Lansing, MI
USA

KATHLEEN EMERY, DVM
Dairy Nutritionist
Mycogen Seeds – DowAgroSciences
Maddison, WI
USA

STEVE ENSLEY, DVM, PhD
Veterinary Toxicologist
Veterinary Diagnostics and Production Animal Medicine
College of Veterinary Medicine
Iowa State University
Ames, IA
USA

CYNTHIA FAUX, DVM, PhD
Diplomate ACVIM (Large Animal)
Assistant Professor
Department of Integrative Physiology and
Neuroscience
College of Veterinary Medicine
Washington State University
Pullman, WA
USA

MARIE-EVE FECTEAU, DVM
Diplomate ACVIM
Associate Professor of Food Animal Medicine
and Surgery
Clinical Studies, New Bolton Center
School of Veterinary Medicine
University of Pennsylvania
Kennett Square, PA
USA

MARIA SOLEDAD FERRER, Vet, MS
Diplomate ACT
Associate Professor
Department of Large Animal Medicine
College of Veterinary Medicine
University of Georgia
Athens, GA
USA

ANNA M. FIRSHMAN, BVSc, PhD
Diplomate ACVIM (Large Animal)
Diplomate ACVSMR (Sports Medicine &
Rehabilitation)
Associate Clinical Professor
Department of Veterinary Population
Medicine
College of Veterinary Medicine
University of Minnesota
Saint Paul, MN
USA

BRANDON FRASER, DVM, MS
Diplomate ACVIM (Large Animal)
Head of Production Animal Service
School of Veterinary Science
University of Queensland
Gatton, Queensland
Australia

DENNIS D. FRENCH, DVM
Diplomate ABVP (Equine Practice)
Professor and Interim Department Head
Veterinary Clinical Medicine
College of Veterinary Medicine
University of Illinois
Urbana, IL
USA

A. JACQUES FUSELIER, DVM, DABVP,
DACT
Board Certified Specialist in Food Animal
Practice
Board Certified Theriogenologist
(Reproduction Specialist)
Whittington Veterinary Clinic
Abbeville, LA
USA

STEVEN M. GALLEGO, DVM
Veterinary Medical Officer
California Department of Food & Agriculture
Animal Health Branch
Redding, CA
USA

DAVID GALLIGAN, VMD, MBA
Professor of Animal Health Economics
University of Pennsylvania
School of Veterinary Medicine
Kennett Square, PA
USA

JULIE A. GARD, DVM, PhD
Diplomate ACT
Professor
Department of Veterinary Clinical Sciences
College of Veterinary Medicine
Auburn University
Auburn, AL
USA

EDGAR F. GARRETT, DVM, MS
Clinical Instructor
Department of Veterinary Clinical Medicine
College of Veterinary Medicine
University of Illinois
Urbana, IL
USA

JOHN M. GAY, DVM, PhD
Diplomate ACVPM
Associate Professor, Epidemiology
AAHP Field Disease Investigation Unit
Department of Veterinary Clinical Sciences
College of Veterinary Medicine
Washington State University
Pullman, WA
USA

SUNNY GEISER-NOVOTNY
Cattle Health Staff, Veterinarian
USDA APHIS VS
Surveillance Preparedness & Response
Services
Fort Collins, CO
USA

LAUREL J. GERSHWIN, DVM PhD
Diplomate ACVM
Professor of Immunology
Department of Pathology, Microbiology &
Immunology
School of Veterinary Medicine
University of California, Davis
Davis, CA
USA

JEREMY M. GESKE, MS
Animal Science and Industry
Owner/Operator
JMG Suffolks
New Prague, MN
USA

PHILIPPA GIBBONS, BVetMed(Hons), MS,
MRCVS
Diplomate ACVIM (LA)
Clinical Assistant Professor, Food Animal
Medicine
College of Veterinary Medicine and
Biomedical Sciences
Texas A&M University
College Station, TX
USA

MIKE GOEDKEN, DVM PhD
Diplomate ACVP (Anatomic Pathology)
Director
Research Pathology Services
Translational Science
Rutgers University
Piscataway, NJ
USA

JENIFER R. GOLD, DVM
Diplomate ACVIM, ACVECC
Clinical Associate Professor
Department of Clinical Sciences
College of Veterinary Medicine
Washington State University
Pullman, WA
USA

DIEGO GOMEZ-NIETO, DMV, MSc,
MVSc, PhD
Diplomate ACVIM
Infection Control Officer
Department of Pathobiology
Ontario Veterinary College
University of Guelph
Guelph, Ontario
Canada

SERGIO GONZALES
Veterinary Teaching Hospital
University of Minnesota
Saint Paul, MN
USA

EMMA GORDON, BVSc, MS
Diploma ACVIM (Large Animal)
Clinical Instructor in Large Animal Medicine
Department of Clinical Sciences
Oregon State University
Corvallis, OR
USA

DANIEL L. GROOMS, DVM, PhD, DACVM
Professor and Chair
Department of Large Animal Clinical
Sciences
College of Veterinary Medicine
Michigan State University
East Lansing, MI
USA

TAMARA GULL, DVM, PhD
Diplomate ACVIM (Large Animal)
Diplomate ACVPM
Diplomate ACVM (Immunology &
Bacteriology/Mycology)
Assistant Professor
Department of Veterinary Pathobiology
Center for Veterinary Health Sciences
Oklahoma State University
Stillwater, OK
USA

GAYLE HALLOWELL, MA, VetMB, PhD,
CertVA, DACVIM, DACVECC, PFHEA,
MRCVS
Diplomate ACVIM (LAIM), Diplomate
ACVECC (LA), Associate Diplomate ECVDI
RCVS Specialist in Equine Internal Medicine
and Emergency and Critical Care
Professor in Veterinary Internal Medicine and
Critical Care
School of Veterinary Medicine and Science
Sutton Bonington Campus
University of Nottingham
Nottingham
United Kingdom

NEIL E. HAMMERSCHMIDT
Manager, Animal Disease Traceability
United States Department of Agriculture
Animal and Plant Health Inspection Service
Riverdale, MD
USA

LAURA Y. HARDEFELDT, BSc, BVMS
Diplomate ACVIM (Large Animal)
PhD student
National Centre for Antimicrobial Stewardship
University of Melbourne
Parkville, Victoria
Australia

SCOTT R.R. HASKELL, DVM, MPVM, PhD
Director
Veterinary Technology Program
Yuba College
Marysville, CA
USA

MEERA HELLER, DVM, PhD
DACVIM (Large Animal)
Assistant Professor of Clinical Livestock
Medicine and Surgery
Department of Medicine & Epidemiology
School of Veterinary Medicine
University of California, Davis
Davis, CA
USA

DENNIS HERMESCH
Kansas State University
Manhattan, KS
USA

TROY E.C. HOLDER, DVM
Diplomate ACVS (Large Animal)
Clinical Assistant Professor
Large Animal Surgery
Oregon State University
Veterinary Teaching Hospital
Corvallis, OR
USA

LARRY D. HOLLER, DVM, PhD
Professor
Veterinary and Biomedical Sciences
Department
South Dakota State University
Brookings, SD
USA

RICHARD M. HOPPER, DVM
Diplomate ACT
Professor & Section Head
Food Animal Medicine, Theriogenology &
Ambulatory
Department of Pathobiology & Population
Medicine
College of Veterinary Medicine
Mississippi State University
Starkville, MS
USA

LYNN R. HOVDA, RPH, DVM, MS
Diplomate ACVIM
Director, Veterinary Services
SafetyCall International and Pet Poison
Helpline
Bloomington, MN;
Adjunct Assistant Professor
Department of Veterinary Biological Sciences
College of Veterinary Medicine
University of Minnesota
Saint Paul, MN
USA

EUGENE JANZEN, BA, DVM, MVS
Professor
Department of Production Animal Health
Faculty of Veterinary Medicine
University of Calgary
Calgary, Alberta
Canada

GREGORY W. JOHNSON, DVM
Nutritional Consultant
Cows Come First, LLC
Ithaca, NY
USA

LAURA JOHNSTONE, BVSc MVSc
DACVIM (LAIM)
Department of Medicine
University of Pennsylvania
New Bolton Center
Kennett Square, PA
USA

MEREDYTH L. JONES, DVM, MS
Diplomate ACVIM (Large Animal)
Associate Professor
Food Animal Field Services
Department of Large Animal Clinical
Sciences
Texas A&M University
College of Veterinary Medicine
College Station, TX
USA

SÉRGIO O. JUCHEM, DVM, PhD
Researcher in Ruminant Nutrition
Embrapa Southern Region Animal
Husbandry
Bagé, Rio Grande do Sul
Brazil

RAY M. KAPLAN DVM, PhD
Diplomate ACVM (Parasitology)
Diplomate EVPC
Professor of Parasitology
Department of Infectious Diseases
College of Veterinary Medicine
University of Georgia
Athens, GA
USA

ANREW KARTER, PhD
Senior Investigator
Associate Director
Center for Diabetes Translational Research
Kaiser Permanente – Division of Research
Oakland, CA
USA

PHILIP H. KASS, DVM, PhD
Associate Vice Provost for Faculty Equity and
Inclusion
UC Davis Academic Affairs;
Professor of Analytic Epidemiology
School of Veterinary Medicine and
School of Medicine
University of California, Davis
Davis, CA
USA

J.F. "NIK" KOTERSKI, DVM, PhD, MSS
Diplomate ACVPM
Veterinary Services of Orrtanna,
Pennsylvania
Orrtanna, PA
USA

JENNIFER H. KOZIOL, DVM, MS
Diplomate ACT
Assistant Professor
Department of Clinical Sciences
College of Veterinary Medicine
Purdue University
West Lafayette, IN
USA

AMANDA KREUDER, DVM, PhD
Diplomate ACVIM (Large Animal Internal
Medicine)
Assistant Professor
Food Animal and Camelid Hospital
Iowa State University
College of Veterinary Medicine
Ames, IA
USA

MICHAELA KRISTULA, DVM, MS
Associate Professor
New Bolton Center
Department of Clinical Studies
Section of Field Service
University of Pennsylvania School of
Veterinary Medicine
Kennett Square, PA
USA

THIBAUD KUCA, DVM
Large Animal Medicine Resident
Department of Clinical Sciences
College of Veterinary Medicine
Auburn University
Auburn, AL
USA

REBECCA LADRONKA, MPH, DVM
Graduate Research Assistant
Comparative Medicine and Integrative
Biology Program
College of Veterinary Medicine
Michigan State University
East Lansing, MI
USA

JEFF LAKRITZ, DVM, PhD
Diplomate ACVIM (Large Animal)
Diplomate ACVCP
Vernon L. Tharp Professor of Food Animal
Medicine
Hospital for Farm Animals
Veterinary Medical Center
College of Veterinary Medicine
The Ohio State University
Columbus, OH
USA

STEPHEN H. LEMASTER, PharmD, MPH,
DABT
Pharmacist and Senior Clinical Toxicologist
Safetycall International, PLLC & Pet Poison
Helpline
Bloomington, MN;
Clinical Associate Professor
Department of Experimental and Clinical
Pharmacology
College of Pharmacy
University of Minnesota
Minneapolis, MN
USA

HUICHU LIN, DVM, MS
Diplomate ACVAA (Anesthesia and
Analgesia)
Professor
Department of Clinical Sciences
College of Veterinary Medicine
Auburn University
Auburn, AL
USA

BONNIE R. LOGHRY, BAS, MPH, CPH
Public Health & Safety Specialist
Yuba College
Marysville, CA
USA

KATHARINA L. LOHMANN, MedVet, PhD,
DACVIM (Large Animal)
Associate Professor
Department of Large Animal Clinical
Sciences
Western College of Veterinary Medicine
University of Saskatchewan
Saskatoon, SK
Canada

DAVID M. LOVE, DVM
Conservation Medicine Fellow
Department of Conservation Medicine
The Wilds
Cumberland, OH
USA

KAITLYN A. LUTZ, VMD
Diplomate ABVP (Food Animal)
Consultant in Production Animal
Agriculture – International
Pennsylvania, USA;
Private Practitioner – Dairy
Ashburton
New Zealand

ROBERT J. MACKAY, BVSc, PhD
Diplomate ACVIM
Professor, Large Animal Medicine
University of Florida
Gainesville, FL
USA

ANTOINETTE E. MARSH, MS, PhD, Esq.
Associate Professor
Service Head Veterinary Medical Center
Diagnostic Parasitology
The Ohio State University
College of Veterinary Medicine
Department of Veterinary Preventive
Medicine
Columbus, OH
USA

KYLE G. MATHIS, DVM
Director/Associate Professor
Veterinary Technology Program
Yuba Community College
Marysville, CA
USA

HERRIS MAXWELL, DVM
Diplomate ACT
Clinical Professor
J. T. Vaughan Large Animal Teaching
Hospital
Department of Clinical Sciences
College of Veterinary Medicine
Auburn University
Auburn, AL
USA

KATE MCCARTHY LOTT, DVM
Veterinary Services of Oregon
Tillamook, OR
USA

ERICA C. MCKENZIE, BSc, BVMS, PhD
Diplomate ACVIM
Professor, Large Animal Internal Medicine
Department of Clinical Sciences
College of Veterinary Medicine
Oregon State University
Corvallis, OR
USA

CARLOS E. MEDINA-TORRES, DVM, MSc,
DVSc, PhD
Diplomate ACVIM (LAIM)/Diplomate ECEIM
Cert Uni Teaching Practice
Senior Lecturer – Equine Medicine Specialist
Equine Specialist Hospital
Veterinary Medical Centre
School of Veterinary Science
The University of Queensland
Gatton, Queensland
Australia

RICHARD W. MEIRING, DVM
Diplomate ACVPM
Clinical Professor
Department of Pathobiology and Population
Medicine
College of Veterinary Medicine
Mississippi State University
Mississippi State, MS
USA

PEDRO MELENDEZ, DVM, MS, PhD
Associate Professor
Department of Veterinary Medicine &
Surgery
College of Veterinary Medicine
University of Missouri
Columbia, MO
USA

PAUL E. MENNICK, DVM
Owner
Pacific International Genetics
Los Molinos, CA
USA

JAMES MERONEK, DVM, MPH
Head Veterinarian
ABS Global, Inc
DeForest, WI
USA

NATHAN MEYER, MS, MBA, PhD, DVM
Consulting Nutritionist/Veterinarian (Beef
Cattle)
JBS Five Rivers Cattle Feeding, LLC
Greeley, CO;
Affiliate Faculty
College of Veterinary Medicine & Biomedical
Sciences
Colorado State University
Fort Collins, CO
USA

JOHN R. MIDDLETON, DVM, PhD
Diplomate ACVIM
Professor, Food Animal
Assistant Director
Agricultural Experiment Station
Department of Veterinary Medicine and
Surgery
College of Veterinary Medicine
University of Missouri
Columbia, MO
USA

JOSEPH A. MILLER, BS, MS, JD
Attorney-at-Law
Seymour, IN
USA

ROBERT B. MOELLER Jr., DVM
Diplomate ACVP
Diplomate ABT
California Animal Health and Food Safety
Laboratory, Tulare
University of California, Davis
Tulare, CA
USA

HARRY MOMONT, DVM, PhD
Diplomate ACT
Clinical Associate Professor
Department of Medical Sciences
School of Veterinary Medicine
University of Wisconsin-Madison
Madison, WI
USA

MICHELLE MOSTROM, DVM, MS, PhD
Diplomate ABVT
Diplomate ABT (Toxicology)
Veterinary Toxicologist
Veterinary Diagnostic Laboratory
North Dakota State University
Fargo, ND
USA

MARY E. MOWRER, DVM
Stonehouse Veterinary Service
St. Clairsville, OH
USA

DANIELLE A. MZYK, BS
Graduate Research Assistant
Food Animal Residue Avoidance Databank
Population Health and Pathology
College of Veterinary Medicine
North Carolina State University
Raleigh, NC
USA

DUSTY W. NAGY, DVM, MS, PhD
Diplomate ACVIM (Large Animal)
Associate Teaching Professor
Department of Veterinary Medicine and
Surgery
College of Veterinary Medicine
University of Missouri
Columbia, MO
USA

REGG D. NEIGER, DVM, PhD
Professor
Department of Veterinary and Biomedical
Sciences
Animal Disease Research and Diagnostic
Laboratory
South Dakota State University
Brookings, SD
USA

BENJAMIN W. NEWCOMER, DVM, PhD
Diplomate ACVIM (Large Animal)
Diplomate ACVPM (Epidemiology)
Assistant Professor
Department of Pathobiology
College of Veterinary Medicine
Auburn University
Auburn, AL
USA

ANDREW J. NIEHAUS, DVM, MS
Diplomate ACVS (Large Animal)
Associate Professor
Department of Veterinary Clinical Sciences
College of Veterinary Medicine
The Ohio State University
Columbus, OH
USA

JORGE L. NORICUMBO-SAENZ, MS
(Animal Science)
Milk Quality Specialist
Tular County, CA
USA

AKINYI C. NYAOKE, BVM, MSc, PhD
Assistant Professor
California Animal Health and Food Safety
Laboratory
San Bernardino Branch
University of California, Davis
San Bernardino, CA
USA

LARRY OCCHIPINTI, DVM, MPVM
Owner
Guardsman Veterinary and K9
Reproduction Services
Tidewater, OR
USA

KATE O'CONOR, BS
Consultant at Yodle
Scottsdale, AZ
USA

DUSTIN OEDEKOVEN, DVM
Diplomate ACVPM
State Veterinarian
South Dakota Animal Industry Board
Pierre, SD
USA

ERIK J. OLSON, DVM, PhD
Diplomate ACVP (Anatomic Pathology)
Associate Professor
Veterinary Diagnostic Laboratory and
Department of Veterinary Population
Medicine
College of Veterinary Medicine
University of Minnesota
Saint Paul, MN
USA

DONAL O'TOOLE, MVB, PhD, DipECVP,
FRCPath
Professor
Department of Veterinary Sciences and
Wyoming State Veterinary Laboratory
University of Wyoming
Laramie, WY
USA

ZENHWA BEN OUYANG, VMD, MSE
Department of Clinical Sciences
College of Veterinary Medicine and
Biomedical Sciences
Colorado State University
Fort Collins, CO
USA

LAUREN PALMER, DVM, MPH
Veterinarian
The Marine Mammal Care Center at Fort
MacArthur
San Pedro, CA
USA

LISA K. PEARSON, DVM, MS, PhD
Diplomate ACT
Adjunct Faculty
Department of Veterinary Clinical Sciences
College of Veterinary Medicine
Washington State University
Pullman, WA
USA

KEVIN D. PELZER, DVM, MPVM
Diplomate ACVPM
Professor
Department of Large Animal Clinical
Sciences
Production Management Medicine
Virginia Maryland College of Veterinary
Medicine
Virginia Tech
Blacksburg, VA
USA

ARUN PHATAK
Nutrition and Reproductive
Management Specialist
Reproduction Specialties, Inc.
Modesto, CA
USA

PABLO PINEDO, DVM, PhD
Assistant Professor
Department of Animal Sciences
Colorado State University
Fort Collins, CO
USA

PAUL J. PLUMMER, DVM, PhD
Diplomate, ACVIM (Large Animal)
Diplomate, European College of Small
Ruminant Health Management
Associate Professor
Veterinary Diagnostic and Production Animal
Medicine;
Veterinary Microbiology and Preventive
Medicine
College of Veterinary Medicine
Iowa State University
Ames, IA
USA

ELEONORA PO, DVM, MRCVS, CVA (IVAS)
Resident, ACVIM (LA) Candidate
Department of Veterinary Clinical Medicine
College of Veterinary Medicine
University of Illinois
Urbana-Champaign, IL
USA

SALUNA POKHREL, BVSc & AH, MVSc
(Veterinary Parasitology)
Assistant Professor
Department of Veterinary Microbiology and
Parasitology
Institute of Agriculture and Animal Science,
Tribhuvan University
Nepal

MARIANNE POLUNAS, RPh, PhD
Assistant Research Professor
Department of Pharmacology & Toxicology
Ernest Mario School of Pharmacy
Rutgers University
Piscataway, NJ
USA

KEITH P. POULSEN, DVM, PhD
Diplomate ACVIM
Clinical Assistant Professor
Large Animal Internal Medicine
Section Head, Client Services
Wisconsin Veterinary Diagnostic Laboratory
School of Veterinary Medicine
University of Wisconsin
Madison, WI
USA

EDWARD L. POWERS, DVM, MPVM
California Department of Public Health
Division of Communicable Disease Control
Infectious Diseases Branch
Veterinary Public Health Section
Richmond, CA
USA

MARIA E. PRADO, MV, PhD
Diplomate ACVIM (Large Animal)
Assistant Professor of Practice
Department of Animal Science
University of Tennessee
Knoxville, TN
USA

STEPHEN R. PURDY, DVM
Director, North American Camelid
Studies Program
President
Nunoa Project
Peru;
Adjunct Associate Professor
UMass Amherst
Amherst, MA
USA

BIRGIT PUSCHNER, DVM, PhD
Diplomate ABVT
Professor and Chair
Department of Molecular Biosciences
School of Veterinary Medicine
University of California
Davis, CA
USA

MERL F. RAISBECK, DVM, MS, PhD
Diplomate ABVT
Professor Emeritus, Veterinary Toxicology
Department of Veterinary Sciences
University of Wyoming
Laramie, WY
USA

CHELSEY R. RAMIREZ, DVM
Clinical Instructor
Integrated Food Animal Management
Systems
Department of Veterinary Clinical Medicine
College of Veterinary Medicine
University of Illinois
Urbana-Champaign, IL
USA

JAMES M. RASMUSSEN, DVM
Senior Veterinarian
Minnesota Zoological Garden
Apple Valley, MN
USA

JIM P. REYNOLDS DVM, MPVM
Diplomate ACAW
Vice President of Consulting
Praedium Ventures
Visalia, CA
USA

JERRY R. ROBERSON, DVM, PhD, ACVIM
Professor Food Animal Medicine and Surgery
Lincoln Memorial University-College of
Veterinary Medicine
Harrogate, TN
USA

JENNIFER N. ROBERTS, DVM
Diplomate ACT
Assistant Professor
Department of Large Animal Clinical
Sciences
College of Veterinary Medicine
Michigan State University
East Lansing, MI
USA

NICHOLAS A. ROBINSON, BVSc (Hons),
PhD, MACVSc
Diplomate ACVP (Anatomic Pathology)
Associate Professor
Cummings School of Veterinary Medicine
Tufts University
North Grafton, MA
USA

JOE RODER, DVM, PhD
Diplomate ABVT
Director
Swine Technical Services
Merck Animal Health
De Soto, KS
USA

FRANCISCO C. RODRIGUEZ, DVM
Associate Professor, Large Animal Medicine
and Surgery
Department of Clinical Sciences
School of Veterinary Medicine
St. Matthew's University
Grand Cayman
British West Indies

KEITH A. ROEHR, DVM
State Veterinarian
Colorado Department of Agriculture
Animal Health Division
Broomfield, CO
USA

EMMANUEL ROLLIN. DVM, MFAM
Clinical Assistant Professor, Dairy Production
Medicine
Department of Population Health
College of Veterinary Medicine
University of Georgia
Athens, GA
USA

JENNIFER A. SCHLEINING, DVM, MS
Diplomate, ACVS (Large Animal)
Associate Professor
Department of Veterinary Diagnostic and
Production Animal Medicine
College of Veterinary Medicine
Iowa State University
Ames, IA
USA

DAVID A. SCHNEIDER, DVM, PhD
Diplomate ACVIM (Large Animal)
Research Veterinary Medical Officer
US Department of Agriculture
Agricultural Research Service
Animal Disease Research Unit
Pullman, WA
USA

CLARE M. SCULLY, MA, DVM, MS
Diplomate ACT
Assistant Professor
Department of Veterinary Clinical Sciences
Louisiana State University School of
Veterinary Medicine
Baton Rouge, LA
USA

WILLIAM J. SEGLAR, DVM
Senior Nutritionist/Veterinarian
Global Nutritional Sciences
DuPont/Pioneer Global Forages
Johnston, IA
USA

JAN K. SHEARER, DVM, MS
Diplomate, American College of Animal
Welfare
Professor and Extension Veterinarian
Iowa State University, CVM, VDPAM
Ames, IA
USA

CLIFFORD F. SHIPLEY, DVM
Diplomate ACT (Theriogenology)
Associate Clinical Professor
Attending Veterinarian
Agricultural Animal Care and Use Program
Department of Veterinary Clinical Medicine
College of Veterinary Medicine
University of Illinois
Urbana, IL
USA

SUVASH SHIWAKOTI, BVSc & AH, MSc
(Microbiology)
Veterinary Officer
Government of Nepal
North Dakota State University
Fargo, ND
USA

EGENDRA KUMAR SHRESTHA, BVSc &
AH, MVSc
Associate Academic Director
Associate Professor
College of Agriculture and Veterinary
Sciences
Nepal Polytechnic Institute Ltd
Bharatpur-11, Chitwan
Nepal

KATHARINE M. SIMPSON, DVM, MS
DACVIM
Associate Professor
Food Animal Medicine and Surgery
Large Animal Medicine and Surgery
Department
St. George's University
School of Veterinary Medicine
True Blue, Grenada
West Indies

BILLY I. SMITH, DVM, MS
Diplomate ABVP (Food Animal)
University of Pennsylvania
School of Veterinary Medicine
New Bolton Center
Department of Large Animal Clinical Studies
Section of Field Service
Kennett Square, PA
USA

JACK D. SMITH, DVM
Diplomate ACT
Associate Professor, Theriogenology
Interim, Associate Dean for Academic Affairs
College of Veterinary Medicine
Mississippi State University
Starkville, MS
USA

JOE S. SMITH, DVM, MPS, DACVIM (LAIM)
Clinician
Food Animal and Camelid Hospital
Department of Veterinary Diagnostic and
Production Animal Medicine
College of Veterinary Medicine
Iowa State University
Ames, IA
USA

KEELY A. SMITH, DVM
Private Practitioner
Hudson, FL
USA

JAMIE L. STEWART, DVM, MS
Theriogenology Resident
Department of Veterinary Clinical Medicine
College of Veterinary Medicine
University of Illinois
Urbana, IL
USA

AUDUN STIEN, PhD
Senior Researcher
Norwegian Institute for Nature
Research – NINA
Fram Centre
Tromsø
Norway

KELLY M. STILL BROOKS, DVM, MPH
Diplomate ACVPM
Clinical Assistant Professor
Veterinary Diagnostic and Production Animal
Medicine
College of Veterinary Medicine
Iowa State University
Ames, IA
USA

RICARDO M. STOCKLER, DVM, MS
Diplomate ABVP (Dairy Practice)
Assistant Clinical Professor of Farm Animal
Ambulatory Services
JT Vaughan Large Animal Teaching Hospital
College of Veterinary Medicine at Auburn
University
Auburn, AL
USA

CAROLYN L. STULL, MS, PhD
Diplomate ACAN (Animal Nutrition), ACAWS
(Animal Welfare Science)
Animal Welfare Cooperative Extension
Specialist, Emerita
Department of Population Health and
Reproduction
School of Veterinary Medicine
University of California
Davis, CA
USA

JENNIFER S. TAINTOR, DVM, MS
Diplomate ACVIM (Large Animal)
Diplomate ACVSMR (Equine)
Associate Professor
Department of Clinical Sciences
College of Veterinary Medicine
Auburn University
Auburn, AL
USA

RACHEL H. H. TAN BVSc, DVCS, MACVSc,
CertVetAc, MS, DipACVIM, GradCertEd
Senior Lecturer, Large Animal
College of Public Health, Medical and
Veterinary Sciences
James Cook University
Townsville, Queensland
Australia

AHMED TIBARY, DMV, MS, DSc, PhD
Diplomate ACT
Professor
Department of Veterinary Clinical Sciences
College of Veterinary Medicine
Washington State University
Pullman, WA
USA

FERENC TOTH, DVM, PhD
Diplomate ACVS (Large Animal)
Assistant Professor
Department of Veterinary Population
Medicine
College of Veterinary Medicine
University of Minnesota
Saint Paul, MN
USA

ALEX K. TURNER, DVM
Traceability Veterinarian
Colorado Department of Agriculture
Animal Health Division
Broomfield, CO
USA

TORKILD TVERAA, PhD
Senior Researcher
Norwegian Institute for Nature
Research – NINA
Fram Centre
Tromsø
Norway

JEFFREY W. TYLER (Deceased)
College of Veterinary Medicine
University of Missouri
Columbia, MO
USA

FRANCISCO A. UZAL, DVM, FRVC,
MSc, PhD
Diplomate ACVP
Professor of Veterinary Pathology
California Animal Health and Safety
Laboratory System
San Bernardino Branch
University of California, Davis
San Bernardino, CA
USA

MODEST VENGUST, DVM, DVSc, PhD
Diplomate ACVIM (Large Animal)
Diplomate ACVSMR (Equine)
Veterinary Faculty
University of Ljubljana
Ljubljana
Slovenia

PAUL H. WALZ, DVM, MS, PhD
Diplomate ACVIM (Large Animal)
Professor
Department of Pathobiology
College of Veterinary Medicine
Auburn University
Auburn, AL
USA

MUHAMMAD SALMAN WAQAS,
DVM, M.Phil
Lecturer
Department of Theriogenology
Faculty of Veterinary Science
University of Agriculture
Faisalabad
Pakistan

MATT G. WELBORN, DVM, MPH
Diplomate ACVPM
Professor
Food Animal Health Management
Department of Veterinary Clinical Sciences
LSU School of Veterinary Medicine
Louisiana State University
Baton Rouge, LA
USA

ASHLEY WHITEHEAD, DVM, BSc, DVSc
Diplomate ACVIM (Large Animal)
Assistant Professor
Department of Veterinary Clinical and
Diagnostic Sciences
Faculty of Veterinary Medicine
University of Calgary
Calgary, Alberta
Canada

JEFFREY J. WICHTEL, BVSc, PhD
Diplomate ACT
Professor and Dean
Ontario Veterinary College
University of Guelph
Guelph, Ontario
Canada

AUDREY WIEMAN, DVM
Owner
Ridgeline Veterinary Services, LLC
Lynch, NE
USA

CHRISTINE M. WINSLOW, DVM
Diplomate, ACT
Assistant Professor
Animal Health Institute
Midwestern University
Glendale, AZ
USA

AMELIA WOOLUMS, DVM, MVSc, PhD
Diplomate ACVIM
Diplomate ACVM
Professor
Department of Pathobiology and Population
Medicine
College of Veterinary Medicine
Mississippi State University
Mississippi State, MS
USA

ALAN YOUNG, PhD
Professor of Veterinary and Biomedical
Science
South Dakota State University
Brookings, SD
USA

ABOUT THE COMPANION WEBSITE

This book is accompanied by a companion website:

www.fiveminutevet.com/ruminant

The website includes:

• Additional topics not found in the book
• Client education handouts
• The figures from the book in PowerPoint

CONTENTS

 Published online, see www.fiveminutevet.com/ruminant

Published online, see www.fiveminutevet.com/ruminant

Published online, see www.fiveminutevet.com/ruminant

Published online, see www.fiveminutevet.com/ruminant

xxiii

Published online, see www.fiveminutevet.com/ruminant

Published online, see www.fiveminutevet.com/ruminant

Published online, see www.fiveminutevet.com/ruminant

Published online, see www.fiveminutevet.com/ruminant

xxvii

Published online, see www.fiveminutevet.com/ruminant

Published online, see www.fiveminutevet.com/ruminant

Published online, see www.fiveminutevet.com/ruminant

*Published online, see www.fiveminutevet.com/ruminant

CONTENTS *by Subject*

 Published online, see www.fiveminutevet.com/ruminant

DIGESTIVE

 *Published online, see www.fiveminutevet.com/ruminant

EPIDEMIOLOGY AND DIAGNOSTIC METHODS

HEMOLYMPHATIC

 Published online, see www.fiveminutevet.com/ruminant

MAMMARY

METABOLIC

 Published online, see www.fiveminutevet.com/ruminant

MULTISYSTEMIC

MUSCULOSKELETAL

 Published online, see www.fiveminutevet.com/ruminant

NEUROLOGY

 Published online, see www.fiveminutevet.com/ruminant

NUTRITION

Published online, see www.fiveminutevet.com/ruminant

Published online, see www.fiveminutevet.com/ruminant

Published online, see www.fiveminutevet.com/ruminant

RESPIRATORY

THERIOGENOLOGY

 Published online, see www.fiveminutevet.com/ruminant

xli

Published online, see www.fiveminutevet.com/ruminant

TOXICOLOGY

 Published online, see www.fiveminutevet.com/ruminant

Published online, see www.fiveminutevet.com/ruminant

URINARY

 Published online, see www.fiveminutevet.com/ruminant

ABOMASAL EMPTYING DEFECT IN SHEEP

 BASICS

OVERVIEW

Abomasal emptying defect (AED) is a syndrome of mature Suffolk sheep characterized by chronic, progressive weight loss and abomasal dilatation in the absence of mechanical obstruction.

INCIDENCE/PREVALENCE

Unknown

GEOGRAPHIC DISTRIBUTION

N/A

SYSTEMS AFFECTED

Digestive

PATHOPHYSIOLOGY

• The pathogenic mechanism is unclear. Neurotoxicosis has been suggested.
• The syndrome shares some characteristics with chronic idiopathic intestinal pseudo-obstruction of humans. Affected individuals have clinical signs suggesting partial or complete gastric obstruction, when none is present.
• Morphologic investigations of human patients indicate degenerative changes in the smooth muscle or the tunica muscularis and/or neurons of the enteric plexus.

HISTORICAL FINDINGS

• Condition occurs sporadically, typically affecting a single individual. Flock management is usually excellent despite affected individuals within it.
• Owners may report weight loss in affected animals despite providing extra attention, nutrition, and anthelmintic treatment. Owners may note that the animal appears "bloated" despite inappetence.

SIGNALMENT

• AED affects sheep, with an anecdotal report in a cross-bred dairy type goat.
• Predominantly affects Suffolks; also reported in the Hampshire, Dorset, and Texel breeds.
• Affected animals are typically over 2 years old and of either gender.

PHYSICAL EXAMINATION FINDINGS

• Body temperature is within normal limits unless concurrent disease is present. Heart and respiration rates may be normal to increased. Fecal consistency usually normal, but volume often decreased.
• Abdominal conformation may be normal; bilateral, asymmetrical abdominal distention may occur (distension of the left paralumbar fossa and right ventrolateral abdomen when the animal is viewed from behind); unilateral distension may be present (right ventrolateral aspect of the abdomen).
• Rumen contractions are variable. Rumen hyperactivity can be dramatic in affected sheep and the left paralumbar fossa appears to be in constant motion, reflecting almost constant rumen activity.
• Sheep with AED are in varying stages of cachexia and their abdominal wall feels "thin" due to muscle wasting. Abdominal organs may also lack tone or give the impression of being fluid filled. In some instances, the caudal border of the abomasum may be visible and palpable as it extends beyond the last rib on the ventrolateral aspect of the abdomen. The distended abomasum usually feels fluid filled rather than the doughy or firm consistency often associated with abomasal impaction in cattle.

GENETICS

• Information regarding genetic predisposition is limited. Pedigree analysis of a flock in which 11/92 Suffolks were affected during a 5-month period did not identify a hereditary pattern.

CAUSES AND RISK FACTORS

Unknown

 DIAGNOSIS

DIFFERENTIAL DIAGNOSES

• Differential diagnoses for chronic weight loss in adult sheep include caseous lymphadenitis and other chronic infections including scrapie, Johne's disease, malnutrition, dental problems, parasitism, neoplasia.
• Historical and clinical findings are fairly specific to AED.
• Vagal indigestion with resulting ruminal distension is uncommon in sheep.

CBC/BIOCHEMISTRY/URINALYSIS

• Hematology and serum chemistry analysis are usually normal.
• Metabolic alkalosis with hypochloremia and hypokalemia observed with proximal GI obstruction in cattle is not consistently noted with AED.
• Elevations in liver enzymes (AST, SDH, GGT) may be noted.
• Increased intra-abdominal pressure from a distended abomasum may lead to secondary liver congestion and ischemia and can precipitate leakage of hepatic enzymes.
• Urinalysis usually unremarkable.

OTHER LABORATORY TESTS

• Elevated rumen chloride concentration is useful in supporting a diagnosis of AED.
• Normal rumen chloride in sheep is ≤15 mEq/L. Affected sheep will have at least a two-fold increase. Rumen fluid samples are easily obtained by percutaneous aspiration of the rumen from a site in the ventrolateral aspect of the left paralumbar fossa.

IMAGING

• Abdominal radiography may be helpful; however, unless the animal can be positioned for an oblique abdominal radiographic view, results will be difficult to interpret.
• Abdominal ultrasonography may be more useful than radiographic imaging. A 3 to 5 MHz linear or convex array can provide adequate images of the abomasum. When placed on the lower right abdomen, the normal abomasum will not extend beyond the last rib. In animals with AED the abomasum will usually appear 2 to 4 times normal size.

OTHER DIAGNOSTIC PROCEDURES

N/A

PATHOLOGIC FINDINGS

• Gross necropsy reveals a greatly distended abomasum and patent pylorus.
• Abomasal contents are usually liquid but may be dry. Histopathologic changes in the abomasum include smooth muscle degeneration, vacuolation, and varying degrees of necrosis. Degenerative changes have been reported in the celiacomesenteric ganglia.

 TREATMENT

THERAPEUTIC APPROACH

• The prognosis for recovery with intensive treatment is variable and dependent upon the duration of abomasal dysfunction and distention. Medical therapy using cathartics and laxatives, and surgical therapy (abomasotomy) have had limited success.
• In animals that are good surgical candidates, abomasotomy followed by metoclopramide and supportive fluid therapy has provided some success.

SURGICAL CONSIDERATIONS AND TECHNIQUES

An abomasotomy is best performed under general anesthesia, although a local line block can be used. The animal is placed in left lateral recumbency and a right paracostal approach provides excellent access to the abomasum. Subsequently the abomasum is opened and its contents removed, and the organ is flushed and closed in a routine manner. Treatment with metoclopramide should be used as an adjunct to the surgery. Concurrent fluid replacement and electrolyte correction therapy is critical to survival and success.

 MEDICATIONS

DRUGS OF CHOICE

Metoclopramide (0.1 mg/kg, q8h, SQ) as an adjunct to abomasotomy has been reported to improve abomasal motility. This medication should not be used if GI obstruction is suspected.

A **ABOMASAL EMPTYING DEFECT IN SHEEP** (CONTINUED)

Erythromycin (8.8 mg/kg, IM) increased abomasal emptying rate in dairy calves; pre-operative administration (10 mg/kg, IM) increased abomasal emptying after surgical correction of left displaced abomasum in dairy cows. Erythromycin may therefore provide some benefit in treatment of AED.

CONTRAINDICATIONS
Neostigmine should not be used in affected animals since it increases frequency rather than strength of rumen contractions.

PRECAUTIONS
Appropriate milk and meat withdrawal times apply to all compounds administered to food-producing animals.

POSSIBLE INTERACTIONS
N/A

 FOLLOW-UP

EXPECTED COURSE AND PROGNOSIS
• The earlier that AED is recognized and treated, the better the prognosis; however, prognosis is guarded for long-term recovery regardless.
• In certain circumstances such as a ram completing a breeding season, or a late gestation ewe completing her pregnancy, a fair to good short-term prognosis may be offered if intensive treatment is provided early.

POSSIBLE COMPLICATIONS
• Complications related to abomasotomy: surgical dehiscence of the abomasal incision (especially if the abomasal wall has undergone degenerative changes) and dehiscence of the abdominal incision may occur (more likely in a debilitated patient).
• Once the condition is recognized, if treatment is declined, euthanasia should be offered as a humane resolution.

CLIENT EDUCATION
Owners of Suffolk sheep should be familiar with the breed predisposition for AED and educated regarding the clinical presentation.

PATIENT CARE
If intensive therapy is undertaken, the animal should be observed for attitude, appetite, fecal production, and abdominal conformation. Signs of improvement following abomasotomy and during metoclopramide therapy may include improvement in attitude and appetite, increased fecal production and decreased abdominal distention.

PREVENTION
Because the underlying cause and heritability of AED is unknown, recommendations cannot be made.

 MISCELLANEOUS

ASSOCIATED CONDITIONS
Other concurrent conditions may occur with AED. Pneumonia and other organ failure can be secondary to any chronic debilitating disease.

AGE-RELATED FACTORS
AED usually occurs in mature sheep.

ZOONOTIC POTENTIAL
N/A

PREGNANCY
In spite of treatment, pregnant animals may abort. Pregnant animals (especially mid- to late-term) represent an increased surgical risk.

BIOSECURITY
N/A

PRODUCTION MANAGEMENT
AED is usually observed in a single animal from a well-managed flock.

SYNONYMS
• Abomasal dilatation and emptying defect
• Abomasal impaction

• Acquired dysautonomia
• Functional pyloric stenosis
• Ovine abomasal enlargement

ABBREVIATIONS
• AED = abomasal emptying defect
• AST = aspartate transaminase
• GGT = gamma-glutamyltransferase
• SDH = sorbitol dehydrogenase

SEE ALSO
Abomasal Impaction

Suggested Reading
Kopcha, M. Abomasal dilatation and emptying defect in a ewe. J Am Vet Med Assoc 1988, 192:783–4.

Nouri M, Hajikolaee MR, Constable PD, Omidi A. Effect of erythromycin and gentamicin on abomasal emptying rate in suckling calves. J Vet Intern Med 2008, 22: 196–201.

Pruden SJ, McAllister MM, Schultheiss PC et al. Abomasal emptying defect of sheep may be an acquired form of dysautonomia Vet Pathol 2004, 41:164–9.

Ruegg PL, George LW, East NE. Abomasal dilatation and emptying defect in a flock of Suffolk ewes. J Am Vet Med Assoc 1988, 193:1534–6.

Wittek T, Tischer K, Gieseler T, Fürll M, Constable PD. Effect of preoperative administration of erythromycin or flunixin meglumine on postoperative abomasal emptying rate in dairy cows undergoing surgical correction of left displacement of the abomasum. J Am Vet Med Assoc 2008, 232: 418–23.

Author Dennis D. French
Consulting Editor Erica C. McKenzie
Acknowledgment The author and book editors acknowledge the prior contribution of Michelle Kopcha.

ABOMASAL IMPACTION

BASICS

OVERVIEW
• Abomasal impaction occurs when there is obstruction to the passage of fluid and ingesta from the abomasum through the pylorus by feed, sand, gravel or other foreign bodies, or as a result of neurologic dysfunction from various conditions.
• Pyloric obstruction from improperly placed percutaneous fixation of left-displaced abomasum ("roll and toggle") can also result in abomasal impaction in cattle.
• Clinical signs can be acute or chronic and are characterized by anorexia, decreased or scant feces, abomasal distension, weakness, dehydration, and signs of abdominal pain.
• Abomasal impaction typically occurs in cattle and occasionally in sheep. It is usually sporadic, but morbidity can be associated with feeding of low-quality forages.
• This disorder has a high mortality rate.
• Abomasal emptying defect (AED) is a disorder that primarily affects Suffolk sheep and is characterized by distension and impaction of the abomasum.

INCIDENCE/PREVALENCE
Low morbidity.

GEOGRAPHIC DISTRIBUTION
Worldwide. Occurs more commonly in regions where low quality roughage or low energy diets are fed.

SYSTEMS AFFECTED
Digestive

PATHOPHYSIOLOGY
• Physical obstruction of outflow from the abomasum into the duodenum occurs. This may be due to packing of straw or other poor-quality roughages, or sand or gravel in the abomasum.
• Damage to branches of the vagus nerve as a result of traumatic reticuloperitonitis, lymphoma or other disorders can decrease the emptying ability of the abomasum.
• Failure of fluid to move from the abomasum into the intestines results in dehydration and starvation.
• Sequestration of hydrochloric acid in the abomasum can result in metabolic alkalosis.
• In sheep, no histologic lesion has been consistently associated with AED, and the etiology is unknown. In one study, histologic examination of celiacomesenteric ganglia from affected sheep revealed scattered chromatolytic or necrotic neurons, without inflammation. Chromatolytic neurons were observed more frequently in AED-affected sheep than in healthy Suffolk sheep. Neuronal necrosis was not observed in any of the healthy sheep. Neuronal lesions of AED resemble dysautonomic diseases of humans and other animals.

HISTORICAL FINDINGS
• Abomasal impaction often affects cattle on poor-quality pasture or that are fed chopped, low-quality forages with low dietary energy, especially in cold weather. Beef cattle are more prone due to management characteristics.
• The disorder may also arise in cattle eating from sand or gravel surfaces, or if excessive gravel from the feed storage area contaminates the feed.
• Animals may also develop the condition as a result of pica.

SIGNALMENT
• This disorder typically affects cattle and sometimes sheep.
• Suffolk sheep may be predisposed compared to other ovine breeds due to the higher prevalence of AED in this breed. Abomasal impaction affects juvenile to adult animals; AED affects sheep >2 years old.
• Abomasal impaction may be more prevalent in pregnant females.

PHYSICAL EXAMINATION FINDINGS
• Anorexia, depression, and decreased rumen motility are typical.
• Distension of the abomasum may be identified by visualization, palpation, and ballottement of the lower right flank.
• Affected animals eventually display weight loss, reduced fecal production, and dehydration.

GENETICS
A hereditary pattern has not been demonstrated for abomasal impaction or for AED.

CAUSES AND RISK FACTORS
• Physical blockage of the abomasum in cattle fed low-quality chopped forages, or consuming sand or gravel.
• As a result of "roll and toggle" sutures inadvertently placed in or near the pylorus.
• From conditions that damage the vagus nerve.
• Late pregnancy may predispose.
• Suffolk sheep with AED are predisposed.

DIAGNOSIS

DIFFERENTIAL DIAGNOSES
• Include other disorders that may cause signs of inappetance, scant fecal production, and abdominal distension including abomasal displacement, reticuloperitonitis, lymphoma, and vagal indigestion.

CBC/BIOCHEMISTRY/URINALYSIS
• CBC is usually normal.
• Hypochloremic, hypokalemic metabolic alkalosis may be present in chronic cases.
• Sheep with AED do not typically demonstrate the hypochloremic, hypokalemic metabolic alkalosis commonly found in cattle with outflow obstruction disorders.

OTHER LABORATORY TESTS
Elevated rumen chloride concentrations in sheep (>15 mEq/L) indicate reflux of abomasal contents into the rumen.

IMAGING
• Ultrasonography may be useful to determine distension of the abomasum and to assist detection of potential inciting causes such as traumatic reticuloperitonitis and lymphoma.
• Radiography may be useful to detect traumatic reticuloperitonitis or the presence of excessive sand or gravel within the gastrointestinal tract.

OTHER DIAGNOSTIC PROCEDURES
• Measurement of rumen chloride using fluid samples obtained by orogastric tube or rumenocentesis.
• Laparotomy.
• Abdominocentesis can identify elevated nucleated cell counts, elevated total protein concentration, and/or abnormal cellular morphology in animals with underlying causative disorders that are inflammatory or neoplastic in nature.

PATHOLOGIC FINDINGS
Distension of the abomasum with packing of roughage, gravel or sand is confirmed via laparotomy or necropsy. Concurrent traumatic reticuloperitonitis, lymphoma, and other predisposing causes may also be recognized by these techniques.

TREATMENT

THERAPEUTIC APPROACH
• Surgical therapy likely provides the greatest chance of resolution depending on the underlying cause.
• Medical therapy best accompanies surgical therapy and can consist of administration of cathartics and laxatives daily for 2 to 4 days.
• Correction of metabolic alkalosis may be indicated in severe or chronic disease.

SURGICAL CONSIDERATIONS AND TECHNIQUES
• Impaction may be resolved by abomasotomy with removal of roughage or foreign material. Surgical approaches that allow access to the abomasum include right paracostal, right paramedian and right paralumbar.

MEDICATIONS

DRUGS OF CHOICE
• Cathartics and laxative options include dioctyl sodium sulfosuccinate (50 mg/kg/day), magnesium sulfate (2.5 g/kg/day), mineral oil (8 mL/kg/day), and magnesium hydroxide (1 g/kg/day).

• Metabolic alkalosis can be readily corrected via administration of intravenous sodium chloride preparations.

CONTRAINDICATIONS
• Gastrointestinal motility agents should be considered only after surgical or medical correction of impaction to reduce the risk of abomasal rupture.

PRECAUTIONS
• Lactated Ringer's solution should be used cautiously due to the possibility of inducing or exacerbating metabolic alkalosis.
• Abomasal motility agents (neostigmine, metoclopramide, erythromycin, etc.) should be used with great caution to avoid abomasal rupture.
• Appropriate milk and meat withdrawal times must be followed for all compounds administered to food-producing animals.

POSSIBLE INTERACTIONS
N/A

FOLLOW-UP

EXPECTED COURSE AND PROGNOSIS
Grave prognosis. Death from dehydration, metabolic alkalosis or peritonitis if intervention does not occur.

POSSIBLE COMPLICATIONS
Abomasal rupture and peritonitis.

CLIENT EDUCATION
Feed cattle to meet energy requirements and avoid feeding chopped poor-quality forages with low energy, particularly in cold weather.

PATIENT CARE
Affected animals should be assessed for signs of pain and suffering (lethargy, inappetance, signs of abdominal pain), reduced fecal output, hydration status, and electrolyte balance.

PREVENTION
• Feed good-quality, long fiber-length forage with adequate energy supplementation.
• Avoid feeding on sand or gravel.

MISCELLANEOUS

ASSOCIATED CONDITIONS
Reticuloperitonitis, lymphoma, displaced abomasum.

AGE-RELATED FACTORS
More common in adult and pregnant animals, and mature Suffolk sheep.

ZOONOTIC POTENTIAL
N/A

PREGNANCY
Pregnancy predisposes to abomasal impaction as a result of increased energy requirements, appetite, and the possible effect of size and weight of the gravid uterus on abdominal organs.

BIOSECURITY
N/A

PRODUCTION MANAGEMENT
This disorder is largely preventable through appropriate dietary management.

SYNONYMS
Abomasal emptying defect in sheep

ABBREVIATION
AED = abomasal emptying defect

SEE ALSO
• Abomasal Emptying Defect in Sheep
• Displaced Abomasum
• Lymphosarcoma
• Traumatic Reticuloperitonitis

Suggested Reading
Belknap EB, Navarre CB. Differentiation of gastrointestinal diseases in adult cattle. In: Helman RG ed, The Veterinary Clinics of

Vet Clin North Am Food Anim Pract, Diagnosis of Diseases of the Digestive Tract. Philadelphia: W.B. Saunders Company. Vol. 16, No. 1, March 2000.
Kline EE, Meyer JR, Nelson DR, Memon MA. Abomasal impaction in sheep. Vet Rec 1983, 113: 177–9.
Melendez P, Krueger T, Benzaquen M, Risco C. An outbreak of sand impaction in postpartum dairy cows. Can Vet J 2007, 48: 1067–70.
Pruden SJ, McAllister MM, Schultheiss PC, O'Toole D, Christensen DE. Abomasal emptying defect of sheep may be an acquired form of dysautonomia. Vet Pathol 2004, 41: 164–9.
Radostits OM, Gay CC, Blood DC, Hinchcliff KW eds, Veterinary Medicine: A Textbook of Diseases of Cattle, Sheep, Pigs, Goats and Horses, 9th ed. London: Saunders, 2000, pp. 332–5.
Rings DM, Welker FH, Hull BL, Kersting KW, Hoffsis GF. Abomasal emptying defect in Suffolk sheep. J Am Vet Med Assoc 1984, 185: 1520–2.
Ruegg PL, George LW, East NE. Abomasal dilatation and emptying defect in a flock of Suffolk ewes. J Am Vet Med Assoc 1988, 193: 1534–6.
Smith BP. Large animal internal medicine, 5th ed. St. Louis: Elsevier Mosby, 2015, pp. 818–20.
Wittek T, Constable PD, Morin DE. Abomasal impaction in Holstein-Friesian cows: 80 cases (1980–2003). J Am Vet Med Assoc 2005, 227: 287–91.
Author Jim P. Reynolds
Consulting Editor Erica C. McKenzie

BASICS

OVERVIEW
• Abomasal ulceration represents damage to the abomasal mucosa ranging from mucosal erosion to complete perforation. Often subclinical depending on the severity of disease.
• Abomasal ulceration can be classified as type I (nonperforating ulcers), type II (nonperforating with severe blood loss), type III (perforating with localized peritonitis), and type IV (perforating with diffuse peritonitis).
• When present, clinical signs reflect abdominal pain, blood loss, and peritonitis. The etiology is not clear, but may be associated with stress. There is no demonstrated association with specific bacterial pathogens.

INCIDENCE/PREVALENCE
• Low, likely below 1–2%. May be higher in some types of calf raising systems, and in cattle in the first month postpartum, particularly with concurrent disease.
• Rare occurrence in sheep and goats.

GEOGRAPHIC DISTRIBUTION
N/A

SYSTEMS AFFECTED
Digestive

PATHOPHYSIOLOGY
• Injuries to the protective mucosal layer of the abomasum allow gastric acid and pepsin to diffuse into the mucosa.
• Type I nonperforating ulcers have incomplete penetration, little local reaction, and minimal bleeding.
• Type II bleeding ulcers erode into a major blood vessel in the submucosa. There may be distension of the abomasum and reflux of abomasal contents into the rumen. Melena is typically observed.
• Type III ulcers completely perforate the wall with leakage of fluid and local peritonitis. Adhesions form to viscera, localizing the peritonitis.
• Type IV ulcers also completely perforate the wall; however, the subsequent fluid leakage is not contained by adhesions, resulting in generalized peritonitis.

HISTORICAL FINDINGS
Changes in feeding, such as transition from milk to solid feed in calves or change from a high roughage prepartum diet to high concentrate postpartum diets may be involved.

SIGNALMENT
• This disorder affects cattle, and rarely sheep and goats.
• There are no breed or gender predilections; however, dairy cattle may have a higher prevalence.
• Occurs in calves and adults.

PHYSICAL EXAMINATION FINDINGS
• Melena or occult blood is observed in feces.
• Possible distension of the abomasum detected by ballottement of the ventral right abdomen.
• Pale mucus membranes and tachycardia in cases with severe blood loss or septic shock.
• Anorexia, depression, pyrexia, and abdominal pain (bruxism).
• Peracute death common in adult cattle but not calves.

GENETICS
N/A

CAUSES AND RISK FACTORS
• This disorder has been associated with physical irritation from straw ingestion in veal calves and high grain diets in feedlot cattle.
• May be related to postpartum conditions in dairy cattle.
• Not definitively associated with bacteria such as *Clostridium*, *Salmonella* or *Helicobacter* sp. Recent gene pyrosequencing suggests limited involvement of bacteria in abomasal ulcers.
• No association with hairballs in veal calves.
• Risk factors might include sudden transition from milk diet to dry feed in calves, straw feeding in milk-fed calves, high concentrate diets, recent parturition, and peak milk production.

DIAGNOSIS

DIFFERENTIAL DIAGNOSES
• Lymphoma
• Left displaced abomasum
• Abomasal volvulus or torsion
• Intussusception
• Duodenal ulcers
• Hemorrhagic bowel syndrome

CBC/BIOCHEMISTRY/URINALYSIS
• Acute hemorrhagic anemia in cases of severe gastric hemorrhage, elevated fibrinogen, altered total protein concentration.
• Serum chemistry might reflect chronic inflammation in type III and IV ulceration reflected by high total protein concentrations and possibly neutrophilia on CBC.

OTHER LABORATORY TESTS
• Abdominocentesis may identify peritonitis, with increased leukocyte count, phagocytosed or free bacteria, and possibly feed particles in some cases.
• Testing for occult blood in feces may detect blood in the feces before melena is visible.

IMAGING
Ultrasonography may show free fluid and fibrin in the abdomen.

OTHER DIAGNOSTIC PROCEDURES
• Exploratory surgery.
• Peritoneal emphysema may be detected during per rectum examination.

• Positive withers pinch test may be evident (type III and IV).

PATHOLOGIC FINDINGS
• Ulcers are most commonly found along the greater curvature and usually in the fundic area. Ulcers can be a few millimeters to several centimeters in size. They are often filled with debris or clotted blood. Perforating ulcers are usually adhered to the omentum.
• Cattle with bleeding ulcers have signs of anemia with blood in the distal GI tract.
• Diffuse fibrinous peritonitis may be evident with defects in the serosal surface of the abomasum.

TREATMENT

THERAPEUTIC APPROACH
• Treatment is typically unrewarding but should target correction of management issues (dietary, stress related), correction of concurrent disease, and addressing clinical problems related to abomasal ulceration.
• Medical therapy may include provision of antacids to protect the abomasal mucosa, removal of high energy feedstuffs, and stall confinement.
• Blood transfusion may be beneficial if bleeding ceases or can be controlled, and is indicated if hematocrit declines to ≤14%.
• Broad-spectrum antibiotic therapy is indicated to prevent or address septic peritonitis.

SURGICAL CONSIDERATIONS AND TECHNIQUES
Surgical intervention for perforated ulcers might be attempted for valuable cattle.

MEDICATIONS

DRUGS OF CHOICE
• Magnesium oxide (500 g/400 kg body weight daily for 2–4 days), or a kaolin and pectin mixture (2–3 liters twice daily to mature cattle).
• Treatment options in calves include oral administration of antacids (25–50 mL q8h), ranitidine (50 mg/kg q8h) and omeprazole (4 mg/kg q24h).

CONTRAINDICATIONS
NSAIDs that interfere with the production of prostaglandin E series via the arachidonic acid cascade are not recommended, to avoid compromise of the protective coating of the abomasal mucosa.

PRECAUTIONS
• Avoid NSAIDs and corticosteroid drugs, particularly in susceptible populations.
• Appropriate milk and meat withdrawal times must be followed for all compounds administered to food-producing animals.

A   ABOMASAL ULCERATION   (CONTINUED)

POSSIBLE INTERACTIONS
N/A

FOLLOW-UP

EXPECTED COURSE AND PROGNOSIS
Recovery for type I and type III ulcers is considered likely or possible; type II ulcers are fatal if severe hemorrhage occurs; type IV ulcers carry a guarded prognosis.

POSSIBLE COMPLICATIONS
• Septic peritonitis as a result of abomasal leakage or perforation.
• Hepatic lipidosis as a result of anorexia, particularly in cattle in early lactation.

CLIENT EDUCATION
Gradual introduction of dry feed to calves is preferred over abrupt exposure to dry feed during the milk-fed period.

PATIENT CARE
Serial assessments of CBC, anemia, and pain are used to determine recovery over time.

PREVENTION
• Avoid rapid change from liquid to dry feed in calves.
• Avoid excessive concentrate diets in feedlot or dairy cattle.
• Cull animals infected with bovine leukosis virus to eliminate lymphosarcoma as a cause of abomasal ulceration.

MISCELLANEOUS

ASSOCIATED CONDITIONS
Lymphoma

AGE-RELATED FACTORS
Affects all ages

ZOONOTIC POTENTIAL
N/A

PREGNANCY
N/A

BIOSECURITY
N/A

PRODUCTION MANAGEMENT
Avoid sudden dietary changes, rather, gradually introduce dry feed to calves.

SYNONYMS
N/A

ABBREVIATION
NSAIDs = nonsteroidal anti-inflammatory drugs

SEE ALSO
• Displaced Abomasum
• Hemorrhagic Bowel Syndrome
• Lymphosarcoma

Suggested Reading
Braun U, Bretscher R, Gerber D. Bleeding abomasal ulcers in dairy cows. Vet Rec 1991, 129: 279–84.

Hund A, M, S, Wittek T. Characterization of mucosa-associated bacterial communities in abomasal ulcers by pyrosequencing. Vet Microbiol 2015, 177: 132–41.
Jelinski MD, Ribble CS, Chirino-Trejo M, Clark EG, Janzen ED. The relationship between the presence of *Helicobacter pylori*, *Clostridium perfringens* type A, *Campylobacter* spp, or fungi and fatal abomasal ulcers in unweaned beef calves. Can Vet J 1995, 36: 379–82.
Jelinski MD, Ribble CS, Campbell JR, Janzen ED. Investigating the relationship between abomasal hairballs and perforating abomasal ulcers in unweaned calves. Can Vet J 1996, 37: 23–6.
Palmer JE, Whitlock RH. Bleeding abomasal ulcers in adult dairy cows. J Am Med Assoc 1983, 183: 448–51.
Palmer JE, Whitlock RH. Perforated abomasal ulcers in adult dairy cows. J Am Med Assoc 1984, 184: 171–4.
Radostits OM, Gay CC, Blood DC, Hinchcliff KWeds, Veterinary Medicine: A Textbook of Diseases of Cattle, Sheep, Pigs, Goats and Horses, 9th ed. London: Saunders, 2000, pp. 335–9.
Smith BP. Large animal internal medicine, 5th ed. St. Louis: Elsevier Mosby, 2015, pp. 815–17.

Author Jim P. Reynolds
Consulting Editor Erica C. McKenzie

BASICS

OVERVIEW
Pregnancy loss between 42 days and term, caused by bacterial infection

INCIDENCE/PREVALENCE
• Abortion rates depend on the pathogen and immunologic status of the herd.
• Abortion rates range from <10% (serovar Hardjo of *Leptospira*, listeriosis) to 50–70% (serovar Pomona of *Leptospira*, brucellosis, epizootic bovine abortion).

GEOGRAPHIC DISTRIBUTION
• Worldwide
• Epizootic bovine abortion: California, Nevada, and Oregon

SYSTEMS AFFECTED
• Reproductive
• Other systems depending on cause

PATHOPHYSIOLOGY
• Infection occurs venereally, orally, via inhalation or across conjunctival mucosa.
• Ticks act as vectors for epizootic bovine abortion, *Anaplasma* spp., and *Coxiella burnetii*.
• Conceptus infection via hematogenous spread, ascending infection through the cervix, or descending infection from the abdomen through the oviducts.
• Bacteria may cause placentitis and fetal septicemia via the umbilical veins or by ingestion of amniotic fluid.
• Fetal death occurs secondary to placental insufficiency, fetal septicemia, lysis of the corpus luteum (CL) or failure of the diseased fetoplacental unit to produce progesterone to support pregnancy (after 200 days).
• A delay in fetal expulsion leads to autolysis or maceration.
• Dams may shed bacteria in urine, milk, feces, oronasal secretions, or uterine discharge. The abortus is an important source of infection.
• Gram-negative bacteria causing maternal systemic disease may also lead to abortion associated with luteolysis secondary to endotoxemia.

HISTORICAL FINDINGS
• Abortions
• Inappropriate vaccination
• Introduction of new animals

SIGNALMENT
• Ruminants, bovine (epizootic bovine abortion)
• Breeding age females
• Epizootic bovine abortion more common in naïve heifers

PHYSICAL EXAMINATION FINDINGS
• Physical examination is usually unremarkable.

• Illness and fever may develop secondary to retained fetal membranes (RFM) or a retained macerated fetus and metritis.
• *Campylobacter fetus venerealis*: Infertility, pregnancy loss between 15 and 80 days' gestation, or abortion at 4 to 6 months.
• *Leptospira* spp.: Last trimester abortion, stillbirth, weak calves, and infertility. Severe acute disease with hemolytic anemia, hemoglobinuria, and mastitis with serovar Pomona.
• *Brucella abortus*: Abortion after 5 months' gestation, weak or premature calves, RFM, metritis, infertility, carpal hygromas, regional lymphadenitis.
• *Listeria monocytogenes* and *L. ivanovii*: Abortion in the last trimester, meningoencephalitis, metritis, weight loss, maternal and neonatal septicemia.
• *Histophilus somni*: Pneumonia, arthritis, myocarditis, meningoencephalitis, sporadic abortions in the second half of gestation.
• *Salmonella enterica* serovar Dublin: Enteritis, dysentery, pneumonia, polyarthritis, pyrexia, abortion during the second half of gestation.
• *Trueperella pyogenes* (formerly *Arcanobacterium pyogenes*): Organ abscessation with varying signs, pyometra, abortion at any time.
• *Ureaplasma diversum*: Embryonic death, last trimester abortion, stillbirth, weak calves, neonatal pneumonia, endometritis, granular vulvovaginitis, salpingitis, endometritis.
• *C. burnetii*: late abortions, stillbirth, weak calves.
• *Mycobacterium bovis*: Organ granulomas with variable signs, late abortion, purulent to caseous vaginal discharge.
• *Anaplasma marginale*: Pale mucus membranes, icterus, fever, weakness, abortion during the acute phase of maternal disease.
• *A. phagocytophilum*: Fever, cough, nasal discharge, abortion during the acute phase of maternal disease.
• Epizootic bovine abortion: Last trimester abortion, premature births.
• *Chlamydophila abortus*: Abortions at 6 to 8 months' gestation, stillbirths, weak calves, RFM, mastitis, infertility.

GENETICS
N/A

CAUSES AND RISK FACTORS

Contagious bacteria
B. abortus, *C. fetus* (subsp. venerealis or fetus), *C. jejuni*, *Leptospira* spp., *L. monocytogenes*, *H. somni*, *Salmonella* spp., *Y. pseudotuberculosis*, *M. bovis*, *C. abortus*

Tick-borne infection
C. burnetii, *A. marginale*, *A. phagocytophilum*, epizootic bovine abortion

Mollicute infection
M. bovis, *M. bovigenitalium*, *M. canadense*, *M. leachii*, *Ureaplasma diversum*

Opportunistic bacteria
Bacillus spp., *E. coli*, *Pasteurella* spp., *Pseudomonas* spp., *Staphylococcus* spp., *Streptococcus* spp.

Mode of infection
• Inappropriate biosecurity measurements and vaccination schedules
• Nutritional, social or environmental stress
• Seasonal presence of ticks and vectors
• Exposure to wildlife and rodents

DIAGNOSIS

DIFFERENTIAL DIAGNOSES
• Vaginitis, metritis, endometritis
• Other causes of abortion

CBC/BIOCHEMISTRY/URINALYSIS
• Hemolytic anemia and hemoglobinuria (*L. interrogans* serovar Pomona)
• Anemia or leukopenia (*Anaplasma* spp.)

OTHER LABORATORY TESTS
• Bacterial culture from aborted tissues (lung, abomasal contents, placenta) and dam's milk (brucellosis).
• Dam and fetal serology.
• Immunohistochemistry and/or immunofluorescence on fetal tissues (leptospirosis, listeriosis, campylobacter, *C. burnetii*, *C. abortus*).
• PCR on aborted tissues (leptospirosis, *Brucella* spp., *Mycoplasma* spp., *Ureaplasma*, campylobacteriosis, *C. burnetii*, *Anaplasma* spp., *C. abortus*).
• Direct identification on Giemsa-stained blood smears (*Anaplasma* spp.).
• Pathognomonic microscopic lesions in the thymus (epizootic bovine abortion).

IMAGING
N/A

OTHER DIAGNOSTIC PROCEDURES
Fetal necropsy

PATHOLOGIC FINDINGS
• *C. fetus*: Fetal fibrinous pleuritis, pericarditis and peritonitis. Intercotyledonary placentitis, necrotic cotyledons.
• *Leptospira* spp.: Autolyzed and icteric fetus, cholestasis, intercotyledonary edema, diffuse cotyledonary necrosis.
• *B. abortus*: Fetus (autolysis, fibrinous pleuritis, pericarditis, peritonitis, pneumonia); placentitis.
• *Listeria* spp.: Fetus (autolysis, white foci of liver necrosis, abomasal erosions, pneumonia, polyarthritis); multifocal cotyledonary necrosis and intercotyledonary placentitis.
• *H. somni*: Autolytic fetus, necrosis of cotyledons.
• *Salmonella* spp.: Fetus (autolysis, emphysema, liver necrosis); placentitis.
• *T. pyogenes*: Fetus (autolysis), suppurative bronchopneumonia); cotyledonary and intercotyledonary placentitis.

• *Mycoplasma* spp.: Placentitis, fetal bronchopneumonia, and myocarditis.
• *U. diversum*: Fetus (fresh); thickening and fibrosis of the amnion and chorioallantois, mineralization, necrosis, hemorrhage.
• *C. burnetii*: thick leathery intercotyledonary spaces, multifocal mineralization, and pericotyledonary necrosis.
• Epizootic bovine abortion: Fetus (fresh, ascites, excessive fibrin, enlarged liver, spleen and lymph nodes, petechial hemorrhage on mucosal membranes and thymus, focal necrotizing lesions in lymphatic tissues, depletion of cortical thymocytes, and infiltration with macrophages in the thymus).
• *C. abortus*: Fetus (subcutaneous edema, ascites, thymic and subcuticular petechiae, serofibrinous pleuritis and peritonitis, nodular mottled liver, and enlarged lymph nodes); necrotizing placentitis with leathery, reddish, opaque intercotyledonary patches and multifocal cotyledonary necrosis.

TREATMENT

THERAPEUTIC APPROACH
• Treatment of systemic disease, RFM, metritis or hypocalcemia as needed.
• Vaccination can be curative (*Campylobacter* spp.).
• Supportive as needed.

SURGICAL CONSIDERATIONS AND TECHNIQUES
N/A

MEDICATIONS

DRUGS OF CHOICE
• *H. somnus*: β-lactams, florfenicol, tetracycline, and sulfonamides
• *Leptospira* spp: oxytetracycline, erythromycin, tiamulin, tylosin, tilmicosin, tulathromycin, ceftiofur
• *Listeria* spp.: tetracycline
• *U. diversum* and *Mycoplasma* spp.: tetracycline, tylosin
• *C. abortus*: tetracycline
• Epizootic bovine abortion: chlortetracycline

CONTRAINDICATIONS
N/A

PRECAUTIONS
Milk and meat withdrawal times should be followed.

POSSIBLE INTERACTIONS
N/A

FOLLOW-UP

EXPECTED COURSE AND PROGNOSIS
Infected or exposed cows may develop natural immunity to some bacteria, with lower rates of abortion in subsequent breeding seasons.

POSSIBLE COMPLICATIONS
• Dystocia
• RFM
• Metritis
• Infertility

CLIENT EDUCATION
• Zoonotic potential. Wear protective gloves and clothes when handling aborted tissues and animals.
• Pregnant women, children, elderly and immunosuppressed people should not handle aborting animals or tissues.
• Keep aborted tissues refrigerated and call a veterinarian.
• Proper disposal of aborted tissues.

PATIENT CARE
• Monitor cow for RFM and metritis.
• Monitor herd for further abortions, stillbirths, or birth of weak calves.
• Change silage source (listeriosis).
• Adjust diet to eliminate ruminal acidosis and bacterial translocation.

PREVENTION
• Appropriate immunization program, nutrition, and environmental management.
• Test and quarantine new animals.
• Test and cull positive animals.
• Use virgin bulls and heifers for replacement.
• Use artificial insemination.
• Reduce contact with wildlife and rodents.
• Cure silage properly and avoid feeding spoiled material.
• Use fall calving season to prevent exposure of pregnant cows to ticks.
• Expose cows to ticks prior to breeding to stimulate natural immunity.

MISCELLANEOUS

ASSOCIATED CONDITIONS
N/A

AGE-RELATED FACTORS
N/A

ZOONOTIC POTENTIAL
Brucellosis, leptospirosis, listeriosis, *Coxiella burnetii*, *Chlamydophila abortus*, and salmonellosis

PREGNANCY
N/A

BIOSECURITY
• Brucellosis and tuberculosis are reportable diseases.
• See "Prevention."

PRODUCTION MANAGEMENT
See "Prevention."

SYNONYMS
N/A

ABBREVIATIONS
• CL = corpus luteum
• RFM = retained fetal membranes

SEE ALSO
• Abortion: Bovine
• Abortion: Viral, Fungal, and Nutritional
• Brucellosis
• Campylobacter
• Chlamydiosis
• Listeriosis
• Q Fever (Coxiellosis)
• Vaccination Programs: Beef Cattle
• Vaccination Programs: Dairy Cattle

Suggested Reading
Baumgartner W. Fetal disease and abortion: diagnosis and causes. In: Hopper R ed, Bovine Reproduction. Ames: Wiley Blackwell, 2015.
Yaeger MJ, Holler LD. Bacterial causes of bovine infertility and abortion. In: Youngquist RS, Threlfall WR eds, Current Therapy in Large Animal Theriogenology, 2nd ed. St. Louis: Saunders Elsevier, 2007.
Author Maria Soledad Ferrer
Consulting Editor Ahmed Tibary
Acknowledgment The author and book editors acknowledge the prior contribution of Walter Johnson and Alex Estrada.

BASICS

OVERVIEW
Abortion in cattle is defined as loss of the fetus from 42 days to term. Prior to 42 days, pregnancy loss is considered embryonic mortality.

INCIDENCE/PREVALENCE
• Should be <5% on a herd basis (<1–2% ideal). • Abortion storms may occur in the case of specific infectious diseases. • In a 10-year study on bovine abortions and stillbirths, bacteria were determined to be the cause of 14.49% of the cases. The five bacteria most commonly associated with bovine abortion in the study were *Trueperella pyogenes*, *Bacillus* spp., *Listeria* spp., *E. coli*, and *L. interrogans*.

GEOGRAPHIC DISTRIBUTION
Worldwide

SYSTEMS AFFECTED
• Reproductive • Other systems depending on cause

PATHOPHYSIOLOGY
• Cattle rely primarily on the corpus luteum (CL) for production of progesterone for the first 180–200 days of gestation, followed by a shift to production of progesterone by the placenta in late gestation. • Abortion may be caused by infectious or noninfectious etiologies. ○ Infectious causes of abortion include bacteria, viruses, fungi, and protozoa. ■ Bacteria involved in abortion can be grouped into contagious and opportunistic. ■ Ability of a pathogen to damage the conceptus is influenced by the dam, stage of fetal development, and virulence of the infectious agent. ■ The time between fetal death and expulsion may be characteristic for a pathogen. ○ Noninfectious causes of abortion include nutritional imbalance, exogenous drug administration, malnutrition, stress, environmental toxins, teratogenic compounds, hormone imbalances, and genetic abnormalities. • Abortion may result due to fetal death following: ○ Invasion by microorganisms through hematogenous spread, ascending infection or presence of organism in the uterus prior to conception. ○ Placental disease or insufficiency due to hematogenous (umbilical veins) or amniotic fluid (i.e., fungal infections) contamination. Some pathogens may cause severe placentitis leading to fetal hypoxia and death. ○ Maternal compromise (mastitis, pneumonia, circulatory disorder, hypoxia, endotoxemia, etc.). ○ Severe congenital malformations in some etiologies.

HISTORICAL FINDINGS
• Introduction of new animals • Return to receptivity after confirmation of pregnancy • Bloody or mucopurulent vaginal discharge in the pregnant cow • Protrusion/expulsion of the placenta or fetus • Premature development of the mammary gland and lactation
A complete history should be taken from each aborting case and include the following information:
• Age, breed, lactation/parity, clinical signs of the aborting female. • Reproductive history (i.e. breeding technique, breeding dates). • Individual case vs herd outbreak ○ Number of animals ○ Health problems/body condition ○ Herd abortion history • Treatments and vaccination administered in the preceding 2 weeks. • Animal movement within the last month. • Previous abortions and any workup performed. • Feeding/nutritional management, quality of pasture (toxic plants). • Layout of the facilities (water sources, proximity to other operations, etc.). • Contact with wildlife or feral cats and dogs.

SIGNALMENT
Females of breeding age

PHYSICAL EXAMINATION FINDINGS
• Physical examination findings and evidence of abortion will depend on the stage of gestation and the cause of abortion. • Clinical examination of the cow(s) should be taken into consideration: ○ Body condition score. ○ Thorough physical examination including temperature, pulse, respiration, mucus membrane color, hydration status, presence of vaginal discharge, etc. ○ Demeanor. ○ Visual abnormalities.

GENETICS
N/A

CAUSES AND RISK FACTORS
• Causes of abortion can be classified as infectious (viral, bacterial, protozoal, fungal) or noninfectious (iatrogenic, maternal, fetal/placental, nutritional). • Noninfectious causes of abortion may be sporadic or affect several animals in the herd (nutritional deficiencies or administration of certain drugs). Infectious abortions are more likely to affect several animals within the herd simultaneously. • Risk factors include lack of biosecurity measures, presence of vectors or toxins, overcrowding, etc.

DIAGNOSIS

• The etiology of abortion is often difficult to determine and can be frustrating for owners and practitioners. Even when all required samples are submitted, the diagnostic rate is only 30%. • Abortion frequently results from an event that occurred weeks to months prior to the abortion event, making the diagnosis difficult in many cases. • Evaluation should include: ○ Uterine cytology and culture (indicated in some cases) ○ Serology ■ Samples should be taken from the fetus (cardiac blood), from the aborting dam (paired samples) at abortion and 2 to 3 weeks later, and from at-risk pregnant females in the face of an outbreak. ■ Samples from 10% of the herd will make serological assessment more meaningful. ○ Bacteriology/Virology ■ Samples should be taken from the fetus (stomach content, fetal fluids both thoracic and abdominal, kidney, liver, lung, spleen, and thymus), from the dam (vaginal discharge, uterine swab), and from the placenta. ■ Samples should be collected using aseptic technique into sterile bags, refrigerated, and submitted to the diagnostic laboratory for further evaluation. ○ Necropsy/Histopathology ■ Digital photographs are helpful for documenting lesions. ■ A complete set of tissues should be collected in every case. ■ Fetal necropsy: Measurement of the crown–rump length and weight. External evaluation of the fetus for developmental abnormalities or lesions and evidence of autolysis, maceration, or mummification. Internal evaluation of the fetus. Either the entire fetus (optimal) or samples from the liver, brain, thymus, heart, spleen, kidney, stomach, lungs, skeletal muscle should be submitted fixed in formalin and fresh chilled to a diagnostic laboratory for further evaluation. Collection of ocular fluid (freeze) for nitrate/nitrite levels. ■ Placental evaluation: External examination of the chorioallantois (including the cotyledons) and amnion. External examination for signs of placentitis (thickening, degradation, exudate). Examination for developmental abnormalities or lesions of the umbilical cord. Make impression smears of any lesions. Either the entire placenta or samples of both uterine horns and uterine body (cotyledons and intercotyledonary areas), along with any subjective abnormal areas, should be submitted fixed in formalin and fresh chilled for further evaluation.

DIFFERENTIAL DIAGNOSES
Infectious Causes of Abortion
• Viral causes of abortion: ○ Bovine viral diarrhea virus (BVDV). ○ Bovine herpesvirus 1 (BHV-1, infectious bovine rhinotracheitis; abortion storms affecting 25–60% in naïve pregnant cattle). ○ Bovine herpesvirus 4 (BHV-4, often associated with other pathogens). ○ Bluetongue virus (BTV). ○ Epizootic hemorrhagic disease virus (EHDV). ○ Rift Valley fever phlebovirus (RVF; mortality range 10–70% and abortion occurring at any gestational age reaching 80–90%). ○ Akabane virus. ○ Schmallenberg virus. • Bacterial causes of abortion: ○ Brucellosis (*B. abortus*; in susceptible herds, abortion rates may be as high as 70%). ○ Listeriosis (*L. monocytogenes*, *L. ivanovii*; abortions sporadic and rarely >15%). ○ Campylobacteriosis (*C. fetus* subsp. *venerealis* (abortions <10% in infected herds), *C. fetus* subsp. *fetus*, *C. jejuni*). ○ Leptospirosis (*L. interrogans* serovars Hardjo and Pomona most important causes of abortion, losses of

up to 50% may be experienced in some outbreaks). ° Tuberculosis (*Mycobacterium bovis, M. caprae*). ° Epizootic bovine abortion. ° *Histophilus somni* (formerly *Haemophilus somnus*). ° *Salmonella* spp. ° *Trueperella pyogenes* (formerly *Arcanobacterium pyogenes*). ° *Mycoplasma bovis, Ureaplasma diversum*. ° *Chlamydophila abortus* (lesser extent *C. psittaci*. ° *Coxiella burnetii*. ° Anaplasmosis (*Anaplasma phagocytophilum* has been known to cause abortion storms during first exposure to infected ticks during late pregnancy). ° Other opportunistic bacteria: *Escherichia coli, Pasteurella* spp., *Pseudomonas* spp., *Staphylococcus* spp., *Streptococcus* spp., *Bacillus* spp. • Protozoal causes of abortion: ° *Neospora caninum* (abortion only clinical sign in cattle). ° *Tritrichomonas foetus.* • Fungal causes of abortion: ° *Aspergillus* spp. (*A. fumigatus*; reported most common cause of mycotic abortion in cattle). ° *Candida* spp. ° *Zygomycetes.*

Noninfectious Causes of Abortion
• Iatrogenic causes of abortion: Administration of PGF2$_\alpha$ or glucocorticoids. • Maternal causes of abortion: ° Stress ° Systemic disease ° Hormonal imbalances, adrenal gland dysfunction (particularly in fiber-producing animals) ° Uterine/cervical pathology ° Trauma (hemorrhage during pregnancy). • Environmental/nutritional causes of abortion: ° Nutritional/trace mineral deficiencies. ° Toxic plants: pine needle; broom snakeweed; locoweeds; hairy vetch (sporadic abortions); poison hemlock (cattle surviving acute poisoning generally abort); high plant estrogens; plants that accumulate nitrates. ° Aflatoxins° *Fusarium graminearum* (zearalenone) ° Organophosphates ° Nitrate fertilizer ° Vitamin A, selenium deficiency/toxicosis, iodine deficiency. • Fetal/placental causes of abortion: ° Twinning ° Umbilical cord torsion ° Congenital anomalies

CBC/BIOCHEMISTRY/URINALYSIS
May be indicated in some cases

OTHER LABORATORY TESTS
See "Diagnosis"

IMAGING
N/A

OTHER DIAGNOSTIC PROCEDURES
See "Diagnosis"

PATHOLOGIC FINDINGS
See "Diagnosis"

TREATMENT

THERAPEUTIC APPROCH
Depends on systemic involvement and other complications

SURGICAL CONSIDERATIONS
N/A

MEDICATIONS

DRUGS OF CHOICE
Depends on systemic involvement and other complications

CONTRAINDICATIONS
N/A

PRECAUTIONS
N/A

POSSIBLE INTERACTIONS
N/A

FOLLOW-UP

EXPECTED COURSE AND PROGNOSIS
Dependent on the cause of abortion

POSSIBLE COMPLICATIONS
Dystocia, retained placenta, metritis, mastitis, infertility.

CLIENT EDUCATION
• Establish good preventative programs: biosecurity measures, immunization programs, adequate nutrition, parasite control. • Producers should have an intervention plan in case of abortion (isolation of affected females, collection of aborted materials for submission to veterinarian, examination of female and abortus). • Segregation of animals based on sex, age, and pregnancy status may help reduce transmission of infectious organism.

PATIENT CARE
• Dependent on the cause of abortion. • Isolation of affected cow(s) from remainder of the group. • Adequate nutrition, including balanced trace minerals, for the herd is important for elimination of some of the causes of abortion.

PREVENTION
• General prevention program for abortion (guidelines for biosecurity): ° Quarantine new animals (4 to 6 weeks) ° Nutrition ° Immunization program ° Keep feed, pasture, and water sources free from contamination ° Control rodent, bird, and feral animal populations. • Observe strict hygiene during parturition, keep good calving facilities. • Reduce stress due to poor nutrition, unsanitary environment, crowded conditions.

MISCELLANEOUS

ASSOCIATED CONDITIONS
N/A

AGE-RELATED FACTORS
N/A

ZOONOTIC POTENTIAL
• Brucellosis (*Brucella abortus*) • Campylobacteriosis (*C. jejuni*) • Chlamydial organisms • Q fever (*Coxiella burnetii*) • *Mycobacterium bovis* • Leptospirosis • Listeriosis

PREGNANCY
N/A

BIOSECURITY
See "Prevention"

PRODUCTION MANAGEMENT
N/A

SYNONYMS
N/A

ABBREVIATIONS
• CL = corpus luteum • PGF2$_\alpha$ = prostaglandin F2$_\alpha$

SEE ALSO
• Abortion: Bacterial • Abortion: Viral, Fungal, and Nutritional

Suggested Reading
Anderson M. Infectious causes of bovine abortion during mid- to late-gestation. Theriogenology 2007, 68: 474–86.
Anderson M. Disorders of cattle. In: Njaa BL ed, Kirkbride's Diagnosis of Abortion and Neonatal Loss in Animals, 4th ed. Singapore: John Wiley & Sons, 2012, pp. 13–48.
Baumgartner W. Fetal disease and abortion: diagnosis and causes. In: Hopper R ed, Bovine Reproduction. Oxford: John Wiley & Sons, pp. 481–517.
BonDurant R. Selected diseases and conditions associated with bovine conceptus loss in the first trimester. Theriogenology 2007, 68: 461–73.
Cooper E, Laing I. The clinicians' view of fetal and neonatal necropsy. In: Keenling JW, Yee Khong T eds, Fetal and Neonatal Pathology, 4th ed. London: Springer-Verlag, 2015, pp. 1–19.
Nietfeld J. Field necropsy techniques and proper specimen submission for investigation of emerging infectious diseases of food animals. Vet Clin North Am Food Anim Pract 2010, 26: 1–13.
Whittier W. Investigation of abortions and fetal loss in the beef herd. In: Anderson DE, Rings M eds, Current Veterinary Therapy: Food Animal Practice, 5th ed. St. Louis: Saunders, 2009, pp. 613–18.

Author Alexis Campbell
Consulting Editor Ahmed Tibary

BASICS

OVERVIEW
Abortion is defined as loss of the fetus from 42 days to term. Prior to 42 days, pregnancy loss is considered embryonic mortality.

INCIDENCE/PREVALENCE
• Pregnancy loss ranges from 2 to 17%.
• Losses of up to 60% may be experienced in some leptospirosis outbreaks (i.e., leptospirosis, brucellosis).
• Loss of 40–50% have been reported in maiden females under some management systems.

GEOGRAPHIC DISTRIBUTION
Worldwide with some regional differences

SYSTEMS AFFECTED
• Reproductive
• Other systems depending on cause and complications

PATHOPHYSIOLOGY
• Camelids rely primarily on the corpus luteum (CL) for production of progesterone and maintenance of pregnancy for the entire gestation.
• Abortion is caused by any factor that causes directly or indirectly luteolysis:
  ◦ Treatment with prostaglandin F2$_\alpha$
  ◦ Inflammatory or infectious process
  ◦ Endotoxemia
  ◦ Stress such as heat stress or transport
  ◦ Debilitating diseases
• Abortion can be caused by compromised fetal viability or placental integrity:
  ◦ Placentitis
  ◦ Placental insufficiency (endometrial fibrosis, uterine capacity in maiden females, twinning)
  ◦ Direct insult to the fetus (mechanical or infectious)
  ◦ Fetal malformation/abnormal pregnancy
  ◦ Hormonal insufficiency or imbalance

HISTORICAL FINDINGS
• Presenting complaints may include:
  ◦ Return to receptivity after confirmation of pregnancy
  ◦ Bloody or mucopurulent vaginal discharge in the pregnant female
  ◦ Protrusion/expulsion of the placenta or fetus
  ◦ Premature development of the mammary gland and lactation
• A complete history of the aborting female(s) should include the following information:
  ◦ Age
  ◦ Reproductive history (breeding technique, pregnancy diagnosis, breeding dates)
  ◦ Treatments and vaccination administered in the preceding 2 weeks
  ◦ Animal movement within the last month
  ◦ Possibility of heat stress
  ◦ Feeding management
  ◦ Layout of the facilities (i.e., proximity to stagnant water, run-offs from dairy or swine operations)
  ◦ Contact with wildlife, feral cats

SIGNALMENT
Females of breeding age

PHYSICAL EXAMINATION FINDINGS
• Physical examination findings and evidence of abortion will depend on the stage of gestation and the cause of abortion.
• Anorexia or poor appetite.
• Increased rectal temperature, pulse and respiration are seen in some infectious conditions.
• Signs of colic are often reported prior to abortion particularly in late gestation.
• Emaciated or obese females.
• Mucopurulent or bloody vaginal discharge.

GENETICS
N/A

CAUSES AND RISK FACTORS
• Causes may be infectious or noninfectious (iatrogenic, fetal/placental abnormalities, nutritional, environmental, management).
• Abortion of noninfectious origin is usually sporadic. However, several animals in the herd may be affected in the case of nutritional deficiencies or administration of certain drugs.
• Infectious abortions are more likely to affect several animals within the herd simultaneously.

Infectious Causes of Abortion
• Viral causes:
  ◦ Bovine viral diarrhea virus (most common serotype affecting alpacas and llamas is noncytopathic BVDV-1b)
  ◦ Equine herpes virus-1 (potential)
  ◦ Blue tongue virus (potential)
• Bacterial causes:
  ◦ Brucellosis (*B. meletensis* and *B. abortus*)
  ◦ Listeriosis
  ◦ Chlamydiosis (*Chlamydophila abortus*)
  ◦ Leptospirosis
  ◦ Q fever (*Coxiella burnetii*, well-established cause of abortion in camels)
  ◦ Hemorrhagic disease (*Bacillus cereus*, camels)
• Protozoal causes of abortion:
  ◦ *Neospora caninum*
  ◦ Toxoplasmosis
  ◦ Trypanosomiasis (camels)

Noninfectious Causes of Abortion
• Iatrogenic causes of abortion:
  ◦ Administration of PGF2$_\alpha$
  ◦ Administration of corticosteroids (even topical) in the second half of pregnancy
  ◦ Some multivalent vaccines (8-way vaccines against *Clostridium* spp.)
  ◦ Ecbolic drugs
• Maternal causes of abortion:
  ◦ Hypoluteoidism (luteal insufficiency)
  ◦ Stress
  ◦ Systemic disease
  ◦ Hormonal imbalances, adrenal gland dysfunction (particularly in fiber-producing animals)
  ◦ Uterine/cervical pathology
  ◦ Trauma (hemorrhage during pregnancy)
• Nutritional causes of abortion:
  ◦ Nutritional/trace mineral deficiencies (selenium)
  ◦ Toxic plants (limited information available in camelids)
• Fetal/placental causes of abortion:
  ◦ Twinning
  ◦ Umbilical cord torsion
  ◦ Congenital anomalies
  ◦ Placental insufficiency

DIAGNOSIS

DIFFERENTIAL DIAGNOSES
Evaluation of the female should include:
• Transabdominal ultrasonography
• Vaginal speculum examination
• Uterine cytology, culture, and biopsy may be indicated in some cases.
• Serology
  ◦ Samples should be taken from the fetus (cardiac blood), from the aborting dam (paired samples) at abortion and 2 to 3 weeks later, and from at-risk pregnant females in the face of an outbreak.
• Bacteriology
  ◦ Samples should be taken from the fetus (stomach content, fetal fluids both thoracic and abdominal), from the dam (vaginal discharge, uterine swab), and from the placenta.
• Necropsy/Histopathology
  ◦ Fetal necropsy:
    ▪ Measurement of the crown–rump length.
    ▪ External evaluation of the fetus for developmental abnormalities or lesions.
    ▪ Either the entire fetus or samples from the liver, brain, spleen, kidney, stomach, and lungs should be submitted fixed in formalin and fresh chilled to a diagnostic laboratory for further evaluation.
  ◦ Placental evaluation:
    ▪ External examination of the chorionic surface for lack of villi (placental insufficiency) or signs of placentitis (thickening, degradation, exudate).
    ▪ The umbilical cord is examined for abnormalities or inflammatory lesions.
    ▪ The entire placenta or samples of both uterine horns and uterine body, along with any abnormal areas, should be submitted fixed in formalin and fresh chilled for further evaluation.
• Endocrinology
  ◦ In cases of habitual abortion, progesterone determination during pregnancy may be indicative of possible luteal insufficiency. Pregnant females with progesterone levels

ABORTION: CAMELID

<2 ng/mL should be considered suspicious. However, some females may be able to carry a pregnancy to term even if progesterone levels are 1.5–2 ng/mL.

CBC/BIOCHEMISTRY/URINALYSIS
May be indicated depending on disease condition

OTHER LABORATORY TESTS
See "Diagnosis"

IMAGING
N/A

OTHER DIAGNOSTIC PROCEDURES
See "Diagnosis"

PATHOLOGIC FINDINGS
• Studies on pathological findings in camelid abortion are scarce.
• Placentitis is a common feature in bacterial and fungal abortions.
• Placental insufficiency is often suspected if large avillous areas are seen on the placenta.
• Fetal abnormalities are common.

TREATMENT
THERAPEUTIC APPROACH
• Dependent on the cause of abortion
• Abortion due to hypoluteoidism
  ○ Requires progesterone supplementation (injections of progesterone or hydroxyprogesterone caproate, norgestomet implant). Altrenogest is not active orally in camelids.
  ○ Hydroxyprogesterone caproate 250 mg, IM, every 3 weeks with treatment discontinued at 300 days to allow normal parturition.
  ○ Fetal viability should be monitored regularly if progesterone supplementation is implemented.
• Placental insufficiency
  ○ Early diagnosis and termination of twins.
  ○ Early diagnosis of uterine fibrosis (uterine biopsy) and sexual rest.

SURGICAL CONSIDERATIONS AND TECHNIQUES
N/A

MEDICATIONS
DRUGS OF CHOICE
N/A

CONTRAINDICATIONS
Appropriate milk and meat withdrawal times must be followed.

PRECAUTIONS
N/A

POSSIBLE INTERACTIONS
N/A

FOLLOW-UP
EXPECTED COURSE AND PROGNOSIS
See specific disease/condition

POSSIBLE COMPLICATIONS
Dystocia, metritis, endometritis, retained placenta, infertility

CLIENT EDUCATION
• Pregnancy should be monitored in the first 60–90 days of gestation.
• Producers should have a plan if an abortion occurs (isolation of affected females, collection of aborted materials for submission to veterinarian, examination of female and abortus).
• Adequate nutrition, parasite control, and immunization programs for the herd are important for preventing some causes of abortion. Segregation of animals based on sex, age, and pregnancy status may help reduce transmission of infectious organism.
• Adequate nutrition, including balanced trace minerals, for the herd is important for elimination of some of the causes of abortion.

PATIENT CARE
• Depends on the cause of abortion and complications.
• Supportive care is important in debilitated animals.

PREVENTION
• Observe strict hygiene in breeding management.
• Set up guideline for biosecurity: quarantine new animals; during movement of animals between shows and ranch, visiting animals for breeding.
• Isolate any aborting female until diagnosis is established.
• Vaccination for leptospirosis (4 times a year in high-risk situations).

MISCELLANEOUS
ASSOCIATED CONDITIONS
• Infertility, dystocia, poor systemic health
• Fetal abnormalities

AGE-RELATED FACTORS
N/A

ZOONOTIC POTENTIAL
Possible for brucellosis (*B. meletensis, B. abortus*), *Chlamydophila abortus*, leptospirosis, Q fever

PREGNANCY
N/A

BIOSECURITY
See "Prevention"

PRODUCTION MANAGEMENT
N/A

SYNONYMS
N/A

ABBREVIATION
• CL = corpus luteum
• PGF2$_\alpha$ = prostaglandin F2$_\alpha$

SEE ALSO
• Abortion: Bacterial
• Abortion: Viral, Fungal, and Nutritional
• Camel Diseases
• Congenital Defects: Camelids
• Pregnancy Toxemia: Camelids

Suggested Reading
Pearson LK, Rodriguez JS, Tibary A. 2014. Disorders and diseases of pregnancy. In: Cebra C, Anderson DE, Tibary A, Van Saun AJ, Johnson LW eds, Llama and Alpaca Care: Medicine, Surgery, Reproduction, Nutrition, and Herd Health. St Louis: Saunders, pp. 256–73.
Schaefer DL, Bildfell RJ, Long P, Lohr CV. Characterization of the microanatomy and histopathology of placentas from aborted, stillborn, and normally delivered alpacas (*Vicugna pacos*) and llamas (*Lama glama*). Vet Pathol 2012, 49: 313–21.
Tibary A, Fite C, Anouassi A, Sghiri A. Infectious causes of reproductive loss in camelids. Theriogenology 2006, 66: 633–47.
Van Amstel S, Kennedy M. Bovine viral diarrhea infections in new world camelids: a review. Small Rum Res 2010, 91: 121–6.
Author Alexis Campbell
Consulting Editor Ahmed Tibary
Acknowledgment The author and book editors acknowledge the prior contribution of Ahmed Tibary.

BASICS

OVERVIEW
• Definition: Loss of an embryo or fetus
• Causes may be infectious, environmental, congenital or idiopathic

INCIDENCE/PREVALANCE
The incidence of pregnancy loss in farmed deer is relatively low.

GEOGRAPHIC DISTRIBUTION
N/A

SYSTEMS AFFECTED
• Reproductive • Others depending on cause

PATHOPHYSIOLOGY
• Pathophysiology depends on etiology.
• Infectious: organism spreads to gravid uterus and may cause death of the embryo/fetus or placentitis, which leads to placental separation; absorption or expulsion of the conceptus. • Environmental: as in other ruminant species, stress, malnutrition, or toxins can adversely affect oocyte or embryo quality or hormonal regulation in the female. • Congenital: placental dysfunction or fetal abnormalities usually result, leading to premature expulsion of the fetus.

HISTORICAL FINDINGS
• If fetus is resorbed early in gestation, there may be no findings except missed due date from an expected or confirmed pregnancy. • If pregnancy had been confirmed early in the season, a female may come back into estrus. • If abortion occurred early in the season, the female may give birth much later than the rest of the herd if re-mating occurred. • If abortion occurred late in the pregnancy, discovery of expulsed fetus. • Female may show signs of imminent parturition (i.e., seeking isolation, restlessness) before expected due date.

SIGNALMENT
• Commonly studied species include those within the genera *Cervus* (red deer, wapiti), *Dama* (fallow deer), *Axis* (chital deer), *Rangifer* (reindeer), *Odocoileus* (white-tailed deer, black-tailed deer, mule deer), *Alces* (moose), *Capreolus* (roe deer), *Ozotoceros* (Pampas deer), *Elaphurus* (Père David's deer), *Rucervus* (swamp deer, Barasingha). • Females of breeding age.

PHYSICAL EXAMINATION FINDINGS
• Likely no visible signs if fetal resorption occurred early in gestation. • If suspected, fetal/embryonic loss can be confirmed by transrectal palpation (in wapiti) or transrectal ultrasonography. • A female with an impending or unobserved late-term abortion may exhibit the following clinical signs:
◦ Bloody or purulent vaginal discharge
◦ Presence of expulsed fetus and/or placenta
◦ Premature udder development and dripping
◦ Nonspecific signs of illness, such as

depression, dehydration, pyrexia, anorexia, or weight loss. • An impending late-term abortion may be suspected if the female begins showing signs of imminent parturition before expected due date. • Late-term abortions in cervids may go unobserved if the female eats the placenta and/or a predator consumes the dead fetus. Observation of alternative clinical signs or ultrasound may be able to confirm the loss of a fetus.
• Brucellosis-induced abortion in female reindeer is characterized by a retained placenta and metritis. • Bovine viral diarrhea virus and cervid herpesvirus 2 can both cause ulceration and/or pustules in oral or vulvar mucosa.

GENETICS
N/A

CAUSES AND RISK FACTORS
The major risk factors for abortion are poor herd management ranging from inadequate nutrition to stressful handling to poor biosecurity protocols.

Metabolic Causes
Febrile or severely stressed animals may abort. This may result from factors ranging from environmental (i.e., temperature) to iatrogenic (i.e., excessive handling).

Nutritional Causes
• Inadequate nutrition: Pregnant white-tailed deer females experience a 16% increase in fasting metabolic rates during gestation, 92% of which is in the 3rd trimester in early spring. Females with adequate body condition entering the winter months are more likely to have adequate fat reserves to fulfill gestational requirements in the event of prolonged winter. Females with inadequate fat reserves or that do not receive adequate nutrition in the spring may abort or give birth to nonviable or underweight calves. • Iodine deficiency: Abortion and stillbirth have been reported in cervid species due to iodine deficiency. The deficiency may be caused by insufficient dietary intake, or be secondary to excessive calcium in the diet, ingestion of toxic plants such as *Brassica* spp., gross bacterial contamination of the feed, continuous intake of feeds containing cyanogenic glucosides (e.g., white clover), or ingestion of canola (rapeseed and canola meal). • Vitamin E and/or selenium deficiency: Congenital white muscle disease has been reported in several deer species and can be fatal to the neonate.

Bacterial Causes
• *Brucella abortus*: Biovars 1 and 4 have been recovered from wild elk in the Yellowstone area of the US. Natural infections have not been reported in axis deer, white-tailed deer, or mule deer, but experimental infections have been established in all three, suggesting potential for interspecies transmission.
• *Brucella suis* biovar 4: Brucellosis is the most common cause of abortion in reindeer and caribou and is endemic in some populations in the Arctic. Natural infection has not been

reported in white-tailed deer or mule deer, but experimental infections have been established in both, suggesting possibility for interspecies transmission. • Leptospirosis: Studies in red deer showed reproductive effects, mostly reduced weaning rates, but no reports of abortions. Abortions following experimental inoculation with *L. pomona* have been demonstrated in white-tailed deer, demonstrating its abortigenic potential in cervid species. • Listeriosis: The septicemic form has been reported to cause placentitis and endometritis in farmed red deer, leading to abortion in late-term pregnancy and birth of weak, full-term young. It should be considered as a potential cause of abortion in any cervid species.

Fungal Causes
Incidence of fungal infections in cervid species is very low.

Parasitic Causes
• *Toxoplasma gondii*: Toxoplasmosis has been associated with encephalitis and placentitis in a full-term stillborn reindeer fetus. In red deer, seropositive females experience adverse effects on fetal development. • *Neospora caninum*: Seroprevalence in asymptomatic animals has also been reported in many cervid species; however, there have been reports associated with full-term stillborn Eld's deer and perinatal death in fallow deer and axis deer following suspected vertical transmission.

Viral Causes
• Bluetongue (BTV; orbivirus): Infection of cervid species generally leads to hemorrhagic disease and death. Under experimental inoculation, early embryonic absorption and fetal death were both reported in white-tailed deer. • Epizootic hemorrhagic disease (EHDV; orbivirus): Usually resulting in widespread hemorrhages, dehydration, and sudden death. EHDV has been reported to cause abortion and congenital lesions in cattle and, therefore, cannot be ruled out as a potential cause of fetal death in deer. • Bovine viral diarrhea virus (BVDV; pestivirus): BVDV has been isolated from many cervid species. A wide seroprevalence to BVDV has also been reported in surveys of wild ruminants in North America. Cervid species experimentally inoculated with cattle-derived BVDV experienced mild or no clinical disease. Experimental inoculation with a deer-derived BVDV strain in white-tailed deer resulted in fetal abortion and resorption and establishment of persistently infected (PI) carrier animals, similar to those effects observed in cattle, indicating a potential for natural infection. • Cervid herpesvirus 2 (CvHV-2; Varicellovirus): Endemic in Norway reindeer populations. Reports of vertical transmission and neonatal death in experimentally infected reindeer suggest an abortogenic potential, though this has yet to be reported in naturally occurring abortions.

Other Causes

• Other causes of abortion or stillbirth include toxicoses, traumatic injuries, congenital abnormalities, and administration of some drugs. • Locoweed causes abortions in sheep and cattle and may be a problem for cervidae as well. • Congenital abnormalities, fetal oversize, or abnormalities of presentation at time of parturition are rare, but may lead to dystocia and subsequent fetal death.
• Prostaglandins and steroids can induce fetal expulsion.

DIAGNOSIS

DIFFERENTIAL DIAGNOSES

• Vaginal discharge ∘ Normal term parturition ∘ Vaginitis ∘ Pyometra ∘ Metritis ∘ Uterine trauma or hemorrhage ∘ Uterine or vaginal neoplasia • Missed due date ∘ Infertility, either male or female (if pregnancy was not confirmed) ∘ Incorrect due date • Signs of impending parturition before due date ∘ Isolation: may indicate neurologic disease ∘ Abdominal straining: colic due to bloat (frothy vs. free gas) or other GI disease.

CBC/BIOCHEMISTRY/URINALYSIS

Little data is available on routine analyses but may be extrapolated from domesticated ruminants based on cause of abortion.

OTHER LABORATORY TESTS

Pregnancy Diagnosis and Monitoring

Maternal pregnancy-specific protein B (PSPB): Bovine pregnancy-specific protein B antibody cross reacts with caribou, red, fallow, and white-tailed deer PSPB and, therefore, commercial radioimmunoassay developed for cattle can be used for pregnancy diagnosis and monitoring in cervids.

IMAGING

• Transrectal ultrasonography: Used for early pregnancy detection (30–60 days) and fetal monitoring. • Transabdominal ultrasonography: Can be performed in smaller cervid species as early as 35 days and used to count the number of fetuses if performed within the first 2 trimesters.

OTHER DIAGNOSTIC PROCEDURES

Necropsy and sample collection of aborted fetus and placenta should occur as soon as possible to minimize secondary bacterial overgrowth. It may be difficult to obtain the placenta as the female usually ingests it. In herd outbreaks, it may be worthwhile to sacrifice a female for postmortem diagnosis if fetal tissues are inconclusive. Paired serology that shows rising antibody titers in the female may also be beneficial for antemortem diagnosis in some cases.

Bacterial Abortions

• Brucellosis: Four serological tests available – card test, standard plate agglutination test

(SPT), complement-fixation (CF) test, and rivanol test. ∘ Positive serology requires that a confirmatory test be performed. This includes culture and isolation of *Brucella* from tissues, secretions, or excretions. ∘ Test results must be reported to state and federal animal officials.
• Leptospirosis: ∘ Paired serology: Microscopic agglutination test (MAT) and enzyme-linked immunosorbent assays (ELISAs); MAT will evaluate response to a selection of serovars.
∘ Immunohistochemistry (IHC) staining or polymerase chain reaction (PCR) on aborted tissue. • Listeriosis: ∘ In captive species, cerebrospinal fluid analysis can show a markedly elevated protein concentration and neutrophilic pleocytosis. These results combined with neurologic manifestations are almost pathognomonic for listeriosis, though no pre-mortem confirmatory test is currently available. ∘ Anti-Listeria IHC from the brainstem in deceased animals is quick and most effective for verifying the diagnosis.

Parasitic Abortions

• Toxoplasmosis or Neospora: ∘ Serology: Indirect or direct hemagglutination, indirect immunofluorescent antibody test, ELISA. ∘ Real-time PCR or IHC on aborted tissue.

Viral Abortions

• BTV or EHDV: Serology (competitive ELISA, agar gel immunodiffusion, microtiter virus neutralization (MVN)); IHC, PCR, virus isolation of aborted tissue. • BVDV: Paired serology (MVN; ELISA); virus isolation from blood or nasal secretions; IHC of aborted tissue. • CvHV-2: Serology (ELISA); PCR from tissues samples, nasal swabs, trigeminal ganglia samples.

PATHOLOGIC FINDINGS

Depends upon etiology.

Bacterial Abortions

• Brucellosis: Necrotizing placentitis characterized by a thickened placenta covered with a purulent exudate. • Leptospirosis: Gross lesions in aborted white-tailed deer fetuses (following experimental inoculation with *L. pomona*) included swollen, hemorrhagic, pulpy kidneys, liver, and lymph nodes. • Listeria: Evidence of fibrinopurulent to necrotizing placentitis on histopathology; fetuses may have either have no gross lesions or suppurative pneumonia and meningitis.

Parasitic Causes

Toxoplasmosis: Necrotizing placentitis and multifocal nonsuppurative encephalitis of the fetus with presence of tissue cysts histologically in sections of brain and tachyzoites in placenta and myocardium that stain positive with *T. gondii* antibodies.

Viral Causes

• BVDV: Abortion patterns are similar to those observed in cattle with fetal death occurring at variable stages of gestation, resulting in variable autolysis or

mummification and a variety of dysplastic lesions. • CvHV-2: No specific gross pathologies have been described in aborted fetuses, but severe autolysis has been noted. Affected reindeer cows have demonstrated mild to moderate interstitial verminous pneumonia.

Fungal Causes

Granulomas (gross), fungal hyphae (histopathology) on affected organs.

TREATMENT

THERAPEUTIC APPROACH

N/A

SURGICAL CONSIDERATIONS AND TECHNIQUES

N/A

MEDICATIONS

DRUGS OF CHOICE

• Dependent upon etiology. • Broad-spectrum antibiotics: Indicated for specific bacterial diseases; long-acting antibiotics require less frequent dosing and will help to minimize stress of handling. • Anti-inflammatories: Flunixin meglumine (1.1–2.2 mg/kg IV) or meloxicam (0.5 mg/kg PO) can be administered once daily.

CONTRAINDICATIONS

N/A

PRECAUTIONS

N/A

POSSIBLE INTERACTIONS

N/A

FOLLOW-UP

EXPECTED COURSE AND PROGNOSIS

• Dependent upon underlying cause. • BTV and EHDV are most likely to cause rapid, acute death. • CvHV-2 may become latent and recrudesce during periods of stress. • BVDV may lead to persistently infected animals that can shed the virus throughout their lifetime.

POSSIBLE COMPLICATIONS

• Decreased fertility, increased morbidity in females • Dystocia, uterine infection

CLIENT EDUCATION

See "Biosecurity" and "Production Management"

PATIENT CARE

• In cases of single abortion, important to watch entire herd to ensure no outbreak ensues. • Appropriate health care should be provided based on the underlying etiology. • Supportive care (IV fluids, anti-inflammatories ± antibiotics) for systemic illness. • If suspected nutritional issue, have feed analysis performed to determine underlying deficiency or toxicity. Change feed or supplement nutrients as necessary. • If listeriosis or mycotoxins are suspected, make appropriate changes to silage feeding practices.

PREVENTION
Establish a good nutritional and preventive health program.

Brucellosis
• USDA-APHIS have published minimum program standards and procedures to eradicate and monitor brucellosis in farm or ranch-raised deer. Required cervid surveillance identification tests include: ○ Interstate movement tests: All sexually intact animals 6 months of age or older must test negative for brucellosis within 30 days prior to interstate movement, with a 90-day post-movement test strongly recommended. ○ Slaughter establishment tests: All test-eligible animals are blood-sampled at slaughter and tested for brucellosis. • Certified brucellosis-free cervid herds are exempt from testing requirements for interstate movement. • In infected herds, test and removal programs may be practical for intensively managed deer farms but not for game or wildlife parks. • No recommended vaccine is currently available for most cervid species. • *Brucella suis* biovar 4 (killed) vaccine has been shown to be useful for providing protection in reindeer.

Leptospirosis
Extra-label use of cattle vaccine available in the US.

Bluetongue and EHD
• Parasite control should be implemented to decrease the number of arthropod vectors (e.g., *Culicoides* spp. or gnats). • Autogenous vaccines are available through Newport Laboratories.

BVDV
Fencing of adequate height and double fencing are recommended in order to prevent direct contact and disease transmission between captive and wild cervids.

 MISCELLANEOUS

ASSOCIATED CONDITIONS
Dystocia, infertility

AGE-RELATED FACTORS
N/A

ZOONOTIC POTENTIAL
Brucellosis, toxoplasmosis, leptospirosis, and listeriosis are all zoonotic diseases; appropriate precautions should be taken when handling fetal or placental tissues.

PREGNANCY
N/A

BIOSECURITY
• Quarantine newly acquired animals for 30 days minimum. • Pre-shipment testing for infectious diseases. • Double fences to minimize direct contact with wildlife species.

PRODUCTION MANAGEMENT
• Monitoring birthweight and growth of young animals and keeping records of previous reproductive performance of females will allow owners to make appropriate herd management decisions. • Habituating animals to gates and chutes makes handling during physical exams and other routine procedures less stressful on the animals. • Adequate nutritional management is crucial. Females should have a body condition score of 3–5 out of 9 to even be considered for breeding. Overweight females may be at increased risk for dystocia whereas underweight females are at an increased risk for abortion. • Close monitoring during gestation will be beneficial in the event of an abortion.

SYNONYMS
N/A

ABBREVIATIONS
• BTV = bluetongue virus • BVDV = bovine viral diarrhea virus • CF = complement fixation • CvHV = cervine herpesvirus • EHDV = epizootic hemorrhagic disease virus • ELISA = enzyme-linked immunosorbent assay • IHC = immunohistochemistry • MAT = microscopic agglutination test • PDG = pregnanediol-3alpha-glucuronide • PI = persistently infected • PSPB = pregnancy-specific protein B • SPT = standard plate agglutination test

SEE ALSO
• Abortion: Bacterial • Abortion: Small Ruminant • Abortion: Viral, Fungal, and Nutritional • Bovine Viral Diarrhea Virus • Brucellosis • Cervidae: Biosecurity • Cervidae: Breeding Soundness Examination • Cervidae Reproduction • Cervidae: Vaccination Programs

Suggested Reading
Basso W, Moré G, Quiroga MA, et al. *Neospora caninum* is a cause of perinatal mortality in axis deer (*Axis axis*). Vet Parasitol 2014, 199: 255–8.

das Neves CG, Mørk T, Thiry J, et al. Cervid herpesvirus 2 experimentally reactivated in reindeer can produce generalized viremia and abortion. Virus Res 2009, 145: 321–8.

Dieterich RA., Morton JK. Reindeer Health Aide Manual, 2nd ed. Agricultural and Forestry Experiment Station and Cooperative Extension Service, University of Alaska Fairbanks and US Dept. of Agriculture Cooperating, 1990. AFES Misc. Pub. 90–4 CES 100H-00046.

Dubey JP, Lewis B, Beam K, Abbitt B. Transplacental toxoplasmosis in a reindeer (*Rangifer tarandus*) fetus. Vet Parasitol 2002, 110: 131–5.

Formenti N, Troqu T, Pedrotti L, et al. *Toxoplasma gondii* infection in alpine red deer (*Cervus elaphus*): its spread and effects on fertility. PloS one 2015, 10: e0138472.

Osburn B, Aradaib I, Schore C. Comparison of bluetongue and epizootic hemorrhagic disease complex. Bov Pract 1995, 29: 106–9.

Passler T, Ditchkoff SS, Givens MD. Transmission of bovine viral diarrhea virus among white-tailed deer (*Odocoileus virginianus*). Vet Res 2010, 41: 1–8.

Pekins PJ, Smith KS, Mautz WW. The energy cost of gestation in white-tailed deer. Can J Zool 1998, 76: 1091–7.

Pourliotis K, Gladinis ND, Sofianidis G, et al. Congenital nutritional myodegeneration (white muscle disease) in a red deer (*Cervus elaphus*) calf. N Z Vet J 2009, 57: 244–7.

Rideout BA. Disorders of nondomestic mammals. In: Njaa BL ed, Kirkbride's Diagnosis of Abortion and Neonatal Loss in Animals. John Wiley & Sons, 2011, pp. 201–20.

Ridpath JF, Driskell EA, Chase CC, et al. Reproductive tract disease associated with inoculation of pregnant white-tailed deer with bovine viral diarrhea virus. Am J Vet Res 2008, 69: 1630–6.

Thomas FC, Trainer DO. Bluetongue virus:(1) in pregnant white-tailed deer (2) a plaque reduction neutralization test. J Wildl Dis 1970, 6: 384–8.

Trainer DO, Karstad L, Hanson RP. Experimental leptospirosis in white-tailed deer. J Infect Dis 1961, 108: 278–86.

Wilson PR, Bell M, Walker IH, Quinn A, Woolderink IA. Iodine and deer calf survival. Proc Deer Branch N Z Vet Assoc Conf 2002, 19: 105–12.

Authors Jamie L. Stewart and Clifford F. Shipley

Consulting Editor Ahmed Tibary

ABORTION: SMALL RUMINANT

BASICS

OVERVIEW
• Fetal loss, fetal wastage: conceptus loss at any time during pregnancy. • Most commonly observed in the last 2 months of pregnancy.

INCIDENCE/PREVALENCE
• Flock pregnancy loss should be <5% (<2% ideal). • Abortion storms may occur in the case of specific infectious diseases.

GEOGRAPHIC DISTRIBUTION
• Worldwide • Some diseases processes may be regional (presence of vector)

SYSTEMS AFFECTED
• Reproductive • Other systems depending on etiology

PATHOPHYSIOLOGY
• Abortion results from: ○ Fetal death from invasion by microorganisms or subsequent to placental disease (placentitis, vasculitis) and placental insufficiency. ○ Fetal expulsion or premature parturition may result from maternal compromise. ○ Reabsorption, maceration, mummification, and autolysis may be observed in some cases. ○ Fetal abnormalities are often a feature of some viral infections. • Causes include a variety of infectious and noninfectious agents.
• Infectious causes of abortion are the most economically significant. • Common bacterial causes are *Chlamydophila abortus, Coxiella burnetii, Toxoplasma gondii,* and *Campylobacter* spp. • Common viral causes include caprine herpesvirus (CpHV-1), bluetongue virus, BDV, Cache Valley virus.

GENETICS
• Angora goat may be a habitual aborter.
• Some breeds of sheep are more susceptible to viral bluetongue (Merino, British breeds).

HISTORICAL FINDINGS
• Introduction of new animals • Repeat breeding or return to estrus • Premature udder development • Presence of expelled fetuses • Premature/stillbirths • Increased congenital abnormalities in neonates or fetuses

SIGNALMENT
Nonspecific; females of breeding age that were exposed to the male or inseminated.

PHYSICAL EXAMINATION FINDINGS
• Mucopurulent or hemorrhagic vaginal discharge containing fetal membranes in early pregnancy loss. • Signs of abortion: vaginal discharge vulvar edema, retained placenta.
• Systemic signs such as fever, anorexia may be present. • Other signs in flock: abnormal fetuses, sick or ill-thrift lambs and kids).
• Clinical signs in the aborting female vary depending on the cause. • Complications depend on cause (deterioration of health, retained placenta, metritis).

Clinical Signs
• Several infectious abortions are subclinical in the dam (Cache Valley, Border disease, caprine herpesvirus, Schmallenberg, Q fever).
• Bluetongue: Febrile, swollen tongue, ear or face, lameness, ulcerative lesions on month.
• Campylobacteriosis: Aborting goats may show diarrhea. • Chlamydiosis: Pneumonia, keratoconjunctivitis, epididymitis, and polyarthritis. Anorexia, fever, bloody vaginal discharge 2 to 3 days before abortion.
• Brucellosis (*B. melitensis*) in goats: weak kids and mastitis. Aborting goats may experience fever, depression, weight loss, mastitis, and lameness. • *B. ovis* in sheep: Rarely a cause of abortion but is responsible for poor reproductive performance and in the ram contagious epididymitis. • Leptospirosis: Anorexia, fever, marked jaundice, hemoglobinuria, anemia, neurological signs, abortion, occasionally may be fatal.
• Salmonellosis: Abortion, retained placenta, metritis, and various systemic signs (fever, depression, diarrhea). Mostly in overcrowded flocks. • Toxoplasmosis: Generally no clinical signs; immunocompromised females may present a neurologic form of the disease.
• Leptospirosis: Septicemia, fever, decreased appetite, reduced milk production, abortion, and meningoencephalitis. • Mycoplasmosis (goats): Mastitis, arthritis, keratoconjunctivitis, vulvovaginitis, and abortion in the last 3rd of pregnancy.

CAUSES AND RISK FACTORS
• Causes of abortion include: ○ Viruses: bluetongue, BDV, CpHV-1, CVV, RVF, Akabane, Nairobi, Wesselsbron ○ Bacteria: *Brucella* spp. (*B. ovis, B. melitensis*), *C. fetus* subsp. *fetus, C. jejuni* subsp. *Jejuni, Chlamydophila abortus, Francisella tularensis, Leptospira* spp., *Listeria monocytogenes* and *L. ivanovii, Salmonella abortus-ovis* ○ Rickettsia: *Coxiella burnetii* ○ Protozoa: *Sarcocystis, Neospora caninum, Toxoplasma gondii* ○ Toxic plants: annual ryegrass, *Gutierrezia microcephala* (broomweed, snakeweed), locoweed, subterranean clover, *Veratrum californicum* (skunk cabbage) ○ Mineral deficiencies: copper, iodine, selenium • Risk factors include: ○ Lack of biosecurity measures ○ Vector or reservoir population: bluetongue, CVV, Rift Valley fever, Akabane, Nairobi sheep disease, Wesselsbron disease virus, *Coxiella burnetii* (ticks), *Leptospira* spp., *Neospora, T. gondii* ○ Overcrowding ○ Pasture type

DIAGNOSIS

DIFFERENTIAL DIAGNOSES
Brucellosis
• Isolation: Best samples are vaginal discharges and milk, stomach contents. • Indirect

diagnosis: Complement fixation, agglutination, and precipitation tests may help identify carrier animals.

Chlamydiosis (Enzootic Abortion)
• *C. abortus*, Gram-negative intracellular organism. • Abortion and other clinical signs in neonates. • Aborting females become immune. • Females infected after 100 days of pregnancy may not abort. • Diagnosis: ○ Generalized placentitis, abortion in the last month of pregnancy, high incidence in newly infected flocks. ○ Demonstrations of characteristic inclusion bodies on smear from cotyledons, vaginal discharge, fetal stomach content. ○ Culture from vaginal discharge, placenta and fetal tissue, PCR. ○ Serology: paired samples from dam and fetal serum. ○ ELISA or indirect inclusion fluorescence antibody tests (IIFA).

Toxoplasmosis
• Goats more susceptible than sheep
• Diagnosis: ○ Cotyledons are gray-white to yellow and present small 1–3 mm focal area of necrosis and calcification. Intercotyledonary areas are generally normal. Macroscopic lesions: 2–3 mm necrotic foci on cotyledons, intercotyledonary allantochorion are generally normal. Fetus may be mummified or decomposed. Chalky white necrotic brain lesions. ○ Samples: placenta, fetal brain, fetal fluids, maternal blood, precolostral blood. ○ Isolation from cotyledons, brain and fetal fluids, tissues (shipped packed in ice). ○ Histopathology: fixed cotyledons, fetal brain. ○ Serology: presence of antibodies in fetal fluids or precolostral serum is the preferred diagnostic technique and indicated transplacental infection.

Q Fever (Coxiella burnetii)
• Placentitis, placental necrosis, thickening of the intercotyledonary areas. Abortion and stillbirth. • Isolation: Placenta, vaginal discharges, fetal stomach content. • PCR techniques are available. • Demonstration of organism by Ziehl-Neelsen staining.
• Complement fixation: Need samples from several animals. • Fluorescent antibody test may be used to identify organism in frozen section of placenta.

Campylobacteriosis
• Campylobacter fetus subsp. fetus, C. jejuni subsp. jejuni, and Campylobacter lari.
• Gram-negative microaerophilic rods.
Symptoms
• Late term abortion, stillbirths and weak lambs, retained fetal membranes. • Placentitis, placental edema. • Fetal lesions: Hepatomegaly, hemorrhagic liver, necrotic foci of 1–3 cm, subcutaneous edema, sero-sanguinous fluid in abdominal and thoracic cavity, bronchopneumonia.
• Histopathology: Necrotic areas of the chorionic villi, arterioles and thrombosis of the hilus of the placentomes.

Isolation and Identification
• Samples: Placenta and vaginal discharges, frozen fetal stomach content (–20°C).
• Transport medium required. • Isolation from placenta, vaginal discharge, fetal stomach content.

Salmonellosis
• *Salmonella abortus-ovis, S. barndenburg, S. typhimurium, S. dublin, S. montevideo, S. arizona, S. oranienburg.* • Early, mid or late term abortions, septic metritis, peritonitis in aborting females. Fetuses are often autolyzed. Lambs may be born weak or develop bronchopneumonia. Placentitis, placental edema. • Direct diagnosis: Culture from fetal tissues taken aseptically may be preserved at –20°C, placenta and uterine discharges. • Indirect diagnosis: Seroagglutination.

Listeriosis (Listeria monocytogenes)
• Gram-positive, non-acid-fast facultative microaerophilic organisms. *L. monocytogenes* affects sheep and goats; *L. ivanovii* affects sheep only. • Females may show fever, depression, and anorexia prior to abortion mid to late pregnancy. Stillbirths, birth of weak lambs, and retained placenta are common. Fetuses may be mummified. • Direct diagnosis: Placenta, fetal liver and spleen, fetal stomach content, vaginal discharge within 48 hours of abortion. Samples may be refrigerated if not cultured immediately. • Indirect diagnosis: Histopathology on placenta, fetal liver and spleen- microabscesses (white pinpoint spots), necrosis, and infiltration of macrophages and neutrophils. Gram stain reveals numerous Gram-positive rods.

Leptospirosis
• Sheep and goats are generally less susceptible to leptospirosis than other species. Goats are more susceptible than sheep. • Sheep: mostly *L. hardjo*, sometime *L. pomona, L. ballum* and *L. bratislava*, late term abortion, stillbirths, and ill-thrifty lambs. • Goat: *L. icterohaemrrhagiae, L. pomona, L. grippotyphosa.* • Affected flocks are mostly reared indoors. • Clinical signs in case of acute infection include fever and agalactia. Abortion occurs in late pregnancy. • Direct diagnosis: Fetal tissue, fetal fluids, and placenta. ○ Isolation is difficult. ○ Demonstration by dark-field microscopy, immunofluorescence, and silver stain. • Indirect diagnosis: ○ Serology: macroscopic agglutination test.

Border Disease
• Goats are fairly resistant. • Viremic animals may show fever. Fetal death and resorption when infected in the first 2 months of pregnancy. Infection after 60 days results in fetal death, mummification or abortion, and fetal abnormalities. • Virus isolation (buffy coat) and antigen demonstration: Heparinized blood from dam or hairy shaker lambs, fetal tissue (thyroid, kidney, spleen,

cerebellum, placenta), hairy shakers (thyroid, kidney, spleen, cerebellum, intestine, lymph nodes). • Histopathology: Cerebellum (white matter necrosis and gliosis), spinal cord. • Serology: Flood from dam and hairy shakers. • Clinical: Small cotyledon with focal necrosis, hairy shakers.

Bluetongue
• Viral isolation: Blood, semen, fetal brain and spleen. Unlikely cause of abortion in goats.

Akabane Disease
• Fetal malformation, positive antibody titer in liveborn and aborted fetuses.

Cache Valley Virus
• Congenital abnormalities. • Detection of antibodies in fetal fluids or precolostral serum.

Mycoplasmosis
• Mycoplasma abortions (*M. mycoides, M. agalactiae*) are significant in goats.
• Diagnosis: Culture and serotyping of the isolate from milk, fetal fluids, and placenta.

Noninfectious Causes of Abortion
• Genetic (goat) may be a habitual aborter ○ Angora goats with fine mohair ○ Abortion at 100 days ○ Adrenal dysfunction • Energy protein deficiency • Phenothiazine and levamisole in the last 2 months of pregnancy
• Corticosteroids in late gestation
• Prostaglandin $F2_\alpha$ or analogues (goats)
• Plants that accumulate nitrates

CBC/BIOCHEMISTRY/URINALYSIS
May be indicated if aborting dams are clinically sick.

OTHER LABORATORY TESTS
• Sampling is critical for the proper diagnosis of abortion. • Placenta ○ Ideal for the isolation of most abortion-causing agents. ○ Ideal for identification using specific staining techniques on histological section or impression smears. • For isolation need 5 or 6 cotyledons and section of intercotyledonary spaces both from healthy appearing and diseased areas. ○ These tissues may be rinsed with sterile saline. ○ For isolation need a transport medium ▪ Viruses ▪ *Campylobacter* FBP/glycerol ▪ Leptospirosis 100 mL extender with 1% BSA ○ For histopathology ▪ 0.5 cm section of tissue in 10% formalin 1:10 ○ For bacteriology ▪ Impression smears • Vaginal discharges ○ Collect in sterile manner ○ Vaginal/uterine swabs ○ Use of specific transport medium is preferred if a specific microorganism is suspected. • Fetal tissues ○ Tissue samples from all fetal organs (spleen, liver, kidneys, brain, lymph nodes, spinal cord) should be taken in an aseptic manner immediately after abortion or death. ○ Handle in the same manner as for placenta. • Fetal fluids ○ If fetus is not autolyzed ○ Stomach content ○ Peritoneal/thoracic fluids ○ Blood from the cardiac cavity • Milk ○ Samples of milk are taken from both glands using aseptic techniques (clean the mammary gland,

disinfect teats, and eliminate the first 2 jets).
• Blood ○ For isolation: immediately after/during abortion. ○ For serology: paired samples immediately after abortion and 2 to 3 weeks later ○ In case of an outbreak, blood should be collected from aborting females as well as from lambs/kids before colostral intake.

IMAGING
N/A

PATHOLOGIC FINDINGS
Abortion Associated with Deformities
• Bluetongue: Hydranencephaly. • Akabane disease: Arthrogryposis (dystocia), hydranencephaly, and mummification.
• Cache Valley virus: Arthrogryposis, brachygnathia, hydranencephaly, microencephaly, spinal cord hypoplasia, and mummification. • Border disease virus: Cerebellar hypoplasia, hydranencephaly, brachygnathia, arthrogryposis. Dark pigmentation of the fleece, hairy shaker.
• Toxic plants: Lupine, skunk cabbage, locoweed, and Sudan grass. • Iodine, copper, manganese deficiency.

TREATMENT
THERAPEUTIC APPROACH
Depends on etiology and complications following abortion

SURGICAL CONSIDERATIONS AND TECHNIQUES
N/A

MEDICATIONS
DRUGS OF CHOICE
• Depends on etiology and complications following abortion. Daily tetracycline treatment of the flock may help with some of the abortion-causing diseases.
• Broad-spectrum antibiotics and anti-inflammatory therapy. • *Campylobacter*: Penicillin or streptomycin or tetracycline in feed some strains are resistant. • Chlamydiosis: Tetracycline, Tylosin • Leptospirosis: Tetracycline • Toxoplasmosis: Decoquinate, monensin • Leptospirosis: Tetracycline
• Mycoplasma: Tetracycline and tylosin

CONTRAINDICATIONS
Appropriate milk and meat withdrawal times must be followed.

PRECAUTIONS
N/A

POSSIBLE INTERACTIONS
N/A

FOLLOW-UP

EXPECTED COURSE AND PROGNOSIS
Dependent upon underlying cause.

POSSIBLE COMPLICATIONS
Dystocia, retained placenta, metritis, mastitis, male infertility (brucellosis, chlamydiosis), female infertility, poor lactation, neonatal losses.

CLIENT EDUCATION
• Establish good preventive program (biosecurity measures, vaccination, good nutritional programs). • Consider every case of abortion as a possible outbreak. • Act quickly and help collect appropriate samples to be examined by a veterinarian. • Zoonotic risk awareness.

PATIENT CARE
• Frequent monitoring of late term females in the entire herd or flock. • Correct nutritional deficiencies if suspected. • Avoid toxic plants and mycotoxins if suspected.

PREVENTION
• Assess disease risk and set up preventive measures. ○ Toxoplasmosis: cat population. ○ Leptospirosis: rodent population, humid hot environment, proximity to dairy and swine operation. ○ Salmonellosis: source of infection: bird, cattle, wildlife, predisposing conditions: overcrowding, shipping, climatic changes ○ Chlamydiosis ▪ Infection transmission: placenta, fetal fluids ▪ Pigeon/sparrows are reservoirs, ticks or insects may play a role ▪ Vaginal discharge in goat up to 2 weeks before abortion ▪ Reservoir: young maiden females ○ Listeriosis ▪ Organisms grow in poorly fermented silage ▪ Can survive in soil and feces for extended period of time ○ Bluetongue: *Culicoides* gnat (cattle may be a reservoir) ○ Akabane virus diseases: gnats and mosquito population ○ Cache Valley virus: mosquitoes • General prevention program for abortion ○ Quarantine new animals (4 to 6 weeks) ○ Nutrition ○ Vaccination: *Chlamydia*, *Campylobacter* (2 months and last month of pregnancy) • Feed chlortetracycline

(200–400 mg/head/day), monensin (15 mg/head/day) during gestation ○ Keep feed, pasture and water source free from contamination by run-off, particularly from cattle and hogs. ○ Control rat, bird, cat population. ○ Act quickly on any abortion and assume it is an outbreak. ○ Submit complete samples. ○ Separate pre-partum from postpartum females. ○ Keep good lambing/kidding facilities. • Reduce stress due to poor nutrition, unsanitary environment, crowded conditions.
• Vaccination ○ Bluetongue: questionable ○ Akabane virus: effective ○ Cache valley: effective ○ *Campylobacter*: helpful ○ *Chlamydia*: helpful ○ Q fever: autogenous vaccines in conjunction with chlortetracycline may help ○ *B. ovis*: poor efficacy of killed vaccine ○ *B. melitensis*: live attenuated good when permitted ○ Salmonellosis: autogenous vaccine may be helpful ○ Toxoplasmosis: may be helpful

 MISCELLANEOUS

ASSOCIATED CONDITIONS
N/A

AGE-RELATED FACTORS
N/A

ZOONOTIC POTENTIAL
• *Campylobacter jejuni* (aborted fetus, stomach content, fetal membranes) • *C. abortus* (fetal membranes, vaginal discharges) • Q fever (influenza-like symptoms, myalgia, endocarditis) • Brucellosis (*B. melitensis*), Malta fever, undulating fever, joint pain • Leptospirosis • Toxoplasmosis (milk, fetal membranes) • Listeriosis: aborted fetuses

PREGNANCY
N/A

BIOSECURITY
See "Prevention"

PRODUCTION MANAGEMENT
• Cull infertile animal • Quarantine measures

SYNONYMS
N/A

ABBREVIATIONS
• ELISA = enzyme linked immunosorbent assay
• IIFA= indirect inclusion fluorescence antibody
• PCR= polymerase chain reaction
• BDV = Border disease virus
• CpHV-1 = caprine herpesvirus-1
• RVF = Rift Valley fever

SEE ALSO
• Abortion: Bacterial
• Abortion: Viral, Fungal, and Nutritional
• Akabane
• Arthrogryposis
• Bluetongue Virus
• Cache Valley Virus
• Campylobacter
• Chlamydiosis
• Congenital Defects: Small Ruminants
• Iodine Deficiency and Toxicity
• Leptospirosis
• Listeriosis
• Neosporosis
• Rift Valley Fever
• Schmallenberg Virus
• Selenium Toxicity
• Toxicology: Herd Outbreaks
• Vitamin E/Selenium Deficiency
• Wesselsbron Disease

Suggested Reading
Menzies PI. Control of important causes of infectious abortion in sheep and goats. Vet Clin North Am Food Anim Pract 2011, 27: 81–93.
Moller RB. Disorders of sheep and goats. In: Njaa BL ed, Kikbride's Diagnosis of Abortion and Neonatal Loss in Animals, 4th ed. Wiley-Blackwell, 2012, pp 49–87.
Rodolakis A. Zoonoses in goats: How to control them. Small Rum Res 2014, 121: 12–20.
Van den Brom R, Van Englen E, Roest HIJ, et al. *Coxiella burnetii* infection in sheep or goats: an opinionated review. Vet Microbiol 2015, 181: 119–29.
Author Ahmed Tibary
Consulting Editor Ahmed Tibary

 Client Education Handout available online

BASICS

OVERVIEW
Pregnancy loss during the fetal stage, between 42 days and term, caused by viral or fungal infection of the fetus or placenta, or nutritional problems.

INCIDENCE/PREVALENCE
• BHV-1: sporadic abortions in vaccinated or previously exposed herds, up to 60% in naïve herds. • BVDV: up to 40% in susceptible herds. • Fungal: sporadic, <10% of the herd, can vary from 2 to 20% depending on environment and season. • Selenium deficiency: 4–5% of aborted fetuses in a Canadian study.

GEOGRAPHIC DISTRIBUTION
• Potentially worldwide • Seasonal occurrence of bluetongue virus abortions due to vector cycle (late summer and early autumn in temperate areas) • Seasonal occurrence of fungal abortion (winter and spring) • Seleniferous areas for selenium toxicosis

SYSTEMS AFFECTED
• Reproductive • Other systems depending on etiology

PATHOPHYSIOLOGY
Viral Abortion
• Maternal infection occurs venereally, orally, via inhalation or across conjunctival mucosa. • Vector transmission occurs with BTV (*Culicoides* spp.) and Cache Valley virus (multiple mosquitoes). • Viruses replicate in local lymphoid tissue and spread hematogenously to secondary organs. • Viruses invade the placenta hematogenously from the dam's systemic circulation and cause fetal infection. • Fetal death occurs secondary to fetal infection and direct organ damage, or placental damage. • Fetal expulsion can occur before or immediately after death, with expulsion of a fresh or live fetus. More commonly, a delay in fetal expulsion leads to autolysis. • Fetal mummification may occur with some viral infections. • In the bovine, fetal infection between 100 and 150 days leads to congenital neurologic abnormalities (BVDV, BTV, BPV). • Fetal infection with noncytopathic BVDV strains between 1 and 4 months' gestation leads to birth of persistently infected immunotolerant calves. • In small ruminants, infection with BTV and Border disease virus during the first 40 to 60 days results in fetal death and resorption. Later infection results in abortion, weak neonates, and congenital abnormalities (hydranencephaly, retinal dysplasia). • Depending on the pathogen, dams may shed virus in ocular, oral, nasal, or vaginal secretions. • Latency is established with BHV-1 in the trigeminal nerve or the sacral spinal ganglia. Recrudescence and shedding may occur after stress.

Fungal Abortion
Fungi are thought to cause primary maternal respiratory or gastrointestinal disease and spread to placentomes hematogenously. Fetal infection occurs by extension of amniotic fluid infection.

Nutritional Abortion
• Selenium deficiency results from grazing plants growing in low-selenium soils. Development of congenital white muscle disease is thought to lead to fetal cardiac failure and death. • Ingestion of selenium-accumulating plants or contaminated water in areas with high-selenium soils or with environmental contamination, or iatrogenic overdose or oral or injectable selenium causes toxicosis. The toxic dose of selenium is uncertain, ranging from 2.2 to >20 mg/kg in the literature. • Iodine deficiency has been associated with premature delivery, weak lambs and kids, and congenital goiter.

HISTORICAL FINDINGS
• A herd history of abortions or maternal and neonatal signs (described above) • Inappropriate vaccination schedules • Introduction of new animals to the herd • Ataxic, blind or small calves in the herd (BVDV)

SIGNALMENT
• Ruminants of all breeds • Breeding age females

PHYSICAL EXAMINATION FINDINGS
• Maternal physical examination is usually unremarkable at the time of abortion. • Maternal illness and fever may develop secondary to retained fetal membranes (RFM). • BHV-1: Abortion between 4 and 8 months' gestation, usually 2 weeks to 3 months after maternal clinical disease, respiratory disease, fever, conjunctivitis, nasal lesions, encephalomyelitis, neonatal disease, severe and painful pustular vaginitis. • BVDV: Variable depending on host and virus characteristics: infertility, embryonic death, abortion, mummification, small calves, persistently infected calves, congenital defects, fever, ocular and nasal discharge, oral ulcers, diarrhea, decreased milk production, epithelial erosions at the interdigital spaces, coronary bands, teats or vulva, hemorrhagic syndrome. • BTV: Maternal ulcers in mouth, tongue, muzzle and coronary bands, sloughing of hooves, abortion, stillbirth, embryonic death, fetal malformations. • BPV: first and second trimester abortions, congenital malformations, infertility. • Fungal: abortion between 6 to 8 months' gestation, RFM. • Selenium toxicosis: Abortion, infertility, respiratory distress, lethargy, anorexia, diarrhea, fever, teeth grinding, death. In the chronic form: depression, weakness, anorexia, diarrhea, anemia, hair loss, hoof deformities, lameness.

GENETICS
N/A

CAUSES AND RISK FACTORS
Viral Causes
• Bovine herpes virus 1, 4, and 5, bovine viral diarrhea virus, bluetongue virus, bovine parvovirus. • The most common viral causes of abortion in small ruminants are Akabane, bluetongue, Border disease, Cache Valley virus, caprine herpesvirus-1 (goats).

Fungal Causes
Aspergillus spp., *Mucor* spp. *Absidia* spp., *Rhizopus* spp., *Mortierella* spp., *Candida* spp., *Pseudallescheria boydii*.

Nutritional Causes
Selenium toxicity or deficiency, toxic plants

Risk Factors
• Inappropriate biosecurity measurements and vaccination schedules. • Nutritional, social or environmental stress. • Seasonal presence of vectors. • Poorly ventilated moist environment, high animal density, animal confinement, and feeding moldy hay and feedstuffs (fungal). • Selenium-deficient soil.

DIAGNOSIS

DIFFERENTIAL DIAGNOSES
• Additional viral abortions: Bovine enterovirus, pseudorabies virus, parainfluenza virus 3, lumpy skin capripoxvirus, malignant catarrhal fever, bovine leucosis virus, foot and mouth disease virus; emerging or geographically restricted viruses (Kasba virus in Africa, Asia and Australia, Rift Valley fever in sub-Saharan Africa and Madagascar, Akabane virus in Asia, Australia, Middle East and Kenya, Schmallenberg virus in Germany and the Netherlands, Wesselsbron virus in Africa). • Bacterial abortion: Brucellosis, *Campylobacter* spp., *Leptospira* spp., *Listeria monocytogenes*, *Histophilus somni*, *Salmonella* spp., *Trueperella pyogenes*, *Mycobacterium bovis*, *Chlamydophila abortus*, *Coxiella burnetii*, epizootic bovine abortion, *Mycoplasma* spp., *Ureaplasma diversum*. • Protozoal abortion: *Neospora caninum*, *Tritrichomonas foetus*. • Toxic abortion: Nitrate/nitrite poisoning, Ponderosa pine, broom snakeweed, sumpweed, moldy sweet clover, locoweed, poison hemlock, annual ryegrass infected with *Clavibacter rathayi*, snakeweed, stinkweed, turpentine weed, wild pea, sweet pea, subterranean clover, skunk cabbage mycotoxins, iatrogenic administration of teratogenic or luteolytic drugs. • Vaginal discharge: Vaginitis, metritis, endometritis, pyometra, hemorrhage. • Ulcers: Foot and mouth disease, bovine papular stomatitis, vesicular stomatitis. • Respiratory disease: Bovine respiratory disease complex.

CBC/BIOCHEMISTRY/URINALYSIS
N/A

OTHER LABORATORY TESTS
• Virus isolation from aborted tissues (lung, liver, spleen, kidney, adrenal glands, placenta). • Virus isolation from maternal or neonatal buffy coat (BVDV). • Antigen detection (ELISA or IHC) or PCR on maternal or neonatal ear skin biopsies, serum, whole blood, milk, and nasal swabs (BVDV). • Dam, fetal or pre-colostral calf serology (BVDV, BTV, BPV). • Immunohistochemistry and/or immunofluorescence on fetal tissues (BHV-1, BVDV). • PCR on aborted tissues (BHV-1, BVDV) or whole blood (BVT). • Gross lesions in fetal skin and placenta (fungal). • Fungal culture from aborted tissues (placenta, abomasal fluid, lung). • Direct microscopic examination of skin or placental scrapings or histopathology (fungal).

IMAGING
N/A

OTHER DIAGNOSTIC PROCEDURES
• Fetal necropsy (see finding below) • Determination of selenium content in fetal and maternal liver

PATHOLOGIC FINDINGS
• BHV-1: Autolytic fetus, pinpoint white foci of necrosis in liver, pulmonary and renal hemorrhage and necrosis, diffuse placentitis, and yellow/brown amniotic fluid. • BVDV: Calves with congenital abnormalities (hydranencephaly, hydrocephalus, cerebellar hypoplasia, microphthalmia, retinal dysplasia, cataracts, thymic hypoplasia, hypotrichosis, brachygnathism, arthrogryposis, pulmonary or renal hypoplasia or dysplasia), necrotizing myocarditis, hepatic congestion, ascites. Autolyzed fetuses with rarely recognizable lesions, typically necrotizing inflammation with mononuclear infiltrations and lymphoid depletion, and no placental lesions. • BTV: Congenital abnormalities (hydranencephaly, hydrocephalus). • Fungal: Minimal fetal autolysis with numerous epidermal plaques, emaciation, placentitis with severe thickening of cotyledons and intercotyledonary areas with a leathery appearance; cotyledons may contain attached necrotic caruncular tissue. • Selenium deficiency: Fetal ascites, cardiac dilation and nodular liver, myocardial necrosis and mineralization, necrosis of skeletal muscle.

TREATMENT

THERAPEUTIC APPROACH
• Treatment of systemic disease, RFM, or metritis as needed. • Decrease environmental exposure to fungi by decreasing confinement and cow density, and improving ventilation and feed quality.

SURGICAL CONSIDERATIONS AND TECHNIQUES
N/A

MEDICATIONS

DRUG(S) OF CHOICE
N/A

CONTRAINDICATIONS
Use of modified live virus or attenuated vaccines against BVDV and BTV in pregnant cattle is associated with congenital malformations.

PRECAUTIONS
Latency may result after vaccination with modified live virus or attenuated vaccine against BHV-1.

POSSIBLE INTERACTIONS
N/A

FOLLOW-UP

EXPECTED COURSE AND PROGNOSIS
• Infected or exposed cows may develop natural immunity to some viruses, with lower rates of abortion in subsequent breeding seasons. • 25% of cows with *M. wolfii*-associated abortions may develop post-abortion pneumonia with death within 72 h.

POSSIBLE COMPLICATIONS
• Dystocia • RFM • Metritis • Viral spread to herd mates • Infertility • Secondary bacterial infections

CLIENT EDUCATION
• Wear protective gloves and clothes when handling aborted tissues and animals. • Pregnant women, children, elderly and immunosuppressed people should not handle aborting animals or tissues. • Keep aborted tissues (fetus and placenta) refrigerated and call a veterinarian as soon as abortion was noticed for appropriate diagnostic tests. • Remove additional aborted tissues from the pasture to prevent disease transmission. • Work with a veterinarian to design an appropriate biosecurity and vaccination program. • Follow milk and meat withdrawal times if medications are administered.

PATIENT CARE
• The cow should be monitored to ensure the fetal membranes are expelled and metritis does not develop. • Supportive care as needed. • The rest of the herd should be monitored for further abortions, stillbirths or birth of weak or abnormal calves. • Tests dams of PI calves (BVDV). • Prevent feeding moldy hay or low-quality silage to pregnant animals (fungal).

PREVENTION
• Optimize the herd's health status by providing appropriate nutritional, stress and environmental management. • Test and quarantine new additions to the herd. • Buy replacement animals from BVDV-free herds. • Test and cull positive animals for eradication. • Where vaccines are available, vaccinate breeding stock. • Avoid modified live or attenuated virus vaccines in pregnant cattle.

MISCELLANEOUS

ASSOCIATED CONDITIONS
N/A

AGE-RELATED FACTORS
N/A

ZOONOTIC POTENTIAL
N/A

PREGNANCY
Infection in pregnant animals leads to abortion.

BIOSECURITY
See "Prevention"

PRODUCTION MANAGEMENT
Avoid nutritional, social and environmental stress by using proper management practices.

SYNONYMS
N/A

ABBREVIATIONS
• BHV-1 = bovine herpes virus 1 • BPV = bovine parvovirus • BTV = bluetongue virus • BVDV = bovine viral diarrhea virus • ELISA = enzyme-linked immunosorbent assay • IBR = infectious bovine rhinotracheitis • IHC = immunohistochemistry • PCR = polymerase chain reaction • PI = persistently infected • RFM = retained fetal membranes

SEE ALSO
• Abortion: Bacterial • Abortion: Farmed Cervidae • Abortion: Small Ruminants • Akabane • Bluetongue Virus • Bovine Viral Diarrhea Virus • Infectious Bovine Rhinotracheitis • Rift Valley Fever • Schmallenberg Virus • Selenium Toxicity • Vaccination Programs: Beef Cattle • Vaccination Programs: Dairy Cattle

Suggested Reading
Austin F. Infectious agents: mycotic abortion. In: Hopper R ed, Bovine Reproduction. Ames: Wiley Blackwell, 2015.
Baumgartner W. Fetal disease and abortion: diagnosis and causes In: Hopper R ed, Bovine Reproduction. Ames: Wiley Blackwell, 2015.
Kelling CL. Viral diseases of the fetus. In: Youngquist RS, Threlfall WR eds, Current Therapy in Large Animal Theriogenology, 2nd ed. St. Louis: Saunders Elsevier, 2007.
Author Maria Soledad Ferrer
Consulting Editor Ahmed Tibary
Acknowledgment The author and book editors acknowledge the prior contribution of Walter Johnson and Alex Estrada.

ACTINOBACILLOSIS: WOODEN TONGUE

BASICS

OVERVIEW
Actinobacillosis is caused by *Actinobacillus ligniersii* infection of the soft tissues, usually in the tongue.

INCIDENCE/PREVALENCE
Seen in up to 3% of cattle tongues at slaughter

GEOGRAPHIC DISTRIBUTION
Worldwide

SYSTEMS AFFECTED
• Digestive
• Musculoskeletal
• Integument
• Hemolymphatic

PATHOPHYSIOLOGY
• *Actinobacillus ligniersii* is a Gram-negative rod, which normally inhabits the alimentary tract of domestic ruminants, and is also found on plant awns.
• Mucosal lesions anywhere on the body, typically in the mouth, can be invaded by these bacteria, causing a localized lesion. Bacteria can also spread to different parts of the body via lymphatic drainage.
• A typical site of bacterial invasion is through small ulcers in the sulcus lingualis at the base of the tongue, leading to hard, painful, diffuse lesions of the tongue interfering with prehension of food, hence the synonym "wooden tongue." The bacteria initially cause an acute diffuse myositis of the muscles of the tongue, followed by development of granules and fibrosis.
• Lesions other than "wooden tongue" are usually uncommon; however, actinobacillosis should be included as a differential diagnosis for cutaneous diseases such granulomatous dermatitis and lymphadenitis.

HISTORICAL FINDINGS
Abrasive feeds and crowded conditions may lead to sporadic herd outbreaks or endemic disease. Lesions outside the oral cavity may be associated with previous wounds or needle punctures.

SIGNALMENT
• Mainly cattle and sheep, occasionally goats
• All ages

PHYSICAL EXAMINATION FINDINGS
Cattle generally present with hypersalivation and tongue may protrude from mouth. Weight loss can be seen in more chronic cases due to inability to prehend feed. Tongue may be diffusely firm and immovable and nodular swellings may be present on the tongue or lips or within the pharyngeal region. If present in atypical sites, signs will vary.

CAUSES AND RISK FACTORS
Caused by infection of soft tissues by *Actinobacillus ligniersii*. Abrasive feeds, crowded conditions, surgical lesions, and other sources of trauma.

DIAGNOSIS

DIFFERENTIAL DIAGNOSES
• Pharyngeal trauma and abscessation
• Retropharyngeal lymphadenitis or lymphosarcoma
• Oral foreign bodies
• Dental disease
• Parasitic or foreign body granuloma
• Exuberant granulation tissue
• Contagious ecthyma and caseous lymphadenitis in sheep and goats

CBC/BIOCHEMISTRY/URINALYSIS
Chronic inflammatory profile

OTHER LABORATORY TESTS
• Acute lesions: Culture and cytology of aspirates.
• Chronic: Biopsy/histopathology and culture of lesions.
• Microscopic examination of pus compressed between two glass slides shows "sulfur granule" or clublike rosette appearance with a central mass of Gram-negative rods.

PATHOLOGIC FINDINGS
Firm, pale, gritty, granulomatous abscesses with multifocal necrotic foci containing mononuclear cells, neutrophils, eosinophils, and plant fibers.

TREATMENT

THERAPEUTIC APPROACH
• Sodium iodide 20%: 70 mg/kg IV, once, repeat at least once at 7–10-day intervals.
• Organic iodides: 1 oz/450 kg PO daily following first IV administration above.
• Antibiotics may be used alone or in conjunction with iodide treatment for severe cases.
• Use of a soft feed will aid prehension during treatment.

SURGICAL CONSIDERATIONS AND TECHNIQUES
May need surgical debulking of lesions in severe cases; however, note that access to the surgical lesion and close proximity to major vessels limit feasibility in some cases.

MEDICATIONS

DRUGS OF CHOICE
• Sodium iodide IV
• Daily organic iodides PO
• Antibiotics: sulfonamides, tetracyclines, ampicillin, streptomycin

CONTRAINDICATIONS
• Use sodium iodide with caution in pregnant cattle; see "Precautions."
• Extra-label use of sulfonamides is restricted in lactating dairy cattle.
• Streptomycin is not labeled for use in food-producing species in some countries.
• Appropriate milk and meat withdrawal times must be followed for all compounds administered to food-producing animals. Consult the Food Animal Residue Avoidance Database (www.farad.org) for current withdrawal times. As of August 2015, suggested Milk and Meat withdrawal times for cattle treated with NaI as above were 96 hours and 1 day, respectively.

PRECAUTIONS
Anecdotal reports of association with abortion in cattle at high doses of sodium iodide.

POSSIBLE INTERACTIONS
N/A

FOLLOW-UP

EXPECTED COURSE AND PROGNOSIS
• Good prognosis if only the tongue is involved and lesions are acute. Expect dramatic response to therapy in this case.
• Fair to guarded prognosis if atypical sites are involved or lesions are chronic.

POSSIBLE COMPLICATIONS
Anecdotal reports of association with abortion in cattle at high doses of sodium iodide. If signs of iodism seen (dandruff, excessive lacrimation, inappetence, coughing, diarrhea), halt therapy until signs disappear.

CLIENT EDUCATION
Make aware of risk factors.

PREVENTION
Reduce access to abrasive feed and pastures with hard penetrating plant awns or thistles.

MISCELLANEOUS

ZOONOTIC POTENTIAL
Bite wounds from ruminants can contain *Actinobacillus ligniersii*, but rarely result in actinobacillosis.

PREGNANCY
Anecdotal reports of association with abortion in cattle at high doses of sodium iodide.

SYNONYMS
• Wooden tongue
• Woody tongue

ABBREVIATIONS
• IV = intravenous
• NaI = sodium iodide
• PO = per os

SEE ALSO
• Caseous Lymphadenitis
• Oral Disorders
• Orf (Contagious Ecthyma)
• Tongue Trauma

Suggested Reading
Divers TJ, Peek SF eds, Rebhun's Diseases of Dairy Cattle, 2nd ed. St. Louis: Saunders Elsevier, 2008.
Margineda CA, Odriozola E, Moreira AR et al. Atypical actinobacillosis in bulls in Argentina: granulomatous dermatitis and lymphadenitis. Pesquisa Veterinária Brasileira 2013, 33, 1–4. http://www.scielo.br/pdf/pvb/v33n1/01.pdf.
Pugh DG, Baird AM eds. Sheep and Goat Medicine, 2nd ed. Philadelphia: Saunders Elsevier, 2011.
Radostits OM, Gay CC, Hinchcliff KW, Constable P eds. Veterinary medicine, 10th ed. London: W. B. Saunders, 2006.
Smith BP ed, Large animal internal medicine, 5th ed. St. Louis: Mosby, 2015.

Author Kaitlyn A. Lutz
Consulting Editor Christopher C.L. Chase
Acknowledgment The author and book editors acknowledge the prior contribution of David McKenzie.

ACTINOMYCOSIS: LUMPY JAW

BASICS

OVERVIEW
Common, sporadic, chronic granulomatous osteomyelitis of cattle caused by non-spore-forming, filamentous, Gram-positive, anaerobic bacterium *Actinomyces bovis*.

INCIDENCE/PREVALENCE
Common, sporadic

GEOGRAPHIC DISTRIBUTION
Worldwide

SYSTEMS AFFECTED
• Musculoskeletal, typically confined to the mandible and maxilla • Potential for hematogenous spread to other organs

PATHOPHYSIOLOGY
• *Actinomyces bovis* is part of the normal flora of the bovine oral cavity. It has low virulence and only causes disease when mucosal barriers are compromised. • Trauma to the oral mucosa from rough feed or foreign objects permits entrance of *Actinomyces* into buccal tissues. The organism may also enter through the dental alveolus. • The organism grows best in anaerobic conditions associated with devitalized tissues where there is a lack of phagocyte delivery. • Disease is typically of the mandible or maxilla, beginning as a painless, hard, immobile swelling. It is possible for teeth to become involved. In the following weeks to months, abscess/granuloma formation with necrotic foci may occur. As the disease progresses lesions may become painful. • Discharge of viscous, sticky, "honey- or whey-like," odorless, yellowish pus from openings may occur. The pus contains sand-like, firm, yellowish granules. The granule contains microcolonies of *Actinomyces* in an eosinophilic, amorphous matrix made of calcium phosphate/antigen-antibody complexes. • Occasional involvement of soft tissues, especially of esophageal groove with spread to lower esophagus, anterior wall of reticulum, may occur. Trauma to the digestive tract could allow for disease in regions distal to the oral cavity. • Hematogenous spread to other organs is rare. • Local lymph nodes are usually not involved. • Severe swelling, particularly of the maxilla, may cause dyspnea.

SIGNALMENT
• Primarily cattle; potentially all ruminant species • Often young with erupting teeth, but may affect any age • No sex or breed predilection

PHYSICAL EXAMINATION FINDINGS
• Hard, immovable swelling of the mandible or maxilla • Draining, fistulous tracts with a yellow, odorless pus • Missing or malaligned teeth with difficulty masticating • Weight loss, intermittent diarrhea, chronic bloat • Dyspnea • Rarely, partial tracheal obstruction, orchitis, brain/lung abscesses

CAUSES AND RISK FACTORS
• Eruption of teeth in young cattle • Rough feeds containing awns, foreign objects • Procedures causing oral lacerations

DIAGNOSIS

DIFFERENTIAL DIAGNOSES
• Tooth root abscess • Osteomyelitis from cause other than *Actinomyces bovis* • Cheek abscess from cause other than *Actinomyces bovis* (movable, located in soft tissue) • Impacted feed/foreign body between cheek and teeth (soft, movable) • Lymphosarcoma/fibrosarcoma (soft)

OTHER LABORATORY TESTS
• Culture: Deep samples should be taken and placed in anaerobic transport media. • Microscopic examination of purulent debris: mix sample with saline and crush granules between slides. Gram stain will reveal Gram-positive organisms that may be branching, filamentous, coccoid or diphtheroid.

IMAGING
Osteomyelitis of the affected area; teeth may be involved. Important to differentiate from tooth root abscess.

PATHOLOGIC FINDINGS
Osteomyelitis with organisms present

TREATMENT

Difficult to treat. Antibiotics and sodium iodide have been historically used. Surgical debridement and drainage may be necessary.

MEDICATIONS

DRUGS OF CHOICE
• Penicillin, streptomycin, sulfonamides, erythromycin, and isoniazid have been used. • Sodium iodide: 70 mg/kg IV every 3 to 5 days until signs of iodism occur (scaling skin, lacrimation, cough, anorexia).

CONTRAINDICATIONS
• Iodine therapy may cause abortion. • Appropriate meat and milk withdrawal times must be followed for all compounds administered to food-producing animals. • Many historically used antibiotics are no longer approved in the United States.

FOLLOW-UP

EXPECTED COURSE AND PROGNOSIS
• If untreated, disease will progress until the animal is no longer able to appropriately prehend food. • Difficult to treat. Early, aggressive treatment provides the best outcome.

POSSIBLE COMPLICATIONS
• Some animals become distressed with iodine infusion (restlessness, dyspnea, tachycardia). • Subcutaneous iodine causes severe irritation.

PATIENT CARE
• Lesions will slowly remodel after successful treatment. The affected areas may never return to normal. • Recrudescence is possible, even after prolonged periods of time.

PREVENTION
• Avoid feeds or procedures that could cause oral lacerations. • Monitor young cattle for swelling of mandible, especially following tooth eruptions. • Isolate cattle with discharging lesions. • There is no vaccine.

MISCELLANEOUS

AGE-RELATED FACTORS
Young cattle with erupting teeth

PREGNANCY
Iodine treatment during pregnancy may cause abortion.

ABBREVIATION
IV = intravenous

SEE ALSO
• Actinobacillosis: Wooden Tongue • Caseous Lymphadenitis • Oral Disorders • Orf (Contagious Ecthyma)

Suggested Reading
Bertone AL, Rebhun WC. Tracheal actinomycosis in a cow. J Am Vet Med Assoc 1984, 185: 221–2.
Radostits, OM, Gay CC, Hinchcliff KW, Constable PC eds, Actinomycosis. In: Veterinary Medicine, 10th ed. Philadelphia: Saunders, 2007.
Seifi HA, Saifzadeh S, Farshid AA, Rad M, Farrokhi F. Mandibular pyogranulomatous osteomyelitis in a Sannen goat. J Vet Med A Physiol Pathol Clin Med 2003, 50: 219–21.
Smith BP. Actinomycosis (lumpy jaw). In: Large Animal Internal Medicine, 5th ed. St. Louis: Mosby, 2015.
Strohl WA, Harriet R, Fisher BD eds, Lippincott's Illustrated Reviews: Microbiology. Philadelphia: Lippincott, Williams & Wilkins, 2001.
Watts TC, Olson SM, Rhodes CS. Treatment of bovine actinomycosis with isoniazid. Can Vet J 1973, 14: 223–4.
Watts TC, Olson SM, Rhodes CS. Letter: Use of isoniazid in cattle. Can Vet J 1974, 15: 28.
Author Dusty W. Nagy
Consulting Editor Christopher C.L. Chase
Acknowledgment The author and book editors acknowledge the prior contribution of Karen Carberry-Goh.

ACUPUNCTURE

 BASICS

OVERVIEW
• Acupuncture is one of the four branches of traditional Chinese veterinary medicine (TCVM) and has been practiced for over 2,000 years.
• The twelve regular channels and the eight extraordinary channels connect acupoints all over the body. These pathways, known as meridians, relate to different organ systems and conduct the acupuncture signal and life energy, known as Qi.
• Techniques for stimulating acupoints include dry needling, aquapuncture, electroacupuncture, hemoacupuncture, and moxibustion.
• In 1997 the NIH (USA) released a consensus statement stating that acupuncture was proven to be effective for treatment of musculoskeletal pain, some gastrointestinal diseases, pulmonary disease, immunomodulation, and reproductive disorders in humans.
• Acupuncture is appropriate for use in organic production systems which are otherwise limited in their choice of treatment options.
• The practice of veterinary acupuncture is restricted to licensed veterinarians, or under the supervision of a licensed veterinarian, in most states and provinces in the US and Canada.

 DIAGNOSIS

OTHER DIAGNOSTIC PROCEDURES
A full Western veterinary physical examination should be performed prior to initiating treatment. Both the Western and TCVM examination results are taken together to formulate a diagnosis. Additional TCVM procedures which are not part of the traditional Western examination can include:
• Determination of the patient's temperament type and element association.
• Inspection of the tongue: Tongue color, coating, and degree of moisture.
• Pulse diagnosis: Relative strength of the pulse at different points. In cattle, the pulse is taken at the coccygeal artery; in small ruminants the pulse is taken from the right and left carotid arteries, allowing for comparison between the two.
• Palpation along the meridians to find areas of sensitivity.

 TREATMENT

THERAPEUTIC APPROACH
• Dry needle (DN): Insertion of sterile needles into an acupoint.
• Electroacupuncture (EA): Electrical stimulation of an acupoint; electrical leads are connected to the handles of the metal needles and either low or high frequency current sent into the points and along the associated channels. Provides greater, longer-lasting stimulation of a point or channel than dry needling alone.
• Aquapuncture (AA): Injection of sterile saline, vitamin B12, or the patient's own blood into an acupoint. Provides longer-lasting stimulation of a given point than dry needling alone.
• Hemoacupuncture (HA): Release of blood from an acupoint; the point is pricked with a sterile hypodermic needle and allowed to bleed. Used to release excess heat or relieve stagnation.
• Acupressure: Applying pressure to an acupoint or along a meridian without insertion of a needle or other method of stimulation.
• Moxibustion (moxa): Sticks or cones of dried mugwort are burned and held near an acupoint or touched to a dry needle to stimulate the point. Used to break up stagnation or warm the point.

Protocols
Treatment protocols should take into account the Western diagnosis, TCVM pattern diagnosis, patient's temperament, and the owner's primary concern for each individual case. As such there is no true "cookbook" protocol for any particular condition. That said, the most frequently used points for common Western medical diagnoses are given below along with suggested techniques. For explanation of the channel names and point locations, see "Suggested Reading." It is strongly recommended that one completes a formal training program prior to performing any acupuncture treatment.
Please note that for emergencies (e.g., dystocia) acupuncture should not be used as the sole treatment, and the practitioner must adapt his or her approach as the case develops.
• Anestrus: Bai-hui, Yan-chi, GV-1, GV-2, CV-1, BL-23, BL-26, Shen-shu, Shen-peng and Shen-jiao; can use DN, EA, or moxa.
• Retained fetal membranes: Bai-hui, Ba-jiao, GV-1, BL-31/32/34; EAP recommended daily until resolution.

• Infertility/subfertility: Bai-hui, Shen-peng/shu/jiao, Yan-chi, CV-1; DN, EA, or AA.
• Dystocia: SP-6, BL-60/67 to promote normal labor, add GB-21 for dystocia; DN or AA.
• Resuscitation, esp. of neonates: GV-26; DN.
• Heat stress: Er-jian, Wei-jian, Tai-tang (GB-1), GV-14; DN for GV-14, HA for others; EA between GV-14 and Bai-hui.
• Hemorrhage: Duan-xue (GV-6), Tian-ting; DN or AA; can be administered 2 hours prior to surgical procedures (e.g. castration, enucleation) for prevention.
• Diarrhea: GV-1, ST-36, BL-20/21/25; DN or AA.
• Anorexia: Shan-gen (use hypodermic needle), Mi-jiao-gan, ST-36; DN.
• Calving paralysis: Bai-hui, GB-29/30, BL-54, GV-3 and KID-1; EA or AA.

 MEDICATIONS

DRUGS OF CHOICE
Chinese herbal medications are sometimes given as a complement to acupuncture. Because of metabolism in the rumen and first compartment, oral doses should be 2 to 3 times greater than those listed for horses. Alternatively, the equine dose can be administered per rectum as a slurry.

PRECAUTIONS
These medications have not been evaluated by the FDA and there are no established withdrawal times for any food-producing species.

 FOLLOW-UP

EXPECTED COURSE AND PROGNOSIS
• Improvement should be seen by the third treatment. Chronic or severe conditions will often require multiple treatments over an extended period (weeks to months).
• Although acupuncture can be used symptomatically, being able to make a Chinese medical diagnosis allows the practitioner to target the treatment towards the underlying pathologic process and will enhance results.
• Prognosis depends heavily on the severity and chronicity of the disease process, the patient's temperament and demeanor, and the patient's tolerance of acupuncture treatment.

(CONTINUED)   **ACUPUNCTURE**   **A**

POSSIBLE COMPLICATIONS
• Acupuncture should be used with caution during pregnancy. Avoid points around the abdomen, mid to lower back, and hips. Any points which move blood or Qi should be avoided, as well as potent points such as ST-36, LI-4, BL-67, and SP-6. The CV channel (along ventral midline) should not be stimulated during gestation.
• Very old or debilitated patients (See "Age-Related Factors").
• Although extremely rare, needles can break off and become lodged in the muscle. To prevent breakage, use appropriately sized needles for each point, avoid using hypodermic needles except as a guide or for HA, and do not insert the needle completely up to the handle.
• Concurrent use of sedatives or dexamethasone will blunt the response to acupuncture and should be used only when necessary.

PATIENT CARE
For complicated or severe conditions, multiple treatments over an extended period of time should be expected. As the primary condition improves, other symptoms and disease patterns may become more obvious and treatment protocols adjusted accordingly.

 MISCELLANEOUS

AGE-RELATED FACTORS
• Neonates and juvenile patients respond readily to acupuncture and may not need extensive treatment.
• Very old patients may not have enough energy or Qi left to tolerate a full acupuncture session. Since acupuncture moves energy around the body, it may deplete what little is left for these patients, leading to death. Short treatments with very few needles should be used.

PREGNANCY
• Acupuncture should be used with caution during pregnancy (see "Possible Complications"). Points which are both safe to use and can promote a healthy pregnancy include Bai-hui, Shen-peng/shu/jiao, and BL-20/21/22/23/24/25/26.

BIOSECURITY
• Acupuncture needles are single use only and should be disposed of properly in a sharps container.
• Use of blood for AA should only be performed with the patient's own blood, injected immediately after being drawn from the jugular or coccygeal vein.

ABBREVIATIONS
• AA – aquapuncture
• DN – dry needle technique
• EA – electroacupuncture
• HA – hemoacupuncture
• Moxa – moxibustion
• TCVM – Traditional Chinese Veterinary Medicine
See "Suggested Reading" for full explanation of acupuncture point abbreviations

SEE ALSO
Alternative Medicine (see www.fiveminutevet.com/ruminant)

Suggested Reading
Acupuncture. NIH Consensus Statement Online. 1997 November 3–5; 15(5): 1–34.
Chan WW, Chen KY, Liu H, et al. Acupuncture for general veterinary practice. J Vet Med Sci 2001, 63: 1057–62.
Fry LM, Neary SM, Sharrock J, Rychel JK. Acupuncture for analgesia in veterinary medicine. Top Companion Anim Med 2014, 29: 35–42.
Habacher G, Pittler MH, Ernst E. Effectiveness of acupuncture in veterinary medicine: systematic review. J Vet Intern Med 2006, 20: 480–8.
Kim DH, Cho SH, Song KH, et al. Electroacupuncture analgesia for surgery in cattle. Am J Chin Med 2004, 32: 131–40.

Memon MA, Sprunger LK. Survey of colleges and schools of veterinary medicine regarding education in complementary and alternative veterinary medicine. J Am Vet Med Assoc 2011, 239: 619–23.
Schoen AM. Veterinary Acupuncture: Ancient Art to Modern Medicine, 2nd ed. St. Louis: Mosby, 2001.
Xie H, Preast V. Xie's Chinese Veterinary Herbology. Hoboken, NJ: Wiley-Blackwell, 2010.
Xie H, Preast V. Traditional Chinese Veterinary Medicine: Fundamental Principles, 2nd ed. Reddick, FL: Chi Institute Press, 2013.
Internet Resources
• American Academy of Veterinary Acupuncture: http://www.aava.org/
• American Association of Traditional Chinese Veterinary medicine: http://www.aatcvm.org/index.php/en/
• Association of British Veterinary Acupuncturists (training available): http://www.abva.co.uk/
• Association of Veterinary Acupuncturists of Canada: http://www.avacanada.org/
• Australian College of Veterinary Acupuncture (training available): http://vetacupcollege.com.au/blog/
• Australian Veterinary Acupuncture Group: http://acuvet.ava.com.au/
• Chi Institute (training available): http://www.tcvm.com/
• International Veterinary Acupuncture Society (training available): https://www.ivas.org/
• OneHealth SIM (training available): https://www.onehealthsim.org/
• World Association of Traditional Chinese Veterinary Medicine: http://www.watcvm.org/

Author Christine M. Winslow
Consulting Editor Kaitlyn A. Lutz
Acknowledgment The Book Editors acknowledge the editorial contribution of Sharon Sherman in this topic.

A

ACUTE RENAL FAILURE

BASICS

OVERVIEW
Acute renal failure (ARF) is common in ruminants experiencing hemodynamic changes or exposed to nephrotoxins.

PATHOPHYSIOLOGY
• Dehydration, endotoxemia, hemorrhage, and shock could result in ARF due to sustained decrease in renal perfusion (hypoperfusion and ischemia) and release of endogenous inflammatory and pressure mediators. • Infarction of the renal cortex and destruction of the base membrane of tubular cells in cases of decreased renal perfusion results in nephron dysfunction. • Direct injury to tubular cells caused by exposure to nephrotoxins.

SIGNALMENT
There is no predisposition of ruminant species, breed, sex, or age to develop ARF.

PHYSICAL EXMINATION FINDINGS
• Signs of acute renal failure are nonspecific and signs of primary disease may mask renal affection. • Anuria, oliguria, or polyuria may be observed. • Affected animals may present with dehydration, depression, anorexia, and diarrhea. • Oral ulcerations might be observed in uremic animals. • Severe cases develop muscular weakness and recumbency due to electrolyte and acid-base abnormalities. • Rectal palpation in cattle may reveal left renal enlargement.

CAUSES AND RISK FACTORS
• Conditions that result in systemic compromise, dehydration, and hypotension such as diarrhea, septicemia, endotoxemia, disseminated intravascular coagulopathy, and acute blood loss. • Nephrotoxic agents include heavy metals, aminoglycosides and tetracyclines, NSAIDs, toxic plants such as pigweed and oaks, vitamin C and D, hemoglobin, myoglobin, and calcium oxalate among others. • Infectious agents such as *Leptospira* spp. and urolithiasis are less common causes of ARF.

DIAGNOSIS

DIFFERENTIAL DIAGNOSIS
The nonspecific nature of clinical signs in cases of ARF in ruminants makes it difficult to develop a differential diagnosis list. Many primary disease conditions might result in ARF.

CBC/BIOCHEMISTRY/URINALYSIS
• Azotemia (increased BUN and creatinine). • Isosthenuria in the face of azotemia is a strong indicator of ARF. • Proteinuria, glucosuria, and granular casts may be present in urine. • Metabolic alkalosis, hypochloremia, hyponatremia, hypocalcemia, hyperphosphatemia, and hypermagnesemia are common findings with ARF. • Increased liver enzymes (SDH and GGT) values may be observed.

OTHER LABORATORY TESTS
Fractional excretion of sodium may be evaluated but the test should be compared to a normal animal (e.g., herd mate) of similar age, physiologic state, and nutritional status.

IMAGING
Ultrasonographic evaluation may reveal loss of detail of cortico-medullary junction, dilation of renal pelves and perirenal edema.

DIAGNOSTIC PROCEDURES
• Glomerular filtration rate assessment provides precise information of renal function. • Renal biopsy may provide diagnostic as well as prognostic information in cases of ARF.

PATHOLOGIC FINDINGS
Renal tubular degeneration and necrosis is a consistent histopathologic finding.

TREATMENT

THERAPEUTIC APPROACH
• The animal should be removed from the source of the nephrotoxins or exposure discontinued. • Isotonic, sodium-containing IV fluids with added calcium and potassium are indicated to correct acid-base and electrolyte abnormalities, increase renal perfusion, and promote diuresis. IV fluids should be maintained until the serum creatinine has returned to normal (usually 2–3 weeks). • Oral fluid therapy may be used if IV administration is impractical. • IV or oral fluids should be administered at a rate of two times the adult maintenance rate of 60 mL/kg/day. • Hydration and plasma protein should be monitored to avoid overhydration. • Supportive care should include broad-spectrum antibiotics, rumen transfaunations, and nutritional support.

MEDICATIONS

DRUGS OF CHOICE
• Furosemide (1 mg/kg IV or IM, q12h) administered every 2–3 hours to promote diuresis in anuric animals. • A dopamine drip (2 µg/kg/min IV) should be considered if diuresis is not achieved.

CONTRAINDICATIONS
• With repeated use of furosemide, the patient's serum sodium and potassium must be monitored carefully. • Drug withdrawal times need to be determined and maintained in food-producing animals.

FOLLOW-UP

EXPECTED COURSE AND PROGNOSIS
• ARF due to ischemic episodes generally results in a grave prognosis. • Renal failure due to toxic causes may have a more favorable prognosis. • Failure to produce urine in the face of high volume IV fluids and diuretics carries a grave prognosis.

MISCELLANEOUS

ABBREVIATIONS
• ARF = acute renal failure • BUN = blood urea nitrogen • GGT = gamma glutamyl transferase • IM = intramuscular • IV = intravenous • NSAIDs = nonsteroidal anti-inflammatory drugs • SDH = sorbitol dehydrogenase

SEE ALSO
• Diarrheal Disease: Bovine • Diarrheal Diseases: Camelid • Diarrheal Diseases: Small Ruminants • Oak (*Quercus* spp.) Toxicity • Pyelonephritis

Suggested Reading
Anderson DE, Constable PD, Yvorchuk KE, Anderson NV, St-Jean G, Rock L. Hyperlipemia and ketonuria in an alpaca and a llama. J Vet Intern Med 1994, 8(3):207–11.
Chamorro MF, Passler T, Joiner K, Poppenga RH, Bayne J, Walz PH. Acute renal failure in 2 adult llamas after exposure to Oak trees (*Quercus* spp.). Can Vet J 2013, 54: 61–4.
Gerspach C, Bateman S, Sherding R, Chew DJ, Besier AS, Grieves JL, Lakritz J. Acute renal failure and anuria associated with vitamin D intoxication in two alpaca (*Vicugna pacos*) cria. J Vet Intern Med 2010, 24: 443–9.
Pugh DG. Sheep and Goat Medicine. Philadelphia: Saunders, 2002.
Schlumbohm C, Harmeyer J. Hyperketonemia impairs glucose metabolism in pregnant and nonpregnant ewes. J Dairy Sci 2004, 87: 350–8.

BASICS

OVERVIEW
• Defined by the 1971 Agricultural Chemicals Regulation Law as "chemical agents such as fungicides and insecticides that are used to control crop-harming organisms (e.g., fungi, nematodes, mites, insects, and rodents) or viruses (hereinafter collectively referred to as 'diseases and pests')." Also included are plant growth regulators and germination inhibitors.
• EPA regulates pesticides in the USA; it must find that a pesticide poses a "reasonable certainty of no harm" before it can be registered for use on food or feeds.
• Residual agricultural chemicals are those remaining in the crops after application. They may become part of livestock feed and end up in meat or milk, harming ruminant animals (fetus and neonates in particular) and human beings.
• Agricultural chemicals are best classified by their specific application target.
  ○ Insecticides—control pests; includes ovicides and larvicides.
  ○ Fungicides—control diseases that damage feeds, field crops, and fruit trees.
  ○ Insecticides/fungicides—act together to control harmful pests and diseases that damage field crops.
  ○ Herbicides—control weeds; may be selective for a specific plant or group of plants or be totally nonselective.
  ○ Plant growth regulators—either inhibit or stimulate growth of crops.
  ○ Attractants—attract insect pests.
  ○ Repellants—repel birds and small mammals that may damage crops.
  ○ Spreaders—substances mixed with other chemicals to enhance adherence.
  ○ Rodenticides—control mice, rats, and other small rodents.
• Ruminants are exposed through ingestion of contaminated feeds, treated seeds, or stored chemicals as well as oral and dermal exposure to recently treated fields or pastures.
• Many banned or cancelled products such as arsenicals and organochlorines may not have been properly disposed of, posing a hazard to ruminants that may ingest them.
• Newer insecticides (i.e., pyrethrins and pyrethroids, fipronil, and neonicotinoids) are safer and have replaced organophosphate and carbamates, but they are not without some harm to animals and the environment.

INCIDENCE/PREVALENCE
Sporadic; may be a single isolated animal or entire herd.

SYSTEMS AFFECTED
• Multisystemic, depending on chemical encountered

PATHOPHYSIOLOGY
• Toxicity:
  ○ Variable depending on the product.
  ○ Acute toxicity occurs within a few hours to a day.
  ○ Chronic toxicity develops over time and is much more difficult to diagnose.
• Systemic absorption may result in accumulation in fat, liver, brain, kidney, and milk; some products result in transplacental transmission.
• Insecticides: Older products
  ○ Old insecticides such as DDT, most organochlorines, and arsenicals are no longer registered in the USA, but may be used worldwide.
    ▪ Highly toxic; many are carcinogens and some have associated reproductive defects.
    ▪ Primarily lipid soluble, non-biodegradable, and accumulate in fat resulting in contamination of milk and meat.
    ▪ Persist in the environment for very long periods of time.
    ▪ High potential for bioaccumulation (absorption occurs more rapidly than excretion) and biomagnification (tissue concentrations of a contaminant increase as it passes up the food chain).
  ○ Organophosphate (OP) and carbamate compounds
    ▪ OPs: diazinon, dichlorvos, malathion, parathion, others.
    ▪ Carbamates: aldicarb, carbaryl, carbofuran, methomyl, others.
    ▪ Inhibit the enzyme acetylcholinesterase at cholinergic junction.
    ▪ Many are highly toxic and no longer registered in the USA; still widely used worldwide.
• Insecticides: Newer products
  ○ Pyrethrins and pyrethroids
    ▪ Cyhalothrin, cypermethrin, deltamethrin, others.
    ▪ Slow the opening of sodium channels causing hyperexcitability.
    ▪ Most are highly lipophilic.
    ▪ Generally safe.
    ▪ Salivation, vomiting, tremors, seizures, dyspnea, prostration, death.
  ○ Phenylpyrazole (fipronil)
    ▪ Inhibits $GABA_A$ chloride channels resulting in hyperexcitation and neurotoxicity.
    ▪ Generally safe unless exposed to highly concentrated product.
    ▪ Buffalo and their calves may have increased risk of toxicosis.
    ▪ Anorexia, twitching, tremors, ataxia, seizures.
  ○ Neonicotinoids
    ▪ Acetamiprid, dinotefuran, imidacloprid, nitenpyram, others.
    ▪ Imidacloprid widely used worldwide in crop production.
    ▪ Act on postsynaptic nicotinic receptors in insects CNS; little effect on mammalian receptors.
    ▪ High margin of safety; not carcinogenic, mutagenic, or teratogenic.
    ▪ Adult buffalo and their calves may have an increased risk of toxicity.
    ▪ Lethargy, tremors, ataxia, hypothermia, death with high concentrations.
• Fungicides
  ○ Less acute toxicity; may be due to decreased oral absorption.
  ○ Respiratory and ophthalmic irritation from aerosolized products.
• Herbicides
  ○ Toxicity varies by compound.
  ○ Dinitro compounds
    ▪ Highly toxic to ruminants.
    ▪ Fever, dyspnea, tachycardia, seizures, death.
    ▪ Methemoglobinemia, intravascular hemolysis.
    ▪ Dinitrophenol compounds may cause yellow staining of the skin, conjunctiva, or hair.
  ○ Paraquat
    ▪ Highly toxic when wet; very low toxicity once dry and bound to vegetation.
    ▪ Restricted use, nonspecific herbicide that kills all vegetation.
    ▪ Widely used worldwide, less so in USA.
    ▪ Dyspnea, anuria, muscle tremors, ataxia, salivation, recumbency, death.
  ○ Sodium chlorate
    ▪ Dyspnea, recumbency, seizures, abortion
    ▪ Methemoglobinemia
  ○ Glyphosate—considered less toxic, but controversial

HISTORICAL FINDINGS
Toxic ingestion may be known or suspected based on thorough history taking.

SIGNALMENT
• Very young and old.
• Neonates without functioning rumen are at a greater risk of toxicity from pyrethroids, OPs, and carbamates.
• Buffalo calves may be more susceptible to fipronil and neonicotinoids (acetamiprid).

PHYSICAL EXAMINATION FINDINGS
• General nonspecific signs include:
  ○ Anorexia, hypersalivation, decreased rumen motility and bloat, abdominal pain, diarrhea (SLUDGE with OPs and carbamate insecticides)
  ○ Stimulation or depression; lethargy, ataxia, hyperexcitation, tremors, seizures, recumbency, coma
  ○ Tachypnea, dyspnea, respiratory arrest (paraquat)
  ○ Polyuria, anuria (paraquat)
  ○ Methemoglobinemia (chlorate and nitrate herbicides); cardiac arrest
  ○ Hypo/hyperthermia
  ○ Paresthesia, dermal irritation, inflammation (pyrethrins/pyrethroids; paraquat)
  ○ Ophthalmic irritation (aerosolized products)

- See "Pathophysiology" for specific signs.
- Generally occur within 4–24 hours.
- May differ with individual animals, but specific system abnormalities are normally recognized in a herd situation.

CAUSES AND RISK FACTORS
- Improper storage or labeling of chemicals
- Equipment not cleaned well (e.g., ammonium nitrate residue in tank later used to fill water tanks)
- Access to a newly treated pasture or feed batch

DIAGNOSIS

DIFFERENTIAL DIAGNOSES
- Gastrointestinal—bloat, grain overload, coccidiosis
- Nervous– lead poisoning, nervous ketosis, polioencephalomalacia, rabies (single animal)
- Respiratory—bloat, infectious diseases

CBC/BIOCHEMISTRY/URINALYSIS
Often unremarkable

OTHER LABORATORY TESTS
Gas or liquid chromatography on fresh or frozen samples

OTHER DIAGNOSTIC PROCEDURES
- Variable
- Urine or milk analysis helpful for some exposures

PATHOLOGIC FINDINGS
Often unremarkable, especially with sudden death.

TREATMENT

THERAPEUTIC APPROACH
- Remove animals from suspected source.
- Activated charcoal or mineral oil within 10–12 hours of oral exposure.
  ○ Contraindicated: digestible oils such as corn oil may increase absorption and should not be used as a cathartic.

- Symptomatic and supportive
  ○ Dermal exposure— bathe with grease cutting dish detergent (wear gloves)
  ○ Respiratory exposure—fresh air
  ○ Seizures —barbiturates, diazepam
  ○ Methemoglobinemia—methylene blue
  ○ SLUDGE—atropine; pralidoxime not cost effective for larger animals

FOLLOW-UP

EXPECTED COURSE AND PROGNOSIS
Specific agent and response to therapy guide prognosis.

POSSIBLE COMPLICATIONS
Chronic poor production

CLIENT EDUCATION
See "Prevention"

PATIENT CARE
Milk and meat testing for clearance time

PREVENTION
- Proper labeling and storage of chemicals
- Disposal of older products
- Effective cleaning of multiple use equipment

MISCELLANEOUS

AGE-RELATED FACTORS
Pre-ruminants are more susceptible to chemicals degraded in the rumen.

ZOONOTIC POTENTIAL
- Meat and milk contamination.
- Movement and/or marketing of animals poisoned with agricultural chemicals varies by state; consult with board of animal health or diagnostic laboratory.

ABBREVIATIONS
- CNS = central nervous system
- DDT = dichloro-diphenyl-trichloroethane
- EPA = Environmental Protection Agency

- OPs = organophosphate insecticides
- SLUDGE = salivation, lacrimation, urination, diarrhea, gastroenteritis

Suggested Reading
Bera AK, Rana T, Das S, et al. Ground water arsenic contamination in West Bengal, India: A risk of sub-clinical toxicity in cattle as evident by correlation between arsenic exposure, excretion and deposition. Toxicol Indust Health 2010, 26: 709–16.
Kazemi M, Tahmasbi AM, Valizadeh R, et al. Organophosphate pesticides: a general review. Agric Sci Res J 2012, 2: 512–22.
Ktolel SB, Kumar P, Paril R. Environmental pollutants and livestock health: a review. Vet Res Int 2013, 1: 1–13.
Mrema EJ, Rubino FM, Brambilla G, et al. C. Persistent organochlorinated pesticides and mechanisms of their toxicity. Toxicology 2013, 307: 74–88.
Oliver CE, Craigmill AL, Caton JS, et al. Pharmacokinetics of ruminally dosed sodium [36Cl] chlorate in beef cattle. J Vet Pharm Therap 2007, 30: 358–6.
Shridhar NB. Toxicity of imidacloprid in buffaloes. Indian J Anim Res 2010, 44: 224–5.
Tamuli SM, Pegu SR, Tamuli MK, et al. Pathology of acute paraquat toxicity in ruminants. Indian J Vet Path 2009, 33: 156–9.

Internet Resources
- Agricultural Chemicals. Available at: http://toxics.usgs.gov/topics/agchemicals.html.
- Suspended, restricted, and cancelled pesticides. http://nepis.epa.gov/Exe/ZyPURL.cgi?Dockey=20011E0G.TXT.
Author Lynn Rolland Hovda
Consulting Editor Kaitlyn A. Lutz
Acknowledgment The author and book editors acknowledge the prior contribution of Alejandro Ramirez.

BASICS

OVERVIEW
• Akabane virus (AKAV) is an arthropod-borne virus of ruminants.
• The virus is transmitted by small biting midges (or gnats) of *Culicoides*. Some species may carry both AKAV and bluetongue virus.
• AKAV infects a wide range of domesticated and wildlife ruminants. The disease has been reported in cattle, buffalo, sheep, and goats.
• Infection of pregnant animals results in abortion and stillbirth due to variable defects of the fetal nervous system and arthrogryposis, with no clinical signs in the dam.

INCIDENCE/PREVALENCE
• In endemic areas, the disease has a seasonal pattern, with peak vector activity in summer and diagnosis of outbreak made the subsequent winter.
• Most female animals are infected prior to reproductive age.
• Disease is seen in naïve animals which become infected during pregnancy, either due to "spillover" of the vector from its region, or movement of naïve animals into endemic areas.
• Surveys indicate that more than 80% of adult cattle in an endemic area are seropositive for AKAV. However, following years of drought or times of reduced vector populations, native livestock may not be exposed prior to breeding age and therefore become susceptible.
• Data from Japanese and Australian outbreaks suggest that the fetus is infected in 30–40% of pregnant cows which are infected with AKAV.

GEOGRAPHIC DISTRIBUTION
• The virus is widespread throughout Asia, Australia, Africa, and the Middle East.
• The virus is considered a foreign animal disease in the United States.

SYSTEMS AFFECTED
• Reproductive
• Musculoskeletal
• Nervous

PATHOPHYSIOLOGY
• AKAV is a single-stranded negative sense tripartite RNA virus. It is a member of the genus Orthobunyavirus, family Bunyaviridae, and serogroup Simbu. Four genotypes are identified (I, II, III, IV).
• After infection via the *Culicoides* vector, viremia occurs in the host 1–6 days later.
• Antibodies are detectable 14 days after infection.
• The virus crosses the placenta and infects the fetus, leading to the clinical signs.
• A fetus may be infected months prior to abortion, premature birth, or stillbirth.
• Akabane virus is a potent teratogen and affects the limbs (arthrogryposis) and central nervous system (porencephaly, hydranencephaly).
• Type of fetal abnormalities depend on stage of pregnancy. Susceptible periods range from 28 to 56 days in small ruminants and 3 to 6 months in cattle.
• Long-term carriers of the disease are not believed to occur.

HISTORICAL FINDINGS
• Severe epizootics or smaller outbreaks are associated with movement of naïve pregnant animals into an endemic area, or "spillover" of the vector into naïve populations outside the endemic area.
• Abortion outbreak of abnormal fetuses between 4 and 6 months of gestation.

SIGNALMENT
• Disease occurs only in cattle, sheep, and goats but antibodies have been found in several other large animal species.
• Manifestations of infection depend on the gestational age at the time of infection.
• In cattle:
  ◦ Infection between days 79–104 of gestation results in hydranencephaly.
  ◦ Infection between days 103–174 results in arthrogryposis with focal Wallerian-type degeneration of the brain and spinal cord.
  ◦ Infection in late gestation can result in encephalomyelitis.
  ◦ Infection in few postnatal calves and adult cows has been diagnosed in Japan, which manifested as encephalomyelitis.
• In sheep, infection at 32–48 days' gestation resulted in fetal abnormalities.
• In goats, infection at approximately 40 days' gestation resulted in fetal abnormalities.

PHYSICAL EXAMINATION FINDINGS
• Infections in adult ruminants are typically asymptomatic. However, the Iriki strain (Japan and Korea) has been associated with encephalitis.
• The hallmark of AKAV is congenital abnormalities of the neurologic and muscular systems. Effects on the fetus depend on time of infection during gestation.
• One group of investigators divided the gestational effects of AKAV into 5 groups (1 = late gestation infection; 5 = early gestation infection). Group 1 abnormalities included microscopic non-suppurative encephalomyelitis. Group 2 lesions included loss of ventral horn spinal cord neurons and Wallerian-type degeneration of ventral spinal nerves which resulted in ataxia, flaccid paralysis, and mild arthrogryposis. Group 4 lesions included arthrogryposis and hydranencephaly. Groups 3 and 5 were more severe manifestations of group 2 and 4 signs, respectively.
• Dystocia may occur at parturition or abortion due to fetal abnormalities.

GENETICS
N/A

CAUSES AND RISK FACTORS
• Clinical signs of AKAV are caused by exposure of ruminant fetuses to the virus by dam infection via *Culicoides* midges. Outbreaks are related to seasonal factors and vector distribution.
• Exposure of naïve pregnant animals to the virus-borne vector.

DIAGNOSIS

AKAV can be suspected based on clinical appearance of the fetus and knowledge of endemic areas; however, confirmation of the diagnosis by a diagnostic laboratory is required because gross appearance of AKAV is the same as many other vector-borne viruses.

DIFFERENTIAL DIAGNOSIS
• Bluetongue virus
• Bovine viral diarrhea virus
• Border disease virus
• Schmallenberg virus
• Cache Valley virus
• Aino virus
• Toxic, nutritional, or genetic causes of fetal neuromuscular defects

CBC/BIOCHEMISTRY/URINALYSIS
N/A

OTHER LABORATORY TESTS
• Serology can be performed in affected dams and precolostral serum of the offspring.
• Collection of fetoplacental tissues at necropsy can be diagnostic via several molecular techniques, including reverse transcriptase real-time PCR, competitive ELISA, and immunohistochemistry/immunofluorescence.

IMAGING
N/A

OTHER DIAGNOSTIC PROCEDURES
N/A

PATHOLOGIC FINDINGS
• The most common lesions are arthrogryposis and hydranencephaly.
• Other neurologic abnormalities may include porencephaly and microencephaly.
• In the brain, degenerative and necrotic neurons as well as perineuronal and perivascular edema has been described.
• There may be loss of ventral horn spinal cord neurons and Wallerian-type degeneration of ventral spinal nerves.
• Other findings in calves include: gliosis, demyelination, hepatitis, nephritis, and myodegeneration/polymyositis.
• In sheep, there can be a marked loss of the ventral horns of the spinal cord which leads to hypoplastic spinal cord and muscle atrophy (e.g., torticollis). Pulmonary hypoplasia may also be noted.

TREATMENT

THERAPEUTIC APPROACH
• There is no treatment for AKAV.
• Most fetuses born alive die or are euthanized due to effects of the virus.
• Subsequent pregnancies of the dam will not be affected.

SURGICAL CONSIDERATIONS AND TECHNIQUES
N/A

MEDICATIONS

DRUGS OF CHOICE
N/A

CONTRAINDICATIONS
N/A

PRECAUTIONS
N/A

POSSIBLE INTERACTIONS
N/A

FOLLOW-UP

EXPECTED COURSE AND PROGNOSIS
• Most offspring born alive are either euthanized or die shortly after birth.
• Subsequent pregnancies of the dam will not be affected.

POSSIBLE COMPLICATIONS
• Dystocia
• Infertility

CLIENT EDUATION
• In endemic areas, clients should be aware of repercussions of introducing naïve pregnant animals into the herd.
• Vaccination should also be considered in areas where it is available.

PATIENT CARE
• Specific treatment and supportive care if there are any complications following abortion.

PREVENTION
• Prevention of AKAV includes vector control and vaccination.
• Vector control should include elimination of vector breeding sites, and repellents for pregnant animals.
• Naïve pregnant animals should not be introduced during seasons of high vector activity (summer and autumn).
• Naïve animals should be introduced to endemic areas prior to breeding to develop immunity.
• Breeding season may be altered to avoid period of highest risk.
• Live (Japan) and inactivated (Japan, Australia, Korea) vaccines are available for the prevention of AKAV and are to be administered prior to breeding.

MISCELLANEOUS

ASSOCIATED CONDITIONS
Dystocia, retained placenta

AGE-RELATED FACTORS
AKAV affects fetal ruminants.

ZOONOTIC POTENTIAL
There are no indications that AKAV is zoonotic.

PREGNANCY
Effects of AKAV are dependent on the gestational age of the fetus at the time of infection. However, most affected neonates die or are euthanized after birth due to effects of the virus irrespective of time of infection in utero.

BIOSECURITY
Suspected cases or outbreaks of AKAV outside its endemic areas (see "Geographic Distribution") should immediately be reported to the proper governmental veterinary authorities (i.e., state or federal veterinarian).

PRODUCTION MANAGEMENT
• In endemic areas, avoid introduction of naïve pregnant animals in the summer and autumn months.
• Implement vector control programs to reduce potential transmission of AKAV.
• Consider vaccination protocols prior to breeding.

SYNONYM
Arthrogryposis-hydranencephaly syndrome (AH syndrome)

ABBREVIATION
AKAV = Akabane virus

SEE ALSO
• Abortion: Viral, Fungal, and Nutritional
• Arthrogryposis
• Bluetongue Virus
• Border Disease
• Bovine Viral Diarrhea Virus
• Cache Valley Virus
• Congenital Defects: Bovine
• Lupine Toxicity
• Schmallenberg Virus

Suggested Reading
Agerholm JS, Hewicker-Trautwein M, Peperkamp K, Windsor PA. Virus-induced congenital malformations in cattle. Acta Vet Scand 2015, 57: 54.
Haligur M, Hasircioglu S, Ozmen O, et al. Immunohistochemial evaluation of akabane virus infection in aborted and new-born calves. Vet Med Czech 2014, 59: 230–8.
Horne KM, Vanlandingham DL. Bunyavirus–vector interactions. Viruses 2014, 6: 4373–97.
Kessell AE, Finnie JW, Windsor PA. Neurological diseases of ruminant livestock in Australia. IV: viral infections. Aust Vet J 2011, 89: 331–7.
Kirkland PD. Akabane virus infection. Rev Sci Tech Off Int Epiz 2015, 34: 403–10.
Author Lisa Pearson
Consulting Editor Ahmed Tibary
Acknowledgment The author and book editors acknowledge the prior contribution of Glenda Dvorak.

BASICS

OVERVIEW

An anaphylactic reaction is a pathologic immune response that occurs following exposure of a sensitized animal to a specific antigen. This exposure results in urticaria, pruritus, and angioedema, followed by vascular collapse, shock and often life-threatening respiratory distress. Anaphylaxis has now been included under type I (immediate) hypersensitivity.

INCIDENCE/PREVALENCE

Sporadic, dependent on exposure to inciting antigen. Tetanus antitoxin is one of the major vaccine antigens associated with anaphylaxis.

SYSTEMS AFFECTED

• Cardiovascular • Respiratory • Urinary
• Digestive • Integument

PATHOPHYSIOLOGY

Anaphylaxis is an acute systemic manifestation of the interaction of an antigen (allergen) binding to IgE antibodies, which are bound to mast cells and basophils. This binding of antigens to cell-bound IgE antibodies triggers the release of chemical substances from the mast cells and basophils. The major biologically active mediators produced by mast cells and basophils include histamine, leukotrienes, the eosinophilic chemotactic factor, platelet-activating factor, kinins, serotonins, and proteolytic enzymes. These chemicals directly affect both the vascular system, causing vasodilatation and increased vascular permeability, and smooth muscles, causing contraction of the bronchi and respiratory distress.

SIGNALMENT

Bovine, ovine, and caprine; also reported in many other species of ruminants.

PHYSICAL EXAMINATION FINDINGS

Sudden, severe dyspnea, muscle tremors, anxiety, occurs within a few to 10–15 minutes following exposure to the antigen; muscle tremor may be severe and temperature may rise to 105°F. History of injection in the previous hour. Occasionally profuse salivation, mild bloat, diarrhea, urticaria, angioneurotic edema, and rhinitis. Laminitis rarely occurs in ruminants. Auscultation of the chest—vesicular murmur, crackling if edema is present, and emphysema in the later stages if dyspnea was severe.

GENETICS

There have been reports of higher incidence in certain lines and breeds of cattle (Holstein-Friesian and Angus) and Saanen goats.

CAUSES AND RISK FACTORS

Common agents causing anaphylaxis include blood transfusions, vaccines, horse sera, insect bites, heterologous enzymes and hormones, and certain drugs, such as penicillin and lidocaine. Milk allergy occurs occasionally in cows. This can happen when there is increased intramammary pressure to a point that normally sequestered milk components, notably casein, gain access to the circulation; these "foreign" proteins induce a type I hypersensitivity. Previous exposure to antigens (i.e., previous treatment with blood or blood products or vaccines).

DIAGNOSIS

DIFFERENTIAL DIAGNOSES

• Acute Bloat • Acute Bronchopneumonia

CBC/BIOCHEMSTRY/URINALYSIS

Increase in PCV, high plasma K^+, neutropenia

PATHOLOGIC FINDINGS

Lungs—severe pulmonary edema in calves and lambs; pulmonary edema and emphysema without blood engorgement.

TREATMENT

THERAPEUTIC APPROACH

• Ancillary support of blood pressure (IV fluids) and respiration may be necessary. • In dairy cattle that have been recently dried off, recovery usually is prompt once the gland is emptied.

MEDICATIONS

DRUGS OF CHOICE

• Anaphylactic shock is treated with an injection of epinephrine. Epinephrine (1/100) subcutaneously or intravenously at a dose of 1 mL per 100 lb. of body weight is the drug of choice and can literally be a lifesaver. A second dose can be given in 15–20 minutes if needed. • In addition, flunixin meglumine (50 mg/mL) can be given at a rate of 1–2 mL per 100 lb. body weight IV or IM as well.
• Corticosteroids potentiate the effects of epinephrine and may be given following the administration of epinephrine.
• Antihistamines have no effect once signs are present.

FOLLOW-UP

EXPECTED COURSE AND PROGNOSIS

Animals treated promptly usually return to normal within 12–24 h.

POSSIBLE COMPLICATIONS

Emphysema may result from severe dyspnea and violent muscle spasms. Following anaphylaxis, animals may spontaneously abort.

PATIENT CARE

Animals need to have their respiratory system monitored for the next 24 hours to detect any emphysema.

PREVENTION

Discuss the situation associated with the onset with the producer. Certain products may need to be avoided.

MISCELLANEOUS

ABBREVIATIONS

• IgE = immunoglobulin E
• IV = intravenous
• PCV = packed cell volume

SEE ALSO

• Bloat
• Plants Producing Acute Respiratory Distress Syndrome
• Respiratory Disease: Bovine

Suggested Reading

Gershwin LJ. Immunoglobulin E-mediated hypersensitivity in food-producing animals. Vet Clin North Am Large Anim Pract 2001, 17: 599–619.

Meeusen E.N. Immunology of helminth infections, with special reference to immunopathology. Vet Parasitol 1999, 84: 259–73.

Omidi A. Anaphylactic reaction in a cow due to parenteral administration of penicillin-streptomycin. Can Vet J 2009, 50: 741–4.

Ruby KW, Griffith RW, Gershwin LJ, Kaeberle ML. *Haemophilus somnus*-induced IgE in calves vaccinated with commercial monovalent *H. somnus* bacterins. Vet Microbiol 2000, 76: 373–83.

Ruby KW, Griffith RW, Kaeberle ML. Histamine production by *Haemophilus somnus*. Comp Immunol Microbiol Infect Dis 2002, 25: 13–20.

Schultz KT. Type I and type IV hypersensitivity in animals. J Am Vet Med Assoc 1982, 181: 1083–7.

Author Christopher C. L. Chase
Consulting Editor Christopher C. L. Chase

A **ANAPLASMOSIS**

BASICS

OVERVIEW
Anaplasma is a hemoparasite of ruminants.

INCIDENCE/PREVALENCE
Anaplasmosis is the most prevalent tickborne disease of cattle.

GEOGRAPHIC DISTRIBUTION
Worldwide

SYSTEMS AFFECTED
Hemolymphatic

PATHOPHYSIOLOGY
• *Anaplasma marginale* is the most common cause of clinical disease in cattle; *A. centrale* causes mild disease. *A. ovis* causes mild disease in sheep. • *Anaplasma* is transmitted by many ticks including *Dermacentor* (USA) and *Rhipicephalus* spp. (other regions). • Iatrogenic transmission can occur. • Infected erythrocytes are destroyed by the monocyte macrophage system leading to extravascular hemolysis and anemia.

HISTORICAL FINDINGS
N/A

SIGNALMENT
Clinical disease primarily occurs in cattle over 3 years.

PHYSICAL EXAMINATION FINDINGS
• Calves generally display no clinical signs; cattle 6 months to 3 years of age may have mild to moderate signs. • Cattle over 3 years can have severe clinical disease. • Acute disease provokes fever, lethargy and anorexia. • Anemia results in tachypnea, tachycardia, pallor, icterus, exercise intolerance, ataxia, and death. • Hemoglobinemia and hemoglobinuria do not occur. • Survivors generally become subclinical carriers.

GENETICS
Bos indicus cattle may be more resistant to *A. marginale* infection than *Bos taurus* breeds.

CAUSES AND RISK FACTORS
• Disease is spread naturally by ticks and mechanically by *Tabanid flies*, needles, and blood-contaminated instruments. • Moving naïve adults to endemic areas or carrier animals to non-endemic areas may precipitate outbreaks.

DIAGNOSIS

DIFFERENTIAL DIAGNOSES
• Bleeding abomasal ulcer • Babesiosis • Leptospirosis • Bacillary hemoglobinuria • Hepatotoxic plants • Copper toxicity (sheep)

CBC/BIOCHEMISTRY/URINALYSIS
• CBC shows decline in PCV with regeneration indicated by anisocytosis, basophilic stippling, poikilocytosis, polychromasia, and reticulocytosis. On blood smears stained with Wright's, new methylene blue, or Giemsa stain, organisms will appear darkly stained on erythrocytes. • Increased hepatobiliary values. • No hemoglobinemia or hemoglobinuria.

OTHER LABORATORY TESTS
• cELISA is a widely used serologic test for identifying infected cattle. • Rapid card agglutination and complement fixation tests. • PCR more reliable for diagnosing acute infection.

IMAGING
N/A

OTHER DIAGNOSTIC PROCEDURES
N/A

PATHOLOGIC FINDINGS
• Pallor or icterus • Splenomegaly • Hepatomegaly • Prominent erythrophagocytosis in reticuloendothelial organs

TREATMENT

THERAPEUTIC APPROACH
• Minimize stress • Blood transfusion if significant signs of anemia and low PCV

SURGICAL CONSIDERATIONS AND TECHNIQUES
N/A

MEDICATIONS

DRUGS OF CHOICE
• Long acting oxytetracycline 20 mg/kg, IM or SQ, once to twice q 72 h. • Imidocarb efficacious but not approved in Europe or USA.

CONTRAINDICATIONS
N/A

PRECAUTIONS
Appropriate milk and meat withdrawal times must be followed for all pharmaceutical agents administered to food-producing animals.

POSSIBLE INTERACTIONS
N/A

FOLLOW-UP

EXPECTED COURSE AND PROGNOSIS
• Mildly affected animals may recover and become carriers. • Severely affected animals often die within hours to days.

POSSIBLE COMPLICATIONS
• Old protocols to clear the carrier state are ineffective. • New carrier state protocols violate AMDUCA. • Clearing carrier animals makes them susceptible to reinfection.

CLIENT EDUCATION
N/A

PATIENT CARE
Monitor for clinical indications that transfusion is required.

PREVENTION
• Arthropod control. • Chemoprophylaxis can be achieved with 20 mg/kg of long-acting oxytetracycline every 21–28 days from the start of the vector season until 30–60 days after vector season ends, or with chlortetracycline in feed at 1.1 mg/kg daily during the vector season. • Live and killed vaccines are variably available, and decrease the severity of clinical signs.

MISCELLANEOUS

ASSOCIATED CONDITIONS
N/A

AGE-RELATED FACTORS
See "Signalment"

ZOONOTIC POTENTIAL
N/A

PREGNANCY
Abortion can occur

BIOSECURITY
N/A

PRODUCTION MANAGEMENT
Can cause significant loss in endemic areas.

SYNONYMS
N/A

ABBREVIATIONS
cELISA = competitive ELISA

SEE ALSO
• Babesiosis
• Bacillary Hemoglobinuria
• Leptospirosis

Suggested Reading
Aubry P, Geale DW. A review of bovine anaplasmosis. Transbound Emerg Dis 2010, 58: 1–30.
Kuttler KL. Anaplasma infections in wild and domestic ruminants: a review. J Wildl Dis 1984, 20: 12–20.
Reinbold JB, Coetzee JF, Hollis LC et al. The efficacy of three chlortetracycline regimens in the treatment of persistent *Anaplasma marginale* infection. Vet. Microbiol 2010, 145: 69–75.

Author Dusty W. Nagy
Consulting Editor Erica C. McKenzie
Acknowledgment The author and book editors acknowledge the prior contribution of Dawn J. Capucille.

BASICS

OVERVIEW
• Anemia is defined as a decrease in the red blood cell (RBC) count, hemoglobin (Hb) concentration, and/or packed cell volume (PCV)
• Nonregenerative anemia is caused by reduced or defective erythropoiesis.
• Nonregenerative anemia is suspected when signs of bone marrow regeneration (reticulocytosis, polychromasia, and basophilic stippling of RBCs) are minimal to absent.

SYSTEMS AFFECTED
• Multisystemic

PATHOPHYSIOLOGY
• Anemia is characterized by a reduced capacity of the blood to transport oxygen, leading to systemic tissue hypoxia and increased erythropoietin (EPO) production.
• Most clinical signs associated with anemia result from poor tissue oxygen delivery.

Nonregenerative Anemia Caused by Reduced Erythropoiesis
• Chronic inflammation, chronic renal disease, or bone marrow failure can lead to reduced erythropoiesis
• Chronic inflammation is associated with increased liver expression of hepcidin liver, causing alterations in iron metabolism and bone marrow responsiveness to EPO.
• Chronic renal disease can be associated with decreased EPO production by the kidneys.
• Destruction of hematopoietic stem cells due to damage by toxicants, irradiation, immune-mediated mechanisms, or infiltration of the marrow with abnormal cells can lead to bone marrow failure.

Nonregenerative Anemia Caused by Defective Erythropoiesis
• Disorders of Hb or DNA synthesis can lead to defective erythropoiesis.
• Iron (Fe) and copper (Cu) deficiencies can impair Hb synthesis.
• Iron is crucial to Hb synthesis because each Hb molecule is made up of four heme groups, each group being composed of an Fe molecule and a porphyrin.

• Iron deficiency is usually caused by chronic blood loss but can also be secondary to dietary Fe deficiency in young milk-fed animals.
• Copper deficiency can lead to Fe deficiency because several Cu-containing proteins are required for Fe transport.
• Dietary Cu deficiency and/or excessive dietary intake of molybdenum, sulfate, or zinc can cause decreased Cu absorption and lead to Cu deficiency.
• Dietary cobalt (Co) deficiency can cause Co deficiency and lead to vitamin B12 deficiency and defective DNA synthesis

HISTORICAL FINDINGS
• Weakness, lethargy, anorexia, weight loss, exercise intolerance, or syncopes.

SIGNALMENT
Bovine, ovine, caprine, and camelid species.

PHYSICAL EXAMINATION FINDINGS
• Clinical signs are less overt when the anemia progresses slowly.
• Lethargy, weakness, or obtundation.
• Pale mucus membranes.
• Tachycardia and tachypnea.
• Heart murmur (due to reduced blood viscosity).

GENETICS
• Congenital dyserythropoiesis is an autosomal recessive trait in polled Hereford cattle.
• Myelofibrosis is an autosomal recessive trait in pygmy goats

CAUSES AND RISK FACTORS

Nonregenerative Anemia Caused by Reduced Erythropoiesis
• Common causes of chronic inflammation include pneumonia, peritonitis, deep digital sepsis, liver abscesses, paratuberculosis, and lymphoma
• Causes of chronic renal disease include pyelonephritis, urolithiasis, amyloidosis, and glomerulonephritis.
• Causes of bone marrow failure include bracken fern toxicosis, bovine neonatal pancytopenia, irradiation, myelofibrosis, and neoplasia

Nonregenerative Anemia Caused by Defective Erythropoiesis
• Causes of defective erythropoiesis include congenital dyserythropoiesis and deficiencies in Fe, Cu, and Co.

° Chronic blood loss: GI ulcers, hematuria, hereditary coagulation factor deficiencies, parasitism, dietary Fe deficiency in milk-fed ruminants

DIAGNOSIS

DIFFERENTIAL DIAGNOSES
• Normocytic, normochromic anemia with normal to increased neutrophil and platelet counts can be caused by chronic inflammation or renal disease.
• Normocytic, normochromic anemia with decreased neutrophil and/or platelet counts can be caused by bone marrow failure.
• Microcytic, hypochromic anemia with variable neutrophil and platelet counts can be caused by iron or copper deficiencies.
• Macrocytic, normochromic anemia with variable neutrophil and platelet counts can be caused by cobalt deficiency or congenital dyserythropoiesis.

CBC/BIOCHEMISTRY/URINALYSIS
• The PCV is the easiest and most accurate method to identify anemia.
• The PVC should be interpreted with consideration of the animal's hydration status and any potential cause of splenic contraction (excitement, exercise, handling, or transportation).

Severity of anemia	PCV (%)
Mild	20–26
Moderate	14–19
Severe	10–13
Very severe	<10

• Blood should be analyzed within 30–60 minutes of collection or stored at refrigerator temperature (4°C) and analyzed within 24 hours
• Delayed analysis may result in marked cellular swelling and therefore a false increase in MCV
• Hypochromasia and microcytosis are hallmarks of iron and copper deficiencies.
• Hyperfibrinogenemia, hypoalbuminemia, and hyperglobulinemia are often present in with chronic inflammation.

	Chronic inflammation or renal disease	Bracken fern toxicosis	Iron and copper deficiencies	Cobalt deficiency
Mechanism	Increased hepcidin or decreased EPO production	Cytotoxic damage to bone marrow	Defective	Defective DNA synthesis
Plasma protein	N - ↑	N - ↓	N - ↓	N - ↓
PCV	↓ - ↓↓	↓ - ↓↓	↓ - ↓↓↓	↓ - ↓↓
MCV	N	N	N - ↓	N - ↑
MCHC	N	N	N - ↓	N
Neutrophil count	N - ↑	N - ↓	N - ↑	N - ↑
Platelet count	N - ↑	N - ↓	N - ↑	N - ↑

N = normal, ↓ = slightly decreased, ↓↓ = moderately decreased, ↓↓↓ = markedly decreased, and ↑ = slightly increased

• Azotemia, hypoalbuminemia, and proteinuria are often present with chronic renal disease.

OTHER LABORATORY TESTS
Chronic Inflammation and Iron Deficiency

	Chronic inflammation	*Iron deficiency*
Serum ferritin	N - ↑	↓
Bone marrow iron content	N - ↑	↓
Total iron binding capacity	N - ↓	N - ↑

N = normal, ↓ = decreased, and ↑ = increased

• Hepatic Fe concentration: <40 ppm on a wet matter basis with Fe deficiency anemia

Copper Deficiency
• Plasma Cu concentration: <0.5 μg/mL
• Hepatic Cu concentration: <35 ppm on a dry matter basis

Cobalt Deficiency
• Serum vitamin B_{12} concentration: <0.2 mg/mL
• Hepatic vitamin B_{12} concentration: <0.2 ppm (dry matter basis)

Parasitism
• Examination of the skin and coat
• Fecal flotation

OTHER DIAGNOSTIC PROCEDURES
• Bone marrow examination is indicated when the cause of a nonregenerative anemia remains undetermined and/or atypical or unexplained immature cells are observed on the peripheral blood smear.

TREATMENT
THERAPEUTIC APPROACH
• Treatment must primarily address the underlying cause(s) of the anemia.
• Blood transfusion is indicated in valuable animals with overt clinical signs of anemia and/or PCV <12%.

• Activity and stress should be minimized.
• Routine care procedures should be delayed (deworming, hoof trimming …).

MEDICATIONS
DRUGS OF CHOICE
• Oral iron supplementation is indicated with iron deficiency anemia.
• Oxygen therapy may be beneficial in hypoxemic animals (PaO_2 <80 mmHg).

CONTRAINDICATIONS
• Iron supplementation is contraindicated in animals with chronic inflammation.
• Appropriate milk and meat withdrawal times must be followed for all compounds administered to food-producing animals.

FOLLOW-UP
EXPECTED COURSE AND PROGNOSIS
• Clinical course and prognosis is dependent on the underlying disease process.

PATIENT CARE
• Heart rate, respiratory rate, mucus membrane color, blood lactate, and arterial blood gas analysis can be used to monitor systemic tissue oxygen delivery.
• CBC or PCV with blood smear examination should be repeated every 1–2 days until evidence of bone marrow regeneration is present.
• Reevaluation is indicated after 7–10 days in stabilized animals.

PREVENTION
• Feeding of trace mineral supplements with label claims for the species that are being supplemented is recommended.
• Diet should contain 4–10 ppm of Cu, 0.1–0.2 ppm of Co, and 30–40 ppm of Fe.
• The dietary copper/molybdenum ratio should be maintained between 5:1 and 10:1.

MISCELLANEOUS
ASSOCIATED CONDITIONS
• A congenital syndrome characterized by dyserythropoiesis and progressive alopecia has been described in polled Hereford cattle.

AGE-RELATED FACTORS
N/A

SYNONYMS
• Anemia of inflammatory disease

ABBREVIATIONS
• CBC = complete blood count
• Co = cobalt
• Cu = copper
• DNA = deoxyribonucleic acid
• EPO = erythropoietin
• Fe = iron
• Hb = hemoglobin
• MCHC = mean corpuscular hemoglobin concentration
• MCV = mean corpuscular volume
• PaO_2 = partial pressure of oxygen in arterial blood
• PCV = packed cell volume
• RBC = red blood cell

SEE ALSO
• Anemia, Regenerative
• Bracken Fern Toxicity
• Copper Deficiency and Toxicity
• Molybdenum Toxicity
• Parasite Control Programs

Suggested Reading
Balcomb C, Foster D. Update on the use of blood and blood products in ruminants. Vet Clin North Am Food Anim Pract 2014, 30: 455–74.
Tvedten H. Laboratory and clinical diagnosis of anemia. In: Weiss DJ, Wardrop KJ ed, Schalm's Veterinary Hematology, 6th ed. Ames: Blackwell, 2010, pp. 152–61.
Author Thibaud Kuca
Consulting Editor Christopher C.L. Chase

BASICS

OVERVIEW
• Anemia is defined as a decrease in the red blood cell (RBC) count, hemoglobin (Hb) concentration, and/or packed cell volume (PCV). • Regenerative anemia is caused by blood loss and/or accelerated RBC destruction. • Signs of bone marrow regeneration include reticulocytosis, polychromasia, and basophilic stippling of RBCs.

INCIDENCE/PREVALENCE
• Extravascular hemolysis is more common than intravascular hemolysis. • Chronic copper toxicosis occurs most commonly in sheep. • Neonatal isoerythrolysis (NI) has been described in calves born to cows immunized with *Anaplasma* or *Babesia* vaccines. • NI has been described in lambs and kids following ingestion of bovine colostrum.

SYSTEMS AFFECTED
• Multisystemic

PATHOPHYSIOLOGY
• Anemia is characterized by a reduced capacity of the blood to transport oxygen, leading to systemic tissue hypoxia and increased erythropoietin production. • 2–3 days are necessary for signs of bone marrow regeneration to be evident in the blood. • Reticulocytosis usually peaks about 7–10 days after bone marrow stimulation.

Regenerative Anemia Caused by Blood Loss (Hemorrhagic Anemia)
• Causes of blood loss include trauma, surgery, coagulation factor deficiencies, thrombocytopenia, parasitism, and neoplasia. • Regenerative response is usually higher with internal than external hemorrhage because some RBCs are reabsorbed by lymphatics and iron (Fe) is recycled. • Chronic blood loss is usually associated with mild regenerative response and can lead to Fe deficiency.

Regenerative Anemia Caused by Accelerated RBC Destruction (Hemolytic Anemia)
• Accelerated RBC destruction (hemolysis) can occur within the blood vessels (intravascular) and/or outside of the blood vessels (extravascular). • Extravascular hemolysis is more common than intravascular hemolysis. • Reticulocyte counts are usually higher in hemolytic anemias than in hemorrhagic anemias. • Onset of clinical signs is usually peracute to acute with intravascular hemolysis and more progressive with extravascular hemolysis. • Icterus may develop in animals with hemolytic anemia secondary

to increased Hb degradation and bilirubin formation. • Intravascular hemolysis is characterized by hemoglobinemia (free Hb in the plasma) that can lead to red discoloration of plasma and/or increased MCHC. • Hemoglobinuria can develop if the plasma free Hb concentration exceeds the capacity of renal tubular reabsorption. • Causes of intravascular hemolysis include bacterial infections, erythrocytic parasites, oxidative damage to the RBC membrane, primary immune-mediated disorders, osmotic lysis, envenomation, and congenital disorders. • Extravascular hemolysis results from sequestration and phagocytosis of RBCs in spleen or liver due to decreased RBC deformability or immune-mediated mechanisms. • Extravascular hemolysis does not cause hemoglobinemia or hemoglobinuria. • Causes of extravascular hemolytic anemias include erythrocytic or endothelial parasites and congenital disorders.

SIGNALMENT
• Bovine, ovine, caprine, and camelid species. • Neonatal isoerythrolysis (NI) can occur in calves born to cows immunized with Anaplasma or Babesia vaccines and in lambs fed bovine colostrum. • Chronic copper (Cu) toxicosis occurs most commonly in sheep • Hereditary factor VIII and IX deficiencies almost always occur in males. • Anaplasmosis and babesiosis occur most commonly in adults.

PHYSICAL EXAMINATION FINDINGS
• Lethargy, obtundation, weakness, or syncope • Pale mucus membranes • Tachycardia and tachypnea • Heart murmur (due to reduced blood viscosity) • Icterus • Hemoglobinuria (with intravascular hemolysis)

GENETICS
• Hereditary factor VIII deficiency is an autosomal recessive trait in Hereford and Japanese Brown cattle. • Hereditary factor XI deficiency is an autosomal recessive trait in Holstein and Japanese Black cattle. • Hereditary afibrinogenemia is an incompletely dominant trait in Saanen goats. • Hereditary spherocytosis is an autosomal dominant trait in Japanese Black cattle. • Congenital erythropoietic porphyria is an autosomal recessive trait in Holstein cattle.

CAUSES AND RISK FACTORS
Regenerative Anemia Caused by Acute Blood Loss
• Coagulation factor deficiencies
  ◦ Disseminated intravascular coagulation (DIC) ◦ Hereditary afibrinogenemia and factor VIII or XI deficiencies ◦ Moldy sweet clover and rodenticide toxicosis
• Gastrointestinal ulcers
• Hemorrhagic bowel syndrome

• Thrombocytopenia
  ◦ Bovine viral diarrhea virus infection ◦ DIC ◦ Snake envenomation
• Trauma
• Surgery

Regenerative Anemia Caused by Chronic Blood Loss
• Gastrointestinal ulcers
• Chronic hematuria
  ◦ Bracken fern toxicosis ◦ Urolithiasis ◦ Pyelonephritis
• Hereditary afibrinogenemia and factor VIII or XI deficiencies
• Parasites
  ◦ Internal (*Haemonchus* spp., *Bunostomum* spp., *Eimeria* spp.) ◦ External (blood sucking lice, fleas, ticks)

Regenerative Anemia Caused by Accelerated RBC Destruction
Causes of Extravascular Hemolysis
• Intraerythrocytic parasites
  ◦ *Anaplasma centrale* and *A. marginale* in cattle ◦ *Theileria annulata*, *T. buffeli*, *T. mutans*, and *T. parva* in cattle ◦ *A. ovis* and *T. lestoquardi* in small ruminants
• Epierythrocytic parasites
  ◦ *Candidatus Mycoplasma haemolamae* in camelids ◦ *Mycoplasma wenyonii* in cattle and *M. ovis* in small ruminants
• Extraerythrocytic parasites
  ◦ *Trypanosoma congolense*, *T. brucei*, and *T. vivax* in cattle
• Endothelial parasites
  ◦ *Sarcocystis* spp. in cattle, and small ruminants
• Hereditary RBC membrane defects
  ◦ Hereditary spherocytosis
Causes of Intravascular Hemolysis
• Bacterial infections
  ◦ *Clostridium haemolyticum* in cattle and sheep ◦ *Clostridium perfringens* type A in cattle and sheep ◦ Leptospirosis
• Osmotic lysis
  ◦ Overuse of hypotonic intravenous fluids ◦ Water intoxication
• Intraerythrocytic parasites
  ◦ *Babesia bigemina*, *B. bovis*, *B. divergens*, and *B. major* in cattle ◦ *B. motasi* and *B. ovis* in small ruminants
• Oxidative damage
  ◦ *Brassica* spp. ingestion ◦ Chronic Cu toxicosis ◦ Oak leaves and acorns ingestion ◦ Onion or garlic ingestion ◦ Red maple leaf ingestion ◦ Selenium deficiency ◦ Zinc toxicosis
• Primary immune-mediated disorders
  ◦ Neonatal isoerythrolysis ◦ Incompatible blood transfusion
• RBC membrane alterations due to other mechanisms
  ◦ Congenital erythropoietic porphyria
  ◦ Postparturient hemoglobinuria ◦ Snake envenomation

DIAGNOSIS

CBC/BIOCHEMISTRY/URINALYSIS

• The PCV is the easiest and most accurate method to identify anemia. • The PVC should be interpreted with consideration of the animal's hydration status and any potential cause of splenic contraction (excitement, exercise, handling, or transportation).

Severity of anemia	PCV (%)
Mild	20–26
Moderate	14–19
Severe	10–13
Very severe	<10

• Blood should be analyzed within 30–60 minutes of collection or stored at refrigerator temperature (4°C) and analyzed within 24 hours. • Delayed analysis may result in marked cellular swelling and a false increase in MCV.

	Acute blood loss	Chronic blood loss	Intravascular hemolysis	Extravascular hemolysis
Plasma protein	N - ↓	N - ↓	N - ↑	N - ↑
PCV	↓ - ↓↓	↓ - ↓↓↓	↓↓ - ↓↓↓	↓ - ↓↓↓
MCV	N - ↑	N - ↓	N - ↑	N - ↑
MCHC	N - ↓	N - ↓	↑	N - ↓
Reticulocyte count	N - ↑↑	N - ↑	N - ↑↑↑	N - ↑↑↑
Neutrophil count	N - ↑	N - ↑	N - ↑	N - ↑
Platelet count	N - ↑	N - ↑	N - ↑	N

N = normal, ↓ = slightly decreased, ↓↓ = moderately decreased, ↓↓↓ = markedly decreased, ↑ = slightly increased, ↑↑ = moderately increased, and ↑↑↑ = markedly increased

Intravascular versus Extravascular Hemolysis

	Intravascular hemolysis	Extravascular hemolysis
Hyperbilirubinemia	can be present	usually present
Hemoglobinemia	Yes	No
Plasma color	pink to red	straw to yellow
Hemoglobinuria	usually present	No
Urine color	pink to red	straw to yellow
Blood reagent strip	positive	usually negative
Bilirubinuria	can be present	usually present
RBCs in urine sediment	No	No

• Abnormal RBC morphology or RBC inclusions may suggest the mechanism of hemolysis. • Heinz bodies suggest oxidative damage. • Spherocytes suggest immune-mediated hemolysis. • Keratocytes and schistocytes DIC.

OTHER LABORATORY TESTS

Hemorrhagic Anemia

• Examination of the skin and coat (external parasites) • Fecal flotation (internal parasites) • Fecal occult blood test (gastrointestinal ulcers) • Coagulation tests (coagulation factor deficiencies)

	aPTT	PT	TT
Afibrinogenemia	↑	↑	↑
DIC	↑	↑	↑
Factor VIII deficiency	↑	N	N
Factor XI deficiency	↑	N	N
Sweet clover toxicosis	↑	↑	N
Rodenticide toxicosis	↑	↑	N

aPTT = activated partial thromboplastin time, PT = prothrombin time, TT = thrombin time, N = normal, and ↑ = increased

Immune-Mediated Hemolytic Disorders

• Positive autoagglutination and direct antiglobulin (Coombs') test

Chronic Copper Toxicosis

• Serum or plasma Cu concentration: >2 μg/mL • Hepatic Cu concentration >350 ppm (dry matter basis) • Renal Cu concentration >100 ppm (dry matter basis) (most reliable)

Lead Toxicosis

• Lead toxicosis should be suspected when basophilic stippling if RBCs is accompanied by signs of inappropriate bone marrow regeneration (minimal polychromasia with nucleated RBCs).

Selenium (Se) Deficiency

• Blood Se concentration <50 ng/mL • Blood glutathione peroxidase (GSH-Px) activity <15 m/min/mg of Hb

PATHOLOGIC FINDINGS

• Extravascular hemolysis is usually associated with splenomegaly.

TREATMENT

THERAPEUTIC APPROACH

• Treatment must primarily address the underlying cause(s) of the anemia. • Blood transfusion is indicated in valuable animals with overt clinical signs of anemia PCV <12%. • Activity and stress should be minimized. • Routine care procedures should be delayed (deworming, hoof trimming ...).

MEDICATIONS

DRUGS OF CHOICE

• Oral iron supplementation is indicated with chronic blood loss. • Oxygen therapy may be beneficial in hypoxemic animals (PaO$_2$ <80 mmHg). • Fluid therapy is indicated with hypovolemia to support cardiovascular function and with intravascular hemolysis to prevent renal damage.

CONTRAINDICATIONS

• Appropriate milk and meat withdrawal times must be followed for all compounds administered to food-producing animals.

FOLLOW-UP

EXPECTED COURSE AND PROGNOSIS

• Clinical course and prognosis is dependent on the underlying disease process. • Return to reference intervals is expected in 1–2 weeks following a single acute blood loss. • Chronic blood loss should be suspected if reticulocytosis persists >3 weeks.

POSSIBLE COMPLICATIONS

• Iron deficiency anemia loss develops more quickly in young milk-fed animals because they have limited Fe stores.

PATIENT CARE

• Heart rate, respiratory rate, mucus membrane color, blood lactate, and arterial blood gas analysis can be used to monitor systemic tissue oxygen delivery. • CBC or PCV with blood smear examination should be repeated every 1–2 days until stabilization of the PVC. • Reevaluation is indicated after 7–10 days in stabilized animals.

PREVENTION
• Cross-matching is indicated in animals receiving more than one blood transfusion.
• Feeding of trace mineral supplements with label claims for the species that are being supplemented is recommended. • Diet should contain 4–10 ppm of Cu and not less than 0.1 ppm of Se. • The dietary copper/molybdenum ratio should be maintained between 5:1 and 10:1
• Prevention programs of vector-borne diseases should be implemented in endemic areas.

MISCELLANEOUS
ABBREVIATIONS
• aPTT = activated partial thromboplastin time
• CBC = complete blood count

• Cu = copper
• DIC = disseminated intravascular coagulation
• Fe = iron
• GSH-Px = glutathione peroxidase
• Hb = hemoglobin
• MCHC = mean corpuscular hemoglobin concentration
• MCV = mean corpuscular volume
• NI = neonatal isoerythrolysis
• PaO$_2$ = partial pressure of oxygen in arterial blood
• PCV = packed cell volume
• PT = prothrombin time
• RBC = red blood cell
• Se = selenium
• TT = thrombin time

SEE ALSO
• Anaplasmosis
• Anemia, Nonregenerative
• Babesiosis
• Bracken Fern Toxicity
• *Brassica* spp. Toxicity

• Copper Deficiency and Toxicity
• Haemonchosis
• Parasite Control Programs
• Parasitic Skin Diseases
• Rodenticide Toxicity
• Selenium Deficiency
• Sweet Clover Poisoning
• Trypanosomiasis
• Zinc Deficiency and Toxicity

Suggested Reading
Balcomb C, Foster D. Update on the use of blood and blood products in ruminants. Vet Clin North Am Food Anim Pract 2014, 30: 455–74.
Allison RW. Anemia caused by rickettsia, mycoplasma, and protozoa. In: Weiss DJ, Wardrop KJ eds, Schalm's Veterinary Hematology, 6th ed. Ames: Blackwell, 2010, pp. 199–210.
Author Thibaud Kuca
Consulting Editor Christopher C.L. Chase

ANESTHESIA: INHALATION

BASICS

OVERVIEW
• Most ruminants tolerate surgical procedures with appropriate physical restraint, local or regional anesthesia, and sedation (if necessary).
• Inhalational anesthesia requires specialized equipment including: an anesthetic machine, oxygen source, oxygen regulator, oxygen flow meter, agent-specific vaporizer, breathing circuit, and a gas scavenging system.
• Ruminants <60 kg can be anesthetized with a conventional small animal machine. Ruminants 60–250 kg can be anesthetized with a human or small animal anesthetic machine with expanded carbon dioxide absorbent canisters. Ruminants >250 kg should be anesthetized with a conventional large animal anesthetic machine.
• Endotracheal intubation and proper cuff inflation are recommended.
• Inhalational anesthetics do not provide analgesia.
• Inhalant anesthetics are off-label drugs in food-producing animals. These agents are primarily eliminated through the lungs so accumulation within tissues is unlikely.

SYSTEMS AFFECTED
• Nervous
• Musculoskeletal
• Respiratory
• Cardiovascular

PATHOPHYSIOLOGY
• General anesthesia is defined as a state of controlled but reversible depression of the CNS not arousable by noxious stimuli. The sensory, motor, and autonomic functions of the body are attenuated to different degrees based on type of drugs used and the dose administered.
• Inhalant anesthetics are administered and removed primarily through the lungs.
• The mechanism of inhalant anesthetic actions is still largely unknown.

Minimum Alveolar Concentration
• Inhalant anesthetic doses are based on the calculation of MAC in healthy animals anesthetized without other drugs (Table 1).
• MAC is the minimum alveolar concentration of inhalant anesthetic that

produces immobility in 50% of patients from responding to a supramaximal stimulus (electrical stimulation of oral mucus membrane). This is equivalent to the ED_{50} and corresponds to a light plane of anesthesia.
• The ED_{95} is equal to 1.2 to $1.4 \times MAC_{agent}$ and corresponds to a moderate plane anesthesia in 95% of patients.
• There is some individual variation in MAC and inhalant dose should be titrated based on evaluation of the patient's monitored anesthetic depth and physiologic parameters.
• If adjunctive anesthetics or analgesics are used, the MAC requirements may be reduced, therefore the inhalant dose should be titrated as stated above.

SIGNALMENT
Potentially all ruminant species

PHYSICAL EXAMINATION FINDINGS
• Palpebral reflexes disappear at minimal anesthetic depth in ruminants but corneal reflexes remain intact.
• Cattle demonstrate eye globe rotation at different depths of anesthesia. When awake, the globe is positioned between the eyelids. At induction, the globe rotates ventrally and may be partially hidden below the lower eyelid. As anesthetic depth increases, the globe can be completely hidden under the lower eyelid. At the surgical anesthetic plane, the globe rotates dorsally between the eyelids again.
• Any purposeful movement will indicate an insufficient plane of anesthesia and adjustment should be made as necessary (i.e., administer intravenous anesthetic agent, increase vaporizer setting, administer additional analgesics).

CAUSES AND RISK FACTORS
• Minor procedure or surgery like hernia repair or fracture stabilization.
• Complicated procedures like abdominal exploratory, arytenoidectomy, or bladder repair.

DIAGNOSIS

CBC/BIOCHEMISTRY/URINALYSIS
• May be included as routine preoperative workup.
• Recommended for sick patients with an ASA status of III or higher.

OTHER LABORATORY TESTING
Blood gas analysis (arterial or venous) if suspect respiratory disease or patient is not appropriately fasted.

TREATMENT

THERAPEUTIC APPROACH
Inhalational Anesthetics in Ruminants
• Often not required if adequate restraint plus local or regional anesthesia is provided.
• Fasting is recommended for all ruminants to minimize complications associated with recumbency and general anesthesia (i.e., tympany, regurgitation, aspiration pneumonia, ventilation/perfusion mismatch). The food and water fasting recommendations for calves, sheep, and goats are 12–18 hours and 8–12 hours respectively. The food and water fasting recommendations for adult cattle are 18–48 hours and 12–24 hours respectively. Neonates should not be fasted before anesthesia to avoid hypoglycemia.
• Airway protection with a cuffed endotracheal tube is essential for injectable or inhalational anesthesia. Intubation in adult cattle is usually performed with a blind or digital palpation technique whereas small ruminants and calves can be intubated with a laryngoscope with a 250–300 mm blade.
• The head and neck should be positioned to allow free flow of regurgitation from the mouth.
• Padding and positioning of the patient are critical to prevent complications associated with neuropathy, myopathy, and injuries to the eyes.
• An IV catheter is recommended for administration of analgesic drugs or supplemental injectable drug doses.
• Ruminants usually have smooth, controlled recoveries from inhalational anesthetics as they do not experience emergence delirium like their equine counterparts. Extubation should only take place when swallowing reflexes have returned.

MEDICATIONS

DRUGS OF CHOICE
Isoflurane
• The most common anesthetic agent used today.
• Isoflurane is less arrhythmogenic than halothane and is not dependent on metabolism for elimination.

Sevoflurane
• Currently widely available but not used in food animal anesthesia, often due to cost.
• Sevoflurane is less arrhythmogenic than halothane and is not dependent on metabolism for elimination.

Halothane
• Limited availability but may still be available in some areas.

Table 1

Minimum Alveolar Concentration of Inhalant Anesthetics			
Species	Isoflurane	Sevoflurane	Halothane
Cow	1.14	—	0.76
Sheep	1.58	—	0.97
Goat	1.2–1.5	2.33	1.29–1.3

• Halothane is associated with increased risk of cardiac arrhythmias in patients with high amounts of circulating catecholamines (i.e., stressed animals, septic shock).
• A preservative, thymol, is added to the halothane to prevent degradation. Thymol can concentrate within a vaporizer over time so frequent cleaning is recommended.

CONTRAINDICATIONS
• Caution in non-fasted animals.
• Caution in patients with compromised airways, respiratory systems, or systemic hypotension.

PRECAUTIONS
Meat and milk withholding: No current published withholding times. Suggested withholding times may be obtained by contacting FARAD.

POSSIBLE INTERACTIONS
N/A

FOLLOW-UP

CLIENT EDUCATION
Discuss the risks associated with general anesthesia with clients prior to performing on the client's animal(s).

PATIENT CARE
• Ruminants tend to hypoventilate under general anesthesia and require mechanical ventilation for procedures >90 minutes or if hypercapnic and/or hypoxemic.
• Other potential complications include: bradycardia, hypotension, hypothermia, hypoxemia, and hypoventilation. Monitoring for these complications is important, especially in compromised patients, and can be assisted by use of EKG, blood pressure monitoring, thermometer, and arterial blood gas analysis when available.

MISCELLANEOUS

AGE-RELATED FACTORS
• Neonatal and geriatric animals will have exaggerated drug effects if standard drugs are used; therefore it is recommended to reduce the drug doses.
• Both have decreased respiratory and cardiac reserves so support of oxygenation, ventilation, and chronotropic or inotropic support should be expected.

PREGNANCY
• There are several physiologic alterations in pregnant animals including an increase in cardiac output, blood volume, oxygen consumption, and minute ventilation.
• In addition, gastrointestinal motility and esophageal sphincter tone can decrease as well as functional residual capacity.
• Therefore the anesthetist should be prepared to intubate with a cuffed endotracheal tube, ventilate, and support the pregnant animal.

ABBREVIATIONS
• ASA = American Society of Anesthesiologists
• CNS = central nervous system
• ED50 = effective dose 50
• ED95 = effective dose 95
• FARAD = Food Animal Residue Avoidance Databank
• IV = intravenous
• MAC = minimum alveolar concentration

SEE ALSO
• Alternative Medicine (see www.fiveminutevet.com/ruminant)
• Anesthesia: Injectable
• Anesthesia: Local and Regional Analgesia
• Pain Management (see www.fiveminutevet.com/ruminant)

Suggested Reading
Carroll GL, Hartsfield SM. general anesthetic techniques in ruminants. Vet Clin North Am Food Anim Pract 1996, 12: 627–62.
Galatos AD. Anesthesia and analgesia in sheep and goats. Vet Clin North Am Food Anim Pract 2011, 27: 47–59.
Greene SA. Protocols for anesthesia of cattle. Vet Clin North Am Food Anim Pract 2003, 19: 679–93.
Grubb TL, Perez Jimenez TE, Pettifer GR. Neonatal and pediatric patients. In: Greene SA, et al. eds, Veterinary Anesthesia and Analgesia, 5th ed. Ames: Blackwell, 2015, pp. 988–92.
Grubb TL, Perez Jimenez TE, Pettifer GR. Senior and geriatric patients. In: Greene SA, et al. eds, Veterinary Anesthesia and Analgesia, 5th ed. Ames: Blackwell, 2015, pp. 983–7.
Lin H. Comparative anatomy and analgesia of ruminants and swine. In: Greene SA, et al eds, Veterinary Anesthesia and Analgesia, 5th ed. Ames: Blackwell, 2015, 743–53.
Papich MG. Drug residue considerations for anesthetics and adjunctive drugs in food-producing animals. Vet Clin North Am Food Anim Pract 1996, 12: 693–706.
Raffe MR. Anesthetic considerations during pregnancy and for the newborn. In: Greene SA, et al eds, Veterinary Anesthesia and Analgesia, 5th ed. Ames: Blackwell, 2015, pp. 708–719.
Riebold TW. Ruminants. In: Greene SA, et al. eds, Veterinary Anesthesia and Analgesia, 5th ed. Ames: Blackwell, 2015, pp. 912–927.
Steffey EP, Mama KR, Brosnan RJ. Inhalational anesthetics. In: Greene SA, et al. eds, Veterinary Anesthesia and Analgesia, 5th ed. Ames: Blackwell, 2015, pp. 297–331.

Author Jennifer L Bornkamp
Consulting Editor Kaitlyn A. Lutz

A

ANESTHESIA: INJECTABLE

BASICS

OVERVIEW
• General anesthesia produces unconsciousness, analgesia, and muscle relaxation for surgical or diagnostic procedures.
• To prevent complications associated with regurgitation, it is important to protect anesthetized ruminants' airways by placement of a cuffed endotracheal tube and positioning the head to allow regurgitant to flow out of oral cavity during lateral or dorsal recumbency.
• Injectable anesthetics may be administered via intravenous (IV) or intramuscular (IM) injection.
• An IV catheter, placed in jugular or auricular vein, is recommended for anesthesia maintained with continuous IV infusion.
• During recovery, ruminants should be placed in sternal recumbency and the endotracheal tube removed with cuff inflated when the patient regains swallowing and coughing reflexes.

INCIDENCE/PREVALENCE
N/A

GEOGRAPHIC DISTRIBUTION
Worldwide

SYSTEMS AFFECTED
Multisystemic

PATHOPHYSIOLOGY
N/A

SIGNALMENT
All ruminant species

GENETICS
N/A

CAUSES AND RISK FACTORS
N/A

DIAGNOSIS

CBC/BIOCHEMISTRY/URINALYSIS
May be indicated as preoperative workup.

TREATMENT
N/A

MEDICATIONS

DRUGS OF CHOICE

α₂ Agonists (Xylazine, Detomidine, Medetomidine, Romifidine)
• Classified as sedatives/analgesics.

• Produce profound sedation, analgesia and central muscle relaxation by binding to α_2 receptors in the CNS and spinal cord.
• Often use with an injectable anesthetic to produce general anesthesia.
• Ruminants are more sensitive to xylazine's effect and only one tenth of the dose used in horses should be used.
• Doses required for detomidine, medetomidine, and romifidine to produce sedation in ruminants are similar to the doses required for horses.
• At higher recommended doses, α_2 agonists induce analgesia, recumbency, and immobilization suitable for minor procedures.
• Order of breed variation of sensitivity to xylazine in cattle: Brahman > Hereford > Holstein; in small ruminants: goats > sheep; in camelids: llamas > alpacas.
• Recommended dose ranges of xylazine are 0.1–0.2 mg/kg IV for cattle, sheep, and goats, 0.15–0.25 mg/kg IV for llamas and alpacas.
• Recommended dose ranges of medetomidine are 0.02 mg/kg IV for cattle and 0.025–0.05 mg/kg IV for llamas and alpacas.
• A α_2 antagonist (atipamezole, tolazoline, or yohimbine) can be given to reverse an α_2 agonist's pharmacological effect.
• Recommended dose ranges of atipamezole are 0.02–0.06 mg/kg IV for cattle, 0.05–0.2 mg/kg IV for sheep and goats, and 0.125 –0.5 mg/kg IV for llamas and alpacas.
• Recommended dose ranges of tolazoline are 0.2–2 mg/kg IV for cattle and 1–2 mg/kg IV for sheep, goats, llamas, and alpacas.
• Recommended dose ranges of yohimbine are 0.12–0.2 mg/kg IV for cattle and 0.125–0.22 mg/kg IV for sheep, goats, llamas, and alpacas.

CONTRAINDICATIONS
Animals with severely compromised cardiopulmonary functions

PRECAUTIONS
• Side effects: bradycardia, hypotension, decreased respiratory rate, cardiac arrhythmias, decreased gastrointestinal (GI) motility, hypoinsulinemia, hyperglycemia, increased urine output, and oxytocin-like effect.
• Premature parturition has occurred in pregnant ruminants with xylazine during the last trimester.
• Severe hypoxemia and pulmonary edema can occur in sheep.
• In animals with urethral obstruction, rupture of bladder can result from increased urine output.
• Ruminants and camelids are more sensitive to tolazoline's toxicity effect. Low recommended dose and slow IV injection should be used.

POSSIBLE INTERACTIONS
Additive or synergistic effect with other anesthetics.

Benzodiazepines (Diazepam, Midazolam, Zolazepam)
• Primary use for their anxiolytic, anticonvulsant, and central muscle relaxing effects.
• Have little or no analgesic effect.
• Produce minimal cardiovascular depression, used in animals with high anesthetic risk.
• Use with an injectable anesthetic to produce general anesthesia and improve muscle relaxation.
• Diazepam has 40% propylene glycol as solvent in the injectable solution. May precipitate if mix with water soluble solution.
• Midazolam is water soluble with two to three times more potency than diazepam.
• Diazepam or midazolam is used in goats with urethral obstruction, when the effect of increasing urine output is contraindicated.
• Immobilization with good analgesia is produced when diazepam is combined with xylazine in cattle.
• Recommended dose ranges of diazepam are 0.1 mg/kg IV for cattle, 0.23–0.3 mg/kg IV for sheep and goats, and 0.1–0.2 mg/kg IV for llamas and alpacas.
• Recommended dose of midazolam is 0.4 mg/kg IV.

CONTRAINDICATIONS
N/A

PRECAUTIONS
Propylene glycol may cause hypotension if diazepam is administered IV rapidly.

POSSIBLE INTERACTIONS
Additive or synergistic effect with other anesthetics.

Dissociative Anesthetics (Ketamine, Tiletamine)
• Dissociative anesthesia is characterized by unconsciousness while maintaining eye reflexes (palpebral and corneal reflexes) and pharyngeal–laryngeal reflexes (swallowing reflex).
• Dissociative anesthetics cause direct CNS stimulation leading to increased sympathetic outflow and increased heart rate and arterial blood pressures.
• Respiratory pattern is characterized by an apneustic, shallow, and irregular pattern.
• Ketamine is the most popular injectable anesthetic for large animal species.
• Ketamine induces rapid onset and short duration of anesthesia and analgesia. When administered alone, muscle relaxation is inadequate for more painful surgery. Often combine with xylazine or diazepam for their central muscle relaxing effect.
• Subanesthetic doses of ketamine produce profound analgesia by blocking N-methyl-D-aspartate receptors.
• Recommended dose ranges of ketamine are 2.2–4.5 mg/kg IV for cattle, 1–5.5 mg/kg IV for sheep and goats, and 3–5 mg/kg IV for llamas and alpacas.

Table 1

	Drugs Used for Injectable Anesthesia in Cattle, Small Ruminants, and Camelids.			

	Dosages (mg/kg)			
Drugs	*Cattle*	*Sheep & Goats*	*Alpacas & Llamas*	*Comments*
Diazepam Xylazine	0.1, IV 0.2, IV	— 	— 	Immobilization with good analgesia for 30 min Total recumbency 60 min
Diazepam Ketamine	0.1, IV 4.5, IV	Mix 1 mL D (5 mg), 1 mL K (100 mg), give 1 mL/18–22 kg, IV	0.1–0.2, IV 4, IV	Anesthesia 10–15 min Total recumbency 30 min
Medetomidine Ketamine	0.02, IV 2.2, IV	0.02, IV 1–2, IV	0.025, 0.035, or 0.05, IM 1–1.5, IM	Anesthesia 70–120 min in calves Light anesthesia for 30–60 min in camelids
Midazolam Ketamine	— 	0.4, IM 4, IV	— 	Anesthesia 15 min

Xylazine
Ketamine
 	
Xylazine
Ketamine
	0.1–0.2, IV
	2, IV
		0.1, IV Sheep
		2.2, IV 0.2, IM
		     3–5, IM
		     Goats
		     0.1, IM
		     3–5, IM
			Alpacas
			0.35–0.8, IM 5–8, IM
			    Llamas
			0.15–0.25, IV 0.25, IM
			3–5, IV 5–8, IM
				Anesthesia 30 min
				Preferred combination for adult large ruminants

BKX Butorphanol Ketamine Xylazine	0.0375, IM 3.75, IM 0.375, IM	1 mL/23 kg, IM; 1 mL/45 kg, IV	Alpacas: 1 mL/18 kg, IM Llamas: 1 mL/23 kg, IM	Anesthesia 20–30 min Mixture: add 1 ml LA X (100 mg), 1 mL B (10 mg) into 10 mL K (1,000 mg), give 1 mL/20 kg IM
Modified BKX Butorphanol Ketamine Xylazine	—	0.02 mL/kg, IV 0.03, IV 1.6, IV 0.03, IV	—	Mixture: add 8 mg of X, 8 mg of B into 400 mg (4 mL) of K For debudding in young animals
Bovine Triple Drip Xylazine (0.1 mg/mL) Ketamine (1–2 mg/mL) into 5% Guaifenesin	Induction: 0.67–1.1 mL/kg Maintenance: 2.2 mL/kg/hr	Induction: 0.67–1.1 mL/kg Maintenance: 2.2 mL/kg/hr	Induction: 0.67–1.1 mL/kg Maintenance: 2.2 mL/kg/hr	Adjustable dose for induction & maintenance Stable plane of anesthesia Smooth recovery
Propofol	4–6, IV	Induction: 3–4, IV or 4–8, IV Maintenance: 18–40 mg/kg/hr	Induction: 2–3.5, IV Maintenance: 24 mg/kg/hr	Anesthesia 5–10 min, single dose Apnea may occur CRI: 24 mg/kg/hr for maintenance of light anesthesia
Telazol	4, IV	2–4, IV	2, IV or 4.4, IM	Anesthesia 45–60 min Smooth but prolonged recovery
Xylazine Telazol	0.1, IM 4, IM	—	0.25, IV 1, IV	Anesthesia 60 min Standing in 130 min
TKX-Ru Telazol Ketamine Xylazine	1.25–1.5 mL/125 kg, IM for small cattle 1 mL/125 kg IM for large, adult cattle	—	1.25–1.5 mL/kg, IM for smaller patients 1 mL/110–115 kg, IM for larger patients	Mixture: Add 2.5 mL (250 mg) of K and 1 mL (100 mg) of X into 500 mg of Telazol Allow 20 min to reach peak effect Effective for capture wild ruminants Deep sedation, recumbency and chemical restraint in camelids; awake and assume sternal recumbency in 40–60 min

• Telazol® is a combination of a tiletamine and zolazepam, in a 1:1 ratio by weight base.
• Telazol® comes as 500-mg powder, and is reconstituted with 5 mL sterile water into 100 mg/mL solution. Telazol® can be reconstituted with a smaller volume of sterile water with higher concentration, like adding 2.5 mL sterile water into 500-mg powder, resulting in a final concentration of 200 mg/mL.
• The pharmacologic effect of Telazol® is predominated by tiletamine. Similar to diazepam and midazolam, zolazepam produces minimal cardiovascular depression. Thus, Telazol® anesthesia is characterized by that of ketamine anesthesia, but better muscle relaxation, more profound analgesia, and longer duration of anesthesia.
• Recovery from Telazol® anesthesia tends to be smooth but prolonged in ruminant as a result of slower metabolism and elimination of zolazepam.
• Recommended dose ranges of Telazol® are 4–6 mg/kg IV for cattle, 2–4 mg/kg IV for sheep and goats, and 1–2 mg/kg IV for llamas and alpacas.

CONTRAINDICATIONS
N/A

PRECAUTIONS
• Ketamine increases salivation and mucus secretion in the respiratory tract, which can be reduced by administration of an anticholinergic, e.g., atropine.
• Prolonged recovery may follow Telazol® anesthesia.

POSSIBLE INTERACTIONS
Additive or synergistic effect with other anesthetics.

Guaifenesin (Glycerol Guaiacolate; GG)
• Administered alone, GG produces muscle relaxation, ataxia, and recumbency.
• Minimal changes on respiratory muscle activity and respiratory function at recommended doses of GG. Respiratory muscle paralysis occurs at doses 3–4 times higher than that required to induce recumbency.
• GG can be reconstituted with 5% dextrose to make up 5% or 10% injectable solution.
• Xylazine, ketamine, and GG combination ("bovine triple drip") for induction and maintenance of anesthesia (see Table 1).

CONTRAINDICATIONS
GG does not produce anesthesia or analgesia. It should always be used with an anesthetic.

PRECAUTIONS
Thrombophlebitis can occur with the administration of 5% solution. Hemolysis, hemoglobinuria, and venous thrombosis may occur with a solution of 10% or higher.

POSSIBLE INTERACTIONS
Additive or synergistic effect with anesthetics.

Propofol
• Short-acting hypnotic/anesthetic.
• Propofol is not water soluble, the injectable solution comes as a white, oil-in-water emulsion. This emulsion contains no preservative, the contents should be used or discarded within 8 hours. New formulation, PropoFlo 28, uses 20 mg/mL of benzyl alcohol as preservative, thus the 28 days of shelf life.
• A single dose of propofol induces 10 minutes of general anesthesia. Complete recovery without residual sedation and ataxia occurs within 20 minutes.
• Side effects include absence of analgesic effect at subanesthetic doses, apnea following bolus injection, and hypotension due to peripheral vasodilation.
• Recommended dose ranges of propofol are 4–6 mg/kg IV for cattle, 3–8 mg/kg IV for sheep and goats, and 2–3.5 mg/kg IV for llamas and alpacas.

CONTRAINDICATIONS
• Do not use in animals with preexisting hypotension.
• Cost is prohibitive for most large animal patients.

PRECAUTIONS
Apnea and hypotension may occur after bolus.

POSSIBLE INTERACTIONS
Additive or synergistic effect with other anesthetics.

 FOLLOW-UP

POSSIBLE COMPLICATIONS
Severe CNS and cardiopulmonary depression which may result in death if overdose.

PATIENT CARE
Closely monitor vital signs: eye reflexes, heart rate, rhythm, respiratory rate and depth, and arterial blood pressures.

 MISCELLANEOUS

PREGNANCY
• Premature parturition has occurred in pregnant ruminants with xylazine during the last trimester.
• Reduced anesthetic requirement in pregnant animals.

ABBREVIATIONS
• CNS = central nervous system
• GG = guaifenesin (glycerol guaiacolate)
• GI = gastrointestinal

SEE ALSO
• Anesthesia: Inhalation
• Anesthesia: Local and Regional
• Common Pharmacologic Therapies: Adult Dairy Cattle (see www.fiveminutevet.com/ruminant)
• Pain Management (see www.fiveminutevet.com/ruminant)

Suggested Reading
Craigmill A, Rangel-Lugo M, Damian P, et al. Extralabel use of tranquilizers and general anesthetics. J Am Vet Med Assoc 1997, 211: 302–4.
Lin HC. Standing sedation and chemical restraint. In: Lin HC, Walz P eds, Farm Animal Anesthesia: Cattle, Small Ruminants, Camelids, and Pigs. Ames: Wiley/Blackwell, 2014, pp. 38–59.
Lin HC. Injectable anesthetics and field anesthesia. In: Lin HC, Walz P eds, Farm Animal Anesthesia: Cattle, Small Ruminants, Camelids, and Pigs. Ames: Wiley/Blackwell, 2014, pp. 60–94.
Passler T. Regulatory and legal considerations of anesthetics and analgesics used in food-producing animals. In: Lin HC, Walz P eds, Farm Animal Anesthesia: Cattle, Small Ruminants, Camelids, and Pigs. Ames: Wiley/Blackwell, 2014, pp. 228–47.
Internet Resources
• AMDUCA. Animal Medicinal Drug Use Clarification Act of 1994 (AMDUCA). http://www.fda.gov/AnimalVeterinary/ GuidanceComplianceEnforcement/ ActsRulesRegulations/ucm085377.htm
• FARAD. Food Animal Residue Avoidance Databank, 2015. www.farad.org/ amduca/amduca_law.asp
Author HuiChu Lin
Consulting Editor Kaitlyn A. Lutz

BASICS

OVERVIEW
• Local or regional anesthesia with appropriate patient restraint provides the most cost-effective method of humane anesthesia and analgesia in ruminants. Fractious animals may also require sedation.
• Local or regional analgesia causes a reversible loss of sensation to an area without loss of consciousness. Some techniques (i.e., LS epidural) can affect motor function if motor nerves are targeted.
• These techniques should not be used as the sole source of analgesia but can be used in conjunction with NSAIDs and/or systemic opioids for optimal analgesia.

SYSTEMS AFFECTED
• Nervous
• Musculoskeletal

PATHOPHYSIOLOGY
• All LA will block sodium channels and can be infiltrated near a nerve, epidural space, or in areas near planned surgical sites.
• Signs of LA toxicity include sedation, muscle twitching, convulsions, cardiopulmonary depression, coma, and death.

CAUSES AND RISK FACTORS
Variety of procedures from castration or dehorning to abdominal exploratory procedures.

DIAGNOSIS

CBC/CHEMISTRY/URINALYSIS
Routine blood work may be performed but is not commonplace for routine procedures.

TREATMENT

THERAPEUTIC APPROACH

Anesthesia for Dehorning and Castration
It is well documented that LA should be used in conjunction with NSAIDs for optimal analgesia in these procedures.

Dehorning, Bovine
There are 1 or 2 nerves to block in cattle, depending on horn size.
• *Cornual branch of zygomaticotemporal nerve*: 2.5–3.8 cm, 20G needle with 5–10 mL 2% lidocaine injected SQ ventral to the frontal ridge and halfway between the lateral canthus and the base of the horn.
• *Cutaneous branches of the second cervical nerve*: 2.5 cm, 20G needle with 5–10 mL 2% lidocaine injected SQ along the caudal aspect of the base of the horn. *Note*: this is only necessary in adult cattle with larger horns.

Dehorning, Ovine and Caprine
There are two nerves to block in sheep and goats.
• *Cornual branch of the lacrimal nerve*: 2.5 cm, 22G needle with 2–3 mL 2% lidocaine injected SQ halfway between the lateral canthus and lateral edge of the horn base.
• *Cornual branch of the infratrochlear nerve*: 2.5 cm, 22G needle with 1–2 mL 2% lidocaine inject SQ halfway between the medial canthus and the medial edge of the base of the horn.

Castration, Bovine, Ovine, Caprine
Infiltrate LA into the skin at the proposed incision site to desensitize the skin. Inject LA into the center of the testicle until it feels firm to the touch. The LA will migrate into the spermatic cord.

Anesthesia of the Eyelid and Eye
• *Auriculopalpebral block, bovine, ovine, caprine*: 2.5 cm, 22G needle with 5 mL (2 mL in ovine and caprine) 2% lidocaine injected SQ on the dorsal zygomatic arch about 5–6 cm behind the supraorbital process.
• *Retrobulbar block, bovine*: 9 cm, 18 or 20G curved needle with 5–10 mL 2% lidocaine at each of 4 sites. The needle is passed thru the eyelids at the 12, 3, 6, and 9 o'clock positions around the eye. *Ovine and caprine*: 3.8 cm, 20 or 22G needle curved is inserted as above but only at sites (6 & 12 or 3 & 9 o'clock) with 2–3 mL 2% lidocaine per site.
• *Peterson block, bovine*: 10–12 cm, 20G needle with 15–20 mL of 2% lidocaine. The needle is passed in front of the rostral border of the coronoid process of mandible but caudal to the zygomatic arch and supraorbital process. *Ovine and caprine*: 6.3 cm, 20G needle with 3–4 mL 2% lidocaine using the technique described for cattle.

Anesthesia of the Nasal Passages
• *Infraorbital block, bovine, ovine, caprine*: 3.8 cm, 18G needle with 5–10 mL 2% lidocaine is injected SQ at the infraorbital canal. The foramen is located 5 cm above the second premolar.

Anesthesia of the Flank and Paralumbar Fossa
• *Proximal paravertebral block, bovine*: The area should be prepped from the last rib to the TP of L4 about 4–5 cm from midline. A 3.8 cm, 16G needle is used as a guide for a 8.9 cm, 20G spinal needle. The cannula needle is placed thru the skin at anterior edge of TP of L1, 4–5 cm from dorsal midline. The spinal needle is passed until it contacts the L1 TP and walked off the cranial edge; as it passes thru the transverse ligament inject 6–8 mL for the ventral branch. Then withdraw the needle to 2.5 cm over the fascia and deposit an additional 6–8 mL for the dorsal branch. Continue this at the other sites. *Ovine and caprine*: Same technique with a 2.5–3.8 cm, 20G needle with 0.5–1 mL for the dorsal branch and 2–3 mL for the ventral branch

with 2% lidocaine. Do not exceed 5–6 mg/kg total.
• *Distal paravertebral block, bovine*: The area of the block is clipped and prepped from T13 to L3 on the lateral aspect. A 3.5–5.5 cm, 18G needle is inserted ventral to the TP and 10 mL of LA is infused in a fan pattern. The needle is then redirected or reinserted dorsally and LA is infused caudally in a fan pattern as well. Repeat at the other sites.

Anesthesia of the Linea Alba and Paramedian Region
• *Cranial (lumbosacral) epidural block*, bovine: Not recommended as LA infiltration will cause motor blockade of the pelvic limbs preventing ability to stand. *Ovine and caprine*: 3.8 cm or 7.5 cm, 20 or 22G spinal needle is inserted on midline between L6 and S1. Confirmation of correct placement is usually done with the hanging drop technique where saline will be pulled by negative pressure into the epidural space. A dose of 0.4–0.6 mL/kg of 2% lidocaine will provide anesthesia up to the navel region.

Anesthesia of Pelvic Area
• *Caudal (sacrococcygeal or intercoccygeal) epidural, bovine*: The space is located between S5-Co1 or Co1-Co2 and is easily palpable while moving the tail up and down. You will feel this as the space between the last anchored and first movable vertebrae. A 3.8 cm, 20 or 18G needle is passed on midline at a slight cranial angle into the vertebral space. Check placement with hanging drop technique. A dose of 0.01–0.02 mL/kg of 2% lidocaine can be used. *Ovine and caprine*: The same technique as above with 2.5 and 3.8 cm, 20G needle at S4-Co1 or Co1-Co2 with an injection volume of 0.01–0.03 mL/kg. The needle is directed at a 45° angle in small ruminants.

Anesthesia of the Teats and Udder
See "Suggested Reading" for these techniques including a ring block, inverted "V" block, and teat sinus infusion blocks. A proximal or distal paravertebral block extending from T13 to L4 can be used to block a majority of the udder.

SURGICAL CONSIDERATIONS AND TECHNIQUES
The type of block used will largely depend on clinician preference, position and temperament of the animal, and length of procedure.

MEDICATIONS
DRUGS OF CHOICE
Lidocaine
• Only approved LA for use in cattle and sheep in the United States and Canada.
• The maximal effect occurs within 2–5 minutes of injection and lasts 90 minutes.

• The addition of epinephrine (0.01 mg/mL) was found to increase the duration of activity to 304 minutes. However, epinephrine cannot be used in limb blocks or wound edges due to the potential risk of ischemia and tissue necrosis.
• The maximum dose is 6 mg/kg for ruminants.

Bupivacaine and Mepivacaine
• Off-label use
• The maximal effect occurs within 20–30 minutes and lasts 5–8 hours for bupivacaine. Mepivacaine behaves similarly to lidocaine.
• Bupivacaine exhibits the most cardiotoxic effects of all the LA and should be only used for SQ or infiltrative techniques.
• The maximum dose is 2 (bupivacaine) and 5–6 (mepivacaine) mg/kg. No withdrawal times have been established.

CONTRAINDICATIONS
• Regulatory restrictions: See "Suggested Reading" for links to the FDACVM and AMDUCA or recommendations for the use of LA in ruminants.
• Meat and milk withholding: See "Suggested Reading" for the link to FARAD and withdrawal times recommended.

FOLLOW-UP
N/A

MISCELLANEOUS

ABBREVIATIONS
• AMDUCA = Animal Medical Drug Use Classification Act

• FARAD = Food Animal Residue Avoidance Databank
• FDACVM = Food and Drug Administration Center for Veterinary Medicine
• LA = local anesthetics
• LS = lumbosacral
• NSAIDs = nonsteroidal anti-inflammatory drugs
• SQ = subcutaneous
• TP = transverse process

SEE ALSO
• Alternative Medicine (see www.fiveminutevet.com/ruminant)
• Anesthesia: Inhalation
• Anesthesia: Injectable
• Castration/Vasectomy: Bovine
• Castration/Vasectomy: Camelids
• Castration/Vasectomy: Small Ruminants
• Dehorning
• Enucleation/Exenteration (see www.fiveminutevet.com/ruminant)
• Pain Management (see www.fiveminutevet.com/ruminant)

Suggested Reading
Anderson DE, Edmondson MA. Prevention and management of surgical pain in cattle. Vet North Am Food Anim Pract 2013, 29: 157–84.

Carroll GL, Hartsfield SM. General anesthetic techniques in ruminants. Vet Clin North Am Food Anim Pract 1996, 12: 627–62.

Coetzee JF. Assessment and management of pain associated with castration in cattle. Vet Clin North Am Food Anim Pract 2013, 29: 75–101.

Couture Y, Mulon PY. Procedure and surgeries of the teat. Vet Clin North Am Food Anim Pract 2005, 21: 173–204.

Edmondson MA. Local and regional anesthesia in cattle. Vet Clin North Am Food Anim Pract 2008, 24: 211–26.

Fajit VR. Drug Laws and regulations for sheep and goats. Vet Clin North Am Food Anim Pract 2011, 27: 1–21.

Garcia ER. Local anesthetics. In: Greene SA, et al. eds, Veterinary Anesthesia and Analgesia, 5th ed. Ames: Blackwell, 2015, pp. 332–54.

Greene SA. Protocols for anesthesia of cattle. Vet Clin North Am Food Anim Pract 2003, 19: 679–93.

Papich MG. Drug residue considerations for anesthetics and adjunctive drugs in food-producing animals. Vet Clin North Am Food Anim Pract 1996, 12: 693–706.

Stock ML, Baldridge SL, Griffin D, Coetzee JF. Bovine dehorning: assessing pain and providing analgesic management. Vet Clin North Am Food Anim Pract 2013, 29: 103–3.

Valverde A, Sinclair M. Ruminant and swine local anesthetic and analgesic techniques. In: Greene SA, et al. eds, Veterinary Anesthesia and Analgesia, 5th ed. Ames: Blackwell, 2015, pp. 941–62.

Internet Resources
• AMDUCA. Animal Medicinal Drug Use Clarification Act of 1994 (AMDUCA). http://www.fda.gov/AnimalVeterinary/GuidanceComplianceEnforcement/ActsRulesRegulations/ucm085377.htm
• FARAD. Food Animal Residue Avoidance Databank, 2015. www.farad.org/amduca/amduca_law.asp

Author Jennifer L. Bornkamp
Consulting Editor Kaitlyn A. Lutz

BASICS

OVERVIEW
• Anestrus is the absence of estrus behaviors in female animals.
• Anestrus is physiological before puberty, between estrus periods, for a variable time after parturition or during lactation, during pregnancy, and seasonally in sheep and goats.
• Pathologic anestrus is the absence of estrus during a time when it would normally be expected to occur.
• Pathologic anestrus results from a disruption of the reproductive axis and typically involves the absence of both the behavioral signs of estrus and the underlying normal ovarian events associated with cyclic activity, although follicular waves may still occur.
• The most common clinical manifestation of anestrus is a delayed return to ovular cycles after parturition. Anestrus is also used to describe animals undergoing normal ovular cycles where the signs of estrus are missed, due either to deficiencies in management (unobserved estrus), subtle or absent signs of estrus (silent heat/substrus), or both. The intensity and duration of estrus behavior may also be reduced or absent altogether at the first postpartum, seasonal or postpubertal ovulation in ruminants.
• Animals experiencing pathologic anestrus are usually anovular though some cases are associated with prolonged luteal function (CL retention).
• Follicular growth may be arrested at any stage of development as reflected in the size of structures found on the ovaries. Growth and persistence of follicular structures beyond the normal ovulatory size and duration is defined as OCD.

INCIDENCE/PREVALENCE
• The incidence of anestrus varies widely with the specific condition on the farm and the species affected.
• In dairy cows, for example, the incidence of delayed return to estrus after parturition in four recent reports ranged from 29 to 54% in primiparous cows and from 15 to 32% in multiparous cows.

GEOGRAPHIC DISTRIBUTION
Worldwide

SYSTEMS AFFECTED
Reproductive

PATHOPHYSIOLOGY
• Pathologic anestrus may be the result of a primary disruption or disease at the level of the hypothalamus, pituitary, or ovary.
• Commonly, anestrus is secondary to disease or derangement in some other body system. Examples include nutritional deficiencies, especially energy; chronic severe illness, pain or stress resulting in a loss of body condition;

heat stress; and uterine disease with or without retention of a CL.
• The endocrine basis for profound anestrus associated with very small follicles is unclear. Anestrus associated with follicular growth to the point of deviation and beyond appears to be related to inadequate LH pulses for follicular development and the absence of an LH surge sufficient to cause ovulation.
• Anestrus occurring in association with prolonged luteal function is likely the result of inadequate uterine $PGF2_\alpha$ production, secretion, or transport to the ovary.
• Management deficiencies related to estrus detection can lead to a mistaken diagnosis of anestrus in otherwise normally cycling animals.
• In high-producing dairy cattle, increased liver metabolic rates related to high feed intake result in lower circulating levels of gonadal steroids with a subsequent depression of the length and intensity of estrus.
• In heat-stressed cattle, follicular steroidogenic capacity is reduced leading to lower blood estradiol concentration and diminished or absent signs of estrus.
• On rare occasion, anestrus in cattle may be iatrogenic due to inadvertent feeding of a progestational agent (e.g., MGA).

HISTORICAL FINDINGS
• Individual animals: Absence of cyclicity (estrus) beyond 60 days postpartum. Absence of estrus after a negative pregnancy diagnosis.
• Herd or flock: Reduced mating activity, decreased pregnancy rates, increased interval from calving to first insemination, poor heat detection.

SIGNALMENT
• Sexually mature (postpubertal) female animals.
• Specific conditions vary with species and breed depending on nutrition, milk production levels, reproductive management systems, suckling intensity, seasonal (photoperiodic) influences, and the occurrence of systemic or uterine diseases.
• Suckled beef cattle will have a postpartum anestrus period 2 to 3 times as long as beef or dairy cattle that are milked.

PHYSICAL EXAMINATION FINDINGS
• Absence of sexually receptive behavior.
• Poor body condition score or other condition preventing expression of estrus.

GENETICS
• Ovarian agenesis, ovarian hypoplasia, and premature ovarian failure are rare examples of profound anestrus conditions and all probably have a genetic basis.
• The role of inheritance in the more common types of anestrus is uncertain.

CAUSES AND RISK FACTORS
• Poor nutritional management, especially in the transition period.

• High milk production and increased feed intake.
• Heat stress.
• Systemic disease.
• Lameness.
• Loss of body condition.
• Postpartum uterine infections (see chapter, Endometritis) can delay the resumption of normal cycles and increase the incidence of OCD.
• Long dry periods.
• Twin calving/Freemartinism.
• Primary uterine or fetal disease (e.g., pyometra, hydrometra [goats], mummified fetus, prolonged gestation).
• Early postpartum ovulation (<25 days) is associated with a persistent or retained CL.
• Rarely, ovarian tumors, segmental aplasia, ovarian hypoplasia, mycotoxins, and micronutrient deficiencies.

DIAGNOSIS

DIFFERENTIAL DIAGNOSES
• Physiological anestrus (pregnancy, sexual immaturity, lactation, or seasonal).
• Ruling out pregnancy should be the first consideration, otherwise diagnostic and therapeutic procedures could potentially result in iatrogenic abortion.
• Freemartinism.
• Inadequate estrus detection/reproductive management deficiencies.

CBC/BIOCHEMISTRY/URINALYSIS
N/A

OTHER LABORATORY TESTS
Consistently low progesterone concentrations in serum or milk may confirm anovular (lacking ovulation) anestrus.

IMAGING
• Transrectal ultrasonography reveals persistently small inactive ovaries or failure to ovulate when larger follicles or cystic structures are present.
• Repeated examination may be necessary to confirm the diagnosis. A CL will be absent in most cases but, if present, the uterus should be carefully examined for evidence of pyometra or other uterine disease.

OTHER DIAGNOSTIC PROCEDURES
• Records analysis/history.
• Transrectal ultrasonography or palpation per rectum in cattle.
• Serum progesterone analysis.
• Observation for sexual activity as appropriate for each species.

PATHOLOGIC FINDINGS
N/A

TREATMENT

THERAPEUTIC APPROACH
• Correct nutritional deficiencies or other primary problems (e.g., lameness).
• Hormonal induction of estrus and/or ovulation.
• Heat abatement.

SURGICAL CONSIDERATION AND TECHNIQUE
Ovariectomy in case of GTCT.

MEDICATIONS

DRUGS OF CHOICE
• GnRH or hCG
• PG600 (combination of FSH and hCG) in sheep and goats
• PGF2$_\alpha$ for retained/persistent CL, pyometra and hydrometra
• Ovulation synchronization (Ovsynch®) protocol with the addition of a CIDR
• Ovulation presynchronization protocols that include an injection of GnRH before the breeding Ovsynch®.

CONTRAINDICATIONS
PGF2$_\alpha$ should not be given to pregnant animals.

PRECAUTIONS
N/A

POSSIBLE INTERACTIONS
N/A

FOLLOW-UP

EXPECTED COURSE AND PROGNOSIS
• Estrous cycles will resume once nutritional, reproductive, and management issues are addressed.
• Delay in initiating treatment increases the risk of culling for reproductive reasons.

POSSIBLE COMPLICATIONS
• Pyometra
• Delayed conception

CLIENT EDUCATION
Use appropriate methods for estrus detection and monitoring of breeding activity.

PATIENT CARE
Monitor body condition score and behavioral activity.

PREVENTION
• Sound nutritional management, especially in the transition period, to avoid excessive loss of body condition.
• Minimize the incidence of dystocia, retained fetal membranes, and metritis/endometritis.
• Heat abatement.
• Decreased dry period length for older cows.

MISCELLANEOUS

ASSOCIATED CONDITIONS
• Pyometra
• Endometritis
• Twinning
• Lameness
• Starvation
• Heat stress

AGE-RELATED FACTORS
In cattle, prolonged postpartum anestrus is more common in primiparous than in multiparous cows.

ZOONOTIC POTENTIAL
N/A

PREGNANCY
• Pregnant animals experience a normal, physiological anestrus.
• PGF2$_\alpha$ will invariably (goats and camelids) or frequently (sheep and cattle) cause abortion.

BIOSECURITY
N/A

PRODUCTION MANAGEMENT
• Persistently anestrus females in well-monitored operations with strong management and husbandry protocols should be considered for culling.

ABBREVIATIONS
• CIDR = controlled intravaginal drug release device for delivery of progesterone
• CL = corpus luteum
• FSH = follicle stimulating hormone
• GnRH = gonadotropin-releasing hormone
• GTCT = granulosa-theca cell tumor
• hCG = human chorionic gonadotropin
• LH = luteinizing hormone
• MGA = melengestrol acetate
• OCD = ovarian cystic degeneration
• PGF2$_\alpha$ = prostaglandin F2$_\alpha$

SEE ALSO
• Artificial Insemination: Bovine
• Artificial Insemination: Small Ruminant
• Body Condition Scoring (see www.fiveminutevet.com/ruminant)
• Endometritis
• Estrus Synchronization: Bovine
• Estrus Synchronization: Small Ruminants
• Freemartinism
• Heat Stress
• Ovarian Cystic Degeneration
• Ovarian Hypoplasia, Bursal Disease, Salpingitis
• Pyometra
• Uterine Anomalies

Suggested Reading
De Rensis F, Garcia-Ispierto I, Lopez-Gatius F. Seasonal heat stress: Clinical implications and hormone treatments for the fertility of dairy cows. Theriogenology 2015, 84: 659–66.
Gumen A., Rastani RR, Grummer RR, Wiltbank MC. Reduced dry periods and varying prepartum diets alter postpartum ovulation and reproductive measures. J Dairy Sci 2005, 88: 2401–11.
Sangsritayong S, Combs DK, Sartori R, Armentano LE, Wiltbank MC. High feed intake increases liver metabolism of progesterone and estradiol-17*beta* in dairy cattle. J Dairy Sci 2002, 11: 2831–42.
Wiltbank MC, Gumen A, Sartori R. Physiological classification of anovulatory conditions in cattle. Theriogenology 2002, 57: 21–52.
Authors Harry Momont and Celina Checura
Consulting Editor Ahmed Tibary
Acknowledgment The author and book editors acknowledge the prior contribution of John Gibbons.

BASICS

OVERVIEW

• Angular limb deformity (ALD; "bent-leg") is a deviation from the normal axis of a limb (in the frontal plane) and is defined by the joint involved and the direction that the distal aspect of the limb is deviated.

  ○ **Valgus** deformity: The limb distal to the lesion deviates *laterally.*
  ○ **Varus** deformity: The limb distal to the lesion deviates *medially.*
  ○ ALDs are further described by the location of the pivot point (axis of deviation) and by the location of the site of defective growth.

• Some ALDs are caused by asymmetrical lesions involving an active growth plate (e.g., distal radius), but growth plate damage is not always the underlying cause.

• Related conditions include flexural deformities, tendon injuries, joint luxations/joint instability caused by laxity of supporting structures, and rotational/torsional deformities.

• Hereditary chondrodysplasia (HC), or spider lamb syndrome, is a hereditary condition in young lambs characterized by a number of skeletal deformities, including angular limb deformities.

INCIDENCE/PREVALENCE

• Valgus and varus ALDs are common and well documented in horses, but are relatively rare in ruminants. • Congenital limb abnormalities are reported to account for 6.9% of all congenital abnormalities in cattle.

GEOGRAPHIC DISTRIBUTION

Worldwide.

SYSTEMS AFFECTED

Musculoskeletal

PATHOPHYSIOLOGY

• ALDs are considered multifactorial in origin and have congenital/perinatal and developmental predisposing factors.

• Congenital ALDs may arise from environmental factors, genetic factors, or both. These include: toxins, placentitis, laxity of periarticular soft tissues, and intrauterine or perinatal physical factors (e.g., twinning, trauma). • Contributions to the formation of ALDs in immature and mature animals can stem from a low plane of nutrition, trauma, and excessive limb loading. • In llamas, the distal ulnar epiphysis fuses with the distal radial epiphysis. This unique development of the distal portion of the ulna is associated with forelimb valgus deformities in crias. The ulnar epiphysis extends distally, crosses the radial physis, and fuses with the radial epiphysis. This early fusion demands synchronous growth to ensure normal limb development. • Most calves have a mild carpal valgus deformity of approximately 7 degrees, which does not require treatment. Varus

deformities in cattle are abnormal and often need treatment.

HISTORICAL FINDINGS

A complete history including current age, birthing details, age at which the deformity was noticed, course and progression of the deformity, and diets of affected animal and dam should be obtained.

SIGNALMENT

Species

• Bovine, ovine, caprine, South American camelids (especially llama crias), cervids—including fallow deer (*Dama dama*), red deer (*Cervus elaphus*), white-tailed deer (*Odocoileus virginianus*)—and a single case report of ALD in a giraffe calf (*Giraffa camelopardalis*).

Breed Predilections

• ALDs have been described in many different beef and dairy cattle breeds. • HC primarily affects black-faced breeds of sheep (Suffolk, Hampshire, Southdown, Shropshire, and Oxford). • Varus/valgus deformities have been described in the distal radial physis of yearling farmed male red and wapiti-red crossbred (elk) deer in New Zealand.

Mean Age and Range

• ALDs primarily affect young growing animals up to 7 months of age, but can be seen in older animals (e.g., trauma-induced ALD). • HC has two distinct clinical entities: lambs are either grossly abnormal at birth or develop the abnormal conformation at 4–6 weeks of age. Radiographic changes at birth are similar for both.

Predominant Sex

No apparent sex predisposition.

PHYSICAL EXAMINATION FINDINGS

• Conformation should be assessed first by having the animal stand in a symmetrical manner on a firm, flat surface and observing it from multiple angles. Affected animals may appear to be knock-kneed or bowlegged. All limbs should be palpated and affected limbs should be manually manipulated. Clinical signs such as abnormal bending of the affected limb, increased laxity, muscle atrophy, swelling, heat, pain on manual pressure, abrasions on lateral or medial side of hoof wall, presence of orthopedic injury, and abnormal gait and locomotion are indicative of ALD. • Compensatory deviation (opposite that of the affected limb) is relatively common in the contralateral limb. • If varus deformity is found unilaterally, the contralateral limb should be examined for a significant orthopedic injury as a cause of excessive weight bearing in the deformed limb/joint.

• Since cattle are considered to have a "normal" degree of medial deviation at the level of the carpus and hock, as well as normal external rotation of the lower limb, ALDs tend to be missed in the early stages of development. • Most bovine ALDs occur at

the level of the mid-diaphysis of long bones.

• In sheep affected with HC, various degrees of ALDs of fore- and/or hindlimbs will be noted. Other physical examination findings include severe scoliosis/kyphosis of the thoracic spine, pectus excavatum, retarded growth rates, facial deformities such as angular deviation and/or shortening of maxilla, rounding of the dorsal silhouette, and Roman-shaped noses.

GENETICS

• The questions of heritability in ALDs have not been definitively answered; the details of some syndromes are known. • ALDs in Jersey calves are genetically transmitted as a simple autosomal recessive trait. • HC of Suffolk and Suffolk-cross sheep is inherited as a single, autosomal recessive gene that has been localized to the distal end of chromosome 6. A defect in the gene encoding fibroblast growth factor receptor 3 (FGFR3) is suspected. DNA tests (blood or semen) are available to identify homozygous and heterozygous animals.

CAUSES AND RISK FACTORS

• ALDs are often related to asymmetrical growth of the physis, ligament rupture, or orthopedic injuries.

Congenital Predisposing Factors

• Incomplete cuboidal bone ossification (carpal and/or tarsal). • Physiologic immaturity at birth. • Uterine malpositioning. • In utero bending stress and bone remodeling early in gestation. • Twin (or triplet) pregnancy. • Reduced intrauterine space may limit fetal movement and subsequently cause congenital angular and/or flexural limb deformities. • Laxity of periarticular supporting structures.

• Disproportionate osseous growth of medial and lateral aspects of long bones (e.g., distal radius, tibia, metatarsus). • Nutritional imbalance during gestation. • Genetic causes.

Developmental Predisposing Factors

• Conformational defects (causing abnormal weight distribution across a joint).

• Nutritional disorders (e.g., improper dietary calcium and phosphorus ratios; copper, zinc, manganese, iron, and molybdenum concentrations). • External trauma (e.g., compression of or trauma to growth plate; Salter-Harris fractures, malunion of fractures, inflammation of growth plate). • Iatrogenic (e.g., assisted delivery). • Excessive exercise.

• Hematogenous osteomyelitis involving the physeal region. • Rapid weight gain in heavy breeds (high energy rations and rapid growth).

• Often, no specific cause is identified.

Camelids

• May see ALDs (usually carpal valgus) in growing camelids with hypophosphatemic rickets syndrome. • Ill-thrift syndrome in llamas may be associated with ALDs as well as anemia, low serum iron concentrations, and metabolic disorders (hypothyroidism). Underlying cause not established.

DIAGNOSIS

DIFFERENTIAL DIAGNOSES
• Physiologic deformities. • Metabolic bone disease (e.g., rickets). • HC may be confused with arthrogryposis-hydranencephaly syndrome (AHS) in lambs, in which there is characteristic hyperflexion of forelimbs, cranial overextension of hindlimbs, with a corkscrew deviation of the spine. In lambs with AHS, severe deformities result from primary abnormalities of the CNS (including hydranencephaly and others) and not of the skeleton.

Camelids
True ALDs in llamas must be differentiated from valgus deformities of the forelimbs in newborn crias that self-correct without surgical treatment.

CBC/BIOCHEMISTRY/URINALYSIS
• There are usually no associated laboratory abnormalities with ALDs. • HC results in slightly elevated serum alkaline phosphatase activity; insufficient for diagnostic purposes.

Camelids
• Ill-thrift syndrome: Serum vitamin D (25-hydroxycholecalciferol) concentrations are often diagnostic. • May also see hypothyroidism, anemia, erythrocyte dyscrasias, hypophosphatemia, and low serum iron concentrations.

OTHER LABORATORY TESTS
N/A

IMAGING
• Radiographs are critical in diagnosing ALDs—at least two views, 90 degrees apart, should be taken of the affected joint, including joints immediately proximal and distal to the affected joint. • The dorsopalmar/dorsoplantar (DP) view is needed for examination of the anatomical location of the deformity and for measurements. The pivot point is defined as the intersection between lines drawn through the long axis at the center of the proximal and distal long bone using the dorsopalmar view. Location of the pivot point identifies the type of deformity. Measure the angle of deviation with a protractor. • HC: Most consistent lesions include multiple islands of ossification of the anconeal process and malformed, displaced sternebrae. The anconeal lesions of HC are progressive, whereas similar lesions in other skeletal conditions of lambs regress.

OTHER DIAGNOSTIC PROCEDURES
• Bacterial cultures may be indicated in cases of septicemia, arthritis, or osteomyelitis.
• Toxicology (heavy metal and mineral analysis) and feed analysis may assist in diagnosis.

PATHOLOGIC FINDINGS
• Histology: Focal or segmental thickening of the physis (expansion of the hypertrophic zone) with extension into the proximal metaphysis; closely resembles physeal manifestations of osteochondrosis.
• Histology associated with HC (vertebrae and long bones): Increase in width of the zone of proliferation and hypertrophy and unevenness of growth cartilage; failure to form or maintain orderly columns of chondrocytes.

TREATMENT

THERAPEUTIC APPROACH
• Treatment of neonatal animals with incomplete ossification involves the application of tube casts or splints to the affected limb(s) until ossification is complete (based on repeated radiographs). • Many cases of ALD will resolve without surgery if the underlying cause(s) can be identified and addressed and if the animal does not damage the affected physis or joints with vigorous exercise. • Specific treatment methods are selected on the basis of age, degree of angulation, remaining growth potential of the involved physis, and experience of the veterinarian. • Minor limb deviations may be conservatively treated by manual alignment and external support of the limb (e.g., rigid splinting, bandaging, or casting/tube casts) and/or hoof (claw) trimming. • Hoof manipulations create growth plate response to stress applied opposite the deformity, and self-correction occurs. The hoof tends to turn in the direction of the longer claw or toward the side of the wider wall, resulting in straightening and de-rotation of the limb.
• Medial (varus) deformities can be treated by trimming the medial claw shorter than the lateral claw and by placing an acrylic (methyl methacrylate) wing on the weight-bearing surface of the lateral claw (to increase lateral contact with the ground). • Treatment should be directed at the orthopedic injury when varus deformity is present secondary to a contralateral limb injury.

SURGICAL CONSIDERATIONS AND TECHNIQUES
• Surgery is recommended for older animals (near the end of active physeal growth), for those that do not respond to conservative treatments, and for animals with bone malformations that require realignment (via osteotomy). • The choice of surgical technique should take into consideration the economic value and age of the animal, severity of the deformity, and the joint involved.

Treatment Strategies Include the Following:
Growth Acceleration (Periosteal Stripping/ Elevation)
In young calves and lambs with early cases of ALD, surgical growth stimulation via periosteal stripping on the concave aspect (shorter side) of the deformity has been used successfully. Based on the remaining growth potential in the physis, allow the animal to correct the deviation by physeal growth.

Growth Retardation (Transphyseal Bridging)
• Transphyseal bridging is indicated for severe cases of ALD or in animals past the rapid growth phase of the radius and ulna (often recommended for animals older than 5 months of age). • By creating a temporary transphyseal bridge on the convex side of the deformity using staples or screws and wires, limb growth is slowed by restricting growth and allows the other side to continue growing, resulting in limb straightening. • The surgical implants must be removed when the limb achieves normal conformation to prevent overcorrection. This can be used in combination with periosteal stripping to increase the likelihood of full correction in animals with severe deviations.

Corrective Wedge Osteotomy
• This procedure is indicated in mature animals with ALD and in neonates with congenital fracture malunion. If the growth plates are closed or if the growth plate is not involved in an ALD, a corrective osteotomy is recommended. This requires more experience and equipment and often is reserved for valuable animals when response to other therapies has failed. • The site and orientation of the wedge should be determined by clinical and radiographic examination. • The limb needs to be stabilized by internal fixation with a plate and screws for an extended postoperative period.

Camelids
An ulnar osteotomy must be done in conjunction with the periosteal transection because the ulna spans the radial physis.

MEDICATIONS

DRUGS OF CHOICE
Nonsteroidal anti-inflammatory agents (NSAIDs) are recommended to reduce inflammation in some cases of ALD.

CONTRAINDICATIONS
Prolonged NSAID administration has been associated with gastrointestinal (abomasal or C3) ulcers.

PRECAUTIONS
• Many of these affected animals are young; precautions regarding drug choices must take age into consideration. • Appropriate milk

and meat withdrawal times must be followed for all compounds administered to food-producing animals.

POSSIBLE INTERACTIONS

N/A

 FOLLOW-UP

EXPECTED COURSE AND PROGNOSIS

• Prognosis is guarded, yet reasonable for ALDs associated with growth plate imbalances, such as most valgus deformities. • The prognosis for ALDs secondary to contralateral orthopedic injury (such as most varus deformities) is generally poor because it is usually centered over a joint and is dependent on the prognosis of the primary orthopedic injury. • HC-affected individuals rarely survive the neonatal period. • Camelids: The prognosis for ill-thrift syndrome in llamas is poor; etiologic agent often not identified.

POSSIBLE COMPLICATIONS

• In cases of valgus deformity, efforts should be taken to prevent compensatory varus in the contralateral limb. Persistence of hoof distortion is possible if the angular deformity is not corrected. • Surgical: transphyseal bridging—overcorrection of the physis is possible. Owner cooperation is required to determine when limb has regained its normal conformation. • Possible ALD surgical complications include muscle, tendon, and ligament atrophy/laxity, hyperextension of limbs, fibrous scar tissue development, and postoperative infection.

CLIENT EDUCATION

• Examination and intervention of young animals with congenital ALDs should be done as early as possible. • Due to the possible hereditary link with ALDs, breeding of affected animals is not recommended.

PATIENT CARE

• Severely affected animals may be unable to rise to nurse and require additional supportive care. Protect limbs with thick, soft bandages that fit well. • Care should be taken to maintain a soft (padding), clean, and dry environment and to minimize decubital/pressure sores, open arthritis, muscle atrophy, umbilical infections, and septicemia. • Physical confinement (stall) is recommended for the management of ALDs to limit stresses placed on affected limbs.

• Nutritional imbalances have been implicated, such as ill-thrift in llamas. Treatment for this condition includes appropriate vitamin D supplementation. • Other dietary imbalances should be corrected while treating cases of ALD. • Frequent physical monitoring and repeated radiographs should be done to assess the efficacy of corrective measures and to monitor progress. • In cases of transphyseal bridging surgery, owner cooperation is required to determine when the limb has regained its normal conformation, at which time the implants must be removed to prevent overcorrection.

PREVENTION

Avoid breeding affected animals.

 MISCELLANEOUS

ASSOCIATED CONDITIONS

• Conditions associated with ALDs include osteochondrosis of the physis, epiphysitis, and incomplete ossification of the cuboidal carpal bones. • Hyena disease (premature physeal closure) has been reported in calves due to overdose of vitamins A, D3, and E. • Congenital lethal chondrodysplasia in Australian Dexter cattle = "Dexter bulldog calves". • Congenital chondrodysplastic dwarfism in Holstein calves. • Complex vertebral malformation is a familial syndrome of Holstein calves. • Syndrome known as "bentleg" or "bowie" associated with ingestion of *Trachymene glaucifolia* (wild parsnip) by pregnant ewes in Australia and New Zealand.

AGE-RELATED FACTORS

The majority of ALDs occur during the active growth phase of the affected bone/joint.

ZOONOTIC POTENTIAL

N/A

PREGNANCY

• Many of the causes of ALDs are congenital diseases in which the in utero environment is somehow disturbed (hormones, vascular supply, teratogens, mechanical factors, or prenatal viral infections). • Cases of ALDs in goats pregnant with triplets have been reported. • Contributing factors likely include stress and in utero malpositioning.

BIOSECURITY

N/A

PRODUCTION MANAGEMENT

N/A

ABBREVIATIONS

• AHS = arthrogryposis-hydranencephaly syndrome
• ALD = angular limb deformity
• CNS = central nervous system
• DP = dorsopalmar/dorsoplantar
• FGFR3 = fibroblast growth factor receptor 3
• HC = ovine hereditary chondrodysplasia
• NSAIDs = nonsteroidal anti-inflammatory drugs

SEE ALSO

• Arthrogryposis
• Congenital Defects: Bovine
• Hereditary Chondrodysplasia: Ovine
• Lameness (by species)

Suggested Reading

Aiello SE ed. The Merck Veterinary Manual. 2015. Retrieved from http://www.merckvetmanual.com/mvm/index.html

Ducharme NG. Angular deformities. In: Fubini SL, Ducharme NG eds, Farm Animal Surgery. Philadelphia: Saunders, 2004.

Ferguson JG. Angular deformity of radiocarpal and tibiotarsal joints. In: Greenough PR ed, Lameness in Cattle, 3rd ed. Philadelphia: Saunders, 1997.

Kaneps AJ. Orthopedic conditions of small ruminants, llama, sheep, goat, and deer. Advances in ruminant orthopedics. Vet Clin North Am Food Anim Pract 1996, 12: 211–31.

Maxie GM. Jubb, Kennedy and Palmer's Pathology of Domestic Animals, vol. 1, 6th ed. New York: Saunders Elsevier, 2015.

Paul-Murphy JR, Morgan JP, Snyder JR, Fowler ME. Radiographic findings in young llamas with forelimb valgus deformities: 28 cases (1980–1988). J Am Vet Med Assoc 1991, 12: 21107–11.

Radostits OM, Gay CC, Hinchcliff KW, Constable PD eds, Veterinary Medicine: A Textbook of the Diseases of Cattle, Horses, Sheep, Pigs, and Goats, 10th ed. New York: Elsevier Saunders, 2008.

Schleining JA, Bergh MS. Surgical correction of angular and torsional metatarsal deformity with cylindrical osteotomy and locking compression plates in a calf. Vet Surg 2014, 43: 563–8.

Authors Erik J. Olson and Nicholas A. Robinson
Consulting Editor Kaitlyn A. Lutz
Acknowledgment The authors and book editors acknowledge the prior contribution of Cathy S. Carlson.

A

ANTHELMINTIC RESISTANCE

BASICS

OVERVIEW
Gastrointestinal nematodes are common and may cause pathology that impacts health and welfare of infected animals. Infestation with these nematodes decreases production parameters. Control measures have relied predominantly on periodic administration of anthelmintic drugs to the entire herd or flock. Their continual use has led to the selection of populations of drug-resistant worms worldwide. Multi-drug resistance has now been reported in sheep and cattle. Anthelmintic resistance by *Haemonchus contortus* in sheep has been well documented and in cattle recent reports of resistance in *Cooperia* spp. and to a lesser extent in *Ostertagia ostertagi* are now documented.

INCIDENCE/PREVALENCE
Each farm may have different levels of resistant parasite populations. The level of resistance is dependent on how frequently the herd has been treated with anthelmintics and how effective those compounds have been in reducing luminal burdens.

GEOGRAPHIC DISTRIBUTION
Worldwide

SYSTEMS AFFECTED
Gastrointestinal, which may lead to pathology of other organ systems with significant infections.

PATHOPHYSIOLOGY
Individual nematodes that survive an anthelmintic treatment have a reproductive advantage in the absence of competition by susceptible worms in the intestine. This advantage persists until lifecycle features prevail or anthelmintic levels decrease and allow reestablishment of susceptible parasites. Resistant worms transmit their unique, heritable traits to the next generation and by doing so they increase the frequency of their genetic alleles in the general population. Depending upon the parasite, the clinical significance of the infection may be greater than would be present if the treatment was more effective. Resistant worms have no particular advantage until the selection pressure of anthelmintic treatment is applied. Once this happens, a great way to accentuate this advantage is to repeatedly use the same anthelmintic. Individual worms are initially resistant to only one class of anthelmintics, so when "drug A" is used, they survive, but if "drug B" were introduced, the worms would be removed like the rest of the susceptible population. Thus, the reproductive advantage of resistant worms would be favored if "drug A" were used exclusively.

HISTORICAL FINDINGS
Lack of efficacy of anthelmintic treatment evidenced by poor fecal egg count reductions and increased clinical signs of parasitism.

SIGNALMENT
All ruminants may be affected.

PHYSICAL EXAMINATION FINDINGS
The signs of parasitism may be variable depending upon the pathogenicity of the resistant parasites.

GENETICS
All ruminants may be affected, but it is most common to find that 20% of a herd will harbor 80% of the parasites. This fact suggests that a genetic component exists within a population of animals that allows the majority of the herd to have some level of resistance to internal parasites. The issue then becomes identifying those individuals within the herd that are most susceptible to continued infection and providing them with effective treatment.

CAUSES AND RISK FACTORS
Anthelmintic resistance in a nematode population is a phenotypic manifestation of a heritable, genetic trait within that population. The genetic basis and modes of inheritance of resistance are quite complex and differ widely among the various classes of compounds, but positive selection occurs whenever worms carrying resistant alleles are exposed to an anthelmintic to which they have lost their susceptibility.

DIAGNOSIS

DIFFERENTIAL DIAGNOSES
Any cause of weight loss may be considered as a differential for chronic parasitism. In sheep with *Haemonchus contortus* infections anemia and hypoproteinemia are predominate signs.

OTHER LABORATORY TESTS
The standard by which parasite loads are measured is the assessment of fecal egg counts per gram of feces (EPG). Fecal EPG of cattle tend to be less reflective of the adult worm burden when compared to sheep. This fact leads to a great deal of uncertainty in the detection of anthelmintic resistance in cattle. Resistance can be defined as a measurable decrease in efficacy of a compound against parasitic species and its larval stages that were previously susceptible.

OTHER DIAGNOSTIC PROCEDURES
The use of fecal EPGs on a herd basis is important to obtain knowledge of the efficacy of any anthelmintic. It is important to obtain an adequate sample size, although the number of animals with an adequate infection for enrollment can be limited. Recommendations

to minimize diagnostic uncertainty include the use of arithmetic means over geometric means to calculate anthelmintic efficacy, the use of individual based group means with pre- and post-treatment individual fecal egg counts, and the preferred use of diagnostic methods with higher analytic sensitivity to minimize inaccuracies in populations with low baseline fecal egg count.

PATHOLOGIC FINDINGS
The pathology associated with internal parasites is variable and dependent on the genus.

TREATMENT

THERAPEUTIC APPROACH
The key to parasite control is either to prevent egg shedding and/or prevent larval uptake. For the last 50 years we have tried to prevent egg shedding by routine anthelmintic treatments. Managing animals to prevent larval uptake can be accomplished by co-grazing different species, removal of feces or clever use of available pasture lands. The assessment of the drug disposition in the host and increased knowledge of the mechanisms of drug interaction in the targeted parasites has increased our understanding of how these anthelmintics actually work. It is clear that we need additional scientific knowledge on how to improve the use of available molecules to avoid or delay development of resistance.

MEDICATIONS
- See "Follow-Up"
- See chapters, Parasite Control Programs

FOLLOW-UP

EXPECTED COURSE AND PROGNOSIS
This is a life-threatening aspect of small ruminant production and serious consequences will occur if solutions are not forthcoming.

POSSIBLE COMPLICATIONS
Very limited information is available on the potential additive or synergistic effects occurring after co-administration of two (or more) drugs with different modes of action.

CLIENT EDUCATION
A change in treatment philosophy is necessary to combat or delay the development of anthelmintic resistance in ruminant nematodes. Producers have used dewormers in a very cavalier manner over the past 40

years and been taught that when deworming, all animals in the herd must be treated. New knowledge and evidence point out that this technique has helped to create the resistance that is now present. Educating producers on how to address parasite problems must be done and this knowledge needs to encompass feed stores and pharmaceutical supply houses as well.

PATIENT CARE
The individual monitoring within a herd will be necessary to allow for identification of those that have the highest parasite loads.

PREVENTION
• Integrated management and pharmacologic intervention.
• Treatment targeted at those individuals that harbor the most parasites and are at risk for the development of adverse clinical signs.
• Different pharmacokinetic-based approaches to enhance parasite exposure.
• Mixed-class anthelmintic treatment.

MISCELLANEOUS
PREGNANCY
Chronic parasitism may significantly affect gestating dams, especially in small ruminants infected with *H. contortus*.

BIOSECURITY
Anytime a new animal is brought on to a property they should be evaluated for their internal parasite load. This is especially critical in small ruminant populations with *Haemonchus contortus*. Purchased additions should be screened and quarantined to evaluate their existing infestation and, if they are infected, their response to treatment.

PRODUCTION MANAGEMENT
Production is imperative to success in ruminants and internal parasites are a major contributor to production losses. Control of these parasites is critical for success in rearing young stock.

ABBREVIATION
• EPG = egg count per gram of feces

SEE ALSO
• Parasite Control Programs: Beef
• Parasite Control Programs: Camelid
• Parasite Control Programs: Dairy
• Parasite Control Programs: Small Ruminant

Suggested Reading
Coles GC, Jackson F, Pomroy WE, et al. The detection of anthelmintic resistance in nematodes of veterinary importance. Vet Parasitol 2006, 136: 167–85.
Demeler J, Van Zeveren AM, Kleinschmidt N, et al. Monitoring the efficacy of ivermectin and albendazole against gastro intestinal nematodes of cattle in Northern Europe. Vet Parasitol 2009, 160: 109–15.
Dobson RJ, Hosking BC, Jacobson CL, et al. Preserving new anthelmintics: a simple method for estimating faecal egg count reduction test (FECRT) confidence limits when efficacy and/or nematode aggregation is high. Vet Parasitol 2012, 186: 79–92.

Gasbarre LC, Smith LL, Lichtenfels JR, Pilitt PA. The identification of cattle nematode parasites resistant to multiple classes of anthelmintics in a commercial cattle population in the US. Vet Parasitol 2009, 166: 281–5.
Lanusse C, Alvarez L, Lifschitz A. Pharmacological knowledge and sustainable anthelmintic therapy in ruminants. Vet Parasitol 2014, 204: 18–33.
Leathwick DM, Miller CM. Efficacy of oral, injectable and pour-on formulations of moxidectin against gastrointestinal nematodes in cattle in New Zealand. Vet Parasitol 2013, 191: 293–300.
McArthur MJ, Reinemeyer CR. Herding the US cattle industry toward a paradigm shift in parasite control. Vet Parasitol 2014, 204: 34–43.
Smith LL. Combination anthelmintics effectively control ML-resistant parasites; a real-world case history. Vet Parasitol 2014, 204: 12–17.
Sutherland IA, Leathwic DM. Anthelmintic resistance in nematode parasites of cattle: a global issue? Trends Parasitol 2011, 27: 176–81.
Author Dennis D. French
Consulting Editor Kaitlyn A. Lutz

 Client Education Handout available online

ANTHRAX

BASICS

OVERVIEW
• Anthrax is a bacterial disease that many animals are susceptible to including humans.
• In ruminants it causes acute bacteremia, septicemia, and usually death. It is caused by *Bacillus anthracis* which is present in the soil.
• It is seen most often in and is highly pathogenic for most wild and domestic herbivores.
• In most areas anthrax is a reportable disease and the regional veterinary authorities should be notified of an outbreak.
• In the USA, *Bacillus anthracis* is listed in the Federal Select Agent Program.

INCIDENCE/PREVALENCE
• Anthrax spores are endemic in parts of the United States, where occurrence of clinical disease is usually sporadic.
• Both sporadic cases and outbreaks are often associated with disruption of the soil.
• Morbidity varies widely but case mortality is 90–95%.

GEOGRAPHIC DISTRIBUTION
• Anthrax is found worldwide but certain regions have higher occurrence of disease.
• Anthrax spores favor areas with neutral to alkaline soils with high levels of calcium and manganese and are organically rich.

SYSTEMS AFFECTED
• Hemolymphatic
• Multisystemic

PATHOPHYSIOLOGY
• Soil-borne spores are the infective form of the bacteria.
• In ruminants the main source of infection is consuming spore-contaminated pasture or feed. However, spores can enter the host via the cutaneous or respiratory systems also.
• Once in the host, the spores germinate and produce the vegetative form of the bacterium which rapidly proliferate.
• These rapidly dividing bacteria produce capsule and toxins. Early in the infection these toxins help the bacteria to evade the immune system resulting in systemic infection. Later in the infection with large numbers of bacteria in the blood, the toxins enter cells of other systems resulting in vascular shock and death.
• Late in the course of the disease and at death all animal excretions contain large numbers of bacteria and sporulate when contacting air. This exposes additional animals and contaminates the environment.

SIGNALMENT
Goats, sheep, cattle, and bison are more susceptible than other species such as horses, pigs, and dogs.

PHYSICAL EXAMINATION FINDINGS
• Commonly animals will be found dead and clinical signs not observed.

• Clinical signs include fever up to 107°F (41.5°C), congested mucus membranes, excitement, depression, stupor, dyspnea, ataxia, muscle tremors, collapse, convulsions, and death. Younger animals will have less severe signs.
• If the animal lives long enough bloody diarrhea, hematuria, and localized swellings maybe seen as well as abortion.

CAUSES AND RISK FACTORS
• Anthrax is caused by *Bacillus anthracis* which is a large (1 μm by 3–5 μm) Gram-positive rod that is rectangular with square ends and commonly forms chains.
• *Bacillus anthracis* exists in two forms: the spore and vegetative cell.
• Once the spore infects the animal it germinates into the vegetative form. The vegetative form in infected tissues of the dead animal only survives up to 1–2 weeks. However, when exposed to air vegetative bacteria will sporulate in several hours. Sporulation is oxygen dependent.
• It is important not to necropsy the carcass to limit the spore formation and therefore keeping contamination of the environment to a minimum.
• Scavengers and biting insects may mechanically disseminate anthrax after feeding on affected carcasses.
• Risk factors include:
  ◦ Animals residing in endemic pastures or range.
  ◦ Exposure to disturbed soil in endemic areas. Disturbances can be due to flooding, excavations, cattle disturbing soil around wet pastures, or shrinking surface water sources.
  ◦ Grazing plants close to the ground, as seen in overstocking range or pasture or drought in endemic areas.

DIAGNOSIS

DIFFERENTIAL DIAGNOSES
Anthrax, because of the nonspecific history and clinical appearance, can be confused with many other causes of acute death in ruminants including clostridial infections (blackleg, malignant edema), lightning strike, acute toxicosis (cyanobacterium), and bloat.

OTHER DIAGNOSTIC PROCEDURES
• Samples must be submitted for a definitive diagnosis.
• The laboratory should be forewarned of a suspected anthrax case submission due to the zoonotic risk.
• Collections of samples are recommended at or soon after death when bacterial numbers are at their highest.
• Blood is the main and best sample for diagnostic submission. Bloody fluids and

tissues are also useful; however, opening the carcass is strongly discouraged.
• To prevent contamination of the environment collection of blood sample from a superficial vein using a large gauge needle and syringe is recommended.
• Microscopic examination of blood smears, bacterial cultures, and PCR are a few of the examinations laboratories use to identify *Bacillus anthracis*.

PATHOLOGIC FINDINGS
• If the carcass is inadvertently opened the lesions are those of septicemia.
• Rigor mortis is commonly not present or incomplete.
• Cattle that die of anthrax decompose rapidly and are found gas distended with bloody exudates coming from any of the body orifices.
• Blood is usually thick and dark red with little or no clotting. Any clotted blood found is not well formed.
• Multifocal hemorrhages are common on mucosal and serosal surfaces as well as subcutaneously.
• Gelatinous fluid accumulates in loose connective tissue and serous cavities and could be blood tinged.
• Parenchymatous organs are congested, swollen, and soft. The spleen can be greatly enlarged and bloody.
• The heart has a dull appearance and is flaccid.
• In cattle the lesions at the site of bacterial entry can be more severe, such as ulcerative hemorrhagic enteritis.
• If the bacteria come in through the oropharynx there will be hemorrhage and swelling of local lymph nodes as well as edema in adjacent connective tissue and throat.
• Likewise if there is a case of pulmonary anthrax in cattle, lesions would be most severe in lung and mediastinum.
• Sheep and goats are more susceptible to anthrax than cattle. The course of the disease is more rapid so some of the lesions maybe less prominent or missing.

TREATMENT

THERAPEUTIC APPROACH
Often no therapeutic approach is available as the disease is peracute. Sick animals are treated with antibiotics (see "Drugs of Choice").

MEDICATIONS

DRUGS OF CHOICE
B. anthracis is generally antibiotic-sensitive but some strains can be resistant to penicillin. *B. anthracis* is susceptible to many antibiotics,

including but not limited to penicillin and tetracycline. However, eliminating the bacteria may not increase survival: once the toxins have entered cells in sufficient quantity, they can still manifest their lethal effects.

CONTRAINDICATIONS

Because the Sterne strain vaccine must replicate to effectively stimulate an immune response, antibiotic treatment should not be given in conjunction with or shortly after the administration of vaccine in healthy animals. However, field conditions may dictate a combination of vaccine and antibiotics as a practical course of action.

 FOLLOW-UP

EXPECTED COURSE AND PROGNOSIS

In ruminants the incubation period is 1–5 days and the course of the disease is from hours to 2 days and the usual outcome is death.

PREVENTION

• Affected premises are quarantined to prevent further spread of the disease.
• Consideration should be given to limiting access to suspected sources of exposure in affected herds. This may include moving livestock to a different pasture, fencing livestock away from low-lying water sources, where spores may recently have been exposed due to drought conditions, providing insect control, and proper disposal of affected carcasses.
• Hygiene and carcass disposal are of paramount importance in halting an outbreak and preventing future disease occurrence.
• Autolysis of the carcass destroys the vegetative forms of *B. anthracis* and, therefore, if carcasses are not opened up, the potential for contamination of the environment is minimized.

• Carcasses must be disposed of in accordance with state or local regulations.
• Livestock in endemic areas should be vaccinated with Sterne-strain spore vaccine at least 2–4 weeks prior to the expected seasonal onset. Booster vaccination is given 4–5 weeks following the initial vaccination, and then annually thereafter.
• The vaccine is a live nonencapsulated organism and therefore antibiotics should not be given within 7–10 days of vaccine administration.
• Following vaccination, there is a 60-day withdrawal time for the carcass, and milk should be discarded for at least 72 hours.

 MISCELLANEOUS

AGE-RELATED FACTORS

There are some reports of males being more susceptible than females and older animals being more susceptible than young animals, but these probably reflect differences in grazing behavior rather than inherent differences in susceptibility.

ZOONOTIC POTENTIAL

Anthrax can infect humans and precautions should be taken to avoid contamination with infected animal tissues, contaminated animal products, and anthrax spores.

BIOSECURITY

• Once anthrax is diagnosed, the farm will be quarantined. No movement of animals on or off the premises should occur during the quarantine period.
• Animals surviving an outbreak may be moved to uncontaminated pastures or holding pens in order to reduce the possibility of additional cases.
• Scavenger and insect control is important to prevent the spread of the disease.

• All equipment, vehicles, and working facilities used in an outbreak must be cleaned and disinfected.

PRODUCTION MANAGEMENT

Vaccination of livestock is an important consideration in anthrax endemic areas.

ABBREVIATION

PCR = polymerase chain reaction

Suggested Reading

A History of Anthrax. Centers for Disease Control and Prevention, http://www.cdc.gov/anthrax/resources/history/

Anthrax. In: Merck Veterinary Manual on line. http://www.merckvetmanual.com/mvm/generalized_conditions/anthrax/overview_of_anthrax.html?qt=Anthrax&alt=sh

Anthrax. In: Spickler AR, Roth JA, Gaylon J, Lofstedt J eds, Emerging and Exotic Diseases of Animals, 4th ed. Ames: Iowa State University, 2010.

Clothier KA. Anthrax. In: Smith BP ed, Large Animal Internal Medicine, 5th ed. St. Louis: Elsevier, 2015, pp. 1077–8.

Moayeri M, Leppla SH, Vrentas C, Pomerantsev A, Liu S. Anthrax pathogenesis. Annu Rev Microbiol online 2015, 69: 185–208.

Stewart GC, Thompson BM. Bacillus. In: McVey DS, Kennedy M, Chengappa MM eds, Veterinary Microbiology, 3rd ed. Ames: Wiley-Blackwell, 2013, pp. 206–11.

Valli VEO. Hematopoietic system: Anthrax. In: Maxie MG ed, Pathology of Domestic Animals vol 3, 5th ed. New York: Saunders Elsevier, 2007, pp. 294–6.

Authors Regg D. Neiger and Dustin Oedekoven
Consulting Editor Christopher C.L. Chase

 Client Education Handout available online

ARSENIC TOXICOSIS

BASICS

OVERVIEW
• Arsenic is the second most common cause of heavy metal intoxication of cattle, after lead.
• Arsenic is still used in herbicides, defoliants, wood preservatives, and other products; however, alternative products with lower toxicity and less environmental persistence are becoming progressively more available.

INCIDENCE/PREVALENCE
Unknown

GEOGRAPHIC DISTRIBUTION
Worldwide

SYSTEMS AFFECTED
• Digestive
• Urinary

PATHOPHYSIOLOGY
• Poisoning most often results from exposure to inorganic arsenic compounds contained in commercial products including herbicides, insecticides, and pressure-treated wood.
• Inorganic arsenic products can be trivalent (arsenite) or pentavalent (arsenate), with the arsenites being more soluble and toxic.
• Organic arsenic compounds are aliphatic or aromatic, and aromatic compounds can also be trivalent or pentavalent in nature.
• Ingestion of soluble arsenic compounds results in distribution of arsenic to many organs, with tissues rich in oxidative enzymes being the most vulnerable to damage, including the lungs, liver, kidneys, endothelium, and gastrointestinal tract.
• Mechanism of toxicity and toxic dose depend upon the formulation, route of exposure, and duration of exposure.
• Arsenates uncouple oxidative phosphorylation and trivalent arsenicals disrupt the citric acid cycle, creating damage to metabolically active tissues.

HISTORICAL FINDINGS
Deliberate or incidental exposure to products containing arsenic.

SIGNALMENT
Any ruminant species of any age, breed, or gender can be affected.

PHYSICAL EXAMINATION FINDINGS
• Signs typically reflect acute toxicosis and can include sudden death.
• Signs of acute or subacute toxicosis occur within 3–12 hours of exposure and reflect shock associated with gastrointestinal and cardiovascular damage.
• Colic, dehydration, weakness, anorexia, and severe watery diarrhea, which may be hemorrhagic, are observed.

GENETICS
N/A

CAUSES AND RISK FACTORS
• Exposure or access of animals to arsenic-containing products or residues such as herbicides, insecticides, and the ashes of pressure-treated wood.
• Grazing animals in areas of high environmental contamination which can result from residue from livestock dip, mining waste, and sources of industrial contamination.
• Ruminants are particularly sensitive to the aliphatic arsenicals MSMA and DSMA which are used as herbicides.

DIAGNOSIS

DIFFERENTIAL DIAGNOSES
• Bovine viral diarrhea virus (BVDV) could take out
• Bacterial enteritis (*Salmonella* spp.)
• Organophosphate insecticide exposure
• Other heavy metal toxicoses (lead)
• Urea toxicosis

CBC/BIOCHEMISTRY/URINALYSIS
Changes are not specific to arsenic toxicosis, but are consistent with dehydration, shock, gastrointestinal damage, and hemorrhage.

OTHER LABORATORY TESTS
• Arsenic concentration can be chemically determined in tissues including the liver and kidney (>3 ppm wet weight associated with toxicity); however, tissue concentrations may be normal in animals suffering peracute death.
• Arsenic can be measured in gastrointestinal content and blood for 24–48 hours after poisoning, and for several days in urine.
• Chemical determination of arsenic in water (>0.25 ppm potentially toxic) or feedstuffs can be performed.
• Skin or hair can be tested in animals exposed for more than 2 weeks.

IMAGING
N/A

OTHER DIAGNOSTIC PROCEDURES
N/A

PATHOLOGIC FINDINGS
• Gross findings include pale, swollen liver and kidneys, and generalized or localized reddening of the gastrointestinal mucosa with hemorrhage, erosions, submucosal edema, and sloughing of the mucosal lining into the gut lumen. In ruminants, the abomasum is often the most severely affected region.
• Peracute cases may have no abnormalities on gross inspection.
• Histopathologic findings include hepatic and renal tubular necrosis; dilation of intestinal capillaries, submucosal congestion and edema, and intestinal epithelial necrosis.

TREATMENT

THERAPEUTIC APPROACH
• Recently exposed animals may benefit from maneuvers to reduce further ingestion and absorption of arsenic from the gastrointestinal tract.
• Effective treatment of clinically affected animals relies on supportive medical care in addition to targeted chelation therapy.
• Fluid support and blood transfusion may be required in severely affected animals.

SURGICAL CONSIDERATIONS AND TECHNIQUES
N/A

MEDICATIONS

DRUGS OF CHOICE
• Absorption from the rumen after recent ingestion may be reduced via administration of mineral oil, or by rumen gavage or rumenotomy.
• Chelation therapy can be attempted using:
  ○ Thioctic acid (lipoic acid)—50 mg/kg, IM, q8h (20% solution divided into two to three injection sites).
  ○ Thioctic acid should be used in combination with dimercaprol at 3 mg/kg, IM, q4h for 2 days, q6h on day 3, then q12h for 10 days. Dimercaprol is also known as British anti-lewisite (BAL) and is recommended for treating trivalent inorganic or aliphatic organic arsenic toxicity.
  ○ Sodium thiosulfate—IV: 30–40 mg/kg; PO: 20–30 g in 300 mL water (cattle) or 5–7.5 g in sheep and goats given q12h or q8h for 3–4 days.
  ○ d-penicillamine (may be cost prohibitive)—10–50 mg/kg, PO, q8h–q6h for 3–4 days.
  ○ 2,3-dimercaptosuccinic acid (DMSA, a water-soluble analog of dimercaprol)—10 mg/kg, PO, q8h has been recommended in small animals.

CONTRAINDICATIONS
N/A

PRECAUTIONS
• The source of arsenic exposure should be identified to reduce human risk.
• Carcasses should be disposed of carefully to avoid environmental contamination.
• Appropriate milk and meat withdrawal times must be followed for all compounds administered to food-producing animals.

POSSIBLE INTERACTIONS
N/A

(CONTINUED) | **ARSENIC TOXICOSIS** | **A**

FOLLOW-UP

EXPECTED COURSE AND PROGNOSIS
Death can occur within the first 3–5 days of clinical signs; surviving animals may demonstrate slow recovery over several weeks.

POSSIBLE COMPLICATIONS
• Bacteremia/septicemia from severe gastrointestinal damage
• Renal failure

CLIENT EDUCATION
Avoid access by ruminants to heavy metals.

PATIENT CARE
Fluid and nutritional support, and nursing care are indicated to optimize survival.

PREVENTION
Avoid access by ruminants to heavy metals.

MISCELLANEOUS

ASSOCIATED CONDITIONS
• Colic
• Renal failure
• Anemia

AGE-RELATED FACTORS
N/A

ZOONOTIC POTENTIAL
N/A

PREGNANCY
Pregnant animals may abort.

BIOSECURITY
N/A

PRODUCTION MANAGEMENT
N/A

SYNONYMS
N/A

ABBREVIATIONS
• BAL = British anti-lewisite
• BVDV = bovine viral diarrhea virus
• DMSA = 2, 3-dimercaptosuccinic acid
• DSMA = disodium methane arsenate
• MSMA = monosodium methane arsenate

SEE ALSO
Toxicology: Herd Outbreaks

Suggested Reading
Dash JR, Datta BK, Sarkar S, Mandal TK. Chronic arsenicosis in cattle: possible mitigation with Zn and Se. Ecotoxicol Environ Saf 2013, 92: 119–22.
Faires MC. Inorganic arsenic toxicosis in a beef herd. Can Vet J 2004, 45: 329–31.
Garland T. Arsenic. In: Gupta RC ed, Veterinary Toxicology, Basic and Clinical Principles, 2nd ed. New York: Elsevier, 2012, pp. 499–502.

Hullinger G, Sangster L, Colvin B, Frazier K. Bovine arsenic toxicosis from ingestion of ashed copper-chrome-arsenate treated timber. Vet Hum Toxicol 1998, 40: 147–8.
Selby LA, Case AA, Osweiler GD, Hayes HM. Epidemiology and toxicology of arsenic poisoning in domestic animals. Environ Health Perspect 1977, 19: 183–9.
Stair EL, Kirkpatrick JG, Whitenack DL. Lead arsenate poisoning in a herd of beef cattle. J Am Vet Med Assoc 1995, 207: 341–3.
Thatcher CD, Meldrum JB, Wikse SE, Whittier WD. Arsenic toxicosis and suspected chromium toxicosis in a herd of cattle. J Am Vet Med Assoc 1985, 187: 179–82.
Valentine BA, Rumbeiha WK, Hensley TS, Halse RR. Arsenic and metaldehyde toxicosis in a beef herd. J Vet Diagn Invest 2007, 19: 212–15.

Author Marianne Polunas
Consulting Editor Erica C. McKenzie
Acknowledgment The author and book editors acknowledge the prior contribution of Joe Roder.

ARTHROGRYPOSIS

 BASICS

OVERVIEW

• Arthrogryposis is not a specific diagnosis, but rather a clinical finding of congenital contractures; these may be present in numerous disorders.

• Congenital arthrogryposis ("crooked joint") is defined as a syndrome of persistent joint flexure or contracture present at birth and may involve one or multiple limbs (forelimbs and/or hindlimbs).

• The carpal and phalangeal joints are most commonly affected, followed by metacarpophalangeal and metatarsophalangeal joints.

• Arthrogryposis is often associated with cleft palate and primary CNS lesions such as hydranencephaly and syringomyelia. Severely affected animals may also have scoliosis, kyphosis, and torticollis; with rotation, abduction, or curled limbs.

• The arthrogryposis-hydranencephaly syndrome (AHS) is usually associated with flexural contracture of the limbs rather than angular limb deformities (ALDs).

• In contrast with contracted tendons, arthrogryposis involves improper articular alignment or rotational deformity.

• Crooked calf disease (CCD) is a congenital deformity condition widely recognized in western North America, characterized by arthrogryposis, scoliosis, torticollis, and cleft palate. CCD is observed in calves after maternal ingestion of lupines containing the quinolizidine alkaloid anagyrine during gestation days 40–100.

• Congenital arthrogryposis may be associated with denervation muscle atrophy.

• The terms "arthrogryposis multiplex congenita" and "congenital articular rigidity" have been introduced to describe cases in which the rigidity may be due to lack of extensibility of muscles, tendons, ligaments, or other tissues around the joint, or to deformity of articular surfaces, or to fusion between bones at the articular surface.

INCIDENCE/PREVALENCE

• For CCD, there are reports of up to 40% of calves from a single herd being affected. The incidence of disease varies with year, area, and herd.

• Cattle records reveal that the disease usually affects <10% of a herd.

GEOGRAPHIC DISTRIBUTION

• Arthrogryposis is thought to occur worldwide. Depending on the etiologic cause and based on the distribution of vectors, viruses, and plants, the geographic distribution of individual syndromes may vary (e.g., CCD is most common in western North America).

• Calf arthrogryposis has been reported from most parts of the world and in many breeds of cattle.

SYSTEMS AFFECTED

Musculoskeletal

PATHOPHYSIOLOGY

• Congenital arthrogryposis is considered multifactorial in origin and has multiple predisposing factors and etiologies, including inherited defects. The causes are often not clear.

• Can be caused by a number of etiologic agents including: plant teratogens, spinal dysraphism, prenatal viral infections that affect the nervous system, and in utero hormonal and vascular defects.

• May also be attributed to a decrease or lack of motion of the fetus during critical stages of development, such as malpositioning and overcrowding caused by the size of the fetus relative to the dam.

• Ingestion of teratogenic plants such as *Astragalus* or *Oxytropis* spp. (locoweed); *Verratrum californicum* (skunk cabbage); piperidine alkaloid-containing plants such as *Lupinus, Conium,* and *Nicotiana* species.

  ○ Repeated dosing or continuous low-level ingestion over time may result in cumulative intoxication and/or teratogenesis.

  ○ Teratogenic plant alkaloids may be transferred to the placenta and induce a sedative or anesthetic effect in the fetus.

• In CCD, there is often a lesion in the CNS that may result in reduced or absence of movement of the affected body parts in the developing fetus, especially during the period of rapid growth. Alpha-motor neurons in the cervical spinal cord are significantly reduced.

• May cause disruption in normal innervation of muscles leading to paresis and instability of the limb, or may result in hypotonic condition of extensor muscle and dysfunction of the radial nerve.

HISTORICAL FINDINGS

A complete history including age, birthing details, age at which the deformity was noticed, course and progression of deformity, diets of affected animal and dam should be obtained. The animal may be normal at birth and develop the flexural deformity within hours or days.

SIGNALMENT

Species

Bovine, ovine, caprine, and camelid species

Breed Predilections

• Certain syndromes are predominantly reported to occur in certain breeds (e.g., congenital arthrogryposis in Charolais cattle). CCD has been observed in most dairy breeds and in all breeds of beef cattle common to western North America.

• No breed predilection or genetic susceptibility in cattle to the lupine-induced condition has been determined.

Mean Age and Range

• Arthrogryposis tends to affect young, growing animals. The incidence of CCD is highest in heifers at first calving, but the disease has been observed in calves from cows of all ages.

• For each species (cattle, sheep, and goats), there are specific periods of gestation when the fetus is susceptible to plant teratogens. The critical gestational period for exposure of cattle to lupines is 40–70 days with susceptible periods extending to 100 days.

Predominant Sex

No apparent sex predisposition

PHYSICAL EXAMINATION FINDINGS

• The animal's conformation should be assessed first by having the animal stand in a symmetrical manner on a firm, flat surface and observing it from multiple angles.

• Arthrogryposis in CCD is characterized by deformities of the limbs (rigid flexion of elbows and carpal joints) and spinal column (scoliosis, lordosis, kyphosis), and rib cage abnormalities. Affected calves occasionally have torticollis and cleft palate.

• The joints are often flexed and cannot be extended even after the flexor tendons are cut—distinguishing the disease from contracted tendons.

GENETICS

• Some genetic patterns have been worked out, for example, the arthrogryposis multiplex anomaly of Angus cattle is thought to be a simple autosomal recessive pattern.

• Syndromes in the Charolais, Friesian, Swedish, and Red Danish breeds of cattle are consistent with a simple recessive or modified recessive characteristic.

• Dominant defect traits are inherited as well and are sometimes selected for.

• Lambs: A congenital arthrogryposis exists in pedigree Suffolk and Australian Merino lambs as an inherited limb deformity.

CAUSES AND RISK FACTORS

A number of etiologic agents such as intrauterine infection with Border disease virus, BVDV, Akabane virus, Cache Valley virus, bluetongue virus, Aino virus, Kasba (Chuzan) virus, Rift Valley Fever virus, Schmallenberg virus, and Wesselsbron virus, as well as teratogenic plant ingestion have been implicated in the pathogenesis of arthrogryposis in ruminants.

Congenital Predisposing Factors

• Uterine malpositioning

• Genetic causes

• Ingestion of teratogenic plants by pregnant dam such as *Astragalus* or *Oxytropis* spp. (locoweed); *Verratrum californicum* (skunk cabbage); piperidine alkaloid-containing plants such as *Lupinus, Conium,* and *Nicotiana* species.

• Conditions associated with arthrogryposis include CCD/congenital arthrogryposis, HC (hereditary chondrodysplasia or spider lamb

syndrome), ill-thrift syndrome in llamas, metabolic, and neurovascular disorders.
• Leg deformities in young calves are most commonly associated with congenital contraction of the tendons. Flexural deformities involving contracted tendons and ligaments may be seen in many breeds of cattle and small ruminants.

Risk Factors
Predisposing factors for congenital arthrogryposis include male calves, posterior intrauterine presentation, and double muscling.

DIAGNOSIS

DIFFERENTIAL DIAGNOSES
• Arthrogryposis and CCD differ from contracted tendons; in animals with contracted tendons, the joints are usually properly aligned and the legs are not rotated. In calves with arthrogryposis, the articular and osseous changes are usually permanent and worsen as the calf grows.
• Fracture malunion.
• See "Causes and Risk Factors" (viruses and toxic plants).
• Arthrogryposis-hydranencephaly syndrome (AHS) in lambs may be confused with HC.

CBC/BIOCHEMISTRY/URINALYSIS
N/A

OTHER LABORATORY TESTS
N/A

IMAGING
• Radiographs can be used to diagnose ALDs; at least two views, 90 degrees apart, should be taken of the affected joint.
• The dorsopalmar/dorsoplantar (DP) view is needed for examination of the anatomic location of the deformity and for measurements. Shoot with radiographic beam in line with the claws.

OTHER DIAGNOSTIC PROCEDURES
• Serology and virologic diagnostic assays may aid in ruling out in utero viral infections (e.g., Cache Valley virus).
• Feed analysis and assessment of the availability of potentially toxic plants in the environment (pasture) may assist in diagnosis.

PATHOLOGIC FINDINGS
• No consistent primary lesion in CCD; a number of varied tissue responses are observed. It is likely that these findings are at least in part due to the animal's inability to stand.
• CCD histology: Few lesions, restricted to muscles of the forelimb, external intercostalis muscle, or radial and femoral nerves—myositis, myodegeneration, muscle necrosis and atrophy, cellulitis, and perineuritis.

TREATMENT

THERAPEUTIC APPROACH
• Severely affected animals may be unable to rise to nurse and require additional supportive care.
• Protect limbs with thick, soft bandages that fit well. Minor deformities may be corrected by manual alignment and external support of the limb (e.g., rigid splinting, bandaging, or casting/tube casts).
• Provide good footing and allow for stretching of flexor tendons.
• Maintain a soft (padding), clean, and dry environment to minimize decubital/pressure sores, open arthritis, muscle atrophy, umbilical infections, and septicemia.
• Restrict activity until it is certain that the deformity is improving; however, some degree of exercise allows for stretching and lengthening of affected limb structures. Weight bearing provides the necessary physical exercise to strengthen and lengthen affected tendons and musculature.
• Dietary imbalances should be addressed while treating cases of arthrogryposis.

SURGICAL CONSIDERATIONS AND TECHNIQUES
• Surgery may be required for animals with severe deformities and for animals that do not improve with age or conservative management.
• Treatment of arthrogryposis includes surgery to improve the animal's posture sufficient for it to obtain slaughter weight (a salvage procedure).
• Surgical procedures include transection of flexor tendon and suspensory ligament, joint capsule release, flexor tendon lengthening procedures, and joint arthrodesis.
• May require postoperative splinting or casting for support.

MEDICATIONS

DRUGS OF CHOICE
N/A

CONTRAINDICATIONS
N/A

PRECAUTIONS
N/A

POSSIBLE INTERACTIONS
N/A

ALTERNATIVE DRUGS
N/A

FOLLOW-UP

EXPECTED COURSE AND PROGNOSIS
• The prognosis is guarded, depending on the severity of the flexural deformity. Severe deformities requiring surgery often have a poor prognosis.
• For arthrogryposis in cattle, approximately 80% of surgically treated animals can be kept until they reach normal slaughter weight.

POSSIBLE COMPLICATIONS
Some severe cases of arthrogryposis cannot be corrected and full extension may not be possible postoperatively.

CLIENT EDUCATION
• Examination of young animals with congenital arthrogryposis should be done as early as possible to assess the degree of manual correction possible.
• Because of a possible hereditary component associated with some forms of arthrogryposis, breeding of affected animals is not recommended.
• Many affected animals are stillborn or die shortly after birth. Others may fail to thrive and euthanasia should be considered.

PATIENT CARE
Frequent physical examinations and assessing the efficacy of corrective measures should be done to monitor progress.

PREVENTION
• CCD/HC: Avoid breeding affected animals.
• Coordinate grazing times and alter breeding dates to minimize exposure. Avoid grazing potentially teratogenic plants when pregnant cows are at the susceptible stage of pregnancy.
• Control teratogenic plant populations with herbicides.

MISCELLANEOUS

ASSOCIATED CONDITIONS
A syndrome known as "bentleg" or "bowie" has been associated with ingestion of *Trachymene glaucifolia* (wild parsnip) by pregnant ewes in Australia and New Zealand.

AGE-RELATED FACTORS
Majority of cases occur during the active growth phase of the affected bone/joint.

ZOONOTIC POTENTIAL
N/A

PREGNANCY
In cases of congenital arthrogryposis, the teratogenic plants are ingested by the pregnant dam and the compounds are passed to the fetus through the placenta.

BIOSECURITY
N/A

ARTHROGRYPOSIS

PRODUCTION MANAGEMENT
• Producers should be aware of the association between certain toxic plants (e.g., lupines) and angular limb deformities such as CCD.
• To reduce the incidence of CCD, graze lupines during their least hazardous growth period and reduce exposure of pregnant cows. Lupines are most hazardous when they are young or in the mature seed stage.
• Fence off heavily infested pasture areas and use intermittent, short-term grazing of lupine pastures.

SYNONYMS
N/A

ABBREVIATIONS
• AHS = arthrogryposis-hydranencephaly syndrome
• ALD = angular limb deformity
• BVDV = bovine viral diarrhea virus
• CCD = crooked calf disease/syndrome
• CNS = central nervous system
• DP = dorsopalmar/dorsoplantar
• HC = hereditary chondrodysplasia
• IBR = infectious bovine rhinotracheitis virus

SEE ALSO
• Akabane
• Angular Limb Deformities
• Brain Assessment and Dysfunction (see www.fiveminutevet.com/ruminant)
• Cache Valley Virus
• Lameness: Bovine
• Lameness: Camelid
• Lameness: Small Ruminants
• Lupine Toxicity
• Schmallenberg Virus
• Wesselsbron Disease

Suggested Reading
Aiello SE ed. The Merck Veterinary Manual, 2015. Retrieved from http://www.merckvetmanual.com/mvm/index.html
Maxie GM. Jubb, Kennedy, and Palmer's Pathology of domestic animals, vol. 1, 6th ed. New York: Saunders Elsevier, 2015.
Panter KE, James LF, Gardner DR. Lupines, poison-hemlock and *Nicotiana* spp: toxicity and teratogenicity in livestock. J Nat Toxins 1999, 8: 117–34.
Panter, K.E., Keeler RF, Bunch TD, Callon RJ. Congenital skeletal malformations and cleft palate induced in goats by ingestion of *Lupinus, Conium,* and *Nicotiana* species. Toxicon 1990, 28: 1377–85.
Peperkamp NH, Luttikholt SJ, Dijkman R, et al. Ovine and bovine congenital abnormalities associated with intrauterine infection with Schmallenberg virus. Vet Pathol 2015, 52: 1057–66.
Radostits OM, Gay CC, Hinchcliff KW, Constable PD eds. Veterinary Medicine: A Textbook of the Diseases of Cattle, Horses, Sheep, Pigs, and Goats, 10th ed. New York: Elsevier Saunders, 2008.
Steiner A, Anderson DE, Desrochers A. Diseases of the tendons and tendon sheaths. Vet Clin North Am: Food Anim Pract 2014, 30: 157–75.
Van Huffel X, De Moor A. Congenital multiple arthrogryposis of the forelimbs in calves. Compend Food Anim 1987, 9: F333–9.
Washburn KE, Streeter RN. Congenital defects of the ruminant nervous system. Vet Clin North Am: Food Anim Pract 2004, 20: 413–34.

Authors Erik J. Olson and Nicholas A. Robinson
Consulting Editor Kaitlyn A. Lutz
Acknowledgment The authors and book editors acknowledge the prior contribution of Cathy S. Carlson.

BASICS

OVERVIEW
Artificial insemination (AI) is the aseptic delivery of viable spermatozoa into the female reproductive tract (uterus).

INCIDENCE/PREVELENCE
AI is more prevalent in dairy cattle than beef cattle.

GEOGRAPHIC DISTRIBUTION
Worldwide

SYSTEMS AFFECTED
Reproductive

PATHOPHYSIOLOGY
• Improvements in semen extenders, implementation of protocols for estrus synchronization and timed insemination, and availability of sex-sorted semen have increased the use and importance of AI in cattle.
• Advantages of AI over natural service:
  ◦ Efficient use and dissemination of valuable bull genetics
  ◦ Eliminate cost associated with bull maintenance
  ◦ Decreased risk of sexually transmitted diseases
  ◦ Fewer breeding-related injuries
  ◦ Enables evaluation of semen before insemination
• AI success is dependent on semen quality and handling, timing, site of deposition, and female fertility.
• Acceptable fertility in an AI program involves excellent management of all phases of the program.

HISTORICAL FINDINGS
• Estrus synchronization and timed AI
• Cows selected based on estrus detection

SIGNALMENT
Females of breeding age

PHYSICAL EXAMINATION FINDINGS
• Estrus behavior and observations:
  ◦ Standing to be mounted (cardinal sign of estrus)
  ◦ Cervical mucus discharge
  ◦ Mounting other cattle
  ◦ Increased locomotion and vocalization
  ◦ Decreased feed intake/milk production

Semen Collection and Cryopreservation
• Semen used for AI is commonly collected using an artificial vagina (AV) (most common in commercial AI bull centers) or by electroejaculation (custom freezing of bulls not trained to an AV, salvage of genetics from terminally ill bulls).
• Epididymal spermatozoa may be collected to salvage genetics from bulls following catastrophic injury or terminal illness.
• Semen collected with an AV presents better post-thaw motility than semen collected with electroejaculation.

• Although fresh/cooled semen may be used in some ranches, most AI in the bovine uses frozen-thawed semen.
• Semen is frozen after dilution in various commercial extenders in the presence of antibiotics, egg yolk, and glycerol.
• Bovine sperm is usually frozen in 0.25 or 0.5 mL straws. The majority of sex-sorted (gender-selected) semen is packaged in 0.25 mL straws.
• In general, the total dose per straw is 10 to 20 million motile spermatozoa. However, this dose is considerably lower for elite bulls and sex-sorted semen. Higher doses are used for bulls with lower fertility or in custom freezing of beef bulls.
• The cryopreservation process varies slightly depending on extender and technique used.

Factors Affecting AI Success
Quality of Semen
• The quality of frozen-thawed semen depends on initial quality at production, handling during storage, thawing procedures, and interval until deposition into the uterus.
• Quality at production is affected by initial quality of the ejaculate, method of collection used, the inherent freezability, and methods of processing used for cryopreservation.
• Repeated exposure to temperature above −80°C may cause changes in liquid/frozen phase and damage to the sperm membrane. This can occur during handling or transfer of straws between tanks or may be due to faulty tank performance and lack of verification of LN level. To prevent these problems, the following points should be observed:
  ◦ LN tank management:
    ▪ Keep in a cool, dry, well-ventilated area away from direct sunlight.
    ▪ Check LN level frequently. Presence of frost on the surface of the LN tank is a sign of leakage.
    ▪ Place LN tanks on a wooden or plastic dolly above concrete or wet floors to prevent corrosion.
    ▪ Keep a precise inventory for quick identification of straws to be used.
    ▪ Attach LN refill date logs to the tank.
  ◦ Removing straws from the tank:
    ▪ Remove straws quickly without exposing other straws to air.
    ▪ Do not raise canisters higher than 10 cm above the neck of the LN tank; do not raise the top of the goblet in the canister above the frost line in the neck of the tank.
    ▪ Ensure that the goblet is always filled with LN.
    ▪ Always use forceps to remove straws from the goblets.
  ◦ Handling at the time of use:
    ▪ Use recommended thawing temperature and time. Recommendation of the NAAB is immersion in the water bath at 30–35°C for at least 40 seconds. Others recommend thawing at 70°C for 6 seconds or 35–37°C for 30 seconds.

Thawing at high temperatures may be very difficult to observe in field conditions.
  ▪ Thawing procedures should be strictly observed.
  ▪ Check water baths for temperature control accuracy.
  ▪ Use a stopwatch for the timing of thawing.
  ▪ In cold areas, it is preferable to keep straws in the water bath, at 35°C, until use.
  ▪ Prevent exposure of the straw to low temperatures after thawing: use a pre-warmed insemination gun; protect prepared gun from exposure to low temperature.
  ▪ Thaw out straws and prepare insemination guns in a sheltered area when ready to inseminate.
  ▪ Clean and dry straws before loading in the AI gun.
  ▪ Straws should be cut using straw cutters to prevent backflow of semen during insemination.
  ▪ Time period from removal of straw from the tank to insemination should not exceed 15 minutes.

Timing of Insemination
• Insemination timing is important to maximize conception rates. Ovulation occurs 28–32 hours after the beginning of estrus. Optimum fertility of the oocyte is 6–12 hours after ovulation and the viable lifespan of spermatozoa in the reproductive tract is estimated to be between 24 and 30 hours.
• The optimal time for insemination is 12 hours after first observed estrus. This has led to the AM/PM rule: if a cow is observed in estrus in the morning she is inseminated in the afternoon, and vice versa.
• Several schemes for timed insemination have been developed.
• Double insemination at a 12-hour interval is sometimes performed in cows with decreased fertility, when using semen straws with lower concentration, or in cows that have been superstimulated for embryo collection.

Insemination Technique
• Semen should be deposited at the proper site without excess manipulation.
• People who inseminate cows periodically cannot achieve a high level of expertise.
• Semen is deposited in the body of the uterus by transrectal manipulation of the insemination gun for cervical catheterization.
• Deep horn insemination may reduce conception rates in the hands of untrained people due to irritation of the uterus.
• Deep uterine insemination may be important when low spermatozoa numbers are used (i.e., sexed semen).
• Good inseminators should be able to pass the cervix rapidly and with a high degree of reliability. Cervical catheterization is particularly difficult in some breeds of cattle (e.g., Santa Gertrudis).

• Strict hygienic measures should be observed during insemination to prevent vaginal or uterine contamination.
• Use a protective plastic sheath (cannula or chemisette) to help prevent contamination.

GENETICS
Semen is selected based on specific selection criteria.

CAUSES AND RISK FACTORS
N/A

DIAGNOSIS

DIFFERENTIAL DIAGNOSIS
N/A

CBC/BIOCHEMISTRY/URINALYSIS
N/A

OTHER LABORATORY TESTS
• Serum progesterone concentration <2 ng/mL may confirm estrus activity.
• Diagnosis of pregnancy can be performed by detection of serum pregnancy associated glycoproteins.

IMAGING
• Ultrasonography of the reproductive tract in an estrus female should reveal a dominant follicle (>10 mm diameter), regressing or absent CL, and uterine edema.
• Diagnosis of pregnancy as early as 28 days post-ovulation.

DIAGNOSTIC PROCEDURES
N/A

PATHOLOGIC FINDINGS
N/A

TREATMENT

APPROPRIATE HEALTH CARE
N/A

SURGICAL CONSIDERATIONS AND TECHNIQUES
N/A

MEDICATIONS

DRUGS OF CHOICE
N/A

CONTRAINDICATIONS
N/A

PRECAUTIONS
N/A

POSSIBLE INTERACTIONS
N/A

ALTERNATIVE DRUGS
N/A

FOLLOW-UP

EXPECTED COURSE AND PROGNOSIS
• Pregnancy rates depend on many factors: breed, quality of semen, site of semen deposition, nutrition, milk production (dairy), environmental conditions, parity, type of synchronization program, and human factors.
• Conception rates following artificial insemination range between 40 and 50% in cows and 60 to 70% in heifers. However, in dairy cattle, pregnancy rates 35 to 40 days following AI are generally between 20% and 30% due to a high early embryonic loss.
• In addition to the factors already mentioned, other factors involved in decreased conception rate in dairy cows are:
  ○ Insemination of non-estrous cows
  ○ Heat stress prior to artificial insemination
  ○ Incidence of postparturient diseases
  ○ Clinical mastitis

POSSIBLE COMPLICATIONS
Perforation of the vagina or uterus by unskilled or inexperienced technicians.

PATIENT CARE
Appropriate estrus detection and handling to reduce stress.

PREVENTION
N/A

MISCELLANEOUS

ASSOCIATED CONDITIONS
N/A

AGE-RELATED FACTORS
Normal conception rates have been achieved with as low as 2 million spermatozoa in heifers.

ZOONOTIC POTENTIAL
N/A

PREGNANCY
See "Expected Course and Prognosis"

BIOSECURITY
• Use semen from bulls routinely tested for brucellosis, IBR, BVD, trichomoniasis, and campylobacteriosis, as well as bluetongue virus (Certified Semen Service).
• Bacteriologic quality of semen is ensured by strict hygiene during collection and use of specific guidelines for antimicrobials in the extenders (Certified Semen Service).
• All straws are properly labeled, identifying the semen center, bull, breed, and date on which semen was collected.

PRODUCTION MANAGEMENT
Use a professional inseminator.

SYNONYMS
N/A

ABBREVIATIONS
• AI = artificial insemination
• AV = artificial vagina
• BVD = bovine viral diarrhea
• CL = corpus luteum
• IBR = infectious bovine rhinotracheitis
• LN = liquid nitrogen
• NAAB = National Association of Animal Breeders

SEE ALSO
• Beef Bull Management (see www.fiveminutevet.com/ruminant)
• Estrus Synchronization: Bovine
• Reproductive Pharmacology
• Reproductive Ultrasonography: Bovine (see www.fiveminutevet.com/ruminant)

Suggested Reading
Chebel RC, Santos JEP, Reynolds JP et al. Factors affecting conception rate after artificial insemination and pregnancy loss in lactating dairy cows. Anim Reprod Sci 2004, 84: 239–55.

Kaproth M, Rycroft H, Gilbert G, et al. Effect of semen thaw method on conception rate in four large commercial dairy heifer herds. Theriogenology 2005, 63: 2535–49.

Kasimanickam R. Artificial insemination. In: Hopper R (ed) Bovine Reproduction, Wiley Blackwell, 2015; pp. 295–303.

Lopez-Gatius, F. Site of semen deposition in cattle: a review. Theriogenology 2000, 53: 1407–14.

Rath D, Johnson LA. Application and commercialization of flow cytometrically sex-sorted semen. Reprod Dom Anim 2008; 43: 338–46.

Author Alexis Campbell
Consulting Editor Ahmed Tibary
Acknowledgment The author and book editors acknowledge the prior contribution of Ahmed Tibary, Paul E Mennick, and John Gibbons.

BASICS

OVERVIEW
• Artificial insemination (AI) is used in sheep and goat herds to improve genetics, improve reproductive efficiency of males, reduce disease transmission, and permit out-of-season breeding.
• Success of an AI program is affected by several factors including timing, semen quality, and semen placement.
• For economic reasons, except in a few cases (dairy goat), most AI is performed at a fixed time following synchronization of estrus.

INCIDENCE/PREVALENCE
• AI using fresh or cooled semen is a common procedure in several countries.
• AI with frozen-thawed semen is more common in dairy goats.

GEOGRAPHIC DISTRIBUTION
Worldwide

SYSTEMS AFFECTED
Reproductive

PATHOPHYSIOLOGY
• Adequate fertilization rates are achieved when sperm form a reservoir at the level of the isthmus of the uterine tube and remain viable until ovulation occurs.
• Fertilization rates are dependent on quality of semen, adequate transport to the fertilization site, and proper timing in relationship to ovulation.
• In small ruminants, semen is deposited onto the cervix after natural mating. Sperm is selectively transported through the cervix into the uterus and only highly motile, morphologically normal sperm is found in the isthmus.
• With AI the number of sperm used is significantly lower than in natural mating. In addition, processing and cryopreservation reduces sperm viability. Therefore, timing and site of deposition of sperm are critical in achieving acceptable fertilization rates.
• Oocyte viability is extremely reduced beyond 12 hours post-ovulation. AI should be performed within 12 hours after onset of estrus.
• The number of viable spermatozoa per insemination required for adequate fertilization rates depends on quality and site of semen deposition. Ideally, preserved semen (chilled or frozen-thawed) should be deposited into the uterine cavity.
• In sheep and small breeds of goats, TCI is extremely difficult due to the tortuous anatomy of the cervical canal. To bypass the cervix, insemination is performed laparoscopically.

HISTORICAL FINDINGS
• Flock or herd desiring to improve genetics
• Out-of-season breeding

SIGNALMENT
Postpubertal female sheep and goats

PHYSICAL EXAMINATION FINDINGS
• Females to be inseminated should be in estrus.
• Estrus detection may be performed with a teaser male (sheep and goat) or by visual observation (goats).
• Females in estrus will show typical receptive behavior. Does express estrus more intensely than ewes (tail fanning, mounting other females, and standing to be mounted).
• Females in estrus show variable degrees of vulvar swelling and mucus discharge. Mucus is clear and runny at the beginning of estrus and becomes thick and whitish near ovulation.
• On vaginoscopy, the cervix is hyperemic and open.

Artificial Insemination Techniques
Semen Source and Processing
• Semen is collected from selected males using an artificial vagina (preferred) or electroejaculation.
• Only high-quality ejaculates are used. Semen is diluted in one of a variety of available commercial extenders (milk-based, egg yolk-based, or new chemically defined soybean lecithin-based).
  ○ Milk-based extenders are commonly used for fresh, chilled (4°C) or cooled (15°C) semen insemination. Skim-milk or UHT-treated milk is used in order to remove lactenin which is spermicidal.
  ○ Tris-based egg yolk extenders are used routinely for cryopreservation. However, egg yolk is toxic to buck semen because of the presence of lipase produced by the bulbourethral gland (*BUSgp60*). Buck semen needs to be washed prior to addition of egg yolk-based extender. An alternative is to use a minimal quantity of egg yolk in the extender.
  ○ Chemically defined media have been shown to be effective for the cryopreservation of small ruminant sperm. They offer the advantage of not containing any additional animal products, which guarantee its biosecurity for international movement of semen.
  ○ Additional improvement in preservation of semen has been achieved by addition of antioxidants.
• Small ruminant sperm is cryopreserved in either 0.25 mL or 0.5 mL straws and rarely in pellet form. Semen handling and thawing procedures (time and temperature) are critical for viability.

Timing of Insemination
• Natural estrus: AI is performed 12 hours after detection of estrus. A second insemination is often needed 12 hours later if frozen-thawed semen is used.
• Fixed time after synchronization:
  ○ TCI insemination: Sheep – 55 hours (1 dose) or 50 and 60 hours (2 doses) after progesterone removal. Goats – 45 to 65

hours (1 dose) or 30 and 48 hours (2 doses) after progesterone removal.
  ○ Laparoscopic AI: 54 to 60 hours after progestogen removal (6 to 8 hours earlier for frozen-thawed semen) in sheep, and 43 to 46 hours after progesterone removal in goats.
Method of Insemination
• Blind vaginal insemination—At least 400 million sperm are blindly deposited around the external cervical os. This technique is useful only when fresh, extended semen is used.
• Intracervical—At least 200 million sperm are deposited into the cervical canal as far as the AI gun can advance.
• TCI—Between 50 and 100 million spermatozoa are required. TCI is used more in goats as the cervix is more easily catheterized. In sheep, TCI is limited by the morphology of the sheep cervix, which is long, tortuous, and narrow, with nonconcentric rings. However, several techniques have been proposed to improve TCI in sheep; these include the use of special cradles for restraint, and the use of flexible AI guns.
• Laparoscopic—Semen is injected directly into the uterus via laparoscopic portals. Between 20 and 40 million sperm are required (15–20 million if sex-sorted). Drawbacks to this technique include the need for sedation or anesthesia of the animal, laparoscopic equipment, increased labor time and costs, and postoperative monitoring.

GENETICS
AI is the best method for rapid genetic improvement of a flock or herd.

CAUSES AND RISK FACTORS
N/A

DIAGNOSIS

DIFFERENTIAL DIAGNOSIS
N/A

CBC/BIOCHEMISTRY/URINALYSIS
N/A

OTHER LABORATORY TESTS
Semen analysis

IMAGING
Transrectal or transabdominal ultrasonography for pregnancy diagnosis following artificial insemination.

OTHER DIAGNOSTIC PROCEDURES
Pregnancy diagnosis using serum concentration of pregnancy associated glycoproteins.

PATHOLOGIC FINDINGS
N/A

TREATMENT

THERAPEUTIC APPROACH
• Estrus should be synchronized using approved hormonal methods of synchronization.
• Several treatments (oxytocin, estrogen, ß-adrenergic blocking agents, relaxin, and PGE) have been used in sheep to induce cervical relaxation for TCI but were not very successful.

SURGICAL CONSIDERATIONS AND TECHNIQUE
• Estrus animals displaying systemic illness should not be selected for surgical insemination. Obese and non-fasted animals present surgical challenges.
• Animals should be fasted for 18–24 hours prior to laparoscopic AI (LAI).
• LAI is performed under sedation and local block in sheep. Heavy sedation or general anesthesia is preferred in goats. The animal is placed in dorsal recumbency on a cradle in a Trendelenburg position. The ventral abdomen is clipped and prepared for surgery.
• Two portals are created on each side (about 5 cm) of the linea alba and about 6–10 cm from the cranial border of the mammary gland. The laparoscope is inserted into the abdominal cavity from one portal. The uterus is visualized and the insemination gun is inserted through the other portal using a cannula. The uterine horn is stabbed with the needle of the insemination gun and semen is deposited in the lumen.
• Skin incisions are usually closed with staples or absorbable suture.

MEDICATIONS

DRUGS OF CHOICE
• Sedation and anesthesia: xylazine and ketamine.
• Administration of antibiotics and anti-inflammatories is recommended.

CONTRAINDICATIONS
Appropriate milk and meat withdrawal times must be followed.

PRECAUTIONS
N/A

POSSIBLE INTERACTIONS
N/A

FOLLOW-UP

EXPECTED COURSE AND PROGNOSIS
• Pregnancy rates depend on many factors: species and breed, type of semen used,

extender type, site of deposition of semen, nutrition, season, environmental conditions, parity, the synchronization program used, and human factors.
• Expected conception rates when semen quality and number of spermatozoa are adequate are:
  ◦ Vaginal AI: fresh semen 60–75%; frozen semen 5–30%
  ◦ Intracervical AI: fresh semen 50–80%; frozen semen 35–60%
  ◦ TCI: fresh semen 40–80%; frozen semen 30–70%
  ◦ Laparoscopic AI: fresh semen 40–80%; frozen semen 40–70%.

POSSIBLE COMPLICATIONS
• For surgical complications see "Patient Care."
• TCI in sheep may result in cervical trauma or laceration.

CLIENT EDUATION
• Clients should be aware of factors affecting fertility and the expected pregnancy rates for the type of semen and AI used.

PATIENT CARE
• Animals should be handled with minimal stress.
• After laparoscopic AI, animals should be monitored for complications, including incisional infection or dehiscence, fever, peritonitis, and adhesion formation. Animals should be vaccinated against *Clostridium tetani*. Administration of antibiotics and anti-inflammatories is recommended.
• Pregnancy diagnosis should be performed after an AI program.

PREVENTION
N/A

MISCELLANEOUS

ASSOCIATED CONDITIONS
N/A

AGE-RELATED FACTORS
TCI is more difficult in young maiden females.

ZOONOTIC POTENTIAL
N/A

PREGNANCY
N/A

BIOSECURITY
• All males used for semen collection and AI should have a health screening and infectious disease testing prior to use.
• Hygienic semen collection and processing of semen should be performed according to guidelines described by the Office International des Epizooties.
• Diseases that can be transmitted by semen include: Bluetongue, Border disease,

brucellosis, leptospirosis, paratuberculosis, Q fever, contagious caprine pleuropneumonia, ovine enzootic abortion, Lentivirus infection, peste des petit ruminants, *Salmonella* serotype abortus-ovis, sheep and goat pox.

PRODUCTION MANAGEMENT
• AI with fresh semen allows more efficient use of top sires, particularly after synchronization of estrus.
• Use of frozen semen allows genetic improvement.
• AI after a synchronization program can allow predictable parturition dates and allow segregation of animals on the farm by physiologic status.
• AI can allow for accelerated lambing programs or out-of-season breeding.

SYNONYMS
N/A

ABBREVIATIONS
• AI = artificial insemination
• PGE = prostaglandin E
• TCI = transcervical insemination

SEE ALSO
Estrus Synchronization: Small Ruminants

Suggested Reading
Cseh S, Faigl V, Amiridis GS. Semen processing and artificial insemination in health management of small ruminants. Anim Reprod Sci 2012, 130: 187–92.
Bartlewski PM, Candappa IRR. Assessing the usefulness of prostaglandin E2 (Cervidil) for transcervical artificial insemination in ewes. Theriogenology 2015, 84: 1594–602.
Khalifa T, Lymberopoulos A, Theodosiadou E. Association of soybean-based extenders with field fertility of stored ram (*Ovis aries*) semen: a randomized double-blind parallel group design. Theriogenology 2013, 7: 517–27.
Mata-Capuzzano M, Alvares-Rodriguez M, Tamayo-Canul J, Lopez-Uruena E, Paz PD, Martinez-Pastor F, Alvarez M. Refrigerated storage of ram sperm in presence of Trolox and GSH antioxidants: effect of temperature, extender and storage time. Anim Reprod Sci 2014, 151: 137–47.
Paramio MT, Izquierdo D. Assisted reproductive technologies in goats. Small Rumin Res 2014, 121: 21–6.
Palcin I, Yaniz JL, Fantova E, Blasco ME, Quintin-Casarran FJ, Sevilla-Mur E, Santolaria P. Factors affecting fertility after cervical insemination with cooled semen in meat sheep. Anim Reprod Sci 2012, 132: 139–44.

Author Lisa Pearson
Consulting Editor Ahmed Tibary
Acknowledgment The author and book editors acknowledge the prior contribution of Ahmed Tibary.

BASICS

OVERVIEW
Aspiration pneumonia arises from the inhalation or accidental administration of liquids, pastes, gels or foreign bodies (plant debris, dirt) which can result in inflammatory, gangrenous or granulomatous pneumonia, or in the case of oil aspiration, lipid or lipoid pneumonia. Some substances directly insult the respiratory tissues, while others may induce vigorous inflammatory responses associated with nondegradable foreign material. Secondary bacterial infection is a common sequela.

INCIDENCE/PREVALENCE
Uncommon

GEOGRAPHIC DISTRIBUTION
N/A

SYSTEMS AFFECTED
Respiratory

PATHOPHYSIOLOGY
• The disorder often arises following the accidental or forceful administration of substances and medication by unskilled personnel, or after inappropriate regurgitation/aspiration associated with heavy sedation, anesthesia, or oropharyngeal and esophageal disorders.
• Lung tissue in the cranioventral thorax is most commonly affected after inhalation or instillation of a foreign substance.
• The affected lung tissue is irritated, inflamed, and loses capacity for appropriate clearance, immune function, and oxygenation. Secondary bacterial invasion frequently occurs.

HISTORICAL FINDINGS
Consistent with a primary illness or management activity prompting treatment with oral medications or substances, or preexisting signs of upper gastrointestinal dysfunction.

SIGNALMENT
• Varies with different inciting conditions.
• Young ruminants and crias may suffer aspiration from accidental orotracheal intubation during provision of colostrum or milk; from inhalation of meconium in fetal fluids during difficult parturition; from poorly performed bottle feeding; from congenital disorders such as cleft palate and aortic arch defects; and from acquired disorders such as selenium deficiency and necrotic laryngitis.
• Mature ruminants and camelids may suffer aspiration due to pharyngeal and esophageal dysfunction related to trauma, abscessation, choke, or megaesophagus; infectious diseases (botulism, listeriosis); heavy sedation or anesthesia; toxicities (ingestion of lead, crude oil, fuel oil, natural gas condensate, rhododendron); and from oral medication administration or severe hypocalcemia (lactating cattle).

PHYSICAL EXAMINATION FINDINGS
• Acute-onset depression, tachypnea, coughing, and fever.
• Large volume aspiration can produce dyspnea, tachypnea, tachycardia, nasal discharge, and malodorous breath.
• Thoracic auscultation can reveal adventitious lung sounds, pleural friction rubs, or reduced audibility of ventral lung sounds if pleural fluid accumulates.
• Shock and sudden death may occur.
• Milk or feed material may be seen coming from the nostrils in cases where dysphagia or esophageal disorders are the initiating cause.

GENETICS
N/A

CAUSES AND RISK FACTORS
• Accidental or forceful administration of substances and medication orally or orogastrically by unskilled personnel.
• Heavy sedation or general anesthesia.
• Oropharyngeal and esophageal disorders.
• Submergence dipping of livestock.
• Exposure to poorly cured silage (*Listeria*) or specific toxins in the feed or environment.

DIAGNOSIS

DIFFERENTIAL DIAGNOSES
• Acute bronchopneumonia due to infectious agents or causes other than aspiration.
• Systemic sepsis, particularly in neonates.

CBC/BIOCHEMISTRY/URINALYSIS
• Complete blood count may demonstrate leukocytosis or leukopenia with left shift, elevated total plasma protein, and hyperfibrinogenemia.
• Serum chemistry may demonstrate hyperglobulinemia and azotemia, and/or specific electrolyte abnormalities such as hypocalcemia.

OTHER LABORATORY TESTS
N/A

IMAGING
• Radiographs typically show alveolar-interstitial pattern that is most pronounced in the cranioventral lung fields. Pleural fluid lines or pulmonary abscesses may be evident.
• Ultrasonography reveals cranioventral consolidation with or without pleural effusion.
• Pharyngeal abscessation or trauma, and esophageal dilation, stricture or obstruction may be evident on radiographs (contrast enhancement can be performed if indicated).

OTHER DIAGNOSTIC PROCEDURES
• Endoscopic or transtracheal wash can be performed to obtain samples for cytologic examination and aerobic and anaerobic bacterial culture and sensitivity procedures.
• Endoscopy of the upper gastrointestinal tract is appropriate to investigate pharyngeal and esophageal disorders.

PATHOLOGIC FINDINGS
• Reflect acute bronchopneumonia with cranioventral distribution, with or without accompanying fibrinous pleuropneumonia.
• In early disease the main findings may include pulmonary congestion and edema, and the bronchi may be hyperemic and contain froth and potentially foreign material. As disease progresses affected areas of lung become suppurative, necrotic and soft, and fibrinous pleuritis is evident. Chronic cases may have pulmonary abscesses and fibrous adhesions between the visceral and parietal pleura.

TREATMENT

THERAPEUTIC APPROACH
• Commences with identification of the reason or cause for aspiration to protect the airway from further damage, and to determine the prognosis (e.g., treatment may be futile with large volume oil aspiration).
• Treatment is aimed at neutralizing secondary bacterial infection by Gram-positive and Gram-negative aerobic and anaerobic bacterial agents and should start as soon as possible after the aspiration event is recognized, typically regardless of whether clinical signs exist.
• Steroidal and/or nonsteroidal anti-inflammatory agents can be utilized to control shock and inflammation.

SURGICAL CONSIDERATIONS AND TECHNIQUES
N/A

MEDICATIONS

DRUGS OF CHOICE
• Broad-spectrum antibiotic therapy is indicated to cover Gram-positive and Gram-negative bacterial agents. In severe cases anaerobic bacterial coverage is also indicated.
• Appropriate antibiotic coverage can be achieved using combinations of antibiotics, or one antibiotic depending on the desired spectrum and duration of coverage; drugs should be given at recommended doses and dosing intervals.

CONTRAINDICATIONS
Oral administration of medications during treatment is likely contraindicated if deficits in pharyngeal and esophageal function are present.

ASPIRATION PNEUMONIA

PRECAUTIONS

Appropriate milk and meat withdrawal times must be followed for all compounds administered to food-producing animals.

POSSIBLE INTERACTIONS

N/A

FOLLOW-UP

EXPECTED COURSE AND PROGNOSIS

• Animals with relatively minor aspiration events that receive prompt therapy are expected to survive.
• Aspiration events that are large volume, promote gangrenous pneumonia, have delayed recognition and treatment, or are associated with congenital or poorly reversible disorders have a poor prognosis.
• Fibrosing alveolitis (oil aspiration), pulmonary abscessation, and pulmonary granulomas are chronic sequelae that typically reduce prognosis.

POSSIBLE COMPLICATIONS

• Chronic respiratory disease related to fibrosing alveolitis or ongoing pulmonary inflammation and infection.
• Septicemia and multiorgan failure.

CLIENT EDUCATION

Personnel should be thoroughly instructed in the correct techniques for administering medications by mouth or orogastric tube.

PATIENT CARE

• Monitor for worsening of respiratory function, fever and any other associated clinical signs.
• Provide a soft and palatable ration.
• Intermittent orogastric feeding may be indicated for animals with upper gastrointestinal dysfunction.

PREVENTION

• Education regarding medication administration is the most important method of preventing aspiration events.
• Fasting of animals combined with careful head positioning, ± intubation during sedation and general anesthesia reduces the risk of inducing aspiration.

MISCELLANEOUS

ASSOCIATED CONDITIONS

N/A

AGE-RELATED FACTORS

Young animals are prone to aspiration events associated with feeding management, or with congenital disorders and selenium deficiency.

ZOONOTIC POTENTIAL

N/A

PREGNANCY

N/A

BIOSECURITY

N/A

PRODUCTION MANAGEMENT

• Avoid unnecessary oral medications and instruct personnel to deliver oral medications or drenches at a measured rate to allow the animal to swallow, with the head positioned level or down, and with great caution during periods of struggling and vocalization.
• Caustic or inflammatory substances (calcium chloride, mineral oil) are often best given by orogastric tube versus oral drench.

SYNONYMS

N/A

ABBREVIATIONS

N/A

SEE ALSO

• Atypical Interstitial Pneumonia
• Calf Diphtheria/Necrotic Stomatitis
• Enzootic Pneumonia of Calves
• Respiratory Disease: Bovine
• Respiratory Disease: Camelids
• Respiratory Disease: Small Ruminant

Suggested Reading

Adler R, Boermans HJ, Moulton JE, Moore DA. Toxicosis in sheep following ingestion of natural gas condensate. Vet Pathol 1992, 29: 11–20.

Davidson HP, Rebhun WC, Habel RE. Pharyngeal trauma in cattle. Cornell Vet 1981, 71: 15–25.

Lopez A, Bildfell R. Pulmonary inflammation associated with aspirated meconium and epithelial cells in calves. Vet Pathol 1992, 29: 104–11.

Lopez A, Lofstedt J, Bildfell R, Horney B, Burton S. Pulmonary histopathologic findings, acid-base status, and absorption of colostral immunoglobulins in newborn calves. Am J Vet Res 1994, 55: 1303–7.

Smith BL, Alley MR, McPherson WB. Lipid pneumonia in a cow. N Z Vet J 1969, 17: 65–7.

Toofanian F, Aliakbari S, Ivoghli B. Acute diesel fuel poisoning in goats. Trop Anim Health Prod 1979, 2: 98–101.

Author Jeff Lakritz

Consulting Editor Erica C. McKenzie

BASICS

OVERVIEW

• Atypical interstitial pneumonia (AIP) is a loosely defined term that covers a variety of respiratory disorders with different etiologies. These disorders typically present with acute respiratory distress and are characterized by the microscopic findings of pulmonary congestion or edema, hyaline membrane formation, epithelial hyperplasia, and interstitial emphysema.

• Specific causes include intoxication of cattle with 3-methyl-indole (3-MI), 4-ipomeanol (4-IP), and perilla ketone. A form of AIP also affects feedlot cattle, and other potential causes include noxious gases, *Brassica* spp. plants, perennial ryegrass intoxication and lungworm infestation.

INCIDENCE/PREVALENCE

Variable; high morbidity and mortality can occur in cattle herds when AIP is related to toxicity.

GEOGRAPHIC DISTRIBUTION

• Widespread, but specific causes have some degree of regional distribution.

• AIP related to 3-MI toxicity has been reported in the United Kingdom, Canada, and the western United States. Moldy sweet potato toxicity and perilla ketone toxicity occur in southeastern USA. Feedlot cattle in the USA, Canada and other countries can develop AIP of unknown etiology.

SYSTEMS AFFECTED

Respiratory

PATHOPHYSIOLOGY

• 3-MI toxicity results from ruminal conversion of L-tryptophan to 3-MI which is absorbed from the rumen and further metabolized in the lung, resulting in bronchiolar, alveolar epithelial and endothelial damage with pulmonary edema, hyaline membrane formation, alveolar epithelial hyperplasia, and interstitial emphysema resulting in hypoxemia and distress. Most often this arises after movement of cattle from sparse, dry feed, to lush green pastures without significant time for acclimation or feed additives provided to prevent AIP.

• 4-IP toxicity arises with the formation of furanoterpenoid toxins by sweet potatoes infected with the fungus *Fusarium solani*. Ingestion of moldy sweet potatoes by cattle allows these compounds to be absorbed from the rumen and converted in the lungs to toxic metabolites that produce bronchiolar, alveolar epithelial, and endothelial injury by irreversible binding to cellular proteins.

• Perilla ketone toxicity occurs in cattle grazing on sparse pastures in late summer in the southeastern USA (*Perilla frutescens*) and New Zealand (*Perilla maculatta*). The tall, green plants are found along the edge of wooded areas in pastures and grow well in later summer when other plants are dry. Intoxication commonly occurs in drought years when forage is limited. Consumption of volatile oil in these plants, including perilla ketone and two other substituted furans, results in comparable lung injury to 3-MI and 4-IP toxicity.

• AIP in feedlot cattle has not been fully elucidated but typically occurs in the late feeding period when animals have been consuming a high concentrate diet for some time. This is considered a multifactorial condition and specific features of feedlot rations and rumen metabolism may contribute to the formation of 3-MI and other metabolites. Mortality is highest in summer and fall, when on finishing diets. Heifers are far more susceptible than males which may relate to the use of melengestrol acetate to control estrus.

HISTORICAL FINDINGS

• Management factors relevant to these disorders include feeding of moldy sweet potatoes, access to toxic plants, exposure to noxious gases, or finishing stages in a feedlot environment. Pasture-related AIP develops within 2 weeks of sudden movement to a variety of lush pastures.

SIGNALMENT

• Adult cattle are most susceptible; typically brood cows or bulls over two years of age

• Nursing calves are generally not affected and yearlings are less susceptible

• Feedlot cattle, particularly heifers, nearing the end of their feeding period are predisposed

PHYSICAL EXAMINATION FINDINGS

• Sudden onset of severe expiratory dyspnea with open mouth breathing, ptyalism, extension of the head and neck, distress, and anxiety.

• Quiet lung sounds are noted on auscultation; coughing is uncommon.

• Collapse and sudden death can occur with exertion.

• Subcutaneous emphysema may occur.

GENETICS

• No breed predilection.

• Heifers are >3 times as likely to develop AIP in feedlot situations.

CAUSES AND RISK FACTORS

• Movement of cattle from dry summer range onto irrigated or fertilized pastures in fall.

• Feedlot environment and ration.

• Female gender (feedlot AIP).

• Mature age (>2 years).

• Access to toxic plants in times of limited feed availability.

• Consumption of moldy sweet potatoes.

DIAGNOSIS

DIFFERENTIAL DIAGNOSES

• Intoxication with 3-MI, 4-IP, and perilla ketone may appear clinically similar to one another but can usually be readily separated on review of management factors.

• Infectious respiratory diseases (particularly bovine respiratory syncytial virus).

• Hypersensitivity pneumonitis of confined adult cattle (extrinsic allergic alveolitis).

• Verminous pneumonia (*Dictyocaulus viviparus*).

CBC/BIOCHEMISTRY/URINALYSIS

Stress leukogram may be evident; however, restraint and sampling can be fatal and is not usually justified.

OTHER LABORATORY TESTS

N/A

IMAGING

Not typically indicated

OTHER DIAGNOSTIC PROCEDURES

Necropsy

PATHOLOGIC FINDINGS

• Typically lesions are confined to the respiratory system. The lungs are heavy, wet and rubbery, and do not float. The lungs may fail to collapse and maintain rib impressions after the thorax is opened. Petechial hemorrhages may be evident in the upper respiratory tract, with foamy fluid in the large airways. Incriminating feedstuffs (Perilla mint, moldy sweet potatoes) may be present in the rumen.

• Microscopic pulmonary lesions include congestion, edema, hyaline membranes, interstitial emphysema, and proliferation of alveolar epithelial cells.

TREATMENT

THERAPEUTIC APPROACH

Largely limited to preventing further exposure to offending pasture, feed, or toxins, and avoiding stress or exertion that exacerbates respiratory distress.

SURGICAL CONSIDERATIONS AND TECHNIQUES

N/A

MEDICATIONS

DRUGS OF CHOICE

• Treatment should be considered carefully and performed with caution due to associated stress.

ATYPICAL INTERSTITIAL PNEUMONIA (CONTINUED)

• Furosemide (1 mg/kg IM or IV, q24h or q12h).
• Flunixin meglumine (1.1–2.2 mg/kg IV, q24h or divided q12h).
• Dexamethasone (0.05 to 0.2 mg/kg IM or IV, once or twice).
• Antibiotics may be indicated to prevent secondary bacterial pneumonia.

CONTRAINDICATIONS
N/A

PRECAUTIONS
• Any stress or exertion, including treatment, can precipitate fatal collapse.
• Appropriate milk and meat withdrawal times must be followed for all compounds administered to food-producing animals.

POSSIBLE INTERACTIONS
N/A

FOLLOW-UP

EXPECTED COURSE AND PROGNOSIS
• Most fatalities from toxic interstitial pneumonia are likely to occur in the first two days of clinical signs. Animals with severe disease may display chronic emphysema or signs of cardiac failure related to cor pulmonale.
• Moderately to mildly affected animals often improve substantially and spontaneously after 72 hours and continue to recover over 10 days.
• Feedlot AIP typically has a poor prognosis.

POSSIBLE COMPLICATIONS
Secondary bacterial pneumonia

CLIENT EDUCATION
Focus on preventive management factors relevant to the various disorders.

PATIENT CARE
• Exertion should be minimized; it is generally best to leave affected animals in their location and to provide alternative sources of safe feed (hay).

• Monitor progression of disease or improvement, so animals in severe distress can be euthanized before undue suffering occurs.

PREVENTION
• Management practices that prevent abrupt exposure of animals to suspect pasture can include gradually increasing pasture time over 10–12 days (commencing with 2 hours/day); strip grazing; or using other species or young stock to graze pasture down before adult cattle. Delaying use of lush pastures until after a hard frost, or cutting and windrowing pasture before turning cattle out is also preventive.
• Prophylactic administration of monensin or lasalocid (200 mg/head/day) for 1 day or 6 days respectively, prior to placing adult cattle on lush pasture can prevent disease if maintained for at least 10 days after introduction to pasture. These drugs reduce the conversion of L-tryptophan to 3-MI.
• Provide sufficient feed and minerals during late summer to limit consumption of toxic plants.
• Do not feed moldy sweet potatoes to livestock.
• Fence off access to toxic plants.

MISCELLANEOUS

ASSOCIATED CONDITIONS
• Secondary bacterial bronchopneumonia
• Viral respiratory infections

AGE-RELATED FACTORS
Young animals are resistant.

ZOONOTIC POTENTIAL
N/A

PREGNANCY
N/A

BIOSECURITY
N/A

PRODUCTION MANAGEMENT
Management has the greatest influence on the occurrence of these disorders, hence attention

should be paid to minimizing all associated causes and risk factors, or where possible, employing specific preventive strategies.

SYNONYMS
• Fog fever
• Acute bovine pulmonary emphysema
• Pulmonary adenomatosis
• Acute respiratory distress syndrome

ABBREVIATIONS
• AIP = atypical interstitial pneumonia
• 3-MI = 3-methyl-indole
• 4-IP = 4-ipomeanol

SEE ALSO
Respiratory Disease: Bovine

Suggested Reading

Breeze R. Respiratory disease in adult cattle. Vet Clin North Am Food Anim Pract 1985, 1: 311–46.
Carlson JR, Dickinson EO, Yokoyama MT, et al. Pulmonary edema and emphysema in cattle after intraruminal and intravenous administration of 3-methylindole. Am J Vet Res 1975, 36: 1341–47.
Doster AR. Bovine atypical interstitial pneumonia. Vet Clin North Am Food Anim Pract 2010, 26: 395–407.
Hammond AC, Carlson JR, Breeze RG. Effect of monensin pretreatment on tryptophan-induced acute bovine pulmonary edema and emphysema. Am J Vet Res 1982, 43: 753–6.
Jensen R, Pierson RE, Braddy PM, et al. Atypical interstitial pneumonia in yearling feedlot cattle. J Am Vet Med Assoc 1976, 169: 507–10.
Kerr LA, Linnabary RD. A review of interstitial pneumonia in cattle. Vet Human Toxicol 1989, 31: 247–54.
Peckham JC, Mitchell FE, Jones OH Jr, et al. Atypical interstitial pneumonia in cattle fed moldy sweet potatoes. J Am Vet Med Assoc 1972, 160: 169–72.

Author Jeff Lakritz
Consulting Editor Erica C. McKenzie

BASICS

OVERVIEW
• There are approximately 150 species of avocado (*Persea*). Of these, *Persea americana* and its races and cultivars are of toxicologic importance. Races and cultivars most commonly encountered include Guatemalan and its hybrid ("Fuerte"), Mexican, and West Indies.
• The tree or shrub has a dense crown with brown to gray bark.
• Leaves, fruit, and seeds are toxic with leaves being the most toxic.
• Leaves alternate and crowd near the end of the twig. Leaf blades are ovate-elliptical with single primary vein.
• Flowers are perfect, greenish yellow.
• Fruit are ovoid to pyriform with thick glossy green to dark green skin.
• Seeds are large and light brown.

GEOGRAPHIC DISTRIBUTION
Cultivated primarily in Mexico, California and Florida, but can also be found as an ornamental in the Gulf coast areas.

SYSTEMS AFFECTED
• Mammary
• Cardiovascular

PATHOPHYSIOLOGY
• Suspected toxin is a R-enantiomer of persin. However, the mechanism of action is unknown.
• Toxin targets the mammary gland and myocardium depending on the amount of plant consumed.

HISTORICAL FINDINGS
Exposure to avocado groves

SIGNALMENT
Bovine, ovine, caprine (especially). Goats are highly susceptible to the mammary-induced effects of avocado poisoning, although all lactating animals can develop noninfectious mastitis and agalactia. With respect to cardiotoxic effects of avocado, all animal species are considered susceptible.

PHYSICAL EXAMINATION FINDINGS
• Mammary gland effects present as mastitis 24 hours post-ingestion with a 75% decrease in milk production. Milk appears to be watery and curdled.

• Myocardial effects present as edema of the neck and brisket, infrequent cough, depression, reluctance to move, leading to respiratory distress and cardiac arrhythmias.

CAUSES AND RISK FACTORS
• Presumed exposure to R-enantiomer of persin.
• Toxic dose:
  ○ Mammary effects are seen with ingestion of 20 g of fresh leaves/ bwt (kg) in lactating goats.
  ○ Myocardial effects were seen with ingestion of:
    ▪ 30 g of fresh leaves/bwt (kg) in lactating goats
    ▪ 25 g fresh leaves/bwt (kg) for 5 days in sheep (severe signs)
    ▪ 5.5 g fresh leaves/bwt (kg) for 21 days in sheep (chronic signs)
    ▪ 2.5 g fresh leaves/bwt (kg) for 32 days in sheep (mild signs)

DIAGNOSIS

DIFFERENTIAL DIAGNOSIS
Other causes of mastitis and cardiac disease

CBC/BIOCHEMISTRY/URINALYSIS
• No characteristic changes on CBC
• Elevation of liver enzymes such as AST and LDH
• Elevated CK

OTHER DIAGNOSTIC PROCEDURES
Finding of plant material within gastric contents on gross pathology

TREATMENT

THERAPEUTIC APPROACH
• Remove from source
• Treatment of mastitis
• Supportive care

MEDICATIONS

N/A

CONTRAINDICATIONS
N/A

FOLLOW-UP

EXPECTED COURSE AND PROGNOSIS
• Recovery possible
• Death

PREVENTION
Avoid feeding avocado plant material or grazing near avocado trees.

MISCELLANEOUS

ASSOCIATED CONDITIONS
N/A

PRODUCTION MANAGEMENT
Restrict grazing of livestock from avocado groves

ABBREVIATIONS
• AST = aspartate aminotransferase
• CK = creatine kinase
• LDH = lactate dehydrogenase

SEE ALSO
• Mastitis: No Growth
• Toxicology: Herd Outbreaks

Suggested Reading
Burrows GE, Tyrl RJ. Lauraceae, Chapter 45. In: Burrows GE, Tyrl RJ eds, Toxic Plants of North America, 2nd ed. Ames: Wiley-Blackwell, 2013, pp. 743–6.
Knight AP, Walter RG. Plants affecting the cardiovascular system. In: Knight AP, Walter RG eds, A Guide to Plant Poisoning of Animal in North America. Wyoming: Teton NewMedica, 2002.
Author Jennifer S. Taintor
Consulting Editor Christopher C.L. Chase
Acknowledgment The author and book editors acknowledge the prior contribution of Joe Roder.

BABESIOSIS

 BASICS

OVERVIEW
• Eradicated from the USA for 60 years, babesiosis remains an important disease in cattle throughout the world where the tick vector is prevalent.
• The causative agent is an intraerythrocytic protozoan that produces intravascular hemolysis in the ruminant host.

INCIDENCE/PREVALENCE
• Widespread in endemic areas.
• Asymptomatic carriers obscure the true prevalence.

GEOGRAPHIC DISTRIBUTION
• Worldwide, eradicated from the USA.
• Endemic in tropical climates where tick vectors flourish.

SYSTEMS AFFECTED
• Hemolymphatic
• Cardiovascular
• Nervous

PATHOPHYSIOLOGY
• Babesiosis is contracted via inoculation of infected blood, principally by tick vectors, and via blood-contaminated needles or instruments.
• The organism is transmitted by several one-host ticks; the genus *Boophilus* is particularly important.
• Female ticks are infected during feeding on infected cattle, with subsequent replication of *Babesia* in the tick's embryos. As the embryos develop into larvae, nymphs, and adults, the *Babesia* persist and can be transmitted to new mammalian hosts during tick feeding. For *B. bigemina,* only nymph or adult ticks are capable of transmitting the disease. The infection does not persist beyond the larval stage in *B. bovis.*
• Although rare, vertical transmission in mammalian hosts has been reported.
• The incubation period is 2–3 weeks.
• In endemic areas, where passive humoral immunity is transferred from dam to offspring, clinical disease is uncommon in cattle <6 months old.
• Immunosuppressed or immunologically naïve individuals are susceptible to parasitemia and clinical signs. If an animal survives initial infection, active immunity rapidly ensues, thereby controlling parasitemia.
• Immunity after natural exposure may last 1–2 years, but may be insufficient to completely eliminate the organism, allowing for persistence without clinical signs of disease (premunition).
• Subclinical "carriers" of *Babesia* serve as a silent reservoir for persistent infection within a herd.

• Carriers also may experience episodic clinical signs of recrudescence as protective immunity and parasitemia wax and wane.
• Some individuals may eventually eliminate the infection; other chronic carriers eventually succumb to the disease.
• Upon inoculation, infective sporozoites enter red blood cells wherein binary fission occurs within 14 days of inoculation. When replication is complete, the organisms are released by erythrolysis to propagate infection in new red blood cells.
• The predominant clinical signs of disease are fever and intravascular hemolysis. Other factors that may contribute to hemolysis include increased red blood cell fragility, removal of infected cells by the mononuclear phagocytic system, and the development of secondary autoimmune hemolytic anemia.
• Anemia develops, and in severe cases, death from hypoxemia may ensue.
• With *B. bovis* infection, release of inflammatory mediators in response to infection may also lead to intense hypotension, cardiovascular shock, and disseminated intravascular coagulation.
• *B. bigemina* may also replicate within the endothelium of the cerebrum, causing local hypoxemia and the development of "cerebral babesiosis," characterized by acute onset of signs of cerebral disease.

HISTORICAL FINDINGS
Concurrent illness; progressive depression, weakness, and lethargy; poor growth; separation from the herd; anorexia; tick infestation; hemoglobinuria; fever; and icterus.

SIGNALMENT
• Cattle and small ruminants are the principal hosts, but cases have been reported in other ruminants, such as water buffalo, reindeer, and the American bison.
• Any age may be affected, but younger calves in endemic areas rarely develop infection prior to 6 months of age due to passive immunity.
• Immunosuppressed, debilitated, stressed, or immunologically naïve adult ruminants are more susceptible to infection and often are more severely affected by the disease.

PHYSICAL EXAMINATION FINDINGS
• Onset of clinical signs depends on the size of the inoculum.
• Signs can develop within 1 week of inoculation, but may not be apparent for 2–3 weeks.
• High fever, depression, anorexia, and progressive weakness occur first.
• The predominant clinical signs develop with the onset of intravascular hemolysis that occurs as reproducing merozoites destroy erythrocytes in the circulation.
• Tachycardia and tachypnea may be profound and depend on the degree and rate at which the anemia develops. A low-grade

systolic murmur may be present over the heart base as blood viscosity decreases.
• Hemoglobinemia and membrane pallor precede hemoglobinuria and icterus.
• Pregnant cows often abort.
• In severe cases, death results from hypoxemic shock. If the infected animal survives the initial episode of hemolysis, convalescence is prolonged until anemia has regenerated (weeks to months).
• Emaciation, poor condition, failure to thrive, and the existence of the carrier stage are common developments during convalescence.
• Infection of the endothelium of the central nervous system in cattle with *B. bigemina* may result in clinical signs of cerebral disease, including maniacal behavior, hyperexcitability, seizures, bruxism, opisthotonus, blindness, ataxia, and coma, with a grave prognosis.
• A unique phenomenon of anal sphincter spasm in cattle infected with *B. divergens* may produce the additional clinical sign of pipestream feces.

GENETICS
Zebu, Afrikaner, and Santa Gertrudis cattle are less susceptible to babesiosis than other breeds of cattle.

CAUSES AND RISK FACTORS
• Babesiosis is caused by infection with protozoa from the phylum Apicomplexa, order Piroplasmida, genus *Babesia*.
• At least six species of *Babesia* affect cattle and two species affect small ruminants (see Table 1). *B. bovis* is the most pathogenic; *B. major* and *B. ovate* are less pathogenic to nonpathogenic.
• Immunologically naïve, immunosuppressed, or otherwise debilitated individuals in endemic areas are most at risk for infection.

 DIAGNOSIS

DIFFERENTIAL DIAGNOSES
• Causes of intravascular hemolysis include leptospirosis, bacillary hemoglobinuria, Heinz body anemia (onion, rape, kale toxicity), theileriosis, postparturient hemoglobinuria, and autoimmune hemolytic anemia.
• Causes of extravascular hemolysis should also be considered.
• Copper toxicity should be considered in sheep.

CBC/BIOCHEMISTRY/URINALYSIS
• Regenerative anemia 5–7 days after onset (signs of regeneration include an increased MCV, anisocytosis, polychromasia, basophilic stippling, reticulocytes, Howell Jolly bodies, nucleated red blood cells).
• Hemoglobinemia (pink plasma, increased MCH and MCHC).

Table 1

Distribution and Vectors for *Babesia* in Ruminants			
Species	*Geographic location*	*Reported vectors*	*Infective stage of tick vector*
B. bigemina	South America, Europe, Africa, Australia, Middle East, Asia, West Indies	*Boophilus annulatus, B. decoloratus, B. microplus, B. calcaratus, Rhipicephalus evertsi, R. bursa, R. appendiculatus, Haemaphysalis punctata*	Nymphs and adults
B. bovis (also includes *B. berbera*, or *B. argentina*)	South America, Europe, Russia, Africa, Asia, Australia	*B. annulatus, B. microplus, Ixodes* spp., *Rhipicephalus bursa*	Larvae
B. divergens	Europe, Africa	*Ixodes ricinus*	Larvae
B. major	Europe, Russia, North Africa, Middle East	*Haemaphysalis punctata*	Adults
B. jakimovi	Siberia, Asia	*Ixodes ricinus*	
B. ovata	Japan	*Haemaphysalis longicornis*	
B. motasi (sheep and goats)	Europe, South America, Africa	*Dermacentor silvarum, Haemaphysalis, Rhipicephalus bursa*	Adults
B. ovis (sheep and goats)	Europe, Russia, Asia, Middle East	*Ixodes ricinus, Rhipicephalus bursa, Dermacentor reticulatis*	Adults

• Hemoglobinuria (red-brown urine, dipstick positive for blood; positive for hemoglobin with saturated ammonium sulfate test).
• Hyperbilirubinemia (unconjugated).
• Hypokalemia.
• Thrombocytopenia.
• Metabolic acidosis.

OTHER LABORATORY TESTS
• *Babesia* species may be seen within erythrocytes in a peripheral Wright- or Giemsa-stained blood smear. *B. bovis* is often difficult to find in the peripheral blood.
• The organisms are non-pigmented, pyriform to irregular, round or amoeba-shaped.
• Often, the protozoa appear in groups of two, with the "tops" of the pear-shaped organisms joined at an angle to form a "V."
• Parasitemia is often low, or affected cells are removed from circulation, so absence of visible protozoa does not preclude the diagnosis.
• The humoral response to *Babesia* can usually be detected within a week of infection. Many serologic assays exist, but the complement fixation and the indirect fluorescent antibody tests are most commonly used. Other tests include the rapid card agglutination, gel precipitation, latex agglutination, and enzyme-labeling immunoassay.
• Because humoral immunity post-infection is long lived, it may be difficult to distinguish active infection from previous exposure.
• Highly sensitive and specific molecular biology techniques are useful for diagnosis and surveillance of active infection in ticks and cattle. Nested PCR, RTqPCR and reverse line blotting technique are considerably more sensitive at detecting infection than traditional PCR.

IMAGING
N/A

OTHER DIAGNOSTIC PROCEDURES
N/A

PATHOLOGIC FINDINGS
• Depending on the stage of the disease, diffuse pallor of the tissues or icterus is present.
• Splenomegaly, hepatomegaly, edema, body cavity effusion, petechial and ecchymotic hemorrhages on the heart and gastrointestinal tract, thin blood, thrombi, gallbladder distension, and the presence of red-brown urine in the urinary bladder are common.
• In chronically infected cattle, emaciation also occurs.
• *B. bigemina* tends to proliferate in peripheral vessels, whereas *B. bovis* multiplies in visceral blood vessels.
• Direct fluorescent antibody staining and PCR assay of blood or tissues are the most specific tests used to confirm the diagnosis postmortem.

 TREATMENT

THERAPEUTIC APPROACH
• If anemia is severe and clinical or laboratory evidence of hypoxemia is evident (intense lethargy or weakness, profound tachycardia or tachypnea, severe anemia, acidosis, increased anion gap), a whole blood transfusion is indicated.
• The normal total blood volume is approximately 8% of the body weight (i.e., 0.08 × body weight in kilograms equals the total blood volume in liters). Typically,

transfusing one-fourth to one-third of the total blood volume is adequate.

SURGICAL CONSIDERATIONS AND TECHNIQUES
N/A

 MEDICATIONS

DRUGS OF CHOICE
• The most commonly used drugs include diminazene diaceturate (Berenil or Ganeseg; 3–5 mg/kg IM), phenamidine diisethionate (Lomadine; 8–13 mg/kg, SQ or IM), imidocarb dipropionate (Imizol; 1–3 mg/kg, SQ or IM), and amicarbalide diisethionate (Diampron; 5–10 mg/kg IM). Imidocarb therapy may prevent reinfection for up to 2 months.
• Concern over tissue residues, particularly with imidocarb, has resulted in withdrawal of some of these products in certain countries.
• Overzealous use of babesiocidal drugs may abruptly reduce parasitemia to a level that is inadequate for establishment of protective immunity.

CONTRAINDICATIONS
N/A

PRECAUTIONS
Appropriate milk and meat withdrawal times must be followed for all compounds administered to food-producing animals.

POSSIBLE INTERACTIONS
N/A

B

FOLLOW-UP

EXPECTED COURSE AND PROGNOSIS
• Carriers are common in endemic areas. Infection with *B. bovis* is generally more severe than infection with other species.
• Cerebral babesiosis warrants a grave prognosis.
• The mortality rate is high in adult immunologically naïve or immunosuppressed individuals.

POSSIBLE COMPLICATIONS
• Death from hypoxemic anemia or cerebral babesiosis.
• Treatment frequently does not eliminate the carrier state.

CLIENT EDUCATION
• See "Prevention."
• Immunologically naïve cattle moving into endemic areas should be vaccinated prior to movement.

PATIENT CARE
Monitor heart rate, respiratory rate, attitude, appetite, PCV, body weight of affected animals.

PREVENTION
• Most control programs are tailored to individual herds.
• Complete eradication from a herd within an endemic area leaves that herd susceptible to future reinfection from surrounding herds.
• Thus most control programs are aimed at balancing infection with an appropriate level of immunity. This is most effectively achieved by reducing the tick population with acaricides and cattle tick vaccines and vaccination with live or live-attenuated *Babesia* organisms produced by either in vivo inoculation or in vitro culture to establish a state of premunition. There is little cross protection between species of *Babesia*. The

shelf life of live and live-attenuated vaccines is short (approximately one week) unless ultra-frozen.
• Calves are typically vaccinated between 4 and 10 months of age.
• As older animals are more sensitive to the effects of infection, vaccination with live organisms is often followed with babesiostatic or babesiocidal drugs.
• Newer vaccines using recombinant proteins are promising but not commercially available.
• Selection of cattle that are resistant to the tick vector and/or the disease is another method of control.

MISCELLANEOUS

ASSOCIATED CONDITIONS
N/A

AGE-RELATED FACTORS
Younger cattle in endemic areas are rarely infected.

ZOONOTIC POTENTIAL
Rare. Immunosuppressed humans may be susceptible to infection.

PREGNANCY
Immunization of pregnant cows with live or live-attenuated vaccines may induce neonatal isoerythrolysis.

BIOSECURITY
N/A

PRODUCTION MANAGEMENT
N/A

SYNONYMS
• Bovine malaria
• Piroplasmosis
• Redwater
• Texas fever
• Tick fever
• Tristeza

ABBREVIATIONS
• MCH = mean corpuscular hemoglobin
• MCHC = mean corpuscular hemoglobin concentration
• MCV = mean corpuscular volume
• RTqPCR = real-time quantitative polymerase chain reaction

SEE ALSO
• Anemia, Regenerative
• Bacillary Hemoglobinuria
• Copper Deficiency and Toxicity
• Leptospirosis
• Postparturient Hemoglobinuria

Suggested Reading
Regassa A, Penzhorn BL, Bryson NR. Attainment of endemic stability to *Babesia bigemina* in cattle on a South African ranch where nonintensive tick control was applied. Vet Parasitol 2003, 116: 267–74.
Yeruham I, Avidar Y, Aroch I, Hadani A. Intrauterine infection with *Babesia bovis* in a 2-day-old calf. J Vet Med B Infect Dis Vet Public Health 2003, 50: 60–2.
Florin-Christensen M, Suarez CE, Rodriguez AE, Flores DA, Schnittger L. Vaccines against bovine babesiosis: Where we are now and possible roads ahead. Parasitology 2014, 41: 1563–92.
QiSheng L, ZhenBao W, Zhen W, Sen H, YuTing Z. Development of real-time PCR assay for detection of *Babesia bovis* Harbin. Chin J Prevent Vet Med 2013, 35: 58–61.
Guerrero FD, Miller RJ, Pérez de León AA. Cattle tick vaccines: many candidate antigens, but will a commercially viable product emerge? Int J Parasitol 2012, 42: 421–7.
Gohil S, Herrmann S, Gunther S, Cooke BM. Bovine babesiosis in the 21st century: Advances in biology and functional genomics. Int J Parasitol 2013, 43: 125–32.
Author Michelle Henry Barton
Consulting Editor Erica C. McKenzie

BACILLARY HEMOGLOBINURIA

BASICS

OVERVIEW
• Fatal clostridial disease associated with the proliferation of *Clostridium haemolyticum* (*Clostridium novyi* type D) in the liver as a consequence of hepatic damage induced by parasite larval migration, trauma or abscessation of hepatic parenchyma. The fulminant course of the disease is characterized by toxemia, hemoglobinuria, and sudden death.
• Spores of *Clostridium haemolyticum* are normally found in the soil and gastrointestinal tract, liver, feces, and urine of healthy cattle and sheep and accumulate in the environment as a result of fecal shedding by carrier animals.
• Disease results when a hepatic insult or damage creates an area of anaerobiosis in the liver that promotes spore germination and results in vegetative cell multiplication and toxin production.
• Hepatic insult often results from migration of liver flukes (*Fasciola hepatica, Dicrocoelium dendriticum, Fascioloides magna* or *Cysticercus cellulosae*), trauma (iatrogenic or spontaneous) or abscessation of the liver.
• The disease is usually fatal but recovery after treatment of some cases has been reported.
• Endemic in swampy areas with an alkaline soil pH (~8).
• Organism capable to survive in decomposed carcasses and soil for years.
• Outbreaks are seen in cattle fed hay from infected fields and after flooding.

INCIDENCE/PREVALENCE
Herd mortality rate ranges from 5% to 25% and case fatality rate is 95%.

GEOGRAPHIC DISTRIBUTION
This is a disease that affects cattle and sheep all over the world. In the United States, Red Water is found primarily in the western part of the country and occasionally in the southern states.

SYSTEMS AFFECTED
• Digestive
• Hemolymphatic

PATHOPHYSIOLOGY
• *Clostridium haemolyticum* is transported to the liver from the GI tract and persist in Kupffer's cells.
• Asymptomatic but infected cattle harbor the organism in their GI tract, liver, and tissues and may shed it in feces and urine.
• Anaerobiosis resulting from liver damage causes germination of *Clostridium haemolyticum* spores, vegetative growth, and release of exotoxins.
• The β-toxin (phospholipase C) released by the organism causes extensive hepatic necrosis, vasculitis, and intravascular hemolysis.
• Anemia, icterus, hemoglobinuria, and shock result from release of exotoxins.

SIGNALMENT
• Occurs usually in cattle older than 1 year but it is uncommon in young calves.
• Highly conditioned cattle seem most susceptible.
• Mature sheep affected sporadically.
• Uncommonly elk, other ruminants.
• No sex or breed predilection.

PHYSICAL EXAMINATION FINDINGS
• Short course of clinical disease 12–48 h
• Sudden death/found dead
• Rare to see affected animals alive
• Severe depression/affected animals stand apart from the herd
• High fever (103°F–106°F; 39.5°C–41°C)
• Tachycardia
• Abdominal pain
• Rectal bleeding and bloody feces
• Diarrhea
• Shallow breathing/dyspnea
• Hemoglobinuria/dark red urine
• Icteric or pale mucus membranes
• Progressive anemia
• Weakness
• Recumbency

CAUSES AND RISK FACTORS
• Pasturing cattle in wet and swampy pastures that favor liver fluke survival.
• Geographic areas with high soil pH.
• Irrigated and poorly draining alkaline pastures.
• Hepatic insult(s) caused by larval migration, liver abscesses, septicemia, hepatotoxins, trauma, biopsy, and high nitrate diets which create a state of anaerobiosis and promote germination of *Clostridium haemolyticum* spores and toxin production.
• Unvaccinated cattle and sheep.

DIAGNOSIS

DIFFERENTIAL DIAGNOSES
• Leptospirosis
• Postparturient hemoglobinuria
• Enzootic hematuria (bracken fern toxicosis)
• Acute pyelonephritis
• Chronic copper poisoning
• Black disease
• Hemorrhagic cystitis
• Babesiosis

CBC/BIOCHEMICAL/URINALYSIS
• Anemia
• Leukocytosis or leukopenia with left shift
• Neutrophilia/neutropenia with toxic changes
• Increased values of liver enzymes (SDH, AST, GGT, ALP)
• Increased CK
• Hyperbilirubinemia
• Azotemia
• Hemoglobinuria

OTHER LABORATORY TESTS
• Blood culture.

• Nested PCR of whole blood samples for *Cl. haemolyticum.*
• Identification of large, Gram-positive rods on impression smear from liver, spleen, blood, or abdominal fluid.
• Isolation of *Cl. haemolyticum* from tissue from the edge of liver infarcts and from blood of affected animals.
• Fluorescent antibody test (FAT) on impression smears from liver infarcts, or immunohistochemistry on spleen will be positive for the organism.
• Biochemical and toxin (β-toxin) identification tests.
• Definitive diagnosis by culture and GLC confirmation that isolate is *Cl. haemolyticum.*
• Detection of the flagelin gene (*fliC*) sequence of *Cl. haemolyticum* by nested PCR of whole blood samples of affected animals.
• Caution should be exerted when interpreting Gram stains, culture, or FAT of liver lesions or GI tract as *Cl. haemolyticum* could be found in healthy animals and proliferates rapidly after death.
• Clostridial FAT cross reacts with *Clostridium novyi* type B and C.

IMAGING
Hepatic ultrasound:
• Infarct
• Disruption of normal parenchyma
• Vascular changes

PATHOLOGIC FINDINGS
• Subcutaneous edema, petechial and ecchymotic hemorrhages throughout the body.
• Diffuse hemorrhage in GI tract, respiratory tract, and pericardium.
• Red-tinged abdominal and thoracic fluid.
• Large ischemic hepatic infarct is pathognomonic.
• Usually a single infarct but occasionally multiple of varying size.
• Congestion and hemorrhage of lymph nodes
• Pigmented kidneys (blackened kidney)
• Red urine in kidney and bladder
• Icterus
• Anemia
• Splenomegaly

TREATMENT

THERAPEUTIC APPROACH
• Treatment is rarely effective.
• High doses of penicillin (44,000 IU/kg), intravenously preferred (q6h).
• Tetracyclines, cephalosporins, and ampicillin have also been recommended.
• Blood transfusion(s) as indicated; minimum of 6–8 liters for adult cattle.
• Antitoxic serum, if available.
• Intravenous isotonic polyionic fluids.
• Liver fluke treatment.
• Anti-inflammatory therapy.

BACILLARY HEMOGLOBINURIA (CONTINUED)

MEDICATIONS

DRUGS OF CHOICE
- Sodium, potassium or procaine penicillin
- Oxytetracycline
- Cephalosporins
- Blood transfusion
- Antitoxic serum
- Polyionic fluids

CONTRAINDICATIONS
Appropriate milk and meat withdrawal times must be followed for all compounds administered to food-producing animals.

FOLLOW-UP

EXPECTED COURSE AND PROGNOSIS
- Mortality in treated animals is high.
- Heavy mortalities when naïve, unvaccinated cattle brought onto infected pastures.
- Recovered animals may become poor doers: chronic weight loss, poor production.
- Cattle surviving subclinical attacks of disease may act as immune carriers.

MISCELLANEOUS

ASSOCIATED CONDITIONS
- Toxemia, hypovolemia, and severe anemia
- Renal or pulmonary emboli
- Renal infarcts
- Cardiac arrhythmias
- Pigment nephropathy

PRODUCTION MANAGEMENT
- Cattle should not be grazed on liver fluke-infested pastures.
- Liver fluke control is recommended in endemic areas.
- Prevent acute or sub-acute ruminal acidosis in order to decrease the risk of liver abscess formation.
- Vaccinate young animals with bacterin-toxoids of *Cl. haemolyticum* at 3–4 months of age and revaccinate 21 days later.
- Booster vaccination at weaning and every 6 months.
- Time of vaccination should be dictated by liver fluke season exposure.
- Deworm sheepdogs to reduce *Cysticercus tenuicollis* infection.
- Avoid pasture contamination by properly disposing (burn, deep burial, remove from premises) of decomposing carcasses of affected animals.

SYNONYMS
- Icterohemoglobinuria
- Infectious icterohemoglobinuria
- Red water

ABBREVIATIONS
- ALP = alkaline phosphatase
- AST = aspartate transaminase
- CK = creatine kinase
- FAT = fluorescent antibody test
- GGT = gamma-glutamyl transferase
- GI = gastrointestinal
- GLC = gas–liquid chromatography
- IM = intramuscular
- PCT = polymerase chain reaction
- SDH = sorbitol dehydrogenase

SEE ALSO
- Bracken Fern Toxicity
- Brassica spp. Toxicity
- Copper Deficiency and Toxicity
- Infectious Necrotic Hepatitis
- Leptospirosis
- Liver Flukes
- Postparturient Hemoglobinuria
- Pyelonephritis

Suggested Reading
Garry F. Miscellaneous infectious diseases. In: Diseases of Dairy Cattle, 2nd ed. St. Louis: Saunders, 2008.
Shinozuka Y, Yamato O, Hossain MA, et al. Bacillary hemoglobinuria in Japanese black cattle in Hiroshima, Japan: a case study. J Vet Med Sci 2011, 73: 255–8.
Snyder J, Snyder S. Bacillary hemoglobinuria. In: Smith B ed, Large Animal Internal Medicine, 4th ed. St. Louis: Mosby, 2009.
Takagi M, Yamato O, Sasaki Y, et al. Successful treatment of bacillary hemoglobinuria in Japanese Black cows. Vet Med Sci 2009, 71: 1105–8.
Vine N, Fayers J, Harwood D. Bacillary haemoglobinuria in dairy cows. Vet Rec 2006, 159: 160.

Author M. F. Chamorro
Consulting Editor Christopher C.L. Chase
Acknowledgment The author and book editors acknowledge the prior contribution of Susan Semrad and Sheila McGuirk.

BACTERIAL ENDOCARDITIS

B

BASICS

OVERVIEW
• Bacterial endocarditis is the most common valvular or endocardial disease in cattle. Chronic active infections such as rumenitis, mastitis, metritis, abscesses, foot infection, lead to continual bacteremia which predisposes cattle to bacterial endocarditis.
• Bacterial endocarditis can be an acute, subacute, or chronic infection, usually involving one or more heart valves resulting in variably-sized mass-like lesions. Less commonly, lesions may involve the mural endocardium.
• Initial clinical signs can be vague and variable. As lesions progress, valvular insufficiency can lead to heart failure, but heart failure is observed only in advanced disease.
• Clinical signs related to septic thromboembolism can be observed.
• The most common etiologic agents associated with bacterial endocarditis in cattle are *Trueperella pyogenes* and *Streptococcus* spp.
• Tricuspid valve most frequently and severely affected in cattle, but can also involve mitral, aortic, and pulmonic valves. Valves may be affected singly, or multiple valves can be involved.
• Rarely a curable disease. Long-term antimicrobial and supportive therapy required.
• Prognosis is poor for productivity and long-term survival.

INCIDENCE/PREVALENCE
Prevalence of bacterial endocarditis is estimated from slaughterhouse surveys to range from 0.01% to 0.15%.

GEOGRAPHIC DISTRIBUTION
Worldwide distribution

SYSTEMS AFFECTED
Cardiovascular

PATHOPHYSIOLOGY
• Chronic bacterial infection predisposes to bacterial endocarditis. Endocarditis most commonly occurs secondary to a chronic infection at a distant site that results in a recurrent or sustained bacteremia.
• Whether bacteria directly adhere to undamaged valvular endothelium, gain access to valves through damaged valvular surfaces, or enter hematogenously through capillaries at the base of valve is unknown.
• Bacteria proliferate within valve leaflets. Further endothelial damage by bacteria exposes collagen and enhances platelets and fibrin; fibrin is a major component of the vegetative lesion.
• Certain bacteria can adhere directly to endothelium because of their ability to synthesize polysaccharides (dextrans) and fibronectin, thus enhancing their ability to

colonize endothelial surfaces (vascular walls, heart valves).
• Bacteria adhering to valve surface activates coagulation cascade via release of tissue thromboplastin and extrinsic pathway.
• Endothelial surfaces are continuously exposed as a result of persistent bacteremia.
• Heart failure, right-sided more commonly than left-sided, may subsequently develop.
• In cattle, endocarditis most commonly occurs on the tricuspid valve, with the mitral valves the second most common valve affected. If multiple valves, bilateral infection of atrioventricular valves (tricuspid and mitral) is more common.
• Endocardium adjacent to valves can also be affected, especially secondary to congenital heart disease that causes turbulent blood flow.
• Embolic showering to secondary organs is common. Further bacteremia and septic thromboembolism leads to infections in other parts of the body, particularly those sites with high blood flow (lungs, kidney, joints).
• Lesions may be small or can be large enough to occupy most of adjacent heart chamber.
• Three histologic zones in lesions: (1) inner zone composed of fibrous tissue, (2) intermediate zone contains fibrin and bacterial colonies, and (3) superficial zone of fibrin and blood cells.
• Gross necropsy findings: (1) valvular lesions, often vegetative or fibrotic, thickening and distortion of valve leaflet, (2) embolic lesions to other organs, (3) signs of right-sided or congestive heart failure (e.g., hydrothorax, hydroperitoneum, passive congestion of liver, subcutaneous edema).

SIGNALMENT
• Primarily in mature cattle, goats, sheep
• More common in adult than in young
• No sex or breed predilection

PHYSICAL EXAMINATION FINDINGS
• Clinical signs often related to two phenomena: valvular insufficiency and septic thromboembolism.
• Clinical signs are often variable and vague.
• Persistent tachycardia is the most consistent finding in bacterial endocarditis.
• Heart murmur noted in ~50% of cattle cases. Absence of a murmur does not rule out bacterial endocarditis.
• Location, timing, and point of maximum intensity of murmur depends on valve(s) affected. If tricuspid is involved, heart murmur is primarily holosystolic or pansystolic and heard loudest on right side of thorax.
• Frequently, animal has history of temporary remission of clinical signs during antibiotic therapy.
• Ill-thrift, decreased appetite, and weight loss.
• Intermittent or constant fever.
• Lameness, septic arthritis.
• Temporary but dramatic drop in milk production.

• Cardiac arrhythmias (sinus tachycardia, other tachyarrhythmias) in affected cattle.
• Less common signs: weakness, diarrhea, abdominal pain, pale mucus membranes.
• As disease progresses, signs of heart failure, primarily right-sided, develop. Signs of right-sided heart failure include ventral, mandibular, or brisket edema, jugular or mammary vein distention, vein pulsation, tachycardia, hepatomegaly.
• Occasionally, affected cattle die suddenly without observed clinical signs.
• Signs of secondary organ (lung, kidney) involvement (infection, infarction) or embolic disease.

CAUSES AND RISK FACTORS
• Numerous bacterial species have been isolated from cattle with bacterial endocarditis.
• *Trueperella* (formerly *Arcanobacterium*) *pyogenes* is most frequent isolate from bacterial endocarditis cases in cattle with *Streptococcus* spp. second most commonly isolated.
• Other common isolates: *Escherichia coli*, *Micrococcus* spp., *Staphylococcus aureus*, *Pseudomonas* spp., *Klebsiella pneumoniae*, *Proteus mirabilis*, *Clostridium* spp., *Bacterioides* spp., *Fusobacterium necrophorum*.
• Less common isolates: *Mycoplasma mycoides*, *Erysipelothrix rhusiopathiae*, *Helcococcus ovis*.
• Recently, *Bartonella bovis* has been identified with bacterial endocarditis in cattle in the US and Europe. Other etiologic agents will likely be identified with next-generation sequencing technologies.
• Predisposing factors include chronic infection, chronic bacteremia, and underlying damage to valvular or endocardial surface.
• Risk factors include ruminal acidosis (acute, subacute, chronic), thrombophlebitis, distant infection site (mastitis, metritis, septic arthritis, tail infection, pneumonia, omphalophlebitis, abscesses, etc.), hardware disease (traumatic reticuloperitonitis), decubital ulcers, traumatic myocarditis, indwelling intravenous catheter, iatrogenic lesions.

DIAGNOSIS

DIFFERENTIAL DIAGNOSES
• Bacterial, viral, or protozoal myocarditis
• Brisket disease
• Cardiac lymphosarcoma or other neoplasm
• Congenital cardiac abnormalities
• Congestive heart failure
• Cor pulmonale
• Dilated cardiomyopathy
• Endocardiosis
• Nutritional myodegeneration
• Parasitic endocarditis
• Septic pericarditis
• Toxic myocardial necrosis (ionophore toxicity, gossypol toxicity, plant toxicosis)

BACTERIAL ENDOCARDITIS

B

CBC/BIOCHEMISTRY/URINALYSIS
• Clinical pathologic abnormalities can assist with diagnosis: Hyperfibrinogenemia and hypergammaglobulinemia due to infectious or inflammatory processes.
• Complete blood count findings may include a nonregenerative anemia, leukocytosis with or without a left shift and monocytosis.
• May have normal leukogram or leukopenia with left shift.
• Cattle have less consistent leukocyte response compared to other species.
• Marked elevation in cardiac troponin I was observed in a case report of bacterial endocarditis, but elevations may also be observed in myocardial disease.
• Serum chemistry panel often reflects accompanying changes in other organ systems, hydration status, or hypophagia.
• Azotemia.
• Elevated GGT.
• Elevated creatine kinase if recumbent.
• Electrolyte abnormalities from anorexia.
• Urinalysis if renal infection or infarct suspected.

OTHER LABORATORY TESTS
• Electrocardiogram if arrhythmia present.
• Transtracheal wash for cytology and microbiologic cultures if signs of pulmonary disease.
• Thoracic radiographs are of limited value in evaluating cardiac disease in cattle.
• Arterial blood gas to evaluate oxygenation status.
• Venous blood gas to evaluate metabolic status.

IMAGING
• Echocardiography is a sensitive diagnostic tool; however, specific criteria to define endocarditis are lacking. Endocarditis lesions appear as echogenic shaggy, smooth, or cystic masses. Vegetative lesion on or around heart valve can be visualized and measured. Valves are thickened with ventricular hyperkinesis.
• For adult cattle, use a 3.5 megahertz (MHz) (or smaller) transducer. 5.0 MHz can be used for young calves or small ruminants. Scan both sides of the chest.
• Echocardiography: Vegetative lesion on or near one or more heart valves, most commonly tricuspid valve, secondary chamber enlargement (right atrial) may be observed.
• Negative study does not rule out diagnosis of bacterial endocarditis.

OTHER DIAGNOSTIC PROCEDURES
• Field diagnosis is based on history (chronic infection) and clinical findings (murmur, persistent tachycardia) consistent with bacterial endocarditis. A murmur heard over the tricuspid valve area in an adult cow is suggestive of bacterial endocarditis.
• A recent meta-analysis identified that positive blood cultures had the highest sensitivity (86.9%) for diagnosis of bacterial endocarditis, followed by echocardiographic

identification of valvular lesions (84.3%), presence of tachycardia (79.7%), presence of a murmur (60.3%), presence of fever (45.7%), and presence of lameness/polyarthritis (43.5%). In same meta-analysis, presence of clinical signs of heart failure had a sensitivity of 37.3%.
• Aerobic and anaerobic blood cultures and sensitivity should be attempted for valuable livestock. Blood cultures should be obtained prior to initiation of antimicrobial therapy. A minimum of 10 mL of blood should be collected aseptically, with two to three cultures drawn several hours apart from separate venipuncture sites.
• Culture blood at a 1:10 to 1:20 ratio to broth medium. Incubate at 37°C for 24 hours before plating on traditional blood agar plates.
• Antimicrobial removal device (ARD) should be used if animal previously received antimicrobial drugs. Alternatively, if animal's condition permits, withdraw antimicrobial therapy for 24–48 hours before obtaining blood samples for culture.
• Failure to obtain a positive blood culture does not rule out the presence of bacterial endocarditis.
• Examination of buffy-coat smears or leukocyte monolayer preparation stained with Gram or Giemsa stain.

TREATMENT
THERAPEUTIC APPROACH
• Long-term and often costly; compliance and economic issue provide major disadvantages for treating bacterial endocarditis in ruminants.
• Often palliative rather than curative. The bacteria create permanent damage to valvular endocardium.
• Treatment is aimed at sterilizing lesion, halting spread of infection, managing clinical signs of heart failure.
• Antimicrobial therapy should be ideally based on sensitivity of bacteria isolated from blood culture or other site of infection.
• Parenteral administration of bactericidal antimicrobials required for a minimum of 4–6 weeks and often as long as 8–12 weeks.
• Ideally, initial therapy includes broad-spectrum antimicrobials given intravenously (IV) to achieve increased blood levels.
• In cattle, penicillin and beta-lactam drugs are frequently first-choice therapy due to high percentage of Gram-positive organisms isolated from affected animals.
• Early withdrawal of therapy may result in relapse.
• Extra-label use of antimicrobial is required because current antimicrobials are not labeled for bacterial endocarditis and for the duration of therapy required.

• Anti-inflammatory/antipyretic agents: aspirin, flunixin meglumine.
• Anticoagulants to limit enlargement of vegetative lesions and thromboembolic disease; bovine platelets respond poorly to antithrombotic effects of aspirin.
• If signs of heart failure are present, diuretics are added to the therapeutic plan.
• Maintenance of normal blood electrolyte concentrations, acid-base status, and hydration.
• Appropriate treatment of secondary organ disease or dysfunction.
• Correct hypokalemia, hypocalcemia, and other electrolyte abnormalities associated with anorexia and diuretic therapy.
• Oxygen supplementation if hypoxemic.

MEDICATIONS
DRUGS OF CHOICE
• Drug of choice is based upon information collected from blood culture and sensitivity.
• All medications used for treatment of bacterial endocarditis must be used following AMDUCA guidelines.
• Penicillin: 22,000 IU/kg: Aqueous potassium penicillin IV, q6h or procaine penicillin IM, q12h
• Amoxicillin: 10 mg/kg IM, q12h
• Ampicillin: 20 mg/kg IV, q8h; 10–20 mg/kg IM, q12h
• Anti-inflammatories: flunixin meglumine, aspirin
• Furosemide: 0.5–1 mg/kg IV, q12–24h
• Potassium supplement (50–200 g/day PO) if on potassium-wasting diuretics

CONTRAINDICATIONS
Appropriate milk and meat withdrawal times must be followed for all compounds administered to food-producing animals.

FOLLOW-UP
EXPECTED COURSE AND PROGNOSIS
• Most cases die or are culled due to poor prognosis and expense of therapy.
• Long-term survival rate and productivity level is not known.
• Prognosis is generally guarded to poor for recovery and productivity.
• Animals diagnosed early and treated aggressively with small or single lesions have a fair to good prognosis.
• Evidence that lesions or disease are resolving include regression of clinical signs, return of fibrinogen and serum protein concentrations to normal, reduction in size of lesion on echocardiographic examination, negative blood cultures 3–4 days after discontinuing antimicrobial therapy.

(CONTINUED)

• Reasons for therapeutic failure include advanced stage of disease at initiation of therapy, premature withdrawal of therapy, ongoing valvular thrombosis due to endothelial damage, bacterial recolonization of valve, and change in sensitivity or type of infecting bacteria.

 MISCELLANEOUS

ASSOCIATED CONDITIONS
• Cardiac arrhythmias including sinus tachycardia, premature ventricular contractions, and atrial fibrillation.
• Septic arthritis.
• Passive hepatic congestion.
• Congestive heart failure.
• Myocardial disease.
• Most common sequelae include embolic pneumonia, renal infarction, suppurative arthritis, hepatic emboli.
• Less common sequelae: cerebral and adrenal emboli, epididymitis, pleural effusion.

PRODUCTION MANAGEMENT
• Observe appropriate milk and meat withdrawal times for drugs administered.

• Treatment of most animals with bacterial endocarditis is often not undertaken due to costs.
• Genetically valuable animals often treated to enhance options for genetic salvage procedures (e.g., semen collection, embryo collection, cloning).
• Infection results in decreased milk and meat production.

ABBREVIATIONS
• AMDUCA = Animal Medicine Drug Use Clarification Act
• ARD = antimicrobial removal device
• GGT= gamma-glutamyl transferase
• IM = intramuscular
• IV = intravenous
• PO = per os, by mouth
• SC = subcutaneous

SEE ALSO
• Brisket Disease
• Cardiotoxic Plants
• Congential Defects: Bovine
• Gossypol Toxicosis
• Lymphosarcoma
• Monensin Toxicity
• Pericarditis
• Traumatic Reticuloperitonitis

Suggested Reading
Buczinski S, Tsuka T, Tharwat M. The diagnostic criteria used in bovine bacterial endocarditis: A meta-analysis of 460 published cases from 1973 to 2011. Vet J 2012, 193: 349–57.
Diseases of the heart. In: Radostits, Gay, Hinchcliff, Constable eds, Veterinary Medicine: A Textbook of Diseases of Cattle, Horses, Sheep, Pigs, and Goats, 10th ed. New York: Saunders, 2007, pp. 428–30.
Healy AM. Endocarditis in cattle: A review of 22 cases. Irish Vet J 1996, 49: 43–8.
Houe H, Eriksen L, Jungersen G, Pedersen D, Krogh HV. Sensitivity, specificity and predictive value of blood cultures from cattle clinically suspected of bacterial endocarditis. Vet Rec 1993, 133: 263–6.
Reef VB, McGuirk SM. Diseases of the cardiovascular system. In: Smith BP ed, Large Animal Internal Medicine, 5th ed. St. Louis: Elsevier, 2015, pp. 436–41.
Author Paul H. Walz
Consulting Editor Christopher C.L. Chase
Acknowledgment The author and book editors acknowledge the prior contribution of Susan Semrad and Sheila McGuirk.

BACTERIAL MENINGITIS

B

BASICS

OVERVIEW
• Meningitis is defined as inflammation involving one or more layers of the meninges. The meninges function to support, protect, and contribute to nourishment of the brain and spinal cord.
• Bacterial meningitis is more common than viral meningitis and is most commonly seen in neonatal ruminants concomitantly due to bacterial sepsis as a result of poor neonatal colostral intake and/or absorption. Gram-negative enteric bacteria, especially *E. coli,* are the most common pathogens associated with bacterial sepsis and bacterial meningitis.
• Meningitis can also be observed in older animals as a result of osteonecrosis induced by thermal cauterization during dehorning, extension of localized infection from skull fractures or coccygeal vertebrae (poor docking hygiene), or secondary to bacterial endocarditis.

INCIDENCE/PREVALENCE
In general, meningitis is a relatively rare condition in large animals, but is most frequently reported in neonatal farm animals. A recent survey demonstrated that the prevalence of meningitis-meningoencephalitis was 36% in critically ill Piedmontese calves <15 days of age.

SYSTEMS AFFECTED
Nervous

GEOGRAPHIC DISTRIBUTION
Worldwide

PATHOPHYSIOLOGY
• The mechanisms by which bacteria gain entry to the meninges are poorly understood; however, sustained bacteremia in neonatal ruminants may provide a source of bacteria reaching the meninges. This bacteremia, when combined with a highly perfused dural venous system and choroid plexuses, and pathogenic factors including attachment fimbria in some strains of *E. coli,* create an opportunity for bacterial colonization of the meninges.
• Once bacterial colonization occurs, a relative lack of bactericidal and opsonic activities in the CNS allow bacteria to survive and proliferate in the cerebrospinal fluid (CSF).
• The inflammatory response including release of host-derived cytokines and the direct effects of bacterial invasion and replication are responsible for the long-term neurologic sequelae and death associated with bacterial meningitis.
• Defects of CSF drainage occurring secondary to meningeal inflammation lead to hypertensive hydrocephalus.

• Bacterial meningitis can also occur by direct extension of an infectious agent into the calvarium (otitis media, infected skull fracture, sinusitis, thermal osteonecrosis) or by hematogenous spread to the CNS from a distant site (heart valves, lungs, gastrointestinal tract, joints, umbilicus).

SIGNALMENT
Neonates of all species, especially calves

PHYSICAL EXAMINATION FINDINGS
• Earliest clinical signs are often nonspecific.
• Acute meningitis may or may not be accompanied by fever in the neonate. Anorexia and loss of a coordinated suckle reflex in a neonate are common clinical signs.
• Hyperesthesia, stiff neck, depression, seizures, or blindness, with or without a history of another illness, such as enteritis or polyarthritis.
• Depression, omphalophlebitis, polyarthritis, and ophthalmitis are frequent concurrent findings.
• Ataxia, with or without spasticity and mild tetraparesis, depression, wandering, star-gazing, and abnormal vocalization may be seen.
• Lethargy, recumbency, coma, opisthotonus, convulsions, tremors, and hyperesthesia are the common clinical signs in calves with meningitis.

CAUSES AND RISK FACTORS
• Failure in the transfer of maternal antibodies predisposes to hematogenous meningitis.
• *E. coli,* the organism most often associated with neonatal sepsis, is the most common bacterium isolated. Other isolates include *Klebsiella pneumoniae, Salmonella* spp. (*S. dublin* and *S. typhimurium*), *Staphylococcus* spp., *Streptococcus* spp., and *Bacillus* spp. in calves. In sheep and goats, *Klebsiella pneumoniae, Salmonella* spp., *Streptococcus* spp., *Trueperella pyogenes, Erysipelothrix rhusiopathiae,* and occasionally *Leptospira interrogans, Listeria monocytogenes, Mycoplasma* spp., and *Fusobacterium necrophorum* are isolated.
• Both maternal and neonatal factors contribute to the development of sepsis in the neonate. They include bacterial placentitis, perinatal stress, prematurity, dystocia, birth asphyxia, unsanitary or adverse environmental conditions, overcrowding, contamination of the environment with pathogenic bacteria, and the presence of enteritis, omphalitis, or respiratory infections in the neonate.
• There may be a history of trauma, recent dehorning, or tail docking, or there may be information relating to the presence of a wound near the calvarium or vertebrae (usually older ruminants), or an infection of the sinuses, middle ear, or inner ear.
• *Histophilus somni* is a potential cause of meningitis in feedlot cattle.

DIAGNOSIS

DIFFERENTIAL DIAGNOSES
• Cerebral edema
• Encephalitis (e.g., viral)
• Hydrocephalus
• Metabolic disease (e.g., hypoglycemia, hypomagnesemia)
• Toxicity

CBC/BIOCHEMISTRY/URINALYSIS
• Leukocytosis with a left shift is common in calves.
• Respiratory acidosis, hypernatremia, hyponatremia, hyperkalemia, hypomagnesemia, and hypoglycemia may be observed also.

OTHER LABORATORY TESTS
• Low serum immunoglobulin concentrations may be observed.
• In the presence of neurologic signs, a positive blood culture supports a diagnosis of bacterial meningitis secondary to neonatal infection. Other samples, such as synovial fluid, also may culture positive.

IMAGING
Radiographs and/or ultrasound may be indicated when trauma or extension of a localized infection is suspected.

OTHER DIAGNOSTIC PROCEDURES
Definitive diagnosis is based on the presence of a neutrophilic pleocytosis, xanthochromia, turbidity, high total protein concentration in the CSF, and, ideally, positive culture from the CSF. Gram stain and culture should be attempted on CSF.

PATHOLOGIC FINDINGS
On gross necropsy, meningeal vessels appear congested and meninges are swollen and opalescent with petechiae. The CSF is often cloudy and can contain fibrin clots. Microscopic changes can include suppurative inflammation of meningeal vessels with bacterial colonies present in the meninges and brain parenchyma. Hemorrhagic or thrombotic infarcts may also be observed within the CNS.

TREATMENT

THERAPEUTIC APPROACH
• Early diagnosis and aggressive treatment are imperative for a successful outcome. By the time clinical signs are present, treatment is often unrewarding.
• Provision of adequate nutritional support and a clean, comfortable environment; protection from self-inflicted trauma; and maintenance of body temperature, fluid, and

B

acid-base balance are critical for a successful outcome.
• Treatment may be expensive and mortality rate high despite appropriate therapy.

MEDICATIONS

DRUGS OF CHOICE

Antimicrobials
• Antimicrobial therapy is the treatment of choice but is often unrewarding because course of treatment is begun too late and case fatality rate is high. The blood-brain barrier makes achieving therapeutic levels of drug in the CNS difficult.
• Selection of antimicrobial drugs should be based on either smears stained by Gram stain or culture from CSF. If empirical antimicrobial therapy is chosen, the therapy should include Gram-negative and Gram-positive spectrum.
• No drugs are labeled for treatment of bacterial meningitis; thus, treatment of bacterial meningitis in ruminants constitutes an extra-label use.
• Inflammation markedly enhances CSF concentrations of beta-lactams, particularly cephalosporins, which normally penetrate poorly. Meningitis caused by Gram-negative enteric bacteria can be treated with a third- or fourth-generation cephalosporin.
• Selection of an antimicrobial drug in ruminants should also be based on the pharmacokinetics and pharmacodynamics of the drug in neonates, the likelihood of antimicrobial resistance, and the potential for violative antimicrobial tissue residues.
• Bacteriocidal drugs are superior to bacteriostatic drugs.
• Antibiotics should be administered by intravenous routes to attain maximum peak blood and CSF concentrations.
• There is a lack of CSF pharmacokinetic data in ruminants. Specific antimicrobial therapy could include florfenicol (20 mg/kg, IV, q12h), ceftiofur (must be used at labeled dose levels, frequencies, durations, and routes of administration), and sodium ampicillin (10–20 mg/kg, IV, q8h).
• Relapses may occur as meningeal inflammation subsides and CNS concentrations of (nonlipophilic) antimicrobial drug(s) fall.
• Antimicrobial drug therapy should continue for at least 7 days after resolution of all clinical signs.

Anticonvulsants
The following drug doses for neonatal ruminants have been "guess-estimated", based on recommended doses for equine neonates.
• Diazepam (0.1–0.2 mg/kg, slowly IV, repeated every 30 minutes if necessary) is used for short-term control.
• If two to three doses of diazepam fail to control convulsions, a loading dose of phenobarbital (10–20 mg/kg diluted in 30 mL saline, IV over 15 minutes) should be given. Oral therapy (5–10 mg/kg, q8h to q12h) is then used for maintenance for long-term control.

Other Treatments
• Following rehydration, nonsteroidal anti-inflammatory drugs may be beneficial (flunixin meglumine, 0.5–1.0 mg/kg, IV, q12h to q24h)
• A plasma transfusion may be required.
• Additional therapy may be required to resolve secondary complications (i.e., abomasal ulcers due to NSAID usage, corneal trauma, etc.).

CONTRAINDICATIONS
• Acepromazine should not be used as a sedative due to its ability to lower the seizure threshold.
• Drug withdrawal times must be determined for all drugs used to treat food-producing animals.

PRECAUTIONS
Care should be exercised when dosing anticonvulsant drugs in neonates because of the increased permeability of their blood-brain barrier.

FOLLOW-UP

EXPECTED COURSE AND PROGNOSIS
Prognosis in neonatal ruminants with septic meningitis is poor, despite treatment. The key to a successful outcome relies on early recognition of CNS involvement and institution of aggressive, appropriate therapy.

PATIENT CARE
Close monitoring of vital parameters and metabolic indices is warranted during antimicrobial therapy, especially in animals showing seizure activity.

PREVENTION
• The key to prevention of meningitis in neonates is paying attention to the events leading up to and including parturition, and ensuring adequate colostral intake.

• Proper dehorning technique and hygiene during tail docking will decrease the incidence of meningitis in older animals.

MISCELLANEOUS

ASSOCIATED CONDITIONS
Generalized sepsis typically accompanies septic meningitis in neonates.

PREGNANCY
Diseases affecting the dam during gestation may predispose the neonate to partial or complete failure of passive transfer after birth.

PRODUCTION MANAGEMENT
• Measures taken that reduce perinatal stress will reduce the incidence of septic meningitis in the neonate.
• Proper dehorning technique and hygiene during tail docking will reduce the incidence of septic meningitis in older animals.

ABBREVIATIONS
• CNS = central nervous system
• CSF = cerebrospinal fluid
• IV = intravenous
• PO = per os, by mouth

Suggested Reading
Biolatti C, Bellino C, Borrelli A, et al. Sepsis and bacterial suppurative meningitis-meningoencephalitis in critically ill neonatal Piedmontese calves: clinical approach and laboratory findings. Schweiz Arch Tierheilkd 2012, 154: 239–46.
Fecteau G, George L. Bacterial meningitis and encephalitis in ruminants. Vet Clin North Am Food Anim Pract 2004, 25: 363–77.
Fecteau G, Smith BP, George LW. Septicemia and meningitis in the newborn calf. Vet Clin North Am Food Anim Pract 2009, 20: 195–208.
Passler T, Walz PH, Pugh DG. Diseases of the neurologic system. In: Pugh DG ed, Sheep and Goat Medicine, 2nd ed. Maryland Heights, MO: Elsevier Saunders, 2012.
Prescott JF. Infections of the nervous system: meningitis and encephalitis. In: Prescott JG, Baggot JD, Walker RD eds, Antimicrobial Therapy in Veterinary Medicine, 3rd ed. Ames: Iowa State University Press, 2000.
Author: Paul H. Walz
Consulting Editor Christopher C.L. Chase
Acknowledgment The author and book editors acknowledge the prior contribution of Maureen E.G. Wichtel.

BISON: BACTERIAL DISEASES

BASICS

OVERVIEW
The bacterial diseases that bison are susceptible to are similar to those found in cattle, and the disease processes in bison mimic those seen in cattle as well. Different bacterial diseases have implications regarding biosecurity, production efficiency, and clinical health of the herds affected. Further in-depth information for each disease can be found in the pertinent chapter (see pertinent chapter; SPC).

INCIDENCE/PREVALENCE
• *Arcanobacter pyogenes*: Uncommon; top differential for localized abscesses.
• Actinobacillosis: Pathology found in bison.
• Anthrax: Described in bison in the USA and Canada. • Blackleg: Uncommon; unvaccinated bison are susceptible.
• Brucellosis: Endemic in Wood Buffalo National Park, Yellowstone National Park, and Grand Teton National Park. • Foot rot: Incidence lower in bison than in cattle.
• Hemorrhagic septicemia: Uncommon in bison. • Hemophilosis: Isolated in clinically normal bison. • Johne's Disease: Clinical disease reported in bison. • Leptospirosis: ~ 7% of bison in Yellowstone National Park showed titers to leptospirosis. • Listeriosis: Low incidence in bison. • Mannheimiosis: *M. hemolytica* isolated in clinically affected bison. • Mycoplasma: *M. bovis* thought to be spread from cattle to bison. • Necrotic stomatitis: Sporadic in nature with low prevalence. • Pinkeye: Sporadic in bison, with some herds becoming infected more than others. • TB: Prevalence increases with age in endemic herds.

SYSTEMS AFFECTED
Multisystemic.

PATHOPHYSIOLOGY
• *Arcanobacter pyogenes*: This bacterium (aka *Trueperella pyogenes* or *Actinomyces pyogenes*) is present throughout the environment and in ruminant GI tracts, often taking advantage of breaches in the integument or in the oral mucosa (associated with rough/coarse feed). It can also take advantage of injury to the ruminal mucosa due to acidosis or injury. Abscesses often result, and can happen anywhere in the body. Bison develop subcutaneous, soft tissue, and hepatic abscesses caused by this bacterium.
• Actinobacillosis: SPC • Anthrax: *Bacillus anthracis* causes sudden death. Affected bison will be unresponsive, staggering, or reluctant to move. Edematous swellings on the ventrum and serosanguinous fluid seeping from orifices in dead animals can be seen. SPC • Blackleg: *Clostridium chauvei* has been reported to cause this disease in bison. SPC
• Brucellosis: *Brucella abortus* biovar 1 (in

North America) has been reported to cause disease in bison. Male bison can develop orchitis, seminal vesiculitis, and epididymitis, decreasing/eliminating fertility. Chronic infections in males can cause scrotal/testicular abnormalities. In female bison, placentitis, abortions (less frequent than in cattle), and retained placentas have been seen. Other clinical signs in bison include abscesses, chronic septic arthritis, lameness, and hygromas. Bison vaccinated with the RB51 or Strain 19 vaccines are shown to be more prone to abortion. SPC • Foot rot: The organisms responsible for foot rot in bison have not been isolated/reported. SPC.
• Hemorrhagic septicemia: This disease, caused by *Pasteurella multocida,* has not been reported in bison in the USA in the past 30 years. Disease occurs in explosive outbreaks with high mortalities. Disease often associated with high temperature, humidity, and the rainy season. Most bovids are colonized with small numbers of *P. multocida* serotype B:2 or E:2, which shed in periods of stress. Infection begins at the tonsils/nasopharyngeal tissues, with subsequent bacteremia and multi-organ infection, resulting in large release of endotoxins causing organ failure. The disease has a sudden onset, and clinical signs include excessive salivation, mucus membrane hemorrhage, depressed mentation, severe pyrexia, edema/swelling on the ventral aspect of the body, and labored breathing. Death often occurs within 1 day. • Hemophilosis: *Haemophilus somnus* (*Histophilus somni*) has been associated with bronchopneumonia in recently weaned bison calves in feedlots with minimal clinical signs, though sudden death can occur. Outbreaks are associated with cold weather and stressful situations. Thrombotic meningoencephalitis has been found in weaning bison calves, presenting with depression, recumbency, body temperature extremes, partial/complete blindness, seizures, weakness, ataxia, and proprioceptive deficits; death occurs within 1 or 2 days. SPC • Johne's disease: SPC • Leptospirosis: SPC
• Listeriosis: *Listeria monocytogenes* has caused sporadic abortions in bison, usually occurring in the last trimester of pregnancy. SPC
• Mannheimiosis: SPC • Mycoplasma: *Mycoplasma bovis* infections have been associated with a pneumonia-polyarthritis syndrome in calves, young adults, and adult bison. Clinical signs include dyspnea, stridor, coughing, lethargy, isolation from the herd, weight loss, lameness, and abortion. Infection with BVDV increases susceptibility. Cases of pneumonia with high morbidity/mortality have been seen in mature bison cows and bulls on pasture. Recovered animals can often show infertility and ill-thrift. SPC • Necrotic stomatitis: SPC • Pinkeye: The causative agent of infectious keratoconjunctivitis in bison is unknown, but thought to be *Moraxella bovis*. Disease is spread by the face

fly vector. SPC • TB: *Mycobacterium bovis* infection is characterized by granulomatous lymphadenitis affecting the lymph nodes of the head, thorax, and abdominal cavity. Clinical signs include chronic weight loss, cough, and enlarged lymph nodes. Affected bison also suffer from orchitis, metritis, and abortions. SPC

SIGNALMENT
Plains bison (*Bison bison* subsp *bison*) and woods bison (*Bison bison* subsp *athabascae*)

PHYSICAL EXAMINATION FINDINGS
See SPC

CAUSES AND RISK FACTORS
• *Arcanobacter pyogenes*: Breaches in protective epithelial layer (skin/mucosa) due to coarse feeds/high grain diets causing acidosis.
• Actinobacillosis: Breaches in the oral mucosa/tongue epithelium caused from coarse feeds/eruption of teeth. • Anthrax: Ingestions of infective environmental spores. Outbreaks occur during summer months with prolonged wet periods followed by drying conditions. Spores surface after heavy rainfall.
• Blackleg: Ingestion of environmental spores, seeding of spores in muscle in combination with muscle injury/bruising. Unvaccinated individuals are at high risk. • Brucellosis: Susceptible animals that come in contact (from ingestion/mucus membrane contact/skin breaches) with infected herd mates/wildlife and their contaminated bodily fluids (blood, urine, milk, semen, vaginal discharges) or aborted fetuses/placentas from positive females. • Foot rot: Abrasions in interdigital space allow bacterial invasion. Wet weather, rough pasture, stony ground, and unsanitary housing conditions can predispose bison. • Hemorrhagic septicemia: Infection occurs by ingestion of contaminated feed/water or contact with infected oral/nasal secretions from carrier animals/diseased animals, with young immunosuppressed/stressed individuals most at risk. • Hemophilosis: Exposure to diseased animals/carrier animals when individuals are immunocompromised. Handling/processing, weaning, and exposure to cattle can predispose individuals. • Johne's disease: Transplacental transmission, or ingestion of contaminated feed/water. Risk factors include exposure to shedding individuals, especially when young. Rain run-off from cattle farms can be a source of infection. • Leptospirosis: Ingestion/contact with contaminated environment/water sources or with contact with urine, vaginal discharge, post-abortion discharge, or a fetus from a *Leptospira*-induced abortion. • Listeriosis: Ingestion/contact with contaminated environment/feed or clinically/subclinically infected individuals. Stress, pregnancy, and feeding of poorly preserved ensiled forages are risk factors. • Mannheimiosis: Immunocompromise increases susceptibility.

Stressful situations (weaning/transport) can predispose. • Mycoplasma: Exposure to infected animals (domestic cattle/bison) through fence line contact, importation of stock, and concurrent infection with BVDV are risk factors. • Necrotic stomatitis: Injuries/abrasions to the mouth/tongue from the use of balling guns or rough/coarse feeds can allow invasion into oral tissues. • Pinkeye: *Moraxella bovis*, spread by the face fly, is thought to be the most likely cause; herds with face fly issues are at risk. Proximity to endemic cattle herds is a risk factor. • TB: Ingestion of contaminated feed/aerosolized infectious particles from infected/shedding individuals can precipitate disease, especially in the immunocompromised.

DIAGNOSIS

OTHER DIAGNOSTIC PROCEDURES
• *Arcanobacter pyogenes*: SPC
• Actinobacillosis: SPC • Anthrax: SPC
• Blackleg: SPC • Brucellosis: A fluorescence polarization assay with high sensitivity/specificity in bison has been developed and shows promise at differentiating antibodies induced by strain 19 vaccination and true infection. SPC • Foot rot: SPC • Hemorrhagic septicemia: Diagnosis is often made on postmortem examination, with submission of tissues for C/I/S. Antemortem diagnosis is done based on history, vaccination status, environmental conditions, and clinical signs/lesions. Blood/tissues from individuals can be sent off for bacterial isolation by PCR.
• Hemophilosis: Diagnosis is difficult in live bison, and most often diagnosed on postmortem examination. SPC • Johne's Disease: Antemortem tests in cattle can be used in bison, but have poor sensitivity. Fecal PCR/culture are the most reliable diagnostic tests. SPC • Leptospirosis: SPC • Listeriosis: An aborted fetus with the placenta must be submitted to a pathology laboratory for histopathology/bacterial culture (to diagnose listeriosis abortion). SPC • Mannheimiosis: SPC • Mycoplasma: *M. bovis* should be considered in herd disease outbreaks with high morbidity and mortality. Lung tissue culture taken from postmortem examination is best way for definitive diagnosis. Histopathologic lesions can ID the organism by IHC or PCR. Affected and exposed bison have high antibody titers. SPC • Necrotic stomatitis: SPC • Pinkeye: SPC • TB: SPC

PATHOLOGIC FINDINGS
• *Arcanobacter pyogenes*: N/A
• Actinobacillosis: SPC • Anthrax: SPC
• Blackleg: SPC • Brucellosis: Arthritis, retained placenta, placentitis, and pyometra. Histopathology includes necropurulent placentitis, bronchointerstitial pneumonia in

fetuses/neonates, serous arthritis with thickening/distention of the joint capsule, and seminal vesiculitis/orchitis in bulls. SPC • Foot rot: SPC. • Hemorrhagic septicemia: Widespread subcutaneous edema, subserosal hemorrhages of organs/body cavities, and edema/inflammation of the lungs.
• Hemophilosis: Hemorrhagic infarcts in the brain/spinal cord found in bison. SPC
• Johne's disease: SPC • Leptospirosis: SPC
• Listeriosis: SPC • Mannheimiosis: SPC
• Mycoplasma: Affected individuals are generally emaciated with severe fibrinonecrotizing pneumonia, fibrinous pleuritis, epicarditis, and/or chronic pleuropneumonia. Widespread dissemination to the tonsils, pharynx, larynx, mediastinal/abdominal lymph nodes, peritoneum, pericardium, liver, spleen, kidney, mammary gland, endometrium, and joints. Lesions in distant locations from lung are characterized by areas of caseous necrosis. Histopathology includes eosinophilic necrosis with ID of the organism on IHC. Liquefactive necrosis in the lung and inflammatory cell infiltrates of the joint capsules are common. SPC • Necrotic stomatitis: SPC • Pinkeye: SPC • TB: Abscesses or granulomas in the lymph nodes of the head, pharynx, thoracic cavity, and abdominal cavity are seen. Some cases only involve a few or a single lymph node. Generalized tuberculosis has occurred. SPC

TREATMENT

THERAPEUTIC APPROACH
• *Arcanobacter pyogenes*: SPC
• Actinobacillosis: SPC • Anthrax: SPC
• Blackleg: SPC • Brucellosis: SPC • Foot rot: SPC • Hemorrhagic septicemia: Antimicrobial treatment is successful if enacted early in the disease. • Hemophilosis: Disturbing newly weaned bison calves to examine/treat is very stressful and can predispose other calves to the disease. Sick calves should be removed from the group, treated, and returned to the group; SPC
• Johne's disease: SPC • Leptospirosis: SPC
• Listeriosis: SPC • Mannheimiosis: Broad-spectrum antibiotics; supportive care (decreasing stress/overexertion, providing high-quality nutrition/free choice water); surveillance of calves at risk with little or no intervention is critical to minimize mortalities; sick calves should be removed from the group, treated, and returned to the group; SPC • Mycoplasma: Recrudesces after cessation of antibiotic therapy, indicating persistent nature of infection; SPC • Necrotic stomatitis: Broad-spectrum antibiotics, anti-inflammatories (to aid respiration); SPC
• Pinkeye: Spontaneous recovery occurs; small volumes of penicillin injected into bulbar

conjunctiva/eyelid conjunctiva; not recommended to suture the eyelids closed/use third eyelid flaps, bison will remove these sutures shortly after placement; bison with pinkeye can be very dangerous to themselves and to handlers; SPC • TB: SPC

MEDICATIONS

DRUGS OF CHOICE
Note: No medications have been approved or licensed for use in bison, and minimal efficacy trials performed; all use must be done extra-label and generally at cattle dosages unless otherwise stated. Appropriate milk and meat withdrawal times must be followed for all compounds: contact FARAD. Please follow BQA guidelines regarding injections.
• *Arcanobacter pyogenes*: N/A
• Actinobacillosis: Shown sensitivities to tetracyclines/erythromycin. Sodium iodide at 70 mg/kg as a 10–20% solution must be administered IV, which is problematic in bison. • Anthrax: N/A • Blackleg: N/A
• Brucellosis: N/A • Foot rot: Long-acting antibiotic preparations are the practical choice for bison, SPC • Hemorrhagic septicemia: Sulfonamides, tetracyclines, penicillin, ceftiofur, enrofloxacin, and tilmicosin. Some strains (B:2) show resistance to tetracyclines and penicillins. • Hemophilosis: Long-acting oxytetracycline or florfenicol have been used for neurologic disease. • Johne's disease: N/A
• Leptospirosis: SPC • Listeriosis: Penicillin/oxytetracycline. Frequency of administration of these medications may be prohibitive in bison. • Mannheimiosis: SPC
• Mycoplasma: Oral tetracyclines and tylosin have been used with variable results. SPC
• Necrotic stomatitis: SPC • Pinkeye: SPC
• TB: N/A

FOLLOW-UP

PREVENTION
Note: No vaccinations have been approved or licensed for use in bison, and minimal efficacy trials performed; all use must be done extra-label.
• *Arcanobacter pyogenes*: Feeding high forage/low concentrates, allowing most nutrition to come from pasture/quality hay.
• Actinobacillosis: Pasture grazing/offering quality hay. • Anthrax: SPC. • Blackleg: Recommended to administer a commercial cattle multivalent *Clostridium* vaccination annually to all bison. • Brucellosis: *B. abortus* eradication programs instituted: serologically positive or infected bison are slaughtered. Other surveillance measures include farm testing, slaughterhouse testing, and monitoring movement of bison. Vaccination

B

of bison is not recommended (not permitted in Canada). • Foot rot: SPC • Hemorrhagic septicemia: Removal of carrier animals; a formalin inactivated vaccine was developed/used in a Montana herd; control programs in wild herds are not currently in use due to the low disease prevalence.
• Hemophilosis: Reduce frequency of elective stressful situations (handling, processing, weaning) in combination with uncontrollable stressful situations (cold weather); recurrence rate in subsequent years is moderate-to-high if disease is found within a herd. Anecdotal evidence suggests that vaccination with a commercially available *H. somnus* cattle vaccine may reduce mortalities in bison calves.
• Johne's disease: Fecal cultures/PCR every 6 months, culling of infected animals and their offspring. Depopulating/repopulating with clean stock in the face of severe disease outbreaks. New arrivals to herd should be tested. SPC • Leptospirosis: No vaccinations recommended; practitioner discretion.
• Listeriosis: SPC • Mannheimiosis: Decrease stressful situations when weaning calves.
• Mycoplasma: Quarantine new arrivals, avoid fence line contact with domestic cattle, routine surveillance in susceptible herds.
• Necrotic stomatitis: SPC • Pinkeye: Due to unknown etiologic agent for pinkeye in bison, efficacy of commercial vaccines questionable, though anecdotal accounts of moderate-to-good efficacy with these vaccines. SPC • TB: Acquiring animals from a TB-free herd/having them tested (caudal tail fold tuberculin skin test) prior to arrival into herd; exclusion of wild reservoir hosts (white-tailed deer) from pastures. SPC

 MISCELLANEOUS

ZOONOTIC POTENTIAL
• Anthrax: SPC • Brucellosis: SPC • Johne's Disease: SPC • Leptospirosis: SPC
• Listeriosis: SPC • TB: SPC

BIOSECURITY
• Anthrax: SPC • Brucellosis: SPC
• Tuberculosis: SPC

PRODUCTION MANAGEMENT
• Thought that bison will respond to antibiotics similarly as cattle, but no pharmacologic studies have been performed in bison. Care should be taken when dosages/meat withdrawal times are recommended. • Often best to use a long-acting preparation as first choice when treating bison; daily handling of sick bison increases risk of injury/stress to both handler and animal. Including a few healthy bison in pen with a sick bison can keep the animal calmer due to herd mentality. • Bison mask clinical signs associated with disease, and often don't show clinical signs until just before death; important to be knowledgeable about normal bison behavior in order to remedy stressful situations and catch disease early.

ABBREVIATIONS
• BQA = Beef Quality Assurance
• BVDV = bovine viral diarrhea virus
• C/I/S = culture/identification/susceptibility
• FARAD = Food Animal Residue Avoidance Databank
• ID = identification
• IHC = immunohistochemistry
• IV = intravenous
• PCR = polymerase chain reaction
• SPC = see pertinent chapter. "SPC" written next to specific disease sections indicates to the reader to "See Pertinent Chapter" of Blackwell's Five-Minute Veterinary Consult: Ruminant. These chapters are listed in the "See Also" section for each disease.
• TB = tuberculosis

SEE ALSO
The following chapters will provide more details on particular diseases:
• Actinobacillosis: Wooden Tongue
• Actinomycosis: Lumpy Jaw
• Anthrax

• Brucellosis
• Calf Diphtheria/Necrotic Stomatitis
• Clostridial Disease: Muscular
• Corneal Disorders
• Foot Rot: Bovine
• *Histophilus somni* Complex
• Johne's Disease
• Leptospirosis
• Listeriosis
• *Mycoplasma bovis* Associated Diseases
• Respiratory Disease: Bovine
• Tuberculosis: Bovine
Also of interest:
• Bison: Clinical Examination and Treatment (see www.fiveminutevet.com/ruminant)
• Bison: Management (see www.fiveminutevet.com/ruminant)
• Bison: Parasitic Diseases
• Bison: Viral Diseases

Suggested Reading
Choquette LPE. Parasites and diseases of bison in Canada. 1. Tuberculosis and some other pathological conditions in bison at Wood Buffalo and Elk Island National Park in the fall and winter of 1959-60. Can Vet J 1961, 2.5: 168–74.
Choquette LPE. Parasites and diseases of bison in Canada IV. Serologic survey for brucellosis in bison in Northern Canada. J Wildl Dis 1978, 14: 329–32.
Heddleston KL. Septicemic pasteurellosis (hemorrhagic septicemia) in the American bison: A serologic survey. Bul Wildl Dis Assoc 1969, 5: 206–7.
Taylor SK. Serologic survey for infectious pathogens in free-ranging American bison. J Wildl Dis 1997, 33: 308–11.
Tessaro SV. Review of the diseases, parasites and miscellaneous pathological conditions of North American bison. Can Vet J 1989, 30: 416–22.
Author David M. Love
Consulting Editor Christopher C.L. Chase
Acknowledgment The author and book editors acknowledge the prior contribution of John Berezowski.

BISON: PARASITIC DISEASES

BASICS

OVERVIEW
• Parasitism is common in bison, but its clinical significance must be judged based on overall condition, environment, stocking density, clinical signs, and other factors.
• Parasites found in bison are also found in cattle, and the treatment is often similar between these species. Many of these diseases generate important economic concerns affecting bison production.

INCIDENCE/PREVALENCE
• Anaplasmosis: Depends on location, local reservoirs (i.e., *A. marginale* positive cattle farms), and tick prevalence. 15.7% of wild bison tested in the National Bison Range in Montana were positive.
• Babesiosis: Depends on location, local reservoirs, and tick prevalence.
• Coccidiosis: Common in ranched/farmed bison; uncommon in free-ranging bison.
• Demodecosis: Minor significance.
• Helminthiasis: Common and prevalent anywhere herds reside.
• Hydatid tapeworms: Isolated from bison, no clinical signs/deaths reported (though potential for disease is present).
• Liver flukes: Fluke eggs have been observed in the feces of bison; clinical disease not commonly reported.
• Lungworm: Occurs in the USA and Canada; often not diagnosed until the bison dies due to nonspecific obscure clinical signs.
• *Parelaphostrongylus tenuis*: Uncommon, but should be considered in bison exhibiting neurologic disease.
• Ticks and tick paralysis: Uncommon, reported in bison from Montana.
• Warbles: Isolated in bison in the USA/Canada; may be more common than clinically noted due to the insidious nature of these parasites.

GEOGRAPHIC DISTRIBUTION
Dependent on distribution of management systems, vectors and hosts.

SYSTEMS AFFECTED
Multisystemic

PATHOPHYSIOLOGY
• The specific pathophysiologic processes of most parasitic infections of bison are described in individual chapters throughout this text that address specific parasitic pathogens.
• Anaplasmosis: Acute infections occur; bison remain infective up to 496 days post-infection, suggesting bison may act as reservoirs; bison thought to be more resistant than cattle.
• Babesiosis: *Babesia bigemina* and *B. major* have both been isolated from bison and fatalities reported.

• Coccidiosis: Various *Coccidia* species have been isolated from bison, with no published reports of clinical disease.
• Demodecosis: The causative species of demodex in bison has not been identified. Mites invade hair follicles/sebaceous glands, and create small (7–9 mm) black nodules filled with pus around the eyes, perineum, ventral aspect of tail, neck, flank, and shoulders.
• Helminthiasis: Type II ostertagiosis causes morbidity/mortality in bison. *Cooperia* is commonly identified in bison, but clinical disease has not been seen.
• Hydatid tapeworms: Adult forms of two tapeworms (*Taenia hydatigina* and *Echinococcus granulosis*) release eggs into the feces of carnivores (ex. domestic dogs) which are consumed by secondary hosts (bison); eggs hatch in the intestinal tract, migrate to the peritoneal cavity/liver/lungs, and form cysts (hydatids/cysticerci). Damage occurs with cyst formation, causing organ failure.
• Liver flukes: Bison develop acute/chronic hepatitis with hepatic fluke migration and biliary damage
• Lungworm: Clinical signs are difficult to recognize at pasture, leading to mortalities; disease is commonly seen in late summer.
• *Parelaphostrongylus tenuis*: Documented aberrant migration of larvae in bison cause various neurologic signs.
• Ticks and tick paralysis: *Dermacentor andersoni* has been implicated in tick paralysis of bison calves/yearlings in Montana.
• Warbles: *Hypoderma* larvae are unable to penetrate through the skin and dense hair of bison; however, numerous bison in the western US have been found with dead larvae underneath the hide along their back.

HISTORICAL FINDINGS
N/A

SIGNALMENT
Bison of any age and gender may be affected.

PHYSICAL EXAMINATION FINDINGS
• Dependent on the specific parasite, its pathogenesis, and parasite burden.
• Signs relate to damage of the liver, intestines, lungs, integument, nervous or hemolymphatic systems.

GENETICS
There is gathering evidence that genetic characteristics are important in host resistance/resilience to parasitic infections.

CAUSES AND RISK FACTORS
• Anaplasmosis and babesiosis: Older bison are more susceptible. No deaths have been reported due to *A. marginale* infection in bison.
• Coccidiosis: Poor sanitation, overcrowding, poor pen design, wet conditions, and stress associated with weaning can all precipitate coccidiosis.

• Demodecosis: Immunocompromised individuals are more susceptible.
• Helminthiasis: Risk factors include wet weather, cool summers/warm winters, high stocking rates, and contaminated pastures.
• Hydatid tapeworms: Risk factors include exposure to carnivore feces on pasture.
• Ticks and tick paralysis: Heavy infestation of ticks can cause anemia in young calves due to sheer volume of blood being removed by the parasites. Risk factors include immunosuppression and *D. andersoni* home range overlap.

DIAGNOSIS

DIFFERENTIAL DIAGNOSES
Differentials should be relevant to the major organ system affected and/or the primary clinical signs displayed.

CBC/BIOCHEMISTRY/URINALYSIS
• Depending on the type of parasite infestation, abnormalities might reflect dehydration, blood loss, protein loss, inflammation, liver damage, etc.

OTHER LABORATORY TESTS
• Fecal analysis by various methods is a useful method for detection of many parasites.
• An array of tests also exists for blood-borne parasites.

IMAGING
N/A

OTHER DIAGNOSTIC PROCEDURES
See individual chapters on specific parasites for additional procedures.

PATHOLOGIC FINDINGS
Strongly dependent on the parasite in question and the systems affected.

TREATMENT

See individual chapters on specific parasites for recommendations.

THERAPEUTIC APPROACH
Pharmaceutical intervention, including anthelmintic agents, may be indicated, along with concurrent supportive care measures in clinically diseased animals.

SURGICAL CONSIDERATIONS AND TECHNIQUES
N/A

MEDICATIONS

DRUGS OF CHOICE
• No medications have been approved or licensed for use in bison, and minimal efficacy trials have been performed; all drugs are

BISON: PARASITIC DISEASES

B

therefore used in an extra-label fashion and generally at cattle dosages unless otherwise stated.
• See individual chapters on specific parasites for treatment recommendations.

CONTRAINDICATIONS
N/A

PRECAUTIONS
• Appropriate milk and meat withdrawal times must be followed for all compounds.
• Advice is to follow BQA guidelines regarding injections.

POSSIBLE INTERACTIONS
N/A

 FOLLOW-UP

EXPECTED COURSE AND PROGNOSIS
See individual chapters on specific parasites for recommendations.

POSSIBLE COMPLICATIONS
N/A

CLIENT EDUCATION
Should focus on establishing appropriate management and prevention protocols, and judicious use of pharmaceutical or anthelmintic agents where necessary.

PATIENT CARE
N/A

PREVENTION
• See individual chapters on specific parasites for recommendations.
• Demodecosis is not a highly contagious ectoparasite so no control programs are reported.
• Hydatid tapeworms: Prevent contamination of bison pasture/feed areas with carnivore feces; screen and treat suspect domestic carnivores around ranches/farms.
• Liver flukes: Consider treating bison in early spring to reduce contamination of pasture during summer.

• Lungworm: Set up a two-pasture rotation system; administer anthelmintics prior to pasture turnout/rotation; perform surveillance of fecal samples in early spring to identify individuals shedding larvae.

 MISCELLANEOUS

ASSOCIATED CONDITIONS
N/A

AGE-RELATED FACTORS
Young and old bison are likely more susceptible to specific parasitic infections.

ZOONOTIC POTENTIAL
N/A

PREGNANCY
N/A

BIOSECURITY
N/A

PRODUCTION MANAGEMENT
• The importance of most gastrointestinal parasites in bison is uncertain, therefore the economic value of routine deworming is questionable. Anecdotal evidence suggests that many of these parasites contribute to poor growth rate and clinical disease in farmed bison.
• Commercially available deworming pellets are not recommended due to the hierarchical structure of bison herds and inability to ensure proper dosing of all individuals. Their use can allow low-level anthelmintic exposure within most individuals in the herd, promoting parasite resistance.
• Delaying spring grazing of infected pastures until overwintered larvae have died on pasture is highly recommended. Pasture rotation and management is crucial in reducing parasite burdens.

SYNONYMS
N/A

ABBREVIATION
• BQA = Beef Quality Assurance

SEE ALSO
• Anaplasmosis
• Babesiosis
• Coccidiosis
• Coenurosis
• Haemonchosis
• Liver Flukes
• Nematodirus
• Ostertagiasis
• Parasite Control Programs: Dairy
• Parasitic Pneumonia
• Tick Paralysis

Suggested Reading
Choudary C. Hydatidosis in lungs and liver of an American bison (*Bison bison*). Ind Vet J 1987, 713–14.
Haigh JC, Mackintosh C, Griffin F. Viral, parasitic and prion diseases of farmed deer and bison. Rev Sci Tech 2002, 21: 219–48.
Kohls GM. Tick paralysis in the American buffalo, *Bison bison*. Northwest Sci 1952, 26: 61–4.
Locker B. Parasitism of Bison in Northwestern USA. J Parasitol 1953, 39: 58–9.
Tessaro S. Review of the diseases, parasites and miscellaneous pathological conditions of North American bison. Can Vet J 1989, 30: 416–22.
Van Vuren D, Scott CA. Internal parasites of sympatric bison, *Bison bison*, and cattle, *Bos taurus*. Can Field Nat 1995, 4: 467–9.
Vestweber JG, Ridley RK, Nietfeld JC, Wilkerson MJ. Demodicosis in an American bison. Can Vet J 1999, 40: 417–18.
Author David M. Love
Consulting Editor Erica C. McKenzie
Acknowledgment The author and book editors acknowledge the prior contribution of John Berezowski.

BASICS

OVERVIEW
Many of the viral diseases that bison are susceptible to are similar to those found in cattle, and certain viral disease processes in bison mimic those seen in cattle, with a few notable exceptions. Other cattle viral diseases have shown to stimulate bison to produce antibodies against the virus, but clinical disease has not been reported. Different viral diseases have implications regarding biosecurity, production efficiency, and clinical health of the herds affected. Further in-depth information for each disease can be found in the pertinent chapter (see pertinent chapter; SPC).

INCIDENCE/PREVALENCE
• BVDV/Mucosal disease: Acute BVDV has been seen in bison, but none of the other forms (mucosal disease, persistent infection, or thrombocytopenic forms) have been reported in bison. It has been shown that in some herds in the western USA, up to 55% of adult bison were seropositive for BVDV.
• Neonatal viral diarrhea (rotavirus): Not as common as in cattle, but is seen in overcrowded holding pens or overstocked production systems.
• Infectious bovine rhinotracheitis (IBR): Clinical disease in bison is not reported to be common, but up to 44% of bison screened in the western USA and Canada were seropositive for the virus, indicating exposure.
• Malignant catarrhal fever (MCF): Bison are very susceptible if exposed to sheep shedding the virus. Multiple epizootics have been reported in the USA.
• Parainfluenza-3 (PI-3): In Yellowstone National Park, 36% of all bison tested showed antibodies to this virus. No clinical disease has been reported.

SYSTEMS AFFECTED
• Respiratory
• Digestive
• Cardiovascular
• Musculoskeletal
• Reproductive

PATHOPHYSIOLOGY
BVDV/Mucosal Disease
• BVDV is an RNA virus from the family Togaviridae, genus Pestivirus. BVDV is a very complex disease, and its behavior even in cattle has not completely been established, let alone in bison. It is known that not only is it present within bison herds, but it also causes disease—with both non-cytopathic and cytopathic forms. There are various strains within the cattle population that can cause various maladies, but the strains of the virus that are found in bison have not been reported. There are several different manifestations of the disease that have been seen in cattle: acute BVD, fetal infections, mucosal disease, and the thrombocytopenic form of BVD.
• The acute form of BVD occurs in animals that have not been previously exposed to the virus, and can range from an asymptomatic infection to acute diarrhea associated with anorexia and pyrexia. This form of BVDV infection has been seen in bison and has been shown to cause mortality in bison of all ages.
• Fetal BVDV infections have not been reported in bison, but are entirely possible and usually are seen (in cattle) following an acute BVDV outbreak. Fetal infections can cause abortion, stillbirths, weak calves, persistent infection, and fetal abnormalities. Persistently infected calves can occur if the fetus contracts BVDV in the first 40–120 days of gestation. Persistently infected calves are born infected and continue to be a subclinical shedder the remainder of their lives, infecting others (including their own progeny) with the disease. These animals are generally unthrifty and are poorly developed, with low weaning weights. They can develop diarrhea at any time in their life.
• Mucosal disease has not been reported in bison. The disease only occurs in animals (cattle) that are persistently infected and contract another strain of BVDV. It is often fatal, and clinical signs include ulcerations of the mucus membrane, snout, and the feet, with sloughing of the hooves noted in a few cases. They develop diarrhea, pyrexia, and emaciation before death.
• The thrombocytopenic form of BVDV has also not been reported in bison, but in cattle it had shown to cause hemorrhage in all mucus membranes, blood nasal discharges, bloody diarrhea, and coagulopathies. Mortality from this form is extremely high. SPC.

Neonatal Viral Diarrhea (Rotavirus)
• In calves, there are many possible etiologies of diarrhea, which include some viruses such as rotavirus, coronavirus, calicivirus, parvovirus, and BVDV, as well as many bacterial and protozoal etiologies.
• Rotavirus has been associated with neonatal diarrhea in bison. Though not as common as it is in cattle, stress can predispose neonatal calves to this disease and in bison it has been associated with overcrowding.
• The most common clinical sign is a watery diarrhea, which can predispose the calf to becoming dehydrated, weak, and depressed. They often can be seen staggering and remaining recumbent prior to death, though some bison calves hide their clinical signs until the disease is very severe. Observing the perineal area of bison calves and bedding is important to look for signs of diarrhea. SPC.

Infectious Bovine Rhinotracheitis
• IBR is common in cattle, and caused by bovine herpesvirus-1 (BHV-1). It is spread by nasal secretions, semen, and fetal fluids, and can easily be aerosolized from coughing animals.
• Clinical signs have not been described in bison, but are suspected to be similar to those found in cattle: fever, anorexia, reddening of the nasal mucosa, ocular discharge, nasal discharge, increased respiratory rate, and coughing. It can be very contagious and occurs in large outbreaks in cattle.
• Calves who develop symptoms have been associated with a high mortality rate, and cattle <6 months of age can develop neurologic signs from BHV-1 induced encephalitis, also leading to a high mortality rate.
• Abortion can occur in infected pregnant animals, up to 90 days after infection. SPC.

Malignant Catarrhal Fever
• MCF in bison in North America is caused by ovine herpesvirus type 2, which is endemic in both domestic and wild sheep. When a dead-end host, such as a bison, contracts this virus, it can cause severe disease. It is not, however, contagious between bison.
• Numerous reports have discussed this disease in bison, which is almost always fatal. Bison most often develop an acute fatal form of disease where they die 7–10 days after contracting the virus, but they can also develop a chronic fatal form where it may take up to 156 days for them to die.
• Clinical signs include corneal opacity, keratoconjunctivitis, nasal discharge, ocular discharge, excessive salivation, diarrhea, ulceration of the oral mucosa, anorexia, fever, neurologic signs, melena, and hematuria, with the most common signs being anorexia, depression, and bloody diarrhea. They often separate themselves from herd mates, and become depressed.
• In most reports, this disease is seen in winter, but can occur at any time. Herd mortalities have reached 100% in some instances. It is seen more commonly in animals >6 months of age. SPC.

Parainfluenza-3
• PI-3 is a virus seen commonly in respiratory disease complexes of cattle. Though antibodies have been found in the serum of bison (both wild and farmed), no clinical disease or decrease in productivity have been reported. That being said, any stressed bison can be affected by this virus, and measures should be taken to avoid immunocompromise.
• In cattle, clinical signs include nasal discharge, coughing, and pneumonia, often with secondary bacterial infections. SPC.

SIGNALMENT
Plains bison (*Bison bison* subsp. *bison*) and woods bison (*Bison bison* subsp. *athabascae*)

PHYSICAL EXAMINATION FINDINGS
SPC

B

CAUSES AND RISK FACTORS

• BVDV/Mucosal disease: BVDV is spread from animal to animal through secretions and excretions, such as diarrhea. Fomites can also carry the virus from pasture to pasture, and to different farms. It is thought that the virus can spread from infected cattle to bison. Pregnant animals infected with the non-cytopathic strain of the virus within a specific time period (40–120 days) can cause the calf to become persistently infected and shed the virus its whole life. Bison farms adjacent to cattle farms, poor hygiene within bison facilities, and poor biosecurity practices are all risk factors. SPC.
• Neonatal viral diarrhea (rotavirus): Most transmission occurs through the fecal-oral route, often with ingestion of contaminated feed or water. Young animals, immunocompromised individuals, and high stress environments (like overcrowding) can all predispose bison to rotaviral diarrhea. SPC.
• Infectious bovine rhinotracheitis (IBR): Transmission of the virus through aerosolized secretions is the main way this virus is transmitted. It has a high morbidity, and high mortality in young and immunocompromised animals. Young animals and immunocompromised individuals are at high risk of fatal disease. Proximity to cattle herds, overcrowding, high stress situations, and omitting quarantine protocols for newly acquired animals are potential risk factors. SPC.
• Malignant catarrhal fever (MCF): Exposure to animals (generally sheep), transmitted through direct contact, fomite transmission, or contact with discharge/feces from hosts. Bison have contracted MCF when sheep were grazed as far as 3 km away SPC.
• Parainfluenza 3 virus (PI-3): Exposure to infected cattle is most likely the source of exposure to this virus. Stressed bison can potentially become susceptible to the virulent effects of this viral disease that are seen in cattle. SPC.

DIAGNOSIS

OTHER DIAGNOSTIC PROCEDURES

• BVDV/Mucosal disease: In cattle, blood samples for virus isolation or PCR testing can give reliable results. Immunohistochemistry from an ear skin notch can test for a persistently infected individual. Serial BVDV serology can be performed to determine exposure versus infection titer. Postmortem examination and submission of samples can also be done. SPC.
• Neonatal viral diarrhea (rotavirus): Fecal samples can be submitted to diagnostic pathology laboratories for bacterial culture (to rule out other etiologies) and virus isolation.

Postmortem samples can be sent off for histopathology and virus isolation. SPC.
• Infectious bovine rhinotracheitis (IBR): The virus can be isolated in swabs taken from nasal and ocular exudate. Postmortem examination with histopathology and virus isolation of aborted fetuses or samples can provide a diagnosis as well. Serial antibody testing can be performed 2–3 weeks apart to detect rising titers to BHV-1. SPC.
• Malignant catarrhal fever (MCF): Diagnosis can be made from blood samples or nasal swabs submitted for PCR testing—though this method is not validated in bison. Serum samples from herds can be used for antibody screening via competitive inhibition ELISA tests. Postmortem examination and submission of tissue samples for PCR is the only validated way to establish a diagnosis—pooled tissue samples are best, as ovine herpesvirus type 2 does not infect all tissues consistently. SPC.
• Parainfluenza-3 (PI-3): Serology is the best test to determine exposure to this virus. Virus isolation from nasal swabs or blood can determine active infection. SPC.

PATHOLOGIC FINDINGS

• BVDV/Mucosal disease: In cattle with mucosal disease, postmortem findings include shallow ulcers in the mouth, pharynx, esophagus, rumen, and omasum. There also can be mucosal erythema and hemorrhage within the gastrointestinal tract. SPC.
• Neonatal viral diarrhea (rotavirus): Dehydration, emaciation, and fluid feces within the intestinal tract are often seen on rotavirus-infected bison calf postmortems. SPC.
• Infectious bovine rhinotracheitis (IBR): The pathologic changes have not been reported in bison, but in cattle the lesions are often focused in the nasal cavities, pharynx, larynx, trachea, and on the muzzle. SPC.
• Malignant catarrhal fever (MCF): Ulcerations of the mouth, esophagus, rumen, abomasum, intestinal tract, and trachea are common. Hemorrhages in the urinary bladder, enlarged lymph nodes, injected conjunctiva, and corneal opacity have also been seen in bison. Widespread necrotizing lymphocytic vasculitis without thrombosis is most often seen on histopathology. There can also be vascular hemorrhages, epithelial degeneration, and lymphoid hyperplasia with invasion of lymphoid cells into nonlymphoid tissues— which can sometimes be seen on the kidney at gross necropsy. SPC.
• Parainfluenza-3 (PI-3): SPC.

TREATMENT

THERAPEUTIC APPROACH

• BVDV/Mucosal disease: There has not been any treatment that has shown to be successful

in either bison or cattle. Supportive care is the best option, but often culling infected individuals can decrease chances of spread to other individuals within the herd. SPC.
• Neonatal viral diarrhea (rotavirus): This can be a self-limiting disease, and many bison calves recover spontaneously. Reducing stress and offering supportive care can help, but providing supportive care to bison calves most often results in a calf that must be hand-reared (bison cows will reject the calves after only a few days of separation). Supportive care can include oral or intravenous fluid and electrolyte therapy, correction of acid-base imbalances, and potentially parenteral antibiotics, as the calves can be susceptible to other infections. SPC.
• Infectious bovine rhinotracheitis (IBR): Infected bison should be separated from noninfected bison, and not allowed nose-to-nose contact. No treatment protocols are described, but NSAIDs can potentially lessen the severity of disease. Antimicrobials can help decrease the chances of a secondary bacterial infection. In cattle, vaccinating with a modified-live intranasal vaccine during an outbreak can sometimes help reduce the spread of the disease. SPC.
• Malignant catarrhal fever (MCF): There are no successful treatment protocols established for treating bison, and are usually ineffective. Supportive care can be provided. SPC.
• Parainfluenza-3 (PI-3): No treatment protocols are suggested for bison due to no clinical disease reported. SPC.

PREVENTION

• BVDV/Mucosal disease: In cattle, control of BVDV can be very difficult. Vaccines are available for cattle, but the immunogenicity, safety, or efficacy have not been tested and published in bison. Vaccination may not provide adequate protection against the occurrence of mucosal disease and persistently infected individuals, but may provide adequate protection against acute BVD infection in bison—though none are registered or labeled for use in bison, and should be approached with caution. Certain adjuvants found in killed BVDV vaccines can have unfavorable effects in calves, and modified-live vaccines have shown to not only cause diarrhea in recently weaned bison calves, but also abortion in pregnant beef cattle. Yearling and older adult nonpregnant adult bison have, anecdotally, shown no adverse reactions to these vaccines.
• Neonatal viral diarrhea (rotavirus): At the time of writing, calf scour vaccinations are not generally recommended for use in bison. No studies have been done, and the best prevention is reducing stocking density, increasing facility hygiene, and decreasing sources of stress for neonatal bison calves. SPC.
• Infectious bovine rhinotracheitis (IBR): Currently, there are no approved vaccinations

B

for use against BHV-1/IBR in bison, though there are multiple available modified-live and killed vaccines for cattle. Properly quarantining new animals and infected animals can help reduce introduction and spread of the disease, respectively. SPC.
• Malignant catarrhal fever (MCF): There are no vaccinations available for this virus. Avoid all contact between bison and sheep/goats as well as wildebeest, and keep a safe distance between pastures of these animals. The mean incubation period following exposure to sheep is reported to be 81 days, range 50–220 days. SPC.
• Parainfluenza-3 (PI-3): Avoiding contact with cattle is the best chance of avoiding exposure to this potential pathogen. Some respiratory vaccines also include this in their coverage, but they have not been approved in bison. SPC.

ABBREVIATIONS
• BHV-1 = bovine herpesvirus type 1
• BVD = bovine viral diarrhea
• BVDV = bovine viral diarrhea virus
• ELISA = enzyme-linked immunosorbent assay
• IBR = infectious bovine rhinotracheitis
• MCF = malignant catarrhal fever
• PCR = polymerase chain reaction
• PI-3 = parainfluenza-3
• SPC = see pertinent chapter. "SPC" written next to specific disease sections indicates to the reader to "See Pertinent Chapter" of Blackwell's Five-Minute Veterinary Consult: Ruminant. These chapters are listed in the "See Also" section for each disease.

SEE ALSO
The following chapters will provide more details on particular diseases:

• Bovine Viral Diarrhea Virus
• Infectious Bovine Rhinotracheitis
• Malignant Catarrhal Fever
• Neonatal Diarrhea
• Parainfluenza-3 Virus
• Rotavirus
Also of interest:
• Bison: Bacterial Diseases
• Bison: Clinical Examination and Treatment (see www.fiveminutevet.com/ruminant)
• Bison: Management (see www.fiveminutevet.com/ruminant)
• Bison: Parasitic Diseases

Suggested Reading
Amborski GF. Isolation of a retrovirus from American bison and its relation to bovine retroviruses. J Wildl Dis 1987, 23: 7–11.
Berezowski JA, Appleyard GD, Haigh J, et al. An outbreak of sheep-associated malignant catarrhal fever in bison (*Bison bison*) after exposure to sheep at a public auction sale. J Vet Diagn Invest 2005, 17: 55–8.
Collins JK, Bruns C, Vermedahl TL, Demartini JC. Malignant catarrhal fever: polymerase chain reaction survey for ovine herpesvirus 2 and other persistent herpesvirus and retrovirus infections of dairy cattle and bison. J Vet Diagn Invest 2000, 12: 406–11.
Haigh JC, Mackintosh C, Griffin F. Viral, parasitic and prion diseases of farmed deer and bison. Rev Sci Tech 2002, 21: 219–48.
Heuschele WP, Reid H. Malignant catarrhal fever. In: Williams E, Barker I, eds, Infectious Diseases of Wild Mammals. Ames: Iowa State University Press, 2001, pp. 157–64.

Li H. Prevalence of antibody to malignant catarrhal fever virus in wild and domesticated ruminants by competitive-inhibition ELISA. J Wildl Dis 1996, 32: 437–43.
Li H, Shen DT, O'Toole D, Knowles DP, Gorham JR, Crawford TB. Investigation of sheep-associated malignant catarrhal fever virus infection in ruminants by PCR and competitive inhibition enzyme-linked immunosorbent assay. J Clin Microbiol 1995, 33: 2048–53.
Liggitt HD. Experimental transmission of bovine malignant catarrhal fever to a bison (*Bison bison*). J Wildl Dis 1980, 16: 299–304.
Ruth GR. Malignant catarrhal fever in bison. J Am Vet Med Assoc 1977, 171: 913–17.
Sausker E, Dyer N. Seroprevalence of OHV-2, BVDV, BHV-1, and BRSV in ranch raised bison (*Bison bison*). J Vet Diagn Invest 2002, 14: 68–70.
Schultheiss PC. Malignant catarrhal fever in bison, acute and chronic cases. J Vet Diagn Invest 1998, 10: 255–62.
Taylor SK. Serologic survey for infectious pathogens in free-ranging American bison. J Wildl Dis 1997, 33: 308–11.
Tessaro S. Review of the diseases, parasites and miscellaneous pathological conditions of North American bison. Can Vet J 1989, 30: 416–22.

Author David M. Love
Consulting Editor Christopher C.L. Chase
Acknowledgment The author and book editors acknowledge the prior contribution of John Berezowski.

BLACK LOCUST TOXICITY

BASICS

OVERVIEW
• Black locust (*Robinia pseudoacacia*) may also be known as yellow locust, post locust, locust tree, or false acacia.
• Medium size tree growing up to 80 feet.
• Bark of black locust is dark reddish-brown to black in color. It has an alternate branching pattern with a pair of sharp short thorns at each node.
• Leaves are pinnate, compound measuring approximately 8 to 14 inches in length with 7 to 19 short stalked leaflets. Leaflets are ovoid or oval, 1 to 2 inches long, thin, rough, dull green above and pale below.
• Flowers are creamy white, with five petals arranged in a pyramidal spike, usually blooming in May or June.
• Seeds are produced in a flat, brown to black pod, approximately 2 to 4 inches long with an average of 25,500 seeds per pound.

INCIDENCE/PREVALENCE
Feeding meal composed of 20% locust leaves causes decreased protein digestibility in lambs.

GEOGRAPHIC DISTRIBUTION
• Native to United States from northern Georgia and Alabama to Pennsylvania and westward to Oklahoma but has been transplanted thru much of the US.
• It has been additionally transplanted to areas of Europe, Southern Africa, and Asia.

SYSTEMS AFFECTED
• Digestive
• Cardiovascular

PATHOPHYSIOLOGY
• Toxic compounds include: glycoside robitin, alkaloid robinine, and lectins or toxalbumins robin, ricin, and phasin.
• Toxalbumins inhibit protein synthesis leading to cell death. Rapidly proliferating cells, such as those found within the intestinal wall, are most commonly affected.
• Ricin decreases calcium uptake by the sarcoplasmic reticulum as well as increasing the sodium calcium exchange, leading to a dysfunction of intracellular calcium homeostasis.
• Bark, leaves, and seeds are the primary source of the toxin. Bark is the most toxic. Flowers are nontoxic.
• Toxic dose is not well established; it is approximately 0.5% body weight in cattle.

HISTORICAL FINDINGS
Presence of plant or cuttings of the plant within the pasture.

SIGNALMENT
• Bovine, ovine, caprine, and camelid species.
• Ruminants are one tenth less sensitive than horses.

PHYSICAL EXAMINATION FINDINGS
• Depression; however, cattle can become belligerent
• Anorexia
• Abdominal pain
• Diarrhea (blood may be present)
• Weakness
• Weak pulse
• Congested mucus membranes
• Arrhythmias

CAUSES AND RISK FACTORS
• Gastric irritation and ulceration as a result of toxalbumin effects.
• Cardiac dysfunction as a result of ricin effects on calcium homeostasis.
• Rarely reported intoxication in cattle.

DIAGNOSIS

DIFFERENTIAL DIAGNOSES
Other causes of gastroenteritis

OTHER DIAGNOSTIC PROCEDURES
• History of exposure to the plant
• Finding of plant material within gastric contents on gross pathology

PATHOLOGIC FINDINGS
Gastroenteritis, reddening, edema, and perhaps small hemorrhages of the mucosa of the stomach and small intestine, although degenerative lesions may be found in other organs.

TREATMENT

THERAPEUTIC APPROACH
• Decrease absorption of the toxin thru administration of charcoal.
• Supportive including gastroprotectants, fluid therapy, and pain management.

FOLLOW-UP

EXPECTED COURSE AND PROGNOSIS
• Prognosis depends on the amount of the plant that has been consumed and the time of supportive treatment initiation. Recover may take several weeks.
• Death is rare.

PATIENT CARE
• Dehydration
• Fecal consistency and color

PREVENTION
Restrict grazing of livestock from areas where black locust tress grow.

MISCELLANEOUS

Suggested Reading
Burrows GE. Fabaceae. In: Burrows GE, Tyrl RJ eds, Toxic Plants of North America. Iowa: Wiley, 2013, p. 596.
Vanschandevijl K, van Loon G, Lefere L, et al. Black Locust (*Robina pseudoacacia*) intoxication as a suspected cause of transient hyperammonaemia and enteral encephalopathy in a pony. Eq Vet Educ 2010, 22: 336–9.
Author Jennifer S. Taintor
Consulting Editor Christopher C.L. Chase
Acknowledgment The author and book editors acknowledge the prior contribution of Larry A. Kerr.

BASICS

OVERVIEW
Gas distension of the rumen and reticulum. Primary or frothy bloat occurs when rumen gas is trapped in bubbles/froth, and cannot be eructated. Secondary or free gas bloat occurs because of physical blockage of the esophagus or from decreased vagal nerve function.

INCIDENCE/PREVALENCE
• Normally very low incidence, generally <1%.
• Incidence of primary bloat may be >25% if animals are grazed on immature legumes/clover or fed excessive amounts of highly fermentable carbohydrates, such as finely ground grains.

GEOGRAPHIC DISTRIBUTION
Worldwide

SYSTEMS AFFECTED
• Digestive
• Cardiovascular

PATHOPHYSIOLOGY
• Normal rumen bacterial fermentation produces gases that are eructated from the rumen. Primary or frothy bloat occurs when the gas is trapped in bubbles/froth, and cannot be eructated. Immature legumes and clovers are rapidly fermented by rumen microflora, resulting in release of chloroplast particles that trap gas bubbles and prevent their coalescence.
• Additionally, liquid is trapped in the foam, reducing the passage of liquid from the rumen. This serves to enhance bacterial growth and increase gas and foam production. Feeding finely ground grains can also cause frothy bloat.
• Secondary or free gas bloat occurs because of physical blockage of the esophagus (i.e., feed materials such as potatoes/beets) or from decreased vagal nerve function. Decreased vagal nerve function may be caused by mediastinal masses such as tumors from lymphoma, enlarged lymph nodes from tuberculosis and chronic bacterial pneumonia. Expansion of the rumen within the abdominal cavity eventually compresses the diaphragm, decreasing lung volume, oxygenation and the venous return to the post cava, causing hypovolemia.
• Young calves can bloat from fermentation of milk or milk replacer in the rumen.

HISTORICAL FINDINGS
Sheep and cattle grazing on lush pastures, especially young legumes or clovers. High concentrate diets with finely ground grains. History of chronic pneumonia.

SIGNALMENT
Ruminants, especially cattle

PHYSICAL EXAMINATION FINDINGS
• Distension of the left flank from gas accumulation. Tachycardia from hypoxia. Rumen contractions may decrease but often remain normal. Abdominal discomfort is evident.
• Severe cases may show open mouth breathing and staggering. Animal may become recumbent from hypoxia.
• Distension of the dorsal left flank. Cattle with chronic vagal indigestion may have concurrent distension of ventral right flank due to rumen emptying defect ("papple-shape": right side pear/left side apple).
• Tachycardia often present.

GENETICS
N/A

CAUSES AND RISK FACTORS
• Blockage of the esophagus or interference with the vagus nerve.
• Grazing or feeding early legumes or clovers. Feeding finely ground grains or rapidly fermented carbohydrates.
• Inflammation or masses in the mediastinum can affect vagus nerve function. Factors associated with the spread of tuberculosis, bovine leukemia virus, and chronic bacterial pneumonia can impact the vagus nerve.

DIAGNOSIS

DIFFERENTIAL DIAGNOSES
• Ruminants often bloat postmortem. Necropsy signs of antemortem bloat include compression of blood and lymph flow in the neck and thorax, resulting in enlarged cervical vessels and lymph nodes. There is often a visible "white line" demarcation in the esophagus near the thoracic inlet from compression of the distal esophagus and congestion in the proximal esophagus.
• Lymphoma, enlarged lymph nodes from tuberculosis and chronic bacterial pneumonia.

CBC/BIOCHEMISTRY/URINALYSIS
N/A

OTHER LABORATORY TESTS
N/A

IMAGING
N/A

OTHER DIAGNOSTIC PROCEDURES
Passing a stomach tube differentiates primary (frothy) from secondary (free gas) bloat. Esophageal blockages may often be detected while passing the stomach tube.

PATHOLOGIC FINDINGS
• Distension of the rumen and reticulum with gas.

• Congestion of cervical lymph nodes and vessels.
• "White line" demarcation in esophagus at interface of compressed and congested tissue.

TREATMENT

THERAPEUTIC APPROACH
• Depends on the cause and the degree of hypoxia. Severely hypoxic animals should be intubated to relieve the free gas. The tube often plugs with froth or dips below the fluid level in the rumen, requiring clearing the tube by blowing into it or moving the end within the rumen.
• Mild to moderate cases of frothy bloat often respond to oral surfactants such as poloxalene (25–50 g per animal). Mineral or vegetable oils may act as anti-foaming agents.
• In severe cases it may be necessary to place a rumen trocar in the dorsal left flank. Animals may die from cardiac insufficiency due to collapse of splanchnic venous return.

MEDICATIONS

DRUGS OF CHOICE
Poloxalene (25–50 g per animal) for primary bloat

CONTRAINDICATIONS
N/A

PRECAUTIONS
Administer using an orogastric tube rather than oro-esophageal tube to reduce the risk of aspirating surfactant products.

POSSIBLE INTERACTIONS
N/A

FOLLOW-UP

EXPECTED COURSE AND PROGNOSIS
• Spontaneous recovery in mild cases and those patients sufficiently relieved by stomach tube/trocar or treated with poloxalene.
• Death from hypoxia or hypovolemic cardiac insufficiency in severe cases.

POSSIBLE COMPLICATIONS
• Physical damage to the vagus nerve or branches of the vagus from excessive rumen distension may result in rumen dysfunction and possible recurrence.
• Trocarization may result in localized or diffuse peritonitis.

PATIENT CARE
Watch for recurrence.

BLOAT

B

CLIENT EDUCATION
• Advise clients about the danger of grazing or feeding immature legumes/clovers especially to hungry animals.
• Discuss the importance of a functional rumen mat in cattle on high concentrate diets.
• Discuss early recognition of bloat and treatments such as poloxalene and stomach tubing.

PREVENTION
• Avoid feeding or grazing high-risk plants such as legumes or clovers. If feeding is necessary, ensure a slow transition and always fill cattle with a high dry matter feed such as straw prior to grazing. Do not overfeed finely ground grain or other highly fermentable carbohydrates.
• Avoid feeding apples, potatoes, or feedstuffs that can lodge in the esophagus and block eructation.
• Prevent infections with bovine respiratory disease complex, bovine leukemia virus, and tuberculosis.

MISCELLANEOUS

ASSOCIATED CONDITIONS
• Lymphoma
• Vagal indigestion
• Tuberculosis

AGE-RELATED FACTORS
Young calves may bloat from fermentation of milk or milk replacer in the rumen.

ZOONOTIC POTENTIAL
N/A

PREGNANCY
N/A

SYNONYM
Ruminal tympany

ABBREVIATIONS
N/A

SEE ALSO
• Lymphosarcoma
• Respiratory Disease: Bovine
• Tuberculosis: Bovine
• Vagal Indigestion

Suggested Reading
Majak W, Hall JW, McCaughey WP. Pasture management strategies for reducing the risk of legume bloat in cattle. J Anim Sci 1995, 73: 1493–8.
Radostits OM, Gay CC, Blood DC, Hinchcliff KW eds. Veterinary Medicine: A Textbook of Diseases of Cattle, Sheep, Pigs, Goats and Horses, 9th ed. London: Saunders, 2000, pp. 293–303.
Author Jim P. Reynolds
Consulting Editor Kaitlyn A. Lutz

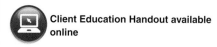

Client Education Handout available online

BLUE-GREEN ALGAE POISONING

BASICS

OVERVIEW

• Over 50 genera of freshwater blue-green algae (also referred to as cyanophytes or cyanobacteria) exist worldwide that produce two major types of toxins: neurotoxic alkaloids, such as anatoxins, and hepatotoxic peptides, such as microcystins.
• Very few cases of anatoxin poisoning (often produced by *Anabaena flos-aquae*) have been reported in cattle with clinical signs resembling organophosphorus insecticide poisoning (depolarizing neuromuscular blocking agent), such as muscle weakness and paralysis.
• Microcystin toxicosis is much more common than anatoxin poisoning and numerous cases have been reported in cattle and sheep worldwide. Therefore, microcystin toxicosis is discussed in detail.
• Microcystins are primarily produced by *Microcystis aeruginosa*, but many other cyanobacteria produce these peptides such as other *Microcystis* spp., *Anabaena* spp., *Oscillatoria* spp., and *Nostoc* spp.
• Microcystins are usually confined within the algal cells and are released only when cells are damaged (e.g., when cells encounter the acidic environment of the stomach).
• Microcystins enter the hepatocytes through a carrier-mediated transport system and cause inhibition of protein phosphatase (1 and 2A) in the hepatocytes. Dissociation and necrosis of hepatocytes lead to intrahepatic hemorrhage and diffuse centrilobular hepatocellular degeneration.
• Sudden death is possible as a result of hemorrhagic shock.
• Death in animals usually occurs within hours to days postexposure.
• Animals that survive the acute phase of poisoning can recover, but may develop clinical signs related to liver disease (e.g., hepatogenous photosensitization; drop in production).
• Respiratory—pulmonary edema and congestion have been reported in acute cases.

SYSTEMS AFFECTED

• Nervous
• Multisystemic

INCIDENCE/PREVALENCE

• Blue-green algae poisoning occurs seasonally during warm weather conditions. The blooms are most common in the summer and fall when bodies of water are stagnant and warm and contain ample nutrients.
• A breeze blowing across the water may help concentrate the organisms near a shore.
• Not all animals in a herd may be affected. Several important factors are related to

occurrence of poisoning. Favorable algae growth conditions are usually required to produce sufficiently high concentrations of algae in water. Nutrient pollution of lakes and ponds with phosphorus and nitrogen leads to eutrophication and accelerated algae growth.
• Long periods of sustained sunshine, which produce warm water temperatures, are usually necessary. A breeze blowing across the water has also been identified as critical in some situations for concentrating algae near a shore where cattle congregate on the leeward side during hot weather.
• Microcystins are the most prevalent hepatotoxins and are produced by several cyanobacteria genera including *Microcystis, Planktothrix, Anabaena,* and *Oscillatoria.* Anatoxins are produced mainly by *Anabaena* spp. in addition to *Aphanizomenon, Microcystis,* and *Oscillatoria* spp. Saxitoxin production is associated with a few specific freshwater cyanobacteria species found in the genera of *Anabaena, Aphanizomenon, Cylindrospermopsis, Lyngbya,* and *Planktothrix.*

GEOGRAPHIC DISTRIBUTION
Worldwide

PHYSICAL EXAMINATION FINDINGS

• Animals exposed to blue-green algae toxins are often found dead near water that has a thick algal bloom. Cattle may have algae on their limbs.
• Abrupt onset of apprehension and distress occurs within hours of microcystin exposure.
• This is quickly followed by pale mucus membranes, ruminal atony, diarrhea, weakness, nervousness, ataxia, and anorexia. In severe cases, the animals become recumbent and comatose.
• Death may occur within 24 hours of exposure, but may be delayed several days.
• Animals that survive the initial toxicosis may develop hepatogenous photosensitization.

SIGNALMENT

• All ruminant species are susceptible to blue-green algae toxins. Microcystin poisoning has been reported in cattle and sheep.
• Dead animals are often found close to water bodies that have a "painted green" or "scumlike" bloom.

CAUSES AND RISK FACTORS

• Exposure to water contaminated with toxin-producing cyanobacteria.
• Warm, dry weather and stagnant water and a breeze that blows across water, allowing the organisms to concentrate near a shore.
• High concentrations of nutrients in the water, such as nitrates and phosphates from sewage, detergents, industrial pollution, and fertilizers increase the risk for a blue-green algae bloom.

DIAGNOSIS

DIFFERENTIAL DIAGNOSES

• Other hepatotoxicants—metals (detection in liver and kidney, histopathologic lesions), aflatoxins (detection in feed, often chronic), pyrrolizidine alkaloids (evidence of plant consumption, histopathologic lesions, chronic disease).
• Cardiotoxic plant exposure, such as oleander, milkweed, and azalea—chemical analysis for plant toxins in gastrointestinal contents, history of presence of plants in the environment.
• Cyanide poisoning—mucus membranes are initially bright cherry red, evidence of exposure to cyanogenic plants, chemical analysis for cyanide in gastrointestinal contents, liver, or muscle.
• Electrocution or lightning strike.
• Grass tetany—hypomagnesemia.
• Hepatopathy—serum clinical chemistry and liver biopsy.
• Larkspur poisoning—mainly found in the western US states; bloat is a common finding, evidence of exposure to *Delphinium* spp.
• Nitrate toxicosis—chocolate-colored blood, exposure to nitrate-accumulating plants.
• Organophosphorus or carbamate insecticide exposure—commonly associated with gastrointestinal irritation and neurologic signs, evaluation of cholinesterase activity, detection of pesticides in gastrointestinal contents.
• Lead poisoning—determination of blood lead concentration.
• Neurotoxic plant exposure, such as poison hemlock, water hemlock, tree tobacco, lupine—chemical analysis for plant toxins in gastrointestinal contents, history of presence of plants in the environment.

CBC/BIOCHEMISTRY/URINALYSIS
Increased GGT, AST, SDH, and GLDH

OTHER LABORATORY TESTS

• Direct microscopic examination of water and gastrointestinal contents.
• Detection of microcystins in water or rumen contents by high-performance liquid chromatography/mass spectrometry.
• Mouse bioassay.
• Analysis of suspect water by direct competitive ELISA or protein phosphatase inhibition assay.

PATHOLOGIC FINDINGS

• Postmortem lesions in animals that died of exposure to microcystins include hepatomegaly, congested and hemorrhagic liver.

BLUE-GREEN ALGAE POISONING   (CONTINUED)

B

• Histopathologically, microcystin toxicosis results in centrilobular hepatocellular degeneration and necrosis; dilatation and engorgement of sinusoids; and loss of hepatic cords.
• Postmortem lesions are generally nonspecific in animals that died of exposure to neurotoxic blue-green algae toxins (e.g., anatoxins).

TREATMENT

THERAPEUTIC APPROACH
• Treatment of animals exposed to blue-green algae toxins is primarily supportive and symptomatic. Supportive therapy should include administration of intravenous fluids, corticosteroids, and calcium.
• Poisoned animals should be removed immediately from the source.
• Poisoned animals should be protected from UV exposure to prevent/minimize secondary photosensitization.
• Adsorption of toxins with activated charcoal has been suggested.
• Rumenotomy or a rumen lavage may be considered in valuable animals.

MEDICATIONS

DRUGS OF CHOICE
• No antidote available
• Activated charcoal, mineral oil, or saline cathartics
• Corticosteroids
• Vitamin E and selenium supplementation
• Hepatic uptake blockers, such as rifampicin and cyclosporin A, may be helpful, but their usefulness in the treatment of microcystin-poisoned ruminants has not been evaluated.

CONTRAINDICATIONS
N/A

POSSIBLE INTERACTIONS
N/A

FOLLOW-UP

EXPECTED COURSE AND PROGNOSIS
• Animals poisoned with microcystins are often found dead.
• Microcystin poisoning progresses rapidly, and treatment is often too late. If animals exhibit clinical signs of liver failure, the prognosis is poor.
• Animals that survive 24–72 hours after exposure usually survive but may develop clinical signs associated with hepatic failure.

POSSIBLE COMPLICATIONS
Hepatogenous photosensitization

CLIENT EDUCATION
• Create awareness for potential of blue-green algae toxicity, especially during sunny, warm weather and other favorable environmental conditions.
• A heavy water bloom of algae producing a surface scum is usually necessary for poisonings to occur.

PATIENT CARE
• Monitoring of liver enzymes is helpful.
• Monitor serum electrolytes.

PREVENTION
• Keep animals away from water bodies with visible algal blooms.
• Precipitation of algal cells:
  ○ Lime (100–250 mg/L) to precipitate cells without rupturing them
  ○ Suspend ferric alum block (1 kg/10,000 L)
  ○ Suspend gypsum block (50 kg/1000 L)
• Algaecide (lysis of algal cells): Copper sulfate at 20–40 g/50,000 L (target concentration: 0.2–0.4 ppm). After treating water body with copper sulfate, animals must be kept away for approximately 7 days.
• Use of straw bales (100 g/1000 L) to control algal blooms has also been reported. Barley straw seems to be more effective when compared to wheat or other straws.

MISCELLANEOUS

ASSOCIATED CONDITIONS
Hepatopathy

SYNONYMS
N/A

ABBREVIATIONS
• AST = aspartate aminotransferase
• ELISA = enzyme linked immunosorbent assay
• GGT = gamma-glutamyl transferase
• GLDH = glutamate dehydrogenase
• SDH = sorbitol dehydrogenase

SEE ALSO
• Carbamate Toxicity
• Cardiotoxic Plants
• Cyanide Toxicosis
• Grass Tetany/Hypomagnesemia
• Lead Toxicosis
• Lupine Toxicity
• Mycotoxins
• Nitrate and Nitrite Toxicosis
• Organophosphate Toxicity
• Poison Hemlock
• Pyrrolizidine Alkaloids
• Tobacco Toxicosis
• Water Hemlock

Suggested Reading
Puschner B, Roegner AF. Cyanobacterial (blue-green algae) toxins. In: Gupta R ed, Veterinary Toxicology: Basic and Clinical Principles, 2nd ed. San Diego: Elsevier, pp. 953–66.
Puschner B, Galey FD, Johnson B, et al. Blue-green algae toxicosis in cattle. J Am Vet Med Assoc 1998, 213: 1605–7.
Roder JD. Blue-green algae. In: Plumlee KH ed, Clinical Veterinary Toxicology. St. Louis: Mosby, 2004.

Authors Birgit Puschner and Adrienne C. Bautista
Consulting Editor Christopher C.L. Chase
Acknowledgment The author and book editors acknowledge the prior contribution of Asheesh Tiwary and Terry W. Lehenbauer.

BASICS

OVERVIEW
- Bluetongue (BT) is an arthropod-borne, noncontagious viral infection of domestic and wild ruminants caused by bluetongue virus (BTV).
- Antibodies against BTV have been detected in a wide variety of domestic and wild ruminants.
- In 2006, the spread of the northern European strain of BTV-8 resulted in one of the major outbreaks in the history of BT.
- In some countries, BTV is a reportable disease of significant economic concern and of major importance for the international trade of animals and animal products.
- The Office International des Epizooties (OIE) includes BT in their A list of diseases.

INCIDENCE/PREVALENCE
- Prevalence of serum BTV antibodies in endemic areas ranges from 1% to >80% in domesticated and wild ruminants.
- Clinical disease varies from <5% to 50–75% when the virus is first introduced into a naïve population of sheep, but once the infection becomes endemic, morbidity and mortality may be as low as 1 to 2%.

GEOGRAPHIC DISTRIBUTION
- Bluetongue is enzootic throughout much of a broad belt encompassing subtropical and tropical areas of the world, from latitude approximately 40° North and 35° South, corresponding to the distribution of specific species of *Culicoides* biting midges. In recent years, BT has spread beyond this traditional range.
- Periodic incursions of the infection occur annually or at longer intervals in latitudes as far as 50° North. With the exception of BTV-8, other BTV serotypes do not persist throughout the winter.
- Outbreaks in Northern Europe are almost exclusively caused by BTV-8.
- In the United States, BTV infection is more prevalent in the southern and western parts of the country; and most infections occur in late summer and fall.
- Currently, twenty-six BTV serotypes (BTV-1 to -26), including Toggenburg virus (BTV-25) and a serotype 26 from Kuwait, are recognized worldwide.
- Four serotypes are endemic in the US (10, 11, 13, 17); BTV-2 has been isolated sporadically in the US. Nonendemic serotypes (1, 3, 5, 6, 9, 12, 14, 19, 22, and 24) have been found in the southeastern US since 1999.
- During the last two decades, BT has spread beyond its normal range due to climate change, deforestation, and increased global commerce.

SYSTEMS AFFECTED
- Cardiovascular
- Musculoskeletal
- Reproductive
- Digestive
- Respiratory
- Nervous

PATHOPHYSIOLOGY
- Bluetongue is caused by BT virus (BTV), of the genus *Orbivirus* in the family Reoviridae. The genus also includes epizootic hemorrhagic disease virus (EHDV), equine encephalosis, and African horse sickness (AHS) viruses.
- The BTV genome consists of ten linear segments of dsRNA encoding seven structural (VP1 to VP7) and four nonstructural (NS1 to NS4) proteins.
- BTV serotype is determined predominantly by VP2, which is the main target of neutralizing antibodies.
- Transmission of BTV among susceptible hosts occurs through the bite of certain species of infected *Culicoides* or biting midges.
- The main vector of BTV in the US is *Culicoides sonorensis* (previously known as *C. varipennis*); in Australia, *C. brevitarsis*; in Africa, Asia, and Europe, *C. imicola*; *C. insignis* is the major vector of multiple BTV serotypes in Central and South America. *C. insignis* also is found in the southeastern US.
- Transmission can also occur transplacentally or by semen.
- Viremia is prolonged but not persistent. In cattle, viremia may last 60 days, occasionally up to 100 days. In sheep and goats, viremia lasts 14–54 days and 19–54 days, respectively.
- BTV RNA can be detected by RT-PCR in blood of some infected animals for over 200 days in the absence of infectious virus.
- After entering the body, BTV disseminates to the regional lymph node to commence replication. It then disperses to many tissues throughout the body, and replicates within the mononuclear phagocytic and endothelial cells and lymphocytes. BTV infection of red cells facilitates infection of insect vectors.
- Replication of BTV in endothelial cells leads to cell death and subsequent injury to small blood vessels. This can create thrombosis, tissue ischemia, and hemorrhage. Endothelial damage in vulnerable species (e.g., white-tailed deer) can provoke disseminated intravascular coagulation (DIC).

HISTORICAL FINDINGS
N/A

SIGNALMENT
- BTV infects a wide range of domestic and wild ruminants. Among domestic animals, severe disease occurs almost exclusively in sheep, and particularly those naïve to the infection.
- White-tailed deer, bighorn sheep and pronghorn antelope are highly susceptible.

Morbidity and mortality in these species can be as high as 100% and 80–90%, respectively.
- Cattle and goats generally develop subclinical infection; however, during the BTV-8 outbreaks in Western and Central Europe, mortality in cattle reached 26% in some areas.
- European BTV-8 is a particularly virulent strain capable of passing the placenta and infecting the fetus.
- BT with high mortality has been reported sporadically in South American camelids.

PHYSICAL EXAMINATION FINDINGS
- BT clinical signs range from inapparent infection to acute fulminant disease.
- The incubation period ranges from 2 to 15 days.
- Clinical disease in domestic ruminants is largely restricted to sheep; the acute fulminant form is characterized by fever up to 107.6°F (42°C), leukopenia, anorexia, weight loss, depression, edema and swelling of the face, lips, muzzle, and ears, reddening of the oral mucosa, and salivation. Pregnant sheep may abort.
- Crusting and accumulation of mucopurulent discharge in the muzzle and nostrils occurs, and in some cases, the tongue appears edematous and purplish-blue (hence the name of the disease) as a result of cyanosis.
- Hemorrhages, erosions, and ulcers of the gums, cheeks, tongue, and nostrils.
- Lameness and stiffness.
- Laminitis manifests as swelling, hyperemia, and hemorrhage of the hoof laminae and coronary band, and may induce "knee walking" or recumbency.
- Death due to bronchopneumonia or secondary bacterial infections may occur 8–10 days after initial signs.
- BTV infection of pregnant sheep or cattle may result in abortion, stillbirths, fetal malformation, or the birth of live but weak offspring (dummy lambs/calves) with minimal systemic signs in the dam. These negative effects have been linked to the use of modified-live vaccines (MLV) and more recently to BTV-8 infection in Europe.

GENETICS
North European breeds of sheep appear to be more susceptible to BTV-induced disease.

CAUSES AND RISK FACTORS
Ruminants living in areas where the vector *Culicoides* and BTV coexist.

DIAGNOSIS

DIFFERENTIAL DIAGNOSES
- Sheep: Foot-and-mouth disease (FMD), orf, sheep pox, peste des petits ruminants, photosensitization, polyarthritis, foot rot, and also toxic (monensin) and nutritional

B

(vitamin E/selenium deficiency) myopathies must be considered.
• Cattle: FMD; vesicular stomatitis; bovine viral diarrhea (BVD); rinderpest; bovine malignant catarrhal fever; Ibaraki disease (in Japan), and photosensitization.
• In white-tailed deer, epizootic hemorrhagic disease (EHD).
• The differential diagnosis for BTV fetal infection, fetal malformations and abortions include infection with Cache Valley virus, Akabane virus, Border disease virus, BVD, Rift Valley fever virus, Nairobi sheep disease virus, Wesselsbron disease virus, and genetic defects, and ingestion of teratogenic plants.

CBC/BIOCHEMISTRY/URINALYSIS
Leukopenia

OTHER LABORATORY TESTS
N/A

IMAGING
N/A

OTHER DIAGNOSTIC PROCEDURES
• Serologic assays include complement fixation, virus neutralization, agar gel immunodiffusion (AGID), and ELISA. Only the AGID and competitive ELISA (cELISA) are recommended by the OIE for international movement of ruminants.
• Virus isolation can be performed by inoculation of susceptible sheep or embryonated chicken eggs with heparinized blood or homogenized lymph nodes, spleen, or lung. Subsequent adaptation to cell culture and serotyping of the virus may be necessary. Blood and tissue samples for diagnosis need to be preserved at 4°C, and not frozen.
• BTV can be isolated from blood of infected sheep and cattle for up to 54 and 60 days post-infection, respectively. BTV nucleic acids can be detected by reverse transcription-polymerase chain reaction (RT-PCR) for up to 222 days post-infection. However, blood from sheep and cattle is infectious for *C. sonorensis* for only 21 days after infection of the ruminant host.
• Real-time RT-PCR is a commonly used diagnostic test with high sensitivity and specificity; however, a positive RT-PCR result does not indicate the presence of infectious virus.

PATHOLOGIC FINDINGS
• Grossly, BTV infection in sheep may result in extensive vascular injury that leads to congestion, edema, hemorrhage, disseminated intravascular coagulation, and tissue necrosis.
• Affected animals may have hyperemia and edema of the eyelids, ears, intermandibular area, muzzle, and other areas of the skin.
• Laminitis and coronitis.
• Lips, gums, and tongue may be edematous, congested, or cyanotic, with ulcerations and hemorrhages of the tongue, oral mucosa, hard palate, dental pad, and sometimes fore-stomachs and intestine.

• Subcutaneous and intramuscular edema and hemorrhages.
• Superficial lymph nodes may be enlarged and edematous.
• The most consistent lesion in sheep is hemorrhage in the tunica media at the base of the pulmonary artery and less often aorta, epicardium, endocardium, and myocardium.
• Pale areas in skeletal and cardiac muscles.
• Pulmonary congestion and edema.
• Pneumonia due to secondary bacterial infections.
• Fetal infection during the first trimester results in hydranencephaly, porencephaly, retinal dysplasia, and/or arthrogryposis.
• Microscopically, affected animals have vascular thrombosis with congestion, edema, hemorrhage, and ischemic necrosis.
• Myofiber necrosis (infarcts) of the left ventricular papillary muscles and other areas of the myocardium.
• Hemorrhages and myodegeneration and necrosis of skeletal muscles.
• Ulceration and crusting of the gastrointestinal tract.
• Pneumonia.

TREATMENT

THERAPEUTIC APPROACH
There are no specific treatments for BT.

SURGICAL CONSIDERATIONS AND TECHNIQUES
N/A

MEDICATIONS

DRUGS OF CHOICE
Broad-spectrum antimicrobials are often used to treat secondary bacterial infections.

CONTRAINDICATIONS
Appropriate milk and meat withdrawal times must be followed for all compounds administered to food-producing animals.

PRECAUTIONS
N/A

POSSIBLE INTERACTIONS
N/A

FOLLOW-UP

EXPECTED COURSE AND PROGNOSIS
The majority of infections are subclinical, but mortality can be high in sheep with severe disease.

POSSIBLE COMPLICATIONS
• Secondary bacterial infections.
• DIC

CLIENT EDUCATION
N/A

PATIENT CARE
Affected animals should be protected from the environment, and provided with clean water and good-quality feed.

PREVENTION
• Both modified-live virus (MLV) and inactivated BTV vaccines are available in some parts of the world for use in sheep and sheep and cattle, respectively.
• MLV vaccines have side effects, including reduced milk production in lactating ewes, and pregnancy loss and fetal teratogenesis when pregnant females are vaccinated during the first half of gestation.
• Recombination of viral genes between vaccine and BTV field strains and reversion to virulence are concerns with the use of BTV MLV vaccines.
• In the US, an MLV vaccine containing serotype 10 is available. In addition, MLV vaccines containing serotypes 10, 11, or 17 can be obtained in California.
• Lambs can be vaccinated close to weaning, and breeding stock 3 weeks before breeding or after lambing. Pregnant animals should not be vaccinated with MLV vaccines.
• To induce protection, the BTV serotype of the vaccine must correspond to the serotype of the virus in the region.
• Monovalent inactivated vaccines directed against serotypes 2, 4, 8, 11 and 16 and a bivalent vaccine directed against serotypes 2 and 4 induce neutralizing antibodies in sheep and in most cases prevent both viremia and clinical disease.
• Autogenous BTV inactivated vaccines have been used successfully in Europe.
• Limiting vector exposure by housing susceptible animals during peak feeding times (from dusk to dawn) may reduce the risk of exposure, but vectors may be active during daytime when overcast.
• Methods of controlling the vector population include approved low-toxicity insecticides, such as synthetic pyrethroids (deltamethrin, cyfluthrin, permethrin, and fenvalerate), housing livestock in enclosed buildings, and making vector habitat unsuitable.
• Many countries impose restrictions to the movement of livestock and germplasm from infected areas.

MISCELLANEOUS

ASSOCIATED CONDITIONS
Abortion and fetal malformation.

AGE-RELATED FACTORS
N/A

ZOONOTIC POTENTIAL
N/A

PREGNANCY
• Modified-live BTV vaccines may cause pregnancy loss and teratogenesis.
• Infection with BTV-8 results in abortions and fetal malformations.

BIOSECURITY
Sheep and cattle whose blood contains BTV nucleic acid detected by RT-PCR, but which have no infectious virus detected by virus isolation, are unlikely to play an important role in the epidemiology of BTV.

PRODUCTION MANAGEMENT
See Prevention.

ABBREVIATIONS
• BT = bluetongue
• BTV = bluetongue virus
• DIC = disseminated intravascular coagulation
• EHD = epizootic hemorrhagic disease
• ELISA = enzyme-linked immunosorbent assay
• MLV = modified-live vaccine
• OIE = Office International des Epizooties
• RT-PCR = reverse transcription-polymerase chain reaction

SEE ALSO
Epizootic Hemorrhagic Disease Virus

Suggested Reading
Bluetongue. World Assembly of Delegates of the OIE, chapter 2.1.3. OIE Terrestrial Manual, 2014, pp. 1–18.
Maclachlan NJ, Drew CP, Darpel KE, Worwa G. The pathology and pathogenesis of bluetongue. J Comp Pathol 2009,141: 1–16.
McVey DS, MacLachlan NJ. Vaccines for prevention of Bluetongue and Epizootic Hemorrhagic Disease in livestock: A North American perspective. Vector Borne Zoonotic Dis 2015, 15: 385–96.
van der Sluijs MT, Schroer-Joosten DP, Fid-Fourkour A, et al. Transplacental transmission of BTV-8 in sheep: BTV viraemia, antibody responses and vaccine efficacy in lambs infected in utero. Vaccine 2013, 31: 3726–31.
Wilson WC, Daniels P, Ostlund EN, et al. Diagnostic Tools for bluetongue and epizootic hemorrhagic disease viruses applicable to North American veterinary diagnosticians. Vector Borne Zoonotic Dis 2015, 15: 364–73.

Author Andrés de la Concha-Bermejillo
Consulting Editor Erica C. McKenzie

BORDER DISEASE

B

BASICS

OVERVIEW
• Congenital disease of sheep resulting from viral infection of the dam during pregnancy. The virus crosses the placenta and infects the fetus.
• Caused by Border disease virus (BDV), a pestivirus closely related to classical swine fever virus (CSFV) and bovine viral diarrhea virus (BVDV).
• Affected lambs are often referred to as "hairy shaker" lambs due to characteristic coat changes and the presence of ataxia or muscle tremors, particularly in the hindlimbs.

GEOGRAPHIC DISTRIBUTION
Worldwide in almost all major sheep-producing countries.

SYSTEMS AFFECTED
• Reproductive
• Musculoskeletal
• Nervous

PATHOPHYSIOLOGY
• Infection of susceptible dams prior to 80 days' gestation with noncytopathic strains of the virus may result in persistent infection in the fetus.
• Persistently infected (PI) animals do not mount an immune response to the virus and consistently shed high levels of virus throughout their lifetime.
• PI animals serve as the main reservoir for the virus.

SIGNALMENT
• Sheep are primarily affected. Goats are affected less commonly.
• Clinical signs in lambs are evident at birth.
• Clinical manifestations in the fetus depend on the stage of gestation when infection occurs. Signs are generally present in neonates at the time of birth but resolve gradually over time so that animals may be clinically normal after 3–6 months of age.
• No breed or sex predilections are described.

PHYSICAL EXAMINATION FINDINGS
• Infection in nonpregnant adult and adolescent sheep is generally subclinical.
• Viral infection in susceptible pregnant sheep results in placentitis and potential infection of the fetus.
• Fetal infection may result in abortion, stillbirth, mummification, and congenital malformations.
• Clinical manifestations in the fetus depend on the stage of gestation when infection occurs. Gestational infections before development of fetal immunocompetence (<80 days' gestation) may result in PI lambs. These lambs are permanent carriers and shedders of the virus, but do not always develop clinical signs of disease.

• Surviving fetuses infected <80 days' gestation that do not become PI may develop the characteristic clinical signs of border disease.
• The fleece of affected lambs appears hairy due to long fibers rising above the fleece. The coat may also be pigmented. Skin and coat changes are apparently absent in coarse-fleeced breeds of sheep and goats.
• Mild muscle tremors to tonic-clonic contraction of skeletal muscles of the body and head.
• Affected lambs may have lower birth weights and decreased crown–rump lengths and may be weak at birth.
• Deficiency of T_3 and T_4 thyroid hormones has been demonstrated in affected lambs.

CAUSES AND RISK FACTORS
The disease is caused by BDV. The main source of infection is the asymptomatic, PI sheep. These animals shed the virus in saliva, respiratory secretions, urine, feces, or semen throughout their lifetime. Transmission occurs across mucus membranes.

DIAGNOSIS

DIFFERENTIAL DIAGNOSES
• Other causes of abortion such as enzootic abortion (ovine chlamydiosis), toxoplasmosis, listeriosis, salmonellosis, and bluetongue.
• In lambs, other neurologic conditions such as enzootic ataxia (swayback), bacterial meningoencephalitis, focal symmetric encephalomalacia. Caprine arthritis and encephalitis (CAE) infection should be considered in affected kids.
• BVDV infection can present with similar clinical signs in sheep.

OTHER DIAGNOSTIC PROCEDURES
• Presumptive diagnosis often made based on clinical signs. Confirmation through detection of the virus or viral antigen and/or histologic demonstration of pathognomonic lesions of the central nervous system.
• Virus isolation from tissues or blood. Leukocytes in the blood buffy coat are recommended sample. Precolostral samples are preferred; colostral antibody can mask virus for up to 2 months.
• RT-PCR also used to detect viral RNA.
• Fluorescent antibody tests for viral antigens performed on tissues of affected lambs. Tissues to be collected for biopsy include: abomasum, pancreas, kidneys, thyroid, testicles, and skin.
• PI animals are seronegative. Serology on dams of affected lambs generally demonstrates high antibody titers. Seronegative dams should be sampled for detection of virus or viral antigen.
• Serology is of limited diagnostic value for abortions as clinical signs generally lag several weeks behind infection. Seropositivity does

not indicate the virus as the cause of abortion; seronegativity rules out a diagnosis of BDV unless the dam is persistently infected.

PATHOLOGIC FINDINGS
• Abnormal "hairy" appearance of birth coat due to enlargement and relative increase in primary hair follicles.
• Cerebellar dysplasia or hypoplasia.
• Hydranencephaly or microcephaly.
• Abnormal skin pigmentation.
• Placentitis and placental necrosis can occur.
• Gross findings may be normal.
• Histopathologic findings may include white matter lesions in the CNS, spinal cord and CNS hypomyelinogenesis. An increase in interfascicular glial cells with myelin-like lipid droplet accumulation.

TREATMENT

THERAPEUTIC APPROACH
No specific or effective treatment. Supportive care for affected lambs although production potential is poor.

MEDICATIONS

DRUGS OF CHOICE
N/A

FOLLOW-UP

EXPECTED COURSE AND PROGNOSIS
Affected lambs that survive the first few months will show gradual resolution of neurologic signs and fleece abnormalities. Permanent identification of affected lambs is recommended as lambs may no longer be clinically recognized as infected after a few months of age.

PREVENTION
• Stimulation of herd immunity and prevention of exposure during pregnancy are keys to prevention.
• To prevent exposure, PI lambs should be identified and culled promptly.
• Not all PI lambs exhibit clinical signs. Routine serologic surveillance in endemic areas or on farms with history of disease is recommended. Seropositive animals are not PI and are immune to further challenge with homologous viral strains. Seronegative animals should be screened to determine PI status.
• There are no approved vaccines for use against Border disease virus in the United States. Field strains of BDV are antigenically distinct from most BVDV strains and, thus, cattle BVDV vaccines are generally not effective for use against BDV in sheep.

(CONTINUED)

• Recovered lambs can be commingled with the herd prior to breeding as a means of natural immunization. Such lambs should be removed from the herd prior to breeding and, if not removed from the farm, quarantined from contact with pregnant animals.
• Serologic monitoring of bulk tank milk samples can be performed in dairy sheep herds.

 MISCELLANEOUS

ASSOCIATED CONDITIONS
• BVDV and CSFV are closely related pestiviruses found primarily in cattle and swine, respectively. Similar clinical signs may be seen in sheep naturally infected with either BVDV or BDV.

AGE-RELATED FACTORS
Age at time of infection determines clinical signs in the individual. Persistent infection only results from congenital infection; exposure to the virus at other times results in subclinical disease except in pregnant animals when infection may result in abortion.

ZOONOTIC POTENTIAL
N/A

PREGNANCY
• Infection of sheep and goats during pregnancy may result in abortion.
• Clinical disease or death in lambs is the result of infection of the dam during gestation.

BIOSECURITY
• Biosecurity is most critical for pregnant ewes during the critical period for formation of PI lambs.
• PI lambs should be identified and removed from the herd prior to the breeding season.

PRODUCTION MANAGEMENT
Affected lambs should not be kept as replacement animals.

ABBREVIATIONS
• BDV = Border disease virus
• BVDV = bovine viral diarrhea virus
• CSFV = classical swine fever virus
• PI = persistently infected
• RT-PCR = reverse transcription-polymerase chain reaction

SEE ALSO
• Abortion: Small Ruminant
• Akabane
• Bacterial Meningitis
• Bovine Viral Diarrhea Virus
• Caprine Arthritis Encephalitis Virus
• Chlamydiosis
• Copper Deficiency and Toxicity
• Enzootic Ataxia

Suggested Reading
Border disease. In: Radostits OM, Gay CC, Hinchcliff KW, Constable PD eds. Veterinary Medicine: A Textbook of the Diseases of Cattle, Horses, Sheep, Pigs, and Goats, 10th ed. Edinburgh: Saunders Elsevier, 2007, pp. 1414–18.
Loken T. Border disease in sheep. Vet Clin North Am Food Anim Pract 1995, 11: 579–95.
Nettleton PF, Gilray JA, Russo P, Dlissi E. Border disease of sheep and goats. Vet Res 1998, 29: 327–40.
Newcomer BW, Givens MD. Approved and experimental countermeasures against pestiviral diseases: Bovine viral diarrhea, classical swine fever and border disease. Antiviral Res 2013, 100: 133–50.
Pratelli A, Bollo E, Martella V, Guarda F, Chiocco D, Buonavoglia C. Pestivirus infection in small ruminants: virological and histopathological findings. New Microbiol 1999, 22: 351–56.

Author Benjamin W. Newcomer
Consulting Editor Christopher C.L. Chase
Acknowledgment The author and book editors acknowledge the prior contribution of Lisa Nashold.

BORNA DISEASE

B

BASICS

OVERVIEW
Borna disease (BD) is sporadic, transmissible, progressive encephalitis. The virus does not have a direct cytopathic effect. Virally infected cells initiate a T-cell immune response, which leads to tissue destruction.

INCIDENCE/PREVALENCE
Up to 20% of a flock can develop the disease. The incubation time is several weeks, and the duration of disease is around 4–10 days, with around 90% mortality.

GEOGRAPHIC DISTRIBUTION
Borna disease was historically endemic to areas of Germany and Switzerland. Confirmed outbreaks of the disease have generally been in middle and eastern Europe and in horses in the Middle East. Clinically normal animals have tested positive for the RNA virus responsible for the disease in many areas of the world including the United States.

SYSTEMS AFFECTED
Nervous

PATHOPHYSIOLOGY
• BDV is neurotropic, with a particular predilection for neurons of the limbic system. The virus ultimately spreads throughout the central, peripheral and autonomic nervous systems infecting astrocytes, Schwann cells and ependymal cells in the central nervous system (CNS); sensory and autonomic ganglia; and nerves to organs. Viral transport is presumably axonal and transsynaptic.
• Following intranasal infection, viral antigen is detected sequentially in olfactory receptor cells, olfactory nerve fibers, cells of the olfactory bulb and olfactory tract. In the hippocampus, viral antigen is localized in axon terminals, which form synaptic contacts with cortical area 1 (CA1) pyramidal cell dendrites, prior to appearing in pyramidal cell bodies.
• Borna disease is an immune-mediated multiphasic syndrome where the immune response to viral antigens after BDV infection does not elicit protective immunity but rather an immunopathologic reaction where T cells play an important role in causing disease. The critical role of T cells in the pathogenesis of BD was demonstrated in adoptive transfer experiments: transfer of BDV-specific major histocompatibility complex class II-restricted TH 1 cell lines resulted in acute meningoencephalitis and disease. Consequently, conventional immunization with inactivated virus preparations or purified virus-specific antigens did not confer protective immunity against clinical BD, despite detectable levels of virus-specific antibodies after immunization.

SIGNALMENT
• Natural infections occur in sheep and horses. Goats and cattle are rarely affected.
• BDV has been experimentally transmitted to a wide range of animals including chickens, rabbits, rats, guinea pigs, and monkeys.
• BDV antibodies have been identified in monkeys, humans, and birds.

PHYSICAL EXAMINATION FINDINGS
• Borna disease is a progressive neurologic disease.
• Initial signs in sheep are generally nonspecific including social behavioral changes, apathy and may include anorexia, fever, excessive salivation, yawning, and chewing movements. Early neurologic signs include hyperesthesia, ataxia, head pressing, head tremors, muscle contractions, and depression. Transient signs of irritability, kicking, biting or compulsive movements may occur.
• In later stages of disease, animals may lean against objects or maintain a sawhorse stance. Convulsion or coma is possible. Nystagmus is observed in terminal cases.
• As the disease progresses, decreased feed intake, bruxism and gait disturbances including circular movement are seen. Finally, in some cases paresis or paralysis occurs.
• The incubation time is several weeks, and the duration of disease is around 4–10 days, with around 90% mortality.
• Besides the initial reports of BD in cattle, demonstrated by transmission of the disease to laboratory animals, there seems to be only sporadic occurrence in cattle. Hence, BDV infection of cattle has been considered as a rare event.

CAUSES AND RISK FACTORS
• The etiologic agent of BD, Borna disease virus (BDV), is an enveloped, non-segmented, negative-stranded RNA virus with a genomic size of approximately 9 kb and a nuclear site for replication and transcription. The genomic organization is similar to that of other members of the Mononegavirales order; therefore, BDV is the prototype of the new family *Bornaviridae* within this order. The Mononegavirales also include *Filoviridae* (e.g. Ebola viruses), *Paramyxoviridae* (e.g., rinderpest, bovine respiratory syncytial virus, Newcastle disease virus), and *Rhabdoviridae* (e.g., rabies, vesicular stomatitis virus).
• Actively infected, convalescent, and immune carrier animals shed the virus in nasal secretions, saliva, urine, or milk. Infection often occurs due to contaminated food and water. The virus moves to the CNS by intra-axonal transport via nerves in the nose and throat area. Disease outbreaks are more commonly seen in spring and early summer.
• The virus is transmitted between birds by the tick *Hyalomma anatolicum*. An arthropod vector is not necessary for transmission in

other species. An outbreak of disease in horses in the Middle East was associated with a dense population of infected wild birds. Rodents have also been suspected as a source of infection.

DIAGNOSIS

DIFFERENTIAL DIAGNOSES
• CNS tumor
• Metabolic or digestive disorders—milk fever, nervous ketosis
• *Oestrus ovis* infestations in sheep
• Pseudorabies
• Rabies
• Scrapie, bovine spongiform encephalopathy, chronic wasting disease in elk and deer

OTHER LABORATORY TESTS
In some cases, serum and CSF may contain antibodies to BDV.

OTHER DIAGNOSTIC PROCEDURES
Polymerase chain reaction (PCR) viral amplification and in situ hybridization have been used to demonstrate viral RNA in peripheral blood mononuclear cells (PBMC) neurons, astrocytes, Schwann cells, and ependymal cells.

PATHOLOGIC FINDINGS
• There are no characteristic gross lesions.
• On histologic examination, inclusion bodies in neuronal nucleus known as Joest or Joest-Degen bodies are found in ganglion cells of the hippocampus and olfactory lobes of the cerebral cortex. They are considered pathognomonic for Borna disease.
• Other histologic lesions are characteristic of encephalitis including perivascular cuffing, ganglion cell degeneration, and gliosis.
• Neuronophagic nodules may be found.
• Lesions are typically found in gray matter of the cerebral hemispheres and brainstem. The most severe lesions are found in the olfactory bulbs, caudate nucleus, and hippocampus.

TREATMENT

THERAPEUTIC APPROACH
• No specific treatment is available.
• Supportive therapy with mannitol may temporarily relieve cerebral edema. Anti-inflammatory medications may reduce discomfort.

MEDICATIONS

No specific medications

B

FOLLOW-UP

EXPECTED COURSE AND PROGNOSIS

• Unlike other viral encephalitides, the incubation period can vary from 3 weeks to months or possibly years. The average incubation period is usually 2–3 months. Duration of clinical illness is normally 1–3 weeks.
• Mortality rates can range from 60% to 95% in animals exhibiting clinical signs. Surviving animals may remain permanently neurologically impaired.

PATIENT CARE

Surviving animals may have permanent neurologic deficits.

PREVENTION

There is no vaccine.

MISCELLANEOUS

ASSOCIATED CONDITIONS

• The viruses of Borna disease and Near Eastern encephalitis are indistinguishable.
• BD is serologically distinct from the viruses that cause West Nile virus (WNV), Eastern equine encephalitis (EEE), Western equine encephalitis (WEE), Venezuelan equine encephalitis (VEE).

ZOONOTIC POTENTIAL

BDV antibodies have been found in humans with various neuropsychiatric disorders such as schizophrenia. Although most reports of an association between infection and disease have focused on unipolar depression, bipolar disorder or schizophrenia, BDV has also been implicated in an improbably wide range of disorders, including chronic fatigue syndrome, acquired immune deficiency syndrome (AIDS) encephalopathy, multiple sclerosis, motor neuron disease, and aggressive brain tumor. The actual significance of BDV in these disorders has yet to be determined.

BIOSECURITY

Animals coming into BD areas should not be fed and watered together in large numbers and should be kept separate from horses and sheep. Incoming animals should be quarantined for 2 months due to the long incubation period of the disease, and tested twice during this period for the presence of antibodies. BDV is resistant to drying and other adverse environmental conditions.

ABBREVIATIONS

• AIDS = acquired immune deficiency syndrome
• BD = Borna disease
• BDV = Borna disease virus
• CA1= cortical area 1
• CNS = central nervous system
• CSF = cerebrospinal fluid
• EEE = Eastern equine encephalitis
• PBMC = peripheral blood mononuclear cells
• PCR = polymerase chain reaction
• TH 1= T helper 1 cells
• VEE = Venezuelan equine encephalitis
• WEE = Western equine encephalitis
• WNV = West Nile virus

SEE ALSO

• Bovine Spongiform Encephalopathy
• Cervidae: Chronic Wasting Disease
• Hypocalcemia: Bovine
• Ketosis: Dairy Cattle
• *Oestrus ovis* Infestation
• Pseudorabies
• Rabies
• Scrapie

Suggested Reading
Lipkin WI, Briese T, Hornig M. Borna disease virus: fact and fantasy. Virus Res 2011, 162: 162–72. http://doi.org/10.1016/j.virusres.2011.09.036
Richt JA, Pfeuffer I, Christ M, Frese K, Bechter K, Herzog S. Borna disease virus infection in animals and humans. Emerg Infect Dis 1997, 3: 343–52. http://doi.org/10.3201/eid0303.970311
Wensman J. Borna disease virus and its hosts. Veterinary Sciences Tomorrow, 2011. http://vetscite.org/files/pdf/000106.pdf
Author Christopher C.L. Chase
Consulting Editor Christopher C.L. Chase
Acknowledgment The author and book editors acknowledge the prior contribution of Lisa Nashold.

BOVINE DERMATOLOGY

B

BASICS

OVERVIEW
• The most important skin diseases of cattle are those that are contagious, zoonotic, and/or affect production or animal welfare. • The most common problems are external parasites, bovine papilloma virus, udder cleft dermatitis, digital dermatitis, dermatophytosis, and dermatophilosis.

INCIDENCE/PREVALENCE
Varies depending on the disorder and management factors; contagious disorders can achieve high prevalence in herds.

GEOGRAPHIC DISTRIBUTION
Worldwide; regional distribution varies for specific ectoparasites and infectious disorders.

SYSTEMS AFFECTED
Integument

PATHOPHYSIOLOGY
• Dermatologic disorders cause disease through a variety of mechanisms which can be distinguished to some degree by clinical presentation. • Any dermatologic disorder has the potential to adversely impact animal welfare and productivity which may be reflected by changes in behavior, production variables, and visible alterations to the skin or hair. • Ectoparasites can also facilitate transmission of a variety of infectious disorders including babesiosis, heartwater, and infectious keratoconjunctivitis. • Pruritic conditions create damage due to inflammation associated with the causative agents (typically ectoparasites performing feeding and development activities), compounded by self-trauma. • Nodules or masses may reflect edema/inflammation from allergic response, infestation with particular ectoparasites (*Demodex, Hypoderma*), and cellular proliferation associated with specific viruses (poxviruses) or neoplastic processes. • Papules, pustules, and/or vesicles on the skin often form as the result of allergic or immune conditions, viral or bacterial infections of the skin, and ectoparasite activity. • Ulceration or erosions of the skin arise from a wide range of disorders, some of which are infectious and potentially reportable. • Many infectious and noninfectious disorders can cause scaling and crusting of the skin. Dermatophytosis and dermatophilosis are two of the more significant causes in cattle.

HISTORICAL FINDINGS
• Vary with etiology; however, defining the history of skin disease within the herd, and any relevant treatment or management procedures, is important. • A description of skin lesion appearance and duration, number of animals affected, and the presence or absence of pruritis are important historical factors.

SIGNALMENT
All breeds of cattle, of any age, are at risk of dermatologic disease.

PHYSICAL EXAMINATION FINDINGS
• Many disorders can be diagnosed by lesion characteristics and location on the body; these should be carefully annotated during examination. • The skin should be closely evaluated for characteristics that include sensitivity/pruritis, alopecia, excoriations, lumps, vesicles, and other anomalies. • Signs of anemia or related infectious diseases may be observed. • Ticks and lice are often readily visible on close examination of the skin. • Udder cleft dermatitis is identified by necrosis of skin between the udder and hind leg or between quarters of the udder. Secondary bacterial infection leads to a foul odor and severe cases have skin sloughing and erosion into vessels resulting in hemorrhage. • Photosensitization following ingestion of specific plants or chemicals or secondary to liver disease tends to most severely affect white-haired areas exposed to sunlight. Affected skin appears erythematous, thickened, necrotic, and may slough. • Rain rot (*Dermatophilus congolensis*) typically affects the dorsum; however, any part can be affected if subjected to prolonged or repeated moisture. Lesions are palpable as thick, usually circular, crusts under the hair. When crusts are removed the skin and removed hair form a paintbrush shape. • Dermatophytosis in cattle often invokes circular lesions with alopecia and scaling. Lesions most often affect the face, especially near the eyes and are generally nonpruritic.

GENETICS
• Individual breed differences exist in susceptibility to specific infectious disorders associated with ectoparasite vectors. • Individual breed differences exist in susceptibility to squamous cell carcinoma (Hereford cattle predisposed).

CAUSES AND RISK FACTORS
• The presence of specific parasitic or infectious agents in the region. • Overcrowding and poor nutrition. • Lack of control and treatment procedures for external parasitism. • Udder rot is more prevalent in older or high-producing animals, and is often associated with udder edema. • Dermatophilosis manifests when the hair coat is frequently moist such as during rainy seasons, or in summer if sprinklers are used for cooling. • Lice infestations are more prevalent/problematic in winter.

DIAGNOSIS

DIFFERENTIAL DIAGNOSES
Pruritus
• Lice • Ticks • Mites (*Psoroptes, Sarcoptes, Chorioptes*) • Migrating helminths

(*Strongyloides, Pelodera*) • Flies (*Musca, Stomoxys calcitrans, Culicoides, Tabanus*)

Pustular/Papular/Vesicular Lesions
• Impetigo (*Staphylococcus*) • Contagious ecthyma • Pemphigus foliaceus • Capripox virus (lumpy skin disease) • Foot and mouth disease • Papillomas (bovine papilloma virus) • Hypersensitivity lesions

Nodules with or without Ulcers
• Demodicosis • Staphylococcal dermatitis • Warble flies (*Hypoderma*) • Mycetoma (fungal tumors) • Abscesses: foreign bodies, *Staphylococcus, Streptococcus, Corynebacterium pseudotuberculosis, Trueperella* • Neoplasia: squamous cell carcinoma (SCC), cutaneous lymphosarcoma, fibroma/fibrosarcoma • Tuberculosis • Epidermal inclusion cyst • Cryptococcosis

Erythema and/or Sloughing
• Sunburn • Frostbite • Ergot toxicity • Photosensitization • Vasculitis

Ulcerations, Erosions
• Hypersensitivity • Adverse drug reaction • Contact irritants • Photosensitivity • Vasculitis • Udder cleft dermatitis • Dermatophilosis • *C. pseudotuberculosis* • Viral infections: herpes viruses, malignant catarrhal fever, vesicular stomatitis • Squamous cell carcinoma (SCC)

Scaling, Crusting
• All pruritic disease can cause scaling • Dermatophilosis (*D. congolensis*) • Dermatophytosis (*Trichophyton verrucosum, T. mentagrophytes*) • *Staphylococcus* pyoderma • Stephanofilariosis • Nutritional (zinc deficiency) • Iodism • Immune mediated

CBC/BIOCHEMISTRY/URINALYSIS
Relevant in specific conditions such as when liver disease might be contributing to photosensitization conditions (serum biochemistry can provide supporting evidence of liver damage).

OTHER LABORATORY TESTS
• Bacterial culture and sensitivity are relevant in infections of the skin or ear canals. Avoid surface contamination and obtain samples from underneath crusts or from fresh pustules or vesicles. • Cytologic examination (including Gram stain) can be performed on impression smears of lesions or exudates. *D. congolensis* forms typical "railroad track" cocci, or mincing crusts will reveal filamentous Gram-positive branching organisms.

IMAGING
N/A

OTHER DIAGNOSTIC PROCEDURES
• Skin scraping or microscopic evaluation of crusts can provide a positive diagnosis and species identification in mange mite conditions. • Potassium hydroxide preparation (10–20% KOH), allows identification of dermatophytes from skin

(CONTINUED)

B

scrapings or minced crusts. • Dermatophyte culture. • Skin biopsy is the most effective diagnostic aid for skin diseases where the diagnosis cannot be made clinically or with other diagnostic tests.

PATHOLOGIC FINDINGS

Histologic findings in skin biopsies vary substantially depending on the underlying cause of disease (see individual conditions in this text for more details).

TREATMENT

THERAPEUTIC APPROACH

• Udder rot can be addressed by cleaning the region with mild soap and water and applying a drying agent. Systemic antibiotics may be indicated if there is deep infection, fever, or maggot infestation. Diuretics may help if udder edema is a factor. • Dermatophilosis can be treated by removing crusts and washing animals with iodine-based scrub; systemic antibiotics may be required.
• Photosensitization is addressed by discontinuing exposure to plants or chemicals containing primary photodynamic agents, or determining if liver disease is causative. Animals should be provided shade or moved indoors, and monitored for skin necrosis.
• Dermatophytosis is usually self-limiting in 1–4 months; however, topical treatment with dilute bleach (1:10) and other solutions has been used. • Ectoparasites can be treated with topical or parenteral treatment with insecticides provided via ear tags, residual livestock sprays, pour-on formulations, dust bags, back rubbers, oilers, or wipe-ons.
• Animals should be supported via good management, adequate nutrition, and where relevant, good hygiene procedures. • For reportable conditions, contact appropriate state, provincial, or government bodies to determine specific quarantine requirements and treatments.

SURGICAL CONSIDERATIONS AND TECHNIQUES

• Skin biopsy is a quick and relatively painless procedure that can be achieved using a 6 mm skin biopsy punch with no preceding preparation of the skin or local anesthesia to avoid lesion disruption and artifact. • Do not clean or clip biopsy site; leave crusts in place.
• Take biopsies at a border with normal tissue, without local anesthesia if possible. • Biopsy sites can be left to heal by granulation but should be protected from invasion by external parasites. • Warts can be crushed and pinched off with hemostats or pliers if small, or removed with cryotherapy or surgical excision.

MEDICATIONS

DRUGS OF CHOICE

• Topical insecticide (permethrins or macrocyclic lactones) every 2 weeks for 2 or 3 treatments will treat and prevent lice infestation if bedding, grooming equipment and other fomites are cleaned as well.
• Diazinon, pyrethroids, carbaryl or tetrachlorvinos might be indicated for other ectoparasite disorders. • Dermatophilosis responds to parenteral penicillin or tetracycline. • Corticosteroid agents (dexamethasone, methylprednisolone) are indicated for immune-mediated or hypersensitivity disorders.

CONTRAINDICATIONS

• Corticosteroids should not be used in pregnant animals. • Topical ectoparasiticides that fall under the jurisdiction of the EPA rather than the FDA in the USA cannot be applied in an extra-label manner.

PRECAUTIONS

Appropriate milk and meat withdrawal times must be followed for all compounds administered to food-producing animals.

POSSIBLE INTERACTIONS

N/A

FOLLOW-UP

EXPECTED COURSE AND PROGNOSIS

Depends upon the causative agent; however, most disorders of the integument cause production loss but carry a good to excellent prognosis for recovery and survival.

POSSIBLE COMPLICATIONS

• Secondary bacterial infection and toxemia
• Cutaneous myiasis

CLIENT EDUCATION

Focus on methods of control and prevention to reduce disease related to ectoparasites and infectious disorders.

PATIENT CARE

N/A

PREVENTION

• Quarantine new animals before introduction into the herd, with close inspection for skin lesions. • Remove wet, rotting organic matter to reduce habitat for fly larvae; dragging pastures to break up manure masses is also helpful. • Vaccination for specific disorders (such as papillomas) is possible but might require construction of autogenous vaccine products. • Ensure cleanliness of equipment used in routine procedures such as foot trimming, ear tagging, grooming or tattooing.

MISCELLANEOUS

ASSOCIATED CONDITIONS

• Secondary infection • Cutaneous myiasis

AGE-RELATED FACTORS

• Warts typically occur in cattle <2 years of age. • Dermatophytosis is more common in young animals.

ZOONOTIC POTENTIAL

Sarcoptes scabiei, contagious ecthyma, dermatophilosis, dermatophytosis, and some pox viruses, including some other dermatologic disorders, are potentially zoonotic.

PREGNANCY

N/A

BIOSECURITY

• Quarantine new animals before introducing into the herd/flock. • Isolate affected herd members or whole herds during testing and treatment. • Contact regulatory bodies if reportable conditions are suspected. • Crusts from *D. congolensis* infected animals are a source of contagion, so should be disposed of with caution. • Potential fomites such as grooming equipment and blankets should be cleaned and disinfected between animals.
• Limit exposure and mingling of young naïve animals with older stock.

PRODUCTION MANAGEMENT

• Diseases which cause lameness, pruritis or pain can reduce production and diminish welfare of cattle. • Many of these diseases are contagious and are important to detect when issuing health certificates or screening entrants to fairs or shows.

SYNONYMS

• Dermatophytosis: ringworm
• Dermatophilosis: rain rot, rain scald, mud fever • Mange: mite infestation • Cutaneous myiasis: fly strike • Udder cleft dermatitis: udder rot, udder scald, intertrigo (intertriginous dermatitis)

ABBREVIATIONS

• EPA = Environmental Protection Agency
• FDA = Food and Drug Administration
• KOH = potassium hydroxide

SEE ALSO

• Dermatophilosis • Dermatophytosis
• Lumpy Skin Disease • Orf (Contagious Ecthyma) • Parasitic Skin Diseases: Bovine

Suggested Reading
Scott DW. Large Animal Dermatology. Philadelphia: Saunders, 1984, pp. 71–2.
White SD. Diseases of the skin. In: Smith BP ed, Large Animal Internal Medicine. St. Louis: Elsevier, 2015, pp. 1192–222.
Author Meera Heller
Consulting Editor Erica C. McKenzie

BOVINE DIGITAL DERMATITIS

B

BASICS

OVERVIEW
• Digital dermatitis [DD] has been a well-recognized cause of lameness in dairy cattle for several decades, and is becoming increasingly recognized as a major cause of lameness in feedlot cattle. It is an extremely painful condition associated with severe lameness and reduced milk production.
• DD is highly contagious and can spread rapidly through a herd. Management practices have been developed that aid control and reduce lameness; however, the majority do not eradicate disease. Most herds with DD remain chronically infected.
• Discussion of the condition is hampered by the great variety of names that are used to describe DD (see "Synonyms").
• Affected cattle are often lame and tend to walk on the toes of the feet with lesions.
• Lesions occur most commonly on the plantar surface of the rear feet, adjacent to the interdigital cleft or ridge.
• DD is an important animal welfare concern.

INCIDENCE/PREVALENCE
• Anecdotally, infection spreads rapidly in susceptible cows once introduced into a naïve herd; however, more recent controlled experiments suggest that lesions may require 3–4 months to develop to mature lesions.
• In dairy herds, DD often affects the majority of cows within the first year of infection. Prevalence in endemic herds can vary from <5% to >70% depending on conditions and control programs.
• In feedlots, DD-associated lameness often increases in prevalence when cattle are heavy and close to slaughter.

GEOGRAPHIC DISTRIBUTION
• Worldwide.
• Reports of a similar process in sheep and goats (contagious ovine digital dermatitis) have been confined to Europe but are likely present in other regions.

SYSTEMS AFFECTED
• Integument
• Musculoskeletal

PATHOPHYSIOLOGY
• DD is polybacterial in nature, meaning that no single bacterial organism has been identified as an etiologic agent. Disease occurs when there is an appropriate consortium of organisms present. Mature lesions are predominantly infected with *Treponema* spp. bacteria, however earlier lesions have small numbers and different species of treponemes, suggesting that this family is not exclusively causal for the disease. Viral and fungal etiologies are not considered important.
• Transmission of DD is believed facilitated by constant moisture (hydropic maceration)

and low oxygen tension (anaerobic bacterial involvement is suspected).
• Early lesions vary from small, localized focal to multifocal or coalescing lesions that involve the majority of the plantar skin adjacent to the interdigital cleft. The transition to more mature lesions is characterized by the presence of an ulcerated, hyperemic circular lesion that has the roughened "strawberry-like" appearance of a classical DD lesion. More chronic lesions can become proliferative and papillomatous.
• Most active lesions are 2–6 cm in diameter, circular to oval in appearance, and have clearly demarcated borders with ulceration.
• Lesion borders are often surrounded by true hairs that are 2–3 times the length of normal hairs.
• Chronic lesions may have filiform papillae varying in length from 1 mm to >2 cm (hence, the name "hairy footwarts"). Lesions without the filiform papillae can have a thickened granular appearance.
• Washed lesions vary in color from bright red to gray or brown and are generally very painful to touch or when exposed to water jets.

HISTORICAL FINDINGS
• The main sign of DD is severe lameness (often non-weight-bearing) in one or more limbs.
• The disease is highly contagious and outbreaks are common, with lameness being the predominant herd sign, with multiple cows walking on their toes.

SIGNALMENT
• Digital dermatitis has been reported in all breeds of cattle including dairy and beef breeds.
• Holsteins appear to have a higher incidence among the dairy breeds.
• In dairy herds DD can occur in all ages of cattle. In some cases there is an increased recognition of disease in fresh heifers.
• In feedlots DD is most likely to result in lameness in heavy cattle. Dairy steers, presumably due to exposure prior to entry into the feedlot, may develop lesions earlier in the feeding period than other breeds.
• Sheep and goats in Europe have been reported to suffer from a very similar condition termed contagious ovine digital dermatitis.

PHYSICAL EXAMINATION FINDINGS
• Affected cows may have "club feet" (i.e., longer heels, since they are reluctant to put weight on their heels).
• The classical lesion is found on the caudal aspect of the skin above the heel at the interdigital cleft and may extend to the interdigital skin.
• Lesions are typically on the midline between the heel bulbs and below the accessory digits (dew claws) and are covered in a friable layer of gray, fibrin like material.

• The area should be carefully cleaned to remove any debris so that the lesion can be clearly examined; cleaning should be attempted with great care, as the lesion is extremely painful. In some cases IV and/or regional anesthesia may be necessary.
• Although the majority of cases affect the heels, lesions may occasionally be found on the skin in the interdigital cleft, on the heel bulbs, or on the coronary band on the abaxial aspect of the foot.
• Regardless of the position of the lesion, the characteristic lesion appearance is most diagnostic.

GENETICS
A genetic predisposition has not been clearly established; however, a higher incidence may occur in Holstein cattle.

CAUSES AND RISK FACTORS
• DD is highly contagious between cattle. It is typically brought into a herd through the purchase of an affected animal. However, veterinarians or lay foot trimmers may also play a role in transmission through contaminated hoof trimming equipment.
• Once DD is in a herd it is thought to spread through unsanitary conditions in the barn.
• Muddy or wet conditions and purchasing animals from off-premises locations are the two most common risk factors.
• Poor freestall and bedding management will exacerbate problems since cows will spend more time standing in manure slurry, not allowing the feet to dry out periodically.

DIAGNOSIS

DIFFERENTIAL DIAGNOSES
• Few conditions can be confused with DD; however, laminitis, foot rot, interdigital dermatitis and heel horn erosion, interdigital fibroma, traumatic injury, and thin soles from excessive wear or improper hoof trimming might be considered as causes of lameness.
• DD should also be differentiated from heel erosion ("slurry heel"), interdigital fibroma, traumatic injury to the distal limb, and foot rot (interdigital necrobacillosis).

CBC/BIOCHEMISTRY/URINALYSIS
N/A

OTHER LABORATORY TESTS
N/A

IMAGING
N/A

OTHER DIAGNOSTIC PROCEDURES
• In most cases, the clinical signs of DD are considered diagnostic.
• Definitive diagnosis can be achieved by biopsy using a skin biopsy punch.
• Histopathology using an appropriate stain can demonstrate the presence of spirochete bacteria within the tissue.

• Given the polybacterial nature of the disease, bacterial culture is not widely practiced and is not generally beneficial for diagnosis.

PATHOLOGIC FINDINGS

• Histopathology is helpful but not necessary for diagnosis. Histopathologic findings include a combination of ulcerative and proliferative changes consisting of ulceration of tips of dermal papillae, epidermal hyperplasia with parakeratosis and hyperkeratosis, colonization and invasion by profuse numbers of spirochetes (*Treponema* spp.), and inflammation.

TREATMENT

THERAPEUTIC APPROACH

• One should approach the treatment of DD from two different standpoints: (1) treatment of individual animals that are clinically affected and in severe discomfort, and (2) treatment of the entire herd, which likely contains a large number of subclinically affected individual.
• For individual animals, the affected area should be thoroughly cleaned and the hooves trimmed to ensure no other causes of lameness exist. Hoof testers can be used to ensure that lameness is not due to a claw disorder prior to direct topical treatment of the lesion.
• Herd treatment can be performed via footbath.

SURGICAL CONSIDERATIONS AND TECHNIQUES

N/A

MEDICATIONS

DRUGS OF CHOICE

• Tetracycline derivatives are considered ideal for topical treatment. Most reports show no benefit of systemic antibiotics in therapy and control of DD.
• Individual lesions can be treated with topical oxytetracycline (either 3 mL injectable oxytetracycline or a small volume of tetracycline or oxytetracycline soluble powder) applied topically. No difference in treatment outcomes were observed when comparing lesions treated with a wrap to those with the drug applied as a paste and no wrap. Data suggest that while lesions change appearance shortly after treatment, the majority do not completely heal after a single application and repeated treatments are often necessary.
• Herd treatment of DD can be performed via footbath using formalin (3–5%), copper sulfate (5%) or a wide variety of commercially available products, with cattle forced to walk through the solution. Fecal contamination of footbaths can result in decreased efficacy and

therefore baths should be drained, cleaned, and refilled every 100–300 cow passages depending upon the degree of organic contamination of feet on the dairy.
• Herd treatment using solutions consisting of either 25 g/L oxytetracycline (made using water additive powder) or 8 g/L of lincomycin or a combination lincomycin/spectinomycin (Linco-spectin water-soluble powder) may be prepared and applied to the heels of all cattle using a "garden sprayer." To be effective, the feet should first be cleaned using a high-pressure hose.
• In severe cases, clinicians may consider the use of systemic NSAIDs if severe discomfort is displayed by affected individuals.

CONTRAINDICATIONS

N/A

PRECAUTIONS

• Drugs used for treating DD are not licensed for this use. Appropriate milk and meat withdrawal times must be followed.
• When using aqueous antibiotic sprays in the parlor, care must be taken to avoid spraying the udder or milking machine to avoid violation residues. Antibiotic residues have not been reported from treatment.
• Great care must also be taken to ensure that cattle do not drink footbath solutions as this can also result in residue violations and possible toxicity.
• Copper and zinc are problematic to the environment due to their heavy metal content and formalin is a carcinogen and respiratory irritant.

POSSIBLE INTERACTIONS

N/A

FOLLOW-UP

EXPECTED COURSE AND PROGNOSIS

• Animals typically show increased discomfort immediately after treatment but lameness should resolve almost fully within 48 hours.
• In some cases the disease will affect exposed corium and interfere with normal horn production. A non-healing claw lesion usually results, requiring antibiotic therapy before healing can resume.

POSSIBLE COMPLICATIONS

Some DD lesions will undermine the horn of the heel or wall, which will necessitate removing the loose horn overlying the active lesion and treating it with topical antibiotics.

CLIENT EDUCATION

Clients should be educated regarding this disease, and associated risk factors, and treatment strategies.

PATIENT CARE

• Most individual lame animals treated with topical antibiotics will show rapid improvement in lameness within 24–48

hours. Animals that still have significant lameness after 72 hours should be reexamined for an additional cause of lameness.
• Animals should be monitored for recurrence and retreated as necessary.

PREVENTION

• Due to the high costs associated with DD, prevention is the goal (see "Biosecurity").
• Once DD has become endemic within a herd, good hygiene within the barn (regular scraping of passageways and maintaining clean, dry stalls) will minimize spread.
• Recurrence is common, so control must be ongoing. Monitoring herd prevalence will help to determine how aggressive the control program needs to be.
• It may also be necessary to use prophylactic footbath treatments on a regular basis, and footbaths must be maintained appropriately to keep the treatment solution clean and active.

MISCELLANEOUS

ASSOCIATED CONDITIONS

• Lameness, decreased milk production, decreased longevity in the herd.
• Erosive form: A reddened raw area of granulation tissue.
• Proliferative form: In some chronic cases, there may be proliferation of the epithelial tissue to form hairy, frondlike projections.

AGE-RELATED FACTORS

Generally a disease of maturing or mature animals

ZOONOTIC POTENTIAL

N/A

PREGNANCY

N/A

BIOSECURITY

• Introduction of DD to a group commonly occurs with purchase and introduction of new animals to a herd or feedlot. For this reason, it is prudent to inquire and evaluate potential animals for purchase specifically for the presence of DD prior to introduction.
• Any personnel involved in bovine foot care should ensure equipment is suitably disinfected between farm visits.
• DD-free herds should not buy replacement animals from other premises.

PRODUCTION MANAGEMENT

• Recommendations that pertain to cow comfort, including well-designed and bedded freestalls or open housing, are important.
• Prompt and aggressive treatment of active lesions will help control DD.

SYNONYMS

• Hairy heel warts
• Mortellaro's disease
• Papillomatous digital dermatitis
• Strawberry foot rot

BOVINE DIGITAL DERMATITIS

B

ABBREVIATIONS
• DD = digital dermatitis
• NSAIDs = nonsteroidal anti-inflammatory drugs

SEE ALSO
• Foot Rot: Bovine
• Lameness: Bovine
• Sole Lesions in Dairy Cattle

Suggested Reading
Berry SL. Diseases of the digital soft tissues. Vet Clin North Am Food Anim Pract 2001, 17: 129–42.
Demirkan I, Murray RD, Carter SD. Skin diseases of the bovine digit associated with lameness. Vet Bull 2000, 70: 149–71.
Hernandez J, Shearer JK, Webb DW. Effect of lameness on milk yield in dairy cows. J Am Vet Med Assoc 2002, 220: 640–4.

Krull AC, Shearer JK, Gorden PJ, Cooper VL, Phillips GJ, Plummer PJ. Deep sequencing analysis reveals the temporal microbiota changes associated with the development of bovine digital dermatitis. Infect Immun 2014, 82: 3359–73.
Krull A, Shearer J, Gorden P, Scott HM, Plummer PJ. Digital dermatitis: Natural lesion progression and regression in Holstein dairy cattle over three years. J Dairy Sci 2016, 99: 3718–31.
Milinovich GJ, Turner SA, McLennan MW, Trott DJ. Survey for papillomatous digital dermatitis in Australian dairy cattle. Aust Vet J 2004, 82: 223–7.
Shearer JK, Elliott JB. Papillomatous digital dermatitis: Treatment and control strategies—part I. Compend Cont Educ Pract Vet 1998, 20: S158–73.

Shearer JK, Hernandez J, Elliott JB. Papillomatous digital dermatitis: Treatment and control strategies—part II. Compend Cont Educ Pract Vet 1998, 20: S213–23.
Trott DJ, Moeller MR, Zuerner RL, et al. Characterization of *Treponema phagedenis*-like spirochetes isolated from papillomatous digital dermatitis lesions in dairy cattle. J Clin Microbiol 2003, 41: 2522–9.

Authors Paul J. Plummer and Jan K. Shearer
Consulting Editor Erica C. McKenzie
Acknowledgment The author and book editors acknowledge the prior contribution of Chris Clark and Steven L. Berry.

BASICS

OVERVIEW
Bovine ephemeral fever (BEF) is a seasonal, arthropod-transmitted, viral disease of cattle and water buffalo that occurs in the subtropics or temperate regions of Africa, Australia, and Asia.

INCIDENCE/PREVALENCE
Morbidity rates can be very high (approaching 100%) and mortality rates are typically low (<1%). Typically, most cases are asymptomatic. However, recently, there have been reports from several countries of alarmingly high case-fatality rates, sometimes exceeding 20%. It is not unusual for serologic surveys to have prevalence rates of 70–80%. In some cases, the prevalence of BEFV antibodies in African wildlife including a number of ruminants and also hippopotamus and elephants was quite high (>60% of animals tested), suggesting they may serve as natural reservoirs of infection in which the virus cycles during inter-epizootic periods.

GEOGRAPHICAL DISTRIBUTION
• Since BEFV is recognized as an arthropod-borne virus (arbovirus), geographic distribution is dependent on the presence of competent insect vectors.
• BEF has a wide distribution over subtropics or temperate regions of Africa, Australia, and Asia. It occurs from the southern tip of Africa to the Nile River Delta, across the Middle East through South and South-East Asia, into northern and eastern Australia, and throughout most of China, extending into Taiwan, the Korean Peninsula and southern Japan.
• BEFV does not occur in the islands of the Pacific, Europe (other than in the western regions of Turkey) or in the Americas where, for quarantine purposes, it is considered an important foreign animal disease.

PATHOPHYSIOLOGY
• Inflammation and fever are hallmark features of acute BEF.
• Bovine ephemeral fever virus (BEFV) is not cytolytic so cellular death and necrosis are not responsible for the inflammatory response.
• The direct induction of proinflammatory cytokines by BEF virus is believed to play a significant role in the pathogenesis and clinical expression of the acute disease. The virus uses the cell's signaling pathways to induce high levels of the proinflammatory cytokines, interleukin-1 beta (IL-1β) and interleukin-6. IL-1β is associated with high febrile responses and IL-6 is a major chemotactic cytokine for initiating innate immune responses.
• Interestingly, BEF infection does not induce the other major proinflammatory cytokine, tumor necrosis factor-alpha (TNF-α), and it

also induces the anti-inflammatory cytokine, IL-10. This production of anti-inflammatory cytokine IL-10 may explain the biphasic nature of the febrile response.

SIGNALMENT
• Bovine and water buffalo.
• BEF is a seasonal disease whose severity varies from year to year and region to region. Epidemics may occur periodically and are characterized by rapid onset within days or a few weeks in many animals in a region.
• Ephemeral fever is most prevalent in the wet season in the tropics and in summer to early autumn in the subtropics or temperate regions when conditions favor the presence of biting arthropods. BEF disappears abruptly in winter.
• Morbidity may be as high as 80%; overall mortality is usually 1–2%, although it is higher in well-conditioned cattle (10–20%).

PHYSICAL EXAMINATION FINDINGS
• The clinical signs occur suddenly and vary in severity. They include biphasic or polyphasic fever, shivering, inappetence, lacrimation, serous nasal discharge, drooling, dyspnea, atony of the fore stomachs, depression, stiffness and lameness, and a sudden decrease in milk yield. Cattle may also become recumbent and paralyzed for 8 hours to >1 week.
• After recovery, milk production often fails to return to normal levels until the next lactation.
• Abortion, with total loss of the season's lactation, occurs in ~5% of cows pregnant in months 8 and 9 of the last trimester.
• Bulls, market cattle, and heavily producing dairy cows are the most severely affected, but even so, spontaneous recovery usually occurs within a few days.

CAUSES AND RISK FACTORS
• The disease is caused by ephemeral fever virus, a Rhabdovirus (single-stranded, negative sense RNA in the same family as rabies virus). BEFV displays typical rhabdovirus bullet-shaped morphology, although appears to be more tapered at one end than the rounded forms that are observed for vesicular stomatitis virus (VSV) or rabies virus (RABV). The 14.9 kb BEFV genome is much larger and more complex than those of VSV or RABV. Since the G protein is a major antigenic determinant there is only a single serotype. The G gene is a useful genotyping marker as it displays reliable alignment with adequate sequence variation to obtain precision and resolution, and the absence of genetic recombination suggests it is likely to be is representative of the entire genome. Using the G gene ectodomain, three lineages have been identified: East Asia, Australia, and Middle East.
• The major transmission route of BEFV is by hematophagous insects. The virus has been recovered from some *Culicoides* (biting midge)

and mosquito species (*Anopheles, Culex,* and *Culicine* spp.) collected in the field and has been shown to multiply in *Culicoides* and *Culex* mosquitoes in the laboratory. The role of the insect in biologic transmission appears to be very limited as only a small proportion of insects become infected (~20%) and the virus does not survive in them for more than 10 days. The virus can be mechanically transmitted by IV inoculation of blood from infected viremic cattle to susceptible cattle.
• Transmission by contact or fomites does not occur, and the virus does not appear to persist in recovered cattle.

DIAGNOSIS

DIFFERENTIAL DIAGNOSES
Parturient paresis (milk fever, hypocalcemia)

CBC/BIOCHEMISTRY/URINALYSIS
Clinical cases have a neutrophilia with bands.

OTHER LABORATORY TESTS
Viral serum neutralization, complement fixation, and the blocking ELISA tests are used for serology. Virus isolation can also be done but isolation usually requires mouse inoculation.

OTHER DIAGNOSTIC PROCEDURES
• Diagnosis of BEF is usually based on history and clinical signs (rapid onset of febrile signs for 2–5 days with spontaneous recovery).
• The clinical outbreak is confirmed by serology in paired serum samples collected during illness and 2–3 weeks later with a fourfold rise in antibodies.

PATHOLOGIC FINDINGS
• The gross lesions of BEF include polyserositis affecting joint, pleural, and peritoneal surfaces. Some lung edema is evident, atelectasis, cellulitis, and focal necrosis of skeletal muscle. The lymph nodes are edematous.
• The histologic findings include neutrophilia, leukocytosis, and high fibrinogen deposition.
• Hemosiderosis of the lymph nodes and spleen from loss of erythrocytes early in infection has been observed.
• The venules and capillaries of the tendon sheath, synovial membranes, muscle, and fascia have perivascular neutrophilic infiltration, focal or complete necrosis of vessel walls, thrombosis, and perivascular fibrosis.

TREATMENT

THERAPEUTIC APPROACH
• Complete rest is the most effective treatment, and recovering animals should not be stressed or worked because relapse is likely.

BOVINE EPHEMERAL FEVER (CONTINUED)

B

• Isotonic fluids can be administered IV to treat dehydration. Oral dosing should be avoided unless the swallowing reflex is functional.

MEDICATIONS

DRUGS OF CHOICE
• Anti-inflammatory drugs can be given early and in repeated doses for 2–3 days.
• IV or subcutaneous administration of calcium borogluconate has been found to be beneficial in some animals.
• Antibiotics can be administered to prevent secondary bacterial infections.

CONTRAINDICATIONS
During acute illness, no oral therapy should be given, to avoid inhalation pneumonia due to the inability of the animal to swallow.

FOLLOW-UP

EXPECTED COURSE AND PROGNOSIS
A complete recovery occurs in 95–97% of cases. BEF virus infection confers life-long immunity to cattle.

POSSIBLE COMPLICATIONS
Pneumonia, mastitis, hindlimb paralysis, abnormal gait, abortion in late pregnancy, and temporary (up to 6 months) infertility in bulls.

PATIENT CARE
• Animals should be encouraged to stand within 2–5 days. The animals should be rolled over several times a day to help avoid loss of circulation to the underside limbs, which will result in permanent muscle damage.
• The heavier the animal is, the more critical it is to get it back on its feet as quickly as possible.

PREVENTION
A modified-live vaccine is available that confers good protection. An inactivated vaccine is also available but it gives only 6 months of protection.

MISCELLANEOUS

ASSOCIATED CONDITIONS
Pneumonia, mastitis, hindlimb paralysis, abnormal gait, abortion in late pregnancy.

PREGNANCY
Infection in the last trimester can result in abortion.

BIOSECURITY
The virus cannot be spread by direct animal-to-animal contact. However, it can be spread from infected animals to susceptible animals by injection, so single-use needles should be used.

SYNONYMS
• Dengue fever of cattle
• Lazy man's disease
• Stiff sickness
• Three-day fever
• Three-day sickness

ABBREVIATIONS
• BEF = bovine ephemeral fever
• BEFV = bovine ephemeral fever virus
• ELISA = enzyme-linked immunosorbent assay
• IL-1β = interleukin-1 beta
• IL-6 = interleukin-6
• IL-10 = interleukin-10
• IV = intravenous
• TNF-α = tumor necrosis factor-alpha

SEE ALSO
• Abortion: Bovine
• Hypocalcemia: Bovine
• Mastitis: No Growth
• Postparturient Paresis/Hypocalcemia
• Respiratory Disease: Bovine

Suggested Reading
Barigye R, Melville LF, Davis S, et al. Kinetics of pro-inflammatory cytokines, interleukin-10, and virus neutralising antibodies during acute ephemeral fever virus infections in Brahman cattle. Vet Immunol Immunopathol 2015, 168: 159–63. http://doi.org/10.1016/j.vetimm.2015.09.004

Kirkland PD. Akabane and bovine ephemeral fever virus infections. Vet Clin North Am Food Anim Pract 2002, 18: 501–14.

Walker PJ, Klement E. Epidemiology and control of bovine ephemeral fever. Vet Res 2015, 46: 124. http://doi.org/10.1186/s13567-015-0262-4

Author Christopher C.L. Chase
Consulting Editor Christopher C.L. Chase

BOVINE LEUKEMIA VIRUS

BASICS

OVERVIEW
Bovine leukemia virus (BLV) is the causative agent of enzootic bovine leukosis (EBL), which is a chronic progressive lymphoproliferative disease of cattle.

INCIDENCE/PREVALENCE
• In the United States, approximately 80% of dairy herds have some level of BLV infection and 30–50% of all US dairy cattle are infected. Approximately 40% of beef cow/calf herds have some level of BLV infection. Incidence of new cases within a herd is highly dependent on current within-herd prevalence and management conditions. The cumulative incidence of lymphoma among infected cattle is estimated to be 1–2% per year, but may reach 5% in high-prevalence herds.

GEOGRAPHIC DISTRIBUTION
• BLV is present on all continents and is endemic in many countries where control programs have not been implemented. In the European Union, 21 countries are officially BLV free; 3 have BLV free regions. New Zealand and Western Australia have eliminated BLV from their dairy herds, though it is still present in low levels in beef herds.

PATHOPHYSIOLOGY
BLV is a delta retrovirus which preferentially infects B lymphocytes. Like other retroviruses, infection is persistent and life-long. Transmission occurs through transfer of lymphocytes with integrated provirus from infected to susceptible animals. There are 4 stages of infection.
• Primary infection: Upon initial infection there is a short period of virus replication during which the virus infects new B lymphocytes. Infected cattle may experience flu-like symptoms. As the immune system responds to infection, expression of virus particles ceases and further expansion of the population of infected lymphocytes occurs via polyclonal proliferation.
• Aleukemic (AL) infection: The majority (50–70%) of animals will remain subclincally infected with normal lymphocyte counts. Immune dysregulation occurs which makes animals susceptible to a variety of infections and impairs their response to vaccination.
• Persistent lymphocytosis (PL): Approximately 30–50% of infected cattle will develop persistent lymphocytosis, with circulating lymphocyte levels elevated above normal physiologic levels. These animals are immune suppressed and prone to opportunistic infections.
• Lymphoma: <5% of infected animals will eventually develop lymphoma. Tumors occur in a variety of organs, most commonly the superficial, visceral and retrobulbar lymph nodes, heart (right atrium), abomasum, uterus, liver, spleen, kidneys, and extradural spine.

SIGNALMENT
• Natural infection has been confirmed in *Bos taurus* and *Bos indicus* cattle, and in water buffalo. Experimental infection has been induced in many other species, most notably sheep.
• Infection is more common in dairy cattle than in beef cattle. Animals can be infected at any age. Decreased milk production and increased premature culling are more common in dairy cows in their second and later lactations. Lymphoma is typically seen in cattle >3 years of age.

PHYSICAL EXAMINATION FINDINGS
• No physical examination findings are specific to the AL or PL stages. However, nonspecific clinical signs associated with immune dysregulation may be present, including: weakness, more frequent infections, delayed recovery from infections, decreased milk production, and increased premature culling.
• Physical examination findings due to lymphoma include enlarged lymph nodes and palpable masses, variable signs of organ dysfunction depending on the organs involved, and generalized weakness and loss of body condition. Signs of organ dysfunction that may be noted include: jugular pulses, tachycardia, murmurs, and/or arrhythmias; dyspnea and/or tachypnea; anorexia, constipation, and/or diarrhea; pelvic limb weakness or paralysis; jaundice; keratitis and/or proptosis. Splenic lymphoma can result in rupture and sudden death.

GENETICS
• There is a genetic component to BLV susceptibility and disease progression. The major histocompatibility complex of cattle—bovine leukocyte antigen (BoLA)—is highly polymorphic. Certain polymorphisms in the genes for BoLA have been associated with higher risk of seropositivity, resistance/susceptibility to PL, the number of BLV-infected peripheral B lymphocytes, and high/low proviral load.
• The genetics of BoLA are complex and may potentially be linked to genes controlling milk production, therefore the utility of genetic selection for BLV control is limited.

CAUSES AND RISK FACTORS
• Purchase of infected animals is the main risk factor for introduction of BLV into a previously negative herd.
• Risk factors for new infections of individual animals within an infected herd include: calves born to a positive dam; feeding of fresh, raw colostrum and milk from infected cows to calves; shared use of blood-contaminated equipment including dehorners, tattoo pliers, needles, and rectal palpation sleeves; bull breeding; lack of fly control; and use of milking machines.
• The relative importance of various risk factors and the mechanisms by which they result in transmission are not completely understood and are an area of ongoing research.

DIAGNOSIS

DIFFERENTIAL DIAGNOSES
• For opportunistic infections in AL/PL stages: Various primary infections, unrelated to underlying BLV.
• For lymphoma: Visceral lymphoma may feel similar to abdominal fat necrosis on rectal palpation. Keratitis due to retrobulbar lymphoma should be differentiated from pink eye. Pelvic limb weakness or paralysis due to extradural spinal lymphoma may mimic nerve damage from calving. Lumpy jaw (*Actinomyces bovis*) causes hard swellings on the jaw and neck, similar to enlarged lymph nodes. Other tumors of affected organs can be differentiated based on histology. Sporadic lymphoma can only be differentiated from BLV-induced lymphoma by PCR.

CBC/BIOCHEMISTRY/URINALYSIS
Cows with PL will have an increased absolute lymphocyte count. Biochemistry and urinalysis may reflect dysfunction of lymphoma-affected organs.

OTHER DIAGNOSTIC PROCEDURES
• AGID and antibody capture ELISA are commercially available for antibody detection; however, ELISA is the test of choice for routine diagnosis of BLV. ELISA tests have higher sensitivity than AGID and can be performed on milk as well as serum. Sensitivity and specificity of commercially available ELISA tests vary from 97–100% and 78–100%, respectively. These tests will miss early infections, prior to onset of antibody production, and cannot differentiate between maternal antibody and active immunity in calves <6 months of age. ELISA can be performed on pooled milk samples for screening, and is used on bulk tank milk for herd-level screening in many countries with control programs.
• RT-PCR for provirus can be used to identify early infections and to differentiate between maternal antibody and true infection in young stock. PCR can also be used to confirm infection in cases where ELISA results are equivocal. PCR may be used as a tool to identify highly infectious animals within herds for disease control protocols. PCR on lymphoma tissue is necessary to definitively differentiate between BLV-induced lymphoma and sporadic lymphoma cases.

BOVINE LEUKEMIA VIRUS   (CONTINUED)

B

PATHOLOGIC FINDINGS

• Grossly, lymphoma can be suspected when tumors of the visceral lymph nodes, uterus, abomasum, heart (especially right atrium), liver, spleen, and kidneys are found. These tumors are usually soft and gray-white, and can include friable areas of necrosis.

• Microscopically, massive lymphoid cell infiltration is observed in the affected organs as they replace normal cells. Histopathology cannot differentiate between BLV-associated lymphoma and sporadic lymphoma.

TREATMENT

THERAPEUTIC APPROACH

Infections are life-long. There is no specific treatment.

MEDICATIONS

DRUGS OF CHOICE

N/A

FOLLOW-UP

EXPECTED COURSE AND PROGNOSIS

• Progression from AL to PL occurs in 30–50% of infected animals, and <5% develop lymphoma. Lymphoma develops more commonly in PL animals; however, PL is not a prerequisite for the development of lymphoma.

• Prognosis for AL and PL animals is fair, though the productive lifespan is shortened by premature culling.

• Prognosis for lymphoma cases is poor. Once lymphoma is clinically apparent it is fatal, typically within months of diagnosis.

PREVENTION

• Prevent introduction of BLV into previously negative herds by keeping closed herds, or testing all additions—including breeding bulls.

• Minimize spread of BLV to negative animals within a positive herd by implementing a control program for the herd which may include some combination of routine screening of animals, strict management protocols, segregation, and/or culling of infectious animals.

• Management protocols to minimize transmission of BLV have been successful in reducing within-herd prevalence, but have not

been demonstrated to be capable of completely eliminating BLV from a herd without some selective culling. These protocols may include: using single-use needles for injection, single-use sleeves for rectal palpation and AI, heat treating and/or freezing colostrum and milk to be fed to calves, fly control, exclusive use of AI breeding, dehorning via cautery, and cleaning/disinfection of any blood-contaminated equipment.

• There are no commercial vaccines currently available. A promising vaccine is currently in experimental trials.

MISCELLANEOUS

ASSOCIATED CONDITIONS

Sporadic bovine leukosis (SBL) also results in lymphoma, but is not associated with BLV infection.

AGE-RELATED FACTORS

A minority of calves born to infected dams are infected at birth. Incidence of infection increases as heifers enter the milking herd. Lymphoma occurs mainly in cattle 3 years of age and older.

ZOONOTIC POTENTIAL

While some studies have demonstrated an association between BLV exposure and human breast cancer, there is no evidence that BLV plays an etiologic role in human disease.

PREGNANCY

Lymphoma of the reproductive tract can result in reproductive failure. About 10% of calves born to infected cows are infected in utero or perinatally.

BIOSECURITY

• Biosecurity for BLV includes keeping a closed herd and implementing management described under "Prevention."

• Virus is cell-associated and does not survive well outside the host in most environmental conditions. Infected cells can survive outside the host in milk and blood. Infected cells are sensitive to freezing, heat, and UV light.

PRODUCTION MANAGEMENT

• BLV infected dairy cows are estimated to have an average loss of 950–1050 kg of milk per cow per year. Given the high prevalence in many herds and the life-long course of the disease, this can be a significant financial loss over time. BLV-infected dairy cows have shortened productive lifespans within the herd, resulting in a lower return on the investment in raising those animals to the age

when then enter the milking herd. Similar production measures are currently being studied in beef cow/calf herds. Lymphoma is the largest single reason for cattle carcass condemnation at slaughter in the US, accounting for 13.5% of beef condemnations and 26.9% of dairy cattle condemnations.

• The later stages of BLV infection are characterized by a slow deterioration of condition and may be a significant source of animal distress. Efforts should be made to identify and cull or euthanize animals before disease results in suffering.

SYNONYMS

• Bovine leukemia
• Bovine leukosis
• Enzootic bovine leukosis

ABBREVIATIONS

• AGID = agar gel immunodiffusion
• AI = artificial insemination
• AL = aleukemic
• BLV = bovine leukemia virus
• BoLA = bovine leukocyte antigen
• EBL = enzootic bovine leukosis
• ELISA = enzyme-linked immunosorbent assay
• PL = persistent lymphocytosis
• RT-PCR = reverse transcription-polymerase chain reaction
• SBL = sporadic bovine leukosis

SEE ALSO

• Lymphocytosis
• Lymphosarcoma

Suggested Reading
Bartlett PC, Sordillo LM, Byrem TM, et al. Options for the control of bovine leukemia virus in dairy cattle. J Am Vet Me Assoc 2014, 244: 914–22.
European Food Safety Authority Panel on Animal Health and Welfare. Scientific opinion on enzootic bovine leukosis. EFSA J 2015, 13: 4188, 63 pp. doi:10.2903/j.efsa.2015.4188
Frie MC, Coussens PM. Bovine leukemia virus: A major silent threat to proper immune responses in cattle. Vet Immunol Immunopathol 2015, 163: 103–14.
Miyasaka T, Takeshima SN, Jimba M, et al. Identification of bovine leukocyte antigen class II haplotypes associated with variations in bovine leukemia virus proviral load in Japanese Black cattle. Tissue Antigens 2013, 81: 72–82.

Author Rebecca LaDronka
Consulting Editor Christopher C.L. Chase
Acknowledgment The author and book editors acknowledge the prior contribution of Christopher C.L. Chase.

BOVINE PAPULAR STOMATITIS

BASICS

OVERVIEW
Bovine papular stomatitis (BPS) is a mild viral disease of calves characterized by proliferative lesions around the mouth and head caused by bovine papular stomatitis virus (BPSV), a Parapoxvirus. Infections are usually asymptomatic, but raised papules may be observed on nasal planum, hard palate, nares, and occasionally on the esophageal or ruminal mucosa. There are no lesions at the coronary band. Bovine papular stomatitis virus, like other parapoxviruses, can be zoonotic.

INCIDENCE/PREVALENCE
Worldwide distribution

SYSTEMS AFFECTED
Integument

PATHOPHYSIOLOGY
• Viral infection results in early hyperemia and inflammation in focal regions of the nares and mouth. Secondary lesions may occur for up to 4 months. Histopathologic evaluation of lesions demonstrates degeneration of epithelial cells and eosinophilic inclusions in degenerated cells. Hyperplasia of the papillae of the lamina propria is observed. Ulceration of lesions is accompanied by bacterial infection and sloughing of the epithelium.
• A chronic form of BPS has been described associated with more severe clinical signs (salivation, diarrhea, anorexia, and fever). The ulcers in chronic cases become encrusted with an exudate.
• Similar to contagious ecthyma and pseudocowpox in sheep and goats, bovine papular stomatitis is zoonotic and common in veterinary personnel.

SIGNALMENT
• Young dairy calves, feedlot calves shortly after arrival. Commonly observed in calves 1–12 months of age. Rare in adult cattle.
• Also has been seen in sheep and goats.

PHYSICAL EXAMINATION FINDINGS
• Acute lesions consist of 2–4 mm macules on the nares and muzzle that progress rapidly to papules with raised periphery and depressed center. Lesions later develop in the oral cavity. Lesion size may increase to 1 cm in diameter or greater (coalescence of multiple lesions) and regress within several days to weeks. Lesions are not found at coronary band.

• Most animals are afebrile, eat normally, and have no clinicopathologic alterations associated with viral infection.

GENETICS
No association with breed or genetics observed. Commonly observed in dairy calves and recent arrivals in feedlots.

CAUSES AND RISK FACTORS
• The disease is caused by infection with a parapoxvirus, bovine papular stomatitis virus.
• Calves born to cows affected by BPSV when young.
• Adult cows may serve as reservoir for future calf infection.
• Recent introduction of naïve animals to feedlot.

DIAGNOSIS

DIFFERENTIAL DIAGNOSES
• Bovine virus diarrhea virus/Mucosal disease
• Foot and mouth disease
• Pseudocowpox
• Vesicular stomatitis

CBC/BIOCHEMISTRY/URINALYSIS
No abnormalities consistently associated with viral lesions

OTHER DIAGNOSTIC PROCEDURES
Polymerase chain reaction, electron microscopy, and histopathology are useful in the diagnosis of BPS.

TREATMENT

THERAPEUTIC APPROACH
Symptomatic treatment of severely affected animals

MEDICATIONS
N/A

FOLLOW-UP

PREVENTION
Prevention can focus on biosecurity and production of vaccines using locally obtained viral strains.

MISCELLANEOUS

ZOONOTIC POTENTIAL
Bovine papular stomatitis virus, like other parapoxviruses, can be zoonotic. Lesions are usually confined to the hands and have been reported on farm workers who are milkers.

ABBREVIATIONS
• BPS = bovine papular stomatitis
• BPSV = ovine papular stomatitis virus

SEE ALSO
• Bovine Viral Diarrhea Virus
• Foot and Mouth Disease
• Pseudocowpox
• Vesicular Stomatitis

Suggested Reading
Buttner M, Rziha HJ. Parapoxviruses: from the lesion to the viral genome. J Vet Med B 2002, 49: 7–16.

Delhon G, Tulman ER, Afonso CL, et al. Genomes of the parapoxviruses Orf virus and bovine papular stomatitis virus. J Virol 2004, 78: 168–77.

Guo J, Rasmussen J, Wunschmann A, de la Concha-Bermejillo A. Genetic characterization of orf viruses isolated from various ruminant species of a zoo. Vet Microbiol 2004, 99: 81–92.

Inoshima Y, Morooka A, Sentsui H. Detection and diagnosis of parapoxvirus by the polymerase chain reaction. J Virolog Meth 2000, 84: 201–8.

Jeckel S, Bidewell C, Everest D, et al. Severe oesophagitis in an adult bull caused by bovine papular stomatitis virus. Vet Rec 2011, 169: 317.

Schnurrenberger PR, Swango LJ, Bowman GM, Luttgen PJ. Bovine papular stomatitis incidence in veterinary students. Can J Comp Med 1980, 44: 239–43.

Smith BP. Bovine papular stomatitis (proliferative stomatitis). In: Smith BP ed, Large Animal Internal Medicine. St. Louis: Mosby, 2002, pp. 706–7.

Stroebel JC, Gerdes GH. Bovine papular stomatitis: an incidental finding. J S Afr Vet Assoc 1996, 67: 104.

Yeruham I, Abraham A, Nyska A. Clinical and pathological description of a chronic form of bovine papular stomatitis. J Comp Pathol 1994, 111: 279–86.

Author Jeff Lakritz
Consulting Editor Christopher C.L. Chase

BOVINE PETECHIAL FEVER

B

BASICS

OVERVIEW
Bovine petechial fever (Ondiri disease) is an infectious disease of cattle in East Africa characterized by petechial and ecchymotic hemorrhages on mucosal membranes. The disease has not been reported in North America.

SYSTEMS AFFECTED
Hemolymphatic

HISTORICAL FINDINGS
Affected animals have a fluctuating fever. The most consistent signs are petechiation and ecchymosis of mucus membranes. Unilateral conjunctival edema, hyphemia, epistaxis, and anemia are present in some severe cases. Dairy cattle imported into endemic areas often exhibit a profound drop in milk production.

SIGNALMENT
There is no sex or age predisposition. *Bos taurus* breeds are more susceptible than *Bos indicus*.

CAUSES AND RISK FACTORS
• The cause is *Ehrlichia* (*Cytoecetes*) *ondiri*. The organism is endemic in wild animals, particularly the bushbuck (*Tragelaphus scriptus*) of highlands above 5000 feet in East Africa. Cattle acquire the disease when grazing on edges of thick, humid forests particularly when they are grazed in these areas at the end of the dry season.
• Bovine petechial fever is common in cattle that have been recently introduced to these areas while indigenous cattle appear to acquire resistance.
• The disease is thought to be transmitted by an arthropod vector. The vector has yet to be identified, but epidemiologic findings suggest a tick vector. Grazing in or adjacent to thick, high elevation East African forests and the presence of the bushbuck, the reservoir of the organism, are important risk factors. Recently introduced animals are more susceptible.

DIAGNOSIS

DIFFERENTIAL DIAGNOSES
• Bracken fern poisoning.
• Trypanosomiasis occurs in the tropics where the vector, the tsetse (*Glossina* spp.) fly is found.
• Theileriosis is also common in areas where the tick vector *Rhipicephalus* spp. is present.

OTHER LABORATORY TESTS
Ehrlichia ondiri is diagnosed on demonstration of the organism in peripheral blood monocytes and granulocytes after Giemsa staining, but cannot be cultured.

TREATMENT

THERAPEUTIC APPROACH
Tetracyclines are effective as a treatment. Recovered animals are immune to reinfection for at least 2 years.

MEDICATIONS

DRUGS OF CHOICE
Tetracyclines are effective as a treatment.

FOLLOW-UP

EXPECTED COURSE AND PROGNOSIS
• Prognosis is guarded. The mortality is up to 50% in affected animals.
• The disease is important in imported animals introduced into risk areas where significant losses are recorded.

MISCELLANEOUS

PRODUCTION MANAGEMENT
• Bovine petechial fever is common in cattle that have been recently introduced to infected areas, while indigenous cattle appear to acquire resistance.
• Grazing in or adjacent to thick, high elevation East African forests and the presence of the bushbuck, the reservoir of the organism, are important risk factors. Recently introduced animals are more susceptible.

ABBREVIATIONS
N/A

SYNONYM
Ondiri disease

SEE ALSO
• Bracken Fern Toxicity
• Trypanosomiasis

Suggested Reading
Davies G. Bovine petechial fever (Ondiri disease). Vet Microbiol 1993, 34: 103–21.
Radostits OM, Gay CC, Blood DC, Hinchcliff KW. Veterinary Medicine, 10th ed. New York: Saunders, 2007, pp. 1469–70.
Author Munashe Chigerwe
Consulting Editor Christopher C.L. Chase

BOVINE RESPIRATORY SYNCYTIAL VIRUS

BASICS

OVERVIEW
Bovine respiratory syncytial virus (BRSV) induces a mild to severe lower respiratory tract disease in cattle. This viral infection is one of the pathogens associated with bovine respiratory disease complex.

INCIDENCE/PREVALENCE
• BRSV is endemic in cattle.
• Seroprevalence in herds is often >90%.

GEOGRAPHIC DISTRIBUTION
Worldwide

SYSTEMS AFFECTED
Respiratory

PATHOPHYSIOLOGY
• BRSV induces damage to the respiratory epithelium with a concomitant influx of inflammatory cells (neutrophils and lymphocytes) and production of proinflammatory cytokines (IL-6, IL-8) and often also T helper type 2 cytokines, such as IL-4. Arterial oxygen is often reduced by 30–40%.
• Production of anti-BRSV IgE antibodies has been associated with the most severe clinical and pathologic disease.
• The damage to epithelium coupled with inflammatory changes increases the susceptibility of the lung to secondary bacterial infection. Concomitant infection with *Histophilus somni* has been shown to cause synergistic upregulation of inflammatory cytokines and increased severity of disease.
• Severe BRSV infections can cause severe damage to bronchiolar and alveolar epithelial tissue resulting in the formation of bullae and interstitial emphysema.

SIGNALMENT
• Bovine, ovine.
• BRSV is seldom seen in calves <2 weeks of age, and is most prevalent and severe in animals between 1 month and 8 months of age.
• BRSV disease is rarely seen in cattle >9 months of age. Adult cattle can occasionally experience severe disease.

PHYSICAL EXAMINATION FINDINGS
• BRSV infection results in respiratory signs. These respiratory signs can be mild, with increased respiratory rate and increased harshness in respiratory sounds, to severe, with dyspnea, forced expiration, and open-mouth breathing. In severe cases wheezing can be heard on thoracic auscultation.

• Spontaneous cough is always present and induced cough can usually be precipitated by tracheal palpation; cough can vary from dry and nonproductive to moist.
• Nasal discharge can vary from none to serous to mucopurulent.
• Conjunctivitis and lacrimal discharge are seen infrequently. There is an increased rectal temperature (104–108°F; 40–42°C), depression, and decreased feed intake.
• Secondary pneumonia with bacterial pathogens (*Mannheimia haemolytica, Pasteurella multocida, Histophilus somni*) or *Mycoplasma bovis* is a frequent sequela.

GENETICS
Recent studies are showing associations between immune response genes and BRSV resistance.

CAUSES AND RISK FACTORS
• BRSV is an enveloped, negative, single-stranded RNA virus in the pneumovirus group of the paramyxovirus family. The virus is easily inactivated by desiccation, heat, and disinfectants.
• Stress (weaning, shipping, etc.) will increase the risk. Excessive levels of dust have been reported to increase clinical BRSV.
• Maternal antibody will inhibit vaccine response but will not prevent infection. However, it will lessen the clinical course of disease.
• Concurrent infection with other viral agents, particularly bovine viral diarrhea virus (BVDV), exacerbates BRSV clinical disease.

DIAGNOSIS

DIFFERENTIAL DIAGNOSES
• Bovine herpesvirus 1 (BHV-1) is associated with rhinotracheitis and upper respiratory disease. BHV-1-infected calves frequently have mucopurulent discharge and conjunctivitis.
• BVDV is associated with oral ulcers, mucopurulent discharge, and upper respiratory disease.
• Bovine parainfluenza-3 virus (PI-3) infection is usually a mild lower respiratory disease.
• Bovine coronavirus (BCV) has also been associated with respiratory disease. In younger calves, it is seen in calves suffering from enteritis and diarrhea. BCV in 5- to 13-month-old cattle causes symptoms of dyspnea, nasal discharge, and increased respiratory rate.
• Atypical interstitial pneumonia (AIP) is characterized by sudden onset of disease with

subsequent death. AIP animals have labored breathing with loud expiration, frothing at the mouth, and open-mouth breathing. They have harsh respiratory sounds with crackles and rhonchi. These animals usually have a recent history of grazing lush pastures or having a ration change in a feedyard.

CBC/BIOCHEMISTRY/URINALYSIS
BRSV causes a slight lymphopenia 3–10 days post-infection.

OTHER DIAGNOSTIC PROCEDURES
• BRSV is a very difficult virus to detect by virus isolation. Animals need to be sampled in the incubation or acute phase of infection (3–7 days).
• BRSV can often be detected on nasal swabs by quantitative RT-PCR (qPCR) between 4 to 7 days post-infection. Transtracheal washes have also been successful in PCR detection of BRSV. Antigen detection kits have been developed and can detect BRSV antigen.
• Other procedures that have proved useful in detection of BRSV antigen are fluorescent antibody tests of fresh tissue and immunohistochemistry staining of cell cultures or formalin-fixed paraffin-embedded tissues. Staining of lung tissue from cases necropsied late in infection (after day 7) will often be negative for viral antigen.
• Paired serum samples can be used in the diagnosis of BRSV infection. However, the antibody titer of animals with well-developed clinical disease may be higher in acute samples than the samples taken 2–3 weeks later.
• BRSV antibody response often develops rapidly, and clinical signs follow virus infection by up to 7–10 days.
• Single serum samples showing high antibody titers from a number of animals in a respiratory outbreak may be useful in making a diagnosis if coupled with clinical signs.
• Younger calves infected with BRSV in the presence of maternally acquired antibody may not seroconvert.

PATHOLOGIC FINDINGS
• Gross lesions include a diffuse interstitial pneumonia with subpleural and interstitial emphysema along with interstitial edema. These lesions are similar to and must be differentiated from AIP.
• Regional suppurative bronchopneumonia of bacterial origin is usually present.
• Histologic examination reveals necrotizing and proliferative bronchiolitis with alveolitis that is sometimes proliferative along with hyaline membrane formation and edema.
• Syncytial cells are present in bronchiolar epithelium and lung parenchyma.

B

TREATMENT

THERAPEUTIC APPROACH
The therapy for BRSV is supportive. See "Patient Care" for additional information.

MEDICATIONS

DRUGS OF CHOICE
• Corticosteroids or nonsteroidal anti-inflammatory drugs (NSAIDs) may have some benefit to lessen the severity of BRSV disease.
• Antimicrobial treatment is utilized to reduce secondary bacterial infections.

CONTRAINDICATIONS
Appropriate milk and meat withdrawal times must be followed for all compounds administered to food-producing animals.

FOLLOW-UP

EXPECTED COURSE AND PROGNOSIS
• Uncomplicated BRSV infections will resolve in 10–14 days.
• Animals that have secondary infections usually will develop bronchopneumonia with varying levels of morbidity and mortality.

POSSIBLE COMPLICATIONS
• Some formaldehyde-inactivated BRSV vaccines have been shown to increase the severity of BRSV disease. This method of inactivation is not currently used for commercial vaccines.
• Maternal antibodies in calves interfere with development of an effective BRSV immune response with MLV vaccines.

CLIENT EDUCATION
Minimize handling of animals, decrease animal exposure to high levels of dust, and use preventive vaccines.

PATIENT CARE
• Respiratory characteristics along with rectal body temperatures should be frequently monitored to assess BRSV clinical progression and also the development of secondary bacterial infections that would result in bovine respiratory disease complex (BRDC).
• Severely diseased animals that are dehydrated may receive oral and/or intravenous fluids.
• Handling of BRSV-infected animals should be minimized to decrease the risk of secondary bacterial infections.
• Concentrate and silage should not be fed to severely diseased animals.

PREVENTION
• Both modified-live virus (MLV) and inactivated virus BRSV vaccines are available.
• Vaccination is an important part of a BRSV control program.

MISCELLANEOUS

ASSOCIATED CONDITIONS
BRDC is a frequent sequela to BRSV infections.

AGE-RELATED FACTORS
Younger animals (between 1and 8 months of age) are usually affected.

BIOSECURITY
• BRSV survives very poorly in the environment and is susceptible to UV light, desiccation, heat, and disinfectants. The virus will survive better in the winter.
• Animals exhibiting clinical signs of BRSV should be isolated from other cattle as transmission of BRSV occurs by the oronasal route.

• In pens of animals that have had a BRSV outbreak, it would be prudent to clean the water sources.

PRODUCTION MANAGEMENT
In herds with a history of BRSV in their calves, a BRSV vaccine program should be implemented.

ABBREVIATIONS
• AIP = atypical interstitial pneumonia
• BCV = bovine coronavirus
• BHV-1 = bovine herpesvirus 1
• BRDC = bovine respiratory disease complex
• BRSV = bovine respiratory syncytial virus
• BVDV = bovine viral diarrhea virus
• MLV = modified-live virus
• NSAIDs = nonsteroidal anti-inflammatory drugs
• PCR = polymerase chain reaction
• PI-3 = bovine parainfluenza-3 virus

SEE ALSO
• Atypical Interstitial Pneumonia
• Bovine Viral Diarrhea Virus
• Coronavirus
• Parainfluenza-3 Virus
• Respiratory Disease: Bovine

Suggested Reading
Gershwin LJ. Immunology of bovine respiratory syncytial virus infection of cattle. Comp Immunol Micro Infect Dis 2012, 35: 253–7.
Larsen LE. Bovine respiratory syncytial virus (BRSV) review article. Acta Vet Scand 2000, 41: 1–24.
Woolums AR, Anderson ML, Gunther RA, et al. Evaluation of severe disease induced by aerosol inoculation of calves with bovine respiratory syncytial virus. Am J Vet Res 1999, 60: 473–80.
Author Laurel J. Gershwin
Consulting Editor Christopher C.L. Chase
Acknowledgment The author and book editors acknowledge the prior contribution of Christopher C.L. Chase.

BOVINE SPONGIFORM ENCEPHALOPATHY

B

BASICS

OVERVIEW
Bovine spongiform encephalopathy (BSE) is a progressively fatal, neurodegenerative disease of cattle and is a type of transmissible spongiform encephalopathy (TSE).

INCIDENCE/PREVALENCE
• BSE is an OIE-reportable disease.
• Since the inception of the feed ban, there have been noticeable reductions in the incidence of typical BSE diagnosis.
• The incidence of atypical BSE has not changed significantly, further indicating the potential for a spontaneous origin.
• In 2014, a total of 13 cases of BSE were reported among member countries worldwide.
• As of 2014, 11 countries are listed as having a "controlled BSE risk," with a significantly larger number having a "negligible risk." Canada is currently listed as having a controlled BSE risk, with a 2014 incidence rate of 0 cases per million cattle. The United States is listed as having negligible risk. The highest incidence rate in 2014 was 1.2 cases/million cattle, as compared to peak incidence rate of over 6000 cases/million in the United Kingdom in 1992.

GEOGRAPHIC DISTRIBUTION
Infected indigenous cattle have been reported in most countries in Europe and North America, as well as Brazil and Southeast Asia. The majority of recent cases appear to be of the "atypical" form of the disease, and may be spontaneous in nature.

SYSTEMS AFFECTED
Nervous

PATHOPHYSIOLOGY
• Since its first diagnosis in the UK in 1986, different theories about the origin of BSE have been proposed, generally involving the feeding of an initial new "strain" of the prion agent to cattle.
• Addition of rendered material from affected cattle carcasses to make meat and bone meal amplified the agent.
• Origins for the original source case include a single mutated form of sheep scrapie, a spontaneous case of atypical BSE, or contamination with additional prion-contaminated material into the food chain from additional sources.
• A complete ban on the feeding of ruminant-derived products back to cattle has effectively controlled the majority of cases of BSE; however, it appears that there are at least two "types" of apparently spontaneous BSE that may occur, similar to several classical human prion diseases.

• Unlike TSE diseases in other species, there is no significant involvement of the lymphoreticular system in cattle.
• Unlike other TSEs, there appears to be a single "strain" of conventional BSE that is capable of significant cross-species infection. Atypical BSE (classified as either "H" or "L"-type) may be spontaneous in origin, and differs in both age of onset and molecular signature.

HISTORICAL FINDINGS
Usually an insidious onset of neurologic signs in cattle >2 years of age.

SIGNALMENT
• Cattle, bison.
• Generally affects cattle between 3 and 6 years of age and the incubation period ranges from 2 to 12 years.

PHYSICAL EXAMINATION FINDINGS
Slowly progressive, degenerative neurologic disease. Cattle will often be ataxic, primarily on the hindlimbs with hypermetria. They will also have hyperreflexia, muscle fasciculation and tremors, fall down, and behavior changes such as nervousness and frenzy. Over time, the animal will become anorexic and lose weight and body condition; dairy animals will have decreased milk production.

GENETICS
• Offspring of BSE-infected cattle seem to have an increased risk of developing BSE but exact etiology is unknown at this time.
• Vertical or venereal transmission has not been proven, although it may have been demonstrated in transgenic mice using the BSE agent.
• There is no clear genetic linkage to the development of conventional BSE; however, atypical BSE may be partially linked to unique genetic signatures within the bovine prion (PRNP) gene.

CAUSES AND RISK FACTORS
• BSE and other TSEs are believed to be caused by a pathogenic effect on neurons of an abnormal isoform of a host-encoded glycoprotein, the prion protein.
• The pathogenic form of this protein appears to be devoid of nucleic acids and supports its own amplification in the host through conversion of the secondary structure of host prion protein to the pathogenic protein structure. TSEs in animals primarily occur by transmitting the etiologic agent within a species, either naturally or through domestic husbandry practices. A notable exception among the TSEs is the apparent ability of BSE to effectively cross species barriers, affecting most mammalian species including humans (variant Creutzfeldt-Jakob disease; vCJD).
• Cattle consuming prion-infected meat and bonemeal or other ruminant by-products that may be contaminated with the BSE agent. No horizontal transmission has been reported.

DIAGNOSIS

DIFFERENTIAL DIAGNOSES
• Hypomagnesemia
• Intracranial tumors
• Lead poisoning
• Listeriosis
• Nervous ketosis
• Polioencephalomalacia
• Rabies
• Spinal cord trauma

CBC/BIOCHEMISTRY/URINALYSIS
There is no antemortem test for BSE as the host does not mount an immune response to the agent.

PATHOLOGIC FINDINGS
• Gross lesions are restricted to carcass changes such as emaciation and damage to the hide from ataxia and nervousness.
• Histopathologic detection of neurodegeneration lesions in the brain (bilaterally symmetrical spongiform changes in the gray matter) will help confirm the diagnosis. Immunohistochemistry, immunoblotting, and ELISA to demonstrate accumulations of the prion (PrP^{res}) protein are needed for definitive diagnosis.

TREATMENT

THERAPEUTIC APPROACH
There is no treatment for this disease.

MEDICATIONS

DRUGS OF CHOICE
N/A

FOLLOW-UP

EXPECTED COURSE AND PROGNOSIS
This is a progressively fatal neurodegenerative disease and 100% of the cases will die.

PREVENTION
Do not feed ruminant products to ruminants. Restrictions have been put in place in many countries that preclude the feeding of ruminant products back to ruminants, but clients should be made aware of this as a risk factor and prevent contamination of any cattle feed on their farms.

MISCELLANEOUS

AGE-RELATED FACTORS
Most often seen in cattle between 2 and 10 years of age.

BOVINE SPONGIFORM ENCEPHALOPATHY

B

ZOONOTIC POTENTIAL
• There is evidence to suggest that persons consuming BSE-contaminated products may develop a disease called variant Creutzfeldt-Jakob disease.
• The exact incubation period for vCJD is unknown but it is thought to be decades. It too is a progressively fatal neurologic disease with 28 years of age being the mean age at death of those affected.
• Since the first discovery of vCJD in 1996 through November 2006, there have been 200 cases worldwide, with the majority in the UK (164) and France (21). The US has reported 3 cases, but the patients had resided in the UK (2) and Saudi Arabia (1) the majority of their lives.
• There are recommendations regarding blood donations, surgical equipment, and organ transplants from countries where vCJD has been diagnosed, to prevent further spread of this disease.

PREGNANCY
Vertical transmission of BSE has not been documented but offspring of BSE-infected cattle are at higher risk for developing the disease; offspring are usually culled.

SYNONYM
Mad cow disease

ABBREVIATIONS
• BSE = bovine spongiform encephalopathy
• ELISA = enzyme-linked immunosorbent assay
• OIE = Office International de Epizooties
• PrP^{res} = abnormal prion protein
• SE = transmissible spongiform encephalitis
• vCJD = variant Creutzfeldt-Jakob disease

SEE ALSO
• Cervidae: Chronic Wasting Disease
• Grass Tetany/Hypomagnesemia
• Lead Toxicosis
• Listeriosis
• Ketosis: Dairy Cattle
• Rabies
• Scrapie
• Spinal Column and Cord Assessment and Dysfunction (see www.fiveminutevet.com/ruminant)
• Vitamin B Deficiency

Suggested Reading
Aiello SE ed. Merck Veterinary Manual, 8th ed. Whitehouse Station, NJ: Merck & Co., 1998.

Bovine Spongiform Encephalopathy disease card from the OIE website. http://www.oie.int/animal-health-in-the-world/official-disease-status/bse/
Bovine Spongiform Encephalopathy from the United States Department of Agriculture, Animal and Plant Inspection Service website. https://www.aphis.usda.gov/aphis/ourfocus/animalhealth/animal-disease-information/cattle-disease-information/sa_bse/ct_about_bse
Bovine Spongiform Encephalopathy. Chapter 2.3.13. In: Manual of Standards for Diagnostic Tests and Vaccines. Paris: Office International des Epizooties, 2000.
Centers for Disease Control and Prevention: https://www.cdc.gov/prions/bse/

Author Alan Young
Consulting Editor Christopher C.L. Chase
Acknowledgment The author and book editors acknowledge the prior contribution of Danelle Bickett-Weddle and Neal Bataller.

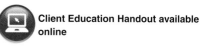 **Client Education Handout available online**

BASICS

OVERVIEW
• Bovine viral diarrhea (BVD) is a viral infection of cattle.
• BVD is caused by the virus bovine viral diarrhea virus (BVDV).
• BVDV is capable of infecting and causing disease in other ruminant species (sheep, goats, camelids, cervids) and swine.
• BVDV is capable of causing pathology in many different organ systems.
• Cattle can become acutely infected with BVDV at any age. This is also referred to as primary infection or transient infection.
• Fetal infection prior to day 125 of gestation can result in the development of immunotolerance to the BVDV and the development of a persistent infection (PI) with the virus. Camelids and cervids can also develop PI.
• Cattle persistently infected with BVDV shed large amounts of virus during their lifetime. They are the major source of virus spread within and between farms.
• Cattle persistently infected with BVDV can develop a fatal form of BVD called mucosal disease.

INCIDENCE/PREVALENCE
BVDV is a ubiquitous pathogen of ruminants with high seroprevalence worldwide. Infections with BVDV are endemic in many countries and are often associated with severe economic losses for the cattle industry. Prevalence of cattle persistently infected with BVDV is low, estimated at generally <0.05% of the cattle population.

GEOGRAPHIC DISTRIBUTION
Worldwide

SYSTEMS AFFECTED
• Digestive
• Hemolymphatic
• Nervous
• Respiratory
• Reproductive

PATHOPHYSIOLOGY
• Two main methods of virus transmission include postnatal horizontal transmission and gestational vertical transmission from a viremic dam to her fetus. Transmission may occur by aerosols, nose-to-nose contact, and via semen.
• Following infection with BVDV, a short incubation period of 3–7 days is followed by viremia, which generally lasts for 1–4 days but may persist for 15 days (Figure 1).
• BVDV can result in immunosuppression (leukopenia, hypoimmunoglobinemia, neutrophil dysfunction, decreased antigen presentation) following acute infection resulting in secondary infections caused by opportunistic pathogens. BVDV has been implicated most often as an

Clinical Forms of BVD

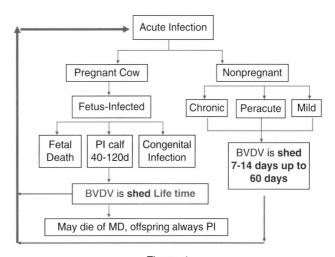

Figure 1.

Outcomes of BVDV Infections.

immunosuppressive component of the bovine respiratory disease complex.
• Following BVDV infection in pregnant animals the virus infects the fetus, resulting in one of several outcomes: early embryonic death occur with infections in the first 45 days of gestation; abortions can occur following infection at any stage of gestation; persistent infection occurs with fetal infection between day 45 and 145; congenital defects can occur with infections in the 2nd and 3rd trimester of gestation and include cerebral hypoplasia, retinal atrophy, cataract, growth retardation, arrested bone development, and pulmonary hypoplasia. Congenital infections are defined as those occurring late in gestation and characterized by the presence of virus-neutralizing antibodies at birth. These congenital infections can result in increased neonatal disease, later sexual maturity and reduced fertility (Figure 1).
• Persistently infected (PI) animals shed high levels of virus in all their secretions, feces, and semen (Figure 2). PI animals are much more efficient transmitters of BVDV than transiently infected animals because they shed large amounts of virus for a long period of time.
• PI animals typically have reduced lifespan with >80% of PI animals dead by 2 years of age.
• The most common sequelae in PI animals is mucosal disease. Mucosal disease is the result of a PI animal developing a superinfection with cytopathic (CP) BVDV (see "Causes and Risk Factors") and results in high mortality. The superinfection is often the result of mutation of the noncytopathic (NCP) BVDV from the PI animal becoming a CP mutant. The superinfection can also be the result of

the vaccination of PI animals with a CP modified live virus (MLV) BVDV vaccine.

SIGNALMENT
BVDV is capable of infecting other ruminant species (sheep, goats, camelids, cervids) and swine. It can cause PI in alpacas, white-tailed deer, camels, llamas, and other wild ruminants

PHYSICAL EXAMINATION FINDINGS
• Acute infections are mostly subclinical in nature.
• Severe acute infections may be characterized by fever, leukopenia, thrombocytopenia, and hemorrhagic disease.
• Other manifestations of acute BVDV infection may include enteric disease, respiratory disease, and immunosuppression. The severity of disease depends upon host and viral factors.
• Reproductive outcomes following fetal infection can include transient infertility, early embryonic death, abortion, congenital defects, congenital infections, and persistent infection.
• A mild, biphasic elevation in body temperature and leukopenia may be evident.
• Lactating cattle may have an associated decrease in milk production.
• Mucosal disease occurs in cattle persistently infected with BVDV and is characterized by fever, anorexia, depression, profuse salivation, nasal discharge, severe diarrhea, hemorrhages and erosions in gastrointestinal tract, and a very high case fatality rate.
• BVDV genotype 2 is usually involved in severe acute BVD characterized by severe thrombocytopenia with hemorrhages (prolonged bleeding from venipuncture sites; hemorrhages on sclera of eye and inner surface of eyelids; hemorrhages on mucosal

B

Pregnant female whose
fetus may become
infected.

Cow and calf that may both
develop acute infections. Cow may
suffer from infertility.

PI calf constantly
shedding BVD virus
to herdmates

Calves exposed to PI calf may develop
pneumonia, diarrhea, etc.

Herd bull that may become acutely infected
and then expose cows while breeding.

Figure 2.

Effects of a PI in the Herd.

surfaces of cheeks, lower gingiva, tongue, and soft palate), fever, pneumonia, diarrhea, and sudden death in 10–100% of infected animals.
• In calves: Pyrexia, leukopenia, anorexia, diarrhea, immunosuppression with secondary infections.
• In pregnant animals: Early embryonic death occurs with infections in the first 45 days of gestation; abortions can occur following infection at any stage of gestation; persistent infection occurs with fetal infection between day 45 and 145; congenital defects can occur with infections in the 2nd and 3rd trimester of gestation and include cerebral hypoplasia, retinal atrophy, cataract, growth retardation, arrested bone development, and pulmonary hypoplasia. Congenital infections are defined as those occurring late in gestation and characterized by the presence of virus-neutralizing antibodies at birth.

CAUSES AND RISK FACTORS
• BVDV is an RNA virus and a member of the genus *Pestivirus* in the family Flaviviridae.
• The BVDV is antigenically related to classical swine fever virus (CSFV) of pigs and Border diseases virus (BDV) of sheep.
• BVDV is further divided into genotypes (1 and 2) and sub-genotypes (a, b, c . . .). The most common sub-genotypes in the USA include BVDV 1a, BVDV 1b, BVDV 2a, and BVDV 2b.
• BVDV can be further divided into two biotypes; cytopathic (CP) or non-cytopathic (NCP). This differentiation is based on the

ability to cause cell cytopathology in cell culture. Only noncytopathic BVDV has been associated with persistent BVDV infection.
• The major risk factor for BVDV being introduced into a farm is the acquisition of new cattle, specifically cattle persistently infected with BVDV. Other risk factors include sharing of pastures with other cattle (direct or fence line) and lack of a BVDV vaccination program.
• The virus is shed in most secretions and excretions of infected animals including tears, milk, saliva, urine, feces, nasal secretions, and semen.
• Virus can survive for several days in a cool, protected environment and hence fomites (nose tongs, halters, etc.) can play a role in virus transmission.
• Flies can also transmit the virus.
• The virus can be present in milk and colostrum.

DIAGNOSIS

DIFFERENTIAL DIAGNOSES
• Differential diagnosis for calves with diarrhea as the result of BVDV includes any pathogen known to cause diarrhea in neonatal calves. In adult cattle, differential diarrheal diagnoses would include winter dysentery and salmonella.
• Differential diagnosis in white-tailed deer includes epizootic hemorrhagic disease of deer and bluetongue.

• Differential diagnosis for abortions caused by BVDV includes BHV-1, Neospora, leptospirosis, and brucellosis.
• Differential diagnosis for thrombocytopenia induced by BVDV includes sweet clover poisoning, coumarol poisoning, and vitamin K deficiency.

CBC/BIOCHEMISTRY/URINALYSIS
• Severe leukopenia is characteristic in the early stages of acute BVD, with total leukocyte count in the range of 1,000–5,000/µL being common.
• Isolates of BVDV associated with hemorrhagic BVDV can result in severe thrombocytopenia and subsequently anemia.

OTHER DIAGNOSTIC PROCEDURES
• Acute infections can be identified by virus isolation from serum, whole blood, nasal swabs, or lymphoid tissue; RT-PCR on serum, whole blood, nasal swabs, or lymphoid tissue; identification of a fourfold increase in virus-neutralizing antibody titers in acute and convalescent serum samples.
• Persistent infection with BVDV can be diagnosed by serial identification of virus 3 weeks apart using virus isolation, antigen detection ELISA, or RT-PCR, in serum, whole blood, milk or skin, or identification of BVDV antigen in skin samples (ear notch biopsies) by immunohistochemistry.
• Because of the high analytical sensitivity of RT-PCR, it can be used on pools of individual samples to reduce costs. Individuals in positive pools are then retested to identify positive animals.

• Herd screening for BVDV infection can be done by testing bulk milk for antibody or virus. Identifying BVDV neutralizing antibodies in young cattle 6–12 months of age that have not been vaccinated for BVDV is highly correlated with virus circulation in the herd. Precolostral screening of newborn calves for BVDV neutralizing antibodies has also been demonstrated to be highly correlated with virus circulation in the herd.

PATHOLOGIC FINDINGS
• In most cases, acute BVDV presents with no gross lesions that are specific.
• Cattle acutely infected with BVDV may have lesions similar to those found with mucosal disease including erosions in the oral cavity, esophagus, rumen, abomasums, and small intestine, especially over areas of the Peyer's patches.
• Widespread petechial and ecchymotic hemorrhages may be present in cattle suffering from hemorrhagic syndrome.
• No specific lesions are seen in aborted fetuses.
• Cerebellar hypoplasia can be seen grossly in congenitally affected calves.
• Histopathologic findings following acute BVDV infections include lymphoid depletion of the Peyer's patches, lymph nodes, spleen, and thymus.
• In PI animals, BVDV immunohistochemistry (IHC) will demonstrate BVDV antigen in all organs. On histologic examination, hair follicles have high levels of BVDV antigen. Ear notches containing hair follicles have been used in IHC assays to identify PI animals.

TREATMENT

THERAPEUTIC APPROACH
• Cattle acutely infected with BVDV typically recover over time.
• In severe cases, supportive therapy is indicated.
• There is no treatment for cattle persistently infected with BVDV.

MEDICATIONS

DRUGS OF CHOICE
N/A

FOLLOW-UP

EXPECTED COURSE AND PROGNOSIS
Most cattle recover within 10–14 days.

POSSIBLE COMPLICATIONS
• The use of modified-live vaccines against BVDV in pregnant cattle is contraindicated unless specified by the product manufacturer.
• Modified-live vaccines may be immunosuppressive and therefore should be used with caution.

CLIENT EDUCATION
• Clients should be educated about the importance of biosecurity in the prevention of BVDV entering an operation.
• Clients should understand the significance of cattle persistently infected with BVDV in bringing the virus onto a farm and serving as the major virus reservoir.
• Clients should understand that vaccination is an important tool in controlling BVDV. However, because of the antigenic diversity of the virus, control programs should not rely on vaccination alone, but should include the implementation of appropriate biosecurity as well.

PREVENTION
• Implementation of a whole-herd vaccination program against BVDV is recommended.
• Vaccinations should include antigens against both type 1 and type 2 BVDV.
• Newly acquired cattle should be quarantined for a minimum of 3 weeks and screened for persistent infection.
• Vaccination of breeding age females is important for reducing the risk of fetal infections and subsequent adverse outcomes, most importantly the birth of calves persistently infected with BVDV.
• Vaccination of young stock is important for reducing risk of syndromes associated with acute infections including respiratory disease and hemorrhagic disease.
• Effective vaccines against infectious agents must account for both antigenic and genetic diversity, and they should provide fetal protection.
• Both modified-live (MLV) and killed vaccines are available.

MISCELLANEOUS

ASSOCIATED CONDITIONS
• BVDV infection frequently is a predisposing factor to bovine respiratory disease (shipping fever).
• Mucosal disease occurs in cattle persistently infected with BVDV following a superinfection with an antigenically related cytopathic BVDV strain.
• Cytopathic BVDV may also arise by mutation of the infecting noncytopathic virus.

AGE-RELATED FACTORS
Colostral antibodies can protect newborn calves for 2–4 months.

ZOONOTIC POTENTIAL
BVDV is not considered a zoonotic agent.

PREGNANCY
• Infections during gestation can result in early embryonic deaths, abortion, congenital defects, persistent infection, or congenital infection. The result of fetal infection is dependent on the virus strain, biotype, and the stage of gestation when fetal infection occurs.
• In utero infection of the fetus with noncytopathic BVDV prior to 125 days' gestation leads to immune tolerance and the birth of persistently infected (PI) calves that are usually unthrifty and poor doers and act as a source of virus for the rest of the herd.

BIOSECURITY
• Biosecurity is a central pillar in the prevention of BVDV in a cattle operation. This includes quarantine and testing of animals prior to entering the herd.
• Purchased pregnant animals are a huge threat to introduce BVDV through the birth of a PI calf. There is no simple test of the pregnant animal that can be used to detect a PI calf in utero.
• The role of wild ruminants as a reservoir host or as a dead-end host in BVDV epidemiology is not clear. Controlling contact between cattle and wildlife is advisable if possible.

PRODUCTION MANAGEMENT
• Vaccination is an important tool in controlling BVDV. To be the most successful at preventing PI animals, animals need to be vaccinated prior to breeding.
• Because of the antigenic diversity of the virus, control programs should not rely on vaccination alone, but should include the implementation of appropriate biosecurity programs as well as monitoring and testing for BVDV PI.
• Purchased pregnant animals pose a large threat to any BVDV prevention program. Their offspring need to be immediately tested for PI following calving.

ABBREVIATIONS
• BDV = Border diseases virus of sheep
• BHV = bovine herpes virus
• BT = bovine turbinate
• BVD = bovine viral diarrhea
• BVDV = bovine viral diarrhea virus
• CP = cytopathic
• CSFV = classical swine fever virus
• ELISA = enzyme-linked immunosorbent assay
• IHC = immunohistochemistry
• NCP = noncytopathic
• PBL = peripheral blood leukocytes
• PCR = polymerase chain reaction
• PI = persistent infection
• RT-PCR = reverse transcription polymerase chain reaction

BOVINE VIRAL DIARRHEA VIRUS

B

- SN = serum neutralization
- VN = virus neutralization

SEE ALSO
- Bluetongue Virus
- Bovine Papular Stomatitis
- Brucellosis
- Epizootic Hemorrhagic Disease Virus
- Leptospirosis
- Neosporosis
- Salmonellosis
- Sweet Clover Poisoning
- Winter Dysentery

Suggested Reading
Baker JC, Houe H eds. Bovine viral diarrhea virus. Vet Clin North Am Food Anim Pract 1995, 11(3).

Brock KV eds. Bovine viral diarrhea virus. Vet Clin North Am Food Anim Pract 2004, 20(1).

Lanyon SR, Hill FI, Reichel MP, Brownlie J. Bovine viral diarrhoea: pathogenesis and diagnosis. Vet J 2014, 199: 201–9.

Nelson DD, Duprau JL, Wolff PL, Evermann JF. Persistent bovine viral diarrhea virus infection in domestic and wild small ruminants and camelids including the mountain goat (*Oreamnos americanus*). Front Microbiol 2016, 6: 1–7. http://doi.org/10.3389/fmicb.2015.01415

Passler T, Ditchkoff SS, Walz PH. Bovine viral diarrhea virus (BVDV) in white-tailed deer (*Odocoileus virginianus*). Front Microbiol 2016, 7: 1–11. http://doi.org/10.3389/fmicb.2016.00945

Ridpath JF. Immunology of BVDV vaccines. Biologicals 2013, 41: 14–19.

Schweizer M, Peterhans E. Pestiviruses. Annu Rev Anim Biosci 2014, 2: 141–63.

Author Daniel L. Grooms
Consulting Editor Christopher C.L. Chase
Acknowledgment The author and book editors acknowledge the prior contribution of Sagar Goyal

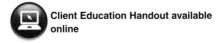 **Client Education Handout available online**

BRACKEN FERN TOXICITY

BASICS

OVERVIEW
• All ruminant species are at risk of developing toxicosis. Most cases of poisonings have been reported in cattle.
• Bracken fern (*Pteridium aquilinum*) is a native perennial fern found throughout the United States and is the source of intoxication. *Pteridium* species in other parts of the world have also been shown to contain the toxic principle.
• Disease in ruminants is generally seen following ingestion of high quantities of the plant over a period of several months.
• Diseases reported in ruminants include bone marrow suppression, bovine enzootic hematuria, bladder and gastrointestinal neoplasias, and progressive retinal degeneration.
• Key to controlling the disease is prevention. Bracken fern is susceptible to a wide variety of herbicides.

INCIDENCE/PREVALENCE
Sporadic and relatively uncommon

GEOGRAPHIC DISTRIBUTION
Worldwide

SYSTEMS AFFECTED
• Hemolymphatic
• Digestive
• Nervous
• Urinary

PATHOPHYSIOLOGY
• Ptaquiloside is the main toxic principle. Other toxic metabolites include quercetin and shikimic acid. The species of animal exposed, and the dose and duration of exposure, are thought to be the determining factors in which clinical syndrome is observed.
• Bone marrow suppression has been observed in clinically affected animals; there is suppression of all cell lines (radiomimetic effect).
• Clinically affected animals generally present with signs associated with thrombocytopenia and neutropenia; anemia may occur as a result of blood loss or later as the red cells disappear from circulation (longer lifespan).
• Toxicosis is often complicated by bacteremia. Neutropenia due to myelosuppression allows bacterial invasion through ulcerations of the gastrointestinal (GI) tract and may result in infarction of the liver or other bodily organs.
• Under alkaline conditions, ptaquiloside is converted to dienone, an active carcinogen, which alkylates DNA and leads to tumor formation. Because ruminant urine is usually alkaline, tumors are commonly found in the bladder and result in bovine enzootic hematuria.
• Quercetin and papilloma virus type 4 act as co-carcinogens to produce malignant tumors

in the upper GI tract, most commonly from the tongue to the rumen.
• Bracken fern also contains a thiaminase which rarely results in clinical signs in ruminants, given the ample production of thiamine by the ruminal microflora. However, intoxication results in neurologic disease more commonly in monogastric species.

SIGNALMENT
• Cattle are most commonly affected; but there are reports of sheep, llamas, and other ruminants being affected.
• All ruminants appear susceptible; most poisonings have been reported to occur in cattle. Natural outbreaks have occurred in sheep. Monogastric livestock species (horses and swine) may also be affected.
• Enzootic hematuria and tumors are generally observed in older animals, following months or years of exposure. The toxin is excreted in the milk and suckling animals may be affected secondarily.

PHYSICAL EXAMINATION FINDINGS
• Cattle afflicted with bone marrow suppression generally present with bloody nasal discharge, petechiation and ecchymoses, and weakness. Thrombocytopenia may result in hyphema or bleeding from the external orifices. Hemorrhagic diarrhea, melena, and hematuria may also be present.
• Secondary bacterial infections are common (e.g., lung), and signs of dyspnea, decreased appetite, and hyperthermia can be observed.
• Bovine enzootic hematuria ("red water") has been reported in cattle chronically exposed to bracken fern. This syndrome is linked to the development of bladder lesions, some of which are neoplastic. Bovine papillomavirus types 2 and 4 may play a role in the development of neoplastic lesions.
• Red to brown urine is a common sign in those cattle suffering from enzootic hematuria.
• Experimentally, bracken fern exposure for 4–12 months has been associated with progressive retinal degeneration in sheep. Sheep suffering from retinal degeneration show bilateral pupil dilatation and have a glassy-eyed appearance ("bright blindness").

CAUSES AND RISK FACTORS
• Bracken ferns (*Pteridium* spp.) are perennial ferns found throughout much of the world, 1–6 feet tall, with triangular, coarse, pinnately compound fronds. Other species of fern may also contain ptaquiloside.
• Bracken fern has a deep-seated, black, elongate, branched, hairy, horizontal rhizome. Spores develop late in the summer and are found rolled under the blade edges.
• Poisonings can occur as a result of grazing the fresh plant (thought to be unpalatable) or following chronic consumption of contaminated hay.
• The plant is toxic green or dry; the most toxic parts of the plant are the young

developing fronds (fiddleheads or crosiers) and rhizomes.
• The plant prefers moist to dry woods and open slopes, with good drainage. It tends to occur naturally in very dense stands.
• Clinical disease is generally seen when animals consume significant amounts of plant material (up to 20% of their diet) for 30 days or more.
• Clinical cases may continue to emerge for up to 6 weeks after cessation of exposure.

DIAGNOSIS

DIFFERENTIAL DIAGNOSES
• Other hemorrhagic diseases of cattle include anthrax, BVDV infection, furazolidone poisoning, sweet clover intoxication, and radiation injury.
• Cases of bovine enzootic hematuria need to be differentiated from other causes of hematuria such as cystitis, pyelonephritis, and other toxicants.

CBC/BIOCHEMISTRY/URINALYSIS
• Thrombocytopenia and leukocytosis; polymorphonuclear leukocytes are the most severely affected.
• The presence of anemia depends on the stage of disease and the amount of blood loss by the patient.
• Inflammatory leukogram, hyperproteinemia, elevated fibrinogen can be due to secondary infectious processes.
• Hematuria and the increased presence of epithelial cells may be seen on urinalysis.

OTHER LABORATORY TESTS
• Prolonged bleeding times
• Normal prothrombin times

OTHER DIAGNOSTIC PROCEDURES
• Bone marrow biopsy may reveal pancytopenia. Caution is warranted as this procedure is not without risks in compromised patients.

PATHOLOGIC FINDINGS
• Petechiation and ecchymoses, multiple hemorrhages throughout the tissues, pale bone marrow, edematous and ulcerated GI tract.
• Numerous neoplastic conditions of the GI and urinary tracts—papillomas, transitional cell carcinomas, squamous cell carcinomas, adenocarcinomas, hemangiomas.
• Retinal degeneration in affected sheep.

TREATMENT

THERAPEUTIC APPROACH
• No primary treatment.
• Supportive care includes removal of the animal from contaminated pastures or

BRACKEN FERN TOXICITY (CONTINUED)

B

forages, broad-spectrum antibiotics, blood transfusion, and good nursing care.
• Most animals respond poorly to treatment. Animals with neoplastic changes should be culled or humanely euthanized.

MEDICATIONS

N/A

FOLLOW-UP

EXPECTED COURSE AND PROGNOSIS
Animals suffering from bone marrow suppression almost never recover.

POSSIBLE COMPLICATIONS
N/A

PATIENT CARE
• Monitor platelet, neutrophil, and red blood cell values.
• Check for onset of secondary infections.

PREVENTION
• Recognition of bracken fern in the field or in hay.
• When removal of exposure is not possible, avoid excessive grazing and provide alternate feedstuffs to limit intake.
• Herbicide application can be successful in eliminating the plant.

MISCELLANEOUS

ASSOCIATED CONDITIONS
Monogastric animals exposed to bracken fern suffer from thiamine deficiency due to thiaminases present in bracken fern.

ZOONOTIC POTENTIAL
Since ptaquiloside is a direct-acting carcinogen, people conceivably can be affected through direct consumption of the plant or ingesting milk from exposed animals.

PRODUCTION MANAGEMENT
• Avoid grazing in bracken-dense areas, provide adequate forage, and instill appropriate stocking densities.
• Avoid feeding contaminated hay.

SYNONYMS
• Bovine enzootic hematuria
• Bright blindness

ABBREVIATIONS
• BVDV = bovine viral diarrhea virus
• GI = gastrointestinal

SEE ALSO
• Anthrax
• Bovine Viral Diarrhea Virus
• Rodenticide Toxicity
• Sweet Clover Poisoning
• Toxicology: Herd Outbreaks

Suggested Reading
Burrows GE, Tyrl RJ. Dennstaedtiaceae Ching. In: Burrows GE, Tyrl RJ eds, Toxic Plants of North America, 2nd ed. Ames: Wiley-Blackwell, 2013, pp. 408–20.
Gava A, da Silva Neves D, Gava D, de Moura ST, Schild AL, Riet-Correa F. Bracken fern (*Pteridium aquilinum*) poisoning in cattle in southern Brazil. Vet Hum Toxicol 2002, 44: 362–5.
Knight AP, Walter RG. Plants affecting the blood. In: Knight AP, Walter RG eds, A Guide to Plant Poisoning of Animals in North America. Jackson, WY: Teton NewMedia, 2001, pp. 186–203.
Perez-Alenza MD, Blanco J, Sardon D, Sanchez Moreiro MA, Rodriguez-Bertos A. Clinico-pathological findings in cattle exposed to chronic bracken fern toxicity. N Z Vet J 2006, 54: 185–92.
Plumlee KH, Nicholson SS. Ptaquiloside. In: Plumlee KH ed, Clinical Veterinary Toxicology. St. Louis: Mosby, 2004, pp. 402–3.
Author Benjamin W. Newcomer
Consulting Editor Christopher C.L. Chase
Acknowledgment The author and book editors acknowledge the prior contribution of Patricia Talcott.

BRASSICA SPP. TOXICITY

BASICS

OVERVIEW
- Forages, seeds, and the roots of plants of the genus *Brassica* (e.g., kale, rape, turnips, mustards, cabbage, Brussel sprouts) contain S-methyl-L-cysteine sulfoxide (SMCO), a rare sulfur-containing amino acid, and glucosinolates which upon metabolism yield toxic principles.
- Syndromes associated with *Brassica* poisoning in ruminants include congenital hypothyroid goiter (enlarged thyroid), enteritis, Heinz-Ehrlich body anemia, polioencephalomalacia (PEM; "rape blindness"), nitrate poisoning, photosensitization, hypotrichosis, decreased libido in bulls, delayed estrus in cows, and acute bovine pulmonary emphysema and edema (ABPEE).
- Severe hemolytic anemia is associated with SMCO intake. Although the SMCO content in culinary vegetables is too low to induce hemolysis, ill-thrift is commonly observed.
- Dependent on their composition, glucosinolate metabolites will become either intestinal irritants (isothiocyanates) or goitrogens (thiocyanate ion and thiones such as vinyloxazolidine-2-thione).
- Isothiocyanate, a metabolite of the mustard oil contained in plant seeds, causes enteritis.
- Thiocyanate ions cause goiter when small amounts are chronically ingested along with iodine-deficient forages. *Brassica* plants also tend to be iodine-deficient. This syndrome is iodine-responsive.
- Thiones also arise from the seeds and are more potent than thiocyanates. They interfere with T4 formation and are unresponsive to iodine therapy. Treatment with iodine is clinically ineffective.
- Instead of being a direct cause of ABPEE, it is believed that fog fever is precipitated by the intake of *Brassica* spp.

INCIDENCE/PREVALENCE
Outbreaks of glucosinolate poisoning vary with the weather, variety, and growth stage of the plants. Grazing of SMCO-containing plants yields high morbidity and case fatality rates.

GEOGRAPHIC DISTRIBUTION
Worldwide

SYSTEMS AFFECTED
- Digestive
- Hemolymphatic
- Integument
- Nervous
- Reproductive
- Respiratory

PATHOPHYSIOLOGY
- Hemolytic anemia usually develops 1–3 weeks after exposure and occurs as a result of the conversion of SMCO to dimethyl disulfide (DMDS) by rumen microbes. Irreversible oxidization and denaturation of hemoglobin leads to Heinz body formation which, concurrent with membrane phospholipid peroxidation, contributes to cell lysis.
- Glutathione reductase (GR) deficiency in cattle, and reduced erythrocyte glucose-6-phosphate dehydrogenase (G6PD) activity in some sheep breeds, contribute to cell fragility.
- Thiocyanates are released by both plant and rumen microbial enzymes during mastication and fermentation, respectively, and are five times more concentrated in the smaller younger leaves than the larger more mature ones. Reduced iodide uptake and hence tyrosine iodination within the thyroid of the developing fetus results in the birth of goitrous neonates which exhibit signs of hypothyroidism. In Japan, the calves of gestating beef cows fed iodine-deficient forages and water concurrent with cruciferous plants alternatively developed diffuse hyperplastic goiter.
- Thiones interfere with the incorporation of iodine into thyroxine (T4) precursors and block its secretion from the thyroid gland.
- "Rape blindness," which is believed to be either a mild form of PEM or hepatotoxicity, is hypothesized to be the result of sulfate poisoning.
- The mechanism of photosensitization remains unclear.

HISTORICAL FINDINGS
- Animals will quickly ingest large quantities of highly palatable *Brassica* spp. which are used to supplement pastures in poor growth.
- Poisonings are more likely to occur when rumen microbes have had little time to adapt.
- Chronic ingestion by pregnant dams in iodine-deficient settings gives rise to a high incidence of neonatal goiter.
- Except for rape, all other varieties of kale yield high concentrations of rumen thiocyanate.
- Drought or high inorganic fertilizer content will amplify clinical signs.

SIGNALMENT
- Bovine, caprine, and ovine.
- Sheep and cattle breeds deficient in G6PD and GR activity, respectively, are especially susceptible to SMCO toxicosis.
- Goiter and clinical hypothyroidism are observed in neonates.
- Heinz body anemia is more likely to occur in ruminating animals.

PHYSICAL EXAMINATION FINDINGS
- Outbreaks of *Brassica*-induced hypothyroidism are characterized by abortions, stillbirths and the prolonged parturition of weak, lethargic and recumbent goitrous newborns with varying degrees of hypotrichosis. Kids are often more severely affected than lambs.
- A "thyroid thrill," the result of increased vascularity, is often palpated and auscultated within the jugular furrow.
- Neonatal mortality rates tend to be high during inclement weather.
- Clinical disease is rare in adults, despite palpably enlarged glands.
- Hypersalivation, colic, diarrhea, dysentery, and occasionally scant and sticky feces are observed in cases of rapeseed poisoning.
- Animals in hemolytic crisis may exhibit lethargy, pallor, icterus, dyspnea, coffee-colored urine (Figure 1a), hypoxic abortion, shock, and death.
- Erythema, edema, vesicles, and blindness may develop in photosensitive animals.
- Animals may develop methemoglobinemia and other signs of acute nitrite poisoning post-exposure. Stillbirths and stunted neonatal growth occur with chronic ingestion.
- Severe dyspnea and subcutaneous emphysema are signs of ABPEE.

CAUSES AND RISK FACTORS
- *Brassica* poisoning is possible whenever ruminants consume either *Brassica* plants or their by-products.
- Although glucosinolates are present in all plant components, seeds are the most toxic.
- SMCO content is highest in seeds, flowers, and secondary growth.
- Lightly pigmented animals are likely to develop photosensitivity after ingesting mature plants.
- During droughts and fertilizer overuse, higher levels of nitrates accumulate in *Brassica* leaves.

DIAGNOSIS

DIFFERENTIAL DIAGNOSES
- Nutritional iodine deficiency and the ingestion of couch grasses (*Cynodon aethiopicus*, *C. nlemfuensis*) or white clover (*Trifolium repens*) also result in goiter.
- Hemolytic anemia secondary to immune-mediated disease, onion or red maple toxicosis, chronic copper poisoning, hemo-parasites, leptospirosis, and bovine postparturient hemoglobinuria, should be considered.
- Viable alternatives for enteritis include infectious agents and the ingestion of oak and oleander species.
- Plants such as St John's wort and blue-green algae also cause photosensitization.

CBC/BIOCHEMISTRY/URINALYSIS
Results vary with the observed syndrome and include leukopenia, macrocytic, hyperchromic anemia with Heinz bodies in up to 100% of erythrocytes; elevated serum GGT and bilirubin; bilirubinuria and hemoglobinuria.

BRASSICA SPP. TOXICITY (CONTINUED)

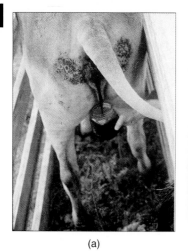
(a)

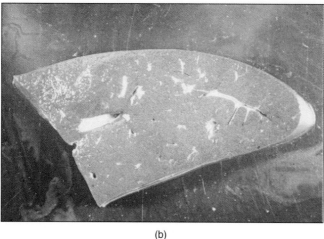
(b)

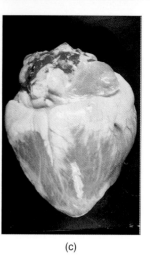
(c)

Figure 1.

Rape and Kale Poisoning. (a) Passage of Dark Urine (Hemoglobinuria) (b) Jaundiced Liver (c) Pale Jaundiced Heart. Reproduced with permission of Elsevier.

OTHER LABORATORY TESTS
• Blood glucosinolate assay.
• Determination of milk, serum or plasma iodine to assess T4 status.
• Chromatographic detection of blood dimethyl disulfide.
• Arterial blood gas and pulse oximetry.

OTHER DIAGNOSTIC PROCEDURES
Skin and liver biopsy

PATHOLOGIC FINDINGS
• Goiter; mean fresh thyroid weight is 6.5 g and 2 g in full-term calves and lambs, respectively.
• Thyroid follicles are infolded, depleted of colloid, and lined with columnar epithelium.
• Pallor, jaundiced organs (Figures 1b, 1c; see www.fiveminutevet.com/ruminant), darkened kidney, and hypoxia-induced hepatocellular necrosis.

TREATMENT

THERAPEUTIC APPROACH
• In all cases, further access to *Brassica* spp. should be restricted; provide shade and apply balm to skin lesions as needed.
• Iodine supplementation of pregnant dams is key in cases of thiocyanate-induced neonatal goiter.
• Supportive therapy may include colostrum administration and warmth to weak newborns, blood transfusions, and fluid and electrolyte therapy.

MEDICATIONS

DRUGS OF CHOICE
• Methylene blue
• Zinc-containing ointments

PRECAUTIONS
Adhere to appropriate milk and meat withdrawal times.

FOLLOW-UP

EXPECTED COURSE AND PROGNOSIS
Fair to guarded if exposure is restricted.

PREVENTION
Control livestock access to *Brassica* plants and by-products. Iodine supplementation either in the form of potassium iodide or weekly applications of tincture of iodine inside the flank of animals, has been effective.

MISCELLANEOUS

PREGNANCY
Feeding *Brassica* spp. to pregnant dams predisposes neonates to goiter.

PRODUCTION MANAGEMENT
The ingestion of *Brassica* plants and feedstuffs must be closely monitored.

SYNONYMS
N/A

ABBREVIATIONS
• ABPEE = acute bovine pulmonary emphysema and edema
• DMDS = dimethyl disulfide
• G6PD = glucose-6-phosphate dehydrogenase
• GR = glutathione reductase
• PEM = polioencephalomalacia
• SMCO = S-methyl-L-cysteine sulfoxide
• T4 = thyroxine

SEE ALSO
• Anaplasmosis
• Babesiosis
• Blue-Green Algae Poisoning
• Copper Deficiency and Toxicity
• Iodine Deficiency and Toxicity
• Leptospirosis
• Oak (*Quercus* spp.) Toxicity
• Photosensitization

Suggested Reading
Bell JM. Nutrients and toxicants in rapeseed meal: a review. J Anim Sci 1984, 58: 996–1010.
Bray TM, Kirkland JB. The metabolic basis of 3-methylindole-induced pneumotoxicity. Pharmacol Ther 1990, 46: 105–18.
Burrows GE, Tyrl RJ. Brassicaceae Burnett. In: Burrows GE, Tyrl RJ eds, Toxic Plants of North America, 2nd ed. Iowa: Wiley-Blackwell, 2013, pp. 280–9.

Gonzalez JM, Yusta B, Garcia C, Carpio M. Pulmonary and hepatic lesions in experimental 3-hydroxymethylindole intoxication. Vet Hum Toxicol 1986, 28: 418–20.

Morton JM, Campbell PH. Disease signs reported in south-eastern Australian dairy cattle while grazing *Brassica* species. Aust Vet J 1997, 75: 109–13.

Radostits O. Special Medicine: Diseases associated with nutritional deficiencies. In: Radostits OM, Gay CC, Hinchcliff KW, Constable PD eds, Veterinary Medicine: A Textbook of the Diseases of Cattle, Horses, Sheep, Pigs and Goats, 10th ed. Edinburgh: Saunders Elsevier, 2007, pp. 1691–783.

Radostits O. Special Medicine: Diseases associated with toxins in plants, fungi, Cyanobacteria, plant-associated bacteria, and venoms in ticks and vertebrate animals. In: Radostits OM, Gay CC, Hinchcliff KW, Constable PD eds, Veterinary Medicine: A Textbook of the Diseases of Cattle, Horses, Sheep, Pigs and Goats, 10th ed. Edinburgh: Saunders Elsevier, 2007, pp. 1851–920.

Stoewsand GS. Bioactive organosulfur phytochemicals in *Brassica oleracea* vegetables—a review. Food Chem Toxicol 1995, 33: 537–43.

Taljaard TL. Cabbage poisoning in ruminants. J S Afr Vet Assoc 1993, 64: 96–100.

Author Maisie E. Dawes

Consulting Editor Christopher C.L. Chase

Acknowledgment The author and book editors acknowledge the prior contribution of Natalie Coffer.

BREEDING SOUNDNESS EXAMINATION: BULL

 BASICS

OVERVIEW
• The aim of a breeding soundness examination (BSE) is to identify satisfactory potential breeding males and to remove unsatisfactory breeding males from the herd.
• Major emphasis is placed on physical attributes that affect the bull's ability to locate females in estrus, mount, achieve intromission, and deliver good-quality semen.
• Libido or serving capacity testing is sometimes included as part of a BSE.

INCIDENCE/PREVALENCE
Common procedure in beef bulls

SYSTEMS AFFECTED
• Reproductive
• Musculoskeletal
• Ophthalmic
• Behavioral

GEOGRAPHIC DISTRIBUTION
Worldwide

PATHOPHYSIOLOGY
N/A

HISTORICAL FINDINGS
• General history should include purchase/travel, health/nutritional, and vaccination and deworming.
• Reproductive history should include previous BSE findings, breeding records for previous breeding seasons, and the breeding management of the farm.

SIGNALMENT
• BSE should be performed prior to the breeding season, prior to sale, for insurance purposes, or as part of a herd fertility investigation.
• BSE is particularly important in young bulls prior to their first breeding season.
• Standards set forth by the SFT for minimum scrotal circumference to be classified as a potential satisfactory breeder are based on a minimum age of 15 months.
• Bulls should be examined annually.

PHYSICAL EXAMINATION FINDINGS
• BCS: Bulls should be slightly overconditioned heading into the breeding season. Bulls that are thin may not be able to maintain condition throughout the breeding season and bulls that are obese may experience reduced fertility due to impaired thermoregulation of the testicles from increased fat deposition within the scrotum.
• Eyes: Normal eyesight is required; bulls primarily use eyesight to detect cows in estrus.
• Conformation: A bull must be able to cover large distances to search out and find cows in estrus. Serving capacity is reduced by lameness or pain. Breeding bulls should be free of heritable conformation abnormalities.

• Reproductive examination should include:
  ○ Evaluation of the scrotal contents and palpation of the testes/epididymides
    ▪ Visual inspection of the scrotum for symmetry, size, and shape. The scrotum should have a distinct neck above the testes to allow for adequate thermoregulation.
    ▪ The scrotal skin should be free of dermatitis or frostbite lesions.
    ▪ The testes should be equal in size, shape, and consistency. They should be freely movable within the scrotum and turgid/resilient on palpation.
    ▪ The epididymides should be palpated for symmetry and any abnormalities including enlargement, heat, or pain. The head of the epididymis can be palpated on the craniodorsal aspect of the testis and the tail of the epididymis can be palpated at the ventral aspect of the testis.
  ○ Scrotal circumference
    ▪ SC is measured at the greatest diameter by grasping the neck of the scrotum and firmly pulling the testes down into the scrotum. Care should be taken not to place the thumb or fingers between the spermatic cords, which can falsely enlarge the SC diameter.
  ○ Penis and prepuce
    ▪ The prepuce should be palpated from the base of the scrotum to the preputial orifice. Special attention should be paid to the reflection of the prepuce onto the glans penis, as this is a common site of preputial injury.
    ▪ The penis should be thoroughly evaluated during exteriorization at the time of semen collection.
  ○ Transrectal palpation
    ▪ The internal genitalia that are readily palpated transrectally consist of the pelvic portion of the penis, body of the prostate, ampullae, and seminal vesicular glands. The bulbourethral glands are imbedded in the urethralis muscle and cannot be palpated.
    ▪ Abnormalities are most commonly detected in the seminal vesicular glands (i.e., acute or chronic seminal vesiculitis).
    ▪ Enlarged inguinal rings may predispose a bull to development of a scrotal hernia.
• Serving capacity/libido test
  ○ Serving capacity/libido test is not always included as part of a BSE.
  ○ Bulls are exposed to restrained, estrus cows for a specified time period and observed for sexual behavior and mating activity.

GENETICS
• Onset of puberty and testicular size are age and breed dependent.
• SC is correlated with age at puberty of bull half-sib females and daughters.
• Some spermatozoa abnormalities are hereditary.

CAUSES AND RISK FACTORS
N/A

DIAGNOSIS
• Bulls are classified as satisfactory, unsatisfactory or deferred potential breeders, based on physical examination, scrotal circumference size, progressive motility, and morphology. Any bull with abnormalities of the physical examination should be considered unsatisfactory or deferred.
• Satisfactory potential breeder
  ○ Scrotal circumference: ≥30 cm at <15 months; ≥31 cm at 15–18 months; ≥32 cm at 18–21 months; ≥33 cm at 21–24 months; ≥34 cm at ≥24 months
  ○ Progressive motility: >30%
  ○ Normal morphology: >70%
• Unsatisfactory potential breeder
  ○ Scrotal circumference: <30 cm at <15 months; <31 cm at 15–18 months; <32 cm at 18–21 months; <33 cm at 21–24 months; <34 cm at ≥24 months
  ○ Progressive motility: <30%
  ○ Normal morphology: <70%
• Deferred
  ○ A "deferred" classification may be assigned if the bull does not meet the standards but is likely to improve.
  ○ Bulls classified as deferred should be retested at a later date, typically 60 days, but often earlier based on the judgment of the veterinarian performing the examination.

DIFFERENTIAL DIAGNOSES
N/A

CBC/BIOCHEMISTRY/URINALYSIS
N/A

OTHER LABORATORY TESTS
Semen Collection
• The most common methods for semen collection in bulls in practice are electroejaculation or transrectal massage of the ampullae.
• Semen can also be collected by an artificial vagina in trained bulls.
• Post-mating aspiration from a cow is rarely performed.

Semen Evaluation
• Volume is variable, in the range 1–12 mL.
• Color varies from gray to milk white depending on concentration. Some ejaculates may be yellow (presence of riboflavin).
• Consistency: Ejaculates should be homogeneous.
• Motility: Mass motility or individual motility should be evaluated using clean warm equipment (Table 1).
  ○ Motility is reduced if semen is contaminated with urine, blood, or purulent material.
  ○ A minimum of 30% progressive motility is required for a classification of satisfactory potential breeder.

BREEDING SOUNDNESS EXAMINATION: BULL

Table 1

Evaluation of Motility		
Mass motility	*Description*	*Individual motility*
Very good	Rapid dark swirls	>80%
Good	Slower swirls and eddies	50–69%
Fair	No swirls, individual motility	30–49%
Poor	Little or no individual motility	<30%

- Morphology is assessed on eosin–nigrosin stained smears under oil (1000× magnification) or on formalin-fixed samples under phase contrast (wet mount).
  - A minimum of 70% morphologically normal spermatozoa is required for a classification of satisfactory potential breeder.
- Cytology of the ejaculate is assessed using a differential stain or Wright-Giemsa stain to identify any leukocytes. Presence of PMNs should alert the examiner to the possibility of seminal vesiculitis.

Semen Culture and Sensitivity
May be indicated when disease is suspected.

IMAGING
Testicular or transrectal ultrasonography may be performed if abnormalities are identified. This examination is not part of a routine BSE.

DIAGNOSTIC PROCEDURES
N/A

PATHOLOGIC FINDINGS
Abnormalities detected during a BSE are numerous and may include (but are not limited to): immaturity, poor semen quality, reduced scrotal circumference/testicular size, penile/prepucial injury or abnormality, congenital reproductive anomalies (e.g., persistent penile frenulum), testicular degeneration, infectious processes involving the reproductive tract, lameness, poor or excessive body condition, and ophthalmic abnormalities.

TREATMENT

THERAPEUTIC APPROACH
N/A

SURGICAL CONSIDERATIONS AND TECHNIQUES
N/A

MEDICATIONS

DRUGS OF CHOICE
N/A

CONTRADICTIONS
N/A

PRECAUTIONS
N/A

POSSIBLE INTERACTIONS
N/A

FOLLOW-UP

EXPECTED COURSE AND PROGNOSIS
N/A

POSSIBLE COMPLICATIONS
N/A

CLIENT EDUCATION
Bulls should be submitted for BSE annually.

PATIENT CARE
Breeding activity should be monitored during the mating season.

MISCELLANEOUS

ASSOCIATED CONDITIONS
N/A

AGE-RELATED FACTORS
Young males (<15 months) often fail the BSE because of abnormal morphology due to immaturity.

ZOONOTIC POTENTIAL
Brucellosis

PREGNANCY
Early pregnancy diagnosis is helpful for monitoring breeding activity and fertility of bulls.

BIOSECURITY
Quarantine all new bulls and those returning from shows for a determined period of time to protect herd health.

PRODUCTION MANAGEMENT
- In herds with short breeding and calving seasons, bull BSEs are vital to productivity and economic success.
- Bulls should have a BSE prior to the breeding season.

- BSE is particularly important in young virgin bulls.
- BSE should be performed at least 2 months prior to the intended breeding season to allow for replacement if unsatisfactory. For bulls intended for sale, the BSE should be within a month prior to auction.
- Bull to cow ratio should be 1:25.

SYNONYMS
N/A

ABBREVIATIONS
- BCS = body condition score
- BSE = breeding soundness examination
- PMNs = polymorphonuclear leukocytes
- SC = scrotal circumference

SEE ALSO
- Beef Bull Management (see www.fiveminutevet.com/ruminant)
- Body Condition Scoring: Beef (see www.fiveminutevet.com/ruminant)
- Body Condition Scoring: Dairy Cattle (see www.fiveminutevet.com/ruminant)
- Penile Disorders
- Penile Hematoma
- Seminal Vesiculitis
- Testicular Disorders: Bovine

Suggested Reading
Chenoweth PJ, McPherson FJ. Bull breeding soundness, semen evaluation and cattle productivity. Anim Reprod Sci 2016, 169: 32–6.
Hopper R, King E. Evaluation of breeding soundness: basic examination of the semen. In: Hopper R ed, Bovine Reproduction. Chichester: Wiley Blackwell, 2015, pp. 68–78.
Palmer CW. Management and breeding soundness of mature bulls. Vet Clin North Am Food Anim Pract 2016, 32: 479–95.
Palmer C, Brito L, Arteaga A, et al. Comparison of electroejaculation and transrectal massage for semen collection in range and yearling feedlot beef bulls. Anim Reprod Sci 2005, 87: 25–31.
Author Alexis Campbell
Consulting Editor Ahmed Tibary
Acknowledgment The author and book editors acknowledge the prior contribution of John Gillam.

BREEDING SOUNDNESS EXAMINATION: CAMELIDS

 BASICS

OVERVIEW
• Male breeding soundness examination (BSE) is performed as a routine management procedure, for pre-purchase or work-up of cases of infertility.
• BSE is not a measure of fertility but helps identify males with reproductive problems.
• The male camelid reproductive system presents several anatomic and physiologic peculiarities, making some aspects of the BSE unique.

INCIDENCE/PREVALENCE
• Common procedure in alpacas and llamas.
• The procedure is not yet well established in camels (except for highly valuable racing dromedaries).

GEOGRAPHIC DISTRIBUTION
Worldwide

SYSTEMS AFFECTED
• Digestive
• Reproductive
• Multisystemic

PATHOPHYSIOLOGY
• Male fertility is the culminating point of intricate endocrine and physiologic events regulating the behavior and function of the reproductive system.
• Testes are in scrotal position at birth. However, they may not be visible or palpable in camels until 1 year of age.
• Rise in testosterone determines onset of sexual behavior and maturation of the reproductive system (detachment of the penis from the prepuce).
• Spermatogenesis is initiated after puberty (15–18 months SAC, 2–4 years in camels).
• Camels are seasonal breeder but SAC can breed all year around. However, semen quality in SAC is lower in hot summer months. Rutting season in camels is signaled by increased poll gland secretions, marking behavior, and exteriorization of the soft palate (dulla).
• Camelids mate with the female sitting in a sternal position.
• Mating lasts 5–20 minutes in camels and 5–60 minutes in SAC.
• Erection is achieved by extension of the sigmoid flexure which is cranial to the scrotum. The penis penetrates through the cervix and semen is deposited deep into the uterine horns.
• Ejaculation occurs throughout the mating period in a dribbling manner. The ejaculate is very viscous and composed of spermatozoa and secretion from the bulbourethral glands and prostate (camelids do not possess seminal vesicles).
• Seminal plasma contains ß-nerve growth factor which, combined with uterine

inflammation caused by mating, induces ovulation in the female.

GENETICS
Some defects may have genetic origin (e.g., testicular hypoplasia, cryptorchidism, cystic rete testis).

HISTORICAL FINDINGS
• Selection of male for breeding
• Neonatal examination of a male
• Infertility or abnormal behavior

SIGNALMENT
• Differences exist among the four domesticated species of camelids: dromedaries (*C. dromedaries*), Bactrian (*C. bactrianus*), alpaca (*Vicugna pacos*), and llama (*Lama glama*).
• BSE should be performed on animals that have reached the appropriate age for breeding (3 year for alpacas and llamas, 4–5 years for camels).
• Age, origin, breeding records, and previous health problems should be recorded.
• Reasons for examination should be clearly stated.
  ○ Define exactly the problem(s) to be addressed: existence of visible lesions, suspicion of infertility due to many unsuccessful breedings, or a change in the reproductive behavior (reduced libido).
  ○ An approximate date of the onset of the problem should be obtained as well as conditions: did the problem appear suddenly or was it a slow, progressive process?

PHYSICAL EXAMINATION FINDINGS
• Reproductive performance can be affected by diseases of other systems. Prolonged febrile conditions or debilitating diseases affect spermatogenesis.
• Clinical signs depend on the reason for examination.
• A general physical examination should be performed including general appearance and BCS. Attention should be given to contagious diseases and presence of congenital or potentially heritable conditions.
• Prepuce and penis
  ○ Prepuce abnormalities such as pendulous, edema, laceration, and prolapse should be noted. Sedation may be required for further evaluation.
  ○ Penile attachment to the prepuce is normal in young, prepuberal animals but can signal the presence of adhesions in the mature male. In SAC, the penis should be completely free at 3 years of age.
• Scrotum and testes
  ○ The scrotal region is examined from a distance to evaluate testicular descent and integrity of the skin in the area. Lacerations due to bites are common.
  ○ Both testes should be present and visible within the scrotum in the perineal region. One of the testicles is usually situated slightly more ventral than the other but

both should be nearly equal in size (difference less than 15%).
  ○ In older males, the scrotum may sometimes be pendulous.
  ○ Palpation of the scrotum and its contents is necessary to appreciate the regularity of the contour of the testes as well as their consistency.
  ○ The surface of the testes should be smooth and regular. The testes are normally resilient. They become hard and fibrotic or very soft in the case of degenerative changes.
  ○ The scrotal sac should be free from fluid.
  ○ The tail of the epididymis is palpable as a small hard nodule.
  ○ Testicular length and width should be determined using precision calipers. In the llama, length should be least 1.1 cm in a yearling and 3.2 cm by 2–3 years of age. In alpacas the testes long axis should be at least 3.5 cm in order to achieve good fertility in a herd. The length and width of the testicle in adult males should be 5–7 cm and 3–4 cm respectively in llamas and 4–5 cm and 2.5–3 cm respectively in alpacas. In camels, the adult testis during the rutting season should be at least 4 cm in width and 7 cm in length.
• Examination of the accessory sex glands is not performed as a routine.
• Evaluation of mating behavior
  ○ Mating ability of the male is observed in the presence of a receptive female.
  ○ The succession of normal behavioral patterns as well as the times needed for each step (chasing, flehmen response, forcing down, mating, intromission, and duration of copulation) are recorded.
  ○ Behavioral problems at mating can be due to shyness, inexperience, or lack of libido.

CAUSES AND RISK FACTORS
• Infertility in male camelids is primarily due to inadequate sperm production or sperm quality (impotentia generandi) and inability to physically complete mating (impotentia coeundi).
• Impotentia generandi is primarily due testicular hypoplasia, degeneration, fibrosis, or neoplasia. Testicular degeneration occurs following severe loss of body condition, persistent high fever, or direct trauma to the testis.
• Impotentia coeundi is primarily due to penile adhesions, musculoskeletal disorders, or debilitating diseases.

 DIAGNOSIS

Diagnosis of causes of infertility requires complete physical examination and systematic evaluation of all the reproductive organs and semen.

DIFFERENTIAL DIAGNOSIS

• Scrotal enlargements may be due to edema, hydrocele, orchitis, testicular hemorrhage or neoplasia. Differential diagnosis requires imaging and further testing.
• Inability to exteriorize the penis may be due to adhesions.

CBC/BIOCHEMSTRY/URINALYSIS

Baseline CBC, biochemistry, and urinalysis are highly recommended in valuable males and for prepurchase examinations.

OTHER LABORATORY TESTS

• Fecal analysis for parasites.
• Testing for contagious diseases: Tuberculosis, brucellosis, BVD, trypanosomiasis where endemic.
• Endocrine evaluation
  ○ Information on endocrinologic evaluation of the infertile male camelid is scarce.
  ○ Presence of testicular tissue in bilaterally cryptorchid male or castrated males suspected to be cryptorchid is ascertained if there is at least a twofold increase in serum testosterone level within 8–24 hours after IV administration of hCG (3000 IU for alpacas, 5000 IU for llamas, 10,000 IU for camels).

IMAGING

• Ultrasonography of the testis is highly recommended to differentiate among causes of testicular enlargement and to evaluate the testicular parenchyma. The parenchyma should be homogeneous and the rete testis hyperechoic. Cystic rete testis is common in alpacas.
• Transrectal ultrasonography may be indicated in some cases in order to evaluate the bulbourethral glands, pelvic urethra and penis, and prostate.

OTHER DIAGNOSTIC PROCEDURES

Semen Collection

• Semen collection is challenging due to the nature of copulatory behavior and the slow (dribbling) process of ejaculation.
• Use of an AV is possible but requires training and the use of a specially designed dummy mount fitted with a collection apparatus. Modified ruminant AVs work well if they are adapted to camelid by simulating the presence of cervical rings.
• Electroejaculation, using ram probes in SAC and bovine probes in camels, is possible under general anesthesia.
• Response to the electrical stimulus varies greatly from one individual to another.
• The ejaculate obtained by electroejaculation is often of poor quality and contaminated with urine and cellular debris.
• Postcoital vaginal aspiration is commonly used in general practice in SAC. The male is mated to a receptive female. Upon completion of the mating an infusion pipette is introduced vaginally and the seminal fluid is aspirated using a 12 mL syringe.

Semen Evaluation

• The major problem in interpreting semen analysis in the camelid is the lack of standard methods for collection and for examination.
• Ejaculate volume varies greatly depending on the method of collection used, duration of copulation, and male variation.
• Ejaculate volume is in the range 0.4–12.5 mL. Postcoital aspiration yields volumes in the range 0.25–0.5mL in SAC.
• Ejaculates are gray to creamy white depending on sperm concentration. Ejaculates collected by vaginal aspiration may be pink or red because of contamination with blood from the cervix.
• Ejaculate may be heterogeneous with some translucent material mixed with cloudy areas. This is due to its viscous nature.
• Camelid semen is viscous and requires time to liquefy. The degree of viscosity depends on the individual male and on the proportion of seminal plasma, which tends to decrease with number of ejaculates.
• The time required for liquefaction varies from one male to another and from one ejaculate to another. Viscosity is attributed to the presence of secretions of the bulbourethral glands.
• Liquefaction of camelid semen can be obtained by addition of collagenase to the ejaculate.
• Concentration of semen is best estimated after liquefaction using a hemocytometer.
• Sperm concentration is highly variable (82,000–250,000/mm^3) and is affected by age, method of collection, and ejaculate rank.
• The pH of semen varies between 7.5 and 8.1. Semen pH is affected by method of collection and rank of ejaculate.
• Motility of semen is appreciated on nondiluted samples (mass activity) and on diluted samples (individual sperm motility). Mass activity is generally poor in camelid semen unless the ejaculate is constituted exclusively by the sperm-rich fraction. In fresh nondiluted samples, only oscillatory movements are observed. Initial motility is very low (5%) and increases as the ejaculate liquefies. Progressive motility can only be estimated after liquefaction and dilution with a suitable extender. Normal males should have at least 50% oscillatory or progressive motility.
• Morphology of the spermatozoa can be evaluated on smears stained with eosin–nigrosin stain or DiffQuick® (Giemsa) stains.
• A total of at least 200 sperm cells from different fields should be evaluated from each sample. Morphological evaluation is done under phase contrast microscopy (1000×) as for other species. The morphologic abnormalities should be reported according to type and location.
• Effect of various types of abnormalities on fertility has not yet been determined. Total abnormalities should not exceed 50%.

• The most common abnormalities are proximal and distal droplets, knobbed or swollen acrosome, mid-piece reflex, and coiled tails.

Testicular Biopsy

• Testicular biopsy should be considered in subfertile males and in cases of testicular asymmetry or abnormal testicular ultrasonography that is not consistent with hematoma or orchitis. This technique is useful for diagnosis of spermatogenic arrest, oligospermatogenesis, hypogonadism, inflammation, and neoplasm.
• Several techniques of testicular biopsy have been described.
  ○ *Wedge biopsy:* An incisional or open biopsy requires general anesthesia. After surgical preparation of the scrotum, an incision (0.5 cm) is made over the skin, parietal vaginal tunic and the exposed tunica albuginea avoiding vascular areas. Testicular tissue allowed to protrude from the rent in the tunica albuginea is ablated using a scalpel blade. The tunica albuginea, parietal vaginal tunic, and the scrotal skin are closed with absorbable suture.
  ○ *Tru-Cut:* Use under sedation or anesthesia. After surgical preparation of the testicles, the scrotum is incised using a sterile #10 surgical blade (alpacas) or #11 scalpel (llamas). The trucut (14 gauge self-firing) biopsy needle is inserted in the testicle through the tunica albuginea. The scrotum is closed with two skin sutures using 2-0 Vetafil®. Results obtained with this technique are more reliable but hemorrhage at the biopsy site is more frequent.
  ○ *"Core" biopsy:* A needle "core" biopsy can be performed using a 1½ inch 16 gauge needle after heavy sedation of the animal. After surgical preparation of the scrotal skin, the needle is introduced into the testicular parenchyma and redirected by a gentle push-pull movement into two different sites. The needle is retracted from the tissue while a finder is placed over the hub to maintain the core sampled. A direct smear is prepared from the sample obtained.
  ○ *Fine-needle aspirate:* Fine-needle aspirate cytology is a commonly used technique for the evaluation of azoospermia and testicular neoplasm in humans. It is rapid, simple, and inexpensive. Testicular tissue is aspirated with a 20-gauge needle and 12 mL syringe. A puncture is made and aspirates are taken in three to four directions making sure not to include the epididymis. Cytologic smears stained with DiffQuick® are interpreted based on the different types of spermatogenic cells.
• Interpretation
  ○ Interpretation should be done by an individual familiar with the technique and histology of camelid testis.
  ○ Fine-needles aspirates are difficult to interpret. The relative frequency of cell

B

types provides a differential diagnosis between hypospermatogenesis, spermatogenic arrest, and normal spermatogenesis. A fine-needle aspirate from azoospermic animals consists of Sertoli cells alone, a few mature spermatozoa, and scant cell material or spermatid but no spermatozoa.
○ Tru-Cut or self-firing biopsy instruments are safe and provide a good amount of tissue for examination of seminiferous tubule spermatogenic activity. Presence of normal spermatogenic activity in cases of azoospermia may suggest the presence of segmental aplasia or other forms of obstructive azoospermia. Atypical spermatogenic cells are usually associated with testicular neoplasm (seminoma). No spermatogenic cells are obtained from atrophic testicles.
• Complications
○ Hematoma or hemorrhage.
○ Adhesions and inflammation.
○ Autoimmune reactions (development of antisperm antibodies).
○ Degeneration of germinal epithelium and tubules.
○ Transient decrease in sperm output that lasts for several months.
○ Wedge biopsy is the most unsafe of all methods.
○ Complication risk increases if the technique is not performed correctly and quickly.

PATHOLOGIC FINDINGS
• Penile/preputial disorders
○ Prolapse prepuce, penile-preputial adhesions
○ Phimosis
○ Persistent frenulum
○ Abscesses
• Testis
○ Testicular hypoplasia or degeneration
○ Segmental aplasia of the epididymis
○ Epididmal cysts or rete testis cysts
○ Orchitis/epididymitis
○ Testicular degeneration/fibrosis and calcification of the testicular parenchyma
○ Testicular trauma or neoplasia
○ Cryptorchidism

TREATMENT
THERAPEUTIC APPROACH
Treatment depends on the complaint and diagnosis. It is important to note that restauration of normal testicular function is very difficult.

SURGICAL CONSIDERATIONS AND TECHNIQUES
• Surgical correction of preputial prolapse.
• Hemicastration in cases of acquired testicular pathologies (orchitis, hemorrhage, neoplasia).
• Males with congenital defects should be castrated.
• Camels with impacted dulla should undergo palatectomy.

MEDICATION
DRUGS OF CHOICE
• GnRH (camels 100 μg, IM; SAC 50 μg, IM) prior to breeding to increase libido
• Other depending on underlying condition

CONTRAINDICATIONS
• Appropriate milk and meat withdrawal times must be followed.
• Testosterone should not be used to increase libido.

PRECAUTIONS
N/A

POSSIBLE INTERACTIONS
N/A

FOLLOW-UP
EXPECTED COURSE AND PROGNOSIS
• Males with congenital defects or abnormal development of the reproductive organs should be eliminated (castrated or culled) from reproduction.
• Fertility prognosis is good after hemicastration in unilateral acquired conditions of the testis.
• Poor fertility prognosis in cases of testicular degeneration or severe musculoskeletal impairment.

POSSIBLE COMPLICATIONS
Urinary complications (urethral or bladder rupture) in cases of preputial trauma/adhesion.

CLIENT EDUCATION
• Introduction of breeding males constitutes one of the major biosecurity breaches for the herd.
• BSE should be performed on all males prior to breeding.
• BSE should be performed annually.
• Detailed breeding records should be kept including behavior and pregnancy results of bred females.

• Handling techniques should be implemented to ensure safety for personnel and females.

PATIENT CARE
• Dependent on condition.
• Breeding males, particularly camels, can be dangerous during the rutting season. Exercise should be provided. Male should be in separate enclosure to avoid fighting and accidental injuries.
• Weight loss is common during the breeding season. Males should be supplemented accordingly nda special attention should be given to trace mineral supplementation.
• Avoid obesity and emaciation.

PREVENTION
• Prevention of acquired disorders of the reproductive tract relies on good management practices and biosecurity measures.
• Breeding males should be in top health at all times. Vaccination and deworming program should be designed appropriately.
• Routine wellness checks should be performed including dental and foot care.

MISCELLANEOUS
ASSOCIATED CONDITIONS
Infertility, behavioral problems

AGE-RELATED FACTORS
Breeding schedule should take into consideration age and testicular size.

ZOONOTIC POTENTIAL
Brucellosis is a major concern when collecting semen.

PREGNANCY
Early pregnancy diagnosis allows monitoring of male fertility.

BIOSECURITY
• Test all males for contagious diseases and diseases that can spread by vectors.
• Provide a quarantine area for outside female breeding.
• Quarantine males that have traveled to shows.

PRODUCTION MANAGEMENT
• Breeding male management requires special attention in order to avoid loss of fertility.
• Males should be easy to handle and undergo BSE every year.
• Males should be in top health condition before the breeding season.

SYNONYMS
N/A

ABBREVIATIONS
- BSE = breeding soundness examination
- HCG = human chorionic gonadotropin
- IU = international units
- IV = intravenous
- SAC = South American camelids

SEE ALSO
- Artificial Insemination: Camelid (see www.fiveminutevet.com/ruminant)
- Body Condition Scoring: Alpacas and Llamas (see www.fiveminutevet.com/ruminant)
- Body Condition Scoring: Camels (see www.fiveminutevet.com/ruminant)
- Camel Diseases
- Camel Management and Health Programs
- Camelid: Reproduction
- Congenital Defects: Camelid
- Orchitis and Epididymitis
- Parasite Control Programs: Camelid
- Penile Disorders
- Reproductive Prolapse
- Testicular Disorders: Camelid
- Vaccination Programs: Camelid

Suggested Reading
Ali A, Derar D, Al Sobyil FA, et al. Phymosis in male dromedary camels: clinical findings and changes in the hemogram, nitric oxide metabolites, and testosterone concentration. Theriogenology 2016, 85: 1576–81.
Tibary A, Pearson LK, Anouassi A. Applied andrology in camelids. In Chenoweth P, Lorton S eds, Animal Andrology: Theories and Applications. Wallingford, UK: CABI, 2014, pp. 418–49.
Waheed MM, Ghoneim IM, Hassieb MM, Alsumait AA. Evaluation of the breeding soundness of male camels (*Camelus dromedaries*) via clinical examination, semen analysis, ultrasonography and testicular biopsy: A summary of 80 clinical cases. Reprod Domest Anim 2014, 49: 790–6.

Author Ahmed Tibary
Consulting Editor Ahmed Tibary

B

B

BREEDING SOUNDNESS EXAMINATION: CERVIDAE

 BASICS

OVERVIEW
• BSE in cervids is used to select breeding animals or to investigate herd or individual fertility problems.
• Chemical (sedation, anesthesia) and/or physical (squeeze chute) immobilization is necessary. This presents several inherent risks that must be considered.
• A complete BSE includes the following:
  ◦ Physical examination for anatomic and structural soundness (eyes, mouth, feet, legs, external genitalia, body condition, and overall wellness)
  ◦ In the male, a reproductive evaluation includes
    ▪ Testicle palpation and scrotal circumference (SC) measurement
    ▪ Exteriorization and evaluation of the penis
    ▪ Collection of a semen sample for sperm motility and morphology assessment
  ◦ In the female, transrectal ultrasonography (US) or laparoscopic evaluation of the uterus and ovaries may be necessary.

INCIDENCE/PREVALENCE
N/A

GEOGRAPHIC DISTRIBUTION
Worldwide

SYSTEMS AFFECTED
Reproductive

PATHOPHYSIOLOGY
Male Reproductive Function and Infertility
• Seasonality is pronounced in most species. BSE should be performed early in the breeding season. Atrophy of the testes (i.e., SC can decrease by up to 50%) with a decline in sperm quality occurs outside of the breeding season.
• SC varies with species and age. It is strongly correlated with sperm production and quality.
• Endocrine regulation of seasonality is similar to sheep and goats with increasing luteinizing hormone (LH) and testosterone (T) production as day length decreases.
• Libido is almost completely absent outside the breeding season (exception: *Axis*, which manifest a strong sex drive and produce sufficient sperm to impregnate females regardless of season).
• Male infertility may be due to congenital (hypoplasia), inflammatory (orchitis, epididymitis), degenerative (testicular degeneration or atrophy) or neoplastic processes.

Female Reproductive Function and Infertility
• Most species are seasonally polyestrous. Females breed in the autumn and give birth in the summer. Exceptions include tropical species (i.e., *Axis*), which are reproductively active year-round, and *Capreolus*, which are monovulatory.
• Hormonal control of the estrous cycle and ovulation is similar to that of small ruminants.
• Estrous cycle length varies by species, but tends to average around 18–24 days.
• Monotocous species include those that are larger-bodied, longer-living, and later-maturing, such as those within the genera *Cervus* (red deer, wapiti), *Dama* (fallow deer), *Axis* (chital deer), and *Rangifer* (reindeer, caribou).
• Polytocous species include those that are smaller-bodied, shorter-lived, and early-maturing, such as those within the genera *Odocoileus* (white-tailed deer, black-tailed deer, mule deer), *Alces* (moose), and *Capreolus* (roe deer).
• Female infertility may be due to severely pathologic processes. Freemartinism, gonadal hypoplasia, nabothian cysts in the cervix, cystic ovarian disease, pyometra, and metritis have all been reported as causes of infertility in various cervid species and may be detected with a thorough physical examination.

HISTORICAL FINDINGS
• Lack of sexual activity during the breeding season
• Excessive return to estrus
• Poor pregnancy rate
• Poor birthing rate

SIGNALMENT
• The family Cervidae represents close to 40 species and 200 subspecies.
• Commonly studied species include those within the genera *Cervus* (red deer, wapiti), *Dama* (fallow deer), *Axis* (chital deer), *Rangifer* (reindeer, caribou), *Odocoileus* (white-tailed deer, black-tailed deer, mule deer), *Alces* (moose), *Capreolus* (roe deer), *Ozotoceros* (Pampas deer), *Elaphurus* (Père David's deer), *Rucervus* (swamp deer, Barasingha).

PHYSICAL EXAMINATION FINDINGS
Male Reproductive Anatomy and Examination
• Scrotum is extra-abdominal, bifurcated, symmetrical, and similar in tone, shape, location, and function to that of domestic ruminants. An exception is the Pampas deer, whose scrotum is located in the inguinal region.
• Each testicle should be palpated to check for orchitis, epididymitis, masses, hypoplasia, or degeneration.
• In general, SC >18 cm in an adult male during the breeding season is indicative of normal sized testicles in white-tailed deer and mule deer.
• The penis is fibroelastic and held within the prepuce by the retractor penis muscle. The sigmoid flexure, if present, can readily be palpated through the skin posterior to the scrotum. The sigmoid flexure is not present in some species, such as *Cervus* and *Ozotoceros*. The penis should be exteriorized to inspect for adhesions, ulcerations, masses, or other pathologies that may prevent normal intromission.
• In species that display "thrash urination" during rut (e.g., *Cervus, Elaphurus*), the position of the urethral orifice is more dorsal on the glans to allow for upward expulsion of urine and sperm onto the ventral abdomen, neck, and throat. The glans varies, depending on species, from blunt and rounded to narrow and tapered.
• Though the anus and rectum are too small to allow for thorough manual palpation of the internalized reproductive organs, prominent abnormalities of the prostate and seminal vesicles may be palpable with a gloved, lubricated finger. If indicated, transrectal US may also aid in evaluation of the accessory sex glands.

Female Reproductive Anatomy and Examination
• Reproductive anatomy and function is similar to that of domestic ruminants. Similar protocols in evaluating reproductive fitness apply.
• Most females have 4 teats. There are reports of congenital absence of active teats, which should be suspected if sudden neonatal death occurs in a maiden female. Teats should also be inspected for signs of mastitis.
• A vaginal speculum can be used on medium and large cervid females to evaluate the vestibule, vagina, and caudal cervix for pathologies.
• The anus and rectum are too small to allow manual palpation of the internal reproductive organs except in the larger cervids; however, transrectal US may be employed for evaluation of the uterus and ovaries.

GENETICS
There are species differences.

CAUSES AND RISK FACTORS
N/A

 DIAGNOSIS

DIFFERENTIAL DIAGNOSES
Differential diagnosis of poor reproductive performance requires a thorough evaluation of breeding record and examination of the males and females.

CBC/BIOCHEMISTRY/URINALYSIS
May be indicated in specific cases.

OTHER LABORATORY TESTS
Serology, bacteriology, and biopsy (endometrial and testicular) may be indicated in specific cases.

B

IMAGING
• Trasrectal US is indicated for the evaluation of ovarian function and uterine health.
• In the male, testicular US and transrectal evaluation of the accessory sex gland may be helpful.

OTHER DIAGNOSTIC PROCEDURES
Semen Collection and Evaluation
• Methods of collection include EE, AV, and manual stimulation. Higher quality samples are obtained using AV; however, due to the need for chemical or physical immobilization, EE is most common.
• Fractionation of the ejaculate is difficult but should be attempted to minimize the amount of seminal plasma and avoid urine contamination.
• Volume varies with relative size of species (e.g., *Odocoileus* 0.5–2 mL; *Rucervus* 1–2 mL; *Rangifer* 3–5 mL, *Elaphurus* 6–10 mL).
• Concentration ranges from 1.5 billion to 4 billion spermatozoa per mL (e.g., *Elaphurus, Rucervus, Odocoileus*).
• Overall sperm motility should be 30–50% at minimum.
• Morphologic defect classifications are similar to those of domestic ruminants. There should be a minimum of 80% normal sperm to be classified as reproductively sound.

PATHOLOGIC FINDINGS
N/A

TREATMENT
THERAPEUTIC APPROACH
N/A
SURGICAL CONSIDERATIONS AND TECHNIQUES
N/A

MEDICATIONS
DRUGS OF CHOICE
N/A
CONTRAINDICATIONS
N/A

PRECAUTIONS
N/A

POSSIBLE INTERACTIONS
N/A

FOLLOW-UP
EXPECTED COURSE AND PROGNOSIS
N/A
POSSIBLE COMPLICATIONS
N/A
CLIENT EDUCATION
N/A
PATIENT CARE
N/A
PREVENTION

MISCELLANEOUS
ASSOCIATED CONDITIONS
Infertility, epididymitis, orchitis, vesiculitis, testicular degeneration, ulcerative posthitis (pizzle rot), vaginitis, metritis
AGE-RELATED FACTORS
N/A
ZOONOTIC POTENTIAL
Many reproductive diseases are zoonotic. Care should be maintained when collecting and processing semen.
PREGNANCY
Herd fertility should be closely monitored using an early and accurate method of pregnancy diagnosis
BIOSECURITY
CWD, TB, and brucellosis
PRODUCTION MANAGEMENT
• Decreased fertility or serving capacity of the buck can have drastic economic implications in affected herds.
• Tropical species have longer breeding seasons than cold-adapted species and may reproduce year round (e.g., *Axis*).
• In temperate environments, allowing tropical species to birth during the winter months may result in high perinatal mortality. Mating management should be employed to ensure birthing in the spring or summer, when there are optimal pasture conditions.

SYNONYMS
N/A

ABBREVIATIONS
• AV = artificial vagina
• BSE = breeding soundness examination
• CWD = chronic wasting disease
• EE = electroejaculation
• LH = luteinizing hormone
• SC = scrotal circumference
• T = testosterone
• TB = tuberculosis
• US = ultrasound

SEE ALSO
• Biosecurity: Cervidae (see www.fiveminutevet.com/ruminant)
• Cervidae: Reproduction

Suggested Reading
Geist V. Deer of the World: Their Evolution, Behavior, and Ecology, 1st ed. Mechanicsburg: Stackpole Books, 1998.
Jacobson H. Reproduction management of white-tailed deer. In: Youngquist RS, Threlfall WR eds, Current Therapy in Large Animal Theriogenology. Elsevier Health Sciences, 2006, pp. 965–9.
Portillo T, Wemmer C. Estrous cycle, estrus, and gestation in Pere David's deer. Proc 63rd Ann Conf Am Soc Mammal, 1983.
Sathe S, Shipley CF. Applied andrology in sheep, goats and selected cervids. In: Chenoweth PJ, Lorton S eds, Animal Andrology: Theories and Applications. Wallingford: CABI, 2014, pp. 226–53.
Wemmer C, Grodinsky G. Reproduction in captive female brow-antlered deer (*Cervus eldi thamin*). J Mammal 1988, 69: 389–92.
Wemmer C, Halverson T, Rodden M, Portillo T. The reproductive biology of female Pere David's deer (*Elaphurus davidianus*). Zoo Biol 1989, 8: 49–55.

Authors Jamie L. Stewart and Clifford F. Shipley
Consulting Editor Ahmed Tibary
Acknowledgment The author and book editors acknowledge the prior contribution of Timothy P. Portillo.

BREEDING SOUNDNESS EXAMINATION: SMALL RUMINANT

BASICS

OVERVIEW
• Breeding soundness examination (BSE) is a screening method to identify satisfactory potential breeding males.
• It is not a measure of fertility.
• The BSE is a quick, inexpensive screening test which can help identify unsuitable breeding males for a herd or flock.
• Animals should be presented at least 2 months prior to the intended breeding period such that identification of any abnormalities in the spermiogram may be addressed prior to breeding. Animals which are found unsatisfactory and for which treatment is not available or elected can be replaced.
• BSE in sheep includes four classifications: excellent, satisfactory, questionable, and unsatisfactory. There are no standards for goats; however, the sheep requirements are often used (minimum scrotal circumference, sperm motility and morphology, and physical examination findings).

INCIDENCE/PREVALENCE
10–20% of males are eliminated from breeding.

GEOGRAPHIC DISTRIBUTION
Worldwide.

SYSTEMS AFFECTED
• Reproductive
• Multisystemic

PATHOPHYSIOLOGY
• Ram/buck fertility depends on normal spermatogenesis, sperm production ability, and delivery.
• Sperm production is positively correlated to testicular volume.
• Sperm production is compromised if the male is in poor health or due to local pathologic processes such as degenerative or inflammatory changes.
• Semen delivery to the female can be hindered by poor health, poor vision, lameness, or penile and preputial abnormalities.

HISTORICAL FINDINGS
• History of the male should include purchase/travel history, general health history, vaccination and deworming history, and details of the nutritional program.
• Reproductive history should include previous BSE findings, results of previous breeding seasons (pregnancy rates), and the breeding management of the farm (multiple or single male herds/flocks).

SIGNALMENT
• Rams and bucks of breeding age.
• The BSE should be performed on all males prior to joining, or on any male for which a herd reproductive problem is identified (i.e.,

poor pregnancy rates or high rate of return to estrus).
• Prospective sires should be examined prior to or at weaning for major abnormalities (cryptorchidism, split scrotum, etc.). The first BSE should be performed at 6–8 months of age, prior to introduction to females.

PHYSICAL EXAMINATION FINDINGS
Physical Examination
The physical examination should include specific attention to the following:
• Teeth – There is an association between dental health and BCS in breeding rams. Animals with poor dentition may not be able to maintain weight during the breeding season.
• BCS – Males should be slightly overconditioned heading into the breeding season (BCS 3.5–4). Obese animals may have reduced fertility due to fat deposits causing increased temperature of the scrotum. Thin animals may not be able to maintain condition to serve females.
• Eyes – Normal eyesight is required of breeding males.
• Conformation –It is important that correct traits are passed to future generations. Any conformational defects may hinder the male's ability to serve females.
• Feet – males should be checked for common causes of lameness.
• Males should also be examined for any evidence of contagious diseases (mange, contagious lymphadenitis).

Reproductive Examination
The reproductive examination should include the following:
• Palpation of the scrotal contents. Males with enlarged, thickened tails of the epididymis should be suspected of epididymitis, sperm granuloma, or other pathology.
• Palpation of the testes. Outside of the breeding season, testes may palpate smaller or softer than normal. There can be up to 30% seasonal variation in testicular volume. In the breeding season, the testes should be turgid and resilient on palpation.
• Measurement of the scrotal circumference. Minimum circumference is required for satisfactory classification.
• Examination of the prepuce. Ulcerative balanoposthitis (pizzle rot) is a common finding, particularly in males on a high concentrate, high protein diet.
• Examination of the penis. The penis may be exteriorized prior to semen collection with the ram seated, or may be examined during electroejaculation for any pathologies.

Semen Collection and Evaluation
• Semen is collected by electroejaculation unless the male is trained to serve an artificial vagina.
• The volume, color, and consistency are noted. The color and consistency can give a rough idea of the concentration of

spermatozoa per mL (thick and creamy > 1 billion, milky 0.5–1 billion, watery <0.5 billion).
• Motility can be assessed by either mass motility (on a scale from 0–5) or by individual motility (as a percentage).
• Morphology is assessed on eosin-nigrosin stained smears under oil (1000x magnification) or by examination of formalin-fixed samples under phase contrast (wet-mount).
• Cytology of the ejaculate is assessed using a differential stain or Wright-Giemsa to identify any leukocytes. Presence of PMNs should alert the possibility of infection with *B. ovis* in sheep.

GENETICS
In goats, the polled characteristic is associated with abnormalities of the reproductive tract.

CAUSES AND RISK FACTORS
• There are multiple causes of infertility or poor reproductive performance in the male. BSE is not intended to make a diagnosis but to screen males and eliminate those that are not suitable for breeding.
• Risk factors for infertility include general poor health, specific reproductive infectious diseases, and poor nutrition.

DIAGNOSIS

• There are four classifications for rams, based on scrotal size, sperm motility, and morphology. Any rams positive for *B. ovis* are automatically unsatisfactory. Bucks are considered satisfactory with a minimum of 30% motility and 70% normal morphology, with scrotal size dependent on breed.
• The classifications are as follows:
  ○ Excellent
    ▪ Scrotal circumference: >35 cm for adults; >33 cm for rams < 1 year of age
    ▪ Sperm motility: >50%
    ▪ Sperm morphology: >90% normal
  ○ Satisfactory
    ▪ Scrotal circumference: >33 cm for adults; >30 cm for rams < 1 year of age
    ▪ Sperm motility: >30%
    ▪ Sperm morphology: >70% normal
  ○ Questionable
    ▪ Scrotal circumference: <33 cm for adults; <30 cm for rams < 1 year of age
    ▪ Sperm motility: <30%
    ▪ Sperm morphology: <70% normal
  ○ Unsatisfactory
    ▪ Scrotal circumference: <33 cm for adults; <30 cm for rams < 1 year of age
    ▪ Sperm motility: <30%
    ▪ Sperm morphology: <50% normal

DIFFERENTIAL DIAGNOSIS
N/A

CBC/BIOCHEMISTRY/URINALYSIS
N/A

(CONTINUED) BREEDING SOUNDNESS EXAMINATION: SMALL RUMINANT

OTHER LABORATORY TESTS
Serologic testing for *Brucella ovis* should be included as part of the ram BSE.

IMAGING
• Testicular ultrasonography may be performed if abnormalities of the scrotum are identified. This examination is outside of the BSE.

DIAGNOSTIC PROCEDURES
N/A

PATHOLOGIC FIDINGS
• In a study of more than 11,000 rams, 20.7% were classified as excellent, 50.4% as satisfactory, 10.8% as questionable, and 18.1% as unsatisfactory.
• The most common reasons for unsatisfactory classification were poor semen quality (43.8%), inflammatory causes (20%), physical abnormalities (15.5%), emaciation (14.2%), and ulcerative posthitis (4.6%).

TREATMENT

THERATPEUTIC APPROACH
N/A

SURGICAL CONSIDERATIONS AND TECHNIQUES
N/A

MEDICATIONS

DRUGS OF CHOICE
N/A

CONTRAINDICATIONS
N/A

PRECAUTIONS
N/A

POSSIBLE INTERACTIONS
N/A

FOLLOW-UP

EXPECTED COURSE AND PROGNOSIS
• Males classified as questionable should be reexamined within 30–60 days.

• Prognosis for fertility is favorable if the diagnosed condition is treatable.

POSSIBLE COMPLICATIONS
N/A

CLIENT EDUCATION
• Clients should present the male for BSE annually prior to the joining period, and if any abnormalities are noted (decreased pregnancy rates in the flock, abnormalities of the scrotum or prepuce, etc.).
• All new rams to a flock should be tested for *B. ovis*.

PATIENT CARE
• Breeding activity should be monitored using marking harnesses.
• The diet should be monitored such that males do not lose too much body condition over the course of the joining period. The protein content should be reduced in males that have a history or diagnosis of ulcerative balanoposthitis (pizzle rot). Obesity should be avoided.

PREVENTION
N/A

MISCELLANEOUS

ASSOCIATED CONDITIONS
• Contagious epididymitis is due to *B. ovis*.
• Polled character is associated to segmental aplasia and spermastasis in goats.

AGE-RELATED FACTORS
• Testicular degeneration can occur in older males or which have sustained thermal injury (high fever or hyperthermia).
• In one large study, 36.7% of rams >6 years were unsatisfactory, which was significantly higher than all rams <6 years of age.

ZOONOTIC POTENTIAL
B. ovis is not zoonotic.

PREGNANCY
Early pregnancy diagnosis on joined females provides more accurate information on male fertility.

BIOSECURITY
All rams or bucks introduced into a flock/herd should be quarantined prior to introduction to the resident population. They should also be screened for infectious diseases, vaccinated, and treated with antiparasite medications.

PRODUCTION MANAGEMENT
• Producers should have all males examined at least 2 months prior to the intended breeding period in order to find replacements for any unsatisfactory animals, or to treat any that may subsequently become satisfactory (cases of ulcerative posthitis, inappropriate body condition, etc.).
• All females joined to the male should be examined for pregnancy. The male should be examined annually.
• All rams positive for *B. ovis* should be culled.

SYNONYMS
N/A

ABBREVIATIONS
• BSE = breeding soundness examination
• BCS = body condition score

SEE ALSO
• Body Condition Scoring: Goats (see www.fiveminutevet.com/ruminant)
• Body Condition Scoring: Sheep (see www.fiveminutevet.com/ruminant)
• Reproductive Ultrasonography: Small Ruminant (see www.fiveminutevet.com/ruminant)
• Testicular Disorders: Small Ruminant

Suggested Reading
Gouletsou PG, Fthenakis GC. Clinical evaluation of reproductive ability of rams. Small Rumin Res 2010, 92: 45–51.
Ridler AL, Smith SL, West DM. Ram and buck management. Anim Reprod Sci 2012, 130: 180–3.
Van Metre DC, Rao S, Kimberling, CV, Morley PS. Factors associated with failure in breeding soundness examination of Western USA rams. Prev Vet Med 2012, 105: 118–26.

Author Lisa Pearson
Consulting Editor Ahmed Tibary
Acknowledgment The author and book editors acknowledge the prior contribution of Larry D. Holler.

BRISKET DISEASE

BASICS

OVERVIEW
Brisket disease is a form of right-sided heart failure that affects susceptible cattle grazing at high elevations (>2,000 m). Synonyms are: bovine pulmonary hypertension, high mountain disease, high-elevation disease, and *cor pulmonale*. A similar disease affects captive exotic species maintained at high elevation, and includes maras (*Dolichotis patagonum*), cotton-top tamarins (*Saguinus oedipus oedipus*), capybaras (*Hydrochaeris hydrochaeris*), Bennet's wallaby (*Macropus rufogriseus*), nilgai antelope (*Boselaphus tragocamelus*), and scimitar-horned oryx (*Oryx dammah*).

INCIDENCE/PREVALENCE
• The disease is common and well-recognized at elevations >2,000 m.
• Prevalence tends to be herd-specific. It can be as high as 5%. It is higher when susceptible animals, including breeding stock, are introduced from low elevations. A low annual incidence (0.5%) is more common. Sporadic cases can continue to occur even when the bull battery is PAP (pulmonary arterial pressure)-tested annually and only bulls with low m-PAP scores are retained.
• Introduction of carrier bulls will increase the incidence of the disease.
• Large numbers of cases can be seen when non-acclimated cattle from predisposed pedigrees are moved from lowland to montane zones.

GEOGRAPHIC DISTRIBUTION
• Elevations >2,000 m. This cut-off is not absolute. Low rates of brisket disease are seen at or below elevations of 1,500 m.
• The disease occurs worldwide wherever domestic cattle are raised at high elevations. Most published accounts of brisket disease originate from affected areas of the United States (esp. Wyoming, Utah, New Mexico, and Colorado), and from Peru.
• Unexplained cases of brisket disease-like syndromes occur in feedlots in the American Midwest. At least some of these appear to represent animals that entered the feedlot in the early clinical stages of the disease, since they originated in high altitude herds.

SYSTEMS AFFECTED
• Cardiovascular
• Respiratory
• Digestive

PATHOPHYSIOLOGY
• Susceptible cattle at high elevations develop an inappropriate (high) pulmonary vasopressor response to alveolar hypoxia, leading to hypoxic arteriolar vasoconstriction. This is attributed in part to the relatively small size of the lungs relative to body weight in cattle. Increased vascular resistance results in pruning of portions of the pulmonary capillary bed, muscular hypertrophy of pulmonary arterioles, thickened tunica adventitia of small and medium caliber pulmonary arteries, and varying degrees of pulmonary thrombosis. The result is pulmonary hypertension. Increased vascular load leads to compensatory right ventricular hypertrophy. If this pulmonary hypertension is sustained, cattle develop right-sided heart failure.
• The disease has a distinct yet poorly defined inherited component. Inheritance is thought to involve a small number of dominant genes.
• Progression to clinical disease is accelerated by cold ambient temperatures, toxic plants such as *Astragalus* and *Oxytropis* spp. (locoweeds), and intercurrent pneumonia. A relationship exists between elevation (e.g. 2,000 m vs. 3,000 m) and likelihood of developing the condition.

HISTORICAL FINDINGS
Chronic poor-doing, heavy cattle at high altitude.

SIGNALMENT
Brisket disease is a syndrome of older calves and yearlings.

PHYSICAL EXAMINATION FINDINGS
• Cattle present with clinical signs typical of right-sided heart failure: enlarged jugular veins with or without jugular pulse; palpably large subcutaneous abdominal veins; hepatic enlargement that extends beyond the posterior costochondral margin (chronic passive congestion); lethargy and anorexia (terminally); weight loss; subcutaneous edema of the brisket area and submandibular tissue; tachycardia, often with cardiac murmur; weakness and collapse, especially when trailed; bulging eyes.
• Some degree of ascites is present. It may not be obvious clinically. Pleural or pericardial effusion is generally present.
• A common terminal event is diarrhea, associated with ascites, hepatomegaly, and mesenteric-mesocolonic edema.

GENETICS
• There is an appreciable genetic component. At the time of writing, no genetic test is available to identify carriers and to facilitate culling.
• All domestic cattle breeds are susceptible. It is sometimes stated that Angus cattle are particularly predisposed. This is probably related to the current predominance of the breed in the Rocky Mountain area of the United States.

CAUSES AND RISK FACTORS
• Disease is due to a combination of genetic predisposition, combined with residence at high elevation. The higher the elevation, the more rapid the onset. Contributing factors are cold temperatures, some toxic plants (esp. locoweeds), and (in feedlots) feeding for rapid weight gain.
• There is a strong suspicion that animals on high carbohydrate rations, including cattle at low elevations, are more prone to develop brisket disease.
• Cattle with naturally high pulmonary blood pressure. Cattle of any age with an mPAP of 49 mmHg at any elevation are at high risk.

DIAGNOSIS

DIFFERENTIAL DIAGNOSES
Other causes of heart failure in cattle <1 year old. Common rule-outs are interventricular septal defects, other major congenital cardiac defects, bacterial valvular endocarditis, heart failure due to chronic bacterial papillary myocarditis, and pericarditis (e.g., due to traumatic reticulopericarditis).

CBC/BIOCHEMSTRY/URINALYSIS
Hepatic enzyme concentrations are elevated. Terminally, myocardial necrosis develops, resulting in elevated myocardial enzyme activities.

OTHER LABORATORY TESTS
• PAP testing
• The sensitivity of PAP testing depends on the altitude at which it is performed, combined with the experience of the veterinarian who performs the test. The higher the altitude, the greater the sensitivity of the test. This creates a dilemma for vendors living at low elevations: they may not wish to risk moving valuable bulls to high elevations so that they can be tested, as brisket disease may develop. Some veterinarians in Wyoming, Colorado, Utah, and New Mexico are proficient at performing PAP tests on bull batteries, and this constitutes a sizable portion of their practice.
• There is a need to develop a validated genetic test for one or more dominant genes thought to predispose cattle to brisket disease.

IMAGING
N/A

OTHER DIAGNOSTIC PROCEDURES
Thorough physical examination with focus on cardiac auscultation.

PATHOLOGIC FINDINGS
• Grossly, HMD is characterized by myocardial hypertrophy affecting the free wall of the right ventricle and atrium, combined with dilation of the pulmonary trunk. The heart is abnormally globular. Serous atrophy of fat is generally present systemically in chronic cases. Fibrin tags on the epicardial surfaces are common. Associated lesions are hepatomegaly with chronic passive congestion ("nutmeg liver"), ascites, and edema of mesentery, mesocolon, and perirenal adipose tissue. The name "brisket disease"

B

notwithstanding, and although subcutaneous edema over sternum is found at necropsy, swelling of the brisket may not be clinically prominent in affected cattle. Many animals develop anteroventral pneumonia, most often due to *Pasteurella multocida* and other members of the bovine respiratory disease complex.

• Confirming the diagnosis at necropsy is straightforward. Dissect free the right and left ventricular myocardial free walls, along with interventricular septum (i.e., remove and discard atrial tissues and the great vessels). Separately weigh the right and left ventricular walls, and interventricular septum. The following ratio is found in healthy cattle: RVFW/(RVFW + LVFW + IVS) = 0.25 (i.e., the right ventricular free wall is no more than one-quarter the combined weight of ventricular muscles). By contrast, in brisket disease the ratio is >0.30, and in typically chronic terminal cases it is 0.40–0.50. Ventricular ratios, determined by weight, are more reliable than ventricular wall thickness.

• A definitive diagnosis can be made postmortem. If histologic confirmation is desired, the diagnostic laboratory should receive, at a minimum, samples of the following: lung (non-pneumonic); right and left ventricular free wall (separately identified); and liver. Pathologists who are inexperienced in the appearance of pulmonary arteries and arterioles in brisket disease should consult a standard veterinary textbook for the characteristic lesions. These can be missed, particularly when concurrent pneumonia is present in the submitted samples of lung. If in doubt, submit the entire pluck unfixed on ice packs for the laboratory pathologist to examine. Cardiocyte hypertrophy is diffuse in the right ventricular myocardium, so that measurements of their diameter—and comparison with those of left ventricular myocardium—may be needed to diagnose hypertrophy histologically.

TREATMENT

THERAPEUTIC APPROACH
• Some affected cattle early in the clinical course may be salvaged by moving them to lower elevations.
• Cattle with brisket disease should not be exercised or excited unnecessarily, or trailed long distances.
• Supportive treatment of affected animals may include diuretics, thoracocentesis, vitamin B complex (appetite stimulant), ± antimicrobial therapy.

SURGICAL CONSIDERATIONS AND TECHNIQUES
N/A

MEDICATIONS

DRUG(S) OF CHOICE
• Furosemide and digoxin
• Vitamin B complex

CONTRAINDICATIONS
Overdosing or chronic use of diuretics can cause electrolyte disturbances and dehydration.

PRECAUTIONS
N/A

POSSIBLE INTERACTIONS
N/A

ALTERNATIVE DRUGS
N/A

FOLLOW-UP

EXPECTED COURSE AND PROGNOSIS
• The prognosis for cattle with advanced heart failure is poor. Some can be salvaged by a combination of furosemide treatment and movement to low elevations.
• Some producers are proficient at recognizing affected cattle early in the clinical course. Such animals can be sold, on the principle of caveat emptor, thereby introducing the disease and its susceptibility trait(s) into other herds.

POSSIBLE COMPLICATIONS
N/A

CLIENT EDUCATION
Brisket disease is a herd problem. The best management tool at present is to use sires with low PAP scores (bulls with mPAP of <42 mmHg). Control is by testing introduced pedigrees for pulmonary arterial pressures.

PATIENT CARE
N/A

PREVENTION
• Exercise care when introducing pedigrees of unknown PAP status to high elevation operations.
• Trailing calves long distances (classically, from Forest Service land in late summer, to native range) is a common situation in which brisket disease is recognized. Producers performing necropsies themselves may diagnose the problem to their veterinarians as an outbreak of "peritonitis," due to fluid effusion in the abdomen.

MISCELLANEOUS

ASSOCIATED CONDITIONS
Pneumonia (of any cause) precipitates clinical onset of terminal brisket disease.

AGE-RELATED FACTORS
Disease is typically seen in cattle <1 year of age.

ZOONOTIC POTENTIAL
No risk

PREGNANCY
N/A

BIOSECURITY
N/A

PRODUCTION MANAGEMENT
• Obtain PAP measurements of all incoming bulls. Use only bulls that have a mPAP of <42 mmHg.
• If AI is used, solicit from vendors where the bulls were PAP-tested and use test results as part of sire selection.

SYNONYMS
• High-altitude disease
• *Cor pulmonale*
• Bovine pulmonary hypertension

ABBREVIATIONS
• AI = artificial insemination
• HMD = high mountain disease
• mPAP = mean pulmonary arterial pressure
• PAP = pulmonary arterial pressure

SEE ALSO
Cardiac Failure

Suggested Reading
Holt TN, Callan RJ. Pulmonary arterial pressure testing for high mountain disease in cattle. Vet Clin North Am Food Anim Pract 2007, 23: 575–96.
Juan-Sallés C, Martínez LS, Rosas-Rosas AG, et al. Pulmonary arterial disease associated with right-sided cardiac hypertrophy and congestive heart failure in zoo mammals housed at 2,100 m above sea level. J Zoo Wildl Med 2015, 46: 825–32.
Malherbe CR, Marquard J, Legg DE, Cammack KM, O'Toole D. Right ventricular hypertrophy with heart failure in Holstein heifers at elevation of 1,600 meters. J Vet Diagn Invest 2012, 24: 867–77.
Shirley KL, Beckman DW, Garrick DJ. Inheritance of pulmonary arterial pressure in Angus cattle and its correlation with growth. J Anim Sci 2008, 86: 815–19.
Stenmark KR, Fasules J, Hyde DM, et al. Severe pulmonary hypertension and arterial adventitial changes in newborn calves at 4,300 m. J Appl Physiol 1987, 62:821–30.

Author Donal O'Toole
Consulting Editor Kaitlyn A. Lutz

BRUCELLOSIS

B

BASICS

OVERVIEW
• Brucellosis refers to disease states induced by infection with one of several *Brucella* species.
• Economic losses in livestock are associated with reproductive failure in both males and females.
• In much of the world brucellosis remains an economic and public health concern.
• Zoonotic concerns have led to eradication or control programs in many developed countries.
• Efforts to prevent and/or control infection can impact regional and international trade.
• *Brucella* are Gram-negative bacteria and infect a wide range of mammalian hosts.
• Brucellosis is a cause of abortion in females and infertility in males.

INCIDENCE/PREVALENCE
• In much of the world, *Brucella* infection in domestic ruminant species is common.
• Targeted control programs have reduced the incidence of bovine brucellosis due to *B. abortus*.
• *B. abortus* is uncommon in North America, northern Europe, Australia, New Zealand, and Japan.
• Bison and elk in Yellowstone National Park remain infected with *B. abortus*.
• *B. abortus* control programs rely on widespread surveillance, slaughter, and herd-level eradication.
• Similar control and eradication programs have reduced *B. melitensis* in some developed countries.
• *Brucella ovis* infections occur in sheep-producing areas of the world.
• In North America *B. ovis* infection is most common in western range flocks.

GEOGRAPHIC DISTRIBUTION.
• Ruminant brucellosis has historically been seen worldwide.
• Control and eradication programs implemented to reduce human exposure have reduced the incidence of *B. abortus* and *B. melitensis* in many developed countries.
• *B. melitensis* is uncommon in North America and Northern Europe.

SYSTEMS AFFECTED
• In ruminants, infection commonly affects the reproductive system.
• Pregnant females often abort.
• Infectious organisms are shed in milk.
• Infection in males can result in epididymitis and orchitis.
• Arthritis and diskospondylitis occur less commonly in ruminants than in dogs and pigs.

PATHOPHYSIOLOGY
• Transmission of most ruminant *Brucella* species occurs through direct contact.

• Ingestion and aerosol exposure are efficient methods of transmission.
• Infectious organisms are most often ingested.
• Fluids or tissues associated with abortion or infected neonates are infectious.
• Placental tissues and fetal fluids are particularly heavily contaminated.
• Vertical transmission occurs through the milk of infected females.
• Following transmission, *Brucella* spp. establish long-term infection in many tissues.
• Recrudescence of infection with bacteremia is a hallmark of the disease.
• Localization of infection in the gravid uterus may be followed by abortion or delivery of a weak neonate.

HISTORICAL FINDINGS
Endemic herd infection is characterized by poor reproductive performance.

Brucella abortus
• Causes epizootic and endemic abortion in cattle.
• Abortion, weak neonates, retained fetal membranes, and reduced milk production are characteristic.
• Abortion due to *B. abortus* in cattle occurs in the second half of gestation.
• Epidemic abortion (*abortion storms*) can follow introduction of infection in a naïve herd.

Brucella melitensis
Abortions in goats usually occur from 4 months until term.

SIGNALMENT
• All ruminant species and many nonruminant species are susceptible.
• No breeds are considered resistant or immune.
• Disease is usually recognized in adult animals.
• *B. melitensis* infection occurs in goats and less commonly in sheep and cattle.
• *B. ovis* causes epididymitis and orchitis in rams and less commonly goats and cattle.

PHYSICAL EXAMINATION FINDINGS
Brucella abortus:
• Late-term abortion is associated with severe placentitis and retention of fetal membranes in cattle.
• Cotyledonary and intercotyledonary necrosis are typical findings but not pathognomonic.

Brucella melitensis:
• Infection in goats closely resembles *B. abortus* infection of cattle.
• Least species specific of the classical *Brucella* species.

Brucella ovis:
• Principally manifests as infectious epididymitis in breeding-age rams.
• Epididymitis is a serious cause of reduced fertility in endemic flocks.
• Occasional cause of abortion in the ewe.

GENETICS
• No breeds are resistant to infection.
• Host-adapted species create persistent reservoirs of infection.
• Infections with non-host-adapted species occur when multiple species are maintained in close proximity.

CAUSES AND RISK FACTORS
• Infection with various *Brucella species* follows contact with fluids, discharges, fetal membranes from infected females, and aborted fetuses or infected neonates.
• Group housing of rams is a risk factor for *B. ovis* infection.
• Vertical transmission occurs following ingestion of milk from infected animals.
• Venereal transmission is rare in cattle.

Brucella abortus:
Following an abortion, infected females may carry subsequent pregnancies to term, shedding infectious organisms at each parturition.

Brucella melitensis:
• Naïve herds are most often infected by introduction of an infected animal.
• Infected females efficiently transmit disease at the time of abortion or subsequent parturitions.

Brucella ovis:
Infection in ewes is not considered a major factor in persistence of flock-level infection.

DIAGNOSIS

DIFFERENTIAL DIAGNOSES
• Other infectious causes of abortion
  ○ In cattle, *Leptospira* spp., *Campylobacter fetus*, *Listeria monocytogenes*, *Trueperella pyogenes*, *Histophilus somni*, epizootic bovine abortion, mycotic abortion, bovine herpesvirus 1, bovine viral diarrhea virus, bluetongue virus, *Neospora caninum*, *Tritrichomonas foetus*, others
  ○ In sheep, *Campylobacter fetus*, *Campylobacter jejuni*, *Chlamydophila abortus*
• Noninfectious causes of abortion
  ○ Stress
  ○ Toxins
  ○ Heritable anomalies
• Other causes of epididymitis and orchitis: e.g., *Histophilus somnus*, *Actinobacillus seminis*

CBC/BIOCHEMISTRY/URINALYSIS
N/A

OTHER LABORATORY TESTS
• Bacterial culture provides definitive diagnosis.
• Serologic tests are commonly used for diagnostic screening and for surveillance programs.
• The Milk Ring Test provides a convenient method of screening dairy herds.

• Various confirmatory serologic tests are run by accredited diagnostic laboratories.

IMAGING
N/A

OTHER DIAGNOSTIC PROCEDURES
• Serologic testing at the time of abortion is valuable. Paired serology is not usually required.
• Serologic screening of cattle entering commerce and the Milk Ring Test often detect infected herds.
• Bacteriologic culture of fetal tissues, associated membranes and vaginal discharges confirm infection.

PATHOLOGIC FINDINGS
• Severe placentitis is common in cattle and most other species.
• Placentitis following *B. melitensis* abortion in goats is reportedly less severe.
• Aborted fetuses often have bronchopneumonia.
• Epididymitis and orchitis in males.

TREATMENT

THERAPEUTIC APPROACH

B. abortus:
• Regulatory programs require slaughter or euthanasia of infected animals.
• Treatment is not allowed.
• Clearing a herd from quarantine requires serial whole-herd testing.

B. melitensis:
• Treatment not recommended.
• Quarantine and serial testing similar to *B. abortus* control necessary to clear a herd/flock infection.

B. ovis:
• Treatment of infected rams is seldom recommended.
• Success is limited and infected animals are the major reservoir.

SURGICAL CONSIDERATIONS AND TECHNIQUES
N/A

MEDICATIONS

DRUGS OF CHOICE
N/A

CONTRAINDICATIONS
N/A

PRECAUTIONS
• Bovine brucellosis is a reportable disease in the United States.
• State and federal animal health agencies must be notified following diagnosis.

FOLLOW-UP

EXPECTED COURSE AND PROGNOSIS
N/A

POSSIBLE COMPLICATIONS
N/A

CLIENT EDUCATION
See "Prevention"

PATIENT CARE
N/A

PREVENTION
• Avoid introduction of disease into uninfected herds/flocks.
• Maintain closed herds when possible.
• Test and isolate herd additions.
• Prevent interaction with established wildlife reservoirs.
• Vaccination of calves limits disease in cattle but will not replace appropriate biosecurity.
• Vaccination of adult bovines in infected herds requires regulatory approval.

MISCELLANEOUS

AGE-RELATED FACTORS
• Disease (abortion) is seen in adults.
• Infection at a young age may be followed by abortion many months later.

ZOONOTIC POTENTIAL
• Brucellosis is a major zoonotic infection seen worldwide.
• Brucellosis in humans can be associated with consumption of unpasteurized milk products.
• Contact with aborted fetuses, placentas, and uterine discharges can result in human infection.
• Human disease can be debilitating if not recognized and treated.
• Cattle and wild ruminants are the principal reservoirs for human infection with *B. abortus.*

PREGNANCY
Abortion is a common result of infection in ruminants.

BIOSECURITY
• Effective biosecurity protocols are necessary to prevent introduction into uninfected herds and flocks.

• Surveillance by regulatory agencies is a necessary part of an effective control or eradication program.
• Mandatory testing of animals at the time of slaughter is required in many countries.
• Routine milk testing using the Brucellosis Ring Test readily detects infection in dairy herds.

PRODUCTION MANAGEMENT
• In cattle, vaccination of female calves can be useful to increase herd resistance and marketability.
• In much of the world, RB-51 *B. abortus* vaccine has replaced Strain 19 as the vaccine of choice in cattle.
• Calfhood vaccination is allowed only in females between 4 and 12 months of age in the United States.
• Vaccination is regulated by the government in many countries.
• Vaccination of adult cattle is allowed only in special circumstances and only carried out by regulatory officials.
• *B. melitensis* Rev 1 vaccine for sheep and goats is available in some countries.

SYNONYMS
Bangs

ABBREVIATIONS
N/A

SEE ALSO
• Biosecurity: Beef Cow/Calf (see www.fiveminutevet.com/ruminant)
• Biosecurity: Dairy (see www.fiveminutevet.com/ruminant)
• Vaccination Programs: Dairy Cattle

Suggested Reading
Brucellosis Eradication: Uniform Methods and Rules. United States Department of Agriculture, Animal and Plant Health Inspection Service. APHIS 91–45–013.
Seleem MN, Boyle SM, Sriranganathan N. Brucellosis: A reemerging zoonosis. Vet Microbiol 2010, 140: 392–8.
Olsen S, Tatum F. Bovine brucellosis. Vet Clin North Am Food Anim Pract 2010, 26: 15–27.
Blasco JM, Molina-Flores B. Control and eradication of *Brucella melitensis* infection in sheep and goats. Vet Clin North Am Food Anim Pract 2011, 27: 95–104.
Author Herris Maxwell
Consulting Editor Kaitlyn A. Lutz
Acknowledgment The author and book editors acknowledge the prior contribution of Danelle Bickett-Weddle.

BUCKEYE (*AESCULUS* SPP.) TOXICITY

BASICS

OVERVIEW
• Approximately 13 species with the most commonly encountered being:
  ○ California buckeye (*A. californica*)
  ○ Sweet or yellow buckeye (*A. flava*)
  ○ Western, white, Ohio, Texas, or fetid buckeye (*A. glabara*)
  ○ Red buckeye (*A. pavia*)
  ○ Georgia or painted buckeye (*A. sylvatica*)
  ○ Horse chestnut (*A. hippocastanum*).
• Deciduous tree or shrub.
• Bark is gray or dark brown and can be either rough or smooth. It has an alternate branching pattern with a pair of sharp short thorns at each node.
• Leaves are palmate, compound, and opposite with 5 to 11 serrated leaflets. Blades of leaves are elliptical to ovoid, pinnate venation, and acute to acuminate apices.
• Flowers are white, yellow or red with four petals that are free and clawed, usually blooming in May or June.
• Seeds are glossy brown, bearing a large conspicuous, light-brown scar, approximately 2.5 cm in diameter.

GEOGRAPHIC DISTRIBUTION
• Throughout the United States.
• It is also native to Greece, Balkans, the Caucasus mountains, and northeast Turkey.
• It has been cultivated throughout Europe.

SYSTEMS AFFECTED
Nervous

PATHOPHYSIOLOGY
• Toxic compounds include: alkaloids, glycoside (aesculin), and saponins (escin).
• Aesculin or esculin, a lactone glycoside, is additionally a derivative of coumarin.
• Escin is a mixture of various saponins and has neurotoxic as well as hypoglycemic effects.
• Presumed neurotoxin is aglycone, which is a result of the hydrolysis of escin.

SIGNALMENT
• Bovine, ovine, caprine, and camelid species.
• Ruminants are most sensitive likely as a result of the reducing environment of the rumen.

PHYSICAL EXAMINATION FINDINGS
• Sawhorse stance
• Reluctance to move
• Incoordination, stilted gait
• Seizure and collapse

CAUSES AND RISK FACTORS
• History of exposure to the plant.
• Nuts or seeds, dried fruit, bark, leaves, flowers, and young growth including stump sprouts are the primary source of the toxin.
• Presence of plant or cuttings of the plant within the pasture.
• Toxic dose is not well established, it is approximately 1% body weight.

DIAGNOSIS

DIFFERENTIAL DIAGNOSES
• Botulism.
• Gossypol toxicity.
• Hypocalcemia, hypomagnesemia, and hypokalemia: There is a decreased chance of an acute outbreak involving multiple animals with a deficiency of calcium, magnesium or potassium.
• Monensin/other ionophore toxicities.
• Organophosphate and carbamate toxicity.
• Chlorinated hydrocarbon organochlorine insecticides.
• Other neurologic disorders, e.g., tick paralysis, paralytic rabies, louping ills, West Nile virus (sheep and goats), and other encephalitic agents.

CBC/BIOCHEMISTRY/URINALYSIS
• No characteristic changes.
• Hyperglycemia in experimentally induced toxin in calves.

PATHOLOGIC FINDINGS
No lesions but finding of plant material within gastric contents on gross pathology.

TREATMENT

THERAPEUTIC APPROACH
• Decrease absorption of the toxin thru administration of charcoal.
• Clinical signs are usually self-limiting.
• Recovery occurs within a few days.
• Supportive care required for severe cases.

MEDICATIONS

DRUGS OF CHOICE
N/A

FOLLOW-UP

EXPECTED COURSE AND PROGNOSIS
• Recovery usually within 12–48 hours post-exposure.
• Death is rare.

PREVENTION
Avoid feeding buckeye plant material or grazing near buckeye trees.

MISCELLANEOUS

ASSOCIATED CONDITIONS
N/A

PRODUCTION MANAGEMENT
Restrict grazing of livestock near buckeye trees.

SEE ALSO
• Carbamate Toxicity
• Gossypol Toxicosis
• Grass Tetany/Hypomagnesemia
• Hypocalcemia
• Monensin Toxicity
• Organophosphate Toxicity
• Ovine Encephalomyelitis (Louping Ill)
• Rabies
• Tick Paralysis

Suggested Reading
Burrows GE, Tyrl RJ. Aesculus. In Burrows GE, Tyrl RJ eds, Toxic Plants of North America. Wiley-Blackwell, 2013, pp. 1111–14.
Casteel SW, Johnson GC. *Aesculus glabra* intoxication in cattle. Vet Hum Toxicol 1992, 34: 55.
Author Jennifer S. Taintor
Consulting Editor Christopher C.L. Chase
Acknowledgment The author and book editors acknowledge the prior contribution of Larry A. Kerr.

BASICS

OVERVIEW

- Burns in livestock are one of the most devastating forms of trauma:
  - Thermal—fire (barn, brush, forest), heat (heat lamps, heating pads), hot solutions
  - Electrical—lightning, electrocution
  - Frictional—rope burns, abrasions
  - Chemical—caustic agents, topical medications
  - Ultraviolet—sunburn
  - Radiation
  - Freeze "burns"
- Burns in livestock commonly occur over back, face, udder, and teats, and over ventrum with brush fires.
- Classification of burns is based on depth to which burn penetrates skin and extent of body surface involved.
  - First-degree burn involves superficial layers of epidermis; characterized by erythema, transient edema, and pain, and generally heals without complication or extensive scarring. Prognosis is good.
  - Second-degree burn: Partial-thickness burns involving all epidermal layers but sparing hair follicles and sweat glands; characterized by erythema, pain, and vesicles (blisters), necrosis, and sloughing with superficial and eschar with deep second-degree burns; usually re-epithelialized with proper care, some scarring.
  - Third-degree burn: Full thickness burns involving entire epidermis, dermis, and appendages and exposing deeper structures; local blood vessels and hair follicles destroyed; characterized by necrosis, ulceration, anesthesia, eschar, and extensive scarring. Require extensive wound care ± skin grafting.
  - Fourth-degree burn involves entire skin, subcutis, underlying fascia, muscle, and tendon.
- The full extent of the thermal burn is difficult to predict immediately after injury.
- Burns are usually complex with body areas being affected to different degrees.
- The development of blisters, fluid separation of epidermis and dermis, and eschars may not appear for several days.
- Thermal injuries caused by fire are often associated with more than skin pathology:
  - Fluid shifts, hypovolemia
  - Electrolyte abnormalities (especially sodium)
  - Hypoproteinemia (loss of plasma is maximal in first 12–24 hours)
  - Extreme stress
  - Smoke inhalation
  - Immune suppression

- Extracutaneous complications of burns may be cardiopulmonary, ocular, hematologic, and renal.
- Animals suffering burns and/or smoke inhalation need to be closely monitored and repeatedly examined as signs and lesion development may be delayed. This is especially so with fluid therapy, which may precipitate pulmonary edema with fluid overload.
- Wound or burn infection is common in cattle and *Pseudomonas aeruginosa* is the most common organism to establish infection.
- Infection under eschars is a common problem.
- Animals with second-degree and third-degree burns over 50% of their body have a guarded prognosis.
- Poor prognosis if second-degree and third-degree burns affect more than 10–15% of body surface.
- Sequelae to burn injuries:
  - Hypoproteinemia from protein exudate from wounds
  - Progressive edema
  - Hyperkalemia
  - Burn-induced immunosuppression
  - Progressive anemia
  - Secondary infections; pneumonia, skin infections
  - Multiple system involvement, i.e., renal shut down, eye damage
  - Scarring
  - Damage to eyelids, conjunctiva, cornea, anterior uveitis, exfoliation of lens capsule
- Sunburn
  - White and light-skinned animals, lateral aspects of teats, ears, nose, areas covered with little hair are most susceptible to ultraviolet light, 290–320 nm.
  - White-faced sheep, especially ears and face.
  - Exposure to sunlight is associated with skin tumor development, especially on udder of white goats.
  - Erythema, pain, swelling, blisters, erosions.
- Complications of teat burns include obstruction of teat orifice, distorted teats, and mastitis.

INCIDENCE/PREVALENCE
Usually sporadic

GEOGRAPHIC DISTRIBUTION
N/A

SYSTEMS AFFECTED
- Integument
- Musculoskeletal, depending on degree of burn

PATHOPHYSIOLOGY
- Thermal burns can result from scalding with hot liquids, contact with hot objects, or exposure to flames or radiant heat (sunburn).
- The three zones of a burn are the zones of coagulation, stasis, and hyperemia respectively. The zone of coagulation is the

point of maximum damage. There is irreversible tissue loss due to coagulation of the constituent proteins. The zone of stasis has decreased tissue perfusion. The tissue in this zone is potentially salvageable. The goal in burn resuscitation would be to increase tissue perfusion to prevent any damage becoming irreversible. Pathology resulting from prolonged hypotension, infection or edema can convert this zone to an area of complete tissue loss. The zone of hyperemia is the outermost zone where tissue perfusion is increased. This tissue invariably recovers unless there is severe sepsis or prolonged hypotension.
- The release of cytokines and other inflammatory mediators at the site of the injury usually can have a systemic effect when approximately 30% or more of the body surface area is affected.
- Cardiovascular changes: Capillary permeability is increased, leading to loss of intravascular proteins and fluids into the interstitial compartments.
- Metabolic changes: The basal metabolic rate can increase up to 3 times the original rate. Without intervention there will be increased catabolism and compromise of the gut integrity.
- Respiratory changes: Inflammatory mediators cause bronchoconstriction which can result in respiratory distress.
- Immunologic changes: Nonspecific downregulation of the immune response, affecting both cell-mediated and humoral pathways.
- Electrical injuries: The current will travel from one point of the body to another, creating an entry and exit point. The tissue between these two points can also be damaged by its passage. The amount of heat generated is dependent on the voltage the animal is exposed to.
- Chemical injuries: They tend to be deep, as corrosive agents continue to cause coagulative necrosis until completely removed. Alkalis tend to penetrate deeper and cause more severe burns than acids.

HISTORICAL FINDINGS
Source of trauma is not always known and thorough history should be taken in order to better treat and provide an accurate prognosis.

SIGNALMENT
- No age, sex, or breed predilection
- Sunburn: light-skinned or white animals, white-faced sheep

PHYSICAL EXAMINATION FINDINGS
- Severity of burn determines signs present and may range from mild erythema and superficial scabbing to extensive tissue damage and necrosis with severe protein exudation.
- Wool is fire-retardant; burns on sheep most commonly found on legs and around face.
- Goats and cattle are likely to have burns on any part of body.

BURN MANAGEMENT   (CONTINUED)

B

- Signs of sunburn:
  - Erythema, swelling, crusting of skin
  - Headshaking, pruritus
  - Discomfort during milking or nursing if udder or teats burned.
- Teat burns:
  - Mild burns: erythema, sloughing of outer, white, paper-thin tissue; areas of sloughing, crusting, and discoloration of tissue; milk appears normal; teat pliable on palpation.
  - Severe burns: teats tend to be dull brown or black, dry, and often corrugated; thick layer of tissue is sloughed, underneath is red hemorrhagic tissue; teat is leather-like and lacks pliability ± distorted.
- Healing lesions may be very pruritic causing animals to scratch or lick at affected sites.
- Non-dermatologic signs occur about 7 days after the onset of skin lesions: pyrexia.

GENETICS
N/A

CAUSES AND RISK FACTORS
See "Overview"

DIAGNOSIS

DIFFERENTIAL DIAGNOSIS
Differentiate sunburn from photosensitivity.

CBC/BIOCHEMISTRY/URINALYSIS
N/A

OTHER LABORATORY TESTS
N/A

IMAGING
N/A

OTHER DIAGNOSTIC PROCEDURES
N/A

TREATMENT

- Initial overall assessment of survivors—recumbent, severely burned animals who are suffering should be euthanized.
- Evaluation of animal's systemic and local injuries is essential. The main aim is to control decreasing circulatory volume.
- Repeat examination is necessary to determine response to therapy and development of delayed signs and lesions.

THERAPEUTIC APPROACH
Treatment is aimed at care of initial injuries, cardiovascular support, respiratory support, and prevention of secondary infection. The goal of treatment is epithelialization of the wound. First- and mild second-degree burns should heal well by epithelialization, while severe second-degree and most third-degree burns may require skin grafts. Burn patients are extremely heterogeneous with significant inter and intra-patient variation with regard to

treatment and drug choice. Below are general guidelines for treatment of burn patients.
- Cool affected body areas to reduce heat retention and limit necrosis.
  - Hosing with cool water for 15 minutes (also removes burnt hair, crust, and debris)
  - Wet cool towels.
- Burn wound care:
  - Thorough cleaning with irrigation or dilute chlorhexidine solution (controversial); repeat 2 or 3 times daily.
  - Daily hydrotherapy.
  - Topical antimicrobial; use water-soluble emollient antimicrobial cream, silver sulfadiazine (Silvadene).
  - Use of hydrogel and nonadherent, absorbent dressings, which are not constrictive, may be indicated in some cases but must be kept clean and changed at appropriate intervals.
  - Avoid occlusive dressings, which produce a closed wound with bacterial proliferation and delayed healing.
  - Eschar over large second- or third-degree burns should be left undisturbed until natural sloughing occurs or if infection develops under eschar.
  - Blisters should be allowed to remain in place for 1–2 days on second-degree burns.
  - Wound debridement after 24–36 hours if necessary.
  - Wound allowed to heal by granulation.
- Systemic support:
  - Analgesia as needed—nonsteroidal anti-inflammatory drugs (concern these may delay healing).
  - Correct hypovolemia: rule of thumb—give 3–4 mL/kg of body weight for each percentage body surface involved. Very important to not overhydrate as it can precipitate development of pulmonary edema or generalized edema.
  - Maintenance of electrolyte and acid-base balance.
  - Plasma administration if severe hypoproteinemia.
  - Tetanus booster if indicated.
- Eye damage:
  - Cornea and eyelid damage are of particular concern.
  - With burns on face, cornea should be treated with artificial tears.
  - Gently remove debris from eye with saline-soaked cotton swab.
  - Inspect and fluorescein stain eye for ulcers.
  - Apply topical antibiotics with atropine.
  - Third eyelid flap if necessary to protect eye.
- Teat burns:
  - Soothing, softening burn ointments, lanolin ointments, aloe vera
  - Antimicrobial ointment if skin surface sloughs
  - Maintain open teat orifice.
  - Healing is slow, takes many weeks to months.

- Sunburn
  - Remove from exposure to sunlight.
  - Provide shelter.
  - Soothing burn ointments, topical human sunburn medications, or aloe vera, topical steroids.
  - Application of pigmented teat dips.
  - Contamination of milk should be avoided.
  - For secondary bacterial infection, use topical or systemic antimicrobial agents.

SURGICAL CONSIDERATIONS AND TECHNIQUES
Third-degree burns may require skin grafting.

MEDICATIONS

DRUGS OF CHOICE
Many different medications and products are used in wound management and their use is highly case dependent and dependent on clinician preference. See "Therapeutic Approach."

CONTRAINDICATIONS
Systemic antimicrobials fail to penetrate local burn wound infections and may permit growth of resistant organisms; therefore, they should be reserved for use when there is documentation of a secondary site of infection (e.g., pneumonia).

PRECAUTIONS
Appropriate milk and meat withdrawal times must be followed for all compounds administered to food-producing animals.

POSSIBLE INTERACTIONS
N/A

FOLLOW-UP

EXPECTED COURSE AND PROGNOSIS
Lesions can persist for up to 12 weeks.

POSSIBLE COMPLICATIONS
- Complications will vary depending on specific etiology and location.
- Infections beneath eschars are common in cattle secondary to burn wounds.
- Chronic mastitis or teat obstruction may occur after damage to the skin of teats. When the face is involved, chronic vision impairment due to corneal opacity is possible.
- In general, complications are more common with severe burns where systemic support and further surgical interventions are required.

CLIENT EDUCATION
Advise clients of preventive measures (i.e., proper chemical storage, electrical safety, etc.) as well as the possible secondary wound complications.

PATIENT CARE
Monitor for signs of secondary infection and systemic involvement. See "Associated

Conditions" for information on fire-related burns specifically.

PREVENTION
See "Production Management"

 MISCELLANEOUS

ASSOCIATED CONDITIONS
Smoke Inhalation
Involves carbon monoxide toxicity and smoke toxicity.

Three Mechanisms of Injury to Respiratory System
• First stage: Heat damage to upper respiratory tract, injury from toxic chemicals in smoke and carbon monoxide toxicity; usually signs within first 6 hours.
  ◦ Inflammation, edema, and necrosis of nasal passages, pharynx, and larynx lead to airway obstruction ± laryngospasm.
  ◦ Bronchoconstriction of lungs; inhalation of soot, noxious gases.
  ◦ Carbon monoxide toxicity: hypoxemia and tissue hypoxia in all organs, especially brain; level above 10% carbon monoxide is consistent with toxicity.
  ◦ Shock.
• Second stage: Formation of pulmonary edema
  ◦ Within 12–72 hours after exposure.
  ◦ Damage due to inflammatory mediators (cytokines, proteolytic enzymes, oxygen free radicals).
  ◦ Obstruction of small airway from deposition of smoke material and inflammatory debris.
• Third stage: bronchopneumonia
  ◦ Result of impaired immune system and exposure to pathogens.
  ◦ May occur within 24–48 hours or 1–3 weeks after initial injury.

Clinical Signs
• Many signs may not be apparent for 1–2 days after fire.
• Oral burns, nasal mucosal swelling, pharyngeal swelling, laryngospasm, conjunctivitis.
• Hoarseness, expiratory wheezes, cough, stridor, tachypnea.
• Tachycardia.

• Bright mucus membranes with carbon monoxide toxicity may mask cyanosis.
• ±Cyanosis.
• Signs of hypovolemia.
• Signs of shock.
• Depression, disorientation, irritability, ataxia, or even comatose.
• ± Signs of septicemia or pneumonia.

Treatment
• Depends on stage and severity of injury.
• Oxygen support.
• Maintenance of airway: Tracheotomy if upper airway obstruction.
• Keep airways clean.
• Bronchodilators to counteract bronchoconstriction.
• Diuretics and anti-inflammatory agents (nonsteroidal anti-inflammatory drugs) to reduce edema and inflammation. Use of corticosteroids is controversial.
• Analgesics.
• Fluid therapy if hypovolemic, electrolyte imbalances, or acid-base derangements. Caution not to fluid overload if ongoing protein loss through burns or from vasculature.
• Plasma therapy if hyperproteinemia.
• Strict hygiene, nursing care, and optimal nutritional support.
• Appropriate antimicrobials based on culture and sensitivity from documented site of infection. Prophylactic antimicrobials are not recommended.

PRODUCTION MANAGEMENT
• Recovery time is prolonged with teat burns and extensive burns.
• Need to determine which animals to be euthanized or culled due to poor prognosis for successful recovery:
  ◦ Animals with second- and third-degree burns over extensive area.
  ◦ Burnt teats that will not withstand milking; mastitis is inevitable.
  ◦ Badly burned feet may slough claws.
  ◦ Facial burns involving cornea may lead to permanent stromal opacities.
• Teat burns:
  ◦ Mild lesions have good prognosis.
  ◦ Severe lesions have variable prognosis due to mastitis and secondary occlusion of teat canal and distortion of teat.
  ◦ Mature adult cows are more likely to return to full function than heifers.

• Prevention of sunburn:
  ◦ Gradual acclimation to exposure to sunlight.
  ◦ Provide shade.
  ◦ Application of sun blocking screens or ointments; use sunblocks with highest SPF available and those that are suitable for use in children; avoid PABA as it is not recommended as safe in children and little is known about its safety in animals.
  ◦ Iodophor teat dips.
  ◦ Pet animals may wear fly nets on ears, or hats or bonnets.

ABBREVIATION
PABA = para-aminobenzoic acid

SEE ALSO
• Frostbite
• Lightning Strike
• Pain Management (see www.fiveminutevet.com/ruminant)
• Wound Management

Suggested Reading
Knottenbelt, DC. Management of burn injuries. In: Robinson NE ed, Current Therapy in Equine Medicine 5. Philadelphia: Saunders, 2003.
Marsh P. Smoke inhalation. In: Smith BP ed, Large Animal Internal Medicine, 3rd ed. St. Louis: Mosby, 2002.
Pugh D. Diseases of the integumentary system. In: Sheep and Goat Medicine. Philadelphia: Saunders, 2002.
Rebhun WC. Skin diseases. In: Diseases of Dairy Cattle. Baltimore: Williams & Wilkins, 1995.
Scott DW. Environmental skin diseases. In: Howard JL, Smith RA eds, Current Veterinary Therapy 4: Food Animal Practice. Philadelphia: Saunders, 1999.
Smith MC, Sherman DM. Environmental insults. In: Goat Medicine. Philadelphia: Lea & Febiger, 1994.
Author Troy E.C. Holder
Consulting Editor Kaitlyn A. Lutz
Acknowledgment The author and book editors acknowledge the prior contribution of Susan Semrad and Karen A. Moriello.

CACHE VALLEY VIRUS

C

BASICS

OVERVIEW
• Cache Valley virus (CVV) is an arthropod-borne viral infection that belongs to the genus *Orthobunyavirus* in the family Bunyaviridae. CVV afflicts a variety of domestic and wild ruminants, and humans.
• The majority of CVV infections in ruminants are subclinical; however, embryonic mortality, fetal teratogenesis, and stillbirth occur in sheep, goats, and possibly other ruminants.
• Infected deer have 1–3 days of viremia and are considered amplifying hosts.
• In the southwestern United States, lambs and goat kids born in December, January, and February are more likely to show CVV-induced teratogenesis. This period coincides with increased rainfall and mosquito activity during the breeding season.
• Fetal susceptibility to CVV-induced pathology in sheep is higher when infection occurs during the first 48 days of pregnancy.

INCIDENCE/PREVALENCE
Serologic surveys in North America show widespread prevalence of CVV antibodies in domestic and wild ruminants.

GEOGRAPHIC DISTRIBUTION
CVV is endemic throughout the United States, Canada, Mexico, and some countries of Central America.

SYSTEMS AFFECTED
• Nervous
• Musculoskeletal

PATHOPHYSIOLOGY
• The CVV genome is composed of three negative sense, single-stranded RNA segments: large (L), medium (M), and small (S).
• CVV transmission to vertebrates occurs via the bite of infected mosquitoes, including several species of *Aedes, Psorophora, Anopheles, Coquillettidia, Culex,* and from *Culiseta inornata.*
• The virus circulates in an enzootic cycle involving mammal-biting mosquitoes and deer hosts.
• After infection, there is transient viremia, during which the virus can cross the placenta, inducing embryonic mortality or fetal malformation in small ruminants.
• Fetal malformation in experimentally CVV-inoculated pregnant ewes occurs during a narrow window of susceptibility before the ovine fetus becomes immunocompetent, an event which occurs at approximately 70–75 days of gestation.
• Infection of pregnant ewes before 32 days of pregnancy results in early embryonic death. Infection between 32 and 37 days causes musculoskeletal and CNS lesions. Infection

between 37 and 48 days results mainly in musculoskeletal lesions.
• After 60 days of pregnancy, fetal infection results in production of fetal neutralizing antibodies and innate immune responses that clear CVV without malformation.
• There is no cross-protection against other related orthobunyaviruses.
• Ewes that are CVV seropositive at breeding are resistant to reinfection with CVV.

HISTORICAL FINDINGS
N/A

SIGNALMENT
• CVV infects a variety of wild and domestic ungulates and other animals, including sheep, goats, deer, cattle, pigs, horses, raccoons, woodchuck, mouflon, caribou, turtles, rabbits, and foxes.
• In sheep there is a positive relationship between seropositivity to CVV and age.
• In pregnant sheep and goats, CVV can cross the placenta causing embryonic death, mummification, or fetal malformation.
• No gender or breed predilection to infection.

PHYSICAL EXAMINATION FINDINGS
• In most adult animals, CVV infection is subclinical.
• In pregnant sheep and goats, CVV infection may result in embryonic mortality, fetal mummification, and various musculoskeletal or central nervous system anomalies.
• Dystocia may occur in ewes that deliver full-term malformed offspring.

GENETICS
N/A

CAUSES AND RISK FACTORS
• Excessively wet summers preceded by years of drought result in high vector populations and outbreaks of CVV-induced fetal malformation.
• Ecologic modification of the environment, such as constructions of dams or the presence of rice fields, has been associated with an increased risk of vector-borne viral infections.
• The prevalence of CVV antibodies in sera of animals increases with age and reduces the risk of fetal malformation occurring in pregnant ewes.

DIAGNOSIS

DIFFERENTIAL DIAGNOSES
• Main Drain, La Crosse, and San Angelo viruses induce similar fetal pathology.
• Bluetongue virus (BTV) serotype 8 or BTV of vaccine origin, and Border disease virus also may result in CNS malformations in sheep.
• Schmallenberg virus, Akabane, Rift Valley fever, Nairobi sheep disease, and Wesselsbron viruses are exotic to North America, but may cause similar fetal pathology.

• Other causes of teratogenesis include ovine hereditary chondrodysplasia (spider lamb syndrome) and teratogenic plants (*Lupinus, Oxytropis, Astragalus*).

CBC/BIOCHEMISTRY/URINALYSIS
N/A

OTHER LABORATORY TESTS
N/A

IMAGING
N/A

OTHER DIAGNOSTIC PROCEDURES
• CVV can be isolated from the blood of infected animals during acute viremia, though viremia is short-lived and in most cases virus isolation is unsuccessful.
• CVV serum antibodies can be demonstrated by serum neutralization, ELISA, complement fixation, and hemagglutination-inhibition.
• In adult animals, serum antibodies indicate previous exposure, but do not provide information regarding the infectious status of those individuals.
• Malformed fetuses that survive in utero for some time develop neutralizing antibodies and eliminate the virus. In these cases, assaying pre-colostral fetal serum for CVV antibodies establishes the diagnosis.
• In experimentally infected fetuses, CVV can be isolated up to approximately day 69 of pregnancy.
• In full-term malformed fetuses or neonates, virus isolation is always unsuccessful; however, viral nucleic acid can be detected by real-time PCR for some time after clearance of infectious virus.
• Lack of CW antibodies in sera of ewes lambing malformed fetuses rules out CVV as the cause.
• A recent duplex real-time RT-PCR for the California serogroup viruses serogroup and CVV has been reported but has not been validated.

PATHOLOGIC FINDINGS
• CVV infection of ewes during early pregnancy may result in embryonic mortality, fetal teratogenesis, stillbirth, and/or oligohydroamnios (deficiency of amniotic fluid).
• Congenital abnormalities of the fetus include arthrogryposis, hydranencephaly, hydrocephalus, microcephaly, porencephaly, cerebellar hypoplasia, scoliosis, torticollis, and lordosis.
• In multiple pregnancies, the degree and type of fetal pathology may be different in each fetus. In some cases, one fetus may be normal while others may have malformations.
• Fetal mummification occurs in some infected fetuses.
• In other ruminants, fetal abnormalities caused by CVV are less well documented.
• Histologic lesions are more frequently observed in the brain, spinal cord, and skeletal muscle of malformed fetuses.

C

• Multifocal areas of necrosis with accumulation of necrotic debris are seen in the gray matter of the brain of affected fetuses.
• Brain cavities containing blood and evidence of neurophil rarefaction and malacia may be present.
• In the spinal cord, there is progressive cellular and parenchymal loss with micromyelia.
• Skeletal muscles of CVV-infected fetuses with arthrogryposis show loss of myofibers with scattered inflammatory infiltrates.
• Affected lambs often have meconium in pulmonary alveoli due to intrauterine stress.

 TREATMENT

THERAPEUTIC APPROACH
N/A

SURGICAL CONSIDERATIONS AND TECHNIQUES
N/A

 MEDICATIONS

DRUGS OF CHOICE
N/A

CONTRAINDICATIONS
N/A

PRECAUTIONS
N/A

POSSIBLE INTERACTIONS
N/A

 FOLLOW-UP

EXPECTED COURSE AND PROGNOSIS
Affected fetuses are born dead or die shortly after birth.

POSSIBLE COMPLICATIONS
N/A

CLIENT EDUCATION
N/A

PATIENT CARE
N/A

PREVENTION
• There are no vaccines available.
• Ewes and does seropositive to CVV at the time of breeding are protected from subsequent infection and its adverse effects on pregnancy; however, they are susceptible to infection by bunyaviruses of different serogroups, some of which may induce similar fetal pathology.
• Insect control is difficult because of the wide range of mosquito vectors and vertebrate hosts, and because insecticides may not be ecologically admissible.
• Breeding ewes or does after the first frost of the fall or early winter once mosquitos subside reduces the risk of fetal infection.
• The use of insecticide ear tags and topical permethrin reduces insect blood feeding in experimental sheep.
• Other insect control methods such as removing standing water sources may reduce abundance of vectors.

 MISCELLANEOUS

ASSOCIATED CONDITIONS
N/A

AGE-RELATED FACTORS
Developing fetuses are most susceptible to clinical disease with infection.

ZOONOTIC POTENTIAL
• CW is an indirect zoonosis; humans are infected by infected mosquitoes, but not directly from infected vertebrate animals.
• Infection can occur through accidental puncture with infected needles.
• The great majority of CVV infections in humans are subclinical; however, fever, myalgia, chills, headache, vomiting, and death occasionally occur. At least three cases of CVV-associated neurologic disease have been reported in humans.

• There is no conclusive evidence that CVV infection in humans causes fetal malformation.

PREGNANCY
Infection during pregnancy may result in embryonic death, abortion, and fetal malformation in ruminants.

BIOSECURITY
N/A

PRODUCTION MANAGEMENT
N/A

SYNONYMS
N/A

ABBREVIATIONS
• BTV = bluetongue virus
• CNS = central nervous system
• CVV = Cache Valley virus
• ELISA = enzyme-linked immunosorbent assay

SEE ALSO
• Akabane
• Bluetongue Virus
• Border Disease
• Nairobi Sheep Disease
• Rift Valley Fever
• Schmallenberg Virus
• Teratogens
• Wesselsbron Disease

Suggested Reading
de la Concha-Bermejillo A. Cache Valley virus is a cause of fetal malformation and pregnancy loss in sheep. Small Rum Res 2003, 49: 1–9.
Rodrigues-Hoffmann A, Welsh CJ, Varner PW, et al. Identification of the target cells and sequence of infection during experimental infection of ovine fetuses with Cache Valley virus. J Virol 2012, 86: 4793–800.
Rodrigues Hoffmann A, Dorniak P, Filant J, et al. Ovine fetal immune response to Cache Valley virus infection. J Virol 2013, 87: 5586–92.

Author Andrés de la Concha-Bermejillo
Consulting Editor Erica C. McKenzie

CALF DIPHTHERIA/NECROTIC STOMATITIS

BASICS

OVERVIEW
• Necrobacillosis is a term used to describe any lesion associated with the Gram-negative, strictly anaerobic bacterium *Fusobacterium necrophorum*, including hepatic abscesses in cattle, foot abscesses, and infections of the oral cavity.
• Oral necrobacillosis is a term used to describe infections of the mouth and larynx with *F. necrophorum*.
• This includes "necrotic stomatitis" in which the lesions are restricted to the oral cavity and "calf diphtheria" in which the lesions are largely confined to the larynx, buccal, and pharyngeal mucosa.
• *F. necrophorum* is a ubiquitous bacterial organism commonly found in the environment (soil); and it is considered part of the normal flora of the oral cavity, respiratory tract, gastrointestinal tract, and urogenital tract of many omnivores and herbivores. The organism is commonly isolated from the soil of feedlots.
• Because of the lack of availability of suitable immunoprophylaxis, the control of *F. necrophorum* infection has depended mainly on the use of antimicrobial agents and management strategies.

INCIDENCE/PREVALENCE
• Sporadic, often with a higher incidence in fall and winter.
• Feedlot cattle are estimated to have a prevalence of 1–2%.

GEOGRAPHIC DISTRIBUTION
• Worldwide.
• More common in countries where animals are housed indoors in the winter (confined quarters), maintained in feedlots, or housed in unsanitary environments.

SYSTEMS AFFECTED
• Digestive
• Respiratory

PATHOPHYSIOLOGY
• *F. necrophorum* is a Gram-negative, non-spore-forming anaerobe that is a normal inhabitant of the respiratory and alimentary tracts of many species of animals.
• Two types of *F. necrophorum*, subspecies *necrophorum* (biotype A) and subspecies *funduliforme* (biotype B), have been recognized. These two biotypes differ morphologically, biochemically, and biologically. Subspecies *necrophorum* is more virulent in nature.
• Injury to the mucosa of the oral cavity, pharynx and larynx allows *F. necrophorum* to invade and infect the tissues. Inflammation, necrosis, and edema can subsequently constrict the larynx, causing dyspnea and painful swallowing.

• *F. necrophorum* is encountered frequently in mixed infections and, therefore, synergism with other pathogens may play an important role in infection.
• Laryngeal contact ulcers provoked by a variety of respiratory pathogens (viral and bacterial) might serve as an important factor in laryngeal invasion.
• Several toxins produced by *F. necrophorum*, including leukotoxin, endotoxin, hemolysin, hemagglutinin and adhesin, have been implicated as virulence factors.
• Leukotoxin and endotoxin are believed to be particularly important in overcoming the host's defense mechanisms and allowing infection to establish.
• Leukotoxin is known to be cytotoxic and causes vascular thrombosis.
• Infection leads to localized inflammation and edema of the laryngeal mucosa and cartilage; however, bacteremia and dissemination of organisms to the liver and other organs can occur in some cases.

HISTORICAL FINDINGS
Intensively managed cattle consuming rough or abrasive feeds, exposed to unsanitary feeding areas or feeding practices, or receiving recent oral bolus medication are at risk.

SIGNALMENT
• Necrotic stomatitis tends to occur in calves <3 months of age, most commonly between 2 weeks and 3 months of age.
• Necrotic laryngitis typically affects cattle <3–18 months of age.

PHYSICAL EXAMINATION FINDINGS
• Fever: temperature tends to be higher for calf diphtheria (106°F), and moderately elevated for necrotic stomatitis (103–104°F).
• Swollen (edematous) and hyperemic oral, pharyngeal, and/or laryngeal mucus membranes.
• The pharyngeal region may be painful on external palpation.
• The laryngeal opening is often reduced by edema and inflammation.
• Inspiratory dyspnea progressing to open-mouth breathing and stertor with extended head and neck.
• Necrotic erosions and ulcers (with diphtheritic membranes) are usually visible in the larynx/pharynx.
• Other signs include painful or difficult swallowing, salivation, a moist cough, anorexia, and depression. Fetid breath and bilateral nasal discharge might be noted.
• Chronic cases of laryngitis may display roaring respiration and a harsh, dry cough.

GENETICS
N/A

CAUSES AND RISK FACTORS
• The etiologic agent is *F. necrophorum*, though many cases involve mixed infections.
• *F. necrophorum* invades into abraded or damaged mucosa of the oral cavity, larynx or pharynx.

• Risk factors include rough or abrasive feeds, unsanitary conditions, administration of oral bolus medications, and infection with viral or bacterial respiratory pathogens.
• The incidence of disease tends to be highest in groups of animals that are kept in confined quarters under unsanitary conditions (housed cattle and feedlot cattle).
• Cattle <18 months of age are at higher risk.

DIAGNOSIS

DIFFERENTIAL DIAGNOSES
• Pharyngeal trauma, cellulitis or abscessation
• Severe viral laryngitis/tracheitis (e.g., BVD, IBR)
• Aspiration
• Actinobacillosis
• Pharyngeal neoplasia
• Mycotic stomatitis
• Dental abscess
• Maxillary or mandibular fracture
• Foreign body

CBC/BIOCHEMISTRY/URINALYSIS
CBC changes can include leukopenia resulting from neutropenia in acute cases; or leukocytosis with neutrophilia, monocytosis, and hyperfibrinogenemia in chronic cases.

OTHER LABORATORY TESTS
• Bacterial cultures can be obtained from deep within the oral and laryngeal lesions.
• Most specimen cultures contain a single *Fusobacterium* species (usually *F. necrophorum*).
• Specimen cultures will also commonly contain other obligate anaerobes together with facultative and obligate aerobes.

IMAGING
• Direct examination of the oral cavity can be aided with use of an oral speculum and a good light source.
• Laryngoscopy or endoscopy of the pharynx allows visual observation of the pharynx and larynx to identify inflamed and necrotic mucosa, but may exacerbate respiratory distress.
• Radiography or ultrasonography of the pharynx might also be useful to delineate differential diagnoses.

OTHER DIAGNOSTIC PROCEDURES
Postmortem examination of affected animals is recommended to confirm diagnosis and to rule out other diseases.

PATHOLOGIC FINDINGS
• Acute cases typically display edema and hyperemia of the larynx and/or pharynx which may surround centers of necrotic mucosa.
• Lesions are typically identified at the vocal processes and medial angles of the arytenoid cartilages. They may extend along the vocal folds and into the dorsal laryngeal musculature.

(CONTINUED)

CALF DIPHTHERIA/NECROTIC STOMATITIS

C

• The tongue, buccal mucosa, pharynx, cheeks, gums, palate, and trachea may also be involved.
• The regional lymph nodes may be swollen and/or hyperemic. May see necrosis of the palatine and pharyngeal tonsils.
• Chronic cases may present with tissue tracts extending into regions of necrotic cartilage, and may have deformed or misshapen arytenoid cartilages.
• On histopathology, areas of coagulation necrosis are surrounded by a zone of vascular reaction, leukocytes, and granulation tissue.
• The bacteria are typically arranged in long filaments (sometimes as rods or cocci), but are relatively difficult to demonstrate in tissue sections.

TREATMENT

THERAPEUTIC APPROACH
• Affected animals are typically treated with antibiotics and supportive medical care, which is best instituted early in disease to optimize success.
• Broad-spectrum systemic antimicrobial therapy should be provided for several days using short- or long-acting preparations according to acceptable standards for food animal practice.
• Cases with significant dyspnea may require tracheotomy.
• Fluids and nutritional support may be necessary for particularly compromised and valuable animals.

SURGICAL CONSIDERATIONS AND TECHNIQUES
• In severe cases, a tracheotomy can be performed if necessary to obtain a patent airway.
• Severe, chronic cases may require surgical debridement to remove necrotic and/or granulation tissue and to drain laryngeal abscesses.
• Subtotal arytenoidectomy may be indicated in severe cases involving chronic chondritis (inflammation of the cartilage).

MEDICATIONS

DRUGS OF CHOICE
• Antibiotic options include:
  ○ Procaine penicillin: 22,000 U/kg, IM, q24h or q12h
  ○ Oxytetracycline: short-acting preparation: 11 mg/kg, IV or SC, q24h; long-acting preparation: 20 mg/kg, SC, q72h
  ○ Sulfonamide agents: Sulfamethazine - initial/loading dose of 140 mg/kg IV, followed by 70 mg/kg IV q24h OR 150 mg/kg PO q24h for 3–5 days. Treatment not to exceed 5 days.

• Nonsteroidal anti-inflammatory drugs can reduce fever, inflammation and pain; options include aspirin (100 mg/kg, PO, q12h); flunixin meglumine (1.1–2.2 mg/kg, IV, q24h or divided q12h); or ketoprofen (3 mg/kg, IM or IV, q24h).
• In significantly dyspneic animals, a single dose of dexamethasone (0.05–0.2 mg/kg, IV or IM) may help to reduce laryngeal edema.
• The use of mild topical disinfectants and antiseptics (e.g., Lugol's or povidone iodine) has been described.

CONTRAINDICATIONS
Oral medications should be avoided initially if possible to prevent additional damage to the irritated oropharynx and larynx and because affected animals have reduced ability to swallow.

PRECAUTIONS
Appropriate milk and meat withdrawal times must be followed for all pharmaceutical compounds administered to food-producing animals.

POSSIBLE INTERACTIONS
N/A

FOLLOW-UP

EXPECTED COURSE AND PROGNOSIS
• If the condition is detected early and treated aggressively, the prognosis is guarded to good. Case mortality has been reported as approximately 15–20%.
• The disease course for acute cases is in the range of 7–10 days, but may be as long as 2–3 months for chronic cases.
• Severe complications can occur, especially if diagnosis is delayed. Several reports suggest that approximately 20% of affected animals progress to chronic disease. The prognosis for chronic cases (especially cases with bilateral involvement) is guarded to poor.
• Untreated calves tend to die from toxemia, upper airway obstruction/asphyxia, and pneumonia, usually within 2–7 days.
• A 60% success rate for surgical intervention in severe and chronic cases has been reported.
• Involvement of the laryngeal cartilage (ulcers and necrosis) often leads to a delay in healing or failure to recover.
• It is recommended that chronic, unresponsive cases be culled.

POSSIBLE COMPLICATIONS
• Systemic toxemia and disease.
• Chronic infection of the laryngeal cartilages leading to chronic coughing.
• Pneumonia (aspiration or hematogenous spread).

CLIENT EDUCATION
• Provide good-quality forage and minimize abrasive materials such as sticks and cockleburs in hays and pastures.

• Keep feed areas, mangers, and feeding equipment clean.
• Early recognition is essential for successful treatment.

PATIENT CARE
• Monitor the ability to breathe and swallow appropriately while diseased.
• Provide soft and palatable food sources, water, and shelter from the elements.

PREVENTION
• Maintain sanitary feeding areas and equipment (minimize exposure to dust and inhaled irritants).
• Avoid rough feeds.
• Apply control measures for viral and respiratory pathogens.
• Identify infected animals early to prevent spread.

MISCELLANEOUS

ASSOCIATED CONDITIONS
Aspiration pneumonia

AGE-RELATED FACTORS
Most commonly cattle 3–18 months old are affected, with necrotic stomatitis usually observed in calves <3 months and necrotic laryngitis in calves >3 months.

ZOONOTIC POTENTIAL
N/A

PREGNANCY
N/A

BIOSECURITY
• Although the organism is fairly ubiquitous, measures to control other respiratory diseases may reduce the incidence of necrotic laryngitis.
• Proper hygiene precautions and disinfection of potential fomites in calf pens and feeding/drinking places.

PRODUCTION MANAGEMENT
• Observation and early diagnosis of cases is critical to minimize the impact on a feedlot.
• Preventive measures and early treatment can reduce the total number of animals affected.
• Management of feeding protocols and practices, and control of respiratory pathogens in intensively managed cattle, can be used to reduce the incidence of this disease.
• This disease is usually sporadic in nature and the economic losses are primarily due to reduced live weights, inefficient feed conversion, expensive treatments, and fatalities.

SYNONYMS
• Necrotic/necrotizing stomatitis, necrobacillary stomatitis, oral necrobacillosis.
• Calf diphtheria, necrotic/necrotizing laryngitis, laryngeal necrobacillosis.

C

• *Fusobacterium necrophorum* was previously named *Sph(a)erophorus necrophorus*, *Actinomyces necrophorum, Corynebacterium necrophorum*, and *Fusiformis necrophorus*.

ABBREVIATIONS
• BVD = bovine viral diarrhea
• IBR = infectious bovine rhinotracheitis

Suggested Reading
Howard JL, Smith RA. Current Veterinary Therapy: Food Animal Practice, 4th ed. Philadelphia: WB Saunders, 1999.
Jang SS, Hirsh DC. Characterization, distribution, and microbiological associations of *Fusobacterium* spp. in clinical specimens of animal origin. J Clin Microbiol 1994, 32: 384–7.
Maxie GM. Jubb, Kennedy and Palmer's Pathology of Domestic Animals, vol. 2, 6th ed. New York: Saunders Elsevier, 2015.
Nagaraja TG, Narayanan SK, Stewart GC, Chengappa MM. *Fusobacterium necrophorum* infections in animals: Pathogenesis and pathogenic mechanisms. Anaerobe. 2005, 11: 239–46.
Radostits OM, Gay CC, Blood DC, Hinchcliff KW eds. Veterinary Medicine: A Textbook of Diseases of Cattle, Sheep, Pigs, Goats and Horses, 9th ed. London: Saunders, 2000, pp. 961–2.
Smith BP. Large Animal Internal Medicine, 5th ed. St. Louis: Elsevier Mosby, 2015, pp. 580–1.
Tan ZL, Nagaraja TG, Chengappa MM. *Fusobacterium necrophorum* infections: virulence factors, pathogenic mechanism and control measures. Vet Res Commun 1996, 20: 113–40.

Authors Erik J. Olson, Jim P. Reynolds, and Nicholas A. Robinson
Consulting Editor Erica C. McKenzie

C

BASICS

OVERVIEW
• With a few exceptions, camel diseases are similar those of domestic ruminants. Diagnostic approach is also similar, although physical examination and interpretation of laboratory data may present some challenges for veterinarians not familiar with these species. • Some diseases of critical importance to camel production are region specific (e.g., trypanosomiasis, theileriosis, hemorrhagic disease, tuberculosis, brucellosis, camel pox).

INCIDENCE/PREVALENCE
• Incidence of various infectious diseases in countries where camels are important production animals shows that the most important are: trypanosomiasis, brucellosis, camel pox, gastrointestinal and external parasites, hydatidosis, caseous lymphadenitis (*Corynebacterium pseudotubeculosis*), clostridial diseases, mastitis, and tuberculosis. • Neonatal and juvenile disorders are dominated by infectious enteritis (collibacillosis, salmonellosis), respiratory disorders (pasteurellosis), and parasite infestation (coccidiosis). • In a Jordanian study, intestinal parasite ova were detected in 98% of camels; one or more species of external parasites were found on the skin of all camels; 33% of animals had nasal myiasis; and hydatid cysts were identified in 44% of the slaughtered animals. Sarcoptic mange (*Sarcoptes scabiei* var. cameli) and trypanosomiasis were diagnosed in 83% and 33% of examined camels, respectively. Rabies virus was detected in eight camels by fluorescent antibody examination. • Noninfectious diseases are dominated by nutritional deficiencies (selenium deficiency, energy and protein deficiency) and foreign body accumulation within the first and second stomach compartments.

GEOGRAPHIC DISTRIBUTION
• Worldwide, specific diseases vary depending on environment and management. • Regional differences exist and depend on environment, type of management (nomadic vs. sedentary), and epidemiologic situation.

SYSTEMS AFFECTED
Multisystemic

PHYSIOPATHOLOGY
Pathophysiologic processes for specific disease are similar to those described for ruminants.

HISTORICAL FINDINGS
• The ability to obtain a thorough history depends on the type of management. Nomadic herds are particularly challenging. Individual animals or specialized operations (dairies, individual pleasure animals, racing animals) may have a more complete history.

• History should take into account any animal movement, environment and management.

SIGNALMENT
• Both species of *Camelus* (dromedary camel or *C. dromedarius*, Bactrian camel or *C. bactrianus*) are affected by the same diseases. • Racing animals are more predisposed to gastrointestinal and renal disorders as well as musculoskeletal problems. • Dairy camels are more predisposed to hypocalcemia, mastitis, and postpartum disorders. • Neonates and juvenile animals are predisposed to infectious or gastrointestinal problems.

PHYSICAL EXAMINATION FINDINGS
Physical examination is similar to that of other large animal species. The process starts with a thorough history, signalment, and management.

Temperature
• Camel body temperature is affected by ambient temperature, state of hydration, and seasonal variations. • Morning rectal temperature may vary between 35.5 and 37.5°C while afternoon temperature varies between 38.5 and 41°C. • Young camels (<6 months) have a 0.5 to 1.0°C higher rectal temperature than adults. • Temperatures >39°C should be considered suspect and indicative of fever on cool days or when taken in the morning.

Respiratory Frequency
• Determined by visual observation, palpation of the chest or flank or auscultation. • In cool environments respiratory frequency is 5 to 8 breaths per minute. • On hot summer days respiratory frequency increases to 10 to 12 per minute.

Pulse
• Heart rate is best determined by auscultation. • Normal resting heart rate is 30 to 36 beats per minute. • Heart rate may increase to 40 to 44 bpm in excited animals. • Heart rates above 45 bpm are significant findings in febrile animals or animal with severe pain or intoxication.

CRT and Mucus Membrane Color
Evaluated similarly to ruminants. It may be difficult to appreciate in pigmented animals.

Lymph Nodes
The major lymph nodes can be palpated for reaction as in cattle. The palpable external lymph nodes include the parotid, maxillary, prescapular (superficial cervical), inferior cervical, thoracic, cubital, ilial, and popliteal.

Symptoms
• A systemic disease state may be suspected if the animal has poor appetite and reduced activity. • Specific clinical signs depend on the disease, but sick camels often display a depressed look and prolonged sternal or lateral recumbence. Increased lacrimation is often observed.

GENETICS
There are differences in disease incidence between dairy camels and racing or riding camels.

CAUSES AND RISK FACTORS
Common causes of disease in camels include • Viral (camel pox, rabies) • Bacterial (brucellosis, hemorrhagic disease, anthrax, salmonellosis, tuberculosis, caseous lymphadenitis) • Parasites (trypanosomiasis, coccidiosis, echinococcosis, helminths) • Nutritional: selenium deficiency
Risk factors include
• Geographic location, age, type of management, animal concentration

DIAGNOSIS

DIFFERENTIAL DIAGNOSES
Abdominal Pain (Colicky Syndrome)
• Abdominal pain is recognized by behavioral changes such as excessive rolling, kicking at the belly, stretching or overextension of the hind legs, loss of appetite or selective eating and vocalization. • Severe pain is generally accompanied by an increased heart rate and reluctance to rise or move. • The most common reasons for abdominal pain in camels include: ○ Impeding abortion, parturition or dystocia (uterine torsion) ○ Gastrointestinal obstruction; can occur at any level of the GI tract (e.g., sand impaction, fecolith/enterolith, intestinal torsion, volvulus or intussusception) ○ Gastric ulcers ○ Traumatic reticulitis/pericarditis ○ Rumen acidosis/grain overload ○ Rumen tympany, bloat ○ Enteritis ○ Peritonitis ○ Nephritis ○ Urolithiasis (males)

Abortion and Early Pregnancy Loss
• Trypanosomiasis • Brucellosis • Q-fever • Chlamydia • Toxoplasmosis • Neosporosis • Twining • Starvation • Iatrogenic (prostaglandin F 2 alpha, steroidal anti-inflammatory drugs) • Trauma

Anemia
• Heavy parasitism (e.g., coccidiosis, trypanosomiasis, haemonchosis, tick infestation) • Theileriosis • Chronic illnesses such as paratuberculosis and neoplasia • Bleeding disorder; ulcers, trauma, coagulopathy

Coughing/Dyspnea
• Dust • Respiratory viral infection/influenza • Pneumonia (bacterial or aspiration) • Camel pox • Hemorrhagic disease • Lung worm • Melioidosis • Tuberculosis • Soft palate trauma, impaction • Nasal bots • Toxoplasmosis • Pneumothorax • Cardiac dysrhythmias

Diarrhea, Adult
• Stress, nervous camels • Dietary • Internal parasites • Paratuberculosis • Salmonellosis

CAMEL DISEASES

C

• Trypanosomiasis (some countries)
• Hemorrhagic septicemia (clostridial)

Diarrhea, Young Animal
• Neonatal viral diarrhea (i.e., rotavirus, coronavirus) • Colibacillosis • Dietary (poor quality milk replacer) • Salmonellosis
• Coccidiosis • Internal parasite

Dysphagia
• Tongue laceration • Fractured mandible
• Tooth abscesses • Lump jaw (actinomycosis)
• Soft palate impaction/trauma in rutting male • Cranial never paralysis • Rabies
• Pharyngitis

Head Tilt
• Ear infections • Wry neck (torticollis, often traumatic) • Head injuries

Lacrimation/Photophobia
• Keratoconjunctivitis • Corneal ulcers
• Myasis • Occluded nasolacrimal duct

Lameness
• Arthritis (common in old animals particularly in wet areas) • Upward fixation of the patella • Racing or riding camel myopathy
• White muscle disease • Sole ulcers
• Pododermatitis • Cracked or worn foot pads
• Fractures • Tendonitis (racing or working camels)

Nasal Discharge
• Nasal bots, rhinitis • Camel pox • Head trauma • Hemorrhagic disease

Neurologic Signs
• Polioencephalomalacia • Hemorrhagic disease • Head trauma • Meningitis
• Envenomation • Anthrax • Botulism
• Rabies

Skin Diseases
• Contagious ecthyma • Camel pox • Various ectoparasite (mange, tick infestation)
• Dermatophilosis • Ring worm
• *Corynebacterium pseudotuberculosis* abscesses

Sudden Death
• Heart failure • Vitamin E/selenium deficiency • Monensin toxicosis • Anaphylaxis
• Enterotoxaemia • Botulism

Weight Loss/Failure to Thrive
• Failure of passive transfer • Malnutrition
• Vitamin E/selenium deficiency • Heavy parasitism • Chronic diseases (paratuberculosis, renal failure) • Dysphagia (due to swollen soft palate or teeth abscesses, broken jaw)

Common Infectious Diseases
• Rinderpest • Rift Valley fever • Pasteurellosis
• Rabies • Anthrax • Tuberculosis • Camel pox
• Contagious ecthyma • Ringworm
• Staphylococcal dermatitis (contagious skin necrosis) • Dermatophilosis • Hemorrhagic disease (*Bacillus cereus* intoxication) • Tetanus
• Lymphadenitis (*Corynebacterium pseudotuberculosis*) • Brucellosis (abortion, orchitis) • Leptospirosis • Q fever

Common Parasitic Diseases
• Mange • Tick infestation (tick paralysis)
• Lice • Nasal bots (*Cephalipina titilator*)
• Lungworms (*Dictyocaulus* filarial, *D. viviparous*) • Hydatidosis (echinococcosis, hydatid cysts) • Coccidiosis

Common Nutritional/Metabolic Disease
• Hypocalcemia (retained placenta, uterine prolapse) • Grain overload/acidosis
• Hyperlipemia (pregnancy toxemia)
• Vitamin A deficiency • White muscle disease (selenium and vitamin E deficiency)
• Hypomagnesemia • Cooper deficiency

CBC/BIOCHEMSTRY/URINALYSIS
• Blood samples can be easily collected from the jugular vein. • Interpretation of CBC and blood biochemistry should take into account age and state of hydration of the animal (see Table 1 for reference ranges). • Urine production is highly variable. Samples are collected by free catch in males or females or by catheterization in the female. ○ Urine is clear and pale yellow. ○ Specific gravity varies from 1.020 to 1.070 and depends on the degree of hydration. ○ Urine pH ranges from 6 to 7 in resting animals and 8 to 9 after effort (work, racing). ○ Other constituents: Urea 0.18 to 3.6 g/dL (1.95±0.38 g/dL), uric acid 60.41 ±10.46 mg/dL, creatinine 0.58 ± 0.128 g/L, chloride (4.5 ± 1.3 g/dL), phosphate (1.71 ± 0.22 mg/dL), sulfate (77.6 ± 12.4 mg/dL). ○ Protein is low (1+) but increases after prolonged exercise.
○ Calcium oxalate, calcium hydrogen phosphate, ammonium urate, and triple phosphate may also be present in up to 30% of the samples.

OTHER LABORATORY TESTS
• Fecal analysis: Fecal balls should be well-formed, shiny and free of mucus. Diarrhea may be a response to high stress or training. ○ Obstruction should be suspected if no feces are produced in a 24 hour period.
○ Fecal sample should be taken from a fresh defecation or removed from the rectum.
○ Feces can be analyzed for parasite eggs using the standard methods. • Serology and microbiology are indicated if specific infectious diseases are suspected.

IMAGING
• Transabdominal ultrasonography is very helpful in colic or reproductive problems.
• Percutaneous flank ultrasonography for renal disorders. • Percutaneous thoracic ultrasonography for lung evaluation.
• Transrectal ultrasonography for urogenital and caudal GI evaluation. • Radiography, computed tomography, and ultrasonography are used for musculoskeletal disorders.

OTHER DIAGNOSTIC PROCEDURES
• Serology for disease testing • Skin biopsy

PATHOLOGIC FINDINGS
Pathologic findings depend on cause and course of the disease.

TREATMENT

THERAPEUTIC APPROACH
Depends on the diagnosis but is generally similar to that applied to bovine and other camelids.

SURGICAL CONSIDERATIONS AND TECHNIQUES
Depends on the diagnosis but is generally similar to that applied to bovine and camelid with some adjustment of medication choices and doses.

MEDICATIONS
• Information on the pharmacokinetics of common veterinary drugs in camels is limited.
• There are no established withdrawal times for pharmaceuticals used in camels. It is important to keep in mind that camels are food-producing animals (milk and meat) in many areas of the world.

Antimicrobials
• Most antimicrobials used in veterinary medicine have been used in camels without any overt adverse effects. • In general the route of administration and dosage are based on recommended guidelines for the bovine.
• Sulfonamides are safe in the camel due to the lower degree of acetylation compared with domestic ruminants. Sulfadimidine or sulfamethoxypyridazine are used at the dose of 55–70 mg/kg bw IV q24h. • Penicillin G dosage: 10,000–20,000 IU per kg bw, SQ or IM, q24h. • Long-acting penicillin (Procaine penicillin 150 mg/mL and benzathine penicillin 115 mg/mL) 20–30 mL/500 kg q72h. • Ampicillin: 4–8 mg/kg bw IV, q24h.
• Enrofloxacin 1.6–3 mg/kg bw, q12h (oral solution is used at 2.5 mg/kg). maximum dose of 5 mg/kg is used in cases of pasteurellosis or salmonellosis.
• Oxytetracycline: 5–10 mg/kg bw IM q24h; long-acting tetracycline can be used at 20 mg/kg q48h. • Chloramphenicol: 10–30 mg/kg bw IM, q12h (not approved in many countries; illegal in Canada and the United States). • Streptomycin: 8 mg/kg bw IM, q12h. • Rifampin and erythromycin have also been used in camels for specific conditions at the same dosage and length of treatment as equines. • Gentamycin 3–4 mg/kg bw IM, q12h. Gentamycin is known to be extremely nephrotoxic in young camels and dehydrated animals. • Tylosin 10 mg/kg bw q8h.
• Metronidazole: 5–10 mg/kg • Griseofulvin: 0.25 g/45 kg (not available in some countries; illegal for use in Canada and US).
• Trimethoprim (2.7 mg/kg bw)/Sulfadiazine (13.3 mg/kg bw) daily IM or IV.

Table 1

Hematologic and Serum Biochemistry References Values for Camels (Abu Dhabi Veterinary Research Center)			
Parameter (unit)	Neonate at birth	Neonate after colostrum intake	Adult
White blood cells ($\times 10^3$/µL)	13.9 ± 0.3	12.9 ± 0.3	7–18
Neutrophils (%)	—	—	35–60
Lymphocytes (%)	—	—	30–60
Monocytes (%)			<4
Eosinophils (%)			<6
Basophils (%)			Rare
Red blood cells ($\times 10^6$/µL)	14.0 ± 0.1	14.2 ± 0.2	7–13
Hemoglobin (g/dL)	45.1 ± 01	45.5 ±0.2	10–17
PCV (%)	31.1 ± 0.3	31.1 ±0.3	25–36
Mean Cell Volume (fL)	30.8 ± 0.7	27.7 ± 0.8	27–33
MCH (pg)	9.9 ± 0.2	8.9 ± 0.2	12.5–15
MCHC (g/dL)	26.1 ± 1.1	21.9 ± 1.1	44–55
Platelets ($\times 10^3$/µL)	—	—	240–320
GOT/AST (IU/L)	55.4 ± 5.2	95.7 ± 20.5	40–120
LDH-L (IU/L)	368 ± 31	664 ± 104	275–450
CK (IU/L)	307.2 ±57.2	154.1 ± 26.8	40–120
Gamma GT(IU/L)	12.4 ± 1.2	67.4 ± 13.1	3–25
SGPT/ALT (IU/L)	5.8 ± 0.7	12.7 ± 3.5	3–20
ALP (IU/L)	3324 ± 436	3381± 579	114–406
Creatine (mg/dL)	3.7 ± 0.9	1.8 ± 0.1	1.1–2.2
BUN (mg/dL)	25.7 ± 1.2	18.3 ±0.1	5–21
Total Protein (g/dL)	4.4 ± 0.1	5.2 ±0.2	5.5–7.8
Albumin (g/dL)	3.0 ± 0.1	2.6 ± 0.1	3.0–4.8
Globulin (g/dL)	1.4 ± 0.1	2.6 ± 0.1	1.7–3.0
Glucose (mg/dL)	60–150	60–130	60–130
Fibrinogen (mg/dL)	—	—	250–300
Iron (µg/dl)	20.6.4 ± 16.7	75.7 ± 14.1	82–135
Calcium (mg/dL)	11.2 ± 0.3	9.7 ± 0.5	8.5–11
Magnesium (mg/dL)	—	—	1.8–2.9
Phosphorus (mg/dL)	—		3.9–6.8
Sodium (mmol/L)			129–161
Potassium (mmol/L)	—	—	2.9–5.9
Chloride (mmol/L)	—	—	114–120
pH	—	—	7.3–7.8

Anthelmintics and Other Antiparasitic Drugs

• All types of bovine anthelmintics can be used safely in camels at the same or slightly higher dosage. • Levamisole has been reported ineffective and possibly toxic in camels.
• Oral: albendazole 7.5 mg/kg, oxfendazole 5–7.5 mg/kg, fenbendazole (6–7.5 mg/kg, morantel tartrate 35 g/500 kg bw).
• Subcutaneous: ivermectin (0.2 mg/kg), moxidectin 0.15 mg /kg bw (helminths, suckling lice, and mange mites). • Pour On: ivermectin 5 mg/10 kg bw. • Monensin is very toxic and can be fatal in camels.

Antiinflammatory Drugs

• Methylpredinosolone: 200 mg IM for allergic reactions in adult camel; can cause abortion in the last half of pregnancy.
• Dexamethasone: same dose as the bovine. Do not use in pregnant animals.

• Flunixin meglumine: 1 mg /kg IV q24h.
• Phenylbutazone: use with care in food-producing animals.

Hormones

• Progesterone: 100 mg/day for synchronization of follicular waves (14 days) and for maintenance of pregnancy (throughout pregnancy). • HCG: induction of ovulation 1,500–3,000 IU IV. • $PGF2_\alpha$ and analogues: dinoprost (25–35 mg, IM), cloprostenol (500–750 µg, IM). • Oxytocin: 5–20 IU for milk letdown, 20–40 IU for retained placenta, IM or IV. • GnRH: buserelin 10 µg, for induction of ovulation.

Sedatives and Anesthetics

• Propofol: 2 mg/kg alone or 0.25–1 mg/kg if premedicated with xylazine and valium.
• Detomidine: 0.01–0.08 mg/kg bw, IM or slow IV. • Ketamine: 2–5 mg/kg in association with xylazine. • Reserpine for long-distance transport 1.5–2 mg initially and then on alternate days. • Xylazine: 0.2–1 mg/kg (reversed by yohimbine hydrochloride 0.125 mg/kg IV mixed with 4-aminopyridine 0.3 mg/kg).

Other drugs

• Polysulfated glycosaminoglycan, glucosamine, chondroitin: see horse dosage.
• Vitamin B complex for polioencephalomalacia, same dosage as for the bovine. • Anti-diarrhea agents: use same product and dosage as for the bovine.
• Laxatives: methylcellulose, magnesium sulfate, same dosage as for the bovine.
• Diuretics: furosemide 0.25–1 mg/kg in the adult. • Topical ointments: similar dosages as in cattle. • Buparvaquone, treatment of theileriosis (125 mg/kg bw, IM repeat in 48–72h if necessary). • Trypanocide: bis(aminoethylthio)-4 metaminophenylarsine dihydrochloride (Cymelarsan®): 25 mg/100 kg bw IM, safe in pregnant animals.

CAMEL DISEASES

C

CONTRAINDICATIONS
• Appropriate milk and meat withdrawal times must be followed. • Levamisole has been reported ineffective and possibly toxic in camels. • Ionophores (monensin) are toxic to camels.

PRECAUTIONS
• Be aware of nephrotoxic drugs. • Individual reactiosn have been observed with some antibiotics and trypanocides.

POSSIBLE INTERACTIONS
Depend on drugs

FOLLOW-UP

EXPECTED COURSE AND PROGNOSIS
• Varies depending on disease. Prognosis is often guarded in major outbreaks of camel pox, trypanosomiasis, brucellosis, and tuberculosis. • Herd nutritional and parasite problems have a favorable prognosis if treatment plan and corrective measured are developed early. • Individual cases may justify advanced medical treatment when animals are very valuable (breeding males, racing animals, embryo transfer donors).

POSSIBLE COMPLICATIONS
Dependent on disease

CLIENT EDUCATION
• Proper nutrition and health care • Early recognition of signs of illness

PATIENT CARE
Dependent on disease or disorder

PREVENTION
• Major contagious disease should be monitored by regular testing and elimination of positive animals. • Implement a thorough herd health, nutrition and immunization program that is appropriate for the region. • Regular deworming and treatment against external parasites.

MISCELLANEOUS

ASSOCIATED CONDITIONS
Depends on disorder

AGE-RELATED FACTORS
• Depends on disorders

ZOONOTIC POTENTIAL
Brucellosis, Q fever, rabies, anthrax, camel pox, toxoplasma, *Salmonella* spp., contagious ecthyma, ringworm, and tuberculosis are zoonotic diseases.

PREGNANCY
• Methylprednisolone causes abortion in the last half of pregnancy. • Dexamethasone: Do not use in pregnant animals.

BIOSECURITY
• Testing and quarantine of new animals • Segregation of breeding stock from performance or show animals • Regular testing of farm hands (tuberculosis) • Reduce movement of animals and humans between herds

PRODUCTION MANAGEMENT
N/A

SYNONYMS
N/A

ABBREVIATIONS
• BPM = beats per minute
• BW = body weight
• GI = gastrointestinal
• IM = intramuscular
• IV = intravenous
• SQ = subcutaneous

SEE ALSO
• Body Condition Scoring: Camels (see www.fiveminutevet.com/ruminant)
• Camel Management and Health Programs
• Camelid: Reproduction
• Trypanosomiasis

Suggested Reading
Manefield GW, Tinson AH. Camels: A compendium. The TG Hungerford Vade Mecum Series for Domestic Animals, University of Sydney Post Graduate Foundation, Sydney NSW, Australia, 1997.
Wernery U, Fowler ME, Wernery R. Color Atlas of Camelid Hematology. Blackwell Wissenschafts-Verlag Berlin, Wien, 1999.
Wernery U, Kinne J, Schuster EK. Camelid infectious diseases. OII (World Organization for Animal Health) Publication. Paris France, 2014.

Author Ahmed Tibary
Consulting Editor Ahmed Tibary

CAMEL MANAGEMENT AND HEALTH PROGRAMS

BASICS

OVERVIEW
• Camels belong to the family Camelidae, genus: *Camelus*, species *C. dromedarius* (dromedary camel) and *C. bactrianus* (Bactrian camel).
• Some *C. bactrianus* populations or subspecies are endangered.
• *C. dromedarius* and *C. bactrianus* can interbreed and produce a fertile first generation.
• Mature weight in males and females varies from 600–750 kg and 450–650 kg, respectively.
• Birthweights vary according to breeds (dromedary: 30–45 kg, Bactrian: 35–55 kg).
• Camel production systems include intensive sedentary and nomadic herds. Milk, meat, hair, and hide are the main products. Camels are also used for draught, transportation, and riding. Camel racing is a highly specialized business in the Middle East.
• Dairy camels can produce 3–10 kg of milk/day with some breeds in intensive production systems reaching 25 kg/day. Lactation length varies between 300 and 450 days with a total production of 2,500–5,000 kg (8,000–10,000 in high-producing breeds).
• Carcass dressing percentage averages 40% (some breeds may reach 77% at young age).
• Fiber production: 2.5–4.5 kg/year for dromedaries, 5–15 kg/year for Bactrians.

INCIDENCE/PREVALENCE
Incidence of disease depends on region and production system.

GEOGRAPHIC DISTRIBUTION
• Dromedary: Northern and Saharan Africa, Middle East, India, Pakistan, and Australia (feral).
• Bactrian camel: Central Asia and Iran.

SYSTEMS AFFECTED
Multisystemic

PATHOPHYSIOLOGY
• Production camel medicine is an evolving field as production systems are changing from nomadic production to intensive sedentary production.
• Herd production medicine approach is similar to beef cattle for camel meat production and dairy cattle for dairy camels.
• Herd preventive medicine has focused on immunization against the major infectious diseases and preventive treatment against internal and external parasites. Nutritional requirements have not yet been fully studied and adapted to production systems.
• The major production-limiting diseases are: neonatal losses, trypanosomiasis, brucellosis, tuberculosis, camel pox, nutritional deficiencies, and poor reproductive performances (infertility and abortion).

Nutritional Requirements
• Camels are browsers
• The voluntary food intake of camels is about 50–75% that of cattle.
• Dry matter intake is 1.5–1.7% of body weight per day.
• Maintenance energy requirements are estimated to be 75–90 kcal ME per $kg^{0.75}$ daily.
• Maintenance protein requirements are estimated to be 320–370 mg DP per $kg^{0.75}$ daily.
• Camels have an extremely efficient urea recycling ability and they are better equipped than other ruminants to handle protein-deficient diets.
• To allow for energy-protein interactions, the recommended "allowances" for maintenance would be 104 kcal ME and 368 mg DP per $kg^{0.75}$ daily.
• Various feed sources have been used in camels including green alfalfa, barley, Rhodes grass, commercial pellets and mixed grains.
• Traditional systems are based mainly on pasture with a little supplementation with grass or alfalfa hay.
• Grass and alfalfa hay mix is sufficient nutritionally provided that animals have access to mineral and vitamin supplementation.
• Intake should be increased by 25% during the last 3 months of pregnancy and the first 8 weeks of lactation.
• Working camels (600 kg) in traditional management (India) generally receive 9–18 kg of green feed, 7 kg of straw or hay, and 2 kg of grain per day.

Minerals, Trace Elements, and Vitamins
• Copper deficiency has been reported. Normal plasma level is comparable to cattle (70–120 mg/100 mL). Camels are more tolerant to copper excess than sheep and goats. However, death has resulted following intakes of 200 mg of copper daily for 8 days.
• Camels appear to maintain lower zinc levels than other ruminants (<60 µg/100 mL).
• Zn and Cu requirements can be maintained by as little as 15–20 mg $CuSO_4$ and 18–20 mg of $ZnSO_4$. However, up to 100 mg $CuSO_4$ and 750 mg of $ZnSO_4$ has been suggested by some authors.
• Vitamin E and selenium deficiency (white muscle disease) can be a serious problem in camels. Daily allowance should be 100 mg for vitamin E and 0.1–0.5 mg/kg of diet for selenium.
• Camels appear to be more sensitive to iodine deficiency than domestic ruminants.
• Crystalline salt is often fed ad lib (120–150 g per day).
• No data is available for cobalt status in camels.
• Thiamine deficiency/polioencephalomalacia have been described.

Reproductive Management
• Camels have a slow reproductive rate due to a delayed age at puberty (2 and 3 years of age for females, 3 and 4 years of age for males) and a long lactation anestrus (one year if the calf is not weaned).
• Breeding season depends on nutrition in both the female and the male and on temperature in the male. Males enter the rutting season in the fall through the spring.
• Male to female ratio ranges from 1:15 to 1:50.

Calf Management
• In nomadic herding systems, calves wean themselves at 15–18 months of age. Calves are generally allowed to nurse (in a controlled manner) so that the female can also be used for human milk supply.
• Early weaning, at 3 months, is used in some areas to increase reproductive ability (i.e., decrease the length of lactational anestrus).
• Weaning can be done as early as 2 days postpartum and calves are raised on milk replacers. (The author has used equine and bovine milk replacers successfully.)
• Calves should be introduced to solid food by 4 weeks of age. Creep feeding should contain 12% good-quality hay.

HISTORICAL FINDINGS
Poorly managed herds present the following features:
• Poor reproduction rate: <70% calving rate due to infertility, early or late pregnancy loss
• Poor weaning rate and weight: Neonatal losses >10% (may reach in some instance up to 50%)
• High morbidity and mortality
• Poor BCS

PHYSICAL EXAMINATION FINDINGS
• Docile/trained adult camels may be examined in horse stocks and will tolerate with minimal discomfort procedures such as transrectal palpation.
• Untrained animals should be examined while hobbled in a sternal (cush) position. Sedation may still be required for some procedures.
• Young calves (<6 months) can be restrained by two persons.
• Sedation: Xylazine, detomidine or xylazine and butorphanol. Combination of xylazine with ketamine is useful in untrained or feral animals.
• Vaginal examination or minor surgeries (e.g., draining abscesses, castration, vulvar sutures, and suture of superficial lacerations) require a combination of sedation and physical restraint.
• In the dromedary a simple method for estimation of body weight is:
  ○ Weight (kg) = height at the shoulder (m) × chest girth (m) × body girth at the hump (m) × 50
• Management and examination of the camel neonate is similar to other domestic species.

CAMEL MANAGEMENT AND HEALTH PROGRAMS   (CONTINUED)

○ Normal birthweights vary from 26 to 52 kg depending on the breed of camel and nutrition.

○ Camel calves should be able to stand and nurse on their own within the first hour after birth.

○ Urination and passage of meconium should be observed in the first 24 hours after birth.

○ Colostrum (10–15% of body weight) should be taken in the first 18 hours of life. Passive transfer can be verified by camelid RAPD or by total protein.

○ Administration of vitamin E and selenium is recommended at 3 days of age and again at weaning.

Common Physical Findings in Neonates

• *Congenital defects:* goiter, umbilical hernia, angular limb deformities, atria ani, ventricular septal defect, cleft palate

• *Common problems of the first 48 hours:*
  ○ Prematurity (extreme laxity, small birthweight)
  ○ Inability to nurse (dysmaturity "dummy")
  ○ Hypothermia (exposure, hypoglycemia, weak calf, septicemia)
  ○ Hyperthermia (exposure, septicemia)
  ○ Colic (meconium impaction, atresia coli, ruptured bladder)

Physical Findings in Lactating Females

• In traditionally managed herds the interval between calving is in the range 18–36 months (average 2 years).

• Early weaning reduces the calving interval by decreasing lactational anestrus.

• Agalactia is seen sometime in maiden females.

• Mastitis is a major production disease. Diagnosis and treatment are based on the same principles used in cattle.

GENETICS

Dairy camels are more susceptible to postpartum disorders (hypocalcemia, uterine prolapse, retained placenta) and mastitis.

SIGNALMENT
N/A

CAUSES AND RISK FACTORS
N/A

DIAGNOSIS

DIFFERENTIAL DIAGNOSES

Herd disease investigation requires a systematic approach based on historical data, clinical signs, and epidemiology of specific diseases in the region.

CBC/BIOCHEMSTRY/URINALYSIS

CBC and biochemistry on a subset of animals may be helpful in detection of trypanosomiasis and severe mineral deficiencies.

OTHER LABORATORY TESTS

• Periodic fecal analysis for parasitology
• Serology for the major diseases (brucellosis, trypanosomiasis, camel pox, chlamydiosis, Q fever)
• Neonates: IgG or total protein for determination of passive transfer of immunity
• Lactating animals: California mastitis test (CMT) and somatic cell count to monitor mastitis

IMAGING
N/A

OTHER DIAGNOSTIC PROCEDURES
N/A

PATHOLOGIC FINDINGS
Depend on disorder investigated

TREATMENT

THERAPEUTIC APPROACH

• External and internal parasites can be controlled or prevented using the same strategies devised for domestic ruminants.

• Strategies should be developed for the specific geographic region.

• Most drugs used in cattle can be used at the same dosage in camels for the control of most parasites.

• Injectable ivermectin is efficacious on most external and internal parasites in camels, but injection site reactions are common.

• Ionophores are very toxic in camelids.

SURGICAL CONSIDERATIONS AND TECHNIQUES

• The most common surgical technique in camels is castration. It may be performed as early as 6 months of age but most breeders will wait until 2 years. Standing and recumbent techniques are used depending on tractability. Methods of castration are similar to those used in the bovine for calves or equine for adults.

• Racing intact males are subjected to palatectomy (surgical excision of the soft palate) to improve breathing. Surgery is performed under heavy sedation or injectable anesthesia with xylaxine and ketamine.

  ○ The oral cavity is washed with a weak antiseptic solution and a mouth gag is placed with the tongue exteriorized to one side.

  ○ The soft palate is grasped with long forceps and exteriorized, then clamped as close to the base as possible. Large blood vessels are cauterized and the soft palate is excised.

  ○ Postoperative care includes long-acting antibiotics (3–4 days), anti-inflammatories and fasting for 24 hours. Soft feed (mash or chopped fresh alfalfa) is given for 2–3 days. Animals should be monitored for a few days for dysphagia.

MEDICATION

DRUGS OF CHOICE

• Sedation and anesthesia
  ○ Xylazine 0.25–0.5 mg/kg IM (0.1–0.25 mg/kg IV)
  ○ Ketamine (3–5 mg/kg, IV) with xylazine
  ○ Detomidine (25–75 μg/kg, IV)
  ○ Butorphanol (0.05–0.1 mg/kg, IM).

• Antiparasites: similar to bovine, do not use ionophores.

• Antibiotics: similar to bovine, avoid aminoglycosides.

CONTRAINDICATIONS

Appropriate milk and meat withdrawal times must be followed for food-producing animals.

PRECAUTIONS
N/A

POSSIBLE INTERACTIONS
N/A

FOLLOW-UP

EXPECTED COURSE AND PROGNOSIS
N/A

POSSIBLE COMPLICATIONS
N/A

CLIENT EDUCATION

Work with veterinarian to design a herd health program.

PATIENT CARE
N/A

PREVENTION

Mandatory Vaccines

• Clostridial vaccines (*C. tetani, C. perfringens* types A, B, C, D, *Cl. chauvoei, septicum, novyi*) initially given at 2–3 months of age, booster 4 weeks later and then annual re-vaccination is recommended.

• *C. perfringens* types C and D and *C. tetani* (tetanus toxoid) (combined as CDT vaccine) should be given to pregnant females 4–6 weeks prior to parturition.

• Rabies vaccination at 3 months, booster in 4 weeks, then annual re-vaccination is recommended.

• Anthrax (*Bacillus anthracis*) at 2–3 months and then annually in endemic countries **(considered a foreign disease in some countries)**.

• Camel pox (Orthopoxvirus): Vaccinate at 6 months of age and booster 4 weeks later. Adults are given 2 injections before 4 years of age. Lifelong immunity develops **(considered a foreign disease in some countries)**.

Optional Vaccines

• Leptospirosis (5-way) may need to repeat vaccination 3–4 times per year.

• *E. coli* (for calf diarrhea), oral for calves in the first 10 days of life, pregnant females 6–8 weeks prior to parturition.
• Salmonella: oral for calves in the first 10 days of life; pregnant females 6–8 weeks prior to parturition.
• Neonatal viral diarrhea (i.e., rotavirus, coronavirus): Dams are vaccinated 4 and 2 weeks before parturition.
• Botulism (*Clostridium botulinum* types C and D) may be indicated.

MISCELLANEOUS

ASSOCIATED CONDITIONS
N/A

AGE-RELATED FACTORS
N/A

ZOONOTIC POTENTIAL
• MERS (Middle East respiratory syndrome) due to coronavirus
• Brucellosis (*B. meletensii* and *B. abortus*)
• Q fever (*Coxiella burnetii*)
• Tuberculosis
• Anthrax

PREGNANCY
• Pregnancy diagnosis is performed by teasing at 14 days post breeding.
• Pregnancy length varies from 340 to 412 days (majority between 375 and 395 days).
  ○ The factors affecting pregnancy length are season and nutrition.

○ Adjusting nutrition in the last trimester of pregnancy and booster vaccination improves neonatal survival.

BIOSECURITY
• Test personnel for tuberculosis (dairy camels).
• Avoid comingling with unknown herds.
• Quarantine all newly introduced animals.
• Separate performance animals from breeding stock.
• Regularly test for trypanosomiasis, brucellosis, and tuberculosis.

PRODUCTION MANAGEMENT
• Working camels (600 kg) in traditional management (India) generally receive 9–18 kg of green feed, 7 kg of straw or hay, and 2 kg of grain per day.
• External and internal parasites can be controlled or prevented using the same strategies devised for domestic ruminants.
• Strategies should be developed for a specific geographic region and based on the most commonly found parasite using suitable pharmaceuticals.

SYNONYMS
N/A

ABBREVIATIONS
• CDT = clostridial vaccine combining types C and D with tetanus toxoid
• CMT = California mastitis test
• DP = digestible protein
• IM = intramuscular
• IV = intravenous
• ME = metabolizable energy
• RAPD = random amplified polymorphic DNA analysis

SEE ALSO
• Body Condition Scoring: Camels (see www.fiveminutevet.com/ruminant)
• Breeding Soundness Examination: Camelids
• Camel Diseases
• Camelid: Reproduction
• Castration/Vasectomy: Camelid
• Testicular Disorders: Camelid
• Trypanosomiasis

Suggested Reading
Higgins AJ, Kock RA. A guide to the clinical examination, chemical restraint and medication of the camel. Br Vet J 1984, 140: 485–504.
Kamber R, Farah Z, Rusch P, Hassig M. Studies on the supply of immunoglobulin G to newborn camel calves (*Camelus dromedarius*). J Dairy Res 2001, 68: 1–7.
Tefera M. Observations on the clinical examination of the camel (*Camelus dromedarius*) in the field. Trop Anim Health Prod 2004, 36: 435–49.
Tibary A, Anouassi A, Sghiri A. Factors affecting reproductive performance of camels at the herd and individual level. In: Faye B, Esenov P eds, Desertification combat and food safety: the added value of camel producers, Ashkabad, Turkmenistan, 19–21 April 2004. Amsterdam, Netherlands: IOS Press, 2005, pp. 97–114.
Wernery U, Kinne J, Schuster EK. Camelid infectious diseases. OII (World Organization for Animal Health) Publication. Paris France, 2014.

Author Ahmed Tibary
Consulting Editor Ahmed Tibary

CAMELID: DENTISTRY

BASICS

OVERVIEW
Camelids suffer an array of dental diseases, and require routine care. Retained deciduous incisors, incisor malocclusion, and tooth root abscess are more common anomalies. Trimming of fighting teeth in males is a common routine procedure.

INCIDENCE/PREVALENCE
Tooth root abscesses are a common occurrence, particularly in aged camelids. Mandibular molars 1 and 2 are most often affected and maxillary teeth are rarely affected. The incidence in canine teeth appears to be decreasing with change in methods for trimming fighting teeth.

GEOGRAPHIC DISTRIBUTION
Worldwide

SYSTEMS AFFECTED
• Digestive
• Musculoskeletal

PATHOPHYSIOLOGY
• The adult camelid dental formula is: (I 1/3, C 1/1, PM 1-2/1-2, M 3/3) × 2 for 30 to 32 teeth.
• The upper incisors are found caudally in the region of the canine teeth.
• Cheek teeth can be numbered from 1 to 5 (rostral to caudal), or labeled according to the dental chart (PM 1 and PM 2, M 1 to M 3).
• The upper premolars have three roots each; the lower have two roots each.
• The upper molars have four roots each; lower M 1 and M 2 have two roots, M 3 has three roots, but two are fused.
• Dental points on the buccal side of the maxillary cheek teeth and the lingual side of the mandibular cheek teeth are normal due to the orientation of the maxilla and mandible. These are rarely a problem and should not be reduced.
• Retained deciduous incisors occur when eruption of the permanent incisor is misaligned and fails to push out the deciduous tooth. Typically, retained teeth are smaller and rostrally located.
• Incisor malocclusion occurs when the mandibular incisors fail to meet the dental pad. Malocclusion may cause abnormal prehension and abnormal wear of the molars.
• Tooth root abscesses can arise from tooth fracture, gingival penetration, or infundibular decay and infection. Often the source is unknown.
• Periostitis and osteitis of the mandible secondary to tooth root abscesses can spread extensively along the mandibular canal.
• Fighting teeth; the upper I 3 and canine, and lower canines in males, are sharp and used as weapons. Routine trimming is performed to reduce risk of trauma to other animals.

HISTORICAL FINDINGS
N/A

SIGNALMENT
All camelids can be affected; however, retained deciduous incisors are commonly noted in young animals with erupting teeth; incisor malocclusion is most common in adults; and tooth root abscesses rarely occur in animals <12 months of age (median age 5 years).

PHYSICAL EXAMINATION FINDINGS
• Retained deciduous incisors present as smaller incisors located rostral to the permanent teeth.
• Incisor malocclusion creates protrusion of the upper lip and incisors do not meet the dental pad.
• Tooth root abscesses may produce firm swelling of the jaw, drainage of exudates from the mandible or maxilla, reluctance to eat, quidding, abnormal chewing, weight loss, and nasal discharge if the sinus is affected.

GENETICS
N/A

CAUSES AND RISK FACTORS
Tooth root abscesses can arise after tooth fracture, gingival penetration, or infundibular decay and infection.

DIAGNOSIS

DIFFERENTIAL DIAGNOSES
Differentials are most relevant to tooth root abscesses, in which case other possibilities include mandibular osteitis/osteomyelitis, subcutaneous abscessation/cellulitis, fracture, sinusitis, neoplasia, actinomycosis, salivary gland disease, and caseous lymphadenitis.

CBC/BIOCHEMISTRY/URINALYSIS
Mild elevation in white blood cell count may occur in severe chronic tooth root abscesses with chronic periostitis/osteitis.

OTHER LABORATORY TESTS
Culture of exudates may rule in or out other causes of facial swelling in cases of suspected tooth root abscess.

IMAGING
• Radiography or computed tomography (CT) can be used to evaluate bony anomalies of the jaw, including suspected tooth root abscesses. Contrast agent may be injected into a draining tract if the affected root is not obvious, or can be given IV (during CT).
• Imaging helps determine the severity and extent of disease and identifies how many and which specific teeth are involved. Relevant findings can include bone lysis, periodontal sclerosis, abscesses, and fistulous tracts.
• Adequate imaging is particularly critical if surgical interventions are anticipated.

OTHER DIAGNOSTIC PROCEDURES
N/A

PATHOLOGIC FINDINGS
At necropsy, localized purulent exudates, necrotic bone and alveolus, fistulous tracts, loose teeth, and bony proliferation may be apparent in affected areas.

TREATMENT

THERAPEUTIC APPROACH
Medical therapy alone can suffice for treatment of tooth root abscesses; however, surgical interventions are often needed for dental disorders of camelids.

SURGICAL CONSIDERATIONS AND TECHNIQUES
• Retained deciduous incisors are resolved by extraction of the retained teeth. If they are loose they can be readily pulled. Teeth that are more firmly attached may require sedation/anesthesia and the use of a periosteal elevator.
• Incisor malocclusion is resolved by trimming incisors to meet the dental pad. This is best accomplished with a rotary trimmer, and may require sedation.
• Tooth root abscesses can be addressed with medical care, or with surgical intervention followed by medical care. Oral extraction may be appropriate for premolars, canines, and incisors; however, elevation from the alveolus may be difficult via an oral approach due to the limited excursion of the jaws in these species.
  ○ Some curettage of the alveolus will help remove necrotic bone.
  ○ Repulsion of the cheek teeth has also been recommended.
  ○ Care must be taken due to the fragility of the mandible and maxilla, which can be easily fractured.
  ○ Motorized burr has been successful for removal of affected teeth, especially mandibular teeth.
  ○ Incision is made along the ventral or ventrolateral aspect of the mandible, resecting draining fistulas if possible.
  ○ Periosteum and overlying musculature are elevated along the lateral aspect of the mandible to the level of the gingival attachment.
  ○ Following removal of the overlying bone, the tooth and roots are carefully elevated and removed.
  ○ In some cases, resection of the single affected root using the burr can be effective in resolving the problem without complete extraction.
  ○ A ventral opening in the incision is left for drainage, closing the remainder of the incision.
  ○ The empty alveolus can be packed with gauze or acrylic if desired, which may be necessary in the maxilla, but is not necessary in the mandible.

(CONTINUED)

C

○ Following surgery, flushing of the tract with dilute chlorhexidine solution can help remove food particles.
○ Diet changes are not necessary and most animals will begin eating within hours of anesthetic recovery.
• Fighting teeth should be trimmed leaving 2–3 mm above the gum line, which is most safely accomplished with a rotary trimmer and may require sedation.

MEDICATIONS

DRUGS OF CHOICE
• Tooth root abscesses are often treated with anti-inflammatory medications and long-term antibiotics.
• Anti-inflammatory medications can include flunixin meglumine 1.1 mg/kg IV q24h, typically for postsurgical pain.
• Antibiotics that might be appropriate for tooth root abscesses include procaine penicillin G (20,000 U/kg IM, q12h for 5–10 days or longer if indicated); oxytetracycline (200 mg/mL formulation, 18 mg/kg SC, q48h for 5–10 days); ampicillin (11 mg/kg IM, q24h for 5–10 days); and florfenicol (20 mg/kg SQ, q48h for 10 days of treatment).

CONTRAINDICATIONS
• Wire saws can generate excessive heat and damage the pulp cavity of teeth, particularly the incisors.
• Cutting tools may fracture teeth and predispose to tooth root abscesses.
• Nephrotoxic drugs (flunixin, oxytetracycline) are contraindicated in dehydrated or azotemic animals.

PRECAUTIONS
Appropriate milk and meat withdrawal times must be followed for all compounds administered to food-producing animals.

POSSIBLE INTERACTIONS
N/A

FOLLOW-UP

EXPECTED COURSE AND PROGNOSIS
• Retained deciduous incisors, incisor malocclusion, and routine trimming of fighting teeth carry an excellent prognosis.
• Tooth root abscesses often heal over several weeks, though the presence of significant bony infection can reduce the success rate. Surgical removal of an infected tooth generally results in a good prognosis, particularly in short-term disease, though additional abscesses can arise at adjacent teeth if the extent of the disease was not accurately identified at the initial examination.

POSSIBLE COMPLICATIONS
Tooth root abscesses can be affiliated with ongoing osteitis, discomfort, and drainage in spite of treatment.

CLIENT EDUCATION
Instruct clients on signs of dental disease, and good herd management.

PATIENT CARE
Provide a high-quality, palatable diet.

PREVENTION
Avoiding stemmy hay and foxtail contamination may be helpful for tooth root abscesses.

MISCELLANEOUS

ASSOCIATED CONDITIONS
N/A

AGE-RELATED FACTORS
N/A

ZOONOTIC POTENTIAL
N/A

PREGNANCY
N/A

BIOSECURITY
N/A

PRODUCTION MANAGEMENT
Regular assessment of body condition and dental health of animals in the herd can help facilitate identification of animals with dental issues.

SYNONYMS
N/A

ABBREVIATIONS
• C = canine teeth
• CT = computed tomography
• I = incisor teeth
• IM = intramuscular
• IV = intravenous
• M = molar teeth
• PM = premolar teeth
• SC = subcutaneous

SEE ALSO
• Body Condition Scoring: Alpacas and Llamas (see www.fiveminutevet.com/ruminant)
• Body Condition Scoring: Camels (see www.fiveminutevet.com/ruminant)

Suggested Reading
Cebra C, Anderson DE, Tibary A, Van Saun RJ, Johnson L. Surgical Disorders in Llama and Alpaca Care, 1st ed. St. Louis: Elsevier, 2014, pp. 725–30.
Cebra ML, Cebra CK, Garry FB. Tooth root abscesses in New World camelids: 23 cases (1972–1994). J Am Vet Med Assoc 1996, 209: 819–22.
Fowler ME. Surgery. In: Fowler ME ed, Medicine and Surgery of Camelids, 3rd ed. Ames: Wiley-Blackwell, 2010, pp. 13–41.
Kock MD. Canine tooth extraction and pulpotomy in the adult male llama. J Am Vet Med Assoc 1984, 185: 1304–6.
Long P. Llama herd health. Vet Clin North Am Food Anim Pract 1989, 5: 227–32.
Author Dusty W. Nagy
Consulting Editor Erica C. McKenzie
Acknowledgment The author and book editors acknowledge the prior contribution of Jennifer M. Ivany Ewoldt.

CAMELID: DERMATOLOGY

C

BASICS

OVERVIEW
- A variety of diseases of the skin have been described in camelid species, and they vary in presentation with respect to their inciting cause. Parasitic, infectious, nutritional, idiopathic, neoplastic, and congenital diseases have all been reported.
- Parasitic: Biting and sucking lice both affect camelids; biting lice are thought to be more common. Mites are also common in camelids.
- Viral: Bluetongue virus, vesicular stomatitis virus, contagious ecthyma, papilloma viruses, and papilloma viruses have all been described in camelid species.
- Bacterial: Dermatophilosis and folliculitis are commonly encountered skin diseases in camelids.
- Fungal: Dermatophytosis ("ringworm") has been described in camelid species.
- Neoplastic: Squamous cell carcinoma, fibrosarcoma, papilloma, fibropapilloma, fibroma, melanocytoma, hamartoma, and mast cell tumors have all been described in camelid species.
- Congenital ichthyosis (excessive dry skin scaling) has been reported in llamas.
- Camelid skin can be organized into several layers:
  - Stratum corneum: The thickest, outermost layer, composed of the remnants of keratinized cells pushing outward from lower layers.
  - Stratum lucidum: An eosinophilic layer immediately below the stratum corneum.
  - Stratum granulosum: Keratinocytes migrating from underlying layers develop in this layer. They have distinct keratohyalin granules that are thought to bind keratin filaments together.
  - Stratum spinosum: Composed of polyhedral keratinocytes, the cells of this layer are active in synthesizing proteins which ultimately contribute to the desmosomes that arise from between adjacent keratinocytes.
  - Stratum basale: This layer is composed of what are considered the stem cells of the epidermis.
- There are several large glands that are normal anatomic features in camelid species, but which are absent or less pronounced in traditional ruminants.
  - Metatarsal gland: Oval-shaped glands located on both the medial and lateral aspects of the metatarsus of the pelvic limbs. Glandular secretions can accumulate and flake off from these glands.
  - Interdigital gland: Found in the interdigital space of all four feet.
  - Poll gland: A feature of old world camelids. This scent gland is used for marking by bulls in rut.

INCIDENCE/PREVALENCE
Varies by inciting causative agent. Contagious disorders can achieve high prevalence within a group.

GEOGRAPHIC DISTRIBUTION
Worldwide; regional distribution influenced by causative agent and relevant management factors.

SYSTEMS AFFECTED
Integument

PATHOPHYSIOLOGY
- Bacterial disorders:
  - Dermatophilosis ("rain rot") is caused by *Dermatophilus congolensis*, a Gram-positive coccoid organism that can appear in branching filaments. The causative organism requires a break in the skin and moisture to spread.
  - Folliculitis is most commonly caused by *Staphylococcus intermedius*.
- Fungal:
  - Multiple fungal species have been described as causing dermatophytosis in camelids, predominantly *Trichophyton* and *Microsporum*.
- Parasitic:
  - Chewing lice (*Damalinia breviceps*) feed on debris of the superficial skin.
  - Sucking lice (*Microthoracius* spp.) feed on blood and lymph fluid.
  - Mites (mange) cause clinical signs by several mechanisms. The action of burrowing into the skin leads to thickening and reduced local immune response. Some mites stimulate an immune response with their mouthparts that leads to serum loss at the bite sites.
  - *Psoroptes* mites, most commonly found in the pinna and ear canal, induce head shaking due to local irritation.
  - *Chorioptes* mite (*C. bovis*) infestation is common and may be asymptomatic or create pruritis and alopecia of the feet and tail base.
  - *Sarcoptes scabiei* var *auchinae* can cause severe pruritis, particularly in fiberless areas.
- Idiopathic:
  - Munge, or "idiopathic hyperkeratotic dermatitis," is assumed to have an underlying immunodeficiency as the cause.
- Neoplastic:
  - Pathophysiology varies by tumor type.
- Burns:
  - Thermal burns: Severity can range from reddened skin (first-degree burn) to swelling and blistering (second-degree burn) to tissue charring and deep damage (third-degree burn). The pathophysiology of burn injuries is a combination of thermal destruction of tissues, decreased resistance to infection of damaged skin, as well as loss of fluid and protein (albumin) through damaged skin.
  - Chemical burns: Vary considerably depending on the agent involved. Where possible contact the local Poison Control

Center or National Poison Control Hotline (1-800-222-1222 in the USA) for information about specific chemical agents.
- Viral:
  - Several parapox viruses can cause skin lesions in camelid species. Contagious ecthyma ("orf") and camel pox have been observed in camelids. Cowpox virus, an orthopoxvirus, has also been noted. Immunosuppression is thought to play a role in the development of clinical cases.
- Zinc-responsive dermatosis:
  - As a significant trace element, zinc plays a role in modulation of the immune response as well as management of inflammation.
  - Disease can arise as a result of poor absorption, binding of zinc with other minerals (calcium), or decreased dietary zinc in the ration. Phytases present in grains may limit zinc absorption in some cases.

HISTORICAL FINDINGS
- Vary with the underlying etiology but defining the history of skin disease within the herd, and any relevant treatment or management procedures, is important.
- A description of skin lesion appearance and duration, number of animals affected, and the presence or absence of pruritis are important historical factors.

SIGNALMENT
All species and breeds of camelids, of any age or gender, are at risk of dermatologic disease.

PHYSICAL EXAMINATION FINDINGS
- Vary depending on the inciting cause of disease.
- Dermatophilosis is most commonly observed on the dorsum, ears, feet, and neck. Lesions can be non-pruritic or pruritic, and erythema may be noted on affected skin.
- Dermatophytosis tends to affect the legs, perineum, and head. Lesions tend to be hyperkeratotic crusts that are not pruritic.
- Lice typically cause pruritis with affected camelids exhibiting scratching, traumatic loss of fiber, excoriation, and restlessness.
- Mange
  - Affected skin may be reddened, or potentially moist from serum leakage.
  - Head shaking and incoordination have been reported as signs of psoroptic mange.
  - Sarcoptic mange is typically localized to the thorax, ventrum, limbs, perineal region, and interdigital space; regions with limited fiber.
  - *Chorioptes* commonly affects the feet and tail base, but can become more extensive.
- Munge is most common in animals <2 years of age and is reflected by crusting and hyperkeratosis of the muzzle, eyes, and ears.
- Neoplasia can present as skin thickening, cutaneous nodules or masses, or superficial ulceration of affected regions.
- Parapox viruses typically cause disease at mucocutaneous junctions, most commonly on the lips. Painful, clumped, raised, alopecic,

C

crusty, and ulcerated masses in younger animals are suggestive.
• Signs of zinc-responsive dermatosis are most notable on the muzzle, pinnae, neck, ventrum, and thighs where thickening of the skin, alopecia, and scaling may be noted. Hyperpigmentation may occur in chronic cases.

GENETICS
There are few known dermatologic conditions of camelids with a genetic basis. Crooked nails, teat abnormalities, aural hematomas, rolling or "wrinkled" skin, and chondritis are all thought to have a genetic component or to occur more commonly in certain breeding lines.

CAUSES AND RISK FACTORS
• Increased stocking density is likely a risk factor for parasitic skin disease.
• Fiber and skin color may be associated with increased risk of zinc-associated dermatitis.
• Dermatophilosis typically occurs in areas with high rainfall where the fiber of camelids is moist frequently or for extended periods of time.
• Operations with poor biosecurity, management and parasite control measures may be predisposed to contagious, parasitic or nutritional dermatologic disorders.

DIAGNOSIS

DIFFERENTIAL DIAGNOSES
Differential diagnoses encompass all of the listed disorders; another approach is to consider possible differentials based on the anatomic region in which lesions occur:
• Heavily fleeced areas: Lice, dermatophilosis, neoplasms, shearing injuries ("clipper burn").
• Lightly fleeced areas: Dermatophytosis, mange, photosensitization, folliculitis, hyperkeratotic disorders, coccidioidomycosis, and solar dermatitis should all be considered.
• Mucocutaneous junctions: Contagious ecthyma, parapox virus infections (camel pox, cowpox), and skin neoplasms should be considered.

CBC/BIOCHEMISTRY/URINALYSIS
N/A

OTHER LABORATORY TESTS
• Bacterial culture can be performed directly on skin swabs or on skin biopsies. Susceptibility testing should also be considered to guide antimicrobial selection. Contact the laboratory to determine what antibiotic trays will be used for sensitivity: some laboratories use default trays containing drugs that are not available in a formulation suitable for camelids.
• Cytologic examination of smears of exudates or lesions can help distinguish bacterial, fungal, and neoplastic etiologies.

• Gram staining of roll smears and cytology samples can aid antimicrobial selection in pyoderma and folliculitis.

IMAGING
N/A

OTHER DIAGNOSTIC PROCEDURES
• Skin biopsies can be obtained for histologic examination and/or bacterial culture.
  ○ Collection of several samples from an affected animal is recommended, ideally with healthy and affected skin contained within each sample.
  ○ Select fully developed lesions without secondary trauma or infection.
  ○ Avoid disturbing the skin surface; rigorous preparation of the skin can disrupt cellular architecture.
  ○ The skin should be undermined with 1–2 mL of local anesthetic solution if necessary.
  ○ 4–8 mm biopsy punches can be utilized with care: roll the punch in one direction (instead of alternating back and forth) during sample collection to minimize crush artifact.
  ○ The sample should be lifted off the biopsy punch with a needle or iris scissors to avoid crush artifact and immediately placed in a fixative, such as 10% buffered formalin, since architectural changes will begin shortly after collection.
• Fiber microscopy using a light microscope can help identify *Demodex* mites adhered to the hair follicle or lice eggs attached to the fiber. If the end of the hair shaft appears to be broken, or sharply cut, this suggests a pruritic lesion.
• Fungal culture can be achieved using commercial Dermatophyte Test Media "DTM" culture kits.
  ○ When dermatophytes metabolize the culture medium, an alkaline pH is created that will turn the phenol red dye in the medium red.
  ○ False positives can occur with benign fungal species; after they metabolize the carbohydrates in the medium, they will break down the protein components of the medium, which will shift the pH to alkaline. The color of the media should therefore be recorded when the colony is first noted to avoid false-positive results.
  ○ The media should be stored loosely to allow for aeration, as well as at room temperature, and examined daily. Black or greenish-black colonies should be regarded as contaminants since dermatophyte colonies typically appear fluffy and light colored.
  ○ *Trichophyton verrucosum* and some other species do not grow on DTM media.
• Plasma zinc can be measured on blood collected into a lithium heparin ("green top") tube, kept upright, and immediately spun down and plasma removed. Hemolysis or use of tubes with zinc in the container or stopper can artificially elevate concentrations.

• Skin scraping is useful for diagnosis of *Psoroptes, Sarcoptes, Chorioptes,* and *Demodex* infections.
  ○ A no. 10 scalpel blade can be used; excessive damage to the skin can be prevented by dulling the blade by passing it over a hard surface several times.
  ○ Several drops of mineral oil are placed on the dulled blade, a microscope slide, and the areas of the skin to be scraped.
  ○ The dull blade is scraped over the sampling area and the debris is placed on the mineral oil on the microscope slide. The sample can then be viewed with a coverslip. Care should be taken not to press the blade into the skin as this may cause a laceration.
  ○ Since false-negative scrapings are common, samples should be taken from multiple sites. It is often necessary to scrape deeply enough to draw blood to achieve a diagnostic sample.
  ○ Digestion with potassium hydroxide may be necessary to clear debris from the visual field.
  ○ Mites may be visualized at lower magnification, but 100× is often required for identification; 400× may be required for *Psoroptes*.
  ○ Alternatively an acetate tape test may be useful for identifying surface mites, but will not be effective for mites that burrow into the skin.
• Skin surface cytology
  ○ Samples can be gathered by directly pressing the slide onto the lesion, aspiration of pustules, rubbing the slide on the interdigital space, or rolling a sterile swab on the lesion.
  ○ Cytology samples can be heat fixed and stained (Gram stain or Diff-Quick) for improved visualization of cellular changes and structures.
• Wood's lamp visualization
  ○ When dermatophytes are suspected, lesions can be screened with a 253.7 nm wavelength ultraviolet light (Wood's lamp). Due to the reaction of the light with a tryptophan metabolite, some species of dermatophytes will fluoresce under the lamp.
  ○ A negative Wood's lamp screening does not verify absence of dermatophytes as numerous species do not fluoresce and false-positive results can occur in previously treated animals.
  ○ Battery-powered lamps may not have sufficient power to cause fluorescence, so where possible, lamps that draw outlet power should be utilized.

PATHOLOGIC FINDINGS
• Dermatophilosis causes infiltration of the skin with neutrophils, hyperkeratosis, and a "railroad track"-appearing double chain of Gram-positive coccoid organisms.
• Ichthyosis appears as hyperkeratinization on biopsy with minimal to no inflammation.

CAMELID: DERMATOLOGY (CONTINUED)

- Zinc-responsive dermatosis
  - Plasma zinc concentration <0.5 mg/dL may be suggestive. Clinically affected animals can have normal plasma zinc concentrations.
  - Biopsy demonstrates hyperkeratosis, potentially with perivascular infiltrates of white blood cells.
  - Often a diagnosis of exclusion and response to supplemental zinc.

TREATMENT

THERAPEUTIC APPROACH
- There are no labeled drugs for use in camelid species. As such, in some countries treatment of camelid conditions is considered "extra-label" drug use and may come with additional restrictions or responsibilities for the prescribing veterinarian.
- Whenever possible evidence-based approaches utilizing the current literature should be employed for therapy considerations.

SURGICAL CONSIDERATIONS AND TECHNIQUES
Neoplastic lesions including fibromas, fibrosarcomas, fibropapillomas, and papillomas may be managed by surgical excision. Where possible wide surgical excision, with margins checked for completeness, should be employed. Clients should be aware that regrowth is a possibility with surgical removal of these lesions. Surgical excision appears to be curative for mast cell tumors, hamartomas, and melanocytomas.

MEDICATIONS

DRUGS OF CHOICE
- Coccidioidomycosis (systemic) has been treated with fluconazole (2.27 mg/kg, PO). For topical infection, agents such as nystatin or thiabendazole may be useful.
- Dermatophilosis responds to ceftiofur, penicillin, or oxytetracycline given for a minimum of 5–7 days. Topical cleaning of crusts with disinfectants such as dilute chlorhexidine (25 mL per liter of saline) can also be performed.
- Dermatophytosis is primarily managed with shearing affected regions to increase air flow and light exposure, after which, treatment with topical antiseptics such as chlorhexidine (scrub solution or shampoo), iodine (2%, or 0.5% povidone), captan, lime sulfur, or a topical antifungal cream such as clotrimazole or miconazole can be tried. Topical treatments may need to be applied once to several times daily for up to 2 weeks or longer.
- Lice are responsive to macrocyclic lactone compounds (ivermectin, moxidectin,

doramectin, eprinomectin). Topical livestock products can be useful; pyrethrin or permethrin compounds are safer than carbamate or organophosphate compounds. Lice burden can be further reduced by shearing and exposure to sunlight.
- Munge has been addressed using combination therapies ("Witches Brew"), typically involving a mixture of mineral oil, dimethyl sulfoxide (DMSO), gentamicin and ivermectin (e.g. 317 mL of mineral oil, mixed with 95 mL of DMSO, 8 mL of ivermectin, and 5 mL of 50 mg/mL gentamicin. The solution can be applied every 3 days for 2–3 weeks, and clients should wear gloves.
- *Psoroptes*: Ivermectin (eardrop) and fipronil spray to the affected pinnae.
- *Sarcoptes*: Ivermectin (0.2 mg/kg, SQ) is often required as topical treatment and is often ineffective.
- *Demodex*: Ivermectin (parenteral), permethrin (topical), fipronil spray (total dose not to exceed 2–3 mL/kg of 2.5% solution), and lime sulfur (2% topical) can be used.
- *Chorioptes*: Ivermectin and topical therapies as described for other mites.
- For squamous cell carcinoma, cisplatin injections as well as topical 5-fluorouracil have been reported along with cryotherapy.
- Antiviral drugs are not indicated for parapox or orthopox viruses. Treatment should focus on supportive care with analgesics, anti-inflammatories, and potentially antibiotics to treat or manage secondary infections.
- Zinc-responsive dermatosis has been treated by ensuring dietary zinc at 100–200 parts per million of the ration, or supplemental administration of oral zinc methionine (4 grams/day) or oral zinc sulfate (2 g/day). Supplementation with zinc methionine is thought to reach greater tissue concentrations, and treatment may be necessary for 60 days or longer.

CONTRAINDICATIONS
Corticosteroids should not be used in pregnant female camelids.

PRECAUTIONS
- Appropriate milk and meat withdrawal times must be followed for all compounds administered to food-producing animals.
- Topical ectoparasiticides that fall under the jurisdiction of the EPA rather than the FDA in the USA cannot be applied in an extra-label manner.

POSSIBLE INTERACTIONS
N/A

FOLLOW-UP

EXPECTED COURSE AND PROGNOSIS
- Varies depending on cause.

- Most skin diseases take several weeks to resolve once therapy is initiated.

POSSIBLE COMPLICATIONS
Secondary infection

CLIENT EDUCATION
Focus on methods of control and prevention to reduce disease related to ectoparasites and infectious disorders.

PATIENT CARE
- Mange: Follow-up may be required for weeks to months to monitor for recurrence.
- Neoplasia: Camelids with neoplastic masses should be observed for regrowth, and where possible screened for potential metastasis.

PREVENTION
- External parasites can be prevented by decreasing stocking density, shearing fiber, dusting, minimizing sharing of brushes and coats, as well as monitoring frequently.
- Quarantine new animals before introduction into the herd, with close inspection for skin lesions.

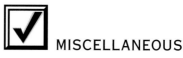

MISCELLANEOUS

ASSOCIATED CONDITIONS
N/A

AGE-RELATED FACTORS
Younger animals are more prone to munge, contagious ecthyma, and ichthyosis.

ZOONOTIC POTENTIAL
- Dermatologic diseases in large animals should be considered zoonotic until proven otherwise. Clients should be advised to wear gloves and other barrier clothing when handling animals with a potential zoonosis.
- Dermatophytes, *Dermatophilus*, *Sarcoptes*, contagious ecthyma, camel pox, cowpox, and other skin disorders are all considered potential zoonoses.

PREGNANCY
N/A

BIOSECURITY
- Several mite species can persist in the environment. Common items such as brushes, blankets, and halters should not be shared between individuals when an animal is suspected of having an infectious condition.
- For the disinfection of facilities where dermatophytosis is suspected, chlorhexidine or bleach can be used.

PRODUCTION MANAGEMENT
While the majority of skin conditions are not immediately-life threatening, these conditions can contribute to decreased fiber yield and quality, as well as decreased reproduction.

SYNONYMS
Munge: idiopathic nasal dermatitis or hyperkeratotic dermatitis

C

ABBREVIATIONS
- DMSO = dimethyl sulfoxide
- DTM = Dermatophyte Test Media
- EPA = Environmental Protection Agency
- FDA = Food and Drug Administration

Suggested Reading

Cebra C, Anderson DE, Tibary A, Van Saun RJ, Johnson LW. Llama and Alpaca Care: Medicine, Surgery, Reproduction, Nutrition, and Herd Health. Elsevier Health Sciences, 2014.

Fowler ME. Medicine and Surgery of Camelids. Wiley, 2011.

Köhler-Rollefson I, Mundy P, Mathias E. A Field Manual of Camel Diseases: Traditional and Modern Health Care for the Dromedary. ITDG Publishing, 2001.

Author Joe S. Smith

Consulting Editor Erica C. McKenzie

CAMELID: GASTROINTESTINAL DISEASE

C

BASICS

OVERVIEW
• New world camelids (NWC) or South American camelids (SAC) include the guanaco, llama, alpaca, and vicuna.
• NWC can subsist on a lower plane of nutrition than other domestic herbivores due to unique gastric anatomy and physiology permitting utilization of less digestible feedstuffs.
• Common GI diseases of camelids include third compartment (C3) ulceration, dental disease, enteritis, peritonitis, intestinal accidents, parasitism, and neoplasia.
• Assessment of body condition, ration analysis, and herd management procedures are important in preventing GI disease in NWC.

INCIDENCE/PREVALENCE
N/A

GEOGRAPHIC DISTRIBUTION
Worldwide

SYSTEMS AFFECTED
Digestive

PATHOPHYSIOLOGY
• Camelids are considered pseudo-ruminants with three stomach compartments: C1, C2, and C3.
• C1, the largest compartment in the adult, contains 83% of the content and lies predominantly on the left side of the abdomen. While C1 is analogous to the true rumen given its role is fermentation, it contains a homogeneous mixture of partially digested feed, while the rumen is stratified and contains a fluid layer, topped with a fibrous mat and gas cap.
• C2 is much smaller and primarily involved in mixing and fermentation.
• C1 and C2 contain saccules that secrete bicarbonate to buffer the environment for resident microorganisms.
• C3 has two functional parts: the proximal 4/5^{ths} controls absorption of nutrients and the distal 1/5th is glandular and secretes acid.
• Camelids absorb most nutrients in the small intestine and form fecal pellets in the large intestine. They have a spiral colon, which is a common site for obstruction.
• GI disease in camelids can result from parasitism (nematodes, protozoa, helminths, flukes), intestinal obstruction (bezoar, gastroliths), compartment ulceration (C1, distal C3), neoplasia (adenocarcinoma, lymphosarcoma, round cell tumor, squamous cell carcinoma), infection (*Streptococcus zooepidemicus* peritonitis or abdominal abscess; viral and bacterial enteritis), esophageal dysfunction (megaesophagus, vascular ring anomalies; VRA), and other disorders.

HISTORICAL FINDINGS
Signs of colic, weight loss, tenesmus, or abnormal fecal passage or consistency are common complaints.

SIGNALMENT
• Any age, species, gender of camelid.
• Neonatal alpacas are most likely to present with VRA.
• Young camelids are more likely to have bezoars.

PHYSICAL EXAMINATION FINDINGS
• Vary depending on the disorder.
• Salivation, regurgitation, or staining around the mouth may indicate oral or esophageal disease.
• Unusual esophageal activity (fluctuations, billowing, distension) can occur with esophageal disorders.
• Signs of colic reflected by abnormal cush, restlessness, lateral recumbency; vocalization and rolling if severe pain occurs.
• Abdominal distension.
• Empty rectum or diarrhea on digital rectal examination.
• Tachycardia: Usually indicates shock or hypovolemia rather than pain.
• Poor body condition suggests chronic disease or poor management.

GENETICS
N/A

CAUSES AND RISK FACTORS
Poor management procedures related to hygiene, nutrition and parasite control.

DIAGNOSIS

DIFFERENTIAL DIAGNOSES
• Enteritis (viral, bacterial, parasitic)
• Ileus or atony
• Toxicity (rhododendron or other)
• GI obstruction (bezoar, intussusceptions, adhesions)
• Peritonitis
• Compartment ulceration
• Neoplasia
• Mesenteric root torsion

CBC/BIOCHEMISTRY/URINALYSIS
• Neutrophilia or neutropenia reflect inflammatory or infectious disease.
• Hypoalbuminemia suggests parasitic disease.
• Hypochloremic metabolic alkalosis can occur in GI obstruction located near the pylorus or duodenum.
• Increased gamma-glutamyltransferase (GGT) and aspartate aminotransferase (AST) activity may be noted in animals with hepatic disorders or secondary lipidosis due to reduced feed intake.
• Elevations of nonesterified fatty acids and beta-hydroxybutyrate may occur in animals

with anorexia and can be used to determine the need for supplemental nutrition.

OTHER LABORATORY TESTS
Fecal samples can be submitted for bacterial culture, parasite detection, and virus detection if indicated.

IMAGING
• Ultrasonography is excellent for imaging the abdomen of camelids and can often be achieved by applying alcohol and spreading the fiber without clipping.
• Radiography is useful to evaluate esophageal disorders and to detect gastroliths.
• Computed tomography 3 hours after orogastric administration of contrast agent (± IV contrast) provides an excellent abdominal study to identify obstruction, neoplasia, and other anomalies.

OTHER DIAGNOSTIC PROCEDURES
• Abdominocentesis can be readily performed in the right paracostal region ~ 2–3 cm caudal to the last rib and level with the costochondral junction. Fluid total protein should be <2.5 g/dL and total nucleated cell count <3,000/μL.
• Exploratory laparotomy may be necessary when uncontrollable pain or diagnostic procedures do not identify the problem, but should be avoided if possible due to risk and the low likelihood of a surgically amenable issue in the vast majority of cases.

PATHOLOGIC FINDINGS
Vary with underlying cause

TREATMENT

THERAPEUTIC APPROACH
• Most GI disease in camelids is medical in nature, and the underlying issue should be correctly identified and addressed as promptly as possible.
• Intensive supportive care may be needed which can include delivery of fluids, nutrition, pain relief, and specific therapeutic medications; this must be balanced against the stress of handling and medicating these animals.

SURGICAL CONSIDERATIONS AND TECHNIQUES
• Most GI disorders in camelids are medical in nature.
• Surgery should only be performed where surgical intervention is confirmed to be appropriate (bezoar or other obstruction), or surgical exploration is considered a necessary diagnostic step.
• C3 is highly vascular with an extensive anastomotic capillary network at the luminal surface. Branching vessels provide extensive collateral circulation. Incisions into C3 should be oriented parallel to the longitudinal plane.

(CONTINUED) CAMELID: GASTROINTESTINAL DISEASE

C

MEDICATIONS

DRUGS OF CHOICE
• Nonsteroidal anti-inflammatory drugs provide analgesia in camelids; flunixin meglumine is often used (1.1 mg/kg IV, q24h or q12h).
• Opioids including morphine (0.05–0.2 mg/kg IV), butorphanol (0.05–0.1 mg/kg IM or IV), buprenorphine (5 –10 µg/kg IM), and fentanyl (1–5 µg/kg IV) or fentanyl (1–2 µg/kg/hr via transdermal patch) are analgesic but have variable adverse effects on GI motility.
• Constant rate IV infusion of lidocaine, butorphanol, or ketamine have been used to control severe discomfort.
• Orally administered proton pump inhibitors and H-2 receptor antagonists are ineffective in camelids. Pantoprazole (1 mg/kg IV or 2 mg/kg SC, q24h) is effective at increasing the pH of C3.
• Partial parenteral nutrition can be provided by supplementation of isotonic crystalloid fluids with dextrose (1–2%) and amino acids.
• Thiamine (10 mg/kg, q24h) is indicated in animals with prolonged anorexia.
• Provision of 500 mL of fresh rumen fluid via orogastric tube once or twice daily is helpful in anorexic animals unless the procedure causes excessive distress.
• Plasma transfusion (5–10 mL/kg of llama plasma) is indicated for severe hypoproteinemia (albumin ≤1.5 mg/dL, total protein ≤3.5 mg/dL).
• Mineral oil can be given by orogastric tube as a mild laxative (5–10 mL/kg).

CONTRAINDICATIONS
Nephrotoxic drugs should be avoided in dehydrated, azotemic animals.

PRECAUTIONS
Appropriate milk and meat withdrawal times must be followed for all compounds administered to food-producing animals.

POSSIBLE INTERACTIONS
N/A

FOLLOW-UP

Variable by underlying disease

MISCELLANEOUS

ASSOCIATED CONDITIONS
• Renal failure
• Peritonitis
• Septic shock

AGE-RELATED FACTORS
Young camelids are more likely to have congenital disorders or bezoar obstruction.

ZOONOTIC POTENTIAL
Some causes of enteritis in camelids are potentially zoonotic, including *Salmonella*, *Giardia*, and *Cryptosporidium*.

PREGNANCY
N/A

BIOSECURITY
Careful hygiene precautions and potential isolation procedures are recommended for infectious disorders and zoonotic pathogens.

PRODUCTION MANAGEMENT
N/A

SYNONYMS
• Colic
• Diarrhea
• Endoparasitism

ABBREVIATIONS
• C1, C2, C3 = compartments of the stomach
• NSAIDs = nonsteroidal anti-inflammatory drugs
• NWC = new world camelids
• SAC = South American camelids
• VRA = vascular ring anomaly

SEE ALSO
• Camelid: Parasitology
• Parasite Control Programs: Camelid

Suggested Reading
Bickers RJ, Templer A, Cebra CK, Kaneps AJ. Diagnosis and treatment of torsion of the spiral colon in an alpaca. J Am Vet Med Assoc 2000, 216: 380–2.
Cebra CK, Cebra ML, Garry FB, Belknap EB. Forestomach acidosis in six New World camelids. J Am Vet Med Assoc 1996, 208: 901–4.
Cebra CK, Mattson DE, Baker RJ, Sonn RJ, Dearing PL. Potential pathogens in feces from unweaned llamas and alpacas with diarrhea. J Am Vet Med Assoc 2003, 223: 1806–8.
Cebra CK, Tornquist SJ, Bildfell RJ, Heidel JR. Bile acids in gastric fluids from llamas and alpacas with and without ulcers. J Vet Intern Med 2003, 17: 567–70.
Christensen JM, Limsakun T, Smith BB, Hollingshead N, Huber M. Pharmacokinetics and pharmacodynamics of antiulcer agents in llama. J Vet Pharmacol Ther 2001, 24: 23–33.
Drew ML, Ramsay E, Fowler ME, Kass PH. Effect of flunixin meglumine and cimetidine hydrochloride on the pH in the third compartment of the stomach of llamas. J Am Vet Med Assoc 1992, 201: 1559–63.
Smith BB, Pearson EG, Timm KI. Third compartment ulcers in the llama. Vet Clin North Am Food Anim Pract 1994, 10: 319–30.
Smith BB. An overview of selected diseases and drug needs in the llama and alpaca industries. Vet Hum Toxicol 1998, 40 Suppl 1: 29–34.
Van Hoogmoed LM, Harmon FA, Snyder J. Microvascular anatomy of the third compartment of the stomach of llamas. Am J Vet Res 2003, 64: 346–50.
Yarbrough TB, Snyder JR, Harmon FA. Laparoscopic anatomy of the llama abdomen. Vet Surg 1995, 24: 244–9.

Author Andrew J. Niehaus
Consulting Editor Erica C. McKenzie

CAMELID: HEAT STRESS

C

BASICS

OVERVIEW
Disease syndrome in South American camelids exposed to excessively high ambient temperature or combined high ambient temperature and high humidity.

INCIDENCE/PREVALENCE
N/A

GEOGRAPHIC DISTRIBUTION
Heat stress can occur in any part of the world where ambient temperature rises above 80°F (27°C).

SYSTEMS AFFECTED
- Cardiovascular
- Respiratory
- Digestive
- Hemolymphatic
- Urinary
- Reproductive
- Nervous

PATHOPHYSIOLOGY
- The preoptic area of the anterior hypothalamus receives and processes information from thermosensors throughout the body.
- Hyperthermia arises from thermoregulatory malfunction. In heat stress, malfunction arises due to an elevated thermal burden that the body is incapable of handling.

HISTORICAL FINDINGS
High environmental temperatures ± high humidity prior to the animal displaying signs suggestive of heat stress.

SIGNALMENT
Typically adult camelids in full fiber.

PHYSICAL EXAMINATION FINDINGS
- Signs vary depending on severity.
- Typically there is an elevated rectal temperature that may vary with ambient temperature. If animals are examined early in the course of disease or at a cooler time of day, rectal temperature may not be excessively high.
- Tachycardia and tachypnea.
- Sweating and open mouth breathing are common as disease progresses. Weakness and incoordination occur and can progress to recumbency.
- Ventral edema, particularly scrotal edema in males, is common in affected individuals.
- In severely affected animals, petechial and ecchymotic hemorrhages are associated with disseminated intravascular coagulation (DIC), and a uremic smell to the breath and ulcers in the mouth can occur with secondary renal failure.
- Cyanosis, droopy lip with froth at the commissures, depression, marked weakness, colic, and multi-organ failure (kidney, liver) may occur.

GENETICS
N/A

CAUSES AND RISK FACTORS
- Failure of thermoregulatory function due to exposure to high heat ± high humidity combined with a variety of factors.
- Environmental factors include temperature, humidity, and air movement.
- Animal factors include dehydration, exertion, heavy dark fleece, obesity, pregnancy, lactation, and current or recent illness.
- Nutritional factors include high concentrate diet, high protein hay, selenium-deficient diets, and vitamin- and mineral-deficient diets.
- Management factors include availability of fresh drinking water, shade, and cooling water as well as the presence of fans and the timing of stressful activities.

DIAGNOSIS

DIFFERENTIAL DIAGNOSES
Vary depending on the observed clinical signs, and can include:
- Infectious diseases that generate fever
- Polioencephalomalacia
- Tick paralysis
- Parelaphostrongylosis
- GI causes of colic
- Urethral rupture (animals with severe ventral edema)
- Testicular abscess or hydrocele (males with scrotal swelling)

CBC/BIOCHEMISTRY/URINALYSIS
- CBC often shows a mature neutrophilia; platelet count may decrease with time.
- Biochemistry abnormalities depend on the organ systems involved. Increases can occur in creatinine, urea nitrogen, AST, CK, bilirubin, and SDH. Hypoproteinemia may be present. Serum sodium and chloride may be decreased. Whole body potassium is often depleted; however, serum concentrations may be elevated in the presence of metabolic acidemia. Metabolic and respiratory acidosis also may be present.
- Urinalysis: Initially increased specific gravity that may become isosthenuric if renal failure ensues; tubular casts may be present in individuals with severe disease; blood and protein also may be present.

OTHER LABORATORY TESTS
Clotting times (may be increased)

IMAGING
N/A

OTHER DIAGNOSTIC PROCEDURES
CSF analysis can be performed to rule out other neurologic diseases.

PATHOLOGIC FINDINGS
- Gross necropsy identifies autolysis that is advanced with respect to the time of death; hemorrhages and other findings consistent with DIC might be present, and serous atrophy of fat.
- Histopathologic changes include renal and hepatic necrosis, coagulative necrosis of neurons, and vascular congestion in the lungs, liver, spleen, and myocardium.

TREATMENT

THERAPEUTIC APPROACH
- Animals should be cooled to achieve a normal rectal temperature, but with caution as they may lack the ability to warm themselves if overcooled. Cooling efforts should focus on the ventral body surface where evaporative cooling is optimal. Intact fleece will help insulate the animal even when wet, so water must soak through to the skin, and shearing can be performed to improve heat loss if shearing is not unduly stressful.
- IV fluids are indicated for correction of dehydration, electrolyte disturbances, and acidosis. Adult camelids require 30–40 mL/kg/day of fluid and crias require 80–120 mL/kg/day. Camelids are prone to pulmonary edema with rapid infusion rates, so administration rate should not exceed 20 mL/kg/h.
- Intranasal oxygen if indicated.
- The extent of body system damage is dependent upon the severity of the exposure.
- Animals that have undergone prolonged severe heat stress may have systemic complications that far outlast the inciting hyperthermic incident.

SURGICAL CONSIDERATIONS AND TECHNIQUES
N/A

MEDICATIONS

DRUGS OF CHOICE
- Anti-inflammatory agents
  - Corticosteroids can be given to address shock, including dexamethasone (0.05–0.1 mg/kg, IV or SQ, q48h for 2 treatments) and prednisolone sodium succinate (0.5–1.0 mg/kg IV or SQ, q12–24h).
  - Flunixin meglumine (1.1 mg/kg): should be used cautiously because many heat-stressed animals have renal compromise at presentation.
- Antimicrobial agents to prevent secondary infection
  - Ceftiofur hydrochloride: 2.2 mg/kg IM or SC, q24h; ceftiofur sodium can be used IV at the same dose, q12h.
  - Ampicillin trihydrate: 10 mg/kg IM q24h; sodium ampicillin can be used q8h at the same dose.

(CONTINUED)

C

○ Penicillin: 22,000 IU/kg IM or SC, q12h; potassium penicillin can be used IV q6h at the same dose.
- Antioxidant agents
  ○ Vitamin E provides immediate antioxidant activity: 1 mL/100 lbs SC or IM (of 300 IU/mL formulation).
  ○ Selenium (antioxidant activity will take 7–10 days for effect): Bo-Se® at 1 mL/50 lb or Mu-Se® at 1 mL/200 lb.

CONTRAINDICATIONS
NSAIDs and other nephrotoxic drugs are contraindicated in animals with severe renal compromise.

PRECAUTIONS
- Even after regaining normal rectal temperature, heat-stressed animals may have ongoing poor thermoregulation and may be more susceptible to heat stress in future.
- Appropriate milk and meat withdrawal times must be followed for all compounds administered to food-producing animals.
- None of the drugs listed are approved for use in camelids and none have established withdrawal times.

POSSIBLE INTERACTIONS
N/A

FOLLOW UP

EXPECTED COURSE AND PROGNOSIS
- Prognosis varies from good to grave depending on presenting condition.
- Early heat stress with no systemic complications will often resolve with cooling and several days in a cooler environment.
- Individuals with organ failure and other serious manifestations may not survive despite aggressive therapy.

POSSIBLE COMPLICATIONS
- Affected animals are more predisposed to heat stress in the future.
- Infertility:
  ○ Male—excessive heat is spermicidal to primary spermatocytes.
  ○ Female—ovarian activity will decrease in times of high heat.
- Pregnancy loss.
- Congenital abnormalities in the fetus.

CLIENT EDUCATION
Management steps to reduce the risk of heat stress during hot weather in problematic climates.

PATIENT CARE
- Rectal temperature should be monitored regularly (every 30 mins) until stable, then several times daily.
- Serum biochemistry should initially be monitored every 1–2 days depending on severity of disease to assess progress and provide a basis for alteration in fluid therapy.
- Limit exertion as muscle activity increases heat production.

PREVENTION
- Clients should be educated on risk factors and prevention techniques as well as early recognition of affected animals.
- Use the comfort index (CI; ambient temperature + % humidity) to anticipate problems.
  ○ CI <120—Problems are unlikely.
  ○ CI 120–180—Caution. Problems are possible.
  ○ CI >180—Danger. Problems are likely, observe animals closely.
  ○ Shear animals prior to hot humid months.
- Adequate access to clean drinking water.
- Adequate access to a mineral and salt supplement.
- Provide shade, fans, and other cooling mechanisms for animals during high heat and humidity.
- Observe animals and institute immediate treatment at signs of trouble.
- It is important to avoid overfeeding as it predisposes to obesity and the necessity to process the excess energy at a metabolic level.
- High-quality forages should be fed during warmer times of the year to decrease the heat increment of digestion.

MISCELLANEOUS

ASSOCIATED CONDITIONS
N/A

AGE-RELATED FACTORS
N/A

ZOONOTIC POTENTIAL
N/A

PREGNANCY
- Corticosteroid use during pregnancy may induce abortion.
- Thermal damage to the developing fetus may result in congenital abnormalities, particularly of the CNS.

BIOSECURITY
N/A

PRODUCTION MANAGEMENT
See "Prevention"

SYNONYMS
- Hyperthermia
- Heat stroke

ABBREVIATIONS
- AST = aspartate aminotransferase
- CI = comfort index
- CK = creatine kinase
- CNS = central nervous system
- CSF = cerebrospinal fluid
- DIC = disseminated intravascular coagulation
- GI = gastrointestinal
- SDH = sorbitol dehydrogenase

SEE ALSO
- Body Condition Scoring: Alpacas and Llamas (see www.fiveminutevet.com/ruminant)
- Body Condition Scoring: Camels (see www.fiveminutevet.com/ruminant)

Suggested Reading
Cebra C, Anderson DE, Tibary A, Van Saun RJ, Johnson L. Llama and Alpaca Care, 1st ed. St. Louis: Elsevier, 2014.
Evans CN. Veterinary llama field manual, 2nd ed. Madisonville, KT. Self-published by author.
Fowler ME. Hyperthermia in llamas and alpacas. Vet Clin North Am Food Anim Pract 1994, 10: 309–17.
Fowler ME. Medicine and Surgery of Camelids, 3rd ed. Ames: Wiley-Blackwell, 2010.
Middleton JR, Parish SM. Heat stress in a llama (*Lama glama*): a case report and review of the syndrome. J Camel Pract Res 1999, 6: 265–9.
Strain MG, Strain SS. Handling heat stress syndrome in llamas. Vet Med 1998, 83: 494–8.
Author Dusty W. Nagy
Consulting Editor Erica C. McKenzie

CAMELID: PARASITOLOGY

C

BASICS

OVERVIEW
• Camelids are susceptible to strongyle-type nematodes, coccidia, protozoa, cestodes, trematodes, and a range of ectoparasites, like other ruminants. *Haemonchus contortus* (barberpole worm) and *Parelaphostrongylus tenuis* (meningeal worm) are economically important nematode parasites of llamas and alpacas in North America. Monthly systemic doses of ivermectin to prevent CNS damage associated with migrating *P. tenius* larvae is thought to contribute to anthelminthic resistance exhibited by *H. contortus* and other gastrointestinal nematodes. Other disease-causing parasites seen in adult camelids include *Nematodirus* sp, *Marshallagia* sp, and *Eimeria macusaniensis*. *Lamanema chavezi*, a nematode of NWC, was identified in an animal from an Oregon herd. In dromedaries and Bactrian camels, *Trichuris* sp. can cause weight loss, ill health, and even death in severe cases. Other parasites such as *Monezia* (tapeworm) are less frequently associated with disease or clinical presentation in adult animals. Nonetheless, as in other ruminants, any one parasite may reduce productivity or cause disease.
• Where trematodes are present, *Fascioloides magna*, *Fasciola hepatica* and *Dircocoelium dendriticum* can infect new world camelids. The latter two are associated with pathology.
• In young camelids, coccidia, *Giardia*, *Cryptosporidium* and *Mycoplasma haemolaema* can be associated with illness. *Eimeria macusaniensis* is a coccidian that can infect and cause disease in all ages.

INCIDENCE/PREVALENCE
• Nematode parasitism is common wherever camelids are pastured.
• *Mycoplasma haemolamae* infections are most commonly subclinical, with varying incidences in individual herds. In one Ohio herd, 40/100 males housed on pasture containing a mud bottom pond were blood PCR positive. On this same farm, the breeding female herd had a blood PCR positive rate of 18%. Other studies indicate infection prevalence rates of 10–20%.

GEOGRAPHIC DISTRIBUTION
• Worldwide for most nematodes, trematodes, and coccidia.
• *P. tenuis* is found in the Eastern USA and Canada where white-tailed deer and the molluscan intermediate hosts reside.
• *Lamanema chavezi* is common in South America. Recent descriptions of this parasite in Oregon and in New Zealand herds suggests it may parasitize NWCs outside South America.

SYSTEMS AFFECTED
• Digestive
• Hemolymphatic
• Nervous

PATHOPHYSIOLOGY
• *Haemonchus contortus* adults are blood feeders, causing anemia and loss of iron into feces, leading to hypoferremia. As with other ruminant gastrointestinal nematodes, hypobiosis may occur with its importance to the pathophysiology of nematodiasis to be determined in the camelid. *Trichuris* pathophysiology has been described in camelids; the morbidity and occasional mortality is associated with host inflammatory responses to parasites (larval and adult) interwoven within the cecum and large bowel. This response is commonly associated with diarrhea. The importance of trichuroids in camelids is suggested by the requirement for higher dosages of avermectin-type anthelmintics and susceptibility to fenbendazole.
• *Parelaphostrongylus tenuis* causes inflammatory tracts within the CNS. For greater detail, see chapter, *Parelaphostrongylus tenuis* (Meningeal Worm).
• Liver flukes cause cirrhosis, abscesses, and granulomas. Reports of *F. magna* are not common whereas *F. hepatica* or *D. dendriticum* can develop into acute and chronic forms and potentially fatal forms of infection.
• Pathology associated with coccidian parasites occurs in association with the reproductive stages occurring within the gastrointestinal cells causing their rupture and cellular death. As parasite multiplication within hosts progress, hemorrhagic enteritis with diarrhea may result. In severe cases, denudation of the intestinal epithelia may result in anemia and hypoproteinemia.
• *Giardia*, as in other host species, may cause a malabsorptive and maldigestive disorder due to the physical presence of the protozoa on the small intestinal microvilli and the influx of lymphocytes due to small intestinal barrier dysfunction associated with enterocyte apoptosis and disruption of epithelial tight junctions.

SIGNALMENT
• Nematodes are most common in pregnant and nursing dams due to periparturient immunosuppression.
• Coccidial species are most common in juvenile crias in confinement.
• *P. tenuis* can be found in any grazing animal cohabiting with white tail deer.

PHYSICAL EXAMINATION FINDINGS
• *Haemonchus contortus:* Anemia, hypoproteinemia, weakness, weight loss, sire's inability to breed, malnourished cria of nursing dam, and death.
• *Lamanema chavezi:* Anemia, eosinophilia, and focal granulomatous liver lesions.

• *Parelaphostrongylus tenuis:* Ataxia, progressive paralysis (rear limb generally), and recumbence.
• *Fasciola hepatica:* Anemia, progressive weakness, and hypoproteinemia.
• Neonatal GI protozoal disease: Diarrhea, anorexia, dehydration and weakness.
• *Eimeria macusaniensis* and other coccidia: lethargy, anorexia, weight loss, sudden death, and mild catarrhal to hemorrhagic diarrhea.
• *Mycoplasma haemolaema:* Hypoglycemia, anemia, seizures, and death.

GENETICS
N/A

CAUSES AND RISK FACTORS
• *Haemonchus contortus:* Overstocking, frequent use of systemic or low-dose anthelmintics, warm wet seasons. Periparturient females from approximately 2 weeks before to 8 weeks after parturition have a clinically significant suppression in immunity to GI nematodes and may shed elevated levels of nematode eggs.
• *Trichuris:* Often associated with paddock/dry-lot confinement after prolonged accumulation of ova. Severe infestations (particularly in old world camelids) can occur after prolonged use of individual paddocks with accumulation of eggs.
• *Lamanema chavezi:* Younger animals are reported to be at greater risk.
• *P. tenuis:* Areas where white-tailed deer and the mollusk intermediate hosts are present.
• *Trematodes:* The life cycle is indirect. For *Fasciola hepatica,* it involves the intermediate host, Lymnaeid snails, and a competent definitive host to shed the trematode ova. The snail sheds the infective form which encysts on aquatic plants and is then ingested. In contrast, *D. dendriticum* is shed by snails, ingested by ants whereby the fluke infective stage will encyst within an ant, later to be ingested by a grazing ruminant. Trematodes require multiple factors for their transmission.
• *Coccidia,* including *E. macusaniensis,* and *Giardia:* Contaminated facilities and environment. The reservoir for coccidiosis and gastrointestinal protozoa are primarily younger animals although adults can be a source of contamination.
• *Mycoplasma haemolaema:* In utero transmission and low concentration or drop in protective maternal antibodies acquired through passive transfer. In other species of *Mycoplasma* biting flies and contaminated needles will transmit these agents.

DIAGNOSIS

DIFFERENTIAL DIAGNOSES
• *Haemonchus contortus: Mycoplasma haemolamae*, acute or chronic hemorrhage, neoplasia

C

• *Lamanema chavezi: Mycoplasma haemolamae*, acute or chronic hemorrhage, neoplasia
• *Parelaphostrongylus tenuis:* Trauma, cerebrocortical necrosis, listeriosis
• *Fasciola hepatica:* Hepatic lipidosis
• *Coccidia* and neonatal GI protozoal disease: Viral, bacterial or other protozoal infections; sepsis, hypernatremia hyperosmolar syndrome, selenium deficiency
• *Mycoplasma haemolaema:* Sepsis, cerebrocortical necrosis, listeriosis

CBC/BIOCHEMISTRY/URINALYSIS
Anemia, hypoproteinemia, electrolyte and acid-base abnormalities, azotemia, or hepatic and biliary enzyme elevation may be present depending on etiology.

OTHER LABORATORY TESTS
• Fecal examination for nematode, trematode, and protozoa stages.
• Fecal occult blood positive for coccidia.
• CSF analysis for eosinophilic pleocytosis.
• Blood smear for *M. haemolaema* in acute cases, PCR for survey or more chronic cases.

IMAGING
N/A

OTHER DIAGNOSTIC PROCEDURES
• *Haemonchus contortus:* Double centrifugation (sucrose; >1.26 specific gravity) fecal flotation for strongyle-type ova, followed by fluorescent peanut lectin staining. Larval cultures to identify and distinguish the first stage larvae. PCR is available through specialized diagnostic laboratories.
• *Lamanema chavezi:* Double centrifugation (sucrose; >1.3 specific gravity) fecal flotation for yellow-brown, cylindrical eggs with parallel sides and rounded poles measuring 170 μm × 73 μm, similar to *Marshallagia* except *Lamanema* are often yellow-brown.
• *Parelaphostrongylus tenuis:* Cerebrospinal fluid with eosinophilia.
• *Fasciola hepatica:* Detection of fluke ova can be problematic. Fecal sedimentation of ova or fecal flotation using a high specific gravity (1.30–1.45) can be used.
• *Coccidia* and *Giardia:* Centrifugation fecal flotation analysis to recover ova and cysts. *Giardia* antigen-based detection kits are available but have not been validated for use in camelids. Sugar solutions with specific gravity of 1.27–1.30 or magnesium chloride at 1.30 can be used to recover coccidian oocysts.
• *Mycoplasma haemolaema:* Peripheral blood smears stained with Wright/Giemsa stains to visualize the 2–3 μm cocci-shaped organisms on the peripheral edges of the red blood cells. PCR is also available through specialized diagnostic laboratories.

PATHOLOGIC FINDINGS
Dependent upon the parasite and organ system infected.

TREATMENT
THERAPEUTIC APPROACH
• Anemia, hypoproteinemia: Blood transfusion, iron supplementation, colloid therapies
• Rehydration, replacement/correction of electrolyte and acid-base abnormalities
• Supportive care: Rest, low stress environment; physical therapy with *P. tenuis*
• Selective chemotherapy to remove parasites (requires parasite identification)
• Analgesia, anti-inflammatories

SURGICAL CONSIDERATIONS AND TECHNIQUES
N/A

MEDICATIONS
DRUGS OF CHOICE
Nematodes
• Fenbendazole 10–20 mg/kg PO
  ○ 20 mg/kg PO for 3 consecutive days if *Trichuris*
  ○ 20 mg/kg PO for 5 days if *Nematodirus*
• Albendazole 10 mg/kg PO (**given only once**)
• Ivermectin 0.2–0.3 mg/kg PO; 0.4–0.6 mg/kg if whipworms present
• Levamisole 5–8 mg/kg PO once
• Pyrantel pamoate 25 mg/kg PO for 3 days

Cestodes
• Fenbendazole 50 mg/kg PO for 5 days
• Praziquantal 2–5 mg/kg PO
• Pyrantel pamoate 25 mg/kg PO for 3 days
• Albendazole 10 mg/kg PO (**given only once**)

Trematodes
• Clorsulon 7 mg/kg PO
• Albendazole 10 mg/kg PO (**given only once**)

Coccidia
• Treatment
  ○ Sulfadimethoxine 55 mg/kg orally on day 1, followed by 22.5 mg/kg PO once daily for 5 days
  ○ Ponazuril 20 mg/kg PO once (reportedly used 3 days in a row)
  ○ Toltrazuril 20 mg/kg PO once (metabolized to ponazuril)
• Prevention
  ○ Amprolium 5 mg/kg diluted in water for 21 days
  ○ Decoquinate 0.5 mg/kg orally in feed for 28 days

CONTRAINDICATIONS
Albendazole should not be used in juveniles <6 months of age, pregnant animals or females within 30 days of breeding.

PRECAUTIONS
• Dewormers should be used judiciously and in association with appropriate husbandry and herd management strategies to decrease risk of infection in order to lower risk of increased resistance.
• Albendazole and levamisole have low margins of safety and therefore accurate weight estimation is important.

POSSIBLE INTERACTIONS
Amprolium administration has been associated with development of polioencephalomalacia, although the risk appears to be very low.

FOLLOW-UP
EXPECTED COURSE AND PROGNOSIS
• Blood feeding gastrointestinal parasites may produce acute or more gradual onset of weakness, weight loss, and loss of condition depending upon number of parasites. These clinical signs often go unnoticed until animal becomes recumbent. A hungry cria not gaining weight should trigger evaluation of its dam.
• Cestodes are not associated with obvious clinical signs. Rarely, intestinal impactions may occur associated with routine deworming of younger stock.
• Whipworms and perhaps *Nematodirus* ova in fecal samples should be considered significant in camelids (especially when associated with clinical signs: diarrhea, hematochezia, colic in herds that routinely administer avermectin-type anthelmintics).

POSSIBLE COMPLICATIONS
Nematode-resistant population to common dewormers such as ivermectin and benzimidazoles.

CLIENT EDUCATION
Clients should be made aware of the major parasite risks in their specific geographic location as well as the seasonality and appropriate management practices necessary to decrease risk. Education on proper anthelmintic usage and resistance is also vital.

PATIENT CARE
N/A

PREVENTION
• Periodic fecal egg count reduction tests to monitor the development of nematode resistance. Maintenance of drug-susceptible nematode refugia population.
• Trematodes: Drain or fence off swampy areas.

MISCELLANEOUS
AGE-RELATED FACTORS
Age resistance may develop to some parasites such as coccidia, nematodes, and cestodes.

CAMELID: PARASITOLOGY   (CONTINUED)

Significant susceptibility to nematode infection remains throughout their life.

ZOONOTIC POTENTIAL
Minimal potential and generally only associated with protozoa such as *Cryptosporidium* or *Giardia*.

ABBREVIATIONS
- GI: gastrointestinal
- NWC: New world camelids
- PCR: polymerase chain reaction
- CNS: centran nervous system
- PO: per os, by mouth

SEE ALSO
- Anthelmintic Resistance
- Coccidioidomycosis
- Diarrheal Diseases: Camelid
- Down Camelid
- Haemonchosis
- Liver Flukes
- Parasite Control Programs: Camelid
- *Parelaphostrongylus tenuis* (Meningeal Worm)

Suggested Reading

Ballweber LR. Ecto- and endoparasites of new world camelids. Vet Clin North Am Food Anim Pract 2009, 25: 295–310.

Cebra C, Anderson DE, Tibary A, Van Saun RJ, Johnson LW. Llama and Alpaca Care, 1st ed. St. Louis: Elsevier, 2014.

Pinn TL, Bender HS, Stoko T, Erb HN, Schlafer DH, Perkins GA. Cerebrospinal fluid eosinophilia is a sensitive and specific test for the diagnosis of *Parelaphostrongylus tenuis* in camelids in the northeastern United States. J Vet Diagn Invest 2013, 25: 54–60.

Whitehead CE, Anderson DE. Neonatal diarrhea in llamas and alpacas. Small Rumin Res 2006, 61: 207–15.

Authors Antoinette E. Marsh and Jeff Lakritz
Consulting Editor Kaitlyn A. Lutz
Acknowledgment The authors and book editors acknowledge the prior contribution of Jennifer M. Ivany Ewoldt.

CAMELID: REPRODUCTION

BASICS

OVERVIEW
• Camelid reproductive anatomy and physiology present many peculiarities compared to other domestic species.
• Knowledge of these differences is required in order to provide a comprehensive reproductive medicine and surgery service.

INCIDENCE/PREVALENCE
Congenital abnormalities of the reproductive system are relatively common in SAC.

GEOGRAPHIC DISTRIBUTION
Worldwide

SYSTEMS AFFECTED
Reproductive

PATHOPHYSIOLOGY
Reproductive function is affected by genetics, nutrition, general health, and management.

Female Reproduction
• Puberty: Range is 4–8 months in alpacas, 8–12 months in llamas, 12–24 months in camels. Age at puberty is affected by genetics, nutrition, and early life health and development. • Recommended age at first breeding: 12–15 months in alpacas, 15–18 months in llamas, and 36–48 months in camels. Females should not be bred until they reach 65% of adult weight and height.
• Female camelids are not seasonal if they are in good body condition. • Camelids are induced ovulators. Spontaneous ovulation is very rare (1–5%) and occurs mostly in the postpartum. • Ovulation is induced by seminal plasma (ß nerve growth factor) and uterine inflammation. • In absence of copulation, there is a succession of overlapping follicular waves from both ovaries. Each follicular wave spans 12–23 days and has one or two dominant follicles. Follicles establish dominance when they are 7 mm in diameter in SAC and 8–9 mm in camels. Dominant follicles grow 12 mm in SAC and 25 mm in camels. Dominant follicles regress and become atretic in most cases. In camels, in 25–45% of cases dominant follicles continue to grow and form large anovulatory/hemorrhagic follicles, that may persist for a long time. Anovulatory hemorrhagic follicles may become luteinized and produce progesterone. • In presence of a sterile mating, the preovulatory follicle (7–12 mm in alpacas, 8–13 mm in llamas, 9–25 mm in camels) ovulates 30–48 hours in response to an LH surge which occurs within 30 minutes of copulation. Double ovulations are common. The corpus hemorrhagicum develops into a functional CL over a period of 5–6 days. The CL reaches its maximum diameter (peak progesterone production) by 8 days post-mating. The luteal phase is very short. PGF2$_\alpha$ is released by 10 days and

another period of receptive behavior starts by 14 days. The left uterine horn secretes PGF2$_\alpha$ systemically whereas from the right uterine horn PGF2$_\alpha$ secretion is more localized. In ovulating nonpregnant camelids the cycle length (from mating to another period of receptivity with possibility of ovulation) is 12–14 days.

Reproductive Function in the Male
• Penile-preputial adhesions prevent extension of the penis in the first year of life in SAC and for two years in camels. Preputial detachment is a good indicator of sexual activity. Spermatogenesis is initiated at 12 months in SAC but sexual maturity may not be reached until 2 and 3 years in some males. • Camels reach puberty between 3 and 4 years of age. Testicular size continues to grow until 4 years of age. • Sexual maturity is reached at 5 years of age. • Male camels are seasonal breeders and testicular size decreases during the nonbreeding season (dry/summer season).
• Mating behavior ○ Marking behavior in camels is characterized by smearing poll gland secretion and urine spraying. In SAC marking is limited to rubbing and dusting. ○ Camels exteriorize the soft palate and produce a metallic sound by grinding their teeth during the rutting season. ○ Males seek receptive females by smelling their urine, feces, and perineal area. All camelids display flehmen behavior. ○ Females are chased by the male and forced down by mounting (SAC) or neck pressure (camels). ○ Receptive females sit in the normal sternal position (cush) which is also the mating position. Female receptivity is not always correlated with follicular activity. Females that sit on their side may be submissive rather than receptive.
○ Copulation lasts 5–60 minutes in camelids (average 13–24 minutes). During copulation the male will display characteristic behavior (orgling sound in SAC, metallic teeth grinding and soft palate exteriorization in camels). ○ Semen is deposited in utero in a dribbling manner throughout copulation.

Reproductive Failure in the Female
• Females bred three times to a fertile male without resulting pregnancy should undergo complete evaluation for reproductive function. • The most common manifestations of reproductive disorders in the open female: ○ Repeat breeding ■ Females without follicular activity can display receptivity. Anestrus can be caused by nutritional deficiencies (poor body condition), lactation or development abnormalities. Hypothyroidism and pituitary dysfunction are possible but difficult to diagnose.
■ Ovulation failure: poor follicular development, incomplete mating, lack of LH surge, pituitary or hypothalamic disorders, hypothyroidism. Some males may be at increased risk of failing to induce ovulation.
■ Fertilization failure: caused by a disorder of gamete transport or survival, developmental

abnormalities (persistent hymen, segmental aplasia, double cervix, hydrosalpinx), endometritis, vaginal, cervical or uterine adhesions, endometritis. ■ Early embryonic death generally caused by uterine disorders, luteal insufficiency, chromosomal abnormalities. ○ *Absence of receptivity* ■ Congenital (intersex, gonadal dysgenesis). ■ Painful conditions, persistent hymen, vaginal or cervical adhesions, acquired anestrus). ■ Persistent luteal function (persistent CL). ■ Some females with normal follicular development may continue to refuse the male (behavioral problem). ■ Immature or small male may be rejected by mature aggressive female. ○ *Visible abnormalities of the genital tract* ■ Congenital: persistent hymen with mucometra, vulvar hypoplasia or aplasia, intersex conditions, elongated clitoris. ■ Acquired: bloody or mucopurulent discharge before or after mating due to uterine infection, vaginal adhesions, stenosis. ○ *Male-like behavior* ■ Female camelids may display normal homosexual behavior during the period of receptivity. ■ Clucking, orgling, and aggressive behavior toward the male may be seen in some androgenized females or in females with gonadal development abnormalities. ■ *Females with male-like behavior* should be examined for presence of granulosa-theca cell tumor (GTCT).
• Complaints in the pregnant female: ○ *Repeat pregnancy loss* ■ Incidence is relatively high in the first 60 days of pregnancy. Very young maiden females and females with previous reproductive problems are at risk. Most common causes are poor development (maiden), uterine fibrosis/inflammation, iatrogenic, poor luteal function, congenital abnormalities (uterus unicornis). ■ Infectious or noninfectious abortion. ○ Vaginal prolapse ■ Generally older or obese females ■ Occurs in the last trimester of pregnancy ○ *Uterine torsion* • Occurs in the last 2 months or at term • Common in llamas and alpacas ○ *Pregnancy toxemia/hepatic lipidosis* ■ Often a complication of a stressful condition with development of anorexia • Postpartum disorders: ○ *Retained placenta* ■ The placenta is considered retained if not delivered 6 hours after parturition. ■ Predisposing causes include hypocalcemia, uterine inertia, dystocia, selenium deficiency, uterine tears. ○ *Traumatic injuries to the reproductive tract* ■ Perineal laceration and rectovaginal tear occurs following dystocia and require surgical correction. ■ Vaginal tears are often due to prolonged manipulation. Many females develop a severe necrotic vaginitis and vaginal adhesion. ■ Cervical tears due to poor cervical dilation or early intervention. ○ *Postpartum metritis* ■ Severe puerperal metritis may develop after dystocia or prolonged untreated retained placenta. ■ Endotoxemia may develop. ■ May be complicated by hepatic lipidosis in anorexic females. ○ *Postpartum*

CAMELID: REPRODUCTION   (CONTINUED)

C

hemorrhage ▪ Rupture of the cranial or caudal (vaginal) branch of the uterine artery during parturition (can be fatal). ○ *Agalactia* ▪ Poor lactation is seen in primiparous females and following dystocia. ▪ Obese females are at risk. ▪ Fescue toxicosis is suspected to be a cause in SAC.

Reproductive Failure in the Male
• Reproductive disorders in the male should be approached using a thorough breeding soundness evaluation. • The most common complaints are ○ Poor libido ▪ Age and inexperience ▪ Musculoskeletal disease ▪ Painful conditions of the prepuce, penis (urethra), and testis ▪ Pain due to urolithiasis ▪ Systemic diseases ▪ Megaesophagus in alpacas and llamas may be a major component due to the discomfort caused by orgling (the call of the male). ○ *Erection failure* ▪ Persistent peno-preputial attachment ▪ Persistent frenulum ▪ Preputial adhesions ▪ Neurologic damage to the sacral nerve ▪ Sequelae of neurologic diseases (meningeal worm) ▪ Sequelae of debilitating diseases ○ *Ejaculation failure* ▪ Improper mating conditions: female position or receptivity, failure of cervical dilation, pneumovagina, urovagina ▪ Damaged cartilaginous process of the penis ▪ Painful condition ○ *Oligo- or azoospermia* ▪ Incomplete ejaculation ▪ Immaturity ▪ Testicular hypoplasia ▪ Testicular cysts ▪ Testicular degeneration ▪ Heat stress ▪ Orchitis/epididymitis ▪ Testicular neoplasia ○ *Teratozoospermia* ▪ Immaturity ▪ Testicular degeneration ▪ Testicular insult

HISTORICAL FINDINGS
Depends on complaint

SIGNALMENT
Domestic camelids include alpacas (*Vicugna pacos),* llamas *(Lama glama),* dromedary (*C. dromedarius*), and Bactrian camel (*C. bactrianus*).

PHYSICAL EXAMINATION FINDINGS
• History is critical for the diagnosis of all reproductive disorders. • Management is a common underlying problem in many reproductive disorders. • Physical examination findings depend on the complaint.

GENETICS
Some reproductive parameters may be affected by breed.

CAUSES AND RISK FACTORS
Risk factors for reproductive disorders include age, poor management, poor nutrition, and systemic diseases.

 DIAGNOSIS

DIFFERENTIAL DIAGNOSES
• Differential diagnosis of the cause of infertility in females requires an evaluation combining clinical (palpation and ultrasonography per rectum, vaginal examination), histopathologic (uterine cytology and biopsy), microbiologic (uterine culture), and endocrinologic (hormone assays) techniques. • Differential diagnosis of the cause of infertility in males requires a complete breeding soundness evaluation including clinical (palpation and ultrasonography of the testis), semen collection and evaluation, histopathologic (testicular biopsy), and endocrinologic (hormone assays) techniques. • Other techniques such as hysteroscopy, laparoscopy, exploratory laparotomy, and cytogenetics may be indicated in some cases.

CBC/BIOCHMESTRY/URIANALYSIS
• In the female, CBC and serum biochemistry are indicated if the health of the patient is compromised (uterine torsion, suspected hepatic lipidosis, abortion, postpartum metritis) or the female appears debilitated (downer animals). • In the male, CBC and serum biochemistry are indicated if the male presents for an emergency scrotal or preputial swelling or dysuria.

OTHER LABORATORY TESTS
Serology
Testing for brucellosis, BVD, trypanosomiasis

Bacteriology and Virology
• Diagnosis of uterine infection • Diagnosis of infectious causes of abortion

Endocrinologic Evaluation
Progesterone
In the absence of luteal tissue, serum progesterone should be <1 ng/mL. Concentrations of 1–2 ng/mL are difficult to interpret but suggest presence of luteal tissue. Concentrations >2 ng/mL suggest presence of a normal CL.
• Occurrence of ovulation: samples taken 8 days after mating. • Pregnancy diagnosis: samples taken 14 days and 3 weeks after mating. • Pregnancy loss: luteal insufficiency. Samples <1.5 ng/mL in females confirmed pregnant by ultrasonography are arbitrarily considered suspect for luteal insufficiency.
• Accuracy is affected by: ○ Laboratory errors, sensitivity of method used ○ Sample handling errors ○ High progesterone may indicate persistent CL function or presence of luteinized anovulatory follicles.
Estrogens
• Determination of estradiol 17β or estrone sulfate. • Determination of follicular activity. Not as accurate as ultrasonography.
• Pregnancy: Ultrasonography is easier and more accurate.
FSH Challenge
Administration of FSH or FSH-like hormones (eCG) may be used to determine whether the female is capable of growing follicles (differentiates acquired anestrus from congenital ovarian hypoplasia).

LH or GnRH Challenge
• Administration of LH in the form of hCG or GnRH allows verification of the ability of the female to ovulate. • Administration in males followed by determination of testosterone levels allows verification of presence of testicular tissue (cryptorchid, intersex).
Inhibin and Anti-Mullerian Hormone
• In the male: diagnosis of cryptorchidism
• In the female: diagnosis of GTCT
Testosterone
Presence of testicular tissue (cryptorchid) or interstitial cell tumors
Thyroid Function Evaluation
Testing for hypothyroidism is indicated in cases of absence of ovarian activity, recurrent pregnancy loss, or poor spermatogenesis.

Cytogenetics
• All camelids have 74 chromosomes.
• Karyotyping and chromosome banding is indicated in all cases of congenital abnormalities or in females born co-twin to male (rare but possible). • Cytogenetic abnormalities include: 73 XO, 74XX/73XO, 74XX/73XY, 75XXX, 74XX sex reversal, 74XY testicular feminization. • A minute chromosome has been reported in llamas and alpacas and has been found in females with ovarian dysgenesis.

Semen Collection and Evaluation in Males
See chapter, Breeding Soundness Examination: Camelids.

Trace Mineral Analysis
Trace mineral status should be evaluated in all cases on unexplained infertility, abortion, and recurrent pregnancy loss.

IMAGING
• Ultrasonography ○ In the female: Transrectal ultrasonography (linear 5 or 7.5 MHz transducer) is an important part of any reproductive evaluation of the open or early pregnant female. Transabdominal ultrasonography (3.5 MHz linear or sector transducer) is performed at any stage of pregnancy to determine fetal and placental health in females with compromised health. Transabdominal ultrasonography may be used for the diagnosis of other ovarian and uterine disorders not visualized on transrectal ultrasonography. ○ In the male, ultrasonography is important for the evaluation of testicular parenchyma, and verification of presence of abdominal or inguinal testes. • Radiography ○ Fluoroscopy should be considered for the evaluation of cervical patency.

OTHER DIAGNOSTIC PROCEDURES
• Vaginal examination ○ Indicated for all open females, pregnant females with abnormal vaginal discharge. ○ Use mare tube speculum for camels and llamas, and human sigmoidoscope for alpacas. ○ Look for congenital or acquired vaginal and cervical

abnormalities, origin of discharge. • Uterine culture and cytology ○ Indicated for all females with a history of infertility or presence of abnormal uterine content or vaginal discharge. ○ Use mare double-guarded swabs for bacteriology and cytobrush for endometrial cytology. ○ Ideally done when female is receptive (cervix open). ○ Samples should be taken from the uterine cavity (not the cervix). ○ Combined bacteriology and cytology are very good for the assessment of uterine infection. • Endometrial biopsy ○ Considered the gold standard for prognostication of the ability of a female to maintain a pregnancy to term. ○ It should be performed in all cases of chronic infertility or recurrent pregnancy loss. ○ For camels and llamas, use mare biopsy forceps; use heifer or human rectal biopsy forceps (Turell) for alpacas and llamas. • Laparoscopy/exploratory laparotomy ○ Use techniques similar to sheep and goats for llamas and alpacas. ○ Laparoscopy is difficulty in camels, exploratory flank laparotomy is preferred. ○ Use for the confirmation of abnormalities suspected on palpation and ultrasonography: ■ Periuterine adhesions ■ Ovarian abnormalities (dysgenesis, tumors, cystic structures, adhesions) ■ Segmental aplasia ■ Verification of uterine tube patency. • Hysteroscopy ○ Indications: abnormal echotexture of the uterus, severe bleeding following mating, unexplained infertility. ○ Alpaca and llamas: use pediatric gastroscope. ○ Camels: use adult gastroscope. ○ Animals should be sedated. ○ Each uterine horn should be examined all the way to the uterotubal junction. ○ Findings: uterine tears, intraluminal adhesions, neoplasm, cysts, foreign objects.

PATHOLOGIC FINDINGS
• Ovarian abnormalities include hypoplasia or dysgenesis, ovarian neoplasia (GTCT and teratomas) • Congenital (infantilism, uterus unicornis, mucometra) or acquired uterine abnormalities (fibrosis, inflammation, pyometra, intraluminal adhesions, uterine cysts) • Congenital (cervical aplasia, stenosis) or acquired cervical abnormalities (cervical lacerations, fibrosis, adhesions) • Congenital (duplication, persistent hymen, stenosis) or acquired (adhesions) vestibulo-vaginal abnormalities • Testicular and penile abnormalities in males

TREATMENT

THERAPEUTIC APPROACH
• Treatment protocol depends on the complaint. • Animals with congenital defects should be removed from breeding. • Treatment of endometritis requires uterine lavage followed by proper antimicrobial therapy for 4–5 days. • Acquired ovarian

disorders are treated by proper hormonal management, adjustment of nutrition or surgically.

SURGICAL CONSIDERATIONS AND TECHNIQUES
• In the female ○ Unilateral ovariectomy (laparoscopy or via flank laparotomy) for all acquired ovarian and bursal disorders that cannot be managed by hormonal therapy. ○ Vulvoplasty in cases of postpartum perineal laceration. ○ Uterine torsion may require surgical correction via laparotomy. • In the male ○ Castration (normal) or cryptorchidectomy (parainguinal or laparoscopy-assisted) for nonbreeding quality males. ○ Unilateral castration for unilateral acquired testicular disorders.

MEDICATIONS

DRUGS OF CHOICE
• Hormones
○ Oxytocin (IM): (5–10 IU in llamas and alpacas, 20–40 IU in camels) for retained placenta
○ PGF2$_\alpha$ (Dinoprost tromethamine IM, 5–10 mg in SAC, 20–35 mg for camels) or analogs (Cloprostenol IM, SAC 250 µg, camels 500–750 µg) for retained CL or luteal structures and induction of parturition or abortion.
○ PGE (misoprostol): Cervical dilation within 30–120 minutes after local application of 500 µg–1 mg of PGE in gel.
○ Progesterone for maintenance of pregnancy: natural progesterone daily (50 mg in SAC, 150 mg in camels) or hydroxyprogesterone caproate (250 mg every 3 weeks in alpacas).
○ Human chorionic gonadotropin (hCG) IV, 500–750 IU for SAC, 1,500–3,000 IU for camels for induction of ovulation.
○ GnRH or analogs IM (50 µg in SAC and 100 µg in camels) for induction of ovulation or to increase libido in males.
• Antibiotics
○ Postpartum metritis: Systemic antibiotics.
○ Uterine lavage (make sure that there are no traumatic lesions to the uterus and cervix).
○ Endometritis
■ Uterine flushing with a buffered solution.
■ Intrauterine infusion of antibiotics based on culture and sensitivity for 3–5 days.
■ Some antibiotics such as ceftiofur can be used systemically.

CONTRAINDICATIONS
• Appropriate milk and meat withdrawal times must be followed for food-producing animals. • Anti-inflammatory steroids are contraindicated during pregnancy, particularly in the last half. • Estrogens should not be used to enhance cervical dilation.

• Testosterone or anabolic steroids should not be used in breeding males. • Progesterone therapy is contraindicated in cases of uterine infection.

PRECAUTIONS
• Toxicity (respiratory distress) has been reported with high doses of PGF2$_\alpha$.
• Aminoglycosides are nephrotoxic.

POSSIBLE INTERACTIONS
• Maintenance of pregnancy with exogenous progesterone may result in failure of cervical dilation. • Progesterone therapy should be stopped at 300 days' gestation in SAC.

FOLLOW-UP

EXPECTED COURSE AND PROGNOSIS
• Prognosis for fertility: Good for uterine infections and unilateral ovarian disorders with proper treatment and management of breeding. • Prognosis is poor for females with severe chronic uterine disorders, cervical or vaginal adhesions. Assisted reproductive biotechnologies may be the only course of action. • Prognosis for fertility in males is good if affection is unilateral and no other complications are observed.

POSSIBLE COMPLICATIONS
• Mucometra and pyometra are common complications of congenital abnormalities and severe vaginal or cervical adhesions.
• Peritonitis and periuterine adhesions may occur following ovariectomy or laparoscopy.
• In males, complications of castration.

CLIENT EDUCATION
• All breeding animal should undergo a BSE before initiation of mating. • Animal with congenital defects should be removed from the breeding pool. • Breeding animals should be in top health (adequate nutritional and preventive program). • Females should undergo postpartum examination before rebreeding. • Breeding management practice: Avoid excessive mating.

PATIENT CARE
Varies depending on complaint and diagnosis

PREVENTION
• Prevention of acquired infertility relies on a sound herd health program and good management practice. • Practice strict measures of biosecurity and hygiene in breeding animals, particularly if outside animals are bred.

MISCELLANEOUS

ASSOCIATED CONDITIONS
• Varies according to complaint. • Poor nutrition and contagious infectious diseases may be the underlying cause of infertility.

CAMELID: REPRODUCTION

C

AGE-RELATED FACTORS
• Congenital defects should not be overlooked in young/maiden animals. • Senile changes include poor ovarian activity, uterine degenerative changes in the female, and poor libido and testicular degeneration in males.

ZOONOTIC POTENTIAL
Many abortive diseases are potentially zoonotic.

PREGNANCY
• The left uterine horn is almost always the fetal horn in camelids. • Maintenance of pregnancy relies exclusively on ovarian progesterone. • Administration of PGF2$_\alpha$ or analogs at any stage results in loss of pregnancy.

BIOSECURITY
• Quarantine all breeding animals from other herds and animals participating in shows or other off-farm activity. • Fencing is extremely important when herds are in proximity to each other. • Contact with other ruminants should be monitored and limited.

PRODUCTION MANAGEMENT
• Free mating systems: Practiced in large herds with one male or several males in a group. It does not allow precise record keeping for breeding dates and early identification of infertile males or females. Pregnancy diagnosis is scheduled periodically. Prediction of parturition date requires estimation of gestation age. • Controlled field mating: The male is introduced at a specific time of the day and observed for breeding activity. Some males may display complete breeding behavior but do not complete penetration. Pregnancy diagnosis is scheduled at specific dates after mating. • In-hand mating: This system is commonly used for breeding valuable animals and has several advantages: breeding records and pregnancy stages are more precise. • Controlled breeding: Females are presented to the stud only after veterinary verification of follicular status. This system is recommended for efficient use of males and management of infertile females or visiting females.

SYNONYMS
N/A

ABREVIATIONS
• BSE = breeding soundness examination
• BVD = bovine viral diarrhea
• CL = corpus luteum
• eCG = equine chorionic gonadotropin
• FSH = follicle stimulating hormone
• *GnRH = gonadotropin releasing hormone*
• GTCT = granulosa-theca cell tumor
• hCG = human chorionic gonadotropin
• IM = intramuscular
• IU = international units/intrauterine
• IV = intravenous
• LH = luteinizing hormone
• PGE = prostaglandin E
• PGF2$_\alpha$ = prostaglandin F2$_\alpha$
• SAC = South American camelids

SEE ALSO
• Abortion: Camelid
• Body Condition Scoring: Alpacas and Llamas (see www.fiveminutevet.com/ruminant)
• Body Condition Scoring: Camels (see www.fiveminutevet.com/ruminant)
• Breeding Soundness Examination: Camelid
• Castration/Vasectomy: Camelid
• Cesarean Section: Camelid
• Congenital Defects: Camelid
• Dystocia: Camelid
• Embryo Transfer: Camelid
• Nutrition and Metabolic Diseases: Camelid (see www.fiveminutevet.com/ruminant)
• Parasite Control Programs: Camelid
• Physical Examination: Camelid (Appendix 5)
• Pregnancy Diagnosis: Camelid
• Pregnancy Toxemia: Camelid
• Testicular Disorders: Camelid
• Reproductive Ultrasonography: Camelid (see www.fiveminutevet.com/ruminant)
• Uterine Torsion: Camelid
• Vaccination Programs: Camelid
• Weight Loss: Camelid

Suggested Reading
Pearson LK, Tibary A. Reproductive disorders of male camelids. Clin Theriogenol 2014, 6: 571–7.
Pearson LK, Tibary A. Reproductive failure in female camelids. Clin Theriogenol 2014, 6: 555–70.
Rodriguez JS, Pearson LK, Tibary A. Clinical examination of the female reproductive function. In: Cebra C, Anderson DE, Tibary et al. eds, Llama and Alpaca Care. St. Louis: Saunders, 2014, pp. 168–87.
Rodriguez JS, Pearson LK, Tibary A. Infertility and subfertility in the female camelid. In: Cebra C, Anderson DE, Tibary et al. eds, Llama and Alpaca Care. St. Louis: Saunders, 2014, pp. 216–43.
Tibary A, Pearson LK, Anouassi A. Applied andrology in camelids. Wallingford: CABI, 2014, pp. 418–49.
Author Ahmed Tibary
Consulting Editor Ahmed Tibary

BASICS

OVERVIEW

• *Campylobacter* are Gram-negative, microaerophilic, curved or spiral rods in the family Campylobacteriaceae.
• *Campylobacter jejuni* (formerly known as *C. fetus* subsp. *jejuni*) and *C. coli* are associated with enteritis in domestic animals. *C. fetus* subsp. *fetus* is found in cattle, sheep, and goats. *C. fetus* subsp. *venerealis* is found in cattle.
• *C. jejuni, C. fetus* subsp. *venerealis*, and *C. fetus* subsp. *fetus* (also known as *C. fetus* subsp. *intestinalis* and *Vibrio fetus var intestinalis*) cause infertility and abortions in sheep, cattle, and goats.
• An additional subspecies of *venerealis* was identified as biotype *intermedius* (*C. fetus venerealis intermedius*) which has also been shown to cause fertility issues in cattle.
• *C. fetus* subsp. *fetus* is occasionally isolated from humans with septicemia.
• *C. lari, C. hyointestinalis,* and *C. upsaliensis* have been reported to cause disease but seem to be of minor importance in domestic animals.
• *C. jejuni* can be shed for as long as 2–7 weeks in untreated infections and *C. fetus* subsp. *fetus* can be shed for several days to several weeks.

INCIDENCE/PREVALENCE

• Incidence of *C. jejuni* and *C. coli* enteritis and resultant diarrhea is variable and oftentimes these organisms can be isolated from healthy animals with no apparent signs of disease.
• Bovine infections with *C. fetus* subsp. *fetus* do occur but are considered to be much more sporadic in occurrence in comparison to sheep.

GEOGRAPHIC DISTRIBUTION

• Campylobacteriosis exists worldwide including South-America, Africa, Asia, North America, Europe, and New Zealand.
• The true prevalence of *Campylobacter* in some countries is still questionable due to lack of reporting and reliable testing.

SYSTEMS AFFECTED

• Reproductive
• Digestive

PATHOPHYSIOLOGY

• *C. fetus* subsp. *fetus* is transmitted primarily by ingestion in cattle, sheep, and goats.
• Oral transmission of *C. fetus* subsp. *fetus* occurs and results in bacteremia and subsequent colonization of the gall bladder and intestines of sheep and cattle leading to systemic infections: enteritis, hepatitis and late-term abortion, still births, mostly in sheep and goats and sporadically in cattle.
• Transmission can also occur following contact with contaminated feed, water, feces,

vaginal discharges, aborted fetuses and fetal membranes.
• Venereal transmission of *C. fetus* subsp. *venerealis* as well as an additional subspecies of *venerealis* biotype *intermedius* (*C. fetus venerealis intermedius*) can occur.
• Genital *C. fetus* infections can be spread on fomites including contaminated semen, contaminated instruments and bedding.
• Cattle are considered the primary reservoir of *C. fetus* subsp. *venerealis* and bulls may transmit *C. fetus* for several hours after being bred to an infected cow; some bulls and cows can become chronic or persistent carriers, respectively.
• During coitus contaminated semen gains entrance to the vagina and can live in the cervical mucus for 3 weeks to 3 months.
• The organism can grow and thrive on the penis and prepuce of the bull with the correct microenvironment.
• *C. fetus* subsp. *venerealis* and *C. fetus venerealis intermedius* are confined to the epithelial surface of the glans penis, prepuce, and the urethra.
• Infection is often manifested as infertility, embryonic and fetal death, metritis, placentitis, salpingitis, pyometra, and abortion.

HISTORICAL FINDINGS

In herds with venereal disease, poor conception rates or birth rates may be the first sign noticed.

SIGNALMENT

• Naïve, pregnant ruminants are most often severely affected by *C. fetus* subsp. *venerealis* and *C. fetus* subsp. *fetus*.
• *C. jejuni and C. coli* will affect naïve animal populations as well.

PHYSICAL EXAMINATION FINDINGS

• Enteritis, diarrhea, and dehydration are seen in *C. jejuni* and *C. coli* infections.
• Infertility, placentitis, salpingitis, embryonic and fetal death, abortion, stillbirths, vulvar discharge, metritis, reduced lamb and kid crops, and calf crop, and reduced weaning weights are seen in *C. fetus* subsp. *venerealis* and with *C. fetus* subsp. *fetus*.

GENETICS

N/A

CAUSES AND RISK FACTORS

• Exposure of naïve populations to *C. fetus* subsp. *fetus* and *C. fetus* subsp. *venerealis* is a risk factor.
• Widespread contamination of feed and water troughs and pastures increases the chances for exposure and infection.

DIAGNOSIS

DIFFERENTIAL DIAGNOSES

• There are a number of diseases in sheep and goats that result in abortion infertility and

have similar signs such as trichomoniasis, bluetongue, BVDV, with many being zoonotic including: *Brucella melitensis* (goats), *Brucella ovis* (sheep), *Coxiella burnetii, Chlamydophila abortus, Leptospira* spp., *Listeria monocytogenes, Toxoplasma gondii,* and Rift Valley fever.
• The differentials list for enteritis and diarrhea is a long one and includes: toxic insults, nutritional disturbances, *E. coli* and *Salmonella*, Border disease, BVDV, corona- and rotaviruses, and many others.

CBC/BIOCHEMISTRY/URINALYSIS

• Neutrophilia with a high fibrinogen due to local and systemic infection is often found.
• The hematocrit may be decreased or falsely elevated due to dehydration.

OTHER LABORATORY TESTS

• Fecal and blood cultures may be run on sick animals.
• Uterine/vaginal swabs taken within 3 days of abortion.

IMAGING

N/A

OTHER DIAGNOSTIC PROCEDURES

• *Campylobacter* spp. have an "S," "spiral," or "seagull" shape.
• In order for *Campylobacter* to be detected on culture, it must be incubated at 37°C for at least 3 days in a micro-aerobic atmosphere.
• Discrimination between species and subspecies requires additional biochemical or molecular methods (i.e., PCR).
• A presumptive diagnosis can be made utilizing dark field or phase contrast microscopy if characteristic darting motile organisms are seen.
• Whole or partial placentas are optimal for submission for culture and analysis.
• Acute (at the time of abortion) and convalescent (2–3 weeks post-abortion) serum titers are an important indicator of current and past exposure and can reflect ongoing bacteremia or viremia.
• Diagnosis via collection of cervical mucus from infected cows and heifers at 3 weeks to 3 months post-infection can be made.
• If cervical mucus is collected in metestrus, false-positives can occur at a higher rate.
• Culture results, vaginal mucus agglutination tests, and fluorescent antibody tests can all be questionable so confirmatory PCR is being looked to as a more reliable diagnostic of herd infection.
• Bulls: Preputial scraping or preputial wash performed twice, one week apart, or testing of contaminated semen via culture, fluorescent antibody, and PCR.
• It is imperative that the sample be inoculated into Clark's media soon after collection to allow for maximum survival of the organism.
• The organism can survive for approximately 6–8 hours following collection but when placed in Clark's media it will allow for a longer period of survival up to 48 hours.

PATHOLOGIC FINDINGS
• Whole or partial placentas are optimal for assessment of pathology.
• Abortion, metritis, endometritis, salpingitis, and enteritis can all be seen in the dam during and after infection.
• The fetus may have bronchopneumonia, pleuritis, hepatitis, or peritonitis and may even present as an autolyzed fetus in *C. fetus* abortions in sheep.
• Necrotic yellow to orange foci in the liver, mild placentitis with hemorrhagic cotyledons, and edematous "leathery" intercotyledonary areas may be seen.
• Histologically areas of vasculitis and necrosis are seen.
• Fetal and placental lesions may also be absent.
• The aborted fetus is the best sample for diagnosis of *C. fetus* subsp. *fetus*.
• The aborted fetus and preputial washes are the most likely samples from which to isolate *C. fetus* subsp. *venerealis*.

TREATMENT
THERAPEUTIC APPROACH
• *C. fetus* subsp. *fetus* abortion storms in sheep can be treated with tetracyclines, penicillin, or streptomycin.
• Supportive care including fluids, antibiotics, and anti-endotoxin drugs may be necessary in cases of *C. jejuni* and *C. coli* enteritis.
• Whole herd treatment of *C. fetus* is considered to be impractical due to the lack of overt clinical signs at the initiation of the disease process.
• Bulls may be treated with extra-label administration of one to two treatments of streptomycin given subcutaneously at a dose of 20 mg/kg along with administration of a topical suspension containing 5 g streptomycin to the prepuce and penis for three consecutive days, but resistant strains have been reported.
• Prevention of venereal diseases in the herd is the most practical approach to dealing with *C. fetus*.

MEDICATIONS
DRUGS OF CHOICE
• Tetracyclines, penicillins, and streptomycin.
• Streptomycin is the drug of choice for *C. fetus* subsp. *venerealis* infections but resistance has been reported.

CONTRAINDICATIONS
All animals receiving drugs must undergo the determined milk and meat withdrawal times prior to the meat or milk from the animal entering the food supply.

FOLLOW-UP
EXPECTED COURSE AND PROGNOSIS
• Mortality is low in adult sheep and cattle.
• Morbidity may be up to 90% in outbreaks in sheep but is usually around 5–50%.
• For sheep flocks, there will be some level of convalescent immunity which will decrease infections and abortions for a few years but subsequent abortions and fertility problems will again occur.
• Most cows will clear the infection in approximately 3–6 months and have some immunity to *C. fetus* subsp. *venerealis*.
• Bulls will often develop a chronic infection and carrier state with *C. fetus* subsp. *venerealis* infections due to the organism thriving in the microenvironment of the bull's prepuce and penis.
• Herd immunity can reduce the significant economic losses associated with *Campylobacter* infections but, due to short-lived immunity, losses will continue if strict prevention and control measures are not instituted.

POSSIBLE COMPLICATIONS
Additional complications may include endocarditis, pericarditis, pneumonia, thrombophlebitis, peritonitis, or meningoencephalitis.

CLIENT EDUCATION
See "Biosecurity"

PATIENT CARE
Appropriate monitoring and treatment of all sick animals as well as isolation from other pregnant animals is indicated.

PREVENTION
• Control measures include utilization of AI with non-contaminated semen, testing and culling of infected animals, and vaccination of all bulls, cows, and heifers.
• Utilization of AI exclusively for two breeding seasons is suggested in infected herds.
• The use of AI is impractical in range cattle but most producers utilize management (cull problem cattle and use virgin bulls) and vaccination as their primary means of prevention and control.
• The recommendations for vaccination by the World Organisation of Animal Health (OIE) include vaccination of all infected herds: all breeding animals should be vaccinated twice prior to the breeding season.
• Cows and heifers are often administered an additional vaccine in the middle of the breeding season to enhance their immunity.
• Vaccination reduces the length of the infection but carrier cows may still infect susceptible bulls.
• It has been suggested that bulls should be given double the dose of vaccine at each of two vaccinations annually to assist in terminating established infections.

• Noninfected herds: Bulls should at least be vaccinated initially with two doses given 3–4 weeks apart with the last dose approximately 30 days prior to the start of the breeding season.

MISCELLANEOUS
ASSOCIATED CONDITIONS
Bacteremia, septicemia, hepatitis, dehydration, and death can all be associated with infections.

AGE-RELATED FACTORS
Older flocks and herds might have some protection from previous exposure or vaccination.

ZOONOTIC POTENTIAL
• *Campylobacter* species are readily transmitted between animals or from animals to humans.
• Organisms are present in feces, vaginal discharges, and the products of abortions and can be spread by direct contact, on fomites, and by arthropods acting as mechanical vectors.
• The consumption of raw milk and contaminated meat are the primary sources of infection in humans.

PREGNANCY
Female ruminants may become pregnant but sporadically abort in the case of *C. fetus* subsp. *fetus* and *C. fetus* subsp. *venerealis* results in early embryonic death and repeat breeder syndrome as well as abortion in sheep and cattle.

BIOSECURITY
• Isolation and testing of sick animals and any replacements is necessary to prevent disease transmission to herd animals.
• Disinfectants can be utilized to kill *Campylobacter* species and 1% sodium hypochlorite, 70% ethanol, 2% glutaraldehyde, iodine-based disinfectants, phenolic disinfectants, and formaldehyde are efficacious against the organism.
• Disinfectants have been used to kill *C. jejuni* and *C. fetus* in drinking water.
• Moist heat, dry heat, and gamma irradiation and UV radiation can also kill *C. jejuni* and *C. fetus*.

PRODUCTION MANAGEMENT
• Isolation and testing of sick animals along with vaccination during abortion storms seems the most effective against *C. fetus* subsp. *fetus* abortion storms.
• Use of virgin bulls that are tested negative for *Tritrichomonas* and *Campylobacter*.
• Culling carrier bulls.
• Utilization of AI with antibiotic extenders for 2 years due to the chance of a bull breeding a chronically infected cow.
• Follow guidelines for vaccination.

SYNONYMS
Vibriosis

ABBREVIATIONS
- AI = artificial insemination
- BVDV = bovine viral diarrhea virus
- PCR = polymerase chain reaction

SEE ALSO
Beef Bull Management (see www.fiveminutevet.com/ruminant)

Suggested Reading

OIE. Chapter 2.4.5, http://www.oie.int/ fileadmin/Home/eng/Health_standards/ tahm/2.04.05_BGC.pdf

Chaban B, Chu S, Hendrick S, Waldner C, Hill. Evaluation of a *Campylobacter fetus* subspecies *venerealis* real-time quantitative polymerase chain reaction for direct analysis of bovine preputial samples. Can J Vet Res 2012, 76: 166–73.

Cobo ER, et al. Immunization in heifers with dual vaccines containing *Tritrichomonas foetus* and *Campylobacter fetus* antigens using systemic and mucosal routes. Theriogenology 2004, 62: 1367–82.

Sanderson M, Gnad D. Biosecurity for reproductive diseases. Vet Clin North Am Food Anim Pract 2002, 18: 79–98.

Sanhueza JM, Heuer C, Jackson R, Hughes P, Anderson P, Kelly K, Walker G. Pregnancy rates of beef cattle are not affected by *Campylobacter fetus* subsp. *venerealis* real-time PCR-positive breeding sires in New Zealand. NZ Vet J 2014, 62: 237–43.

Truyers I, Luke T, Wilson D, Sargison N. Diagnosis and management of venereal campylobacteriosis in beef cattle. BMC Vet Res 2014, 10: 280.

Waldner C, Hendrick S, Chaban B, Garcia Guerra A, Griffin G, Campbell J, Hill J. Application of a new diagnostic approach to a bovine genital campylobacteriosis outbreak in a Saskatchewan beef herd. Can Vet J 2013, 54: 373–6.

Yaeger MJ, Holler LD. Bacterial causes of bovine infertility and abortion. In: Younquist RS ed, Current Therapy in Large Animal Theriogenology, 2nd ed. Philadelphia: Saunders, 2007, p. 391.

Author Julie A. Gard

Consulting Editor Kaitlyn A. Lutz

Acknowledgment The author and book editors acknowledge the prior contribution of John M. Adaska.

CANDIDIASIS

C

BASICS

OVERVIEW
• *Candida* is not highly pathogenic and rarely causes disease in healthy animals.
• Various *Candida* species are normal microflora of intestinal, oral, upper respiratory, and reproductive tracts of mammals and are commonly found in feces.
• Causes opportunistic disease in various body systems, especially in immunocompromised or malnourished animals or those that have been extensively treated with antibiotics.

INCIDENCE/PREVALENCE
N/A

GEOGRAPHIC DISTRIBUTION
Candida spp. are found worldwide.

SYSTEMS AFFECTED
• Integument
• Digestive
• Reproductive
• Respiratory

PATHOPHYSIOLOGY
• *Candida* spp. are yeasts that propagate by budding.
• Cells are round to oval, 3.5–6 × 6–10 µm and buds are single or multiple.
• Form blastoconidia, pseudohyphae, and true hyphae in culture and in tissues.
• Form mycelium or pseudomycelium when invading tissue.
• *Candida* spp. produce acid proteinases and keratinases, which degrade the stratum corneum, and phospholipases, which aid in penetration of tissues.
• In systemic mycosis, the alimentary tract is the most common route of entry of the organism, which then spreads hematogenously.

SIGNALMENT
• Cattle, camelids, sheep, and goats.
• Most common in neonatal, debilitated or immunocompromised animals.
• Occurs as a complication of polyantimicrobial therapy.

PHYSICAL EXAMINATION FINDINGS
• Depends on organ systems affected.
• Dermatitis
  ○ Reported in cattle, camelids, sheep, and goats.
  ○ Chronic moisture and skin maceration predispose to yeast invasion.
  ○ Cattle: Ulceration, erosion, scaling, crusting, papules, pustules, and secondary alopecia.
  ○ Goats: Nonpruritic exfoliative dermatitis with alopecia, scales, crusting, greasiness, and lichenification.
  ○ Evaluate affected goats for protein deficiency or trace mineral deficiency.
  ○ Camelids: Nonpruritic crusting, papule formation, and epidermal hyperplasia.

• Alimentary
  ○ Reported primarily in cattle.
  ○ Calves: Oral candidiasis (thrush) is characterized by white pseudomembranous plaque and ulcers over tongue and gingiva.
  ○ Mycotic pharyngitis and gastroenteritis in calves results in white pseudomembranes at back of pharynx and extending down to forestomachs.
  ○ Diarrhea in young calves following prolonged use of antimicrobials.
  ○ Adult cattle: Mycotic omasitis, rumenitis, and enteritis reported; forestomach lesions include acute hemorrhagic mucosal necrosis.
  ○ Cattle with GI candidiasis may show nonspecific signs including lethargy, hypophagia, milk drop, decreased GI motility, ± fever, ± low-grade abdominal pain.
• Abortion
  ○ Rare cause of abortion in cattle and goats.
  ○ Abortion at 6–8 months' gestation in cattle.
  ○ Abortus may have patchy alopecia and/or felted appearance.
• Mastitis
  ○ Reported in cattle, sheep, and goats.
  ○ Milk drop, increased SCC and hard, swollen udder usually resolve spontaneously after 5–6 days.
  ○ Organisms are shed in milk for 1–5 weeks; SCC remains increased for up to 2 months.
  ○ Fever (104–107°F; 40–40.5°C) may be seen acutely.
  ○ May become chronic.
• Pneumonia
  ○ Reported in cattle and sheep.
  ○ Seen in calves and lambs raised indoors.
  ○ Feedlot cattle may show chronic pneumonia, pulmonary abscesses, dyspnea, fever, brownish nasal discharge, diarrhea, and lacrimation; outbreaks have been reported.
• Systemic candidiasis
  ○ Reported in cattle, sheep, goats, and camelids.
  ○ Peracute septicemic infections reported in newborn calves.
  ○ May affect lungs, GI tract, brain, kidney, liver, heart, pancreas, udder, and reproductive tract.
  ○ Signs depend on system(s) affected; fever (104–107°F; 40–40.5°C) may be seen.

CAUSES AND RISK FACTORS
• Prolonged antibiotic therapy, especially if administered orally.
• Immunocompromised.
• Glucocorticoid or immunosuppressive therapy.
• Malnutrition.
• Exposure to chronic moisture.
• Feeding of poorly formulated artificial diets to sucklings.
• Use of intramammary infusions may be a risk for development of mastitis.

DIAGNOSIS

DIFFERENTIAL DIAGNOSIS
• Other fungal, bacterial or parasitic skin infections.
• Other systemic mycoses.
• Common causes of diarrhea, mastitis, or pneumonia in ruminants.

CBC/BIOCHEMISTRY/URINALYSIS
No specific clinicopathologic changes have been noted.

OTHER LABORATORY TESTS
• Isolation of organism from infected material plus histologic evidence of invasion is the gold standard.
• Culture of skin biopsy, lesion swab or feces: Sabouraud dextrose agar incubated at 30°C; also grows readily on potato dextrose agar and blood agar.
• Colonies are white to cream, shiny, convex, 3–5 mm diameter and smell "beery."
• Skin scraping for cytology, impression smears taken from the edge of the lesion, or direct fecal smears: Budding yeast or pseudohyphae may be seen.
• Scrapings/smears may be viewed with 10% KOH, Diff-Quick, Gram or new methylene blue stains.
• Periodic acid-Schiff, Gridley or Gomori methenamine silver techniques make organisms visible in tissue biopsies or necropsy specimens.
• In systemic cases, polymerase chain reaction, immunohistochemistry or serology may be useful.

OTHER DIAGNOSTIC PROCEDURES
• Direct smear or scraping: Cytology of lesion exudate.
• Culture of lesion exudate, tissue or feces.

PATHOLOGIC FINDINGS
• Dependent on system affected.
• Yeasts, pseudohyphae or hyphae demonstrated as invading tissue.

TREATMENT

THERAPEUTIC APPROACH
• Treatment of underlying or predisposing condition.
  ○ Withdrawal of immunosuppressive drugs.
  ○ Withdrawal of antibiotics, if possible.
  ○ Provide adequate and balanced nutrition.
  ○ Treat underlying disease process if present.
  ○ Remove from excessive moisture.
• Dermatitis:
  ○ Focal lesions: clip, dry, and apply topical medication.
  ○ Topical therapies for dermatitis:
    ▪ Nystatin (100,000 U/g).
    ▪ 2% Miconazole.

(CONTINUED)

- 1% Clotrimazole (over-the-counter vaginal cream).
- Potassium permanganate (1:3000 in water).
- Enilconazole 0.2% solution.
- Apply 2–3 times a day until lesions are healed.
- Only use approved drugs in food animals.
  ○ Treatment for severe dermatitis may require administration of oral or parenteral antifungal agents; however, no protocols have been validated.
  - No systemic antifungal agents are approved for use in food animals.
  - Efficacy of oral antifungals in ruminants is not known.
- Alimentary:
  ○ Oral candidiasis: No validated treatment regimens. Human recommendations include nystatin or 1% gentian violet mouthwash.
  ○ Enteric candidiasis: No validated treatments. Transfaunation may be of benefit.
- Abortion:
  ○ No treatments have been reported.
- Mastitis:
  ○ Most cases are self-limiting.
  ○ No antifungal agents are labeled for intramammary infusion.
  ○ Chronic cases should be culled.
- Pneumonia:
  ○ No treatments have been reported.
  ○ If attempted, systemic antifungals should be used.
  ○ None labeled for food animals.
- Systemic mycosis:
  ○ No successful treatments reported for systemic candidiasis.
  ○ Doses must be extrapolated from other species (usually dogs).

MEDICATIONS

DRUGS OF CHOICE
- Systemic mycosis:
  ○ No successful treatments reported for systemic candidiasis.
  ○ Doses must be extrapolated from other species (usually dogs).
  - Amphotericin B 0.6–1 mg/kg/day IV (human dose).
  - Fluconazole 5–10 mg/kg PO, q12h.
  - Itraconazole 5–10 mg/kg PO, q12h.

- Ketoconazole 5–10 mg/kg PO q24h.
- IV azole formulations exist, but no pharmacokinetic data in food animals.
- Up to 10% of *Candida* isolates may be azole-resistant.

CONTRAINDICATIONS
- Many of the suggested drugs for therapy are not approved and therefore should not be used in food animals.
- Confirm safety of drugs in species to be treated before initiating therapy.
- Appropriate milk and meat withdrawal times must be followed for all compounds administered to food-producing animals.

FOLLOW-UP

EXPECTED COURSE AND PROGNOSIS
- Dermatitis usually resolves with appropriate therapy.
- Alimentary candidiasis often resolves in calves but guarded prognosis in adults.
- Chronic *Candida* mastitis is considered incurable.
- No information on future breeding success following *Candida* abortion.
- *Candida* pneumonia or systemic disease cases usually die despite treatment.

POSSIBLE COMPLICATIONS
- Hematogenous spread of fungus.
- Adverse reaction to antifungal therapy.

PATIENT CARE
- If underlying condition is an inherent immunodeficiency, prognosis is guarded to poor.
- Poor prognosis for systemic mycosis.

PREVENTION
- Avoid long-term or high-dose glucocorticoids.
- Avoid polyantimicrobial therapy, especially oral.
- Provide an adequate plane of nutrition.
- Prevent chronic exposure to moisture or wet conditions.
- Use appropriate hygiene when administering intramammary infusions.

MISCELLANEOUS

ASSOCIATED CONDITIONS
- Immunocompromise
- Malnutrition

AGE-RELATED FACTORS
Disease is more severe in neonates.

ZOONOTIC POTENTIAL
Not zoonotic; *Candida* spp. are normal human flora.

PREGNANCY
Abortion in the third trimester has been seen in cattle and goats.

PRODUCTION MANAGEMENT
- Provide adequate and appropriate nutrition.
- Avoid the use of moldy or musty hay or straw.
- Keep animals in a dry environment.
- Avoid prolonged or inappropriate use of antimicrobial agents and corticosteroids.
- Use appropriate hygiene when infusing intramammary medications.

SYNONYMS
- Candidosis
- Moniliasis
- Thrush

ABBREVIATIONS
- PO = per os, by mouth
- SCC = somatic cell count

SEE ALSO
- Abortion: Bovine
- Abortion: Camelids
- Abortion: Small Ruminant
- Mastitis, fungal

Suggested Reading

Jones TC. Diseases caused by fungi. In: Jones TC, Hunt RD, King NW eds, Veterinary Pathology, 6th ed. Philadelphia: Lippincott Williams & Wilkins, 1997.

Prescott JF. Systemic mycoses. In: Howard JL, Smith RA eds, Current Veterinary Therapy 4: Food Animal Practice. Philadelphia: W. B. Saunders, 1999.

Pugh D, Baird AN. Sheep and Goat Medicine, 2nd ed. Philadelphia: Saunders, 2012.

Radostits OM, Gay CC, Hinchcliff KW, Constable PD eds. Veterinary Medicine: A Textbook of the Diseases of Cattle, Horses, Sheep, Pigs and Goats, 10th ed. New York: Saunders, 2007.

Scott DW. Fungal infections. In: Large Animal Dermatology. Philadelphia: Saunders, 1988.

Author Tamara Gull
Consulting Editor Christopher C.L. Chase
Acknowledgment The author and book editors acknowledge the prior contribution of Susan Semrad and Karen A. Moriello.

CAPRINE ARTHRITIS ENCEPHALITIS VIRUS

BASICS

OVERVIEW
- Caprine arthritis encephalitis (CAE) is characterized by chronic degenerative polyarthritis, chronic indurative mastitis, and/or chronic pneumonia in adult goats, and less frequently by acute paralysis in young kids.
- It is one of the most important diseases of dairy goats in industrialized countries.
- The disease is caused by caprine arthritis encephalitis virus (CAEV), a member of the small ruminant lentiviruses (SRLVs) group that also includes maedi visna virus (MVV). Currently, the term SRLVs is widely used to refer to CAEV and MVV.
- Epidemiologic studies have shown that goats comingled with MVV-infected sheep can get infected with MVV and vice versa.
- Cross-species transmission between goats and sheep is influenced by type of farming practiced and is common in places where goats and sheep are raised together in close confinement.
- Economic losses are associated with decreased productivity as a result of clinical disease. Diminished production is related to secondary infections, animal deaths, and the potential loss of international markets due to trade barriers.

INCIDENCE/PREVALENCE
- In the United States, seroprevalence of CAEV antibodies ranges from 38% to 81% in dairy goat herds.
- The prevalence of CAE in some European countries has declined drastically as a result of eradication programs.
- Switzerland started a CAEV eradication program in 1984 and the prevalence has been reduced from 60–80% to <1%; currently cases of clinical disease are rare. However, seroconversions still occur regularly and SRLV has been isolated from different goat and sheep flocks. The main circulating viruses in these goats belong to subtypes A4 and A3, and appear to be of low virulence, with no cases of clinical disease except some cases of mammary gland inflammation.
- In some developing countries, CAE prevalence is high in imported European breeds, but nonexistent in native goats.

GEOGRAPHIC DISTRIBUTION
CAE is widespread among dairy goat herds in most industrialized countries but rare among native goat breeds of developing countries.

SYSTEMS AFFECTED
- Musculoskeletal
- Mammary
- Respiratory
- Nervous
- Hemolymphatic

PATHOPHYSIOLOGY
- CAEV is a *Lentivirus* in the family Retroviridae, subfamily Orthoretrovirinae.
- The genome of CAEV is single-stranded RNA. After infection, the CAEV genome is reverse transcribed into a double-stranded DNA copy that integrates into the host DNA, persisting in infected goats for life.
- SRLV isolates are classified into five main phylogenetic clusters. Genotypes A and B are widely distributed throughout the world, whereas genotypes C–E are geographically restricted.
- Genotype A includes MVV-like strains and genotype B comprises CAEV-like isolates originally isolated from sheep and goats, respectively, from across the world.
- Genotype C includes isolates originally detected in Norway; isolates from Switzerland and Spain are grouped in genotype D. More recently Italian SRLVs isolated from the Roccaverano goat breed have been designated as genotype E.
- Groups A, B and E can be further subdivided into a number of subtypes.
- Group A is highly heterogeneous and contains at least fifteen subtypes (A1–A15), while group B is less complex and contains three subtypes (B1–B3). Group E contains two subtypes (E1 and E2) and has been detected only in Italy.
- SRLVs from groups B–D and most of the group A subtypes (A1–A6, A9, A11–A13) can infect both sheep and goats. The other SRLV groups and subtypes have so far only been described either in sheep (A15) or in goats (A7, A8, A10, A14, E1, and E2). Co-infection with more than one SRLV strain may occur and can result in recombination to form new CAEV-MVV strains.
- Small ruminant lentivirus quasi-species are continuously generated through mutation, recombination, and selection pressure by the host immune system.
- Ingestion of CAEV-contaminated colostrum or milk by neonates is the most common form of transmission.
- Feeding pooled colostrum or unpasteurized milk and bad hygiene practices during milking increase the risk of transmission.
- Transmission by close contact between infected and noninfected goats, particularly during lactation and parturition, may also occur.
- Vertical intrauterine transmission of SRLVs occurs in a small percentage of animals.
- CAEV has been demonstrated in semen, but venereal transmission does not appear an important route of transmission.
- Transmission by contaminated milking machines or buckets is possible.

HISTORICAL FINDINGS
Herd history of disease or introduction of new stock is relevant.

SIGNALMENT
- Goats are the natural host of CAEV, but sheep can also be infected.
- CAE infection rates among meat and hair goat breeds in North America is low. This may reflect differences in management practices between dairy and meat/hair goats that prevent transmission.
- Clinical signs manifest more often in goats ≥2 years of age. Paralysis with a rapid clinical course occurs in kids 2–6 months of age.
- Chronic paralysis has been occasionally described in adult goats.

PHYSICAL EXAMINATION FINDINGS
- In the majority of goats, infection is subclinical.
- In ~25% of seropositive goats, arthritis, mastitis, and/or pneumonia manifest several years after infection. More than one clinical manifestation may be observed in the same animal. Chronic weight loss is common.
- Chronic, proliferative arthritis ("big knee") in mature goats is the most common clinical manifestation and is characterized by swelling of the joints, particularly the carpi and less frequently other joints. The onset of arthritis is insidious. Affected animals show pain, decreased range of articular motion, stiff gait, "knee walking," and chronic weight loss.
- The majority of CAE arthritic female goats also show chronic indurative mastitis ("hard bag"). The udder is firm and symmetrically enlarged. There may be reduction of milk production or agalactia.
- Some CAEV-infected goats develop chronic nonsuppurative interstitial pneumonia with dyspnea, cough, and weight loss.
- Adult goats with CNS involvement show slight aberration in gait, progressing to complete paralysis over the course of several months.
- Once CAEV-infected goats show clinical signs of the disease, death, months or years after primary infection, results from secondary infections.
- A rapid clinical course and afebrile paralysis in kids 2–6 months of age has been described. Paralysis starts in the rear legs and progresses to paresis and quadriplegia. Some kids show head tilt, tremors, and ataxia. Affected kids continue to be alert and eat if hand-fed.

GENETICS
- CAE is more common in dairy goats.
- Host genetics may influence the clinical outcome of CAEV infection.

CAUSES AND RISK FACTORS
- Large herd size, high stocking density, increased age, extended exposure to infected animals, prevalence of bacterial mastitis, high somatic cell counts in milk, and intensive rearing systems are risk factors.
- Close contact with SRLV-seropositive sheep is highly correlated with seroconversion in SRLV-seronegative goat herds.

CAPRINE ARTHRITIS ENCEPHALITIS VIRUS

C

DIAGNOSIS

DIFFERENTIAL DIAGNOSES
• Caseous lymphadenitis, paratuberculosis (Johne's disease), chronic parasitism, and malnutrition.
• Bacterial, chlamydial, mycoplasma polyarthritis, and mastitis (contagious agalactia).
• Bacterial and verminous pneumonia and lung abscesses.
• Trauma or abscesses in the brain or spinal cord, meningitis, parelaphostrongylosis, vitamin E and selenium deficiency; copper deficiency, listeriosis, scrapie, and rabies.

CBC/BIOCHEMISTRY/URINALYSIS
N/A

OTHER LABORATORY TESTS
N/A

IMAGING
N/A

OTHER DIAGNOSTIC PROCEDURES
• Serum antibodies can be detected as early as 3–6 weeks after exposure. Some infected goats may remain seronegative for several months in spite of being virus positive.
• The agar gel immunodiffusion (AGID) test and the enzyme-linked immunosorbent assay (ELISA) are the most commonly used assays. None of these tests are standardized across laboratories, and their sensitivity and specificity vary widely. Confirmation is achieved with Western blot and radioimmunoassay.
• A competitive ELISA (cELISA) with high sensitivity and specificity is commercially available in the US. Several commercially available CAE ELISA tests are available in other countries.
• Goat kids that have received heat-treated colostrum with CAEV antibodies can test positive by serologic methods for several months due to the passive transfer of maternal antibodies.
• Virus isolation has low sensitivity.
• Although PCR is a highly sensitive technique, its usefulness for the detection of CAEV in clinical samples from naturally infected goats still needs validation.
• The sensitivity and specificity of serologic tests and PCR are strongly influenced by the CAEV strains circulating in a particular herd or region.
• A combination of ELISA and real-time PCR increases the likelihood of detecting infected animals.
• Some serologic tests or molecular techniques with high sensitivity and specificity in one country may have lower sensitivity and specificity in another due to genetic and antigenic variability of SRLV subtypes.

PATHOLOGIC FINDINGS
• Gross necropsy findings may include emaciated body condition and swelling of the carpi and less frequently stifle, hock, hip, and atlantooccipital joints in goats with arthritis. In early stages, synovial fluid is increased but remains translucent. Later, fibrin or hard white grains of inspissated fibrin ("rice grains") are evident. Mineralization of periarticular tissues and erosion of articular cartilage are found in advanced cases. Cystic subcutaneous hygromas may be found in the carpi.
• The udder of goats with mastitis is symmetrically enlarged and firm.
• In goats with pulmonary involvement, there is diffuse interstitial pneumonia characterized by firm, gray-pink lungs with numerous 1–2 mm gray-white foci.
• The draining lymph nodes may be enlarged.
• In the neurologic form, there may be asymmetric brown-pink swollen areas in the posterior brain and spinal cord.
• Microscopically, the joints of goats with arthritis exhibit subsynovial infiltration of lymphocytes, plasma cells, and macrophages; formation of lymphoid follicles with germinal centers, and villous synovial hyperplasia. As the disease progresses, there is degeneration of the articular cartilage and mineralization of the joint capsule.
• In the mammary gland, there is infiltration of lymphocytes and plasma cells in the interstitium surrounding lobular ducts.
• Pulmonary lesions consist of lymphoid interstitial pneumonia with mononuclear cell aggregates and lymphoid follicles adjacent to bronchioles and small blood vessels.
• In the neurologic form, there is chronic, nonsuppurative leukoencephalomyelitis in the posterior brain and spinal cord characterized by perivascular infiltration of lymphocytes, macrophages, and demyelination.

TREATMENT

THERAPEUTIC APPROACH
There are no treatments.

SURGICAL CONSIDERATIONS AND TECHNIQUES
N/A

MEDICATIONS

DRUGS OF CHOICE
Broad-spectrum antibiotics are indicated for treating secondary bacterial infections.

CONTRAINDICATIONS
N/A

PRECAUTIONS
Appropriate milk and meat withdrawal times must be followed for all compounds administered to food-producing animals.

POSSIBLE INTERACTIONS
N/A

FOLLOW-UP

EXPECTED COURSE AND PROGNOSIS
• Infected goats remain infected for life.
• Goats often die months or years after initial clinical signs appear.

POSSIBLE COMPLICATIONS
Secondary bacterial infections

CLIENT EDUCATION
Focus on managing the major methods of transmission; colostrum management in newborn kids is particularly critical.

PATIENT CARE
N/A

PREVENTION
• There are no vaccines available.
• Control of CAE depends on limiting transmission and culling infected animals.
• CAEV-free accreditation programs are in existence in some European countries.
• Serologic testing and segregation of positive reactors reduces prevalence and in some cases facilitates eradication of the disease.
• Retesting every 3–6 months and elimination of new positive reactors is necessary until 3 to 5 consecutive tests result in 100% of goats being negative, following which, yearly testing and acquisition of replacements from CAEV-free herds are recommended.
• Reappearance of occasional positive reactors years after eradication has been documented.
• The use of heat-treated colostrum (56–59°C for 1 hour) to raise goat kids from CAEV-infected goats reduces lactogenic transmission, but does not eliminate the risk of transmission.
• Reporting requirements for CAE differ between countries.
• Good biosecurity and hygiene practices should be adopted to minimize transmission of CAEV by contaminated equipment and other sources.
• Lentiviruses are susceptible to environmental factors and are destroyed by disinfectants.

MISCELLANEOUS

ASSOCIATED CONDITIONS
N/A

CAPRINE ARTHRITIS ENCEPHALITIS VIRUS (CONTINUED)

AGE-RELATED FACTORS
• Clinical signs occur more often in goats 2–3 years old or older.
• Acute leukoencephalomyelitis, although uncommon, is more common in 2- to 6-month-old kids.

ZOONOTIC POTENTIAL
N/A

PREGNANCY
N/A

BIOSECURITY
Acquire replacement animals from SRLVs-free herds.

PRODUCTION MANAGEMENT
Should focus on minimizing transmission risks

SYNONYMS
• Big knee
• Infectious leukoencephalomyelitis

ABBREVIATIONS
• AGID = agar gel immunodiffusion test
• CAEV = caprine arthritis encephalitis virus
• ELISA = enzyme-linked immunosorbent assay
• MVV = maedi-visna virus
• OPP = ovine progressive pneumonia
• PCR = polymerase chain reaction
• SRLVs = small ruminant lentiviruses

SEE ALSO
Maedi-Visna (Ovine Progressive Pneumonia)

Suggested Reading

Cardinaux L, Zahno ML, Deubelbeiss M, Zanoni R, Vogt HR, Bertoni G. Virological and phylogenetic characterization of attenuated small ruminant lentivirus isolates eluding efficient serological detection. Vet Microbiol 2013, 162: 572–81.

de la Concha-Bermejillo A. Caprine arthritis encephalitis: an update. Sheep Goat Res J 2003, 18: 69–78.

Larruskain A, Jugo BM. Retroviral infections in sheep and goats: small ruminant lentiviruses and host interaction. Viruses. 2013, 5: 2043–61.

Minguijón E, Reina R, Pérez M, et al. Small ruminant lentivirus infections and diseases. Vet Microbiol 2015, 181: 75–89.

Author Andrés de la Concha-Bermejillo
Consulting Editor Erica C. McKenzie

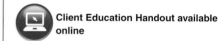 **Client Education Handout available online**

CARBAMATE TOXICITY

BASICS

OVERVIEW
• Carbamates are anticholinesterase insecticides derived from carbamic acid commonly found in crop and animal insecticides.
• The binding of carbamates is reversible and temporary, unlike the mechanism of another class of anticholinesterase insecticide, the organophosphates, which is irreversible.
• Most intoxications are a result of accidental ingestion of insecticide or indirect exposure to plants or water source sprayed by carbamate.

SYSTEMS AFFECTED
• Nervous
• Digestive
• Respiratory
• Musculoskeletal
• Cardiovascular

PATHOPHYSIOLOGY
Anticholinesterase insecticides bind with and inhibit acetylcholinesterase, the enzyme that breaks down the neurotransmitter acetylcholine. These compounds cause acetylcholine to accumulate at nerve junctions and cause excessive synaptic activity. The effects are in the parasympathetic nervous system and at neuromuscular sites.

SIGNALMENT
Any animal can be exposed to toxic levels of carbamate insecticides and all ruminants are susceptible.

PHYSICAL EXAMINATION FINDINGS
Muscarinic Symptoms
Result from stimulation of the parasympathetic nervous system and are described by the acronym SLUD:
• Salivation
• Lacrimation
• Urination
• Defecation

Other Possible Muscarinic Signs
• Vomiting—rare
• Miosis
• Bradycardia
• Dyspnea
• Bloating
• Transient diarrhea

Nicotinic (Neuromuscular) Signs
• Muscle tremors
• Twitching of facial muscles and eyelids
• Hyperthermia
• Ataxia
• Progressive paresis to paralysis
• Tetany

Central Nervous System Signs
• Depression
• Seizures
• Behavioral changes

CAUSES AND RISK FACTORS
• Domestic animals are usually exposed to carbamate insecticides due to accidental ingestion, or improper treatment by owners. Carbamate insecticides are used primarily on crops and other plants but can be used as topical insecticides on animals. They were previously commonly used for ectoparasite control.
• Carbamates are anticholinesterase insecticides commonly found in insecticides.
  ◦ Carbaryl—LD50 in rats is 250 mg/kg orally and >2000 mg/kg dermally.
  ◦ Carbofuran—Minimum toxic dose in sheep and cattle is 4.5 mg/kg, becoming lethal for sheep at 9 mg/kg and for cattle at 18 mg/kg.
  ◦ Methomyl (Golden Malrin)—LD50 in rats is 50 mg/kg orally.
  ◦ Propoxur—LD50 in rats is 0.8 mg/kg orally and in goats is >800 mg/kg orally.

DIAGNOSIS

DIFFERENTIAL DIAGNOSES
• Gastrointestinal causes of diarrhea
• Metabolic disturbances such as nervous ketosis
• Nonprotein nitrogen toxicosis
• Numerous plant toxicities cause tremor or ataxia
• Other pesticides including organophosphates, rodenticides
• Other toxins such as strychnine or lead
• Rabies

CBC/BIOCHEMISTRY/URINALYSIS
N/A

OTHER LABORATORY TESTS
• Prompt testing is necessary due to the temporary binding of carbamate toxins. Cholinesterase activity may return to normal before or during laboratory testing.
• Cholinesterase activity in whole blood, retina, or brain that is 25–50% of normal for the species being tested indicates cholinesterase inhibitor toxicosis. If <25% of normal, clinical correlation of symptoms is required for diagnosis.
• Half of the brain should be submitted for homogenization, as cholinesterase activity varies in different brain regions.

OTHER DIAGNOSTIC PROCEDURES
Diagnosis is often based on known exposure to carbamate and response to treatment with atropine.

PATHOLOGIC FINDINGS
None

TREATMENT

THERAPEUTIC APPROACH
• Provide supportive care for SLUD or secondary clinical signs such as dehydration.
• Wash the animal with soap and water if dermal exposure occurs, to decrease absorption. Clipping may be advisable in long-haired animals.
• Administer activated charcoal PO at a dose of 1–2 lb per 500 kg body weight.
• Atropine injection
  ◦ Atropine sulfate L.A. 15 mg/mL
  ◦ Cattle: 30 mg per 100 lb body weight or 0.1 mg/kg SC to standing animals or for recumbent animals 1/3 dose IV and the remainder SC.
  ◦ Sheep and goats: 50 mg per 100 lb body weight or 0.3 mg/kg SC to standing animals or for recumbent animals 1/3 dose IV and the remainder SC. Give 1/4 of the initial dose IV (watch the pupils and see if they start to return to normal) and the rest SC or IM.
  ◦ Dosage can be repeated in 4–8 hours if clinical signs recur.

MEDICATIONS

DRUGS OF CHOICE
• Activated charcoal.
• Atropine is the primary drug of choice and always should be used first.

CONTRAINDICATIONS
• Oximes such as pralidoxime chloride (2-PAM) that are used to release the acetylcholinesterase-organophosphate bond are *not* used due to the reversible nature of carbamate binding to acetylcholinesterase.
• Appropriate milk and meat withdrawal times must be followed for all compounds administered to food-producing animals.

FOLLOW-UP

EXPECTED COURSE AND PROGNOSIS
Good prognosis if treated promptly

POSSIBLE COMPLICATIONS
Bloating, inhalation pneumonia

PATIENT CARE
• Heart rate
• Respiration
• Fluid and feed intake

C

CARBAMATE TOXICITY (CONTINUED)

PREVENTION
• Closely follow instructions for dilution and application found on carbamate insecticide label.
• Premises should be washed and contaminated soil removed. Runoff can poison fish and aquatic animals.
• Avoid use of carbamate insecticides for ectoparasite control, especially on sick or debilitated animals.

MISCELLANEOUS

ZOONOTIC POTENTIAL
• Carbamate toxicity is not a transmissible disease; however, humans are also susceptible to toxic exposures.
• Follow labeled instructions and precautions when handling carbamate insecticides.
• Use caution when washing poisoned animals.

ABBREVIATIONS
• 2-PAM = pralidoxime chloride
• SLUD = salivation, lacrimation, urination, defecation

SEE ALSO
• Clostridial Disease: Gastrointestinal
• Fungal Tremorgens

• Grass Tetany/Hypomagnesemia
• Ketosis: Dairy Cattle
• Lead Toxicosis
• Metaldehyde Toxicosis
• Nitrate and Nitrite Toxicosis
• Organophosphate Toxicity
• Rabies
• Rodenticide Toxicity
• Strychnine Poisoning
• Toxicology: Herd Outbreaks
• Urea Toxicity

Suggested Reading
Aiello SE., ed. Carbamate insecticides. In: Merck Veterinary Manual, 8th ed. Whitehouse Station, NJ: Merck and Co., 1998.
Beasley V. Toxicants that affect the autonomic nervous system. In: Beasley V ed, Veterinary Toxicology. University of Illinois, 1999.
Budavari S. The Merck Index, 12th ed. on CD-ROM. Version 12:3a. Chapman & Hall/CRCnetBASE. Whitehouse Station, NJ. 2000.
Giadinis ND, Raikos N, Loukopoulos, et al. Carbamate poisoning in a dairy goat herd: Clinicopathological findings and therapeutic approach. NZ Vet J 2009, 57: 392-4.
Lewis RA. Lewis' Dictionary of Toxicology. Boca Raton, FL: Lewis Publishers, 1998.
Lloyd WE. Chemical detection techniques for diagnosing dairy herd health problems. J Dairy Sci 1978, 61: 676–8.
Meister RT. Farm Chemicals Handbook. Willoughby, OH: Meister Publishing Co, 2001.
Osweiler GD. Organophosphorus and carbamate insecticides. In: Toxicology. Baltimore: Williams & Wilkins, 1996.
Pohanish RP. Sittig's Handbook of Toxic and Hazardous Chemicals and Carcinogens, 4th ed. Norwich, NY: Noyes Publications/William Andrew Publishing, 2002.
Smith BP ed. Toxicology of organic compounds. In: Large Animal Internal Medicine, 3rd ed. St. Louis: Mosby, 2002.
Tilley LP, Smith FWK Jr, eds. Organophosphate and carbamate toxicity. In: The Five-Minute Veterinary Consult—Canine and Feline, 3rd ed. Philadelphia: Lippincott, Williams & Wilkins, 2004.

Authors Steve Ensley and Jennifer S. Taintor
Consulting Editor Christopher C.L. Chase
Acknowledgment The authors and book editors acknowledge the prior contribution of Lisa Nashold.

BASICS

OVERVIEW
• Cardiac failure can result from primary cardiomyopathy (myocardial disease and dysfunction) typically characterized by cardiac dilation, or secondary to other cardiovascular and respiratory disorders that ultimately produce congestive heart failure (CHF).
• Causes include viral, bacterial, and parasitic pathogens; acquired and congenital cardiac and respiratory disorders; genetic disorders; nutritional deficiencies; toxicants; and neoplasia.
• CHF reflects the terminal endpoint of many cardiac disorders, where the heart can no longer effectively circulate blood to organs and peripheral tissues, resulting in congestion and edema.

INCIDENCE/PREVALENCE
• Uncommon and sporadic.
• Inbred Holstein-Friesian cattle have a 3–5% incidence of hereditary cardiomyopathy.
• Cattle have ~ 4% prevalence of tricuspid valve endocarditis.

GEOGRAPHIC DISTRIBUTION
Worldwide

SYSTEMS AFFECTED
• Cardiovascular
• Respiratory
• Digestive

PATHOPHYSIOLOGY
• Dependent on the primary disease; however, progressive reduction in myocardial contractility leads to decreased cardiac output.
• Compensatory changes in blood volume and blood pressure occur, and constant sympathetic stimulation of the heart causes arrhythmias and myocyte death.
• Renin-angiotensin-aldosterone release causes vasoconstriction and retention of sodium and water.
• Cumulatively these changes result in dilatation of cardiac chambers and atrioventricular rings, increased ventricular mass, reduced myocardial contractility, and decreased systolic function.
• Signs of CHF develop as disease progresses, with left heart failure reflected by tachypnea, coughing, dyspnea, and exercise intolerance; and right heart failure by submandibular, brisket, or ventral edema, jugular and mammary vein distention, and pleural and peritoneal effusion.
• Cardiomyopathy can be inherited, idiopathic, or secondary to ingestion of ionophores, gossypol, *Cassia occidentalis*, and *Phalaris* spp.; to deficiency of vitamin E, selenium or copper; to cardiac lymphoma; and from myocardial fibrosis.
• Infectious endocarditis is also a common cause of CHF in cattle, and typically affects the tricuspid valve, producing right heart failure.
• Restrictive cardiomyopathy characterized by impeded diastolic relaxation and reduced left ventricular filling can occur secondary to pericardial diseases.

HISTORICAL FINDINGS
Vary with cause, but historical assessment should consider management factors, toxicants, nutritional status, and other relevant topics.

SIGNALMENT
• Congenital cardiac anomalies most commonly affect neonates or juveniles.
• A heritable cardiomyopathy linked to the red gene causes cardiac failure in Holstein cattle 2–7 years of age.
• A heritable cardiomyopathy causes cardiac failure in Japanese Black cattle and Australian polled Herefords in the first weeks to months of life. In Herefords the disorder is associated with a dense, tight, curly haircoat.
• Other causes are more common in mature animals.

PHYSICAL EXAMINATION FINDINGS
• Depend on the primary cause and the severity and duration of cardiac disease.
• Primary cardiac signs include cardiac arrhythmias, murmurs, tachycardia, and muffled heart sounds.
• Secondary signs of cardiac failure include peripheral edema, venous distension, abnormal thoracic auscultation (pulmonary edema and/or pleural fluid), and abnormal abdominal contour and percussion (ascites and hepatomegaly).
• Other findings may reflect causative disorders and include fever, anorexia, stiffness or reluctance to move, signs of thoracic or abdominal pain, and sudden death.

GENETICS
Inherited cardiomyopathy disorders in Holstein-Friesians, Australian polled Herefords, and Japanese Black cattle are autosomal recessive traits.

CAUSES AND RISK FACTORS
• Genetic predisposition
• Stress can precipitate clinical signs
• Pericarditis
• Cardiac lymphoma
• High altitude
• Nutritional deficiency
• Toxicity

DIAGNOSIS

DIFFERENTIAL DIAGNOSES
• Ionophore toxicity
• Gossypol toxicosis
• Selenium deficiency
• Primary or secondary copper deficiency
• Myocarditis
• Endocarditis
• Traumatic reticuloperitonitis/pericarditis
• Cardiac neoplasia
• Idiopathic pericardial hemorrhage
• Cor pulmonale (high altitude or chronic respiratory disease)
• Parasitism

CBC/BIOCHEMISTRY/URINALYSIS
Unremarkable, or findings reflect inflammation (leukocytosis, high total protein), heart failure, reduced feed and water intake, and primary disease, represented by increased liver or muscle enzymes, metabolic alkalosis, low serum electrolytes, and azotemia.

OTHER LABORATORY TESTS
• Cardiac troponin I
• Bovine leukemia virus: AGID, ELISA or PCR
• Whole blood selenium concentration or glutathione peroxidase activity (low in deficiency)
• Serum and urine transferrin concentrations (increased in cattle with dilated cardiomyopathy)

IMAGING
Ultrasonography of the thoracic and abdominal cavities is ideal for evaluating severity of cardiac disease and delineating causes and consequences.

OTHER DIAGNOSTIC PROCEDURES
• Pericardiocentesis
• Feed or rumen content can be tested for ionophores

PATHOLOGIC FINDINGS
• Myocarditis may have minimal gross lesions; histopathologic examination may identify fibrosis, necrosis, or inflammatory cell infiltrates within the cardiac muscle.
• Cardiomyopathy is identified by enlargement of cardiac chambers and the pulmonary artery. Generalized edema, cavity effusions, and vascular congestion of the lung, liver, and spleen can occur. Microscopically myocardial vacuolation and degeneration with necrosis and fibrosis is appreciated.
• Interstitial nephritis has been reported in Holstein-Friesian cattle with dilated cardiomyopathy.
• Other lesions can reflect precipitating causes including muscular lesions with selenium deficiency, pericardial lesions in traumatic reticuloperitonitis, etc.

TREATMENT

THERAPEUTIC APPROACH
• Treat precipitating disorders if feasible.
• Treatment of CHF is palliative and short term, culling is appropriate.
• Supportive care, diuretics, restriction of salt intake, and potentially cardiac medications can transiently reduce severity of clinical signs.

SURGICAL CONSIDERATIONS AND TECHNIQUES
N/A

MEDICATIONS

DRUGS OF CHOICE
• Furosemide: 1.0 mg/kg IV or IM, q12h.
• Digoxin (positive inotrope) must be given IV in ruminants, and requires intensive monitoring. Can be dosed at 0.86 µg/kg per hour (valuable hospitalized animals) or at 3.4 µg/kg IV every 4 hours (greater risk of digoxin toxicity).
• Potassium chloride: 5–10 g per day PO in older calves; 50–200 g daily PO for adult cow/bull.
• Vitamin E/selenium, if indicated, at label dose.

CONTRAINDICATIONS
Digoxin is contraindicated in ionophore toxicosis.

PRECAUTIONS
Appropriate milk and meat withdrawal times must be followed for all compounds administered to food-producing animals.

POSSIBLE INTERACTIONS
N/A

FOLLOW-UP

EXPECTED COURSE AND PROGNOSIS
• Mortality is inevitable long term.
• Short-term prognosis depends on the primary disorder, duration, and severity of disease; severe clinical signs have a guarded short-term prognosis and sudden death is likely.
• Holsteins with hereditary cardiomyopathy may survive 6–7 years, whereas Japanese Black cattle usually die by 1 month of life and Australian polled Herefords by 3 months of life.

POSSIBLE COMPLICATIONS
N/A

CLIENT EDUCATION
• Breeding selection for hereditary disorders
• Provision of safe feed supply with minimal foreign bodies and toxicants
• Appropriate infectious disease protocols to minimize relevant disorders (BLV)

PATIENT CARE
• Restrict exertion.
• Monitor heart rate, rhythm, perfusion and hydration.
• Monitor changes in body condition, edema, and venous distension.
• Measurement of plasma/serum digoxin concentrations is indicated to monitor for toxicity in treated animals.

PREVENTION
• Gossypol toxicity can be avoided by not feeding cottonseed meal or choosing meal with a low gossypol content, especially when feeding pre-ruminants. Concentrations of gossypol should be ≤1–2 g/kg of feed for adult cattle and ≤0.5–1 g/kg of feed for immature cattle.
• Ionophore-containing feeds should be mixed at approved facilities.
• Breeding stock should be selected to avoid propagating heritable diseases.

MISCELLANEOUS

ASSOCIATED CONDITIONS
• Cardiac arrhythmias
• Congestive heart failure
• Diarrhea
• Digoxin toxicity

AGE-RELATED FACTORS
Congenital disorders and specific heritable diseases are often clinically evident early in life, while most other disorders present in mature animals.

ZOONOTIC POTENTIAL
N/A

PREGNANCY
N/A

BIOSECURITY
Relevant to specific disorders such as BLV.

PRODUCTION MANAGEMENT
• Avoid using suspected or known carriers of heritable traits in breeding programs.
• Maintain safe feed supply.
• Selenium supplementation of feed or by injection of neonates is recommended in deficient regions.

SYNONYMS
N/A

ABBREVIATIONS
• BLV = bovine leukemia virus
• CHF = congestive heart failure

SEE ALSO
• Copper Deficiency and Toxicity
• Gossypol Toxicosis
• Lymphosarcoma
• Monensin Toxicity
• Pericarditis
• Selenium/Vitamin E Deficiency

Suggested Reading
Borsberry S, Colloff A. Cardiomyopathy in adult Holstein Friesian cattle. Vet Rec 1999, 144: 735–6.
Dolf G, Stricker C, Tontis A, Martiq J, Gaillard C. Evidence for autosomal recessive inheritance of a major gene for bovine dilated cardiomyopathy. J Anim Sci 1998, 76: 1824–9.
Neary JM, Booker CS, Wildman BK, Morley PS. Right-sided congestive heart failure in North American feedlot cattle. J Vet Intern Med 2016, 30: 326–34.
Reef V, McGuirk SM. Diseases of the cardiovascular system. In: Smith BP ed, Large Animal Internal Medicine, 5th ed. St. Louis: Elsevier Mosby, 2014, pp. 442–5.
Peek SF, McGuirk SM. Cardiovascular diseases. In: Peek SF, Divers TJ eds, Diseases of Dairy Cattle, 2nd ed. St. Louis: Saunders Elsevier, 2008, pp. 43–78.
Author Keith P. Poulsen
Consulting Editor Erica C. McKenzie

CARDIOTOXIC PLANTS

BASICS

OVERVIEW
A large group of unrelated plants can be cardiotoxic to livestock; the majority contain cardiac glycosides. Other cardiotoxic plants that have resulted in livestock poisoning include yew (*Taxus* spp.), grayanotoxin-containing plants, death camas (*Zigadenus* spp.), avocado (*Persea* spp.; see chapter, Avocado Toxicosis) and oleander (*Nerium oleander*).

INCIDENCE/PREVALENCE
Cardiac Glycoside–Containing Plants
• Plants containing cardiac glycosides include oleander (*Nerium oleander*), summer pheasant's eye (*Adonis aestivalis*), foxglove (*Digitalis purpurea*), lily-of-the-valley (*Convallaria majalis*), dogbane (*Apocynum* spp.), and some species of milkweed (*Asclepias* spp.).
• Oleander is cultivated widely in the southern United States and is most commonly associated with plant poisonings in livestock. This plant is common in Florida and widely planted in California. Therefore, oleander is discussed in detail as a representative of plants containing cardiac glycosides.

Death Camas
Many species of death camas occur across the US and are seasonal with the greatest abundance being in the spring.

Grayanotoxin-Containing Plants
• Plants containing grayanotoxins include *Rhododendron* spp. (rhododendron, azalea, rosebay), *Kalmia* spp. (mountain laurel, sheep laurel, lambkill, sheepkill, dwarf laurel, calico bush), *Pieris* spp. (Japanese pieris, mountain pieris), *Leucothoe* spp. (dog hobble, dog laurel, fetter bush, black laurel), and *Lyonia* spp. (fetter bush, maleberry, staggerbush).

Yews
Yews are popular shrubbery used as a hedge or foundation planting. Several *Taxus* species are found in the US with *T. baccata* (English yew) and *T. cuspidata* (Japanese yew) most commonly reported in poisonings. However, all species of *Taxus* including *T. brevifolia* (Pacific or western yew) should be considered toxic.

GEOGRAPHIC DISTRIBUTION
See "Incidence/Prevalence"

SYSTEMS AFFECTED
Cardiovascular

PATHOPHYSIOLOGY
Cardiac Glycoside–Containing Plants
Cardiac glycosides cause poisoning by inhibiting the cellular membrane Na$^+$/K$^+$-ATPase, which results in an indirect increase in intracellular Ca^{2+} concentrations, intracellular sodium, decreased intracellular potassium, and a subsequent positive inotropic effect. In addition, direct effects on the sympathetic nervous system are seen.

Death Camas
Death camas contains steroidal alkaloids, such as zygacine and zygadenine. The alkaloids decrease blood pressure, slow the heart rate, and lead to respiratory depression.

Grayanotoxin-Containing Plants
Grayanotoxins are diterpenes that exert their toxic effect by binding to sodium channels in excitable cell membranes. The resulting increase in membrane permeability to sodium ions maintains excitable cells in a state of depolarization. Accumulation of intracellular sodium results in an exchange with extracellular calcium and plays an important role in the control of transmitter release. The membrane effects caused by grayanotoxins account for the observed responses of skeletal and myocardial muscle, nerves, and central nervous system.

Yews
Yews contain taxine alkaloids (major alkaloids are taxine A and taxine B) that cause an increase in cytoplasmic calcium by interfering with both the calcium and the sodium ion channel conductance across the myocardial cells. This results in the depression of cardiac depolarization and conduction of the heart.

SIGNALMENT
Cattle, sheep, goats, llamas, alpacas, deer

Cardiac Glycoside–Containing Plants
All species are susceptible to cardiac glycoside-containing plants. Oleander poisoning is commonly seen in llamas and alpacas. Severe losses have also been reported in cattle.

Death Camas
Sheep are at highest risk, especially when hungry, because they are most likely to eat the death camas in early spring when little alternative forage is available. However, cattle have also been poisoned.

Grayanotoxin-Containing Plants
Grayanotoxin poisoning has been reported in cattle and sheep, but most reports of poisoning involve goats.

Yew
Most poisonings with yew have involved cattle, but sheep, goats, and wild ruminants are also susceptible. Deer are able to tolerate considerable amounts of yew during the winter months, probably because of lower concentrations of taxine alkaloids in newly grown shoots.

PHYSICAL EXAMINATION FINDINGS
• Animals exposed to cardiotoxic plants are often found dead.
• If animals are presented alive, clinical signs of colic (abdominal pain) are often seen within hours of exposure. Progression of disease is rapid and animals develop weakness, tremors, excessive salivation, incoordination, dyspnea, and sometimes convulsions.
• In cardiac glycoside poisonings, animals often have an irregular, fast pulse with tachycardia, ventricular arrhythmias, or gallop rhythms.
• Animals exposed to avocado develop subcutaneous edema of the neck and brisket, submandibular edema, respiratory dyspnea, and cardiac arrhythmias. Lactating animals exposed to a low dose of avocado develop noninfectious mastitis and agalactia within 24 hours of exposure.

CAUSES AND RISK FACTORS
• Ingestion of cardiotoxic plants presents a great risk to ruminants. Plants most commonly associated with acute poisoning are oleander, yew, and rhododendron.
• Hungry animals are most likely to receive toxic exposures.
• Young and rapidly growing plants often contain highest concentrations of toxins.
• Fresh plant material of cardiotoxic plants is often considered to be of low palatability. However, animals frequently eat the leaves readily, if no other forage is available.

Cardiac Glycoside–Containing Plants
• The median toxic dose of oleander leaves in cattle is 45 mg of plant material per kg body weight or approximately 12 averaged-sized leaves or approximately 15–25 grams of dry leaves.
• In sheep, one to five grams is toxic, or 2 or 3 leaves.
• All parts of oleander are extremely toxic, whether the plant is fresh or dried. Ingestion of dried oleander clippings is a common source of poisoning in livestock.

Death Camus
• Leaves during the early stages of growth pose the greatest risk for poisoning. Seeds and fruits as well as the dried plant in hay are also toxic.
• The minimum lethal dose of the green plant in sheep is approximately 1% of the animal's body weight, but serious illness may be seen with as little as ingestion of 0.2% of an animal's body weight. Cattle are equally or possibly more susceptible than sheep.

Grayanotoxin-Containing Plants
• Toxicosis usually occurs when animals are offered plant trimmings or stray into wooded areas during adverse weather conditions and little else is available to eat.
• In cattle and sheep, ingestion of 0.2–0.6% of an animal's body weight is considered toxic. Goats can be poisoned by the ingestion of fresh foliage in the amount of 0.1% of the animal's body weight.

CARDIOTOXIC PLANTS   (CONTINUED)

Yew
- All parts of the plant, green or dried, with the exception of the red fleshy part surrounding the seed (aril portion), are toxic. Ingestion of yew clippings is most often the cause of poisonings.
- The minimum lethal dose in adult cattle is estimated to be approximately 200 g of dried leaves.
- Green foliage is toxic to ruminants at 0.5% of body weight.

DIAGNOSIS

DIFFERENTIAL DIAGNOSES
- Avocado toxicosis.
- Cyanide poisoning—mucus membranes are initially bright cherry red; evidence of exposure to cyanogenic plants, chemical analysis for cyanide in gastrointestinal contents, liver, or muscle.
- Grass tetany—hypomagnesemia.
- Ionophore antibiotics—history of ionophores (e.g., monensin) in the feed ration, detection of toxic concentrations of ionophores in the feed, histologic lesions.
- Larkspur poisoning—mainly found in the western states; bloat is common finding, evidence of exposure to *Delphinium* spp.
- Lead poisoning—determination of blood lead concentration.
- Exposure to neurotoxic plants, such as poison hemlock, water hemlock, tree tobacco, lupine—chemical analysis for plant toxins in gastrointestinal contents, history of presence of plants in the environment.
- Nitrate toxicosis—chocolate-colored blood, exposure to nitrate-accumulating plants.
- Organophosphorus or carbamate insecticide exposure—commonly associated with gastrointestinal irritation and neurologic signs, evaluation of cholinesterase activity, detection of pesticides in gastrointestinal contents.
- Exposure to the plant "fly poison" (*Amianthium muscaetoxicum*)—found only in the eastern United States, most commonly seen in the spring, history of presence of plants in the environment.
- Exposure to star-of-Bethlehem (*Ornithogalum* spp.)—mainly found in the Northeast and Midwest, severe diarrhea, history of presence of plants in the environment.
- Nonprotein nitrogen (NPN) toxicosis—history of NPN supplements in the feed ration, detection of toxic levels of ammonia in rumen content and blood.

CBC/BIOCHEMISTRY/URINALYSIS
- Serum chemistry changes are limited.

- Myocardial damage may result in hyperkalemia, and elevated LDH, CK, and AST activities.

OTHER LABORATORY TESTS
- Detection of oleandrin, gitoxin, digitoxin, grayanotoxins, strophanthidin, or other cardiac glycosides or aglycones in blood, rumen, cecal, or colon contents, and liver.
- Detection of taxine alkaloids in rumen contents.
- Visual and microscopic examination of rumen or intestinal contents for plant fragments.

PATHOLOGIC FINDINGS
- In peracute cases, no lesions are found.
- Postmortem lesions are generally nonspecific in animals that died of exposure to cardiotoxic plants. Lesions include reddening of the mucosa of the gastrointestinal tract and congestion of organs.
- Cattle with oleander poisoning have evidence of fluid in the bowel and thrombosis and hemorrhage in the heart.
- There are no or very few lesions in cases of yew, grayanotoxin, or death camas poisoning.
- Avocado poisoning can result in fluid accumulation in the pericardial sac and in the thoracic and abdominal cavities. Edema of the gallbladder and perirenal tissues and a flabby, pale heart have been observed. Mammary glands are edematous with clots in the large ducts.

TREATMENT

THERAPEUTIC APPROACH
- Immediate removal of the toxic plant material to prevent further exposure. Provide the animals with good-quality feed.
- Treatment of animals exposed to cardiotoxic plants is primarily supportive and symptomatic. Supportive therapy should include administration of intravenous fluids, antiarrhythmics, and antibiotics if indicated.
- Adsorption of toxins with activated charcoal has been suggested.
- Rumenotomy may be considered in a valuable individual animal if ingestion is known and clinical signs have not yet developed.
- Passing a stomach tube, if necessary, should relieve bloat.
- Any possible stress or trauma should be avoided.
- If edema is present in avocado poisoning, administration of diuretics is recommended.
- Atropine should be considered in cases of severe bradycardia. Additionally, it may be warranted in severely poisoned animals that do not respond to decontamination procedures and fluid therapy alone.

MEDICATIONS

DRUGS OF CHOICE
- Lidocaine, phenytoin, or propranolol to treat tachyarrhythmias
- Atropine to treat bradyarrhythmias
- Activated charcoal
- Alternative drug: Anticardiac glycoside Fab antibodies have been used in humans and small animals, but their usefulness in the treatment of cardiac glycoside-poisoned ruminants has not been evaluated.

CONTRAINDICATIONS
- Do not administer potassium in fluids if hyperkalemia is present.
- Avoid calcium-containing solutions and quinidine.
- Appropriate milk and meat withdrawal times must be followed for all compounds administered to food-producing animals.

FOLLOW-UP

EXPECTED COURSE AND PROGNOSIS
- Animals poisoned with cardiotoxic plants are often found dead.
- Cardiotoxic plant exposure progresses so rapidly that treatment is often too late. In most cases, the affected animals have a poor-to-grave prognosis.
- If treatment is initiated promptly after the onset of clinical signs, the prognosis is fair.
- Animals that survive the acute poisoning may suffer from myocardial damage and may be more prone to stress.

PATIENT CARE
Monitor progression of clinical signs.

PREVENTION
- Prevent hungry animals from accessing new pasture, especially in the spring when only limited (and often toxic) forage is available.
- Animals should be denied access to landscaped yards and discarded clippings.
- Suspect forage should be inspected for the presence of cardiotoxic plants before allowing ruminants to graze.
- Hay should be inspected carefully for weeds, as many cardiotoxic plants remain toxic when dried (oleander, death camas, yew).

MISCELLANEOUS

PRODUCTION MANAGEMENT
In lactating animals poisoned with avocado, the milk production remains reduced even after the mastitis has been controlled.

ABBREVIATIONS
- AST = aspartate aminotransferase
- CK = creatine kinase
- LDH = lactate dehydrogenase
- NPN = nonprotein nitrogen

SEE ALSO
- Avocado Toxicosis
- Carbamate Toxicity
- Cyanide Toxicosis
- Grass Tetany/Hypomagnesemia
- Monensin Toxicity
- Lead Toxicosis
- Lupine Toxicity
- Nitrate and Nitrite Toxicosis
- Oleander and Cardiotoxic Plant Toxicity
- Organophosphate Toxicity
- Poison Hemlock (*Conium* spp.) Toxicity

- Tobacco Toxicosis
- Toxicology: Herd Outbreaks
- Urea Toxicity
- Water Hemlock

Suggested Reading

Burrows GE, Tyrl RJ. In: Burrows GE, Tyrl RJ eds, Toxic Plants of North America, 2nd ed. Ames: Wiley-Blackwell, 2013.

Casteel SW. Taxine alkaloids. In: Plumlee KH ed, Clinical Veterinary Toxicology. St. Louis: Mosby, 2004.

Cheeke P, ed. Natural Toxicants in Feeds, Forages, and Poisonous Plants. Danville, IL: Interstate Publishers, Inc., 1998.

Galey FG. Cardiac glycosides. In: Plumlee KH ed, Clinical Veterinary Toxicology. St. Louis: Mosby, 2004.

Oelrichs PB, Ng JC, Seawright AA, et al. Isolation and identification of a compound from avocado (*Persea americana*) leaves which causes necrosis of the acinar epithelium of the lactating mammary gland and the myocardium. Nat Toxins 1995, 3: 344–9.

Puschner B. Grayanotoxins. In: Plumlee KH ed, Clinical Veterinary Toxicology. St. Louis: Mosby, 2004.

Author Steve Ensley

Consulting Editor Christopher C.L. Chase

Acknowledgment The author and book editors acknowledge the prior contribution of Birgit Puschner.

C

CASEOUS LYMPHADENITIS (CLA)

BASICS

OVERVIEW
Caseous lymphadenitis (CLA) is an endemic, contagious disease caused by *Corynebacterium pseudotuberculosis*, characterized by caseous abscessation of internal and external lymph nodes and visceral organs of sheep, goats, and rarely camelids.

INCIDENCE/PREVALENCE
• Common worldwide in small ruminants
• Flock/herd prevalence may exceed 75% in adults if no control program
• Flock/herd incidence varies depending on management and surveillance, but likely >15%
• Abscesses estimated to affect 17–24% of adult sheep at abattoirs
• Important cause of carcass condemnation and trim

GEOGRAPHIC DISTRIBUTION
• Widely distributed in North America
• Mostly in terminal sire flocks in the UK

SYSTEMS AFFECTED
• Hemolymphatic
• Respiratory

PATHOPHYSIOLOGY
• Bacteria invade via wounds, unbroken or abraded skin, or mucus membranes and can be contracted through contaminated fomites (particularly water, feed, soil, or housing), directly from animals with draining abscesses, or from pulmonary abscesses via coughing.
• Bacteria travel through lymphatics or blood to local lymph nodes and organs.
• Phospholipase D (PLD) exotoxin, secreted by the bacteria, disrupts endothelium and is leukotoxic, facilitating spread of the bacteria through tissues.
• The cell wall is thick with high lipid content, enabling bacteria to resist phagocytosis.
• Abscesses generally form first in the lymph node(s) draining the site of initial infection, but may form anywhere in the body.
• Abscesses may rupture (through skin or into bronchi) or regress. New abscesses may form months later in the same or different location.

HISTORICAL FINDINGS
• Typically producers report a lump under the skin or a ruptured abscess.
• Abscesses can be missed in long wool or hair; it is common to identify lesions during shearing.
• Occasionally, adults may present with chronic weight loss and no external evidence of disease.
• Less commonly, respiratory difficulty or regurgitation may arise from enlarged retropharyngeal nodes or from pulmonary involvement.
• Rarely, animals may present acutely anorexic with cellulitis at the site of primary infection,

or can be found dead with no previous signs of disease (though there is usually a history of CLA in the group).
• Although the disease usually does not adversely affect general health, owners may be concerned with the negative esthetics of abscesses, particularly in show sheep and goats.

SIGNALMENT
• Domestic and wild sheep and goats, and llamas and alpacas.
• Can affect lambs and kids as young as 6 weeks of age but usually animals >3 months, and more often adults than young stock.

PHYSICAL EXAMINATION FINDINGS
• Affected animals are generally bright, alert, and afebrile, with good appetite.
• External abscesses are initially discrete, cool, and firm, but become soft as they mature.
• Prior to rupture, hair is lost from the center of the lesion and the overlying skin thins and darkens.
• Purulent matter expressed from the abscess is thick, cream colored to slightly green, and odorless. In sheep it is often inspissated and may have concentric layers like an onion skin (this feature is absent in goats).
• Internal abscessation can result in nonspecific signs such as weight loss, variable appetite often without fever. Coughing may occur but even with severe pulmonary involvement, there are often no signs referable to the respiratory system.
• Rarely, acute swelling and pain with high fever (>40°C) can occur with initial infection, potentially attributable to PLD exotoxin.
• At the flock level, decreased weight gains and wool growth have been reported.
• In housed sheep and goats in North America and Europe, CLA most commonly affects the parotid, submandibular, and cervical lymph nodes, as well as the respiratory system.
• In range flocks in Australia, CLA usually affects the respiratory system (parenchyma and mediastinal lymph nodes) and popliteal lymph nodes.
• Less commonly abscesses may affect the prescapular, prefemoral, or mammary nodes; or occur in the liver, kidney, adrenals, pituitary, or vertebrae.

GENETICS
N/A

CAUSES AND RISK FACTORS
• *C. pseudotuberculosis* is a small, Gram-positive, facultative intracellular rod that produces PLD exotoxin.
• Two biotypes are classified on nitrate requirements: nitrate-negative types cause CLA and some cases of ulcerative lymphangitis in cattle; nitrate-positive isolates cause ulcerative lymphangitis in horses but do not cause disease in ruminants.
• The bacteria can survive several days in water, several weeks on fomites such as

wooden feeders, and several months in soil. Cool, moist conditions improve its survival.
• Gathering sheep for shearing allows transmission by coughing from animals with pulmonary abscesses, or via skin contamination when abscesses are nicked during shearing. Shearers that do not clean equipment or clothing between flocks can bring the disease to unaffected flocks.
• Broken or abraded skin, which can occur during shearing, increases the risk of transmission, although the bacteria can penetrate unbroken skin.
• Draining abscesses that contaminate feed, water, and feeders are an important source of infection. "Keyhole" type feeders can be particularly problematic for spreading the disease in herds or flocks where lesions occur in the parotid and submandibular lymph nodes.
• Fighting between rams or bucks can also transmit the bacteria.

DIAGNOSIS

DIFFERENTIAL DIAGNOSES
• Many bacteria cause abscesses that may or may not be associated with a lymph node. In small ruminants, these often occur in the cheek or jaw, associated with trauma from feed or other insults. A variety of bacteria have been isolated from these including anaerobes (e.g., *F. necrophorum*), *Mannheimia haemolytica*, *S. aureus*, many species of streptococci, *T. pyogenes*, and *E. coli*. These abscesses may have a watery content, with or without gas, a foul odor, and often do not involve a lymph node.
• Sterile abscesses occur in about one third of animals recently vaccinated with a multivalent clostridial vaccine.
• Abscesses on the back of the neck are often caused by sheep crawling under wooden feeders that then become infected secondarily with *S. aureus*.
• Chronic wasting can arise from conditions affecting a few individuals in the group such as dental disease, competition, paratuberculosis, ovine progressive pneumonia (maedi visna), caprine arthritis encephalitis (goats), and scrapie. Gastrointestinal parasitism and nutritional deficiency should be considered if a large proportion of the group has weight loss.
• Bacterial pneumonia, lungworm (*Dictyocaulus filaria* or *Muellerius capillaris* in goats only), sheep pulmonary adenomatosis, and transmissible nasal adenocarcinoma can cause weight loss.
• Lymphosarcoma may present as external and/or internal masses, cause chronic wasting, and/or be space occupying in the thorax.

CBC/BIOCHEMISTRY/URINALYSIS
Generally, no specific abnormalities

(CONTINUED) CASEOUS LYMPHADENITIS (CLA)

OTHER LABORATORY TESTS
• Culture abscesses prior to rupture by performing sterile aspiration or by lancing with a sterile blade and collecting material into a sterile container. Animals which have had lesions sampled or lanced should be isolated from others until completely healed.
• A variety of serologic tests detect antibodies to important antigens. Most commonly the tests detect antibody to PLD, including the synergistic hemolysin inhibition (SHI) test and different ELISA tests. Sensitivity on a flock basis is good, but only fair on an individual animal level, likely because the bacteria are walled off after initial infection. Titers may be higher and more persistent in goats than in sheep. Vaccines that contain PLD toxoid interfere with interpretation (i.e., reduce specificity).
• IFN gamma ELISA. Using whole blood, this assay detects cell-mediated immunity. Response does not appear to decrease with time post-infection and vaccination will not interfere with interpretation. This test is not widely available on a commercial basis in the US.

IMAGING
In cases of chronic wasting or respiratory disease: Ultrasound or radiographs of the thorax can identify the number and size of abscesses affecting the respiratory system. In cases of upper respiratory stridor or regurgitation, radiographs of the pharyngeal area can identify large retropharyngeal nodes. Computed tomography can be very useful to identify number and size of internal abscesses.

OTHER DIAGNOSTIC PROCEDURES
N/A

PATHOLOGIC FINDINGS
• Abscesses may occur in any lymph node or visceral organ and are grossly evident. Bacterial culture will determine whether *C. pseudotuberculosis* is the causative agent.
• In cases of sudden death, cut down the trachea and bronchial tree to check for evidence of an abscess rupturing into and occluding an airway.

TREATMENT
THERAPEUTIC APPROACH
• Response to therapy is variable at best.
• Many months or years may pass between abscess events in an animal, but once an animal exhibits an abscess, it should generally be considered infected for life.
• Although the bacterium is sensitive to many antibiotics, including penicillin, abscess formation hinders effective therapy.
• One prospective randomized clinical trial compared three treatment options for heavily infected herds: (1) Lancing, flushing, and SC penicillin; (2) Closed-system lavage and

intralesional tulathromycin; and (3) Closed-system lavage with SC tulathromycin. There was no statistically significant difference in outcomes between treatments. However, use of the drugs in this manner constituted extra-label usage and would require veterinary oversight with extended withdrawal times prior to meat or milk consumption.
• To hasten recovery and prevent contamination of the environment, isolate animals with abscesses until healed. Isolation facilities should have the following features:
  ◦ No shared water or feed source with other animals
  ◦ Ideally, separate air space
  ◦ Pen must be dedicated to housing animals with abscesses (e.g., not used for lambing or for housing animals with other diseases).
• Lance abscess with sterile blade when it becomes soft. Wear disposable gloves. Catch all material in a container to prevent environmental contamination. Clean wound with iodine or chlorhexidine. Repeat twice per day until wound is scabbed and dry. In cases of chronic and/or repeated episodes of abscess development, strongly consider culling to reduce the risk of infection to the rest of the flock or herd.

SURGICAL CONSIDERATIONS AND TECHNIQUES
• Retropharyngeal abscesses may be surgically drained under anesthesia if animal value warrants it.
• Surgical removal of external nodes can be performed in select cases.

MEDICATIONS
DRUGS OF CHOICE
Antibiotic treatment is controversial and not widely practiced. Herd-level use is not appropriate. However, treatment with penicillin or tulathromycin may be useful in individual animals (see "Therapeutic Approach"). Use of both drugs in this manner constitutes extra-label drug use and requires veterinary oversight with extended withdrawal times for meat and milk.

CONTRAINDICATIONS
N/A

PRECAUTIONS
N/A

POSSIBLE INTERACTIONS
N/A

FOLLOW-UP
EXPECTED COURSE AND PROGNOSIS
• Most infected animals do not experience severe disease.

• The disease is more important at the herd level where it can cause chronic wasting, sudden death, premature culling, carcass condemnation and trim, and restriction of movement of animals.

POSSIBLE COMPLICATIONS
N/A

CLIENT EDUCATION
Focus on what a positive diagnosis means to the flock or herd so that control measures can be instituted quickly if relevant using prevention measures (see "Prevention").

PATIENT CARE
• If the owner elects not to cull, animals should be checked at least once a month for new abscesses.
• Animals should be kept in isolation until abscesses are healed.

PREVENTION
A control program is based on the following.

Reduction of Environmental Contamination with the Bacteria
• Routine palpation of external nodes whenever animals are handled.
• Isolation of affected animals and appropriate treatment.
• Disinfection of shearing blades and pieces whenever an abscess is nicked.
• Routine washing of hands with chlorhexidine soap when handling infected animals.
• Use feeders that reduce contact of the head and neck with the feeder (e.g., bars or keyhole feeders).
• Cull all affected animals if economics allow.
• Cull all repeat offenders.

Reduction of Risk of Transmission to Uninfected Animals
• Rear young stock away from adults (e.g., remove at birth and rear artificially in another barn).
• Shear young sheep first and older and infected sheep last.
• Milk affected does last and wash down parlor with disinfectant afterward.
• Purchase breeding stock from flocks with known health status.
• Shearers should wear clean clothing (including footwear) that has not been worn to another flock without laundering. Ideally, producers should purchase their own shearing equipment.
• Treat all shearing wounds immediately with iodine or other topical disinfectant.

Improve the Immune Status of Uninfected Animals
• Commercial vaccines that contain PLD toxoid and some cell components are licensed for use in sheep. The vaccines are marketed as a combined clostridial-CLA vaccine.
• In the US there is one conditionally licensed vaccine (must be approved by the state animal health board for use in that state) for use in healthy, nonpregnant and nonlactating goats

C

CASEOUS LYMPHADENITIS (CLA)

C

3 months of age or older. Vaccines approved for sheep have been reported to cause adverse reactions in goats that are already infected, so extreme caution should be used when vaccinating with sheep vaccines.
• The vaccines work best if administered before chance of infection and after colostral immunity has waned (around 3 months of age).
• A vaccination program involves vaccination of young stock with a primary series (e.g., vaccinate at 3 and 4 months of age) and an annual booster.
• For breeding ewes, the booster can be administered 1 month prior to lambing, to optimize transfer of colostral immunity to offspring. Use of the goat vaccine in pregnant animals is not approved and has not been tested.
• The vaccine will not cure existing infection and works best when combined with other control measures as it will reduce risk of infection but will not totally prevent. Routine vaccination, when combined with culling of affected sheep, can reduce flock prevalence to <2%.
• Vaccine efficacy may be improved by increasing the frequency of vaccination to every 3–6 months, particularly if sheep and goats are housed all or part of the year.
• Autogenous vaccines have been employed, but if the PLD toxin is not totally inactivated, severe illness and death may occur.

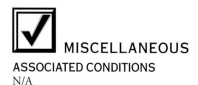

MISCELLANEOUS

ASSOCIATED CONDITIONS
N/A

AGE-RELATED FACTORS
N/A

ZOONOTIC POTENTIAL
C. pseudotuberculosis infection of humans is uncommon. Suppurative granulomatous lymphadenitis may occur secondary to wound contamination when treating or handling infected animals or contaminated materials. It is important to wear gloves when lancing abscesses and to wash hands with chlorhexidine soap after treating this disease.

PREGNANCY
N/A

BIOSECURITY
See "Prevention"

PRODUCTION MANAGEMENT
See "Prevention"

SYNONYMS
Cheesy gland, CL, CLA

ABBREVIATIONS
• CLA = caseous lymphadenitis
• ELISA = enzyme-linked immunosorbent assay
• IFN = interferon
• PLD = phospholipase D exotoxin
• SHI = synergistic hemolysin inhibition

SEE ALSO
• Caprine Arthritis Encephalitis Virus
• Johne's Disease
• Maedi-Visna (Ovine Progressive Pneumonia)
• Scrapie

Suggested Reading
Arsenault J, Girard D, Dubreuil P, et al. Prevalence of and carcass condemnation from maedi-visna, paratuberculosis and caseous lymphadenitis in culled sheep from Quebec, Canada. Prev Vet Med 2003, 59: 67–81.
Baird G, Synge B, Dercksen D. Survey of caseous lymphadenitis seroprevalence in British terminal sire sheep breeds. Vet Rec 2004, 154: 505–6.
Paton MW, Walker SB, Rose IR, Watt GF. Prevalence of caseous lymphadenitis and usage of caseous lymphadenitis vaccines in sheep flocks. Aust Vet J 2003, 81: 91–5.
Prescott JF, Menzies PI, Hwang YT. An interferon-gamma assay for the diagnosis of *Corynebacterium pseudotuberculosis* infection in adult sheep from a research flock. Vet Microbiol 2002, 88: 287–97.
Washburn KE, Bissett WT, Fajt VR, et al. 2009. Comparison of three treatment regimens for sheep and goats with caseous lymphadenitis. J Am Vet Med Assoc 2009, 234: 1162–6.
Author Paul J. Plummer
Consulting Editor Erica C. McKenzie
Acknowledgment The author and book editors acknowledge the prior contribution of Paula I. Menzies.

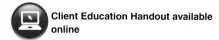

Client Education Handout available online

CASTOR BEAN TOXICITY

BASICS

OVERVIEW

• Castor bean, *Ricinus communis*, is considered to be a native of northern Africa. In the United States it is commonly grown as an ornamental plant.
• Commercially, castor bean is used in the production of castor oil. This oil has been used for centuries for medicinal purposes. It is used in cosmetic products and as an industrial lubricant.
• The entire plant is toxic. The primary toxic principle is ricin and is found in highest concentration in the seeds. Ricin is not found in castor oil.
• Ricinin is another toxin in the castor bean plant. It is concentrated in the leaves.
• A by-product of castor oil manufacturing is castor oil cake. This has been fed to livestock as it is high in protein. It must be heat treated prior to feeding in order to destroy the ricin.
• The castor bean plant is a large, robust erect annual woody herb reaching up to 15 feet in height. Large, serrated leaves are alternate and palmate with 5 to 11 lobes. Leaves range in size from 4 to 36 inches. Fruits are three-lobed, spiny capsules with three seeds. The seeds resemble an engorged, female *Ixodes ricinus* tick.

INCIDENCE/PREVALENCE

• Relative to the availability of the plants.
• Castor bean toxicity is not a common intoxication of ruminants.

GEOGRAPHIC DISTRIBUTION

Castor bean is found throughout the world, primarily in tropical, but also in temperate environments. It is found in the southern portions of the U.S.

SYSTEMS AFFECTED

• Digestive
• Nervous
• Multisystemic

PATHOPHYSIOLOGY

• Ricin is a large molecular weight protein and classified as a toxalbumin.
• After ingestion, ricin is absorbed from the gastrointestinal tract into the blood and is transported to the liver and other organs/tissues to a lesser degree.
• After entering a cell, it inhibits cellular protein synthesis, resulting in cell death.

SIGNALMENT

All ruminants are susceptible to castor bean.

PHYSICAL EXAMINATION FINDINGS

• Clinical signs from ricin intoxication range from a few hours to 2–3 days. The delay may be due to the time necessary for cells to die.
• Anorexia, fever and abdominal pain
• Vomiting and profuse, watery, hemorrhagic diarrhea with subsequent dehydration and hypovolemic shock
• Depression
• Terminally, collapse, convulsions, and death
• Clinical signs in animals from ricinin including weakness, and ataxia are usually short-lived and recovery is seen in a few hours.

CAUSES AND RISK FACTORS

Ricin is concentrated in the seeds. They have a hard shell, making it somewhat difficult to break when chewed. If the seed is unbroken when swallowed, it will pass through the digestive tract intact and will not cause any adverse effects to the animal.

DIAGNOSIS

DIFFERENTIAL DIAGNOSES

• Other causes of enteritis and hemorrhagic diarrhea
• Bovine viral diarrhea virus
• Mucosal disease
• Salmonella
• Winter dysentery

CBC/BIOCHEMISTRY/URINALYSIS

• Elevation of hepatic enzymes: AST, LDH
• Increase in BUN

OTHER LABORATORY TESTS

Evidence of plant consumption in gastrointestinal contents

PATHOLOGIC FINDINGS

• Hemorrhagic gastritis and enteritis
• Edematous mesenteric lymph nodes
• Swelling of the liver and kidney may occur.

TREATMENT

THERAPEUTIC APPROACH

• Supportive: good nursing care
• Symptomatic: correct dehydration and electrolyte abnormalities

MEDICATIONS

DRUGS OF CHOICE

• Activated charcoal: 2–5 g/kg given orally to control absorption of toxins from the gastrointestinal tract (1 g charcoal per 5 mL water).
• Mineral oil administered orally to more rapidly transport plant materials through the gastrointestinal tract.
• Generally, it is considered best to use either activated charcoal or mineral oil, but not both at the same time.

FOLLOW-UP

EXPECTED COURSE AND PROGNOSIS

• Dependent upon amount of seeds/plant material ingested.
• Ruminants are less susceptible to the effects of ricin.

PREVENTION/AVOIDANCE

Prevent animals' access to plants.

MISCELLANEOUS

PRODUCTION MANAGEMENT

Restrict grazing of livestock near castor beans or feeding castor bean plant materials.

ABBREVIATIONS

• AST = aspartate aminotransferase
• BUN = blood urea nitrogen
• LDH = lactate dehydrogenase

SEE ALSO

• Bovine Viral Diarrhea Virus
• Salmonellosis
• Winter Dysentery

Suggested Reading
Burrows GE, Tyrl RJ. Toxic Plants of North America. Ames: Iowa State University Press, 2001.
Burrows GE, Tyrl RJ. Toxic Plants of North America, 2nd ed. Ames: Wiley-Blackwell, 2013.
Knight AP, Walter RG. A Guide to Plant Poisonings of Animals in North America. Jackson, WY: Teton New Media, 2001.

Author Matt G. Welborn
Consulting Editor Christopher C.L. Chase
Acknowledgment The author and book editors acknowledge the prior contribution of Troy E.C. Holder.

CASTRATION/VASECTOMY: BOVINE

BASICS

OVERVIEW
• Castration is a husbandry practice used to remove males from the genetic breeding pool and eliminate aggressive behaviors associated with testosterone during the feeding period prior to animal harvest.
• Unilateral castration may be used in breeding males with acquired unilateral testicular disease.
• Vasectomy preserves testosterone production and creates "teaser" bulls that are used for heat detection in females that will undergo breeding by artificial means and is covered elsewhere in this textbook.

INCIDENCE/PREVALENCE
• Castration of calves is a common procedure in many countries.
• Castration may not be acceptable in some countries.
• Vasectomy is not as common.

GEOGRAPHIC DISTRIBUTION
Worldwide

SYSTEMS AFFECTED
Reproductive

PATHOPHYSIOLOGY
• The major aim of castration is to eliminate behavior and physiologic changes associated with testosterone period.
• Castration improves feed efficiency and reduces risk of accidents to humans or other animals.
• This can be accomplished using bloodless techniques. Elastrator bands cause an ischemic, avascular necrosis followed by sloughing of the distal tissues. Emasculatome applied to the spermatic cord cause atrophy of the testes but preserves the scrotal skin.
• Early (prepubertal) castration is the standard management technique.
• Vasectomized males will retain their male behavioral and anatomic characteristics but will be sterile. Spermatogenesis may continue for a long time but viable sperm disappears from the ejaculate within 2–3 weeks.

HISTORICAL FINDINGS
N/A

SIGNALMENT
• Castration
  ○ Routine management: young calves 2–4 months of age.
  ○ Mature breeding bulls with acquired unilateral testicular disorders.
• Vasectomy: Yearling with normal reproductive tract development and behavior.

PHYSICAL EXAMINATION FINDINGS
• Routine castration and vasectomy are performed on healthy animals.
• Unilateral castration: Animal may have testicular abnormalities.

GENETICS
N/A

CAUSES AND RISK FACTORS
N/A

DIAGNOSIS

DIFFERENTIAL DIAGNOSES
N/A

CBC/BIOCHEMISTRY/URINALYSIS
Indicated for complicated unilateral castration and cryptorchidectomy

OTHER LABORATORY TESTS
N/A

IMAGING
• Ultrasonographic evaluation of the scrotal content is indicated prior to emergency unilateral castration in a breeding bull with sudden increase in scrotal size.
• Transabdominal (inguinal) and transrectal ultrasonography are used to identify cryptorchid testes.

OTHER DIAGNOSTIC PROCEDURES
N/A

PATHOLOGIC FINDINGS
• Unilateral castration: Pathologic finding of diseased testicle (orchitis, periorchitis, inguinal hernia, neoplasia).
• Vasectomy: Histology performed on the excised tissue to ascertain that it is the vas deferens.
• Cryptorchidectomy: Histopathology confirms lack of spermatogenesis and may reveal neoplastic changes.

TREATMENT

THERAPEUTIC APPROACH
• Sedation and analgesia: Bloodless castration techniques are performed on very young animals without analgesia.
• Premedication with antibiotics and post-surgical pain management are required for adult castration and cryptorchidectomy.
• Anti-tetanus prophylaxis is important.

SURGICAL CONSIDERATIONS AND TECHNIQUES

Castration
• Castration is best performed in young animals <3 months of age. At this age, the testicles are smaller, animals are easier to handle, there is less stress when the calf can return to the cow, and there are fewer complications associated with the procedure. Castration can be performed with either open or closed methods. Attention to the animal's environment, fly control, vaccination status, facilities, and cleanliness of the procedure is

warranted to minimize risk of postoperative morbidity.
• *Open castration*
  ○ Restraint: Calf chute or, if the animal is small enough, in lateral recumbency.
  ○ Local anesthesia: 2% lidocaine can be used in a pistol grip syringe to accommodate rapid injection of 4–5 mL of anesthetic into the base of the scrotum and 2 mL into each spermatic cord.
  ○ Scrotal incision: Various methods are used. The use of a Newberry castration knife is common. The testicles are displaced proximally into the neck of the scrotum with one hand.
  ○ The Newberry Knife is applied with the other hand in the frontal plane of the scrotum, closed, and forcefully pulled distally to incise both sides of the scrotum at the same time. If a local block in the spermatic cords was used, both testicles should descend through the incisions.
  ○ An alternative method is to grasp the base of the scrotum with one hand or a surgical instrument (e.g., Allis Tissue Forceps) and transect it using a scalpel blade. The advantage of using the Newberry Knife is that the operator's hands are out of the way of the sharp instrument if the calf kicks during the incision.
  ○ Removal of the testes. The operator grasps one testicle (potentially two if the animal is very small), and place gentle, steady traction on the testicle(s) with one hand while stripping fascial attachments proximally with the other hand. An emasculator or other instrument, such as the Henderson Bloodless Castration Tool, is applied to emasculate the cord and provide hemostasis of the testicular vessels. Alternatively, a transfixation ligature of appropriately sized absorbable suture material can be used. Because of the increased amount of time and expense in using suture material, this is often not done in practice for routine castrations.
  ○ In young calves, the cords may be stretched until they break. The vas deferens may need to be transected with a scalpel. This technique is less desirable because of the increased incidence of postoperative bleeding, greater discomfort to the animal, and a higher potential of bleeding into the abdomen.
  ○ Any adipose tissue or extraneous fascia should be sharply removed from the surgical site.
• *Closed castration*
  ○ Emasculotomes (Burdizzo) should be the appropriate size for the age of the animal and size of the scrotum.
  ○ The emasculotome is applied across each spermatic cord separately in the neck of the scrotum with two applications of the crush approximately 2 cm apart. It is important that the tension of the emasculotome is set

appropriately to effectively crush the cord within the scrotum without damaging the scrotal skin. The instrument should not be applied across the entire neck of the scrotum as this will cause crushing of the blood vessels that supply the scrotum, resulting in postoperative development of a large, necrotic, painful mass.
○ Advantage: No postoperative monitoring required.
○ Disadvantage: The scrotum remains intact, which may lead people to believe that the calves are still intact.
○ Closed castration may be achieved with tight rubber band (e.g., Callicrate Bander) placed around the neck of the scrotum. This method is popular for castration of large bulls in a feedlot. Disadvantages include a higher degree of pain and development of severe scrotal edema and/or clinical tetanus. The entire scrotum and its contents often fall off within 7–10 days.

Vasectomy
• Restraint: Standing or in lateral recumbency. The incision site is blocked with lidocaine.
• A 2 cm vertical incision is made in the caudomedial aspect through the skin and parietal layer of the tunica vaginalis just above the vascular cone. The ductus deferens is identified by palpation and isolated by blunt dissection. A 3–4 cm segment is ligated and removed. The skin is closed with absorbable suture. The procedure is repeated on the other side.

MEDICATIONS

DRUGS OF CHOICE
Meloxicam (1 mg/kg PO) should be considered to reduce inflammation.

CONTRAINDICATIONS
Appropriate meat withdrawal times must be followed.

PRECAUTIONS
N/A

POSSIBLE INTERACTIONS
N/A

FOLLOW-UP

EXPECTED COURSE AND PROGNOSIS
Vasectomized males should undergo semen collection and evaluation 2–3 weeks after surgery to make sure that there are no viable spermatozoa in the ejaculate.

POSSIBLE COMPLICATIONS
• Hemorrhage and wound infection, especially at the peak of the fly season or when muddy or very dry, dusty conditions exist.
• Clinical tetanus can be a complication of closed castration.

CLIENT EDUCATION
• Welfare issues regarding castration
• Use proper technique

PATIENT CARE
Patients should be closely monitored for the first 24–48 hours for lethargy, inappetence, fever, and/or severe swelling of the surgical site.

PREVENTION
• Proper technique insuring both testicles are within the scrotum distal to the band.
• Avoid banding the sigmoid flexure of the penis.
• Appropriate restraint, environmental control, and good vaccination protocols.

MISCELLANEOUS

ASSOCIATED CONDITIONS
Testicular disorders

AGE-RELATED FACTORS
Choice of castration technique depends on age of animal

ZOONOTIC POTENTIAL
N/A

PREGNANCY
N/A

BIOSECURITY
Males to be used as teasers after vasectomy should be free of contagious diseases and selected from known herds or flocks.

PRODUCTION MANAGEMENT
• Welfare questions have risen regarding these practices.
• Noncastrated males should be separated from females before onset of puberty.

SYNONYMS
N/A

ABBREVIATIONS
N/A

SEE ALSO
• Teaser Preparation
• Testicular Disorders: Bovine

Suggested Reading
Gilbert RO, Cable C, Fubini SL, et al. Surgery of the bovine reproductive system and urinary tract. In: Fubini SL, Ducharme NG eds, Farm Animal Surgery, 2nd ed. St. Louis: Saunders Elsevier, 2014, pp. 439–50.
Morgan G. Surgical correction of abnormalities of the reproductive organs of bulls and preparation of teaser animals. In: Youngquist RS, Threlfall WR eds, Current Therapy in Large Animal Theriogenology, 2nd ed. St. Louis: Saunders Elsevier, 2007, pp. 243–4.
Author Jennifer A. Schleining
Consulting Editor Ahmed Tibary

Client Education Handout available online

CASTRATION/VASECTOMY: CAMELID

BASICS

OVERVIEW
• Castration or orchiectomy is the most common method to remove males from the genetic pool.
• Vasectomy is often considered when the male is intended as a teaser for heat detection or to induce ovulation in a sterile mating (mostly for research purposes).
• Other methods for sterilization, including immunologic castration by GnRH vaccine, have been examined but results are variable.
• Unilateral castration is required for the removal of a diseased testicle in a breeding male.

INCIDENCE/PREVALENCE
Castration is the most common surgical procedure in camelid practice.

GEOGRAPHIC DISTRIBUTION
Worldwide distribution

SYSTEMS AFFECTED
Reproductive

PATHOPHYSIOLOGY
• Male aggression is often a problem when a large group of males is housed together. Additionally, intact males are often poor fiber producers (alpacas and llamas) and are not suitable for riding or work (camels).
• Male sexual behavior is more pronounced in camels than in alpacas or llamas, and includes extrusion of the soft palate, tail flapping, secretion from the poll glands, and aggression (which may become directed at humans).
• Male camelids can become very aggressive towards humans, particularly if they were bottle raised (berserk male syndrome). In llamas, castration was shown to decrease human-directed aggression in 73% of cases.
• Castration also removes the source of testosterone, and therefore the majority of sexual behaviors. However, some behaviors may persist, particularly after castration of a sexually mature, breeding male. These may include interest in females, and ability to achieve intromission.
• Vasectomy allows sterilization of males while preserving the ability to mate and induce ovulation.

GENETICS
• Unilateral cryptorchid males and males with congenital testicular disorders should be eliminated from breeding.
• Bilateral cryptorchidism is associated with cytogenetic and developmental abnormalities.

SIGNALMENT
• The current recommendations are to castrate a male after puberty (12–15 months in SAC, 2 years in camels). Prepubertal castration can result in orthopedic disorders.
• Camels intended for food may be castrated earlier. However, testicular descent is often delayed in some individuals, making early castration difficult.

HISTORICAL FINDINGS
• Castration or vasectomy may be elective procedures.
• Treatment of testicular pathologies in breeding males (hemicastration).

PHYSICAL EXAMINATION FINDINGS
• For elective procedures, the animal should be healthy, with no clinical signs of disease.
• Animals submitted for castration should be examined for the presence of both testes in the scrotum.
• Unilateral cryptorchidism and ectopic testis are not uncommon in alpacas and llamas. The abnormal testicle should be removed before the normally descended testicle.

CAUSES AND RISK FACTORS
N/A

DIAGNOSIS

DIFFERENTIAL DIAGNOSES
Differential diagnosis between abnormal male behavior in a gelding and cryptorchidism can be achieved by testing for testosterone levels.

CBC/BIOCHEMISTRY/URINALYSIS
May be indicated in breeding males undergoing emergency unilateral castration or before cryptorchidectomy.

OTHER LABORATORY TESTS
• Serum testosterone levels may indicate presence of testicular tissue in cases of cryptorchidism or intersex.
• A rise in testosterone levels is observed within 8 hours of IV administration of hCG (3000 IU for SAC; 10,000 IU for camels).

IMAGING
Percutaneous, transabdominal, or inguinal ultrasonography may help locate retained testes in cryptorchid animals.

DIAGNOSTIC PROCEDURES
N/A

PATHOLOGIC FINDINGS
The most common reasons for unilateral castration are orchitis, neoplasia (seminoma), testicular hemorrhage/trauma.

TREATMENT

THERAPEUTIC APPROACH
• Animals should be fasted if general anesthesia is considered.
• Tetanus toxoid vaccination prior to surgery.
• Perioperative antimicrobials and anti-inflammatory medications.

SURGICAL CONSIDERATIONS AND TECHNIQUES

Castration
• Castration can be performed in the standing, sedated animal (camels, llamas) or under injectable anesthesia.
• Combinations of xylazine, butorphanol, and ketamine are often used for sedation and anesthesia.
• Two techniques have been described: A prescrotal technique with primary closure, or scrotal technique, with placement of the incisions directly over the testes, and healing by second intention.
  ○ For both techniques, the testis is removed through the skin incision. Fascia is stripped away from the spermatic cord. A transfixation ligature may be placed around the spermatic cord. Emasculators or crushing forceps are used to achieve hemostasis and the testis is removed. The procedure is repeated on the other side, removing the testis from either the same incision (prescrotal) or an additional incision (scrotal).
  ○ Closed or open castration may be performed.
  ○ Analgesia may be enhanced by intratesticular injection of lidocaine or bupivacaine.
  ○ Animals which have second intention healing should be monitored for fly strike, particularly in hot weather.

Cryptorchidectomy
• Removal of abdominally retained testes may be performed via an abdominal parainguinal approach or laparoscopic assisted technique under general anesthesia with the animal placed in dorsal recumbency.
• For a parainguinal approach, a skin incision is made parallel to the external inguinal ring and the abdominal cavity is penetrated by blunt dissection of the abdominal wall. The testis is retrieved using a spay hook and excised after placement of a transfixation ligature.
• For the laparoscopy-assisted approach, a laparoscopic portal is created at the umbilical scar. A second grasping instrument portal is created parainguinal on the side of the retained testis. The testis is visualized, grasped, and elevated to the second portal, which is enlarged for exteriorization. The testis is excised as already described.

Vasectomy
• Vasectomy is performed under general anesthesia.
• Two techniques have been described: a laparoscopic, intra-abdominal approach, and a prescrotal, extra-abdominal technique.
• For the laparoscopic approach, the ductus deferens is identified using a laparoscope and long-handled forceps. For the prescrotal approach, it is found after dissection between

the external inguinal ring and the scrotum. In both cases, a 2–4 cm segment is removed.
• For the prescrotal approach, the ductus deferens may be ligated after folding over the incised aspect, to reduce risk of sperm granuloma formation at the incision site.
• Intradermal skin sutures at the incision sites remove the need to handle the animals for suture removal.

MEDICATIONS

DRUGS OF CHOICE
• Standing castration sedation: Xylazine (0.2 mg/kg IM) and butorphanol 0.1 mg/kg IM
• Field anesthesia:
  ◦ Llamas and alpacas: Xylazine (0.22–0.55 mg/kg), butorphanol (0.08–0.11 mg/kg) and ketamine (0.22–0.55 mg/kg IM) in combination for llamas and alpacas.
  ◦ Camels: Xylazine (0.25 mg/kg IV or 0.35 mg/kg IM), ketamine (5–8 mg/kg IM, 3–5 mg/kg IV)
• Broad-spectrum antimicrobials

CONTRAINDICATIONS
• Unhealthy animals should not be submitted for surgery.
• Appropriate meat withdrawal times must be followed.

PRECAUTIONS
N/A

POSSIBLE INTERACTIONS
N/A

FOLLOW-UP

EXPECTED COURSE AND PROGNOSIS
• Following castration, serum testosterone levels drop to baseline within 24 hours. However, sexual behaviors may persist in some males.
• Semen samples collected at 15 and 30 days postoperatively had non-viable spermatozoa present.
• Vasectomized males have been successfully used for several years postoperatively with no alterations in sexual behavior. Postmortem examination demonstrated small sperm granulomas at the incision site of the ductus deferens but no other abnormalities.

POSSIBLE COMPLICATIONS
• Castration: Complications are possible, particularly in older males or those with diseased testes, and include surgical site infection, scirrhous cord, and hemorrhage.
• Cryptorchidectomy: peritonitis.
• Vasectomy: Surgical site infection. Excision of the vas deferens should be verified by histology in order to avoid fertility.

CLIENT EDUATION
Clients should be aware that males which undergo vasectomy will still maintain male sexual behavior and be able to achieve intromission in females.

PATIENT MONITORING
Animals should be monitored postoperatively for complications, including fever, inappetence, and incisional infection, dehiscence, or seroma formation. For incisions left to heal by second intention, monitoring for swelling, edema, hemorrhage, and fly strike should be performed.

PREVENTION
N/A

MISCELLANEOUS

ASSOCIATED CONDITIONS
• Testicular disorders
• Abnormal behavior

AGE-RELATED FACTORS
• Males which are castrated too young have been shown to develop orthopedic disorders.
• Males which are castrated after sexual maturity and breeding activity may continue to display those behaviors after castration.

ZOONOTIC POTENTIAL
N/A

PREGNANCY
Pregnancy may occur if vasectomy is not performed correctly.

BIOSECURITY
Vasectomized males can still transmit disease through intromission. Males should be examined for general health prior to use in a breeding program.

PRODUCTION MANAGEMENT
• Vasectomized males may be used to detect estrus in females.
• Castrated males are often used as guard animals for the herd.

SYNONYMS
• Orchiectomy
• Deferentectomy

ABBREVIATIONS
N/A

SEE ALSO
• Breeding Soundness Examination: Camelid
• Camelid: Reproduction
• Testicular Disorders: Camelid

Suggested Reading
Nickell J, Barter LS, Dechant JE. Effects of intratesticular and incisional local anesthetic administration for castration of alpacas anesthetized with intramuscular ketamine-xylazine-butorphanol. Vet Surg 2015, 44: 168–73.
Pearson LK, Campbell AJ, Sandoval S, Tibary A. Effects of vasectomy on seminal plasma alkaline phosphatase in male alpacas (*Vicugna pacos*). Reprod Domest Anim 2013, 48: 995–1000.
Tibary A, Anouassi A. Standing castration in camels. J Camel Pract Res 2004;11:125–7.
Tibary A, Anouassi A. Surgery of reproductive tract in camels. In: Adams G, Skidmore J eds, Recent Advances in Camelid Reproduction. Ithaca, NY: International Veterinary Information Service, 2000; A1008.1100.
Author Lisa Pearson
Consulting Editor Ahmed Tibary

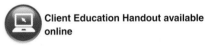
Client Education Handout available online

C

CASTRATION/VASECTOMY: SMALL RUMINANT

BASICS

OVERVIEW
• Castration is the most common management surgical procedure performed in small ruminants.
• Castration improves fiber production and carcass yield.
• Castration age may be delayed in show or pet animals to avoid risk for urolithiasis.
• Most castrations are performed by the producers themselves except for adult or complicated cases.
• Castration techniques may be bloodless (elastrator bands and Burdizzo emasculatome); alternatively there is surgical excision.
• There is increasing concerns about the welfare of lambs and kids when castration is used without pain management.
• Unilateral castration may be performed on breeding animals to remove a diseased testicle and preserve breeding ability.
• Vasectomy is the bilateral excision of a portion of the vas deferens. It is used to sterilize males for use as estrus teasers. Epididymectomy (cauda epididymis excision) is an alternative but is not as esthetic.

INCIDENCE/PREVALENCE
Common in sheep and goat production

GEOGRAPHIC DISTRIBUTION
In some areas of the world castration is not acceptable for religious reasons or consumer preference.

SYSTEMS AFFECTED
• Reproductive
• Urinary

PATHOPHYSIOLOGY
• The major aim of castration is to eliminate behavior and physiologic changes associated with testosterone during the postpubertal period. In goats, castration eliminates male odor (male taint of meat).
• Bloodless techniques such as elastrator bands cause an ischemic, avascular necrosis followed by sloughing of the distal tissues. An emasculatome applied to the spermatic cord causes atrophy of the testes but preserves the scrotal skin.
• Surgical techniques are preferable in adult males in order to reduce complications.
• Early castration has been associated with increased risk for urolithiasis due to poor development of the penis and small diameter of the urethra.
• Vasectomized males retain their male behavioral and anatomic characteristics but are sterile. Spermatogenesis may continue for a long time but viable sperm disappears from the ejaculate within 2–3 weeks. Development of sperm granuloma is common in vasectomized males.

HISTORICAL FINDINGS
N/A

SIGNALMENT
• Males of various age
• Unilateral castration: Valuable males with acquired testicular disorders

PHYSICAL EXAMINATION FINDINGS
Routine castration is performed on healthy animals.

GENETICS
N/A

CAUSES AND RISK FACTORS
N/A

DIAGNOSIS

DIFFERENTIAL DIAGNOSES
N/A

CBC/BIOCHEMISTRY/URINALYSIS
Indicated for complicated unilateral castration and cryptorchidectomy

OTHER LABORATORY TESTS
N/A

IMAGING
Transabdominal ultrasonography to identify cryptorchid testes

OTHER DIAGNOSTIC PROCEDURES
N/A

PATHOLOGIC FINDINGS
• Unilateral castration: Orchitis, periorchitis, neoplasia.
• Vasectomy: Histology performed on the excised tissue to ascertain that it is the vas deferens.
• Cryptorchidectomy: Histopathology confirms lack of spermatogenesis and may reveal neoplastic changes.

TREATMENT

THERAPEUTIC APPROACH
• Sedation and analgesia: Bloodless castration techniques are performed on very young animals (24 hours to 1 week) without analgesia.
• Premedication with antibiotics and post-surgical pain management are required for adult castration and cryptorchidectomy.
• Anti-tetanus prophylaxis is important.

SURGICAL CONSIDERATIONS AND TECHNIQUES
• Elastrator bands
  ○ Usually performed on kids and lambs <1 week of age but can be used up to 4 months of age.
  ○ Very young animals: Restrained physically by one person. The elastrator band, previously soaked in an antiseptic, is placed

around the neck of the scrotum, making sure that both testicles are distal to the band.
  ○ Sloughing of the scrotum and its contents occurs 7–10 days later.
• Burdizzo emasculatome is used to crush the testicular cord.
  ○ The emasculatome is applied to each testicular cord separately at different levels if the scrotal skin is to be preserved.
  ○ This technique has been shown to be less stressful than surgical excision.
  ○ Reduction of pain may be achieved by administration of bupivacaine in the spermatic cord.
• Surgical excision
  ○ Sedation and local anesthesia is a subject of debate but it is required in animals 6 weeks or older.
  ○ General anesthesia is recommended in adult rams and bucks.
  ○ A crude technique of cutting off the bottom of the scrotum and forced rupture of the testicular cord by traction is commonly used by producers.
  ○ Alternately, the bottom third of the scrotum is removed with a scalpel or transected with a Newberry knife. The testes are exteriorized. The testicular cord is ligated by transfixing using absorbable suture, then transected with a scalpel or an emasculator.
• Unilateral castration in breeding animal
  ○ Animal is placed under general anesthesia in lateral or dorsal recumbency.
  ○ The scrotum is clipped and prepared for surgery.
  ○ A longitudinal elliptical incision is made on the lateral aspect of the scrotum and continued through the subcutaneous tissue. For closed castration the vaginal tunic is left intact. The cord is ligated with a circumferential suture proximal to a transfixation suture using absorbable #1 or #2 suture material. The testis is removed using an emasculator.
  ○ The elliptical incision allows removal of as much skin as possible. The subcutaneous tissue is closed with absorbable material to eliminate dead space and the skin is closed using a Ford interlocking pattern.
• Crypotorchidectomy
  ○ This surgery is often considered for pet animals.
  ○ The retained testis is removed under general anesthesia following laparotomy or laparoscopy-assisted technique.
  ○ Food is withheld for 24–36 hours depending on size of the animal.
  ○ The abdomen is prepared for surgery. The abdominal cavity may be explored through a flank laparotomy. The retained testis is identified by following the vas deferens as it crosses the ureter.
  ○ Laparoscopy: A laparoscope portal is placed either in a paramedian site or at the umbilical scar. Another portal, to introduce

(CONTINUED)   ## CASTRATION/VASECTOMY: SMALL RUMINANT

grasping forceps, is placed parallel to the inguinal canal ipsilateral to the retained testis or paramedian to the penis in bilateral cases. The retained testis is identified, grasped, and lifted toward the portal, then exteriorized and excised after transfixing ligation of the vascular cone and the gubernaculum separately.

- Vasectomy
  ○ Bilateral vasectomy is the preferred method for preparation of teaser animals under field conditions.
  ○ The procedure is done under sedation, general or lumbosacral anesthesia. Caudal epidural may be helpful.
  ○ The animal is placed in a cradle or in a sitting position. A 3–4 cm skin incision is made on the medial aspect of the spermatic cord proximal to the vascular cone. The incision is continued through the vaginal tunic and the vas is identified by palpation and lifted using a hemostat or a spay hook.
  ○ A 4 cm portion of the vas deferens is isolated and transected after ligation.
  ○ The skin is closed using subcuticular suture with absorbable material.

MEDICATIONS

DRUGS OF CHOICE
- Sedation: Butorphanol, xylazine
- Local analgesia: Lidocaine or bupivacaine
- Post-surgical anti-inflammatories: Flunixin meglumin
- Antibiotic therapy: Penicillin

CONTRAINDICATIONS
Appropriate meat withdrawal times must be followed.

PRECAUTIONS
N/A

POSSIBLE INTERACTIONS
N/A

FOLLOW-UP

EXPECTED COURSE AND PROGNOSIS
- Semen evaluation should be performed 60–90 days after surgery in unilaterally

castrated breeding males. Fertility is generally not affected but male to female ratio should be adjusted.
- Vasectomized males should undergo semen collection and evaluation 2–3 weeks after surgery to make sure that there are no viable spermatozoa in the ejaculate.

POSSIBLE COMPLICATIONS
- Error in placement of bands or Burdizzo may result in crushing the penis, severe hematoma (crushing of testis), or maintenance of male characteristic if testes are proximal to crushing site or band.
- Clostridial infections (*Cl. tetani*).
- Excessive traction on the testicular cord may cause herniation.
- Adult castration may result in excessive swelling and scirrhous cord.
- Hemorrhage and peritonitis are the main complications of cryptorchidectomy.

CLIENT EDUCATION
- Welfare issues regarding castration
- Use proper technique

PATIENT CARE
- Animals undergoing general anesthesia and abdominal surgery should be fasted.
- Antimicrobial and anti-inflammatory medication should be administered to males undergoing crypotorchidectomy or unilateral castration.
- Older animals should be monitored for any signs of surgical site infection or hemorrhage.

PREVENTION
- Vaccination against clostridial infections or administration of tetanus antitoxin and tetanus toxoid at the time of castration.

MISCELLANEOUS

ASSOCIATED CONDITIONS
Testicular disorders

AGE-RELATED FACTORS
Choice of castration technique depends on age of animal.

ZOONOTIC POTENTIAL
N/A

PREGNANCY
N/A

BIOSECURITY
Males to be used as teasers after vasectomy should be free of contagious diseases and selected from known herds/flocks.

PRODUCTION MANAGEMENT
- In production system castration of lambs is performed at the same time as docking in the first week of life.
- Welfare questions have arisen regarding these practices.
- Noncastrated males should be separated from females before onset of puberty.

SYNONYMS
N/A

ABBREVIATIONS
N/A

SEE ALSO
- Teaser Preparation
- Testicular Disorders: Small Ruminant

Suggested Reading
Melches S, Mellema SC, Doherr MG, et al. Castration of lambs: A welfare comparison of different castration techniques in lambs over 10 weeks of age. Vet J 2007, 173: 554–63.
Stewart M, Beausoleil NJ, Johnson GB, et al. Do rubber rings coated with lignocaine reduce the pain associated with ring castration of lambs? Appl Anim Behav Sci 2014, 160: 56–63.
Tibary A, Pearson LK, Van Metre DC, Ortved K. Chapter 25: Surgery of the sheep and goat reproductive and urinary tract. In: Fubini S, Ducharme N eds, Farm Animal Surgery, 2nd ed. Elsevier, 2016, pp. 571–95.
Author Ahmed Tibary
Consulting Editor Ahmed Tibary

 Client Education Handout available online

CAUDAL VENA CAVAL THROMBOSIS SYNDROME

BASICS

OVERVIEW
• Caudal vena caval thrombosis syndrome represents a metastatic pneumonia characterized by multifocal abscessation, caused by septic emboli that originate from a septic thrombus typically located in the caudal vena cava.
• The septic thrombus may occasionally be located in the cranial vena cava.
• Septic thrombi in the vena cava are most often a sequela of liver abscesses arising from ruminal acidosis.
• Other less common causes of liver abscesses include septic conditions such as foot rot, mastitis, metritis, and jugular phlebitis.

INCIDENCE/PREVALENCE
A large feedlot survey revealed that this syndrome represented 1.3% of feedlot necropsy diagnoses, with 1.6–7.3 cases per 100,000 head on feed. It was also reported that 68% of cases occurred during the first 90 days of feeding.

GEOGRAPHIC DISTRIBUTION
Influenced by distribution of feedlot and dairy management systems

SYSTEMS AFFECTED
• Digestive
• Respiratory

PATHOPHYSIOLOGY
• Feedlot and dairy cattle that are fed rapidly fermentable high-carbohydrate grain diets commonly experience ruminal acidosis.
• Acidosis of the rumen promotes damage to ruminal epithelium.
• Bacteria including *Fusobacterium necrophorum* and *Trueperella pyogenes* penetrate the damaged ruminal epithelium and are transported to the liver in the portal bloodstream.
• Bacteria are filtered in the portal circulatory system resulting in hepatic abscessation.
• A liver abscess may erode through into the caudal vena cava resulting in formation of a septic thrombus.
• Septic emboli detach from the thrombus and metastasize to the lungs through the pulmonary arterial system.
• Emboli lodge in the arterioles where they cause thromboembolism, arteritis, endarteritis, and pulmonary abscesses.
• Arteritis and endarteritis, in combination with pulmonary hypertension, result in formation of aneurysms.
• A perivascular abscess in the lung may erode both the pulmonary arterial wall and a bronchial wall and cause rupture of the aneurysm.
• Blood from the ruptured aneurysm is channeled into the bronchus resulting in hemoptysis, and rupture of aneurysms may

result in pulmonary hematomas; both contribute to anemia in affected animals.
• Large emboli may block lobar and larger arteries, causing acute hypoxemia and death.

HISTORICAL FINDINGS
• Chronic history of weight loss
• Coughing
• History of episodes of epistaxis
• May exhibit acute respiratory distress
• May be found suddenly dead

SIGNALMENT
The syndrome typically occurs in young feedlot cattle and adult dairy cattle consuming high energy rations. It is uncommon in cattle <1 year of age.

PHYSICAL EXAMINATION FINDINGS
• Tachypnea
• Dyspnea
• Tachycardia
• May be febrile
• Thoracic pain on deep palpation of the sternum and intercostal spaces
• Mild expiratory grunt
• Epistaxis
• Hemoptysis
• Pale mucus membranes due to anemia
• Heart murmurs
• Coughing
• Melena caused by coughing up and swallowing of blood
• Subcutaneous emphysema
• Widespread wheezes on auscultation of advanced cases
• Many cases may die suddenly because of acute hemorrhage from the respiratory tract.

GENETICS
N/A

CAUSES AND RISK FACTORS
• Causative bacteria can include
  ○ *Fusobacterium necrophorum*
  ○ *Trueperella pyogenes*
  ○ *Staphylococcus* spp.
  ○ *Streptococcus* spp.
  ○ *Escherichia coli*
• Highly fermentable carbohydrate-based diets
• Sudden increase in the proportion of grain in the diet
• Thrombi may also originate from other sites of infection, such as jugular phlebitis, mastitis, metritis, foot rot.

DIAGNOSIS

DIFFERENTIAL DIAGNOSES
• Interstitial pneumonia
• Anaphylaxis
• Hypersensitivity pneumonitis
• Lungworm
• Suppurative bronchopneumonia
• Aspiration pneumonia

CBC/BIOCHEMISTRY/URINALYSIS
• Changes are nonspecific but anemia and neutrophilic leukocytosis with a left shift may be observed on CBC.
• Hypergammaglobulinemia due to chronic infection.
• Chronic liver congestion results in elevation of serum liver enzyme activities.

OTHER LABORATORY TESTS
N/A

IMAGING
• Ultrasonography is the most reliable method of diagnosing a thrombus of the caudal vena cava.
• Normally, the caudal vena cava appears triangular in cross-section but, with thrombosis, the vein is oval to circular and dilated.
• Although a rare occurrence, detection of a thrombus in the caudal vena cava via ultrasonography is diagnostic.
• Ultrasonography may reveal ascites in some cases.
• Comet tail artifacts and pulmonary abscesses may be observed on thoracic ultrasonography.
• Thoracic radiographs often reveal increase in lung density. Distinct opacities related to embolic infarcts may be evident, and bullae and abscesses may be observed.

OTHER DIAGNOSTIC PROCEDURES
N/A

PATHOLOGIC FINDINGS
• Hepatic abscesses
• Thrombus in caudal vena cava
• Hepatomegaly
• Ascites
• Multiple pulmonary abscesses
• Intrapulmonary hemorrhage
• Swallowed blood evident in rumen

TREATMENT

THERAPEUTIC APPROACH
• The case fatality rate is close to 100% so treatment is rarely indicated.
• Salvage is typically the only realistic option although condemnation of the carcass is highly likely.
• Euthanasia should be considered.
• Antibiotic therapy is largely unsuccessful, but slaughter withdrawal times should be observed if antimicrobials are used.

SURGICAL CONSIDERATIONS AND TECHNIQUES
N/A

MEDICATIONS

DRUGS OF CHOICE
N/A

CONTRAINDICATIONS
N/A

PRECAUTIONS
N/A

POSSIBLE INTERACTIONS
N/A

FOLLOW-UP

EXPECTED COURSE AND PROGNOSIS
Most cases are fatal so the prognosis is grave and euthanasia or slaughter recommended.

POSSIBLE COMPLICATIONS
Death typically relates to acute hemorrhage and hypoxemia.

PATIENT MONITORING
N/A

CLIENT EDUCATION
Discuss potential risk factors and evaluate reasons for the occurrence of ruminal acidosis to try to prevent additional cases.

PATIENT CARE
N/A

PREVENTION
• Slowly adapt ruminants to high-carbohydrate rations.
• Utilize ionophores in rations to modulate feed intake and control acidosis.
• Antimicrobial feed additives such as tylosin, virginiamycin, chlortetracycline, or oxytetracycline have been used to prevent liver abscesses. Changes in regulations may now affect their use.

• Appropriate milk and meat withdrawal times must be followed for all pharmaceutical agents administered to food-producing animals.
• Vaccines for *F. necrophorum* may lower the incidence of liver abscesses.

MISCELLANEOUS

ASSOCIATED CONDITIONS
• Rumenitis or grain overload
• Liver abscessation
• Embolic pneumonia
• Foot rot, metritis, mastitis

AGE-RELATED FACTORS
N/A

ZOONOTIC POTENTIAL
N/A

PREGNANCY
N/A

BIOSECURITY
N/A

PRODUCTION MANAGEMENT
Evaluate feeding regimens to determine methods of reducing the risk of this condition occurring in vulnerable groups.

SYNONYMS
• Embolic pneumonia
• Embolic pulmonary aneurysm

• Metastatic pneumonia
• Pulmonary thromboembolism

ABBREVIATIONS
N/A

SEE ALSO
• Anaphylaxis
• Atypical Interstitial Pneumonia
• Bovine Respiratory Syncytial Virus
• Parasitic Pneumonia
• Plants Causing Acute Respiratory Distress Syndrome
• Respiratory Disease: Bovine

Suggested Reading
Braun U. Clinical findings and diagnosis of thrombosis of caudal vena cava in cattle. Vet J 2008, 175: 118–25.
Gudmundson J, Radostits OM, Doige CE. Pulmonary thromboembolism in cattle due to thrombosis of posterior vena cava associated with hepatic abscessation. Can Vet J 1978, 19: 304–9.
Radostits OM, Gay CC, Blood DC, Hinchcliff KW eds. Veterinary Medicine, 9th ed. London: Saunders, 2000.
Wikse SE. Other pneumonias. In: Smith BP ed, Large Animal Internal Medicine, 3rd ed. St. Louis: Mosby, 2002.
Author Clemence Z. Chako
Consulting Editor Erica C. McKenzie
Acknowledgment The author and book editors acknowledge the prior contribution of John R. Campbell.

C

CECAL DILATION AND VOLVULUS

BASICS

DEFINITION
• Cecal dilation is primarily a disease of adult dairy cattle occurring within the first 1–2 months postpartum.
• It is believed to share similar epidemiologic and physiologic characteristics as abomasal dilation and displacement.
• Cecal dilation is also reported in calves <4 months of age, the majority of which are fed high-concentrate diets for purposes of early slaughter.

INCIDENCE/PREVALENCE
Cecal dilatation is thought to occur with similar prevalence as abomasal displacements.

GEOGRAPHIC DISTRIBUTION
Worldwide

SYSTEMS AFFECTED
Digestive

PATHOPHYSIOLOGY
Cecal Dilation
• The presence of excess gas from the digestion of fermentable substrates and decreased intestinal motility may cause cecal dilation. Experimental models have also implicated motility aberrations in the proximal loop of the ascending colon as a possible cause.
• Diets high in concentrates and with inadequate roughage produce high levels of fermentable carbohydrates that pass into the lower intestine. Lower intestinal flora digest the excess carbohydrates into volatile fatty acids (VFAs), methane, and carbon dioxide. Increased VFAs present in the cecum and ascending colon are believed to cause a reduction in intestinal motility.
• Decreased intestinal motility may also result from decreased levels of ionized calcium.

Cecal Torsion
Cecal torsion is present if a twist of the cecum occurs along its longitudinal axis, leading to increased tension of the ileocecal fold. This then leads to compromised blood flow and innervation of the cecum. The exact cause of cecal torsion is unknown; however, it is believed to be predisposed by, and therefore a sequela to, the occurrence of cecal dilation.

HISTORICAL FINDINGS
• Cattle suffering cecal dilation typically present with mild to moderate anorexia and decreased milk production.
• Cattle suffering cecal torsion typically demonstrate abrupt anorexia, rumen stasis, and significantly decreased milk production.

SIGNALMENT
Predominantly dairy breeds, adult female cattle within 2 months postpartum

PHYSICAL EXAMINATION FINDINGS
• Cattle with cecal dilation have an area of increased resonance ("ping") that is auscultated over the right paralumbar fossa. The right paralumbar fossa may be distended, and cattle may exhibit mild to moderate signs of abdominal pain.
• Fecal output is normal to decreased and fecal consistency is typically more fluid.
• During rectal examination, a gas-distended cecum is usually palpable with the apex located in or near the pelvic inlet.
• Cattle with cecal torsion have moderate to severe abdominal pain and are often tachycardic and tachypneic, with little to no fecal production and a precipitous drop in milk production.
• Rectal examination usually reveals a markedly distended cecum containing both gas and fluid. The apex of the cecum is often not palpable as it is positioned cranially. The area of resonance in the right paralumbar fossa is generally much larger than that noted with simple cecal dilation. Increased resonance may even be noted over the caudal dorsal left paralumbar fossa.

GENETICS
N/A

CAUSES AND RISK FACTORS
Postpartum cattle fed low-roughage, high-concentrate diets, and those suffering from hypocalcemia, metritis, mastitis, or indigestion that could result in gastrointestinal ileus.

DIAGNOSIS

DIFFERENTIAL DIAGNOSES
Right displaced abomasum, abomasal displacement with volvulus, small intestinal obstructions, and intussusception.

CBC/BIOCHEMISTRY/URINALYSIS
• Serum biochemical profile, blood gas analysis, and complete blood count are typically unremarkable, though a stress leukogram may be observed in cecal dilation cases.
• Depending on the severity and duration of cecal torsion, cattle may present with moderate to severe acid-base and electrolyte derangements. Hypochloremic, hypokalemic metabolic alkalosis is most commonly observed, but circulatory compromise is rarely observed. Urinalysis is typically within normal limits.

OTHER LABORATORY TESTS
N/A

IMAGING
Ultrasonography via the right abdominal wall at the level of the tuber coxae may be useful in the diagnosis.

OTHER DIAGNOSTIC PROCEDURES
Rectal palpation is a reliable diagnostic procedure for cecal dilatation coupled with percussion auscultation of the right flank. The distended, displaced, or twisted cecum can be palpated at rectal examination in most affected animals. In the case of a simple dilatation, the cecal apex is easily recognizable as a rounded, dome-shaped structure, with a diameter of approximately 15 cm, extending into the pelvic inlet. If retroflexion is present, the body of the cecum, but not the apex, can be palpated as a large, rounded, tense structure in front of the pelvis. Rectal palpation alone does not always allow for differentiation of cecal dilatation with retroflexion from right abomasal displacement or volvulus. The appearance of the dilated cecum during ultrasound examination from the right flank has been described.

PATHOLOGIC FINDINGS
N/A

TREATMENT

THERAPEUTIC APPROACH
• Cecal dilation in the early stages of the disease, when the general condition of the affected animal remains good, and when some feces are still being passed, can be managed by conservative treatment with prokinetic drugs, purgatives, along with intravenous fluids. Administration of neostigmine (87.5 mg in 5–20 L of isotonic saline solution supplemented with 5% dextrose as a continuous intravenous infusion at a rate of 1–2 drops per second) or bethanechol (0.07 mg/kg subcutaneously, q8h for 2 days) has been advocated. Intravenous or subcutaneous calcium borogluconate solutions (20 g in 500 mL) can be useful in lactating cows. Mineral oil (3 L) or sodium sulfate (300 g in 10 L water) administered per stomach tube have been described as adequate purgatives for conservative or postoperative treatment of cecal dilatation. Large volumes (20 L) of oral fluids containing electrolytes (8 oz NaCl, 2 oz KCl), calcium (12 oz calcium propionate), and cathartics (12 oz Mg-hydroxide, Mg-sulfate) can also be given q12h or q24h.
• Transfaunation with rumen liquor (10–20 L) can be used to stimulate rumen motility and appetite.

SURGICAL CONSIDERATIONS AND TECHNIQUES
• In cattle with recurrent cecal dilation, preventive typhlectomy may be indicated.
• Cattle with cecal torsion typically require surgical intervention along with appropriate fluid therapy to correct fluid, acid-base, and electrolyte abnormalities. A standing right paralumbar approach is typically used. Decompression via typhlotomy may be

necessary to remove excess fluid and gas and to facilitate correction of a volvulus. In the event that ischemic necrosis is severe, a typhlectomy may be required.

MEDICATIONS

DRUGS OF CHOICE
Management of electrolyte and mineral imbalances is important. Antibiotics should be administered preoperatively when decompression of the cecum is necessary as abdominal contamination may occur during the procedure.

FOLLOW-UP

EXPECTED COURSE AND PROGNOSIS
• For patients with normal heart rate, some manure production, a small appetite, no dehydration, and minimal abdominal distension, medical treatment is usually successful.
• Patients with high heart rate, dehydration, and colic signs, are surgical candidates. Post-surgical prognosis is dependent on the degree of ischemic compromise to the cecum and adjacent bowel, successful corrections of acid-base and electrolyte derangements, and appropriate surgical technique.

POSSIBLE COMPLICATIONS
Cecal torsion leading to rupture and peritonitis in severe untreated cases.

CLIENT EDUCATION
Warranted in cases that are induced by inappropriate diet.

PATIENT CARE
Increased appetite and milk production with manure production are all good signs that treatment is working.

PREVENTION
Pre- and postpartum management of dairy cattle to maximize adequate intake of a forage-based diet, minimize infections of the uterus and vagina by calving in a clean environment, and minimizing the risk of gastrointestinal upset.

MISCELLANEOUS

ASSOCIATED CONDITIONS
Mastitis, metritis, hypocalcemia, inappetence

PREGNANCY
Generally, a postpartum condition

PRODUCTION MANAGEMENT
Management of at-risk cattle to maximize intake of a forage-based diet, and minimize the risk of gastrointestinal upset.

SYNONYMS
N/A

ABBREVIATION
VFA = volatile fatty acid

SEE ALSO
Displaced Abomasum

Suggested Reading
Abegg R, Eicher R, Lis J, Lischer CJ, Scholtysik G, Steiner A. Concentration of volatile fatty acids in digesta samples obtained from healthy cows and cows with cecal dilation or dislocation. Am J Vet Res 1999, 60: 1540–5.

Braun U, Amrein E, Koller U, Lischer C. Ultrasonographic findings in cows with dilation, torsion and retroflexion of the caecum. Vet Rec 2002, 150: 75–9.
Braun U, Hermann M, Pabst B. Haematological and biochemical findings in cattle with dilation and torsion of the caecum. Vet Rec 1989, 125: 396–8.
Eicher R, Audige L, Braun U, Blum J, Meylan M, Steiner A. Epidemiology and risk factors of cecal dilation/dislocation and abomasal displacement in dairy cows. Schweiz Arch Tierheilkd 1999, 141: 423–9.
Guard C. Obstructive intestinal diseases. In: Smith BP ed, Large Animal Internal Medicine, 3rd ed. St. Louis: Mosby, 2002.
Meylan, M. Surgery of the bovine large intestine. Vet Clin North Am Food Anim Pract 2008, 24: 479–96.
Stocker S, Steiner A, Geiser S, et al. Myoelectric activity of the cecum and proximal loop of the ascending colon in cows after spontaneous cecal dilatation/dislocation. Am J Vet Res 1997, 58: 961–8.

Author Dennis D. French
Consulting Editor Kaitlyn A. Lutz
Acknowledgment The author and book editors acknowledge the prior contribution of George Barrington.

C

CERVIDAE: CAPTIVE MANAGEMENT

BASICS

OVERVIEW
• Elk (*Cervus canadensis*), red deer (*Cervus elaphus*) and their hybrids are commonly farmed cervid species in North America, Europe, and New Zealand. There are also significant numbers of white-tailed deer (*Odocoileus virgninianus*) which are farmed or kept on hunting preserves. These species are well adapted to North American climate, pasture rearing, and the stress of handling. They also have strong herding instincts and are relatively disease resistant.
• Other deer species that are farmed include fallow deer (*Dama dama*), sika (*Cervus Nippon*), chital (*Axis axis*), rusa (*Cervus timorensis*), sambar (*Cervus unicolor*), and reindeer (*Rangifer tarandus*).
• Cervid species vary in size from the approximately 8 kg pudu to moose that can exceed 800 kg. The males of all but two species of cervids grow antlers, as do females of the genus *Rangifer*.
• The species selected should be based upon the farmer's experience, farm size, handling facilities, and production goals.
• In the United States, deer are marketed mostly for their venison and antlers/velvet.
• In Asian countries, antlers/velvet are used for medicinal products.

INCIDENCE/PREVALENCE
N/A

GEOGRAPHIC DISTRIBUTION
Worldwide

SYSTEMS AFFECTED
N/A

PATHOPHYSIOLOGY
N/A

HISTORICAL FINDINGS
N/A

SIGNALMENT
All cervids

PHYSICAL EXAMINATION FINDINGS
N/A

GENETICS
N/A

CAUSES AND RISK FACTORS
Morbidity and mortality in the herd may be due to noninfectious or infectious causes.

Noninfectious Causes
• A good nutrition program is essential to maintain healthy animals and reduce morbidity and mortality.
• Overcrowding, poor handling facilities, and failure to remove antlers and antler stubs can result in trauma.
• Consideration must be given to the farm's layout, stocking densities, handling facilities, and time of year (rutting season).

• Conditioning animals to the handling facilities will keep stress levels down when performing routine procedures.

Infectious Causes
• Significant infectious diseases of deer can be divided into bacterial, mycobacterial, viral, prion, and parasitic etiologies.
• Bacterial diseases of significance in deer include: *Mycobacterium bovis* (tuberculosis), *Mycobacterium avium paratuberculosis* (Johne's disease), brucellosis, clostridial agents, leptospirosis, yersiniosis, and rarely salmonellosis.
• Malignant catarrhal fever (MCF), a viral infection carried by sheep and goats, can be highly fatal in cervids.
• Other viral diseases of concern include: rabies, bovine viral diarrhea, bluetongue, Eastern equine encephalitis, epizootic hemorrhagic disease, and foot and mouth disease.
• White-tailed deer are asymptomatic carriers of *Babesia odocoilei*, a tick-borne hemoprotozoal parasite that can be fatal in reindeer and other ungulates. They also are the natural host of the meningeal worm *Parelaphostrongylus tenuis* which can cause morbidity and mortality in other cervid and ungulate species.
• CWD is has been identified in white-tailed deer, black-tailed deer, elk, red deer, and moose. It is endemic in wild deer and elk populations in some regions of the US and Canada. It has also been identified in a number of captive cervid herds and there are governmental programs in place to prevent its spread in both captive and wild populations.
• Deer are also susceptible to a number of nematode and trematode infections.
• *Dictyocaulus viviparus*, the lungworm, can cause significant loss of condition in young animals and sometimes death.
• Parasitic gastroenteritis occurs in herds in which stocking densities are too high.
• Ectoparasites such as lice and ticks can cause poor coat condition and weight loss as animals become too pruritic to graze. Ticks and other arthropods are capable of transmitting blood parasites such as babesiosis and anaplasmosis. Maggot infestations can also lead to animal discomfort and subsequent losses from decreased feeding.
• Fecal analysis, strategic deworming, and vector control will help minimize the effects of parasitic infections.

DIAGNOSIS

DIFFERENTIAL DIAGNOSES
N/A

CBC/BIOCHEMISTRY/URINALYSIS
N/A

OTHER LABORATORY TESTS
N/A

IMAGING
N/A

OTHER DIAGNOSTIC PROCEDURES
N/A

PATHOLOGIC FINDINGS
N/A

TREATMENT

THERAPEUTIC APPROACH
N/A

SURGICAL CONSIDERATIONS AND TECHNIQUES
N/A

MEDICATIONS

• Facility design is essential for safe and efficient handling and care of animals (see chapter, Cervidae: Game Park Management, Facilities).
• Drugs may be administered via hand syringe, pole syringe, or immobilization dart.
• There are large differences between species of cervid in their sensitivity to anesthetic agents.
• Excited animals require higher dosages of anesthetics so it is important to keep animals as calm as possible prior to drug administration. During field anesthesia or manual restraint, placing a towel or other cover over the animal's eyes and minimizing noise reduces stimulation and stress for the animal.
• Potent narcotics such as carfentanil, etorphine, and thiafentanil have been successfully used for immobilization of deer, elk, and moose. They provide rapid immobilization but poor muscle relaxation when used as the sole anesthetic agent. The addition of a small amount of xylazine provides better muscle relaxation, but in some species such as moose it needs to be used cautiously as it increases the likelihood of regurgitation and aspiration pneumonia.
• Disadvantages of using potent narcotics include cost, legal requirements, and safety concerns for humans.
• Ketamine/medetomidine or other dissociative/alpha-2 agonist combinations have been used successfully in cervids, but they have a slower onset of action. This is not a significant consideration in a captive situation compared to wildlife immobilization.
• During anesthesia, animal positioning is important to minimize the risk of bloat or regurgitation and aspiration. Sternal

positioning while keeping the neck and head elevated and nose down is safest.
• Upon completion of procedures, the narcotic agents and alpha-2 agonists should be reversed with appropriate antagonists such as naltrexone and atipamazole or tolazoline.
• If IV access is available, ketamine/diazepam or Telazol® works well for short procedures. IV administration may be possible once an animal is in a squeeze chute or alternatively it is possible to condition animals for voluntary blood collection or drug administration. Facilities should be designed appropriately to protect a person doing voluntary injections.
• Smaller animals can also be masked down with inhalant anesthetics once they have been properly restrained.
• Hypoventilation and hypoxemia are not uncommon during anesthesia so it is important to monitor and have supplemental oxygen available. For longer procedures, animals may be intubated and placed on inhalation anesthetics. The injectable agents may be reversed at this point or may allow for a lower concentration of inhalational agent.
• It is beneficial to restrict food intake for 24–36 hours and water intake for 12–24 hours prior to chemically restraining adult cervids, to reduce the likelihood of bloating and regurgitation.

DRUGS OF CHOICE
N/A

CONTRAINDICATIONS
N/A

PRECAUTIONS
N/A

POSSIBLE INTERACTIONS
N/A

 FOLLOW-UP

EXPECTED COURSE AND PROGNOSIS
N/A

POSSIBLE COMPLICATIONS
N/A

CLIENT EDUCATION
N/A

PATIENT CARE
• Good nutrition is essential for reproductive success, calf survival, and disease resistance. Nutrition also plays a key role in maximizing profits from velvet and venison production.
• The natural diet of cervids of the genus *Cervus* (e.g. elk, red deer) consists of a large proportion of grasses, but they also eat browse. Other cervid species such as moose are primarily browse feeders. Browsers require specially formulated diets or access to adequate browse to provide optimal nutrition and health.
• In general, grazing species do well on good-quality pasture or mixed grass/alfalfa

hay. Mineral/vitamin supplementation or addition of a pelleted ration may be necessary depending on forage, environmental conditions, and health status of the animal.
• Weighing animals regularly helps farmers meet target weights and make ration adjustments as necessary.
• Winter feeding helps desensitize deer to the presence of the handlers and makes it easier to work them. While grain supplementation is often required, it should be introduced slowly to reduce risk of acidosis.
• Feed analysis and consultation with an animal nutritionist should be done so that the farmer knows when and with what to supplement. Mineral and trace element supplements can be provided either in concentrate rations or as a free choice block.
• During the fall rut, stags eat little and lose weight. They are much more susceptible to winter mortality than hinds. It is important that stags have access to an adequate amount of appropriate diet following the rut.

PREVENTION
• Herd health programs should increase profits by reducing disease incidence and enabling the farmer to meet and exceed production goals.
• Knowledge of the geographic area and good medical records help the veterinarian and farmer decide which vaccinations and dewormers to administer and when to give them.
• The veterinarian and farm manager should review the feeding program, past production levels, reproductive efficiencies, losses, and other management issues and implement changes if indicated.
• Veterinarians are involved with performing physical examinations, TB tests, and serology on new arrivals and animals to be shipped out.

 MISCELLANEOUS

ASSOCIATED CONDITIONS
N/A

AGE-RELATED FACTORS
• Growth of calves from birth to weaning is critical for winter survival as well as for achieving desirable market weights.
• Calves normally experience little to no weight gain in the winter and are typically unable to eat enough forage to maintain their weight. Supplementation with concentrates or pelleted diets is often indicated.
• During the spring, summer, and fall, young stock have great potential for growth, and feeding programs should be adjusted to take advantage of this natural phenomenon.

ZOONOTIC POTENTIAL
Brucellosis, tuberculosis, lyme disease, leptospirosis, rocky mountain spotted fever, Q

fever, cryptosporidiosis, salmonella, yersiniosis, and anthrax.

PREGNANCY
• Hinds have their greatest energy demands during the summer when they are lactating. If pasture quality is poor, lactating hinds should be supplemented with grain, pelleted ration or high-quality legume hay to ensure adequate milk production.
• The goals for the fall breeding period are to help hinds regain conditioning lost during lactation and build up their fat reserves for winter. Grain supplementation in the fall conditions the hinds and introduces the soon-to-be-weaned calves to feed.

BIOSECURITY
N/A

PRODUCTION MANAGEMENT
• Proper record keeping is essential for good management and compliance with governmental regulations.
• Identification of animals is required to maintain accurate records. To participate in the USDA-APHIS national CWD herd certification program (HCP) all animals must be identified with two forms of permanent identification. The official animal identification must be linked to that animal and herd in the National CWD Database or a state database that is approved by APHIS. The farm must also have a unique national premise identification number assigned by the state, tribal authority or federal authority that is linked to the physical location of the farm.
• The APHIS traceability website provides information on official forms of identification: http://www.aphis.usda.gov/traceability/downloads/ADT_eartags_criteria.pdf
• It is essential to have accurate breeding records including sire and dam and their pedigrees, breeding date(s), previous reproductive history, and related medical problems. Weights should be obtained and recorded any time an animal is handled to maintain growth and body condition information.
• Medical records: Medical procedures, worming dates, vaccination dates, parasitology data, prescription information, anesthesia records, clinical pathology information, necropsy and histopathology data and may also include nutrition and diet-related information.

SYNONYMS
N/A

ABBREVIATIONS
• CWD = chronic wasting disease
• MCF = malignant catarrhal fever
• TB = tuberculosis

SEE ALSO
• Abortion: Farmed Cervidae
• Cervidae: Capture Myopathy
• Cervidae: Game Park Management, Facilities

C

CERVIDAE: CAPTIVE MANAGEMENT

- Cervidae: Mortality
- Vaccination Programs: Cervidae

Suggested Reading
Caulkett N, Haigh JC. Deer (Cervids). In: West G, Heard DJ, Caulkett N eds, Zoo Animal and Wildlife Immobilization and Anesthesia. Ames: Blackwell, 2007.
Haigh JC, Hudson RJ. Farming Wapiti and Red Deer. St. Louis: Mosby, 1993.
Hudson R, Kozak H, Adamczewski J, Olsen C. Reproductive performance of farmed wapiti (*Cervus elaphus nelsoni*). Small Ruminant Res 1991, 4: 19–28.
Kreeger TJ, Arnemo JM. Handbook of Wildlife Chemical Immobilization, 4th ed. Copyright® 2012 Terry J. Kreeger. Amazon.com #0965465209.
Manning EJB. Paratuberculosis in captive and free-ranging wildlife. Vet Clin North Am Food Anim Pract 2011, 27: 621–30.
Miller MW. Chronic wasting disease of cervid species. In: Fowler ME, Miller RE eds, Zoo and Wild Animal Medicine Current Therapy Vol. 6. St. Louis: Saunders Elsevier, 2008.
Noyes JH, Johnson BK, Dick BL, Kie JG. Effects of male age and female nutritional condition on elk reproduction. J Wildl Manage 2002, 66:1301–7.
Thorleifson I, Pearse T, Friedel B. Elk Farming Handbook. St. John, New Brunswick: Abbott Richards Graphic Design, 2000.

Author James M. Rasmussen
Consulting Editor Ahmed Tibary

CERVIDAE: CAPTURE MYOPATHY

BASICS

OVERVIEW
• Capture myopathy (CM) is also known as post-capture myopathy, overstraining disease, transport myopathy, exertional rhabdomyolysis, and exertional myopathy.
• Wild and farmed deer are susceptible to CM. It is reported in animals that have been captured or handled by a variety of methods: short or long distance chases, chemical immobilization, drop netting, net gunning, boma capture, handling, and restraint in chutes.
• CM can be divided into four phases: Capture shock syndrome, ataxic myoglobinuric syndrome, ruptured muscle syndrome, and delayed-peracute syndrome.
• CM is generally undetected at the time of the animal's release, resulting in mortality hours to weeks post-capture.
• If capture-related mortality among deer within farmed settings is >2% of all deaths, new strategies must be implemented for handling and capture.

INCIDENCE/PREVALENCE
N/A

GEOGRAPHIC DISTRIBUTION
Worldwide

SYSTEMS AFFECTED
• Musculoskeletal
• Urinary

PATHOPHYSIOLOGY
• Exerted muscle changes its metabolism from aerobic to anaerobic, leading to lactic acid buildup in the bloodstream.
• Systemic acidosis follows and affects the heart output. Reduced oxygen to the affected muscle causes necrosis and release of myoglobin, which can damage the renal tubules and stress the body further. It also causes the muscle to be prone to rupture.
• The disease process is characterized by metabolic acidosis, muscle necrosis, and myoglobinuria.

HISTORICAL FINDINGS
Recent capture or immobilization

SIGNALMENT
• All cervids are susceptible.
• Capture myopathy can be a significant cause of mortality for white-tailed deer (*Odocoileus virginianus*). In one study, 10% of white-tailed deer caught from net guns died from CM.
• The semimembranosus and semitendinosus muscles are often ruptured in elk suffering from ruptured muscle syndrome.
• Net gun capture causes ataxic myoglobinuric syndrome and death in roe deer.

PHYSICAL EXAMINATION FINDINGS
• Cervids often are hyperthermic, tachycardic, and can develop a stiff or weak gait. Muscle tremors may develop involving few muscles or entire muscle groups, and the animal may just collapse and die.
• Capture shock syndrome: Observed in recently trapped animals or during immobilization. Animals usually die within 1–6 hours post-capture. Clinical signs include depression, tachypnea/dyspnea, tachycardia, hyperthermia, weak pulse, and death.
• Ataxic myoglobinuric syndrome: This is thought to be the most common in cervids. It can be seen several hours to several days post-capture. Clinical signs include ataxia, torticollis, and myoglobinuria, ranging from mild to severe in nature.
• Ruptured muscle syndrome: Animals appear normal at capture but show clinical signs 24–48 hours later, including a marked drop in the hindquarters and hyperflexion of the hock. This is often caused by unilateral or bilateral gastrocnemius, semimembranosus or semitendinosus muscle rupture. This has been seen in wild captured elk.
• Delayed peracute syndrome: Usually seen in animals that have been in a stressful captive situation for >24 hours. The animals appear normal when undisturbed, but if disturbed, handled, or captured, the animals try to escape and stop abruptly, often standing or lying still for several minutes. This is a rare form of CM, and these animals often die from ventricular fibrillation.

GENETICS
N/A

CAUSES/RISK FACTORS
• Several factors can either act alone or, more commonly, in combination, to lead to the development of CM.
• Factors include restraint methodology, overexertion, hyperthermia, isometric exercise, drug effects, alterations in the muscle pump activity, species predisposition, individual variation, seasonal effects, environmental factors, fear/habituation and familiarity with events, environment, and personnel.

DIAGNOSIS

History and clinical signs are important.

DIFFERENTIAL DIAGNOSES
• Enzootic ataxia or acute central nervous system disease
• Selenium deficiency, white muscle disease
• Fractures, other traumatic injuries, and wasting diseases

CBC/BIOCHEMSTRY/URINALYSIS
• Capture shock syndrome: Elevated AST, CPK, and LDH. Increased serum potassium and lactic acid levels may occur during the acute phase.
• Ataxic myoglobinuric syndrome: Elevated AST, CPK, LDH, BUN, and creatinine (due to renal tubular damage).
• Ruptured muscle syndrome: AST, CPK, and LDH levels are extremely elevated. BUN levels are usually normal.
• Delayed peracute syndrome: AST, CPK, and LDH, may be elevated but sometimes death occurs before elevations are observed.

OTHER LABORATORY TESTS
N/A

IMAGING
N/A

OTHER DIAGNOSTIC PROCEDURES
N/A

PATHOLOGIC FINDINGS
Gross Postmortem Findings
• Capture shock syndrome: Congestion and edema of the lungs, severe congestion of small intestine and liver, sometimes frank blood within small intestine.
• Ataxic myoglobinuric syndrome: Renal and skeletal muscle lesions, swollen and dark kidneys, empty urinary bladder occasionally containing brown urine, multifocal pale, soft, dry areas with small white foci found in cervical and lumbar muscles and in flexors and extensors of the limbs. The lesions are often bilateral but not symmetrical, and subtle in animals that die 1–2 days post-capture but more pronounced in animals that survive longer.
• Ruptured muscle syndrome: Massive subcutaneous hemorrhage of the rear limbs and multifocal, small to large, pale, soft lesions in the limbs, diaphragm, cervical and lumbar musculature. Muscular lesions are similar to those described for the ataxic myoglobinuric phase, but are more severe and widespread. Small to large ruptures can be found within necrotic muscles. Commonly ruptured muscles include the gastrocnemius, subscapularis, middle and deep gluteal, semitendinosus, and semimembranosus muscles.
• Delayed peracute syndrome: There are often no visible lesions seen, though there could be a few small pale foci within the skeletal muscles.

Histopathologic Findings
• Capture shock syndrome: Small areas of necrosis occasionally found in skeletal muscle and brain, liver, heart, adrenal glands, lymph nodes, spleen, pancreas, and renal tubules – most prominent when an animal was hyperthermic.
• Ataxic myoglobinuric syndrome: Primarily lesions within the renal cortex and skeletal muscle. Renal lesions are characterized by dilation of tubules, moderate to severe tubular necrosis, and myoglobin casts. Muscular lesions are characterized by acute rhabdomyolysis with swollen myocytes.
• Ruptured muscle syndrome: Most lesions within the skeletal muscles and characterized

C

by massive necrosis. Similar to lesions found in white muscle disease, but there is less mineralization in CM-affected muscles.
• Delayed peracute syndrome: Lesions within muscle are characterized by mild to moderate rhabdomyolysis throughout the skeletal muscle, especially in the hindlimbs.

TREATMENT

THERAPEUTIC APPROACH
• Treatment of capture myopathy in cervids is often unsuccessful.
• In the hyperthermic stage, animals are sedated with anesthetics that provide central muscle relaxation (benzodiazepines and alpha-2 agonists).
• The most important treatment is intravenous fluids to allow for improved blood flow to kidneys to reduce tubular damage by myoglobin, dilute lactic acid within the bloodstream, expand blood volume, address mechanisms of shock, correct acid-base and electrolyte abnormalities, and reverse hyperthermia.
• Administration of vitamins, analgesics, and anti-inflammatory drugs have been tried, with little success.
• Successful treatment depends on the type of CM and the ability to treat without exacerbating existing conditions.

SURGICAL CONSIDERATIONS AND TECHNIQUES
N/A

MEDICATIONS

DRUGS OF CHOICE
Prophylactic use of sedative and tranquilizing drugs have been employed to prevent the development of capture myopathy syndromes in cervids not used to human contact, handling, and captivity. A combination of long-acting neuroleptics (LANs) have been shown to greatly reduce morbidity and enhance capture and translocation of numerous cervid species.

CONTRAINDICATIONS
• Animals released under the influence of LANs into new herd situations are at high risk of being harassed or attacked by other animals.
• Releasing cervids onto hunting ranches with LANs on board can reduce their perceptiveness and increase their risk of predation and self-trauma.

PRECAUTIONS
N/A

POSSIBLE INTERACTIONS
N/A

FOLLOW-UP

EXPECTED COURSE AND PROGNOSIS
Extremely poor prognosis in all forms. Even animals who survive a mild CM event may be debilitated, leading to loss of productivity or failure to breed.

POSSIBLE COMPLICATIONS
Animals that recover have long-term muscle damage (especially cardiac muscle) and can succumb later in times of stress.

CLIENT EDUCATION
• Importance of proper restraint methods and for training of handlers.
• Be aware and be able to identify specific symptoms and behaviors that indicate stress in individuals.

PATIENT CARE
N/A

PREVENTION/AVOIDANCE
• Choice of the most suitable method of restraint and handling for each herd situation is vital, and depends on the needs of each producer, ranch, or farm.
• Ensure that the animals are habituated to human presence, handling, chute and hallway systems, and various enclosure types.
• Cervids should never be rushed through handling situations. It is best to habituate them to the hallway and chute systems by positive reinforcement, such as highly palatable feeds, to decrease apprehensive stress when the processing day arrives.
• Handling, processing, and capture of cervids should be avoided in harsh environmental conditions. Increased ambient temperatures combined with handling can precipitate hyperthermia in most cervids.
• Noise and movement should be kept at a minimum: blindfolds can help decrease stimuli on individuals that are immobilized or restrained in a chute system and help reduce stress.
• Immobilized animals or those restrained for extended periods of time should be monitored for hyperthermia by rectal temperature.
• Transporting cervids should be done in well-suited crates or trailers. Some species are best suited to be transported alone, while others do better in small groups. Ensure crate- or trailer-mates are compatible; do not place mature males together with females or neonates.
• Food and water should be provided to meet the specific needs of the animals during transport, especially during long trips.
• If chemical immobilization is used, ensure appropriate dosages, drugs, and delivery systems for each species.

• When releasing animals into new pens or new herd situations, ensure the individuals already in the enclosure or pen do not harass the new arrivals.

MISCELLANEOUS

ASSOCIATED CONDITIONS
White muscle disease has a very similar symptomatic process with a different etiology.

AGE-RELATED FACTORS
All ages may be affected, but studies in white tailed deer (*Odocoileus virginianus*) show that the very young and very old are more susceptible.

ZOONOTIC POTENTIAL
N/A

PREGNANCY
N/A

BIOSECURITY
N/A

PRODUCTION MANAGEMENT
N/A

SYNONYMS
N/A

ABBREVIATIONS
• AST = aspartate aminotransferase
• BUN = blood urea nitrogen
• CM = capture myopathy
• CPK = creatinine phosphokinase
• LANs = long-acting neuroleptics
• LDH = lactate dehydrogenase

SEE ALSO
Cervidae: Captive Management

Suggested Reading
Beringer J, Hansen LP, Wildling W, Fischer J, Sheriff SL. Factors affecting capture myopathy in white-tailed deer. J Wildl Manage 1996, 60: 373–80.
Dechen Quinn AC, Williams DM, Porter WF, Fitzgerald SD, Hynes K. Effects of capture-related injury on post capture movement of white-tailed deer. J Wildl Dis 2014, 50: 250–8.
Lewis, RJ, Chalmers GA, Barrett MW, Bhatnagar R. Capture myopathy in elk in Alberta, Canada: A report of three cases. J Am Vet Med Assoc 1977, 171: 927–32.
Spraker TR. Stress and capture myopathy in artiodactylids. In: Fowler ME ed, Zoo and Wild Animal Medicine: Current Therapy, vol. 3. Denver: Saunders, 1993, pp. 481–8.
Author David M. Love
Consulting Editor Ahmed Tibary
Acknowledgment The author and book editors acknowledge the prior contribution of Jerry Haigh.

CERVIDAE: CHRONIC WASTING DISEASE

BASICS

OVERVIEW
• Chronic wasting disease (CWD) is a transmissible spongiform encephalopathy (TSE) that affects free-ranging and captive cervids including mule deer, black-tailed deer, white-tailed deer, Rocky Mountain elk, and moose. Exotic cervids may also be susceptible.
• CWD was first recognized in captive mule deer in Colorado in the 1960s and later identified as a TSE in 1978. • TSEs are a group of diseases characterized by the accumulation of a misfolded normal host prion protein in the brain. • Additional TSEs in other species include bovine spongiform encephalopathy (BSE) in cattle, scrapie in sheep and goats, transmissible mink encephalopathy(TME) in mink, kuru, Creutzfeldt-Jakob disease (CJD), and vCJD in humans, and feline spongiform encephalopathy. • Horizontal spread of the disease by oral exposure to infected carcasses, excretions, secretions, contaminated soil, or other tissue source has been proven by epidemiologic studies. The agent is shed in feces, urine, saliva, blood, and antler velvet.
• Clinical signs of CWD include changes in behavior, weight loss, loss of muscle mass, and salivation. The average age of affected animals is in the range 3–5 years.

INCIDENCE/PREVALENCE
• Epidemiologic modeling suggested that chronic wasting disease might have been present among free-ranging animals in some portions of the disease-endemic area several decades before it was initially recognized.
• Incidence varies with the geographic region and species. • It also differs between wild populations and captive herds. This disease can be highly transmissible within captive deer and elk populations. In newly infected herds of farmed cervids, the prevalence may be <1%. However, once the disease has become established, 50% of the herd or more often becomes infected, and in some cases, the incidence may be as high as 100%. Generally, only one animal shows signs of disease at a time. Long-term environmental contamination has been suggested by both biochemical and epidemiologic studies.
• CWD is less common in than farmed cervids. The prevalence is usually <1% in elk; however, it can be as high as 30% in concentrated populations of wild deer. Between 1996 and 1999, 4.7% of mule deer, 2% of white-tailed deer, and 0.5% of elk killed in northeastern Colorado and southeastern Wyoming were infected with the CWD prion overall, although there were "hot spots" where greater numbers of deer were infected. In Wisconsin, up to 13% of the male deer are infected in some areas. In contrast, the estimated prevalence in South

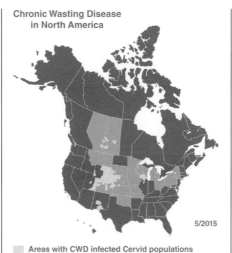

Chronic Wasting Disease in North America

5/2015

☐ Areas with CWD infected Cervid populations

☐ States/Provinces where CWD has been found in captive populations

Figure 1.

The geographic distribution of CWD in free-ranging deer in the United States and Canada (courtesy Chronic Wasting Disease Alliance; www.cwd-info.org).

Dakota in 2003 was 0.001% in white-tailed deer and no cases were reported in elk or mule deer. More than 97% of cases found during the surveillance of wild deer and elk are subclinical. • The low prevalence and lack of large-scale surveys has hampered identifying genetic profiles of susceptible populations and the use of genotyping to identify susceptible populations.

GEOGRAPHIC DISTRIBUTION
• North America, potentially worldwide (see Figure 1). • CWD has been detected in wild populations in at least 17 US states and 2 Canadian provinces, and has been diagnosed in captive populations in numerous other states.

SYSTEMS AFFECTED
• Nervous • Hemolymphatic
• Musculoskeletal

PATHOPHYSIOLOGY
• Transmission of CWD within wild populations appears to be via oral exposure to infected carcasses, secretions, and excretions.
• Dead and decaying carcasses, placenta, and placental fluids are suspected to be common sources of infection, and may contribute to long-term infectivity in soils. • Analysis by immunohistochemical studies of the tissue distribution of prions in CWD-infected cervids identified the agent in the brain, spinal cord, eyes, peripheral nerves, tongue, and lymphoreticular tissues. • Involvement of the mucosal lymphoid tissues and peripheral nerves early in the course of experimental and natural prion infection indicates involvement of the lymphoreticular and peripheral nervous systems in the pathogenesis and transmission of the disease. • A unifying feature of all the

prionoses is their neuropathology. CWD affects the gray matter of the central nervous system (CNS), producing neuronal loss, gliosis, and characteristic spongiform change. In addition, plaques with the typical staining properties of amyloid (e.g., apple-green birefringence after Congo red staining when viewed under polarized light) are observed.

SIGNALMENT
• Both free-ranging and captive white-tailed deer (*O. virginianus*), Rocky Mountain elk (*Cervus elaphus nelsoni*), mule deer (*Odocoileus hemionus*), black-tailed deer (*Odocoileus hemionus columbianus*), and moose (*Alces alces shirasi*) have all been diagnosed with CWD.
• Most affected cervids are >2 years of age and many are 3–5 years old. • In captive cervids, most cases occur in animals 2–7 years of age; however, the disease has been reported in cervids as young as 17 months and as old as >15 years of age.

PHYSICAL EXAMINATION FINDINGS
• Many cervids diagnosed with CWD are asymptomatic. The more chronically affected animals have progressive fat and muscle loss over a period of weeks or months.
• Additional clinical signs include changes in behavior, which can include loss of fear to humans, increased salivation, and atrophy of muscles around the head leading to droopy ears. • Clinical manifestations of CWD include weight loss over weeks or months, behavioral changes, excessive salivation, difficulty swallowing, polydipsia, and polyuria. In some animals, ataxia and head tremors may occur.

GENETICS
• The PRNP (prion) gene may relate to susceptibility to some TSEs. • The PRNP gene is highly conserved among diverse cervid species, with limited polymorphisms. • While no genotype has been absolutely correlated to resistance or susceptibility, genetic data has indicated certain genotypes in white-tail deer, elk, and moose may demonstrate enhanced susceptibility to disease.

CAUSES AND RISK FACTORS
• CWD and other TSEs are believed to be caused by a pathogenic effect on neurons of an abnormal isoform of a host-encoded glycoprotein, the prion protein. • The pathogenic form of this protein appears to be devoid of nucleic acids and supports its own amplification in the host through conversion of the secondary structure of host prion protein to the pathogenic protein structure. TSEs in animals primarily occur by transmitting the etiologic agent within a species, either naturally or through domestic husbandry practices. A notable exception among the TSEs is the apparent ability of BSE to effectively cross species barriers, affecting most mammalian species.
• Although CWD does not appear to occur naturally outside the cervid family, it has been

transmitted experimentally by intracerebral injection to a number of animals, including laboratory mice, ferrets, mink, squirrel monkeys, cattle, and goats. Oral transmission has not been demonstrated to cause diseases in any species but cervids. • The mode of transmission among deer and elk is not fully understood; however, evidence supports lateral transmission through direct animal-to-animal contact or as a result of indirect exposure to the causative agent in the environment, including contaminated feed, soil, and water sources.

DIAGNOSIS

DIFFERENTIAL DIAGNOSES
• Bluetongue • Epizootic hemorrhagic disease • Locoweed • Meningeal worm (*Parelaphostrongylus tenuis*) infection

CBC/BIOCHEMISTRY/URINALYSIS
N/A

OTHER DIAGNOSTIC PROCEDURES
• Immunohistochemical (IHC) staining of the retropharyngeal lymph nodes and obex with a monoclonal antibody is considered the gold standard for postmortem diagnosis of CWD. ELISA-based diagnostic test on fresh retropharyngeal lymph node tissue has been used to test large numbers of wild cervids in a short time frame. • There is currently no approved antemortem test for CWD. • Prion strain diversity is believed to be encoded in the three-dimensional conformation of the protein, which determines the cleavage site and molecular size of proteinase-K–treated prion fragment, indicating that the difference in molecular size may correlate with strain differences. However, one-dimensional immunoblot analysis may not identify more subtle differences that may influence the conformation of different prion strains. • Analysis of the glycoform ratios of prion fragments and application of a two-dimensional immunoblot may help further identify these subtle differences.

PATHOLOGIC FINDINGS
• There are no gross pathognomonic changes in cervids with CWD. Gross examination of the brain is unremarkable in cervids with CWD. Additional postmortem changes in chronically affected animals are nonspecific, but can include emaciation, serous atrophy of fat, abomasal ulcers, and aspiration pneumonia. • Histopathologic lesions of chronic wasting disease include spongiform change of the gray matter; neuronal intracytoplasmic vacuolation, degeneration, and loss; and astrocytosis in the absence of a host inflammatory response.

TREATMENT

THERAPEUTIC APPROACH
N/A

MEDICATIONS

DRUGS OF CHOICE
N/A

FOLLOW-UP

EXPECTED COURSE AND PROGNOSIS
Most animals with the disease die within several months of onset of symptoms, sometimes from aspiration pneumonia. In rare cases, illness may last for ≥1 year.

PREVENTION
In establishing new enclosures for farmed cervids, a "new" uncontaminated area needs to be found. CWD, like other prion proteins, can survive in contaminated environments for many years.

MISCELLANEOUS

AGE-RELATED FACTORS
In captive cervids, most cases occur in animals 2–7 years of age; however, the disease has been reported in cervids as young as 17 months and as old as >15 years of age.

ZOONOTIC POTENTIAL
• There is no plausible link between CWD and BSE in cattle and scrapie in sheep. No known human has been infected with CWD. • CWD appears host specific and will not readily transmit to humans, sheep, swine, cattle, or other wildlife. • Increasing spread of CWD has raised concerns about the potential for increasing human exposure to the CWD agent. The foodborne transmission of bovine spongiform encephalopathy to humans indicates that the species barrier may not completely protect humans from animal prion diseases.

BIOSECURITY
• State and national programs have been implemented to reduce the spread of CWD. • Many states have mandatory identification and postmortem testing of all captive cervids. In addition to testing, some states have restricted movement of deer and elk across state boundaries. • Captive herds with a CWD-positive animal are typically eliminated. • CWD, like other prion proteins, can survive in contaminated environments for many years.

PRODUCTION MANAGEMENT
• Mandatory identification and postmortem testing of all captive cervids. • Captive herds with a CWD-positive animal are typically eliminated. • CWD, like other prion proteins, can survive in contaminated environments for many years.

ABBREVIATIONS
• BSE = bovine spongiform encephalopathy • CJD = Creutzfeldt-Jakob disease • CNS = central nervous system • CWD = chronic wasting disease • ELISA = enzyme-linked immunosorbent assay • IHC = immunohistochemical staining • TME = transmissible mink encephalopathy • TSE = transmissible spongiform encephalopathy • vCJD = variant form of Creutzfeldt-Jakob disease

SEE ALSO
• Body Condition Scoring: Cervidae (see www.fiveminutevet.com/ruminant) • Bovine Spongiform Encephalopathy • Cervidae: Captive Management • Cervidae: Mortality • Scrapie

Suggested Reading

Chronic Wasting Disease. Center for Food Safety and Public Health, 2008, pp. 1–6. http://www.cfsph.iastate.edu/Factsheets/pdfs/chronic_wasting_disease.pdf (accessed June 25, 2016).

Greenlee JJ, Greenlee MHW. The transmissible spongiform encephalopathies of livestock. ILAR J 2015, 56: 7–25.

Miller MW, Williams ES, McCarty CW, et al. Epizootiology of chronic wasting disease in free-ranging cervids in Colorado and Wyoming. J Wildl Dis 2000, 36: 676–90.

Miller MW, Wild MA, Williams ES. Epidemiology of chronic wasting disease in captive Rocky Mountain elk. J Wildl Dis 1998, 34: 532–8.

Robinson SJ, Samuel MD, O'Rourke KI, Johnson CJ. The role of genetics in chronic wasting disease of North American cervids. Prion 2012, 6: 153–62.

Saunders SE, Bartelt-Hunt SL, Bartz JC. Occurrence, transmission, and zoonotic potential of chronic wasting disease. Emerging Infect Dis 2012, 18:369–76.

Williams ES, Miller MW. Chronic wasting disease in deer and elk in North America. Rev Sci Tech 2002, 21: 305–16.

Williams ES, Young S. Neuropathology of chronic wasting disease of mule deer (*Odocoileus hemionus*) and elk (*Cervus elaphus nelsoni*). Vet Pathol 1993, 30: 36–45.

Wolfe, L. L., et al. 2002. Evaluation of antemortem sampling to estimate chronic wasting disease prevalence in free-ranging mule deer. J Wildl Manag 66: 564–73.

Author Alan Young
Consulting Editor Christopher C.L. Chase
Acknowledgment The author and book editors acknowledge the prior contribution of Jeremy Schefers and Dennis Hermesch.

CERVIDAE: GAME PARK MANAGEMENT, FACILITIES

BASICS

OVERVIEW
• All aspects of animal care and husbandry in a captive environment.
• Scale and type of issues faced can vary markedly depending on type of facility, i.e., indoor versus outdoor, zoological garden versus commercial deer farm versus hunting preserve, and type of cervid species.
• There are over 40 species of Cervidae ranging from pudu (*Pudu pudu*) that weigh approximately 7 kg to moose (*Alces alces*) that weigh up to 800 kg.
• Antlers are present in the males of all species except from the genus *Hydropotes*. Females of the genus *Rangifer* also have antlers.

INCIDENCE/PREVALENCE
N/A

GEOGRAPHIC DISTRIBUTION
• Cervids are naturally distributed throughout most of North and South America, Eurasia, and northern Africa.
• Deer have been introduced into wild habitats in Australia, New Zealand, Cuba, New Guinea, and elsewhere.
• Deer are farmed for meat and velvet production in numerous countries.

SYSTEMS AFFECTED
N/A

SIGNALMENT
Captive and farmed cervid species

GENETICS
N/A

PRODUCTION MANAGEMENT

Handling Facilities
• Facility design is important to facilitate animal handling for medical and management procedures.
• Properly designed pens with communicating alleyways allow for loading animals into trailers for transport or into chutes or mechanical restraint devices to allow for physical examinations, hoof trimming, or minor medical procedures.
• Farms need a yard system that will lead animals up to corrals where they can be sorted and moved through a chute. It is best to make a gradual transition from open fencing to solid walls in areas of crowding. Wooden walls are better than metal as they are quieter and do not absorb heat as readily. It is important that animals cannot see escape routes and that facilities and hardware such as hinges stand up to the animals pushing against gates and walls.
• Moving animals through alleyways as part of a normal routine facilitates moving them when necessary for other procedures.
• It is important to have adequate ventilation and shade in handling areas to reduce the likelihood of animals overheating. Nonslip, level substrate that does not retain moisture is important for areas in which animals will be gathered for handling.
• The system design should be based upon the size and number of animals present on the farm.
• In general, deer do best when they are herded around blind bends because this gives them the sense that they are escaping from danger. Therefore, raceways should incorporate turns and curves rather than long straight runs. Raceways should be wide enough to allow passage of tractors or other necessary machinery.
• In handling areas, fences should be solid and a minimum of 8 feet high and probably 9 feet for elk and red deer. Physical restraint may be accomplished with a drop floor chute, or mechanical or hydraulic crush restraints. Covering the animal's eyes with a towel or other cover will help keep it calm while being restrained.
• Areas in which animals are brought in or loaded out should be within a perimeter fence to prevent escape off the farm should an animal break free.
• The loading area should allow for a trailer to pull up without gaps between the trailer and the walls of the loading chute. If there are gaps, wood planks or plywood can be used to fill the void. Having an adjustable floor to allow it to be level with the trailer floor will facilitate loading. It is essential to avoid gaps in the floor between trailer and loading chute where an animal might get a foot or leg caught.
• Operant conditioning of animals for blood collection and voluntary injections of anesthetic agents, vaccines, and medications facilitates care of cervids in captivity. An appropriate barrier system should be in place to protect persons doing these procedures.
• Smaller cervid species such as muntjac or pudu can be run into opaque restraint bags made of canvas or nylon mounted on a metal frame. The dark bag has a calming effect, and having the animal in a bag decreases the risk of injury to the animal and the person(s) restraining the animal.

Housing
• Requirements will depend on species and geographic location of the animal collection.
• In temperate regions, tropical species may require indoor housing during cold seasons.
• Outdoor facilities require adequate shade as well as protection from wind and rain. Animals must have access to a clean reliable source of water in any areas in which they are housed.
• State, provincial, and federal regulations typically dictate minimal fencing requirements for outdoor exhibits. USDA CWD program standards require fencing to be a minimum of 2.4 meters (96 inches) high, complying with any other state regulations or requirements, and that the fence is constructed and maintained in a way that prevents ingress of wild cervids onto the premises and egress of captive cervids to the wild.
• In areas of high snowfall, additional fence height or snow removal may be required to maintain effective fencing.
• A large percentage of animal escapes from deer farms are due to gates not being properly closed. Having well-designed gates with good locking mechanisms and considering double gates in areas of high traffic may be beneficial to reduce this problem.
• Solid fencing and high tensile page wire are commonly used for red deer and elk facilities. Electric fencing is sometime incorporated along with primary fencing, but may be removed by antlered animals as mature antlers are devoid of sensory innervation. Electric fencing inside or outside of the primary fence has been shown to reduce the chance of nose-to-nose contact between the captive animals and wild cervids outside the enclosure.
• Entanglement of antlers or limbs is of concern with chain link or other forms of permeable fencing and it is not recommended to house stags in adjacent pens during rut because they may attempt to fight through the fence.
• It is generally not recommended to house multiple stags in a single enclosure during rut because it will cause fighting and may lead to severe injuries or mortalities. During periods when antlers are shed or are in velvet, stags are not likely to fight. Antlers can be removed to reduce the potential for serious injuries between animals.
• With adequate space, a single stag and multiple hinds (harem) and juveniles are typically housed together, but it is important to have the ability to isolate the stag to manage reproduction.
• Natural dirt substrate typically works well. In outdoor exhibits shelter and windbreaks should be provided in sufficient numbers for all animals.
• Visual barriers/hiding places are important to allow animals to feel secure at certain times such as during calving or for newly introduced animals.
• Cervids will destroy exhibit plants that are not protected, but stags require rubbing posts or trees to clean off velvet.
• It is important to provide multiple food and water sources to allow lower-ranking animals access.
• An isolation/hospital pen should be available for sick or injured animals. Depending on the facility this may also suffice for a quarantine area for new animals or there may be a need for a separate quarantine area. Ideally a quarantine area will be physically separated from the rest of the collection and should have separate staff and equipment to care for these animals (see chapter, Biosecurity: Cervidae).

CERVIDAE: GAME PARK MANAGEMENT, FACILITIES   (CONTINUED)

• If animals are managed on pasture, it is ideal to be able to rotate animals between pastures to maintain quality of pasture forage and to minimize parasite build-up on pastures.

Social Requirements
Most cervid species are social animals and live in herds at least during part of the year.

Laws and Regulations
• Federal regulations under the Animal Welfare Act and Animal Welfare Regulations apply to cervids, and licensure through the USDA is generally required for zoos (except federal facilities), promotional exhibits (use of animals for promotion or advertisement of goods or services, use of animals as prizes, use of animals to promote photography, use of animals in public venues), public exhibitions, and performing animals.
• Licensure is not required for operations raising animals for food and fiber, game preserves, or hunting preserves unless animals from these ventures are sold to other ventures requiring licensure. License fees depend on a number of factors, including the type of license required. In certain situations an exhibitor may be registered rather than licensed and as such no fees apply.
• The Animal Welfare Act and Animal Welfare Regulations are available online: http://awic.nal.usda.gov/government-and-professional-resources/federal-laws/animal-welfare-act
• Both state and federal laws and regulations apply to maintaining a captive cervid population, although federal laws may not apply unless there is interstate movement of the animals. Local zoning ordinances may also apply. Federal regulations apply to any interstate movement of cervids, but state regulations may be more restrictive in relation to allowing cervids to enter a state, if not just passing directly through. In addition to specific testing and various requirements for herd certification, an official certificate of veterinary inspection (CVI) signed by an accredited veterinarian is required for interstate movement of captive cervids.
• Contacts for appropriate state agencies can be found online: http://www.aphis.usda.gov/import_export/animals/animal_import/animal_imports_states.shtml
• Questions regarding international importation and exportation of live cervids can be emailed to: VS.Live.Animal.Import.Export@aphis.usda.gov or can be answered by calling: (301)851-3300.

CAPTIVE CERVID HERD CWD CERTIFICATION PROGRAM
• USDA-APHIS has established a voluntary captive cervid herd CWD certification program (HCP) to reduce the risk of introduction, transmission and spread of chronic wasting disease in captive cervid herds in the United States. The federal CWD

program only covers cervids of the genus *Cervus* (e.g. elk, red deer) *Odocoileous* (e.g. white-tailed deer, mule deer) and *Alces* (moose). A state may oversee its own certification program with the approval of USDA-APHIS. A state's program must at least meet the requirements of the federal HCP, but may be more restrictive and may include all species of cervid.
• All participating cervid farms must have a unique premises identification number (PIN). Captive cervids that are not from a CWD "certified herd" cannot be transported between states. There are special exemptions for animals used for research, wild animals being moved for reintroduction efforts, or animals being taken directly to slaughter facilities.
• Deaths of program animals that are 12 months or older must be reported to state or federal representatives and the animals must be tested for CWD. Exceptions to testing may be permitted by approved state agencies due to extenuating circumstances beyond the herd owner's control.
• In states which allow cervid ownership, but do not have an approved CWD herd certification program, interested parties can enroll directly by applying to APHIS. Herd animals require two forms of positive animal identification. One form of ID must be an officially approved device with a nationally unique animal identification number that is linked to that animal in the CWD national database or in an approved state database.
• An animal must be identified with appropriate methods by the time it is 12 months old or if it leaves the farm. Information about official identification can be obtained at the at the USDA website: http://www.aphis.usda.gov/traceability/downloads/ADT_eartags_criteria.pdf
• A herd reaches "certified" status 5 years after it has been continuously enrolled in the program and has maintained requirements for progressing from first- through fifth-year status.
• Should a CWD-positive animal be detected in a herd, regulatory agents work with the owner to develop a herd plan to eradicate CWD from the infected herd and prevent the introduction of CWD into uninfected herds. The implemented plan is a management program written by a state or federal representative with input from the herd owner, the herd veterinarian, and other affected parties.
• Herd plans take steps to stop the introduction of CWD into uninfected herds, eradicate CWD from infected herds, and control the risk of CWD in suspect herds. A plan could require depopulation of a herd and could prevent cervids from occupying the affected site for a specified period of time if a herd was found to be CWD-positive. Perimeter fencing around the herd must be

adequate to prevent ingress or egress of cervids.
• A herd may be classified as: **CWD positive**—a herd which contains CWD-infected animals; **CWD exposed**—one in which a CWD-positive animal has resided within 5 years prior to that animal's diagnosis as CWD positive as determined by an APHIS employee or state representative; **CWD suspect**—one that has laboratory evidence or clinical signs suggestive of CWD, but has not yet had a conclusive, confirmed diagnosis.
• USDA CWD Program Standards can be found at: https://www.aphis.usda.gov/animal_health/animal_diseases/cwd/downloads/cwd_program_standards_2014.pdf
• Voluntary herd tuberculosis accreditation and brucellosis certification programs are available for cervids and are administered by regulatory agencies in each state. States also regulate importation requirements for cervids and the State Board of Animal Health or similar state or provincial regulatory agency should be contacted prior to making arrangements for interstate movements.

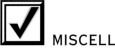 MISCELLANEOUS

ASSOCIATED CONDITIONS
N/A

AGE-RELATED FACTORS
N/A

ZOONOTIC POTENTIAL
Some zoonotic diseases of potential concern in cervids include rabies, plague, anthrax, salmonella, Q fever, cryptosporidiosis, brucellosis, listeriosis, dermatophytosis, tuberculosis, and parapox virus. Care must be taken in the collection of laboratory samples and the diagnosis and treatment of affected animals.

PREGNANCY
N/A

BIOSECURITY
• Isolation and quarantine of new stock entering the herd.
• Treat and/or cull new animals for disease conditions prior to herd introduction.

PRODUCTION MANAGEMENT
N/A

SYNONYMS
• Adult male cervid: stag, bull, buck. Nomenclature depends on species and geographic locale.
• Adult female cervid: hind, cow, doe. Nomenclature depends on species and geographic locale.
• Juvenile cervid: calf, fawn. Nomenclature depends on species and geographic locale.

ABBREVIATIONS
• CWD = chronic wasting disease
• USDA-APHIS = United States Department of Agriculture-Animal Plant Health Inspection Service

SEE ALSO
• Biosecurity: Cervidae (see www.fiveminutevet.com/ruminant)
• Cervidae: Capture Myopathy
• Cervidae: Mortality
• Vaccination Programs: Cervidae

Suggested Reading

Animal Welfare Act and Animal Welfare Regulations. Nov.2013. United States Department of Agriculture.

Flach E. Cervidae and tragulidae. In: Fowler ME, Miller RE eds, Zoo and Wild Animal Medicine, 5th ed. St. Louis: Saunders, 2003.

Haigh JC, Hudson RJ. Farming Wapiti and Red Deer. St Louis: Mosby, 1993.

Miller MW. Chronic wasting disease of cervid species. In: Fowler ME, Miller RE eds, Zoo and Wild Animal Medicine Current Therapy, vol. 6. St. Louis: Saunders Elsevier, 2008.

Thorleifson I, Pearse T, Friedel B. Elk Farming Handbook. St. John, New Brunswick: Abbott Richards Graphic Design, 2000.

VerCauteren KC, Lavelle MJ, Seward NW, Fischer JW, Phillips GE. Fence-line contact between wild and farmed cervids in Colorado: Potential for disease transmission. J Wildl Manage 2007, 71: 1594–602.

VerCauteren KC, Vandeelen TR, Lavelle MJ, Hall W. Assessment of abilities of white-tailed deer to jump fences. J Wildl Manage 2010, 74: 1378–81.

Author James M. Rasmussen
Consulting Editor Ahmed Tibary

C

CERVIDAE MORTALITY

C

BASICS

OVERVIEW
• Mortality among farmed deer is subject to considerable variation according to species, sex, age, season, and location.
• Most deaths are a result of faulty management and are preventable.
• Undiagnosed deaths confound incidence rates of diseases.

INCIDENCE/PREVALENCE
Unknown

GEOGRAPHIC DISTRIBUTION
Worldwide

SYSTEMS AFFECTED
• Musculoskeletal
• Nervous
• Digestive

PATHOPHYSIOLOGY
Depends on the cause of death

HISTORICAL FINDINGS
N/A

PHYSICAL EXAMINATION FINDINGS
N/A

SIGNALMENT
Cervidae of all ages

GENETICS
N/A

CAUSES AND RISK FACTORS
Noninfectious Causes
Trauma and Handling-Related Deaths
• Mortality as a result of trauma was a leading cause of death in adult captive WTD and elk populations surveyed.
• Traumatic injuries related to handling are usually a result of poorly designed handling facilities or improper handling techniques, especially with inexperienced farmers.
• Yearling males tend to have the highest percentage of handling-related injuries.
• Capture myopathy in WTD seems to be a leading cause of handling-related deaths in adult females.
• Traumatic injuries from fighting among animals, especially adult males in rut, can result in perforations (i.e., thoracic, abdominal) if antlers are not removed or head/neck injuries (vertebral/skull fractures, brain abscesses, meningitis) if antlers are removed.
• Darting injuries can result in skeletal fractures, body cavity perforations, and deep tissue damage with subsequent disease.
• Accidental anesthetic overdose can directly cause death.
• Conversely, underdosing with anesthetics can lead to traumatic injuries due to ataxia, prolonged induction, and capture myopathy.

Nutrition
• Starvation in neonates can result from dam agalactia or abandonment.
• Starvation in yearlings and adults occur with improper feed supplementation throughout the winter months or when age groups are mixed such that older, dominant animals monopolize the feed sources.
• Ruminal acidosis ("grain overload") has been reported to affect as many as 25% of adult deer, with more dominant animals being predisposed due to overindulging on supplementary feed.
• Congenital white muscle disease, caused by inadequate vitamin E and selenium intake by pregnant dams, can lead to stillborn or weak neonates that die shortly after birth.
• Chronic vitamin E deficiency in juvenile or adult deer can cause fatal cardiomyopathy.
• Copper deficiency usually manifests as clinical disease (enzootic ataxia and osteochondrosis) and can lead to poor performance, bullying from herdmates, and death.

Infectious Causes
Bacterial Diseases
Necrobacillosis
• Primary etiologic agent is *Fusobacterium necrophorum*; second most common cause is *Trueperella pyogenes*; occasionally *Fusobacterium varium* is isolated in WTD.
• The leading cause of overall death in WTD fawns and most common cause of bacterial death in both fallow and WTD.
• Results in significant morbidity due to the development of foot rot, wooden tongue, and lumpy jaw with secondary multi-organ abscessation and erosion or ulceration of the intestinal wall (esp. rumeno-reticulum).
• Stressors such as heat, cold, overcrowding, mud, and malnutrition predispose deer to infection.
• Good management practices can minimize incidence of clinical disease and include stress prevention, good hygiene, decreasing food coarseness, ensuring adequate nutrition, and choosing substrates that do not retain water.
• Vaccines against *F. necropohorum* have been developed for cattle and may be used in deer, but its efficacy has not been evaluated. Autogenous vaccines may be used in some herds.
Tuberculosis (*Mycobacterium bovis*)
• Has been reported in at least 14 Cervidae species including red deer, fallow deer, elk, and WTD.
• Transmission usually occurs through the mouth or nasal cavity, resulting in subacute to chronic disease.
• Lesions are usually found in retropharyngeal lymph nodes, followed by lung and associated lymph nodes.
• Clinical signs are often nonspecific and include weight loss, emaciation, and rough hair coat, with death usually occurring after the onset of clinical signs.

• Lymphadenopathy occurs commonly, and all abscess-like lesions should be cultured for mycobacteria.
• Testing can be performed antemortem using a tuberculin skin test or a serologic test and is generally required for interstate movement of captive cervids (elk, red deer, WTD, fallow deer, reindeer) in the US.
Johne's Disease (*Mycobacterium avium* subsp. *paratuberculosis*)
• Deer show clinical signs earlier than other ruminants, but only a small proportion exposed become clinically ill.
• Adult deer show chronic loss of condition and weight over a few months (similar to sheep and cattle), and young deer tend to exhibit a much more acute, rapid loss of weight and muscle mass over a few weeks.
• Affected deer also experience diarrhea and death due to poor condition.
Respiratory Diseases
• Pneumonia is the most common respiratory disease associated with mortality.
• Primary etiology commonly unknown, but *T. pyogenes* has been reported most frequently with *Mannheimia haemolytica, Escherichia coli, Pasteurella* spp., *Streptococcus* spp., *Fusobacterium necrophorum*, and *Mycobacterium* spp. also having been reported.
• If untreated, can progress to septicemia, acute hemorrhagic disease, and death.
Gastrointestinal Diseases
• Common bacterial pathogens associated with acute enteritis and mortality include *E. coli, Clostridium perfringens, Salmonella* spp., and *Yersinia pseudotuberculosis*.
• Colibacillosis (*E. coli*)
  ◦ Clinical signs include endotoxic shock and sudden death, acute diarrhea (± hemorrhage), and/or neurologic deficits due to meningitis.
  ◦ Neonates most severely affected with slightly older fawns/calves experiencing mild scours and colic.
  ◦ Vaccine (autogenous/extra-label) may be available for pregnant dams; best prevention strategy is practicing good hygiene and ensuring adequate colostrum intake.
• Clostridial Disease
  ◦ In adults, usually a result of sudden change in feed composition.
  ◦ *C. perfingens* type D has been reported as a cause of acute enteritis and death in young cervids.
  ◦ Vaccination of dams 30–60 days before calving and of calves at weaning and 30 days later is used in preventive programs. However, the efficacy is unproven.
• Salmonellosis
  ◦ Many different *Salmonella* spp. have reportedly caused isolated cases of peracute septicemia, acute enteritis, and sudden death in neonates.
  ◦ The only preventive methods available are practicing good hygiene, reducing stress, and ensuring adequate colostrum intake.

C

• Yersiniosis (*Yersinia pseudotuberculosis*)
  ○ Sudden death is most common initial finding when outbreak occurs.
  ○ Formation of microabscesses of various sizes enveloping large bacterial colonies in the intestinal lamina propria is typical histologic lesion; can be easily isolated from intestine and mesenteric lymph nodes.
  ○ Affected deer tend to be weanlings during inclement weather within their first fall, but other stressors (malnourishment, transport, concurrent diseases) can also predispose them.
  ○ An effective licensed vaccine is available in New Zealand.

Anthrax (*Bacillus anthracis*)
• Severe outbreaks have been reported in red deer, wapiti, moose, and fallow deer.
• Transmission generally through ingestion of contaminated soil or water.
• Septicemia and sudden death may occur <2 days after exposure in acute form.
• Other animals may show nonspecific signs of abdominal pain or have bloody discharge from nostrils and anus.
• Any suspected cases must be reported.
• Vaccine may be available in endemic areas.

Leptospirosis
• Caused by serovars of bacterium *Leptospira interrogans*.
• Young cervids most susceptible, experiencing clinical signs ranging from sudden death in peracute cases to fever, anorexia, and hemoglobinurea in others.

Viral Diseases

Malignant Catarrhal Fever
• The most important viral disease of farmed deer, worldwide.
• Cervid outbreaks are commonly sheep-associated (OvHV-2), but a currently unnamed gammaherpesvirus has been reported in WTD.
• Elk and red deer often develop the chronic "head and eye" form, characterized by excessive salivation, lachrymation, and nasal discharge.
• WTD, axis deer, Père David's deer, and rusa deer are all highly susceptible and may die acutely or peracutely.
• Widespread hemorrhages ± mucosal erosions are most commonly observed.
• Lymphocytic vasculitis with lymphoid hyperplasia is a characteristic histologic finding that can be confirmed using ELISA or PCR.

Hemorrhagic Diseases
• Two closely related Orbiviruses, bluetongue (BT) and epizootic hemorrhagic disease (EHD) of deer, have been reported to cause major epizootic deaths in WTD, with less severe effects in mule deer.
• An adenovirus has also been implemented as a cause of acute hemorrhagic disease and death in several cervid species with similar lesions to those seen in BT and EHD.

• Transmission of BT and EHD are through biting gnats or sandflies of the genus *Culicoides*, whereas adenovirus is transmitted through direct contact.
• Widespread hemorrhages of mucus membranes, pulmonary edema, and enteropathy are often observed, and EHD is usually more acutely fatal.
• Autogenous vaccines have been used with some success for control of EHD and BT.

Rotavirus and Coronavirus
• Frequently associated with enteric disease in young cervids.
• Watery diarrhea is most consistent clinical sign with secondary dehydration and depression.
• Can be managed with appropriate supportive care (oral or IV fluids; ± antibiotics for secondary bacterial infection; tube feeding) as death may occur if no intervention occurs; however, careful monitoring is crucial as hypernatremia has been reported in wapiti calves treated with oral fluids designed for cattle.
• Cattle vaccines are available and have been used with variable success; appropriate management of the dam and environmental conditions are of utmost importance for prevention.

Parasitic Diseases

Lungworms (*Dictyocaulus* spp.)
• Cause a chronic disease in young cervids (3–5 months most susceptible).
• Nonspecific clinical signs such as decreased appetite, weight loss, impaired growth, roughened coat, and sudden death.
• Asphyxia from massed dead adult worms in the airways has been reported after anthelmintic administration.

Gastrointestinal Worms
• Important intestinal parasites of the family Trichostrongylidae include *Ostertagia, Haemonchus,* and *Spiculopteragia*.
• Type II ostertagiasis has been reported in WTD, red deer, and wapiti, causing poor performance and death.
• Hemonchosis has been associated with anemia, emaciation, and death in WTD.
• Infestations can occur concurrently with lungworm.

Liver Fluke (*Fascioloides magna*)
• Also known as the giant liver fluke, has an indirect life cycle involving aquatic snail intermediate hosts.
• Heavily infected wapiti and WTD may die with extensive liver damage.
• Calves and fawns may develop peritonitis and die acutely.

Meningeal worm (*Parelaphostrongylus tenuis*)
• Has an indirect life cycle involving gastropod intermediate hosts.
• Severity of clinical signs varies based on species and seems to be dose-dependent, with WTD being relatively resistant.

• Moose and elk appear to be most susceptible, exhibiting clinical signs that include ataxia, blindness, collapse, and death.

Cryptosporidiosis
• Similar syndrome to that in other livestock.
• Usually only occurs in 2- to 4-week-old animals, especially when hand reared.
• Severe diarrhea can lead to dehydration and death.
• Has occurred in outbreak form.
• Marked zoonotic potential—good hygiene is essential for personnel.

Prion Disease

Chronic Wasting Disease
• Within the group of transmissible spongiform encephalopathies, characterized by abnormal proteinaceous material accumulation in the CNS.
• Has been reported in mule deer, WTD, moose, and elk in the US and Canada, with mule deer being most susceptible.
• Mode of transmission is generally thought to be oral and incubation periods are prolonged.
• Clinical signs include chronic weight loss, polydipsia, polyuria, drooling, and ataxia followed by death.
• Secondary aspiration pneumonia is commonly seen on necropsy.
• Surveillance programs are in place to minimize spread and transmission throughout captive cervid populations and include submission of obex and medial retropharyngeal lymph nodes from dead animals for testing.

 DIAGNOSIS

DIFFERENTIAL DIAGNOSES
See "Causes and Risk Factors"

CBC/BIOCHEMISTRY/URINALYSIS
OTHER LABORATORY TESTS
See "Causes and Risk Factors"

IMAGING
N/A

OTHER DIAGNOSTIC PROCEDURES
See "Causes and Risk Factors"

PATHOLOGIC FINDINGS
See "Causes and Risk Factors"

 TREATMENT

THERAPEUTIC APPROACH
N/A

SURGICAL CONSIDERATIONS AND TECHNIQUES
N/A

CERVIDAE MORTALITY

C

MEDICATIONS

DRUGS OF CHOICE
N/A

CONTRAINDICATIONS
N/A

PRECAUTIONS
N/A

POSSIBLE INTERACTIONS
N/A

FOLLOW-UP

EXPECTED COURSE AND PROGNOSIS
N/A

POSSIBLE COMPLICATIONS
N/A

CLIENT EDUCATION
PATIENT CARE
N/A

PREVENTION

MISCELLANEOUS

ASSOCIATED CONDITIONS
See "Causes and Risk Factors"

AGE-RELATED FACTORS
• Most mortality in young stock occurs in summer or just after weaning.
• The highest mortality rate in yearlings and adults occurs in winter.

ZOONOTIC POTENTIAL
Brucellosis, tuberculosis, leptospirosis, and cryptosporidiosis are all zoonotic in nature.

PREGNANCY
N/A

BIOSECURITY
Many infectious diseases can be prevented by practicing good biosecurity, which includes quarantining new animals and implementing vaccination and treatment protocols.

PRODUCTION MANAGEMENT
• Trauma is a major cause of mortality in all farmed deer, and is usually associated with poorly designed handling systems or improper handling techniques.
• Capture myopathy is a potential sequela, but its incidence can be minimized by vitamin E supplementation, proper handling, and acclimation of animals.
• Nutritional causes are less common causes of death in captive deer populations and can be minimized with proper management.

SYNONYMS
N/A

ABBREVIATIONS
• CNS = central nervous system
• WTD = white-tailed deer

SEE ALSO
• Brucellosis
• Biosecurity: Cervidae (see www.fiveminutevet.com/ruminant)
• Cervidae: Captive Management
• Cervidae: Capture Myopathy
• Cervidae: Chronic Wasting Disease
• Cervidae: Reproduction
• Nutrition and Metabolic Diseases: Cervidae
• *Parelaphostrongylus tenuis* (Meningeal Worm)
• Tuberculosis: Bovine
• Vaccination Programs: Cervidae

Suggested Reading
Haigh JC, Mackintosh C, Griffin F. Viral, parasitic and prion diseases of farmed deer and bison. Revue scientifique et technique-Office international des epizooties 2002, 21: 219–48.

Haigh J, Berezowski J, Woodbury MR. A cross-sectional study of the causes of morbidity and mortality in farmed white-tailed deer. Can Vet J 2005, 46: 507–12.

Hattel AL, Shaw DP, Fisher JS, et al. Mortality in Pennsylvania captive elk (*Cervus elaphus*): 1998–2006. J Vet Diagn Invest 2007, 19: 334–7.

Mackintosh C, Haigh JC, Griffin F. Bacterial diseases of farmed deer and bison. Revue scientifique et technique-Office international des épizooties 2002, 21: 249–64.

Mackintosh CG, Griffin JF. Paratuberculosis in deer, camelids and other ruminants. In: Behr MA, Colins DM eds, Paratuberculosis: Organism, Disease, Control. Wallingford: CABI, 2010, p. 179.

Palmer MV, et al. Tuberculosis in wild and captive deer. In: Mukundan H, Chambers MA, Waters WR, Larsen MH eds, Tuberculosis, Leprosy and Mycobacterial Diseases of Man and Animals: The Many Hosts of Mycobacteria. Wallingford: CABI, 2015, p. 334.

Sanford SE. Outbreaks of yersiniosis caused by *Yersinia pseudotuberculosis* in farmed cervids. J Vet Diagn Invest 1995, 7: 78–81.

Sieber V, et al. Causes of mortality and diseases in farmed deer in Switzerland. Vet Med Internat 2010.

Woodbury MR, Berezowski J, Haigh J. A retrospective study of the causes of morbidity and mortality in farmed elk (*Cervus elaphus*). Can Vet J 2005, 46: 1108.

Authors Jamie L. Stewart and Clifford F. Shipley
Consulting Editor Ahmed Tibary
Acknowledgment The author and book editors acknowledge the prior contribution of Jerry Haigh.

CERVIDAE: REPRODUCTION

BASICS

OVERVIEW
• There are ~40 species in the family Cervidae, many of which vary greatly from one another in their reproductive strategies.
• Most cervid species are of northern temperate origin and are seasonally polyestrous, breeding in the autumn when day length is decreasing.
• The breeding season lasts between 4 and 6 months and is tightly synchronized with gestation length so that birth occurs late spring to mid-summer.
• Tropical species, such as chital deer, have less well-defined seasonal constraints and are able to reproduce year-round.
• Onset of puberty and reproductive success are largely influenced by nutritional availability and BCS.
• Nomenclature depends on species and geographic locale:
  ○ Adult male: stag, bull, buck
  ○ Adult female: hind, cow, doe
  ○ Juvenile: calf, fawn

INCIDENCE/PREVALENCE
N/A

GEOGRAPHIC DISTRIBUTION
Worldwide, depending on species

PATHOPHYSIOLOGY
N/A

SYSTEM AFFECTED
Reproductive

HISTORICAL FINDINGS
N/A

SIGNALMENT
Commonly studied species include those within the genera *Cervus* (red deer, wapiti), *Dama* (fallow deer), *Axis* (chital deer), *Rangifer* (reindeer), *Odocoileus* (white-tailed deer, black-tailed deer, mule deer), *Alces* (moose), *Capreolus* (roe deer), *Ozotoceros* (Pampas deer), *Elaphurus* (Père David's deer), *Rucervus* (swamp deer, Barasingha).

PHYSICAL EXAMINATION FINDINGS
Puberty and the Reproductive Cycle in the Female
• Onset of puberty: red deer, wapiti, fallow deer: between 9–18 months of age; white-tailed deer, reindeer: as early as 6 months of age; chital deer: ~14 months of age; Pampas deer: ~12 months of age; age at onset can vary based on environmental stressors.
• Species of northern temperate origin are seasonally polyestrous, with cycles beginning in Sept/Oct and continuing, if unmated, for 4–6 months.
• Tropical species (e.g., *Axis*) are aseasonal and exhibit estrous cycles year-round.

• The estrous cycle length varies by species but is generally between 18–24 d in length with *Cervus* species being shorter (18–20 d) and *Odocoileus* species being longer (21–27 d).
• Short cycles of 8–10 d with no overt signs of estrus (i.e., "silent ovulation") at the beginning of the season have been reported in most species and help to synchronize the first estrus of the season within a herd.
• One exception is the roe deer, which exhibits estrus as early as July, is monoovulatory, and, subsequently, experiences delayed implantation to allow for birthing to occur in the summer.
• Behavioral estrus tends to be subtle, with females exhibiting increased activity and displaying proceptive behaviors towards the male.
• In some species, overt estrus is terminated following successful copulation and may be as brief as a few minutes. If unmated, duration of standing heat can range from a few hours to >24 h. Ovulation generally occurs ~24 h after onset of estrus.

Pregnancy
• Gestation length varies with species and tends to increase with increasing body mass (e.g., *Odocoileus* 200 d; *Rangifer* 216 d; *Dama* 234 d; *Cervus* 240 d; *Elaphurus* 284 d).
• Variation in gestation lengths are compensated for by adjustments of up to 8 weeks in the onset of mating season between species to allow for parturition to occur mid-summer.
• "R-selected" populations are those species that normally produce twins or triplets, achieve early sexual maturation (<1 year), and experience a short breeding life (<10 years); this includes species within *Odocoileus* and *Capreolus*. The fecundity of these species can be influenced by habitat and nutritional availability.
• "K-selected" populations are those species that normally produce a single offspring, achieve later sexual maturation (>1 year), and experience a long breeding life (10+ years); includes species within *Cervus, Dama, Axis, Elaphurus,* and *Rangifer.*
• Similar to other ruminants, cervids undergo synepitheliochorial placentation. However, cervids have fewer placentomes (6–12) and are considered oligocotyledonary.
• The presence of a functional corpus luteum (CL) is required for pregnancy maintenance in both red deer and white-tailed deer. Conversely, reindeer appear to have some contribution of progesterone from the fetoplacental unit for pregnancy maintenance.

Parturition
• As in domestic ruminants, the mammary development begins about a week before parturition, with the udder becoming noticeably turgid.
• Females become restless and will isolate themselves from the herd in the days preceding parturition.

• The 1st stage of labor is marked by increased pacing of the fence line with a high stepping gait and extended neck, vocalization, and vulvar licking.
• The 2nd stage of labor is initiated with visible abdominal contractions, followed by appearance and subsequent rupturing of the amniotic sac, and is terminated with the expulsion of the fetus. The fetus can be expelled either standing or lying down.
• The progression of parturition can vary in duration among species, but producers should monitor captive females in labor to ensure that some progress is made every 30 min after entering the 2nd stage of labor.
• The placenta is usually expelled within the first hours postpartum (15 min to 4 h).

Puberty and Sexual Activity in the Male
• Puberty onset occurs when testosterone (T) production from the testis begins and development of secondary sex characteristics and accessory sex glands occurs. Onset depends mostly on body weight, but also somewhat on photoperiod.
• In *Cervus* and *Dama* species, males usually reach puberty in the 2nd autumn of life, at ~15 months of age, though they may not be able to breed in the presence of older males.
• Similar to females, white-tailed deer and reindeer males can attain puberty and successfully breed as early as 6 months of age if nutrition is adequate.
• Antler growth ("velvet") from the pedicle occurs during the spring and summer months while T levels are low. In temperate species, testicular atrophy occurs and spermatozoa are not produced during this time.
• As day length decreases, LH and T output increase, modulated through the pineal gland's effect on the hypothalamic-pituitary-gonadal axis (similar to sheep and goats), and the antlers mineralize and shed the velvet (i.e., "hard antler").
• In rut, males are at their most fertile with maximal testicular size, spermatogenesis, and androgenic activity. Adult males undergo rapid mobilization of fat and catabolization of muscle, causing a decrease in live weight of up to 30% that is not regained until the following spring.
• During the rutting season males have an increased neck girth and some species develop a characteristic long shaggy mane. *Cervus* species display urine spraying over the ventral abdomen, thorax, and forelegs, giving the male a strong pungent odor. Other behaviors include increased aggressiveness and special vocalization.

GENETICS
N/A

CAUSES AND RISK FACTORS
Poor reproductive performance may be due to poor management (nutrition, male selection, and pregnancy loss).
Dystocia is rare in cervids.

CERVIDAE: REPRODUCTION   (CONTINUED)

DIAGNOSIS

DIFFERENTIAL DIAGNOSES
• Pre-mating BCS of the female is associated with conception rate, conception date, and weight of weaned offspring.
• Brucellosis and leptospirosis has been reported to cause abortions or infertility in many cervid species.
• Dystocia is rare and usually occurs as a result of an overconditioned female.
• Causes of infertility in the male include epididymitis, orchitis, and cryptorchidism. Ulcerative posthitis (pizzle rot) and prolapsed prepuce are observed frequently in wapiti.

CBC/BIOCHEMISTRY/URINALYSIS
N/A

OTHER LABORATORY TESTS
• Pregnancy specific protein B (PSPB) detection in the serum can also be used efficiently for pregnancy diagnosis past 30 days in all species.
• Serology and bacteriology in cases of abortion.

IMAGING
Pregnancy diagnosis using transabdominal ultrasound is easy and accurate after 35 days' gestation. Number of fetuses can be determined using this method if performed in first two trimesters of pregnancy (mid-Jan to early March).

OTHER DIAGNOSTIC PROCEDURES
Dependent on complaint

PATHOLOGIC FINDINGS
Dependent on complaint

TREATMENT

THERAPEUTIC APPROACH
N/A

SURGICAL CONSIDERATIONS AND TECHNIQUES
N/A

MEDICATIONS

DRUGS OF CHOICE
N/A

CONTRAINDICATIONS
N/A

PRECAUTIONS
N/A

POSSIBLE INTERACTIONS
N/A

FOLLOW-UP

EXPECTED COURSE AND PROGNOSIS
N/A

POSSIBLE COMPLICATIONS
N/A

CLIENT EDUCATION
• Importance of management/nutrition
• Breeding soundness evaluation of males
• Biosecurity measures

PATIENT CARE
N/A

PREVENTION
• Biosecurity measures
• Vaccination

MISCELLANEOUS

ASSOCIATED CONDITIONS
• Infertility
• Abortion

AGE-RELATED FACTORS
• Females >10 years of age may produce offspring with low birthweight.
• Primiparous females tend to begin cycling later in the season than multiparous females, giving birth later in the summer.

ZOONOTIC POTENTIAL
Many reproductive diseases are zoonotic (*Leptospira* spp., *Brucella* spp., etc.). Care should be maintained when diseases are suspected.

BIOSECURITY
Brucellosis testing for susceptible species

PRODUCTION MANAGEMENT
• Hormonal control of the estrous cycle of cervids is similar to that of domestic ruminants and can be manipulated using similar protocols to those used in sheep and goats for artificial insemination.
• Neonatal losses are in the range 5–20% in farmed cervid and are usually due to dystocia, accidental injuries, and starvation (rejection or agalactia).
• Offspring are preferably weaned before the start of the rutting season to allow dry-off and weight gain. However, lactation does not seem to interfere with ovarian activity and ovulation unless the BCS deteriorates.

SYNONYMS
N/A

SEE ALSO
• Abortion: Farmed Cervidae
• Biosecurity: Cervidae (see www.fiveminutevet.com/ruminant)
• Breeding Soundness Examination: Cervidae
• Nutrition and Metabolic Diseases: Cervidae
• Vaccination Programs: Cervidae

ABBREVIATIONS
• BCS = body condition score
• CL = corpus luteum
• LH = luteinizing hormone
• PSPB = Pregnancy Specific Protein B
• T = testosterone

Suggested Reading
Asher GW. Reproductive cycles of deer. Anim Reprod Sci 2011, 124: 170–5.
Church J, Hudson R. Calving behaviour of farmed wapiti (*Cervus elaphus*). Appl Anim Behav Sci 1995, 46: 263–70.
Duquette JF, et al. Comparison of pregnancy detection methods in live white-tailed deer. Wildl Soc Bull 2012, 36: 115–18.
Lincoln GA. Biology of seasonal breeding in deer. In: The Biology of Deer. New York: Springer, 1992, pp. 565–74.
Morales-Piñeyrúa JT, Ungerfeld R. Pampas deer (*Ozotoceros bezoarticus*) courtship and mating behavior. Acta Veterin Scand 2012, 54: 60.
Noyes JH, Johnson BK, Dick BL, Kie JG. Effects of male age and female nutritional condition on elk reproduction. J Wildl Manage 2002, 66: 1301–7.
Youngquist RS, Threlfall WR. Current Therapy in Large Animal Theriogenology. Elsevier Health Sciences, 2006.

Authors Clifford F. Shipley and Jamie L. Stewart
Consulting Editor Ahmed Tibary
Acknowledgment The author and book editors acknowledge the prior contribution of Ahmed Tibary.

BASICS

OVERVIEW

• Indications for C-section in the bovine include dystocia caused by uterine torsion, feto-maternal disproportion, fetal abnormalities, emphysematous fetus, and fetal maldispositions not resolved by obstetric manipulations.
• C-section may be performed electively in high-risk pregnancies.
• Selection of a surgical approach is based on several factors.

INCIDENCE/PREVALENCE

C-section is the second most common abdominal surgery performed in the bovine.

GEOGRAPHIC DISTRIBUTION

Worldwide

SYSTEM AFFECTED

• Reproductive
• Multisystemic depending on complications

PATHOPHYSIOLOGY

C-section is indicated when other obstetric manipulations to resolve a dystocia are not possible.

HISTORICAL FINDINGS

• Signs of parturition without progression
• Unsuccessful obstetric manipulations

SIGNALMENT

Pregnant females at term

PHYSICAL EXAMINATON FINDINGS

• Depend on duration of the dystocia and manipulation attempts. Elevated heart and respiratory rates are common. Abdominal contraction and tenesmus are common. Dehydration is present in protracted cases.
• Dilated and edematous vulva if parturition has progressed to the second stage.
• Presence of discharge or fetal parts at the vulva.
• Vaginal speculum and manual vaginal palpation is performed to determine cervical dilation status and fetal disposition.

GENETICS

• Double muscled breeds (Belgian blue, some Charolais lines are at risk)
• Breeding to bulls with poor calving ease

CAUSES AND RISK FACTORS

• Dystocia
• Severe fetal abnormalities
• Uterine torsion
• Small heifers

 DIAGNOSIS

DIFFERENTIAL DIAGNOSES

Refer to chapter, Dystocia: Bovine

CBC/BIOCHEMISTRY/URINALYSIS

Performed in severely compromised/valuable females. Electrolyte imbalances, hypocalcemia, hypophosphatemia, and elevated liver enzymes are common with pregnancy toxaemia.

OTHER LABORATORY TEST

N/A

IMAGING

N/A

DIAGNOSIC PROCEDURES

N/A

PATHOLOGIC FINDINGS

Vary depending on the cause of dystocia. Large offspring syndrome is encountered in pregnancies from somatic cell nuclear transfer cloned embryos.

 TREATMENT

THERAPEUTIC APPROACH

• C-section may be performed on the farm without need of hospitalization is the patient is stable and the surgery is uncomplicated.
• Complicated cases should be handled in a hospital setting with capability of support (fluid therapy, pain management).

SURGICAL CONSIDERATIONS AND TECHNIQUES

Surgical Considerations

• Choice of approach depends on facilities, animal temperament, the medical condition of the animal, environment, and availability of assistance.
• Surgical approaches include standing paralumbar laparotomy, ventral midline celiotomy, paramedian celiotomy, left oblique celiotomy, and ventrolateral celiotomy.
• The two most common procedures are the standing paralumbar laparotomy and the ventrolateral celiotomy.
• Local anesthesia via an aseptic epidural injection of 2% lidocaine is almost always indicated to prevent straining,
• If the calf is dead and fetotomy is not an option, standing paralumbar laparotomy is performed if the cow is in good health and the fetus is not emphysematous. A ventrolateral celiotomy should be used if the calf is emphysematous, to improve exteriorization of the uterus and reduce risk of contaminating the abdomen.
• The use of preoperative antibiotics and anti-inflammatories should be considered on a case-by-case basis.

Standing Paralumbar Laparotomy

• The left side approach is the most common. The rumen serves as a visceral retainer and the small intestine is less likely to prolapse out of the incision.

• In dairy cattle, a right-sided incision allows to secure the abomasum during the procedure.
• The hair is clipped in the paralumbar fossa and the area cleansed from debris, hair, and gross contamination.
• Local anesthesia is achieved by lidocaine line block, inverted-L block, distal paravertebral (Cakala) block, and proximal paravertebral (Farquharson) block.
• The surgical site is aseptically prepared and a surgical drape placed over the side of the cow. The drape can be secured by towel clamps placed directly on the topline, then at the corners of the drape where local anesthesia is not present or with backtag glue or eyepatch glue at the periphery of the surgical area.
• A vertical incision, 30–50 cm depending, is made in the paralumbar fossa.
• The incision is extended through the skin and external abdominal oblique muscle.
• The internal abdominal oblique muscle and transverse abdominus muscle can then each be separated bluntly parallel to their fiber orientation in a "grid" technique to reduce hemorrhage and provide better apposition during closure.
• The peritoneum can then be bluntly entered or tented with an instrument and incised to gain access to the abdominal cavity.
• The uterus is identified by palpation in the caudal abdomen. Wearing a sterile obstetric sleeve makes manipulation easier and decreases risk for adhesions.
• The fetal horn is identified and grasped around the hock or carpus of the fetus then gently brought to the incision line.
• Exteriorization of the uterine horn is the most difficult step, particularly if the uterus is very contracted or fetus is large.
• A small incision is made between the calf toes, a sterile obstetric chain is placed and handed to an assistant, then incision is extended to allow exteriorization of the other foot, then the entire fetus.
• The incision should be long enough to allow extraction of the calf without tearing the uterus.
• The uterus should be maintained exteriorized during the procedure.
• The uterus is checked for presence of any abnormalities or twins prior to closing.
• Extraneous detached placenta is removed, but the placenta should be left in place if not detached.
• The uterine incision is closed in an inverting pattern (Cushings or Utrecht) using #2 absorbable suture. If the uterus is compromised, two layers are recommended, the first layer being a simple continuous pattern oversewn with an inverting pattern.
• Whenever possible the knots should be buried to prevent adhesion formation.
• The uterus is examined again for tears. The serosal surface is cleaned gently with warm

CESAREAN SECTION: BOVINE   (CONTINUED)

sterile saline the replaced into the abdomen. Aggressive use of gauze sponges on the uterine surface in this process should be avoided as this precipitates adhesion formation.
• The body is closed in three layers (the transverse abdominus and internal oblique layers in one layer followed by the external abdominal oblique) using size 2 or 3 absorbable suture material.
• The skin is closed with nonabsorbable suture in a simple continuous or Ford interlocking pattern. The ventralmost aspect of the incision is closed with 2 or 3 simple interrupted sutures to allow drainage if a postoperative incisional abscess or seroma is formed.

Ventrolateral Celiotomy
• The patient is placed in lateral or oblique-lateral recumbency after casting or placing on tilt table.
• All legs and the head of the cow should be restrained with ropes to maintain recumbency throughout the procedure.
• The uppermost back leg should be secured up and away from the abdomen. Right lateral recumbency is preferred to minimize the risk of small intestinal prolapse during surgery.
• Hair is clipped from the ventral abdomen and the area is cleaned from gross contamination.
• The incision is parallel to and lateral to the milk vein beginning approximately a hand's width caudal to the level of the umbilicus and coursing caudally.
• In dairy cattle the course of the milk vein is traced with a permanent marker as the vein will collapse the longer the animal is in lateral recumbency, and incising this vein should be avoided at all costs.
• Local anesthesia is performed using a generous lidocaine line block. The surgical site is aseptically prepared and draped.
• A linear incision is made through the skin extending through the aponeuroses of the muscle layers. The incision may need to be oriented obliquely to avoid mammary tissue caudally.
• The uterus should then be easily identified in the caudal abdomen.
• The gravid uterine horn should be exteriorized from the incision as much as possible to avoid contamination of the abdomen with uterine fluid. The uterine incision, fetal extraction, and closure are performed as described under "Standing Paralumbar Laparotomy."
• The body wall is closed in at least 3 layers using size 3 synthetic absorbable suture

material (Vicryl), due to the increased tension this incision experiences postoperatively.
• The skin can be closed in a simple continuous or Ford interlocking pattern.

MEDICATIONS
DRUGS OF CHOICE
• Anti-inflammatory: Meloxicam (1 mg/kg orally) or flunixin meglumine IV.
• Patients undergoing ventrolateral celiotomy should also be placed on broad-spectrum antibiotics for 5–7 days perioperatively.

CONTRAINDICATIONS
Appropriate milk and meat withdrawal times must be followed.

PRECAUTIONS
N/A

POSSIBLE INTERACTIONS
N/A

FOLLOW-UP
EXPECTED COURSE AND PROGNOSIS
• Dam survival rate is >80% when fetus is alive, 79% when fetus is dead and 33% when fetus is emphysematous.
• Ventrolateral celiotomies carry a less favorable prognosis because of the condition of the uterus and/or increased risk of gross contamination of the abdomen during surgery.
• Uncomplicated C-sections carry a very good prognosis for future fertility. Females may be bred after 60 days.

POSSIBLE COMPLICATIONS
• The most common complication of paralumbar laparotomy is incisional swelling with possible resultant abscess formation.
• Peritonitis is a common complication of patients undergoing ventrolateral celiotomy.
• Retained placenta is common after C-section.

CLIENT EDUCATION
• Management techniques to prevent dystocia
• Male selection for calving ease

PATIENT CARE
• Dam care
  ○ Animals should be monitored for signs of septicemia and peritonitis.
  ○ Daily monitoring includes rectal temperature, appetite, defecation, urination,

vaginal discharge, maternal behaviour, mammary development, and milk production.
• Neonatal care
  ○ Resuscitation may be necessary after delivery
  ○ Colostrum administration
  ○ Normal care

PREVENTION
N/A

MISCELLANEOUS
ASSOCIATED CONDITIONS
N/A

AGE-RELATED FACTORS
N/A

ZOONOTIC POTENTIAL
N/A

PREGNANCY
N/A

BIOSECURITY
N/A

PRODUCTION MANAGEMENT
N/A

SYNONYMS
N/A

ABBREVIATIONS
• IM = intramuscular
• IV = intravenous

SEE ALSO
• Dystocia: Bovine
• Neonatology: Beef
• Prolonged Pregnancy
• Uterine Torsion: Bovine

Suggested Reading
Fubini SL. Surgery of the uterus. In: Fubini SL, Ducharme NG eds, Farm Animal Surgery. St. Louis: Saunders Elsevier, 2004, pp. 382–7.
Newman KD. Bovine cesarean section in the field. Vet Clin North Am Food Anim Pract 2008, 24: 273–93.
Schultz LG, Tyler JW, Moll HD, Constantinescu GM. Surgical approaches for cesarean section in cattle. Can Vet J 2008, 49: 565–568

Author Jennifer A. Schleining
Consulting Editor Ahmed Tibary
Acknowledgment The author and book editors acknowledge the prior contribution of Loren G. Schultz.

BASICS

OVERVIEW
A surgical procedure involving laparotomy and hysterotomy for the removal of a fetus when obstetric manipulation is unsuccessful or impossible.

INCIDENCE/PREVALENCE
Dystocia in camelids is rare (1–5% of parturitions) but life-threatening for the dam and fetus.

GEOGRAPHIC DISTRIBUTION
Worldwide

SYSTEM AFFECTED
• Reproductive
• Other systems depending on complications

PATHOPHYSIOLOGY
• Camelids present several unique obstetric characteristics compared to ruminants. The epitheliochorial microcotyledonary placentation and short and explosive second stage labor make dystocia a life-threating condition for both the dam and fetus.
• Fetal hypoxia occurs rapidly following placental detachment and may result in death or birth of a severely compromised neonate.
• Immediate C-section in indicated in term pregnancies when a live fetus demonstrates persistent tachycardia (>130 beats/min) or bradycardia (<50 beats/min).
• The narrow pelvis and strong expulsive effort make obstetric manipulation difficult. Lengthy manipulations result in cervical laceration, necrotic vaginitis, and vaginal adhesions.
• C-section is often considered in cases of uterine torsion, uterine inertia, failure of cervical dilation, severe fetal malposition, fetal malformations, twins, and rarely oversized fetuses.

HISTORICAL FINDINGS
• Protracted first stage of labor.
• Rupture of the chorioallantois without expulsion of the fetus, or presence of fetal extremities without progression.
• Excessive abdominal contractions, straining, and rolling.
• Unsuccessful attempted assisted vaginal delivery.

SIGNALMENT
• Term pregnant female. It important to remember that gestation length is extremely variable in camelids.
• Both multiparous and maiden females are equally represented.

PHYSICAL EXAMINATON FINDINGS
• Physical examination of the dam must be performed quickly and efficiently.
• Females may present with tachycardia, tachypnea, and sometimes diarrhea due to stress (camels).

• The degree of dehydration is variable but should be assessed.
• Bloody vaginal discharge may be present, particularly in cases of bilateral hip flexion.
• The mammary gland is well developed and colostrum is present.
• Diarrhea, rectal or vaginal prolapse are not uncommon in protracted cases.

GENETICS
N/A

CAUSES AND RISK FACTORS
• In one study cesarean section was performed due to dystocia (95.8% of cases) or concurrent maternal disease (4.2% of cases).
• The most common dystocia of maternal origin resulting in C-section is uterine torsion and the most common dystocia of fetal origin resulting in C-section is fetal malposition (most commonly bilateral hip flexion).
• Failure of cervical dilation may result from administration of exogenous progesterone.
• Metabolic disorders and obesity (hepatic lipidosis, hypocalcemia, etc.) predispose to uterine inertia.
• Obstetric manipulations are not possible in animals with small stature, small pelvic size, or abnormal pelvis.

DIAGNOSIS

• Fetal viability and uterine integrity should be assessed by transabdominal ultrasonography.
• A protocol of obstetric evaluation should be followed in order to determine the type of dystocia and whether C-section is indicated.
• Suspected uterine torsion must be diagnosed/confirmed by transrectal palpation.

DIFFERENTIAL DIAGNOSES
Abortion and other causes of colic if no evidence of parturition

CBC/BIOCHEMISTRY/URINALYSIS
The most common abnormalities in camelids undergoing C-section are leukophilia due to neutrophilia, elevated creatinine kinase, hypocalcemia, hyperglycemia, and elevated liver enzymes.

OTHER LABORATORY TESTS
N/A

IMAGING
Transabdominal ultrasonography for evaluation of fetal viability and uterine/placental integrity.

OTHER DIAGNOSIC PROCEDURES
N/A

PATHOLOGIC FINDINGS
Variable depending on the cause and duration of the dystocia and systemic condition of the dam at presentation.

TREATMENT

THERAPEUTIC APPROACH
• Cesarean sections can be performed on the farm if the patient is stable and the surgery is uncomplicated.
• Complicated cases should be handled in a hospital with capability of additional supportive care (i.e., fluid therapy, general anesthesia).
• Pre-surgical care includes anti-inflammatory and antibiotic therapy.
• A neonatal resuscitation kit should be available.

SURGICAL CONSIDERATIONS AND TECHNIQUES
• In SAC, both ventral midline and left paralumbar fossa approaches may be used. The left paralumbar or low flank approaches are used in camels.

Ventral Midline Approach
• Indicated in cases of uterine torsion or when the uterus is compromised.
• General anesthesia is required: Induction with propofol (0.6–2 mg/kg IV slowly to effect) and maintenance on isoflurane in oxygen.
• The animal is placed in dorsal recumbency and the ventral abdomen prepared for surgery.
• A 30 cm skin incision is made on midline starting just cranial to the mammary gland.
• The linea alba is incised and the abdominal cavity is penetrated exposing the uterus.
• The left uterine horn is exteriorized and an incision is made over the greater curvature. The fetus is exteriorized.
• The placenta is removed if already detached, otherwise it should be peeled off 2 cm from the edge of the uterine incision to avoid trapping it in the uterine closure. A continuous "whipstitch" with absorbable suture material may be used to stop bleeding before closing the uterus with a 1 or 2 layer inverting pattern (i.e., Utrecht, Cushing, Lembert) using an absorbable suture.
• The abdominal wall and skin are closed.

Left Paralumbar Flank Approach
• The female is restrained in cush position under sedation or injectable anesthesia.
  ○ SAC: butorphanol tartrate 0.05–0.1 mg/kg IM and/or diazepam 0.1–0.2 mg/kg IV, IM; or butorphanol 0.03 mg/kg, xylazine 0.3 mg/kg, ketamine 3 mg/kg, IM ○ Camels: xylazine 0.25 mg/kg IV
• Local analgesia is provided by line or inverted L block, using 2% lidocaine.
• Caudal epidural placement is helpful.
• An oblique skin incision is made parallel to the thigh making sure not to extend too low into the aponeurosis. The abdominal muscles are incised as for the bovine. Care should be taken not to penetrate the abdominal cavity with the scalpel and nick the spleen.

C

• The uterus is exteriorized by firmly grasping it around a fetal limb. The fetus is exteriorized as described for "Ventral Midline Incision."
• Abdominal closure is similar to C-section in other large animal domestic species.

MEDICATIONS

DRUGS OF CHOICE
• Sedation: Benzodiazepines (e.g., diazepam) and/or opioids (e.g., butorphanol). Avoid α_2-adrenergic agonists where possible due to their potential marked sedation/cardiovascular depression in the neonate.
• Anesthesia: Induction with propofol where possible due to more rapid metabolism and reduced depression in the neonate.
• NSAIDs prior to the surgery and postoperatively as needed.
• Broad-spectrum antibiotics for 3–5 days. The most common bacteria isolated from uterine culture include *Escherichia coli*, *Streptococcus equi zooepidemicus*, β-hemolytic streptococci, *Pseudomonas aeruginosa*, *Klebsiella pneumoniae*, and *Arcanobacterium pyogenes*. Therefore, antimicrobial selection should include both Gram-positive and Gram-negative spectrum.
• Oxytocin q4h, IM (5–7.5 IU in alpacas; 10 IU in llamas, 20 IU in camels) to prevent/manage retained placenta.
• Pain management.
• Additional supportive care: IV fluid therapy, correction of electrolyte/trace mineral imbalances, and transfaunation, may need to be considered on a case-by-case basis.

CONTRAINDICATIONS
Appropriate milk and meat withdrawal times must be followed.

PRECAUTIONS
N/A

POSSIBLE INTERACTIONS
N/A

FOLLOW-UP

EXPECTED COURSE AND PROGNOSIS
• Dam survival is high (>90%).

• Neonate survival is highly dependent on duration of dystocia and time from rupture of the allantochorion.
• Uncomplicated C-sections carry a good prognosis for future fertility.

POSSIBLE COMPLICATIONS
• Retained placenta (most common)
• Peritonitis
• Incisional infection/surgical dehiscence
• Abdominal herniation
• Toxic metritis

CLIENT EDUCATION
Recognize signs of normal parturition and early identification of signs of dystocia.

PATIENT CARE
• Dam:
  ∘ Dam should be confined to a small paddock and monitored daily through physical examination, appetite, demeanor, assessment of vaginal discharge, mothering ability, and appropriate lactation.
  ∘ Suture removal and reproductive evaluation 14 days after surgery.
  ∘ Females can be rebred after 60 days of sexual rest if no complications.
• Neonate:
  ∘ Resuscitation kit available at time of cesarean section.
  ∘ Colostrum administration.
  ∘ Physical examination to evaluate for potential congenital abnormalities.
  ∘ Daily monitoring should include through physical examination, appetite, demeanor, appropriate weight gain, ability to ambulate, nursing appropriately.

PREVENTION
N/A

MISCELLANEOUS

ASSOCIATED CONDITIONS
N/A

AGE-RELATED FACTORS
N/A

ZOONOTIC POTENTIAL
N/A

PREGNANCY
N/A

BIOSECURITY
N/A

PRODUCTION MANAGEMENT
N/A

SYNONYMS
N/A

ABBREVIATIONS
• C-section = cesarean section
• IM = intramuscular
• IU = international units
• IV = intravenous
• NSAID = nonsteroidal anti-inflammatory
• SAC = South American Camelids

SEE ALSO
• Camelid: Reproduction
• Dystocia: Camelid
• Neonatology: Camelid
• Pregnancy Toxemia: Camelid

Suggested Reading
Campbell AJ, Pearson LK, Tibary A. Cesarean section in alpacas and llamas at a referral center—technique, survival, and postoperative fertility: 24 cases (2000–2012). Clin Therio 2013, 5: 360 (abstract).
Miller BA, Brounts SH, Anderson DE, et al. Cesarean section in alpacas and llamas: 34 cases (1997–2010). J Am Vet Med Assoc 2013, 242: 670–4.
Pearson LK, Rodriguez JS, Tibary A. Uterine torsion in late gestation alpacas and llamas: 60 cases (2000–2009). Small Ruminant Res 2012, 105: 268–72.
Tibary A, Pearson LK. Reproductive emergencies in camelids. Clin Therio 2014, 6: 579–92.
Tibary A, Anouassi A. Surgery of the reproductive tract in camels. In: Skidmore L, Adams GP eds, Recent Advances in Camelid Reproduction. Ithaca, NY: International Veterinary Information Service (www.ivis.org), last updated: 17-Dec-2000; A1008.1100.
Author Alexis Campbell
Consulting Editor Ahmed Tibary

CESAREAN SECTION: SMALL RUMINANT

BASICS

OVERVIEW
Cesarean section (C-section) is a surgical procedure to remove the fetus from the uterus following laparotomy and uterotomy.

INCIDENCE/PREVALENCE
• C-section is the most common abdominal surgery performed in small ruminants.
• About 7% of dystocia in goats are resolved by C-section.

GEOGRAPHIC DISTRIBUTION
Worldwide

SYSTEM AFFECTED
• Reproductive
• Multisystemic depending on complications

PATHOPHYSIOLOGY
• C-section is indicated when other obstetric manipulations to resolve a dystocia are not possible.
• The most common indications are:
  ○ Failure of cervical dilation (ringwomb)
  ○ Irreducible vaginal prolapse
  ○ Fetopelvic disproportion
  ○ Fetal maldisposition, emphysema, or other abnormalities
  ○ Uterine torsion
  ○ Vulvovestibular stricture
  ○ Metabolic compromise (i.e., pregnancy toxemia, hypocalcemia) and uterine inertia

HISTORICAL FINDINGS
• If breeding date is not available, term pregnancy may be estimated form history (mating period), and presence of colostrum
• Signs of parturition without progression
• Excessive abdominal contraction/straining
• Unsuccessful obstetric manipulations

SIGNALMENT
Pregnant females at term

PHYSICAL EXAMINATON FINDINGS
• Depend on duration of the dystocia and manipulation attempts. Vocalization, elevated heart and respiratory rates are common. Abdominal contraction and tenesmus are common. Dehydration is present in protracted cases.
• Mammary gland development and presence of colostrum.
• Dilated and edematous vulva if parturition has progressed to the second stage.
• Presence of discharge or fetal parts at the vulva.
• Vaginal speculum and manual vaginal palpation is performed to determine cervical dilation status and fetal disposition.

GENETICS
• Small breeds (Pigmy goats) and prolific breeds (Romanov and Finnsheep) are more predisposed
• Meat breeds (selective breeding of heavily muscled animals)

CAUSES AND RISK FACTORS
• C-section is the best approach for resolving dystocia if obstetric manipulation is not possible, particularly if the fetus(es) are alive.
• Ventral wall defect (hernia, prepubic tendon rupture).

DIAGNOSIS

DIFFERENTIAL DIAGNOSES
Abortion should be ruled out from history and physical examination.

CBC/BIOCHEMISTRY/URINALYSIS
• Performed in severely compromised/valuable females. Electrolyte imbalances, hypocalcemia, hypophosphatemia, and elevated liver enzymes are common with pregnancy toxaemia.
• At a minimum, a PCV and TP should be obtained prior to surgery in animals that appear dehydrated.

OTHER LABORATORY TESTS
N/A

IMAGING
Percutaneous transabdominal ultrasonography should be performed in order to evaluate fetal viability and uterine integrity if the cervix is closed.

DIAGNOSIC PROCEDURES
N/A

PATHOLOGIC FINDINGS
Vary depending on the cause of dystocia. Large offspring syndrome is encountered in pregnancies from somatic cell nuclear transfer cloned embryos.

TREATMENT

THERAPEUTIC APPROACH
• C-section may be performed on the farm without need of hospitalization if the patient is stable and the surgery is uncomplicated.
• Complicated cases should be handled in a hospital setting with capability of support (fluid therapy, pain management).

SURGICAL CONSIDERATIONS AND TECHNIQUES
• Small ruminant cesarean section may be done in a hospital setting or on the farm. Clear communication with the clients should include outcome for the dam and fetuses on a case by case basis.
• If surgery is performed on the farm, adequate clean area and help are needed.
• A neonatal resuscitation kit should be available.
• Instrumentation:
  ○ Iodine-based surgical scrub
  ○ 4 sterile towels
  ○ Complete small surgical tray for abdominal surgery
  ○ 4 obstetric straps
  ○ Suture material
  ○ Bucket with antiseptic for the obstetric straps.
• General anesthesia, local anesthesia with light sedation or a combination of general and local anesthesia can be used in sheep and goats.
• Usually a light sedation with xylazine (0.07 mg/kg BW, IM) in addition to a local block with 1% lidocaine (line, inverted "L" or paravertebral blocks) and physical restraint is enough to keep the animal recumbent during the surgery. Anesthesia can be also achieved successfully by lumbosacral or sacrococcygeal epidural in association with a local block.
• Two approaches can be considered: ventral midline or left paralumbar flank technique.

Left Paralumbar Flank Approach
• The left flank is clipped and scrubbed and an inverted L-block is performed with 1% lidocaine.
• The area is draped. A 15–20 cm incision is made through the skin. The external and internal abdominal oblique and transversus abdominis are dissected and gridded or incised with Metzenbaum scissors. The peritoneum is identified and incised using Metzenbaum scissors.
• The abdominal cavity is explored and the uterus identified. The uterine horn is grasped around the fetus and brought to the incision. A stab incision is made between the fetal claws and the uterus is opened with Metzenbaum scissors along the greater curvature. The fetus is removed. Fetus in the other horn is removed through the same incision.
• The placenta is only removed if it is not firmly attached to the uterus.
• The uterine incision is closed with absorbable suture in an inverting pattern (e.g., Utrecht, Cushing, and Lambert).
• The peritoneum and transversus abdominis are closed in a simple continuous pattern with absorbable suture.
• The internal abdominal oblique and the external abdominal oblique are each closed with a simple continous pattern with absorbable suture.
• The skin is closed with a nonabsorbable suture using a Ford interlocking pattern.

Ventral Midline Approach
• This approach offers a better exposure of the uterus but requires general anesthesia or deeper analgesia with better restraint. It should be considered in cases of uterine torsion, uterine rupture or fetal emphysema.
• The patient is placed in dorsal recumbency and prepared for surgery. A skin incision is made just cranial to the mammary gland and extending 20–30 cm towards the umbilical scar.
• The linea alba is incised and the uterus is exposed. Other steps are similar to the flank

C

approach. The linea alba is closed with absorbable suture and the skin is closed according to surgeon's preference.

MEDICATIONS

DRUGS OF CHOICE
• Xylazine (0.05–0.2 mg/kg, IM) and butorphanol (0.2–0.5 mg/kg, IM) provide an excellent option for a deeper sedation.
• General anesthesia may be obtained with xylazine (0.1 mg/kg BW, IM) followed by ketamine (4–8 mg/kg BW, IM).
• Lidocaine 1% is used for local desensitization of the incision site.
• NSAID may be administered as necessary.
• Multiple broad-spectrum antibiotics to prevent peritonitis and other septic conditions (penicillin 22,000 IU/kg SQ or IM q12h for 7 days).
• Energy and mineral supplementation (calcium, magnesium, phosphorus) may be indicated in some cases.
• Oxytocin administration (5–10 IU) a few hours post-surgery is suggested to promote uterine involution and placental delivery.

CONTRAINDICATIONS
• Small ruminants are very sensitive to xylazine, with unpredictable effects, but antipamezole is effective in reversing the effects of xylazine.
• Goats are more sensitive to lidocaine and xylazine than are sheep.
• Appropriate milk and meat withdrawal times must be followed.

PRECAUTIONS
Lidocaine dose should be closely monitored to avoid toxicity (sheep: 10 mg/kg; goats: 5 mg/kg).

POSSIBLE INTERACTIONS
N/A

FOLLOW-UP

EXPECTED COURSE AND PROGNOSIS
• Dam survival rate is higher than 90% when foetuses are fresh but drops to 50% when fetus(es) are autolyzed

• Uncomplicated c-sections carry a very good prognosis for future fertility. Females may be bred after 60 days
• Females with failure of cervical dilation, or severely compromised uterus should be culled after they wean their offsprings

POSSIBLE COMPLICATIONS
• Peritonitis
• Incision site infection and dehiscence
• Retained placenta
• Toxic metritis

CLIENT EDUCATION
• Management techniques to prevent dystocia
  ◦ Breeding age and weight
  ◦ Pregnancy diagnosis and fetal numbering
  ◦ Feeding strategy
  ◦ Male selection
• Early identification of signs of dystocia and need for veterinary assistance

PATIENT CARE
• Dam care
  ◦ On the farm, the patient should be confined for a few days to a warm, clean area and monitored.
  ◦ Animals should be monitored for signs of septicemia and peritonitis.
  ◦ Daily monitoring includes rectal temperature, appetite, defecation, urination, vaginal discharge, maternal behaviour, mammary development and milk production.
  ◦ Transfaunation is indicated in animals that are anorexic.
• Neonatal care
  ◦ Resuscitation may be necessary after delivery
  ◦ Colostrum administration
  ◦ Normal care

PREVENTION
• Culling strategies and genetic selection
• Proper BCS and appropriate diet during pregnancy based on fetal numbers

MISCELLANEOUS

ASSOCIATED CONDITIONS
N/A

AGE-RELATED FACTORS
C-sections are more common in primiparous animals.

ZOONOTIC POTENTIAL
N/A

PREGNANCY
N/A

BIOSECURITY
N/A

PRODUCTION MANAGEMENT
See "Prevention"

SYNONYMS
N/A

ABBREVIATIONS
• IM = intramuscular
• IU = international units
• IV = intravenous
• PCV = packed cell volume
• TP = total protein

SEE ALSO
• Dystocia: Small Ruminant
• Neonatology: Caprine
• Neonatology: Ovine (see www.fiveminutevet.com/ruminant)
• Pregnancy Toxemia: Small Ruminant

Suggested Reading
Brounts SH, Hawkins JF, Baird AN, Clickman LT. Outcome and subsequent fertility of sheep and goats undergoing cesarean section because of dystocia: 110 cases (1981 to 2001). J Am Med Assoc 2004, 224: 275–9.
Ennen S, Scholz M, Voigt K, Failing K, Wehrend A. Puerperal development of ewes following dystocia: a retrospective analysis of two approaches to cesarean section. Vet Rec 2013, doi: 10.1136/vr.101370.
Tibary A, Pearson LK, Van Metre DC, et al. Surgery of the sheep and goat reproductive system and urinary tract. In: Fubini S, Ducharme N eds, Farm Animal Surgery, 2nd ed. Elsevier, 2016, pp. 571–9.
Author Michela Ciccarelli
Consulting Editor Ahmed Tibary

BASICS

OVERVIEW
Chlamydophila abortus is an important cause of abortion in small ruminants around the world. *Chlamydophila pecorum* is a sporadic cause of polyarthritis and conjunctivitis in ruminants. These agents may rarely be associated with pneumonia, enteritis, or encephalomyelitis in individual animals.

INCIDENCE/PREVALENCE
Chlamydophila abortus is a leading cause of third-trimester abortion in small ruminants.
• High rates of abortion (abortion storms) are common when the pathogen is introduced to naïve flocks or herds.
• *C. abortus* causes sporadic third-term abortion in cattle, or abortion outbreaks after 90 days' gestation in sheep and goats.
• In flocks or herds where disease is endemic, a lower rate of abortion occurs, primarily affecting young animals and new introductions.

GEOGRAPHIC DISTRIBUTION
Disease has been reported in most parts of the world

SYSTEMS AFFECTED
• Reproductive
• Ophthalmic
• Musculoskeletal

PATHOPHYSIOLOGY
Death of the fetus occurs primarily due to placentitis, although in utero infection of the fetus can also occur, contributing to fetal death or the birth of infected and clinically ill neonates.

SIGNALMENT AND CLINICAL SIGNS
• All naïve animals are susceptible, but reliable immunity that develops after abortion generally prevents future abortions.
• In a newly infected sheep flock, between 30% and 60% of the pregnant animals may abort. Storms of 60–90% abortions in goats have been reported.
• In an endemic herd or flock, the animals in their first gestation or naïve new introductions are at highest risk to abort.
• Polyarthritis, pneumonia, enteritis, or encephalomyelitis are generally limited to young stock. Conjunctivitis can occur in animals of all ages.

DIAGNOSIS

DIFFERENTIAL DIAGNOSIS
Causes of third-term or late gestation abortion associated with placentitis include toxoplasmosis, Q fever, *Campylobacter jejuni* or *C. fetus fetus*, brucellosis, listeriosis, salmonellosis, aspergillosis, and leptospirosis.

OTHER DIAGNOSTIC PROCEDURES
• Paired serology can indicate a rising titer after recent infection; serologic tests used include complement fixation (CF) and ELISA.
• Ruminants can exhibit titers without clinical disease.
• In most laboratories, CF titers of 1:16 to 1:32 are considered positive. Most animals that have aborted from chlamydiosis will have a titer of 1:80 or higher that peaks 2–3 weeks after abortion.
• Serology is generally not useful for individual animal diagnosis, or identification of latently infected animals.
• Serologic cross reaction between *C. abortus* and *C. pecorum* may complicate diagnosis.
• The agent is difficult to isolate so culture is not routinely used for diagnosis.
• Cytology using impression smears of affected placentas may reveal elementary bodies; these are most easily seen by staining with modified Ziehl-Neelsen or Gimenez stains.

PATHOLOGIC FINDINGS
• Placenta: dark red or gray-brown cotyledons, leathery or opaque intercotyledonary areas.
• Fetus: usually fresh but may be autolyzed. Often excess fluid is seen in the abdominal cavity, as are small necrotic foci in the liver.
• Histopathologic evaluation of placentas with special staining to identify organisms may also be diagnostic.

TREATMENT

THERAPEUTIC APPROACH
After the initial outbreak, good management techniques combined with judicious use of antibiotics should reduce the rate of abortion to negligible levels.

MEDICATIONS

DRUGS OF CHOICE
• Abortions—various protocols suggested
  ○ Long-acting oxytetracycline (OTC) (20 mg/kg) at 10–14-day intervals from midgestation until parturition.
  ○ 400–500 mg OTC/head/day orally.
• General chlamydiosis
  ○ Single dose of long-acting OTC (20 mg/kg).
  ○ Three treatments at 3-day intervals has also been suggested.

FOLLOW-UP

EXPECTED COURSE AND PROGNOSIS
• After the initial outbreak, good management techniques combined with judicial use of

antibiotics and/or vaccines should reduce the rate of abortion to negligible levels.
• Animals that have aborted are generally immune from further abortions.

POSSIBLE COMPLICATIONS
• Following abortion some ewes or does may have retained placenta.
• Perinatally infected neonates may be weak with pneumonia or infection in other organ systems.

PREVENTION
• Vaccines given prior to breeding will significantly reduce abortion but do not eliminate the carrier state or excretion.
• In various parts of the world, different vaccines are available which may be used to limit disease.
• In the midst of an abortion storm, treatment with tetracycline in feed or by injection may help to decrease fetal loss.
• All aborting animals should be segregated from the flock to prevent transmission to other stock. In some herds, individuals which have experienced abortion have been culled.
• Aborted fetuses, placental membranes, bedding, and other contaminated materials should be removed and destroyed.
• As animals that aborted may continue to excrete the organism for several weeks, breeding rams that have been with them should not have access to other clean stock.
• Abortion can be prevented by feeding tetracycline or periodic treatment with long-acting tetracycline by injection in the last 4–6 weeks of gestation.

MISCELLANEOUS

ASSOCIATED CONDITIONS
Rarely, other diseases including conjunctivitis, polyarthritis, pneumonia, enteritis, or encephalomyelitis can be associated with infection by *Chlamydophila abortus* or *Chlamydophila pecorum*.

ZOONOTIC POTENTIAL
• *C. abortus* may cause abortion in pregnant women who should, therefore, not work in a flock with this disease.
• The avirulent live vaccine used in some parts of the world may be zoonotic.

PREGNANCY
High rates of abortion (abortion storms) are common when the pathogen is introduced to naïve flocks or herds.

BIOSECURITY
• All aborting animals should be segregated from the flock to prevent transmission to other stock. In some herds, individuals which have experienced abortion have been culled.
• Aborted fetuses, placental membranes, bedding, and other contaminated materials should be removed and destroyed.

CHLAMYDIOSIS

• As animals that aborted may continue to excrete the organism for several weeks, breeding rams that have been with them should not have access to other clean stock.

PRODUCTION MANAGEMENT
Vaccines given prior to breeding will significantly reduce abortion but do not eliminate the carrier state or excretion.

SYNONYMS
• Enzootic abortion of ewes (EAE)
• Ovine enzootic abortion

ABBREVIATION
OTC = oxytetracycline

SEE ALSO
• Abortion: Small Ruminant
• Aspergillosis
• Brucellosis
• Campylobacter
• Leptospirosis
• Listeriosis
• Q Fever
• Salmonellosis

Suggested Reading
Rodolakis A, Laroucau K. Chlamydiaceae and chlamydial infections in sheep or goats. Vet Microbiol 2015, 181: 107–18.

Stuen S, Longbottom D. Treatment and control of chlamydial and rickettsial infections in sheep and goats. Vet Clin North Am Food Anim Pract 2011, 27: 213–33.
Author Amelia Woolums
Consulting Editor Christopher C.L. Chase
Acknowledgment The author and book editors acknowledge the prior contribution of Michael D. Bernstein and Tina Wismer.

CLOSTRIDIAL DISEASE: GASTROINTESTINAL

BASICS

OVERVIEW
Clostridium perfringens is an important cause of enteric diseases in ruminants. Its virulence is based largely upon toxinogenesis.

INCIDENCE/PREVALENCE
Clostridial enterotoxemia is sporadic, but outbreaks have been reported.

GEOGRAPHIC DISTRIBUTION
• Types A, C, and D are considered a problem in North America.
• Type B is frequently reported in Europe, Africa, and Asia.
• Type E has rarely reported in North America.

SYSTEMS AFFECTED
• Digestive
• Cardiovascular
• Nervous

PATHOPHYSIOLOGY
• Clostridia form part of the gastrointestinal tract of many normal ruminants and can also be found in many soils.
• Factors favoring intestinal clostridial bacteria overgrowth, such as high-carbohydrate diets, result in rapid toxin production with subsequent clinical signs and death.
• Clinical signs depend on the predominate type of toxin produced although there is considerable crossover.
• Clinical isolates are assigned to one of the types (A, B, C, D, E) on the basis of production of the major toxins (*alpha, beta, epsilon and iota*).
• Strains of *C. perfringens* can also produce other recognized soluble antigens of pathogenic importance such as enterotoxin (CPE) and beta-2-toxin.
• *Alpha-toxin (type A)* is a phospholipase that causes lysis of the red blood cells, platelets and leukocytes, vascular permeability through endothelial damage. In the intestines, the toxin causes necrosis and hypersecretion of fluid into the lumen.
• *Beta-toxin (types B and C)*, a trypsin-sensitive toxin, is a potent cytotoxin causing necrosis and hemorrhage of affected tissues, especially the intestine.
• *Epsilon-toxin (types B and D)* alters intestinal mucosal permeability that facilitates absorption into the bloodstream. The toxin subsequently causes widespread vascular damage and increased vascular permeability. Vascular damage in the brain results in characteristic perivascular edema and focal symmetrical encephalomalacia.

SIGNALMENT
• All ruminant species
• Young animals more susceptible

PHYSICAL EXAMINATION FINDINGS
• *C. perfringens* type A is associated with hemorrhagic bowel disease (HBS; jejunal hemorrhagic syndrome) in high-producing dairy cattle. Clinical signs—decreased milk production, scant feces, and colic. Feces can contain partially digested or clotted blood. Rectal examination—distended loops of small intestine.
• In sheep, type A is associated acute enterotoxemia in lambs (yellow lamb disease). Clinical signs—depression, anemia, icterus and hemoglobinuria. Animals usually die within 6–12 h of the onset. In calves, limited reports have associated type A with abomasitis.
• In camelids, type A can cause neonatal enterotoxemia. Clinical signs—severe depression, colic, and sudden death. Diarrhea can be seen if the cria survive >12 h.
• In small ruminants, type B has been associated with lamb dysentery and hemorrhagic enteritis in young animals, whereas type C has been associated with struck in adult sheep. Types B and C produce similar clinical signs including sudden death or acute neurologic signs with or without hemorrhagic diarrhea. In calves, type C has been associated with acute fatal hemorrhagic enteritis in young calves.
• Type D is associated with enterotoxemia (overeating disease) affecting young ruminants. Clinical signs—profuse and bloody diarrhea, ataxia, trembling, stiff limbs, opisthotonus, convulsion, coma and death.
• Regardless of the type, many cases are simply found dead. If affected animals are found alive, most cases present with colic and/or neurologic signs such as convulsions and opisthotonus before death.

CAUSES AND RISK FACTORS
• *Clostridium perfringens* types A, B, C, and D.
• Sudden change of diet—usually from milk/forage to grain, high-grain diet, or offspring of dams that produce abundant milk.
• Ingestion of protein-rich diet in a protease-deficient intestinal tract allows rapid growth of *C. perfringens* organisms.
• Inconsistent feeding practices—feed changes, temperature, mixing, frequency, volume.
• The healthy, rapidly growing young ruminant is most at risk.
• Copper deficiency.
• Heavy tapeworm infestation in sheep.
• Cold weather.
• Stress.
• Concomitant infestation with coccidia.

DIAGNOSIS

C

DIFFERENTIAL DIAGNOSES
• Causes of acute death—anthrax, various poisonings
• Abomasal diseases
• Salmonellosis
• Leptospirosis
• Polioencephalomalacia

CBC/BIOCHEMISTRY/URINALYSIS
• Leukopenia and neutropenia—enterotoxemia.
• Hemoconcentration, metabolic acidosis, hyperglycemia, and glucosuria—lambs with type D enterotoxemia.
• Hyperglycemia, hyponatremia, hypochloremia, and hypokalemia—cattle with HBS.

OTHER LABORATORY TESTS
• Culture and impression smears
• Toxin identification essential for diagnosis

IMAGING
Cattle suffering from HBS—transabdominal ultrasound can reveal distension of small intestine and homogeneous echogenic intraluminal material compatible with intraluminal hemorrhage and clot formation.

OTHER DIAGNOSTIC PROCEDURES
• History, physical examination, gross postmortem examination.
• *C. perfringens* proliferates after death and can invade tissues beyond the gut. Thus, isolation of the bacteria in a postmortem sample is not sufficient basis for a diagnosis.
• Detection of the toxin in intestinal content and histopathologic lesion compatible with the disease are essential for the diagnosis.
• ELISA and counter-immunoelectrophoresis tests for toxins are comparable to the traditional mouse lethality tests.
• Intestinal fluid for toxin evaluation should be frozen until testing.

PATHOLOGIC FINDINGS
• Type A—watery blood, icterus, hemoglobinuria, excessive fluid in abdominal and thoracic cavities, and evidence of hemorrhages on thoracic and abdominal viscera.
• Type B—inflammation, ulceration, and necrosis of the intestinal tract, liver, and adjacent lymphatic.
• Type C—acute hemorrhagic enteritis, bloody diarrhea can be present at death. Swollen and hemorrhagic mesenteric lymph nodes.
• Type D—paintbrush hemorrhages of the subendocardium of the left ventricle are most typical and hydropericardium.

CLOSTRIDIAL DISEASE: GASTROINTESTINAL (CONTINUED)

TREATMENT

THERAPEUTIC APPROACH
• Response to treatment is usually poor.
• Animals with right-sided bloat will benefit from relieving the distention in the abomasum.
• Anecdotal evidence suggests that oral antibiotics such as penicillin or tetracycline can be beneficial.
• Type C and D antitoxin can be beneficial (see below).
• Activated charcoal and mineral oil—anecdotal evidence.
• Fluid therapy. (See chapters, Diarrheal Diseases: Bovine, Diarrheal Diseases: Camelid, Diarrheal Diseases: Small Ruminant for details.)
• If at all possible, eliminate oral nutrition during the first hours of treatment.

MEDICATIONS

DRUGS OF CHOICE
• Procaine penicillin G at doses of 20,000–30,000 IU/kg, IM or SC q12h.
• Type C and D antitoxin can be beneficial at doses ranging from 3 mL in lambs to 30 mL in adult cattle. IV or SC administration. Dosages can be repeated q3–4h.

CONTRAINDICATIONS
Appropriate milk and meat withdrawal times must be followed.

PRECAUTIONS
Type C and D antitoxin—anaphylactoid reactions can occur.

FOLLOW-UP

EXPECTED COURSE AND PROGNOSIS
• The prognosis is fair at best for ambulatory patients. If the patient is recumbent, the prognosis is guarded to grave.
• The prognosis for affected cows with JHS is grave, even with aggressive medical and surgical therapy.
• Mortality approaches 100% regardless of type.

PREVENTION
• Passive transfer of immunity protects against *C. perfringens* types C and D.
• Vaccination strategies should take into consideration the necessity for a booster vaccination approximately 4 weeks after the first vaccination.
• Vaccination of the dams in late gestation using the type C and D toxoid.
• The type C and D toxoid could protect against type B due to overlap of toxins.
• Neonates can be vaccinated as early as 10 days of age and 2 weeks later.
• Outbreaks—antitoxin can be administered to neonates at birth if necessary.
• Preventive measures for type A diseases include proper animal husbandry, sanitation, and feeding (avoid excessive milk intake).
• *C. perfringens* type A autogenous bacterins are being used in many herds with HBS but it is unlikely that a bacterin without toxoid will prevent the disease.
• Vaccines for type B appear to be useful in countries in which the disease occurs.

MISCELLANEOUS

AGE-RELATED FACTORS
Young ruminants, although adults can be affected.

BIOSECURITY
• Environmental hygiene. Cleaning and disinfection of environmental sites.
• Hand and outerwear hygiene. Wash hands and disinfect boots, maintain coveralls free of fecal material.
• Segregating sick animals will reduce the pathogen exposure.
• Clostridial diseases are not spread from animal to animal.
• Carcasses should be disposed of properly by burial or incineration.

PRODUCTION MANAGEMENT
• Consistent feeding practices—adaptation before change.
• Appropriate fiber length, storage, and fermentation of total mixed ration.
• Prevent the occurrence of rumen acidosis.

SYNONYMS
• *C. perfringens* type A in cows; hemorrhagic bowel disease (HBS; jejunal hemorrhagic syndrome JHS)

• *C. perfringens* type A associated acute enterotoxemia in lambs; yellow lamb disease
• *C. perfringens* type B in young animals; lamb dysentery and hemorrhagic enteritis
• *C. perfringens* type C in adult sheep; struck
• *C. perfringens* types C in young calves; acute fatal hemorrhagic enteritis
• *C. perfringens* type D in young ruminants; enterotoxemia, overeating disease

ABBREVIATIONS
• ELISA = enzyme-linked immunosorbent assay
• HBS = hemorrhagic bowel syndrome
• IM = intramuscular
• IV = intravenous
• JHS = jejunal hemorrhagic syndrome
• SC = subcutaneous

SEE ALSO
• Anthrax
• Anaplasmosis
• Atypical interstitial pneumonia
• Blue-green Algae Toxicity
• Carbamate Toxicity
• Clostridial Diseases-Nervous System
• *Histophilus somni* Complex
• Lightening Strike
• Nitrate and Nitrate Toxicosis
• Oleander and Cardiotoxic Plant Toxicity
• Organophosphate toxicity
• Salmonellosis
• Vitamin B Deficiency

Suggested Reading
Dennison AC, VanMetre DC, Callan RJ, Dinsmore P, Mason GL, Ellis RP. Hemorrhagic bowel syndrome in dairy cattle: 22 cases (1997–2000). J Am Vet Med Assoc 2002, 221: 686–9.
Garcia JP, Anderson M, Blanchard P, Mete A, Uzal FA. The pathology of enterotoxemia by *Clostridium perfringens* type C in calves. J Vet Diagn Invest 2013, 25: 438–42.
Kirino Y, Tanida M, Hasunuma H, Kato T, Horii Y, Nonaka N. Increase of *Clostridium perfringens* in association with Eimeria in haemorrhagic enteritis in Japanese beef cattle. Vet Rec 2015. doi: 10.1136/vr.103237.
Uzal FA, Songer JG. Diagnosis of *Clostridium perfringens* intestinal infections in sheep and goats. J Vet Diagn Invest 2008, 20: 253–65.
Author Diego Gomez-Nieto
Consulting Editor Christopher C.L. Chase
Acknowledgment The author and book editors acknowledge the prior contribution of Jerry R. Roberson.

CLOSTRIDIAL DISEASE: MUSCULAR

BASICS

OVERVIEW
Clostridial myositis is a term used to describe two diseases (blackleg and gas gangrene) characterized by a rapid course of myonecrosis and sometimes cellulitis, and high mortality.

INCIDENCE/PREVALENCE
• The incidence is usually low (generally <10%), but lethality (death of affected animals) is always close to 100%. Infrequently, outbreaks of gas gangrene associated with the use of contaminated medical instruments can present with a very high incidence.
• Some herds may go for many years without clostridial myositis cases.
• Most cases of blackleg are seen in the late summer to early winter.
• Cases of gas gangrene may occur any time during the year.

GEOGRAPHIC DISTRIBUTION
Worldwide

SYSTEMS AFFECTED
• Musculoskeletal
• Integument

PATHOPHYSIOLOGY
• Endogenous pathogenesis (blackleg): Spores are ingested, absorbed into the bloodstream and phagocytized by macrophages of skeletal and/or cardiac muscles. The spores can survive for several months in the cytoplasm of the macrophages, but when an area of muscle becomes anaerobic, usually associated with blunt trauma, the spores germinate and the bacteria proliferate and produce exotoxins that produce local necrosis and toxemia.
• Exogenous pathogenesis (gas gangrene; formerly known as malignant edema): Spores enter the organism via skin or mucosal wounds and proliferate in the anaerobic environment produced by those same injuries. Bacterial proliferation and toxin production ensues as described for blackleg.

SIGNALMENT
• Blackleg is typically a disease of young cattle (6 months to 2 years of age), although cases can sporadically occur in animals outside this age range. Rare cases have been reported in sheep.
• Gas gangrene can occur in several animal species (cattle, sheep, goats, pigs, horses, dogs) of any age.

PHYSICAL EXAMINATION FINDINGS
• Blackleg: Most cases are characterized by sudden death. When clinical signs are observed, they include depression, lethargy, anorexia, and reluctance to move, which is quickly followed by death. When superficial muscles are affected, swelling and crepitation of the affected area is evident associated with lameness, most commonly in rear legs. Signs of congestive heart failure may be seen when the heart is affected.
• Gas gangrene: Most cases are acute; subacute and chronic cases can occasionally occur. Clinical signs are similar to those of blackleg, except that skin or mucosal wounds are usually present.

CAUSES AND RISK FACTORS
• Blackleg: *Clostridium chauvoei*
• Gas gangrene: *Clostridium septicum*, *Clostridium chauvoei*, *Clostridium sordellii*, *Clostridium perfringens* type A, *Clostridium novyi* type A, acting alone or in combination of two or more of these microorganisms.
• The organisms survive as spores in the environment. The spores can gain access to the organism by ingestion as in the case of blackleg (endogenous pathogenesis) or via skin or mucosal wounds in cases of gas gangrene (exogenous pathogenesis).
• Animals on high planes of nutrition and in excellent body condition are most likely to develop blackleg.
• No relationship with nutritional level has been found for cases of gas gangrene.
• Unvaccinated herds are most at risk for both diseases.

DIAGNOSIS

DIFFERENTIAL DIAGNOSES
Conditions that result in sudden death in ruminants should be considered as differentials. These include, but are not limited to, gunshot, anthrax, snake bite, toxic plants (oleander, Japanese yew, others), various toxicants (lead, arsenic), nitrate and cyanide poisoning.

CBC/BIOCHEMISTRY/URINALYSIS
Of little benefit

OTHER DIAGNOSTIC PROCEDURES
• Presumptive field diagnosis may be based on characteristic signs and gross lesions. Impression smears of affected tissues or fluids showing large Gram-positive, sporulated rods is helpful, particularly in fresh carcasses.
• Confirmation of the diagnosis must be based on demonstration in affected tissues of the clostridial species involved. This can be achieved by anaerobic culture, PCR, fluorescent antibody testing or immunohistochemistry.

PATHOLOGIC FINDINGS
• Necropsy reveals areas of dark muscle necrosis and subcutaneous edema. In blackleg, the muscular lesions are more significant than those in the subcutaneous tissue and they frequently affect both skeletal and cardiac muscle.
• Gas gangrene is characterized by subcutaneous lesions with less prominent and inconsistent skeletal muscle lesions. In blackleg the affected muscle may have an odor of rancid butter.

TREATMENT

THERAPEUTIC APPROACH
• Because most cases of blackleg and gas gangrene in ruminants are acute, there is frequently not enough time to start treatment.
• Course permitting, procaine penicillin G (PPG) is very effective against the clostridial species involved in these diseases.
• Anti-inflammatory drugs, fluid therapy, and incisions of the skin over the affected muscles to drain exudates and gas, and washing these wounds with hydrogen peroxide and iodine solution is also recommended in valuable animals.

SURGICAL CONSIDERATIONS AND TECHNIQUES
Serial fasciotomy of affected areas to allow aeration and drainage.

MEDICATIONS

DRUGS OF CHOICE
• Procaine penicillin G (PPG) at high doses (24,000 IU/kg), IM.
• Many other antimicrobials may be effective but penicillin is the drug of choice.
• Anti-inflammatory drugs may be administered for pain, shock, and inflammation.

CONTRAINDICATIONS
• Because of the poor prognosis, humane euthanasia should be considered. Slaughter is usually not an option.
• Drug withdrawal time must be determined and maintained for the treated animal.

FOLLOW-UP

EXPECTED COURSE AND PROGNOSIS
Prognosis is guarded to grave at best. Even if the animal survives, it may be permanently disabled.

CLIENT EDUCATION
The most important client education is to convey the need to vaccinate the whole herd preventively.

PREVENTION
• Vaccinate all young stock (<2 years of age) at least twice a year against blackleg and for the life of the animal against gas gangrene. The first vaccination in the life of an animal should be followed by a booster 4–6 weeks later. Protective immunity usually occurs by 2 weeks post-vaccination.

CLOSTRIDIAL DISEASE: MUSCULAR   (CONTINUED)

C

• Vaccinate cows in late gestation to boost colostral immunity for neonates that will not be vaccinated until the next cattle working period.
• When faced with an outbreak, vaccinate all susceptible stock and administer PPG at the same time in an attempt to prevent further cases while waiting for protective titers to develop.
• Vaccines are economical and efficacious.
• Carcasses should be burnt or buried deeply and covered with lime as they represent concentrated areas of clostridial spores.

 MISCELLANEOUS

AGE-RELATED FACTORS
Blackleg appears to be most common among young ruminants between 6 months and 2 years of age. Gas gangrene can occur at any time in the life of an animal.

ZOONOTIC POTENTIAL
Several of the clostridial species involved in gas gangrene may infect humans, particularly if they are immunocompromised.

PRODUCTION MANAGEMENT
Vaccination should help prevent clinical disease.

SYNONYMS
• Black leg: black quarter, clostridial myositis
• Gas gangrene: malignant edema (this term should be abandoned)

ABBREVIATIONS
• IM = intramuscularly
• PCR = polymerase chain reaction
• PPG = procaine penicillin G

SEE ALSO
• Anthrax
• Arsenic Toxicosis
• Cyanide Toxicosis
• Lead Toxicosis
• Management of Gunshot Wounds
• Nitrate and Nitrite Toxicosis
• Oleander and Cardiotoxic Plant Toxicity
• Snakebite
• Yew Toxicity

Suggested Reading
Bagge E, Lewerin SS, Johansson KE. Detection and identification by PCR of *Clostridium chauvoei* in clinical isolates, bovine faeces and substrates from biogas plant. Acta Vet Scand 2009, 51: 8.
De Groot B, Dewey CE, Griffin DD, et al. Effect of booster vaccination with a multivalent clostridial bacterin-toxoid on sudden death syndrome mortality rate among feedlot cattle. J Am Vet Med Assoc 1997, 211: 749–53.
Frey J, Falquet L. Patho-genetics of *Clostridium chauvoei*. Res Microbiol 2015, 166:384–92.
Groseth PK, Ersdal C, Bjelland AM, Stokstad M. Large outbreak of blackleg in housed cattle. Vet Rec 2011, 169: 339.
Kojima A, Uchida I, Sekizaki T, et al. Rapid detection and identification of *Clostridium chauvoei* by PCR based on flagellin gene sequence. Vet Microbiol 2001, 78: 363–71.

Odani JS, Blanchard PC, Adaska JM, et al. Malignant edema in postpartum dairy cattle. J Vet Diagn Invest 2009, 21: 920–4.
Snider TA, Stern AW. 2011. Pathology in practice. Myocarditis and epicarditis. J Am Vet Med Assoc 2011, 238: 1119–21.
Sojka JE, Bowersock TL, Parker JE, et al. *Clostridium chauvoei* myositis infection in a neonatal calf. J Vet Diagn Invest 1992, 4: 201–3.
Troxel TR, Burke GL, Wallace WT, et al. Clostridial vaccination efficacy on stimulating and maintaining an immune response in beef cows and calves. J Anim Sci 1997, 75: 19–25.
Troxel TR, Gadberry MS, Wallace WT, et al. Clostridial antibody response from injection-site lesions in beef cattle, long-term response to single or multiple doses, and response in newborn beef calves. J Anim Sci 2001, 79: 2558–64.
Uzal FA. Evidence-based medicine concerning efficacy of vaccination against Clostridium chauvoei infection in cattle. Vet Clin North Am Food Anim Pract 2012, 28: 71–7.
Uzal FA, Paramidani M, Assis R, et al. Outbreak of clostridial myocarditis in calves. Vet Rec 2003, 152: 134–6.
Weatherhead JE, Tweardy DJ. Lethal human neutropenic enterocolitis caused by *Clostridium chauvoei* in the United States: tip of the iceberg? J Infect 2012, 64: 225–7.

Author Francisco A. Uzal
Consulting Editor Christopher C.L. Chase

CLOSTRIDIAL DISEASE: NERVOUS SYSTEM

BASICS

OVERVIEW
The most significant clostridial nervous diseases are tetanus, botulism, and *Clostridium perfringens* type D enterotoxemia. Occasionally other clostridial diseases may manifest nervous clinical signs. Because each of these diseases are dealt with in different chapters (Clostridial Disease: Gastrointestinal, Clostridial Disease: Muscular) we present here only the most significant features of the clostridial diseases that manifest themselves as neurologic disease.

INCIDENCE/PREVALENCE
The incidence of *C. perfringens* type D enterotoxemia is usually low (generally <5%). Tetanus can present as individual cases, but large outbreaks following procedures with contaminated medical instruments have been reported. Botulism is frequently seen as large outbreaks in mammals, birds, and fish. In some areas of the world (Australia, South Africa, and South America) botulism intoxication is a fairly common occurrence and is considered an endemic problem.

GEOGRAPHIC DISTRIBUTION
• Worldwide for tetanus and *C. perfringens*.
• Various botulinum toxins (BoTx) tend to have a unique geographic distribution.
  ◦ Type B BoTx-producing organisms prefer moist neutral pH soils and commonly found in Europe and the Eastern United States.
  ◦ Type C BoTx-producing organisms prefer slightly acidic soils and commonly found in the Western United States.
  ◦ Type D BoTx-producing organisms prefer alkaline soils and commonly found in South Africa, South America, and Australia.

SYSTEMS AFFECTED
• Nervous

PATHOPHYSIOLOGY
• Tetanus occurs after wound contamination with *C. tetani* spores acquired from the environment. Deep wounds with a little exposure to air and the presence of necrotic tissue favor spore germination. This microorganism produces tetanus toxin (TeTx) and tetanolysin. TeTx is formed in wounds colonized by *C. tetani*. TeTx diffuses in the extracellular fluid and can target all types of nervous endings (sensory, adrenergic neurons and motor neurons), but it is mainly transported retrogradely through the motor neurons.
• Botulism can be caused by one of eight different neuroparalytic toxin subtypes (A to H). These botulinum neurotoxins (BoTxs) are produced by anaerobic Gram-positive clostridia, mainly *Clostridium botulinum*. Two main routes of exposure to BoTxs have been identified: (1) ingestion of preformed toxins

in food, water, or carrion, and (2) in vivo production of BoTxs, so-called toxicoinfection, and is encountered during wound botulism. After diffusion into the extracellular fluid and bloodstream, BoTXs target motor neuron endings. The toxin attaches to the nerve and incorporates into the nerve's cytoplasm where it acts as a metalloprotease that inactivates proteins needed to release the neurotransmitter acetylcholine. Each BoTx affects different areas of the docking proteins needed for the release of acetylcholine. Prevention of neurotransmitter (acetylcholine) release at the neuromuscular junction results in muscle weakness and paralysis.
• *Clostridium perfringens* type D enterotoxemia: This microorganism produces epsilon prototoxin which is proteolytically activated in the intestine. After facilitating its own absorption into the bloodstream, epsilon toxin reaches several internal organs including the brain, where there is vascular damage and also direct action on brain cells, including neurons, astrocytes, and oligodendrocytes.

SIGNALMENT
• Tetanus occurs in multiple species of mammal of any age.
• Botulism occurs in cattle, goats, sheep and in several other mammalian, avian and fish species. Most cases involve adult or young growing animals. Cattle are very sensitive to the toxins (13 times more than mice to BoTx C).
• *C. perfringens* type D enterotoxemia affects mostly sheep and goats and, occasionally, cattle. Most cases occur in animals >2 weeks of age.

PHYSICAL EXAMINATION FINDINGS
Tetanus
• Stiffness and reluctance to move are often the initial signs.
• Twitching and tremors of the muscles.
• Lockjaw.
• Prominent protruding third eyelid.
• Unsteady gait with stiff, held-out tail.
• Affected cattle are usually anxious and easily excited by sudden movements or handling.
• Bloat is common because the rumen stops working.
• Later signs include collapse, lying on side with legs held stiffly out, spastic paralysis and death.

Botulism
• Clinical signs develop usually 48–72 hours after ingestion, but may appear as early as 24 hours and as late as 10–14 days, dependent on the amount of BoTx ingested.
• Animals often first present with a hunched-up appearance and strain to defecate. Owners may say that animals are colicky.
• Affected animals may be weak, stagger about, or go down. Progressive muscle

weakness (paresis) is the hallmark of the disease.
• Over the next 24–48 hours, the animals become weaker with staggering and muscle fasciculation of large muscle groups; they lean against fences or walls for support. When lying down, animals remain in sternal recumbency. Eventually, the animal becomes prostrate.
• Cattle characteristically display flaccid paralysis and occasionally protrusion of the tongue. Tongue is easily removed from the mouth. Once the tongue is released, the animals have difficulty in replacing the tongue back into the mouth. Jaw muscle tone is also reduced.
• Animals will usually lose tail tone as the disease progresses, with the tail easily handled and elevated.
• Signs in sheep and goats are similar to cattle but protrusion of the tongue may not be as obvious. They may bob their head when walking due to muscle weakness.
• Serous nasal discharge and excessive salivation common are due to loss of tongue tone and coordination. In most cases the disease is fatal although some animals may recover.
• When a large amount of toxin has been ingested, the animal may be found dead without having been seen any signs of disease

C. perfringens Type D Enterotoxemia
• Enterotoxemia progresses very rapidly, with death occurring within minutes or a few hours after onset of clinical signs.
• Sudden death may also occur.
• Some lambs will show symptoms of muscle tremors, circling, opisthotonus or convulsions.
• Other nervous system signs are frothing of the mouth, grinding of the teeth, blindness, and oscillations of the eyes. Diarrhea may also be present, although infrequently.
• In goats, the course of disease ranges from peracute to chronic, with signs that vary from watery diarrhea with or without blood to sudden death. The chronic form in goats can result in diarrhea and nervous signs over several weeks, ending in death.
• Affected calves not found dead show convulsions, blindness, and death within a few hours. Subacutely affected calves are stuporous for a few days and may recover.

CAUSES AND RISK FACTORS
• Tetanus: *Clostridium tetani* is the etiologic agent. Risk factors include deep wounds and failure to use tetanus vaccines.
• Botulism: *Clostridium botulinum* is the etiologic agent. There are eight antigenically distinct BoTx (A, B, C$_1$, D, E, F, G, and H). Each toxin is found in different environments and affects different species of animals. Rare cases of botulism in humans have been associated with some strains of *Clostridium baratii* and *Clostridium butyricum*. Risk factors include exposure to decomposed

CLOSTRIDIAL DISEASE: NERVOUS SYSTEM (CONTINUED)

C

carcasses, contaminated feed, feeding poultry litter, phosphorus-deficient diets with associated bone chewing (pica), and lack of botulism vaccination in high risk areas.
• *C. perfringens* type D enterotoxemia: *Clostridium perfringens* type D is the etiologic agent. Risk factors include sudden access to large amounts of highly fermentable carbohydrates and failure to vaccinate animals for *Clostridium perfringens* type D.

DIAGNOSIS
DIFFERENTIAL DIAGNOSES
• Conditions that result in sudden death in ruminants should be considered as differentials. These include but are not limited to gunshot, anthrax, snakebite, toxic plants (oleander, Japanese yew, others), various toxicants (gossypol, lead, arsenic, strychnine, nitrate, monensinn, and cyanide) poisoning.
• Neurologic differentials include listeriosis, rabies, bacterial and viral encephalitides, plant toxicities that cause tremor or ataxia, pesticides including organophosphates, carbamates, and ionophores.

CBC/BIOCHEMISTRY/URINALYSIS
Glycosuria may be observed in a few cases of C. perfringens type D enterotoxemia

OTHER DIAGNOSTIC PROCEDURES
• Tetanus: Clinical signs. Mouse bioassay may also be performed, but it is rarely available.
• Botulism: Clinical signs, toxin detection in feed and/or gastrointestinal content and/or liver. Feed samples from the previous 2–5 days should be evaluated for BoTx contamination. The sample should be closely examined for evidence of animal tissues present in the feed source. Animal samples to submit for BoTx testing are serum, liver, rumen content, and cecal content. Mouse bioassay is still the gold standard. Agar immunodiffusion testing and ELISA testing for the toxin can also be performed. The diagnostic value of isolation of *C. botulism* is questionable as this microorganism can be found, albeit not frequently, in the gastrointestinal content of healthy animals.
• *C. perfringens* type D enterotoxemia: Histopathology of brain (perivascular edema is diagnostic); detection of epsilon toxin in intestinal content by ELISA; PCR for detection of epsilon toxin gene is available for identification of the isolates as type D, although this does not confirm the diagnosis as this microorganism may be present in the intestine of a normal animal.

PATHOLOGIC FINDINGS
• Tetanus: usually no lesions; except for presence of deep wounds
• Botulism: usually no lesions, dilated rectum with dry content sometimes observed

• *C. perfringens* type D enterotoxemia: None or hydropericardium, a few hyperemic areas on the intestine and pulmonary edema in acute cases. Cerebellar vermis herniation and/or focal symmetrical encephalomalacia can be seen in subacute and or chronic cases. Rapid postmortem autolysis of the kidneys has led to the popular name of pulpy kidney disease; however, the diagnostic significance of this finding is questionable. Hemorrhagic or necrotic enterocolitis may be seen in goats.

TREATMENT
THERAPEUTIC APPROACH
• Tetanus: Treatment of valuable animals consists of tranquilization of the animal and tetanus antitoxin in large doses; however, treatment is often unrewarding in animals exhibiting clinical signs. Supportive treatment to prevent dehydration and starvation may need to be given for 1–4 weeks.
• Botulism: Antitoxin in valuable animals.
• *C. perfringens* type D enterotoxemia: Usually none as anti-epsilon toxin is not usually commercially available.

MEDICATIONS
DRUGS OF CHOICE
N/A

FOLLOW-UP
EXPECTED COURSE AND PROGNOSIS
For all three diseases the prognosis is poor and most animals will succumb; and euthanasia should be considered for the welfare of the animal.

PREVENTION
• Tetanus: Vaccination; avoid contamination of surgical wounds.
• Botulism: Vaccination in endemic areas; phosphorus supplementation in areas with phosphorus-deficient soils; removing carcasses from pastures; not feeding poultry litter; insure ensiled feed (rye, oat, and barley silage and hay) has been fermented correctly. No animal parts to be present in the feed.
• *C. perfringens* type D enterotoxemia: Vaccination; avoid sudden changes to diets rich in highly fermentable carbohydrates.

MISCELLANEOUS
ZOONOTIC POTENTIAL
Botulism: Since this is an intracellular toxin bound to the nerves, minimal risk to

individuals working with affected animals. Affected animals should be disposed of by burial or rendering. Animals should not be sent to slaughter for human consumption. Evidence of milk contamination with the toxin from intoxicated cows has been inconclusive.

PRODUCTION MANAGEMENT
See "Prevention"

SYNONYMS
• Tetanus—lockjaw
• Botulism—loin disease, bulbar paralysis, lamsiekte
• *C. perfringens* type D enterotoxemia—pulpy kidney disease, overeating disease

ABBREVIATIONS
• BoTx = Botulinum toxin
• ELISA = enzyme labeled immunosorbent assay
• PCR = polymerase chain reaction
• TeTx = tetanus toxin

SEE ALSO
• Carbamate Toxicity
• Gossypol Toxicosis
• Grass Tetany/Hypomagnesemia
• Hypocalcemia: Bovine
• Hypocalcemia: Small Ruminant
• Hypokalemia
• Monensin Toxicity
• Organophosphate Toxicity
• Ovine Encephalomyelitis (Louping Ill)
• Rabies
• Tick Paralysis

Suggested Reading
Deprez PR. Tetanus and botulism in animals. In: Duchesnes C, Granum PE, Menozzi MG, et al. eds, Clostridia in Medical, Veterinary and Food Microbiology. Brussels: European Commission, 2006, pp. 27–36.
Finnie JW. Pathogenesis of brain damage produced in sheep by *Clostridium perfringens* type D epsilon toxin: A review. Aust Vet J 2003, 81: 219–21.
Garcia JP, Adams V, Beingesser J, et al. Epsilon toxin is essential for the virulence of Clostridium perfringens type D infection in sheep, goats, and mice. Infect Immun 2013, 81: 2405–14.
Garcia JP, Giannitti F, Finnie JW, et al. Comparative neuropathology of ovine enterotoxemia produced by *Clostridium perfringens* type D wild-type strain CN1020 and its genetically modified derivatives. Vet Pathol 2015, 52: 465–75.
Hassel B. Tetanus: pathophysiology, treatment, and the possibility of using botulinum toxin against tetanus-induced rigidity and spasms. Toxins 2013, 5: 73–83.
Le Maréchal C, Woudstra C, Fach P. Botulism. In: Uzal FA, Prescott J, Songer G, Popoff M eds, Clostridial Diseases of Animals. Ames: Wiley Blackwell, 2016, pp. 303–30.

Lindstrum M, Myllykoski J, Sivela S, et al. *Clostridium botulinum* in cattle and dairy products. Crit Rev Food Sci Nutr 2010, 50: 281–304.

Moeller RB, Puschner B. Botulism in cattle: A review. Bovine Practitioner 2007, 41: 54–8.

Moeller RB Jr, Puschner B, Walker RL, et al. Determination of the median toxic dose of type C botulinum toxin in lactating dairy cows. J Vet Diagn Invest 2003, 15: 523–6.

Moeller RB Jr, Puschner B, Walker RL, et al. Attempts to identify *Clostridium botulinum* in milk from experimentally intoxicated Holstein cows. J Dairy Sci 2009, 92: 2529–33.

Popoff MR. Tetanus. In: Uzal FA, Prescott J, Songer G, Popoff M eds, Clostridial Diseases of Animals. Ames: Wiley Blackwell, 2016, pp. 295–302.

Popoff MR, Bouvet P. Clostridial toxins. Future Microbiol 2009, 4: 1021–64.

Prescott FJ. Diseases produced by other clostridia producing neurotoxins. In: Uzal FA, Prescott J, Songer G, Popoff M eds, Clostridial Diseases of Animals. Ames: Wiley Blackwell, 2016, pp. 331–2.

Rossetto O, Megighian A, Montecucco SC. Botulism neurotoxins. Toxicon 2013, 67: 31–6.

Uzal FA, Giannitti F, Finnie JW, García JP. Diseases produced by *Clostridium perfringens* type D. In: Uzal FA, Prescott J, Songer G, Popoff M eds, Clostridial Diseases of Animals. Ames: Wiley Blackwell, 2016, pp. 157–172.

Authors Francisco A. Uzal and Robert B. Moeller Jr

Consulting Editor Christopher C.L. Chase

COCCIDIOIDOMYCOSIS

BASICS

OVERVIEW
• Coccidioidomycosis is a fungal infection caused by the dimorphic soil ascomycete fungi, *Coccidioides immitis* and *C. posadasii*.
• The disease also known as valley fever, California fever, and San Joaquin valley fever, affects many mammalian and some reptile species. Transmission of the fungus is by inhalation of airborne spores (arthroconidia) leading to asymptomatic or symptomatic infection.

INCIDENCE/PREVALENCE
• Clinical cases are rarely seen in cattle or sheep, but asymptomatic infections may be common.
• Lesions have been reported in 5–15% of cattle slaughtered in some parts of Arizona, and in 2.5% of cattle slaughtered in Mexico.
• In some endemic regions of Mexico, 13% of the cattle were seropositive, and approximately 7% of cattle tested positive with the coccidioidin skin test.
• Up to 20% of cattle can be affected in enzootic areas.

GEOGRAPHIC DISTRIBUTION
Southwestern United States and parts of Mexico and Central and South America; the fungus was recently found in south central Washington state.

SYSTEMS AFFECTED
• Respiratory
• Integument
• Multisystemic in cases of dissemination

PATHOPHYSIOLOGY
• *Coccidioides* spp. propagate by two asexual reproductive structures—arthroconidia (arthospores) and endospores.
• Soil mycelial forms release arthroconidia which are dispersed by wind. These can germinate to form new mycelia in appropriate conditions, but can also be infectious to humans and animals.
• Arthroconidia are mainly inhaled and reach alveoli where they form endospore-producing nonbudding spherules.
• Spherules enlarge and rupture to release endospores that can develop into new spherules.
• Dissemination of endospores to other parts of the body is through blood and lymphatics causing disseminated disease. If they reach the environment, endospores can form new mycelial forms.
• Ascending infections via the vagina have been associated with abortions in mares. Though uncommon, arthroconidia can be inoculated directly into skin, bone or other tissues by penetrating objects.

SIGNALMENT
• All domesticated, captive exotic and wild ruminants especially camelids
• No age, sex or breed predilection

PHYSICAL EXAMINATION FINDINGS
• Primarily a respiratory disease, rarely with dissemination to other organs.
• Primary pulmonary infections usually become symptomatic 1–4 weeks after exposure, while disseminated disease can occur months to years later.
• Commonly causes subclinical infections or may manifest as a self-limiting respiratory infection.
• Animals may exhibit persistent cough, anorexia, depression, peripheral lymphadenopathy, chronic weight loss, fever, skin lesions.

CAUSES AND RISK FACTORS
• Coccidioidomycosis is caused by dimorphic soil fungi *C. immitis* and *C. posadasii*. Fungi grow in semiarid regions with sandy alkaline soils, and can grow in environmental extremes including alkaline conditions, extreme temperatures, and high salinity.
• Risk factors include airborne dust containing arthroconidia.

DIAGNOSIS

DIFFERENTIAL DIAGNOSES
• Actinomycosis/bacillosis
• Blastomycosis
• Caseous lymphadenitis (sheep and goats)
• Histoplasmosis
• Nocardiosis
• Tuberculosis

CBC/BIOCHEMISTRY/URINALYSIS
Mild nonregenerative anemia, monocytosis, leukocytosis

IMAGING
Radiographs: The most common lung abnormality is consolidation as solitary or multiple areas of lung, simulating bacterial pneumonia. Osteolytic lesions develop if bone is involved.

OTHER DIAGNOSTIC PROCEDURES
• Cytology: Presence of spherules in affected tissues, exudates, transtracheal or bronchoalveolar lavage fluids, lymph nodes and pleural fluid. Spherules are round, thick-walled, 20–80 μm in diameter, and can be as large as 200 μm, and contain 2–5 μm endospores. Occasionally there may be hyphae in tissues.
• Serology: ELISA, immunodiffusion and CFT.
• Culture of affected body fluids, exudates or tissue specimens.
• Molecular testing (PCR).

PATHOLOGIC FINDINGS
• Raised, miliary to nodular, firm, caseous or liquefactive lesions in lung or disseminated to mediastinum, thoracic lymph nodes, and viscera.
• Abortion, in llamas, with placental and fetal lesions.
• On histology, granulomas and pyogranulomas with fibrosis. Presence of double-contoured spherules 20–200 μm in diameter with or without 2–5 μm diameter endospores in affected tissues.

TREATMENT

THERAPEUTIC APPROACH
• Antifungal drugs including amphotericin B and azole drugs such as ketoconazole, itraconazole and fluconazole for 6–12 months, up to several years in disseminated disease.
• Disease is often self-limiting but relapses can occur.

MEDICATIONS

DRUGS OF CHOICE
Antifungal drugs including amphotericin B and azole drugs such as ketoconazole, itraconazole, and fluconazole.

CONTRAINDICATIONS
Appropriate withdrawal times for meat and milk in all food-producing animals following antifungal administration.

FOLLOW-UP

EXPECTED COURSE AND PROGNOSIS
• Primary pulmonary infections may be symptomatic in 1–4 weeks after exposure; disseminated disease occurs months to years later.
• Decreasing titers are associated with clinical improvement.
• Death in severe pulmonary or disseminated disease.

PATIENT CARE
Serology to test for IgM and IgG

PREVENTION
• Limit animal exposure to large concentrations of arthroconidia, such as in desert soils, areas of soil disturbance, and dusty conditions. Dust storms after a rainy season may contain especially high concentrations of aerosolized spores.
• No vaccine is available.

(CONTINUED)

MISCELLANEOUS

ZOONOTIC POTENTIAL
• Not contagious but disease can occur following cutaneous inoculation or inhalation of arthroconidia.
• Often limited to mild or asymptomatic respiratory tract infection, but may disseminate to other tissues (skin, brain, lymph node, musculoskeletal system) in some instances such as immunosuppression.
• Signs include flu-like illness, coughing, and chest pain.
• Cutaneous lesions and regional lymphadenopathy.

PREGNANCY
• Abortion associated with ascending infections in mares.
• Fetuses can become infected in birth canal during parturition.

BIOSECURITY
The mycelial phase in laboratory culture plates is highly infectious; biosafety level 2 (BSL2) or higher needed for isolation.

SYNONYMS
• California fever
• Desert rheumatism
• San Joaquin valley fever
• Valley fever

ABBREVIATIONS
• CFT = complement fixation test
• ELISA = enzyme-labeled immunosorbent assay
• IgG = immunoglobulin G
• IgM = immunoglobulin M
• PCR = polymerase chain reaction

SEE ALSO
• Actinomycosis: Lumpy Jaw
• Caseous Lymphadenitis (CLA)
• Tuberculosis: Bovine

Suggested Reading
Caswell JL, Williams KJ. Coccidioidomycosis. In: Jubb, Kennedy and Palmer's Pathology of Domestic Animals, 5th ed. Philadelphia: Elsevier, 2007, pp. 644–5.

Center for Food Safety and Public Health. Coccidioidomycosis. 2010. http://www.cfsph.iastate.edu/Factsheets/pdfs/coccidioidomycosis.pdf
Coster ME, Ramos-Vara JA, Vemulapalli R, Stiles J, Krohne SG. *Coccidioides posadasii* keratouveitis in a llama (*Lama glama*). Vet Ophthalmol 2010, 113: 53–7.
Radostits OM, Gay CC, Blood DC, Hinchcliff KW eds. Coccidioidomycosis. In Veterinary Medicine: A Textbook of the Diseases of Cattle, Sheep, Pigs Goats and Horses, 9th ed. London: Saunders, 2000, p. 1281.
Taboada J. Coccidioidomycosis (Valley Fever). Merck Veterinary Manual-Online https://www.merckvetmanual.com/generalized-conditions/fungal-infections/coccidioidomycosis accessed March 14, 2017.

Author Akinyi Carol Nyaoke
Consulting Editor Christopher C.L. Chase
Acknowledgment The author and book editors acknowledge the prior contribution of Karen Carberry-Goh.

COCCIDIOSIS

C

BASICS

OVERVIEW
- Most ruminants are exposed and infected with coccidia. Infection is usually asymptomatic and self-limiting with the development of species-specific immunity.
- Clinical signs develop when large numbers of oocytes are ingested or the host's immune system is suppressed.
- *Eimeria* species infect ruminants. Coccidia are species specific. The most common coccidia in cattle are *E. bovis* and *E. zuernii*, in sheep *E. ovinoidalis*, and in goats *E. arloingi*.

INCIDENCE/PREVALENCE
- Incidence of nervous coccidiosis is highest in the winter.
- Incidence of diarrhea is related to the buildup of infective oocysts within the animals' environment and associated stresses, such as weaning.

SYSTEMS AFFECTED
- Digestive
- Nervous

PATHOPHYSIOLOGY
- Oocysts are shed in the feces of infected animals, either from those with clinical signs or from older carrier animals. The oocysts are not infective until sporulation has occurred. Sporulation occurs within a week. Sporulation time is related to the moisture content and temperature of the environment; warm moist environments promote sporulation.
- Sporulated oocytes are ingested and during the asexual reproductive stage intestinal epithelia are damaged. Oocysts are produced during the sexual phase. The number of infective oocysts ingested is related to the severity of clinical signs.
- Healthy non-immune animals ingesting few oocysts may not show any clinical signs as intestinal damage is not significant and is quickly repaired. If a healthy non-immune animal is exposed to many oocysts, widespread intestinal damage occurs with disruption of the intestinal mucosa.
- Mucosal damage produces diarrhea as a result of alterations in gut function, loss of blood, fluid, protein, and electrolytes into the intestinal lumen. Fecal material may contain pieces of sloughed mucosa and blood. Mucosal damage allows for bacterial invasion into and through the gut wall.
- Animals experiencing stress are more likely to exhibit clinical signs.
- Animals acquire active immunity solely to the species to which they are exposed.
- The pathophysiology of nervous coccidiosis is not fully elucidated but a neurotoxin is suspected to be involved.

HISTORICAL FINDINGS
- Animals were recently weaned, moved from individual to group housing, housed in a crowded area that has a buildup of fecal material, or the housing environment has become wet or muddy.
- Owners may report poor feed intakes and weight gains.
- In cases of nervous coccidiosis, the animal has recently exhibited signs of diarrhea, tenesmus, or hematochezia along with cold environmental temperatures.

SIGNALMENT
- Bovine, caprine, and ovine.
- There is no specific age range for infection. Most clinical signs are observed in animals <1 year of age. Clinical signs may be observed as early as 16 days of age.
- Clinical signs are often associated with the stress of weaning and movement into a feed yard.

PHYSICAL EXAMINATION FINDINGS
- The disease is primarily of young animals managed as groups in unsanitary conditions. Most animals in a group become infected but only a minority may exhibit signs.
- Clinically, animals may have suppressed appetites and poor weight gains for several weeks after enteric signs resolve.
- Impairment of growth is observed in animals with subclinical infection.
- Rough hair coat, poor body condition, and fecal-stained perineum are commonly observed in young animals. Animals have varying degrees of dehydration, anorexia, and weakness.
- Depending on the severity of the infection, feces may contain mucus, strands of mucosa, and blood. Feces may be dark in small ruminants but hematochezia is rarely observed.
- Tenesmus is common with slight rectal prolapse.
- Nervous coccidiosis, initial signs of depression and incoordination are noted, progressing to muscle tremors, hyperesthesia, clonic-tonic convulsions, nystagmus, and blindness.

CAUSES AND RISK FACTORS
- *Eimeria* species infect ruminants. Coccidia are species specific. The most common coccidia in cattle are *E. bovis* and *E. zuernii*, in sheep *E. ovinoidalis*, and in goats *E. arloingi*.
- Changes in feed, weaning, and transport increase the development of clinical signs of disease.
- Housing which encourages buildup of fecal material such as crowded conditions and group housing.
- Exposure to moist environments such as areas around leaking waterers and poorly drained feeding stations.

DIAGNOSIS

DIFFERENTIAL DIAGNOSES
Enteric Coccidiosis
Salmonellosis, BVDV infection, abomasal or intestinal nematode parasitism, cryptosporidiosis

Nervous Coccidiosis
Polioencephalomalacia, lead intoxication, thromboembolic meningitis, rabies.

CBC/BIOCHEMISTRY/URINALYSIS
- Hemoconcentration, although a slight anemia may exist but is masked by dehydration.
- Inflammatory leukogram if mucosal damage is severe.
- Plasma proteins are increased initially due to dehydration; however, plasma protein levels decrease due to leakage into the gut and depressed feed consumption.

OTHER LABORATORY TESTS
- Fecal flotation.
- Diarrhea may be present for 3 or 4 days prior to the presence of oocysts in the feces.
- Checking multiple individuals increases the chances of finding oocysts, as stages of oocyst development will vary among individual animals.
- Presence or absence of oocysts in a single fecal examination is neither diagnostic nor confirmatory for coccidiosis. An animal can shed large numbers of oocysts; yet show no clinical disease because of immune status.

PATHOLOGIC FINDINGS
- Mucosa of the ileum, cecum, colon and rectum may be congested, hemorrhagic and thickened.
- The mucosa may be sloughing and ulcerated in severe cases resulting in blood and pieces of mucosa present within the lumen of the gut.
- The mucosa may also contain small white nodules.

TREATMENT

THERAPEUTIC APPROACH
- Treatment with anticoccidial drugs (see "Drugs of Choice").
- Fluid therapy, consisting of commercial oral or intravenous polyionic fluids, may be needed to correct dehydration and restore electrolytes.

MEDICATIONS

DRUGS OF CHOICE
- Sulfamethazine 110 mg/kg for 5 days, for cattle, may help control bacterial invasion and

C

pneumonia. Resistance to sulfamethazine has been observed.
• Amprolium 10 mg/kg for 5 days, for cattle.
• Amprolium 50 mg/kg for sheep, 100 mg/kg for goats for 5 days; use in goats and sheep is extra-label.

CONTRAINDICATIONS
• Use of amprolium may increase the risk of polioencephalomalacia.
• With the use of medications the meat and milk withdrawal times must be maintained appropriately.

FOLLOW-UP

EXPECTED COURSE AND PROGNOSIS
• Course of diarrhea is dependent on severity of infection. Feces begin to firm after several days of treatment with antimicrobials or amprolium.
• Prognosis is based on how debilitated the animal is at the time of presentation.
• Animals that are severely affected may have long-term reduction in weight gains, especially kids, as a result of damage to the intestinal lining.

POSSIBLE COMPLICATIONS
• Pneumonia has been associated with outbreaks of coccidiosis.
• Bacterial invasion through damaged gut wall may lead to septicemia.

PATIENT CARE
• Monitor attitude, appetite, fecal color and consistency, and hydration status.
• Fluid therapy, consisting of commercial oral or intravenous polyionic fluids, may be needed to correct dehydration and restore electrolytes.

• Because animals tend to be thin, feeding an appropriate amount of grain and high-quality forage is indicated.

PREVENTION
• Cleanliness is the basis of prevention. Clean and disinfect animal holding facilities between groups of animals. Drying and exposure to sunlight increases die-off of oocysts.
• Do not overcrowd animals. Reduce manure buildup. Eliminate muddy areas in the animal's environment. Feed up off the ground.
• Do not allow animals to defecate in water or feed.
• Feeding of coccidiostats in feed or in salt mixes.
  ○ Amprolium 5 mg/kg for 30 days for cattle.
  ○ Amprolium 15 mg/kg for 30 days for sheep and goats.
  ○ Decoquinate 0.5 mg/kg for 30 days, for cattle, sheep, and goats.
  ○ Lasalocid 20–30 g/ton of feed, for cattle and sheep, or 1 mg/kg per head per day.
  ○ Monensin 20 g/ton of feed, for cattle and goats, or 1 mg/kg per head per day.
• Clients should be made aware of the potential shedding of oocysts in feces and contamination of the environment, especially in and around waterers and feed troughs.

MISCELLANEOUS

AGE-RELATED FACTORS
• Clinical signs of disease can occur any time after 16 days of age.
• All ages are susceptible until immunity is developed.

ZOONOTIC POTENTIAL
None

PRODUCTION MANAGEMENT
• Do not overcrowd animals.
• Reduce manure buildup.
• Eliminate muddy areas in the animal's environment.
• Feed up off the ground.

ABBREVIATION
BVDV = bovine viral diarrhea virus

SEE ALSO
• Bovine Viral Diarrhea Virus
• Cryptosporidiosis
• Lead Toxicosis
• Rabies
• Salmonellosis

Suggested Reading
Ballweber LR. Coccidiosis in Food Animals. In: Smith BP ed, Large Animal Internal Medicine, 5th ed. St Louis: Elsevier Mosby, 2015, pp. 1516–17.
Chartier C, Paraud C. Coccidiosis due to *Eimeria* in sheep and goats, a review. Small Ruminant Res 2012, 103: 84–92.
Foreyt W. Coccidiosis and cryptosporidiosis in sheep and goats. Vet Clin North Am Food Anim Pract 1990, 6: 655–70.
Author Kevin D. Pelzer
Consulting Editor Christopher C.L. Chase

COENUROSIS

BASICS

OVERVIEW
• Coenurosis is a condition caused by invasion of the central nervous system (CNS) by the cystic larval stage (*Coenurus cerebralis*) of the tapeworm *Taenia multiceps* (bladder worm). This parasite normally inhabits the intestinal tract of carnivores after they have ingested infected raw sheep brain or cyst-contaminated offal. Coenurosis is most frequently encountered in sheep, but goats, deer, horses, cattle, and humans can also be affected.
• A similar condition results from infection with *Coenurus serialis*, the larval form of *Taenia serialis*. It usually affects lagomorphs, with coenuri most often developing in muscle or subcutaneous tissues.

INCIDENCE/PREVALENCE
In the 1980s, UK slaughterhouse surveys showed regional prevalence ranging from 0.5% to 5.8%. Nowadays the disease is less common.

GEOGRAPHIC DISTRIBUTION
Taenia multiceps is present worldwide in scattered foci, including Africa, Asia, parts of Europe, and the Americas. It is more common in temperate regions.

SYSTEMS AFFECTED
Nervous

PATHOPHYSIOLOGY
The intermediate hosts (sheep, goats, deer, etc.) become infected when they eat forage contaminated with the eggs of *Taenia multiceps*. Eggs hatch in the intestines and the released oncospheres enter the bloodstream and form coenuri primarily in the CNS. Lesions of the CNS may result from:
• The large numbers of immature/migrating worms entering and causing encephalitis
• Interference with cerebrospinal fluid drainage
• Large cerebral cysts compressing surrounding nervous tissue
Most signs are caused by the mature *Coenurus cerebralis*, which may be up to 5 cm in diameter after 6–7 months of development.

SIGNALMENT
• Most common in sheep (can also affect cattle, goats, and wild ruminants).
• Whereas acute coenurosis is most commonly seen in young (6–8 weeks of age) lambs, chronic disease is usually reported in sheep aged 6–18 months, and is rarely seen in sheep >3 years of age.

PHYSICAL EXAMINATION FINDINGS
Acute disease may develop due to larval migration approximately 10 days after ingestion of the eggs of *Taenia multiceps*. It is usually seen after a flock of sheep is introduced in a pasture heavily contaminated with dog feces infested with tapeworm eggs. Signs may include:
• Blindness
• Pyrexia
• Listlessness
• Ataxia
• Muscle tremors
• Nystagmus
Chronically infected animals with mature *Coenurus cerebralis* that have grown over 2–6 months may show signs of:
• Solitude
• Partial or complete unilateral blindness
• Depression
• Head pressing and incoordination
• Gradual development of paresis/paralysis and recumbency if the spinal cord is involved.

CAUSES AND RISK FACTORS
Ingestion of forage contaminated with *Taenia* eggs.

DIAGNOSIS

DIFFERENTIAL DIAGNOSES
• Coenurosis should be differentiated from other space-occupying lesions in the CNS, including abscesses, hemorrhage, and neoplasia and from other infectious agents causing neurologic disease such as listeriosis or louping ill.
• Presumptive diagnosis can be based on clinical signs and knowledge of the presence of *Taenia multiceps* in the area.
• Definitive diagnosis requires locating the metacestode in the brain or spinal cord. In 80–90% of cases, the cyst is located in one cerebral hemisphere.

CBC/BIOCHEMISTRY/URINALYSIS
Concentrations of serum creatine kinase brain iso-enzyme (CK-BB) may be increased with brain injury. Normally there is no serum CK-BB, just serum CK-MM (muscle).

OTHER LABORATORY TESTS
Results of cerebrospinal fluid evaluation may be consistent with increased eosinophil concentrations.

IMAGING
Skull radiographs/CT/MRI may be helpful in identifying the cyst.

PATHOLOGIC FINDINGS
Acute disease:
• Gross lesions include pale yellow tracts that are visible on the surface of the brain and in cut sections of the brainstem and cerebellum.
• Histologically eosinophils and giant cells predominate in the inflammatory reaction surrounding these tracts.
Chronic disease:
• Thin-walled cysts are most commonly found on the external surfaces of the cerebral hemispheres on gross examination.
• Local pressure atrophy of neural tissue is usually apparent.

• Spinal cord lesions usually occur in the lumbar region.

TREATMENT

THERAPEUTIC APPROACH
• Surgical removal is the only therapy with any demonstrated success.
• Anthelmintics may have application in the future (see "Drugs of Choice").

SURGICAL CONSIDERATIONS AND TECHNIQUES
• Surgical drainage of the cyst may prolong life.
• Surgical removal of the cyst may lead to complete recovery.

MEDICATIONS

DRUGS OF CHOICE
No drugs are labeled for treatment. Coenuri are susceptible to praziquantel, and there are reports of human patients treated with the combination of surgical excision and praziquantel. In an experimental study, 100% of lambs afflicted with coenurosis recovered after treatment with albendazole (25 mg/kg) or with the combination of fenbendazole and praziquantel (100 mg/kg) for 6 days.

FOLLOW-UP

EXPECTED COURSE AND PROGNOSIS
Prognosis is poor without surgery. After accurate localization of the lesion, 85% success rate for surgical removal of the coenuros cyst has been reported.

PREVENTION
• The spread of infection with *Taenia multiceps* is best prevented by controlling the mature worms in dogs through effective periodic deworming.
• Carnivores should not be given access to carcasses of animals infested with the intermediate stage of *Taenia multiceps*.
• Carnivores should be prevented from defecating in areas where ruminants graze, to minimize exposure to *Taenia* eggs.

MISCELLANEOUS

ZOONOTIC POTENTIAL
Human infection is rare but can occur after ingestion of eggs of *Taenia multiceps* or *Taenia serialis*. Coenuri of *Taenia multiceps* are usually found in the eyes and/or brain, whereas those of *Taenia serialis* are usually present in the subcutaneous tissue. Proper hygiene (washing

hands and wearing gloves) when handling dog feces helps prevent infection.

BIOSECURITY
Not allowing dogs to defecate on forage to be consumed by ruminants helps decrease exposure to *Taenia* eggs.

SYNONYMS
• Sheep gid
• Staggers
• Sturdy
• Vertigo
• Water brain

ABBREVIATIONS
• CK-BB = creatine kinase brain iso-enzyme
• CK-MM = creatine kinase muscle iso-enzyme
• CNS = central nervous system
• CT = computed tomography
• MRI = magnetic resonance imaging

SEE ALSO
• Listeriosis
• Ovine Encephalomyelitis (Louping Ill)

Suggested Reading
Ghazei C. Evaluation therapeutic effects of antihelminthic agents albendazole, fenbendazole and praziquantel against coenurosis in sheep. Small Ruminant Res 2007, 71: 48–51.

Leontides S, Psychas V, Argyroudis S, et al. A survey of more than 11 years of neurologic diseases of ruminants with special reference to transmissible spongiform encephalopathies (TSEs) in Greece. J Vet Med B Infect Dis Vet Public Health 2000, 47: 303–9.
Scott PR. Diagnosis and treatment of coenurosis in sheep. Vet Parasitol 2012, 189: 75–8.
Author Ferenc Toth
Consulting Editor Christopher C.L. Chase
Acknowledgment The author and book editors acknowledge the prior contribution of Danelle Bickett-Weddle.

COLIC: BOVINE

C

BASICS

OVERVIEW
Acute colic is defined as abdominal pain of ≤48 hours duration.

INCIDENCE/PREVALENCE
Colic is common in all domestic ruminant species, and the incidence and prevalence varies dependent on the etiology.

GEOGRAPHIC DISTRIBUTION
Depends on individual diagnoses

SYSTEMS AFFECTED
- Digestive
- Urinary
- Reproductive
- Cardiovascular

PATHOPHYSIOLOGY
- The GI tract is the most common source of acute abdominal pain; and any abdominal organ can be involved.
- Pain results from distension, displacement, torsion/volvulus, obstruction, smooth muscle spasm, or mesenteric tension, and may involve hypermotility, hypomotility, ischemia, and inflammation.
- GI lesions can be strangulating or non-strangulating.
- Strangulating lesions are associated with reduced blood supply that results in necrosis.
- Non-strangulating lesions result in less circulatory disturbance and are not usually associated with necrosis unless they become chronic.
- Any interference with gastrointestinal function can result in endotoxemia.
- Pain may also arise from the urinary tract, reproductive tract, peritoneum or other abdominal organs.

HISTORICAL FINDINGS
- Historical assessment often identifies information relevant to the clinical complaint, including recent parturition, dietary or other management factors, fecal and urinary output, and attempted treatment.

SIGNALMENT
- Any age or gender.
- Certain etiologies may be more common in specific production groups.

PHYSICAL EXAMINATION FINDINGS
- Abdominal pain may range from mild to severe, reflected by slight depression, restlessness and anorexia, to stretching, treading, bruxism, kicking at the abdomen, straining to urinate or defecate, getting up and down repeatedly, and lying in unusual positions.
- Tachycardia often reflects systemic compromise.
- Abdominal distension.
- Reduced gastrointestinal sounds or hypermotility.
- Tympany in the abdomen (pings audible on percussion) indicate a gas-fluid interface under pressure.
- Lack of urine or feces.
- Palpably distended or displaced viscus on rectal examination.
- Grainy or constricted rectal palpation (peritonitis).
- Vomiting (rare).

GENETICS
N/A

CAUSES AND RISK FACTORS
- Risk factors can include dietary change(s), water restriction, recent parturition, and intestinal parasitism.
- Colic related to the forestomachs can reflect ruminal acidosis, vagal indigestion, traumatic reticuloperitonitis, omasal impaction, ruminal fermentation, and gas or frothy bloat.
- Colic related to the abomasum can reflect ulcers, impaction, right abomasal volvulus, abomasal rupture, vagal indigestion, or abomasal stricture.
- Colic related to the small intestine can reflect enteritis, ileus, impaction, stricture, entrapment, torsion, jejunal flange torsion, jejunal hemorrhage syndrome, intussusception, adhesions, fat necrosis, neoplasia, or herniation (inguinal, umbilical, diaphragmatic).
- Colic related to the large intestine can reflect colitis, impaction, cecal tympany, displacement, torsion, volvulus, adhesions, fat necrosis, neoplasia, intussusception, or atresia coli.
- Peritonitis and hepatic disease can cause colic.

DIAGNOSIS

DIFFERENTIAL DIAGNOSES
Many diseases have signs resembling colic, including choke, rabies, tetanus, myositis, hypocalcemia, septicemia, urolithiasis, and dystocia.

CBC/CHEMISTRY/URINALYSIS
- Increased WBC count with peritonitis or other inflammation
- Increased PCV and TP with dehydration
- Decreased Cl, K, Na with most intestinal obstructive lesions in adult cattle
- Increased fibrinogen in inflammatory conditions
- Metabolic alkalosis in most obstructive lesions in adult cattle
- Acidosis with grain overload or severe, long-standing obstructions
- Azotemia and lactatemia with severe dehydration or urinary obstruction

OTHER LABORATORY TESTS
- Abdominocentesis
  - Increased WBC, TP, turbidity
  - Serosanguineous color indicative of strangulating obstruction
  - Foul smell or plant material indicative of GI rupture or enterocentesis
  - Volume increased with inflammation
- Rumen fluid analysis
  - Decreased protozoal activity with poor rumen function or obstruction
  - Decreased pH with acidosis and abomasal reflux
  - Increased Cl with abomasal reflux
  - Abnormal color or smell with acidosis, ruminal fermentation, rumenitis

IMAGING
- Ultrasound may identify intestinal distention, excessive fluid, masses, urinary tract disorders, and other abnormalities in the abdomen.
- Radiographs and contrast radiology are not usually useful in adult cattle but can be used to evaluate some urinary or gastrointestinal disorders in small ruminants.
- Computed tomography with oral and IV contrast administration can be useful in calves and small ruminants with a variety of abdominal disorders.

OTHER DIAGNOSTIC PROCEDURES
- Liptak test
  - Transabdominal paracentesis of a viscus on the left side of the adult cow to differentiate displaced abomasum from rumen. Low pH = abomasum, high pH = rumen.
- Laparotomy
  - Often used diagnostically in cows. The problem can be identified and repaired in many cases by flank laparotomy.
- Laparoscopy
  - Can be used as diagnostic procedure, but most abdominal problems require laparotomy to repair.

PATHOLOGIC FINDINGS
Depend on individual diagnoses, but necropsy is commonly diagnostic.

TREATMENT

THERAPEUTIC APPROACH
Colic should be considered an emergency. Primary or supporting medical therapy is critical; however, surgical treatment is indicated for severe abdominal pain or distension, tachycardia (HR >80 bpm), abnormal abdominocentesis, or based on some abnormal imaging findings.

SURGICAL CONSIDERATIONS AND TECHNIQUES
- Consider positioning before surgically exploring the abdomen. If the animal is

incapable of standing for the entire procedure, the complications can be dramatic.
• Surgical approach in adult bovines is typically via standing right flank laparotomy. However, in many cases general anesthesia will be required and the animal should be positioned in left lateral recumbency with a hole in the padding into which the rumen can sink. If the desired lesion is located on the left side, a left flank approach can be made, but only limited exploration of the right side of the cow is available.
• In small ruminants, the right flank, paramedian, or midline approaches can be used.

MEDICATIONS

DRUGS OF CHOICE
• Analgesics
  ○ Flunixin meglumine 1.1–2.2 mg/kg IV q24h or divided q12h.
  ○ Butorphanol 0.02–0.04 mg/kg IV.
• Laxatives
  ○ Mineral oil 10 mL/kg via ororuminal tube. Use with caution in surgical candidates, especially if an enterotomy may be needed.
  ○ Magnesium oxide 0.5–1.0 kg per adult cow by ororuminal tube.
  ○ Dioctyl sodium succinate 10–30 mg/kg of 10% solution by ororuminal tube.
• Anti-bloat agents
  ○ Mineral oil.
  ○ Poloxalene 30–60 mL per animal (can be repeated) by ororuminal tube.
  ○ Detergent soap can be used in emergency.
• Prokinetics
  ○ Metoclopramide 0.1 mg/kg SQ q6–12h (abomasal stimulation).
  ○ Erythromycin 10 mg/kg IM (increase abomasal emptying).
  ○ Bethanechol 0.07 mg/kg SQ q8h (cecal stimulation).
• Antibiotics
  ○ For infectious conditions or perioperatively.
• Transfaunation
  ○ 4–8 L of fresh rumen juice for repopulation of rumen.
  ○ Probiotic gels and yeast can be used.
• Endotoxemia
  ○ Flunixin meglumine 0.25–1.1 mg/kg IV, q6–12h.

CONTRAINDICATIONS
Prokinetic drugs should not be used if obstruction is present.

PRECAUTIONS
• Prolonged use of NSAIDs can cause ulceration of the abomasum and renal damage.

• Use of butorphanol or xylazine for pain control may cause ileus.
• Appropriate milk and meat withdrawal times must be followed for all compounds administered to food-producing animals.

POSSIBLE INTERACTIONS
N/A

FOLLOW-UP

EXPECTED COURSE AND PROGNOSIS
Varies depending on the initial condition

POSSIBLE COMPLICATIONS
Peritonitis, adhesions, shock, endotoxemia, gastrointestinal rupture

CLIENT EDUCATION
Clients should be educated that animals with a distended abdomen that are not passing feces have a potentially life-threatening disorder.

PATIENT CARE
• Once stable, refeeding should begin slowly with the animal monitored for passage of manure, recurrence of colic or distension, or deteriorating cardiovascular status.
• Animals with severe rumen bloat require immediate ororuminal intubation to relieve pressure.
• IV fluids are often necessary. Alkalosis is most common so a neutral or acidifying fluid is recommended. In grain overload or other situations of confirmed acidosis, an alkalinizing fluid and/or bicarbonate is needed. IV fluids should be supplemented to correct any electrolyte abnormalities.
• Large volume oral fluids may be administered for impaction and may be combined with hypertonic saline (1 mL/kg/min) to restore vascular volume.

PREVENTION
• Avoid sudden feed changes.
• Ensure access to water in all weather and temperatures.

MISCELLANEOUS

ASSOCIATED CONDITIONS
N/A

AGE-RELATED FACTORS
• Young animals are more likely to have intussusception or strangulating hernias.
• Old animals are more likely to have neoplasia or fat necrosis.
• Pregnant animals have indigestion of pregnancy/pseudo-obstruction.

• Peripartum animals are predisposed to displacements or torsions of the abomasum, and abomasal ulcers.

ZOONOTIC POTENTIAL
N/A

PREGNANCY
Late gestation cows most likely to have indigestion of pregnancy/pseudo-obstruction, uterine torsion

BIOSECURITY
N/A

PRODUCTION MANAGEMENT
N/A

SYNONYMS
• Colic
• Bloat
• Acute abdominal pain

ABBREVIATIONS
• GI = gastrointestinal
• IV = intravenous
• TP = total protein
• WBC = white blood cells

SEE ALSO
• Abomasal Impaction
• Abomasal Ulceration
• Displaced Abomasum
• Fluid Therapy: Intravenous
• Gastrointestinal Surgeries: Laparotomy (see www.fiveminutevet.com/ruminant)

Suggested Reading
Braun U, Eicher R, Hausammann K. Clinical findings in cattle with dilatation and torsion of the caecum. Vet Rec 1989, 125: 265–7.
Cable CS, Rebhun WC, Fortier LA. Cholelithiasis and cholecystitis in a dairy cow. J Am Vet Med Assoc 1997, 211: 899–900.
Farrow CS. Reticular foreign bodies: Causative or coincidence? Vet Clin North Am Food Anim Pract 1999, 15: 397–408.
Fubini SL, Ducharme N. Farm Animal Surgery. Philadelphia: Saunders, 2004, pp. 246–9. [VitalBook file]
Scott PR. Cattle Medicine. Boca Raton: CRC Press, 2011, pp. 84–92. [VitalBook file]
Author Dennis D. French
Consulting Editor Erica C. McKenzie
Acknowledgment The author and book editors acknowledge the prior contribution of Jennifer M. Ivany Ewoldt.

COLIC: SMALL RUMINANT

BASICS

OVERVIEW
• Acute colic represents abdominal pain of <48 hours' duration; chronic pain persists beyond 48 hours' duration or occurs in recurrent bouts.
• A wide variety of disorders cause colic in small ruminants; some require surgical intervention for resolution.
• Signs of acute abdominal pain usually represent gastrointestinal (GI) disease but can also reflect disease of other organs including the urinary and reproductive tracts.

INCIDENCE/PREVALENCE
Colic is usually a sporadic disorder unless associated with a problem that can affect multiple individuals (e.g., grain overload, toxic agents).

GEOGRAPHIC DISTRIBUTION
Worldwide

SYSTEMS AFFECTED
• Digestive
• Urinary
• Reproductive
• Cardiovascular

PATHOPHYSIOLOGY
• Gastrointestinal pain can result from distension, displacement, torsion/volvulus, obstruction, smooth muscle spasm, and mesenteric tension, and may involve hyper- or hypomotility, ischemia, and inflammation. Endotoxemia is a common accompaniment due to the large volume of natural gastrointestinal flora.
• Urinary tract pain can result from obstruction, inflammation, or infection.
• Reproductive tract pain can result from parturition, abortion, dystocia, uterine torsion, inflammation, infection, or neoplasia.

HISTORICAL FINDINGS
Determining the signs of concern, how long clinical signs have been present, events of potential significance (accidental access to grain, procedures), and any treatments administered prior to examination are important historical factors.

SIGNALMENT
• All small ruminant species, breeds, ages, and sexes can be affected.
• Castrated males are more likely to have urolithiasis.
• Young animals are more likely to develop intussusception and bezoars.
• Pre-weaned animals are more likely to have rumen putrefaction, abomasitis, abomasal tympany, and necrotizing enteritis.

PHYSICAL EXAMINATION FINDINGS
• Abdominal pain ranges from mild to severe; early signs may be subtle and easily missed.

• Ruminants are stoic animals that tend to display subtle signs of pain.
• Mild colic is reflected by slight depression, reduced appetite, and restlessness.
• Moderate colic can be reflected by reduced appetite and manure output, restlessness, stretching out (sawhorse stance), teeth grinding, posturing to urinate or defecate without production, and tail flagging.
• Severe colic can provoke kicking at the abdomen, recumbency, obtundation, vocalization, straining to urinate or defecate, profound restlessness (getting up and down repeatedly), and even rolling (unusual).
• Other findings can include increased respiratory rate, changes in temperature, abdominal distension and/or asymmetry, and changes in rumen motility or fill.
• The veterinarian should be familiar with the location of the gastrointestinal components in ruminants, and with associated areas of tympany (pings), which indicate gas distension of a viscus.
• Tachycardia is often present and can indicate endotoxemia, shock, hypovolemia, or pain.
• Vomiting is unusual, and most often associated with grayanotoxicity.
• Fecal production may be absent or feces may have abnormal appearance (loose, hemorrhagic, raspberry jam). The contents of the rectum can be assessed by digital palpation.
• Inguinal, scrotal, umbilical, or abdominal hernias may present as a mass, which may be warm, painful and non-reducible.
• Anuria, stranguria, pollakiuria, hematuria, or pyuria or the presence of blood or sediment on preputial hair can suggest urinary tract disease.
• Vulvar discharge may be evident with reproductive disease.
• Tenesmus may occur, and young neonates should be checked for a patent anal opening.

GENETICS
N/A

CAUSES AND RISK FACTORS
• Disease of the forestomachs can arise due to acidosis (grain overload), grayanotoxicity, gas or frothy bloat, penetrating foreign body, impaction (feed, sand), or blockage of the reticulo-omasal groove by a foreign body.
• Disorders of the abomasum include ulcers, abomasitis, abomasal tympany, impaction (sand, feed), phytobezoars/trichobezoars, abomasal emptying defect, and very rarely, displacement.
• Small intestinal disorders include enteritis (parasites, *Salmonella*), intraluminal obstruction (tricho- or phytobezoar; especially pylorus and duodenum), segmental volvulus, mesenteric root volvulus, intussusception, adhesions, fat necrosis, neoplasia, and entrapment (inguinal, umbilical, diaphragmatic hernia).
• Large intestinal disorders include colitis, impaction, intussusception, cecal tympany,

cecal volvulus, spiral colon volvulus, adhesions, fat necrosis, neoplasia, rectal prolapse, rectal tear, and atresia coli/ani.
• Reproductive disorders causing colic include dystocia, uterine torsion, parturition, abortion, tumor, periuterine abscess, testicular torsion, testicular trauma, seminal vesiculitis, and inguinal/scrotal hernia.
• Urinary tract disorders include urolithiasis, cystitis, nephrolithiasis, pyelonephritis, and ruptured bladder.
• Other causes of colic include peritonitis, umbilical abscess (internal remnant), hepatic disease (lipidosis, cholelithiasis, flukes), and potentially aortic, iliac, or femoral thrombosis.
• Some risk factors include dietary change(s), sand ingestion, water restriction, previous abdominal surgery, pregnancy, NSAIDs, and recent breeding or parturition.

DIAGNOSIS

DIFFERENTIAL DIAGNOSES
• Many diseases can cause signs resembling abdominal pain, including rabies, tetanus, and severe musculoskeletal problems/injuries.
• Differential diagnoses will vary depending on the animal's signalment, clinical signs, and the body system involved. In ruminants, when colic is attributed to the GI tract, additional diagnostic procedures should primarily aim at differentiating between problems that are oral versus aboral to the abomasum.

CBC/CHEMISTRY/URINALYSIS
• CBC changes that might be observed include an increased white cell count and fibrinogen with peritonitis or other inflammatory disorders, and hemoconcentration (increased PCV and protein).
• Hyperlactatemia is common in grain overload, strangulating gastrointestinal disease, severe long-standing obstructions, and any disorder causing severe systemic compromise.
• Hypochloremic metabolic alkalosis is observed in most GI lesions affecting outflow of the abomasum (obstruction, severe ileus).
• With forestomach lesions, chloride and total CO_2 concentrations are typically normal.
• Azotemia can indicate urinary obstruction or severe dehydration.
• Urinalysis may identify increased white cells, red cells, bacteria, or crystals with urinary tract disease.

OTHER LABORATORY TESTS
• Cytologic analysis of peritoneal fluid may identify increased total nucleated cell count (>5,000 cells/μL) and total protein concentrations (>5 g/dL) in inflammatory disease. A serosanguineous character suggests strangulation, and foul smell and plant

material can indicate GI rupture (or enterocentesis). A uriniferous smell can indicate uroabdomen.

• Rumen fluid analysis can be performed on samples obtained by ororuminal tube. Decreased protozoal activity may be observed with poor rumen function or obstruction, rumen pH may be decreased with acidosis and abomasal reflux, rumen chloride may be increased (>30 mEq/L) with abomasal reflux, and an abnormal color or smell can occur with acidosis, indigestion, and ruminitis.

IMAGING

• Ultrasonography is useful for examination of the digestive, urinary, and reproductive tracts. Attention should be paid to the amount and character of peritoneal fluid. Small intestinal or spiral colon distension, abnormal motility, and increased wall thickness can be observed in some disorders. Small intestinal intussusception is rare but may have a characteristic "bullseye" appearance.

• Radiographs can help with detection of radiodense uroliths, or sand impaction or metallic foreign bodies of the GI tract. Contrast radiographs are helpful in the diagnosis of intestinal atresia.

• Computed tomography is useful for evaluating all organ systems that might cause signs of abdominal pain, and can be performed several hours after ororuminal administration of contrast agent to help facilitate identification of GI obstruction.

OTHER DIAGNOSTIC PROCEDURES

Exploratory laparotomy can be used in the diagnosis and repair of some lesions. Surgical approach (right, left, midline, paramedian) must be carefully determined based on signalment, history, clinical signs, and the results of diagnostic tests to determine the most likely differentials to be investigated.

PATHOLOGIC FINDINGS

Vary with respective causes, see relevant chapters.

TREATMENT

THERAPEUTIC APPROACH

• Animals with severe rumen bloat require immediate ororuminal intubation to prevent respiratory compromise and collapse.

• IV fluids are often indicated. GI disease typically provokes alkalosis in adult ruminants and a neutral or acidifying fluid (such as 0.9% NaCl) is recommended. If grain overload or systemic acidosis is confirmed, a neutral or alkalinizing fluid is recommended. Electrolytes should be supplemented according to laboratory anomalies.

• Oral fluids may be administered where finances or disease (impaction) indicate.

• Oral fluids can be combined with hypertonic saline (2–4 mL/kg) to quickly

restore vascular volume in appropriate patients.

• Feed should be withheld until resolution of signs, then re-introduced slowly to avoid recurrence or complications.

• Transfaunation can be beneficial in animals with persistently poor appetite, by providing 2–4 L of fresh rumen juice via ororuminal tube for repopulation of rumen microbes.

SURGICAL CONSIDERATIONS AND TECHNIQUES

• Colic should be considered an emergency; diagnosis and treatment initiated immediately and feed withheld until the cause is determined and addressed.

• Indications for immediate surgical treatment include severe abdominal pain, severe abdominal distension, HR >90 bpm, presence of pings, abnormal abdominocentesis, urinary obstruction, uterine torsion nonresponsive to rolling or manipulation, fetal oversize causing dystocia, and confirmed gastrointestinal torsion, displacement, or obstruction.

• Surgical exploration of the abdomen of small ruminants is typically performed with the animal in lateral or dorsal recumbency, and usually under general anesthesia.

• If the desired lesion is located on the left side (i.e., rumen or uterus), a left flank approach can be made, knowing that exploration of the right side of the animal will be limited. The right flank is otherwise almost always selected for entry.

• A paramedian approach is typically chosen for small ruminants with suspected urolithiasis.

MEDICATIONS

DRUGS OF CHOICE

Analgesics

• Flunixin meglumine: 1.1–2.2 mg/kg IV q24h or divided q12h; also useful for endotoxemia at 0.25–1.1 mg/kg IV q6–12h (off label use in food animals).

• Ketoprofen: 2 mg/kg IM q24h (not labeled for use in food animals in the USA).

• Butorphanol: 0.05–0.1 mg/kg IV, IM or SQ, q6–8h.

• Xylazine: 0.05–0.3 mg/kg IM (may cause recumbency when used at higher dose or IV).

• Lidocaine: 1.3 mg/kg IV slowly over 10–15 minutes, then 0.05 mg/kg/min in saline or LRS over 24 hours (based on equine literature).

Laxatives

• Mineral oil: 5–10 mL/kg by ororuminal tube.

• Magnesium hydroxide: 50 g (for adult goat/sheep) by ororuminal tube.

• Dioctyl sodium succinate: 15–30 mL (for adult goat/sheep) of 10% solution given by ororuminal tube.

Antibloat Agents (Frothy Bloat)

• Mineral oil: 5–10 mL/kg given by ororuminal tube.

• Poloxalene: 30 mL/45 kg (can be repeated) by ororuminal tube.

• Detergent soap can be used in emergency.

Prokinetics

• None are truly effective for promoting forestomach motility.

• Metoclopramide: 0.1 mg/kg SQ q6–12h may provide some abomasal stimulation.

• Bethanechol: 0.07 mg/kg SQ q8h may provide some cecal stimulation.

• Erythromycin: 1 mg/kg in 1 L of saline over 60 minutes may provide stimulation throughout the GI tract.

Antibiotics

Antibiotics are indicated for infection and potentially perioperatively.

CONTRAINDICATIONS

• Prokinetic drugs should not be used if GI obstruction is present.

• Prolonged use of NSAIDs can cause ulceration of the abomasum and renal damage.

PRECAUTIONS

• Appropriate milk and meat withdrawal times must be followed for all compounds administered to food-producing animals.

• Butorphanol or xylazine reduce GI motility.

• Xylazine may cause recumbency when used at the higher dose; small ruminants are extremely sensitive to xylazine, hence it should be used with caution and sound monitoring.

POSSIBLE INTERACTIONS

N/A

FOLLOW-UP

EXPECTED COURSE AND PROGNOSIS

Varies with the causative condition, generally disorders that are acute, nonsurgical, and diagnosed and treated promptly have a good prognosis.

POSSIBLE COMPLICATIONS

• Peritonitis
• Adhesions
• Shock
• Endotoxemia
• Gastrointestinal or bladder rupture
• Fetal loss

CLIENT EDUCATION

Promote good management protocols in regard to dietary management and parasite control.

PATIENT CARE

• Once stable, refeeding should begin slowly and fecal passage monitored.

COLIC: SMALL RUMINANT   (CONTINUED)

C

• If the urinary tract was involved, urination must be monitored.
• Monitor for recurrence of colic or distension, or deteriorating cardiovascular status.

PREVENTION
• Avoid sudden feed changes.
• Ensure access to water in all weather and temperatures.
• Investigate signs of abdominal pain or distension early.
• Investigate dams that are pregnant beyond their due date.

 MISCELLANEOUS

ASSOCIATED CONDITIONS
N/A

AGE-RELATED FACTORS
• Young animals are more likely to develop intussusception and bezoars.
• Pre-weaned animals are more likely to have rumen putrefaction, abomasitis, abomasal tympany, and necrotizing enteritis.

ZOONOTIC POTENTIAL
N/A

PREGNANCY
Late gestation dams may have indigestion of advanced pregnancy/pseudo-obstruction and uterine torsion.

BIOSECURITY
N/A

PRODUCTION MANAGEMENT
N/A

SYNONYMS
Abdominal pain

ABBREVIATIONS
• GI = gastrointestinal
• LRS = Lactated Ringer's Solution
• NSAID = nonsteroidal anti-inflammatory drug

SEE ALSO
• Abomasal Emptying Defect in Sheep
• Bloat
• Diarrheal Diseases: Small Ruminant
• Gastrointestinal Surgeries: Laparotomy (see www.fiveminutevet.com/ruminant)
• Grayanotoxin
• Pain Management (see www.fiveminutevet.com/ruminant)
• Rumen Transfaunation (see www.fiveminutevet.com/ruminant)

Suggested Reading
Francoz D, Fecteau G, Desrochers A. Acute abdomen in ruminants. In: Smith BP ed, Large Animal Internal Medicine, 5th ed. St. Louis: Elsevier, 2015, pp. 799–805.

Haskell SRR. Surgery of the sheep and goat digestive system. In: Fubini SL, Ducharme NG eds, Farm Animal Surgery, 1st ed. St. Louis: Saunders, 2004, pp. 521–6.

Navarre CB, Pugh DG. Diseases of the gastrointestinal system. In: Pugh DG ed, Sheep and Goat Medicine, 1st ed. Philadelphia: Saunders, 2002, pp. 69–105.

Smith BP, Magdesian KG. Alterations in alimentary and hepatic function. In: Smith BP ed, Large Animal Internal Medicine, 5th ed. St. Louis: Elsevier, 201, pp. 88–106.

Smith MC, Sherman DM. Digestive system. In: Smith MC, Sherman DM eds, Goat Medicine, 2nd ed. Ames: Wiley-Blackwell, 2009, pp. 377–500.

Tibary A, Van Metre D. Surgery of the sheep and goat reproductive and urinary tract. In: Fubini SL, Ducharme NG eds, Farm Animal Surgery, 1st ed. St. Louis: Saunders, 2004, pp. 527–47.

Author Marie-Eve Fecteau
Consulting Editor Erica C. McKenzie
Acknowledgment The author and book editors acknowledge the prior contribution of Jennifer M. Ivany Ewoldt.

CONGENITAL DEFECTS: BOVINE

BASICS

OVERVIEW
• Numerous congenital defects have been reported in cattle.
• Congenital defects may be of genetic, toxic, nutritional, or infectious origin and commonly result in abortion, stillbirths, dystocia, or neonatal loss.
• This chapter discusses only defects associated with a known cause and that can be prevented by proper selection and management.

INCIDENCE/PREVALENCE
Some defects are breed specific.

GEOGRAPHIC DISTRIBUTION
Worldwide

SYSTEMS AFFECTED
Multisystemic

PATHOPHYSIOLOGY
• Hereditary congenital defects
  ○ Several genetic disorders have been recently reported to cause congenital defects in cattle.
  ○ Arthrogryposis multiplex in Angus cattle, due to a lethal autosomal recessive gene, commonly referred to as "curly calf syndrome." It results in severe malformations of the spine and limbs due to lack of communication between nerves and muscle tissue (in utero paralysis).
  ○ Complex vertebral malformation is an inherited lethal disorder in Holstein cattle, responsible for increased early embryonic death, abortion, and perinatal death. Affected calves show various skeletal abnormalities.
  ○ Congenital contractural arachnodactyly, due to a nonlethal recessive gene in Angus cattle. Affected calves are born with elongated limbs, congenital proximal limb contracture, and distal limb hyperextension.
  ○ Bovine arachnomelia syndrome, due to an autosomal recessive trait with complete penetrance in brown Swiss and Fleckvieh/Simmental cattle, resulting in skeletal abnormalities and a spidery appearance of the limbs.
  ○ Bovine citrullinemia, due to an autosomal recessive gene in Holstein cattle, causes an impairment of urea cycle resulting in elevated citrulline and ammonia in plasma and a neurologic syndrome.
  ○ Dwarfism or chondrodysplasia has been described in several breeds of cattle and is characterized by shortness and deformities of limbs, head and vertebrae. Some forms have been linked to a recessive (Aberdeen Angus) or incomplete dominant (Dexter) autosomal gene.
  ○ Brachyspina syndrome is a lethal malformation in Holstein cattle.

○ Crooked tail syndrome occurs in Belgian Blue cattle and is due to a deletion in the myostatin gene. Affected animals show growth retardation, abnormal skull, and extreme muscle hypertrophy.
○ Developmental duplication, due to an autosomal recessive gene in Angus cattle, results in birth of calves with supernumerary limb.
○ Neuropathic hydrocephalus, due to a lethal autosomal recessive gene of Angus cattle.
○ Syndactyly or "mule foot" (Holstein, Angus), fusion of digits due to an autosomal recessive gene.
○ Tibial hemimelia (dairy Shorthorn, Maine-Anjou), lethal genetic disease characterized by malformed or absent tibia, long shaggy haircoat, cryptorchidism, and meningocele.
○ Pulmonary hypoplasia with anasarca (Brown Swiss), due a recessive often lethal gene.
○ Goiter (Holstein).
○ Chediak-Higashi syndrome (Hereford, Brangus, Waygu), causes albinism and increased susceptibility to infection.
○ Ehlers-Danlos syndrome. Joint laxity and loss of skin tensile due to disorder of collagen type 1 and 2 formation.
○ Glycogen storage disease. Muscle weakness and inability to rise properly.
○ Epitheliogenesis imperfecta. Autosomal recessive, animal shows discontinuities in the skin or mucus membranes.
• Virus-induced congenital malformations
  ○ BVDV
    ▪ Teratogenic effects occur between 79 and 150 days of pregnancy and affect the CNS which is in the process of growth and differentiation. The virus causes destruction or failure of migration of the neuronal and neuroglial cells, resulting in failure of development and cavitary lesions formation. Inflammation causes vascular lesions and destruction of cerebellar folia resulting in cerebellar hypoplasia. Accumulation of fluids in the cavities results in development of hydranencephaly or hydrocephalus.
    ▪ Other lesions: Ocular lesions (bilateral microphthalmia, cataracts) due to retinal dysplasia and optic neuritis. Alterations of thymus (hypoplasia), bone (brachygnathia inferior, growth retardation), hair coat (hypotrichosis, alopecia, curly hair), lungs (hypoplasia), and kidneys (dysplasia).
  ○ Bluetongue virus
    ▪ Infection between 70 and 130 days of pregnancy results in brain malformations due to effects on neuronal and glial precursor cells and vascular injuries. Later in gestation, the virus may cause encephalitis.
  ○ Akabane and Aino viruses

    ▪ Infection between 79 and 104 days' gestation results in hydranencephaly whereas in infection between 103 and 174 days gestation results in arthrogryposis.
  ○ Schmallenberg virus
    ▪ CNS lesions (brain and spinal cord) depend on the stage of pregnancy (fetal immunocompetency) and virulence of the virus. In early pregnancy severe dyspalastic lesions and in late gestation encephalomyelitis. Arthrogryposis is suspected to be the result of CNS lesions.
• Congenital defects caused by teratogenic plants
  ○ Lupine toxicosis is well documented in North America. Ingestion of the plant between 40 and 70 days or pregnancy results in the "crooked calf syndrome" characterized by various degrees of arthrogryposis, scoliosis, torticollis, lordosis, and cleft palate due to alkaloid-induced fetal movement inhibition resulting from desensitization of skeletal muscle type nicotinic acetylcholine receptors.
  ○ Various other plants (locoweed, poison hemlock, tobacco, *Veratrum californicum*, mimosa) cause a variety of skeletal malformations when ingested by cattle between 30 and 60 days of pregnancy.
• Other causes: Cloning by somatic cell nuclear transfer has been associated with severe abnormalities of the umbilical cord, organomegaly commonly referred to as "abnormal offspring syndrome" and believed to be due to epigenetic errors of development
• Other congenital defects
  ○ Amelia: Absence of a limb or limbs
  ○ Atresia ani or atresia coli
  ○ Brachygnathia
  ○ Cryptorchidism
  ○ Hernias: Umbilical, inguinal, diaphragmatic hernia
  ○ Cardiac abnormalities: Ventral septal defect, ectopic heart, ventricular hypoplasia
  ○ Freemartinism

HISTORICAL FINDINGS
• Presence of an epidemiologic factor such as introduction of new animals (viral infections), change in pasture management (toxic plants), use of the same bull for breeding
• Abortion or stillbirth
• Abnormal pregnancy (hydrops allantois) obtained from cloned embryos
• Dystocia
• Neurologic syndrome, head press, convulsion, ataxia (bovine citrullinemia)
• Visible conformation abnormalities (inability to stand, severe angular deformities)

SIGNALMENT
• Abortus or neonate
• Nonlethal congenital defects, particularly of the reproduction system, are usually discovered upon breeding soundness examination.

CONGENITAL DEFECTS: BOVINE   (CONTINUED)

PHYSICAL EXAMINATION FINDINGS
• Congenital abnormalities are identified upon routine neonatal examination or because of complaints of severe distress of a neonate.
• Several conformational and musculoskeletal congenital abnormalities are evident upon inspection of the animal.
• Behavioral abnormalities, neurologic signs, dummy calf, inability to stand may be seen in animal with genetic disorders.

GENETICS
Some congenital defects have been confirmed to be hereditary.

CAUSES AND RISK FACTORS
Genetics; viral infections during pregnancy; exposure to teratogens; see "Pathophysiology"

DIAGNOSIS

DIFFERENTIAL DIAGNOSES
• Congenital defects often present in similar forms. Differential diagnosis of the cause relies primarily on epidemiologic data, herd history, thorough postmortem examination, and genetic evaluation.
• All malformed aborted fetuses and stillborn calves should be submitted to a diagnostic laboratory and processed as for an abortion investigation.

CBC/BIOCHEMISTRY/URINALYSIS
N/A

OTHER LABORATORY TESTS
• Genetic testing if a hereditary cause is suspected.
• Toxicology and viral investigation on abortus or neonates with severe congenital defects.

IMAGING
• Abdominal ultrasonography for suspected gastrointestinal abnormalities
• Thoracic/cardiac ultrasonography for diaphragmatic hernia, pulmonary and cardiac abnormalities.

OTHER DIAGNOSTIC PROCEDURES
N/A

PATHOLOGIC FINDINGS
• BVDV: Hydranencephaly, porencephaly, cerebellar hypoplasia, hydrocephalus, microencephaly, microphthalmia, cataracts
• Bluetongue: Hydranencephaly, cerebellar defects, porencephaly, hydrocephalus
• Akabane and Aino viruses: Hydranencephaly or arthrogryposis
• Schmallenberg virus: Hydranencephaly, arthrogryposis
• Arthrogryposis multiplex: Arthrogryposis, scoliosis, torticollis, hydroamnion
• Toxic plants: Various degrees of arthrogryposis, cleft palate

TREATMENT

THERAPEUTIC APPROACH
Severe congenital defects warrant humane euthanasia as early as the diagnosis is made.

SURGICAL CONSIDERATIONS AND TECHNIQUES
Surgical correction should be considered for some abnormalities (i.e., congenital hernias, abnormal umbilical stump, atresia ani, atresia vulvi, angular limb deformities) in order to improve the animal's welfare, provided the animal is not used for breeding.

MEDICATIONS

DRUGS OF CHOICE
N/A

CONTRAINDICATIONS
N/A

PRECAUTIONS
N/A

POSSIBLE INTERACTIONS
N/A

FOLLOW-UP

EXPECTED COURSE AND PROGNOSIS
• Animals with severe congenital abnormalities should be humanely euthanized.
• Dam and sire should be tested if hereditary/genetic condition is suspected.

POSSIBLE COMPLICATIONS
N/A

CLIENT EDUCATION
• Examination should be performed on all neonates for early detection of common congenital defects.
• Animal with congenital defects suspected to be hereditary should be eliminated from reproduction.

PATIENT CARE
Depends on the condition

PREVENTION
• Eliminate animals with known hereditary defects from breeding.
• Keep good records on genetics.
• Avoid exposure to toxic plants during critical periods of pregnancy.
• Preventive program for viral causes of abortion and congenital abnormalities.

MISCELLANEOUS

ASSOCIATED CONDITIONS
• Abortion

• Sudden death in neonate
• Ill-thrift

AGE-RELATED FACTORS
Congenital defects are usually detected on abortus, stillborn calves, or neonates.

ZOONOTIC POTENTIAL
N/A

PREGNANCY
N/A

BIOSECURITY
• Prevent introduction of animals from infected areas.
• Test animals for viral diseases before introduction.
• Properly dispose of carcasses from fetuses and dead neonates.
• Isolate and test aborting cows.

PRODUCTION MANAGEMENT
Pasture management to avoid exposure of pregnant cows to teratogenic plants

SYNONYMS
N/A

ABBREVIATION
• BVDV = bovine viral diarrhea virus

SEE ALSO
• Abortion: Bovine
• Akabane
• Bovine Viral Diarrhea Virus
• Freemartinism
• Lupine Toxicity
• Neonatology: Beef
• Schmallenberg Virus
• Teratogens
• Vaccination Programs: Beef Cattle
• Vaccination Programs: Dairy Cattle

Suggested Reading
Agerholm JS, Hewicker-Trautwein M, Peperkamp K, et al. Virus-induced congenital malfromations in cattle. Acta Vet Scand 2015, 57: 54–68.
Farin CE, Barnwell CV, Farmer WT. Abnormal offspring syndrome. In: Hopper RM ed, Bovine Reproduction. Ames: Wiley, 2015, pp. 620–38.
Ganwar AK, Devi KS, Singh AK, et al. Congenital anomalies and their surgical corrections in ruminants. Adv Anim Vet Sci 2014, 2:369–76.
Peperkamp NH, Luttikholt SJ, Dijkman et al. Ovine and bovine congenital abnormalities associated with intrauterine infection with Schmallenberg virus. Vet Pathol 2015, 52: 1057–66.
Whitlock BK, Coffman EA. Heritable congenital defects in cattle. In: Hopper RM ed, Bovine Reproduction. Ames: Wiley, 2015, pp. 609–19.

Author Ahmed Tibary
Consulting Editor Ahmed Tibary

CONGENITAL DEFECTS: CAMELID

BASICS

OVERVIEW
• Congenital defects are abnormalities of development or system function that the animal is born with. They can be recognized before birth (i.e., abortion), at birth, or years after birth (necropsy).
• Congenital defects may be of genetic, toxic, nutritional, or infectious origin. They may be lethal or nonlethal.
• Presence of congenital defects raises ethical questions at breeding.

INCIDENCE/PREVALENCE
Incidence of congenital defects is high in SAC compared to traditional domestic animal species.

GEOGRAPHIC DISTRIBUTION
Worldwide

SYSTEMS AFFECTED
Multisystemic

PATHOPHYSIOLOGY
• Common hereditary congenital defects: Several congenital defects are suspected to be hereditary although the mode of inheritance is often not known. The majority of the known hereditary defects are due to recessive genes or to complex multigenetic origins. The most common defects are:
  ◦ Maxillofacial abnormalities: Choanal atresia, wry face, craniofacial shortening, cleft palate, prognathism, cyclopia
  ◦ Reproductive abnormalities: Cryptorchidism, testicular hypoplasia, ovarian dysgenesis or hypoplasia, segmental aplasia of the tubular genitalia, atresia vulvi, polythelia, or supernumerary teats
  ◦ Gastrointestinal: Atresia ani, atresia coli, megaesophagus
  ◦ Cardiac: Ventricular septal defects
  ◦ Renal: Renal agenesis
  ◦ Musculoskeletal: Tail agenesis, kinked tail or sacro-coccygeal defect, syndactyly, polydactyly, dwarfism, patellar luxation
  ◦ Sensory organs: Blindness, blue eye (auditory nerve degeneration, deafness), nasolacrimal duct aplasia, gopher ears
  ◦ Hernias: Diaphragmatic, umbilical
  ◦ Immune system: Juvenile immunodeficiency syndrome (JIDS)
• Congenital defects suspected to be caused by teratogens
  ◦ Viral infections are suspected to cause congenital defects similar to those described in other species. These include BVDV (microphthalmia, hydrocephalus, impaired immune system), bluetongue virus (arthrogryposis, cerebellar hypoplasia).
  ◦ Arthrogryposis, cleft palate and ankyloses have been suspected to occur following ingestion of locoweed, poison hemlock, lupine, and tobacco. These effects are suspected to be due to a sedative effect of alkaloids on the fetus. Craniofacial malformation seen with *Veratrum californicum* may be due to steroidal alkaloids and inhibition of glucose metabolism by the cephalic primordia.
  ◦ Congenital goiter is common in camels and is suspected to be due to iodine deficiency or a toxic form of congenital hypothyroidism.

HISTORICAL FINDINGS
• Abortion, stillbirth, or sudden death of neonates.
• Visible abnormalities (inability to stand, inability to defecate or urinate, joint laxity or overextension, severe angular deformities), respiratory, circulatory, or metabolic complications.
• History of infertility.
• Poor doer or recurrent infections.

SIGNALMENT
• Abortus or neonate in most severe congenital defects.
• Compromise immunity generally discovered around 2–3 months of age.
• Most nonlethal defects are discovered upon pre-purchase or pre-breeding examination.

PHYSICAL EXAMINATION FINDINGS
• Congenital abnormalities are identified during routine neonatal examination or because of complaints of severe distress of a neonate. Several conformational and musculoskeletal congenital abnormalities are evident on inspection of the animal. Palpation of the tail head reveals various degrees of deviation or kinking of the tail in animals with sacro-coccygeal defects.
• Neonates with respiratory distress (dyspnea, open mouth breathing) should be examined for total or partial choanal atresia or diaphragmatic hernia. Air flow may be verified by fogging of a dry glass slide or a mirror placed under the nostril. Obstruction at the level of the medial canthus may be detected by a Foley catheter placed in each nostril.
• Neonates with cleft palate or maxillofacial abnormalities may present for lack of suckling ability or milk discharge from the nose.
• Animals with gastrointestinal abnormalities may present for bloat, lack of defecation, or straining (atresia ani, atresia coli).
• Animals with cardiovascular abnormalities may present for various signs of lethargy or collapse and respiratory distress. Cardiac auscultation reveals abnormal sounds (murmurs of variable degrees).
• Animals with urogenital abnormalities (ectopic ureters, intersex) may show evidence of dysuria or urine scalding.

GENETICS
Congenital defects confirmed to be hereditary in nature include maxillofacial abnormalities, tail abnormalities, polydactyly, and syndactyly.

CAUSES AND RISK FACTORS
• Genetics
• Viral infections during pregnancy
• Exposure to teratogens

DIAGNOSIS

DIFFERENTIAL DIAGNOSES
• Differential diagnosis between hereditary and nonhereditary congenital defects is important for the management of breeding animals.
• Respiratory distress may be caused by respiratory tract abnormalities, cardiovascular abnormalities, or diaphragmatic hernias. Differential diagnosis requires imaging.
• Lethal congenital disorders require a thorough necropsy evaluation.
• Disorders resulting in infertility may be identified in the external genitalia or after ultrasonographic evaluation.

CBC/BIOCHEMISTRY/URINALYSIS
• Indicated to evaluate the effect of a severe defect and make a decision on euthanasia.
• CBC is helpful in identifying animals with JIDS.

OTHER LABORATORY TESTS
• Genetic testing for animals with suspected intersex or freemartinism.
• Toxicology and viral investigation on abortus or neonates with congenital defects.

IMAGING
• Transabdominal ultrasonography for suspected atresia coli, congenital abnormalities of the kidneys.
• Transrectal ultrasonography to identify all congenital abnormalities of the genitalia in the female.
• Echocardiogram for suspected cardiac defects.
• Radiology to confirm choanal atresia, diaphragmatic hernia, and evaluate the severity of angular limb deformities.

OTHER DIAGNOSTIC PROCEDURES
• Laparoscopic exploration is helpful in the diagnosis of some genital abnormalities (uterus unicornis, ovarian dysgenesis, hypoplasia).
• Brainstem auditory evoked response (BAER) measurement for deafness evaluation in blue-eyed alpacas.

PATHOLOGIC FINDINGS
• Choanal atresia: Lack of or reduced communication between the nasal and pharyngeal cavity.
• Diaphragmatic hernias and various atresia of the gastrointestinal system are evident on postmortem examination.
• Cardiac abnormalities include ventral septal defect, atrial septal defects, tetralogy of Fallot, transposition of the great vessels, persistent right aortic arch, and patent ductus arteriosus.

• Defects of the urogenital system can be lethal (bilateral renal agenesis, bladder agenesis, and complete atresia vulvi).
• Reproductive system disorders: Monorchism is often associated with unilateral renal agenesis. Testicular and ovarian hypoplasia are confirmed by absence or lack of germinal epithelium activity.

TREATMENT

THERAPEUTIC APPROACH
• Most severe congenital defects warrant humane euthanasia as early as the diagnosis is made.
• Less severe congenital defects that do not jeopardize the animal's wellbeing may be managed conservatively (slight angular deformities, slight facial deviations, congenital abnormalities resulting in infertility).

SURGICAL CONSIDERATIONS AND TECHNIQUES
• Surgical correction of some abnormalities should be considered in order to improve the animal's welfare providing the animal is not used for breeding.
• Castration and ovariectomy should be considered for animals with suspected hereditary congenital defects or defects that may jeopardize the welfare of the animal during mating or pregnancy.

MEDICATIONS

DRUGS OF CHOICE
N/A

CONTRAINDICATIONS
N/A

PRECAUTIONS
N/A

POSSIBLE INTERACTIONS
N/A

FOLLOW-UP

EXPECTED COURSE AND PROGNOSIS
• Animals with severe congenital abnormalities should be humanely euthanized.
• Animals with sensory abnormalities can have a good life but their management and behavior can be difficult around people and other animals.
• Animals with slight angular limb deformities have a very good prognosis for normal behavior and life.

POSSIBLE COMPLICATIONS
• Angular limb deformities may result in chronic lameness and osteoarticular disorders.
• Animals with cardiac abnormalities may show lethargy and poor growth. Females may have other systemic complications during pregnancy if mated.
• Non-diagnosed congenital defects of the reproductive system may result in overbreeding, reproductive tract infection, or injury, and jeopardize the animal's welfare.

CLIENT EDUCATION
• All neonates should be examined for common congenital defects.
• Animals with congenital defects suspected to be hereditary should be eliminated from reproduction.

PATIENT CARE
Depends on the condition

PREVENTION
• Eliminate animals with known hereditary defects from breeding.
• Keep good records on genetics to make rational mating decisions.
• Avoid exposure of pregnant animals to toxic plants and viruses known to cause congenital abnormalities in other species.

MISCELLANEOUS

ASSOCIATED CONDITIONS
N/A

AGE-RELATED FACTORS
N/A

ZOONOTIC POTENTIAL
N/A

PREGNANCY
N/A

BIOSECURITY
N/A

PRODUCTION MANAGEMENT
N/A

SYNONYMS
N/A

ABBREVIATIONS
• BVDV = bovine viral diarrhea virus
• JIDS: juvenile immunodeficiency syndrome
• SAC = South American camelid

SEE ALSO
• Breeding Soundness Examination: Camelid
• Neonatology: Camelid
• Physical Examination: Camelid (Appendix 5)

Suggested Reading
Fowler M. Congenital/hereditary conditions. In: Fowler ME ed, Medicine and Surgery of South American Camelids, 3rd ed. Ames: Blackwell, 2010, pp. 525–58.
Tibary A, Johnson LW, Pearson LK, Rodriguez JS. Lactation and neonatal care. In: Cebra C et al. eds, Llama and Alpaca Care: Medicine, Surgery, Reproduction, Nutrition and Health Care. St. Louis: Elsevier, 2014, pp. 285–97.
Tibary A, Picha, Y, Pearson LK. Congenital and possibly hereditary causes of infertility in camelids. Proc North Am Vet Conf 2011, pp. 324–6.
Tibary A, Picha, Y, Pearson LK. Congenital anomalies in crias. Proc North Am Vet Conf 2011, pp. 327–9.
Author Ahmed Tibary
Consulting Editor Ahmed Tibary

CONGENITAL DEFECTS: SMALL RUMINANT

BASICS

DEFINITION
Lethal or sublethal defects present at birth due to genetic or environmental influence on embryonic or fetal development.

INCIDENCE/PREVALENCE
• Defects occur generally sporadically, with <1% newborns affected.
• Prevalence of genetic conditions is higher in inbred herds or flocks.
• Entropion is the most common congenital defect in sheep, with 1–10% of lambs affected, and up to 80% of lambs and 50% of kids in highly inbred herds.
• Prevalence of arthrogryposis is 0.3%, but 58% of lambs were affected with genetic arthrogryposis.
• Intersexes are seen in 2–11% of kids born.
• Testicular hypoplasia was seen in 33% of sterile bucks.

GEOGRAPHIC DISTRIBUTION
Varies with distribution of viruses or their vectors, and toxic plants.

SYSTEMS AFFECTED
Depends on etiology

PATHOPHYSIOLOGY
• Chromosomal abnormalities occur during gametogenesis or fertilization.
• Gene mutations, deletions, or translocations lead to heritable defects.
• Plant toxins cause fetal defects if they cross the placenta at a high dose and at a time of gestation when the fetus is susceptible to their effect.
• Viruses cause congenital defects if the fetus is infected during susceptible stages of gestation.
• Defects may be due to excessive or arrested division, failure of normal fusion, failure or excess of tissue growth or development, failure to assume final form or position, failure of normal persistence, or disappearance of structures.

GENETICS
• Most genetic defects are single autosomal recessive traits.
• Entropion may be caused by several recessive genes with additive effects.
• Cryptorchidism and testicular hypoplasia may have the same genetic basis in sheep.
• Some intersex conditions are associated with the polled trait in goats.

HISTORICAL FINDINGS
• Similar congenital problems in progeny of related animals, affected animals descend from a common ancestor, increased frequency of the defect with inbreeding with genetic defects.
• Sudden increase in the percentage of animals born affected, introduction of new animals to the herd with infectious origin.

• Known presence of toxic plants or mineral/vitamin deficiencies in the area.

SIGNALMENT
• Genetic conditions are more prevalent in certain breeds.
• Fetuses and newborn lambs and kids.

PHYSICAL EXAMINATION FINDINGS
• Bunyavirus: Abortion, maternal fever, neonatal deaths, arthrogryposis, torticollis, scoliosis, lordosis, hydrocephalus, cerebellar abnormalities, muscular hypoplasia, anasarca.
• Bluetongue: Neurologic signs in newborns, arthrogryposis.
• Border disease virus: Abortions, mummified or macerated fetuses, stillbirths, weak lambs with hairy fleece and tremors, ataxia, facial and ocular abnormalities, poor growth, depressed immune system, cerebellar hypoplasia, hydranencephaly, porencephaly, arthrogryposis.
• Schmallenberg virus: Maternal diarrhea, dullness, decreased milk production, fever, infertility, weak lambs with poor vision and neurologic signs, arthrogryposis, torticollis, scoliosis, kyphosis, flattened skull, brachygnathia inferior, porencephaly, hydranencephaly, dysplasia of the cerebellum, brainstem and spinal cord.
• Locoweeds, tree tobacco, and poison hemlock: Abortion, infertility, congenital arthrogryposis, crooked legs, scoliosis, torticollis, hydrops, weak neonates.
• Skunk cabbage: With acute poisoning, maternal salivation, vomiting, fast irregular heart rate, muscle tremors, incoordination, coma. With ingestion at 15 days'f gestation, congenital cyclopia, protruding and twisted mandible, shortened upper jaw and prosboscis ("monkey face"). With ingestion at 30–35 days' gestation, congenital cleft palate, hairlip, shortened legs, tracheal stenosis.
• Cerebellar atrophy: Wide stance, opisthotonos, tremors, ataxia.
• Ceroid lipofuscinosis: Blind lambs, nodding head, twitching of eyelids, lips and muzzle, locomotor disturbance.
• Muscle dystrophy: Poor growth, locomotor problems, inability to forage, in Merinos.
• Spider lamb syndrome or chondrodysplasia: Abnormal limb length, bent legs, flattened rib cages, arthrogryposis, spinal and facial deformities.
• Achondroplasia or dwarfism: Short bowed legs, deformed heads.
• Hypotrichosis congenita: No fleece or only patches of hair. Bilateral hypotrichosis is seen with congenital hypothyroidism.
• Epitheliogenesis imperfecta: Defects in the epithelium, oral cavity, and tongue. In redfoot form, hooves are shed soon after birth.
• Epidermolysis bullosa: Subepidermal bullae, erythematous patches, alopecia, hypopigmentation, erosions, ulcers, crusty or scaly areas over bony prominences, lips, nasolabial plane, mouth, tongue, gums, or palate.

• Collagen dysplasias: Abnormally fragile skin that lacerates easily, oral lesions due to trauma of suckling that infect and cause fatal septicemia, skin laxity.
• Copper deficiency: Poor appetite, weakness, twisted joints, hear tremors, ataxia, paresis and paralysis in goats.
• Entropion: Inverted lower eyelids, blepharospasm, epiphora, protophobia, eye rubbing, keratoconjunctivitis, secondary corneal ulcers.
• Intersex: Nearly normal female or male at birth. After puberty, genitalia are ambiguous with small teats, a short penis or an enlarged clitoris, hypospadias, increased anogenital distance, cryptorchidism, and varying degrees of masculinization. Type of gonadal tissue and tubular genitalia varies with the condition.

CAUSES AND RISK FACTORS
Genetic
Arthrogryposis (Merino, Suffolk), cerebellar atrophy (Border Leicester, Corriedale), dwarfism or achondroplasia (Norwegian, Merino, Southdown, Dorset, Blackface, Cheviot), prognathia, brachygnathia, atresia ani, patent foramen ovale, patent ductus arteriosus, spider lamb syndrome or chondrodysplasia (black-faced breeds), ceroid lipofucsinosis (South Hampshire), muscle dystrophy, muscle hyperplasia, hypotrichosis congenita, congenital hypothyroidism, epitheliogenesis imperfecta, epidermolysis bullosa (Suffolk, North Dorset), collagen dysplasias (Dala, Border-Leicester crosses), hydronephrosis, polycystic kidneys, unilateral agenesis, renal fibrosis (Southdown), mesangiocapillary glomerulonephritis (Finnish Landrace), cryptorchidism, entropion (Boer, Charolais, Texel).

Viral
Bunyavirus (Cache Valley virus, Akabane virus, Rift Valley fever virus, Nairobi sheep disease virus), Border disease virus, Schmallenberg virus, bluetongue virus.

Toxic Plants
Locoweeds (*Astragalus* spp., *Oxytropis* spp.), skunk cabbage (*Veratrum californicum*), tree tobacco (*Nicotiana glauca*), poison hemlock (*Conium maculatum*).

Nutritional
Copper deficiency, selenium/vitamin E deficiency

Risk Factors
• Nutritional, social or environmental stress (viral)
• Seasonal presence of vectors and geographic location (viral)
• Presence of toxic plants (toxic)
• Use of genetic carrier dams or sires in breeding programs (genetic)
• Inappropriate nutrition or soil and plant deficiencies (nutritional)

C

CONGENITAL DEFECTS: SMALL RUMINANT (CONTINUED)

DIAGNOSIS

DIFFERENTIAL DIAGNOSES
• Facial deformities: Bluetongue virus, Bunyavirus, Border disease virus, locoweeds, skunk cabbage, spider lamb syndrome, dwarfism.
• Neurologic signs: Border disease virus, Bunyavirus, Schmallenberg virus, bluetongue virus, skunk cabbage, ceroid lipofucsinosis, genetic cerebellar atrophy, copper deficiency.
• Muscular disorders: Selenium/vitamin E deficiency, muscle dystrophy, muscle hyperplasia.
• Spinal defects: Bunyavirus, bluetongue virus, Schmallenberg virus, skunk cabbage, poison hemlock, tree tobacco, spider lamb syndrome.
• Bowed legs: Chondrodysplasia, dwarfism, locoweeds, parbendazole administration at 12–24 days' gestation, copper deficiency.
• Arthrogryposis: Bunyavirus, bluetongue virus, Border disease virus, Schmallenberg virus, tree tobacco, locoweeds, poison hemlock, spider lamb syndrome, recessive gene in Merinos and Suffolks.
• Skin or hair abnormalities: Hypotrichosis congenita, congenital hypothyroidism, Border disease, epitheliogenesis imperfecta, epidermolysis bullosa, collagen dysplasias.
• Ambiguous sex phenotype or intersex: Male pseudohermaphrodite, true hermaphrodite, freemartinism, persistent Mullerian duct syndrome, polled intersex (XX sex reversal), testicular hypoplasia.

OTHER LABORATORY TESTS
Serology, microbiology

IMAGING
• Hydrops and enlarged fetal heart on transabdominal ultrasound with locoweed toxicity.
• Multiple irregular islands of ossification in the elbow, shoulder, and sternum on radiographs with spider lamb syndrome.

OTHER DIAGNOSTIC PROCEDURES
• Necropsy and gross examination
• Histopathology
• Antibody detection in fetal fluids, maternal serum, or precolostral lamb serum (viral)
• Viral isolation from fetal blood, antigen capture ELISA (Border disease virus)
• PCR on fetal brainstem (Schmallenberg virus)
• Identification of toxic plants
• Detection of swansonine in blood within 2 days of ingestion (locoweeds)
• Karyotype (intersexes)

PATHOLOGIC FINDINGS
• Varies with the condition.
• See "Physical Examination Findings" for gross abnormalities in lambs and kids.

TREATMENT

THERAPEUTIC APPROACH
N/A

SURGICAL CONSIDERATIONS AND TECHNIQUES
• Cesarean section may be indicated due to impossibility to deliver severely malformed fetuses vaginally.
• Entropion may be surgically corrected. Lambs and kids should not be used for reproduction.

MEDICATIONS

DRUGS OF CHOICE
N/A

CONTRAINDICATIONS
Avoid using modified-live virus or attenuated vaccines against BVDV in small ruminants (Border disease virus).

PRECAUTIONS
N/A

POSSIBLE INTERACTIONS
N/A

FOLLOW-UP

EXPECTED COURSE AND PROGNOSIS
• Prognosis is poor for life and normal development with severe malformations.
• Cull affected animals. For genetic conditions, cull dams and sires.

POSSIBLE COMPLICATIONS
Dystocia due to fetal malformations, possibly followed by retained fetal membranes and metritis.

CLIENT EDUCATION
• If >1% of lambs or kids are born with similar congenital defects, call a veterinarian to investigate the cause.
• If a genetic component is identified, the dam and sire of the affected lambs and kids should be culled. Even if normal in appearance, these animals may be carriers of the gene.

PATIENT CARE
N/A

PREVENTION
• Optimize the herd's health status.
• Reduce exposure to vectors (Bunyavirus).
• If available, vaccinate susceptible animals (Bunyavirus).
• Test and cull affected animals.
• Test and quarantine new additions to the herd.
• Separate sheep from cattle (Border disease).
• Keep pregnant animals off pastures with toxic plants.
• Cull dam and sire from animals affected by genetic conditions.
• Nutritional supplementation of pregnant animals.

MISCELLANEOUS

ASSOCIATED CONDITIONS
Depends on condition

AGE-RELATED FACTORS
N/A

ZOONOTIC POTENTIAL
N/A

PREGNANCY
N/A

BIOSECURITY
Depends on cause

PRODUCTION MANAGEMENT
N/A

SYNONYMS
N/A

ABBREVIATIONS
• BVDV = bovine viral diarrhea virus
• ELISA = enzyme-linked immunosorbent assay

SEE ALSO
Abortion: Small Ruminant

Suggested Reading
Angus K. Congenital malformations in sheep. In Practice 1992, 14: 33–8.
Basrur PK. Congenital abnormalities of the goat. Vet Clin North Am Food Anim Pract 1993, 9: 183–202.
Greber D, Doherr M, Drogemuller C, Steiner A. Occurrence of congenital disorders in Swiss sheep. Acta Vet Scand 2013, 55: 27–34.
Author Maria Soledad Ferrer
Consulting Editor Ahmed Tibary

CONGENITAL OCULAR DISORDERS

BASICS

OVERVIEW
• Congenital disorders are abnormalities that exist at birth, regardless of cause.
• These may be inherited, due to incidental errors of development, or result from intrauterine infection, deficiency, or teratogen exposure.

INCIDENCE/PREVALENCE
Typically sporadic and rare; however, disorders with a hereditary component can achieve a high prevalence in poorly managed flocks or herds.

GEOGRAPHIC DISTRIBUTION
Worldwide, although disorders with toxic or infectious influences may be regional.

SYSTEMS AFFECTED
• Ophthalmic
• Nervous
• Musculoskeletal

PATHOPHYSIOLOGY
• Vitamin A: Vitamin A allows regeneration of rhodopsin in the retina and normal function of osteoclasts/osteoblasts, epithelial tissues, and the choroid plexus. Deficiency occurs in cattle consuming poor-quality diets and drought-stressed forages, with restriction of green feed. Vitamin A deficiency during pregnancy causes abnormal cranial development in calves, with narrowing of the optic canals and constriction of the optic nerves. Microphthalmia and limb anomalies can also occur. Thickening of the arachnoid and dura results in impaired CSF absorption, increased CSF pressure, and hydrocephalus.
• Cyclopia, the presence of a single central eye, occurs in sheep ingesting *Veratrum californicum* (California false hellebore) on day 14 of gestation. The plant grows mainly in mountainous areas with moist/swampy conditions above 5,000 ft. The prosencephalon of affected lambs does not cleave; there is one midbrain/optic nerve and optic canal. Systems affected by *V. californicum* depend on the day of gestation that exposure occurs. Spontaneous cyclopia is occasionally reported in crias.
• Entropion describes inversion of the eyelid (typically the lower). This can be congenital, hereditary, or acquired (dehydration). Cornea-lid contact can result in ulceration, blepharospasm, and lacrimation.
• Ectropion describes eversion of the eyelid (typically the lower), and can be congenital, hereditary, or acquired.
• Congenital cataracts describe the presence of lens opacities at birth. The disorder is hereditary in some bovine breeds, with prevalence up to 34%. Accompanying abnormalities include retinal detachment, microphakia, and hydrocephalus. Other

causes include in utero BVDV exposure, and exposure to electromagnetic fields.
• Microphthalmia and anophthalmia occur when one or both eyes are small or absent. Depending on severity, there may not be visual deficits. It is congenital or hereditary, and has been observed with concurrent intraocular anomalies in lambs grazing seleniferous pasture.

HISTORICAL FINDINGS
May reflect exposure to causes and risk factors for congenital ophthalmic disease.

SIGNALMENT
Most congenital ocular disorders are observed at birth or shortly after. Entropion and cyclopia are more frequent in lambs, and congenital cataracts, microphthalmia, and blindness associated with vitamin A deficiency more frequent in calves.

PHYSICAL EXAMINATION FINDINGS
• Calves with vitamin A deficiency show weakness, anorexia, intermittent fever, ill-thrift, blindness, diarrhea, and pneumonia. Dilated, unresponsive pupils and a domed forehead are evident. Papilledema develops and the optic disc becomes pale with indistinct borders.
• Cyclopia is marked by a single central eye, and microphthalmia and cleft palate can occur.
• Entropion induces blepharospasm, epiphora, corneal ulceration, conjunctivitis, and corneal edema with an inverted eyelid; ectropion appears similarly but with an everted eyelid.
• Congenital cataracts create uni- or bilateral white intraocular opacities, typically visible to the naked eye; other congenital disorders may be evident.
• Microphthalmia reflects unusually small palpebral fissures and eyes, typically bilaterally, with entropion and corneal damage.

GENETICS
• A hereditary component for congenital cataracts has been described for Holstein-Friesians, Herefords, Jersey, and Brown Swiss cattle, as well as New Zealand Romney sheep.
• Entropion likely has a heritable component in some breeds, including Boer goats, Simmental cattle, and Hampshire sheep.
• Microphthalmia with a hereditary component is described in Japanese Black cattle, Texel sheep, Hereford cattle, Jersey calves, and White shorthorn cattle.

CAUSES AND RISK FACTORS
• Vitamin A deficiency arises with lack of green feed, poor-quality forages, cereal grains, beet pulp, and cottonseed hulls. Disease conditions and growth increase requirement. Prolonged feeding of mineral oil can decrease vitamin A absorption.

• Exposure to *V. californicum* on day 14 of gestation (cyclopia) or seleniferous pastures (microphthalmia).
• Prematurity, dehydration, sepsis, or eyelid malformation (entropion).
• Intrauterine BVDV exposure between days 79 and 150 of gestation, and exposure to electromagenetic fields influence congenital cataracts in cattle.
• Heritable predispositions.

DIAGNOSIS

DIFFERENTIAL DIAGNOSES
• Vitamin A deficiency can be differentiated from polioencephalomalacia or salt poisoning by assessing pupillary light responses; absent in vitamin A deficiency due to retinal degeneration, and intact in the other disorders.
• Disorders that cause corneal damage or infection (entropion, ectropion) must be differentiated from traumatic ocular injury, corneal infection with *Chlamydia* or *Mycoplasma*, foreign body irritation, and ectopic cilia.
• Schmallenberg virus, bluetongue virus and Akabane virus can cause similar clinical signs in calves to BVDV infection; however, the presence of congenital cataracts is suggestive of fetal BVDV exposure.

CBC/BIOCHEMISTRY/URINALYSIS
N/A

OTHER LABORATORY TESTS
• Assay vitamin A/carotene in plasma and feed or liver samples.
• Culture/sensitivity and cytology of corneal lesions.
• BVD testing (cataracts, microphthalmia).

IMAGING
Ultrasonography and/or computed tomography can assist evaluation of ocular and cranial structures in complicated disorders.

OTHER DIAGNOSTIC PROCEDURES
Complete ophthalmic examination with fluorescein staining and assessment of the fundus where indicated, combined with assessments of cranial nerve function.

PATHOLOGIC FINDINGS
• Gross abnormalities are readily evident in microphthalmia, entropion, ectropion, and cyclopia.
• Calves with vitamin A deficiency have narrowing of bony foramina of the skull, closure of the optic foramen, possibly with transection of optic nerve. Retinal hemorrhage, enlargement of the carpi, and cerebellar/cerebral compression may be evident. Microscopically, the optic nerves display necrosis, demyelination, and fibrosis. Retinal atrophy and gliosis of the ganglion cell layer and the nerve fiber layer may occur.

C

CONGENITAL OCULAR DISORDERS (CONTINUED)

• Congenital cataracts related to BVDV infection may be accompanied by cerebellar hypoplasia, bilateral microphthalmia, retinal degeneration, and optic neuritis with combinations of brachygnathism, hypotrichosis, hydrocephalus, or microencephaly.

TREATMENT

THERAPEUTIC APPROACH
Euthanasia is indicated for severe congenital anomalies that result in blindness or which are associated with other significant disorders.

SURGICAL CONSIDERATIONS AND TECHNIQUES
Rarely indicated with the exception of entropion and ectropion, which may require surgical intervention when severe. Entropion can be corrected with temporary tacking sutures/horizontal mattress sutures, or a modified Hotz-Celsus resection. Ectropion often requires surgical correction, with a V-to-Y blepharoplasty.

MEDICATIONS

DRUGS OF CHOICE
• Adult cattle with vitamin A deficiency may respond to 440 IU/kg of vitamin A parenterally followed by 6,000 IU/kg every 2 months; diet should be enriched.
• Any underlying cause for entropion should be addressed (dehydration). Corneal ulceration in ectropion or entropion can be treated with topical ophthalmic antibiotics and atropine if necessary for miosis. The lid can be everted by injecting 0.5–1 mL of procaine penicillin G subcutaneously immediately below the eyelid margin.

CONTRAINDICATIONS
• Surgical correction is contraindicated for entropion secondary to temporary causes such as dehydration.
• Topical corticosteroids are contraindicated when corneal ulceration is present.
• Surgical correction of any disorder with a possible heritable component is discouraged unless necessary for function or pain relief, and breeding of that animal is contraindicated.

PRECAUTIONS
• Aggressive surgical correction of entropion can create ectropion.

• Appropriate milk and meat withdrawal times must be followed for all compounds administered to food-producing animals.

POSSIBLE INTERACTIONS
N/A

FOLLOW-UP

EXPECTED COURSE AND PROGNOSIS
• Prognosis is poor for severe and complicated congenital ocular disorders.
• Animals with potentially heritable disorders, even if mild (entropion), should ideally be culled or excluded from breeding.

POSSIBLE COMPLICATIONS
Disorders that expose or traumatize the cornea (entropion, ectropion, microphthalmia) can create severe discomfort, corneal ulceration, corneal rupture, and permanent blindness if not addressed promptly.

CLIENT EDUCATION
Focus on breeding management for potentially heritable disorders.

PATIENT CARE
Repeat monitoring of the cornea using intermittent fluorescein stain and evaluation of the lids is indicated for disorders where corneal compromise is likely.

PREVENTION
• Maintain appropriate concentrations of vitamin A in adult and calf rations.
• Avoid exposure to toxic plants and infectious diseases during gestation.
• Monitor neonates and young stock for signs of ocular discomfort and discharge.
• Remove any animals that might have a heritable disorder from the breeding pool.

MISCELLANEOUS

ASSOCIATED CONDITIONS
• Several ocular congenital disorders including cyclopia, vitamin A deficiency, and microphthalmia are accompanied by structural and functional anomalies of the skull, limbs, and CNS. Animals with congenital ocular disorders should be carefully assessed for anomalies of other body systems.

AGE-RELATED FACTORS
Most disorders are evident at birth or in the first week of life.

ZOONOTIC POTENTIAL
N/A

PREGNANCY
A controlled ration with no vitamin deficiencies, and avoiding exposure to toxic plants and infectious diseases is critical during pregnancy.

BIOSECURITY
• Avoid mixing pregnant animals, especially early in gestation.
• Vaccinate appropriately pre-breeding (especially for BVDV), quarantine new arrivals, and purchase from a known source.

PRODUCTION MANAGEMENT
• Prophylactic dietary supplementation with vitamin A should be provided to all cattle lacking green feed access. Recommended concentrations of vitamin A in feed (IU/kg dry matter) are 2,200 IU for feedlot cattle, 2,800 IU for pregnant cows, 3,900 IU for lactating cows, and 11,000 IU in pre-ruminant calf milk replacer.
• Avoid grazing fields with *V. californicum* during the first trimester of pregnancy.
• Breeding combinations that consistently produce offspring with entropion or other anomalies should be avoided.

SYNONYMS
N/A

ABBREVIATION
BVDV = bovine viral diarrhea virus

SEE ALSO
• Bovine Viral Diarrhea Virus
• Corneal Disorders

Suggested Reading
Agerholm JS, Hewicker-Trautwein M, Peperkamp K, Windsor PA. Virus induced congenital malformations in cattle. Acta Vet Scand 2015, 57:54.
George LW, Van Metre DC. Vitamin A deficiency. In: Smith BP ed, Large Animal Internal Medicine 5th ed. St. Louis: Mosby Elsevier, 2015.
Moore CP, Whitley RD. Ophthalmic disease of small domestic ruminants. Vet Clin North Am Large Anim Pract 1984, 6: 641–65.
van der Lugt JJ, Prozesky L. The pathology of blindness in new-born calves caused by hypovitaminosis A. Onderstepoort J Vet Res 1989, 56:99–109.
Author Emma Gordon
Consulting Editor Erica C. McKenzie
Acknowledgment The author and book editors acknowledge the prior contribution of Melissa N. Carr.

CONTAGIOUS BOVINE PLEUROPNEUMONIA

BASICS

OVERVIEW
• Contagious bovine pleuropneumonia (CBPP) is a highly contagious bacterial disease of cattle and related ruminants resulting in severe, acute fibrinous pneumonia and occasionally polyarthritis.
• The causative agent is *Mycoplasma mycoides mycoides* (Mmm), formerly designated as small colony (SC) type.
• In Africa, causes greater economic losses in cattle than any other disease.
• OIE List A disease; reportable.

INCIDENCE/PREVALENCE
• Incidence of CBPP varies by country.
• Two major strain clusters exist; African strains may exhibit 30–90% morbidity and 10–90% mortality, while European strains exhibit 10–50% morbidity and 5–30% mortality.

GEOGRAPHIC DISTRIBUTION
• Endemic in much of subSaharan Africa.
• Also present sporadically in Asia, particularly the Middle East, Malaysia, and Mongolia.
• Europe has been free since 2004.
• North America and the western hemisphere are free of CBPP.
• Reported in 26 countries in 2014.

SYSTEMS AFFECTED
• Respiratory
• Musculoskeletal
• Urinary
• Reproductive

PATHOPHYSIOLOGY
• Transmission is via aerosol droplet from clinically affected or carrier animals.
• Carrier animals can shed the organism intermittently in respiratory secretions for months to years following recovery from clinical disease.
• Mycoplasmas transit the lung and mycoplasmemia distributes organism to multiple organs including kidney, joints, udder, and uterus.
• Mycoplasmas can be shed in respiratory secretions, urine, milk, seminal fluid, and birth fluids.
• Transplacental transmission can occur.
• The incubation period is 3–12 weeks post-exposure.
• Up to 50% of cases are subclinical.

SIGNALMENT
• Bovine: *Bos indicus* and *Bos taurus*
• Other susceptible species: yak, bison, antelope, reindeer, water buffalo
• Rarely, sheep and goats
• Camels are resistant

PHYSICAL EXAMINATION FINDINGS
• Acute disease:
  ○ Fever, depression, anorexia, decreased lactation.
  ○ Cough, exercise intolerance.
  ○ Tachypnea, dyspnea, standing with elbows abducted.
  ○ Pleurisy.
  ○ Friction rubs, dullness or crackles on thoracic auscultation.
  ○ Open-mouth breathing.
  ○ Lameness and joint effusion in calves.
  ○ Death may occur in 1–3 weeks.
• Subacute disease:
  ○ Mild fever, inappetence, mild tachypnea, ± cough.
  ○ Subacute cases usually recover.
• Chronic disease:
  ○ Poor doers, emaciation, chronic cough.
• Subclinical cases also occur.
• Up to one-third of recovered animals may become chronic carriers and shed organism intermittently for years from pulmonary sequestrae.

CAUSES AND RISK FACTORS
• Caused by *Mycoplasma mycoides mycoides* (Mmm), a fastidious mycoplasma maintained in carrier cattle.
• Mmm is never considered a commensal.
• Mmm is not likely to be isolated from routine aerobic culture; index of suspicion must be present and specific testing requested.
• Risk factors include:
  ○ Exposure to carrier or clinically ill animals.
  ○ Crowded conditions.
• Herd movement into an endemic area, common in pastoral and migratory cultures.
• Herd manager knowledge of CBPP is vital for effective control.

DIAGNOSIS

DIFFERENTIAL DIAGNOSES
• Pasteurellosis
• *Mannheimia haemolytica*
• *Mycoplasma bovis*
• *Histophilus somni*
• BVDV
• BRSV
• IBR
• PI3
• Hardware disease/traumatic reticulopericarditis
• East coast fever
• Bovine ephemeral fever
• Bovine farcy
• Hydatid cyst
• Actinobacillosis
• *Mycobacterium bovis*

CBC/BIOCHEMISTRY/URINALYSIS
Inflammatory leukograms are often present in acutely affected animals.

OTHER LABORATORY TESTS
• Mycoplasmas lack cell walls and are too small to see with light microscopy, so conventional staining techniques are unhelpful.
• Mmm is fastidious and slow-growing; fresh clinical samples should be submitted in transport media to a diagnostic laboratory for culture.
• Specific mycoplasma culture must be requested, as Mmm requires specific media and growth conditions not present in routine aerobic culture.
• Culture of the organism from clinical samples is the standard of diagnosis.
• Antemortem samples may include pleural fluid, tracheal wash, bronchoalveolar lavage, urine, milk, synovial fluid, or placental tissue.
• Nasal swabs are not ideal, as many subclinical or chronic cases have negative nasal swabs.
• Postmortem samples may include fresh lung, pleural fluid or tissue, synovium, or kidney.
• Serologic tests are primarily useful on a herd basis.
  ○ Complement fixation test (CFT).
  ○ Dot blot or Western blot may be more sensitive than CFT in some situations.
  ○ Latex agglutination may be more sensitive in early disease.
  ○ An ELISA field test is available.
  ○ No single serologic test reliably detects animals in all stages of disease.
  ○ Acute and convalescent sera should be evaluated.
• Polymerase chain reaction on lung, pleural fluid, urine, and cultured colonies.
• Histopathology.
• Immunohistochemistry.

IMAGING
• Imaging techniques are not commonly used.
• Radiographs could reveal evidence of pleural effusion and pulmonary consolidation.
• Ultrasound could demonstrate pleural fluid and guide transthoracic sampling.

PATHOLOGIC FINDINGS
• Pulmonary lesions are frequently unilateral.
• Acute disease:
  ○ Pleuritis and pneumonia with copious fibrin-rich yellow pleural fluid.
  ○ Lung tissue is marbled in appearance due to distended interlobular septae.
  ○ Mediastinal lymph nodes are enlarged and petechiated.
  ○ Alveolar spaces are infiltrated by edema fluid and accumulations of leukocytes. Fibrin thrombi are evident with intense inflammatory infiltrate and necrosis of alveolar septae.
  ○ Renal infarcts may be seen.
  ○ In polyarthritis, copious fibrinous fluid is found within large joints.
• Chronic lesions:
  ○ Sequestrae in pulmonary tissue are encapsulated with fibrosis.
  ○ Lymphocytic infiltration with thickening along interlobular septae, fibrosis of interlobular septae, and coagulative necrosis of lobules.
  ○ Calves may have endocarditis.

CONTAGIOUS BOVINE PLEUROPNEUMONIA (CONTINUED)

• Acute through chronic stages are common in the same animal.

TREATMENT

THERAPEUTIC APPROACH
• Countries with control programs in place may prohibit the treatment of CBPP; slaughter may be mandated.
• While antibiotic treatment may not cure infected animals, it dramatically reduces transmission to susceptible animals and may have a role in outbreak control.

MEDICATIONS

DRUGS OF CHOICE
• No controlled field studies have been done comparing efficacy of antibiotics in naturally infected herds.
• *Mycoplasma mycoides mycoides* is susceptible in vitro to a variety of antimicrobials, including quinolones, tilmicosin, tetracyclines, tylosin, florfenicol, tulathromycin, and streptomycin.
• Mycoplasmas are universally resistant to beta-lactams because they lack a cell wall.
• Danofloxacin (2.5 mg/kg for three consecutive days) has been demonstrated to reduce shedding and decrease infection rates in in-contact naïve cattle.

CONTRAINDICATIONS
• Treatment of CBPP may be prohibited; many countries mandate slaughter of infected animals.
• Antimicrobial therapy may favor the formation of sequestrae and create a carrier state.

PRECAUTIONS
Always follow local laws regarding use and withdrawal of antimicrobials in food animals.

FOLLOW-UP

EXPECTED COURSE AND PROGNOSIS
Chronically affected animals may be poor doers and become progressively emaciated.

POSSIBLE COMPLICATIONS
Up to one third of recovered animals may become long-term carriers.

PATIENT CARE
Monitor for signs of hypoxia and severe dyspnea; if advanced treatment is not available, euthanasia may be appropriate for distressed animals.

PREVENTION
• Two live attenuated vaccines are available, T1/44 and T1/SR.
• In Africa, vaccination against CBPP remains the primary control option.
• Vaccine performance is suboptimal. Low efficacy (33–67%) and a short duration of immunity (6–12 months) are continuing problems.
• Vaccination often generates an extensive tissue reaction, especially primary vaccination or revaccination after a lapse in coverage. Because of this the vaccine is often given in the tail tip, which may become necrotic and slough. Fatal vaccine reactions have occurred.
• Quarantine of farms with testing and slaughtering of animals can provide effective control in the event of an outbreak.
• In endemic areas, uncontrolled or illegal movement of cattle facilitates the spread of disease.
• Vaccination of at-risk or exposed animals may help control an outbreak.
• Serologic testing and quarantine of animals for importation is recommended.

MISCELLANEOUS

ZOONOTIC POTENTIAL
• CBPP is not zoonotic.
• *M. mycoides mycoides* does not constitute a food safety threat.

PREGNANCY
Transplacental transmission can occur.

BIOSECURITY
• CBPP is reportable in many countries.
• Isolating infected herds and restricting movement of animals is imperative to control the spread of disease.
• Separation between animals of 6 meters is considered sufficient to stop droplet transmission.
• Two negative serologic tests two months apart are recommended to verify negative status; however, carriers may be seronegative.
• Animals recovered from clinical disease may be long-term intermittent shedders of the organism.
• *M. mycoides mycoides* survives well in vivo, but is quickly inactivated by external environmental conditions; fomite transmission is unlikely.
• Mmm is susceptible to all common disinfectants.

SYNONYMS
• Mycoplasmosis
• Lung sickness

ABBREVIATIONS
• BRSV = Bovine respiratory syncytial virus
• BVDV = Bovine viral diarrhea virus
• CBPP = Contagious bovine pleuropneumonia
• ELISA = Enzyme-linked immunosorbent assay
• IBR = Infectious bovine rhinotracheitis
• Mmm = *Mycoplasma mycoides mycoides*
• OIE = Office International des Epizooties, World Organization for Animal Health
• PI3 = Parainfluenza type 3

SEE ALSO
• Bovine Respiratory Syncytial Virus
• Bovine Viral Diarrheal Virus
• Echinococcosis
• *Histophilus somni* Complex
• Infectious Bovine Rhinotracheitis
• *Mycoplasma bovis*-Associated Diseases
• Parainfluenza-3 Virus
• Traumatic Reticuloperitonitis
• Tuberculosis: Bovine

Suggested Reading
Contagious bovine pleuropneumonia. Tech Off Int Epizoot 1991, 6: 565–624.
Hübschle OJB, Aschenborn O, Godinho K, Nicholas R. Control of CBPP – a role for antibiotics? Vet Rec 2006, 159: 464.
Hübschle OJB, Ayling RD, Godinho K, et al. Danofloxacin (Advocin™) reduces the spread of contagious bovine pleuropneumonia to healthy in-contact cattle. Res Vet Sci 2006, 81: 304–9.
OIE Disease Cards. Contagious bovine pleuropneumonia, http://www.oie.int/for-the-media/animal-diseases/animal-disease-information-summaries/ (accessed February 18, 2016).
Radostits OM, Gay CC, Hinchcliff KW, Constable PD eds. Veterinary Medicine: A Textbook of the Diseases of Cattle, Horses, Sheep, Pigs and Goats, 10th ed. New York: Saunders, 2007.
United States Animal Health Association, Foreign Animal Diseases book (gray book) website, Contagious Bovine Pleuropneumonia, http://www.usaha.org/Publications.aspx (accessed February 17, 2016).

Author Tamara Gull
Consulting Editor Christopher C.L. Chase
Acknowledgment The author and book editors acknowledge the prior contribution of Scott R.R. Haskell and Danelle Bickett-Weddle.

CONTAGIOUS CAPRINE PLEUROPNEUMONIA

BASICS

DEFINITION
Contagious caprine pleuropneumonia (CCPP) is an extremely contagious bacterial disease of goats resulting in severe, acute pneumonia with high mortality. CCPP is one of the most devastating diseases of goats worldwide.

INCIDENCE/PREVALENCE
• Incidence for CCPP varies worldwide.
• Morbidity often reaches 100% and mortality may be 70–100% in naïve herds.

GEOGRAPHIC DISTRIBUTION
CCPP is considered endemic in east Africa, Asia, and the Middle East. Isolation of the causative agent is difficult and clinical signs can resemble other pneumonias so the actual distribution in these regions is unknown.

SYSTEMS AFFECTED
Respiratory

PATHOPHYSIOLOGY
The bacterial agent *Mycoplasma capricolum capripneumoniae* (*Mccp*, formerly mycoplasma biotype F-38) is extremely contagious and is spread through respiratory secretions from infected goats, resulting in severe respiratory disease and mortality in a naïve herd. Disease caused by *Mycoplasma capricolum capripneumoniae* is limited to the respiratory system. Infection with *Mycoplasma mycoides capri* or other related organisms can occur but demonstrate additional extrarespiratory signs. Secondary infections with other viral pneumonias complicate disease presentation and diagnosis.

HISTORICAL FINDINGS
A severe respiratory disease in goats with high morbidity (100%) and mortality (may approach 100%) within 7–10 days after clinical disease onset. CCPP may present as peracute (animals die within a few days), acute, subacute, and chronic.

SIGNALMENT
• Caprine.
• Sheep may be affected in mixed herds.
• Wild ruminants have been diagnosed.

PHYSICAL EXAMINATION FINDINGS
• CCPP is limited to the respiratory tract. Animals acutely infected with *Mycoplasma capricolum capripneumoniae* present with high fever (106°F), cough, labored breathing, weakness, and anorexia, leading to exercise intolerance and respiratory distress. Goats will stand with legs spread, neck extended downward, and tongue protruded.
• Frothy nasal discharge and continuous stringy salivation appear shortly before death.
• Infection with *Mycoplasma mycoides capri* results in a more generalized infection with respiratory signs as well as lesions beyond the respiratory system.

CAUSES AND RISK FACTORS
• *Mycoplasma capricolum capripneumoniae* causes CCPP.
• Other related organisms, such as *Mycoplasma mycoides capri*, cause a similar condition, sometimes considered a less common form of CCPP, in goats. However, lesions are not limited to the respiratory tract.
• Disease is spread through direct contact and inhalation of infective aerosols.
• A subclinical carrier state in some survivors is suspected but has not been demonstrated.
• Introduction of infected animals into previously uninfected herds.

DIAGNOSIS

DIFFERENTIAL DIAGNOSIS
Peste des petits ruminants, pasteurellosis, other *Mycoplasma* spp. such as *Mycoplasma mycoides capri* pneumonias, and *Salmonella* spp.

CBC/BIOCHEMISTRY/URINALYSIS
N/A

OTHER LABORATORY TESTS
• Serologic tests such as complement fixation, latex agglutination, indirect hemagglutination, and ELISA can be used, particularly on a herd basis. In an outbreak, animals often die before measurable titers are obtained.
• PCR is the technique of choice for CCPP diagnosis and can be applied to postmortem lung tissues and pleural fluid.
• Confirmatory diagnosis is made by culturing the agent from lung, pleuritic fluid, swabs of major bronchi, and tracheobronchial or mediastinal lymph nodes.

PATHOLOGIC FINDINGS
• With *M. capricolum capripneumoniae* infection, one or both lungs may be affected and may be adhered to the thoracic wall due to thickened pleura, with straw-colored fluid in the thoracic cavity. The lungs will have a fibrinous pneumonia and may have pea-sized, yellow-colored nodules with congestion surrounding the nodules. An entire lobe may become solidified or develop massive hepatization. Thickening of the interlobular septa, as seen in bovine pleuropneumonia, is not usually observed in goats.
• Histopathology reveals serofibrinous to fibrinonecrotic pleuropneumonia with infiltrates in the alveoli, bronchioles, interstitial septae, and subpleural connective tissue.
• Peribronchial lymphoid hyperplasia with mononuclear cell infiltration may also be seen.

TREATMENT

THERAPEUTIC APPROACH
• Veterinarians who suspect this disease should follow the regulatory guidelines for their country/locality. In many countries CCPP is a disease reportable to veterinary authorities.
• Due to the contagious nature of this disease, affected animals should be isolated and the entire herd placed under quarantine.

MEDICATIONS

DRUGS OF CHOICE
• Macrolides, tetracyclines, and quinolones are reportedly active against *M. capricolum* subsp. *capripneumoniae*. However, in many countries, including in North America, CCPP is a reportable disease and treatment may not be an option. It is not known whether treated animals could still spread the disease or develop a subclinical carrier status.

CONTRAINDICATIONS
Observation of drug withdrawal periods for meat and milk are important when using antibiotic agents.

FOLLOW-UP

EXPECTED COURSE AND PROGNOSIS
Acute disease has a morbidity of 70–100% with mortality reaching 100% in some goat herds.

POSSIBLE COMPLICATIONS
It is suspected, but not confirmed, that recovered goats could potentially maintain a subclinical carrier status, leading to exposure of susceptible animals.

CLIENT EDUCATION
Clients should be made aware of the seriousness of CCPP and the contagious aspects and that the disease may have regulatory consequences. Clients can be encouraged to practice good biosecurity practices, such as isolation of new animals, to help prevent introduction of any contagious diseases onto their premises.

PATIENT CARE
• Monitor animals for signs of labored breathing and nasal discharge to ensure a patent airway.
• Affected animals should be isolated and activity restricted because of the exercise intolerance due to the severe respiratory disease.
• Maintain a good plane of nutrition with fresh food and water daily.

CONTAGIOUS CAPRINE PLEUROPNEUMONIA   (CONTINUED)

PREVENTION
• A lyophilized saponin-inactivated *Mccp* vaccine is commercially available. Vaccination is reported to have good to excellent success in preventing disease.
• Testing, slaughter of infected animals, vaccination, cleaning and disinfection of infected premises, animal movement control, and quarantine are some of the strategies used to control the disease in endemic countries.

MISCELLANEOUS

ZOONOTIC POTENTIAL
CCPP is not known to be a zoonotic disease.

BIOSECURITY
Isolating infected animals is imperative for the control of this disease. Testing, slaughter of infected animals, vaccination, cleaning and disinfection of infected premises, animal movement control, and quarantine are some of the strategies used to control the disease in endemic countries.

SYNONYMS
• *Mycoplasma* biotype F-38
• Pleuropneumonie contagieuse caprine
• Bou-frida
• Abu-nini

ABBREVIATIONS
• CCPP = contagious caprine pleuropneumonia
• Mccp = *Mycoplasma capricolum capripneumoniae*
• PCR = polymerase chain reaction

SEE ALSO
• Pasteurellosis
• Peste des Petits Ruminants
• Respiratory Disease: Small Ruminant
• Salmonellosis

Suggested Reading
Aiello SE ed. Merck Veterinary Manual, 10th ed. Whitehouse Station, NJ: Merck & Co. 2012. http://www.merckvetmanual.com/mvm/respiratory_system/respiratory_diseases_of_sheep_and_goats/contagious_caprine_pleuropneumonia.html

The Center for Food Security and Public Health, Iowa State University. http://www.cfsph.iastate.edu/Factsheets/pdfs/contagious_caprine_pleuropneumonia.pdf

Office International des Epizooties. 2000. Manual of Standards for Diagnostic Tests and Vaccines, chapter 2.7.6. Contagious Caprine Pleuropneumonia http://www.oie.int/fileadmin/Home/eng/Health_standards/tahm/2008/pdf/2.07.06_CCPP.pdf

Rurangirwa FR, McGuire TC. Contagious caprine pleuropneumonia: Diagnosis and control, http://www.fao.org/wairdocs/ilri/x5473b/x5473b11.htm

United States Animal Health Association. Contagious Caprine Pleuropneumonia. In: Foreign Animal Diseases Gray Book, 7th Ed, 2008, pp. 219–23. http://www.usaha.org/Portals/6/Publications/FAD.pdf

Author Cynthia Faux
Consulting Editor Christopher C.L. Chase
Acknowledgment The author and book editors acknowledge the prior contribution of Danelle Bickett-Weddle.

COPPER DEFICIENCY AND TOXICITY

BASICS

OVERVIEW
- Copper (Cu) is an essential trace element involved in multiple enzyme systems throughout the body. Failure of these enzyme systems interferes with growth and cellular functions, and can result in significant clinical disease.
- Cu plays a necessary role in iron (Fe) metabolism, elastin and collagen formation, bone formation, melanin production, hemoglobin synthesis, myelination of the spinal cord, and antioxidant functions. It is also necessary for normal reproductive and immune function.
- The liver is considered the key organ in Cu metabolism, storage, and excretion.
- Ruminants store Cu in the liver during periods of excess intake and deplete Cu from the liver when intake is low.
- Cu can be toxic if consumed in excessive or unbalanced amounts in feed, via inadvertent ingestion of other copper sources, or with iatrogenic administration of excessive Cu.
- Several other elements have a negative impact on Cu absorption and metabolism including molybdenum (Mo), sulfur (S), iron (Fe), and zinc (Zn). The negative interactions between Cu and these elements significantly affect Cu availability and animal requirements, and can influence the development of Cu deficiency or toxicity.

INCIDENCE/PREVALENCE
- Cu deficiency is uncommon, but is generally associated with specific geographic regions with suboptimal soil conditions (such as in marshy, peaty, or coastal land).
- Cu toxicity is also uncommon; however, a high prevalence can occur in flocks or herds exposed to excessive dietary Cu or other sources of Cu.

GEOGRAPHIC DISTRIBUTION
- Worldwide, influenced by species distribution, soil factors and management systems.
- Cu deficiency is heavily influenced by soil type and is common under natural grazing conditions in Australia, New Zealand, the Netherlands, and the UK, in areas with sandy and limestone soils, and washed-out soils that have low Cu concentrations, resulting in low plant Cu concentration. Reclaimed swamps or peat bogs are often high in Mo.
- Many areas in the United States and Canada are also Cu deficient; however, there can be tremendous variation in Cu soil content within a small region, and even on a given property.

SYSTEMS AFFECTED
Deficiency:
- Integument
- Nervous
- Digestive
- Musculoskeletal
- Cardiovascular
- Hemolymphatic
- Reproductive

Toxicity:
- Digestive
- Cardiovascular
- Hemolymphatic

PATHOPHYSIOLOGY
- Cu is involved in a variety of critical enzyme systems including superoxide dismutase, cytochrome oxidase, lysyl oxidase, ascorbic acid oxidase, and ceruloplasmin. Adequate Cu is also required for iron metabolism and the prevention of cellular oxidative damage. Decreased function of these systems can propagate a wide variety of clinical syndromes that can vary depending on the species and age of the affected animals.
- Primary Cu deficiency arises due to insufficient copper in the diet of the pregnant ewe/doe (congenital deficiency) and/or the diet of the growing lamb/kid (delayed deficiency). Plant copper concentrations <5 mg/kg DM are dangerous and <3 mg/kg DM are likely to result in primary Cu deficiency. Cu-deficient soils are generally sandy and of poor quality.
- Secondary Cu deficiency occurs when dietary concentrations of molybdenum (most commonly), sulfur (occasionally), or iron or zinc (rarely) are high. These minerals compete with Cu uptake and increase excretion of Cu from the body. Secondary deficiency is more likely to occur in grazing adult animals. Forage concentrations of Mo >10 mg/kg are associated with secondary Cu deficiency. Peaty soils are more often associated with excess Mo. S-containing fertilizers may exacerbate Cu deficiency.
- Acute Cu toxicosis is rare and results from ingestion or administration of a large amount of Cu (usually as a soluble copper salt) in a short period of time. This is most common in cattle and occasionally goats.
- Chronic Cu toxicosis is more common and results from chronic ingestion of excess dietary Cu, or rations with a high Cu : Mo ratio (>10:1 for sheep) resulting in slow accumulation of Cu in the liver. Once a threshold is reached, or alternatively a hepatotoxic incident occurs, large quantities of Cu are suddenly liberated from the liver. High serum Cu concentrations then provoke a hemolytic crisis which results in hemoglobinemia, hemoglobinuria, methemoglobinemia, and anemia, with severe systemic disease and a high likelihood of mortality. This is most likely to occur in sheep.

HISTORICAL FINDINGS
Identifies factors related to soil or plant management that could provoke Cu deficiency, or alternatively, identifies potential sources of exposure to excessive Cu.

SIGNALMENT
- Potentially all ruminant species can suffer from deficiency or toxicity.
- Sheep are most susceptible to Cu toxicity.
- Adult cattle are more resistant to Cu toxicity than younger cattle.
- Young cattle are most susceptible to Cu deficiency.
- Young lambs and kids are susceptible to neurologic disease with Cu deficiency.

PHYSICAL EXAMINATION FINDINGS
Copper Deficiency
- Signs of deficiency are variable and affect a large number of body systems.
- Signs of anemia can arise because decreased ceruloplasmin impairs iron oxidation and decreased delta-aminolevulinic acid dehydratase impairs heme synthesis. This causes alterations of the protein skeleton of the erythrocyte resulting in delayed maturation and decreased lifespan of erythrocytes. Anemia can result in decreased production parameters, lethargy and ill thrift.
- Poor hair/fiber quality occurs because of impaired keratinization of the hair or wool, causing a long rough hair coat, or the formation of poorly crimped, "steely" wool. Hair changes indicate late stage Cu deficiency.
- Hypochromotrichia arises from decreased tyrosinase activity causing morphologic and functional changes in melanocytes with lightening of the hair coat color. It is typically most evident in black cattle with the formation of lighter-colored hair on the face around the eyes, or a reddish-orange tinge may be seen behind the shoulder and on the lower hair coat.
- Ataxia in neonatal or juvenile kids and lambs arises because decreased cytochrome oxidase and superoxide dismutase activity in utero causes oligodendrocyte dysfunction and hypomyelination of nerves.
- Reproductive failure represented by decreased fertility, delayed or depressed estrus, fetal death and resorption, and decreased semen quality can occur.
- Pathologic fractures and lameness can arise from decreased lysyl oxidase activity creating increased bone fragility, irregular thickness of the physis, and joint deformation.
- Increased susceptibility to infectious diseases occurs because a decline in superoxide dismutase and cytochrome oxidase provoke decreased number and function of both neutrophils and lymphocytes.
- Diarrhea occurs because decreased cytochrome oxidase activity leads to mitochondrial changes in the intestine resulting in crypt elongation, goblet cell hyperplasia, and villous and mucosal atrophy.
- Poor growth and/or loss of body weight is observed.

Copper Toxicosis
- Acute Cu toxicosis can present with salivation, colic, diarrhea, convulsions,

C

COPPER DEFICIENCY AND TOXICITY

paralysis and collapse, related to severe irritation to the GI tract. Hemolysis can follow in animals that survive the acute consequences.

• Chronic Cu toxicosis can result in anorexia and weakness, and signs relating to intravascular hemolysis and anemia including hemoglobinuria, weakness, tachycardia, and pallor progressing to jaundice. Death occurs, and is often acute. Signs of renal failure (anuria, oliguria, or polyuria; polydipsia and edema) may occur in animals that survive the initial crisis. Goats with chronic toxicity may display neurologic signs without hemolysis.

GENETICS

• There is a strong breed component to the susceptibility of sheep to Cu deficiency. Scottish Blackface and Finnish Landrace sheep are poor utilizers of Cu and very susceptible to deficiency. Conversely, they are more resistant to Cu toxicity.

• Merino sheep are also more resistant to Cu toxicosis; however, Texel sheep require little Cu and are resistant to Cu deficiency but very susceptible to Cu toxicity.

• Simmental and Charolais cattle appear to have higher Cu requirements than Angus cattle.

CAUSES AND RISK FACTORS

Copper Deficiency

• Cu deficiency is considered a severe limitation to grazing ruminants throughout the world, and is more frequent on pastures than in feedlots.

• Cu deficiency in ruminants can result from low Cu concentration in feeds (i.e., <3 mg/kg DM) but most commonly occurs when Cu concentrations in forages are normal (i.e., 6–16 mg/kg DM) but Cu is less available due to concurrently high concentrations of Mo or S.

• Cu deficiency can occur when forage Mo concentration exceeds 3 mg/kg DM and Cu concentration is <5 mg/kg DM.

• Cu deficiency can occur under dietary conditions of low Cu (i.e., <5 mg/kg DM), low Cu and high Mo (i.e., ratio 2:1), higher Mo (i.e., >20 mg/kg DM), and normal Cu and low Mo but with high levels of soluble proteins from lush pastures.

• Overgrazing and excessive dietary calcium or zinc also decrease Cu absorption.

Copper Toxicity

• An extended period of time (i.e., weeks or months) is usually needed for development of chronic Cu toxicity.

• Sheep are considered the most sensitive domestic animal species in regard to Cu toxicity. Marked elevation of hepatic Cu was demonstrated in sheep fed diets containing Cu at 26–38 mg/kg DM whereas rats tolerated diets containing Cu concentrations as high as 500 mg/kg DM.

• Significant differences have also been shown between sheep and cattle in dietary Cu

tolerance (i.e., 25 vs. 100 mg/kg DM). Adequate dietary Cu for sheep is around 5–8 mg/kg DM, and >8 mg/ kg DM can promote toxicity.

• Chronic Cu toxicity has been reported in dairy cows fed diets containing Cu at 37.5 mg/kg DM during lactation and 22.6 mg/kg DM dry cows. The minimum recommended dietary Cu concentration for cattle is 4–10 mg/kg.

• Inappropriate feeding of sheep with commercial products designed for other species (horses, cows) can result in Cu toxicity, particularly in susceptible breeds. Camelids have developed toxicosis after consuming cattle feed.

• Grazing on plants treated with fungicides, pastures fertilized with manure from Cu-fed swine or poultry, or pastures contaminated by copper smelting can create toxicity.

• Other sources of Cu that can be associated with toxicity include copper sulfate foot bath solution which might be inappropriately ingested if not properly disposed of after use. Calf milk replacer excessively supplemented with Cu can induce toxicity in calves.

• Diets with a high Cu : Mo ratio (>10:1) allow enhanced storage of Cu in the liver, due to reduced formation of Cu : Mo complexes which aid Cu excretion.

• Ingestion of hepatotoxic plants can create hepatocellular damage and increase hepatocyte affinity for Cu, which may result in toxicity even when dietary Cu intake is within acceptable limits.

DIAGNOSIS

DIFFERENTIAL DIAGNOSES

• Differential diagnoses for Cu deficiency can include iodine deficiency, vitamin D deficiency (rickets), sulfur deficiency, and vitamin E/selenium deficiency. Additionally, parasitism (internal and external), poor nutrition, Johne's disease, and other causes of anemia should be considered.

• Acute Cu toxicity must be differentiated from intestinal accidents, enteritis, arsenic and nitrate poisoning, and urethral obstruction.

• Differential diagnoses for chronic copper toxicity include ingestion of hemolyzing toxins or plants, and causes of chronic hepatic failure.

CBC/BIOCHEMISTRY/URINALYSIS

• CBC might reveal microcytic, hypochromic anemia in deficiency, and hemoglobinemia, methemoglobinemia, Heinz bodies and anemia are often evident in toxicity.

• Serum chemistry in animals with Cu toxicity might show hyperbilirubinemia, increased liver enzymes, and azotemia (prerenal and/or renal origin). Both AST and GGT can be elevated in advance of a hemolytic crisis, and can be used to identify affected animals

within a group for chelation therapy prior to development of more severe clinical signs.

• Urinalysis is most likely to be abnormal with hemolytic crisis of Cu toxicity, in which case, darkly discolored urine is evident due to hemoglobinuria, and urine specific gravity may be isosthenuric despite azotemia. Red cells, protein and casts in the urine reflect acute nephrosis from hemoglobin damage to the renal tubules.

OTHER LABORATORY TESTS

• Diagnosis of Cu disorders can be difficult. The liver stores Cu and will release it to maintain blood Cu concentrations and essential host functions. Consequently, measurement of blood Cu concentration overestimates body Cu stores in deficient states and underestimates body Cu stores in Cu toxicity states.

• Deficiency diagnosis—sheep
  ○ Serum or plasma Cu (plasma Cu is ~5% higher)
    ▪ Deficient: <0.4 ppm
    ▪ Marginal: 0.4–0.7 ppm
  ○ Erythrocyte superoxide dismutase activity
    ▪ Short-duration deficiency: youngstock <0.5, adult <0.3 mg/g hemoglobin
    ▪ Prolonged deficiency: youngstock <0.3, adult <0.2 mg/g hemoglobin
  ○ Tissue Cu
    ▪ Liver: deficient <4.0 ppm DW
    ▪ Liver: marginal 5.0–20 ppm DW
    ▪ Fetal liver: deficient <10 ppm DW
    ▪ Wool: deficient 0.5–2.5 ppm DW

• Deficiency diagnosis—goat
  ○ Serum Cu
    ▪ Deficient: <0.5 ppm
    ▪ Marginal: 0.5–0.8 ppm
  ○ Tissue Cu
    ▪ Liver: deficient <10 ppm DW
    ▪ Liver: marginal 15–25 ppm DW
    ▪ Fetal liver: deficient <20 ppm DW
    ▪ Hair: deficient <3 ppm DW

• Toxicity Diagnosis
  ○ Increased whole blood Cu concentration: 50–200 µg/dL normal, and 10–20 fold increase occurs in toxicity.
  ○ Increased liver copper concentrations >250 ppm DM.
  ○ Increased kidney Cu concentration >100 ppm DM.

IMAGING

Radiographs can be relevant to investigation of bony pathology associated with Cu deficiency.

OTHER DIAGNOSTIC PROCEDURES

Forage or soil concentrations of Cu, S, and Mo may be helpful adjuncts in the recognition of copper deficiency.

• Normal soils have Cu concentrations of 18–22 ppm and deficient soils generally have copper concentrations <2 ppm.

• Soil Mo concentrations >10 ppm will often precipitate secondary Cu deficiency.

PATHOLOGIC FINDINGS

• Chronic Cu toxicity results in a pale, friable liver, "gunmetal" kidneys, and splenomegaly. Histopathologically, there is centrilobular hepatic necrosis, hepatic fibrosis, and biliary hyperplasia. Kupffer cells contain pigment, and granules in the liver stain positive for copper on rhodanine stain. Cu concentration should be measured in both liver and kidney, since liver concentrations will decrease once a hemolytic crisis has occurred.
• Acute toxicity is marked by severe gastrointestinal inflammation. Cu concentrations in the liver and kidney may be normal in these animals, but elevated in rumen content and feces.

TREATMENT

THERAPEUTIC APPROACH

• Treating or preventing Cu deficiency can be achieved in juvenile and adult animals through a variety of means. Cu deficiency is corrected by supplementation of Cu in the diet, via inclusion in the concentrate mixture of feedlot diets, or supplementing grazing ruminants with Cu compounds through injections or oral treatments. Chelated forms (organic complexes) of Cu have higher bioavailability than inorganic sources.
• Treatment of Cu toxicity is often unrewarding. A variety of protocols exist with varying intensity of treatment and cost. Most protocols focus on methods to chelate Cu.

SURGICAL CONSIDERATIONS AND TECHNIQUES

N/A

MEDICATIONS

DRUGS OF CHOICE

• For deficiency, oral treatment with 1.5 g of Cu sulfate for ewes and 35 mg for lambs can be given as a single dose; cattle can be injected with Cu glycinate (400 mg SC to adult; 100–200 mg SC to calves) or with copper disodium edetate.
• Treating toxicity can be achieved through a variety of methods to compete with or chelate Cu. These include:
  ◦ Administration of Mo and S
    ▪ Ammonium molybdate (100 mg) and sodium sulfate (1 g) in 20 mL of water or in feed daily for 5–6 weeks (lambs)
    ▪ Sodium thiosulfate 6–20 mg/kg PO once daily for 3 weeks
    ▪ Ammonium molybdate 5–10 mg/kg or 50–500 mg PO daily for 3 weeks
    ▪ Ammonium tetrathiomolybdate 2–7 mg/kg IV or SC every 2–3 days for 3–6 treatments.

  ◦ Sodium EDTA 70 mg/kg IV daily for 2 days
  ◦ D-penicillamine 50 mg/kg PO q24h or divided q12h for 6 days (expensive)
  ◦ Vitamin E 2,000–5,000 IU PO q24h for 3 weeks (antioxidant)
  ◦ Zinc 100–200 mg/kg DM of feed decreases liver Cu accumulation
  ◦ Fluid therapy, oral or IV, should be instituted to help prevent or limit the detrimental effects of hemoglobin on renal tubules.

CONTRAINDICATIONS

• If a diagnosis of deficiency is incorrect (i.e., not supported by analysis of Cu levels in the animal), Cu supplementation may result in toxicity.
• Injectable copper can be very toxic in sheep and goats.

PRECAUTIONS

• Appropriate milk and meat withdrawal times must be followed for all compounds administered to food-producing animals.
• Injectable forms of Cu can cause tissue reactions and even mortality.
• Different forms of Cu have varying availability which must be taken into account when formulating mineral mixes. For example, feed grade Cu sulfate offers 25% Cu on an as-fed basis (40% DM basis) whereas feed grade Cu oxide offers 50% Cu as fed (80% DM). Salt mixtures for sheep should usually only contain 0.0625–0.13% Cu.

POSSIBLE INTERACTIONS

Cu interacts significantly with Mo, Zn, and S; hence the balance of these elements must be assessed during thorough nutritional analysis of ruminant rations.

FOLLOW-UP

EXPECTED COURSE AND PROGNOSIS

• The prognosis for Cu deficiency is dependent on the type and severity of clinical signs. Animals with subclinical deficiency or mild clinical signs will often respond well to direct treatment of the presenting syndrome and Cu supplementation. Severely affected animals with more complicated issues, such as pathologic fractures, may require euthanasia.
• The prognosis for Cu toxicity is guarded. It is very poor in severely affected animals in hemolytic crisis, in spite of aggressive intervention. Affected cohorts with minimal or mild signs can respond to chelation and fluid therapy.

POSSIBLE COMPLICATIONS

• Renal failure is common with hemolytic crisis.
• Injections with Cu glycinate and Cu EDTA solutions can cause tissue reactions or acute death.

CLIENT EDUCATION

Provide accurate information regarding Cu requirements for the species and ages within the production system, and measures to control or prevent deficiency and toxicity (depending on which is the more relevant concern).

PATIENT CARE

N/A

PREVENTION

Deficiency

• Cu is distributed in feeds at various concentrations that can range from 1 to 50 mg/kg of dry matter (DM). The Cu content of feeds depends on geographic location of origin, soil pH, climate, crop management, and plant species, maturity, and yield. Cu concentrations are highest in legumes and clover (i.e., 15 mg/kg DM), lowest for grasses (i.e., 5 mg/kg DM), and intermediate for grains (i.e., 4–8 mg/kg DM).
• Copper oxide wire particles or rods contained within a gelatin capsule can be given orally to ruminants at risk of deficiency. Rods are liberated into the rumen and abomasum to release Cu over 4–12 months. Dosing protocols are as follows:
  ◦ Sheep: 1.25 g Cu to weaned lambs, 2.5 g Cu to adults
  ◦ Goats: 2 g Cu to kids 5 weeks of age, 4 g to does in early pregnancy
  ◦ Cattle: 12.5 g Cu to calves, 25 g for animals ≥500 lb
• Copper heptonate can be administered IM (25 mg Cu to weaned lambs and 37.5 mg Cu to adults) once every 3–9 months, respectively. Cu glycinate and Cu EDTA can also be given by injection at 3- to 6-month intervals to prevent deficiency.
• Copper sulfate can be spread on pasture at 1.5–3.0 kg/ha.
• Dosing ewes 8 and 4 weeks prior to lambing with 200 mg Cu sulfate can prevent congenital Cu deficiency in lambs; does can be given Cu glycinate (150 mg SC) mid gestation for the same effect.
• Cu methionate injection (5 mg) can be given to lambs at 3–10 days of age to prevent delayed deficiency; or Cu glycinate (60 mg SC) can be given at birth.
• Cu also can be offered in a free choice mineral mix containing 0.2–0.6% Cu. Under severe deficiency, Cu sulfate could be increased in the mineral mix to 0.5%.

Toxicity

• Feed appropriate feed and mineral supplements, particularly to sheep.
• Avoid contact with compounds that have high Cu concentrations such as fungicides and foot bath compounds.
• Evaluate dietary elements: Mo at 2–5 mg/kg of the ration, S at 0.4%, and zinc at 200 mg/kg will limit copper absorption in ruminants.

COPPER DEFICIENCY AND TOXICITY

C

 MISCELLANEOUS

ASSOCIATED CONDITIONS
• Cu deficiency can provoke anemia, severe diarrhea, neonatal ataxia, reproductive failure, hypochromotrichia, depressed immune function, poor growth, reduced appetite, keratinization failure in hair and wool, and weak, fragile long bones that break easily.
• Toxic plant ingestion can exacerbate Cu toxicity.

AGE-RELATED FACTORS
In general, young and growing ruminants have higher Cu requirements than older animals and are more susceptible to deficiency.

ZOONOTIC POTENTIAL
N/A

PREGNANCY
Abortion secondary to Cu deficiency has been reported.

BIOSECURITY
N/A

PRODUCTION MANAGEMENT
Nutritional requirements:
• It is difficult to provide exact dietary Cu requirements or to predict potential toxic levels of Cu for ruminants under different feeding programs. This is because Cu concentrations and availability vary significantly among feeds and even within the same feed (e.g., a forage species grown in different environmental conditions). Absorption rates of Cu are also affected by homeostatic controls and many other dietary factors.

• Dietary Mo concentrations have the greatest impact on Cu requirements. High dietary Mo under certain grazing conditions significantly increases Cu requirements.
• High intakes of Zn, Fe, and Ca decrease Cu absorption.
• Dietary Cu concentrations of 8, 10, and 7–11 mg/kg DM were recommended to meet the requirements of beef cattle, dairy cattle, and sheep, respectively.
• Because Cu availability in lush pastures is low and its level decreases with forage maturity, Cu supplementation should be increased at early and late maturity stages of forages to prevent deficiency.

SYNONYMS
• "Teart" or "peat scours" refer to ill thrift and diarrhea in cattle with secondary Cu deficiency.
• "Pine" refers to stiffness, epiphyseal enlargement, and ill thrift in young ruminants with Cu deficiency.
• Enzootic ataxia or "swayback" refers to neurologic signs in neonatal and juvenile goats and lambs with Cu deficiency.

ABBREVIATIONS
• Ca = calcium
• CNS = central nervous system
• Cu = copper
• DM = dry matter
• DW = dry weight
• Fe = iron
• Mo = molybdenum
• S = sulfur
• Zn = zinc

SEE ALSO
• Iodine Deficiency and Toxicity
• Selenium/Vitamin E Deficiency
• Sulfur Toxicity
• Vitamin D Deficiency/Toxicosis
• Zinc Deficiency and Toxicity

Suggested Reading
Corah L. Trace mineral requirements of grazing cattle. Anim Feed Sci Technol 1996, 59: 61–70.
Maas J, Smith B. Copper deficiency in ruminants. In: Smith BP ed, Large Animal Internal Medicine, 4th ed. St. Louis: Mosby Elsevier, 2009, pp. 887–9.
McDowell LR. Minerals in Animal and Human Nutrition. San Diego: Academic Press, 1992, pp. 176–204.
Pugh DG, Baird AN eds. Sheep and Goat Medicine, 2nd ed. Midland Heights, MO: Elsevier, 2012.
Smith M, Sherman D. Goat Medicine, 2nd ed. Ames: Wiley Blackwell, 2009.
Solaiman SG, Maloney MA, Qureshi MA, Davis G, D'Andrea G. Effects of high copper supplements on performance, health, plasma copper and enzymes in goats. Small Ruminant Res 2001, 41: 127–39.
Ward JD, Spears JW, Gengelbach GP. Differences in copper status and copper metabolism among Angus, Simmental, and Charolais cattle. J Anim Sci 1995, 73: 571–7.
Xin Z, Waterman DF, Hemken RW, Harmon RJ. Effects of copper status on neutrophil function, superoxide dismutase, and copper distribution in steers. J Dairy Sci 1991, 74: 3078–85.

Author Dusty W. Nagy
Consulting Editor Erica C. McKenzie

CORKSCREW CLAW

BASICS

OVERVIEW
• Corkscrew claw is a deformity of the claw where overgrowth of the abaxial wall displaces the sole axially and dorsally.
• The result is a claw that has a spiral or corkscrew shape. In an animal with a corkscrew claw, the weight-bearing surface of the affected claw is the abaxial wall instead of the sole.
• The lateral claw of the hindlimb is most often affected and the condition is typically bilateral. The deformity is considered heritable.

INCIDENCE/PREVALENCE
The reported incidence rates vary and range from <1% to 11%, with 3% being most typical.

GEOGRAPHIC DISTRIBUTION
Reports are from North America and Europe; however, the condition is likely worldwide.

SYSTEMS AFFECTED
Musculoskeletal

PATHOPHYSIOLOGY
• Animals with corkscrew claw typically have malalignment of the second and third phalanxes with an 11° rotation of the distal interphalangeal joint in the plantar plane.
• Bone exostosis is commonly found on the lateral aspect of the distal interphalangeal joint. In addition, the third phalanx is abnormally long and narrow and curved on its abaxial margin, resulting in an angled ventral surface of the pedal bone.
• The abnormal conformation is thought to cause abnormal mechanical stresses within the claw, with excessive force being applied in the region of the abaxial white line.
• The growth rate of the abaxial wall is significantly faster than in a normal claw, which causes the abaxial wall to curve and displace the sole axially. The result is the abaxial wall becomes the weight-bearing surface and the sole is partially covered by wall and the remaining, exposed sole faces axially. The result is a claw that appears to have twisted along its long axis, thus giving it a corkscrew appearance.

HISTORICAL FINDINGS
Gait is always abnormal in animals with corkscrew claw but the severity of lameness is variable.

SIGNALMENT
Beef and dairy breeds are both affected. Male and female are both affected. Age is typically 3 years and older but may occur in animals as young as 2 years of age.

PHYSICAL EXAMINATION FINDINGS
Typical findings in corkscrew claw are:
• The abaxial wall is not perpendicular to the ground.
• The abaxial wall is displaced axially and curls under the sole.
• The sole is displaced axially and dorsally.
• The toe is elevated in a clockwise rotation.
• The heel is overgrown and higher than the opposite claw.
• Sole hemorrhages, white line hemorrhages, and white line separation commonly accompany corkscrew claw.

GENETICS
The condition is considered heritable with estimates of heritability ranging from 0.11 to 0.23.

CAUSES AND RISK FACTORS
The condition is heritable and underlying conformation of the animal is the most important risk factor for corkscrew claw. Diet and environment may be contributing factors that affect rate of onset and severity of the deformity.

DIAGNOSIS

Diagnosis is based on the physical appearance of the claw.

DIFFERENTIAL DIAGNOSES
• Chronic laminitis. Abnormal hoof growth is common in chronic laminitis. There may be a long, upturned toe commonly referred to as "slipper toe" but there is not overgrowth of the abaxial wall and deviation of the sole.
• Scissor claw. In some cases, overgrowth of the claws, typically of the front limbs, will result in a curvature of the toe towards the axial plane. This is commonly referred to a "scissor claw." In this case, there is not significant overgrowth of the abaxial wall and deviation of the sole.

CBC/BIOCHEMISTRY/URINALYSIS
N/A

OTHER LABORATORY TESTS
N/A

IMAGING
N/A

OTHER DIAGNOSTIC PROCEDURES
N/A

PATHOLOGIC FINDINGS
Postmortem examination is not performed for clinical cases. See "Pathophysiology" for explanation of changes that are present.

TREATMENT

THERAPEUTIC APPROACH
Corrective Hoof Trimming
• Straighten the dorsal wall and remove the curve in the toe as best as possible but stop if bleeding occurs. A small breech in the dorsal wall will not cause any problems. Straightening the dorsal wall is best done with a sanding disc or chipper wheel.
• Gradually shorten the toe length to approximately 7.5 cm but stop if bleeding occurs. This is best done with hoof nippers.
• Remove the excess wall and sole from the weight-bearing surface of the claw until it is similar in height to the opposite claw. Quarter-round hoof nippers work well to remove the bulk of the material. The remainder of the work is best accomplished with a sanding disc or chipper wheel. The sole is often abnormally thin at the abaxial edge. Proceed with caution and check sole thickness frequently by pressing firmly on the sole to see if it flexes. It may not be possible to achieve a normal balance with the other claw.
• Remove excess horn from the axial aspect of the affected claw and slope the sole on the axial half of the claw.
• Trim the normal claw to achieve as close to normal conformation as possible while maintaining some sense of balance with the affected claw.

MEDICATIONS

DRUGS OF CHOICE
No medications are required.

CONTRAINDICATIONS
N/A

FOLLOW-UP

EXPECTED COURSE AND PROGNOSIS
Gait is typically improved immediately after trimming. The condition is chronic and incurable so the abnormal conformation will recur. The time until significant regrowth occurs is variable but most animals require trimming at least twice per year.

POSSIBLE COMPLICATIONS
It is not uncommon to breech the wall or sole during corrective trimming. Complications as a result of this are unusual.

C

CORKSCREW CLAW

CLIENT EDUCATION
Educate regarding the genetic component of this condition.

PATIENT CARE
Monitor for recurrence, which will usually be evident in 6 months.

PREVENTION
• Affected animals should be removed from the herd when economically feasible. Bulls with corkscrew claw should not be used for breeding.
• Regular hoof trimming every 4–6 months will help maintain relatively normal conformation and help prevent secondary complications that could cause significant lameness.

MISCELLANEOUS

ASSOCIATED CONDITIONS
Sole hemorrhages, sole ulcers, white line hemorrhages, and white line separation can be present in the affected claw.

AGE-RELATED FACTORS
Typically seen in animals 3 years of age and older but can occur as early as 2 years of age.

PRODUCTION MANAGEMENT
At the typical incidence rates, the condition is not an economically significant concern for most producers. Because the condition is heritable, affected cows should be removed from the herd when economically feasible and affected bulls should not be used for breeding.

SEE ALSO
Laminitis in Cattle

Suggested Reading
Greenough PR. Bovine Laminitis and Lameness. London: Saunders 2007, pp. 237–40.
Van Amstel SR, Shearer JK. Abnormalities of hoof growth and development. Vet Clin North Am Food Anim Pract 2001, 17: 73–91.
Author Edgar F. Garrett
Consulting Editor Kaitlyn A. Lutz
Acknowledgment The author and book editors acknowledge the prior contribution of Steven L. Berry.

BASICS

OVERVIEW

• The cornea is transparent and avascular. The cornea is also the most refractive surface of the eye. The cornea is composed of four layers: the epithelium, stroma, Descemet's membrane, and the endothelium.
• Corneal disorders in ruminants include blunt compressive trauma, ulcerative keratitis, corneal lacerations, foreign body penetrations, and congenital dermoids. Occasionally neoplastic lesions (SCC) affect the cornea.
• In food-producing species, infectious disease of the cornea (keratoconjunctivitis) is much more frequently a cause of corneal damage than trauma.
• Treatment of corneal ulceration or infection should ideally be guided by results of ocular examination, cytologic examination, bacterial culture and sensitivity assessments, and topical fluorescein stain.

INCIDENCE/PREVALENCE

• Corneal disorders are common in sheep, goats, and cattle.
• Specific infectious pathogens can cause sporadic herd or flock outbreaks of infectious keratoconjunctivitis that occasionally affect most of the group.
• Infectious bovine keratoconjunctivitis (IBK) is the most common ocular disease of cattle, estimated to affect 5% of beef cattle in the United States and up to 50% of herds.
• Congenital ectropion can reach high prevalence in poorly managed sheep flocks, resulting in a high prevalence of secondary corneal disease.

GEOGRAPHIC DISTRIBUTION

Worldwide

SYSTEMS AFFECTED

Ophthalmic

PATHOPHYSIOLOGY

• Tear film proteases normally provide surveillance and repair functions to detect and remove damaged cells or collagen caused by regular wear and tear on the cornea. These enzymes exist in balance with inhibitory factors to prevent excessive degradation of normal tissue.
• Congenital (entropion) or acquired (trauma, foreign bodies) damage to the cornea can cause significant disruption to the epithelium of the cornea, exposing the underlying stroma and permitting secondary infection.
• Bacterial or fungal pathogens that invade the cornea induce upregulation of cytokines in the tear film and matrix metalloproteinases, and elicit a powerful inflammatory and degradative process.

• In conditions such as ulcerative keratitis, excessive proteases can lead to rapid degeneration of collagen, potentially inducing corneal "melting."
• Significant loss of corneal stroma can lead to exposure of Descemet's membrane and even corneal rupture.
• Common causes of infectious keratoconjunctivitis include *Moraxella bovis* in cattle, and *Mycoplasma conjunctivae* and *Chlamydophila pecorum* in sheep and goats.
• Systemic viral infections such as malignant catarrhal fever and bovine herpesvirus 1 can also induce corneal edema and inflammation in cattle.

HISTORICAL FINDINGS

• Dependent on the condition in question, but acute onset of blepharospasm and ocular discharge is often reported.
• With infectious keratoconjunctivitis disorders, a number of individuals in the group may be reported affected.

SIGNALMENT

• Any species and age of ruminant can develop a corneal disorder.
• IBK tends to be more common in calves and yearling cattle.
• Neoplastic disease (SCC) is most common in mature Hereford cattle.
• Entropion is most common in neonatal sheep, and British breeds such as the Suffolk have a greater predisposition.

PHYSICAL EXAMINATION FINDINGS

• Corneal edema
• Corneal irregularities/infiltrates/defects
• Blepharospasm
• Ocular discharge
• Photophobia
• Eye rubbing
• Lid anomalies (ectropion, laceration, entropion)

GENETICS

• Some sheep breeds have a greater predisposition to congenital entropion.
• Herefords may be more prone to IBK, thought to relate to lack of pigmentation at ocular margins.

CAUSES AND RISK FACTORS

• Exposure to viruses or bacteria associated with corneal disease.
• Crowding and transport can increase potential for traumatic corneal injuries.
• Breed predispositions exist for entropion, IBK, and neoplasia.

DIAGNOSIS

DIFFERENTIAL DIAGNOSES

• Corneal trauma (blunt trauma, penetrations, lacerations, entropion)
• Corneal foreign body
• Uveitis or glaucoma (causing corneal edema)

• Bacterial, fungal, or viral keratoconjunctivitis
• Dermoids (appear as a piece of skin attached to the cornea, may be mistaken for neoplastic lesions)
• Corneal neoplasia

CBC/BIOCHEMISTRY/URINALYSIS

N/A

OTHER DIAGNOSTIC TESTS

• The cornea should be examined as part of a complete ophthalmic examination, using at least a direct ophthalmoscope. A bluish hue is indicative of corneal edema, and white opacities may indicate scarring, calcification, or stretching of Descemet's membrane (Haab's striae). A yellow-white color is usually indicative of white blood cell infiltration of the corneal stroma, which may be epithelialized over the surface (stromal abscess); red linear regions indicate neovascularization.
• Foreign bodies and dermoids can usually be readily appreciated with a light source, preferably a trans-illuminator head attachment.
• The slit beam of a direct ophthalmoscope can be used to assess the depth of corneal defects and the quality of the anterior chamber. Accompanying uveitis will create decreased clarity of the aqueous that can be viewed via the slit beam.
• Any pathologic condition of the cornea warrants fluorescein staining to determine the integrity of the cornea. After topically applying the stain, the cornea is evaluated using a cobalt light to determine the size, depth, and severity of a laceration or ulcer. Very deep lesions are represented by a ring of positive fluorescence around a nonstaining dark central region, indicating exposure of Descemet's membrane (desmetocele) with risk of imminent corneal rupture and iris prolapse.
• A perforated cornea may present with aqueous humor draining from the defect, or fibrin or part of the iris may occlude the perforation. Animals with deep corneal defects need to be handled carefully during diagnostic procedures to prevent globe collapse prior to surgical intervention if it is an option.

IMAGING

N/A

OTHER DIAGNOSTIC PROCEDURES

• Bacterial and fungal cultures can be collected using a cotton swab and should be obtained prior to placing topical anesthetic products on the cornea since these might inhibit pathogen isolation.
• Corneal scrapings allow collection of samples for direct microscopic examination which can facilitate the diagnosis of neoplasia, and fungal or bacterial keratitis. Scraping can be performed using the blunt end of a scalpel blade after topical anesthetic (often 0.5% proparacaine hydrochloride) has been applied

C

to the cornea; the material obtained is placed onto slides that are air dried and stained prior to analysis.

PATHOLOGIC FINDINGS
N/A

TREATMENT

THERAPEUTIC APPROACH
• Therapy is dictated by the type and severity of the corneal injury, the complications encountered, the intended use and economic value of the animal, and other welfare and production considerations.
• Dermoids may be asymptomatic if the abnormal region is small and devoid of hair, and in such cases do not require treatment. Clinical signs can arise as dermoids increase in size or develop hair, which may require surgical intervention.
• Plant material embedded in the epithelium or superficial stroma is the most frequently encountered foreign body in the ruminant eye. Foreign bodies are usually easily removed with a moistened cotton tip applicator or ophthalmic forceps. Topical anesthetic, sedation, and motor or sensory blocks may facilitate removal in animals with significant pain, concerned owners, or intractable nature.
• Confirmed corneal ulceration or incomplete corneal laceration can be managed with medical therapy including topical antibiotic administration q4–8h times daily if feasible (plus topical atropine as needed to control painful ciliary body spasm that can accompany severe corneal disease). Affected eyes must be evaluated q24h until resolved in case of sudden deterioration or lack of improvement. Affected eyes may be protected from rubbing by employing a cup or cover over the eye.
• Antibiotic selection should be based on cytologic assessment and/or bacterial culture and sensitivity results unless the presenting clinical and historical characteristics are strongly suggestive of a specific pathogen.
• Subpalpebral lavage systems can be placed in animals that are reluctant to have direct ocular treatments, that are intractable, or if the severity of the injury warrants frequent and prolonged treatment.
• Topical ointments versus solutions are preferred for direct application due to increased contact time. Ophthalmic solutions are best used in subpalpebral lavage systems.
• Nonsurgical management of severe corneal ulceration may include use of ophthalmic adhesives and soft contact lens application.
• Corticosteroid agents are contraindicated in the treatment of corneal ulceration or laceration, and corneal infection, as they can delay healing and further compromise the diseased cornea.

• Infectious keratoconjunctivitis can be a self-limiting disorder in many animals, with self-cure in 2–3 weeks, which should be considered when determining the need for antibiotic therapy.

SURGICAL CONSIDERATIONS AND TECHNIQUES
• Surgical intervention should be considered for deep corneal ulcerations, especially if the Descemet's membrane is exposed, and particularly in high value, breeding or show animals. Procedures of value include conjunctival pedicle flap and keratoplastic procedures.
• Severe corneal lacerations may warrant surgical repair depending on severity and individual animal value.
• Superficial dermoids can be removed via superficial keratectomy using sharp excision. Surgical anesthesia is recommended to perform a controlled and precise corneal incision without eye movement, particularly for deep or extensive dermoids.
• Enucleation is a sound treatment option if the prognosis is poor, or because of the economic value and expected productivity of the animal. It can be readily performed in standing cattle with manual restraint and appropriate local anesthesia techniques.

MEDICATIONS

DRUGS OF CHOICE
• Most bacterial pathogens of sheep and goats are susceptible to tetracycline. Long-acting tetracycline products can be administered (e.g., oxytetracycline 200 mg/mL given at 20 mg/kg IM or SQ, q72h) and can be combined with an ophthalmic preparation of tetracycline applied q6–8h.
• *M. bovis* is also susceptible to oxytetracycline (20 mg/kg once or twice); penicillin administered subconjunctivally (600,000 IU in 2 mL); florfenicol (20 mg/kg IM, given twice 48 hours apart, or 40 mg/kg SQ once); ceftiofur crystalline-free acid (6.6 mg ceftiofur equivalents/kg given once, SQ, in the posterior aspect of the pinna); and tulathromycin (2.5 mg/kg).
• Atropine can be administered topically to animals displaying significant pain, miosis or with characteristics of uveitis. Ophthalmic ointment preparations or solution (1%) are recommended, or injectable preparations can be diluted to ≤1%.
• Flunixin meglumine can be used at label doses to control pain and inflammation.
• 5% topical hypertonic saline ointment can be applied q6–12h if significant corneal edema is present.
• Identification of fungal hyphae on cytologic examination requires administration of topical antifungal agents (and potentially atropine and systemic NSAIDs). Natamycin,

miconazole, itraconazole, ketoconazole, or fluconazole may be appropriate.

CONTRAINDICATIONS
• Corticosteroids are contraindicated when the integrity of the cornea is compromised by ulceration or laceration.
• Topical NSAID preparations are also typically contraindicated when corneal integrity is compromised.

PRECAUTIONS
• Ophthalmic therapy is often associated with extra-label drug use and should be approached with caution.
• Appropriate milk and meat withdrawal times must be followed for all compounds administered to food-producing animals.

POSSIBLE INTERACTIONS
N/A

FOLLOW-UP

EXPECTED COURSE AND PROGNOSIS
Dependent on etiology and treatment

POSSIBLE COMPLICATIONS
• Permanent corneal scarring
• Blindness
• Corneal rupture
• Decreased weight gain and production

CLIENT EDUCATION
Focus on preventive measures for contagious disorders (IBK) when relevant

PATIENT CARE
• All patients with active corneal disease should have the affected eye or eyes evaluated at least q24h since rapid deterioration can occur, in some cases resulting in blindness and potentially loss of the eye.

PREVENTION
• Infectious keratoconjunctivitis conditions can be controlled by quarantining new arrivals, practicing control of possible vectors (face flies), isolating affected animals, or using a patch over affected eyes.
• Mass medication has been practiced during outbreaks of infectious keratoconjunctivitis with parenteral or oral antibiotic administration to all members of the group.
• Commercial and autogenous vaccines for *M. bovis* exist; variable efficacy reported.

MISCELLANEOUS

ASSOCIATED CONDITIONS
Blindness

AGE RELATED FACTORS
Younger animals are more prone to specific conditions including entropion (sheep) and IBK (cattle).

C

ZOONOTIC POTENTIAL
None

BIOSECURITY
Infectious keratoconjunctivitis conditions benefit from management strategies to reduce spread among a group.

PRODUCTION MANAGEMENT
IBK has a significant economic impact on the cattle industry related to significantly lighter weaning weights in affected calves and treatment-related expense.

SYNONYMS
Pink eye (bacterial keratoconjunctivitis)

ABBREVIATIONS
• IBK = infectious bovine keratoconjunctivitis
• SCC = squamous cell carcinoma

SEE ALSO
Congenital Ocular Disorders

Suggested Reading

Belknap E, Gemensky Metzler A. Diseases of the eye. In: Smith BP ed, Large Animal Internal Medicine,5th ed. St. Louis: Elsevier Mosby, 2015, pp. 1149–91.

Fubini S. Surgical disease of the eye. In: Farm Animal Surgery, 1st ed. St. Louis: Saunders, 2004.

Pugh DG. Diseases of the eye. In: Sheep and Goat Medicine, 2nd ed. St. Louis: Saunders, 2012.

Author Troy E.C. Holder
Consulting Editor Erica C. McKenzie

CORONAVIRUS

BASICS

OVERVIEW
• Disease of neonatal ruminants.
• The causative agent is a coronavirus. All coronaviruses are of the same serotype.
• Pathogenicity is related to load of exposure, level of immunity to the virus, concurrent infection with other neonatal pathogens, and stress. Most infections are concurrent with other neonatal pathogens.
• Virus is ubiquitous with seroprevalence in the adult herd of 80–90%.
• Morbidity of coronavirus is estimated to be 15–25%. Mortality rate in uncomplicated cases is 5–10% but may reach 50% with concurrent bacterial or parasitic infections.

INCIDENCE/PREVALENCE
• Prevalence of coronavirus infections is in the range 15–25% with a great variation in mortality, 5–50% depending on concurrent bacterial and parasitic infections.
• Seroprevalence in the adult herd may be close to 100%.

GEOGRAPHICAL DISTRIBUTION
Worldwide

SYSTEMS AFFECTED
• Digestive
• Respiratory

PATHOPHYSIOLOGY
• The virus is acquired either through the ingestion of fecal contaminated material or inhalation. Initially villous epithelial cells are infected in the proximal small intestine with infection progressing caudally into the colon.
• The infection extends into the colon resulting in infection of the epithelial cells of the ridges as well as the crypts.
• The virus is cytocidal, resulting in sloughing of epithelial cells. Coronavirus may also infect undifferentiated epithelial cells, fibroblasts, and endothelial cells of the lamina propria, resulting in significant damage to the colon. Infected cells contain large numbers of virus and are desquamated into the lumen. Immature crypt cells replace the absorptive epithelium of the small intestine but denuded areas within the colon may take several days to heal.
• The loss of epithelial cells results in a maldigestive as well as a malabsorptive type diarrhea. Maldigestion and malabsorption result in change in bacterial populations which may contribute to the diarrhea.
• Undigested carbohydrates undergo bacterial fermentation resulting in an increase in osmotic pressure and water being drawn into the intestinal lumen.

• Diarrhea results due to increased osmotic pressure and decreased absorption. The physical loss of the epithelial cells results in increased susceptibility to other pathogens because of loss of the villous integrity and decreased secretion of lactoferrin and lysozymes as well as the release of inflammatory mediators.
• Damage predisposes the attachment of ETEC and attaching and effacing *E. coli* to the intestinal villi.
• The loss of electrolytes, bicarbonate, and water leads to dehydration and metabolic acidosis.
• The virus can also infect the respiratory epithelium resulting in a mild respiratory or subclinical respiratory infection.

HISTORICAL FINDINGS
• Sudden onset of diarrhea that spreads rapidly through the neonatal population.
• A few cases may have been noticed initially but the frequency of cases increases as the calving season progresses due to build-up of pathogen load.
• Increased number of cases are observed following periods of stress such as a snowstorm or cold wet weather.

SIGNALMENT
• Bovine, ovine, caprine; potentially all ruminant species.
• Most infections occur <3 weeks of age.
• Calves as old as 3 months of age may be affected.

PHYSICAL EXAMINATION FINDINGS
• Mild to severe watery diarrhea with pieces of milk curd and flecks of blood; color, consistency, and composition will vary with coexisting infections.
• Dehydration and depression with degrees of inappetence or reluctance to nurse. Some animals may be weak to the point of recumbency.
• Bruxism and nasal discharge.
• Clinical signs are more severe than rotavirus-induced diarrhea.
• Acute onset of diarrhea varying from mild to severe, depression, and reluctance to nurse.
• Clinical signs last 3–5 days during which calves become progressively depressed, weak, and experience weight loss.
• Some calves may exhibit signs of abdominal pain. In uncomplicated cases, diarrhea may exist for 2–3 days. In cases of secondary bacterial infection, diarrhea may last 4–6 days.

CAUSES AND RISK FACTORS
• Coronavirus. All cattle coronaviruses are of the same serotype.
• Inadequate colostral transfer of immunoglobulins resulting in

agammaglobulinemia or hypogammaglobulinemia. Lack of local colostral immunity in calves 5 days postpartum or in calves raised on milk replacers.
• Birthing areas contaminated with fecal material containing coronavirus.
• Neonatal housing in which build-up of pathogen load occurs.
• Neonates housed or maintained in a cold wet environment.

DIAGNOSIS

DIFFERENTIAL DIAGNOSES
• *E. coli*
• Rotavirus
• Cryptosporidium
• *Salmonella* spp.
• *Clostridium perfringens* type C
• Nutritional causes: History contains a dietary change or identification of nutritional deficiencies or excesses.

CBC/BIOCHEMISTRY/URINALYSIS
• CBC: Hemoconcentration, increased plasma proteins.
• Serum chemistry: Metabolic acidosis with low plasma bicarbonate. Glucose and electrolyte values will be low depending on severity of diarrhea, prerenal azotemia.
• Urinalysis: Depending on state of dehydration, urine will be concentrated resulting in an increased specific gravity.

OTHER LABORATORY TESTS
• Feces should be collected as soon as diarrhea is noted because exfoliation of virus-laden enterocytes is short-lived and occurs early in the disease process.
• Feces can be submitted for electron microscopy and identification of virus. A few drops of formalin can be added to 10 mL of feces for preservation, or feces can be frozen.
• Serology can detect sero-conversion or a 4-fold increase in serum immunoglobulin levels.
• Fresh sections of the small intestine, preferably mid ileum, and colon tied at the cut ends to contain intestinal contents can be submitted on ice for immunofluorescent microscopy.

PATHOLOGIC FINDINGS
• No specific gross lesions, distended bowel containing undigested milk and fluid. The mucosa may be congested with petechial hemorrhages throughout the intestinal tract.
• Histologically, the villi will be shortened and covered with squamous to cuboidal epithelial cells.

(CONTINUED)   CORONAVIRUS

C

TREATMENT

THERAPEUTIC APPROACH
• Fluid therapy is needed to correct dehydration, circulatory impairment, and electrolyte and metabolic imbalances.
• Fluid deficit should be calculated as well as maintenance requirement, 80–100 mL/kg, and fluid loss in the diarrhea to determine volume of fluids needed during a 24-hour period.
• Fluids may be administered orally or intravenously. Commercial oral electrolyte solutions containing glucose and a non-bicarbonate alkalinizing agent are recommended if the neonate is still nursing. Although oral electrolytes are less likely to be absorbed due to enterocyte pathology, not all enterocytes are affected so some absorption does occur.
• Neonates without a suckle response need IV fluids: isotonic 1.3% sodium bicarbonate solution initially (2 L) followed by Lactated Ringer's Solution.
• Dextrose solution (2.5–5%) is indicated in cases of hypoglycemia. With hypoglycemia and after correcting acid-base status, a 2.5% dextrose and 0.45% saline solution has been recommended.
• Plasma transfusion, although not specific for coronavirus infections, may be warranted in cases of failure of passive transfer and depending on value of the animal.

MEDICATIONS

DRUGS OF CHOICE
• Broad-spectrum antibiotics may be considered because of the potential for mixed infections as well as the loss of mucosal integrity.
• Oral amoxicillin trihydrate 10 mg/kg PO q12h for non-ruminating calves (extra-label in small ruminants), 20-day slaughter withdrawal. Amoxicillin trihydrate-clavulanate potassium 12.5 mg combined drug/kg PO q12h for 3 days (extra-label usage).
• Parenteral ceftiofur 2.2 mg/kg IM q24h for 3 days (extra-label usage).
• Drug withdrawal times must be determined and maintained in the treated animal.

CONTRAINDICATIONS
• Do not use kaolin and pectin as use may increase electrolyte loss.
• Meat and milk withdrawal time periods must be maintained.

FOLLOW-UP

EXPECTED COURSE AND PROGNOSIS
• In uncomplicated infections, diarrhea is present for 2 to 3 days. Prognosis is good, as this infection tends to be self-limiting and generally requires minor supportive care.
• Duration of diarrhea may be 4–6 days with secondary bacterial infections. Prognosis is dependent on the degree of pathology produced by the secondary bacteria.
• Prognosis is good to fair with supportive care. It may take a couple of weeks for animals to fully recover.

POSSIBLE COMPLICATIONS
Hypovolemic shock and death

CLIENT EDUCATION
• Clients need to insure that calves acquire an adequate amount of colostrum. Neonates should be kept dry and in a draft-free environment.
• Animals should be moved and fed in such a way as to reduce the build-up of mud and fecal material in the neonate's environment. Diarrheic animals should be isolated from healthy neonates as they are sources for large numbers of pathogens.
• Owners should work with healthy calves before working with sick calves and should clean equipment, bottles, and nipples adequately between calf usage.
• Owners should be advised as to how to reduce pathogen transfer between calves in regard to equipment, clothing, and shoes/boots.

PATIENT CARE
• Neonates with a suckle response should be left with the dam and allowed to nurse.
• Monitor attitude, suckling response and appetite, fecal color and consistency, and hydration status.
• Monitor age cohorts for signs of diarrhea.
• Animals being reared artificially should remain on their diet or switched to whole milk or colostrum. If the diarrhea becomes worse or the calf becomes depressed, removal from the dam or milk is warranted. In the case of hand-fed neonates that are depressed and not interested in sucking, or neonates not nursing the dam, neonates should receive a high-energy electrolyte solution at a rate of 10% of body weight divided into a minimum of four feedings.
• Calves should also receive 5% of their body weight in electrolyte solutions, spacing 2 hours before or after milk feedings. Milk should not be withheld longer than 24 hours and can be given via an esophageal feeder. No more than 1 liter should be tube-fed at a time.

• Milk and electrolyte solutions can be altered as described previously with a minimum of 10% body weight of fluid per day.
• Oral electrolytes containing bicarbonate should not be fed when calves are receiving milk, as milk digestion maybe disrupted.

PREVENTION
• Reduce exposure, clean maternity areas, move to a clean area after birth. Those handling sick neonates should practice biosecurity measures to reduce exposure to healthy neonates, wash hands and disinfect boots, maintain clothes free of fecal material.
• Vaccination of dams prepartum according to manufacturers' recommendations with a coronavirus vaccine will increase colostral antibody.
• In dairy calves, colostrum management of newborn calves includes the feeding of 2–4 liters of colostrum in the first 24 hours following birth. In beef calves, insure that newborn calves suckle within 1–2 hours after birth.
• Oral vaccination of neonates with a modified-live oral vaccine will produce IgA and IgM. This vaccine is cumbersome for management as it is to be given prior to colostrum consumption, and colostrum must be withheld for several hours after vaccination. This may increase the opportunity for bacterial infections and failure of passive transfer.
• In the case of dairy animals, feed neonates colostrum for 30 days if coronavirus is an endemic problem.
• Eliminate areas of fecal build-up.
• Keep environment dry and draft-free.

MISCELLANEOUS

ASSOCIATED CONDITIONS
A mild respiratory infection may occur simultaneously.

AGE-RELATED FACTORS
• Most cases occur at 7–21 days of age.
• Range is 1 day to 3 months.

ZOONOTIC POTENTIAL
None

BIOSECURITY
• See "Client Education."
• Diarrheic animals should be isolated from healthy neonates as they are sources for large numbers of pathogens.
• Feed youngest animals first and oldest animals last.
• Those handling sick neonates should practice biosecurity measures to reduce

C

exposure to healthy neonates, wash hands and disinfect boots, maintain clothes free of fecal material.
• Disinfect with bleach, a phenolic, or peroxymonosulfate. Surface must be free of organic material and surface contact is a minimum of 10 minutes.

PRODUCTION MANAGEMENT
See "Prevention"

ABBREVIATIONS
• ETEC = enterotoxigenic *E. coli*
• IM = intramuscular
• IV = intravenous
• PO = per os, by mouth
• SC = subcutaneous

SEE ALSO
• Clostridial Disease: Gastrointestinal
• Cryptosporidiosis

• *Escherichia coli*
• Rotavirus
• Salmonellosis
• Winter Dysentery

Suggested Reading
Barrington GM, Gay JM, Evermann JF. Biosecurity for neonatal gastrointestinal diseases. Vet Clin North Am Food Anim Pract 2002, 18: 7–34.
Bendali F, Sanaa M, Bichet H, Schelcher F. Risk factors associated with diarrhoea in newborn calves. Vet Res 1999, 30: 509–22.
Cho Yong-il, Yoon Kyoung-Jin. An overview of calf diarrhea – infectious etiology, diagnosis, and intervention. J Vet Sci 2014, 15: 1–17.

Izzo M, Gunn AA, House JK. Neonatal Diarrhea. In: Smith BP, ed, Large Animal Internal Medicine, 5th ed. St. Louis: Elsevier Mosby, 2015, pp. 314–35.
MacLachlan NJ, Dubovi EJ eds. Fenner's Veterinary Virology, 4th ed. San Diego: Elsevier, 2011, pp. 288–90.
Townsend HG. Environmental factors and calving management practices that affect neonatal mortality in the beef calf. Vet Clin North Am Food Anim Pract 1994, 10: 119–26.
Smith GW. Antimicrobial decision making for enteric diseases of cattle. Vet Clin North Am Food Anim Pract 2015, 31: 47–60.
Smith GW, Berchtold, J. Fluid therapy in calves. Vet Clin North Am Food Anim Pract 2014, 30: 409–27.

Author Kevin D. Pelzer
Consulting Editor Christopher C.L. Chase

BASICS

OVERVIEW
• Cowpox is caused by an orthopoxvirus closely related to but distinguishable from the human orthopoxviruses vaccinia and variola.
• Cattle develop poxlike lesions commonly on the teat and udder in adult animals and on the lips and oral cavity of suckling calves.

INCIDENCE/PREVALENCE
Cowpox affects a broad host range that includes cattle, wild and domestic *Felidae*, dogs, numerous rodents, and some zoo animals.

GEOGRAPHIC DISTRIBUTION
Europe

SYSTEMS AFFECTED
Integument

PATHOPHYSIOLOGY
• While this viral disease carries the name "Cowpox," it is a disease of rodents that occasionally infects domestic cats, which usually pass the disease onto humans and cattle through direct contact.
• Further spread from cattle to other cattle is believed to be by exposure to the infected hands of herdsmen during the milking process or by inoculation with contaminated fomites such as teat dipping cups and milking equipment.
• While most animals develop localized skin lesions, cottontop tamarins (*Saguinus oedipus*) develop generalized disease and die.

SIGNALMENT
• Infections in cattle are uncommon because the virus is not endemic in cattle.
• Virus tends to spread rapidly through a naïve herd, particularly during times of the year when the teats and udders are likely to have abrasions on the surface.
• Heifers, as they are introduced to the milking string, are more likely to become involved in endemic herds.

PHYSICAL EXAMINATION FINDINGS
• Incubation: 3–10 days.
• Typical pox lesions are noted only on the teats and udder. In severe cases, the pox lesions can be identified on the thin skin of the inguinal region and occasionally on the perineum.
• Bulls can develop lesions on the scrotum.
• Nursing calves can develop oral lesions similar to bovine papular stomatitis.
• Lesions progress from circular raised reddened areas of erythema and edema to firm 1–2 cm nodules that form a central vesicle. The vesicle ruptures, forming a central crater that undergoes further necrosis and scab formation if the animal is not being milked.
• Milked animals develop a raised circumscribed lesion with a central umbilicated ulcer that is slow to heal.

CAUSES AND RISK FACTORS
• Disease is endemic in rodents of Europe and Asia with the virus occasionally infecting cattle.
• Voles, mice, and gerbils serve as the natural reservoir for this disease.
• Domestic cats are commonly infected in endemic areas by hunting and eating infected rodents. Infected cats usually develop solitary lesions on the face, neck, or paws. It is believed that these infected cats act as a means of spreading the disease to humans and cattle by direct contact.
• Further spread from cattle to other cattle is believed to be by exposure to the infected hands of herdsmen during the milking process or by inoculation with contaminated fomites such as teat dipping cups and milking equipment.
• Insects are also suspected of transferring the virus from cow to cow.

DIAGNOSIS

DIFFERENTIAL DIAGNOSES
• Bovine papular stomatitis: Virus is a parapoxvirus often associated with proliferative calf lesions on the lip, tongue, and palate. But may observe proliferative targetoid/umbilicated lesions on the teats.
• Bovine fibropapilloma virus: Multiple verrucous proliferative growths on teats and udder; lesions are often scabbed over due to trauma.
• Brazilian vaccinia viruses: Vaccinia-like virus that is an endemic disease in Brazilian cattle with papules that develop into painful ulcers on the teats and udder of the mammary gland.
• Buffalopox virus (India/Pakistan regions): A vaccinia-like virus with lesions similar to cowpox on the teats and udder. Disease is observed in domesticated water buffalo and occasionally cattle. Affected udders and teats are painful, leading to a decrease in milk production.
• Caustic substances that are placed on the teat.
• Foot and mouth disease: Vesicles and ulcers can be observed on the teat and/or udder. Affected animals also have lesions in the mouth and on the feet.
• Herpes mammillitis (bovine herpesvirus-2, Allerton virus): Small, slow-healing ulcers develop on teats and udders. Viral cultures will assist in differentiating poxviruses from herpesviruses.
• Pseudocowpox (milker's nodules): Pseudocowpox is a parapoxvirus with lesions similar to cowpox. Virus is similar to bovine papular stomatitis.
• *Staphylococcus aureus* and *Streptococcus* spp. infections on the teats can cause vesicles which may spread to the udder, resulting in furunculitis and boils.

• Vesicular stomatitis virus: Affected animals develop vesicles/ulcers on the teats and udder. Significant lesions (vesicles and ulcers) are often associated with and most prevalent in the mouth and feet.

CBC/BIOCHEMISTRY/URINALYSIS
N/A

OTHER LABORATORY TESTS
PCR testing to determine specific type of poxvirus

OTHER DIAGNOSTIC PROCEDURES
• Biopsies of the lesions will identify typical poxvirus intracytoplasmic inclusions in the epithelium.
• Electron microscopy of the infected epithelium identifies characteristic poxvirus present in infected keratinocytes.

PATHOLOGIC FINDINGS
• On gross examination, lesions are circumscribed raised firm blanched nodules with a circular basilar area of hyperemia. Nodules form a central vesicle/pustule.
• Lesions undergoes necrosis/collapse causing a central cavitary depression. Scab will form over the necrotic tissue which, once removed, identifies a slow-healing ulcerated surface.
• Lesions are seen primarily on the teats and udder but can also be located in the perineal region and the scrotum of bulls.
• Suckling calves can have lesions in the oral cavity.
• Histologically, the pox lesions consist of edema, congestion, and lymphocytic infiltration of the superficial dermis. The associated epithelium becomes hyperplasic with ballooning degeneration and necrosis of the affected epithelium in the stratum spinosum.
• Eosinophilic intracytoplasmic inclusion bodies are seen in the swollen keratinocytes.
• Epithelial cells of the stratum spinosum separate, forming small vesicles that fill with neutrophils, forming a pustule. Later, the associate epithelium beneath the pustules becomes necrotic, forming an ulcerated epidermis with serocellular debris overlying the lesion.
• Variable numbers of neutrophils are present in the affected dermal connective tissues.

TREATMENT

THERAPEUTIC APPROACH
• No treatment for the pox-associated lesions.
• Keep lesions clean and free of secondary bacterial infections.
• Debris/scabs from wounds should be picked up and disposed of to insure that contaminated materials does not contact other animals.
• Antibacterial ointments may assist in healing.

C

COWPOX

MEDICATIONS

DRUGS OF CHOICE
N/A

CONTRAINDICATIONS
If antibiotics are used for secondary bacterial infections, appropriate milk and meat withdrawal times must be followed for all compounds used.

FOLLOW-UP

EXPECTED COURSE AND PROGNOSIS
Cowpox is considered a mild disease and should cause little discomfort to affected cattle. Most cases resolve without complications.

POSSIBLE COMPLICATIONS
Secondary bacterial infections of the lesions can cause mastitis in affected quarters or a severe dermatitis involving the skin of the affected udder.

PATIENT CARE
• Lesions are usually self-limiting.
• Keep the lesions clean and free of contamination to prevent secondary bacterial infections.

PREVENTION
• Herdsmen with lesions should limit involvement in milking since this is a major method of spreading the disease.
• Cleaning cloths, teat dipping cups, and milking machines should be thoroughly disinfected before use on noninfected animals.

• Quaternary ammonia compounds and teat dipping compounds with viricidal activity should be adequate for preventing the spread of the disease.
• Monitor cats for lesions; remove animals from vicinity of cattle or workers while cat is infected.
• Currently no vaccine is available for use in outbreaks.

MISCELLANEOUS

AGE-RELATED FACTORS
• Young animals, particularly naive heifers coming into an endemic herd, are most susceptible.

ZOONOTIC POTENTIAL
• Handling infected material can lead to lesions on the hands and face. Lesions are usually mild and self-limiting.
• Exposure to infected cats (usually handling these cats) is believed to be the most common source of infection in people.
• Exposure to Buffalopox and Brazilian vaccina viruses from cattle can cause lesions in humans.

BIOSECURITY
Keep infected cats or handlers with lesions away from animals.

ABBREVIATION
PCR = polymerase chain reaction

SEE ALSO
• Bovine Papular Stomatitis
• Foot and Mouth Disease
• Frostbite
• Pseudocowpox
• Teat Lesions
• Vesicular Stomatitis Virus

Suggested Reading
Bennett M, Baxby D. Cowpox. J Med Microbiol 1996, 45: 157–8.
Chapman JL, Nichols DK, Martinez MJ, Raymond JW. Animal models of orthopoxvirus infection. Vet Path 2010, 47: 852–70.
Essbauer S, Pfeffer M, Meyer H. Zoonotic poxviruses. Vet Microbiol 2010, 140: 229–36.
Feuerstein-Kadgien B, Korn K. Images in clinical medicine: Cowpox infection. N Engl J Med 2003, 348: 415.
Goerigk DL Theu T, Pfeffer M, et al. Cowpox virus infection in an alpaca (*Vicugna pacos*): Clinical symptoms, laboratory diagnostic findings and pathological changes. Tierarztl Prax Ausg G Grosstiere Nutztiere 2014, 42: 169–77.
Hazel SM, Bennett M, Chantrey J, et al. A longitudinal study of an endemic disease in wildlife reservoir: Cowpox and wild rodents. Epidemiol Infect 2000, 124: 551–62.
Hoffmann D, Franke A, Jenckel M, et al. Out of the reservoir: Phenotypic and genotypic characterization of a novel cowpox virus isolated from a common vole. J Virol 2015, 89: 1059–69.doi 10.1128/JVI.01195-15.
Kalthoff D, Bock WI, Hühn F, et al. Fatal cowpox virus infection in cotton-top tamarins (*Saguinus oedipus*) in Germany. Vector Borne Zoonotic Dis 2014, 14: 303–5. doi: 10.1089/vbz.2013.1442
McInerney J, Papasouliotis K, Simpson K, et al. Pulmonary cowpox in cats: five cases. J Feline Med Surg 2015, 18: 518–25. doi: 10.1177/ 1098612X15583344
Author Robert B. Moeller Jr.
Consulting Editor Christopher C.L. Chase

BASICS

OVERVIEW
• Cryptococcosis is a noncontagious fungal infection caused by the dimorphic basidiomycete yeasts, *Cryptococcus neoformans* and *C. gattii*.
• Humans and a range of domestic species can be infected, including occasionally sheep, goats, and camelids.
• Distributed in temperate and subtropical climates; in both rural and urban environments.
• Sporadic ruminant cases involve the respiratory tract, CNS, mammary glands and wounds or incisions.
• The major risk arises from inhalation of fungus-contaminated soil/dust, bird (pigeon) excreta, or organic debris from Eucalyptus trees.

INCIDENCE/PREVALENCE
Ruminant infections are rare and sporadic; most cases are subclinical.

GEOGRAPHIC DISTRIBUTION
Worldwide distribution with most infections observed in subtropical and temperate climates. *C. gattii* infection is observed particularly in British Columbia, the Pacific Northwestern US, Australia and Papua New Guinea, and in parts of Africa, Asia, Europe, Mexico, and South America.

SYSTEMS AFFECTED
• Respiratory
• Hemolymphatic
• Nervous
• Integument

PATHOPHYSIOLOGY
• Disease typically arises from inhalation of dust containing basidiospores or desiccated yeast forms.
• Most infections are subclinical, and may persist for months without dissemination.
• Organisms inhaled into the lungs are destroyed by the host, remain dormant with no clinical disease, or precipitate active infection.
• Macrophages phagocytize yeast organisms and transport them to other regions of the body where infections can develop.
• *Cryptococcus* demonstrates significant thermotolerance allowing the yeast to grow in the host.
• The thick polysaccharide capsule of *C. neoformans* inhibits phagocytosis, migration of inflammatory cells to the infected site (poorly immunogenic), complement activation, and release of multiple virulent factors (lactase, phospholipase B-1, and urease) that slow, stop, or degrade inflammatory cells recruited to the infected area.
• Organism thrives in the acidic environment that develops during the inflammatory response involving the release of phagosomal enzymes that macrophages use for organism destruction.
• May cause variably sized respiratory tract granulomas or gelatinous diffuse pulmonary infiltrates. Solitary pulmonary nodules may be confused with carcinoma, and lymph node lesions may mimic fungal or bacterial granulomas.
• Occasional hematogenous spread occurs; the most frequent secondary site of colonization is the meninges.
• Yeast have the potential to disseminate to the skin, bone, liver, kidneys, and other organs.
• Retrograde movement up the teat canal or contaminated udder infusions can cause *Cryptococcus* mastitis; infections of wounds or incisions have also been documented in ruminants.

HISTORICAL FINDINGS
Dependent on system infected; onset of signs can be acute or chronic.

SIGNALMENT
• *C. neoformans* tends to affect debilitated or immunocompromised individuals; *C. gattii* frequently afflicts healthy individuals.
• Cattle, sheep, goats, llamas, alpacas, and other ruminants can be affected, in addition to cats, humans, and other species.

PHYSICAL EXAMINATION FINDINGS
• Vary depending on system involved.
• Signs of upper or lower respiratory tract disease may occur with variable respiratory distress.
• Persistent low-grade fever and weight loss are common in advanced disease.
• CNS infection can induce stiffness, hyperesthesia, blindness, and incoordination.
• Nonhealing skin lesions can occur in ruminants.
• Lymphadenitis.
• Swelling, heat, and pain in the udder can occur with mastitis, and caseous debris in viscid secretions.

GENETICS
N/A

CAUSES AND RISK FACTORS
• *C. neoformans* and *C. gattii* have free-living yeast forms that are present in the soil; contaminated soil is a reservoir for these organisms and inhalation presents the main risk.
• *C. neoformans* is identified in bird (pigeon) guano, decaying wood and other debris; organism growth is enhanced by creatinine, which is often present in bird feces. Bird guano protected from direct sunlight (in lofts and roosts) is most commonly associated with disease.
• *C. gattii* is identified in decaying leaves, debris, and flowers of Eucalyptus trees, but has been observed in debris from over 50 tree species.
• Debilitated/immunocompromised animals are at a higher risk for disseminated disease (more relevant to *C. neoformans* infection).
• Habitation of high-risk areas (British Columbia, Pacific Northwestern US) is relevant to *C. gattii* infection.

DIAGNOSIS

DIFFERENTIAL DIAGNOSES
• Cryptococcosis is a rare diagnosis in ruminants but should be considered as a possible differential for ruminants with acute CNS signs, acute or chronic lower respiratory tract disease, nasal or tracheal masses, nonhealing wounds or incisions that respond poorly to standard treatments, and mastitis or lymphadenitis.

CBC/BIOCHEMISTRY/URINALYSIS
Neutrophilia may be observed if CBC is performed in clinically diseased animals.

OTHER LABORATORY TESTS
N/A

IMAGING
Ultrasonography, radiography, computed tomography, and other forms of imaging have utility in valuable animals for characterizing the location and extent of infections, and potentially in monitoring response to treatment.

OTHER DIAGNOSTIC PROCEDURES
• Latex agglutination testing can define *C. neoformans* antigens in serum, CSF, or urine. False-negative results occasionally observed in animals with localized disease.
• Fungal culture of tissues/fluids with speciation based on differential media, appearance, biochemical testing, DNA sequencing.
• Cytologic examination of smears, swabs or aspirates of exudates, tissues, CSF or respiratory fluids demonstrate yeast forms (4–8 μm) with a thick capsule on India ink wet mounts and a variety of other stains.
• Immunofluorescence or immunohistochemistry techniques are available.

PATHOLOGIC FINDINGS
• Large numbers of poorly staining yeast (4–8 μm) with a thick capsule and narrow-based budding bodies off yeast cells are observed. Yeast are surrounded by few macrophages and multinucleated giant cells.
• Granulomas and other evidence of inflammation may be noted at sites of infection.

TREATMENT

THERAPEUTIC APPROACH
• Infections are frequently self-limiting.
• Treatment of disseminated or severe local disease is often futile due to poor prognosis and limited means of effective therapy.

C

CRYPTOCOCCOSIS   (CONTINUED)

SURGICAL CONSIDERATIONS AND TECHNIQUES

Individual granulomatous lesions may be amenable to resection or removal in valuable animals.

MEDICATIONS

DRUGS OF CHOICE

• There are rare reports of treatment in ruminants; use of oral fluconazole has been reported in a goat. However, information regarding absorption by this route in ruminants is lacking.
• Antifungal drugs used in other species have included amphotericin B, flucytosine, ketoconazole, and itraconazole.

CONTRAINDICATIONS

N/A

PRECAUTIONS

Appropriate milk and meat withdrawal times must be followed for all compounds administered to food-producing animals.

POSSIBLE INTERACTIONS

N/A

FOLLOW-UP

EXPECTED COURSE AND PROGNOSIS

• Clinical disease tends to be chronic and/or progressive, particularly without treatment.
• The prospect of complete recovery is often very poor.

POSSIBLE COMPLICATIONS

Hypoxemia, recumbency, death

CLIENT EDUCATION

Educate clients regarding sources of exposure to these pathogens.

PATIENT CARE

N/A

PREVENTION

• Avoid exposure to soils contaminated with bird (pigeon) excreta or decaying cellular debris from trees.
• Insure proper udder/teat cleanliness prior to infusions with mammary products.

MISCELLANEOUS

ASSOCIATED CONDITIONS

Immunocompromising conditions might be present in individuals with *C. neoformans* infection.

AGE-RELATED FACTORS

N/A

ZOONOTIC POTENTIAL

Cryptococcosis is not considered zoonotic; however, infection potential exists linked with accidental inoculation (such as when handling infected tissues); human-to-human transmission has been reported very rarely (such as with solid organ transplantation and mechanical ventilation near another infected patient).

PREGNANCY

N/A

BIOSECURITY

N/A

PRODUCTION MANAGEMENT

• Contaminated udder infusions/improper teat management has been associated with outbreaks of *Cryptococcus* mastitis in cattle.
• Monitor bedding material and be cautious of using Eucalyptus bark as bedding material.

SYNONYMS

• Pigeon fancier's disease
• Torulosis
• European blastomycosis
• Busse-Buschke disease

ABBREVIATIONS

• CNS = central nervous system
• CSF = cerebrospinal fluid

SEE ALSO

• Coccidioidomycosis
• Mastitis: Fungal

Suggested Reading

Baro T, Torres-Rodrigues, JM, De Mendoza MH, et al. First identification of autochthonous *Cryptococcus neoformans* var. *gattii* isolated from goats with predominantly severe pulmonary disease in Spain. J Clin Microbiol 1998, 32: 458–61.

Byrnes EJ, Bartlett JH, Perfect JR, et al. *Cryptococcus gattii*: an emerging fungal pathogen infecting humans and animals. Microb Infect 2011, 13: 895–907.

Chen ACA, Meyers W, Sorrell TC. *Cryptococcus gattii* infection. Clin Microbiol Rev 2014, 27: 980–1024.

Coelho C, Boca AL, Casadevall A. The tools of virulence of *Cryptococcus neoformans*. Adv Appl Microbiol 2014, 87: 1–41.

Kielstein P, Hotzel H, Schmalreck A, et al. Occurrence of *Cryptococcus spp.* in excreta of pigeons and pet birds. Mycoses 2000, 43: 7–15.

Maestrale C, Masia M, Pintus D, et al. Genetic and pathological characteristics of *Cryptococcus gattii* and *Cryptococcus neoformans* var. *neoformans* from meningoencephalitis in autochthonous goats and mouflons. Vet Microbiol 2015, 177: 409–13.

Singh M, Gupta PP, Rana JS, et al. Clinico-pathological studies on experimental cryptococcal mastitis in goats. Mycopathologia 1994, 126: 147–55.

Stillwell G, Pissarra H. Cryptococcal meningitis in a goat – case report. BMC Vet Res 2014, 10: 84. doi: 10.1186/1746-6148-10-84.

Villarroel A, Maggiulli T. Rare *Cryptococcus gattii* infection in an immunocompetent dairy goat following a cesarean section. Med Mycol Case Rep 2012, 1: 91–4.

Author Robert B. Moeller Jr.
Consulting Editor Erica C. McKenzie
Acknowledgments The author and book editors acknowledge the prior contribution of Karen Carberry-Goh.

BASICS

OVERVIEW
• Cryptosporidiosis in ruminants and camelids is caused by a nonhost-specific and widely distributed coccidian parasite, *Cryptosporidium.*
• Several species of *Cryptosporidium* have been identified in ruminants, varying with geographic location and host species.
• *C. parvum* is typically associated with diarrhea in neonatal ruminants and camelids, inducing disease that is clinically similar to many other causes of neonatal scours.
• Infection with *Cryptosporidium* is also often subclinical, and this pathogen is contagious and zoonotic.

INCIDENCE/PREVALENCE
• *C. parvum* was found in 22.4% of calves in a survey of dairy farms in the United States.
• *C. parvum* has caused outbreaks of diarrhea in neonatal crias within individual alpaca herds in the US.
• Shedding of *Cryptosporidium* has been reported in up to 85% of pre-weaned lambs in some systems.
• Morbidity can reach 80–100% and mortality >50% in affected groups of goat kids.

GEOGRAPHIC DISTRIBUTION
• Worldwide
• The predominant *Cryptosporidium* species isolated varies between geographic regions, particularly in small ruminants

SYSTEMS AFFECTED
Digestive

PATHOPHYSIOLOGY
• There are >20 known species of *Cryptosporidium* within the phylum Apicomplexa.
• *C. parvum* is the most significant species affecting neonatal calves, small ruminants, and camelids.
• *C. andersonii, C. bovis,* and *C. ryanae* have been isolated in cattle but are not considered to be clinically significant.
• *C. xiaoi* has been isolated from diarrheic goat kids, and *C. ubiquitum* from lambs.
• Infected hosts, which can be neonatal or adult animals, shed oocysts into the feces which are sporulated and immediately infective.
• The primary route of transmission is direct and fecal-oral; however, indirect transmission via environmental contamination is common, and *Cryptosporidium* is environmentally resistant.
• The pathogen can complete its life cycle within a single host, including the asexual (merogony) and sexual (sporogony) reproductive cycles; therefore autoinfection of the host can occur.

• Ingested oocysts are activated in the stomach and upper small intestine to release four infective motile sporozoites which are taken into intestinal epithelial cells where they undergo the sexual and asexual multiplication stages that result in the production of oocysts.
• A vacuole is formed between the cytoplasm and cell membrane that causes villous atrophy, villous fusion, and, later, inflammatory changes of the mucosa.
• Clinical diarrhea develops usually 4 days after infection, and arises from a combination of malabsorption and maldigestion. Secretory mechanisms and increased intestinal permeability are also thought to play a role.
• Gastric cryptosporidiosis has been described in cattle. *C. andersonii* (formerly categorized as *C. muris*) can cause gastric cryptosporidiosis by infecting the glands of the abomasum in a small percentage of adult cattle. Animals appear clinically normal but inhibition of acid production in the abomasum can lead to decreased milk production in chronically affected cattle.

HISTORICAL FINDINGS
The onset of diarrhea after 4 days of life and within the first 2–3 weeks of life is the typical complaint.

SIGNALMENT
• Cryptosporidiosis causes diarrhea in a wide range of mammals including humans, cattle, small ruminants, and camelids.
• The highest frequency of infection is seen in neonatal ruminants between 5 days and 3 weeks of age, many of which will be asymptomatically infected.

PHYSICAL EXAMINATION FINDINGS
Diarrhea, dehydration, anorexia, and tenesmus are common findings in affected neonates.

GENETICS
N/A

CAUSES AND RISK FACTORS
• Infection with *Cryptosporidium* spp., most commonly *C. parvum* in domestic neonatal ruminants and camelids.
• Poor hygiene in intensively managed systems can increase pathogen exposure from the environment and between neonates.
• Immunocompromised neonates are at greater risk for severe or multiple infections.
• Multi-pathogen infections are common; the significance of other infectious pathogens in permitting or enhancing *Cryptosporidium* infection is not clear.

DIAGNOSIS

DIFFERENTIAL DIAGNOSES
• Rotavirus
• Coronavirus
• Bovine viral diarrhea (BVD)
• *Clostridium perfringens*

• *Escherichia coli*
• Nutritional diarrhea
• Salmonellosis
• Giardiasis

CBC/BIOCHEMISTRY/URINALYSIS
• Serum chemistry analysis may reflect dehydration (azotemia, hyperalbuminemia), acidosis (low total CO_2), hyperkalemia, and hypoglycemia.
• Mixed infections with bacteria or viruses should be considered in animals that are severely or chronically diseased and that have significant acid-base abnormalities, electrolyte disturbances, hypothermia, and weight loss.

OTHER LABORATORY TESTS
High-power magnification with acid-fast staining can be used on feces or mucosal scrapings to identify the organism.

IMAGING
N/A

OTHER DIAGNOSTIC PROCEDURES
• Sheather's flotation sedimentation staining
• Fluorescent antibody assays
• ELISA assays
• PCR
• Rapid immunochromatographic assay

PATHOLOGIC FINDINGS
• Gross necropsy identifies hyperemic intestinal mucosa with yellow degraded intestinal contents.
• Histologic evaluation of the tissues reveals atrophy, fusion, and inflammation of the intestinal villi with circular, intramembranous, extracytoplasmic organisms contained within the brush border.

TREATMENT

THERAPEUTIC APPROACH
• There are currently no recommended specific medications for cryptosporidiosis; however, diarrhea is usually self-limiting, with a 7-day or shorter course expected in uncomplicated cases.
• Treatment consists of supportive care through provision of appropriate nutrition, fluid and electrolyte replacement, and correction of acidosis and hypothermia.
• Antimicrobial therapy may be indicated in cases with secondary bacterial infection.

SURGICAL CONSIDERATIONS AND TECHNIQUES
N/A

MEDICATIONS

DRUGS OF CHOICE
• Paromomycin sulfate administered at 100 mg/kg/day, PO (for 11 days from day 2

CRYPTOSPORIDIOSIS   (CONTINUED)

of life) reportedly prevented natural disease in goat kids.

• Antimicrobial therapy can be considered if there is evidence of secondary bacterial infection or significant immunocompromise.

• Nonsteroidal anti-inflammatory drugs may be used to reduce pain and discomfort in some cases, with caution indicated in dehydrated animals.

• The addition of lactase products to milk may help subsequent digestion in compromised intestines.

• Compounds that improve fecal consistency (bismuth subsalicylate) may be of value.

CONTRAINDICATIONS
N/A

PRECAUTIONS
Appropriate milk and meat withdrawal times must be followed for all compounds administered to food-producing animals.

POSSIBLE INTERACTIONS
N/A

 FOLLOW-UP

EXPECTED COURSE AND PROGNOSIS
• Diarrhea usually resolves within one week in uncomplicated cryptosporidiosis affecting immunocompetent individuals.

• Asymptomatic infection is a common phenomenon.

POSSIBLE COMPLICATIONS
• Severe dehydration, electrolyte disturbances, and acidosis can lead to weakness, recumbency, and death.

• Acute renal failure can result from severe dehydration in conjunction with administration of nephrotoxic drugs such as NSAIDs and specific antibiotics (including oxytetracycline).

CLIENT EDUCATION
• *Cryptosporidium* is a zoonotic pathogen so it is critical to educate clients regarding appropriate hygiene precautions when handling infected individuals.

• Exposure of children and immunocompromised individuals to neonatal ruminants should be performed with strict attention to hygiene.

PATIENT CARE
• Electrolyte and rehydration therapy must be balanced with appropriate nutritional support through the provision of milk or milk replacer.

• Electrolyte/fluid products can inhibit milk clot formation in the abomasum so they should be administered 1–2 hours after milk feedings.

• Decreasing the volume but increasing the number of feedings may help reduce the osmotic effects of provided fluids in the gut.

PREVENTION
• *Cryptosporidium* is very resistant to destruction. Ammonia products (5%), hydrogen peroxide (3–6%), 10% formol saline, chlorine dioxide, desiccation, and extremes of temperature (freezing or >65°C) can destroy oocyst infectivity and help disinfect the environment.

• Individual housing and sanitation of feeding equipment for neonates helps control exposure.

• Adherence to hygienic practices in maternity areas and cleaning manure from neonatal areas can also decrease exposure.

• Isolate diarrheic neonates as soon as clinical disease is noticed and for at least one week after resolution of signs.

 MISCELLANEOUS

ASSOCIATED CONDITIONS
Acute renal failure

AGE-RELATED FACTORS
• Clinical disease most typically occurs in neonatal ruminants and camelids <3 weeks of age.

• Oocyst shedding in asymptomatically infected ruminants is also strongly age related, and highest in neonates.

ZOONOTIC POTENTIAL
• *C. parvum* is highly contagious and one of the most common causes of clinical cryptosporidiosis in humans.

PREGNANCY
N/A

BIOSECURITY
See "Prevention." Since cryptosporidiosis is a highly contagious disorder with limited targeted treatments, biosecurity is critical for the control of disease within production systems.

PRODUCTION MANAGEMENT
Cryptosporidium is a major agent of neonatal diarrhea and can cause severe production losses through neonatal morbidity and mortality.

SYNONYMS
N/A

ABBREVIATIONS
• BVD = bovine viral diarrhea
• ELISA = enzyme-linked immunosorbent assay
• PCR = polymerase chain reaction

SEE ALSO
• Coccidiosis
• Diarrheal Diseases: Bovine
• Diarrheal Diseases: Camelid
• Diarrheal Diseases: Small Ruminant
• Neonatal Diarrhea

Suggested Reading
Chako CZ, Tyler JW, Schultz LG, Chiquma L, Beerntsen BT. Cryptosporidiosis in people: It's not just about the cows. J Vet Intern Med 2010, 24: 37–43.
Harp JA, Goff JP. Strategies for control of *Cryptosporidium parvum* infection in calves. J Dairy Sci 1998, 81: 289–94.
Izzo M, Gunn AA, House JK. Neonatal diarrhea. In: Smith BP ed, Large Animal Internal Medicine, 5th ed. St. Louis: Mosby, 2014.
Paraud C, Chartier C. Cryptosporidiosis in small ruminants. Small Ruminant Res 2012, 103: 93–7.

Author Clemence Z. Chako
Consulting Editor Erica C. McKenzie
Acknowledgment The author and book editors acknowledge the prior contribution of Noah Barka.

C

BASICS

OVERVIEW
• Cyanide poisoning is characterized by the abrupt onset of severe neurologic signs.
• Many *Prunus* spp. are cyanogenic, but only a few present a serious risk to livestock: Choke cherry (*P. virginiana*), black cherry (*P. serotina*), and cherry laurel (*P. laurocerasus*).
• Other cyanide-containing plants associated with livestock toxicosis are Sudan grass, Johnson grass, milo and sorghum (*Sorghum* spp.), arrow grass (*Triglocin* spp.), bird's-foot trefoil (*Lotus* spp.), vetch (*Vicia* spp.), elderberry (*Sambucus* spp.), cassava and tapioca plant (*Manihot* spp.), corn (*Zea mays*), clover (*Trifolium* spp.), California holly (*Heteromeles arbutifolia*), flax (*Linum spp.*), June berry (*Amelanchior* spp.), fava bean (*Vicia* spp.), and eucalyptus (*Eucalyptus* spp.). Although many grasses contain cyanogenic compounds they are rarely at high enough levels to cause intoxication.

INCIDENCE/PREVALENCE
• Depending on the type of exposure (type of plant, environmental conditions), morbidity and mortality are variable.

GEOGRAPHIC DISTRIBUTION
• Worldwide
• Local occurrence depends on the type of exposure

SYSTEMS AFFECTED
Nervous

PATHOPHYSIOLOGY
• Ruminants are more susceptible to the toxic effects than monogastric animals because rumen microorganisms produce enzymes that facilitate rapid hydrolysis of cyanogenic glycosides.
• Hydrogen cyanide is readily absorbed from the gastrointestinal tract and acts by inhibiting cytochrome oxidase.
• Cyanogenic glycosides commonly present are amygdalin, prunasin, dhurrin, linamarin, and triglocinin.

SIGNALMENT
• All ruminant species are very susceptible. Most reported cases involve goats and cattle.
• Losses in sheep and deer have also been reported.

PHYSICAL EXAMINATION FINDINGS
• Abrupt onset of apprehension and distress occurs within 10–15 minutes of ingestion.
• This is quickly followed by weakness, ataxia, hyperventilation, and hypotension. In severe cases, the animals become recumbent and develop cardiac arrhythmias and tetanic-type seizures.
• Death may occur within 15–60 minutes of exposure.

• Mucus membranes are initially bright cherry red due to the well-oxygenated venous blood.
• Cyanosis may be observed at a later stage of poisoning.

CAUSES AND RISK FACTORS
• Young and rapidly growing plants have the highest concentration of cyanide.
• Plant trimmings remain toxic as long as the leaves are green and have not completely dried.
• All parts of the plants have cyanogenic potential. The highest concentrations of cyanogenic glycosides are found in the leaves, but concentrations are subject to many influences and may vary considerably.
• Insect-, frost-, and drought-damaged cyanogenic plants have been associated with a greater risk for cyanide poisoning.
• Concentrations of greater than 200 µg/g of cyanide in plant material are considered potentially toxic.
• Cyanide in mill tailing ponds at gold mines can present a risk to wild ruminants.

DIAGNOSIS

DIFFERENTIAL DIAGNOSES
• Nitrate/nitrite toxicosis—chocolate-colored blood
• Nonprotein nitrogen toxicosis—exposure to NPN supplements, toxic levels of ammonia in rumen content and blood
• Organophosphorus or carbamate insecticide exposure—gastrointestinal irritation and neurologic signs, evaluation of cholinesterase activity, detection of pesticides
• Lead poisoning—determination of blood lead concentration
• Neurotoxic plants (poison hemlock, water hemlock, tree tobacco, lupine)—analysis for plant toxins in gastrointestinal contents, history of exposure
• Cardiotoxic plants (oleander, milkweeds, and azaleas)—analysis for plant toxins in gastrointestinal contents, history of exposure
• Neurotoxic blue-green algae—identification of algae material in rumen contents
• ABPE—onset of clinical signs usually 1–4 days after an abrupt change to lush pasture, pathologic evaluation of lung

CBC/BIOCHEMISTRY/URINALYSIS
No specific changes

OTHER LABORATORY TESTS
• Detection of cyanide in blood, rumen content, liver, and skeletal muscle
• Samples must be collected promptly and stored frozen in airtight containers until analysis.
• Concentrations in tissues from lethal exposures may be reduced to one third of the initial values within 1 hour of death.

• If liver is not collected within 4 hours of death, skeletal muscle is the preferred sample for analysis.
• Because of the volatility of hydrogen cyanide in biological samples, "toxic" thresholds are not established.

PATHOLOGIC FINDINGS
• There are no clearly distinctive changes.
• Cherry red blood may be evident immediately after death, but the color of blood darkens as postmortem time increases.
• Hemorrhages may occur in the subendocardium, subepicardium, and abomasums.
• There may be mild congestion and edema of the lungs.

TREATMENT

THERAPEUTIC APPROACH
• Immediate removal of the cyanogenic plant material
• Avoid stress
• General supportive care in nonsevere cases
• Administration of antidotes as soon as possible in severe cases

MEDICATIONS

DRUGS OF CHOICE
• The primary antidote for ruminants is thiosulfate. Thiosulfate (20%–40% solution) administered IV at a dose of 25–50 mg/ 100 kg body weight.
• Sodium nitrite can be given concurrently, but may not be of additional benefit in ruminants. If given, the recommended dose is 10–20 mg/kg body weight IV.
• Cobalt compounds, such as cobalt chloride or hydroxycobalamin, have been used successfully in the treatment of cyanide poisoning in Europe, but have not been approved for use in animals in the United States. Recommended doses for cattle, sheep, and goats are 10–15 mg/kg slowly IV, 15 g in 250 mL dextrose 5%.

CONTRAINDICATIONS
• Do not administer methylene blue, as it is ineffective as a producer of methemoglobinemia.
• If there is suspicion that cyanide poisoning is combined with nitrate poisoning, administration of sodium nitrite is contraindicated.
• Meat and milk withdrawal periods for drugs given must be determined.

CYANIDE TOXICOSIS (CONTINUED)

C

FOLLOW-UP

EXPECTED COURSE AND PROGNOSIS
• Animals poisoned with cyanide are often found dead.
• Cyanide poisoning progresses so rapidly that treatment is often too late. In most cases, the affected animals have a poor-to-grave prognosis.
• If treatment is initiated promptly, the prognosis is fair.
• Animals that live beyond 1 hour following intake are likely to survive.

PREVENTION
• Delaying grazing until cyanogenic forage has matured.
• Slow and thorough drying of forage reduces the cyanide concentration.
• Avoid exposure of animals to frost- or insect-damaged cyanogenic plants. After a killing frost, wait for at least 4–6 days before grazing.
• Do not allow hungry cattle to graze cyanogenic plants.
• Feeding material as silage will reduce the risk of poisoning, as correct ensilage for 3 weeks reduces levels of toxin by approximately 50%.
• Suspect forage should be analyzed for cyanide concentrations.

MISCELLANEOUS

ASSOCIATED CONDITIONS
Sorghum spp. often contain toxic nitrate concentrations.

PRODUCTION MANAGEMENT
• Delay grazing until cyanogenic forage has matured.
• Slow and thorough drying of forage reduces the cyanide concentration.
• Avoid exposure of animals to frost- or insect-damaged cyanogenic plants. After a killing frost, wait for at least 4–6 days before grazing.
• Do not allow hungry cattle to graze cyanogenic plants.
• Ruminants are more susceptible to the toxic effects than monogastric animals because rumen microorganisms produce enzymes that facilitate rapid hydrolysis of cyanogenic glycosides.

ABBREVIATIONS
• ABPE = acute bovine pulmonary edema and emphysema
• IV = intravenous
• NPN = nonprotein nitrogen

SEE ALSO
• Blue-Green Algae Poisoning
• Carbamate Toxicity
• Cardiotoxic Plants
• Lead Toxicosis
• Lupine Toxicity
• Nitrate and Nitrite Toxicosis
• Oleander and Cardiotoxic Plant Toxicity
• Organophosphate Toxicity
• Poison Hemlock (*Conium* spp. Toxicity)
• Tobacco Toxicosis
• Urea Toxicity
• Water Hemlock

Suggested Reading
Burrows GE, Tyrl RJ. Rosaceae. In: Burrows GE, Tyrl RJ eds, Toxic Plants of North America, 2nd ed. Ames: Wiley-Blackwell, 2013.

Pickrell JA, Oehme F. Cyanogenic glycosides. In: Plumlee KH ed, Clinical Veterinary Toxicology. St. Louis: Mosby, 2004.

Tegzes JH, Puschner B, Melton LA. Cyanide toxicosis in goats after ingestion of California holly (*Heteromeles arbutifolia*). J Vet Diagn Invest 2003, 15: 478–80.

Terblanche M, Minne JA, Adelaar TF. Hydrocyanic acid poisoning. J S Afr Vet Med Assoc 1964, 35: 503–6.

Authors Birgit Puschner and Adrienne C. Bautista

Consulting Editor Christopher C.L. Chase

DEATH CAMAS

BASICS

OVERVIEW
• Approximately 14 species of *Zygadenus* are present in North America including:
  ○ Black death camas, black snakeroot, crow poison (*Z. densus*)
  ○ Mountain death camas, white camas, elegant death camas (*Z. elegans*)
  ○ Chaparral death camas, star lily (*Z. fremontii*)
  ○ Death camas, sand-bog death camas (*Z. leimanthoides*)
  ○ Poison camas, Nuttall's death camas (*Z. nuttallii*)
  ○ Foothill death camas, panicled death camas, sand corn (*Z. paniculatus*)
  ○ Alcove death camas (*Z. vaginatus*)
  ○ Meadow death camas, grassy death camas (*Z. venenosus*)
• Of these *Z. nuttallii, Z. venenosis,* and *Z. paniculatus* are the most toxic.
• *Zygadenus* spp. are an herbaceous perennial plant.
• Leaves are hairless, grass-like, linear, V-shaped, and parallel-veined. They are not hollow. The leaves are the most frequently ingested part of the plant.
• This species arises from an onion-like bulb that has a black membranous outer layer. The bulb is located 6–8 inches below the soil surface. These become present in early spring. The bulb is the most toxic part of the plant.
• The bulb and leaves can be mistaken for wild onion; however, they lack the onion smell.
• Flowers are small, perfect, greenish white to yellow, that inflorescence with a terminal raceme or panicle blooming typically around June.
• Seeds are fusiform to oblong, smooth, angular and light brown.

INCIDENCE/PREVALENCE
• Poisoning is most likely to occur in early spring when few other plants are available.
• Mortality of 10% occurred in a flock of about 2,400 sheep.

GEOGRAPHIC DISTRIBUTION
Found mainly in mountain valleys, sandy hills, and grass plains of the United States.

SYSTEMS AFFECTED
Cardiovascular

PATHOPHYSIOLOGY
• Toxic compounds are steroidal alkaloids, most notable being zygadine and zygacine. The alkaloids are similar to those found in *Veratrum* spp.
• Alkaloids produce hypotensive effects.

• Toxic compounds are found in variable concentrations depending on growth stage with vegetative and pod stages containing the highest concentration and the flowering stages appearing to be the lowest.
• Seeds and leaves in the early stages of growth are most toxic.
• Toxic dose is estimated at 0.2–1% of body weight.

HISTORICAL FINDING
Presence of plant or cuttings of the plant within the pasture

SIGNALMENT
• Sheep are most commonly affected.
• Also cattle, goats, and camelids.

PHYSICAL EXAMINATION FINDINGS
• Salivation
• Depression and weakness
• Low head carriage, arched back
• Incoordination
• Coma, labored breathing, and death

CAUSES AND RISK FACTORS
• Presumed steroidal alkaloid resulting in hypotension.
• Range fire can result in increased nitrogen levels during regrowth. It is unknown if the increased nitrogen has an effect on the toxic compounds but it may increase the palatability of the plant.

DIAGNOSIS

DIFFERENTIAL DIAGNOSES
• Other cardiovascular toxicities (i.e., cyanide toxicosis, cardiotoxic plants)
• Monensin poisoning

CBC/BIOCHEMISTRY/URINALYSIS
No unremarkable changes

OTHER DIAGNOSTIC PROCEDURES
• History of exposure to the plant
• Finding of plant material within gastric contents on gross pathology

PATHOLOGIC FINDINGS
• No characteristic lesions.
• Pulmonary congestion and edema with scattered small hemorrhages are most likely to be present, although there may also be reddening of the mucosa of the stomach and small intestine.

TREATMENT

THERAPEUTIC APPROACH
• Remove from the source.

• Early treatment with atropine 2 mg and 8 mg picrotoxin in 5 mL of water administered subcutaneously per 50 kg bwt.
• Recovery can occur if removed from source and or treated at the beginning of clinical sign presentation.

MEDICATIONS

DRUGS OF CHOICE
Treatment with atropine 2 mg and 8 mg picrotoxin in 5 mL of water administered subcutaneously per 50 kg bwt.

FOLLOW-UP

EXPECTED COURSE AND PROGNOSIS
• Recovery possible
• Death once recumbent

PREVENTION
Avoid grazing pastures that have *Zygadenus* spp. in the spring.

MISCELLANEOUS

PRODUCTION MANAGEMENT
Identify pasture areas that contain *Zygadenus* spp. that are risk areas.

SYNONYMS
N/A

ABBREVIATION
BWT = body weight

SEE ALSO
Cardiotoxic Plants
Monesin Toxicity

Suggested Reading
Burrows GE, Tyrl RJ. 2013. In: Burrows GE, Tyrl RJ eds, Toxic Plants of North America, 2nd ed. Ames: Wiley-Blackwell, 2013, pp. 787–91, Kindle Edition
Collett S, Grotelueschen D, Smith R, Wilson, R. Deaths of 23 adult cows attributed to intoxication by the alkaloids of *Zygadenus venenosus* (Meadow death camas). Agri-Practice 1996, 17: 5–9.
Author Jennifer S. Taintor
Consulting Editor Christopher C.L. Chase
Acknowledgment The author and book editors acknowledge the prior contribution of Heidi Coker.

DERMATOPHILOSIS

BASICS

OVERVIEW
A common pustular/crusting, nonpruritic disease of ruminants caused by *Dermatophilus congolensis.*

INCIDENCE/PREVALENCE
• Highest in regions with wet weather.
• Morbidity can reach 100%.
• Subclinical infections can be present in endemic areas.

GEOGRAPHIC DISTRIBUTION
Worldwide distribution with significant prevalence in Africa, the Middle East, Mediterranean Europe, and the Americas.

SYSTEMS AFFECTED
Integument

PATHOPHYSIOLOGY
• *D. congolensis* is an aerobic to facultatively anaerobic, non-acid-fast, Gram-positive actinomycete.
• Two morphologic forms exist: filamentous hyphae and motile zoospores.
  ○ Hyphae: branching filaments, divide transversely/longitudinally, mature into flagellated ovoid zoospores.
  ○ Zoospores: infective form, released when scabs are exposed to moisture.
• Disruption of the protective barrier of skin allows bacterial entry, related to ectoparasites, self-trauma, foreign body penetration, or shearing abrasions/burns.
• Serous exudation/crusting due to neutrophilic infiltrate leads to matting of wool/hair after an incubation as short as 2 weeks.

HISTORICAL FINDINGS
Recent wet weather and other predisposing incidents might be reported.

SIGNALMENT
All ruminants of all ages can be affected, but juveniles are predisposed and lambs <5 weeks of age are most susceptible.

PHYSICAL EXAMINATION FINDINGS
• Clinical signs correspond to predisposing factors: Moisture and microtrauma of the skin. Areas of body most often affected are those exposed to trauma.
• Lesions begin with matting of hair/wool and coalesce, forming crusts/scabs. Undersides of scabs have a paintbrush appearance. Accumulations of cutaneous keratinized material form wart-like lesions.
• Cattle: Thick crusts palpable under hair coat, scabs, and/or wart-like lesions on head, chest, dorsum, and upper lateral surface of neck. Lesions may be seen on legs of cattle standing in water, mud or lush pasture; or may be localized to the udder/scrotum.
• Sheep: Serous exudate at base of wool, fleece becomes matted (lumpy wool disease).

Chronic lesions persist as crusts on face, nose, or ears.
• Strawberry footrot in sheep: Proliferative dermatitis affecting skin from the coronet to the carpus/hock. Lesions heal by granulation, observed when crusts are removed (strawberry appearance). Clinical cases are most severe in young stock (<1 year old).
• Lambs may rapidly develop generalized infection on the dorsum. Severe serous exudate can make movement difficult. Secondary bacterial infections or flystrike may lead to death if severe.
• Goats: Wartlike scabs on inner pinnae. Nose, muzzle, feet, scrotum, and tail may be affected.
• Buffaloes/cattle may develop erosive/granulomatous lesions on palate, lips, and tongue.
• Subcutaneous and lymph node abscesses may occur in cattle, sheep, and goats.
• Camelids: Focal subcutaneous swelling in addition to the superficial dermatitis is described in Australia. Loosely fleeced areas (face, neck, distal extremities, inguinal region) are most affected. Syndrome is characterized by the development of local abscesses, granulomas, and regional lymphadenopathy. Plant material found within lesions suggests that penetrating or migrating plant material causes the deep infection.
• New world camelids: Lesions on ears, neck, rump, dorsum and feet; wool rot.

GENETICS
• Breed variability with respect to susceptibility
• Zebu cattle considered more resistant than *Bos taurus*
• West African N'dama, and Muturu breeds highly resistant
• Fine wool sheep breeds more susceptible
• More prevalent in Old World camelids than in New World camelids

CAUSES AND RISK FACTORS
• The most important predisposing factors are chronic wetting, maceration, or microtrauma to the skin. Intact healthy skin is not believed to be susceptible.
• Infected animals, healthy carrier animals and apparently recovered animals may transmit the disease.
• Outbreaks most common after periods of heavy rain/high humidity.
• Long hair may predispose to infection.
• Ectoparasites are an important cause of microtrauma.
• Mechanical transmission can occur via ectoparasites, animal-to-animal contact, and during dipping practices.
• Environment/equipment can be contaminated.
• Dried scabs from infected animals are important sources of infection for susceptible animals and for recurrence of infection.
• Sheep may carry the infection subclinically, acting as carriers of the disease.

• Unpigmented skin may be more susceptible.
• Malnutrition/concurrent disease may predispose animals.
• Zoospores can remain viable in crusts at temperatures of 28–31°C for up to 42 months.
• Zoospores in crusts can remain viable when dried and after being heated to temperatures of 100°C.

DIAGNOSIS

DIFFERENTIAL DIAGNOSES
• Contagious ecthyma
• Crusted mange lesions
• Dermatophytosis
• Malignant catarrhal fever
• Mucosal disease
• Pemphigus foliaceus
• Peste des petits ruminants
• Staphylococcal infections
• Ulcerative dermatosis
• Zinc-responsive dermatosis

CBC/BIOCHEMISTRY/URINALYSIS
N/A

OTHER LABORATORY TESTS
N/A

IMAGING
N/A

OTHER DIAGNOSTIC PROCEDURES
• Cutaneous impression smears of underside of moist scabs: Staining with Gram, Giemsa, Wright or Diff Quik stains demonstrate coccoid/branching filamentous organisms when viewed with oil immersion magnification.
• Cytologic examination of deep layer of crusts adjacent to granulation tissue: coccoid bacteria branching into "railroad track" formation.
• Crust preparation: Mince crusts in sterile water on glass microscope slide; allow to dry; stain and examine with oil immersion. This may prove helpful when only older crusts are available.
• Skin biopsy: see "Pathologic Findings."
• Bacterial culture: Grow organism from crusts/skin biopsy on blood agar in increased carbon dioxide atmosphere.
• Indirect fluorescent antibody and ELISA tests are available for herd investigations.

PATHOLOGIC FINDINGS
Skin biopsy: Folliculitis, intraepidermal pustular dermatitis and intracellular edema. Surface crusting is characterized by alternating layers of ortho- and/or parakeratotic hyperkeratosis and neutrophilic exudates. Organism is seen within keratinous debris.

(CONTINUED)

TREATMENT

THERAPEUTIC APPROACH
• Separate clinically affected animals from normal animals.
• Provide shelter from rain.
• Improve nutrition (protein, energy, mineral) and ectoparasite control.
• Tick control is essential in the control of the disease.
• Protect animals from flystrike.
• Disease is self-limiting over several weeks if affected animals are kept dry.
• Remove infected crusts/tufts of crusted hair or clip matted hair to reduce the number of organisms present.
• Bathe with antibacterial shampoo such as chlorhexidine, or use topical agents such as dilute povidone iodine (1:4) to aid healing.

SURGICAL CONSIDERATIONS AND TECHNIQUES
N/A

MEDICATIONS

DRUGS OF CHOICE
• Parenteral antibiotics for minimum 4–6 days (longer in refractory cases).
• Procaine penicillin G (20,000–70,000 units/kg body weight, IM) q12–24h.
• Ceftiofur at standard doses.
• Oxytetracycline (200 mg/ml) 20 mg/kg body weight, SQ or IM, q72h.
• Polymixin B, bacitracin, and sulfonamides may be effective.
• Copper sulfate 0.2%, lime sulfur 0.2–0.5%, potassium aluminum sulfate 1%, or zinc sulfate 0.5% as topical dips or sprays.

CONTRAINDICATIONS
N/A

PRECAUTIONS
Appropriate milk and meat withdrawal times must be followed for all compounds administered to food-producing animals.

POSSIBLE INTERACTIONS
N/A

FOLLOW-UP

EXPECTED COURSE AND PROGNOSIS
Disease generally resolves in 2–4 weeks if animals are removed from wet, moist conditions.

POSSIBLE COMPLICATIONS
Secondary infection of the skin might occur

CLIENT EDUCATION
Educate clients with regard to risk factors and methods of prevention

PATIENT CARE
N/A

PREVENTION
• Provide shelter from excessive moisture and minimize ectoparasite infestations.
• Isolate affected animals, cull chronically infected animals, and disinfect environment.

MISCELLANEOUS

ASSOCIATED CONDITIONS
• Lameness in sheep
• Mastitis in dairy cows, sheep, and goats

AGE-RELATED FACTORS
Young animals are more susceptible

ZOONOTIC POTENTIAL
• Potential zoonotic disease.
• Wear gloves when handling infected animals, hair, wool or crusts.
• Wash hands with disinfectant soap after handling infected animals.
• Properly dispose of infected hair, wool, and crusts.
• Disinfect all items in contact with affected areas (grooming equipment, clippers, etc.).

PREGNANCY
N/A

BIOSECURITY
N/A

PRODUCTION MANAGEMENT
• Decreased milk production in dairy cows and goats
• Decreased fertility

• Cachexia and death
• Impaired heat resistance in camels
• Hides/skin unsuitable for leather
• Fleece with scabs downgraded in quality
• May predispose animals to flystrike

SYNONYMS
• Cakey wool
• Kirchi (Nigeria)
• Lumpy wool
• Mycotic dermatitis
• Rain rot/scald
• Saria (Malawi)
• Senkobo skin disease (central Africa)
• Strawberry foot rot
• Streptothricosis

ABBREVIATIONS
N/A

SEE ALSO
• Dermatophytosis
• Photosensitization
• Wool Rot

Suggested Reading
Gebreyohannes M, Gebresselassie M. An overview on dermatophilosis of animals: a review. J Anim Sci Adv 2013, 3: 337–44.
Lloyd DH. Dermatophilosis. In: Howard JL, Smith RA eds, Current Veterinary Therapy: Food Animal Practice, 4th ed. Philadelphia: Saunders, 1999, pp. 334–5.
Moriello KA. Overview of dermatophilosis. In: The Merck Veterinary Manual, 2013. http://www.merckvetmanual.com.
Roberson JR, Baird AN, Pugh DG. Diseases of the integumentary system. In: Sheep and Goat Medicine, 2nd ed. Maryland Heights: Saunders, 2012, pp. 265–6.
Sisson D, Cebra C. Disorders of the skin. In: Cebra C ed, Llama and Alpaca Care. St. Louis: Saunders. 2014, p. 381.
Wernery U, Kinne J, Schuster RK. Dermatophilosis. In: Camelid Infectious Disorders. World Organisation for Animal Health. Paris: OIE, 2014, pp. 176–81.
White SD. Bacterial diseases. In: Smith BP ed, Large Animal Internal Medicine, 5th ed. St. Louis: Mosby, 2014, pp. 164, 1198.

Author Keely A. Smith
Consulting Editor Erica C. McKenzie
Acknowledgment The author and book editors acknowledge the prior contribution of Karen A. Moriello and Susan Semrad.

DERMATOPHYTOSIS

BASICS

OVERVIEW
• Fungal infection of the keratinized tissues of the skin; affects the stratum corneum layer of epidermis, hair, hoof, and horns.
• Primary causative agents: *Trichophyton* spp. and *Microsporum* spp.

INCIDENCE/PREVALENCE
Dermatophytosis is one of the most common infectious/contagious skin diseases of large animals.

GEOGRAPHIC DISTRIBUTION
• Worldwide
• Common in areas with high humidity—warm subtropical/tropical geographic regions
• Occurs in winter climates where animals are housed indoors

SYSTEMS AFFECTED
Integument

PATHOPHYSIOLOGY
• Naturally infective state is an arthrospore.
• Exposure to infective spores occurs via direct contact with infected animals and/or exposure to contaminated environments.
• Rodents may be reservoirs of infection for *Trichophyton* spp.
• Exposure does not guarantee infection. Organism must evade natural host defenses. Infective spores are brushed off or fall off.
• Moisture/microtrauma to skin allows organism to gain entry and germinate. The organism invades actively growing hairs, making them fragile. Nutrition source is keratin.
• Incubation 1–3 weeks.
• Recovery occurs when host develops a cell-mediated immune response.
• Disease is generally self-limiting.
• Increased immunity in animals previously exposed. Duration of immunity unknown.

HISTORICAL FINDINGS
N/A

SIGNALMENT
• Sheep and cattle most often affected
• Most common in young, old, or debilitated animals

PHYSICAL EXAMINATION FINDINGS
• Clinical signs highly variable; may be affected by treatments administered by client.
• Pruritus can be absent to severe.
• Variably sized annular rings of alopecia, erythema, scaling, crusting, or thick adherent crusts.
• Cattle: Well-demarcated, tightly adherent, grayish crusts; may develop into severe areas of alopecia, crusting, exudation, and ulceration.
• Calves: Most common around eyes and on head/neck. Cows/heifers: Most common on

the udder. Bulls: Dewlap and in intermaxillary spaces.
• Sheep/goats: Most common on face, neck, thorax, and back; appear as circular areas of alopecia and thick, gray crusts.
• Lesions at coronary band may lead to lameness.
• Kerion reactions are inflammatory reactions, particularly to *M. gypseum,* and may look like an abscess.

GENETICS
N/A

CAUSES AND RISK FACTORS
• *Trichophyton* spp.: *T. verrucosum, T. mentagrophytes, T. equinum, T. quinckenum, T. sarkisovii, T. schoeleinii, T. dankaliense, T. tonurans.*
• *Microsporum* spp.: *M. canis, M. nanum, M. gypseum.*
• Not species-specific.
• Age extremes, pre-existing illness, debilitated or immunocompromised animals.
• Poor nutrition.
• Overcrowding.
• Lack of exposure to sunlight.
• Excessive moisture/warmth leading to maceration/skin damage.
• Adult animals are infected/reinfected when new animals are introduced to herd.
• Parasite infestation may predispose animals to infection.

DIAGNOSIS

DIFFERENTIAL DIAGNOSES
• Demodicosis
• Dermatophilosis
• Dermatomycosis
• External parasites
• Immune-mediated diseases including Pemphigus foliaceus
• Pemphigus foliaceus
• Staphylococcal dermatitis
• Zinc-responsive dermatosis

CBC/BIOCHEMISTRY/URINALYSIS
N/A

OTHER LABORATORY TESTS
N/A

IMAGING
N/A

OTHER DIAGNOSTIC PROCEDURES
• Wood's lamp: Fluorescence is not definitive for diagnosis. Causes of false-positives include scaling, sebum, and medications. Most pathogenic dermatophytes do not fluoresce.
• Potassium hydroxide treated hair/scale may reveal ectothrix spores. This is not cost effective and many artifacts can occur; invasion of hair shafts is most easily seen with *M. canis.*
• Take scrapings/hairs from periphery of lesions (active growth). Organism is aerobic.

Exudate from inflamed epithelial layers, epithelial debris, and fungal hyphae produce crusts, resulting in a more anaerobic environment. Organisms die out in center of lesions under crusts.
• Culture: Wipe lesions with alcohol and allow to dry. Remove crusts or pluck infected hairs/scale and embed in fungal culture media—Sabouraud dextrose agar and DTM dual plate.
  ○ Color change (red) on DTM not pathognomonic for presence of the pathogen, only that rapidly growing colonies are suspect
  ○ *Microsporum* spp. colonies usually grow within 7–10 days. *Trichophyton* spp. may take up to 21 days.
  ○ Pathogens are not grossly or microscopically pigmented.
  ○ Use lactophenol cotton blue stain and clear cellophane tape to identify colonies.
• Skin biopsy is the most cost-effective diagnostic tool. Do not scrub/prep lesion prior to biopsy. Include crusts and sample periphery.
• Diagnosis often based upon history and clinical signs; it may not be cost effective to make a definitive diagnosis in all cases.

PATHOLOGIC FINDINGS
• Primarily focal areas of alopecia. Disease is characterized by folliculitis, furunculosis, hyperkeratosis, intraepidermal pustules, and nodular to diffuse pyogranulomatous infiltrates.
• Definitive diagnosis: Presence of fungal hyphae in nodular reactions, in hair shafts/hair follicles. Fungal elements may be seen with H & E stain, but special stains may allow for easier identification.
• Skin biopsy recommended if lesions are atypical and/or if animal does not respond to therapy.

TREATMENT

THERAPEUTIC APPROACH
• Isolate infected animals.
• Eliminate spread by herd animals, farm personnel, or fomites.
• All exposed animals, environment, and fomites should be treated.
• Many treatments are of unknown efficacy and often represent extra-label use; withdrawal times are unknown with respect to meat and milk.
• Improve nutrition/housing; allow animals to go outside, decrease crowding.
• Clean and disinfect environment repeatedly since infective spores are extremely difficult to eradicate. Reduce contamination of the environment by properly disposing of debris containing infective spores. Must be done

D

repeatedly since spores are difficult to eradicate and remain viable for years.
• Treatment of environment: Sprays such as lime sulfur 5%, sodium hypochlorite 5%, formalin 5%, Captan 3% and Cresol 3% have been used. Enilconazole (Clinafarm®) has also been used as a spray or fogger.

SURGICAL CONSIDERATIONS AND TECHNIQUES
N/A

MEDICATIONS
DRUGS OF CHOICE
• Topical treatments can be applied after patient preparation. Remove crusts/scales and clip infected hairs in a wide margin including lesions. Dispose of material properly. Bathe animal, rinse, and towel dry before treatment. Treat lesion, extending out past periphery.
  ○ Natamycin—animals improve, but cure not achieved.
  ○ Listerine® mouthwash for spot treatment, scrubbed into wound once daily for 7 days.
  ○ Chlorhexidine 0.5% solution reported for show lamb fungus, is inactivated by soap.
  ○ Iodine 7% mixed with emollient Bag Balm® applied once daily for 7 days.
  ○ Topical sprays include Captan 3%, lime sulfur 2–5% topically for 5 days, then weekly for 3–4 weeks. Treat entire animal by thoroughly soaking the hair coat/wool using a vat dip or sprayer. Do not rinse.
  ○ Antifungal spray/dip: Enilconazole 0.2% (Imaverol emulsion) not licensed in the United States. Enilconazole (Clinafarm® in US **only**) 55.6 mL/gal; off-label.
• Systemic antifungal drugs—efficacy unknown. Cost prohibitive.
  ○ Griseofulvin (at published dosages) orally once daily until cured. Expensive. No specified withdrawal time.
  ○ Itraconazole 5–10 mg/kg orally once daily until cured, or use as pulse therapy (week on-week off).
  ○ Sodium iodide 10–20% at 1 g/14 kg IV once a week reported effective.

CONTRAINDICATIONS
Some systemic antifungal drugs are contraindicated in pregnant animals.

PRECAUTIONS
Appropriate milk and meat withdrawal times must be followed for all compounds administered to food-producing animals.

POSSIBLE INTERACTIONS
N/A

FOLLOW-UP
EXPECTED COURSE AND PROGNOSIS
• Disease generally resolves within 70–100 days.
• Consider immunosuppressive conditions or predisposing environmental factors if animals not recovered after 4 months.

POSSIBLE COMPLICATIONS
• Lime sulfur discolors white hair coats.
• Systemic antifungals (especially griseofulvin) are teratogenic and should not be used in pregnant animals.

CLIENT EDUCATION
See "Prevention"

PATIENT CARE
Treat animals until cure achieved—clinical cure occurs before mycologic cure. Minimum period is 4–6 weeks.

PREVENTION
• Provide good nutrition, good housing, and adequate exposure to dry, well-ventilated housing.
• Antifungal vaccines: Clinical signs decreased in cattle and camels in eastern Europe, Scandinavia, Kazakhstan, and United Arab Emirates. However, use is controversial; no evidence to show protection against challenge exposure. Not available in the US.
• Isolate new animals before adding to the herd. Prophylactic dipping with lime sulfur may be useful in preventing introduction of organism in "clean" herd.
• Treat all animals to prevent reinfection and/or spread of the disease.

MISCELLANEOUS
ASSOCIATED CONDITIONS
N/A

AGE-RELATED FACTORS
Young animals more susceptible

ZOONOTIC POTENTIAL
This is a zoonotic disease and animal handlers should take appropriate precautions.

PREGNANCY
N/A

BIOSECURITY
N/A

PRODUCTION MANAGEMENT
• Affected lambs can be barred from shipment and shows.
• Decreased hide value.

SYNONYMS
• Ringworm
• Club lamb fungus

ABBREVIATIONS
• DTM = dermatophyte test medium
• H & E = hematoxylin and eosin stain

SEE ALSO
Wool Rot

Suggested Reading
Fowler ME. Medicine and Surgery of Camelids, 3rd ed. Ames: Wiley-Blackwell, 2010.
Roberson JR, Baird AN, Pugh DG. Diseases of the integumentary system. In: Sheep and Goat Medicine, 2nd ed. Maryland Heights: Saunders, 2012, pp. 271–2.
Sisson D, Cebra C. Disorders of the skin. In: Cebra C ed, Llama and Alpaca Care. St. Louis: Elsevier, 2014, p. 382.
Spickler AR. Dermatophytosis. March 2005 (last updated May 2013). http://www.cfsph.iastate.edu/Factsheets/pdfs/dermatophytosis.pdf
Wernery U, Kinne J, Schuster RK. Dermatophytosis. In: Camelid Infectious Disorders. World Organisation for Animal Health. Paris: OIE, 2014, pp. 327–31.
White SD. Dermatophytosis (Ringworm.) In: Smith BP ed, Large Animal Internal Medicine, 5th ed. St. Louis: Mosby, 2014, pp. 1204–5.

Author Keely A. Smith
Consulting Editor Erica C. McKenzie
Acknowledgment The author and book editors acknowledge the prior contribution of Karen A. Moriello and Susan Semrad.

DIARRHEAL DISEASES: BOVINE

BASICS

OVERVIEW
Diarrhea can be defined as abnormally increased water content in the feces, usually associated with increased frequency of defecation.

INCIDENCE/PREVALENCE
The USDA dairy report (2007) included 2,194 herds—diarrhea was reported (by owners) in 2.5% of the mature cows and 24% of the unweaned heifers.

GEOGRAPHIC DISTRIBUTION
Worldwide

SYSTEMS AFFECTED
• Digestive
• Cardiovascular
• Urinary
• Hemolymphatic

PATHOPHYSIOLOGY
• Diarrhea results from different mechanisms including hypersecretion, abnormal permeability, increased intraluminal osmolality, and abnormal motility; most diarrheic states are caused by more than one mechanism.
• Hypersecretory diarrhea arises from an increase in the amount of fluid being drawn into the lumen of the bowel, overwhelming the absorptive capacity of the intestines. Typically caused by infectious agents.
• Abnormal permeability: Mucosal inflammatory ulceration or necrosis can result in abnormal tight junction functions of the intestinal epithelium, leading to fluid loss (mild cases), and loss of albumin, red blood cells, and globulins (severe cases).
• Osmotic: Presence of poorly absorbed, osmotically active substance causes movement of water from the extracellular fluid into the gut lumen (i.e., loss of lactase activity secondary to damage of the intestinal epithelium).
• Abnormal motility: Hypermotility can result from inflammation of the gastrointestinal tract leading to faster transport of intestinal contents and diarrhea.
• Loss of large volumes of electrolyte-rich fluid can result in electrolyte, fluid, and acid-base disorders.
• Damage to the enteric barrier can result in albumin loss, toxemia, bacteremia, systemic inflammation and multi-organ dysfunction associated with hypovolemic and septic shock.
• Bacteremia/septicemia can result in septic arthritis, pneumonia, and abortion.

HISTORICAL FINDINGS
Epidemiologic information, including age and number of animals affected, management characteristics, season, and clinical course can help distinguish appropriate differentials.

SIGNALMENT
Any age, breed or gender

PHYSICAL EXAMINATION FINDINGS
• Mild cases—loose feces and appear otherwise clinically normal.
• Severe cases—fever, diarrhea, dehydration, weakness, and potentially frank blood in the feces (coccidiosis, coronavirus, salmonellosis, torovirus). Diarrhea and oral erosions (30–50% of the cases) can be seen in acute cases of bovine viral diarrhea virus (BVDV).
• Chronic diarrhea—associated with progressive wasting and loss of body condition.

GENETICS
N/A

CAUSES AND RISK FACTORS
Neonatal Calf Diarrhea
Infectious
• Viral—rotavirus, coronavirus, BVDV, torovirus, norovirus, and nebovirus.
• Bacterial—enterotoxigenic *E. coli*, enteropathogenic *E. coli*, *Salmonella* spp., *C. perfringens* (rarely, type A and type C associated with enteritis and abomasitis).
• Protozoal—*Cryptosporidium parvum, Giardia, Eimeria bovis, Eimeria zuernii,* and *Eimeria alabamensis.*
Noninfectious
• Nutritional diarrhea. Anecdotal evidence suggests that ingestion of large volumes of milk can result in diarrhea. Lactose intolerance secondary to infectious diarrhea.
• Diarrhea and emaciation caused by milk replacer feeding. Inappropriate quality (low protein or fat content) and quantity (usually not enough) of milk replacer.
• Poor clotting ability of the milk is associated with low calcium content.

Adult Cattle
Infectious
• Viral—BVDV, coronavirus (winter dysentery), torovirus (winter-like dysentery), acute malignant catarrhal fever (MCF) can cause severe diarrhea as a prominent sign.
• Bacterial—*Salmonella* spp., *Mycobacterium avium* subsp. *paratuberculosis* (MAP, Johne's disease), *C. perfringens* (type C associated with diarrhea).
Noninfectious
• Arsenic toxicosis
• Oak (acorn) toxicosis
• Copper or cobalt deficiency
• Administration of cathartics

Risk Factors
• Failure of passive transfer of immunity.
• Inappropriate volume, fat, protein, or calcium content of milk or milk replacer.
• High stocking density and poor hygiene.
• Presence of other animals with diarrhea, salmonellosis, or advanced MAP in the herd.
• Pastures or diets deficient in cobalt or copper, or with abundant acorn crops.

• Arsenic—wood preservatives, burn piles, discontinued insecticides and molluscicides.
• Copper—diets low in copper or high in sulfates, zinc, or molybdenum.
• Cobalt—diets deficient in cobalt, heavy fertilization with limestone.

DIAGNOSIS

DIFFERENTIAL DIAGNOSES
• Septicemia
• Peritonitis
• Gastrointestinal parasitism
• Neoplasia

CBC/BIOCHEMISTRY/URINALYSIS
• Normal in mildly affected and clinically stable animals.
• Anemia can reflect dysentery, cobalt or copper deficiency, parasitism, or MAP.
• Hemoconcentration—dehydration.
• Leukopenia with neutropenia, left shift, and toxic changes—severe gastroenteritis and toxemia.
• Hypoproteinemia—loss of albumin, the magnitude of hypoalbuminemia can be attenuated by dehydration.
• More severe acute or chronic disease creates changes reflecting dehydration (hemoconcentration, azotemia), inflammation (leukocytosis or leukopenia with neutropenia, left shift, and toxic changes), protein loss (hypoalbuminemia), and metabolic acidosis (reduced TCO_2, increased lactate).
• Electrolyte abnormalities often include low sodium, potassium and chloride.
• Hyperglycemia and glucosuria occur with type D enterotoxemia.

OTHER LABORATORY TESTS
• Culture of feces—*E. coli*, *Salmonella* spp., MAP
• PCR—*E. coli*, *Salmonella* spp., rotavirus, coronavirus, MCF
• Immunoassays—*C. perfringens* toxins, coronavirus, MCF
• Immunofluorescence assays—*Cryptosporidium* and *Giardia*
• Electron microscopy—rotavirus, coronavirus
• Hepatic concentration of copper (normal 90–200 µg/g)
• Serum vitamin B_{12} (cobalt deficiency)—normal 1–3 ng/mL

IMAGING
Transabdominal ultrasonography and abdominocentesis might be useful for distinguishing differentials.

OTHER DIAGNOSTIC PROCEDURES
N/A

PATHOLOGIC FINDINGS
N/A

(CONTINUED) | **DIARRHEAL DISEASES: BOVINE**

TREATMENT

THERAPEUTIC APPROACH
• Success relies on early identification of the problem, immediate correction of dehydration, metabolic acidosis, and electrolyte abnormalities.
• Determine fluid requirements in terms of replacement, maintenance, and ongoing losses.
• Animals estimated to be >8% dehydrated should be rehydrated IV initially, and then can be maintained on IV or oral fluid therapy. Large volumes of water and rehydration solutions can be administered orally to cattle (20–40 L at a time several times per day to adults).
• The volume (L) of fluids to replace the deficit can be calculated as: *Volume (L) = body weight (kg) × % dehydration*. Balanced crystalloids can be given at 20 mL/kg/h (highest rate reached through a 14 gauge catheter) for fluid replacement.
• Maintenance fluids can be continued at a rate of 2–4 mL/kg/h.
• Cows with mild acidemia (base deficits <10 mmol/L) will usually respond to basic fluid therapy.
• Cows with more severe acidemia (base deficits >10 mmol/L) can benefit from isotonic sodium bicarbonate (156 mEq $NaHCO_3$/L; or 1.3% solution).
• The total bicarbonate deficit can be calculated from base deficit on blood gas analysis or by estimating from the decrease in TCO_2 on serum chemistry (*Bicarbonate deficit (mEq) = body weight (kg) × base deficit (mEq/L) × 0.6*).
• Hypertonic saline (5% or 7.2%) can be administered to dehydrated cows at dose of 4–5 mL/kg, IV, over 5 minutes. The cow must be allowed to drink water, and cows not observed to drink within 5 minutes should receive 20 L of water via orogastric tube.
• Ruminal transfaunation can be beneficial in cases of prolonged anorexia.

SURGICAL CONSIDERATIONS AND TECHNIQUES
N/A

MEDICATIONS

DRUGS OF CHOICE
• Animals with prolonged dysentery can need whole blood transfusion (4–8 L).

• Antimicrobials are recommended when septicemia/bacteremia are suspected—beta-lactam drugs (ceftiofur, amoxicillin, or ampicillin), tetracyclines, or potentiated sulfonamides (where permitted).
• Nonsteroidal anti-inflammatory drugs—beneficial in cattle with toxemia (flunixin meglumine or meloxicam).
• Arsenic toxicity—sodium thiosulfate (40 mg/kg IV q8h and 80 mg/kg PO q24h)
• Copper deficiency—copper glycinate 400 mg SC (calves 100 mg). Cattle can be supplemented with copper in salt mineral mixes at 50 g/cow/day.
• Cobalt deficiency—vitamin B12, 2,000–3,000 µg weekly until improvement.

CONTRAINDICATIONS
Nephrotoxic drugs are contraindicated in severe dehydration and azotemia.

PRECAUTIONS
Dehydrated ruminants can generate profound azotemia which is prerenal in origin, and should not be mistaken for renal failure. Prerenal azotemia is expected to respond rapidly to appropriate fluid therapy.

POSSIBLE INTERACTIONS
N/A

FOLLOW-UP

EXPECTED COURSE AND PROGNOSIS
• Prognosis is good to fair for animals with infectious or nutritional diarrhea receiving supportive care.
• Prognosis is grave for cases of arsenic or oak toxicosis or with severe secondary complications.

POSSIBLE COMPLICATIONS
• Shock and death.
• Intussusception, associated with changes in GI motility.
• Renal failure.

CLIENT EDUCATION
Focus on encouraging protocols for optimizing passive transfer to crias, managing stocking density, and controlling parasitic infestations.

PATIENT CARE
Monitor attitude, fecal consistency, and hydration status.

PREVENTION
• Ensure good-quality colostrum intake to neonates.
• Environmental hygiene.
• Vaccination protocols.

MISCELLANEOUS

ASSOCIATED CONDITIONS
• Septicemia
• Meningitis
• Septic arthritis
• Abortion

AGE-RELATED FACTORS
More common in calves <1 month of age.

ZOONOTIC POTENTIAL
• Ruminants can be considered as a reservoir for pathogenic *E. coli*, *Salmonella* spp., and *Cryptosporidium* spp.

PREGNANCY
N/A

BIOSECURITY
• Environmental and personnel hygiene are critical: gloves, outerwear, hand washing, disinfection.
• Segregate sick animals.

SYNONYM
Scours

ABBREVIATIONS
• BVDV = bovine viral diarrhea virus
• IV = intravenous
• MAP = *Mycobacterium avium paratuberculosis*
• MCF = malignant catarrhal fever
• PCR = polymerase chain reaction
• PO = per os
• TCO_2 = total carbon dioxide
• USDA = United States Department of Agriculture

SEE ALSO
• Coccidiosis
• Coronavirus
• Cryptosporidiosis
• Diarrheal Diseases: Small Ruminant
• Johne's Disease
• Malignant Catarrhal Fever
• Manure Microbiology and Zoonosis (see www.fiveminutevet.com/ruminant)
• Neonatal Diarrhea

Suggested Reading
Roussel AJ. Fluid therapy in mature cattle. Vet Clin North Am Food Anim Pract 2014, 30: 429–39.
Author Diego Gomez-Nieto
Consulting Editor Erica C. McKenzie

D

DIARRHEAL DISEASES: CAMELID

BASICS

OVERVIEW
Diarrhea reflects abnormally increased water content in the feces, usually with increased frequency of defecation.

INCIDENCE/PREVALENCE
• Varies with etiology; often sporadic.
• Specific infectious agents can occur with high prevalence in vulnerable groups.

GEOGRAPHIC DISTRIBUTION
Worldwide, with specific distributions of some infectious agents.

SYSTEMS AFFECTED
• Digestive
• Cardiovascular
• Urinary

PATHOPHYSIOLOGY
• Diarrhea results from mechanisms including abnormal permeability, hypersecretion, abnormal motility, and increased intraluminal osmolality.
• Most diarrheic states are caused by more than one mechanism.
• The colon of camelids has large absorptive capacity; therefore, gastric and small intestinal diseases do not consistently cause diarrhea, except when damage is severe, a systemic complication exists (e.g., hypoproteinemia), or the colon is concurrently diseased.
• Loss of large volumes of electrolyte-rich fluid can result in electrolyte imbalances, dehydration, and acid–base disorders.
• Damage to the enteric barrier can result in albumin loss, toxemia, bacterial translocation, and multi-organ dysfunction associated with hypovolemic and septic shock.

HISTORICAL FINDINGS
Depend on the primary disorder. Epidemiologic information, including age and number of animals affected, management characteristics, season, and clinical course can help distinguish appropriate differentials.

SIGNALMENT
• All breeds and ages are susceptible.
• Some infectious disorders are more common in neonates (*E. coli, Cryptosporidium*).

PHYSICAL EXAMINATION FINDINGS
• Initially, signs of systemic illness—lethargy, anorexia, and possibly fever, but without diarrhea.
• Mild, acute cases—clumped stool or low volume, liquid feces.
• Severe, acute cases—fever, liquid feces, dehydration, weakness, hematochezia (blood in the feces), tenesmus, abdominal distension, and colic.
• Chronic diarrhea—progressive wasting, which may not be noted promptly in large herds, or because of fleece cover, avoidance to handling and stoicism of affected camelids.
• Lymphoma—peripheral lymphadenopathy (occasionally).

GENETICS
N/A

CAUSES AND RISK FACTORS
Neonatal and Juvenile Camelids
• Viral—rotavirus or coronavirus in crias >7 days. Potentially bovine viral diarrhea virus (BVDV) and parvovirus.
• Bacterial—*E. coli* and other pathogens that can cause concurrent septicemia in very young crias; *Salmonella* spp. (rare); *Clostridium perfringens* (type A, C, or D).
• Parasites—*Cryptosporidium* spp. or *Giardia* in crias ≥7 days. Internal parasitism—important cause of diarrhea in crias >4–6 weeks old (heavy infestations of small coccidia, *Eimeria macusaniensis* (E. mac), and also *Trichuris* and *Nematodirus battus* among other nematodes).
• Noninfectious—nutritional diarrhea due to inappropriate quality and quantity of milk or milk replacer, related to mixing errors or the use of alternative milk sources (sheep, cow, goat) with different protein and fat content to camelid milk. In older crias, lush pastures or sudden dietary changes.

Adult Camelids
• Viral—coronavirus.
• Bacterial—*Salmonella* spp. (rare), *C. perfringens.*
• Parasites—*Trichuris, N. battus,* and heavy infestations with other nematode species or small *Eimeria* spp; E. mac.
• Noninfectious—forestomach acidosis, peritonitis.

Chronic Diarrhea and Weight Loss
• Bacterial—*Mycobacterium avium* subsp. *paratuberculosis* (Johne's disease) and *M. avium* subsp. *avium; Yersinia enterocolitica,* and *Y. pseudotuberculosa.*
• Parasites—*Trichuris,* liver flukes, E. mac.
• Noninfectious—inflammatory bowel disease (eosinophilic or lymphocytic-plasmacytic infiltration), neoplasia (lymphoma, squamous cell carcinoma, adenocarcinoma).

Risk Factors
• Failure of passive transfer in crias.
• Inappropriate volume, or fat, protein or calcium content of milk or milk replacer.
• High population density and poor hygiene.
• Presence of other animals with diarrhea.
• *Salmonella, Cryptosporidium,* Johne's disease or E. mac within a herd.

DIAGNOSIS

DIFFERENTIAL DIAGNOSES
• Septicemia
• Peritonitis

CBC/BIOCHEMISTRY/URINALYSIS
• Typically normal in mildly affected, clinically stable animals.
• Anemia—GI hemorrhage, chronic disease, or heavy parasitism.
• More severe acute or chronic disease—dehydration (hemoconcentration, azotemia), inflammation (leukocytosis or leukopenia with neutropenia, left shift and toxic changes), protein loss (hypoalbuminemia) and metabolic acidosis (reduced TCO_2, increased lactate).
• Electrolyte abnormalities—hypernatremia more common than hyponatremia, and can be accompanied by hyperchloremia. Hypokalemia, hypochloremia, and hypocalcemia also possible.
• Hyperosmolar syndrome can arise from diarrhea or be induced during treatment (iatrogenic), usually in crias, with profound elevations in serum glucose, urea nitrogen, and sodium.
• Hypoglycemia—septic crias; hyperglycemia is a more common response of camelids to physiologic stress.

OTHER LABORATORY TESTS
• Fecal culture—*E. coli, Salmonella* spp., *Myocbacterium.*
• PCR—*E. coli, Salmonella* spp., coronavirus, E. mac.
• Immunoassays—*C. perfringens* toxins, coronavirus.
• Fecal egg count (quantitative McMaster technique, sugar centrifugation)—internal parasitism.
• Light microscopy of direct smears—*Giardia, Eimeria, Cryptosporidium.*
• Immunofluorescence assays—*Cryptosporidium* and *Giardia.*
• Sucrose flotation—E. mac.

IMAGING
• Ultrasonography can identify thickening of the small intestine and/or colon due to E. mac, neoplasia, and inflammatory bowel disease.
• Thickening of the gastric compartments (particularly C2, C3) can occur with lymphoma.
• Free peritoneal fluid can indicate neoplasia, peritonitis, or ascites.

OTHER DIAGNOSTIC PROCEDURES
• Abdominocentesis—peritonitis, lymphoma.
• Biopsy—can require exploratory procedures to accomplish safely.

PATHOLOGIC FINDINGS
Depend on the etiology of the disease.

TREATMENT

THERAPEUTIC APPROACH
• Success relies on early identification, diagnosis, and correction of dehydration,

acid-base and electrolyte abnormalities.
• Fluid therapy can be provided by oral, IV, or SC routes depending on severity of dehydration. Intraosseous or intra-peritoneal routes have also been utilized in crias.
• Determine fluid requirements by estimating replacement (*Volume (L) = body weight (kg) × % dehydration*), maintenance (50 mL/kg/day adults, 70–80 mL/kg/day crias), and ongoing losses (variable).
• Replacement volume can be given over approximately 4 h; maintenance and ongoing losses can be attended over time.
• If hypoproteinemia is present, administer half the replacement volume over 4–6 h and the remainder can be incorporated into the ongoing administration.
• Balanced polyionic fluid—recommended for IV administration, and can be supplemented as needed with electrolytes and glucose.
• Bicarbonate—only when significant metabolic acidosis is confirmed and is poorly responsive to fluid supplementation. Half the deficit (calculated as *body weight (kg) × (0.3–0.6) × base deficit*) can be added to non-calcium containing fluids. The value 0.3 is often used in adults, and 0.6 in neonates.
• Oral electrolytes designed for calves can be used for maintenance or rehydration of mildly dehydrated neonates at 2- or 3-fold the recommended dilution for calves, or oral human pediatric solutions can be used.
• Hypoglycemia—add dextrose to IV fluids to a final concentration of 2.5–5%. Severe hypoglycemia (glucose <30 mg/dL)—administer 1 mL/5 kg body weight of 50% dextrose.

SURGICAL CONSIDERATIONS AND TECHNIQUES
N/A

MEDICATIONS
DRUGS OF CHOICE
• Antibiotics to treat or prevent bacteremia/sepsis—ceftiofur; penicillin + aminoglycoside (gentamicin or amikacin).
• Nonsteroidal anti-inflammatory drugs can address colic, inflammation, toxemia—flunixin meglumine or meloxicam. Hypoproteinemia—plasma 5–10 mL/kg IV once to twice; llama plasma can be given to alpacas.

• Coccidiosis—amprolium (10 mg/kg, PO, q24h for 5 d); ponazuril or toltrazuril (20 mg/kg, PO, q24h, for 3 d). Sulfadimethoxine (110 mg/kg, PO, q24h for up to 50 d).
• *Giardia*—fenbendazole (10–50 mg/kg, PO, q24h for 1–3 d).
• Nematodes—fenbendazole; ivermectin (0.3–0.6 mg/kg, PO or SC once).

CONTRAINDICATIONS
• Metronidazole is illegal in food-producing animals.
• Nephrotoxic drugs are contraindicated in severe dehydration and azotemia.

PRECAUTIONS
Appropriate milk and meat withdrawal times must be followed for all compounds administered to food-producing animals.

POSSIBLE INTERACTIONS
N/A

FOLLOW-UP
EXPECTED COURSE AND PROGNOSIS
• Prognosis is good to fair for animals with infectious and nutritional diarrhea receiving supportive care.
• Prognosis is guarded for animals with chronic diarrhea.

POSSIBLE COMPLICATIONS
• Hyperosmolar syndrome can accompany diarrhea or occur during treatment. Monitoring blood glucose, blood sodium, and urea nitrogen is recommended.
• Shock and death.
• Renal failure.

CLIENT EDUCATION
Focus on encouraging protocols for optimizing passive transfer to crias, managing stocking density, and controlling parasitic infestations.

PATIENT CARE
Monitor attitude, fecal consistency, and hydration status.

PREVENTION
• Ensure adequate intake of good-quality colostrum in crias.
• Practice good environmental hygiene.
• Cattle vaccines against enteric pathogens can provide protection; however, antigenic variability is a limitation.
• Periodic herd monitoring of body condition—identify chronic diseases early.

MISCELLANEOUS
ASSOCIATED CONDITIONS
• Septicemia
• Gastrointestinal parasitism

AGE-RELATED FACTORS
Diarrhea can be a life-threatening disorder in young crias.

ZOONOTIC POTENTIAL
Camelids can serve as a reservoir for human infection with *Salmonella* spp., *Cryptosporidium*, and *Giardia*.

PREGNANCY
N/A

BIOSECURITY
• Environmental, hand, and outerwear hygiene.
• Segregate and diagnose sick animals.
• Quarantine new animals, visiting animals, or stock that have left the herd temporarily.

PRODUCTION MANAGEMENT
See "Biosecurity"

SYNONYMS
Scours

ABBREVIATIONS
• BVDV = bovine viral diarrhea virus
• C2, C3 = camelid gastric compartments
• GI = gastrointestinal
• IV = intravenous
• PCR = polymerase chain reaction
• SC = subcutaneous
• TCO_2 = total carbon dioxide

SEE ALSO
• Body Condition Scoring: Alpacas and Llamas (see www.fiveminutevet.com/ruminant)
• Body Condition Scoring: Camels (see www.fiveminutevet.com/ruminant)
• Diarrheal Diseases: Bovine
• Diarrheal Diseases: Small Ruminant

Suggested Reading
Cebra C. Diseases of the digestive system. In: Cebra C, Anderson DE, Tibary A, Van Saun RJ, Johnson LW eds, Llama and Alpaca Care: Medicine, Surgery, Reproduction, Nutrition and Herd Health. St. Louis: Elsevier, 2014, pp. 477–537.
Author Diego Gomez-Nieto
Consulting Editor Erica C. McKenzie

D

DIARRHEAL DISEASES: SMALL RUMINANT

BASICS

OVERVIEW
Diarrhea reflects increased water content in the feces, usually associated with increased frequency of defecation.

INCIDENCE/PREVALENCE
• Diarrhea is the most common and costly disease of neonatal small ruminants, and can contribute to over 40% of mortality.
• Gastrointestinal parasitism is an important cause of diarrhea in any ruminant >6 days old.

GEOGRAPHIC DISTRIBUTION
N/A

SYSTEMS AFFECTED
• Digestive
• Cardiovascular
• Urinary
• Hemolymphatic

PATHOPHYSIOLOGY
• Diarrhea results from different mechanisms—hypersecretion, abnormal permeability, increased intraluminal osmolality, and abnormal motility; most diarrheic states are caused by more than one mechanism.
• Loss of large volumes of electrolyte-rich fluid can result in electrolyte, fluid, and acid-base disorders.
• Damage to the intestinal mucosa can result in hypoproteinemia (albumin loss), toxemia (absorption of toxins), bacteremia (translocation of bacteria), hypovolemia, and septic shock.
• Bacteremia can result in secondary complications including septic arthritis, pneumonia, and abortion.

HISTORICAL FINDINGS
Epidemiologic information, including age and number of animals affected, management characteristics, season, and clinical course can help distinguish appropriate differentials.

SIGNALMENT
Small ruminants of any age, breed, or gender

PHYSICAL EXAMINATION FINDINGS
• Mildly affected cases—clumped or loose feces, appearing otherwise normal.
• Severely affected neonates—dehydration, obtundation, weak or absent suckling reflex, excessive salivation, and liquid diarrhea. Dysentery can reflect specific pathogens (*Salmonella*, enteropathogenic *E. coli*, *Clostridium*).
• Older animals—fever, diarrhea, dehydration, weakness, and frank blood in feces (*Coccidia*, *Salmonella*).
• Internal parasitism in juvenile or adult small ruminants—often asymptomatic. Severely infested animals—diarrhea, anemia, poor growth, submandibular edema, and decreased weight gain and milk production.
• Chronic diarrhea—progressive wasting with reduced body condition score.

GENETICS
N/A

CAUSES AND RISK FACTORS
Neonates
• Viral—rotavirus, coronavirus.
• Bacterial—enterotoxigenic *E. coli* (ETEC), *Salmonella* spp; rarely, enteropathogenic *E. coli*.
• Protozoal—*Giardia* and *Cryptosporidium* spp.
• Noninfectious—nutritional diarrhea due to inappropriate quality and quantity of milk or milk replacer, related to mixing errors or the use of alternative milk sources with different protein and fat content.

Older Lambs and Kids
• Bacterial—*Salmonella* spp., *C. perfringens* (rarely, type A, B, C, D). Type D is associated with enterotoxemia in sheep.
• Internal parasitism—most important cause of diarrhea in sheep <18 months of age. This can relate to infection with *Giardia* or *Eimeria* spp, or a variety of nematode parasites.
• Noninfectious—lush pastures.

Adult Sheep and Goats
• Bacterial—*Salmonella* spp., *Yersinia* spp., *Mycobacterium avium* subsp. *paratuberculosis* (MAP, Johne's disease). Chronic diarrhea only occurs in 20% of cases of Johne's disease; weight loss is more prominent.
• Internal parasitism—*Eimeria* spp. and nematodes, though older animals are often more resistant.
• Noninfectious—ruminal acidosis, arsenic toxicosis, cobalt or copper deficiency.

Risk Factors
• Failure of passive transfer of immunity.
• Inappropriate volume, or fat, protein or calcium content of milk or milk replacer.
• High population density and poor hygiene.
• Presence of other animals with diarrhea or with *Salmonella*, *Cryptosporidium* or MAP within a herd.
• Internal parasitism can be exacerbated by high density stocking, overgrazing, inadequate protein intake, and inappropriate deworming protocols.
• *C. perfringens* type D—associated with high calorie (grain) diets.
• Arsenic—wood preservatives, burn piles, discontinued insecticides and molluscicides.
• Cobalt—diets deficient in cobalt, heavy fertilization with limestone.
• Copper—diets deficient in copper, or excess intake of molybdenum, iron, zinc or calcium.

DIAGNOSIS

DIFFERENTIAL DIAGNOSES
• Septicemia
• Peritonitis
• Neoplasia

CBC/BIOCHEMISTRY/URINALYSIS
• Generally normal in mildly affected and clinically stable animals.
• Anemia can occur with parasitism, dysentery, cobalt or copper deficiency and MAP.
• More severe acute or chronic disease creates changes reflecting dehydration (hemoconcentration, azotemia), inflammation (leukocytosis or leukopenia with neutropenia, left shift and toxic changes), protein loss (hypoalbuminemia), and metabolic acidosis (reduced TCO_2, increased lactate).
• Electrolyte abnormalities often include low sodium, potassium, and chloride.
• Hyperglycemia and glucosuria occur in lambs *Clostridium* with type D enterotoxemia.

OTHER LABORATORY TESTS
• Culture of feces—*E. coli*, *Salmonella* spp., MAP.
• Fecal egg count (quantitative McMaster technique)—internal parasitism.
• PCR—*E. coli*, *Salmonella* spp., rotavirus, coronavirus.
• Immunoassays—*C. perfringens* toxins, coronavirus.
• Immunofluorescence assays—*Cryptosporidium* and *Giardia*.
• Iodine-stained wet mounts of feces—*Giardia*.
• Electron microscopy—rotavirus, coronavirus.
• Liver cobalt or copper content.

IMAGING
N/A

OTHER DIAGNOSTIC PROCEDURES
N/A

PATHOLOGIC FINDINGS
Consistent with gastrointestinal inflammation or disease, evidence of parasitism or other disorders.

TREATMENT

THERAPEUTIC APPROACH
• Success relies on early identification, diagnosis, and correction of dehydration, acid-base and electrolyte abnormalities.
• Fluid therapy can be provided by oral, IV or SC routes depending on severity of dehydration

DIARRHEAL DISEASES: SMALL RUMINANT

• In animals with dehydration judged to be >8%, provide IV fluids initially, followed by IV or oral fluids for maintenance.

• Fluid deficits can be calculated as: *Volume (L) = body weight (kg) × % dehydration*, and can be replaced over 4–6 hours using balanced polyionic solutions.

• Maintenance requirements (50 mL/kg/day adults; 80–100 mL/kg/day neonates) should then be provided continuously IV or by intermittent IV or oral bolus; additional volume (0.5–2 L) is required for estimated ongoing losses per day depending on animal size and severity of diarrhea.

• Severe dehydration and metabolic acidemia can be addressed by administering isotonic sodium bicarbonate (156 mEq $NaHCO_3$/L; or 1.3% solution) at a third to a half of the calculated deficit volume, followed by a balanced crystalloid for remaining deficit, maintenance, and ongoing losses.

• Oral electrolytes designed for calves can be used for maintenance or rehydration of mildly dehydrated kids and lambs at 250–500 mL q6–8h.

• Hypoglycemia can be treated by adding dextrose to IV fluids (final concentration of 2.5–5%).

• Milk and milk replacer should not be withheld for more than 4–6 h.

• Animals with prolonged dysentery or severe anemia (internal parasitism) may need whole blood transfusion (approximately 1–2 L to adults).

SURGICAL CONSIDERATIONS AND TECHNIQUES
N/A

MEDICATIONS

DRUGS OF CHOICE
• Antibiotics to address bacteremia/toxemia can include beta-lactam drugs (ceftiofur, amoxicillin, or ampicillin) and potentiated sulfonamides (where permitted).

• Nonsteroidal anti-inflammatory drugs can address colic, inflammation, toxemia—flunixin meglumine or ketoprofen.

• *C. perfringens* Type D antitoxin (15–20 mL SC) can be administered during outbreaks of enterotoxemia, especially if animals are not vaccinated.

• Cobalt deficiency can be addressed with oral cobalt (1 mg/head/day); methods for addressing copper deficiency are provided elsewhere in this text (see *Copper Deficiency and Toxicity*).

Parasite infestations should be addressed by judicious use of appropriate anthelmintic agents in combination with relevant management methods. See *Parasite Control Programs: Small Ruminant* for anthelmintic drug doses.

CONTRAINDICATIONS
Nephrotoxic drugs are contraindicated in severe dehydration and azotemia.

PRECAUTIONS
Appropriate milk and meat withdrawal times must be followed for all compounds administered to food-producing animals.

POSSIBLE INTERACTIONS
N/A

FOLLOW-UP

EXPECTED COURSE AND PROGNOSIS
• Prognosis is grave for severely diseased animals, or those with protracted diarrhea nonresponsive to treatment.

• Prognosis good to fair for mildly to moderately affected animals receiving appropriate care.

POSSIBLE COMPLICATIONS
• Edema
• Septicemia
• Shock and death
• Renal failure

CLIENT EDUCATION
Focus on encouraging protocols for optimizing passive transfer to lambs and kids, managing stocking density, and controlling parasitic infestations.

PATIENT CARE
Monitor attitude, fecal consistency, and hydration status.

PREVENTION
• Ensure adequate good-quality colostrum intake via good nutrition and vaccination of dams with bovine ETEC and rotavirus vaccines, and *C. perfringens* type C and D toxoid to provide colostral antibodies; lambs and kids can be vaccinated for *C. perfringens* during the first week of life when needed.

• Anecdotal evidence suggests that decoquinate provides some control of cryptosporidiosis, decreasing morbidity and mortality rates.

• Newly introduced individuals should be isolated for 1 month. Fecal culture for *Salmonella* and MAP should be considered but is only useful if positive results are obtained.

MISCELLANEOUS

ASSOCIATED CONDITIONS
• Septicemia
• Abortion

AGE RELATED FACTORS
N/A

ZOONOTIC POTENTIAL
Ruminants can be considered as a reservoir for human pathogenic *E. coli*, *Salmonella* spp., *Cryptosporidium* spp., and *Giardia*.

PREGNANCY
N/A

BIOSECURITY
• Environmental hygiene. Cleaning and disinfection of environmental sites.
• Hand and outerwear hygiene. Wash hands, disinfect boots, and maintain coveralls free of fecal material.
• Segregating sick animals will reduce pathogen exposure.

PRODUCTION MANAGEMENT
N/A

SYNONYM
Scours

ABBREVIATIONS
• ETEC = enterotoxigenic *E. coli*
• IV = intravenous
• MAP = *Mycobacterium avium paratuberculosis*
• PCR = polymerase chain reaction
• SC = subcutaneous
• TCO_2 = total carbon dioxide

SEE ALSO
• Diarrheal Diseases: Bovine
• *Escherichia coli*
• Parasite Control Programs: Small Ruminant
• Salmonellosis

Suggested Reading
Jones M., Navarre C.B. Fluid therapy in small ruminants and camelids. *Vet Clin North Am Food Anim Pract.* 2014;30: 441–53.
Navarre C.B., Baird A.N., Pugh D.G. Diseases of the gastrointestinal system. In: D.G. Pugh and A.N. Baird., ed. Sheep and Goat Medicine. 2nd ed. Maryland Heights: Elsevier, 2012:71–106.
Author Diego Gomez-Nieto
Consulting Editor Erica C. McKenzie

DISPLACED ABOMASUM

BASICS

OVERVIEW
• Displacement of the abomasum (DA) is a very common digestive condition affecting lactating dairy cattle, but has also been reported in sheep, goats, beef cattle, and calves.
• The abomasum lies in a ventral position in the right cranial quadrant of the abdomen between the 7th and 11th ribs.
• Displacement mostly occurs after parturition when more space is available in the abdominal cavity due to fetal expulsion and a rumen with less content. This generates enough space for the abomasum to slide down under the rumen. In addition, the muscular tone of the abomasum is reduced due to hypocalcemia. This creates excess gas buildup and allows for dorsal displacement along the left side (~90% of the time) or right side (~10% of displacements).
• In some right-sided displacements, a life-threatening volvulus may develop.

INCIDENCE/PREVALENCE
Lactational incidence of LDA may range between 0.2% and 15%. The prevalence of DA among dairy herds is variable depending on geographic location, management practices, climate, and other factors.

GEOGRAPHIC DISTRIBUTION
Worldwide in dairy cattle

SYSTEMS AFFECTED
Digestive

PATHOPHYSIOLOGY
See "Causes and Risk Factors"

HISTORICAL FINDINGS
• Decreased DMI and milk production
• Depression
• High ketones detected in blood, urine, or milk
• RDA: Colic and toxemia possible
• Herd level: Elevated NEFA prepartum can be used as metabolic predictor of LDA incidence in lactating dairy cows.

SIGNALMENT
Bovine, predominantly dairy breeds, predominantly female

PHYSICAL EXAMINATION FINDINGS
• High-pitched ping during simultaneous percussion and auscultation over the ipsilateral paracostal area.
• Mild to moderate tachycardia, sometimes bradycardia.
• Ketonuria/ketonemia.
• Scant, pasty manure, but sometimes diarrhea.
• Dehydration may be present but is usually mild unless the displacement is to the right side. Cows with RDA and volvulus may demonstrate tachycardia, rapid dehydration,

and metabolic alkalosis with paradoxical aciduria.
• Different degrees of abdominal distension, especially in the paralumbar fossa corresponding to the side of displacement.

GENETICS
Most commonly affected breed is Holstein; however, DA has been diagnosed in all dairy and some beef breeds. For Holsteins, heritability estimates for DA are between 0.03 and 0.53. Genome-wide significant genomic regions associated with LDA have been determined on bovine chromosomes 1, 3, 11, 20, and 23.

CAUSES AND RISK FACTORS
• DA is a multifactorial syndrome.
• The highest risk period for DA is the early postpartum until 30 DIM. However, DAs do occur throughout lactation and occasionally during the dry period.
• DMI is reduced during the transition period, causing decreased rumen fill.
• After parturition, the smaller rumen moves slightly backwards generating enough space for the distended abomasum to slide under the rumen and move upward between the lateral wall of the ventral and dorsal sac of the rumen and left costal wall. Reduced abomasum motility decreases its emptying rate. Consequently, a diet rich in nonstructural carbohydrates will continue fermenting, producing extra gas that worsens abomasum distension.
• Hypocalcemia is also common right after calving. Subclinical hypocalcemia (<8.0 mg Ca per dL of blood) may even last for 10 days in lactation, especially in multiparous cows. Low calcium levels decrease abomasal outflow rate, causing further abomasal distention.

Risk Factors
• *Cow level*: Hypocalcemia, high BCS at calving, winter season, plasma NEFA concentration >0.3 mEq/L at 35–3 d prepartum, low DMI, high levels of ketone bodies postpartum (>1.2 mmol/L of BHB), other concurrent disease such as metritis that induce fever and affect eating behavior, high predicted transmitting ability (PTA) for milk production, body size and depth.
• *Herd level*: High average BCS of the herd; winter and summer seasons; precalving rations containing energy densities >1.65 Mcal of NE_L/kg of DM; rations high in concentrate and corn silage with not enough effective fiber during the postpartum period causing reduction of chewing activity, ruminal fill, motility, fiber mat formation, and increased ruminal VFA concentration; improper feed bunk management due to reduced bunk space, feed availability and freshness of the feed; excessive pen changes, mixing of primiparous and multiparous cows, overcrowded housing and feeding systems; prolonged confinement in individual maternity pens, excessive heat, mud, or

extreme cold; silages that contain abnormal levels of butyric or acetic acid, mycotoxins, and moldy feed; general deficiencies in cow comfort.

DIAGNOSIS

DIFFERENTIAL DIAGNOSES
• Many differential diagnoses exist for animals with acute decrease in milk production and anorexia. The differentials when a ping is auscultated include: gas in the cecum, spiral colon or duodenum, rumen gas cap with decreased fiber mat (i.e., secondary to ruminal acidosis or anorexia), collapsed rumen, pneumoperitoneum, physometra (i.e., anaerobic bacterial metritis), and other causes less commonly found.

CBC/BIOCHEMISTRY/URINALYSIS
• Hypochloremia, hypokalemia, hypocalcemia, metabolic alkalosis, ketonemia, ketonuria, sometimes paradoxical aciduria, hypoglycemia, and elevated levels of beta-hydroxybutyrate (>1.2 mmol/L) and nonesterified fatty acids (>0.7 mEq/L).
• Normal CBC

OTHER LABORATORY TESTS
N/A

IMAGING
Ultrasound can be used to differentiate the abomasal wall from other viscera; however, this is not commonly performed.

OTHER DIAGNOSTIC PROCEDURES
• Liptak test: performed by aspirating fluid from the viscus present beneath the area where percussion yields the loudest ping. Fluid pH differentiates between abomasum (<3.0) and rumen (>6.0).

TREATMENT

THERAPEUTIC APPROACH
• Supportive therapies are recommended to correct metabolic disturbances, including oral or parenteral calcium and IV dextrose, IV fluids to correct acid-base status, oral fluids containing electrolytes and glucose precursors (calcium propionate, propylene glycol, glycerol), anti-inflammatories such as flunixin meglumine for pain management and fever, and systemic antibiotics for 3–5 days, considering withdrawal periods.
• Each case should be evaluated independently and the decision based on the probability of success and return to lactation, cost of the procedure, and potential compensation based on current lactation numbers, previous/predicted production level, feed cost, and milk price. In some cases, culling instead of surgery is the best decision.

D

• Although surgical repair is the preferred treatment, medical treatment may be attempted in the case of LDA with varying long-term success rates. Medical treatment generally includes casting the animal into right lateral recumbency and rolling into left lateral recumbency to replace abomasum. This is followed by administration of oral fluids, vitamin B, and offering a high-quality forage diet along with the above treatments indicated for ketosis and any underlying disease.

SURGICAL CONSIDERATIONS AND TECHNIQUES

• The most common treatment for LDA is the surgical approach (blind or open). Blind technique is based on the toggle suture. Open techniques may be accomplished by laparoscopic approach or standing left flank abomasopexy, standing right flank omentopexy, and dorsal recumbency right paramedian abomasopexy. The toggle suture technique has a higher complication rate in most circumstances.
• All techniques have good results in the short term; however, cows with DAs have a higher risk for culling during the current and following lactation.

MEDICATIONS

DRUGS OF CHOICE

Dependent on underlying disease.

CONTRAINDICATIONS

Appropriate milk and meat withdrawal times must be followed for all compounds administered to food-producing animals.

FOLLOW-UP

EXPECTED COURSE AND PROGNOSIS

Dependent on underlying cause of DA, chronicity, and concurrent disease.

POSSIBLE COMPLICATIONS

Incisional infections, pyloric strictures (pyloropexy), abomasal fistulas (toggle-pin procedure), omental bursitis (omentopexy), vagal nerve damage (chronic DA), abomasal rupture ± enterotoxemia (abomasal volvulus).

CLIENT EDUCATION

See "Prevention"

PATIENT CARE

• Early treatment of a displaced abomasum will limit severity of secondary complications such as ketosis and rumen stasis.
• The focus during and after initial medical or surgical intervention is to reestablish adequate dry matter intakes and minimize negative energy balance. Patients should be offered good-quality, high fiber feed and water ad libitum along with adequate feed space to decrease competition.
• Supportive care for ruminal health and gastrointestinal motility is imperative and may include calcium supplementation, vitamin B complex, and probiotics.
• Patients should be monitored for possible complications (see "Possible Complications").

PREVENTION

• Prevention of abomasal displacement must be based on controlling the identified risk factors for this condition.
• Proper cow comfort and management is crucial. Avoidance of excessive body condition score during the entire production cycle by using the proper nutritional program during late lactation and the dry period is recommended.
• Balanced rations and uniform mixing of the diet during the prepartum and postpartum period is fundamental. Appropriate fiber in the form of effective NDF (no less than 20% of total dry matter) must be followed as a rule of thumb. Avoid excessive corn silage and provide adequate particle size to decrease the sorting behavior.
• Genetic factors are more difficult to control; therefore manage the cow for her milk production potential but preventing the presence of other diseases.
• Establish a postpartum health monitoring program checking rectal temperature, evaluating uterine size and involution, testing blood, urine or milk ketones, and using daily milk production records if the milking equipment will allow it (drop in milk yield and fat : protein ratio).

MISCELLANEOUS

ASSOCIATED CONDITIONS

Drop in feed intake and milk production and failure of cows to succeed during the postpartum period.

AGE-RELATED FACTORS

Younger animals that are genetically superior in milk production are more likely to have the best opportunity for economic payback from surgical intervention; with older animals having a shorter expected future productive life, or lower producing animals that have a lower predicted return, culling may be considered.

PREGNANCY

Cows with DA are less likely to become pregnant than unaffected cows.

PRODUCTION MANAGEMENT

This disorder causes tremendous economic losses to the dairy industry, mostly due to marked reduction in milk yield among affected cows, substantial treatment costs, and increased culling risks. Estimated cost of LDA has been reported to be $340 per cow. LDA has been linked with increased risk for early lactation culling.

Avoid excessive body condition and stressful conditions such as overcrowding, heat, cold, or mud. Proper nutrition management and cow comfort are the key factors to prevent DAs and other related diseases.

ABBREVIATIONS

• BCS = body condition score
• BHB = beta-hydroxybutyrate
• DA = displaced abomasum
• DIM = days in milk
• DM = dry matter
• DMI = dry matter intake
• GI = gastrointestinal
• IV = intravenous
• LDA = left displaced abomasum
• NDF = neutral detergent fiber
• NEFA = nonesterified fatty acids
• NE_L = net energy for lactation
• PTA = predicted transmitting ability
• RDA = right displaced abomasum
• VFA = volatile fatty acids

SEE ALSO

• Dairy Nutrition: Ration Guidelines for Milking and Dry Cows (see www.fiveminutevet.com/ruminant)
• Heat Stress
• Hypocalcemia: Bovine
• Ketosis: Dairy Cattle
• Metritis
• Milk Cow Nutrition Monitoring (see www.fiveminutevet.com/ruminant)
• Nutrition and Metabolic Diseases: Dairy
• Ruminal Acidosis
• Total Mixed Ration: Dairy (see www.fiveminutevet.com/ruminant)
• Transition Cow Management (see www.fiveminutevet.com/ruminant)

Suggested Reading
Cameron RE, Dyk PB, Herdt TH, et al. Dry cow diet, management, and energy balance as risk factors for displaced abomasum in high producing dairy herds. J Dairy Sci 1998, 81: 132–9.
Constable PD, Nouri M, Sen I, Baird AN, Wittek T. Evidence-based use of prokinetic drugs for abomasal disorders in cattle. Vet Clin North Am Food Anim Pract 2012, 28: 51–70.
Detilleux JC, Grohn YT, Eicker SW, Quaas RL. Effects of left displaced abomasum on test day milk yields of Holstein cows. J Dairy Sci 1997, 80: 121–6.
Goff JP. Major advances in our understanding of nutritional influences on bovine health. J Dairy Sci 2006, 89: 1292–301.

D

Kelton DF, Lissemore KD, Martin RE. Recommendations for recording and calculating the incidence of selected clinical diseases of dairy cattle. J Dairy Sci 1998, 81: 2502–9.

LeBlanc SJ, Leslie KE, Duffield TF. Metabolic predictors of displaced abomasum in dairy cattle. J Dairy Sci 2005, 88: 159–70.

LeBlanc SJ, Lissemore KD, Kelton DF, Duffield TF, Leslie KE. Major advances in disease prevention in dairy cattle. J Dairy Sci 2006, 89: 1267–79.

Niehaus AJ. Surgical management of abomasal disease. Vet Clin North Am Food Anim Pract 2016, 24: 629–44.

Raizman EA, Santos JEP, Thurmond MC. The effect of left displacement of abomasum corrected by toggle-pin suture on lactation, reproduction, and health of Holstein dairy cows. J Dairy Sci 2002, 85: 1157–64.

Rohn M, Tenhagen BA, Hofmann W. Survival of dairy cows after surgery to correct abomasal displacement: 2. Association of clinical and laboratory parameters with survival in cows with left abomasal displacement. J Vet Med A Physiol Pathol Clin Med 2004, 51: 300–5.

Zerbin I, Lehner S, Distl O. Genetics of bovine abomasal displacement. Vet J 2015, 204: 17–22.

Author Pedro Melendez
Consulting Editor Kaitlyn A. Lutz
Acknowledgment The author and book editors acknowledge the prior contribution of Michael W. Overton.

DISSEMINATED INTRAVASCULAR COAGULOPATHY

BASICS

OVERVIEW
Disseminated intravascular coagulopathy (DIC) is a pathologic process characterized by inappropriate activation of the clotting cascade, resulting in consumption of coagulation and fibrinolytic factors leading to disseminated microthrombosis and hemorrhagic diathesis.

INCIDENCE/PREVALENCE
N/A

GEOGRAPHIC DISTRIBUTION
Worldwide

SYSTEMS AFFECTED
• Cardiovascular
• Urinary
• Digestive
• Respiratory
• Nervous

PATHOPHYSIOLOGY
• DIC is not a primary disorder, but occurs secondary to severe systemic diseases including neoplasia, inflammatory or ischemic GI disorders, or overwhelming Gram-negative infection.
• Any disease that activates coagulation or causes blood vessel endothelial injury can result in acquired coagulopathy.
• Severity can range and change over time, producing minimal clinical signs through to diffuse thrombosis, ischemic organ failure, and severe hemorrhagic diathesis.
• Initiation of the coagulation cascade leads to formation of blood clots and fibrin deposition within small vessels (microvascular thrombosis). This promotes ischemia of vital tissues followed by organ dysfunction.
• Coagulation occurs simultaneously with fibrinolysis. As the thrombotic stimulus continues, there is depletion of both coagulation factors and natural anticoagulant factors such as anti-thrombin III.
• Petechial or ecchymotic hemorrhages can occur on mucosae/sclerae along with a tendency to bleed from minor trauma.
• Coagulopathy most commonly occurs in a compensated form in cattle and rarely presents as overt hemorrhage, but rather as microvascular thrombosis.
• Microvascular thrombosis can cause ischemic cortical necrosis and acute tubular necrosis of the kidney, with oliguria, depression, and ileus. GI microthrombosis and ischemia may cause colic secondary to submucosal necrosis, and GI hemorrhage may cause melena. Rarely, microvascular thrombosis of pulmonary arteries causes tachypnea and hypoxia.
• Altered consciousness may occur due to cerebral microvascular thrombosis, but is rare. Affected animals may display delirium, convulsions, and coma.

HISTORICAL FINDINGS
Consistent with a primary disorder capable of eliciting DIC.

SIGNALMENT
Any ruminant species of any age or gender is susceptible.

PHYSICAL EXAMINATION FINDINGS
• Often dominated by signs of the primary disease, and in regard to DIC, depend on extent and location of microvascular thrombosis.
• Colic, melena, ileus, oliguria, tachypnea, tachycardia, and altered consciousness can occur.
• Venous thrombosis or prolonged bleeding may occur following routine venipuncture or IV catheter placement, and petechial or ecchymotic hemorrhages may be evident on the pinnae, sclerae, and mucosal surfaces.
• Compensated DIC is chronic DIC that results from a weak/intermittent activating stimulus. Destruction and production of coagulation factors and platelets are approximately equal. The main sign of compensated DIC might be sudden, inappropriate thrombosis.

GENETICS
N/A

CAUSES AND RISK FACTORS
• DIC occurs secondary to inflammatory or ischemic conditions, particularly where GI mucosal compromise occurs, resulting in endotoxemia.
• Vasculitis, heatstroke, snake envenomation, systemic or localized sepsis (mastitis, pleuritis, peritonitis), neoplasia, renal disease, hemolytic anemia, intestinal strangulation, and other severe GI disorders, thromboembolic infarction, and acute hepatic failure can all evoke DIC.

DIAGNOSIS

DIFFERENTIAL DIAGNOSES
• Warfarin toxicosis.
• Moldy sweet clover toxicosis (dicoumarol).
• Inherited coagulation abnormalities: congenital afibrinogenemia (Saanen goats); hemophilia A (factor VIII deficiency) in Japanese Brown cattle and Swiss White Alpine sheep; factor XI deficiency (Holstein cattle); Chediak-Higashi syndrome (Hereford, Japanese Black, and Brangus cattle); hereditary thrombopathy (Simmental cattle); a Simmental calf has been diagnosed with von Willebrand disease.
• Hepatic failure.
• Immune mediated thrombocytopenia.
• Acute bovine viral diarrhea virus infection.
• Bracken fern toxicosis.
• Familial myelophthisis (pygmy goats).
• Endotoxemia.

HISTORICAL FINDINGS
• Acquired platelet function defects secondary to aspirin, phenylbutazone, sulfonamides, estrogens, or phenothiazines.

CBC/BIOCHEMISTRY/URINALYSIS
• Systemic diseases predisposing to DIC often result in leukopenia, neutropenia, lymphopenia, and thrombocytopenia.
• Hypofibrinogenemia may occur in DIC but is uncommon in large animals. The primary disease usually provokes hyperfibrinogenemia.
• Renal and hepatobiliary involvement may be reflected on serum chemistry.
• Platelet counts below 10,000–20,000/μL are correlated with spontaneous hemorrhage. Hematoma formation following minor trauma can occur when platelet counts fall below 40,000/μL.

OTHER LABORATORY TESTS
• Serial testing may be necessary when clinical suspicion of DIC is present. Diagnosis is supported by evidence of platelet consumption (often the earliest indicator of DIC), in addition to evidence of coagulation factor consumption (prolongation of one or more clotting tests), and evidence of increased fibrinolysis.
• Clotting tests include measurement of prothrombin time (PT), activated partial thromboplastin time (APTT), and TT (thrombin time). Prolonged clotting times are insensitive indicators of early disease. If the only laboratory abnormality is persistently prolonged PTT, a hereditary factor deficiency should be suspected.
• Evidence for increased fibrinolysis includes elevated fibrin degradation products (FDPs). Serum FDP concentrations >40 μg/mL or plasma FDP >20 μg/mL are consistent with DIC. Elevated D-dimers (an FDP that is more specific for fibrinolysis) and decreased antithrombin III also support DIC.

IMAGING
Ultrasonography can be used to assess peripheral large vessel thrombosis.

OTHER DIAGNOSTIC PROCEDURES
As indicated for the primary disorder

PATHOLOGIC FINDINGS
• Reflect the primary disease process.
• Thrombosis/fibrin deposition may be evident in large vessels.
• Petechiae, ecchymoses, and hematomas may be grossly visible.
• Microthrombi may be microscopically visible in the vascular beds of kidneys, lung, spleen, adrenal glands, heart, brain, and liver.

TREATMENT

THERAPEUTIC APPROACH
• Treat the underlying cause.
• Control intravascular coagulation.
• Maintain organ perfusion.
• Replace coagulation factors and proteins.

D

DISSEMINATED INTRAVASCULAR COAGULOPATHY   (CONTINUED)

SURGICAL CONSIDERATIONS AND TECHNIQUES
N/A

MEDICATIONS

DRUGS OF CHOICE
• Intravenous fluid therapy to prevent organ dysfunction due to microthrombosis, and to correct acid-base/electrolyte abnormalities.
• Septic conditions require antimicrobial therapy.
• Flunixin meglumine reduces effects of endotoxemia.
• Fresh plasma (15–30 mL/kg) may be indicated when petechiation or hemorrhage is present, to restore coagulation factors and anticoagulant proteins.
• Heparin therapy is controversial and might be contraindicated if bleeding tendencies are present, but is given to prevent microvascular thrombosis and further consumption of coagulation factors. Heparin is a cofactor of AT III, therefore adequate AT III must be present for heparin to be effective, which can be provided by plasma transfusion.

CONTRAINDICATIONS
• Corticosteroids are contraindicated due to a reduction in phagocytic activity and worsening of vasoconstrictive effects of catecholamines.
• Avoid drugs that cause hypotension (phenothiazines and α_2 agonists).
• Avoid drugs that negatively affect organ systems compromised by DIC, i.e., nephrotoxic or hepatotoxic drugs.
• Hetastarch might be contraindicated in patients with known coagulation deficiencies as it can prolong coagulation times if given at high doses.

PRECAUTIONS
• Correct sample handling is vital for accurate coagulation testing. Samples should be submitted in citrate anticoagulant (blue-top vacutainer) following atraumatic blood collection.
• Consider simultaneous submission of blood from a normal cohort for quality control.

• Appropriate milk and meat withdrawal times must be followed for all compounds administered to food-producing animals.

POSSIBLE INTERACTIONS
N/A

FOLLOW-UP

EXPECTED COURSE AND PROGNOSIS
Prognosis for acute, fulminant DIC is guarded to grave. Prognosis for compensated DIC is better. Prognosis depends on ability to identify and neutralize the underlying cause.

POSSIBLE COMPLICATIONS
Multiple organ failure, large vessel thrombosis, hematoma formation, hemorrhage, shock, and death.

CLIENT EDUCATION
N/A

PATIENT CARE
• Frequent physical examinations during acute disease to monitor heart rate and rhythm, pulse quality, respiratory rate, temperature, urine production, and mucus membrane character. Monitor for development of organ system dysfunction via physical examination and laboratory testing.
• Serial monitoring of CBC and coagulation variables (PT, APTT, FDPs, AT III); interpret in light of patient condition. Serial platelet counts can be particularly useful.

PREVENTION
Detecting and treating underlying disease is imperative to prevention of DIC, particularly inflammatory or ischemic conditions of the GI tract.

MISCELLANEOUS

ASSOCIATED CONDITIONS
• Renal failure
• Multi-organ failure
• Primary disorders

AGE-RELATED FACTORS
N/A

ZOONOTIC POTENTIAL
If *Salmonella* or other infectious pathogens are involved in the primary disorder, zoonotic risks may be present.

PREGNANCY
Abortion may occur due to severe systemic compromise.

BIOSECURITY
N/A

PRODUCTION MANAGEMENT
N/A

SYNONYM
Disseminated intravascular coagulation

ABBREVIATIONS
• APTT = activated partial thromboplastin time
• AT III = anti-thrombin III
• FDP = fibrin degradation product
• PT = prothrombin time
• PTT = partial thromboplastin time
• TP = total protein
• TT = thrombin time

SEE ALSO
• Acute Renal Failure
• Blood Chemistry (see www.fiveminutevet.com/ruminant)
• Fluid Therapy: Intravenous

Suggested Reading
Watson JL, Morris DD. Disorders of coagulation factors. In: Smith BP ed, Large Animal Internal Medicine, 5th ed. St. Louis: Mosby Elsevier, 2015.
Author Emma Gordon
Consulting Editor Erica C. McKenzie
Acknowledgment The author and book editors acknowledge the prior contribution of Benjamin J. Darien.

BASICS

OVERVIEW
• Cattle with the inability to rise unassisted. Affected cattle may be found in sternal or lateral recumbency for prolonged periods of time.
• Down cattle are often grouped into two categories depending on the patient's mental state:
  ○ Alert downers
  ○ Depressed downers

SYSTEMS AFFECTED
• Musculoskeletal
• Nervous

PATHOPHYSIOLOGY
• Many etiologies may result in downer cows (see Table 1).
• Alert downers
  ○ Nerve pathology may result in decreased muscular control. Obturator and/or sciatic nerve involvement may be secondary to dystocia (parturient paresis). Radial nerve damage is also common from prolonged recumbency due to surgical procedures where prolonged pressure is placed on the shoulder area. Spinal cord involvement may be due to instability of the bony spinal column resulting from fracture or luxation or cord compression from tumors.
  ○ Direct musculoskeletal issues such as long bone fractures, luxations, avulsions, or other orthopedic issues can also result in a cow's inability to rise.
• Depressed downers
  ○ Electrolyte imbalances may result in decreased muscle function.
  ○ Toxic mastitis, toxic metritis, or other causes of endotoxemia can result in generalized obtundation and weakness, causing an animal to be recumbent.
• Down cows will have some muscle damage from prolonged pressure on the dependent muscle. Pressure necrosis and compartment syndrome can result and contribute to the weakness and inability to stand. The cow may continue to be down even after correction of the primary problem.
• Muscle damage results in increased circulating CK and myoglobin which can cause renal damage, further compromising the patient.
• Down cows are also susceptible to pneumonia due to poor ventilation, and mastitis because their udder and teats are in constant contact with the ground.
• Secondary orthopedic problems such as gastrocnemius rupture can result from trying to rise. Cattle commonly will develop abrasions over bony prominences. Lacerations can lead to localized infections, or infections of synovial structures.

• Secondary coxofemoral luxation is another potential sequela in downer cattle.

HISTORICAL FINDINGS
Obtaining a good history will aid in diagnosis: age, parity, production level, calving history, length of recumbency, etc.

SIGNALMENT
• Dairy or beef cattle.
• Older, periparturient, high producing, and heavier cattle are most commonly affected.
• Cattle in intensive housing/management operations more common.

PHYSICAL EXAMINATION FINDINGS
• May be alert or depressed depending on the cause of recumbency.
• Alert downers typically have a fair to good appetite.
• Superficial abrasions common.
• Dry manure may progress to diarrhea.
• Urine may be dark due to myoglobinuria.
• If assisted to stand, cattle may make weak attempts or may be able to support themselves for short periods of time but generally appear weak and uncoordinated. Cattle may knuckle on fetlocks and exhibit signs of specific nerve paralysis/paresis (peroneal and radial common).

CAUSES AND RISK FACTORS
• Hypocalcemia, hypokalemia, hypophosphatemia, hypomagnesemia
• Intrapelvic trauma and inflammation (secondary to dystocia)
• Toxic mastitis/metritis
• Trauma induced by falls secondary to being ridden while coming into heat or wet, slippery flooring
• Long bone fractures
• Joint luxations (coxofemoral and scapulohumeral)
• Spinal cord lymphoma

DIAGNOSIS

DIFFERENTIAL DIAGNOSES
• Being "down" is a clinical sign rather than a diagnosis.
• Finding a specific cause for an animal to go down (Table 1) can be challenging.

OTHER LABORATORY TESTS
• CBC and chemistry panel may reveal signs of underlying disease.
• Serum creatinine kinase (CK), a marker for muscle damage, is elevated significantly in the early stages but has a short half-life and is not reliable for prognosis in clinical cases.
• Serum calcium and potassium levels may point to metabolic problems.
• Urine should be examined for color and, if dark or brown, myoglobin levels may be evaluated.

Table 1

Possible causes for the animal being down

Alert downer
• Nerve damage
  ○ Sciatic/obturator (calving paresis/paralysis)
  ○ Radial
  ○ Peroneal
  ○ Spinal cord (vertebral body abscess/fracture/lymphoma)
• Muscle damage
  ○ Trauma
  ○ Pressure necrosis (from being down)
• Joint luxation
  ○ Coxofemoral
  ○ Scapulohumeral
  ○ Others
• Fracture
  ○ Long bone
  ○ Avulsion fracture

Depressed downer
• Metabolic
  ○ Hypocalcemia
  ○ Hypokalemia
  ○ Hypophosphatemia
  ○ Hypomagnesemia
• Endotoxemia/infectious
  ○ Mastitis
  ○ Metritis
  ○ Septicemia

IMAGING
• Radiographs can be useful to confirm musculoskeletal injury such as fracture or coxofemoral luxation. Due to the size of adult patients, this may be impractical.
• Diagnostic ultrasound may be useful to diagnose tendon and ligament injuries and certain fractures.

OTHER DIAGNOSTIC PROCEDURES
• TPR, examination of the udder and uterus for signs of mastitis and metritis.
• Cutaneous testing of hindlimbs for evidence of sensory reflexes.
• Palpation of limbs for luxation or fractures.
• Rectal palpation for pelvic fractures or hip luxation, evidence of crepitus.
• Lifting with hip clamps is useful for musculoskeletal and neurologic examination but should be very brief, to avoid pressure damage of muscles in the tuber coxae region. The clamps should be well padded to minimize tissue damage.
• Some cows may be able to stand unassisted once lifted. Standing these animals will help with assessment of weakness.
• Response to treatment in a floatation tank is useful but labor intensive.

DOWN BOVINE (CONTINUED)

TREATMENT

THERAPEUTIC APPROACH
• The primary objective is to prevent further muscle and nerve damage due to recumbency.
• Soft, clean, and dry bedding is essential. Sand is easier to keep clean than straw bedding. Hard, slippery concrete should be avoided. A dirt lot or a manure pack may provide the patient with good footing.
• Frequent repositioning will reduce pressure damage.
• Hydrofloatation therapy reduces pressure damage and enhances vascular supply to compressed tissues. Warm water (body temperature) is essential for hydrofloatation to be beneficial. Hydrofloatation predisposes to development of cutaneous wounds as it softens the skin. Mastitis in lactating cows, incisional infections in postoperative cattle, and catheter site infections may be a result of hydrofloatation in dirty water.
• Hobbles on the hindlimbs prevent limb abduction which may lead to coxofemoral luxation.
• Hindlimb knuckling can be managed with a cast on the affected lower limb.
• An effort should be made to correct the underlying cause if possible.

SURGICAL CONSIDERATIONS AND TECHNIQUES
Teat amputation provides drainage for a quarter with toxic mastitis.

MEDICATIONS

DRUGS OF CHOICE
• Antibiotic and anti-endotoxin treatment is indicated in the case of metritis, mastitis, or generalized sepsis.
• Pain medication will make the patient more willing to attempt to move and improve appetite.
• Topical ointments for dermatitis and pressure sores.

PRECAUTIONS
Appropriate milk and meat withdrawal times must be followed for all compounds administered to food-producing animals.

FOLLOW-UP

EXPECTED COURSE AND PROGNOSIS
Dependent on etiology and proper management of the down cow. Prognosis is often poorer than one may consider due to secondary problems like muscle damage.

POSSIBLE COMPLICATIONS
• Muscle tearing or avulsion due to struggling to stand
• Hip luxation
• Muscle damage due to excessive use of hip clamps
• Drowning (complication of hydrofloatation)
• Renal compromise due to myoglobinemia

CLIENT EDUCATION
• Owners should be educated that a down cow is an emergency because irreversible pressure damage can occur in as short as 6 hours of recumbency.
• All animal care personnel should be educated in appropriate methods for moving down animals, and farms should develop uniform protocols for down cow management and end-point determinants.

PATIENT CARE
• Successful treatment of down cows is labor intensive and requires frequent monitoring of the patient.
• Keeping the bedding clean and dry is important.
• Providing a constant supply of fresh drinking water is important but difficult when animals move continually. A large rubber tub that is not easily turned over works best. The water should be close enough to the patient so that they can access the water easily; however, care should be taken not to allow the patient to drown.
• Frequent skin cleansing is important to prevent urine scalding.
• Frequent repositioning is helpful to minimize pressure damage.
• Floatation therapy requires frequent monitoring to prevent drowning.

PREVENTION
• Prevention is more efficacious than therapy.
• Dry cow feeding should be aimed at prevention of parturient paresis.
• Provision of clean, well-bedded calving stalls is essential to prevent slipping.

• Periparturient cows should be monitored frequently so that problems can be treated before they get worse.

MISCELLANEOUS

AGE-RELATED FACTORS
• Older animals are more susceptible to periparturient problems.
• Older animals are heavier and more likely to succumb to secondary problems.
• Lymphoma may be more common in aged animals.

ABBREVIATIONS
• CK = serum creatinine kinase
• TPR = temperature/pulse/respirations

SEE ALSO
• Dystocia: Bovine
• Lameness: Bovine
• Physical Examination: Bovine (Appendix 4)

Suggested Reading
Cox VS. Downer cow syndrome. In: Howard JL, Smith RA eds, Current Veterinary Therapy 4: Food Animal Practice. Philadelphia: Saunders, 1999.
Funnell BJ, Hilton WM. Management and prevention of dystocia. Vet Clin North Am Food Anim Pract 2016, 32: 511–22.
Hartnack AK. Spinal cord and peripheral nerve abnormalities of the ruminant. Vet Clin North Am Food Anim Pract 2017, 33: 101–10.
Sielman ES, Sweeney RW, Whitlock RH, Reams RY. Hypokalemia syndrome in dairy cows: 10 cases (1992–1996). J Am Vet Med Assoc 1997, 210: 240–3.
Smith BP, Angelos J, George LW, et al. Down cows: causes and treatments. Proc Ann Conf Am Assoc Bovine Practitioners 1997, 30: 43–5.
Van Metre DC, Callan RJ, Garry FB. Examination of the musculoskeletal system in recumbent cattle. Compen Cont Ed Prac Vet 2001, 23: S5–S13.
Washburn KE. Localization of neurologic lesions in ruminants. Vet Clin North Am Food Anim Pract 2017, 33: 19–25.
Author Andrew J. Niehaus
Consulting Editor Kaitlyn A. Lutz
Acknowledgment The author and book editors acknowledge the prior contribution of Victor S. Cox.

BASICS

OVERVIEW
• Camelids often present with the complaint of being "down," i.e., recumbent.
• Recumbency can be classified as intermittent (animal voluntarily rises and moves but is recumbent more than normal), preferred (animal can be coaxed to rise for short periods), or constant (animal cannot physically rise).
• Thorough history collection and detailed physical examination are critical steps in determining the likely system affected and possible differential diagnoses.

INCIDENCE/PREVALENCE
• Typically recumbency is a sporadic complaint unless related to a disorder that can affect multiple animals in a group.

GEOGRAPHIC DISTRIBUTION
Worldwide; some specific conditions including *Parelaphostrongylus tenuis* (meningeal worm) infestation and *Cryptococcus gattii* meningitis have strongly regional distributions.

SYSTEMS AFFECTED
• Nervous
• Musculoskeletal
• Hemolymphatic
• Cardiovascular
• Respiratory
• Digestive

PATHOPHYSIOLOGY
• A wide range of disorders affecting virtually any body system can result in recumbency by inducing pain, weakness, systemic illness, nervous dysfunction, musculoskeletal damage, or other consequences; pathophysiology is strongly dependent on individual etiology.
• Orthopedic problems including fractures and luxations can result in recumbency from pain and/or loss of function.
• Neurologic conditions are a common cause of recumbency, and in regions in which *P. tenuis* infection is prevalent, aberrant migration of larval parasites through the spinal cord and brain is considered a very common cause of acute recumbency related to inflammation and trauma to the delicate nervous tissues. Other disorders include *Cryptococcus gattii* infection of the central nervous system; bacterial meningitis (most often in crias, and associated with *Listeria*, *E. coli*, *Streptococcus*, *Histophilus* and other organisms); polioencephalomalacia related to anomalies of thiamine metabolism and availability; and vitamin D deficiency which most commonly affects dark-coated crias born in autumn in geographic regions with lower UV exposure, resulting in bone fragility and limb and spinal fractures (rickets). Camelids can also develop viral meningitis from

infection with West Nile virus, Eastern equine encephalitis, equine herpesvirus 1, and rabies.
• Diseases that cause profound anemia often create recumbency due to hypoxia, and include infection with the epierythrocytic parasite *Candidatus Mycoplasma haemolamae* and high burdens of *Haemonchus contortus*.
• Debilitation causing recumbency can result from megaesophagus, round cell neoplasia, chronic peritonitis, abdominal abscesses (*S. zooepidemicus, C. pseudotuberculosis*), chronic renal disease, Johne's disease, and oral pathology.
• Gastrointestinal diseases can result in recumbency from pain, systemic illness and debilitation, including parasitism with gastrointestinal nematodes or *Eimeria macusaniensis*, and a variety of disorders causing abdominal pain related to gastrointestinal torsion, ulceration, perforation, or obstruction.
• Cardiorespiratory disease can result in recumbency due to hypoxemia and/or impaired circulation, and can relate to pneumonia, pleuritis (from *S. zooepidemicus*, or esophageal or thoracic injury), diaphragmatic paralysis, congenital cardiac defects, and thrombotic endocarditis.
• Heat stress typically occurs during hot weather and affects animals in full fiber.
• Toxicities such as tick paralysis and ryegrass staggers cause recumbency from injected or ingested neurotoxins.
• Urogenital disorders can cause recumbency related to pain and systemic illness, including uterine torsion in late gestation females and urinary tract obstruction in male or castrated male camelids.

HISTORICAL FINDINGS
Historical findings of significance will vary with the cause of recumbency but enquiries should include the age and gender of the affected animal(s), how long the animal has been recumbent; any interventions or handling that have occurred, and the anthelmintic, vitamin D and other medication and treatment history of the operation.

SIGNALMENT
Age and gender influence the likelihood of specific disorders causing recumbency including rickets, uterine torsion, urinary obstruction, and congenital cardiac defects.

PHYSICAL EXAMINATION FINDINGS
• Reluctance or inability to stand.
• Obtundation suggests central nervous system disease or significant systemic illness.
• Thorough palpation of the spine, limbs, and thorax may identify causative luxations or fractures, or evidence of rickets (enlarged costochondral junctions, rib fractures).
• Pale mucus membranes and tachycardia suggest profound anemia.
• Cardiac murmurs are typically abnormal in camelids and suggest congenital or acquired

cardiac disease, or can result from significant anemia.
• Peripheral edema (brisket, ventrum) ± jugular venous distension suggests cardiac disease.
• Increased respiratory effort may indicate pleural effusion or other cardiorespiratory disorders; paradoxic respiratory pattern (thoracic movement contradictory to abdominal movement) is common in camelids with diaphragmatic paralysis.
• Abnormal positioning of limbs (stretched out in front or behind, or placed to the side) can suggest abdominal pain or occasionally respiratory difficulty.
• Neurologic examination (proprioception, sensation, spinal reflexes) and ophthalmic assessment form part of a complete examination of a recumbent camelid patient, but can be challenging to perform in some circumstances.

GENETICS
N/A

CAUSES AND RISK FACTORS
• *P. tenuis* (in proximity to its definitive and intermediate hosts)
• Severe anemia (usually parasitism)
• Central nervous system trauma or infection (fungal, bacterial, viral)
• Musculoskeletal trauma
• High environmental temperatures and animals in full fiber
• Poor management procedures (parasitism, rickets, malnutrition, infectious diseases)
• Dental disease

DIAGNOSIS

DIFFERENTIAL DIAGNOSES
Recumbency is a clinical sign rather than a diagnosis. Every attempt should be made via thorough anamnesis and physical examination to determine the likely body systems involved; this subsequently defines the differential list and directs diagnostic procedures.
• Anemia
• Cardiac disease
• Rickets
• Polioencephalomalacia
• Tetanus
• Meningitis (bacterial, viral, fungal)
• *S. zooepidemicus* infection
• Colic
• Trauma
• Tick paralysis
• Uterine torsion
• Debilitation
• Heat stress

CBC/BIOCHEMISTRY/URINALYSIS
The presence and severity of changes are dependent on the underlying disorder but laboratory results should be assessed for anemia, significant acid-base and electrolyte

disturbances, and evidence of causative or accompanying major organ disease (abnormalities of liver, renal or muscle variables).

OTHER LABORATORY TESTS

• Blood gas analysis is useful for evaluating cardiorespiratory disorders and to clarify the severity and characteristics of acid-base disturbances.
• Collection of CSF can be readily achieved at the lumbosacral space, or at the atlanto-occipital space (under anesthesia) for cytologic evaluation ± bacterial culture and other tests to identify conditions including bacterial, viral, and fungal meningitis, and infestation with *P. tenuis*.
• PCR on EDTA blood can detect infection with *Candidatus Mycoplasma haemolamae*.

IMAGING

• Radiographs are useful to evaluate orthopedic and thoracic disorders, and can identify urinary obstruction in areas where calcium carbonate urolithiasis occurs.
• Ultrasonography is useful for evaluating cardiorespiratory disorders and abdominal pain, and for assessing fetal viability.
• CT is a useful diagnostic modality for imaging the skull, spine, and other bony structures. Addition of intravenous contrast greatly enhances imaging of most soft tissues, and provision of orogastric contrast several hours prior to imaging is helpful in evaluation of gastrointestinal disorders.

OTHER DIAGNOSTIC PROCEDURES

• Oral examination (may require sedation and speculum).
• Abdominocentesis and/or thoracocentesis to evaluate cavitary effusions for evidence of infection or neoplasia.

PATHOLOGIC FINDINGS

See individual disorders in this text

TREATMENT

THERAPEUTIC APPROACH

• Management should include strategies to prevent bone, muscle, eye, and nerve damage due to recumbency and handling.
• Soft, deep, clean, and dry bedding is essential. Animals should only be encouraged to stand or move with adequate support.
• Frequent repositioning will reduce pressure damage and will help respiratory function; animals should be maintained in sternal, not lateral, recumbency.
• Floating animals in a water tank reduces pressure damage to musculature and enhances vascular supply to compressed tissues, and can be performed q12–24h. Camelids in full fiber must be adequately dried after removal from the tank to prevent flystrike and dermatitis.

• Slings can be utilized in animals that will tolerate it and which are capable of supporting at least 30–50% of their own weight.
• Hobbles on the hind pasterns can help prevent traumatic limb abduction in weak camelids that splay on slippery surfaces or in deeply bedded stalls.
• The underlying cause of recumbency must be determined and treated if possible, which may require fluid, electrolyte and colloid support, antibiotics, anti-inflammatory drugs, anthelmintics, cavity drainage, fracture repair, or reduction of joint luxations.

SURGICAL CONSIDERATIONS AND TECHNIQUES

• Dependent on the underlying cause of recumbency. Generally recumbent patients are poor surgical candidates unless recumbency relates to a surgically reversible issue (such as pain arising from surgically amenable colic).
• Surgical intervention (cesarean section) is typically avoided in uterine torsion of camelids unless the torsion cannot be corrected by repeated attempts at external manual repositioning (rolling).

MEDICATIONS

DRUGS OF CHOICE

• Dependent on the underlying cause.
• *P. tenuis* infestation is often treated with fenbendazole (50 mg/kg PO q24h for 5 days) and/or ivermectin (0.2–0.3 mg/kg PO or SQ, once or repeated).
• Anti-inflammatory drugs can include flunixin meglumine (1.1 mg/kg IV q12–24h) or meloxicam (1–2 mg/kg PO, followed by 1 mg/kg PO q24h). Corticosteroids are occasionally recommended as adjunct therapy for neurologic disorders and may be of value in individual cases (prednisolone sodium succinate 0.5–1.0 mg/kg IV, IM, or SQ).
• Oxytetracycline can be used to suppress (but will not eradicate) *Candidatus Mycoplasma haemolamae* infection (20 mg/kg SQ or IV, q24h for 3–5 days).
• Vitamin D supplementation is recommended for crias at risk of rickets (1,000–2,000 IU/kg SQ).
• Thiamine supplementation is useful in camelids with prolonged anorexia or suspected polioencephalomalacia (10 mg/kg SQ, q4–24h depending on indication).
• Severe pain may require additional analgesia with opioids: butorphanol (0.05–0.2 mg/kg IV or IM); buprenorphine (2–3 μg/kg IM, q4–6h); or morphine (0.5–1.0 mg/kg IM, q6h). In animals requiring intensive management, topical fentanyl patches or constant intravenous infusions (lidocaine, butorphanol, or ketamine) are useful.
• Animals requiring colloid support can receive llama plasma or hydroxyethylstarch products. Whole blood (llama or alpaca) can

be given to either species if blood transfusion is indicated.
• Seizures can be treated with IV diazepam or midazolam.

CONTRAINDICATIONS

Corticosteroids (even topical) should not be used in any pregnant camelid female due to high risk of abortion or stillbirth.

PRECAUTIONS

Nephrotoxic drugs including oxytetracycline, vitamin D, aminoglycosides, and NSAIDs should be avoided or used very cautiously in azotemic or significantly dehydrated patients.

POSSIBLE INTERACTIONS

Bicarbonate will react with calcium-containing IV fluids.

FOLLOW-UP

EXPECTED COURSE AND PROGNOSIS

Prognosis and course depend upon the reason underlying recumbency; however, the prognosis is typically reduced with chronic diseases, significant neurologic impairment, or secondary complications.

POSSIBLE COMPLICATIONS

• Muscle trauma from compression and struggling
• Aspiration
• Renal compromise
• Corneal ulceration or trauma
• Decubitus ulceration
• Hepatic lipidosis
• Seizures

CLIENT EDUCATION

Focus on herd management and targeted health-related procedures (vitamin D or selenium supplementation, vaccination, parasite management protocols) that are individualized to operations to avoid preventable diseases.

PATIENT CARE

• Monitor for progression during treatment to allow adjustments.
• Slings may be required in animals capable of supporting some of their own weight; the duration of time animals are kept in a sling should be adjusted based on individual tolerance and ability to monitor safely.
• Animals placed into float tanks should be attended at all times to prevent drowning; water should be kept close to body temperature to prevent cold stress. Animals with IV catheters should not be floated, to avoid infection.
• Crias with rickets should be handled with extreme caution due to the risk of inducing major skeletal trauma during routine procedures.
• Intravenous (dextrose, amino acids) or orogastric (transfaunation) nutritional

(CONTINUED)

support is indicated in camelids with poor to absent appetite for prolonged durations.

PREVENTION

• Dependent on underlying cause.
• Routinely supplement crias with vitamin D in areas where rickets occurs.
• Periodic preventive anthelmintic treatment is performed in regions with a high prevalence of *P. tenuis*, though it should be acknowledged that this contributes to resistance issues in a range of parasites.
• Teach owners how to appropriately body condition score individual animals so that they can identify condition loss before it becomes extreme.
• Encourage management practices including vaccination for relevant diseases, supplementation to avoid vitamin and mineral deficiencies, and parasite control programs.

MISCELLANEOUS

ASSOCIATED CONDITIONS
Rhabdomyolysis from prolonged recumbency

AGE-RELATED FACTORS
N/A

ZOONOTIC POTENTIAL
N/A

PREGNANCY
Recumbent late gestation females should be evaluated carefully for evidence of uterine torsion; this can include limited (wrist deep) per rectum examination.

BIOSECURITY
N/A

PRODUCTION MANAGEMENT
N/A

SYNONYMS
• *P. tenuis*: meningeal worm, brain worm, or deer worm
• Rickets: vitamin D deficiency, hypovitaminosis D

ABBREVIATIONS
• CSF = cerebrospinal fluid
• CT = computed tomography
• EDTA = ethylenediaminetetraacetic acid
• IM = intramuscular
• IV = intravenous
• NSAID = nonsteroidal anti-inflammatory drug
• PCR = polymerase chain reaction
• PO = per os
• SQ = subcutaneous

SEE ALSO
• Camelid: Gastrointestinal Disease
• Camelid: Heat Stress
• Cardiac Failure
• Cryptococcosis
• Rumen Transfaunation (see www.fiveminutevet.com/ruminant)

Suggested Reading
Belknap EB, Navarre CB, Pugh DG, et al. Recumbent New World camelids: General diagnostics and types of recumbency. Compend Contin Educ Pract Vet 2000, 22: 36–54.
Whitehead CE, Bedenice D. Neurologic diseases in llamas and alpacas. Vet Clin North Am Food Anim Pract 2009, 25: 385–405.

Author Andrew J. Niehaus
Consulting Editor Erica C. McKenzie

Acknowledgment The author and book editors acknowledge the prior contribution of Natalie Coffer.

D

DOWN SMALL RUMINANT

BASICS

D

OVERVIEW
Inability to stand and/or remain standing without assistance

INCIDENCE/PREVALENCE
Worldwide

GEOGRAPHIC DISTRIBUTION
• Depends on cause.
• Meningeal worm occurs wherever white-tailed deer are in contact with small ruminants.

SYSTEMS AFFECTED
• Musculoskeletal
• Nervous
• Multisystemic

PATHOPHYSIOLOGY
See specific disease chapters

HISTORICAL FINDINGS
History is very important to obtain when assessing a down small ruminant. The signalment, stage of pregnancy and lactation, diet changes, recent treatments, and history of trauma will be very helpful in reaching a diagnosis.

SIGNALMENT
All ovine, caprine

PHYSICAL EXAMINATION FINDINGS
• Sternal or lateral recumbency
• A thorough neurologic examination is important
• See specific disease chapters for specifics

CAUSES AND RISK FACTORS
See "Differential Diagnosis." Many diseases can be minimized through good husbandry, preventive health care, and nutrition.

DIAGNOSIS

DIFFERENTIAL DIAGNOSES

Neurologic Disease
• Polioencephalomalacia
• Listeriosis
• *Parelaphostrongylus tenuis*
• Bacterial meningitis
• Tick paralysis
• Botulism
• Rabies
• Scrapie
• Trauma
• Tetanus
• Neoplasia of CNS or spinal cord
• Abscess of CNS or spinal cord

Alimentary Disease
• Debilitation due to severe gastrointestinal parasitism
• Debilitation due to social starvation

Musculoskeletal Disease
• Peripheral nerve damage
• Trauma
• Infectious arthritis (lambs/kids)
• Laminitis

Metabolic Disease
• Pregnancy toxemia
• Hepatic lipidosis
• Hypocalcemia

Intoxications
Urea (ammonia)

Polioencephalomalacia
Necrosis of cortical gray matter associated with thiamine deficiency, often occurs in conjunction with a sudden feed change. Can occur due to a high sulfur diet or overdose of amprolium.
Clinical Signs
Central blindness (absence of menace with intact PLRs), depression and incoordination progressing to recumbency, and seizures.
Diagnosis
Based on history, clinical signs, and rapid response to therapy, though laboratory tests are available.
Treatment
Thiamine (10 mg/kg) intravenously, followed by IM or SC q6h for the first day, with additional doses q6–12h for the next 2–3 days. Thiamine hydrochloride can cause anaphylaxis if given intravenously, therefore it is recommended that the thiamine dose be diluted and administered slowly.

Listeriosis
Acute meningoencephalitis caused by Gram-positive bacterium *Listeria monocytogenes.*
Clinical Signs
Listeriosis most frequently causes focal encephalitis, usually affecting the cranial nerves but animals frequently present in later stages when they may be recumbent. Trigeminal, facial, and vestibular nerve lesions are most frequent, resulting in inability to eat, weakness of facial muscles, and head tilt. Animals may become dehydrated and acidotic due to loss of salivary secretions.
Diagnosis
• Based on clinical signs (particularly multifocal brainstem lesions) and elimination of other differential diagnoses.
• CSF analysis may demonstrate elevated protein (>40 mg/dL) and >5 mononuclear cells/μL.
Treatment
High doses of penicillin (40,000 U/kg q6–8h or 60,000 U/kg q12h), oxytetracycline (5–10 mg/kg IV q12h), or florfenicol (20 mg/kg IM q48h) in addition to supportive care such as anti-inflammatories, correction of hydration status and electrolyte abnormalities, and supplemental feeding as needed.

Parelaphostrongylus tenuis (Meningeal Worm)
• Nematode found in white-tailed deer and carried by snails and slugs.
• Small ruminant ingests snail or slug carrying larvae.
• Larvae are released in stomach and migrate to spinal cord and mature in gray matter; migrate to brain through the spinal subdural space.
Clinical Signs
• The parasite does not cause clinical signs in white-tailed deer.
• Infection in small ruminants can cause signs of neurologic disease including ataxia, paresis, circling, and recumbency. Lesions are more likely to occur in the spinal cord such that the animal retains normal mentation, but larvae can also migrate to the brain and cause depression and central nervous system signs such as blindness.
Diagnosis
• There is no reliable antemortem diagnostic test; the only definitive diagnostic test is identification of larvae in the spinal cord on histologic examination.
• CSF eosinophilia is supportive of infestation and affected animals may also have a peripheral eosinophilia.
• Other causes of ataxia and recumbency should be ruled out.
Treatment
• Ivermectin (0.2–0.4 mg/kg SQ) for 3 days to kill larvae outside the CNS.
• Fenbendazole at a dose rate of 50 mg/kg PO for 3–5 days to kill larvae inside the CNS.
• Supportive care if needed including intravenous fluids, in addition to anti-inflammatory medication such as flunixin meglumine or corticosteroids (in nonpregnant animals).
• Floatation therapy and/or physical therapy may be beneficial.
Prevention
Limit access to snail habitat, control snail/slug populations with domestic poultry, minimize contact with white-tailed deer. Monthly anthelmintic treatment as a preventive measure against meningeal worm is likely to promote anthelmintic resistance and is not recommended in most cases.

Rabies
Invariably fatal neurologic disease caused by rabies virus
Clinical Signs
• Neurologic signs are variable and include depression, ataxia, and anorexia, and can progress to recumbency, salivation, coma, and convulsions among many other signs.
• Should be considered in any case of nonresponsive central nervous system disease.
Diagnosis
• No clinical diagnostic test is available.
• Postmortem diagnosis is confirmed by histopathology of brain tissue and indirect fluorescent antibody testing of brain sections.

Trauma
• Musculoskeletal or peripheral nerve injury or head trauma may result in inability to stand.
• Vertebral fractures can occur in growing animals with dietary imbalances (e.g., calcium or vitamin D deficiency).
• A complete neuromuscular examination should be performed.

Neoplasia or Abscess of CNS or Spinal Cord
• A neurologic examination should be performed to attempt to localize the lesion. Causes of CNS abscesses in small ruminants include *Corynebacterium pseudotuberculosis*, *Trueperella pyogenes*, and *Staphylococcus*. Lymphosarcoma is the most common spinal cord tumor in small ruminants.
• Diagnosis can be achieved in some cases with head or spinal radiographs, magnetic resonance imaging, or computed tomography.

Haemonchus contortus
A blood-sucking gastrointestinal strongyle parasite. Severe cases may progress to debilitation and recumbency as a result of anemia and hypoproteinemia. This is the main rule-out in a recumbent animal with pale/white mucus membranes.
Clinical Signs
• Pale mucus membranes
• Tachycardia
• Poor body condition
• Ventral edema, bottle jaw
Diagnosis
• Diagnosis is based on clinical signs and presence of large numbers of strongyle eggs on fecal float.
• *Haemonchus* cannot be readily identified by float alone but a diagnostic test using fluorescently-labeled peanut agglutinin that specifically binds *Haemonchus* eggs is available at diagnostic laboratories.
Treatment
• Elimination of *Haemonchus contortus* burdens can be difficult due to widespread resistance to commonly used dewormers.
• See chapter, Parasite Control Programs: Small Ruminant, and chapter, Haemonchosis.

Pregnancy Toxemia
Ewes and does carrying multiple fetuses may develop pregnancy toxemia if their increased nutritional needs are not met. A negative energy balance results in mobilization of fat and can cause excessive production of ketones.
Clinical Signs
• Depression and recumbency in ewes and does in the final trimester of pregnancy

• May progress to tremors, ataxia, opisthotonus
• Elevated blood and urine ketones
• Hypoglycemia
Treatment
• Cesarean section is required in critical cases
• Dextrose and propylene glycol are mainstays of treatment
• See chapter, Pregnancy Toxemia: Small Ruminant, for further information

Hypocalcemia
Usually affects ewes and does in the last 2 weeks of pregnancy.
Clinical Signs
• Ataxia progressing to recumbency
• Bloat (decreased eructation)
• Sluggish pupillary light responses
Treatment
1 g calcium per 45 kg body weight, may be split IV and SQ

TREATMENT
See "Differential Diagnoses"

MEDICATIONS
DRUGS OF CHOICE
See "Differential Diagnoses"

CONTRAINDICATIONS
Appropriate milk and meat withdrawal times must be followed for all compounds administered to food-producing animals.

FOLLOW-UP
EXPECTED COURSE AND PROGNOSIS
Dependent on primary cause of disease

POSSIBLE COMPLICATIONS
Neuromuscular damage due to prolonged recumbency, especially on surfaces with inadequate bedding.

PATIENT CARE
Animals should be assisted to stand 3 or 4 times per day to allow for muscle perfusion and ease of urination. Clean, dry, deep bedding is important to prevent neuromuscular damage.

PREVENTION
Specific recommendations for prevention of disease will depend on the underlying cause. See specific disease chapters for more information.

MISCELLANEOUS
AGE-RELATED FACTORS
Neonates are at higher risk of systemic infectious causes of recumbency such as bacterial meningitis (including ascending infection as a result of tail docking) and infectious polyarthritis.

ZOONOTIC POTENTIAL
Rabies is a zoonotic disease.

PREGNANCY
Pregnant small ruminants are at risk of pregnancy toxemia and hypocalcemia.

ABBREVIATIONS
• CNS = central nervous system
• CSF = cerebral spinal fluid
• IV = intravenous
• PLR = pupillary light response
• PO = per os, by mouth
• SQ = subcutaneous

SEE ALSO
• Bacterial Meningitis
• Clostridial Disease: Nervous System
• Hypocalcemia: Small Ruminant
• Laminitis in Cattle
• Neonatal Septic Arthritis
• Parasite Control Programs: Small Ruminant
• Pregnancy Toxemia: Small Ruminant
• Scrapie
• Tick Paralysis
• Urea Toxicity
• Vitamin B Deficiency

Suggested Reading
Nietfeld JC. Neuropathology and diagnostics in food animals. Vet Clin North Am Food Anim Pract 2012, 28: 515–34.
Pugh DG. Sheep and Goat Medicine, 1st ed. Philadelphia, PA: Saunders, 2002.
Smith BP, ed. Large Animal Internal Medicine, 5th ed. St. Louis: Elsevier Mosby, 2015.
Author Kate O'Conor
Consulting Editor Kaitlyn A. Lutz

DRUG HYPERSENSITIVITIES

BASICS

OVERVIEW
- Hypersensitivity reactions can occur following exposure to any drug.
- These reactions encompass the classic Gell and Coombs I–IV classification system.
- Identifying the type of reaction involved in a case can be challenging, but most reactions represent either type I or type III reactions. Cattle (especially Holsteins) can develop an endotoxin reaction from Gram-negative vaccines as well.
- Due to the rapid onset of type I reactions (often occurring within minutes), recognizing the signs of the reaction and properly responding with appropriate therapeutic agents is critical to help ensure the survival of the animal.

INCIDENCE/PREVALENCE
- Overall incidence is not well documented, but has been estimated at 1 per 10,000.
- Incidence and prevalence is dependent on spontaneous reporting by the animal owner or veterinarian. www.fda.gov/AnimalVeterinary/SafetyHealth/ReportaProblem/ucm055305.htm is an internet portal to the US FDA to report adverse drug reactions.

GEOGRAPHIC DISTRIBUTION
Worldwide

SYSTEMS AFFECTED
- Cardiovascular
- Respiratory
- Integument
- Digestive

PATHOPHYSIOLOGY
- Hypersensitivity reactions typically are a result of either type I (IgE mediated/allergic) or type III (immune complex) reactions and require a pre-sensitized host.
- Type I reactions ("anaphylaxis") result from the antigen binding to various cells including basophils and mast cells, which trigger the release of vasoactive substances (e.g., histamine, leukotrienes, chemotactic factors) resulting in multi-organ effects including systemic shock, which are usually rapid and can be fatal in some cases.
- Type III reactions ("immune complex") result from the continued presence of soluble immune complex molecules becoming lodged in vessels and tissues, initiating the complement cascade and resulting in vasculitis, and can be slower in onset.

HISTORICAL FINDINGS
- Generally, hypersensitivity reactions are sporadic and involve individual animals within a group.
- Determine why a drug was given, dose, how the drug was obtained and handled, if more than one individual might be at risk, and the clinical signs suspected to relate to the drug versus the primary disorder being treated.

SIGNALMENT
All ruminant species and breeds of any age and gender potentially affected, though pre-sensitization is more likely to have developed in mature animals.

PHYSICAL EXAMINATION FINDINGS
- Type I ("allergic") reactions
  - Diffuse swelling/edema of skin (especially the face and head) and udder
  - Salivation and lacrimation
  - Behavioral changes including anxiety, trembling, restlessness, or excitement
  - Open mouth respirations and tongue protrusion due to difficulty breathing
  - Wheezing and/or labored respirations, rhinitis
  - Tachycardia
  - Tachypnea
  - Decreased rumen motility
- Type III ("immune complex") reactions
  - Erythema and swollen joints with lameness or ataxia
  - Changes in behavior
  - Fever, polyuria, polydipsia

GENETICS
N/A

CAUSES AND RISK FACTORS
- Previous exposure to offending agent resulting in sensitization.
- Multiple Gram-negative vaccines administered on the same day may increase risk of endotoxin reaction in Holsteins.

DIAGNOSIS

DIFFERENTIAL DIAGNOSES
- Type I hypersensitivity may be generated as a response to some infections and infestations in cattle or sheep (e.g., *Ostertagia ostertagi* or *Bovicola* [*Damalinia*] *ovis*).
- Hypersensitivity reactions (suspected from drugs) should be differentiated from other agents the animal may have been exposed to (e.g., natural toxins).
- Type I hypersensitivity may need to be differentiated from accidental vascular injection of drugs or other types of adverse drug reactions.
- Type III reactions are often a diagnosis of exclusion; common etiologies for the signs of type III reactions could include chronic infections or malignancies.
- Due to the complexity of exposures that animals may have, identifying the offending agent (which may include feed or other exposures) can be challenging.

CBC/BIOCHEMISTRY/URINALYSIS
- Agranulocytosis, thrombocytopenia, or anemia may be noted on CBC depending on the type of reaction.
- Evidence of nephritis, proteinuria, and markers for inflammation may be evident on standard blood chemistry and urinalysis.

OTHER LABORATORY TESTS
Coombs' test or antinuclear antibody testing may help identify the cause.

IMAGING
N/A

OTHER DIAGNOSTIC PROCEDURES
Cytologic examination and bacterial culture of joint fluid might be relevant to rule out septic arthritis in cases of type III reaction.

PATHOLOGIC FINDINGS
- Postmortem findings following true type I (IgE) reactions may show evidence of inflammation and edema (especially of the lungs). In adult cattle and sheep, bronchial constriction and retained air in alveoli may be present. In juvenile cattle, pulmonary edema and vascular engorgement is more common.
- Pathologic evidence of renal injury including interstitial nephritis may be present.

TREATMENT

THERAPEUTIC APPROACH
- Immediately discontinue or remove the suspected agent involved.
- Aggressive symptomatic management focusing on cardiovascular support and administration of anti-inflammatory agents is indicated for type I reactions.
- Antibiotics (as needed) for suspected or confirmed infections and anti-inflammatory agents and supportive fluid therapy as needed if renal impairment is noted for type III reactions.

SURGICAL CONSIDERATIONS AND TECHNIQUES
- Drainage of infected tissues or abscesses occurring from type III reactions may be necessary.

MEDICATIONS

DRUGS OF CHOICE
- Epinephrine 1:1,000—0.5–1.0 mL/50 kg or /100 lbs SQ or IM (extra-label use)
- Dexamethasone 20 mg IM or IV (extra-label)
- Isoflupredone 10–20 mg (total dose) IM based on size of animal and severity of signs
- Methylprednisolone 100–500 mg IM
- Flunixin meglumine 1.1–2.2 mg/kg slow IV
- Diphenhydramine hydrochloride 0.5–2.0 mg/kg slow IV or IM

CONTRAINDICATIONS
Corticosteroids should be avoided in pregnant animals and used judiciously in animals with an underlying infectious disease.

PRECAUTIONS
• Ensure proper dilution of epinephrine solution prior to administration (ideally to 1:10,000).
• Antihistamine drugs can occasionally cause paradoxic excitement.
• Appropriate milk and meat withdrawal times must be followed for all compounds administered to food-producing animals.

POSSIBLE INTERACTIONS
• Many potential drug and disease-state interactions.
• Refer to the specific drug package insert for details regarding interactions.
• Milk and meat withdrawal times may be impacted based on therapeutic agent(s) administered.

 FOLLOW-UP

EXPECTED COURSE AND PROGNOSIS
Good prognosis if recognized early during development of the reaction and treated appropriately with supportive care including cardiovascular support if needed.

POSSIBLE COMPLICATIONS
• Abortion
• Renal failure

CLIENT EDUCATION
Educate owners on risk for recurrence of hypersensitivity reactions following administration of the same drug or drugs from the same class.

PATIENT CARE
• Monitor heart rate and respiratory status.
• Monitor activity, behavior, demeanor, and appetite to gauge response to therapy.

PREVENTION
Avoid administering suspected offending agent or related agents in the future.

 MISCELLANEOUS

ASSOCIATED CONDITIONS
N/A

AGE-RELATED FACTORS
N/A

ZOONOTIC POTENTIAL
N/A

PREGNANCY
Severe drug reactions in pregnant animals may invoke abortion or still birth

BIOSECURITY
N/A

PRODUCTION MANAGEMENT
Close monitoring of animals following vaccine administration is warranted.

SYNONYMS
• Allergic reactions
• Vaccine reactions
• Drug reactions

ABBREVIATION
IgE = immunoglobulin E

SEE ALSO
• Anaphylaxis
• Drug Interactions
• Drug Toxicities

Suggested Reading
Ellis JA, Yong C. Systemic adverse reactions in young Simmental calves following administration of a combination vaccine. Can Vet J 1997, 38: 45–7.
Omidi A. Anaphylactic reaction in a cow due to parenteral administration of penicillin-streptomycin. Can Vet J 2009, 50: 741–4.
Veterinary Drug Safety: www.fda.gov/AnimalVeterinary/SafetyHealth
Author Stephen H. LeMaster
Consulting Editor Erica C. McKenzie

DRUG INTERACTIONS

BASICS

OVERVIEW
• The impact on the overall activity [including the dissolution, pharmacokinetics (PK) and pharmacodynamics (PD)] that one drug has upon another drug can be termed, generally, as a "drug interaction."
• Drug interactions can result in a wide variety of consequences which can be harmful (even fatal), beneficial, or inconsequential depending upon a variety of factors.
• Drug interactions may lead to therapeutic failures due to specific PK or PD effects between co-administered agents (e.g., competitive binding, enhanced drug elimination).
• Interactions between drugs can occur as a result of a physical incompatibility (e.g., mixing drugs in the same syringe or IV bag) or due to the PK or PD properties of the agents.
• Animal-specific factors, including age or end-organ function, can directly impact the likelihood and severity of some interactions.
• Access to up-to-date clinical or electronic references to identify potential interactions is essential for every practitioner to limit the likelihood of harmful interactions.

INCIDENCE/PREVALENCE
• The overall incidence and prevalence of interactions is not well described.
• Many drug interactions do not produce outward signs.

GEOGRAPHIC DISTRIBUTION
Worldwide

SYSTEMS AFFECTED
Multisystemic

PATHOPHYSIOLOGY

In Vitro Interactions
• Physical or physicochemical incompatibility of agents may occur prior to administration and involve interactions between active ingredients, excipients (e.g., fillers, diluents or bulking agents), IV fluids or administration equipment (e.g., IV bag or syringe).
• Cloudiness, color changes, or visible precipitation may be evident.
• Changes in pH of the agent or inactivation of one or more of the drugs may occur.
• The risk of in vitro interactions can be reduced through utilization of IV drug stability and incompatibility references.

Pharmacokinetic (PK) Interactions
• Pharmacokinetic interactions between drugs impact the absorption, distribution, metabolism, and/or excretion of one or more of the drugs.
• Overall, the impact that PK interactions have may result in higher or lower than expected plasma drug concentrations, potentially resulting in drug toxicity or therapeutic failure, respectively.

• Absorption of tetracycline-class antibiotics can be inhibited by the presence of co-administered drugs high in certain metal ions (e.g., calcium, magnesium) due to formation of chelating complexes.
• Drugs that impact the acid secretion or digestive tract motility may increase or decrease absorption (e.g., H_1/H_2 inhibitors, such as ranitidine or cimetidine; anticholinergic agents such as atropine; opioids).
• Distribution of drugs can be impacted by the presence of co-administered agents due to effects on protein binding (e.g., sulfonamides competing with phenylbutazone for protein binding sites).
• Metabolism of some drugs may be enhanced or inhibited due to the impact that other drugs exert on cytochrome P450 enzyme systems involved with the metabolism of the therapeutic agent.
• Elimination of some agents in the urine can be impacted by changes in the pH of the urine (alkalization or acidification), or through competition for protein carrier sites resulting in either inhibition or prolongation of excretion.

Pharmacodynamic (PD) Interactions
• Pharmacodynamic interactions occur at the level of the receptor site and involve the impact one drug may have on binding, with subsequent inhibition or enhancement of clinical effects.
• Drugs may act as a full or partial antagonist at receptor sites, limiting (or blocking) the effect other agents have at that site (e.g., extra-label use of yohimbine blocking the action of xylazine at α_2 receptor sites).
• Drugs may also act as physiologic antagonists to each other, binding to separate and functionally opposing receptor sites (e.g., extra-label use of doxapram in cattle to reverse respiratory depression from inhaled anesthetics).
• Agents with unique receptor site targets, when administered together, may produce either additive effects (e.g., $1 + 2 = 3$) or synergistic effects (e.g., $1 + 1 = 5$) depending on the agents used.

HISTORICAL FINDINGS
N/A

SIGNALMENT
All ruminant species of any age or gender can be affected by drug interaction.

PHYSICAL EXAMINATION FINDINGS
• Signs of a drug interaction vary widely depending on the specific interaction and the impact on various organ system(s).
• Toxic effects may range from mild depression or inappetence to collapse of the animal.
• Outward signs may indicate enhancement of one of the administered agents or lack of efficacy (therapeutic failure).

GENETICS
• Variations in the expression of the cytochrome P450 system exist between ruminant species, leading to marked differences in metabolism (and toxicity) of some agents between species (e.g., susceptibility to pyrrolizidine alkaloid toxicity of sheep vs. cattle). Even among breeds within a species (conventional farm pig vs. Göttinger minipig) large variations in susceptibility may exist.
• The full impact of this varied expression has not been fully described; caution should be exercised when administering therapeutic agents in an extra-label manner.

CAUSES AND RISK FACTORS
• The risk for interactions to occur increases with the number of drugs administered.
• Animal-specific factors including age or pre-existing end-organ dysfunction can directly impact the likelihood and severity of some interactions.
• Older animals predictably experience changes to drug absorption, distribution, and excretion due to age-related physiologic changes which may result in previously unexpected drug interactions.

DIAGNOSIS

DIFFERENTIAL DIAGNOSES
• The physiologic impact of drug interactions may mimic any number of disease conditions.
• A review of all current therapeutic agents (including dosing schedule in relation to other drugs) should be made.
• Involvement of a drug interaction should be considered when apparent signs of drug toxicity occur or in the event an animal's condition does not improve following the initiation of new drug therapy.

CBC/BIOCHEMISTRY/URINALYSIS
• Variable impact based on specific interaction.
• Toxic effects on the kidneys or liver as a result of a drug-drug interaction may mimic underlying diseases.

OTHER LABORATORY TESTS
N/A

IMAGING
N/A

OTHER DIAGNOSTIC PROCEDURES
N/A

PATHOLOGIC FINDINGS
• Variable depending on specific interactions.
• Most commonly the liver and kidneys are affected if interaction is significant enough to result in end-organ damage.

(CONTINUED) | **DRUG INTERACTIONS**

TREATMENT

THERAPEUTIC APPROACH
• Immediate discontinuation of suspected offending agent(s).
• Gastrointestinal decontamination with intraruminal administration of activated charcoal, cathartics, or rumenotomy should be considered when orally administered drugs may result in a serious or life-threatening toxic event.
• Symptomatic and supportive treatment based on specific expected or resultant injury; fluid therapy and electrolyte support to correct perfusion, cardiovascular function, and metabolic disturbances.

SURGICAL CONSIDERATIONS AND TECHNIQUES
N/A

MEDICATIONS

DRUGS OF CHOICE
N/A

CONTRAINDICATIONS
Refer to the package insert of the individual drugs for details.

PRECAUTIONS
Appropriate milk and meat withdrawal times must be followed for all compounds administered to food-producing animals.

POSSIBLE INTERACTIONS
N/A

FOLLOW-UP

POSSIBLE COMPLICATIONS
Variable complications including end-organ injury (liver, kidney).

EXPECTED COURSE AND PROGNOSIS
• Based on a variety of factors including the specific interaction and any resulting injury, age, and underlying end-organ health.
• Early recognition and appropriate action may improve the expected course and prognosis.

CLIENT EDUCATION
Close observation of animals following the initiation or change in drug therapy to recognize the effects of drug interactions.

PATIENT CARE
Close observation of animals following the initiation or change in drug therapy to recognize the effects of drug interactions.

PREVENTION
• Avoid administering agents with known or high likelihood of interactions.
• Limit overall drug administration (rational drug therapy).
• Stagger drug dosing to limit concomitant exposure to multiple agents.
• Adjust dosing of agents based on individual therapeutic response.
• Micromedix (www.micromedex.com) is a Commercial Drug Interaction Database that can be utilized.

MISCELLANEOUS

ASSOCIATED CONDITIONS
• Renal insufficiency
• Hepatic inflammation or insufficiency

AGE-RELATED FACTORS
Older animals experience changes to absorption, distribution, and excretion due to age-related physiologic changes resulting in previously unexpected drug interactions.

ZOONOTIC POTENTIAL
N/A

PREGNANCY
Changes in end-organ blood flow, apparent volume of distribution (V_d), and protein binding capacity as a result of pregnancy may impact the PK/PD of some agents.

BIOSECURITY
N/A

PRODUCTION MANAGEMENT
N/A

SYNONYMS
N/A

ABBREVIATIONS
• PD = pharmacodynamic
• PK = pharmacokinetic
• V_d = volume of distribution

SEE ALSO
• Drug Hypersensitivities
• Drug Toxicities

Suggested Reading
Fink-Gremmels J. Implications of hepatic cytochrome P450-related biotransformation processes in veterinary sciences. Eur J Pharmacol 2008, 585: 502–9.
Ioannides C. Cytochrome p450 expression in the liver of food-producing animals. Curr Drug Metab 2006, 7: 335–48.
Palleria C, Di Paulo A, Giofrè C, et. al. Pharmacokinetic drug-drug interaction and their implication in clinical management. J Res Med Sci. 2013 Jul;18(7):601–10.
Szotáková B, Baliharová B, Lamka J, et al. Comparison of in vitro activities of biotransformation enzymes in pig, cattle, goat and sheep. Res Vet Sci 2004, 76: 43–51.
Author Stephen H. LeMaster
Consulting Editor Erica C. McKenzie

D

DRUG TOXICITIES

BASICS

OVERVIEW
• The term "drug toxicity" represents a broad spectrum of potential adverse drug reactions (ADRs) associated with drug therapy.
• A "toxic effect" of a drug describes events not typically associated with the normal dosing of a medication. Other reported effects, termed "adverse effects," include all other unwanted effects regardless of mechanism.
• Terminology introduced in the 1970s to describe ADRs has included: type A ("augmented") events which occur based solely on the dose administered; and type B ("bizarre") events which are not connected to the dose administered (e.g., idiosyncratic or immune reactions).
• Other events may be categorized based on the chronic nature or overall duration of therapy or events that encompass a genetic predisposition; all events are considered ADRs.
• Some events may not be identified until substantial post-marketing surveillance has been completed.
• In addition to stand alone drugs, supplemented feed may be involved in some drug toxicities.

INCIDENCE/PREVALENCE
Accurate rates of ADRs are difficult to identify; they are dependent on reporting to the pharmaceutical company or to the US FDA.

GEOGRAPHIC DISTRIBUTION
Worldwide; regional distribution might be influenced by quality control procedures and marketing practices.

SYSTEMS AFFECTED
• Digestive
• Integument
• Musculoskeletal
• Cardiovascular
• Nervous
• Respiratory
• Urinary

PATHOPHYSIOLOGY
• Varies based on the drug involved and the organ system(s) affected.
• Type A reactions are more predictable and are a reflection or extension of the pharmacologic effects of the drug (e.g., the effects of an overdose of xylazine). Often such effects have been identified in pre-market studies.
• Type B reactions involve more unexpected or unpredictable mechanisms of toxicity, often appear to be either immune-related or otherwise idiopathic in nature, and can have a highly variable onset.
• Either the parent compound or a reactive metabolite can be involved in type B events.

• Frequently in type B events, the liver is involved, presumably because of its role in drug metabolism. The skin or bone marrow may also be adversely affected.

HISTORICAL FINDINGS
• Determine why a drug was given, the dose, how the drug was obtained and handled, if more than one individual might be at risk, and the clinical signs suspected to relate to the drug versus the primary disorder being treated.
• Route of drug administration is important when an unexpected reaction is observed; signs might relate to accidental arterial injection, or inadvertent penetration of a vessel during IM administration, rather than a true drug reaction.

SIGNALMENT
All species of any age/gender

PHYSICAL EXAMINATION FINDINGS
• Signs vary based on the underlying mechanism of the reaction (e.g., immunologic, pharmacologic).
• Nonspecific signs such as skin reactions (including photosensitivity), inappetence, apparent lameness, behavior changes, tremors, salivation, or diarrhea may be evident depending on the drug or the organ system involved.
• Outward signs may mimic a variety of injuries or organic diseases. Some may have a characteristic "toxidrome"—a group of signs that constitute the basis for a diagnosis of poisoning (e.g., cholinesterase inhibitors).

GENETICS
N/A

CAUSES AND RISK FACTORS
• Administration of any drug creates risk; administering agents above label doses may increase risk of a type A reaction.
• Feed may be implicated in some cases such as in ionophore toxicity, or if feed is supplemented with selenium or copper.
• Topical application of some agents, such as insecticides, can also provoke adverse reactions.
• Pre-existing disease may induce a higher risk of a toxicity event, for example, drug-associated nephrotoxicity is more likely in hypovolemic animals.
• Due to the infrequent and unpredictable nature of some events, a full list of causes and risk factors is not known.

DIAGNOSIS

DIFFERENTIAL DIAGNOSES
• Depending on clinical signs and clinicopathologic findings, the differential diagnosis list may include a variety of organic diseases including infections or physical injury.

• Pharmaceutical agents as an etiologic cause should be considered as part of the routine evaluation of a diseased animal.
• Common exposures (e.g., feed, natural toxins, plants) should be considered if multiple animals are clinically affected with similar findings.

CBC/BIOCHEMISTRY/URINALYSIS
• Routine laboratory assessments are often indicated and can include a CBC with differential, a blood chemistry profile encompassing renal, hepatic, and muscular indices; and urinalysis.
• Laboratory findings vary based on the degree and duration of the adverse event and any accompanying disorder for which the drug might have been administered. Changes in some end-organ variables (e.g., liver enzymes, creatinine) may evolve over time depending on acute versus chronic injury.

OTHER LABORATORY TESTS
• Bone marrow aspiration can help identify hematopoietic diseases.
• Analysis of stomach/rumen contents for ionophore concentrations.

IMAGING
Ultrasonography can be used to evaluate the liver or kidney in some cases of suspected drug toxicity.

OTHER DIAGNOSTIC PROCEDURES
Percutaneous biopsy of liver or kidney if indicated.

PATHOLOGIC FINDINGS
• Variable based on organ injury.
• Lesions in skeletal and cardiac muscle occur from ionophore toxicity.
• Stomach/rumen contents should be collected for analysis where relevant.

TREATMENT

THERAPEUTIC APPROACH
• Discontinue treatment or exposure to the suspected agent.
• Consult with an animal poison center if a "drug overdose" or poisoning is suspected, to review decontamination and necessary care.
• Appropriate treatment including the use of specific antidotes varies based on the toxic agent.
• Fluid therapy, nutritional support, and corticosteroids can be administered if indicated.

SURGICAL CONSIDERATIONS AND TECHNIQUES
N/A

(CONTINUED)

D

MEDICATIONS

DRUGS OF CHOICE
• Incomplete list; consultation with a poison center is recommended in the event of a drug overdose or suspected poisoning.
• Anti-inflammatory:
  ◦ Dexamethasone (IV) 0.05–0.1 mg/kg body weight
• Digestive tract decontamination:
  ◦ Activated charcoal (extra-label): 1–5 g/kg as a slurry by mouth or ororuminal tube
  ◦ Sodium or magnesium sulfate: 250–500 mg/kg added to the charcoal slurry
• Atropine sulfate (for cholinesterase inhibitor toxicity)—dose varies based on degree of toxicity
• Epinephrine (extra-label, for anaphylaxis): 0.5–1 ml per 100 lbs (45 kg) of bodyweight of 1:1,000 SQ or IM; dilute to 1:10,000 if using IV; repeat every 15 minutes as needed.

CONTRAINDICATIONS
Refer to the package insert of the individual drugs for details.

PRECAUTIONS
• Corticosteroids should be avoided in pregnant animals and used judiciously in animals with underlying infectious disease.
• Appropriate milk and meat withdrawal times must be followed for all compounds administered to food-producing animals.

POSSIBLE INTERACTIONS
• Refer to the package insert of the individual drugs for details.
• Milk and meat withdrawal times may be impacted based on therapeutic agent(s) administered.
• Using combinations of drugs from the same class (e.g., use of more than one NSAID agent at once) may enhance the possibility of toxic effects.

FOLLOW-UP

EXPECTED COURSE AND PROGNOSIS
• Variable course and prognosis depending on timing of recognition, and management, age and underlying health status of the affected animal.

• Animals with ionophore toxicity may have a guarded prognosis due to the possibility of developing chronic cardiac disease.
• Animals suffering severe impact to other systems (bone marrow, kidneys) also have a guarded prognosis depending on response to treatment and progression over time.

POSSIBLE COMPLICATIONS
Chronic end-organ dysfunction from initial insult

CLIENT EDUCATION
Animal owners should be alert for changes in animals following drug administration.

PATIENT CARE
Periodic reevaluation of blood chemistries, urine characteristics, and behavior as needed.

PREVENTION
• Avoid drugs from the same class following previous immune-related events.
• Avoid nephrotoxic drugs in dehydrated patients or those with suspected renal disease.

MISCELLANEOUS

ASSOCIATED CONDITIONS
• Renal failure
• Hepatic failure
• Diarrhea

AGE-RELATED FACTORS
Changes in drug metabolism may occur as the animal ages. Metabolic pathways in young animals may not have fully matured.

ZOONOTIC POTENTIAL
N/A

PREGNANCY
Adverse drug reactions in pregnant animals may invoke abortion or stillbirth.

BIOSECURITY
N/A

PRODUCTION MANAGEMENT
• Refer to drug label or appropriate references for meat and milk withdrawal times for all agents administered.
• www.fda.gov/AnimalVeterinary/SafetyHealth/ReportaProblem/ucm055305.htm is an internet portal to the US FDA to report adverse drug reactions.
• www.farad.org/ Food Animal Residue Avoidance Databank is also a useful resource.

SYNONYMS
• Adverse event
• Drug sensitivity

ABBREVIATIONS
• ADR = Adverse Drug Reaction
• US FDA = United States Food and Drug Administration

SEE ALSO
• Acute Renal Failure
• Anaphylaxis
• Common Pharmacologic Therapies: Adult Dairy Cattle (see www.fiveminutevet.com/ruminant)
• Drug Interactions
• Extra-label Drug Use and Compounding (see www.fiveminutevet.com/ruminant)
• Food Animal Residue Avoidance Databank (FARAD) (see www.fiveminutevet.com/ruminant)
• Monensin Toxicity
• Nonsteroidal Anti-inflammatory Drugs (NSAIDs) (see www.fiveminutevet.com/ruminant)
• Pharmacokinetics and Pharmacodynamics (see www.fiveminutevet.com/ruminant)
• Selenium Toxicity
• Toxicity: Herd Outbreaks

Suggested Reading
Aronson JK, Ferner RE Clarification of terminology in drug safety. Drug Saf 2005, 28: 851–70.
Bradley CH. Copper poisoning in a dairy herd fed a mineral supplement. Can Vet J 1993, 34: 287–92.
McGuirk SM, Semrad SD. Toxicologic emergencies in cattle. Vet Clin North Am Food Anim Pract 2005, 21: 729–49.
Roder, JD. Ionophore toxicity and tolerance. Vet Clin North Am Food Anim Pract 2011, 27: 305–14.
Uetrecht J, Naisbitt DJ. Idiosyncratic adverse drug reactions: Current concepts. Pharmacol Rev 2013, 65: 779–808.
Van Metre DC. A case report of the treatment of an overdose of xylazine in a cow. Cornell Vet 1992, 82: 287–91.
Author Stephen H. LeMaster
Consulting Editor Erica C. McKenzie
Acknowledgements The author and book editors acknowledge the prior contribution of Ronette Gehring.

DYSTOCIA: BOVINE

BASICS

OVERVIEW
• Dystocia, or difficulty calving, occurs when the first or second stage in the parturition process is interrupted or prolonged.
• Varying degrees of intervention may be required to correct the cause of dystocia, provide assistance for delivery of the fetus, and preserve the health and fertility of the cow.

INCIDENCE/PREVALENCE
• Incidence varies depending on herd management, age and size at breeding, size and breed of dam, parity, gender of the fetus, and breed of sire of the fetus.
• In US Holstein-Friesian cattle, the reported incidence is 13.7% (22.6% in primiparous animals).
• In beef cattle, the reported incidence is 17.7% for primiparous and 2.7% for multiparous cows.

GEOGRAPHIC DISTRIBUTION
Worldwide

SYSTEMS AFFECTED
• Reproductive
• Musculoskeletal
• Multisystemic

PATHOPHYSIOLOGY
• Causes of dystocia can be fetal or maternal in origin and may be related to lack of expulsive forces or obstruction of the birth canal.
• The most common cause of dystocia in cattle is feto-maternal size disproportions.
• Fetal causes of dystocia:
 ○ Fetal abnormalities due to congenital or genetic defects frequently result in dystocia.
 ○ Abnormal position, presentation or posture.
  ▪ *Presentation* is defined as the orientation of the spinal axis of the fetus to that of the dam (cranial, caudal, or transverse).
  ▪ *Position* is the orientation of the dorsum of the fetus in relation to the quadrants of the maternal pelvis (dorsosacral, dorsoilial, dorsopubic).
  ▪ *Posture* is the relationship of the fetal extremities with respect to its torso (e.g., left carpal flexion, lateral neck flexion).
• Maternal causes include uterine torsion, uterine inertia, incomplete cervical or vulvar dilation, small pelvic size, obesity, fear, or genetic predisposition.
 ○ Failure of expulsive forces may be due to primary or secondary uterine inertia.
 ○ Primary uterine inertia is failure of the myometrium to contract due to over-stretching (hydrops) or metabolic disease (hypocalcemia).
 ○ Secondary uterine inertia is the result of exhaustion of the myometrium due to prolonged second stage of labor.

HISTORICAL FINDINGS
• Lack of progress after initiation of parturition
• Continuous violent abdominal contractions without visualization of fetal parts
• Unsuccessful attempts by either an owner or herdsman to deliver the calf

SIGNALMENT
• Dystocia may occur in cows of any parity; however, incidence is higher in primiparous than multiparous animals.
• Incidence varies by species and breed.
• Belgian Blue cattle have a higher rate of dystocia with over 90% of calvings reported to result in cesarean section.

PHYSICAL EXAMINATION FINDINGS
• Prior to assisting a dystocia, the minimal requirements are an ample supply of clean warm water, disinfectant, buckets, lubricant (petroleum jelly or methylcellulose-derived products), and two obstetrical chains with handles.
• Transrectal palpation to rule out uterine torsion should be performed if no fetal parts are present at the vulva.
• Vaginal examination should be performed if there has been little progress for 2 hours after the amniotic sac is presented at the vulva.
 ○ The presentation, position, and posture of the fetus are determined and fetal viability and birth canal integrity are assessed.
 ○ The fetus can live up to 10 hours within the birth canal after the amniotic sac is ruptured.
 ○ If the head is accessible in cranial presentation, the swallowing reflex may be elicited by inserting a finger into the mouth; if the fetus is alive, swallowing will occur.
 ○ The pedal reflex may be assessed by applying pressure between the hooves; a responsive fetus will retract its leg.
 ○ A blink reflex may also be elicited by applying pressure over the globe.
• The fetus must be in dorsosacral position with a normal posture prior to extraction.
• The final step is to determine whether or not there is sufficient space and lubrication to achieve vaginal delivery of the fetus.
• Fetal traction requires correct placement of chains above the fetlock and below the dewclaws of the fetus.

Anterior/Cranial Presentation
• The front limbs are identified by the flexion of the fetlock and carpus joints in the same direction.
• The head of the fetus should be extended and rest on both knees of the extended front limbs with the legs fully presented in the birth canal.
• Vaginal delivery is possible if one person can pull the first leg presented until the pastern is 6 inches (12 cm) outside the vulva and, while holding the first leg in this position, the second leg can be extended equally far outside the vulva.

• At these distances, both shoulders of the fetus will have passed the bony entrance to the maternal pelvis.
• Pulling alternately on the forelimbs during delivery will decrease the width of the shoulders as the fetus moves through the maternal pelvis.

Posterior/Caudal Presentation
• About 5% of parturitions occur with a fetus is in posterior presentation.
• Both hind legs should be extended. The hindlimbs are identified by the opposite direction of the fetlock and hock flexion.
• Vaginal delivery is possible if both hocks can be exteriorized.
• Passage of the fetal pelvis through the maternal pelvis may be facilitated by rotating the fetus approximately 90 degrees.

GENETICS
The rate of dystocia increases with inbreeding in Holstein cattle.

CAUSES AND RISK FACTORS
• Obesity
• Twins
• Hypocalcemia
• Small frame size
• Oversized fetus

DIAGNOSIS

DIFFERENTIAL DIAGNOSES
N/A

CBC/BIOCHEMISTRY/URINALYSIS
May be indicated if the cow is depressed or showing signs of metabolic compromise.

OTHER LABORATORY TESTS
N/A

IMAGING
N/A

DIAGNOSTIC PROCEDURES
See "Physical Examination Findings"

PATHOLOGIC FINDINGS
N/A

TREATMENT

THERAPEUTIC APPROACH
• Caudal epidural analgesia helps with obstetric manipulations.
• Epinephrine can be administered to help relax the uterus during manipulation of the fetus.
• Rules of obstetric manipulations should always be followed (i.e., ample lubrication, correct diagnosis, retropulsion, mutation, and traction).
• Uterine torsion may be corrected by rolling, use of detorsion rod if the fetus is accessible, or cesarean section.

D

• In anterior presentation, the abnormal limb flexion is corrected and the head is extended with the help of a snare before applying traction.
• Unilateral or bilateral (breech) hip flexions are corrected by pushing the rump forward and grasping a rear foot and flexing it at the fetlock and hock to reorient the legs to coxo-femoral extension. The procedure is repeated on the other limb, then the fetus is extracted.
• Abnormal position due to failure of rotation of the fetus requires the use of the detorsion rod.
• Manipulation time should be kept to a minimum. Fetotomy may be performed if the fetus is dead, the cervix is completely dilated, and there is enough room.

SURGICAL CONSIDERATION
• Cesarean section may be indicated if a live calf cannot be delivered vaginally.
• Dead emphysematous calves or fetal monsters may require a fetotomy.

 MEDICATIONS

DRUGS OF CHOICE
• Activation of β2 receptors in the myometrium via administration of epinephrine (1 mL 1:1000 epinephrine IV or 10 mL IM) will result in uterine relaxation.
• Systemic antibiotics.
• Oxytocin (10–20 IU, IM or IV) administered within 48–72 hours may enhance myometrial contractions and aid in evacuation of uterine contents following dystocia.
• Uterine lavage is recommended if the fetus is dead.

CONTRAINDICATIONS
• Sedatives may cause recumbency and may reach fetal circulation.
• Appropriate milk and meat withdrawal times must be followed.

PRECAUTIONS
Obstetric manipulation should be performed in a safe area for the dam and examiner.

POSSIBLE INTERACTIONS
N/A

 FOLLOW-UP

EXPECTED COURSE AND PROGNOSIS
Prognosis depends on severity of dystocia, degree of trauma suffered by the dam's reproductive tract during forced fetal extraction, and occurrence of other postpartum diseases.

POSSIBLE COMPLICATIONS
• Retained fetal membranes
• Trauma and lacerations to the genital tract
• Downer cow syndrome (due to damage to sciatic or obturator nerves)
• Metritis
• Necrotic vaginitis

CLIENT EDUCATION
• Management practices to prevent risk factors for dystocia.
• Calving management and techniques for prompt and correct handling of dystocia.

PATIENT CARE
• Cows should be monitored for appetite, demeanor and fever.
• Character, odor, and amount of vaginal discharge should be noted.
• Administration of antibiotics, NSAIDs, and calcium supplements may be indicated.
• Walking or movement should be limited in those animals that are weak after parturition.

PREVENTION
• Proper nutrition to prevent obesity, negative energy balance, and hypocalcemia.
• Sire selection for calving ease.
• Heifer selection (pelvimetry).

 MISCELLANEOUS

ASSOCIATED CONDITIONS
N/A

AGE-RELATED FACTORS
• Obese primiparous animals.
• Risk of dystocia increases if dam is <24 months of age.

ZOONOTIC POTENTIAL
N/A

PREGNANCY
Prognosis for future fertility may be lower in complicated cases.

BIOSECURITY
N/A

PRODUCTION MANAGEMENT
Appropriate management of the transition period and periparturient animal.

SYNONYMS
N/A

ABBREVIATIONS
• IM = intramuscular
• IV = intravenous
• NSAIDs = nonsteroidal anti-inflammatory drugs

SEE ALSO
• Cesarean Section: Bovine
• Congenital Defects: Bovine
• Down Bovine
• Metritis
• Reproductive Pharmacology
• Retained Placenta

Suggested Reading
Dargatz DA, Dewell GA, Mortimer RG. Calving and calving management of beef cows and heifers on cow-calf operations in the United States. Theriogenology 2004, 61: 997–1007.
Drost M. Dystocia and accidents of gestation. In: Hopper RM ed, Bovine Reproduction. Ames: John Wiley, 2015, pp. 409–15.
Walters K. Obstetrics: Mutation, forced extraction, fetotomy. In: Hopper RM ed, Bovine Reproduction. Ames: John Wiley, 2015, pp. 416–23.
Zaborski D, Grzesiak W, Szatkowska I, Dybus A, Muszynska M, Jedrzejczak M. Factors affecting dystocia in cattle. Reprod Dom Anim 2009, 44: 540–51.
Author Jennifer N. Roberts
Consulting Editor Ahmed Tibary

DYSTOCIA: CAMELID

BASICS

OVERVIEW
• Dystocia is an abnormal prolongation of the first or second stage of parturition requiring assistance for delivery of the fetus.
• Urgent attention should be given to any complaint of dystocia in camelids as the prognosis for survival of the fetus and the female decrease rapidly.
• Obstetric approaches for fetal extraction vary depending on the cause and include assisted vaginal delivery, controlled vaginal delivery, cesarean, or fetotomy.

INCIDENCE/PREVALENCE
Dystocia is rare in camelids. Less than 5% of parturition requires advanced obstetric manipulations by the veterinarian.

GEOGRAPHIC DISTRIBUTION
Worldwide

SYSTEMS AFFECTED
• Reproductive
• Other systems depending on complications

PATHOPHYSIOLOGY
• Normal parturition in camelids is faster than that of ruminants. Premonitory signs include mammary gland enlargement and pelvic ligament relaxation 2–3 weeks prior to parturition. Vulvar edema and bulging of the perineal area appear a few days prior to parturition. The first stage of labor lasts 3–48 hours and is characterized by frequent urination and defecation, discomfort, and signs of colic. The expulsion of the fetus takes 5–90 minutes (average 20 minutes) from rupture of the chorioallantoic sac.
• Dystocia is suspected if there is no progression of labor with increased signs of colic, depression, abnormal perineal or vaginal discharge.
• The cause of dystocia may be maternal or fetal in origin.
• The most common maternal causes are: uterine torsion, uterine inertia, uterine rupture, failure of cervical or vestibular dilation. Primary uterine inertia is frequent in dairy camels and may be due to hypocalcemia.
• Fetal causes include maldispositions or malpostures which are common due to the length of the neck and legs in camelids. Fetal abnormalities (contracted tendons, hydrocephalus, neck and limb ankyloses, schistosomus reflexus) have been reported in cases of dystocia.
• Fetomaternal disproportion and twinning are possible but rare.
• Prognosis for fetal survival decreases rapidly after rupture of the chorioallantois because of rapid detachment of the epitheliochorial, microcotyledonary diffuse placenta resulting in fetal asphyxia.

HISTORICAL FINDINGS
• Normal pregnancy length (320–375 days in SAC, 315–440 days in camels).
• Clinical signs of preparation for delivery 2–3 weeks prior (relaxation of the pelvic ligaments, udder development, vulvar elongation).
• Increasingly violent abdominal contractions without visible fetal parts at the vulva or progression.
• Initiation of stage 2 of parturition with no progression and excessive rolling, kicking at the belly, and vocalization.
• Owner reporting abnormalities (bloody vaginal discharge, fetal or birth canal abnormalities) or lack of success after attempting to assist.

SIGNALMENT
Pregnant female at term or later abortion

PHYSICAL EXAMINATION FINDINGS
• General demeanor and health of the female is usually normal. The only sign present may be abdominal contractions. Protracted cases may show severe vulvar edema, dehydration, and injected sclera. Diarrhea is not uncommon in distressed camels.
• Transrectal palpation is indicated if no fetal parts are visible at the vulva. Sedation and epidural analgesia are required for this evaluation.
• Examination per vaginam is performed as aseptically as possible using ample lubrication to determine presentation, position, and posture of the fetus and assess integrity of the birth canal.
• Clinical assessment of fetal viability in camelids is very difficult. The fetus should only be considered dead if there is evidence of autolysis or lack of cardiac activity.
• Uterine torsion is a common cause of dystocia and can be ruled in or out by transrectal palpation.
• Cranial presentation is the most common (98%). The front limbs should be fully extended with one slightly more advanced than the other and the head resting at the level of the carpi. The most common fetal maldispositions in this presentation are carpal or shoulder flexion and lateral or ventral head deviations. In maiden females, failure of progression may be due to lack of dilation of the vestibular area.
• Caudal presentation is less common (2%). The hind legs should be completely extended. The most common fetal malpostures are unilateral or bilateral hock or hip flexions.
• Transverse presentation is rare.

GENETICS
N/A

CAUSES AND RISK FACTORS
• Obesity
• Progesterone supplementation to maintain pregnancy
• Injuries to the birth canal

DIAGNOSIS

DIFFERENTIAL DIAGNOSES
Other causes of colic. Verify accuracy of breeding date to ascertain that the female is at term.

CBC/BIOCHEMISTRY/URINALYSIS
Indicated if a decision is made to perform a cesarean section on a compromised female.

OTHER LABORATORY TESTS
N/A

IMAGING
N/A

OTHER DIAGNOSTIC PROCEDURES
N/A

PATHOLOGIC FINDINGS
Postmortem examination of dead fetus may confirm abnormalities that caused the dystocia.

TREATMENT

THERAPEUTIC APPROACH
• Caudal epidural analgesia is sufficient for simple obstetric manipulations (correction of carpal or hock flexion, vestibular dilation).
• Sedation with butorphanol in addition to caudal epidural is helpful for the correction of uterine torsion by rolling and for assisted vaginal delivery in cases of shoulder flexion or slight lateral head deviations.
• Heavy sedation or general anesthesia is required for controlled vaginal delivery. Large llamas and camels should be hobbled in sternal position with the hindquarter elevated to allow manipulation.
• Manipulation time should be <30 minutes in order to minimize complications (necrotic vaginitis).
• Obstetric manipulations require fetal repulsion, mutation, then extraction. These are facilitated by administration of a tocolytic.
• Partial fetotomy may be considered in large llamas and camels but should be avoided in alpacas as the risks for vaginal adhesions are very high.
• Uterine lavage should only be performed if indicated (dead autolyzed fetus or lengthy manipulation).
• Pain management and antimicrobial therapy should be considered on a per case basis.
• Vulvar swelling can be reduced by application of cold compresses (ice) for a few minutes every couple of hours.
• Prevention of adhesions from necrotic vaginitis may be prevented by placement of vaginal tampons covered with protective ointment (lanolin and oxytetracycline).
• Neonatal resuscitation and care should be immediately provided.

D

SURGICAL CONSIDERATIONS AND TECHNIQUES

Cesarean section should be considered if manipulation is not possible.

MEDICATIONS

DRUGS OF CHOICE

- Epidural: Lidocaine 2% (1 mL/100 kg)
- Sedation: Xylazine (0.1 mg/kg), butorphanol (0.05 mg/kg)
- Anesthesia: In the field use combination of xylazine, ketamine, and butorphanol
- Tocolytic: Clenbuterol IM (300 μg in camels, 100 μg in SAC), epinephrine IV (1:1000 IU per mL, 5 mL in SAC, 10 mL in camels), N-butylscopolammonium bromide (4 mg/10 kg, camels)
- Uterotonic: Oxytocin IM (5–10 IU in SAC, 20–30 IU in camels)
- Antimicrobials: Ceftiofur (2.2. mg/kg IM), procaine penicillin G IM (22,000 IU/kg)
- NSAID: Flunixin meglumine (1.1 mg/kg IV or SQ)

CONTRAINDICATIONS

Appropriate meat and milk withdrawal times must be followed.

PRECAUTIONS

Do not handle camel dystocia with the camel in a standing position.

POSSIBLE INTERACTIONS

Ketamine has a severe depressing effect on the fetus and should be avoided if the fetus is alive.

FOLLOW-UP

EXPECTED COURSE AND PROGNOSIS

- Recovery and prognosis for fertility depends on length of manipulation. Normal fertility is expected in females with no postpartum complications.
- Delayed involution and decreased fertility is expected following prolonged manipulations, retained placenta or uterine infections.

- Prognosis for dam survival is poor if the uterus or broad ligaments are compromised.
- Prognosis for fetal survival is poor if not extracted within 90 minutes of rupture of the chorioallantois.

POSSIBLE COMPLICATIONS

- Retained placenta
- Necrotic vaginitis
- Uterine, cervical, or vagina tears
- Toxic metritis and peritonitis

CLIENT EDUCATION

- Keep good breeding record.
- Learn the normal signs of parturition and how to recognize obstetric situations.
- Avoid excessive manipulations and call for veterinary help as soon as possible.

PATIENT CARE

- Provide good-quality hay and water and an area of exercise.
- Monitor appetite and any signs of depression.
- Monitor mothering behavior and lactation.
- Perform a postpartum evaluation 10–15 days after delivery.

PREVENTION

- Proper feeding and exercise during pregnancy.
- Observe rules for age, weight, and height at mating for maiden females.

MISCELLANEOUS

ASSOCIATED CONDITIONS

n/A

AGE-RELATED FACTORS

- Older primiparous females are at high risk (failure of vestibular dilation)
- Age at first mating

ZOONOTIC POTENTIAL

Wear protective gear for manipulation if brucellosis, chlamydiosis, and Q fever are endemic.

PREGNANCY

N/A

BIOSECURITY

N/A

PRODUCTION MANAGEMENT

- Close monitoring of females at term.
- Increase frequency of observation near term (parturition barn with webcam).
- Use electronic alerting devices (i.e., vulvar devices) in extremely valuable camels.

SYNONYMS

N/A

ABBREVIATIONS

- IM = intramuscular
- IV = intravenous
- NSAIDs = nonsteroidal anti-inflammatory drugs
- SAC = South American camelids

SEE ALSO

- Camelid: Reproduction
- Cesarean Section: Camelid
- Uterine Torsion: Camelid

Suggested Reading

Rodriguez JS, Pearson LK, Tibary A. Parturition and obstetrics. In: Cebra et al. eds, Llama and Alpaca Care: Medicine, Surgery, Reproduction, Nutrition, and Herd Health. Philadelphia: Elsevier, 2014, pp. 274–86.

Tibary A, Anouassi A: Obstetrics in camels. In: Adams GP, Skidmore L eds, Advances in Camelid Reproduction. International Veterinary Information Service, 2001, A1005.0501.

Tibary A, Rodriguez JS, Anouassi A, et al. Management of dystocia in camelids. Proc Am Assoc Bov Pract 2008, 41: 166–76.

Tibary A, Rodriguez J, Walker P, et al. Neonatal care and neonatal emergencies in camelids. Proc Am Assoc Bov Pract 2008, 41: 177–84.

Author Ahmed Tibary
Consulting Editor Ahmed Tibary

DYSTOCIA: SMALL RUMINANT

BASICS

OVERVIEW
• Difficult parturition characterized by prolongation of stage 1 or stage 2 of labor.
• Early recognition of dystocia and appropriate assistance make the difference in the life of the fetus and of the dam.

INCIDENCE/PPREVALENCE
• Incidence is highly variable (3–34%).
• Difference between sheep and goat is controversial.
• Certain breeds (pygmy goats, Dorset sheep, and crossbred Texel sheep) are overrepresented in some studies.
• There is a reported higher incidence of dystocia with twins (11%) and triplets (14%) versus that seen in singleton births (10%).
• Incomplete cervical dilation is the most common cause of dystocia (up to 43.5%).
• Incidence of fetal maldispositions are the most common fetal causes of dystocia in ewes (25%) and does (19.1%).

GEOGRAPHIC DISTRIBUTION
Worldwide

SYSTEMS AFFECTED
• Reproductive
• Musculoskeletal

PATHOPHYSIOLOGY
• Dystocia can be due to fetomaternal disproportion, fetal maldisposition (abnormal presentation, position, or posture), uterine inertia, or failure/incomplete cervical dilation.
• Uterine torsion, hydrops conditions, conditions secondary to vaginal prolapse (especially in sheep), and perineal herniation can result in dystocia in a low percentage of cases.
• Management, genetics, nutrition, and/or metabolic state of the animal can predispose to dystocia.
• Stage 1 of labor and cervical dilation lasts 6–12 hours for doelings and ewe lambs and 4–8 hours in adults.
• Stage 2 of labor begins with rupture of the allantochorion and ends with expulsion of a fetus. It lasts 1–4 hours in doelings and ewe lambs and 30 minutes to 1 hour in adults.

HISTORICAL FINDINGS
No apparent progress within an hour of first seeing the fetal membranes, or 70 min in doelings and ewe lambs.

SIGNALMENT
Periparturient females

PHYSICAL EXAMINATION FINDINGS
Fetal membranes, fluid and or bloody to serosanguinous discharges from the vagina, abdominal contractions with straining, anorexia, and colicky behavior.

GENETICS
• Small or prolific breeds

• Bucks and rams size, especially when mating to doelings and ewe lambs.
• Bucks and rams that are known to produce excessively large offspring (fetal oversize).

CAUSES AND RISK FACTORS
• Breed predisposition: Pygmy goats, Dorset sheep and crossbred Texel sheep
• Poor BCS
• Pregnancy toxemia or other metabolic disorders
• Oversized singleton fetuses
• Clover pasture may predispose to failure of cervical dilation

DIAGNOSIS

DIFFERENTIAL DIAGNOSES
• Abortion, uterine torsion, bloat, cystitis, hydrops conditions as well as displacement and/or torsion of the abomasum, cecum, or mesentery may all present with similar clinical signs of colicky behavior and straining.
• Abortion and cystitis may also have a similar looking serosanguinous discharge from the vagina.

CBC/BIOCHEMISTRY/URINALYSIS
• Hypocalcemia, and pregnancy toxemia (ketosis with an elevated anion gap).
• Elevated creatinine kinase, and lactic acidosis (uterine torsion, and exhaustion).
• Anemia (uterine rupture). Loss of blood and parasites can cause a ewe or doe to be very anemic and weak and hence predispose to dystocia as well.
• Neutrophilia and increased fibrinogen (inflammatory/infectious process).
• Urinalysis: Ketonuria (pregnancy toxemia), presence of bacteria and neutrophils (cystitis), increased protein (amyloidosis).

OTHER LABORATORY TESTS
N/A

IMAGING
• Imaging may help determine proper management of dystocia.
• Radiographs for determination of fetal number.
• Ultrasonography to determine fetal viability and uterine integrity.

OTHER DIAGNSTIC PROCEDURES
• Accurate history and physical examination are imperative in appropriate management of dystocia.
• Vaginoscopy is helpful if no fetal parts are visible at the vulva (incomplete cervical dilation) and in very small patients.
• Vaginal examination with sterile obstetric lube and gloved hand to assess cervical dilation and fetal abnormalities and abnormalities of presentation, position, and posture.

PATHOLOGIC FINDINGS
Incomplete cervical dilation, abnormalities of presentation, position and posture, fetal oversize, fetal anasarca, congenital abnormalities, ruptured uterus, metritis, vaginal lacerations, peritonitis are all pathologic findings of dystocia.

TREATMENT

THERAPEUTIC APPROACH
• Medical management of dystocia includes standard therapies such as analgesia, fluids, oxytocin, and antibiotics.
• Hypertonic saline, steroids, dextrose, and blood transfusions may be warranted if shock, pregnancy toxemia, and anemia are present.
• Tetanus prophylaxis if no recent history of tetanus vaccination.
• Correction of fetal malpresentation, position, and posture may be possible if complete cervical dilation has been achieved.
• Caudal epidural analgesia helps with obstetric manipulations.
• Epinephrine can be administered to help relax the uterus during manipulation of the fetus.
• Adequate lubrication should be provided during manipulation.
• There are a multitude of fetal maldispositions but similar principles apply and rules of obstetric manipulations should always be followed (i.e., ample lubrication, correct diagnosis, retropulsion, mutation, and traction).
• It is important to ascertain that fetal parts belong to the same fetus and there are both anterior or posterior before traction is initiated.
• Elevation of the patient's hind legs may provide more room for manipulation.
• Traction should be moderate in a downward fashion and synchronized with the dam's contractions. Slight rotation of the fetus during traction is helpful.
• In anterior presentation, once the forelimbs are extended, the head will often flex back. Extension of the head may be aided by grasping the bony orbits or placing a head snare.
• In cranial longitudinal presentation, dorso-sacral position with forelimbs extended posture and downward flexion of the head, elevation of the hindlimbs before repulsion helps to provide space for correction. A head snare or grasping of the orbits may be necessary to prevent the head from flexing again.
• A caudal/posterior longitudinal presentation, dorso-sacral position with coxofemoral extension is not considered abnormal but risk for premature umbilical rupture and incomplete cervical dilation are increased.

(CONTINUED)

• Bilateral hip flexion (breech) must be corrected by pushing the rump forward and grasping a rear foot and flexing it at the fetlock and hock to reorient the legs to coxo-femoral extension. The procedure is repeated on the other limb, then the fetus is extracted.
• Cranial longitudinal presentation, dorso-pubic position with flexion of the forelimb is best corrected by mutation into a caudal longitudinal presentation and dorso-sacral position by reaching for the hind feet over the head.
• Manipulation time should be kept to a minimum. Fetotomy may be performed if the fetuses are dead, the cervix is completely dilated, and there is enough room.

SURGICAL CONSIDERATIONS AND TECHNIQUES
Cesarean section should be considered if the fetuses are alive.

MEDICATIONS

DRUGS OF CHOICE
• Antiobitic: Pencillins, cephalosporins, tetracyclines, florfenicol.
• Supportive therapy: Flunixin meglumine, intravenous fluids (dextrose, hypertonic saline, calcium, phosphorus, magnesium).

CONTRAINDICATIONS
• Aminoglycosides and enrofloxacin should not be used in cases of dystocia.
• Meat and milk withdrawal times should be followed.

PRECAUTIONS
N/A

FOLLOW-UP

EXPECTED COURSE AND PROGNOSIS
• Prognosis for life and fertility is good with early intervention, especially when there are no metabolic disorders.
• About half of obstetric situation will require surgery (57.3% in ewes and 47.7% in does).

POSSIBLE COMPLICATIONS
• Metritis, vaginitis, peritonitis, cystitis, nerve injury, anemia, and shock in the dam
• Neonatal loss from sepsis or respiratory compromise

CLIENT EDUCATION
• Recognition of signs of labor and dystocia
• Welfare aspects of obstetric manipulations

PATIENT CARE
• Monitor dam for signs of anemia, septicemia, shock, and infection.
• Monitoring neonates for adequate consumption of colostrum and milk.

PREVENTION
• Adequate nutrition and assessment of BCS
• Appropriate breeding management including correct pairings to avoid fetal oversize
• Close monitoring of preparturient females (use of gestation charts and observation).

MISCELLANEOUS

ASSOCIATED CONDITIONS
Pregnancy toxemia, anemia due to parasites, metritis, vaginitis, peritonitis, and shock

AGE-RELATED FACTORS
• Primiparous females at high risk.
• Older dairy does and ewes need to be watched closely for metabolic problems.

ZOONOTIC POTENTIAL
Several bacterial diseases that cause abortion are zoonotic and risk is increased during dystocia management.

PREGNANCY
N/A

BIOSECURITY
Testing and quarantine of new animals to prevent abortion

PRODUCTION MANAGEMENT
• Timely pregnancy diagnosis, monitoring of BCS, and adequate nutrition to prevent pregnancy toxemia.
• Proper facilities for management of lambing/kidding.
• Close monitoring of parturient females.
• Improper nutrition during gestation negatively influences survival rate, postpartum interval, milk production, and weaning weights.

SYNONYMS
N/A

ABBREVIATION
BCS = body condition score

SEE ALSO
• Abortion: Small Ruminant
• Cesarean Section: Small Ruminant
• Neonatology: Caprine
• Neonatology: Ovine (see www.fiveminutevet.com/ruminant)

Suggested Reading
Brounts S, Hawkins J, Baird A, Glickman L. Outcome and subsequent fertility of sheep and goats undergoing cesarean section because of dystocia: 110 cases (1981–2001). JAVMA 2004, 224: 275–9.
FAZD Center. Major Zoonotic Disease of Sheep and Goats. http://iiad.tamu.edu/wp-content/uploads/2012/06/Meat-Goat-and-Sheep-Part-2-English.pdf
Gimenez D, Rodning S. Reproductive management in sheep and goats. aces.edu/pubs/docs/A/ANR-1316/ANR-1316.pdf. 2007: 1–12.
Purohit G. Dystocia in the sheep and goat – A review. Ind J Small Rumin 2006, 12: 1–12.
Sobiraj A. [Birth difficulties in sheep and goats–evaluation of patient outcome from seven lambing periods in an obstetrical clinic]. Dtsch Tieraztl Wochenschr 1994, 101: 471–6.
Author Julie A. Gard
Consulting Editor Ahmed Tibary

 Client Education Handout available online

ECHINOCOCCOSIS

BASICS

OVERVIEW
Echinococcosis is a zoonotic disease condition caused by infection with larvae of *Echinococcus* spp. tapeworms.

INCIDENCE/PREVALENCE
N/A

GEOGRAPHIC DISTRIBUTION
Worldwide with the exception of Iceland and Greenland. Each species has a distinct geographic range.

SYSTEMS AFFECTED
- Nervous
- Cardiovascular
- Musculoskeletal
- Digestive
- Urinary
- Respiratory

PATHOPHYSIOLOGY
- *Echinococcus* spp. have an indirect life cycle. In many cases, the parasite cycles through specific predators or scavengers, and their prey.
- The definite hosts of *Echinococcus* are canines and intermediate hosts are herbivores and small rodents.
- The final hosts are canines which become infected by ingesting the muscles and organs containing cysts of the intermediate hosts. The protoscolex evaginates and attaches to the intestinal wall and develops into adult stages in 32–80 days. Later, gravid proglottids release eggs which are passed into feces. Under favourable conditions, these eggs remain viable for several weeks or months in pastures or on fomites. If exposed to sunlight, they are viable for a short period of time.
- The intermediate hosts are domesticated and wild herbivores.
- The intermediate hosts ingest eggs while grazing or scavenging depending on their feeding habits. The oncospheres of eggs hatch and penetrate into the intestinal wall. Later, they migrate to various organs including the liver, lungs, heart, brain, bones, kidney, skeletal muscles, and spleen through the circulatory system and develop into a hydatid cyst. The cyst contains protoscolices and daughter cysts which fill the cyst interior.

HISTORICAL FINDINGS
- History will vary depending on location of cysts.
- A small liver cyst may not produce any symptoms for 10–20 years until it gets large enough to be felt by physical examination.

SIGNALMENT
- The intermediate hosts of *E. granulosus* are sheep, goat, swine, cattle, horses, and camels where the final hosts are canids, felids, and hyaenids. Sheep and goats are the most commonly affected ruminant species.
- The intermediate hosts of *E. multilocularis* are small rodents and the final hosts are canids, felids, coyotes, and wolves. Dogs may also act as an intermediate host by ingesting eggs shed in feces or through autoinfection and mechanical vector by carrying feces on their fur. The larvae proliferate indefinitely, resulting in excessive invasion of surrounding tissues.
- The larval stage of *E. vogeli* develops in both external and internal parts of organs, resulting in multiple vesicles. The intermediate hosts associated are rodents and the final hosts are bush dogs. *E. vogeli* may undergo exogenous and endogenous proliferation, resulting in multi-chambered cysts in accidental hosts such as primates. But the natural hosts seem to develop exogenous proliferation.
- The intermediate hosts for *E. oligarthrus* are rodents and the final hosts are wild felids.

PHYSICAL EXAMINATION FINDINGS
Pain in upper right part of the abdomen, chest pain, bloody sputum, cough, fever, severe skin itching, diarrhea.

GENETICS
Traditionally, the *Echinococcus* spp. have been divided into different strains, named G1 to G10.

CAUSES AND RISK FACTORS
- *Echinococcus* spp.
- Cattle, deer, pigs, sheep
- Feces of dogs, wolves, or coyotes

DIAGNOSIS

DIFFERENTIAL DIAGNOSES
Gastrointestinal parasitism, multifocal tumors, CNS diseases

CBC/BIOCHEMISTRY/URINALYSIS
N/A

OTHER LABORATORY TESTS
ELISA, PCR (copro-DNA assay), indirect immunofluorescence, indirect hemagglutination, immunoblotting, latex agglutination, and rarely complement fixation.

IMAGING
Imaging techniques such as MRI or CT scan followed by serologic tests.

OTHER DIAGNOSTIC PROCEDURES
Direct examination of intestine during postmortem

PATHOLOGIC FINDINGS
- When liver cyst ruptures, marked and transient elevation of cholestatic enzyme levels occurs. It is often associated with hyperamylasemia and eosinophilia.
- Brain cyst or eye cyst and calcified cysts often induce no or low antibody titers.

TREATMENT

THERAPEUTIC APPROACH
Treatment is not commonly pursued in food-producing animals due to a low rate of diagnosis and prolonged treatment course. The following are based off of the human literature.
- Therapeutic treatment with anthelmintics is effective.
- Percutaneous treatment of the hydatid cysts with the PAIR (puncture, aspiration, injection, re-aspiration) technique.

SURGICAL CONSIDERATIONS AND TECHNIQUES
Surgical removal of cysts may also be practiced but this is complicated.

MEDICATIONS

DRUGS OF CHOICE
The following anthelmintics and dose rates are based off of the human literature. Literature involving treatment of echinococcosis in ruminants is scarce at the time of publication.
- Albendazole at 10–15 mg/kg body weight q12h for 1–6 months. For patients weighing <60 kg, total dose should not exceed 800 mg/day.
- Mebendazole can also be used at 40–50 mg/kg body weight for several months.
- Postoperative chemotherapy with praziquantel and albendazole or mebendazole long term (around 2 years), may be practiced.

CONTRAINDICATIONS
N/A

PRECAUTIONS
Appropriate withdrawal times must be observed after compounds are administered to food-producing animals.

POSSIBLE INTERACTIONS
N/A

FOLLOW-UP

EXPECTED COURSE AND PROGNOSIS
Cystic echinococcosis caused by *E. granulosus* is the most common form of disease in comparison to alveolar echinococcosis caused by *E. multilocularis* though the latter is more pathogenic and difficult to treat.

POSSIBLE COMPLICATIONS
When the cyst ruptures there is a high chance of spreading infection to multiple organs.

Cyst rupture may cause allergic reactions, fever, low blood pressure, and shock.

CLIENT EDUCATION
• Anthelminthic calendar and training should be provided.
• Avoid contact with infected dogs and provide regular deworming for dogs.

PATIENT CARE
N/A

PREVENTION
• Regular examination of dogs, sheep, and goats, and treatment with anthelmintic drugs.
• The on-farm slaughter of small ruminants should be abandoned.
• Humans should avoid consuming raw meat.

 MISCELLANEOUS

ASSOCIATED CONDITIONS
• Inflammatory nodules or tumors
• Other intestinal parasites

ZOONOTIC POTENTIAL
Humans are infected by hand-to-mouth transfer of *Echinococcus* eggs. Humans are the dead end host. Transmission from humans to humans does not occur. However, human echinococcosis occurs in four forms: mainly cystic echinococcosis caused by *E. granulosus*; alveolar echinococcosis caused by *E. multilocularis*; polycystic echinococcosis caused by *E. vogeli*; and unicystic echinococcosis caused by *E. oligarthrus*. The most important forms of disease in humans are cystic echinococcosis and alveolar echinococcosis. Cystic echinococcosis is also referred to as alveolar hydatidosis.

SYNONYM
Hydatid disease

ABBREVIATIONS
• CNS = central nervous system
• CT = computed tomography
• ELISA = enzyme-linked immunosorbent assay
• MRI = magnetic resonance imaging
• PCR = polymerase chain reaction

SEE ALSO
• Brain Assessment and Dysfunction (see www.fiveminutevet.com/ruminant)
• Parasite Control Programs: Small Ruminant

Suggested Reading
Ammann RW, Eckert J. Cestodes: Echinococcus. Gastroenterol Clin North Am 1996, 25: 655–89.
Internet Resources
• http://www.cdc.gov/parasites/echinococcosis/biology.html
• http://www.cfsph.iastate.edu/Factsheets/pdfs/echinococcosis.pdf
• http://www.who.int/mediacentre/factsheets/fs377/en/
Author Saluna Pokhrel
Consulting Editor Kaitlyn A. Lutz

E

EMBRYO TRANSFER: BOVINE

BASICS

OVERVIEW
• Embryo transfer (ET) is an advanced reproductive technology in which embryos from a superstimulated female are collected and transferred to recipient females.
• Embryos can be produced in vivo or in vitro and may be transferred fresh or after cryopreservation.
• Embryo transfer is used to improve genetics, improve reproductive efficiency of females, and reduce disease transmission.

INCIDENCE/PREVALENCE
N/A

GEOGRAPHIC DISTRIBUTION
Worldwide

SYSTEMS AFFECTED
Reproductive

PATHOPHYSIOLOGY
• ET is a multifactorial process that depends on a series of carefully orchestrated sequential steps.
• Poor performance in any of the steps could directly affect the success rate and final outcome of any program.

SIGNALMENT
• Females of breeding age
• Some techniques (oocyte collection and IVF) may use prepubertal calves

HISTORICAL FINDINGS
• Genetically superior females
• Infertility or inability to maintain pregnancy
• Animals with oviductal problems may be used as oocyte donors

PHYSICAL EXAMINATION FINDINGS
Donor Selection
• Criteria: genetic merit and reproductive soundness
  ◦ Insure genetic progress for selected traits
  ◦ Avoid genetic diseases
  ◦ Cycling regularly with no abnormalities of the reproductive tract, normal conception rates (ideal)
• Other considerations: good body condition, free of contagious/systemic disease, minimum of 50–60 days postpartum, current on vaccinations

Recipient Selection
• Criteria to consider:
  ◦ Reproductive performance/ability to calve
  ◦ Disposition/mothering ability
  ◦ Udder conformation/milking ability
• Other considerations: body condition score, adequate nutrition, free of contagious/systemic disease, minimum 50–70 days postpartum (first calf heifers >70 days postpartum), virgin heifers cycling and minimum 13–14 months of age, current on vaccinations

GENETICS
• Genetic selection/improvement is the primary goal of ET and associated biotechnologies.
• There is a significant variation in response to superovulation between *Bos taurus* and *Bos indicus* cattle.
• The embryos of some breeds (Jersey) do not tolerate cryopreservation because of high fat content.

CAUSES AND RISK FACTORS
N/A

DIAGNOSIS

DIFFERENTIAL DIAGNOSES
N/A

CBC/BIOCHEMISTRY/URINALYSIS
N/A

OTHER LABORATORY TESTS
• Serum AMH concentrations may be used to indicate the ovarian follicular reserve and help predict a donor's response to a superstimulation protocol.
• Pregnancy diagnosis using PSPB 25 days following transfer.

IMAGING
Transrectal ultrasonography for pregnancy diagnosis 20–25 days following transfer.

DIAGNOSTIC PROCEDURES
• See "Treatment/Donor Management/Embryo collection, evaluation, and handling."
• Embryo cryopreservation: Conventional slow freezing (requires specialized equipment) or vitrification.

PATHOLOGIC FINDINGS
N/A

TREATMENT

Donor Management
• Single embryos or multiple embryos may be collected from naturally ovulating or superstimulated (superovulated) donors. Ideally 2–4 donors are prepared in order to share cost of recipient management if fresh ET is considered.
• Superstimulation
  ◦ Superstimulation is achieved using FSH.
  ◦ Superstimulation protocols are most successful if initiated during the mid-luteal phase (day 8–12) of the donor's estrous cycle.
  ◦ An alternative is to start superstimulation after CIDR treatment. A simple protocol consists of (Day 0 = Start FSH, 36 hours after GnRH):
    ▪ Day -8: PGF2$_\alpha$ and insert CIDR
    ▪ Day −1: GnRH injection

▪ Day 0: FSH pm
▪ Day 1: FSH am/pm
▪ Day 2: FSH am/pm
▪ Day 3: FSH am/pm, PGF2$_\alpha$ am
▪ Day 4: FSH + remove CIDR + PGF2$_\alpha$ am
▪ Day 5: GnRH am and AI pm
▪ Day 6: AI am
▪ Day 12: embryo collection am
  ◦ Response is variable and depends on age, breed, lactational status, nutritional status, and stage of the cycle at which treatment is initiated.
• Artificial insemination
  ◦ AI should be performed twice with a 10–12 hour interval to cover the range of time over which ovulations may occur.
  ◦ AI performed 4–6 hours after the onset of estrus and repeated once 10–12 hours later.
  ◦ Timed AI at 48 hours after progesterone removal and repeated once 60 hours after progesterone removal.
  ◦ Double insemination dose may be used at each insemination.
• Embryo collection, evaluation, and handling
  ◦ Embryo collection is performed nonsurgically 6–8 days after insemination.
  ◦ The uterine horns can be flushed individually or both at the same time.
  ◦ Caudal epidural analgesia is placed and a Foley catheter is introduced using the rectovaginal technique. The balloon is placed at the base of one horn and inflated.
  ◦ Flushing medium used is Dulbecco's PBS with added fetal calf serum or a commercially prepared variant.
  ◦ Flushing medium should be warmed to body temperature and protected from ultraviolet light and contaminants.
  ◦ The flushing medium is recovered into embryo filters and the embryos quality graded based on stage of development and morphology according to IETS guidelines.
  ◦ Embryos should be kept in a holding medium, washed according to IETS recommendation then loaded in straws (0.25 mL French straws) for fresh ET or submitted to cryopreservation if Grade I or II.

Recipient Management
• Fresh ET requires preparation of 8–10 recipients per donor.
• Pregnancy rates following ET are best when the recipient is in estrus from 36 hours before to 12 hours after the donor.
• With fresh embryos, pregnancy rates were similar if the donor and recipient estrus were −1.0 to +1.0 days.
• For transfer of frozen embryos, the recipient must be synchronous with the stage of development of the embryo.
• Recipients can be selected from a large pool based on heat detection or synchronized in order to match the stage of development of the embryo.
• Embryo transfer procedure

○ Nonsurgical transfer (may consider placement of caudal epidural).
○ Transrectal palpation (or ultrasonography) should be performed to confirm the presence and side of CL at the time of transfer.
○ Embryo is deposited approximately one third of the way up the uterine horn ipsilateral to the CL.
○ A negative correlation has been demonstrated between the time spent manipulating the cervix/uterine horn and pregnancy rates.

SURGICAL CONSIDERATIONS
N/A

MEDICATIONS

DRUGS OF CHOICE
• pFSH for superstimulation: in decreasing dose, total dose (400 mg NIH-FSH-P1 or 700 IU)
• PGF2$_\alpha$ (dinoprost tromethamine 25 mg, IM) or cloprostenol (500 µg, IM)
• CIDR (1.3 mg of progesterone)
• GnRH (100 µg, IM)

CONTRAINDICATIONS
Appropriate milk and meat withdrawal times must be followed.

PRECAUTIONS
N/A

POSSIBLE INTERACTIONS
N/A

FOLLOW-UP

EXPECTED COURSE AND PROGNOSIS
• Pregnancy rates are in the range 55–80% with fresh embryos. A reduction of 10–20% is observed with frozen-thawed embryos.
• Success of an ET program can be measured by the following:
○ Number of CL from superstimulation (measures response)
○ Number of embryos obtained per CL (measures donor selection and flushing technique)
○ Number of fertilized embryos (measures donor selection, semen quality, semen handling, and AI technique)
○ Number of recipients that become pregnant (measures embryo quality, recipient selection, management, and transfer technique)

○ Number of embryos transferred that produce calves (measures embryo quality, recipient selection/management, and transfer technique)

POSSIBLE COMPLICATIONS
• Perforation of the vagina or uterus may occur if the practitioner is unskilled or inexperienced.
• Uterine infection is possible if the technique is not performed cleanly.

CLIENT EDUCATION
Clients should be aware of the expected pregnancy rates and factors affecting success in an ET program.

PATIENT CARE
• Donors:
○ PGF2$_\alpha$ or analogs are administered following embryo collection in order to prevent pregnancy.
○ Donors can be superstimulated at 2-month intervals for 3 treatments without any appreciable decrease in embryo recovery rate.
• Recipients:
○ Pregnancy diagnosis should be performed and confirmed at a later date.
○ Pregnant recipients are managed similar to any pregnant cow.

PREVENTION
N/A

MISCELLANEOUS

ASSOCIATED CONDITIONS
Increased early embryonic loss and abnormal pregnancies (hydrallantois, abnormal offspring syndrome) are associated with transfer of SCNT embryos.

AGE-RELATED FACTORS
N/A

ZOONOTIC POTENTIAL
N/A

PREGNANCY
Check for early embryo loss.

BIOSECURITY
• Donors and recipients should have health screening and infectious disease testing prior to use in an ET program.
• Bull studs are subjected to strict health requirements and disease control.

PRODUCTION MANAGEMENT
• ET enables acceleration of the proliferation of genetic material from the dam as well as the sire.

• ET is beneficial for preservation of genetics, transport of genetics internationally, and disease control/biosecurity.

SYNONYMS
N/A

ABBREVIATIONS
• AI = artificial insemination
• AMH = anti-Mullerian hormone
• CIDR = controlled internal drug release
• CL = corpus luteum
• ET = embryo transfer
• FSH = follicle stimulating hormone
• GnRH = gonadotropin releasing hormone
• IETS = International Embryo Technology Society
• IVF = in vitro fertilization
• PBS = phosphate buffered saline
• PGF2$_\alpha$ = prostaglandin F2$_\alpha$
• PSPB = pregnancy-specific protein B
• SCNT = somatic cell nuclear transfer

SEE ALSO
• Artificial Insemination: Bovine
• Estrus Synchronization: Bovine
• Reproductive Ultrasonography: Bovine (see www.fiveminutevet.com/ruminant)

Suggested Reading

Blondin P. Status of embryo production in the world. Anim Reprod 2015, 12: 356–8.
Farin PW, Moore K, Drost M. Assisted reproductive technologies in cattle. In: Youngquist R ed, Current Therapy in Large Animal Theriogenology, 2nd ed. Ames: Saunders, 2007; pp. 496–508.
Givens MD, Marley SD. Approaches to biosecurity in bovine embryo transfer programs. Theriogenology 2008, 69: 129–36.
Hasler JF. Forty years of embryo transfer in cattle: A review focusing on the journal Theriogenology, the growth of the industry in North America, and personal reminiscences. Theriogenology 2014, 81: 152–69.
International Embryo Technology Society. Manual of the IETS, 4th ed. http://www.iets.org/pubs_educational.asp
Sa Filho MF, Nichi M, et al. Sex-sorted sperm for artificial insemination and embryo transfer programs in cattle. Anim Reprod 2014, 11: 217–24.

Author Alexis Campbell
Consulting Editor Ahmed Tibary

E

EMBRYO TRANSFER: CAMELID

BASICS

OVERVIEW
- Embryo transfer (ET) is an important reproductive biotechnology to propagate genetically superior females and significantly reduce generation interval.
- ET offers other advantages such as reproduction of females that can no longer carry pregnancy to term because of acquired reproductive pathologies or systemic and musculoskeletal disorders that may be exacerbated by pregnancy.
- ET is an even more powerful tool for genetic improvement when combined with other biotechnologies such as in vitro production of embryos by in vitro fertilization, intracytoplasmic sperm injection, or somatic cell nuclear transfer.
- Interspecies transfer within camels (Bactrian camel embryos in dromedary) or SAC (i.e., alpaca embryos in llamas) is possible and can be used for the preservation of endangered species such as the Bactrian camel, vicuna, or guanaco.
- Use of frozen-thawed embryos in ET programs is still limited by the poor pregnancy rate.

INCIDENCE/PREVALENCE
ET is commercially used in racing camels and in llamas and alpaca.

GEOGRAPHIC DISTRIBUTION
Worldwide, depending on breed association regulations

SYSTEMS AFFECTED
Reproductive

PATHOPHYSIOLOGY
- Following ovulation and fertilization, the camelid embryo develops until the morula stage in the uterine tube. The embryo passes through the uterotubal junction and descends into the uterine cavity around 7 days after fertilization at the hatched blastocyst stage.
- Recovery of blastocysts from the uterine cavity is best performed between 8 and 9 days after mating as the embryo grows quickly and collapses after this time.
- The corpus luteum (CL) is mandatory for maintenance of pregnancy. Therefore recipients should be synchronous with the stage of embryo development and maintain their CL after transfer.
- Synchronization between donors and recipients is often difficult to achieve unless a large pool of females is available.
- Blastocysts are collected nonsurgically by uterine flushing using a Foley catheter (12–16 Fr in SAC, 18–22 Fr in camels) inserted through the cervix and manipulated trransrectally to place the balloon just cranial to the cervix. Uterine horns can be flushed separately or at the same time using

commercial embryo collection medium (DPBS or its variants).
- Flushing medium is filtered and the embryos are identified, washed using a holding medium, loaded in 0.25 or 0.5 mL straws, and transferred nonsurgically into the uteri of synchronous recipients.
- Factors affecting pregnancy rate following transfer include embryo quality, health of the recipient, and CL maintenance.
- CL maintenance (i.e., prevention of PGF2$_\alpha$ release and luteolysis) is highly dependent on technical ability of the operator.

HISTORICAL FINDINGS
- Donors are selected based on their genetic potential or performance abilities.
- Recipient should be parous and in good general and reproductive health.
- Old and maiden females are not good recipient candidates.

SIGNALMENT
N/A

PHYSICAL EXAMINATION FINDINGS
- Donors should undergo a complete physical examination and reproductive evaluation to determine their ability to ovulate and achieve fertilization and early embryo development.
- Recipient should have the following characteristics:
  - Good body condition
  - Good general health
  - Normal reproductive function
  - Normal mammary gland development and evidence of at least one normal pregnancy and lactation

GENETICS
Only genetically superior females should be used as embryo donors.

CAUSES AND RISK FACTORS
N/A

DIAGNOSIS

DIFFERENTIAL DIAGNOSES
N/A

CBC/BIOCHEMISTRY/URINALYSIS
N/A

OTHER LABORATORY TESTS
- Serum progesterone level determination is useful for screening potential recipients in large-scale ET programs.
- Serology for the most common infectious diseases is warranted for recipients.

IMAGING
Transrectal ultrasonography is required for monitoring of superovulation, mating, and induction of ovulation in donors and for selection of recipient for induction of ovulation and synchronization with donors and determination of CL quality at the time of transfer.

OTHER DIAGNOSTIC PROCEDURES
N/A

PATHOLOGIC FINDINGS
- Turbidity of the recovered flushing fluid is an indicator of possible uterine infection.
- Cytologic evaluation is recommended if return fluid contains mucus or purulent material.

TREATMENT

THERAPEUTIC APPROACH
- Embryo collection may be performed with or without prior ovarian superstimulation.
- Superstimulation of follicular development is obtained by the use of FSH, eCG, or their combination. The best results are obtained when treatment is commenced at the beginning of follicular recruitment.
- Control of follicular wave development is obtained by daily progesterone treatment for 7–14 days or by initiation of treatment 2 days after induction of ovulation.
- Ovulation is induced in donors after mating when follicles reach mature size (8–10 mm in SAC, 15–18 mm in camels) using hCG or GnRH. Ovulation is induced in the same manner in recipients.

SURGICAL CONSIDERATIONS AND TECHNIQUES
Surgical collection and transfer of embryos is possible but not common.

MEDICATIONS

DRUGS OF CHOICE
- Control of follicular wave development:
  - Camels: Daily progesterone injection (150 mg IM) for 10–14 days.
  - Llamas and alpacas: Progesterone injection (50 mg IM) or vaginal inserts for 7–14 days.
- Superstimulation:
  - FSH: Porcine FSH is administered q12h for 3–5 days in decreasing doses (total dose 150–300 mg in SAC, 300–450 mg in camels).
  - eCG: A single IM injection (1500–6000 IU in camels, 500–2000 IU in llamas, 500–1000 IU in alpacas).
  - Some protocols use one injection of eCG followed by FSH.
- Induction of ovulation:
  - hCG: IV injection (camels 1,500 IU, llamas and alpacas 750–1000 IU).
  - GnRH: IM injection (camels 100 μg, alpacas and llamas 50 μg) or buserelin (4–8 μg).
- Induction of luteolysis:
  - Donors should be given a dose of PGF2$_\alpha$ or its analogs after embryo collection (dinoprost tromethamine 25 mg in camels,

cloprostenol 500 μg in camels, 250 μg in SAC).
• Epidural analgesia: Lidocaine 2% in caudal epidural to reduce straining particularly in llamas, alpacas, and young maiden camels.
• Sedation: Xylazine (0.1 mg/kg IM) and butorphanol (0.05 mg/kg) is often necessary for sedation of alpacas.

CONTRAINDICATIONS
Appropriate meat and milk withdrawal times must be followed.

PRECAUTIONS
• Females may become refractory to superstimulation treatments
• Overstimulation of the ovaries is common problem in donors resulting is poor embryo recovery
• Some donors may fail to ovulate and develop large anovulatory follicles following superstimulation

POSSIBLE INTERACTIONS
N/A

FOLLOW-UP

EXPECTED COURSE AND PROGNOSIS
• Embryo recovery rate in absence of superstimulation varies from 60% to 80% and depends on donor fertility.
• Embryo recovery rate following superstimulation is highly variable (0–70%). The average number of transferable embryos obtained following superstimulation is 3 in SAC and 5 in camels.
• Embryo collection may be performed every 2–3 weeks in absence of superstimulation.
• Superstimulation may be repeated every 2 months.
• Pregnancy rate per transferred embryo varies between 20% and 60%.
• Pregnancy rate is optimized by using good-quality embryos transferred to recipients that ovulated on the same day or one day after the donor.
• External factors affecting pregnancy rate in recipients include general health, body condition score, and lactation status.
• The effect of side of transfer of the embryo in relationship to the CL is still controversial.

POSSIBLE COMPLICATIONS
• Uterine perforation
• Rectal perforation
• Cervical damage
• Uterine infection

CLIENT EDUCATION
• Clients should be informed about the high variability of the results of superovulation, the importance of donor fertility, male fertility, recipients' quality (health and fertility), and recipient management.
• It is important to stress that this manipulation require veterinary care and supervision and that the welfare of the animal may be compromised if not done properly.

PATIENT CARE
• Donors should be provided exercise and a nutritional plan to avoid obesity. They should be observed following flushing for any signs of discomfort or abnormal vaginal discharge.
• Recipients should be handled without stress before and after embryo transfer.

PREVENTION
• Herd health program to prevent abortive diseases
• Laboratory procedures to prevent embryo contamination

MISCELLANEOUS

ASSOCIATED CONDITIONS
Infertility, IVF

AGE-RELATED FACTORS
Embryo quality is affected by age of the donor.

ZOONOTIC POTENTIAL
Brucellosis, Q-fever

PREGNANCY
N/A

BIOSECURITY
• Male used in ET should be regularly tested for brucellosis and other potentially venereal diseases particularly if they are used in natural mating of other females.

• Some infectious disease may potentially be transmitted by the embryos.
• Quarantine should be applied to all potential embryo recipients and donors before entering an ET program.
• Embryo handling (evaluation, washing) should be performed in a clean room preferably under a hood. Embryos should be loaded and transferred aseptically.

PRODUCTION MANAGEMENT
N/A

SYNONYMS
N/A

ABBREVIATIONS
• CL = corpus luteum
• eCG = equine chorionic gonadotropin
• ET = embryo transfer
• FSH = follicle stimulating hormone
• GnRH = gonadotropin releasing hormone
• hCG = human chorionic gonadotropin

SEE ALSO
• Camelid: Reproduction
• Pregnancy Diagnosis: Camelid
• Reproductive Ultrasonography: Camelid (see www.fiveminutevet.com/ruminant)

Suggested Reading
Anouassi A, Tibary A. Development of a large commercial camel embryo transfer program: 20 years of scientific research. Anim Reprod Sci 2013, 113: 211–21.
Ratto MH, Silva ME, Huanca W, et al. Induction of superovulation in South American camelids. Anim Reprod Sci 2013, 136: 164–9.
Sumar JB. Embryo transfer in domestic South American camelids. Anim Reprod Sci 2013, 136: 170–7.
Trasorras V, Giuliano S, Mirayaga M. In vitro production of embryos in South American camelids. Anim Reprod Sci 2013, 136: 187–93.
Vaughan J, Mihm M, Wittek T. Factors influencing embryo transfer success in alpacas: A retrospective study. Anim Reprod Sci 2013, 136: 194–204.

Author Ahmed Tibary
Consulting Editor Ahmed Tibary

EMBRYO TRANSFER: SMALL RUMINANT

BASICS

OVERVIEW
• Embryo transfer (ET) is an important reproductive biotechnology to propagate genetically superior females, import new genetics, and reduce biosecurity risks.
• Cryopreservation of embryos allows easy transport around the world.
• Although other biotechnologies such as in vitro production of embryos by in vitro fertilization, intracytoplasmic sperm injection, or somatic cell nuclear transfer are available, most of ET in sheep and goats still uses embryos produced in vivo.

INCIDENCE/PREVALENCE
ET is primarily used in high-end purebred sheep and goat operations.

GEOGRAPHIC DISTRIBUTION
Countries where sheep and goat production are well developed

SYSTEMS AFFECTED
Reproductive

PATHOPHYSIOLOGY
• ET in sheep and goats relies on hormonal manipulation of the cycle for the synchronization of estrus and superovulation.
• Superstimulated donors are mated naturally or inseminated artificially at specific times after progesterone withdrawal.
• Factors affecting response to superovulation include health, individual animal, age, breed, nutritional status, and season.
• Embryo recovery from the uterine cavity is performed surgically (laparotomy or laparoscopy-assisted) 5–7 days after ovulation when the embryos are at the late morula or early blastocyst stage. Nonsurgical (transcervical) collection of embryos is possible in some large breeds of goat but is not routinely used.
• Early luteolysis is a common problem after superovulation in goats. Donors should receive another CIDR 2 days after ovulation to maintain high levels of progesterone and avoid embryo loss.
• Embryos are washed and transferred surgically to synchronous recipients. Each recipient receives two embryos in the horn ipsilateral to the CL.
• Factors affecting success of ET program include: embryo quality, health of the recipient, nutritional management, and CL maintenance.
• Surgical embryo collection may be repeated during the same season but it is preferable to allow the donor to carry a pregnancy in between 2 or 3 flushes.

HISTORICAL FINDINGS
• Donors are selected based on their genetic potential or performance.

• Recipient should be parous and have good general and reproductive health history.

SIGNALMENT
N/A

PHYSICAL EXAMINATION FINDINGS
• Donors should undergo a complete physical examination and reproductive evaluation to determine their ability to ovulate and achieve fertilization and early embryo development.
• Females should be in good health in order to undergo general anesthesia.
• Recipient should have the following characteristics:
  ○ Body condition score: 3–3.5
  ○ Good general health and current on vaccination and deworming program
  ○ Normal reproductive function
  ○ Normal mammary gland development and evidence of at least one normal pregnancy and lactation

GENETICS
Only genetically superior females should be used as embryo donors.

CAUSES AND RISK FACTORS
N/A

DIAGNOSIS

DIFFERENTIAL DIAGNOSES
N/A

CBC/BIOCHEMISTRY/URINALYSIS
Total protein and packed cell volume should be determined before anesthesia.

OTHER LABORATORY TESTS
Serology for common infectious diseases is recommended for selection of recipients.

IMAGING
• Transrectal ultrasonography is helpful in identifying number and side of ovulation in donors and recipient prior to surgery.
• Transabdominal ultrasonography for pregnancy diagnosis at 45 days.

OTHER DIAGNOSTIC PROCEDURES
N/A

PATHOLOGIC FINDINGS
Periuterine adhesions may develop after multiple surgeries.

TREATMENT

THERAPEUTIC APPROACH
• Ovarian follicular superstimulation is obtained using FSH or eCG at the end of a progesterone (CIDR) treatment.
• Several protocols have been described. A classical protocol for sheep is to start FSH on day 12 of the CIDR treatment and continue FSH q12h for 3–4 days.

• An example of a short superovulation protocol is:
  ○ Day 0, place CIDR
  ○ Day 4, FSH (36 mg pm)
  ○ Day 5, FSH (36 mg am, 24 mg pm)
  ○ Day 6, FSH (24 mg am, 24mg pm) then PGF2$_\alpha$ or analog and removal of the CIDR
  ○ Day 7, FSH (24 mg am, 16 mg pm), estrus detection and mating
  ○ Day 8, FSH (16 mg am), GnRH and estrus detection and mating
  ○ Day 14: Embryo collection
• Superstimulated females are joined to males 24–36 hours after removal of the CIDR and mating recorder. Alternatively, females can be inseminated 12–24 hours after onset of estrus (fresh semen) or 45–50 hours after CIDR removal if frozen semen is used laparoscopically. Donors are given GnRH 30–36 hours after CIDR removal.
• Recipients are synchronized in the same manner as donors and given either eCG (200 IU in season, 400–500 IU out of season) or PG 600. Estrus detection is performed after CIDR removal.

SURGICAL CONSIDERATIONS AND TECHNIQUES
• Laparoscopy-assisted technique for embryo collection and transfer is the best approach in order to minimize risks for surgical complications.
• Ewes and does should be fasted for 24 hours and water withheld for 12 hours.
• Anesthesia is obtained by administration of xylazine and ketamine. A local block with lidocaine at the portal site is recommended.
• The donor is placed in dorsal recumbency in a Trendelenburg position. An endoscope portal is placed about 5 cm lateral to midline and 10–15 cm from the base of the mammary gland. A second portal for grasping forceps is placed on midline about 4 cm from the base of the mammary gland.
• The abdominal cavity is penetrated with a trocar after insufflation with CO_2. The ovaries and uterus are visualized and CLs are counted. The grasping forceps is used through the second portal to hold and elevate the tip of one horn to the body wall. The midline incision is extended to allow exteriorization of both uterine horns.
• A Foley catheter (size 8–10 Fr) is placed at the base of the horn through a small stab incision in the serosa and blunt penetration through the muscularis and endometrium. The balloon is inflated (2–3 mL depending on size) and the uterine horn is flushed by injecting embryo collection medium (30–50 mL) from the tip of the horn towards the base.
• The procedure is repeated on the other side and the uterus is replaced and incision sites closed as per routine.
• For transfer the recipients are handled in the same manner for surgery. Only a small

proximal loop of the uterine horn ipsilateral to the CL is exteriorized and the embryos are injected in the lumen through a small tomcat catheter.

MEDICATIONS

DRUGS OF CHOICE
• Synchronization: CIDR-G (0.3 mg progesterone, vaginal)
• Superstimulation
  ○ FSH: porcine FSH, q12h for 3–4 days in decreasing doses (total dose 150–250 mg depending on breed and size)
• Induction of ovulation
  ○ GnRH: IM injection (100 μg, IM)
• Induction of luteolysis
  ○ Donors should be given a dose of PGF2$_\alpha$ (10 mg IM) or cloprostenol (250 μg, IM) after embryo collection
• Anesthesia: Xylazine (0.2 mg/kg, IM) followed 5–10 minutes later with ketamine (5–10 mg/kg, IM). Inhalation anesthesia is another option if available. Xylazine may be reversed with talazoline (2–4 mg/kg slow IV or IM) or yohimbine (0.125 mg/kg, slow IV or IM)
• Antibiotics: Procaine penicillin (20,000 IU, IM daily for 3 days)
• Anti-inflammatory: Flunixin meglumine (1.1–2.2 mg/kg IV or IM)

CONTRAINDICATIONS
Appropriate meat and milk withdrawal times must be followed.

PRECAUTIONS
Females may become refractory to superstimulation treatments.

POSSIBLE INTERACTIONS
N/A

FOLLOW-UP

EXPECTED COURSE AND PROGNOSIS
• Embryo recovery rate following superstimulation is highly variable. The average number of transferable embryos obtained following superstimulation is 5–6.

• Pregnancy rate per transferred embryo varies between 50% and 60% in well-managed programs.

POSSIBLE COMPLICATIONS
• Periuterine adhesions, broard ligament tears
• Gastrointestinal perforation
• Peritonitis

CLIENT EDUCATION
• Clients should be informed about the high variability of the results of superovulation, the importance of donor fertility, male fertility, recipients' quality (health and fertility), and recipient management.
• It is important to stress that this manipulation requires veterinary care and supervision and that the welfare of the animal may be compromised if not done properly.

PATIENT CARE
Donors and recipients should be monitored for 2–3 days for any signs of pain, loss of appetite, colic, or evidence of surgical site infection.

PREVENTION
• Herd health program to prevent abortive diseases
• Laboratory procedures to prevent embryo contamination

MISCELLANEOUS

ASSOCIATED CONDITIONS
N/A

AGE-RELATED FACTORS
Superovulation response and embryo quality is affected by age of the donor.

ZOONOTIC POTENTIAL
Brucellosis, Q fever, chlamydiosis

PREGNANCY
Pregnancy diagnosis, and fetal number determination should be performed at 45 days.

BIOSECURITY
• Males used in ET should be regularly tested for potentially venereal diseases, particularly if they are used in natural mating of other females.

• The risk for disease transmission via embryos is very limited.
• Quarantine should be applied to all potential embryo recipients and donors before entering an ET program.
• Embryo handling (evaluation, washing) should be performed in a clean room preferably under a hood. Embryos should be loaded and transferred aseptically.

PRODUCTION MANAGEMENT
• The success of ET programs is extremely dependent on excellent management of the donor and recipient animals.
• All animals should have adequate BCS and an increased nutritional plan.
• Preventive treatment should be administered at least 6 weeks prior to breeding.

SYNONYMS
N/A

ABBREVIATIONS
• CIDR = controlled intravaginal drug release
• CL = corpus luteum
• eCG = equine chorionic gonadotropin
• ET = embryo transfer
• FSH = follicle stimulating hormone
• GnRH = gonadotropin releasing hormone

SEE ALSO
• Artificial Inscmination: Small Ruminant
• Estrus Synchronization: Small Ruminant
• Pregnancy Diagnosis: Small Ruminant
• Reproductive Ultrasonography: Small Ruminant (see www.fiveminutevet.com/ruminant)

Suggested Reading
Gibbons A, Cueto M. Embryo transfer in sheep and goats: A training manual. Bariloche Experimental Station, National Institute for Agricultural Technology, Argentina, 2011.
Tibary A, Pearson LK, Van Metre DC, et al. Surgery of the sheep and goat reproductive system and urinary tract. In: Fubini S, Ducharme N eds, Farm Animal Surgery, 2nd ed. St. Louis: Elsevier, 2016, pp. 571–9.
Author Ahmed Tibary
Consulting Editor Ahmed Tibary

EMESIS

BASICS

OVERVIEW
• Emesis, or vomiting, is a centrally mediated event originating in the medulla.
• Emesis is a reflex action that results in expulsion of gastric and proximal small intestinal content through the mouth.
• Emesis is an unusual occurrence in ruminant species, and tends to be most commonly observed in goats.

INCIDENCE/PREVALENCE:
N/A

GEOGRAPHIC DISTRIBUTION
N/A

SYSTEMS AFFECTED
• Digestive
• Nervous

PATHOPHYSIOLOGY
• The medullary vomiting center receives humoral, neural, and chemical input from visceral afferent stimuli derived in the gastrointestinal tract, urogenital tract, heart, liver, and peritoneum; from the chemoreceptor trigger zone in the area postrema of the medulla; from the vestibular system; and from the cerebral cortex and limbic system.
• In ruminant species, activation of the chemoreceptor trigger zone most often results from stimulation via toxins.

HISTORICAL FINDINGS
Dependent upon the cause of disease; history should query exposure to plant and chemical toxins, dietary changes or other signs of GI disturbance. Questioning regarding potential exposure to various toxins or poisonous plants is especially pertinent when multiple animals are showing signs.

SIGNALMENT
There is no breed, gender, or age predilection, although goats are likely most often affected as a result of toxic plant ingestion (e.g., rhododendron).

PHYSICAL EXAMINATION FINDINGS
• Anorexia, hypersalivation, and retching typically precede the powerful abdominal contractions characteristic of emesis.
• Emesis involves coordinated contractions of the abdominal and diaphragmatic muscles with concurrent relaxation of the cardia, and forceful expulsion against a closed glottis to increase intra-abdominal pressure.
• The active nature of gastric content expulsion differentiates emesis from the passive process of regurgitation.
• Additional clinical signs that may accompany emesis associated with intoxication can include bloat, depression,

colic, diarrhea, ptyalism, fever, recumbency, seizures, tachycardia, fasciculations, and seizures, depending on the inciting toxin.

GENETICS
N/A

CAUSES AND RISK FACTORS
• Toxins that can cause emesis include methanol, ethanol, copper, phosphorus, arsenic, nitrates, snake venom, and petroleum products.
• Numerous poisonous plants can cause emesis with exposure dependent on plant availability. A partial list of plants includes *Solanum* spp., *Melia* (chinaberry), *Delphinium* (larkspur), cyanogenic plants (arrow grass, Johnson grass, Sudan grass, chokecherry, elderberry, etc.), nitrate accumulators (pigweed, lamb's quarter, Jimson weed, fireweed, dock, Johnson grass, oats, millet, rye, corn, sorghum, etc.), *Zigandenus* spp. (death camas), castor bean, oleander, cocklebur, *Veratrum* (hellebore), and laurel.
• Azalea/rhododendron ingestion (grayanotoxin) is a common cause of vomiting in small ruminants, particularly goats.
• Deoxynivalenol (vomitoxin) is a mycotoxin produced by toxigenic *Fusarium* species infesting corn, wheat, and barley.

DIAGNOSIS

DIFFERENTIAL DIAGNOSES
• Most cases of feed returning to the mouth of ruminants is due to regurgitation (i.e., reflux of esophageal or rumen contents into the mouth or nose).
• Excessive regurgitation typically results from physical blockage of the esophagus, cardia, or rumenoreticular outflow.
• Common conditions resulting in regurgitation include foreign bodies, tumors, papillomas, granulomas, abscesses, diaphragmatic hernia, or esophageal irritation.
• Pharyngeal lesions (e.g., balling gun injury) may also cause gagging or retching, but not true emesis.
• Soft palate lacerations or deformities may present with nasal regurgitation of water and feed material and tracheal aspiration of this material.

CBC/BIOCHEMISTRY/URINALYSIS
N/A

OTHER LABORATORY TESTS
N/A

IMAGING
No modalities are directly applicable to emesis; however, ultrasound, radiology (plain or contrast), endoscopy, or CT may be useful to investigate pharyngeal or esophageal disease.

OTHER DIAGNOSTIC PROCEDURES
Passage of a stomach tube may aid in determining if the normal passage of ingesta from mouth to the cardia is impeded.

PATHOLOGIC FINDINGS
• Toxins or toxic plants present in forestomachs
• CNS lesions involving medulla
• Additional lesions such as GI hemorrhage or erosions depending on inciting toxin

TREATMENT

THERAPEUTIC APPROACH
• Remove exposure to offending toxin or toxic plants.
• Specific antidotes or treatments for various toxins may be indicated.
• The use of laxatives, charcoal or ruminotorics to decrease toxin absorption, increase forestomach motility and passage of ingesta is unlikely to be of practical benefit in an animal that is actively vomiting.
• Transfer of fresh rumen fluid from a healthy donor is likely to restore rumen flora and function once vomiting has ceased.

SURGICAL CONSIDERATIONS AND TECHNIQUES
Rumenotomy may be indicated to remove toxicants after recent ingestion.

MEDICATIONS

DRUGS OF CHOICE
• The use of antiemetic agents in ruminant species is not well documented.
• Theoretically antiemetic drugs that can be administered IV, IM, or SC may potentially be effective in ruminants, which could include phenothiazine tranquilizers, diphenhydramine, maropitant, and metoclopramide.

CONTRAINDICATIONS
• It may be contraindicated to chemically block the elimination of toxicants from the forestomach of an animal that is actively vomiting.
• Drugs with prokinetic tendencies (metoclopramide, erythromycin) are likely contraindicated in animals that are actively vomiting.

PRECAUTIONS
• Appropriate milk and meat withdrawal times must be followed for all compounds administered to food-producing animals.

POSSIBLE INTERACTIONS
N/A

(CONTINUED)

FOLLOW-UP

EXPECTED COURSE AND PROGNOSIS
• Depending on the type, dose, and duration of a toxic insult, prognosis is guarded to good if animals are immediately removed from the source of the toxin.
• Complications including metabolic derangements, renal failure, neurologic damage, and aspiration pneumonia worsen the prognosis.

POSSIBLE COMPLICATIONS
• Complications associated with emesis (or regurgitation) include aspiration pneumonia, dehydration, electrolyte derangements, and acid-base abnormalities.
• The term "internal vomiting" has been used to describe a form of vagal indigestion whereby abomasal outflow is blocked and the abomasal contents are refluxed into the reticulorumen. Hypochloremic metabolic alkalosis often results from internal vomiting and could conceivably occur with prolonged emesis.

CLIENT EDUCATION
Identification of toxicants to which ruminants may be exposed is crucial to prevention.

PATIENT CARE
• Activity should be reduced to allow animals to recover.
• Provision of highly palatable good-quality forage can help restore normal rumen function.
• Monitor patient for continued signs of emesis and possible complications.

PREVENTION
Avoid exposure to poisonous plants or toxic compounds by maintaining a safe and clean environment and providing adequate feed to reduce the likelihood of ingestion of inappropriate plants.

MISCELLANEOUS

ASSOCIATED CONDITIONS
N/A

AGE-RELATED FACTORS
• In young animals congenital anomalies such as persistent aortic arch or esophageal diverticula/dilation may result in suspected emesis (regurgitation).
• Young animals are also more prone to diseases such as meningitis and potentially trauma to the central nervous system.

ZOONOTIC POTENTIAL
N/A

PREGNANCY
N/A

BIOSECURITY
N/A

PRODUCTION MANAGEMENT
• Pharyngeal lesions (e.g., balling gun injury) may also cause gagging or retching, but not true emesis.
• Restricting access to toxic plants and chemicals, and providing adequate good-quality feed prevents common intoxications.

SYNONYMS
Vomiting

ABBREVIATIONS
• CNS = central nervous system
• GI = gastrointestinal

SEE ALSO
• Aspiration Pneumonia
• Bloat
• Grayanotoxin
• Rumen Transfaunation (see www.fiveminutevet.com/ruminant)

Suggested Reading
Bizimenyera ES. Acute poisoning of Friesian heifers by *Solanum macrocarpon* L. ssp *dasyphyllum*. Vet Hum Toxicol 2003, 45: 222–3.
Galey FD, Holstege DM, Plumlee KH, et al. Diagnosis of oleander poisoning in livestock. J Vet Diagn Invest 1996, 8: 358–64.
Plumlee K ed. Clinical Veterinary Toxicology. St. Louis: Mosby, 2003.
Porter MB, MacKay RJ, Uhl E, Platt SR, de Lahunta A. Neurologic disease putatively associated with ingestion of *Solanum viarum* in goats. J Am Vet Med Assoc 2003, 223: 501–4, 456.
Scott, PR. Cattle Medicine. Boca Raton, FL: CRC Press, 2011, pp. 67–9. VitalBook file.
Smith BP ed. Large Animal Internal Medicine, 3rd ed. St. Louis: Mosby, 2002, p. 114.
Author Dennis D. French
Consulting Editor Erica C. McKenzie
Acknowledgment The author and book editors acknowledge the prior contribution of George Barrington.

E

ENDOCRINE DISORDERS

BASICS

OVERVIEW
• The endocrine system consists of several glands that produce substances (hormones) that are released into the circulatory system having effect in different organs.
• Endocrine glands include the hypothalamus, pituitary, gonads, adrenal, uterus, placenta, pineal, thyroid, parathyroid, and pancreas. Other organs such as the liver and kidney can produce substances with hormonal action.
• Hormones are chemically polypeptides, steroid, tyrosine derivatives (catecholamine and iodothyronine) or fatty acids.
• The endocrine system coordinates multiple mechanisms responsible for maintenance of homeostasis, mechanism of defense (immune system), metabolism, and reproduction during external and internal changes.
• Hormones and neurotransmitters in the hypothalamus and hormones synthesized in the pituitary gland control reproductive, metabolic, urinary, and digestive function.
• Endocrine disorders can be originated by primary or secondary hyperfunction of a gland, hypersecretion of hormones or hormone-like substances by non-endocrine tumors, iatrogenic syndromes, or consumption of toxic plants.

INCIDENCE/PREVALENCE
Reproductive endocrine disorders are common in dairy cows.

GEOGRAPHIC DISTRIBUTION
Worldwide

SYSTEMS AFFECTED
• Multisystemic
• Digestive
• Reproductive
• Urinary

PATHOPHYSIOLOGY
• Alterations in calcium metabolism in bulls
• Milk fever or hypocalcemia causing postpartum paresia, uterine prolapse, delayed uterine involution, and predisposing to abomasum displacement.
• Deficiency in thyroglobulin (congenital dyshormonogenetic goiter in sheep, goats, and cattle) causing subnormal growth, sparse hair coat, myxedema, weakness, and sluggish behavior (most die shortly after birth).
• The thyroid hormones influence thermoregulation and energy/protein metabolism but low T_3 may be also involved in ovarian function and postpartum diseases such as ketosis, mastitis, and endometritis in dairy cows.
• Hyperestrogenia by consumption of estrogenic plants is suspected to cause infertility and failure of cervical dilation.
• Ovarian cysts in cattle are due to lack of or poor release of LH.

• In high producing dairy cattle, increased liver metabolism is responsible for sub-physiologic levels of estradiol and progesterone, resulting in alteration of the cycle, poor estrus expression, and increased early pregnancy loss.
• Pituitary abscesses may cause neurologic signs due to secondary meningitis/encephalitis.
• Adenoma of lactotroph cells with excess of prolactin are reported in nonpregnant lactating goats.
• Prolonged gestation in cattle (up to 11 months) due to genetic failure of adenohypophysis to develop with the consequent lack of development of the adrenal cortex of the fetus.
• Prolonged gestation in sheep by consumption of toxic plants that affect development of central nervous system and hypothalamus of the lamb.
• Hypoluteoidism has been reported anecdotally as a cause of recurrent pregnancy loss in camelids. The pathophysiology of this phenomenon is not known.
• Spontaneous ovulation or luteinization of anovulatory follicle with elevated progesterone levels is suspected to be the cause of nonreceptivity in nonmated camelids.

HISTORICAL FINDINGS
• Poor health—ill thrift
• Abnormal behavior
• Poor reproductive performance
• Prolonged gestation

SIGNALMENT
• Age of onset and reproductive stage depends on disorder.
• In goats, abnormal development of the mammary gland and undesirable lactation is common in older, companion animals.

PHYSICAL EXAMINATION FINDINGS
• Most animals with reproductive endocrine disorders will not show any outward clinical signs.
• Ovarian disorders may be accompanied by abnormalities of estrous cycle and behavior.
• Animal with abnormalities of thyroid function may show poor body condition or obesity, goiter, abnormal growth, or abnormal hair coat.

GENETICS
• Autosomal recessive disorder in some breeds of sheep, goats, and cattle for congenital dyshormonogenetic goiter.
• Aplasia of the adenohypophysis is a genetic defect in Guernsey and Jersey cattle; results in hypoplasia of adrenal cortex, cessation of fetal development after 7 months, and prolonged gestation.

CAUSES AND RISK FACTORS
• Thyroid C-cell adenoma or carcinoma inducing hypercalcitoninism and osteosclerosis in bulls (excess of calcium and vitamin D in the diet).

• Pituitary abscesses are sporadic in ruminants.
• Low T_3 syndrome in cattle.
• Reduced response of parathyroids due to high calcium diets prepartum, together with high milk production and reduced dry matter intake end up in milk fever postpartum.
• Consumption of estrogenic plants (e.g., clover, alfalfa).
• High milk production, low progesterone levels, and stress predispose to ovarian cysts in dairy cattle.
• Ingestion of the toxic plant *Veratrum californicum* by ewes in early pregnancy causes craniofacial deformity and aplasia/hypoplasia of the fetal pituitary; results in hypoplasia of the adrenal cortex, fetus continues to grow but prolonged gestation.

DIAGNOSIS

DIFFERENTIAL DIAGNOSES
• Diseases or conditions affecting hormonal levels
• Postpartum diseases in dairy cattle
• Metabolic disorders

CBC/CHEMISTRY/URINALYSIS
Calcium and vitamin D levels

OTHER LABORATORY TESTS
Hormone assays:
• Hormonal assays are rarely performed in production animals except in research setting or for very valuable animals.
• Progesterone assays can confirm the presence of luteal tissue. Serum progesterone levels in animals with recurrent pregnancy loss may be indicative of poor luteal function.
• Inhibin and anti-Mullerian hormone determination are both helpful in the confirmation of diagnosis of granulosa-theca cell tumors (GTCT).
• Thyroid hormones determination may be helpful in the diagnosis of hypothyroidism. However, the interpretation of these hormones is difficult.

IMAGING
Ultrasonography of genital tract for ovarian cysts or tumors

OTHER DIAGNOSTIC PROCEDURES
• Biopsy
• Histopathology and immunohistochemistry

PATHOLOGIC FINDINGS
• The thyroid C-cell adenoma in bulls is characterized by tumor masses in the thyroid gland including polyhedral to spindle shaped with scanty cytoplasm, lightly eosinophilic and indistinctly outlined. Oval or elongate nuclei with one or more nucleoli and evenly distributed chromatin.
• Hypoplasia of pituitary gland and ACTH-dependent part of the adrenal cortex (prolonged gestation in cattle).

• Ovarian cysts are characterized by persisting multiple follicles, lack of corpus luteum, and uterine tonicity.
• Ovarian tumors.

TREATMENT

THERAPEUTIC APPROACH
• Prostaglandin F2$_\alpha$ and dexamethasone for prolonged gestation.
• GnRH/hCG or synchronization of ovulation for ovarian cysts.
• Progesterone supplementation may be considered for animals with recurrent pregnancy loss due to hypoluteoidism.
• Calcium metabolism disturbances may be addressed by oral or IV calcium supplementation in cases of hypocalcemia.

SURGICAL CONSIDERATIONS AND TECHNIQUES
• Ovariectomy for persistent ovarian cysts or GTCT.
• Mastetectomy should be considered in companion goats with severely enlarged mammary gland.

MEDICATIONS

DRUGS OF CHOICE
• PGF2$_\alpha$ IM (25 mg in cattle and camels, 5–10 mg in small ruminants)
• Cloprostenol IM (500 µg in cattle and camels, 125 mg in small ruminants and SAC)
• Dexamethasone IM (20 mg/kg in cattle and sheep)
• Gonadorelin acetate IM (100 µg in cattle, 50 µg in goats and camelids)

CONTRAINDICATIONS
Appropriate milk and meat withdrawal times must be followed.

POSSIBLE INTERACTIONS
N/A

FOLLOW-UP
N/A

MISCELLANEOUS

ASSOCIATED CONDITIONS
Metabolic and immune disorders may also be associated with endocrine disorders.

AGE-RELATED FACTORS
N/A

ZOONOTIC POTENTIAL
N/A

PREGNANCY
• Pregnancy loss (hypoluteoidism)
• Prolonged gestation in sheep and cattle

BIOSECURITY
N/A

PRODUCTION MANAGEMENT
N/A

SYNONYMS
N/A

ABBREVIATIONS
• ACTH = adrenocorticotropic hormone
• GnRH = gonadotropin releasing hormone
• GTCT = granulosa-theca cell tumor
• hCG = human chorionic gonadotropin
• IM = intramuscular
• IV = intravenous
• LH = luteinizing hormone
• PGF2$_\alpha$ = prostaglandin F2$_\alpha$
• SAC = South American camelid
• T$_3$ = triiodothyronine

SEE ALSO
• Abortion: Bovine
• Abortion: Camelid
• Hypocalcemia: Bovine
• Hypocalcemia: Small Ruminant
• Nutrition and Metabolic Diseases: Camelid (see www.fiveminutevet.com/ruminant)
• Nutrition and Metabolic Diseases: Dairy
• Nutrition and Metabolic Disorders: Beef
• Ovarian Cystic Degeneration
• Postpartum Disorders
• Postparturient Paresis (Hypocalcemia)
• Reproductive Pharmacology

Suggested Reading
Buczinski S, Bélanger AM, Fecteau G, Roy JP. Prolonged gestation in two Holstein cows: transabdominal ultrasonographic findings in late pregnancy and pathologic findings in the fetuses. J Vet Med A Physiol Pathol Clin Med 2007, 54: 624–6.
Cornillie P, Van den Broeck W., Simoens P. Prolonged gestation in two Belgian blue cows due to inherited adenohypophyseal hypoplasia in the fetuses. Vet Rec 2007, 161: 388–91.
Fraser CM, Mays A. The Merck Veterinary Manual. 6th ed. Rahway, NJ: Merck & Co., 1986.
Hanna P. Pathology of the Endocrine System, 2012. http://people.upei.ca/hanna
Huznica GY, Kulcsar M, Rudas P. Clinical endocrinology of thyroid gland function in ruminants. Vet Med – Czech 2002, 47: 199–210.
Seimiya YM, Takahashi M, Furukawa T, Mizutani K, Kimura K, Haritani M. An aged bull with concurrent thyroid C cell carcinoma, adrenal pheochromocytoma and pituitary chromophobe adenoma. J Vet Med Sci 2009, 71: 225–8.
Van Kampen KR, Ellis LC. Prolonged gestation in ewes ingesting *Veratrum californicum*: morphological changes and steroid biosynthesis in the endocrine organs of cyclopic lambs. J Endocrinol 1972, 52: 549–60.

Author Julián A. Bartolomé
Consulting Editor Ahmed Tibary

E

ENDOMETRITIS

BASICS

OVERVIEW
- Endometritis is an inflammation of the lining of the uterus (endometrium) without signs of systemic illness. It is associated with chronic bacterial infection of the uterus beyond 3 weeks postpartum.
- Clinical endometritis is characterized by the presence of a purulent vaginal discharge (PVD).
- In subclinical endometritis, visible purulent exudate is absent and case confirmation is by finding an abnormal increase in the proportion of neutrophils in uterine cytology samples collected 21 or more days postpartum.
- PVD, while frequently associated with endometritis, is more a sign rather than a specific disease process and refers to the presence of a purulent or mucopurulent discharge in the cranial vagina that also occurs with vaginitis or cervicitis.
- Endometritis is a significant disease to the extent that it causes impaired fertility. Both clinical and subclinical endometritis reduce reproductive efficiency by lowering conception rate and increasing the incidence of embryonic loss.
- Most information is generated from and applicable to dairy cattle populations. Camelids are also commonly affected while the condition is rarely diagnosed or treated in sheep or goats.

INCIDENCE/PREVALENCE
- The reported incidence of postpartum endometritis in dairy cattle varies widely, depending on the case definition, diagnostic methodology, and the interval postpartum at examination.
- Using validated diagnostic criteria, between 3 and 5 weeks postpartum, the incidence in dairy cattle was 17%, varying from 5% to 26%.
- Endometritis, as defined here, is primarily a postpartum disease, therefore the prevalence in any given population will vary with the relative distribution of reproductive cycle stage.

GEOGRAPHIC DISTRIBUTION
Worldwide

SYSTEMS AFFECTED
Reproductive

PATHOPHYSIOLOGY
- This chapter deals with inflammation resulting from nonspecific infectious agents that are opportunistic contaminants of the tubular genital tract, primarily during the postpartum period but also affecting immune-compromised or anatomically incompetent animals at other stages of the reproductive cycle.

- Infection and inflammation of the reproductive tract is also a feature of the acute phase of many specific genital diseases (e.g., see brucellosis, toxoplasmosis, and IBR). These are, however, contagious diseases that can infect animals at any stage of the reproductive cycle and are not covered here.
- All animals experience a transient bacterial contamination of the genital tract during and after parturition. The key elements in the pathophysiology of endometritis are an impairment of the immune response of the uterus and of the physical involution and repair of the tubular genital tract required to clear bacterial infection.
- The primary mechanisms of bacterial clearance are local immunity, phagocytosis, and physical clearance as the uterus involutes. By 3–4 weeks postpartum, the number of bacteria and the variety of species have diminished substantially in healthy animals.
- Intact and functional physical barriers (i.e., vulva, vestibulovaginal sphincter, and cervix) and normal estrous cyclicity are necessary to prevent recurrent contamination of the genital tract. Estrus and estrogens appear to promote bacterial clearance while progesterone delays it.
- In dairy cattle, the negative energy balance in early lactation results in metabolic disruptions (e.g., elevated NEFA) that contribute to the inflammatory cascade and suppressed immunologic efficacy.
- Historically, in cows with endometritis the most common bacteria cultured in association with impaired reproductive function were *Truperella pyogenes*, *E. coli*, *Prevotella* spp., and *Fusobacterium necrophorum*. More recent studies using FTIR spectroscopy, RAPD and 16S ribosomal DNA PCR strongly suggest that the bacterial flora of healthy and infected postpartum cattle is both more diverse and more dynamic than previously believed. Specific bacterial involvement may also vary with farm, species, and geography. Organisms isolated from camelidae are similar to those found in cows and mares, with *E. coli* and *Strep. equi* ssp. *zooepidemicus* found most commonly.
- Toxins and enzymes from these bacteria cause inflammation of the endometrium, which may impair ovarian function, delay resumption of normal ovulatory cycles, and inhibit establishment of pregnancy.
- In camelids, the long duration of mating and the site of semen deposition (deep in utero) predisposes to severe inflammatory reaction and establishment of infection if breeding is not managed correctly.

HISTORICAL FINDINGS
- Postpartum females, generally with a history of dystocia, retained placenta, or metabolic disorders.
- Abnormal mucupurulent discharge
- In camelids, often a history of infertility and repeat breeding.

SIGNALMENT
- Postpartum females; predominantly dairy cattle 3–8 weeks after calving
- All species of camelidae
- Less commonly sheep and goats

PHYSICAL EXAMINATION FINDINGS
- Clinical signs often lacking
- Mucopurulent or purulent discharge from the vulva (PVD)
- Repeat breeder syndrome

GENETICS
N/A

CAUSES AND RISK FACTORS
- Delayed clearance of opportunistic organisms allows them to establish an infection in the uterine lumen.
- RP, dystocia, twins, metritis, anestrus, OCD, and clinical ketosis are risk factors for endometritis.
- Traumatic injury to the birth canal during breeding or parturition, as well as poor perineal and pelvic conformation, are likely contributors to chronic contamination and inflammation of the genital tract.
- Repeated (excessive) mating is reportedly the most common cause of uterine disease in camelidae.

DIAGNOSIS

DIFFERENTIAL DIAGNOSES
- Metritis
- Pyometra
- Vaginitis
- Cervicitis
- Pelvic abscess
- Uro-/pneumovagina

CBC/BIOCHEMISTRY/URINALYSIS
N/A

OTHER LABORATORY TESTS
- Uterine bacteriologic culture (collected transcervically using a guarded swab or brush) and uterine biopsy are the definitive antemortem diagnostic tests but are not timely enough and are far too costly for routine use in production animals. Their use is generally restricted to camelidae.
- Subclinical endometritis is diagnosed by uterine cytology obtained by transcervical scraping (cytobrush) or uterine lavage. A sample taken more than 3 weeks postpartum with >5% PMNs is considered positive.

IMAGING
Transrectal ultrasonography can be used to detect uterine enlargement or small amounts of abnormal luminal fluid present in some cases of endometritis. It is also useful for assessing ovarian structures to determine cyclic status of individual animals.

(CONTINUED)   **ENDOMETRITIS**

OTHER DIAGNOSTIC PROCEDURES

• For reproductive examinations before the breeding period to have value, they must identify animals at increased risk of failure to become pregnant in a timely way so that they may benefit from treatment.
• Cows with endometritis will frequently have been affected with one or more risk factors early in the current lactation.
• Transrectal palpation of the uterus has traditionally been the means of diagnosis of endometritis, but this method is subjective and has poor sensitivity and specificity for identifying cows with impaired fertility.
• Vaginoscopy can improve the sensitivity and specificity of the diagnosis but may be impractical for use in cattle.

PATHOLOGIC FINDINGS

Histologically, disruption of the endometrial epithelium, infiltration of inflammatory cells, and accumulations of lymphocytes with vascular congestion, and stromal edema.

TREATMENT

THERAPEUTIC APPROACH

• Spontaneous resolution commonly occurs as dairy cows return to a positive energy balance and resume estrous cycles. Concurrently address any nutritional issues that may be promoting inflammation, delaying involution, or suppressing immune function.
• Intrauterine infusion of cephapirin has been shown to improve the reproductive performance of cows with PVD.
• Camelids are frequently treated with uterine lavage during estrus followed by repeated daily infusion of an antibiotic dictated by culture and sensitivity testing. Systemic antibiotic therapy may replace local infusion or be used as an adjunct.
• It is well established that estrus occurrence has a restorative effect on the postpartum uterus. Treatments that increase the number of estrus periods prior to mating should in theory be beneficial to animals with endometritis. Repeated use of PGF2$_\alpha$ products to cause luteolysis and return to estrus are indicated for cycling females. Anovular females should be treated with GnRH with or without progesterone to hasten the onset of ovulatory cycles.

SURGICAL CONSIDERATIONS AND TECHNQUES

Perineal and vaginal trauma at delivery, often associated with pneumovagina and occasionally with urovagina, may contribute to chronic contamination of the uterus. For valuable cows and camelidae, appropriate surgical repair is indicated.

MEDICATIONS

• The general principle of therapy for endometritis is to reverse inflammatory changes that impair fertility by reducing the load of pathogenic bacteria and enhancing the processes of uterine defense and repair.
• There are limited reports of well-designed studies that confirm an advantage for medical treatment of endometritis in cattle. Treatment in camelids is primarily based on clinical impression.

DRUGS OF CHOICE

• Intrauterine (IU) antibiotic
  ◦ The principle is to reduce the load of pathogens. There are two valid studies showing that one treatment of 0.5 g cephapirin benzathine IU at approximately 30 days in milk reduced time to pregnancy relative to untreated cases.
  ◦ In camelids, antibiotic choice is based on culture and sensitivity. Aminoglycosides should be buffered for IU use.
• PGF2$_\alpha$—the principle is to induce luteolysis and, in turn, estrus. Reducing or removing the influence of progesterone on the uterus increases uterine tone and promotes physical clearance, potentially resolving cases of endometritis. There is little evidence suggesting that PGF2$_\alpha$ causes myometrial contraction or provides any other benefits for treatment of endometritis in the absence of a CL. Although clearcut data are lacking, IM injection of PGF2$_\alpha$ (0.5 mg cloprostenol or 25 mg dinoprost) after approximately 30 DIM is likely beneficial as treatment for endometritis. A second administration of PGF2$_\alpha$ 14 days later may provide additional benefit, although clinical trial data are lacking.

CONTRAINDICATIONS

• Appropriate milk and meat withdrawal times must be followed.
• Use of PGF before approximately 26 DIM is controversial. Some studies suggest beneficial effects, many suggest no benefit, and a few report a deleterious effect on subsequent reproductive performance of cows with endometritis.
• Cephapirin benzathine is approved for use in lactating cows in Canada and the European Union, but not in the United States.
• There are reports of treatment of endometritis by IU infusion of oxytetracycline, crystalline penicillin G, and numerous other antibiotics, as well as Lugol's iodine, povidone iodine, and other disinfectants, and systemically administered estradiol, tetracycline, penicillin, and ceftiofur. There is little evidence that any of these improve reproductive performance, and several of the IU substances may cause damage to the endometrium or to uterine defenses.

PRECAUTIONS

Catheterization of the cervix is difficult in camelids.

POSSIBLE INTERACTIONS

N/A

FOLLOW-UP

EXPECTED COURSE AND PROGNOSIS

• Affected cows take longer to conceive, and are at increased risk of failure to become pregnant.
• Clinical signs will be resolved by 60 DIM in >95% of cases after one (or in a minority of cases, two) treatment with cephapirin IU or PGF.
• It is unknown how many of these are truly cured as opposed to cases of ongoing subclinical endometritis.
• In camelids, females treated for endometritis are at a higher risk for developing a new episode if breeding is not managed correctly.

POSSIBLE COMPLICATIONS

• Given the case definition of a localized uterine condition, there is no mortality attributable to endometritis, and no direct loss of milk production. Reports have shown an increase in the mean calving to pregnancy interval from 7 to 48 days for cows with endometritis compared to unaffected herd mates, despite various treatments administered to affected animals.
• A meta-analysis of 23 studies found that endometritis increased mean days open by 15, decreased the relative risk of pregnancy by 150 DIM by 31%, and reduced the rate at which cows became pregnant by 16%.
• Cows with mucopurulent or purulent cervical discharge or cervical diameter >7.5 cm at approximately 4 weeks postpartum had an increase of 32 days in median time to pregnancy over unaffected cows.
• In camelids, the main complication is iatrogenic damage to the cervix or uterus during treatment if not performed correctly.

CLIENT EDUCATION

• In cattle, record keeping of all reproduction disease and production parameters.
• Development of a herd health program with the veterinarian.
• In camelids, follow sound practices in management of breeding.

PATIENT CARE

• Follow-up examination and repeated treatment 2 weeks after initial diagnosis and treatment (i.e., at approximately 45 DIM) might be useful to identify refractory cases.
• However, in almost 80% of cases, clinical signs will be resolved by this time, even if untreated.

E

ENDOMETRITIS

PREVENTION
• The key element in preventing establishment of chronic uterine infection appears to be the effectiveness of uterine defense mechanisms in clearing the inevitable postpartum or post-breeding infection. However, there is little information on preventive measures specific to endometritis.
• Management and nutritional practices that prevent dystocia, RP, metritis, and ketosis will enhance peripartum immune function (i.e., appropriate diet and adequate bunk space) and potentially reduce the incidence of endometritis in dairy cows.
• Effective breeding management will reduce or eliminate overbreeding in camelidae.

MISCELLANEOUS

ASSOCIATED CONDITIONS
• Infertility/Subfertility
• Pyometra
• Repeat breeding

AGE-RELATED FACTORS
N/A

ZOONOTIC POTENTIAL
N/A

PREGNANCY
N/A

BIOSECURITY
In camelids, outbreaks of endometritis due to *Pseudomonas aeruginosa* have been observed following mating to the same male.

PRODUCTION MANAGEMENT
N/A

SYNONYM
Uterine infection

ABBREVIATIONS
• CL = corpus luteum
• DIM = days in milk
• FTIR = Fourier-transformed infrared
• GnRH = gonadotropin releasing hormone
• IM = intramuscular
• IU = intrauterine
• NEFA = non-esterified fatty acids
• OCD = ovarian cystic degeneration
• PCR = polymerase chain reaction
• PGF2$_\alpha$ = prostaglandin F2$_\alpha$
• PMN = polymorphonuclear leukocytes
• PVD = purulent vaginal discharge
• RAPD = random amplification of polymorphic DNA
• RP = retained placenta

SEE ALSO
• Anestrus
• Infertility and Subfertility Issues
• Metritis
• Postpartum Disorders
• Pyometra
• Repeat Breeder Management
• Reproductive Prolapse
• Uterine Prolapse

Suggested Reading
de Boer MW, LeBlanc SJ, Dubuc J, et al. Invited review: Systematic review of diagnostic tests for reproductive-tract infection and inflammation in dairy cows. J Dairy Sci 2014, 97: 3983–99.
LeBlanc SJ. Reproductive tract inflammatory disease in postpartum dairy cows. Animal 2014, 8:s1: 54–63.
Pascottini OB, Dini P, Hostens M, Ducatelle R, Opsomer G. A novel cytologic sampling technique to diagnose subclinical endometrial cytology samples in dairy cows. Theriogenology 2015, 84: 1438–46.
Risco CA, Youngquist RS, Shore MD. Postpartum uterine infections. In: Youngquist RS, Threlfall WR eds, Current Therapy in Large Animal Theriogenology, 2nd ed. Philadelphia: Saunders, 2007, pp. 339–44.
Sheldon IM, Lewis GS, LeBlanc S, Gilbert RO. Defining postpartum uterine disease in cattle. Theriogenology 2006, 65: 1516–30.
Tibary A, Fite C, Anouassi A, Sghiri A. Infectious causes of reproductive loss in camelids. Theriogenology 2007, 66: 633–47.
Authors Celina Checura and Harry Momont
Consulting Editor Ahmed Tibary
Acknowledgment The authors and book editors acknowledge the prior contribution of Stephen LeBlanc.

BASICS

OVERVIEW
Copper deficiency in the dam may lead to neuronal degeneration and demyelination in the fetus/neonate, resulting in symmetrical ascending posterior paresis in newborn or young lambs or goat kids.

INCIDENCE/PREVALENCE
Unknown

GEOGRAPHIC DISTRIBUTION
Worldwide

SYSTEMS AFFECTED
• Musculoskeletal
• Nervous
• Integument

PATHOPHYSIOLOGY
• Hypomyelinogenesis occurs in utero or shortly after birth in affected kids and lambs resulting in a progressive ataxia, muscle atrophy, paresis, and paralysis.
• Affected animals often have stiffness of the back and legs and are reluctant to rise. When individuals do stand, there may be a characteristic swaying of the hindquarters.
• Other neurologic signs can include blindness, obtundation, and head tremor.
• Abnormal bone growth and increased fragility of bones predisposing to fractures of long bones is apparently due to defects in development of connective tissue and growth plates.
• There may be persistent diarrhea, unthriftiness, and poor fleece in lambs.
• The pathogenesis is not known.

HISTORICAL FINDINGS
Copper-deficient diet with lack of supplementation

SIGNALMENT
• Sheep, goats, Bactrian camels, beef calves, piglets, blesbok (*Damaliscus dorcas phillipsi*), black wildebeest (*Connochaetes gnou*), sika deer (*Cervus nippon Temminck*), and red deer (*Cervus elaphus*) may be affected.
• In the neonatal form, clinical signs are present at birth; in the delayed form, clinical signs often appear at 14–30 days of age.

PHYSICAL EXAMINATION FINDINGS
• Progressive symmetrical ataxia and ascending posterior paresis or paralysis with associated muscle atrophy, ultimately resulting in permanent recumbency if left untreated.
• Most cases occur in lambs or kids that are 1–2 months of age.
• Severity of clinical signs decreases with increasing age at onset.
• Majority of affected lambs/kids are normothermic, bright, alert, and maintain the ability to suckle and vocalize.
• Hypermetric gait may be seen in animals with cerebellar involvement.

• Adult animals with copper deficiency are often asymptomatic, but signs may include ill thrift, diarrhea, anemia, and depigmentation of hair/wool.
• Ewes of affected lambs may have a loss of crimp resulting in a straight and "steely" appearance to the wool.
• Depigmentation of the wool is more noticeable in ewes with black wool.
• Osteoporosis, which can result in long bone fractures, may also occur with copper deficiency.

GENETICS
There is a possible familial predisposition. Dwarf goats have been reported to be overrepresented. Breed or family line may play a role in ewes, possibly through altered intestinal absorption and copper storage efficiency.

CAUSES AND RISK FACTORS
• Copper deficiency in the maternal diet is responsible for the clinical signs; however, the pathogenesis is not known. It is speculated that copper deficiency results in altered phospholipid metabolism and reduced synthesis of myelin.
• Animals raised on pasture with copper-deficient soil are at greater risk of disease.
• There is a possible familial predisposition.

DIAGNOSIS

DIFFERENTIAL DIAGNOSES
Neonatal Form
• Hydrocephalus
• Congenital vertebral or spinal anomalies
• Trauma resulting in vertebral luxation/subluxation or fracture
• Protozoal encephalitis or myelitis, including *Sarcocystis*, *Neospora*, or *Toxoplasma* spp.

Delayed Form
• Trauma resulting in vertebral luxation/subluxation or fracture
• Vertebral abscess or osteomyelitis, ± associated pathologic fracture
• Protozoal myelitis, including *Sarcocystis*, *Neospora*, or *Toxoplasma* spp.
• Neurologic form of caprine arthritis and encephalitis (CAE) virus infection in kids
• Nutritional muscular dystrophy (white muscle disease)
• Listeriosis
• Rabies

CBC/BIOCHEMISTRY/URINALYSIS
Ewes may have a microcytic anemia.

OTHER LABORATORY TESTS
Liver biopsy or collection at necropsy is the most reliable method to determine true copper status. Serum or plasma copper levels may also be low. Analysis of feed, water, and

possibly soil may facilitate diagnosis on a flock or herd level.

IMAGING
N/A

OTHER DIAGNOSTIC PROCEDURES
Generally diagnosed based on clinical signs with possible decreased blood or liver copper levels. Definitive diagnosis is based on low liver copper levels and necropsy and histopathologic lesions. Analysis of CSF and/or spinal radiographs may rule out other differential diagnoses.

PATHOLOGIC FINDINGS
Gross
• Possible symmetric cavitations in the subcortical white matter can lead to marked internal hydrocephalus.
• In severe cases, little is left of the hemispheres except the cortical shell of gray matter.
• Severe osteoporosis and long bone fractures may be present.

Histopathologic
• Neuronal degeneration in the form of chromatolysis, neuronal necrosis, or both may be found in the central portions of the cerebral hemispheres, brainstem, cerebellum, and/or spinal cord.
• Demyelination occurs in the brainstem and spinal cord. Myelinated tracts may have a spongy appearance with some collections of gitter cells.
• Chromatolysis of neurons in the red nucleus may occur.

TREATMENT

THERAPEUTIC APPROACH
Evaluate copper status of the herd and soils where animals are pastured. Copper supplementation should be provided as needed to dams. Administration of parenteral copper glycinate has reportedly been an effective treatment in affected goat kids; however, treatment is generally unrewarding.

MEDICATIONS

DRUGS OF CHOICE
• Oral
  ◦ Copper sulfate
  ◦ Copper oxide wire particles (as a bolus)
• Parenteral
  ◦ Copper glycinate (must be compounded, consider AMDUCA prior to administering)

CONTRAINDICATIONS
Oversupplementation or supplementation of copper in animals with normal liver copper levels could lead to copper toxicity, particularly in sheep.

E

ENZOOTIC ATAXIA   (CONTINUED)

FOLLOW-UP

EXPECTED COURSE AND PROGNOSIS
• Prompt supplementation with copper may improve signs, but complete recovery is uncommon.
• Severely affected animals usually have permanent neurologic deficits.
• Prognosis is guarded to poor.

POSSIBLE COMPLICATIONS
N/A

PATIENT CARE
N/A

PREVENTION
Provide appropriate copper/mineral supplements. Supplements can be administered in various forms such as a top dressing to pasture or feed, or a weekly drench given to individual animals.

MISCELLANEOUS

ASSOCIATED CONDITIONS
Copper supplementation can be toxic to treated animals.

AGE-RELATED FACTORS
Onset of clinical signs usually occurs between birth and 6 months of age. Average age of onset in goat kids with the delayed form is reported to be 13 weeks.

ZOONOTIC POTENTIAL
None

PREGNANCY
Maternal copper deficiency is the cause of clinical signs in lambs and kids.

BIOSECURITY
N/A

PRODUCTION MANAGEMENT
• Etiology is copper deficiency in the ewe/doe.
• Making a definitive diagnosis of copper deficiency in a single animal indicates the need for judicious copper supplementation in animals managed similarly.
• More than one form of copper supplementation may be required in herds/flocks with severe copper deficiency.

SYNONYM
Swayback (often applied to the neonatal form of this condition)

ABBREVIATIONS
• AMDUCA = Animal Medicinal Use Clarification Act of 1994
• CAE = caprine arthritis encephalitis
• CSF = cerebrospinal fluid

SEE ALSO
Caprine Arthritis Encephalitis Virus

Suggested Reading
Allen AL, Goupil BA, Valentine BA. A retrospective study of brain lesions in goats submitted to three veterinary diagnostic laboratories. J Vet Diag Invest 2013, 25: 482–9.

Crilly JP, Rzechorzek N, Scott P. Diagnosing limb paresis and paralysis in sheep. In Practice 2015, 37: 490–507.
Jones TC, Hunt RD, King NW eds. Congenital demyelinating disease of lambs (swayback, enzootic ataxia). In: Veterinary Pathology. 6th ed. Baltimore: Williams & Wilkins, 1997.
Lofstedt J, Jakowski R, Sharko P. Enzootic ataxia and caprine arthritis/encephalitis virus infection in a New England goat herd [corrected]. J Am Vet Med Assoc 1988, 193: 1295–8.
Millar M, Barlow A, Gunning R, Cosser J. Enzootic ataxia in farmed red deer. Vet Rec 2003, 152(13): 408.
Penrith ML, Tustin RC, Thornton DJ, Burdett PD. Swayback in a blesbok (*Damaliscus dorcas phillipsi*) and a black wildebeest (*Connochaetes gnou*). J S Afr Vet Assoc 1996, 67: 93–6.
Suttle NF. The role of comparative pathology in the study of copper and cobalt deficiencies in ruminants. J Comp Pathol 1988, 99: 241–58.

Author Katharine M. Simpson
Consulting Editor Kaitlyn A. Lutz
Acknowledgment The author and book editors acknowledge the prior contribution of Lisa Nashold.

ENZOOTIC PNEUMONIA OF CALVES

BASICS

OVERVIEW
Respiratory disease of young calves <6 months of age caused by multiple etiologic agents, a decreased host defense system, and environmental risk factors such as poor ventilation and overcrowding.

INCIDENCE/PREVALENCE
• Based on producer diagnosis, 7.4–11% of dairy calves
• Based on veterinary diagnosis, 25.6–29% of dairy calves

SYSTEMS AFFECTED
Respiratory

PATHOPHYSIOLOGY
• Enzootic pneumonia of calves is part of the bovine respiratory disease complex that also includes shipping fever of feedlot cattle and pneumonia of adult cows.
• The bacterial pathogens involved with this disease are normal inhabitants of the nasal and pharyngeal mucosa.
• Host and environmental factors combine to weaken the normal pulmonary defense mechanisms.
• Viral infections cause damage to the mucosal lining of the upper respiratory tract and may reduce the mucociliary clearance and production of secretory defenses.
• Viral infections may also have an effect on alveolar macrophages or neutrophils, which can enhance bacterial adherence.
• Factors such as failure of passive transfer and nutritional deficiency, stressors such as overcrowding and mixing, poor ventilation, and high relative humidity also allow the proliferation of these opportunistic bacteria.

HISTORICAL FINDINGS
• Multiple animals depressed and febrile
• Partial anorexia
• Increased respiratory rates
• Coughing
• Nasal discharge
• Lacrimation
• Decreased weight gains
• Rough hair coats
• High morbidity
• Low mortality

SIGNALMENT
• Most common in housed dairy calves and veal calves
• Beef calves in crowded conditions
• Calves <6 months of age
• Peak incidence at 5–6 weeks of age

PHYSICAL EXAMINATION FINDINGS
• Not pathognomonic, but used for decades in the treatment management.
• DART: Depression; Appetite loss; Respiratory distress; Temperature elevation.
• Fever (39.5–40.5°C)

• Polypnea
• Mild to severe dyspnea
• Abnormal cranioventral lung sounds such as loud harsh breath sounds, crackles, and wheezes
• Harsh, dry, cough response on tracheal compression
• Intensity of heart sounds is increased dorsal to heart base

CAUSES AND RISK FACTORS
Multifactorial disease that involves animal stress frequently with co-infections with bacteria and/or viruses.

Bacterial Agents
• *Mannheimia haemolytica*
• *Pasteurella multocida*
• *Histophilus somni*
• *Bibersteinia trehalosi*
• *Mycoplasma bovis*

Viral Agents
• Bovine respiratory syncytial virus
• Parainfluenza-3 virus
• Bovine herpesvirus-1
• Bovine coronavirus

Secondary Bacterial Agents
Trueperella (formerly *Arcanobacterium*) *pyogenes* (considered as an opportunistic agent)

Stressors
• Bovine viral diarrhea virus infection
• Low colostral immunity
• Abrupt weaning
• Mixing of social/ age groups
• Adverse climatic conditions (precipitations and rapid change of environmental temperature)
• Poor air quality in calf barns
• High relative humidity
• Housing calves together in large groups
• Overcrowding
• Poor nutrition: Vitamin E, selenium, zinc and/or copper deficiency

DIAGNOSIS

DIFFERENTIAL DIAGNOSES
• Aspiration pneumonia
• Congenital cardiac defects
• Septicemia (*E coli*, *Salmonella* spp.)

CBC/BIOCHEMISTRY/URINALYSIS
The measurement of serum haptoglobin can serve as an indicator of inflammatory disease and a measure of disease severity.

OTHER LABORATORY TESTS
Isolation and identification of organisms
• Nasopharyngeal swabs
• Transtracheal washes
• Lung lavage samples
• Serologic tests for confirmation of BRSV infections
• Immunohistochemistry, PCR, virus isolation or antigen capture ELISA for

identification of persistently infected BVDV calves
• Necropsy findings, histopathology, aerobic bacterial culture, fluorescent antibodies (BRSV, IBR) and/or PCR

IMAGING
Ultrasonography of the thorax is being proposed as an accurate and sensitive method for the detection and diagnosis of bronchopneumonia in calves, compared to thoracic auscultation.

OTHER DIAGNOSTIC PROCEDURES
New methods for diagnosis are being proposed, such as a computer-aided lung auscultation system (Whisper Veterinary Stethoscope System®) which, when used properly, increase the proportion of cattle accurately diagnosed with bovine respiratory disease.

PATHOLOGIC FINDINGS
• Extensive cranioventral lung consolidation.
• Suppurative bronchopneumonia, with or without fibrinous pleuritis, pus in airways, areas of necrosis (lytic and/or coagulative), with sequestrae and abscess formation.
• Interstitial pneumonia and inflammation of nasal mucosa associated with viral infections.

TREATMENT

THERAPEUTIC APPROACH
• Medical management: Identification of the pathogen followed by use and selection of appropriate antibiotics.
• Appropriate selection and treatment of cases.
• Sick calves should be isolated from healthy calves.

MEDICATIONS

DRUGS OF CHOICE
• Ideally bacterial cultures and antibacterial sensitivity test will be performed on symptomatic, nontreated calves. These may include, among others:
  ○ Short-acting or long-acting oxytetracyclines
  ○ Tilmicosin
  ○ Trimethoprim-potentiated sulfonamides
  ○ Ceftiofur
  ○ Florfenicol
  ○ Enrofloxacin (beef calves only)
• Efficacy of NSAIDs in these cases is questionable.

PRECAUTIONS
• Failure to respond to treatment may indicate predominantly viral infections, *Mycoplasma* infections, or late selection and treatment of cases.

E

ENZOOTIC PNEUMONIA OF CALVES   (CONTINUED)

• Drug withdrawal times must be determined and maintained for treated animals.

FOLLOW-UP

EXPECTED COURSE AND PROGNOSIS
• Response to antimicrobial therapy should be evident within 48 hours if the primary pathogen is bacterial.
• *Mycoplasma* and viral infections may not respond to antimicrobial therapy.
• Calves that are selected early in the course of the disease for treatment will generally have a very low case fatality rate.
• Case fatality rates have been reported at 2.25%.

CLIENT EDUCATION
• Discuss probable causes and risk factors.
• Warn that viral or *Mycoplasma* pneumonias may not respond to antimicrobial therapy.

PATIENT CARE
• Fluid therapy such as oral electrolyte solutions or intravenous fluids may be indicated in dehydrated animals.
• Well-ventilated, draft-free environment provided.
• DART may be utilized as a measure of response to therapy. Calves that are still febrile after 3 days of therapy could be categorized as a relapse and considered for an alternative antimicrobial.

PREVENTION
• Improving air quality is an important criterion for control.
• Dairy calves should not share the same air space as adult animals.
• Rearing dairy calves in calf hutches is an excellent method for reducing the potential risk factors associated with enzootic calf pneumonia.
• Alternatively, use group housing in cold well-ventilated facilities.

• Humidity levels between 55% and 75% are optimal.
• Avoid mixing of various age groups of calves.
• Utilize all-in–all-out approach in group housing, if possible.
• Avoid overcrowding.
• Ensure that calves have high levels of passive immunity by ensuring adequate colostrum ingestion shortly after birth.
• This is a multifactorial disease. Recent studies regarding vaccination provide encouraging results, especially with BRSV vaccines. Further investigation is needed to support the use of vaccines in young calves and their benefit in preventing enzootic pneumonia.

MISCELLANEOUS

ASSOCIATED CONDITIONS
Neonatal diarrhea may be associated with enzootic pneumonia, as many of the same risk factors are shared.

ZOONOTIC POTENTIAL
N/A

BIOSECURITY
• Keeping age groups of calves separate is a significant preventive measure.
• Avoid mixing of calves from various sources.
• Purchased calves may be persistently infected with BVDV, which may predispose infected animals to enzootic pneumonia.

PRODUCTION MANAGEMENT
• Heifers that do not experience enzootic pneumonia are twice as likely to calve and will calve 6 months earlier than heifers that did have enzootic pneumonia.
• Enzootic pneumonia cases are at an increased risk of culling.

SYNONYM
Bovine respiratory disease complex

ABBREVIATIONS
• BRSV = bovine respiratory syncytial virus
• BVDV = bovine viral diarrhea virus
• ELISA = enzyme-linked immunosorbent assay
• IBR = infectious bovine rhinotracheitis
• NSAIDs = nonsteroidal anti-inflammatory drugs
• PCR = polymerase chain reaction

SEE ALSO
• Aspiration Pneumonia
• Congenital Defects: Bovine
• *Histophilus somni* Complex
• Respiratory Disease: Bovine

Suggested Reading
Caswell JL. Failure of respiratory defenses in the pathogenesis of bacterial pneumonia of cattle. Vet Pathol 2014, 51: 393–409.
Caswell JL, Hewson J, Slavic D, et al. Laboratory and post mortem diagnosis of bovine respiratory diseases. Vet Clin North Am Food Anim Pract 2012, 28: 419–41.
Griffin D, Chengappa MM, Kuszak J, Scott McVey D. Bacterial pathogens of the Bovine Respiratory Complex. Vet Clin North Am Food Anim Pract 2010, 26: 381–94.
Griffin D. Bovine pasteurellosis and other bacterial infections of the respiratory tract. Vet Clin North Am Food Anim Pract 2010, 26: 57–71.
Woolums AR. The bronchopneumonias (respiratory disease complex of cattle, sheep and goats). In: Smith BP ed, Large Animal Internal Medicine, 5th ed. St. Louis: Elsevier, 2015, pp. 584–617.
Author Francisco R. Carvallo
Consulting Editor Christopher C.L. Chase
Acknowledgment The author and book editors acknowledge the prior contribution of John R. Campbell.

EPIZOOTIC HEMORRHAGIC DISEASE VIRUS

BASICS

OVERVIEW

• Epizootic hemorrhagic disease (EHD) is an important noncontagious arthropod-borne, viral infection of white-tailed deer (WTD) that often results in epidemic outbreaks of hemorrhagic fever in North America during periods of high vector activity at the end of the summer and early fall.
• An abnormally large number of EHD cases were reported in WTD and cattle in the United States in the summer and Fall of 2012.
• Severe outbreaks of EHD clinical disease have been reported in cattle in Japan, Réunion Island, Israel, Morocco, Algeria, Jordan, and Turkey. In the United States, the majority of EHD infections in cattle are subclinical, but vesicular lesions and pregnancy loss have been reported.
• Since the report of outbreaks of EHD in cattle in four Mediterranean countries, EHD is considered an emerging disease in cattle and has been added to the OIE list of reportable diseases.
• EHDV shows immunologic cross-reactivity with the bluetongue virus (BTV).
• Ibaraki disease (ID) is a noncontagious viral disease of cattle caused by EHD in Japan and other countries, characterized by fever, anorexia, lacrimation, salivation, nasal discharge, conjunctival hyperemia, and dysphagia. Original reports indicated that ID was caused by EHD-2 but recent phylogenetic analysis of an isolate from an outbreak in Japan indicates that ID virus is less related to EHDV serotype 2 and should be classified as EHDV serotype 7.

INCIDENCE/PREVALENCE

• In endemic areas, outbreaks tend to occur every 2–3 years and in epidemic areas every 8–10 years. Most outbreaks of the disease in WTD are seasonal, occurring from mid-summer to late autumn.
• In the US, the disease has been reported sporadically in cattle, with morbidity as high as 7%.
• Serum EHDV antibodies have been found in black-tailed deer, red deer, wapiti, fallow deer, and roe deer.

GEOGRAPHIC DISTRIBUTION

• The distribution of EHDV coincides with areas where the vector is active, usually in tropical and subtropical areas approximately between latitudes 35°S and 49°N.
• Outbreaks of the disease have been reported in North America, Africa, Asia, Australia, and more recently in countries surrounding the Mediterranean basin including Morocco, Algeria, Tunisia, Israel, Jordan, and Turkey.
• Seropositive animals have been found in South America.

• In North America, EHD clinical disease is generally more severe in more northern latitudes, where EHD occurs sporadically and where the EDHV naïve population is high. In contrast, in the southwestern US, where the infection is endemic, clinical disease is less common.

SYSTEMS AFFECTED

• Cardiovascular
• Hemolymphatic
• Digestive
• Musculoskeletal

PATHOPHYSIOLOGY

• EHD is caused by epizootic hemorrhagic disease virus (EHDV), an *Orvivirus* in the Reoviridae family. EHD is closely related to BTV, African horse sickness virus, and equine encephalosis virus. Currently, seven EHDV serotypes are recognized worldwide.
• EHD is a double-stranded RNA virus with a 10-segmented genome.
• EHD serotype is determined by the interaction of virus proteins 2 and 5 (VP2 and VP5) with neutralizing antibodies.
• Currently EHDV has 7 serotypes (EHDV-1 to -7) as determined by sequencing of the VP2 region of the genome.
• In the US, EHDV serotypes 1, 2, and 6 have been identified.
• The virus is transmitted by insects of the genus *Culicoides* and can infect the majority of domestic and wild ruminants. Clinical disease is observed in WTD and to a lesser extent in mule deer and pronghorn antelope.
• In North America, *Culicoides sonorensis* is the primary vector of EHDV.
• Intrauterine transmission and abortion can occur in cattle with EHDV-2 (Ibaraki).
• Viremia can be detected as early as 2 days post-infection and usually lasts for 3 weeks; in some animals, EHDV can be isolated from the blood for over 50 days post-infection.

HISTORICAL FINDINGS

N/A

SIGNALMENT

• All ages of deer are susceptible. Passive immunity may be protective in fawns, but this has not been sufficiently evaluated.
• Morbidity may reach 90% and mortality 60% or higher.
• There is no sex predilection.
• Goats and sheep do not appear to be susceptible to natural infection.

PHYSICAL EXAMINATION FINDINGS

• Infection with EHDV in WTD can be subclinical or can result in high morbidity and mortality.
• Clinical disease can be hyperacute, acute, and chronic.
• In the hyperacute form, sudden death is often reported. In deer where clinical signs are observed, there is swelling of the head, neck, tongue, and eyelids. Death may occur 1–3 days after the initial clinical signs.

• Fever, depression, weakness, respiratory distress, salivation, ulceration of the oral mucosa, anorexia, subcutaneous edema of the head and neck, swelling of the tongue or eyelids, and lameness are observed in the acute form. Death may occur 7–9 days after infection.
• In the chronic form, affected deer may show signs for several weeks but generally recover. Affected deer lose weight; develop coronitis, cracks in the hooves, and exhibit lameness. The hoof sloughs off in some animals resulting in prostration or knee-walking.
• In North American cattle, EHDV infection is generally subclinical or characterized by a mild-to-moderate transient febrile disease. In some animals, there is fever, respiratory distress, anorexia, salivation, decreased milk production, conjunctivitis, nasal and ocular discharge, oral and nasal erosions, and lameness. Affected cattle usually recover. Death may occur in a few cases as a result of secondary bacterial infections.
• EHD infection of cattle can result in fetal loss or fetal hydranencephaly when pregnant cows are infected between 70 and 120 days of gestation.
• Severe clinical disease has been reported in cattle in Japan, Israel, Morocco, Algeria, Jordan, Tunisia, and Turkey.

GENETICS

N/A

CAUSES AND RISK FACTORS

WTD, mule deer, pronghorn antelope, and cattle living in areas where the vector, *Culicoides,* and EHDV coexist are at risk.

DIAGNOSIS

DIFFERENTIAL DIAGNOSES

• EHD in WTD needs to be differentiated from BTV, malignant catarrhal fever (MCF) and adenovirus infection.
• In cattle EHD can be confused with other vesiculo-ulcerative diseases such as foot and mouth disease (FMD), vesicular stomatitis (VS), and MCF.

CBC/BIOCHEMISTRY/URINALYSIS

• Thrombocytopenia and lymphopenia
• Increased creatine kinase, lactate dehydrogenase, and aspartate aminotransferase

OTHER LABORATORY TESTS

N/A

IMAGING

N/A

OTHER DIAGNOSTIC PROCEDURES

• Diagnostic samples include serum, heparinized blood, or chilled unfixed spleen or other blood-rich tissues.

EPIZOOTIC HEMORRHAGIC DISEASE VIRUS (CONTINUED)

• Serum is used for the detection of EHDV antibodies by the AGID test, virus neutralization, or ELISA.
• EHDV can be isolated in cell culture from heparinized blood and from the spleen and other blood-rich tissues.
• Numerous real-time RT-PCR formats for the detection and serotyping of EHDV are used in diagnostic laboratories.

PATHOLOGIC FINDINGS

• Gross findings in the hyperacute and acute forms include severe subcutaneous edema in the head, neck and limbs, and hyperemia of the sclera, conjunctiva and oral mucosa.
• The tongue may be swollen and dark red with hemorrhages or mucosal ulceration.
• Widespread petechiae and ecchymoses are common in mucus membranes, subcutis, and internal organs including the heart and gastrointestinal tract.
• There is severe pulmonary congestion and edema, and straw-colored pericardial fluid.
• Erosions and ulcerations of the rumen and omasum are common.
• Paintbrush hemorrhages occur in the epicardium and papillary muscles.
• The main microscopic lesion consists of disseminated vasculitis and thrombosis, multifocal areas of hemorrhage, and ischemic necrosis in various organs.

TREATMENT

THERAPEUTIC APPROACH

There are no specific treatments for EHD.

SURGICAL CONSIDERATIONS AND TECHNIQUES
N/A

MEDICATIONS

DRUGS OF CHOICE

Broad-spectrum antimicrobials are used to treat secondary bacterial infections.

CONTRAINDICATIONS
N/A

PRECAUTIONS

Appropriate milk and meat withdrawal times must be followed for all compounds administered to food-producing animals.

POSSIBLE INTERACTIONS
N/A

FOLLOW-UP

EXPECTED COURSE AND PROGNOSIS

• The majority of infections are subclinical.
• Mortality is high in clinically affected deer.

POSSIBLE COMPLICATIONS

Secondary infections or recumbency due to limb lesions

CLIENT EDUCATION
N/A

PATIENT CARE
N/A

PREVENTION

• In the US, there are no commercially available vaccines to prevent EHD.
• The use of autogenous EHDV inactivated vaccines is permitted in the US. Two or in some cases one dose of inactivated vaccine can provide considerable immunity against EHDV.

MISCELLANEOUS

ASSOCIATED CONDITIONS
N/A

AGE-RELATED FACTORS
N/A

ZOONOTIC POTENTIAL
N/A

PREGNANCY

Reproductive problems; abortions and fetal resorptions in pregnant cows

BIOSECURITY
N/A

PRODUCTION MANAGEMENT
N/A

SYNONYMS
N/A

ABBREVIATIONS

• AGID = agar gel immunodiffusion
• BTV = bluetongue virus
• EHD = epizootic hemorrhagic disease.
• EHDV = epizootic hemorrhagic disease virus
• ELISA = enzyme-linked immunosorbent assay
• FMD = foot and mouth disease
• ID = Ibaraki disease
• MCF = malignant catarrhal fever
• OIE = Office International des Epizooties
• RT-PCR = reverse transcription-polymerase chain reaction
• VS = vesicular stomatitis
• WTD = white-tailed deer

SEE ALSO

Bluetongue Virus

Suggested Reading

Garrett EF, Po E, Bichi ER, Hexum SK, Melcher R, Hubner AM. Clinical disease associated with epizootic hemorrhagic disease virus in cattle in Illinois. J Am Vet Med Assoc 2015, 247: 190–5.

McVey DS, MacLachlan NJ. Vaccines for prevention of bluetongue and epizootic hemorrhagic disease in livestock: A North American perspective. Vector-Borne Zoonot Dis 2015, 15: 385–96.

Wilson WC, Daniels P, Ostlund EN, et al. Diagnostic tools for bluetongue and epizootic hemorrhagic disease viruses applicable to North American veterinary diagnosticians. Vector-Borne Zoonot. Dis 2015, 15: 364–73.

Author Andrés de la Concha-Bermejillo
Consulting Editor Erica C. McKenzie

ERYTHROCYTOSIS (POLYCYTHEMIA)

BASICS

OVERVIEW
• Erythrocytosis is defined as an increase in the red blood cell (RBC) count, hemoglobin (Hb) concentration, and/or packed cell volume (PCV).
• Polycythemia and erythrocytosis are commonly considered synonyms.
• Polycythemia indicates erythrocytosis with concurrent leukocytosis and thrombocytosis.
• Therefore, the term erythrocytosis should be used when referring specifically to the RBC population.

INCIDENCE/PREVALENCE
• Relative erythrocytosis is the most common form of erythrocytosis.
• Absolute erythrocytosis is less common and is usually due to chronic diseases causing systemic tissue hypoxia.

GEOGRAPHIC DISTRIBUTION
• Cattle and sheep can develop erythrocytosis at 6,000 ft (1,800 m) above sea level.

SYSTEMS AFFECTED
• Cardiovascular
• Nervous
• Multisystemic

PATHOPHYSIOLOGY
• Relative erythrocytosis is defined as a relative increase in total RBC mass caused by hemoconcentration or splenic contraction.
• Hemoconcentration is due to a decrease in plasma volume usually caused by dehydration or endotoxemia.
• Dehydration is usually caused by reduced water intake and/or excessive loss or sequestration of body fluids.
• Endotoxemia is due to the endogenous release of mediators in response to Gram-negative bacterial cell wall components (endotoxins).
• Splenic contraction is due to an increase in blood catecholamine concentration caused by transportation, handling or exercise.
• Absolute erythrocytosis is defined as an absolute increase in total RBC mass caused by increased proliferation of erythroid precursors (erythropoiesis).
• Absolute erythrocytosis may be classified as either primary or secondary.
• Primary absolute erythrocytosis is caused by increased erythropoiesis in the absence of increased erythropoietin (EPO) production.
• Secondary absolute erythrocytosis is caused by increased erythropoiesis due to increased EPO production.
• Increased EPO production may be appropriate (due to systemic tissue hypoxia) or inappropriate (due to EPO-secreting neoplasms or renal tissue hypoxia).

• Erythropoiesis can also be stimulated by hormones other than EPO including cortisol, androgen, thyroxin, and growth hormone.
• Absolute erythrocytosis is characterized by an increase in blood volume and viscosity.
• Hypervolemia interferes antidiuretic hormone release, leading to polyuria and polydipsia.
• Hyperviscosity interferes with tissue oxygen delivery and distends capillaries, leading to an increased risk of thrombosis and rupture of these vessels.

HISTORICAL FINDINGS
Relative Erythrocytosis
• Excitement, exercise, handling, or transportation

Absolute Erythrocytosis
• Weakness, lethargy, anorexia, weight loss, or exercise intolerance

SIGNALMENT
• Cattle and sheep appear more susceptible to high altitude hypoxia.
• Camelids have small ellipsoid RBCs, resulting in fewer problems of sludging.
• Camelids and small ruminants have higher RBC counts than cattle but similar PCV.
• Camelids have higher blood Hb concentration than cattle and small ruminants.

GENETICS
• Familial absolute erythrocytosis has been described in Jersey cattle.

PHYSICAL EXAMINATION FINDINGS
• Relative erythrocytosis is usually mild to moderate and of no clinical significance.
• Most clinical signs associated with absolute erythrocytosis result from blood hyperviscosity.

Relative Erythrocytosis
• Signs of dehydration: Sunken eyes, reduced skin turgor, and dry mucus membranes.
• Signs of endotoxemia: Fever, tachycardia, tachypnea, scleral injection, pale or congested mucus membranes, and cold extremities.

Absolute Erythrocytosis
• Lethargy, ataxia, seizures, central blindness, or behavioral changes.
• Congested brick-red mucus membranes and dilated retinal blood vessels.
• Dyspnea, tachypnea, or harsh bronchovesicular sounds (due to pulmonary congestion).
• Retinal hemorrhage, epistaxis, hematemesis, hematochezia, melena, or hematuria.
• Polyuria and polydipsia (due to hypervolemia).

CAUSES AND RISK FACTORS
Relative Erythrocytosis (Most Common)
• Common causes of splenic contraction include exercise, transportation, and handling.

• Common causes of dehydration include decreased water intake, diarrhea, polyuria, and upper gastrointestinal stasis.
• Common causes of endotoxemia include coliform mastitis, puerperal metritis, and salmonellosis.

Secondary Absolute Erythrocytosis Caused by Appropriate EPO Production (Common)
• Residence at high altitude.
• Congenital heart defects leading to right-to-left shunting including tetralogy of Fallot and double outlet right ventricle.
• Severe chronic pulmonary disease.

Secondary Absolute Erythrocytosis Caused by Inappropriate EPO Production (Rare)
• EPO-secreting neoplasms including renal and hepatic carcinomas.
• Causes of chronic renal disease include pyelonephritis, urolithiasis, amyloidosis, and glomerulonephritis.

DIAGNOSIS

DIFFERENTIAL DIAGNOSES
• The first step is to identify causes of relative erythrocytosis including splenic contraction, dehydration, or endotoxemia.
• Another blood sample should be collected under less stressful conditions in excitable animals.
• Another blood sample should be collected after administration of intravenous fluids in animals with dehydration or hypovolemia.
• In the absence of response to fluid therapy, absolute erythrocytosis should be suspected.
• The second step is to differentiate primary and secondary absolute erythrocytosis.
• Systemic tissue hypoxia should be investigated using arterial blood gas analysis.
• Thoracic auscultation, radiography, and ultrasonography may help identify congenital heart defect or severe chronic pulmonary disease.
• In the absence of hypoxemia and cause of appropriate secondary erythrocytosis, the next step is to investigate causes of inappropriate EPO production.
• Abdominal radiography and ultrasonography may help identify EPO-secreting neoplasm or chronic renal disease.

CBC/BIOCHEMISTRY/URINALYSIS
Sample Collection and Handling
• Blood collected in a tube containing EDTA is the sample of choice for a CBC.
• Blood tubes should be filled to completion to ensure the proper blood-to-EDTA ratio and gently inverted several times immediately after filling.

E

ERYTHROCYTOSIS (POLYCYTHEMIA)

• Blood should be analyzed within 30–60 minutes of collection or stored at refrigerator temperature (4°C) and analyzed within 24 hours.

CBC Interpretation Principles (see Table 1)
• Primary absolute erythrocytosis can ultimately cause sludging of blood and leading to systemic tissue hypoxia and increased EPO production.
• Secondary absolute erythrocytosis is not always associated with increased EPO production if the erythrocytosis has resolved tissue hypoxia.

OTHER LABORATORY TESTS
• PaO_2 <80 mmHg indicates hypoxemia.
• Bone marrow examination should reveal erythroid hyperplasia in animals with absolute erythrocytosis.
• Determination of serum EPO activity has been traditionally recommended to distinguish the two types of absolute erythrocytosis.
• Increased serum EPO activity is expected with secondary absolute erythrocytosis.
• Thorough evaluation is still needed given the overlap in serum EPO activity between animals with primary and secondary erythrocytosis and the absence of validated assays in ruminants.

IMAGING
• Thoracic radiography and ultrasonography may help identify a cause of appropriate absolute erythrocytosis including congenital heart defect or severe chronic pulmonary disease.
• Abdominal radiography and ultrasonography may help identify a cause of inappropriate absolute erythrocytosis including EPO-secreting neoplasm or chronic renal disease.

PATHOLOGIC FINDINGS
N/A

TREATMENT

THERAPEUTIC APPROACH
Relative Erythrocytosis
• Fluid therapy is indicated in animals with dehydration or endotoxemia and the underlying cause(s) should be addressed.

Absolute Erythrocytosis
• Oxygen therapy is indicated in animals with severe chronic pulmonary disease.
• PCV should be maintained <60% to minimize effects of hyperviscosity.
• Phlebotomy (5–10 mL/kg) might be used to control blood hyperviscosity.
• Simultaneous administration of intravenous fluids is indicated to prevent severe hypotension and cardiovascular collapse.
• Excessive phlebotomy (PCV<50%) may worsen systemic tissue hypoxia in animals with secondary appropriate erythrocytosis.
• Surgery may be indicated in animals with EPO-secreting neoplasms.

MEDICATIONS

DRUGS OF CHOICE
• Radioactive phosphorus and chemotherapy drugs including hydroxyurea, doxorubicin, and busulfan have been used in small animals with absolute erythrocytosis with some benefit.

CONTRAINDICATIONS
• Phlebotomy may be contraindicated in patients with secondary appropriate erythrocytosis.

PRECAUTIONS
• Appropriate milk and meat withdrawal times must be followed for all compounds administered to food-producing animals.

FOLLOW-UP

COURSE AND PROGNOSIS
• Long-term prognosis of ruminants with absolute erythrocytosis depends on underlying cause.
• Primary erythrocytosis may be managed by repeated phlebotomy, but evidence on long-term prognosis is lacking.
• Secondary erythrocytosis caused by congenital heart defect or chronic pulmonary or renal disease usually has a poor prognosis.
• EPO-secreting neoplasms may have a better prognosis if surgical removal is successful.

POSSIBLE COMPLICATIONS
• Blood hyperviscosity is associated with increased risk of thrombosis and hemorrhage.
• Iron deficiency anemia may develop after repeated phlebotomy and warrant a decrease in the frequency of phlebotomy and iron supplementation.
• Chemotherapy drugs may cause leukopenia, thrombocytopenia, and/or anemia.

PATIENT CARE
• Heart rate, respiratory rate, mucus membrane color, blood lactate, and arterial blood gas analysis can be used to monitor systemic tissue oxygen delivery.

Table 1

	CBC Interpretation Principles			
	Relative erythrocytosis	*Primary absolute erythrocytosis*	*Appropriate secondary erythrocytosis*	*Inappropriate secondary erythrocytosis*
Mechanism	Splenic contraction, dehydration, or endotoxemia	Neoplastic or non-neoplastic proliferation of erythroid precursors	Systemic tissue hypoxia and increased EPO production	EPO-secreting neoplasms or chronic renal disease
PCV	↑ - ↑↑	↑↑ - ↑↑↑	↑↑ - ↑↑↑	↑↑ - ↑↑↑
Plasma protein	N - ↑	N	N	N
EPO	N	N - ↑	↑↑	↑↑ - ↑↑↑
PaO_2	N	N	↓	N
WBC count	N - ↓	N - ↑	N	N
Platelet count	N - ↑	N - ↑	N - ↑	N

N = normal, ↑ = slightly increased, ↑↑ = moderately increased, ↑↑↑ = markedly increased, ↓ = slightly decreased

ERYTHROCYTOSIS (POLYCYTHEMIA)

• PCV and total solids should be monitored daily in animals with dehydration or hypoproteinemia.
• PCV and total solids should be monitored after repeated phlebotomy to allow for frequency adjustment.
• CBC should be performed weekly in animals receiving chemotherapy drugs.

PREVENTION
N/A

 MISCELLANEOUS

ABBREVIATIONS
• CBC = complete blood count
• EDTA = ethylenediaminetetraacetic acid
• EPO = erythropoietin
• Hb = hemoglobin
• PaO_2 = partial pressure of oxygen in arterial blood
• PCV = packed cell volume
• RBC = red blood cell
• WBC = white blood cell

SEE ALSO
• Brisket Disease
• Fluid Therapy: Oral

Suggested Reading
Randolph JF, Peterson ME, Stokol T. Erythrocytosis and polycythemia. In: Weiss DJ, Wardrop KJ eds, Schalm's Veterinary Hematology, 6th ed. Ames: Blackwell, 2010, pp. 162–6.
Author Thibaud Kuca
Consulting Editor Christopher C.L. Chase
Acknowledgment The author and book editors acknowledge the prior contribution of Frederick S. Almy.

E

ESCHERICHIA COLI

BASICS

OVERVIEW
Escherichia coli (*E. coli*) is the most common cause of diarrhea and septicemia in newborn ruminants.

INCIDENCE/PREVALENCE
• *E. coli* can be isolated in >50% of bacteremic calves.
• Enterotoxigenic *E. coli* (ETEC) is the most common cause of diarrhea in calves <3 days old.

GEOGRAPHIC DISTRIBUTION
Worldwide

SYSTEMS AFFECTED
• Cardiovascular
• Urinary
• Hemolymphatic
• Digestive
• Cardiovascular

PATHOPHYSIOLOGY
• Commensal *E. coli* organisms can be found in soil and the GI tract of most mammals.
• A small number of *E. coli* are distinguished into pathovars (bacterial strains with the same or similar characteristics differentiated at infrasubspecific level).
• Pathotyping is based on the presence of two virulence factors: K99 fimbriae (F) and heat stable toxin (thermolabile [LT] and thermostable [STa and STb]).
• Enterotoxigenic *E. coli* (ETEC) causes neonatal calf diarrhea. ETEC possesses K99 fimbriae that mediate attachment to the intestinal epithelium, while LT, STa, and STb induce a secretory response resulting in diarrhea.
• The capacity of ETEC to bind to the intestinal epithelium is age dependent. Calves >3–5 days are resistant.
• Enteropathogenic *E. coli* (EPEC) include attaching and effacing *E. coli* (AEEC) and Shiga-like toxin-producing *E. coli* (SLTEC) which have been associated with diarrhea and dysentery in calves due to cytotoxic damage to intestinal epithelium.

HISTORICAL FINDINGS
Acute onset of systemic illness and/or diarrhea in young ruminants

SIGNALMENT
• All ruminant species can be affected.
• Septicemic disease occurs in ruminants <2 weeks of age.
• ETEC affects neonates 1–5 days old.
• AEEC and SLTEC affect calves 2–30 days old, but calves up to 4 months old can be affected.

PHYSICAL EXAMINATION FINDINGS
• Septicemic neonates display tachycardia, tachypnea, dehydration, obtundation, weakness, and reduced suckle. Pyrexia is uncommon but hypothermia due to dehydration and SIRS can occur. Swollen joints, diarrhea, pneumonia, meningitis, cloudy eyes, and/or a large, tender navel can develop.
• Diarrhea related to ETEC ranges from mild to severe. Mild signs include loose feces or mild diarrhea and weak suckle. Severe cases have diarrhea and dehydration that progresses rapidly to circulatory shock and death (and can resemble *E. coli* septicemia).
• Bradycardia and cardiac arrhythmias can develop in compromised animals with hyperkalemia, hypoglycemia, and hypothermia.
• Depression, dehydration, weakness, diarrhea, and frank blood in the feces are observed with AEEC and SLTEC.

GENETICS
N/A

CAUSES AND RISK FACTORS
• Sepsis can occur due to a multitude of strains of *E. coli*.
• Diarrhea relates to infection with enterotoxigenic *E. coli* (ETEC), or enteropathogenic *E. coli* (EPEC) including AEEC and SLTEC.
• The main risk factor for *E. coli* septicemia and diarrhea is failure of passive transfer of immunity which can arise from a range of factors including being born to a compromised, dirty, or maiden dam, dystocia, being born into extreme weather, or incidental separation from the dam.
• High animal density and poor hygiene in feeding, housing, and maternity areas.
• Inappropriate volume, fat or protein content of milk or milk replacer.

DIAGNOSIS

DIFFERENTIAL DIAGNOSES
• Septicemia can occur due to a variety of pathogens in neonatal ruminants, which are often hard to differentiate without appropriate diagnostics.
• Diarrhea in neonatal ruminants can relate to rotavirus, coronavirus, cryptosporidiosis, giardiasis, salmonellosis, and clostridiosis.

CBC/BIOCHEMISTRY/URINALYSIS
• CBC findings reflect hemoconcentration (dehydration), inflammation (leukopenia, neutropenia, left shift, and toxic changes) and hypoproteinemia (protein loss or suboptimal passive transfer of immunity).
• Serum chemistry can reveal metabolic acidosis (low TCO_2), hypoglycemia (sepsis and reduced milk intake), and electrolyte disturbances (hypokalemia, hyponatremia, and hypochloremia). Hyperkalemia can be observed in severely dehydrated and acidemic calves.

OTHER LABORATORY TESTS
• Blood culture is essential for confirming bacteremia or sepsis; ideally three samples are obtained over 24 hours to improve the chance of success. Bacteremia occurs in approximately 30% of diarrheic calves and *E. coli* is most commonly isolated (>50% of calves).
• Sepsis score is useful to predict bacteremia/sepsis in a clinical setting.

IMAGING
N/A

OTHER DIAGNOSTIC PROCEDURES
• ETEC—feces and/or ileum content, or ileum tissue can be submitted for histopathology, immune-chromatography assay, atomic emission spectroscopy, latex agglutination, PCR, or slide agglutination.
• EPEC—ileum and colon tissue can be submitted for histopathology and culture, PCR typing of intimin (eae) genes, or toxin detection.
• Mixed infections are common, therefore feces or intestinal content should be analyzed for other possible pathogens.

PATHOLOGIC FINDINGS
• ETEC—distension of the colon with watery, yellow fluid.
• EPEC—colonic mucosa can be normal or have reddening, roughening, and petechial hemorrhages. Frank hemorrhage and fibrin can also be evident.
• Histopathologic findings consistent with sepsis and disseminated intravascular coagulation can occur in septicemic neonates.

TREATMENT

THERAPEUTIC APPROACH
• Fluid therapy (oral, IV or SC) is a cornerstone of therapy.
• Oral electrolytes can be administered to diarrheic neonates that are standing and appear strong, and can be fed as an extra meal.
• In neonates with dehydration judged to be >8%, provide IV fluids initially, followed by IV or oral fluids for maintenance.
• Fluid deficits can be calculated as: *Volume (L) = body weight (kg) × % dehydration*, and can be replaced over 4–6 h.
• Maintenance requirements (50–100 mL/kg/day) should be provided continuously IV or by intermittent IV or oral bolus; additional volume (1–4 L) is required for estimated ongoing losses per day and is dependent on species and severity of diarrhea.
• Fluid resuscitation is typically adequate to reverse mild to moderate acidemia, particularly if a lactate- or acetate-containing solution is used.
• Severe metabolic acidosis in calves can be addressed by administering isotonic sodium bicarbonate (156 mEq $NaHCO_3$/L; or 1.3%

(CONTINUED)

E

solution), at 1–4 L over 4–6 h, or until deficits are mostly resolved.
• The total bicarbonate deficit can be calculated from base deficit on blood gas analysis or by estimating from the decrease in TCO$_2$ on serum chemistry (*Bicarbonate deficit (mEq) = body weight (kg) × base deficit (mEq/L) × 0.6*). Alternatively it can be estimated from depression score charts available online. Typically, half of the deficit is administered if bicarbonate supplementation of fluids is performed, and can be repeated if necessary.
• Dextrose can be added to IV fluids to a final concentration of 2.5–5% for hypoglycemia.
• Milk and milk replacer should not be withheld for more than 8–12 h. Milk should be reintroduced in small amounts starting with 1 L q6–12h.

SURGICAL CONSIDERATIONS AND TECHNIQUES
N/A

MEDICATIONS

DRUGS OF CHOICE
• Antibiotics to treat or prevent bacteremia or sepsis can include beta-lactam drugs (ceftiofur, amoxicillin, or ampicillin) and potentiated sulfonamides (where permitted).
• Combining a beta-lactam with an aminoglycoside (gentamicin or amikacin) can be used in neonatal camelids.
• Nonsteroidal anti-inflammatory drugs (flunixin meglumine or meloxicam) may be beneficial, suggested by results in experimental calves orally challenged with heat-stable *E. coli* enterotoxin.

CONTRAINDICATIONS
Nephrotoxic drugs are contraindicated in severe dehydration and azotemia.

PRECAUTIONS
Appropriate milk and meat withdrawal times must be followed for all compounds administered to food-producing animals.

POSSIBLE INTERACTIONS
N/A

FOLLOW-UP

EXPECTED COURSE AND PROGNOSIS
• The prognosis is grave for septic, obtunded, and hypothermic neonates.
• Prognosis is good to fair for diarrheic cases receiving supportive care.

POSSIBLE COMPLICATIONS
• Septicemia
• Meningitis
• Septic arthritis
• Pneumonia
• Renal failure

CLIENT EDUCATION
Focus on hygiene and passive transfer protocols to reduce prevalence.

PATIENT CARE
Monitor attitude, suckling response, fecal consistency, and hydration status.

PREVENTION
• Ensure good-quality colostrum intake (3–4 L for calves) during the first 2–4 h after birth.
• Calves receiving colostrum from cows vaccinated 6 and 3 weeks before calving have high levels of antibodies and are effectively protected from ETEC diarrhea.

MISCELLANEOUS

ASSOCIATED CONDITIONS
• Septicemia
• Meningitis
• Septic arthritis

AGE-RELATED FACTORS
GI disease with *E. coli* is a neonatal phenomenon.

ZOONOTIC POTENTIAL
• Ruminants are a reservoir for human pathogenic *E. coli*, including EPEC and enterohemorrhagic *E. coli* (EHEC).
• EHEC O157:H7 is commonly associated with hemorrhagic enteritis and hemolytic uremic syndrome in humans.

PREGNANCY
N/A

BIOSECURITY
• Environmental and personnel hygiene are critical; gloves, outerwear, hand washing, disinfection.
• Segregate sick animals.

PRODUCTION MANAGEMENT
Vaccination protocols can be efficacious in preventing neonatal calf scours including *E. coli*-related diseases.

SYNONYM
Scours

ABBREVIATIONS
• AEEC = attaching and effacing *E. coli*
• EPEC = enteropathogenic *E. coli*
• ETEC = enterotoxigenic *E. coli*
• IV = intravenous
• SC = subcutaneous
• SIRS = systemic inflammatory response syndrome
• SLTEC = Shiga-like toxin-producing *E. coli*

SEE ALSO
• Diarrheal Diseases: Bovine
• Diarrheal Diseases: Camelid
• Diarrheal Diseases: Small Ruminant
• Neonatal Diarrhea

Suggested Reading
Blanchard PC. Diagnostics of dairy and beef cattle diarrhea. Vet Clin North Am Food Anim Pract 2012, 28: 443–64.
Dolente BA, Lindborg S, Palmer JE, Wilkins PA. Culture-positive sepsis in neonatal camelids: 21 cases. J Vet Intern Med 2007, 21: 519–25.
Fecteau G, Van Metre DC, Paré J, et al. Bacteriological culture of blood from critically ill neonatal calves. Can Vet J 1997, 38: 95–100.
Smith GW, Berchtold J. Fluid therapy in calves. Vet Clin North Am Food Anim Pract 2014, 30: 409–27.
Author Diego Gomez-Nieto
Consulting Editor Erica C. McKenzie

ESOPHAGEAL DISORDERS

 BASICS

OVERVIEW
- Esophageal disorders are any conditions that disrupt the normal function of the esophagus.
- Esophageal disorders in ruminants and camelids are relatively uncommon.
- The esophagus may be affected by obstruction (choke), inflammation, trauma, stricture, viral/parasitic infections, and megaesophagus.
- Choke is the most common esophageal condition and is defined as the partial or complete obstruction of the esophageal lumen resulting in the inability to effectively move a bolus from the pharynx to the rumen (or C1). The obstruction may be caused by an intraluminal obstruction such as feed material or foreign body, or by an extraluminal obstruction, such as abscess or neoplasia.
- The esophageal muscles in camelids differ from ruminants due to a circular muscle layer surrounding an internal longitudinal muscle layer. This muscle pattern allows active regurgitation of ingesta.

INCIDENCE/PREVALENCE
- Esophageal obstruction is most common in cattle due to their indiscriminant eating habits, and least common in camelids due to their ability to actively regurgitate.
- Megaesophagus is rare in ruminants and camelids.

PATHOPHYSIOLOGY
N/A

SYSTEMS AFFECTED
Digestive

SIGNALMENT
There does not appear to be any age, breed, or sex disposition.

PHYSICAL EXAMINATION FINDINGS
The presence of clinical signs varies with the duration (acute to chronic) and severity of the lesion(s), and may include:
- Ptyalism
- Extension of the head and neck
- Anxiety and restlessness
- Dysphagia
- Regurgitation
- Coughing
- Feed staining on muzzle or mandible
- Nasal discharge
- Repeated attempts to swallow
- Continuous chewing
- Bruxism
- Bloat
- Tachycardia/tachypnea
- Respiratory distress
- Dehydration
- Poor body condition score
- Loss of body condition
- Decreased interest in feed

GENETICS
A genetic inheritance of megaesophagus in camelids has been proposed but not proven.

CAUSES AND RISK FACTORS
Esophageal Obstruction
- Usually caused by impaction of feed material in the esophagus or ingestion of foreign bodies.
- Ingestion of large items such as corncobs, apples, and potatoes can be the sole cause of the obstruction.
- Foreign material (e.g., glass or metallic objects).
- Consuming dry or pelleted feeds if the bolus is not moist enough to allow passage through the esophagus. This is most common in sheep.
- Extraluminal space-occupying mass (abscess, granuloma, or neoplasia). Peri-esophageal hematomas obstructing the esophageal lumen have been reported in camelids.
- Secondary to other disorders of the esophagus such as pre-existing strictures (including vascular ring anomalies, VRA) or diverticula, intraluminal neoplasia, such as squamous cell carcinoma or papillomas, or by underlying neurologic dysfunction.

Esophagitis
- Ingestion of irritants including toxic plant material (rhododendron or oleander).
- Secondary to ingestion of sharp feedstuffs or foreign objects, or iatrogenically with use of esophageal/gastric tubes or during administration of oral boluses.
- Erosive or ulcerative esophagitis may occur in cases of BVDV, bovine malignant catarrhal fever, vesicular stomatitis, papular stomatis, FMD, and after parasite death in infections with *Hypoderma lineatum*.
- Esophageal parakeratosis has been described in camelids after prolonged treatment with sodium EDTA and in individuals with zinc deficiency.

Megaesophagus
- Most cases are idiopathic. Congenital and acquired causes have also been reported in ruminants and camelids.
- VRA have been reported in camelids, cattle, and bison. Most cases present with esophageal dilation proximal and sometimes distal to the VRA stricture point.
- Primary nerve or muscle dysfunction in the neck (including vagal nerve) or secondary to chronic partial obstruction of the esophagus.

 DIAGNOSIS

DIFFERENTIAL DIAGNOSES
- Botulism, tetanus, listeriosis, and rabies can all cause bloat, dysphagia, and ptyalism. Toxic plants, such as milkweed, larkspur, sneezeweed, *Rhizoctonia leguminicola,* and infected red clover, also cause ptyalism.

- Traumatic damage to the pharynx can also cause ptyalism and localized cellulitis.
- Bloat can be caused by vagal indigestion or trauma and inflammation associated with the vagal nerve.

CBC/BIOCHEMISTRY/URINALYSIS
- Packed cell volume and serum protein level may be elevated due to dehydration.
- Metabolic acidosis, hyponatremia, hypophosphatemia, and hypokalemia may be present due to the loss of saliva.
- The leukogram and fibrinogen concentration may be altered due to inflammatory changes associated with the primary disease process or secondary aspiration pneumonia.

IMAGING
Radiography
- Both survey and contrast radiography may be helpful to determine the etiology and severity of esophageal lesions. Contrast material should not be administered until an obstruction is relieved due to risks associated with aspiration of the material.
- The cervical and thoracic esophagus can be easily visualized by radiography in calves, small ruminants, and camelids. In most cases, adult cattle require specialized radiology systems to obtain diagnostic images of the thoracic esophagus.
- Fluoroscopy may be helpful to diagnose motility disorders.
- Computed tomography has been used to investigate causes of extraluminal esophageal obstructions including identifications of VRA.

Ultrasonography
- May be useful to identify intra- or peri-esophageal masses in the cervical region and can occasionally identify intraluminal obstructions.
- May aid in diagnosis of aspiration pneumonia.

OTHER DIAGNOSTIC PROCEDURES
- In small ruminants and camelids, the object may be palpated in the cervical esophagus. This is often not possible in the bovine patient due to overlying musculature.
- Passage of an orogastric tube can establish the location of the obstruction. The tube should be passed through an oral speculum and should be advanced gently to avoid damage to affected mucosa.

Endoscopy
- Esophagoscopy will aid in localizing and characterizing lesions, as well as determining the severity of esophageal damage.
- A 2–3-m endoscope may be necessary to visualize the extent of the bovine esophagus, however, a 1-m or pediatric endoscope is adequate for the small ruminant and many camelids. Use of an oral speculum is necessary to prevent damage to the endoscope. Insufflation with air will help advance the endoscope and allow visualization of the

esophagus, especially in cases where a large amount of saliva is present.

PATHOLOGIC FINDINGS

N/A

TREATMENT

THERAPEUTIC APPROACH

Esophageal Obstruction

• Some cases of esophageal obstruction will resolve spontaneously. Acute cases can be monitored for resolution of the choke in an area free of any feed, bedding or water. If not resolved in a few hours, the animal should be treated.
• Sedation may be given to reduce anxiety and promote relaxation of esophageal spasms; however, this increases risk of aspiration and thus low head carriage should be encouraged.
• If obstruction is palpable within the cervical esophagus, it may be manually extracted by applying gentle and steady pressure in the jugular groove aboral to the obstruction, pushing it orally. Once in the proximal esophagus, it may be propelled into the pharynx or grasped and removed. Sedation, a speculum, and manipulation of the tongue are helpful.
• Thoracic obstructions may be corrected by pushing the object into the rumen and foreign bodies can then be retrieved via rumenotomy. This should not be performed if the object has sharp edges as identified by endoscopy.
• Objects in the cervical esophagus should not be pushed aborally due to the narrowing of the esophagus at the thoracic inlet.
• For persistent obstructions, the animal should be sedated to allow low head carriage. An orogastric tube can be passed to the level of the obstruction, and obstructions that are feed material based may be broken down with a gentle lavage of warm water.
• Aspiration of lavage material can be prevented by placement of a large-bore ET tube into the esophagus, cuff inflated, and the smaller oroesophageal tube inserted through the ET tube. This allows lavage material and fluid to pass through the ET tube and reduce risk of aspiration. Several attempts may need to be made to break down the obstruction, and it may take a significant amount of time. Breaks should be taken to allow the animal to rest.
• If the obstruction cannot be relieved with the animal standing, general anesthesia may be required. The patient is placed in lateral recumbency with the head lowered and the same lavage techniques are used. If this does not allow relief of the obstruction, esophagotomy may be required.
• Rumen or C1 decompression through trocarization or surgical decompression may

be required in cases of complete esophageal obstruction leading to free-gas bloat.

Megaesophagus

• There are no specific treatments for megaesophagus. If an underlying disease process is identified, neuromuscular function of the esophagus may improve after resolution of the inciting cause.
• Elevation of feed and inclined footing to raise the animal's fore-end may help with movement of the feed bolus through gravity.

General Management of Esophageal Disorders

• In cases of dehydration, the patient may require intravenous fluid therapy.
• Diet recommendations are dependent on type and severity of the disease present.
• Ruminants with minimal esophageal mucosal damage and no decrease in motility can be fed frequent small amounts for the first 24–72 hours.
• More severe esophageal damage, decreased motility, or surgical correction will require alternative alimentation.
  ◦ Temporary rumenostomy cannula.
  ◦ Placement of an esophagostomy tube distal to the esophageal lesion is best reserved for pre-ruminant calves, as the regurgitated feed material and saliva will leak around the tube. Daily passage of an orogastric tube can be used for feeding if done cautiously to avoid further mucosal damage.

SURGICAL CONSIDERATIONS AND TECHNIQUES

• Esophageal surgery carries a high complication rate.
• If there is evidence of esophageal rupture, surgical management may be necessary. In acute cases, survival with surgery is possible.
• If the rupture is long-standing, involves contamination of the thorax, or involves extensive soft tissue contamination, the prognosis is extremely guarded.

MEDICATIONS

DRUGS OF CHOICE

• Xylazine (sedation and esophageal relaxation)
  ◦ Cattle, small ruminants: 0.01–0.02 mg/kg, IV
  ◦ Camelids: 0.1–0.15 mg/kg, IV or 0.2–0.3 mg/kg, IM or SQ
• Acepromazine (anxiolytic, antispasmotic)
• Butorphanol may be used in camelids for restraint during procedures with limited sedative effects
  ◦ Camelids: 0.1 mg/kg, IV or IM
• Flunixin meglumine (inflammation and pain)
  ◦ Cattle, small ruminants: 1.1 mg/kg, IV
  ◦ Camelids: 1 mg/kg, IV

• Broad-spectrum antimicrobials should be given in cases of esophageal necrosis, aspiration pneumonia, or esophageal surgery.
• Sucralfate (camelids and pre-ruminants) or bismuth subsalicylate may be used to improve animal comfort while esophageal ulcerations heal.
• Oxytocin is not effective for treatment of esophageal obstruction in ruminants (unlike its possible use in Equidae) due to the presence of striated muscle for the length of the esophagus.

CONTRAINDICATIONS

The use of lubricants, such as mineral oil or surfactants (DSS) to relieve an esophageal obstruction, is contraindicated due to the risk of aspiration.

PRECAUTIONS

• Drug choices should be made with regard to meat and milk withdrawal times.
• NSAIDs should be given judiciously to the dehydrated patient due to the risk of nephrotoxicity.

FOLLOW-UP

EXPECTED COURSE AND PROGNOSIS

• Prognosis is dependent on duration and severity of the lesion and occurrence of complications.
• Prognosis is good for esophageal obstructions if resolution of the obstruction occurs spontaneously or with minimal manipulation and mucosal damage. Prognosis is guarded with more aggressive manipulation or if surgical correction is required, and grave to poor with prolonged obstruction and rupture of the esophagus.
• Prognosis for esophagitis is dependent on underlying cause of the esophageal lesions.
• Megaesophagus can be managed in some animals through diet change and feeding conditions. Some camelids have been reported to live years after diagnosis though most animals are euthanized or culled after diagnosis.

POSSIBLE COMPLICATIONS

• Rumenal or 1st compartment (C1) bloat
• Esophageal perforation
• Esophageal stricture
• Esophageal diverticulum
• Recurrent obstructions
• Aspiration pneumonia
• Altered esophageal motility

PATIENT CARE

See "Treatment"

PREVENTION

Dependent on underlying cause. The diet should be thoroughly evaluated for risk factors (see "Causes and Risk Factors").

ESOPHAGEAL DISORDERS (CONTINUED)

MISCELLANEOUS

ASSOCIATED CONDITIONS
- Aspiration pneumonia
- Bloat
- Regurgitation

ABBREVIATIONS
- BVDV = bovine viral diarrhea virus
- C1 = 1st gastric compartment in camelids
- DSS = dioctyl sodium sulfosuccinate
- EDTA = ethylene diamine tetraacetic acid
- ET = endotracheal tube
- FMD = foot and mouth disease
- IM = intramuscular
- IV = intravenous
- NSAIDs = nonsteroidal anti-inflammatory drugs
- SQ = subcutaneous
- VRA= vascular ring anomaly

SEE ALSO
- Bloat
- Camelid: Gastrointestinal Disease
- Clostridial Disease: Nervous System
- Colic: Bovine
- Colic: Small Ruminant
- Gastrointestinal Surgeries: Rumenotomy/Rumenostomy (see www.fiveminutevet.com/ruminant)
- Listeriosis
- Oleander and Cardiotoxic Plant Toxicity
- Rabies
- Vagal Indigestion

Suggested Reading

Anderson R, Bath GF, Thompson PN, Stadler MM. Oesophageal obstruction in Dorper ewes caused by impaction of a pelleted ration. J S Afr Vet Assoc 2010, 81: 118–20.

Baird AN, Pugh DG. Oro-esophageal diseases. In: Baird AN, Pugh DG eds, Sheep and Goat Medicine, 2nd ed. Maryland Heights: Elsevier, 2012, pp. 69–70.

Braun U, Schwarzwald C, Ohlerth S, Frei S, Hilbe M. Abnormal regurgitation in three cows caused by intrathoracic perioesophageal lesions. Acta Vet Scand 2014, 56: 14–19.

Cebra CK. Disorders of the digestive system: Esophageal disorders. In: Cebra CK, Anderson DE, Tibary A, Van Saun RJ, Johnson LW eds, Llama and Alpaca Care. St. Louis: Elsevier, 2014, pp. 491–4.

Franz S, Baumgartner W. A retrospective study of oesophageal endoscopy in cattle – Oesophagoscopy for diagnosis of mucosal disease. Vet J 2002, 163: 205–10.

Haven ML. Bovine esophageal surgery. In: Surgery of the bovine digestive tract. Vet Clin North Am Food Anim Pract 1990, 6: 359–69.

McKenzie EC, Seguin B, Cebra CK, Margiocco ML, Anderson DE, Lohr CV. Esophageal dysfunction in four alpaca crias and a llama cria with vascular ring anomalies. J Am Vet Med Assoc 2010, 237: 311–16.

Radostits OM, Gay CC, Hinchcliff KW, Constable PD. Diseases of the alimentary tract – 1: Diseases of the pharynx and esophagus. In: Veterinary Medicine: A Textbook of the Diseases of Cattle, Sheep, Pigs, Goats, and Horses, 10th ed. New York: Elsevier Saunders, 2007, pp. 209–15.

Watrous BJ, Pearson EG, Smith BB, et al. Megaesophagus in 15 llamas: A retrospective study (1985–1993). J Vet Intern Med 1995, 9: 92–9.

Author Ashley Whitehead
Consulting Editor Kaitlyn A. Lutz
Acknowledgment The author and book editors acknowledge the prior contribution of Laura M. Riggs.

ESTRUS SYNCHRONIZATION: BOVINE

BASICS

OVERVIEW
• Estrus synchronization is a management technique involving scheduled hormonal treatment which allows synchronized follicle growth, controlled CL regression, predictable estrus expression, and ovulation within a narrow window of time.
• Synchronization of estrus and ovulation allows artificial insemination at a predetermined time.
• Synchronization of estrus improves efficiency of insemination by reducing or eliminating the need for heat detection.

INCIDENCE/PREVALENCE
Common

GEOGRAPHIC DISTRIBUTION
Worldwide

SYSTEMS AFFECTED
Reproductive

PATHOPHYSIOLOGY
• Synchronization protocols rely on simulation of a luteal phase using progestogens or interruption of the natural luteal phase using PGF2$_\alpha$ or its analogs. Progestogens and PGF2$_\alpha$ may also be used in combination.
• Follicular wave dynamics can be controlled by estrogens or GnRH.
• Ovulation is induced with administration of GnRH which induces an LH surge.
• Combined treatment with estrogens and progesterone causes:
  ○ A transitory decrease in plasma FSH, decreases LH pulse frequency, and reduces growth and estradiol activity in the largest follicle.
  ○ Atresia of the follicular wave present at the time of treatment and emergence of a new follicular wave 3–6 days later.
  ○ Estrogens are luteolytic when administered during the early part of the estrus cycle.
• Effects of GnRH
  ○ Induces an LH and FSH surge of variable magnitude depending on days postpartum, progesterone concentration, and stage of the follicular wave.
  ○ GnRH injection causes either ovulation or luteinization of a dominant follicle (≥10 mm in diameter with sufficient LH receptors) with emergence of a new follicular wave 2 days later.
  ○ Injection of GnRH before dominance does not affect the follicular wave.
• Effects of PGF2$_\alpha$ or analogs:
  ○ Luteolysis is induced in presence of a mature CL (day 5 to day 17 of the cycle).
  ○ Progesterone decreases to basal levels within 24 hours after injection. LH pulse frequency increases, causing a significant increase in estradiol from the dominant

follicle and induction of estrus and ovulation.
  ○ The interval from PGF2$_\alpha$ until estrus depends on the stage of the follicular wave and size of the dominant follicle at the time of injection. Cows treated in presence of dominant follicle will display estrus 2–3 days later, whereas cows treated at the beginning of a follicular wave and those whose dominant follicle has become atretic, will require more time (4–6 days) for a dominant follicle to emerge and ovulate.

HISTORICAL FINDINGS
• Dairy cattle: Poor heat detection, increased interval from calving to first ovulation, poor pregnancy rates.
• Beef cattle: Implementation of an artificial insemination program.

SIGNALMENT
Breeding age heifers or mature cows

PHYSICAL EXAMINATION FINDINGS
• Heifers should meet requirement for breeding age and maturity (height and weight) and be cycling. Reproductive tract scoring may be used to select mature heifers.
• Mature cows should be cyclic and at least 50 days (beef cattle) or 30 days postpartum (dairy).

GENETICS
N/A

CAUSES AND RISK FACTORS
N/A

DIAGNOSIS

DIFFERENTIAL DIAGNOSES
N/A

CBS/BIOCHEMSTRY/URIANALYSIS
N/A

OTHER LABORATORY TESTS
• Serum progesterone determination may help determine cyclicity status and monitor response.
• PSPB or PAG1 may be used as pregnancy diagnosis test.

IMAGING
Transrectal ultrasonography helps determine cyclicity status and response.

OTHER DIAGNOSTIC PROCEDURES
Heat detection aids may be used to determine response.

PATHOLOGIC FINDINGS
N/A

TREATMENT

THERAPEUTIC APPROACH
• Estrus synchronization with progestogens:

  ○ MGA, an orally active steroid with progestin activity, fed at a rate of 0.5 mg/day/cow for 14–18 days is used to synchronize estrus.
  ○ Estrus is exhibited 3–7 days after progestin withdrawal. However, conception rates following long-term MGA treatment are low. Subsequent heats show normal fertility. Injection of PGF2$_\alpha$ 16–17 days after MGA treatment will induce a fertile estrus.
  ○ Decreased fertility at the first estrus after MGA treatment may be due to ovulation of an aged oocyte from a persistent follicle, the prolonged period of chronically elevated concentrations of estradiol, reduced weight of corpora lutea, changes in cervical mucus quantity and quality, interference of gamete transport and function, abnormal timing of ovulation, or alteration of the histology and function of the endometrium.
  ○ Short-term MGA (5–7 days) followed by injection of PGF2$_\alpha$ did not improve synchrony and conception rate.
• Estrus synchronization with PGF2$_\alpha$ or analogs:
  ○ These protocols are only effective in cyclic animals.
  ○ Two injections 11 or 12 days apart increase the percentage of cows exhibiting estrus within 2–4 days.
  ○ Heifers tend to show estrus and ovulate earlier than cows.
  ○ In multiparous cows, 2 injections of PGF2$_\alpha$ administered 12 hours apart may be necessary to induce complete luteolysis. Cows with incomplete luteolysis are unlikely to show estrus and have lower conception rates to TAI.
  ○ AI is performed 12 hours after standing estrus.
• Estrus synchronization combining progestogen and PGF2$_\alpha$:
  ○ These protocols decrease the length of required progestogen treatment. They are easy to implement and offer substantial savings in time and labor in large herds.
  ○ Progesterone is delivered as a CIDR or PRID™ Delta® implant.
  ○ CIDR is a T-shaped silicone intravaginal insert impregnated with 1.38 g of progesterone.
  ○ CIDR protocols of 5 and 7 days' duration have been described with similar conception rates.
  ○ A high proportion of cows (>80%) display estrus within 36–60 hours after progesterone removal.
  ○ Administration of PGF2$_\alpha$ or analogs 24 hours before removal of progestogen induces luteolysis and improves estrus synchrony.
  ○ Cows are observed for estrus 2–6 days following CIDR removal and inseminated 12 hours after onset of standing estrus.
  ○ FTAI may be performed 56–72 hours following removal of the progestin insert with concurrent administration of GnRH.

E

ESTRUS SYNCHRONIZATION: BOVINE   (CONTINUED)

○ CIDR inserts have also been used in combination with GnRH-based protocols to improve synchrony by preventing early ovulation.

○ PRID™ Delta® is a triangular shaped device made from a polyethylene spine and ethyl vinyl acetate impregnated with 1.55 g of progesterone.

○ PRIDs™ are left in the vagina for 7 days. PGF2$_\alpha$ is administered 24 hours prior to removal in all cattle. Noncycling cattle receive an injection of eCG on the day of PRID™ removal.

○ All animals are inseminated at 48 hours and 72 hours or at 56 hours after PRID™ removal.

• Ovulation synchronization (Ovsynch®):

○ Ovulation synchronization eliminates need for heat detection and increases AI submission rate of cows eligible for AI.

○ The standard protocol consists of an injection of GnRH followed 7 days later by an injection of PGF2$_\alpha$ or analog to induce luteolysis. A second injection of GnRH is administered 48–56 hours after PGF2$_\alpha$ to induce ovulation of the newly emerged dominant follicle. Cows are inseminated 16 hours after the second GnRH injection.

○ A Co-synch protocol, used to decrease labor and animal handling, consists of a FTAI concurrently with the second GnRH injection. There is a tendency for lower conception rates compared to Ovsynch®.

○ The Ovsynch® protocol is less successful in heifers because of differences in their follicular wave patterns compared to adult cows. There are several variations of this scheme to further improve synchrony and pregnancy rates.

○ The success rate (overall pregnancy rate) of the Ovsynch® program depends on:

■ *Cyclicity of cows treated.* Progesterone supplementation for 7 days between the first GnRH and PGF2$_\alpha$ injections of Ovsynch® may improve fertility in anovular cows.

■ *Complete regression of CL after PGF2$_\alpha$ injection.* Incomplete luteolysis has been reported in 10–25% of cows during Ovsynch® protocols. Two injections of PGF2$_\alpha$ given 12 hours apart will enhance CL regression, especially in multiparous cows, and improve fertility.

■ *The stage of the estrous cycle of treated cows.* Cows enrolled in Ovsynch® between days 12 to 21 of the cycle may experience early CL regression prior to PGF2$_\alpha$ injection and ovulate prior to the second GnRH injection, resulting in lower conception rates. Cows receiving their first injection of GnRH between days 1 and 4 of the estrous cycle will not ovulate in response to the GnRH injection and will not be synchronized to ovulate at the appropriate time for FTAI.

■ *Rate of ovulation to the first GnRH injection.* Only cows that ovulate in response to the first GnRH of Ovsynch® will be at the correct stage of the estrous cycle to respond to subsequent injections. Cows at day 6 of the cycle have the highest rate of ovulation (85–94%) to the first injection of GnRH.

• Presynchronization protocols:

○ These protocols are aimed at ensuring cows are at a phase of the estrous cycle associated with optimal response to Ovsynch®.

○ Presynch-Ovsynch: Cows receive two PGF2$_\alpha$ injections 14 days apart followed by an Ovsynch® protocol 11–12 days after the second PGF2$_\alpha$. This approach improves pregnancy rates by 12–18% in cycling lactating dairy cows.

○ G6G: Cows receive an injection of PGF2$_\alpha$ then GnRH 2 days later and Ovsynch® is initiated 6 days following GnRH injection.

SURGICAL CONSIDERATIONS AND TECHNIQUES
N/A

MEDICATIONS

DRUGS OF CHOICE
• PGF2$_\alpha$ (dinoprost tromethamine, 25 mg IM) or cloprostenol sodium (500 μg, IM)
• GnRH (100 μg, IM)

CONTRAINDICATIONS
• Appropriate milk and meat withdrawal times must be followed.
• Estrogens are not approved in some countries.
• PRID™ implants are not approved in the United States.

POSSIBLE INTERACTIONS
N/A

FOLLOW-UP

EXPECTED COURSE AND PROGNOSIS
Results depend on cyclicity, health, and compliance.

POSSIBLE COMPLICATIONS
N/A

CLIENT EDUCATION
• Compliance is critical for success of estrus synchronization programs and schedules for hormone treatments should be followed closely.
• CIDR or PRID™ implants may cause mild vaginitis in some cows. Insertion of implants should be done in a clean manner.
• Insemination in the absence of estrus is more difficult due to the absence of cervical mucus.

• Reproductive hormones must be handled with caution. Handling of PGF2$_\alpha$ by asthmatics and women of child-bearing age should be avoided.

MISCELLANEOUS

ASSOCIATED CONDITIONS
Infertility

AGE-RELATED FACTORS
N/A

ZOONOTIC POTENTIAL
N/A

PREGNANCY
Administration of PGF2$_\alpha$ will cause abortion.

BIOSECURITY
N/A

PRODUCTION MANAGEMENT
• For improved efficiency of all estrus synchronization treatment, animals should be in good body condition and cyclic.
• Partial weaning may be beneficial in late-calving beef cows.

SYNONYMS
N/A

ABBREVIATIONS
• AI = artificial insemination
• CIDR = controlled intravaginal delivery devices
• FSH = follicle stimulating hormone
• FTAI = fixed time artificial insemination
• GnRH = gonadotropin releasing hormone
• IM = intramuscular
• LH = luteinizing hormone
• MGA = melengestrol acetate
• PAG1 = pregnancy associated glycoprotein 1
• PGF2$_\alpha$ = prostaglandin F2$_\alpha$
• PRID™ = Progesterone Releasing Intravaginal Device
• PSPB = pregnancy specific protein B

SEE ALSO
• Artificial Insemination: Bovine
• Reproductive Pharmacology

Suggested Reading
Colazo MG, Mapletoft RJ. A review of current timed-AI (TAI) programs for beef and dairy cattle. Can Vet J 2014, 55: 772–80.
Wiltbank MC, Pursley JR. The cow as an induced ovulator: Timed AI after synchronization of ovulation. Theriogenology 2014, 81: 170–85.
Author Jennifer N. Roberts
Consulting Editor Ahmed Tibary
Acknowledgment The author and book editors acknowledge the prior contribution of Ahmed Tibary.

ESTRUS SYNCHRONIZATION: SMALL RUMINANT

BASICS

OVERVIEW
• Estrus synchronization protocols are treatments that allow manipulation of the estrous cycle and concentration of females in heat over a specific period of time to allow
  ◦ Artificial insemination
  ◦ Concentration of the lambing period
  ◦ Preparation for recipients for embryo transfer
• Synchronization of estrus may be achieved by hormonal treatment, modification of the photoperiod, or the male effect
• Synchronization protocols are also helpful for out-of-season breeding
• Important components of synchronization programs are:
• A good preventive health program (vaccination/deworming)
• Appropriate nutrition
• Ideal BCS (3 out of 5)
• Estrus detection if artificial insemination is used

INCIDENCE/PREVALENCE
N/A

GEOGRAPHIC DISTRIBUTION
Worldwide

SYSTEMS AFFECTED
Reproductive

PATHOPHYSIOLOGY
• Male pheromones may induce an LH surge if the animals are in the transition to the breeding season. However, cycles induced are shorter than normal (poor luteal activity).
• Direct manipulation of response to light using artificial photoperiod or by hormonal treatment (melatonin) can induce cyclicity but this is not widely used.
• The hormonal protocol simulates a luteal phase using progesterone delivery devices or interrupts the normal luteal phase with $PGF2_\alpha$ if the animal is cycling. The combined use of progestogens and $PGF2_\alpha$ allows shortening of the treatment period.
• Response to hormonal treatment depends on normal reproductive function, health, and nutrition status.

HISTORICAL FINDINGS
Desire by owner to implement artificial insemination, concentrate lambing, or breed out of season.

SIGNALMENT
• Sheep and goats of breeding age.
• Animals must be reproductively sound and in adequate health and body condition.
• Maiden females should be at least 65% of mature body weight and size.

PHYSICAL EXAMINATION FINDINS
N/A

GENETICS
• There is great variation in seasonality among breeds.
• Dose of eCG should be adjusted to the breed and season.

CAUSES AND RISK FACTORS
N/A

DIAGNOSIS

DIFFERENTIAL DIAGNOSES
N/A

CBC/BIOCHEMISTRY/URINALYSIS
N/A

OTHER LABORATORY TESTS
N/A

IMAGING
Transrectal ultrasonography to assess the reproductive status; however, this is not used routinely.

OTHER DIAGNOSTIC PROCEDURES
• Male breeding soundness examination if natural mating
• Semen evaluation if artificial insemination

TREATMENT

THERAPEUTIC APPROACH
Male (Ram or Buck) Effect
• Females that are separated (smell, sight, and contact) from males for at least 3–4 weeks will show estrus between 2 and 6 days after the sudden introduction of a male. Ovulation occurs in response to an LH surge in a large proportion of females.
• Males used for induction of estrus and ovulation are usually vasectomized or fitted with an apron.
• Induced estrus may result in short cycles.
• The best results using this technique are achieved during the transition season.
• The male effect provides good synchronization of sheep and goats for natural breeding.
• Synchronization is not tight enough to use artificial insemination.

$PGF2_\alpha$ or Analogs
• $PGF2_\alpha$ causes luteolysis and return to estrus during the breeding season.
• Treated females should be cyclic and at least 5 days after ovulation.
• A single injection induces estrus 3–6 days after treatment in about 60% of the females.
• A two-injections protocol allows more females (>85%) to be synchronized about 48 hours after the second injection. The interval between injection is different for sheep and goats because of the difference in cycle length.
• In sheep, the injections are given 9–11 days apart.

• In goats, the injections are given 11–12 days apart.
• This system is efficient for AI if combined with heat detection.

Progestogens
• Progestogens are delivered using vaginal insert (sponges or silicone) devices (progesterone, subcutaneous implants (Norgestomet) or oral administration (MGA)
• The most commonly used treatment for synchronization of estrus in sheep in the United States is progesterone CIDR
• During the breeding season, length of treatment without use of $PGF2_\alpha$ is 14 days for sheep and 17 days for goats.
• Outside of the breeding season, length of treatment is shortened.
• Shorter treatments may be used during the breeding season but require administration of a luteolytic dose of $PGF2_\alpha$ at progestogen withdrawal.
• Administration of an FSH-like hormone (eCG or PG 600) the day before or on the day of progesterone withdrawal improves estrus synchrony and promotes follicular development, especially in the non-breeding season.
• Estrus can be expected approximately 54 and 48 hours after progestogen withdrawal in ewes and does, respectively.
• Administration of $PGF2_\alpha$ 24 hours before progestogen withdrawal and introduction of a teaser male 24 hours later further tightens estrus synchrony.

Other Methods
• Photoperiod manipulation can be used for out-of-season breeding but does not provide a good synchronization and is seldom used because of the facilities requirements.
• Melatonin treatment (18 mg SQ for 35 days) in combination with photoperiod manipulation, CIDRs or ram effect has been effective in advancing the breeding season and synchronizing estrus.

SURGICAL CONSIDERATIONS AND TECHNIQUES
N/A

MEDICATIONS

DRUGS OF CHOICE
$PGF2_\alpha$ and Analogs
• $PGF2_\alpha$ (dinoprost tromethamine) IM: Sheep: 15 mg/animal, Goats: 10 mg/animal
• Synthetic analog (cloprostenol): Sheep: 125–150 µg/animal Goats: 50–150 µg/animal

Progestogens
• Vaginal implants
  ◦ CIDR: Progesterone 330 mg
  ◦ FGA: 30–40 mg
  ◦ MAP: 60 mg
• Subcutaneous implants: Norgestomet 3 mg

E

ESTRUS SYNCHRONIZATION: SMALL RUMINANT (CONTINUED)

Gonadotropins
- eCG: 400 IU out of the breeding season and 200 IU during the breeding season.
- PG 600: 400 IU eCG and 200 IU hCG

Melatonin
Melatonin subcutaneous implant has been used to increase ovulation rate and anticipate the breeding season (not available in US).

CONTRAINDICATIONS
- Some synchronization treatments are not approved in some countries.
- Progestogens are not approved for dairy animals in some countries.
- Appropriate milk and meat withdrawal times must be followed.

PRECAUTIONS
Hormones should not be handled by pregnant women. Protective wear is advised during administration.

POSSIBLE INTERACTION
N/A

 FOLLOW-UP

EXPECTED COURSE AND PROGNOSIS
- Response rate in terms of estrus induction is excellent (>90%) with progestogen protocols.
- Fertility after natural breeding depends on the male : female ratio.
- Fertility after fixed-time insemination ranges from 50% to 80%.
- Prolificacy depends on the season and dose of eCG.

POSSIBLE COMPLICATIONS
- Vaginitis may be observed at progestogen withdrawal but subsides within a couple of days.
- Loss of the vaginal insert will result in poor response.

CLIENT EDUCATION
- Instruction on appropriate methods of injections and placement/removal of CIDR.
- Compliance in treatment schedule and dosing.
- Ram/buck breeding soundness examination and male power prior to synchronization.

PATIENT CARE
- Monitoring for signs of heat
- Monitoring for CIDR loss

PREVENTION
N/A

 MISCELLANEOUS

ASSOCIATED CONDITIONS
Vaginitis

AGE-RELATED FACTORS
N/A

ZOONOTIC POTENTIAL
N/A

PREGNANCY
N/A

PRODUCTION MANAGEMENT
- Appropriate preparation for the breeding season should be implemented 4 weeks prior to synchronization
  - Nutrition flushing with adequate BCS (3 out of 5)
  - Vaccination and deworming
- Heat detection
  - Preparation of teaser animals
- Record keeping
- Pregnancy diagnosis timing and fetal number

SYNONYMS
N/A

ABBREVIATIONS
- AI = artificial insemination
- BCS = body condition score
- CIDR = controlled internal device release
- eCG = equine chorionic gonadotropin
- FGA = fluorogestone acetate
- FSH = follicle stimulating hormone
- MAP = 6α-methyl-6-dehydro-16-methylene-17α-acetoxy-preg-1,6-diene-3, 20-dione, megestrol acetate
- $PGF2_\alpha$ = prostaglandin $F2_\alpha$

SEE ALSO
- Artificial Insemination: Small Ruminant
- Breeding Soundness examination: Small Ruminant
- Castration/Vasectomy: Small Ruminant
- Embryo Transfer: Small Ruminant
- Parasite Control Programs: Small Ruminant
- Pregnancy Diagnosis: Small Ruminant
- Vaccination Programs: Small Ruminant

Suggested Reading
Abecia JA, Forcada F, Gonzalez-Bulnes A. Pharmaceutical control of reproduction in sheep and goats. Vet Clin North Am Food Anim Pract 2011, 27: 67–9.
Abecia JA, Forcada F, Gonzalez-Bulnes A. Hormonal control of reproduction in small ruminants. Anim Reprod Sci 2012, 130: 173–9.
Deligiannis C, Valasi I, Rekkas CA, et al. Synchronization of ovulation and fixed time intrauterine insemination in ewes. Reprod Domest Anim 2005, 40: 6–10.
Dowson LJ. Manipulating the estrous cycle in a doe. In: Youngquist RS, Threlfall WR eds, Current Therapy in Large Animal Theriogenology, 2nd ed. St. Louis: Sanders-Elsevier, 2007, pp. 540–7.
Author Michela Ciccarelli
Consulting Editor Ahmed Tibary

FAILURE OF PASSIVE TRANSFER

BASICS

OVERVIEW
• Newborn ruminants are born hypogammaglobulinemic due to the nature of their placentation.
• Although immunocompetent at birth, neonatal ruminants are immunonaïve and dependent on maternally derived immunoglobulin and other factors absorbed from colostrum.
• Neonates that fail to acquire adequate passive immunity are said to suffer failure of passive transfer.
• Failure of passive transfer is not a disease, but a condition that predisposes animals to contracting infectious diseases.

INCIDENCE/PREVALENCE
• May vary by species, farm, and production system employed on the farm.
• An association exists between higher IgG levels and lower disease incidence.
• This association appears to have a greater influence in herds with high disease incidence compared to herds with low disease incidence.

GEOGRAPHIC DISTRIBUTION
Worldwide

SYSTEMS AFFECTED
• Multisystemic
• Digestive
• Musculoskeletal
• Respiratory

PATHOPHYSIOLOGY
• Composition and formation of colostrum
  ○ Colostrum is a complex fluid that contains immunoglobulins, immune cells, immunoactive substances such as cytokines, and nutritional elements.
  ○ While all of these components are important, we often focus on immunoglobulins because they are a large constituent of colostrum and they are the most thoroughly studied component.
  ○ Immunoglobulin G1 (IgG1) is the primary immunoglobulin in bovine colostrum.
  ○ Colostral IgG1 originates from maternal serum and is transferred by active, IgG1-specific, Fc receptors into colostrum during the last 4–6 weeks of gestation.
• Colostral cellular makeup
  ○ Colostrum contains >1 × 10⁶ cells per milliliter.
  ○ Lymphocytes make up approximately 20–30% of colostral cells in sheep and cattle and differ from those in maternal circulation. They function by modulating the neonatal immune system and the secretion of various cytokines, as well as the secretion of immunoglobulin A.
  ○ Macrophages and neutrophils make up the remainder of colostral cells.

○ Macrophages are thought to serve as cytokine-producing and antigen-presenting cells.
○ The neutrophils are likely involved in the protection of the mammary gland rather than the neonate.
○ While interleukin-2 (IL-2) and tumor necrosis factor (TNF) have been found in colostrum, their role as yet is unknown.
○ Colostrum is rich in insulin-like growth factor-1 (IGF-1), which helps regulate newborn growth and may enhance the early neonatal immune response.
○ Transforming growth factor is present in high concentrations in bovine colostrum but decreases by 30 days postpartum.
• Absorption of colostrum
  ○ Absorption and transfer across the neonatal intestinal epithelial cells occur via nonselective pinocytosis initiated by the presence of macromolecules.
  ○ The efficiency of immunoglobulin absorption declines to zero over the first approximately 24 hours of life.
  ○ The term "closure" is used to define the point at which absorption of immunoglobulins by the gut ceases.
  ○ The absorptive process across the gut epithelium appears to be saturable. That is, a finite capacity exists for the absorption of all macromolecules.
  ○ The presence of high levels of non-immunoglobulin molecules fed during the first 24 hours of life may adversely compete with the absorption of colostral immunoglobulins.

SIGNALMENT
Neonates of any ruminant species

PHYSICAL EXAMINATION FINDINGS
• Failure of passive transfer is not a disease, but a condition that predisposes to the development of infectious diseases.
• Affected animals are at increased risk for the development of diseases such as septicemia, enteritis, diarrhea, omphalitis, arthritis, and respiratory disease.
• Animals with FPT may be clinically normal in a low infection pressure environment.

CAUSES AND RISK FACTORS
• An association exists between higher IgG (or protein) levels and lower disease incidence.
• This association appears to have a greater influence in herds with high disease incidence compared to herds with low disease incidence.
• The rate of disease occurrence is obviously a balance between a calf's ability to resist disease and the severity of disease challenging the calf.
• Serum immunoglobulin concentration is only one factor that contributes to disease resistance. Other factors that influence disease resistance might include the less-studied non-immunoglobulin components of colostrum (cells, cytokines, etc.).
• Additional factors to consider in assessing disease risk include general hygiene, pathogen

virulence, pathogen concentration, physical environment (e.g., temperature, humidity, wind chill), nutritional status, and miscellaneous stresses (e.g., transportation, handling, surgery).

DIAGNOSIS

DIFFERENTIAL DIAGNOSES
N/A

CBC/BIOCHEMISTRY/URINALYSIS
• Results of these tests may be indicative of clinical disease as a result of FPT.
• Serum protein >5.5 g/dL is indicative of adequate passive transfer.

OTHER LABORATORY TESTS
• Many methods are available to measure immunoglobulin concentrations in calf serum after absorption from colostrum.
• Serum IgG1 concentration of 10 mg/mL at 48 hours of age is the objective value for defining the threshold between adequate passive transfer and failure of passive transfer.
• The various tests for immunoglobulin concentration vary in their speed, accuracy, and equipment required for operation.
• Single radial immunodiffusion (SRID) and the enzyme-linked immunosorbent assay (ELISA) are the only tests that directly measure serum IgG concentration. Other tests including zinc sulfate turbidity, sodium sulfite precipitation, whole blood glutaraldehyde coagulation, total serum solids by refractometry, and gamma-glutamyl transferase activity indirectly estimate serum IgG concentration based on colostral total proteins.
• The techniques for performing these tests and the values used for their interpretation can be found in numerous manuscripts and texts (see "Suggested Reading").
  ○ Test endpoints for many assays can be manipulated depending on the goals of the individual producer.
• Results of the various testing methods on any particular operation must be kept in perspective and their use not over-interpreted.
• Test accuracy
  ○ Accurate measurement of serum immunoglobulin in a particular calf does not necessarily guarantee protection from disease, for the following reasons:
    ■ The tests only quantify a calf's serum immunoglobulin concentration. They do not determine specific protective capabilities of the absorbed immunoglobulins.
    ■ The tests cannot determine if the absorbed immunoglobulins will reach the appropriate site of challenge in a calf in sufficient concentrations to neutralize a particular pathogen.
  ○ These two points are not meant to conclude that there is no benefit in

measuring serum immunoglobulin levels as an indicator of passive transfer of immunity. They illustrate the potential limitations of measuring immunoglobulin levels.

PATHOLOGIC FINDINGS
N/A

TREATMENT
In cases of failure of passive transfer and depending on the value of the animal, plasma transfusion may be warranted.

MEDICATIONS
DRUGS OF CHOICE
N/A

FOLLOW-UP
EXPECTED COURSE AND PROGNOSIS
• Approximately 70% of animals with FPT will survive, but may have long-term production losses when compared to their peers.
• In animals that become sick, clinical course and prognosis vary and are associated with the underlying disease process. Without aggressive therapy in sick animals, failure of passive transfer warrants a guarded to poor prognosis.

PREVENTION
• Proper colostral management
  ○ Dairy calves should get a minimum of 3 L of good-quality colostrum within 6 hours after birth.

○ Beef calves, kids, lambs, and cria typically will achieve adequate passive transfer if the dam has colostrum and the neonate stands and nurses within the first 2–4 hours.
• Only first milking colostrum should be fed to the newborn during the first 12 hours of life.

MISCELLANEOUS
ASSOCIATED CONDITIONS
Septicemia, enteritis, diarrhea, omphalitis, arthritis, and respiratory disease

AGE-RELATED FACTORS
First 24–48 hours of life

BIOSECURITY
• Do not pool colostrum. Feed colostrum from an individual preselected dam to individual young stock.
• Minimize disease transfer via colostrum (e.g., Johne's disease, CAE, BLV) by preselecting negative dams.

PRODUCTION MANAGEMENT
• Young stock whose dam produces inadequate colostrum should be fed colostrum from a preselected donor.
• Frozen colostrum should be stored from individual donors, identified, and marked prior to freezing.
• Maintain a bank of frozen, high-quality colostrum for use in emergency situations.
• Feed young stock within 2 hours of birth and again within 12 hours of birth.

ABBREVIATIONS
• CAE = caprine arthritis encephalitis
• ELISA = enzyme-linked immunosorbent assay

• Fc = IgG1-specific Fc receptors
• IGF-1 = insulin-like growth factor-1
• IgG1 = immunoglobulin G1
• IL-2 = interleukin-2
• SRID = single radial immunodiffusion
• TNF = tumor necrosis factor

Suggested Reading
Barrington GM, Parish SM. Bovine neonatal immunology. Vet Clin North Am Food Anim Pract 2001, 17: 463–76.
Butler JE. Bovine immunoglobulins: an augmented review. Vet Immunol Immunopathol 1983, 4: 43–152.
Weaver DM, Tyler JW, Marion RS, et al. Evaluation of assays for determination of passive transfer status in neonatal llamas and alpacas. J Am Vet Med Assoc 2000, 216: 559–63.
Weaver DM, Tyler JW, VanMetre DC, Hostetler DE, Barrington GM. Passive transfer of colostral immunoglobulin in calves. J Vet Intern Med 2000, 14: 569–77.
Author Dusty W. Nagy
Consulting Editor Christopher C.L. Chase
Acknowledgment The author and book editors acknowledge the prior contribution of George Barrington.

 Client Education Handout available online

BASICS

OVERVIEW
• Fatty liver is a pathologic fat accumulation resulting from high concentrations of blood NEFA, especially in cows with a high BCS or excessive abdominal fat at calving. Obesity occurs when dry cows are overfed during the prepartum period, or are dried off in an overconditioned state.
• Fatty liver is related to other diseases occurring during the postpartum period such as ketosis, RFM, metritis, hypocalcemia, and displaced abomasum.
• Fatty liver may be a slow, insidious process or may develop abruptly within 48 hours after parturition. Consequently, clinical signs may range from mild decreased milk production to sudden death in a few days post parturition.

INCIDENCE/PREVALENCE
In the United States, incidences ranging from 10% to 20% have been reported.

GEOGRAPHIC DISTRIBUTION
Worldwide

SYSTEMS AFFECTED
Multisystemic

PATHOPHYSIOLOGY
• At calving and beyond, catecholamines and glucagon are increased and insulin is reduced. As a result, hormone-sensitive lipase is activated. Particularly in cows with excessive body fat stores, a large amount of NEFA are released from the TG. This process continues during the postpartum period driven by the process of milk production and the low dry matter intake characterizing the early postpartum cow.
• The cow progresses to a negative energy balance during the postpartum period, which is a normal process. However, obese animals or cows experiencing other postpartum disease may experience a more severe fat mobilization.
• TGs are broken down and released as NEFA and glycerol, which are directed to the liver via the bloodstream.
• The liver of the cow takes up NEFA from the blood. Inside the hepatocyte, they are either oxidized to acetate or re-esterified to TG. If NEFA are in excess, re-esterification is the leading process. Because the bovine liver has a reduced capacity to synthesize and export back to the blood the excess of TG in the form of VLDL, the net result is the accumulation of TG in the cytosol of the cells. If this accumulation is profound, severe liver damage occurs.

HISTORICAL FINDINGS
• Obesity at calving ± history of overfeeding during the dry period.

• Concurrent postparturient disorders such as metritis, retained fetal membranes, milk fever, ketosis, and/or displaced abomasum.

SIGNALMENT
• Primarily high-producing dairy cows, particularly with high BCS at parturition.
• Heifers fed high-energy diets, thus calving while extremely obese, may experience severe fatty liver.
• May be individual animal case or a herd problem.
• Fatty liver has been commonly diagnosed in Holstein cattle; however, it has also been reported in Jersey, Guernsey, and Ayrshire breeds.

PHYSICAL EXAMINATION FINDINGS
Clinical signs are related to the degree of liver damage:
• Overcondition
• Anorexia
• Depression and weakness
• Decreased milk production
• Occasionally sudden death
• These signs can persist even after the levels of hepatic TG decrease back to baseline.

GENETICS
There are no heritability estimates for fatty liver. However, for the related diseases of ketosis and displaced abomasum, heritability estimates are low to moderate.

CAUSES AND RISK FACTORS
Risk factors for fatty liver are obesity at calving (>3.75/5), severe feed restriction during the prepartum close to calving, feeding excess energy during the entire dry period, and long calving intervals. During lactation, risk factors include periparturient disease, anorexia, ketogenic diets, sudden feed changes, dystocia, stress, and poor cow comfort.

DIAGNOSIS

DIFFERENTIAL DIAGNOSES
• Concurrent postpartum diseases
• Secondary differentials include other types of hepatitis such as toxic, infectious (salmonellosis and clostridiosis), parasitic (fluke), and miscellaneous (cholestasis, hepatic encephalopathy, and abscesses).

CBC/BIOCHEMISTRY/URINALYSIS
CBC
Changes may be nonspecific but frequently include leukopenia, neutropenia, lymphopenia, and a degenerative left shift. Fibrinogen, haptoglobin, and serum amyloid A may be increased.

Biochemistry
The common biochemical profiles are variable depending on the degree of liver damage.
• Marked increase: Glutamate dehydrogenase, γ-glutamyl transferase, aspartate

aminotransferase, malondialdehyde, cholic acid, bile acids and bilirubin, albumin.
• Mild to moderate increase: Lactate dehydrogenase, sorbitol dehydrogenase, alkaline phosphatase, and ornithine carbamoyl transferase.
• Decrease: Albumin, α-tocopherol, VLDL, HDL, and LDL.

OTHER LABORATORY TESTS
• Increased NEFA, BHB, and acetoacetate
• Decreased glucagon, insulin, glucocorticoids, IGF-I, and thyroid hormones

IMAGING
Ultrasonography of the liver will show increased echogenicity and possibly enlargement depending on severity.

OTHER DIAGNOSTIC PROCEDURES
Liver biopsy is the definitive diagnostic test for fatty liver. The sample can be evaluated either chemically or histologically.

PATHOLOGIC FINDINGS
• On necropsy, the liver is enlarged with rounded edges, greasy to the touch, extremely friable, and has different degrees of yellow color depending on the amount of TG accumulated. In addition, excessive subcutaneous, abdominal, and omental fat can be observed. Other findings may be toxemia, metritis, RFM, mastitis, and displacement of abomasum.
• Histologic evaluation of liver biopsy shows fatty cysts in parenchyma, increased volume of hepatocytes, mitochondrial damage, and decreased volume of nuclei and other organelles.

TREATMENT

Treatment of fatty liver depends on the degree of fat infiltration, signs and origin of the problem.

THERAPEUTIC APPROACH
• Mild to moderate fatty liver can be challenging to diagnose. Consequently, treatments may be similar to those for preventing hepatic lipidosis.
• Stimulation of feed intake should be done by offering fresh, high-quality diets several times a day. Transfaunation of rumen fluid from healthy cows is complementary.
• Supportive therapy must aim to correct the negative energy balance, reduce fat mobilization, and promote carbohydrate metabolism. The use of feed additives such as ionophores (sodium monensin 300 mg per cow daily), gluconeogenic precursors such as glycerol (200 g/d), propylene glycol (300 g/d), calcium propionate (500 g/d), and vitamins such as protected choline (60 g/d) and niacin (12 g/d), protected methionine and chromium as Cr-methionine, both prepartum and postpartum are recommended.

F

FATTY LIVER

SURGICAL CONSIDERATIONS AND TECHNIQUES
N/A

MEDICATIONS

DRUGS OF CHOICE
• Most treatments are aimed at controlling ketosis.
• Dextrose IV at 50%, 250–500 mL. Repeat for 3 days.
• Glucocorticoids (10–30 mg dexamethasone; 2–5 mg flumethasone, or 100–200 mg prednisolone). Be aware glucocorticoids also depress immunity.
• Glucagon SQ at 15 mg/day for 14 days.

CONTRAINDICATIONS
Appropriate milk and meat withdrawal times must be followed for all compounds. Corticoids in pregnant animals are contraindicated.

FOLLOW-UP

EXPECTED COURSE AND PROGNOSIS
The prognosis is very poor in severe and complicated cases of fatty liver. Early diagnosis and treatment of fatty liver and underlying health conditions will markedly improve the outcome.

CLIENT EDUCATION
See "Production Management"

PREVENTION
• The most effective tool for preventing fatty liver is to avoid an overconditioned dam at calving and to improve overall cow comfort and management. During lactation, the goal is to minimize the negative energy balance.
• Overall proper nutritional and feeding management during the entire transition period is a must.

MISCELLANEOUS

ASSOCIATED CONDITIONS
Clinical signs and the fate of fatty liver are related to the degree of liver damage and to other calving-related disorders that may be simultaneously present.

AGE-RELATED FACTORS
Generally, animals in their second through fourth lactation; however, overconditioned heifers can be a real problem in certain herds.

ZOONOTIC POTENTIAL
N/A

PREGNANCY
Prepartum fatty liver is likely and consequently it may affect the pregnancy status. In addition, fatty liver and ketosis may compromise further fertility of the current lactation.

BIOSECURITY
N/A

PRODUCTION MANAGEMENT
Good transition cow management, in all areas, is imperative to preventing fatty liver. This includes nutrition, health, and facilities management. See chapter, Transition Cow Management (www.fiveminutevet.com/ruminant) for more information.

SYNONYM
Hepatic lipidosis

ABBREVIATIONS
• BCS = body condition score
• HDL = high density lipoprotein
• LDL = low density lipoprotein
• NEFA = non-esterified fatty acid
• RFM = retained fetal membranes
• TG = triglyceride
• VLDL = very low density lipoprotein

SEE ALSO
• Body Condition Scoring: Dairy Cattle (see www.fiveminutevet.com/ruminant)
• Dairy Nutrition: Ration Guidelines for Milking and Dry Cows (see www.fiveminutevet.com/ruminant)
• Displaced Abomasum
• Hypocalcemia: Bovine
• Ketosis: Dairy Cattle
• Metritis
• Nutrition and Metabolic Diseases: Dairy

Suggested Reading
Bobe G, Young JW, Beitz DC. Pathology, etiology, prevention, and treatment of fatty liver in dairy cows. J Dairy Sci 2004, 87: 3105–24.
Esposito G, Irons P, Webb E, Chapwanya A. Interactions between negative energy balance, metabolic diseases, uterine health and immune response in transition dairy cows. Anim Reprod Sci 2014, 144: 60–71.
Goff JP. Major advances in our understanding of nutritional influences on bovine health. J Dairy Sci 2006, 89: 1292–301.
Grummer RR. Nutritional and managment strategies for the prevention of fatty liver in dairy cattle. Vet J 2008, 176: 10–20.
LeBlanc SJ, Lissemore KD, Kelton DF, Duffield TF, Leslie KE. Major advances in disease prevention in dairy cattle. J Dairy Sci 2006, 89: 1267–79.
Ospina PA, McArt JA, Overton TR, Stokol T, Nydam DV. Using nonesterified fatty acids and β-hydroxybutyrate concentrations during the transition period for herd-level monitoring of increased risk of disease and decreased reproductive and milking performance. Vet Clin North Am Food Anim Pract 2013, 29: 387–412.
Author Pedro Melendez
Consulting Editor Kaitlyn A. Lutz
Acknowledgment The author and book editors acknowledge the prior contribution of J. Jerry Kaneko.

BASICS

OVERVIEW
• Tall fescue (*Festuca arundinacea*) is a cool season perennial grass grown worldwide.
• The grass itself is not the cause of toxicity, but rather an endophytic fungus that infects it, *Neotyphodium coenophialum* (endophyte-infected).
• *N. coenophialum* produces several ergot-type alkaloids, which cause the clinical signs associated with fescue toxicity.
• Three syndromes are seen in ruminants: fescue foot, summer slump, and fat necrosis.
• Another syndrome causing severe reproductive abnormalities in pregnant mares is seen less commonly in ruminants.

INCIDENCE/PREVALENCE
Unknown

GEOGRAPHIC DISTRIBUTION
• Tall fescue is a cool season perennial grass grown worldwide.
• Over 40 million acres of tall fescue are used for livestock grazing in the United States. Tall fescue is the predominant pasture grass east of the Mississippi River. Cases of fescue toxicity have been reported throughout the country.

SYSTEMS AFFECTED
• Cardiovascular
• Musculoskeletal
• Reproductive
• Hemolymphatic

PATHOPHYSIOLOGY
• *N. coenophialum* produces several ergot-type alkaloids, namely ergovaline, which are responsible for the clinical signs of fescue toxicity.
• Ergovaline acts as a D2 dopaminergic receptor agonist resulting in inhibition of prolactin secretion and imbalances of progesterone and estrogen.
• Decreased prolactin secretion causes reduced lactation or agalactia and also inhibits function of the hypothalamic thermoregulatory center.
• The toxin also causes peripheral vasoconstriction, resulting in inadequate blood flow to the extremities in cold weather and inhibited thermoregulatory capacity in hot weather.

SIGNALMENT
• This toxicosis affects cattle, sheep, and goats, as well as horses.
• All ruminant species are potentially affected.
• Any animal that is grazing or consuming fescue hay can be affected.
• Cases of exotic ruminants in zoos and wildlife parks have been reported.

PHYSICAL EXAMINATION FINDINGS
• Fescue foot:
  ○ Signs usually develop within 10–14 days after being introduced to contaminated pasture in cool weather.
  ○ Progressive lameness, particularly in rear limbs.
  ○ Redness and swelling around coronary band.
  ○ Cold extremities.
  ○ Gangrenous necrosis of the distal limbs below the level of the pastern or fetlock.
  ○ Tips of ears and switch of tail may also necrose.
  ○ Affected animals are often underweight but remain alert.
• Summer slump:
  ○ Period of poor production (decreased feed intake, growth, milk production) due to heat intolerance when the ambient temperature exceeds 75–80°F.
  ○ Hirsutism, retention of winter coat.
  ○ Elevated temperature and respiratory rate.
  ○ Animals seek shade or wet spots and spend increased amounts of time lying down.
  ○ Hypersalivation.
  ○ Lowered reproductive performance: Delayed puberty; decreased conception and pregnancy rates.
• Fat necrosis:
  ○ Most often an incidental finding at rectal palpation or on necropsy.
  ○ When present, signs are related to obstruction of abdominal organs (e.g., bloat, colic).

CAUSES AND RISK FACTORS
• Consumption of tall fescue that is infected with *N. coenophialum*.
• The fungus has a symbiotic relationship with the fescue, providing insect resistance, drought tolerance, and increased nitrogen utilization to the plant.
• Noninfected varieties of tall fescue are available but they do not withstand extreme environmental conditions so well as the endophyte-infected varieties.
• *Neotyphodium coenophialum* is present within the seed and throughout the plant.
• Summer slump is seen in warm to hot ambient temperatures.
• Fescue foot is more commonly seen in cold ambient temperatures.
• Fescue foot follows introduction to contaminated pasture; cattle permanently pastured on the field are rarely affected.

DIAGNOSIS

DIFFERENTIAL DIAGNOSES
• Fescue foot:
  ○ Ergot toxicosis/*Claviceps purpurea* toxicity
  ○ Foot rot
  ○ Frostbite
  ○ Trauma
  ○ Selenium toxicity
• Summer slump:
  ○ Ergot toxicosis/*Claviceps purpurea* toxicity
  ○ Heat stress
  ○ Nutritional deficiencies
  ○ Water deprivation
  ○ Gastrointestinal parasitism
• Fat necrosis:
  ○ Lymphosarcoma
  ○ Intestinal obstruction

CBC/BIOCHEMISTRY/URINALYSIS
N/A

OTHER DIAGNOSTIC PROCEDURES
• High index of suspicion is provided by observation of classic clinical signs.
• History of consuming fescue (pasture or in hay).
• Clinical signs (with the exception of fat necrosis) may be indistinguishable from those of *Claviceps purpurea* toxicity. As the associated ergotoxins may also be present in tall fescue, a definitive diagnosis may not be achieved.
• Exclusion of other differentials for poor production (e.g., poor nutrition, parasitism) is recommended when summer slump is suspected.
• Microscopic examination of fescue for fungus; the fungus is found throughout the plant, including the seeds, stems, and leaf sheaths.

PATHOLOGIC FINDINGS
• All syndromes
  ○ Poor body condition
  ○ Rough hair coat
• Fescue foot: Gangrenous tissue on extremities, particularly rear limbs, with a line of demarcation from normal tissue.
• Fat necrosis: Presence of calcified fat in abdomen.
• Histologic lesions seen with fescue foot include vascular thrombosis, tissue necrosis in lower limbs.

TREATMENT

THERAPEUTIC APPROACH
• Removal from affected pasture or removal of contaminated hay.
• Early treatment of fescue foot with antibiotics and nursing care may be beneficial. Treatment is generally unrewarding after the onset of tissue necrosis.

MEDICATIONS

DRUGS OF CHOICE
Fescue foot: Broad-spectrum antibiotic therapy may be warranted for secondary bacterial infections.

F

FESCUE TOXICITY

FOLLOW-UP

EXPECTED COURSE AND PROGNOSIS
Gangrenous lesions associated with fescue foot are irreversible and are associated with a poor prognosis for return to production.

PREVENTION
• Avoid grazing fescue pastures when ambient temperature rises.
• Avoid grazing animals in heavy lactation or within 60 days of parturition in affected pastures when possible.
• Gradually introduce animals to fescue pastures by limiting time spent on pastures or by providing hay or alternate forage sources to limit intakes.

MISCELLANEOUS

ASSOCIATED CONDITIONS
• Reproductive effects of fescue toxicity are seen primarily in mares grazing affected pastures. Clinical signs of toxicity include agalactia, prolonged gestation, dystocia, and thickened or retained placenta.
• Classic ergotism, caused by *Claviceps purpurea* toxicity, can produce clinical signs identical to fescue foot and summer slump.

PREGNANCY
Toxicity less commonly results in complication of pregnancy in ruminants than in mares.

PRODUCTION MANAGEMENT
• Pasture dilution with clovers or other grasses can be used to control or limit fescue toxicity.
• Avoid overfertilization of tall fescue with nitrogen as this often precipitates endophyte growth and intoxication.
• Ammoniation of hay removes the toxicity.
• Nontoxic varieties of endophyte-infected fescue have been developed and appear to be hardier than noninfected fescue but with a much lower potential to cause the untoward effects seen with toxic endophyte-infected varieties.
• Recent research suggests that treatment of fescue or direct feeding of seaweed extract (*Ascophyllum nodosum*) may decrease the toxic effects of endophyte-infected fescue.

SYNONYMS
• Fescue foot
• Summer slump

ABBREVIATIONS
N/A

SEE ALSO
• Foot Rot: Bovine
• Foot Rot: Small Ruminant
• Frostbite
• Heat Stress
• Lameness: Bovine
• Lameness: Small Ruminant
• Lymphosarcoma
• Nutritional Assessment (see www.fiveminutevet.com/ruminant)
• Parasite Control Programs: Beef
• Parasite Control Programs: Dairy
• Parasite Control Programs: Small Ruminant
• Selenium Toxicity
• Selenium/Vitamin E Deficiency

Suggested Reading
Brendemuehl JP. Fescue toxicosis. In: Smith BP ed, Large Animal Internal Medicine, 3rd ed. Philadelphia: Mosby, 2002, pp. 221–2.
Davis EW. Fescue foot. In: Smith BP ed, Large Animal Internal Medicine, 3rd ed. Philadelphia: Mosby, 2002, 1126–7.
Mostrom MS, Jacobsen BJ. Ruminant mycotoxicosis. Vet Clin North Am Food Anim Pract 2011, 27: 315–44.
Osweiler GD. Fescue poisoning. In: Kahn CM ed, The Merck Veterinary Manual. Kenilworth, NJ: Merck & Co., 2010. http://www.merckvetmanual.com/mvm/toxicology/mycotoxicoses/fescue_poisoning.html
Riet-Correa F, Rivero R, Odriozola E, Adrien M de L, Medeiros RM, Schild AL. Mycotoxicoses of ruminants and horses. J Vet Diagn Invest 2013, 25: 692–708.
Author Benjamin W. Newcomer
Consulting Editor Christopher C.L. Chase
Acknowledgment The author and book editors acknowledge the prior contribution of Dawn J. Capucille.

BASICS

OVERVIEW
• Floppy kid syndrome (FKS) is a type of acute-onset metabolic acidosis observed in 3- to 10-day-old goat kids and characterized by severe weakness and flaccid paresis.
• The syndrome was first documented in Canada in 1981, and was subsequently recognized in the United States and Europe.
• A major outbreak of FKS occurred in the mid-1990s in west Texas after introduction of the Boer goat and changes in husbandry related to this breed of goat.
• Although confirmation of FKS can be achieved by demonstrating metabolic acidosis on venous blood gas analysis, in the majority of cases, the diagnosis is established on the basis of clinical history, response to treatment, and necropsy findings in nonsurvivors.

INCIDENCE/PREVALENCE
• The incidence of FKS in a given herd varies from year to year.
• Morbidity can reach 10 to >50%.
• If untreated, mortality can be as high as 30–50% of affected kids.

GEOGRAPHIC DISTRIBUTION
The disease has been recognized in Canada, the United States and Europe.

SYSTEMS AFFECTED
Musculoskeletal

PATHOPHYSIOLOGY
• The exact cause of FKS is not well understood.
• Some infectious agents including *Clostridium botulinum*, *Escherichia coli*, *Cryptosporidium* and caprine herpes virus have been suspected as contributing to the syndrome but this has not been definitively confirmed.
• Clinical disease results from metabolic acidosis without dehydration.

HISTORICAL FINDINGS
• In affected herds, recent management changes are often reported which might include improving nutrition of the does prior to or during pregnancy, and greater confinement of doe-kid pairs.
• Affected kids usually have a history of normal birth and no signs of disease for the first few days of life.

SIGNALMENT
• Clinical signs of FKS appear in kids between 3 and 10 days after birth.
• There is no sex or breed predilection.

PHYSICAL EXAMINATION FINDINGS
• At 3–10 days of age, affected goat kids display severe depression, weakness, decreased muscle tone, somnolence, and flaccid tetraparesis without accompanying diarrhea, dehydration, or fever.
• Affected kids are generally presented in sternal or lateral recumbency with carpal flexion and inability to rise.
• Once clinical signs appear, affected kids are unable to suck but they can swallow.
• Abdominal distension is a commonly reported clinical sign in affected kids.
• The signs of depression and paralysis in affected kids can fluctuate in severity over minutes to hours, and affected kids can give the appearance of being dead. Spontaneous transient recovery can occur, often followed by a return to severe depression and coma.
• Affected animals that are not treated may die within a few days.
• Signs of aspiration pneumonia can accompany the condition in kids that are force-fed, due to aspiration of milk during inadequate suckling.

GENETICS
N/A

CAUSES AND RISK FACTORS
• Goat kids raised in pens, with continuous access to milk, are at high risk of FKS.
• Goat kids that are bottle-fed with excessive amounts of pasteurized or unpasteurized milk are also at risk.

DIAGNOSIS

DIFFERENTIAL DIAGNOSES
Diseases that cause weakness, recumbency, and/or abdominal distension should be considered including nutritional myopathy (vitamin E/selenium deficiency), abomasal bloat, neonatal septicemia, colibacillosis, enterotoxemia (pulpy kidney disease), and enzootic ataxia (copper deficiency).

CBC/BIOCHEMISTRY/URINALYSIS
• All affected animals have metabolic acidosis.
• Floppy kids have a significantly larger anion gap than healthy kids (31.2 ± 3.7 versus 21.5 ± 8.5 mM); decreased serum bicarbonate, normal to increased chloride, and occasional hypokalemia.
• The concentration of L-lactate is lower in floppy kids than in healthy kids (0.67 ± 0.49 versus 1.60 ± 1.02 mM), but the concentration of D-lactate is higher in floppy kids (7.43 ± 2.71 versus 0.26 ± 0.24 mM in healthy kids).
• The serum concentration of urea is increased in goat kids with FKS.

OTHER LABORATORY TESTS
N/A

IMAGING
N/A

OTHER DIAGNOSTIC PROCEDURES
N/A

PATHOLOGIC FINDINGS
• The most characteristic gross lesion found in affected kids is a severely distended abomasum that is full of coagulated milk with a very strong acid smell.
• Some affected kids have evidence of secondary bacterial or aspiration pneumonia.
• There are no characteristic microscopic findings in goat kids affected with FKS.

TREATMENT

THERAPEUTIC APPROACH
• Recognition of the disease during the early stages with adjustment of base deficits and provision of good supportive care are critical.
• Under ideal conditions affected kids should be treated with isotonic sodium bicarbonate solution intravenously, sufficient to replace the calculated base deficit determined as body weight (kg) × 0.5 × base deficit, and delivered over 1–3 hours.
• Administration of intravenous fluids can result in dramatic clinical improvement.
• Alternatively, affected kids can be denied milk for 24–36 hours, and administered a solution of sodium bicarbonate using one teaspoon of baking soda dissolved in one cup of water and delivering 10–20 mL of this solution orally at 2- to 3-hour intervals.
• When treatment is initiated early, most kids will show clear improvement within 6–10 hours. Treated kids first become more active and will initially pass very solid feces that subsequently turn into diarrhea.
• Diarrhea is usually self-limiting and considered a positive indication of returning GI peristalsis.

SURGICAL CONSIDERATIONS AND TECHNIQUES
N/A

MEDICATIONS

DRUGS OF CHOICE
• The condition does not seem to respond to antibiotics; however, administration of broad-spectrum antibiotics can be used to prevent secondary bacterial infections, particularly pneumonia.
• Vitamin E and selenium should be supplemented if inadequate.

CONTRAINDICATIONS
N/A

PRECAUTIONS
• Appropriate milk and meat withdrawal times must be followed for all compounds administered to food-producing animals.
• Because the clinical appearance is that of very weak animals "lacking energy," most producers try to solve the problem by force feeding affected kids. This exacerbates disease since it seems to result from overconsumption

FLOPPY KID SYNDROME

of milk, and increases the potential for GI distension, bloat, and aspiration.

POSSIBLE INTERACTIONS
N/A

FOLLOW-UP

EXPECTED COURSE AND PROGNOSIS
Affected kids treated early during the course of the disease generally recover.

POSSIBLE COMPLICATIONS
Secondary bacterial infections and/or pneumonia, the latter resulting from aspiration of milk when kids are bottle fed, are common.

CLIENT EDUCATION
Early recognition and treatment of this condition are critical to optimize successful recovery.

PATIENT CARE
After 36 hours of treatment and monitoring, affected kids can be placed back with their dams. Kids that are rejected after treatment will need to be raised on a milk substitute.

PREVENTION
• Can be attempted by managing factors that promote the overconsumption of milk.
• In dairy goat herds, does should be milked before putting them back with the kids. In meat or Angora goats this is difficult to accomplish.
• Hand-raised kids should be provided appropriate amounts of cool milk or milk substitutes more frequently, to avoid gorging.

• When environmental conditions allow, it is better to allow does to kid on pasture. The constant movement of does under pasture conditions prevents kids from ingesting large quantities of milk in a short time. Kids that are kept constantly penned with their dams often suck frequently, leading to overconsumption of milk.
• FKS has been prevented by separating kids from does and raising them on bovine colostrum/milk.

MISCELLANEOUS

ASSOCIATED CONDITIONS
N/A

AGE-RELATED FACTORS
Most affected goat kids are 3–10 days old at the time of clinical onset.

ZOONOTIC POTENTIAL
N/A

PREGNANCY
N/A

BIOSECURITY
N/A

PRODUCTION MANAGEMENT
Management factors (see "Prevention") play an important role in reducing the prevalence of this condition.

SYNONYMS
• Fading kid syndrome
• Neonatales Lähmungssyndrom
• Glangger-Krankheit
• Syndrome chevreau mou

ABBREVIATION
FKS = floppy kid syndrome

SEE ALSO
• Abomasal Emptying Defect
• Clostridial Disease: Gastrointestinal
• Enzootic Ataxia
• Neonatology: Caprine
• Nutrition and Metabolic Diseases: Small Ruminant
• Selenium/Vitamin E Deficiency

Suggested Reading
Bleul U, Schwantag S, Stocker H, et al. Floppy kid syndrome caused by D-lactic acidosis in goat kids. J Vet Intern Med 2006, 20: 1003–8.
Gufler H. Prevention of floppy kid syndrome: A long-term clinical field study conducted on a goat farm in South Tyrol/Italy. Small Rum Res 2012, 108: 113–19.
Rowe JD, East NE. Floppy Kid Syndrome. Western Veterinary Conference, Small Ruminants for the Mixed Animal Practitioner 1998, 986: 135–6.
Rowe J, East N. Floppy kid syndrome. Dairy Goat J 1996, 74: 350.
Tremblay RRM, Butler DG, Allen JW, Hoffman AM. Metabolic acidosis without dehydration in seven goat kids. Can Vet J 1991, 32: 308–10.

Author Andrés de la Concha-Bermejillo
Consulting Editor Erica C. McKenzie
Acknowledgment The author and book editors acknowledge the prior contribution of M.S. Gill.

FLUID THERAPY: INTRAVENOUS

BASICS

OVERVIEW
• Intravenous fluid therapy is indicated when patients are severely dehydrated or unable or unwilling to ingest oral fluids.
• General goals are to replace fluid and electrolyte deficits and meet ongoing needs and losses.

SYSTEMS AFFECTED
Hemolymphatic

SIGNALMENT
All ruminant species

PHYSICAL EXAMINATION FINDINGS
• The degree of patient dehydration is typically determined by physical examination.
• Skin turgor and elasticity, position of the eye within the orbit, tenacity of mucus within the oral cavity, capillary refill time, and patient demeanor are all indicators of patient hydration status.
• As a general rule of thumb, fluid deficits <6% of body weight cannot be detected on clinical examination and deficits >12% of body weight are fatal. Table 1 summarizes expected clinical signs of dehydration in cattle.
• Clinical demeanor also has been associated with acid-base status in neonatal calves with diarrhea.
• Table 2 summarizes expected base deficits in calves of varying ages. It should be emphasized that this information is relevant only in neonatal calves with primary uncomplicated gastrointestinal disease.
• Calves with septicemia will have highly variable acid-base status. Furthermore, these

rules of thumb are not appropriate in adult ruminants.
• Under ideal circumstances, fluid and electrolyte disorders are confirmed by inexpensive, minimally invasive laboratory procedures (see "CBC/Biochemistry/Urinalysis").

DIAGNOSIS

CBC/BIOCHEMISTRY/URINALYSIS
• Hematocrit and serum protein concentration are readily determined in most veterinary practices.
• These procedures are useful adjuncts to physical examination in confirming the presence of dehydration.
• Serum chemistry analyzers suitable for clinic and ambulatory practice are becoming more common.
• Although panel composition varies with instrument and test kit, patient-side confirmation of azotemia, acid-base status, and serum calcium and potassium is now possible. It should be noted that many of these instruments have not been validated for use in ruminants; however, most practitioners find them useful adjuncts in the development of fluid therapy protocols.

TREATMENT

THERAPEUTIC APPROACH
General Rules
1. Oral fluids are generally preferred unless medically contraindicated. Oral fluids are

inexpensive and safe and can be administered rapidly in field conditions.
2. Hypoglycemia is rare in adult ruminants, but occurs occasionally in neonates. Diseases of adult ruminants, which result in hypoglycemia, include fatty liver, ketosis, and pregnancy toxemia.
3. Mild hypocalcemia is common in anorectic adult cattle.
4. Mild metabolic alkalosis is common and expected in anorectic adult cattle.
5. Metabolic alkalosis and increased serum concentrations of albumin may decrease serum-ionized calcium. Metabolic acidosis and hypoalbuminemia may increase serum-ionized calcium. Many laboratories measure total calcium; however, animals recognize and regulate serum-ionized calcium. Correction factors developed for companion animals are inaccurate in ruminants.
6. Sodium bicarbonate administration is appropriate only for correction of metabolic acidosis. Metabolic acidosis is common in neonates with diarrhea, grain engorgement, and salivary loss, but rare in most other conditions of ruminants.
7. Maximum short-term IV fluid administration rates should not exceed 80–90 mL/kg/h (20 mL/kg/h in llamas).
8. Maximum long-term IV fluid administration rates for cattle should not exceed 20 mL/kg/h.
9. Hypokalemia is common in anorectic adult cattle.
10. Neonates with diarrhea often have hyperkalemia (increased serum potassium concentrations); however, body stores of potassium (intracellular potassium) are often very low.

F

Table 1

Assessing Hydration Status in Ruminants			
% Dehydration	*Demeanor*	*Sunken Eye*	*Skin Tenting*
<6%	Normal	−	−
6–8%	Depressed	+	+/−
8–10%	Depressed	++	2–5 sec
10–12%	Comatose	+++	5–10 sec
>12%	Dead	++++	>10 sec

Table 2

Estimating Base Deficit (mmol/L) in Calves of Various Ages with Diarrhea		
Calf Demeanor	*≤8 days*	*≥8 days*
Bright, alert, ambulatory	0	5
Depressed, stands only with assistance	5	10
Unable to stand, suckling reflex intact	10	15
Comatose, suckling reflex absent	10	20

FLUID THERAPY: INTRAVENOUS (CONTINUED)

11. Potassium administration rates should not exceed 0.5 mmol/kg/h unless the patient is severely hypokalemic, or glucose and/or bicarbonate are administered concurrently. Glucose and bicarbonate administration will cause extracellular potassium to shift to the intracellular space.

12. Near isotonic (300 mOsm/L) fluids should be used under most conditions.

13. Fluid deficit is generally calculated as follows: Body weight (kg) × (% dehydration/100) = deficit (L).

14. Estimates of daily maintenance requirements vary from 60 to 120 mL/kg/day, depending on severity of ongoing losses (diarrhea, renal losses). The values above include ongoing losses. Maintenance requirements are calculated as follows: Body weight (kg) × [(60–120 mL/kg/day)/1,000 mL/kg] = requirement (L).

15. Total daily fluid needs are calculated by adding deficits and daily maintenance requirements.

16. Base deficit is typically calculated as follows: Body weight (kg) × [measured deficit (mmol/L)] × [bicarbonate space]. Bicarbonate space is typically estimated as 0.5–0.6 in cattle. Bicarbonate replacement is used to replace 50–100% of base deficit. Higher percentages of deficit replacement, approaching 100%, are appropriate in neonates with diarrhea.

17. The core electrolyte abnormalities in calves with diarrhea include dehydration, acidosis, low systemic potassium with serum hyperkalemia due to acidosis, and hypoglycemia.

18. Isotonic = 300 mOsm/L. Isotonic sodium bicarbonate = 1.3% = 1.3 g/100mL = 13 g/L. Isotonic sodium chloride = 0.9% = 0.9 g/100 mL = 9 g/L.

19. Do not withhold milk from calves with diarrhea. Do not feed beef calves more than 1 L/feeding. Beef calves are acclimated to small, frequent meals.

20. Oral fluids are probably adequate in mildly dehydrated calves (≤8%). Severely dehydrated calves probably require at least short-term intravenous fluids.

Clinical Approach

In general, fluid therapy can be reduced to the following set of questions:
1. What is the fluid deficit?
2. What is the daily maintenance requirement for fluids?
3. What will the total fluid needs be over the next 24 hours?
4. What is the base deficit?
5. What volume of isotonic sodium bicarbonate will replace this deficit?
6. How would you prepare this volume of isotonic sodium bicarbonate solution?
7. What is the maximum rate of fluid administration in the first hour?

8. How much 50% dextrose will we add to the first hour's fluids to create a 1% solution?
9. What is the theoretical maximum concentration of potassium for fluids administered in the first hour of therapy?
10. Based on the above answers, design a fluid therapy protocol for the patient.

Example

You are examining a 50-kg Holstein heifer calf with profuse diarrhea. The calf is 15 days old. On physical examination, the calf is severely dehydrated (estimate 10%) and is comatose.

1. **What is the calf's fluid deficit?**
Body weight (kg) × (% dehydration)/100 = 50 kg × 10/100 = 5 L

2. **What is the calf's daily maintenance requirement for fluids?**
Body weight (kg) × 100 mL/kg = 50 kg × 100 mL/kg = 5,000 mL = 5 L

3. **What will the calf's total fluid needs be over the next 24 hours?**
Deficit + Maintenance = 5 L + 5 L = 10 L

4. **What is the calf's base deficit?**
Body weight (kg) × (estimated base deficit) × bicarbonate space = base deficit. Estimated deficit based on the calf's demeanor (comatose) and age (>8 days) is 20 mmol/L, so 50 kg × 20 mmol/L × 0.6 = 600 mmol HCO_3^-.
Alternatively, base deficit can be calculated from measured blood bicarbonate. For purposes of this calculation, we will assume the calf has a pure metabolic acidosis and serum bicarbonate of 5 mmol/L, and that normal is 25 mmol/L.
Body weight (kg) × (normal bicarbonate minus measured bicarbonate) × 0.6 = 50 kg × (25 − 5) × 0.6 = 600 mmol/L HCO_3^-

5. **What volume of isotonic sodium bicarbonate (1.3%) will replace this deficit?**
Each liter of an isotonic solution has 300 mOsm/L. In the case of isotonic sodium bicarbonate, half the particles in solution are Na^+ and half are HCO_3^-. Therefore, each liter of isotonic sodium bicarbonate contains 150 mmol/L of HCO_3^-. [Calculated deficit (mmol)]/150 mmol/L = [600]/150 = 4 L 1.3% sodium bicarbonate ($NaHCO_3$)

6. **How would you prepare this volume of isotonic sodium bicarbonate solution?**
1.3% = 1.3 g/100 mL = 13 g/L. Volumes required × 13 g/L = 4 L × 13 g/L = 52 g $NaHCO_3$ in 4 L sterile water It is important that base deficit be corrected using isotonic solutions.

7. **What is the maximum rate of fluid administration in this calf for the first hour?**
Calves may be administered as much as 40–80 mL/kg during the first hour of therapy without creating an inordinate risk of pulmonary edema. Thereafter, administration rates should be reduced to maintenance fluid rates, which in calves is approximately 4 mL/kg/h. If ongoing losses are great, fluid

rates may remain higher but should not exceed 20 mL/kg/h. Body weight (kg) × 80 mL/kg/h = 50 kg × 80 mL/kg/h = 4,000 mL = 4 L

8. **How much 50% dextrose will we add to the first hour's fluids to create a 1% solution?**
We desire a 1% dextrose solution. Standard solutions, which we carry in our truck, are 50% solutions. Consequently, we will need to make a 1:50 dilution to create a 1% solution. 1 L = 1,000 mL, 1,000 mL/50 = 20 mL. Therefore, we add 20 mL of 50% dextrose to each of the 4 L we administer in the first hour. Remember, not all calves with diarrhea are hypoglycemic and excessive glucose supplementation will cause serum glucose to exceed the renal threshold, causing an osmotic diuresis, an undesirable effect in a dehydrated patient.

9. **What is the theoretical maximum concentration of potassium for fluids administered in the first hour of therapy?**
Generally, we limit potassium administration to a maximum of 0.5 mmol/kg/h. (Body weight (kg) × 0.5 mmol/kg)/volume administered, so (50 × 0.5)/4 = 6.25 mEq/L. Having performed this calculation, we recognize that the concurrent administration of bicarbonate and glucose will cause potassium to move intracellularly, resulting in a precipitous decline in serum potassium. Consequently, we will typically administer 8 to 12 mmol/L potassium in bicarbonate-containing fluids.

10. **Based on the above answers, we design a fluid therapy protocol for a calf.**
Obviously, these are not exact calculations. Here is a rough plan.
a. Hour 1: 4 L isotonic sodium bicarbonate, each liter supplemented with 10 mmol K/L. Each of the first 2 L is supplemented with 20 mL 50% dextrose.
b. Hour 2: 2 L of a commercially available oral electrolyte solution (total volume 6 liters).
c. Hour 8: 2 L whole milk (total volume 8 liters).
d. Hour 14: 2 L of a commercially available oral electrolyte solution (total volume 10 liters).
If the calf is readily nursing, alternate oral electrolytes and milk at 6-hour intervals. If hydration appears normal, one or both daily electrolyte feedings may be discontinued. Do not use stool characteristics as criteria for administration of milk.

 FOLLOW-UP

In animals receiving extensive fluid therapy, the need to reassess hydration and acid-base status at frequent intervals should be considered.

MISCELLANEOUS

• Many practitioners use hypertonic fluids. These solutions can be rapidly administered in an ambulatory setting.
• As general rule, 7–8% sodium chloride solution is administered at a rate of 5 mL/kg IV.
• When using such protocols, oral fluids should be provided or administered.

ABBREVIATIONS

• IV = intravenous
• NaHCO₃ = sodium bicarbonate

SEE ALSO

• Colostrum and Milk Replacers (see www.fiveminutevet.com/ruminant)
• Fluid Therapy: Oral

Suggested Reading

Naylor JM. Neonatal ruminant diarrhea. In: Smith BP ed, Large Animal Internal Medicine, 2nd ed. St. Louis: Mosby, 1996, pp. 396–417.
Radostits OM, Gay CC, Hinchcliff KW, Constable P eds. Veterinary medicine, 10th ed. London: W. B. Saunders, 2006.
Roussel AJ. Fluid therapy in mature cattle. Vet Clin North Am Food Anim Pract 2014, 30: 429–39.
Roussel AJ, Cohen ND, Holland PS, et al. Alterations in acid–base balance and serum electrolyte concentrations in cattle: 632 cases (1984–1994). J Am Vet Med Assoc 1998, 212: 1769–75.
Smith GW, Berchtold J. Fluid therapy in calves. Vet Clin North Am Food Anim Pract 2014, 30: 409–27.

Author Adapted from the work of the late Jeffrey W. Tyler
Consulting Editor Kaitlyn A. Lutz

F

FLUID THERAPY: ORAL

BASICS

OVERVIEW
• Oral fluid therapy is a practical and economical approach in ruminants with mild to moderate dehydration or electrolyte and acid-base imbalances.
• Intravenous (IV) fluid therapy is indicated in ruminants with hypovolemia or severe electrolyte or acid-base imbalances.
• Oral fluid therapy can often be used in conjunction with IV fluid therapy.
• Fluid therapy can be beneficial and life-saving and should be considered as important as other medications in the management of ill ruminants.

INCIDENCE/PREVALENCE
N/A

GEOGRAPHIC DISTRIBUTION
N/A

SYSTEMS AFFECTED
• Multisystemic

PATHOPHYSIOLOGY
• Daily maintenance water requirement is about 6% of body weight (BW) in adults and 8% of BW in neonates, and varies with activity level, ambient and body temperatures, and physiologic status (lactation, pregnancy).
• Dehydration is defined as a decrease in total body water and usually leads to a decrease in extracellular fluid volume.
• Extracellular fluid is distributed between interstitial and intravascular fluid compartments.
• Hypovolemia is defined as a decrease in intravascular fluid volume and leads to decreased cardiac output and tissue perfusion.
• The rumen acts as a water reservoir in adults, but can also be a site of fluid sequestration in GI disorders such as grain overload or vagal indigestion.

HISTORICAL FINDINGS
• Lack of access to palatable water
• Evidence of body fluid losses including diarrhea, polyuria, sweating, and prolonged tachypnea.

SIGNALMENT
N/A

PHYSICAL EXAMINATION FINDINGS
• Dehydration can be estimated by assessing skin elasticity, mucus membranes, capillary refill time (CRT), and eyeball recession (degree of enophthalmos) (see Table 1).
• Enophthalmos can also be caused by emaciation and decreased skin elasticity can be normal in geriatric ruminants.

Table 1

Assessing Hydration in Ruminants				
Dehydration (% of BW)	Skin tent (seconds)	Mucus membranes	CRT (seconds)	Enophthalmos (mm)
Mild (5–7)	2–5	moist	<2	2–3
Moderate (8–10)	6–7	tacky	2–4	4–6
Severe (>10)	>7	dry	≥5	7–8

• Signs of hypovolemia include tachycardia, pale mucus membranes, prolonged CRT, cold extremities, weak peripheral pulses, obtundation, and reduced jugular fill.
• Bradycardia can be caused by hypothermia, hypoglycemia, or hyperkalemia.
• Cardiac arrhythmias are usually caused by severe hyperkalemia in neonates and upper GI obstruction in adults.
• Sucking reflex and body position can aid in assessing metabolic acidosis in calves with diarrhea (see Tables 2 and 3).

GENETICS
N/A

CAUSES AND RISK FACTORS
• Dehydration is usually caused by reduced water intake and/or excessive loss or sequestration of body fluids.
• Common causes of excessive loss or sequestration of body fluids include diarrhea, polyuria, heat stress, upper GI obstruction or stasis, and grain overload.
• Common causes of upper GI obstruction include abomasal displacement or volvulus, vagal indigestion, and intestinal volvulus or intussusception.

• Common causes of reduced water intake include lack of access to palatable water, esophageal obstruction, and dysphagia.

DIAGNOSIS

DIFFERENTIAL DIAGNOSES
N/A

CBC/BIOCHEMISTRY/URINALYSIS
• Serum biochemistry and blood gas analyses are indicated in critically ill ruminants to evaluate and monitor electrolyte and acid-base imbalances.
• Diarrhea is often associated with hypoglycemia, hyponatremia, hypochloremia, hyperkalemia, and metabolic acidosis in neonates.
• Upper GI obstruction is often associated with hypokalemia, hypochloremia, hyponatremia, hypocalcemia, and metabolic alkalosis in adults.
• Grain overload is often associated with azotemia, hyperphosphatemia, hypocalcemia, and metabolic acidosis.

Table 2

Assessing Metabolic Acidosis in Diarrheic Calves <8 Days of Age		
Base deficit (mmol/L)	Suckling reflex	Body position
0	strong	standing
5	weak	standing
10	weak or absent	recumbency

Table 3

Assessing Metabolic Acidosis in Diarrheic Calves ≥8 Days of Age		
Base deficit (mmol/L)	Sucking reflex	Body position
5	strong	standing
10	weak	standing
15	weak or absent	sternal recumbency
20	absent	lateral recumbency

OTHER LABORATORY TESTS
N/A

IMAGING
N/A

OTHER DIAGNOSTIC PROCEDURES
N/A

PATHOLOGIC FINDINGS
N/A

TREATMENT

THERAPEUTIC APPROACH
• Total volume of fluids to administer should account for dehydration, maintenance daily water requirement, and losses through GI, urinary, or respiratory tracts.
• Volume of fluids required to correct dehydration can be calculated as follows:
  ○ Volume (L) = BW (kg) × dehydration (%).
• Daily maintenance requirement is about 6% of BW in adults and 8% of BW in neonates
  ○ Volume (L) = BW (kg) × maintenance requirement (%).
• Ongoing losses are usually estimated (1–4 L per day in calves with diarrhea).
• For example, a 40-kg calf with severe dehydration (10%) and diarrhea (1L per day) should receive over 24 hours:
  ○ Volume (L) = 40 × 0.1 + 40 × 0.08 + 1 = 8.2
• Volume should not exceed 5% of BW per oral administration:
  ○ Volume (L) = BW (kg) × 0.05.
• For example, a 40-kg calf can be given safely 2L of oral fluids at one time.
• Neonates with a strong sucking reflex can be offered oral fluids via nipple bottle.
• Drenching syringes can be used in small ruminants and camelids to administer small volumes of oral fluids.
• Care must be taken in recumbent or weak animals due to increased risk of aspiration.

SURGICAL CONSIDERATIONS AND TECHNIQUES
N/A

MEDICATIONS

DRUGS OF CHOICE
Oral Fluid Therapy in Neonatal Ruminants
• Alkalinizing fluids are indicated in calves with metabolic acidosis
  ○ 13 g NaHCO₃ + 1L water
  ○ 150 mL 8.4% NaHCO₃ + 1L water

• Amount of bicarbonate required to correct metabolic acidosis in neonates can be calculated as follows:
  ○ HCO_3^- (mEq) = BW (kg) x base deficit (mmol/L) × 0.6
• Base deficit can be estimated from clinical signs or calculated using blood gas results as follows:
  ○ Base deficit (mmol/L) = 30 − (T_{CO2})
• Amount of sodium bicarbonate to administer can be calculated knowing that 1mL 8.4% NaHCO₃ contains 1mEq HCO_3^- and 1g NaHCO₃ contains 12mEq HCO_3^-
• Commercial electrolyte solutions containing 50–80 mmol/L of acetate, propionate, or citrate can also be used to treat calves with metabolic acidosis.
• Bicarbonate has a direct alkalinizing effect compared to acetate, proprionate, and citrate, and may have a more rapid and profound effect.
• As opposed to bicarbonate, acetate and propionate can be administered with milk and facilitate sodium and water intestinal absorption.
• Commercial electrolyte solutions should contain 90–130 mmol/L of sodium and 40–80 mmol/L of chloride.
• Electrolyte feedings should not replace milk feedings but be given in addition to them to provide adequate fluid and energy intake.
• Diarrheic calves should ideally be offered small feedings of milk 3–4 times a day.
• Calves that are not interested in nursing can be given an electrolyte solution rich in glucose instead of milk.

Oral Fluid Therapy in Adults
• Acidifying fluids are indicated in adults with metabolic alkalosis
  ○ 180g NaCl + 20L water
  ○ 140g NaCl + 50g KCl + 10g CaCl₂ + 20L water
  ○ 2.5L 7.2% NaCl + 20L water
• Alkalinizing fluids are indicated in adults with metabolic acidosis
  ○ 250 g NaHCO₃ + 20L water
• Amount of bicarbonate required to correct metabolic acidosis in adults can be calculated as follows:
  ○ HCO_3^- (mEq) = BW (kg) × base deficit (mmol/L) × 0.3
• Addition of calcium to the fluids is indicated in ruminants with hypocalcemia (<2 mmol/L)
  ○ 500mL of calcium 23% solution per 20L of oral fluids
• Oral administration of KCl is indicated in ruminants with severe hypokalemia (<2.5 mmol/L)
  ○ 10-20 g KCl per 100 kg of BW q8-12h
• Oral administration of phosphate salts is indicated in ruminants with severe hypophosphatemia (<0.5 mmol/L)
  ○ 150–200 g NaH₂PO₄ for an adult cow

CONTRAINDICATIONS
• Commercial solutions containing more than 40 mmol/L of bicarbonate or citrate are likely to interfere with milk clotting
• Commercial electrolyte solutions intended to be mixed with hundreds of liters of water are not suitable for diarrheic calves as they are too dilute.

FOLLOW-UP

EXPECTED COURSE AND PROGNOSIS
• Rapid reversal of hypovolemia is expected after administration of IV fluids in ruminants with severe dehydration.
• Maintenance fluid requirements and ongoing losses can be addressed with oral fluids once hypovolemia has been corrected.
• Correction of dehydration and restoration of the renal function may address mild electrolyte or acid-base imbalances.
• Diarrheic calves with concurrent infections usually have a poor prognosis.

POSSIBLE COMPLICATIONS
• Careful thoracic auscultation is essential to identify ruminants at risk for fluid overload.
• Oral fluids with high osmolality (>650 mOsm/L) can cause reduced abomasal emptying and abomasal bloat in calves.
• Commercial electrolyte solutions do not always have an energy source, and therefore neonates should not be held off milk for more than 24 hours.

CLIENT EDUCATION
• Clients administering oral fluids via esophageal feeder or orogastric tube should be trained to prevent complications

PATIENT CARE
• Mentation, heart rate, CRT, mucus membranes, extremity temperature, peripheral pulses, and jugular fill should be monitored.
• Urine output and urine specific gravity can be used to monitor hydration and renal function.
• PCV and total solids can be used to monitor hydration and prevent fluid overload, especially in calves, small ruminants, and camelids.
• Blood lactate and blood gas analysis can be used to monitor tissue perfusion and electrolyte and acid-base imbalances.
• Blood glucose monitoring is often indicated in neonates, camelids, and ruminants with pregnancy toxemia.

PREVENTION
• Colostrum management is essential to reduce the incidence of neonatal diarrhea in ruminants.
• Incidence of GI disorders in adult ruminants can be decreased by improving

FLUID THERAPY: ORAL

overall herd management, specifically feeding management, and biosecurity measures to decrease enteric pathogens.

MISCELLANEOUS

ASSOCIATED CONDITIONS
• Neonates with diarrhea should be examined carefully for signs of concurrent infections including omphalitis, otitis, arthritis, and pneumonia.

ABBREVIATIONS
• BW = body weight
• $CaCl_2$ = calcium chloride
• CRT = capillary refill time
• GI = gastrointestinal
• HCO_3^- = bicarbonate
• IV = intravenous
• KCl = potassium chloride
• mEq = milliequivalent
• NaCl = sodium chloride
• $NaHCO_3$ = sodium bicarbonate
• NaH_2PO_4 = monosodium phosphate
• PCV = packed cell volume
• T_{CO2} = total carbon dioxide

SEE ALSO
• Blood Chemistry (see www.fiveminutevet.com/ruminant)
• Diarrheal Diseases: Bovine
• Diarrheal Diseases: Camelid
• Diarrheal Diseases: Small Ruminant
• Neonatal Diarrhea
• Parenteral Nutrition
• Rumen Transfaunation (see www.fiveminutevet.com/ruminant)
• Ruminal Acidosis

Suggested Reading
Roussel JR. Fluid therapy in mature cattle. Vet Clin North Am Food Anim Pract 2014, 30: 429–39.
Smith GW, Berchtold J. Fluid therapy in calves. Vet Clin North Am Food Anim Pract 2014, 30: 409–27.
Author Thibaud Kuca
Consulting Editor Kaitlyn A. Lutz
Acknowledgment The author and book editors acknowledge the prior contribution of John Gilliam.

BASICS

OVERVIEW
• Fluoride (F⁻) is absorbed by the gastrointestinal tract and lungs depending on the form.
• Clinical signs associated with chronic F⁻ exposure are manifest primarily in skeletal and dental abnormalities and may take months to years to become apparent depending on the solubility of the fluoride compound, amount of F⁻ absorbed, and duration of exposure.

INCIDENCE/PREVALENCE
Usually chronic and can affect large percentage of the herd. Occurs in areas with fluoride emissions or contamination.

GEOGRAPHIC DISTRIBUTION
Occurs in areas with high levels of fluorides in the soil, water or air.

SYSTEMS AFFECTED
• Cardiovascular
• Digestive
• Mammary
• Musculoskeletal
• Nervous

PATHOPHYSIOLOGY
• Exposure to fluorides delays and alters mineralization by replacing hydroxyapatite in the crystalline structure of bone and mostly affects the matrices supporting formation of enamel, dentine, cementum, and bone. Teeth are affected during development due to damage from the failure to accept minerals normally. Skeletal fluorosis interferes with formation of adequate matrix and mineralization by osteoblasts, resulting in a dysfunction of normal sequences of osteogenesis, acceleration of bone remodeling, production of abnormal bone (exostosis, sclerosis).
• Effects of fluorosis may include brittle bones, calcification of ligaments, and joint pain.
• Fluorosis in cattle has been associated with lameness and spontaneous fractures.
• Chronic fluorosis is commonly due to ingestion of mineral supplements with high F⁻ content or consumption of contaminated forage and water by industrial emissions containing F⁻.
• Acute toxicity is rare but may result from inhalation of gases containing fluoride or ingestion of highly toxic rodenticides containing fluoride. In acute cases, clinical signs are referable to the nervous system and death results from respiratory or cardiac failure. These acute symptoms are the result of a direct effect on serum calcium.

SIGNALMENT
All ruminant species are susceptible. Dairy cattle are considered more at risk of chronic toxicity due to their longer lifetime in production. There is no breed, sex predilection, or genetic basis for fluorosis.

PHYSICAL EXAMINATION FINDINGS
• Dental abnormalities occur only if animals are exposed during permanent tooth development prior to eruption and include dullness, mottling, pitting, and discoloration of tooth enamel, and abnormal tooth wear and loss, particularly in pairs of teeth that erupt at the same time.
• Dental problems may result in decreased feed and water intake, difficulty with mastication, weight loss, and general unthriftiness.
• Other clinical signs include decreased milk production and skeletal abnormalities; lameness, arthritis, fractures of the pedal bones; bilateral enlargement and roughening of metatarsals, metacarpals, ribs, and mandible; and abnormal hoof wear resulting from altered gait with elongated toe, especially on hind feet.

CAUSES AND RISK FACTORS
• >40–100 mg F⁻/kg feed cattle, >60 mg F⁻/kg feed ewes, >150 mg F⁻/kg feed lambs.
• Rock phosphate deposits, nondefluorinated or inadequately defluorinated mineral supplements, monoammonium, diammonium, and gypsum phosphate fertilizers or other sources of phosphorus containing <100:1 parts phosphorus to fluoride, contaminated forage and water from industrial aerial emissions, deep well and thermal spring water, fluorinated municipal water, sewage effluent from municipalities using fluorinated water, forage and water contamination by volcanic gas and ash pose a risk.
• Forage usually has a low level of fluoride but levels are variable and should be considered.
• A calcium-deficient diet may increase F⁻ accumulation. Animals in poor body condition may be more susceptible.
• Rodenticides containing sodium monofluoroacetate (1080) or fluoroacetamide are highly toxic and may account for acute toxicity. Due to the highly lethal nature of these compounds, their use is restricted in the United States.
• Fluoride absorption is related to solubility; sodium fluoride > rock phosphate > dicalcium phosphate > defluorinated phosphate.

DIAGNOSIS

Clinical signs, history of exposure/mineral supplementation, radiography, and feed/bone/urine F⁻ levels.

DIFFERENTIAL DIAGNOSES
Arthritis; osteoporosis; deficiencies in calcium, phosporus, or vitamin D; traumatic injury

CBC/BIOCHEMISTRY/URINALYSIS
Eosinophilia, anemia, hypoglycemia, increased ALP. F⁻ can be detected in urine.

OTHER LABORATORY TESTS
• F⁻, Ca²⁺, P concentrations in forage, mineral supplements, soil, and water
• F⁻ content in bone (normal content will vary with bone selected), antler, kidney, serum
• >10 ppm F⁻ in urine
• T4, T3 hypothyroidism

IMAGING
Radiography: periosteal hyperostosis, exostosis, sclerosis in metacarpals, metatarsal, mandible, and ribs

PATHOLOGIC FINDINGS
• Gross—teeth: pitting, discoloration, chalkiness of enamel, irregular wear, and tooth loss
• Skeletal—exostoses, sclerosis, arthritis, stunted growth
• Histopathologic—abnormal remodeling of bone, atrophy of osteoblasts and bone marrow cells, retardation of cartilage cell differentiation

TREATMENT

THERAPEUTIC APPROACH
Remove from source. Treatment is symptomatic and supportive. Provide feeds that are easily masticated, symptomatic treatment for osteoarthritis/lameness.

MEDICATIONS

DRUGS OF CHOICE
None

FOLLOW-UP

EXPECTED COURSE AND PROGNOSIS
In mild cases, improvement may be seen over weeks to months as fluoride body stores are depleted. In severe cases of lameness or inability to consume adequate forage, euthanasia may be required as some bony lesions are irreversible.

PREVENTION
• Aluminun sulfate, aluminum chloride, calcium aluminate, and calcium carbonate reduce absorption of fluorides.
• Use only feed-grade sources of phosphorus supplements.

FLUORIDE TOXICITY

 MISCELLANEOUS

AGE-RELATED FACTORS

Young animals with growing bones are most severely affected. Exposure of adult animals will result in normal dentition with skeletal lesions.

PREGNANCY

Congenital fluorosis has been reported in calves born to fluoride-intoxicated cows.

ABBREVIATIONS

- ALP = alkaline phosphatase
- Ca²⁺ = calcium
- F = fluoride
- P = phosphorus
- ppm = parts per million

SEE ALSO

- Phosphorus Deficiency/Excess
- Vitamin D Deficiency/Toxicosis

Suggested Reading

Bourke CA, Ottaway SJ. Chronic gypsum fertiliser ingestion as a significant contributor to a multifactorial cattle mortality. Aust Vet J 1998, 76: 565–9.

Jubb TF, Annand TE, Main DC, Murphy GM. Phosphorus supplements and fluorosis in cattle—a northern Australian experience. Aust Vet J 1993, 70: 379–83.

Osheim DL, Rasmusson MC. Determination of fluoride in bovine urine. J AOAC Int 1998, 81: 839–43.

Osweiler G. In: Plumlee K ed, Clinical Veterinary Toxicology. St. Louis: Mosby, 2004.

Patra RC, Dwivedi SK, Bhardwaj B, Swarup D. Industrial fluorosis in cattle and buffalo around Udaipur, India. Sci Total Environ 2000, 253: 145–50.

Schultheiss WA, Van Niekerk JC. Suspected chronic fluorosis in a sheep flock. J S Afr Vet Assoc 1994, 65: 84–5.

Shupe JL, Olson AE, Peterson HB. In: Howard JL ed, Current Veterinary Therapy: Food Animal Practice 2. Philadelphia: Saunders, 1986.

Vikøren T, Stuve G, Frøslie A. Fluoride exposure in cervids inhabiting areas adjacent to aluminum smelters in Norway. I. Residue levels. J Wildl Dis 1996, 32: 169–80.

Author Steve Ensley
Consulting Editor Christopher C.L. Chase

Acknowledgment The author and book editors acknowledge the prior contribution of Lauren Palmer.

FOOT AND MOUTH DISEASE

BASICS

OVERVIEW
Foot-and-mouth disease (FMD) is a highly contagious viral disease of cloven-footed domestic and wild animals. The disease is characterized by fever and vesicular lesions in the mouth, tongue, nostrils, feet, and teats. Sheep and goats are maintenance hosts showing very mild signs while pigs are amplifying hosts as they produce extremely high concentrations of virus particle in aerosols. Cattle are indicators of this disease as they generally are the first species to show signs of infection; the lesions are more severe and progress more rapidly than in other animals.

INCIDENCE/PREVALENCE
Morbidity reaches to almost 100% in susceptible populations. Mortality usually ranges from 1% to 5%, although may be higher in young animals.

GEOGRAPHIC DISTRIBUTION
FMD is a transboundary animal disease distributed worldwide. Various types of FMDV have been identified in Asia, Africa, and South America. Chile, North Central America, Australia, and New Zealand have been free of FMD for many years.

SYSTEMS AFFECTED
- Integument
- Respiratory
- Reproductive
- Cardiovascular
- Urinary

PATHOPHYSIOLOGY
- FMD virus usually enters the host via the respiratory and oral route.
- Infected animals secrete virus in all the secretions, so contact and consumption of animal products such as meat, milk, bones, glands, and cheese can spread the disease.
- Incubation time of the virus is in the range 2–14 days depending on the susceptibility of the host and infecting dose. Clinical signs generally develop in 3–5 days.
- Diseased animals usually recover in 1–3 weeks. Skin lesions usually heal in 7 days after recovery but secondary bacterial infection may complicate the healing process.

SIGNALMENT
- Predominant in cattle, pigs, sheep, goats, water buffalo, deer, elk, bison, antelopes, and wildebeest.
- Other susceptible animals include elephants, nutrias, armadillos, reindeer, mouse, antelopes, chamois, gazelles, impala, giraffe, and hedgehogs and may serve as sources of transmission to ruminants.
- South American camelids are less susceptible to FMDV, whereas camels are resistant to natural infection.

GENETICS
Genetic variation as a predisposing factor of FMD within the same species has not been well documented but, in experimental infection, susceptibility differed within the species. High-yielding European breeds are also found to be more susceptible than low-yielding Asian breeds.

PHYSICAL EXAMINATION FINDINGS
- Best-known signs of FMD are fever together with vesicles (blisters) in the mouth, nares, muzzle, hooves, and teats which progress to erosions and sloughing, leading to lameness and anorexia.
- Sticky, foamy, and stringy drooling saliva from the mouth, serous nasal discharge, and decreased milk production.
- Young animals may die without clinical signs and abortion occurs in pregnant animals.

CAUSES AND RISK FACTORS
- FMD is caused by *Aphthovirus* belonging to the Picornaviridae family. Various strains have been identified under seven immunologically and serologically distinct types: O, A, C, Southern African Territories (SAT)-1, SAT-2, SAT-3, and Asia-1. Immunity to one type or subtype does not confer immunity against other types and subtypes.
- Risk factors include naïve population exposed to exotic serotypes, unvaccinated population in endemic areas, poor biosecurity, and feeding contaminated feed to susceptible animals.

DIAGNOSIS

DIFFERENTIAL DIAGNOSES
The disease is confused with other diseases which show lesions in the mouth. These diseases include vesicular stomatitis, papular stomatitis, bovine viral diarrhea-mucosal disease, malignant catarrhal fever, foot rot, herpes mammillitis, pseudocowpox, rinderpest, bluetongue, contagious ecthyma (orf) in sheep, infectious bovine rhinotracheitis, and chemical and thermal burns.

CBC/BIOCHEMISTRY/URINALYSIS
N/A

OTHER LABORATORY TESTS
- Samples to collect for diagnosis: Vesicular fluid, epithelium that covers vesicles, whole blood, serum, and esophago-pharyngeal fluid from convalescent animals in cell culture fluid.
- Samples must be kept in PBS of pH 7.4 in order to maintain the pH to protect the virus.
- Antigen detection: Virus isolation (gold standard), complement fixation, ELISA.
- Nucleic acid detection: PCR.
- Antibody detection: Virus neutralization, ELISA.

PATHOLOGIC FINDINGS
- Vesicles in foot and mouth ranges from 2 mm to 10 cm in size, sometimes joining with adjacent lesions. The vesicles rupture leaving a red, eroded area, which is then covered with a gray fibrinous coating. This coating becomes yellow, brown, or green, replaced by new epithelium.
- Denuded rumen papillae and a gray or yellow streaking in the myocardium ("tiger heart") can be seen in young animals that die acutely, caused by degeneration and necrosis.

TREATMENT

THERAPEUTIC APPROACH
Supportive treatment of infected individuals is warranted. Milking time hygiene is of utmost importance. In areas where FMD is exotic, health care is usually swift and terminal.

MEDICATIONS

DRUGS OF CHOICE
Drugs are not available to treat FMD. But broad-spectrum antibiotics are intended to control bacterial secondary infection so that the lesions in the mouth and hoofs heal fast.

FOLLOW-UP

EXPECTED COURSE AND PROGNOSIS
FMD is self-limiting disease with fair prognosis for recovery in 2–3 weeks. Prognosis for young animals is sometime grave depending on the strains of the virus associated with the disease. Animals vaccinated with the epidemic strains have good prognosis.

POSSIBLE COMPLICATIONS
Long-term infection leads to severe loss of production. Sloughing of the hoofs causes secondary bacterial infection and takes a long time to heal. Possibility of tetanus infection through the sloughed hoofs in case of delayed healing.

PATIENT CARE
Diseased animals should be carefully monitored for fever and vesicular lesions. Continuous fever and anorexia for a long time leads to the collapse of the animal, so fluid therapy and dexamethasone are indicated in severe cases.

PREVENTION
- Strict biosecurity procedures, good animal husbandry practices (e.g., restriction of high-risk visitors, quarantine of high-risk animals and animal products, etc.) aids in the exclusion of FMDV.

F

FOOT AND MOUTH DISEASE

• Vaccines against FMD are available but cross-protection between different serotypes is limited. Therefore, it is important that the vaccine contain the same subtype of virus as is in the area. This necessitates frequent checking of the serotype and subtype during an outbreak as FMD virus frequently changes during its natural passage through various species. At the time of outbreak, ring vaccination with the same strains can protect against a possible epidemic.

MISCELLANEOUS

AGE-RELATED FACTORS
All ages of animal are susceptible to infection with FMD. Neonates and the young are more susceptible to fatal cardiac disease related to FMD infection.

ZOONOTIC POTENTIAL
FMD has been isolated from only about 40 human cases, despite widespread occurrence of the disease in animals. Vesicular lesions can be seen, but signs are mild. Because of this, FMD is not considered an important public health concern.

PREGNANCY
Some pregnant animals may abort.

BIOSECURITY
• Stringent quarantine rules and regulations prevent the transmission of FMDV over a wide geographic area.

• Sodium hydroxide (2%), sodium carbonate (4%), and citric acid (0.2%) are effective disinfectants. FMDV is resistant to iodophors, quaternary ammonium compounds, hypochlorite, and phenol, especially in the presence of organic matter.

ABBREVIATIONS
• ELISA = enzyme-linked immunosorbent assay
• FMD = foot and mouth disease
• FMDV = foot-and-mouth disease virus
• OIE = Office International des Epizooties
• PBS = phosphate buffered saline
• PCR = polymerase chain reaction
• SAT = South African Territories

SEE ALSO
• Bluetongue Virus
• Bovine Papular Stomatitis
• Burn Management
• Foot Rot: Bovine
• Foot Rot: Small Ruminant
• Infectious Bovine Rhinotracheitis
• Malignant Catarrhal Fever
• Orf (Contagious Ecthyma)
• Vesicular Stomatitis

Suggested Reading
Barteling SJ. Development and performance of inactivated vaccines against foot and mouth disease. Rev Sci Tech 2002, 21: 577–88.
Grubman MJ. New approaches to rapidly control foot-and-mouth disease outbreaks. Expert Rev Anti Infect Ther 2003, 1: 579–86.

Grubman MJ, Baxt B. Foot-and-mouth disease. Clin Microbiol Rev 2004, 17: 465–93.
Mebus CA, House J. Foot and mouth disease. In: Foreign Animal Diseases Book ("The Gray Book"), 6th ed. Richmond: United States Animal Health Association, 1998.
Musser JM. A practitioner's primer on foot-and-mouth disease. J Am Vet Med Assoc 2004, 224: 1261–8.
Paton DJ, et al. Selection of foot and mouth disease vaccine strains–a review. Revue scientifique et technique-Office international des epizooties 2014, 24.3.
Perez AM, Ward MP, Carpenter TE. Epidemiological investigations of the 2001 foot-and-mouth disease outbreak in Argentina. Vet Rec 2004, 154: 777–82.
Wernery U, Kaaden OR. Foot-and-mouth disease in camelids: a review. Vet J 2004, 168: 134–42.
The Merck Veterinary Manual, 10th ed. Whitehouse Station, NJ: Merck & Co. Available at http://www.merckvetmanual.com/mvm/generalized_conditions/foot-and-mouth_disease/overview_of_foot-and-mouth_disease.html. Accessed January 8, 2016.
Author Suvash Shiwakoti
Consulting Editor Christopher C.L. Chase
Acknowledgment The author and book editors acknowledge the prior contribution of Daniel L. Grooms and Daryl V. Nydam.

BASICS

OVERVIEW
Interdigital phlegmon (foot rot) is an opportunistic, acute to subacute, necrotizing infection of the soft tissues of the digit in cattle. Bacteria enter through damaged skin of the interdigital space and the infection extends into the underlying tissues resulting in diffuse digital swelling and moderate to severe lameness. Prompt treatment with antibiotics has a high cure rate.

INCIDENCE/PREVALENCE
• Beef cattle: 1–3%; dairy cattle: 2–4% (range of 0–36% reported).
• Occurrence is usually sporadic but can be epidemic under some conditions.

GEOGRAPHIC DISTRIBUTION
Worldwide

SYSTEMS AFFECTED
• Integument
• Musculoskeletal

PATHOPHYSIOLOGY
• Foot rot is caused by an opportunistic mixed bacterial infection of the soft tissue of the foot. The bacteria typically involved are *Fusobacterium necrophorum*, *Porphyromonas levii*, and *Prevotella intermedia*. *F. necrophorum* is thought to be the dominant pathogen with other bacteria playing synergistic roles.
• The bacteria involved are normal inhabitants of the rumen and thus are common in the environment of cattle.
• Compromise of the integrity of the interdigital skin through chronic wetting or trauma allows colonization of the tissues of the interdigital space. After gaining entry, the bacteria liberate proteases and leukotoxins which cause extensive local tissue damage. The damage to local tissue can be severe and will cause acute lameness.
• There are variations in the virulence of *F. necrophorum* which appear to be predominantly related to the quantity of leukotoxin produced. In addition, some strains are resistant to some antibiotics.
• Lameness can occur <24 hours after infection. Progression of symptoms can be rapid. Most infections are confined to the soft tissue of the digit; however, some cases can progress to involve tendons, joints, and bones of the digit.

HISTORICAL FINDINGS
• Significant decrease in milk production.
• Reduced feed intake or reluctance to come to the bunk.
• Weight loss is not usually evident at the onset of the condition.

SIGNALMENT
All production types are affected. The incidence may be higher in *Bos taurus* than in *Bos indicus*.

PHYSICAL EXAMINATION FINDINGS
• Acute lameness, usually unilateral.
• Symmetrical swelling in the pastern region (may extend to the fetlock if treatment is delayed). There is often separation of the claws due to the swelling in the interdigital region.
• Necrotic defect in the skin of the interdigital space with malodorous material.

GENETICS
Heritability for susceptibility to foot rot is low (estimated to be 0.14). Incidence may be higher in *Bos taurus* than in *Bos indicus*.

CAUSES AND RISK FACTORS
Presence of causative bacteria in the environment along with loss of integrity of interdigital skin due to mechanical trauma or hydropic maceration due to constant moisture.

DIAGNOSIS

DIFFERENTIAL DIAGNOSES
• Septic arthritis, osteomyelitis, deep digital sepsis of the heel region, and white line disease: usually asymmetrical swelling over affected claw.
• Fracture, luxation, and other trauma: Usually lack significant cellulitis as seen with foot rot.
• Foreign body: Likely to have an associated wound track but may be difficult to definitely rule out on physical examination alone.

IMAGING
Radiographs may be indicated for cases with extensive swelling or that have not responded to treatment.

OTHER DIAGNOSTIC PROCEDURES
Physical examination is usually sufficient to make the diagnosis. Microbiologic culture is seldom used due to the time and expense involved in culturing anaerobic organisms.

PATHOLOGIC FINDINGS
There is cellulitis and necrosis of the interdigital skin and subcutaneous tissue of the digit. Postmortem examination or tissue biopsy is rarely done.

TREATMENT

THERAPEUTIC APPROACH
• Prompt treatment with antibiotics is essential. A wide variety of antibiotics are labeled for treatment of foot rot in cattle. Most cases respond well to treatment so criteria such as cost, convenience, and withholding time should be considered in the selection.
• Amputation of a claw may be necessary if septic arthritis or osteomyelitis occurs secondary to interdigital phlegmon.

• Animals should be housed in an area with easy access to feed and water, a comfortable resting surface, and flooring with good traction.

SURGICAL CONSIDERATIONS AND TECHNIQUES
N/A

MEDICATIONS

DRUGS OF CHOICE
• Antibiotics approved for treatment of foot rot that also have clinical evidence to support their use include ceftiofur, florfenicol, tulathromycin, and oxytetracycline. Tylosin and sulfadimethoxine are also labeled for treatment of foot rot. There is evidence indicating ampicillin is efficacious but it is not labeled for treatment of foot rot. Readers should refer to drug labels for doses and withholding times.
• Topical antibiotics are not of use and the foot should not be bandaged.
• Nonsteroidal anti-inflammatory drugs are commonly used as an adjunct to therapy with antimicrobial drugs. While flunixin meglumine is commonly used, meloxicam (0.5 mg/kg PO) is a reasonable alternative for ongoing treatment because animals will often voluntarily consume the tablets when mixed with grain. Injectable meloxicam (0.5 mg/kg), ketoprofen (3 mg/kg), and carprofen (1.4 mg/kg) are effective alternatives in countries where they are labeled for use in food-producing animals. There is no published data to support improved outcome with the use of NSAIDs; however, the use of pain-relieving drugs in cases with significant lameness is justifiable for animal welfare.

PRECAUTIONS
Appropriate milk and meat withdrawal times must be followed for all compounds administered to food-producing animals.

FOLLOW-UP

EXPECTED COURSE AND PROGNOSIS
Recovery is usually uneventful if the disease is diagnosed and treated promptly. Treatment within 24 hours of the onset of symptoms typically results in recovery in 2–4 days. Delaying treatment can prolong the recovery period by 10 days or more. Some strains of *F. necrophorum* are multi-drug resistant and may not be responsive to treatment with antibiotics.

POSSIBLE COMPLICATIONS
Septic arthritis, septic tenosynovitis, rupture of the flexor tendon, abscessation of the interdigital space, and osteomyelitis.

F

FOOT ROT: BOVINE

CLIENT EDUCATION
See "Prevention"

PATIENT CARE
Monitor affected cattle during treatment for indications that pain and swelling are abating. Improvement should be seen within 72 hours of initiating treatment with antibiotics. If improvement is not seen, an alternative class of antibiotic may be used. Radiographs may be justified in these cases.

PREVENTION
• Management of the environment is key to controlling foot rot. For confined cattle, a dry, comfortable resting surface must be provided and the facility stocked such that cattle are able and willing to lie down for at least 10 hours per day. Feeding and traffic areas need to have manure removed regularly to avoid constant wetting of the feet. For pastured cattle, animals should have access to dry ground during wet seasons. Watering and feeding areas should be well drained and be cleaned of manure regularly. Handling facilities should have alleyways that are free of debris (stones, sticks, etc.) that would likely damage the feet of the cattle.
• Footbaths with antiseptic solutions are commonly used on dairies to prevent new cases of infectious foot diseases including interdigital phlegmon. Commonly used footbath compounds are copper sulfate or zinc sulfate (5–10%) or formalin (3%–5%). It is commonly recommended that the footbath be drained, cleaned, and refilled after every 100–300 animals pass through.
• A commercial vaccine (Fusogard®) is available and has a label claim to aid in the reduction of clinical signs of foot rot in cattle 6 months of age and older. There is little data to support the use of the vaccine. There is one published study that showed a reduction in the incidence of foot rot in cattle on a forage diet but not in cattle on a grain diet.
• Feed additives: Chlortetracycline is labeled to aid in the prevention of foot rot in cattle and may be useful in situations where the incidence of foot rot is expected to be high or when several cases are identified in a short period of time. The feeding rate is far below the therapeutic rate and thus should not be used to treat animals clinically affected with foot rot. The product cannot be fed at a rate higher than on the label.

✓ MISCELLANEOUS

ASSOCIATED CONDITIONS
Other infectious causes of lameness exacerbated by poor foot hygiene or wet or muddy conditions, such as interdigital dermatitis, digital dermatitis, and heel horn erosion.

AGE-RELATED FACTORS
Found in all ages

ZOONOTIC POTENTIAL
None

BIOSECURITY
Introduction of new cattle onto a facility may introduce new, highly virulent strains of the bacteria and cause outbreaks of interdigital phlegmon.

PRODUCTION MANAGEMENT
• For dairy cattle, estimates of milk production loss are up to 3,500 lbs per lactation. The risk of culling is up to 5 times greater that of non-lame herdmates. An additional 15 days open is expected if onset occurs at <70 days in milk. Economic losses are estimated to be up to $240 per case, depending on milk production and pregnancy status.
• An estimate of the economic losses associated with foot rot in beef cattle is not available.

ABBREVIATION
NSAID = nonsteroidal anti-inflammatory drug

SEE ALSO
• Bovine Digital Dermatitis
• Lameness: Bovine

Suggested Reading
Apley MA. Clinical evidence for individual animal therapy for papillomatous digital dermatitis (hairy heel wart) and infectious bovine pododermatitis (foot rot). Vet Clin North Am Food Anim Pract 2015, 31: 81–95.
Berry SL. Diseases of the digital soft tissues. Vet Clin North Am Food Anim Pract 2001, 17: 129–42.
Greenough PR. Bovine Laminitis and Lameness. London: Saunders, 2007, pp. 199–204.
Step DL, Smith RA. Non-respiratory diseases of stocker cattle. Vet Clin North Am Food Anim Pract 2006, 22: 413–34.
Stokka GL, Lechtenberg K, Edwards T, et al. Lameness in feedlot cattle. Vet Clin North Am Food Anim Pract 2001, 17: 189–208.

Author Edgar F. Garrett
Consulting Editor Kaitlyn A. Lutz
Acknowledgment The author and book editors acknowledge the prior contribution of Steven L. Berry.

FOOT ROT: SMALL RUMINANT

BASICS

OVERVIEW
• Widespread, economically important, disease of sheep.
• Caused primarily by *Dichelobacter nodosus*.
• Characterized by interdigital swelling, progressive lameness, and separation of the horny portions of the hoof from underlying tissues.
• Footrot is classified as benign or virulent based on pathogen characteristics and severity of clinical signs.
• Treatment includes removal of underrun horn and administration of topical or parenteral bactericidal agents.
• Carrier sheep serve as reservoirs of *D. nodosus*; transmission is enhanced in wet conditions.

INCIDENCE/PREVALENCE
Common problem wherever sheep are exposed to wet conditions.

GEOGRAPHIC DISTRIBUTION
Worldwide in major sheep-producing countries with the exception of arid and semi-arid areas where sheep do not have access to wet areas.

SYSTEMS AFFECTED
Musculoskeletal

PATHOPHYSIOLOGY
• Invasion of the foot by *D. nodosus* is aided by *Fusobacterium necrophorum*. Other bacteria, including a *Treponema* spirochete, are often present but have not been demonstrated in the development of the disease.
• Carrier sheep serve as reservoirs for *D. nodosus*. Such animals may not show symptoms but carry a pocket of infection beneath underrun horn. Survival by *D. nodosus* in the environment is generally limited to a few days and certainly no more than 2 weeks.
• Prolonged wet conditions allow colonization by *F. necrophorum* resulting in a local dermatitis called "ovine interdigital dermatitis" or "foot scald."
• Resultant hyperkeratosis facilitates infection with *D. nodosus*.
• Pili of *D. nodosus* allow attachment to foot epithelium.
• Benign footrot results from *D. nodosus* strains with little keratinolytic ability; virulent footrot is caused by keratinolytic strains resulting in more severe clinical signs.

SIGNALMENT
• Footrot is primarily a disease of sheep.
• Similar clinical signs may be seen in goats infected with *D. nodosus* but hoof separation is generally less severe than in cases of virulent footrot in sheep.
• Cattle can also be affected but lesions are primarily limited to the interdigital space.

• Incidence and lesion severity increase with increasing age although all ages are susceptible to infection.
• No sex predilection.

PHYSICAL EXAMINATION FINDINGS
• Sheep usually present for acute onset of severe lameness.
• Multiple legs are often affected. Animals may graze or walk on their knees.
• Redness, swelling, and moistness of the interdigital epithelium.
• Foul-smelling exudate in the interdigital space.
• The outer wall of the hoof becomes underrun and separated from underlying tissues. In severe cases, attachment of the hoof is limited to the toe and lateral coronary band.
• Benign footrot is limited to interdigital lesions but may be hard to distinguish from early cases of the virulent form.

GENETICS
• Merino-type sheep are the most susceptible to infection. British breeds are more resistant and exhibit milder signs of disease.
• Individual variation within flocks is believed to be genetically determined, and selection for resistance by selective breeding has been demonstrated.

CAUSES AND RISK FACTORS
• The disease is caused by *D. nodosus* in conjunction with *F. necrophorum*.
• Wet and warm conditions are a major risk factor for transmission and development of clinical signs. Thus, disease is often seasonal when environmental conditions are conducive to pathogen transmission.
• Environments conducive to irritation or abrasions of the interdigital space.
• Congregation of sheep in small areas (e.g., handling areas, communal feeding and drinking areas).
• Introduction of carrier sheep.

DIAGNOSIS

DIFFERENTIAL DIAGNOSES
• Bluetongue
• Contagious ecthyma (orf)
• Contagious ovine digital dermatitis (CODD)
• Foot abscess
• Foot and mouth disease
• Laminitis
• Strawberry foot rot

CBC/BIOCHEMISTRY/URINALYSIS
N/A

OTHER LABORATORY FINDINGS
Gram's stain of the interdigital exudate can be performed to tentatively identify *D. nodosus*.

OTHER DIAGNOSTIC PROCEDURES
• Underrunning and separation of the hoof wall accompanied by interdigital

inflammation and malodorous exudate is diagnostic for contagious footrot.
• PCR tests can be used to identify particular bacterial strains.
• Fluorescein-stained antibody assay is available.
• Diagnostic assays are often not available at diagnostic laboratories outside major sheep-producing areas.

PATHOLOGIC FINDINGS
Necropsy is not warranted for diagnosis of foot rot.

TREATMENT

THERAPEUTIC APPROACH
• Treatment is aimed at temporary control or complete eradication.
• Antibiotic therapy is most effective early in the course of disease before development of horn lesions.
• Long-acting parenteral antibiotic therapy in conjunction with topical therapy improves recovery.
• Individual animal topical therapy requires complete removal of underrun horn although some research has questioned the value of hoof trimming.
• Footbaths are commonly used for treatment and control of herd outbreaks. Effective solutions include 10% zinc sulfate, 5% copper sulfate, and 5% formalin.
• Feet should be soaked for 30–60 min.
• Aerosol sprays have been used in lieu of footbaths but are generally less effective than foot soaking.

MEDICATIONS

DRUGS OF CHOICE
N/A

FOLLOW-UP

EXPECTED COURSE AND PROGNOSIS
• Most cases respond to appropriate treatment.
• Nonresponders should be identified and culled to decrease environmental pathogen load and the source of future infections.

PATIENT CARE
• Repeated treatments may be necessary to clear infection from the herd.
• Animals that do not respond to several treatments should be culled.

PREVENTION
• Introduction of outside animals is discouraged and should only occur after quarantine.

F

FOOT ROT: SMALL RUMINANT (CONTINUED)

- Facilities or vehicles used to hold or transport affected animals should be disinfected or avoided.
- Vaccination is used in both treatment and control. Efficacy of vaccination is dependent on the homology of field and vaccine strains.
- Routine foot baths at 10-day intervals during the transmission season will help prevent outbreaks.
- Limit congregation of animals in wet areas.
- Separate affected animals during outbreaks.
- Previous disease does not provide immunity against further infection. Thus, returning treated animals to contaminated environments will result in further outbreaks of disease.

MISCELLANEOUS

ASSOCIATED CONDITIONS

CODD is an emerging disease of sheep characterized by acute-onset lameness and extensive underrunning of hoof horn. In contrast to footrot, interdigital lesions are absent but proliferative or ulcerative lesions are seen at the coronet. Response to traditional footrot treatments is poor. *D. nodosus* and *F. necrophorum* are often present but the primary cause of CODD is believed to be a spirochete similar to bovine digital dermatitis.

AGE-RELATED FACTORS

All ages are susceptible to infection; incidence and lesion severity increase with increasing age.

BIOSECURITY

- Quarantine new arrivals and introduce to the herd only after inspection of the feet for underrun horn and evidence of infection with *D. nodosus*.
- Separate affected and unaffected animals during outbreaks and house in separate pastures.

PRODUCTION MANAGEMENT

- Eradication can be attempted in sufficiently dry areas (annual precipitation <20 inches).
- Eradication hinges on the identification of all affected animals. Examine the feet of all animals and separate the affected and unaffected sheep.
- Unaffected animals are run through a footbath and placed in clean pasture, with or without long-acting antibiotic treatment.
- Affected animals may be culled immediately or treated with antibiotic therapy and weekly footbaths. After at least three soakings, the feet are reexamined and affected animals culled.
- Any animals not showing lameness during the subsequent wet period can be reintroduced to the clean flock.

ABBREVIATION

CODD = contagious ovine digital dermatitis

SEE ALSO

- Bluetongue Virus
- Foot and Mouth Disease
- Foot Rot: Bovine
- Lameness: Small Ruminant
- Orf (Contagious Ecthyma)

Suggested Reading
Bennett GN, Hickford JG. Ovine footrot: new approaches to an old disease. Vet Microbiol 2011, 148: 1–7.
Frosth S, König U, Nyman AK, Pringle M, Aspán A. Characterisation of *Dichelobacter nodosus* and detection of *Fusobacterium necrophorum* and *Treponema* spp. in sheep with different clinical manifestations of footrot. Vet Microbiol 2015, 179: 82–90.
Green LE, George TR. Assessment of current knowledge of footrot in sheep with particular reference to *Dichelobacter nodosus* and implications for elimination or control strategies for sheep in Great Britain. Vet J 2008, 175: 173–80.
Kennan RM, Han X, Porter CJ, Rood JI. The pathogenesis of ovine footrot. Vet Microbiol 2011, 153: 59–66.
Radostits OM, Gay CC, Hinchcliff KW. Infectious foot rot in sheep. In: Radostits OM, Gay CC, Hinchcliff KW, Constable PD eds, Veterinary Medicine: A Textbook of the Diseases of Cattle, Horses, Sheep, Pigs, and Goats, 10th ed. Edinburgh: Saunders Elsevier, 2007, pp. 1070–7.

Author Benjamin W. Newcomer
Consulting Editor Christopher C.L. Chase

BASICS

OVERVIEW
- A disorder of sexual development which occurs in pregnancies with male and female fetuses.
- The condition has been reported in several species of ruminant and camelid. However, it is mainly a production problem in cattle.
- 80–95% of female calves born co-twin to a male are affected.
- Affected female calves may be born singleton if the male twin perished in utero.
- In sheep and goats, it is more likely to occur with increased numbers of fetuses (i.e., 4 or 5) compared to twin and triplet pregnancies.

INCIDENCE/PREVALENCE
- Unknown but suspected to be increasing as the rate of twin pregnancy in cattle has increased.
- Although multiple mixed-sex births are common, incidence is rare in small ruminants (<2%). Reported incidence in sheep varies (0.8–1.9% in Romanov ewes and up to 7% in other breeds).
- In camelids, the condition is extremely rare.

GEOGRAPHIC DISTRIBUTION
Worldwide

SYSTEMS AFFECTED
Reproductive

PATHOPHYSIOLOGY
Vascular anastomoses lead to blood chimerism (XX/XY) and variable effects on each sex. In the female, effects of anti-Mullerian hormone and testosterone lead to variable masculinization of the external and internal reproductive tract. Effects on the male have been sporadically reported, with diagnoses of spermatozoa defects, decreased fertility, and testicular degeneration described.

HISTORICAL FINDINGS
- Female born co-twin to a male.
- Ambiguous external genitalia or abnormal urination.
- Abnormality of the reproductive tract discovered during AI (bovine).
- Male-like behavior has been described in ewes.

SIGNALMENT
Freemartinism has been reported in cattle, sheep, goats, camelids, and cervids.

PHYSICAL EXAMINATION FINDINGS
- The degree of masculinization of female offspring is highly variable.
- In many females, the external genitalia may appear normal. In other cases, abnormalities may include increased anogenital distance, enlarged clitoris, and coarse hair around the vulva.
- Internal genitalia may be characterized by a short blind vagina, small underdeveloped uterus, hypoplastic ovaries, ovotestes, and varying degree of development of male reproductive tract structures, including epididymides, ductus deferens, pampiniform plexus, and cremaster muscle. The gonads may be located abdominally, inguinally, or subcutaneously in the inguinal region. Affected females may show persistent estrus, anestrus, or male-like behavior. Affected males typically do not show outward abnormalities in anatomy or behavior.

GENETICS
Suspected in small ruminants. The risk for freemartinism is increased in breeds with high fecundity genes which carry litters of 4 or more lambs.

CAUSES AND RISK FACTORS
Twin pregnancies

DIAGNOSIS

DIFFERENTIAL DIAGNOSES
- Other causes of abnormal sexual differentiation
- Physical examination of external genitalia

CBC/BIOCHEMISTRY/URINALYSIS
N/A

OTHER LABORATORY TESTS
- Cytogenetics (karyotype) to diagnose blood chimerism (XX/XY)
- Molecular studies (PCR) to diagnose Y-chromosome specific genes (*SRY, AMELY, ZFY*)
- Serology for anti-Mullerian hormone

IMAGING
- Transrectal ultrasonography may be used for the evaluation of the uterus and gonads in large heifers suspected to be freemartin.
- In one study on ewes, ultrasonography of the gonads showed an echotexture of the gonads varying from normal testicular tissue to pseudohermaphrodite appearance with various degree of calcification or cystic anomalies.

OTHER DIAGNOSTIC PROCEDURES
Vaginal canal length and presence of the cervix can be examined in female calves.

PATHOLOGIC FINDINGS
Most affected ewes have small vaginal length and gonads that resemble testicles with degenerating sex cords or testicular tissue with defined tubular structures and interstitial regions.

TREATMENT

THERAPEUTIC APPROACH
N/A

SURGICAL CONSIDERATIONS AND TECHNIQUES
N/A

MEDICATIONS

DRUGS OF CHOICE
N/A

CONTRAINDICATIONS
N/A

PRECAUTIONS
N/A

POSSIBLE INTERACTIONS
N/A

FOLLOW-UP

EXPECTED COURSE AND PROGNOSIS
Culling or raising for slaughter

POSSIBLE COMPLICATIONS
N/A

CLIENT EDUCATION
- Testing of all heifers born co-twin to a male calf
- Examination of purchased females of unknown breeding history

PATIENT CARE
N/A

PREVENTION
N/A

MISCELLANEOUS

ASSOCIATED CONDITIONS
N/A

AGE-RELATED FACTORS
Congenital condition

ZOONOTIC POTENTIAL
N/A

PREGNANCY
N/A

BIOSECURITY
N/A

F

FREEMARTINISM

PRODUCTION MANAGEMENT
• Do not use affected animals for breeding
• Affected females may be used for heat detection (i.e., teaser animal)

ABBREVIATION
A.I. = artificial insemination

SEE ALSO
• Anestrus
• Congenital Defects: Bovine
• Congenital Defects: Camelid
• Congenital Defects: Small Ruminant
• Uterine Anomalies

Suggested Reading
Harikae K, Tsunekawa N, Hiramatsu R, et al. Evidence for almost complete sex-reversal in bovine freemartin gonads: formation of seminiferous tubule-like structures and transdifferentiation into typical testicular cell types. J Reprod Develop 2012, 58: 654–60.

Kozubska-Sobocinska A, Rejduch B, Slota E, et al. New aspects of degenerative changes in reproductive system of freemartin heifers. Ann Anim Sci 2011, 11: 229–39.
Martinez-Royo A, Dervishi E, Alabart JL, et al. Freemartinism and *Fec*X^R allele determination in replacement ewes of the Rasa Aragonesa sheep breed by duplex PCR. Theriogenology 2009, 72: 1148–52.
Padula AM. The freemartin syndrome: an update. Anim Reprod Sci 2005, 87: 93–109.
Remnant JG, Lea RG, Allen CE, et al. Novel gonadal characteristics in an aged bovine freemartin. Anim Reprod Sci 2014, 146: 1–4.
Smith KC, Parkinson TJ, Pearson GR, et al. Morphological, histological and histochemical studies of the gonads of ovine freemartins. Vet Rec 2003, 152: 164–9.

Smith KC, Parkinson TJ, Long SE, Barr FJ. Anatomical, cytogenetic and behavioural studies of freemartin ewes. Vet Rec 2000, 146: 574–8.
Szczerbal I, Kociucka B, Nowacka-Woszuk J, et al. A high incidence of leukocyte chimerism (60,XX/60,XY) in single born heifers culled due to underdevelopment of internal reproductive tracts. Czech J Anim Sci 2014, 59: 445–9.

Author Lisa Pearson
Consulting Editor Ahmed Tibary
Acknowledgment The author and book editors acknowledge the prior contribution of Simon F. Peek.

BASICS

OVERVIEW
• Frostbite represents damage or injury to the skin and body tissues resulting from their freezing following exposure to excessive cold or windchill.
• Severe frostbite is a grave physiologic condition with potentially life-threatening consequences.
• Frostbite may be primary, or secondary to debilitating disease or malnutrition.
• The ears, tail, teats, scrotum, and distal extremities (hindlimbs > forelimbs) are most often affected.
• Tissue damage is substantially exaggerated if thawing is followed by refreezing.
• Tissue previously damaged by freezing is more prone to injury on subsequent exposure to cold temperatures.

INCIDENCE/PREVALENCE
Unknown

GEOGRAPHIC DISTRIBUTION
More common in geographic regions with temperatures that drop below freezing

SYSTEMS AFFECTED
Integument

PATHOPHYSIOLOGY
• Exact mechanism of tissue damage is difficult to define and reflects multiple pathologic mechanisms.
• Frostbite involves direct cellular injury from freezing, injury from progressive vasoconstriction and subsequent arterial thrombosis, and ischemic necrosis.
• Four phases describe the mechanisms of cell damage during freezing:
  ◦ Phase I (pre-freeze phase): congestion and leakage of fluid from vascular compartment due to arterial constriction and venous dilation.
  ◦ Phase II (freeze-thaw phase): extracellular ice crystal formation causes cell membrane rupture or cellular dehydration.
  ◦ Phase III (vascular stasis phase): more severe and persistent arterial spasm and venous dilation leading to arteriovenous shunting and tissue hypoxia.
  ◦ Phase IV (ischemia phase): neural tissue damage due to prolonged tissue hypoxia.
• Additional injury occurs during rewarming with return of blood flow and warming of affected tissue.
• Direct cellular destruction, release of catecholamines, and tissue anoxia have potentially significant secondary effects in severe frostbite, resulting in damage to other organs.

HISTORICAL FINDINGS
• Frostbite is uncommon in well-nourished animals when environmental temperatures are above 10°F (−12.2°C).

• Frostbite can occur when temperatures are at or below 0°F (−17.8°C) or when windchill provokes such low temperatures.

SIGNALMENT
Any species, breed, age, or gender can be affected; however, neonates are at greatest risk due to wet, thin skin at birth, minimal subcutaneous fat, and a high surface area : volume ratio.

PHYSICAL EXAMINATION FINDINGS
• Signs of chilling including piloerection, shivering, and peripheral vasoconstriction.
• Mild frostbite causes blanching of tissue and reduced sensation followed by painful erythema, scaling, and alopecia.
• Severe frostbite results in necrosis, dry gangrene, and sloughing of affected part(s); affected skin is usually anesthetic.
• Death can result from hypothermia if not reversed before vital organs are compromised.
• Frozen teats will initially appear reddened or pale, which can progress to scab formation over the distal half of the teat. As the teat heals the milk duct may become occluded.
• Milk-fed calves may show superficial muzzle sloughing.
• Pain occurs with rewarming of affected areas.
• A line of demarcation between viable and nonviable tissue usually appears within 3 days of rewarming affected areas. This line is initially diffuse and becomes more distinct within 7 days, but may take weeks to become clearly defined.
• Vesicles and blisters develop on affected areas.
• After sloughing, ears are rounded, alopecic, and have pinnae of variable length.

GENETICS
N/A

CAUSES AND RISK FACTORS
• Exposure to subnormal temperatures and wetness.
• Windchill accelerates evaporation and cooling of exposed areas.
• Wet neonates or adults with wet udders, teats, or testicles.
• Heifers with severe periparturient udder edema and reduced perfusion to teats.
• Poor nutrition.
• Hypoglycemic neonates.
• Previous tissue damage due to cold injury.
• Debilitated, sick, or dehydrated animals with reduced metabolic heat generation.
• Animals with heavily pigmented skin.
• Milking cattle and goats turned outside in cold weather with inadequately dried udders and teats.
• Animals with pre-existing vascular damage (e.g., ergotism, fescue toxicosis, vasculitis).

DIAGNOSIS

DIFFERENTIAL DIAGNOSES
• Inherited, small pinna of American La Mancha goat
• Traumatic injury
• Previous tissue damage from ergot toxicosis

CBC/BIOCHEMISTRY/URINALYSIS
Findings might be consistent with metabolic acidosis, dehydration, hypoglycemia (neonates), secondary infection, organ compromise, and hypoalbuminemia (if a large area of tissue is damaged),

OTHER LABORATORY TESTS
N/A

OTHER DIAGNOSTIC PROCEDURES
Skin biopsy

IMAGING
N/A

PATHOLOGIC FINDINGS
• Gross necropsy might define decreased subcutaneous and perirenal fat deposits, subcutaneous hemorrhage of the tarsal region, edema, vesicles, or bullae over affected tissue, or skin and tissue necrosis.
• Histology identifies adipocytes filled with eosinophilic cytoplasm instead of lipid; tissue microthrombosis, vasculitis.

TREATMENT

THERAPEUTIC APPROACH
• Rewarming should be initiated as soon as possible once it is known that refreezing can be prevented; thawing and refreezing increases tissue damage.
• Incomplete or partial rewarming decreases chances for successful recovery.
• Rapid rewarming is painful but results in less cellular and tissue damage than slow rewarming.
• Thaw tissue rapidly in warm water (plain or with a dilute antiseptic solution).
  ◦ Recommended water temperature range: 100.2–111.1°F (38–44°C), ideally 104–106°F (40–41°C).
• Rewarming process should be repeated twice daily for 2–3 days.
• Application of lanolin or other bland, protective ointments or creams after rewarming completed.
• Leave damaged area exposed during healing and protect animal from cold until healing has occurred.

SURGICAL CONSIDERATIONS AND TECHNIQUES
• If necessary, debride necrotic tissue to facilitate healing and limit secondary infection.

FROSTBITE

• Postpone debridement or surgical excision of limbs until boundary between viable and nonviable tissue is clearly obvious, which may take 8 weeks.
• Frostbitten teats may require surgery to keep the teat duct patent.

MEDICATIONS

DRUGS OF CHOICE
• Nonsteroidal anti-inflammatory drugs provide analgesia and systemic anti-inflammatory effects, including flunixin meglumine; 1.1 mg/kg IV, q12–24h; or ketoprofen: 2.2 mg/kg/day IV or IM.
• Epidural analgesia during rewarming period may help with hindlimb pain.
• Broad-spectrum antibiotics may be indicated to prevent secondary infection.
• IV or oral fluids help correct dehydration and metabolic acidosis, assist rewarming, provide vascular support, reduce hyperviscosity, improve capillary circulation, and prevent hypovolemic shock that may occur after peripheral rewarming and subsequent fluid shifts.
• Apply aloe vera topically (anti-thromboxane, anti-inflammatory, and analgesic effects).
• Tetanus immunization is indicated in animals with extensive frostbite.
• A single dose of glucocorticoids may decrease capillary permeability, maintain microcirculation, stabilize cell membranes, and reduce induced histamine.

CONTRAINDICATIONS
N/A

PRECAUTIONS
• Avoid massaging or rubbing tissue during warming as this can prolong edema and recovery.
• Do not use occlusive bandages over damaged areas.
• Avoid premature debridement of affected areas; more tissue may be more viable than initially apparent.
• Appropriate milk and meat withdrawal times must be followed for all compounds administered to food-producing animals.

POSSIBLE INTERACTIONS
N/A

FOLLOW-UP

EXPECTED COURSE AND PROGNOSIS
Dependent on severity of injury

POSSIBLE COMPLICATIONS
Secondary infection, sloughing of extremities, organ failure

CLIENT EDUCATION
Frostbite may occur at less extreme environmental temperatures in compromised animals despite adequate housing and nutrition.

PATIENT CARE
• Provide a palatable high-protein, high-calorie diet with a vitamin supplement.
• Restrain to avoid self-mutilation.
• Edges of healthy and gangrenous tissue should be kept clean, protected, and allowed to slough naturally.

PREVENTION
• Avoid or adjust for the listed risk factors (see "Causes and Risk Factors").
• Dry off calves, kids, and lambs born in cold environments.
• Ensure susceptible body parts remain dry during exposure to subnormal temperatures.
• Provide adequate, clean, dry bedding to neonates to minimize heat loss by convection and evaporation.
• Provide easily accessible shelter and consistent feeding management.

MISCELLANEOUS

ASSOCIATED CONDITIONS
Secondary bacterial infection

AGE-RELATED FACTORS
Neonates are at higher risk

ZOONOTIC POTENTIAL
N/A

PREGNANCY
N/A

BIOSECURITY
N/A

PRODUCTION MANAGEMENT
• With ambient temperatures below 32°F (0°C) management should include:
  ◦ Dry udder and teats completely before animal leaves parlor.
  ◦ Provide adequate windbreaks and shelter.
  ◦ Dip just the teat end during very cold weather.
• Provide windbreaks and bedding for calving cows when windchill temperatures are below 10–20°F (–12 to –10°C).
• House calving cows and calves <1 day old when windchills are below 10°F (–12°C) and calves cannot be kept dry because of rain or snow.
• Keep dairy animals clean, dry, and out of the wind with adequate dry bedding daily when temperatures are subnormal.

SYNONYM
Cold-induced injury

ABBREVIATIONS
N/A

SEE ALSO
• Fescue Toxicity
• Wound Management

Suggested Reading
Pelton JA, Callan RJ, Barrington GM, Parish SM. Frostbite in calves. Comp Cont Ed Vet Pract 2000, 22: S136–41.
Pugh D. Diseases of the integumentary system. In: Sheep and Goat Medicine. Philadelphia: Saunders, 2002.
Rebhun WC. Skin diseases. In: Diseases of Dairy Cattle. Baltimore: Williams & Wilkins, 1995.
Scott DW. Environmental skin diseases. In: Howard JL, Smith RA eds, Current Veterinary Therapy 4: Food Animal Practice. Philadelphia: Saunders, 1999.
Smith MC, Sherman DM. Skin. In: Goat Medicine. Philadelphia: Lea & Febiger, 1994.
White SD. Diseases of the skin. In: Large Animal Internal Medicine, 5th ed. St. Louis: Mosby, 2015.
Author Joe S. Smith
Consulting Editor Erica C. McKenzie
Acknowledgment The author and book editors acknowledge the prior contribution of Susan Semrad and Karen A. Moriello.

F

BASICS

OVERVIEW

• Tremorgens are mycotoxins that have been reported to cause tremoring conditions in cattle, goats, sheep, deer, horses, and camelids.
• Clinical signs associated with ingestion of these neurotoxins are collectively known as "staggers" and include ataxia, muscle tremors, rigid stance, recumbency, and paddling convulsions. The tremors are accentuated by exercise and can lead to tetany and collapse.
• The mycotoxins are produced by fungal genera such as *Neotyphodium, Claviceps, Penicillium,* and *Aspergillus,* and are often associated with specific grasses, such as perennial ryegrass, dallisgrass, bahiagrass, and Bermuda grass (Table 1).

INCIDENCE/PREVALENCE
Unknown

GEOGRAPHIC DISTRIBUTION
Worldwide where affected pastures are used for grazing livestock. Cases have been reported in Australia, New Zealand, Europe, South America, and throughout the United States.

SYSTEMS AFFECTED
Nervous

PATHOPHYSIOLOGY
• Grass staggers is a syndrome caused by a group of related mycotoxins found in toxic stands of various pasture grasses.
• The toxins exert their effects by inhibiting the inhibitory neurotransmitter, gamma-aminobutyric acid (GABA). The mycotoxins are structurally similar to GABA and bind to GABA receptors in the internuncial neurons, resulting in receptor inactivation.
• Loss of inhibitory neurotransmitters leads to increased neurotransmission and prolonged

depolarization, resulting in the neurologic signs of incoordinated movements, ataxia, and muscle tremors.

SIGNALMENT
• All species can be affected. Reports of tremogenic mycotoxin intoxication have occurred in cattle, horses, goats, sheep, deer, and camelids.
• There are no species or breed predilections.
• While there are no age predilections per se, most cases occur in adult cattle and to a lesser extent, weaned animals.

PHYSICAL EXAMINATION FINDINGS
• Signs are initially mild and may be limited to fine head tremors.
• Signs may be minimal or absent at rest but are exacerbated by noise and sudden movements.
• Coarse and fine muscle fasiculations, particularly in the shoulder and flank areas, develop as the disease progresses.
• Stiff, hypermetric gait. When forced to run, movements appear jerky and uncoordinated.
• In severe cases, animals may collapse with opisthotonus, nystagmus, and flailing of the limbs. Generally, the attack subsides in a few minutes and the animal is able to regain its feet.

CAUSES AND RISK FACTORS
• Risk factors and inciting conditions vary between tremorgenic compounds.
• Perennial ryegrass staggers is caused by the endophyte *Neotyphodium lolii* which produces tremorgenic toxins known as lolitrems, notably lolitrem B. Late seasonal growth, warm ambient temperatures, and closely grazed pastures favor toxicity. Clinical cases are seen between June and September in the northern hemisphere.
• The seed heads of dallis- and bahiagrasses can be infected by *Claviceps paspali.* The fungus produces alkaloids including indole compounds derived from lysergic acid known as paspalitrems. Wet conditions following seed head formation result in increased toxin formation.
• Annual ryegrass staggers is caused by a corynetoxin. Toxin levels are highest as the plant dries and seeds ripen in the summer. Outbreaks are commonly seen after outbreaks of stormy weather.

DIAGNOSIS

DIFFERENTIAL DIAGNOSES
• Many of the fungal tremorgens present similarly. Diagnosis is based on forage identification in affected pastures.
• Other conditions that can cause similar neurologic signs include hypomagnesemia, rabies, tetanus, tremetol intoxication, yew toxicity, and selenium poisoning.

CBC/BIOCHEMISTRY/URINALYSIS
No specific changes in clinical pathology. An elevation in serum creatinine kinase or aspartate aminotransferase may be seen due to muscle cell damage from ataxia or incoordination.

OTHER DIAGNOSTIC PROCEDURES
• Presumptive diagnosis is made based on clinical signs and demonstration of exposure to susceptible forages.
• Analysis of forage to identify specific mycotoxins can be performed by most state diagnostic laboratories; but it is not commonly performed, and obtaining a forage sample with adequate mycotoxin levels is difficult.
• Extracts of the fungus-infected feed material can be analyzed by thin-layer chromatography, high-performance liquid chromatography, or bioassay.

PATHOLOGIC FINDINGS
• Mortality due to the fungal tremorgens is low. When deaths do occur, they often result from misadventure such as drowning.
• Pathologic findings reflect the cause of death and are not specific for the fungal tremorgens.

TREATMENT

THERAPEUTIC APPROACH
• There is no specific treatment or antidote for tremorgenic mycotoxin intoxication.
• Removal from affected pastures or contaminated forages and supportive care usually allows for recovery in 1–2 weeks.

MEDICATIONS

DRUGS OF CHOICE
N/A

FOLLOW-UP

EXPECTED COURSE AND PROGNOSIS
• Removal from affected pastures at the time of development of clinical signs generally allows complete recovery within 1–2 weeks.
• Longer recovery times have been noted in cases of annual ryegrass staggers where neurologic deficits have resolved over a period of several months.

POSSIBLE COMPLICATIONS
Though mortality is low, severely affected animals may collapse into bodies of water or cast themselves, resulting in traumatic injury or death.

PREVENTION/AVOIDANCE
• Pasture management is key to preventing grass staggers.

Table 1

Grass Forages Associated with Staggers Syndrome due to Fungal Endophytes	
Cynodon dactylon	Bermudagrass
Hilaria mutica	Tobosagrass
Lolium perenne	Perennial ryegrass
Paspalum	
P. dilatatum	Dallisgrass, large watergrass
P. distichum	Knotgrass, jointgrass
P. scrobiculatum	Indian paspalum, monagrass, kodo millet
Phalaris spp.	Canarygrasses

Source: Burrows, George E., Tyrl, Ronald J. Toxic Plants of North America (p. 902). Wiley. Kindle Edition.

FUNGAL TREMORGENS

• Disease can be avoided by removal from affected pastures.
• Overgrazing of perennial ryegrass increases the likelihood of toxicity.
• *Claviceps paspali* infects the seedheads of dallis- and bahiagrasses. Removal of the seedheads by mowing can prevent intoxication.

 MISCELLANEOUS

AGE-RELATED FACTORS
Though no specific age predilection exists, most cases occur in adults and weaned animals.

PREGNANCY
Abortion is not a common sequela of disease.

BIOSECURITY
N/A

PRODUCTION MANAGEMENT
N/A

SYNONYM
Grass staggers

ABBREVIATION
GABA = gamma-aminobutyric acid

SEE ALSO
• Clostridial Disease: Nervous System
• Grass Tetany/Hypomagnesemia
• Rabies
• Selenium Toxicity
• Tremetol: White Snakeroot and Rayless Goldenrod
• Yew Toxicity

Suggested Reading
Bourke CA, Bunker EC, Reece RI, Whittaker SJ. Cerebellar ataxia in sheep grazing pastures infested with *Romulea rosea* (onion grass or Guildford grass). Aust Vet J 2008, 86: 354–6.
Burrows GE, Tyrl RJ eds. Toxic Plants of North America, 2nd ed. Ames: Wiley-Blackwell, 2013, p. 902.
di Menna ME, Finch SC, Popay AJ, Smith BL. A review of the *Neotyphodium lolii/Lolium perenne* symbiosis and its associated effects on animal and plant health, with particular emphasis on ryegrass staggers. N Z Vet J 2012, 60: 315–28.
Grass Staggers. In: Smith BP ed, Large Animal Internal Medicine, 3rd ed. Philadelphia: Mosby, 2002, pp. 966–71.
Mostrom MS, Jacobsen BJ. Ruminant mycotoxicosis. Vet Clin North Am Food Anim Pract 2011, 27: 315–44.
Thom ER, Waugh CD, Minneé EM, Waghorn GC. Effects of novel and wild-type endophytes in perennial ryegrass on cow health and production. N Z Vet J 2013, 61: 87–97.

Author Benjamin W. Newcomer
Consulting Editor Christopher C.L. Chase
Acknowledgment The author and book editors acknowledge the prior contribution of Natalie Coffer.

BASICS

OVERVIEW
• Gossypol is a toxic phenolic substance that occurs naturally in the cotton plant (*Gossypium* spp.).
• Whole cottonseed (WCS) and cottonseed meal (CSM) are a widely used source of energy, fiber, and protein in diets of adult cattle, calves, and sheep.
• Signs of gossypol toxicity are primarily manifested in the cardiac system and include anorexia, weakness, cardiac failure, and sudden death.
• Gossypol also causes reproductive failure, particularly in males.

INCIDENCE/PREVALENCE
Unknown

GEOGRAPHIC DISTRIBUTION
Worldwide in areas feeding cottonseed meal

SYSTEMS AFFECTED
• Musculoskeletal
• Cardiac
• Reproductive
• Hemolymphatic
• Multisystemic

PATHOPHYSIOLOGY
• Gossypol is contained in variable amounts in whole cottonseed and cottonseed meal. Free gossypol is readily absorbed from the gastrointestinal tract.
• Gossypol binds to cellular constituents including phospholipids and lysine, inhibits dehydrogenases, and uncouples cellular phosphorylation.
• Spermatogenesis is impaired through inhibition of lactic dehydrogenase in testicular Leydig cells and acrosomal plasminogen activator in the sperm.

SIGNALMENT
• Potentially all ruminants feeding on cottonseed meal can be affected.
• Mature ruminants are more resistant to gossypol toxicosis as gossypol can be neutralized in the rumen by binding to soluble proteins. However, the protein-binding detoxifying mechanism in adult cattle can be overwhelmed if the total gossypol content is excessive, or low protein content is present in the rumen.
• Preruminant cattle such as lambs and calves are commonly affected.
• The reproductive effects are primarily seen in male animals although high levels of gossypol can also cause impaired reproductive performance in cows.

PHYSICAL EXAMINATION FINDINGS
• The clinical signs of gossypol toxicity include sudden death as well as physiologic and reproductive effects without death.
• Preruminant calves exhibit anorexia and signs related to congestive heart failure including dyspnea, coughing, jugular distension, brisket edema, and weakness.
• Adult cattle have reduced milk production, anorexia, weakness, and respiratory stress.
• Reduced spermatogenesis and impaired sperm motility associated with morphologic aberrations of the sperm midpiece.
• Reproductive signs in females are not regularly seen clinically but include irregular cycling and potentially early embryonic death.

CAUSES AND RISK FACTORS
• Consumption of diets containing excessive amounts of gossypol from whole cottonseed and cottonseed hulls or meal is the route of exposure that causes toxicity.
• The level predisposing the animal to toxicity depends on the species, rumen function, level of protein in the diet, and duration of consumption.
• Two isomers of gossypol exist in all cotton plants: the (+) isomer acts as an insect deterrent but is more toxic than the (-) isomer. Upland cotton, the predominant strain in the southeastern US, has a higher ratio of the (+) isomer than Pima cotton, which predominates in the western US.
• Solvent extraction of cottonseed oil leaves more free gossypol than heat extraction.

DIAGNOSIS

DIFFERENTIAL DIAGNOSES
• Monensin toxicity
• Vitamin E and selenium deficiency
• Toxic plants such as *Senna* spp., oleander, white snakeroot, and yew

CBC/BIOCHEMISTRY/URINALYSIS
• Elevations in liver-specific isoenzymes are the most consistent change in the serum biochemical profile.
• Minimal changes in erythrocyte parameters are expected during toxicity. However, hemoglobinuria, anemia, and a decrease in hemoglobin content have been reported.

IMAGING
Imaging is rarely undertaken but abdominal or thoracic radiographs and ultrasound will demonstrate the presence of free fluid in the body cavities.

OTHER DIAGNOSTIC PROCEDURES
• Diagnosis is supported by demonstration of elevated gossypol levels in feedstuffs being consumed, clinical signs consistent with gossypol toxicity, and typical pathologic findings.
• Send representative samples of the cotton by-product (WCS or CSM) to a qualified laboratory for total and free gossypol analysis. Note that the standard analytic method will not give accurate results of gossypol levels in a total mixed ration (TMR) sample; therefore, the cotton by-products should be analyzed individually.
• High performance liquid chromatography (HPLC) can be used to detect gossypol levels in some tissue samples.
• Gossypol accumulates in the liver and kidneys which are the preferred tissue samples for postmortem analyses.

PATHOLOGIC FINDINGS
• Generalized edema.
• Gelatinous, yellow proteinaceous fluid in the thoracic and peritoneal cavities.
• Hepatomegaly secondary to congestive heart failure.
• Degeneration of the skeletal and cardiac muscle.
• Histologically there is centrilobular hepatic congestion and necrosis related to hepatic anoxia. There is also myocardial degeneration and necrosis.

TREATMENT

THERAPEUTIC APPROACH
• No specific treatment is available for acute gossypol toxicity. Prognosis depends on the severity of clinical signs and supportive care may not be warranted in the case of advanced disease.
• Administration of vitamin E may ameliorate some clinical signs but will not prevent gossypol toxicity.
• Experimentally, selenium supplementation alleviates the effect of gossypol toxicity in breeding males.

MEDICATIONS

DRUGS OF CHOICE
N/A

FOLLOW-UP

EXPECTED COURSE AND PROGNOSIS
Because of the cumulative nature of the toxicant and the type of pathologic changes, deaths will often continue for several days following cessation of feeding of the toxic ration.

PREVENTION
• Avoid overfeeding of WCS and CSM. Consult a nutritionist for specific dietary recommendations for different species and production classes.
• Testing of gossypol levels in cotton-based commodities is available but not routinely performed. Knowledge of free gossypol levels in feedstuffs may assist in ration planning.

G

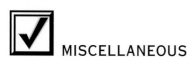

MISCELLANEOUS

AGE-RELATED FACTORS
Stage of rumen development is critical in detoxifying gossypol. While the young ruminant is being fed milk, rumen development and function are minimal. During this time, the animal functions essentially as a preruminant and tolerable levels of free gossypol in the diet are similar to nonruminant species, which is 200 ppm.

ZOONOTIC POTENTIAL
Humans are susceptible to gossypol toxicity but the toxicity is not considered transmissible through milk or meat products.

PRODUCTION MANAGEMENT
• Consumption of diets containing excessive amounts of gossypol from whole cottonseed and cottonseed hulls or meal is the route of exposure that causes toxicity.
• The level predisposing the animal to toxicity depends on the species, rumen function, level of protein in the diet, and duration of consumption.
• When considering toxicity levels of free gossypol in ruminants, the source—whole cottonseed vs. cottonseed meal—should be considered. Detoxification of free gossypol in the rumen appears to be more efficient with whole cottonseed.
• Stress lowers the toxic threshold for gossypol toxicity. Thus, signs of toxicity may be seen when feeding gossypol at recommended levels if the animals are subjected to increased external stressors (e.g., poor nutritional plane, overcrowding).
• Guidelines for safe levels of gossypol intake should not exceed 20 g/day for lactating dairy cows, 8 g/day for breeding bulls.
• Detoxification can be achieved by cooking the CSM or by the addition of 1% calcium hydroxide or 0.1% ferrous sulfate.

ABBREVIATIONS
• CSM = cottonseed meal
• HPLC = high performance liquid chromatography
• TMR = total mixed ration
• WCS = whole cottonseed

SEE ALSO
• Monensin Toxicity
• Oleander and Cardiotoxic Plant Toxicity
• Selenium/Vitamin E Deficiency
• Senna Species
• Yew Toxicity

Suggested Reading
Burrows GE, Tyrl RJ. In: Burrows GE, Tyrl RJ eds, Toxic Plants of North America, 2nd ed. Ames: Wiley-Blackwell, 2013, pp. 813–17.
Galey FD. Gossypol. In: Smith BP ed, Large Animal Internal Medicine, 3rd ed. Philadelphia: Mosby, 2002: pp. 1622–3.
Garland T. Gossypol poisoning. In: Kahn CM ed, The Merck Veterinary Manual. Kenilworth, NJ: Merck & Co. 2010 (online) http://www.merckvetmanual.com/mvm/toxicology/gossypol_poisoning/overview_of_gossypol_poisoning.html
Mena H, Santos JE, Huber JT, Tarazon M, Calhoun MC. The effects of varying gossypol intake from whole cottonseed and cottonseed meal on lactation and blood parameters in lactating dairy cows. J Dairy Sci 2004, 87: 2506–18.
Rogers GM, Poore MH, Paschal JC. Feeding cotton products to cattle. Vet Clin North Am Food Anim Pract 2002, 18: 267–94.

Author Benjamin W. Newcomer
Consulting Editor Christopher C.L. Chase
Acknowledgment The author and book editors acknowledge the prior contribution of Carlos A. Risco.

GRASS TETANY/HYPOMAGNESEMIA

BASICS

OVERVIEW
• Magnesium (Mg) deficiency affects the central nervous system of ruminants.
• Mg is absorbed from the rumen and excreted in urine.
• High dietary potassium decreases absorption of Mg.
• Rapidly growing grasses may contain relatively high concentrations of potassium and most always have low concentrations of Mg.

INCIDENCE/PREVALENCE
Unknown

GEOGRAPHIC DISTRIBUTION
Worldwide

SYSTEMS AFFECTED
• Nervous
• Musculoskeletal

PATHOPHYSIOLOGY
• Mg is necessary for most major cellular metabolic pathways and is vital to maintenance of resting membrane potentials at synapses.
• Because adenosine triphosphate (ATP) requires Mg to form the high-energy bond between phosphates, Mg is required for all enzymatic reactions requiring ATP.
• Mg is also necessary for ATPase activity; therefore, myofibril contractions are sustained in hypomagnesemia, leading to tetanic spasms.
• Most Mg is present in teeth and bones, which is not readily mobilized.
• There is no direct hormonal control of Mg uptake, so daily intake is necessary.

SIGNALMENT
• Cattle, sheep, and goats; potentially all ruminant species.
• Most commonly seen in lactating beef cattle within the first 2 months of calving, particularly if grazing cool season grasses.
• Lactating dairy cattle are affected less commonly because of differences in nutritional management. Grazing dairy cattle would be at greater risk.
• A winter tetany associated with cattle in a dry lot with dry feeds.
• Ewes and dairy goats are also susceptible.
• Calves on all milk diets without added Mg may develop the disease as well.

PHYSICAL EXAMINATION FINDINGS
• Affected animals are often found dead.
• Anorexia and separation from the herd.
• Early in the course, ears will be erect and twitching and hyperesthesia will be noted.
• Alert, hyperexcitable, may be aggressive.
• Muscle fasciculations and head tremors may be noted.
• Nystagmus and fluttering of the eyelids.
• Ataxia.

• Recumbency.
• Clonic convulsions, opisthotonus, or tetanic muscle spasms.
• Elevated body temperature because of excess muscle activity.
• Increased heart and respiratory rate.

CAUSES AND RISK FACTORS
• Magnesium deficiency that can be result of low intake of Mg and/or higher output of Mg, particularly during lactation.
• Mature ruminants just prior to calving and during early lactation have the highest demand for Mg.
• Periods of rapid grass growth, particularly cool season grasses and cereal crops, are the most common time for clinical signs to occur (spring and/or fall).
• Heavy fertilization of pastures with increased potassium increases the risk of grass tetany. Use of recycled poultry bedding as a feed supplement or fertilizer has commonly been associated with an increased incidence of hypomagnesemia.

DIAGNOSIS

DIFFERENTIAL DIAGNOSES
• Hypocalcemia (serum Ca)
• Nervous ketosis (urine ketones)
• Urea toxicosis
• Nervous coccidiosis (fecal float)
• Heavy metal toxicities: for example, arsenic and lead (history of exposure to heavy metals, elevated blood, kidney or liver concentration of heavy metal)
• Salt poisoning (history, necropsy)
• Tetanus (response to therapy, necropsy)
• Rabies (necropsy)
• Viral encephalitides (history of herd and surrounding area, increasing antibody titers)

CBC/BIOCHEMISTRY/URINALYSIS
• Serum Mg <1.2 mg/dL
• Cerebrospinal fluid Mg <1.45 mg/dL
• Urine Mg <2.5 mg/dL
• Postmortem ocular Mg <1 mg/dL (within 24 hours of death)
• Affected animals are often hypocalcemic.
• After episodes of tetany, animals will often have elevated potassium, aspartate aminotransferase (AST), and creatinine phosphokinase (CK) due to muscle damage.

OTHER DIAGNOSTIC PROCEDURES
• Diagnosis is most often made on the basis of clinical signs or history because of the need for immediate treatment.
• Decreased serum, CSF, ocular or urine Mg concentrations are confirmatory.

PATHOLOGIC FINDINGS
• Grossly may note evidence of thrashing on ground around where the animal died.
• No gross findings directly attributable to hypomagnesemia.

• Trauma and bruising are common findings because of seizures.
• Rumen contents may be aspirated into lungs.
• Ecchymotic hemorrhages.
• Agonal pulmonary emphysema.
• Histologically, calves dying of hypomagnesemia may have microscopic calcium deposits in arterial walls of the heart, lungs, and spleen.

TREATMENT

THERAPEUTIC APPROACH
• Minimize handling to decrease the chance of initiating tetanic seizures.
• It may be necessary to administer intramuscular sedation prior to initiating Mg therapy to control seizure activity. Avoid intravenous sedative administration.
• Heart rate should be monitored closely while administering Mg solutions and treatment should be slowed or discontinued if heart rate drops substantially.
• Respiratory failure may occur if Mg solutions are given too quickly due to medullary depression.

MEDICATIONS

DRUGS OF CHOICE
• Animals with hypomagnesemia are often hypocalcemic as well and should receive therapy containing calcium.
• Administer intravenous calcium borogluconate solution containing 5% Mg (500 mL for adult cattle; 50–100 mL for calves and small ruminants).

CONTRAINDICATIONS
• Avoid potassium-containing solutions for therapy because they will interfere with Mg absorption.
• Appropriate milk and meat withdrawal times must be followed for all compounds administered to food-producing animals.

FOLLOW-UP

EXPECTED COURSE AND PROGNOSIS
Therapy is often unrewarding, especially in cases where seizures have already occurred.

CLIENT EDUCATION
• Allowing animals access to only hay or mature grass for a portion of the day will increase Mg in the diet and may prevent further cases.
• Mg is unpalatable and will not be consumed in significant quantities unless mixed with some other dietary component.

G

GRASS TETANY/HYPOMAGNESEMIA

• Mg can be added to feed or water to encourage intake:
  ◦ If feeding Mg in water, animals must be given access to only supplemented water to ensure intake of Mg.
  ◦ Spraying or dusting pastures with Mg fertilizers in the spring will increase dietary Mg.
  ◦ Mg will be readily consumed in concentrate mixtures or molasses licks.

PATIENT CARE
• Many animals relapse several hours after treatment, so an additional source of Mg should be provided with initial treatment.
  ◦ Oral Mg salts: (1) 50% Mg sulfate solution (125–150 mL for adult cattle). (2) Mg oxide (60 g in gelatin capsule for adult cattle).
  ◦ Subcutaneous injection of 100–200 mL (for adult cattle) of a 20%–50% Mg sulfate solution. Limit to 50 mL per site to avoid tissue damage.
• Mg enema—60 g of Mg in 250–500 mL of water. Solution should not be more concentrated than this to avoid mucosal sloughing.

MISCELLANEOUS

AGE-RELATED FACTORS
• Most commonly seen in lactating beef cattle within the first 2 months of calving, particularly if grazing cool season grasses.

• Lactating dairy cattle are affected less commonly because of differences in nutritional management. Grazing dairy cattle would be at greater risk.
• Calves on all-milk diets without added Mg may develop the disease as well.
• Calves dying of hypomagnesemia may have microscopic calcium deposits in arterial walls of the heart, lungs, and spleen.

ZOONOTIC POTENTIAL
Hypomagnesemia is neither contagious nor zoonotic.

PRODUCTION MANAGEMENT
• Periods of rapid grass growth, particularly cool season grasses and cereal crops, are the most common times for clinical signs to occur (spring and/or fall).
• Heavy fertilization of pastures increases the risk of grass tetany. Use of recycled poultry bedding as a feed supplement or fertilizer has commonly been associated with an increased incidence of hypomagnesemia.

SYNONYMS
• Grass staggers
• Hypomagnesemia
• Tetany
• Winter tetany

ABBREVIATIONS
• AST = aspartate aminotransferase
• ATP = adenosine triphosphate
• Ca = calcium
• CK = creatinine phosphokinase
• CNS = central nervous system

• CSF = cerebral spinal fluid
• Mg = magnesium

SEE ALSO
• Clostridial Disease: Nervous System
• Coccidiosis
• Heavy Metal Toxicosis
• Hypocalcemia: Bovine
• Hypocalcemia: Small Ruminant
• Ketosis: Dairy Cattle
• Rabies
• Sodium Disorders: Hypernatremia

Suggested Reading
Blackwelder JT, Hunt E. Disorders of magnesium metabolism. In: Smith BP ed, Large Animal Internal Medicine. Philadelphia: Mosby, 2002.
Goff JP. Ruminant hypomagnesemic tetanies. In: Howard JL, Smith RA eds, Current Veterinary Therapy 4: Food Animal Practice. Philadelphia: Saunders, 1999.
Wilson GF. Metabolic diseases of grazing cattle: from clinical event to production disease. N Z Vet J 2002, 50: S85–7.
Author Steve Ensley
Consulting Editor Christopher C.L. Chase
Acknowledgment The author and book editors acknowledge the prior contribution of Dawn J. Capucille.

G

BASICS

OVERVIEW
• This toxin is found in members of the heath or *Ericaceae* family. This family is known for showy ornamentals that characteristically grow in acidic soils.
• All parts of the plant contain the toxin.
• Leaves are simple and alternate, rarely opposite.
• Flowers in variety of colors.
• Fruits can be berries or capsules.
• Seeds are small.

INCIDENCE/PREVALENCE
N/A

GEOGRAPHIC DISTRIBUTION
Worldwide

SYSTEMS AFFECTED
• Nervous
• Cardiovascular

PATHOPHYSIOLOGY
• Grayanotoxins are heterocyclic diterpenes that exert their effects thru binding to sodium channels within the cell membrane leading increased sodium permeability of excitable membranes within the neurologic, cardiac, and muscular systems.
• Effects on sodium channels results in easily triggered depolarization and thus persistent action.
• Accumulation of intracellular sodium also results in exchange for extracellular calcium which is needed in neurotransmitter release.
• Toxins are found within leaves especially, as well as stems, flowers, and nectar.
• The amount of toxin within various members and the growing stage is unknown.

HISTORICAL FINDING
History of exposure to plants

SIGNALMENT
Bovine, ovine, and especially caprine

PHYSICAL EXAMINATION FINDINGS
• Develop within 6 hours of exposure
• Depression
• Severe salivation
• Abdominal pain
• Regurgitation, can be projectile
• Severe toxicosis
  ◦ Cardiac arrhythmia
  ◦ Hypotension
  ◦ Opisthotonus
  ◦ Pyrexia (reported as high as 106°F or 41.1°C)
  ◦ Seizures

CAUSES AND RISK FACTORS
• This toxin is found in members of the heath or *Ericaceae* family. Most common members of this family include:
  ◦ Azaleas and rhododendrons (*Rhododendron*)
  ◦ Heaths (*Erica*)
  ◦ Mountain laurels (*Kalmia*)
  ◦ Heathers (*Calluna*)
  ◦ Madrones (*Arbutus*)
• Members of this family exist as shrubs, subshrubs, herbs, and small trees. They can be evergreen or deciduous.
• The toxins are found in all parts of the plants, including nectar from the flowers.

DIAGNOSIS

DIFFERENTIAL DIAGNOSES
• Oleander
• Foxglove

CBC/BIOCHEMISTRY/URINALYSIS
• No characteristic changes on full blood count
• No characteristic changes on serum biochemistry/urinalysis

OTHER LABORATORY TESTS
Identification of grayanotoxin in feces and urine through use of liquid chromatography-mass spectrometry

OTHER DIAGNOSTIC PROCEDURES
• History of exposure to the plants
• Clinical signs
• Identification of plant in GI contents

TREATMENT

THERAPEUTIC APPROACH
• There are no specific antidotes.
• Atropine has been used with some success either alone or as reported in goats and cattle with a combination of atropine sulfate and sodium camphorsulfonate (see "Drugs of Choice").
• Because of the acute nature of the disease, oral administration of charcoal may be of some benefit in limiting absorption of the toxins.
• Supportive treatment.

MEDICATIONS

DRUGS OF CHOICE
10–20 mg atropine sulfate and 15–20 mL of 10% sodium camphorsulfonate given subcutaneously.

FOLLOW-UP

EXPECTED COURSE AND PROGNOSIS
Recovery possible even with severe toxicosis

POSSIBLE COMPLICATIONS
Aspiration pneumonia

PREVENTION
Avoidance of the plant materials

MISCELLANEOUS

ASSOCIATED CONDITIONS
N/A

SYNONYMS
N/A

ABBREVIATIONS
N/A

SEE ALSO
Oleander and Cardiotoxic Plant Toxicity

Suggested Reading
Burrows GE. Ericaceae. In: Burrows GE, Tyrl RJ eds, Toxic Plants of North America. Ames: Iowa State University Press, 2001, pp. 439–44.
Burrows GE, Tyrl, RJ. Toxic Plants of North America. Wiley. Kindle Edition, pp. 432–9.
Puschner B. Grayanotoxin poisoning in three goats. J Am Vet Med Assoc 2001, 218: 573–5.
Author Jennifer S. Taintor
Consulting Editor Christopher C.L. Chase
Acknowledgment The author and book editors acknowledge the prior contribution of Benjamin R. Buchanan.

HAEMONCHOSIS

BASICS

OVERVIEW
• *Haemonchus* is a voracious blood-sucking, single-host parasite that causes anemia, hypoproteinemia, and death in ruminants (particularly small ruminants).
• In warm, moist environments, *Haemonchus* is typically the dominant gastrointestinal nematode of pasture production systems.
• *Haemonchus* species (*H. contortus*, *H. placei*, and *H. similis*) tend to be host-specific, with some potential for cross-infection.
• Populations of *Haemonchus* have developed resistance to almost all currently available anthelmintics.

INCIDENCE/PREVALENCE
When conditions are suitable for transmission, nearly 100% of pastured ruminants will be infected, but the prevalence of clinical disease will vary with the number of worms that are able to establish in specific individuals.

GEOGRAPHIC DISTRIBUTION
Animals grazing in humid tropical regions and regions with summer rainfall, with daily mean temperatures >15°C (>59°F) and monthly rainfall >50 mm.

SYSTEMS AFFECTED
• Digestive
• Hemolymphatic

PATHOPHYSIOLOGY
• Adult *Haemonchus* females have great fecundity, and an individual can release more than 5,000 eggs per day into the host feces.
• L1 and L2 stages survive on bacteria within manure; the L2 sheds its cuticle during development to the infective L3 stage, 5–10 days after eggs are released onto pasture.
• Ruminant hosts are infected by ingesting the L3 from pasture; this stage can only exit the fecal pellet and ascend vegetation in a film of moisture.
• The L3 stage exsheaths in the rumen and moves to the abomasum, enters gastric pits, and molts to L4.
• The L4 feeds on blood and molts to the L5 and then the adult stage which can mate and produce eggs approximately 3 weeks after being acquired. Adult worms can live for months in susceptible hosts.
• Adult worms produce so many eggs that some offspring will survive unfavorable conditions within or outside of the host. The L3 larvae maintain a protective cuticle that helps them avoid desiccation, and they can

survive on pasture for weeks to months, depending on conditions.
• During prolonged periods of drought or winter weather, ensheathed larvae survive in the fecal pellet; they are inactive and apparently do not utilize stored energy; when rain occurs they rapidly exit the fecal pellet.
• The early L4 stage can undergo hypobiosis (arrested development) within the abomasum. These larvae are in a state of inactivity and are not affected by the host's immune system. They survive until conditions within the host or environment are more favorable before resuming their life cycle.
• Adults and developing larvae possess a buccal lancet that allows laceration of capillaries in the abomasal mucosa to facilitate feeding, and they have prolyl-carboxypeptidases which can act as anticoagulants to facilitate feeding.
• Loss of erythrocytes and serum protein causes clinical signs of anemia and hypoproteinemia which can be profound, to the point of causing severe morbidity and mortality.

HISTORICAL FINDINGS
• Clinical signs can vary from peracute, to acute or chronic in nature, and reflect variably severe anemia and hypoproteinemia.
• Diarrhea is an infrequent clinical sign.

SIGNALMENT
• All ages of sheep, goats, camelids, deer, and cattle can become infected but recently weaned and lactating small ruminants are at greater risk of disease.
• Until young ruminants have been exposed to *Haemonchus* and maturation of the immune system occurs (4–7 months), they do not develop resistance to the parasite.
• Affected hosts can vary depending on environment and vegetation consumed. Where sheep and goats graze on short grass and legumes, clinical disease is more often seen in goats. When there is plentiful browse, goats are unlikely to be exposed to large numbers of infective larvae.

PHYSICAL EXAMINATION FINDINGS
• Clinical signs primarily reflect anemia and hypoproteinemia.
• Peracute disease is typically reflected by sudden weakness, pallor, recumbency, and death, as the PCV falls to <10%. Typically only a few individuals in the flock will be affected in this manner; soft stool or melena may be observed.
• In acute disease, a larger number of individuals in the flock will be affected. Anemia, pale mucus membranes, and hypoproteinemia (bottle jaw) are the most

common clinical signs. Constipation can occur, and wool break often occurs in sheep several weeks after acute clinical signs.
• Chronic disease is often reflected by ill thrift with poor-quality wool, weight loss or failure to gain, and anemia can become unresponsive due to iron depletion.

GENETICS
• There is genetic host resistance to haemonchosis, which usually manifests as acquired protective immunity (after exposure), with fewer worms establishing in these individuals, and established worms producing fewer eggs.
• The genetic aspects of resistance to gastrointestinal parasitism are not well understood. It appears that multiple genes are involved in the protective response and different genes may be more important at different times during the course of infection.
• Ruminant breeds and species that evolved in humid tropical areas are more likely to have genetic traits increasing resistance to infection, including Barbados sheep.
• Factors such as lactation, age, or nutritional status influence the course of disease in individuals.
• Production traits should be carefully measured against parasite resistance. There is no evidence that traits associated with increased production are linked to increased susceptibility, but caution is warranted when selecting animals for breeding.
• Genetic selection can be employed by choosing individual animals with a level of resistance to *Haemonchus* or those that have the capacity to rebound from the effects of parasitism. The offspring of resistant hosts have a higher likelihood of being more resistant.

CAUSES AND RISK FACTORS
• Warm, humid climactic conditions.
• Young or lactating animals; when animals are producing at their genetic maximum they are at greater risk of parasitic disease because they are immunologically and nutritionally challenged.
• Female ruminants are unable to mount a protective immune response against helminths during the periparturient period.
• Heavily stocked and grazed pastures.

DIAGNOSIS

DIFFERENTIAL DIAGNOSES
• Anemia related to other endoparasites, bacterial infections or toxic agents.
• Chronic copper poisoning in sheep may be differentiated by time of the year, age of

affected animals, presence of icterus, and access to sources of copper.
• Poisoning caused by sweet clover, pokeweed, or plants that cause intestinal or other bleeding may resemble haemonchosis. History of access, age of animals, and time of year may help differentiate.

CBC/BIOCHEMISTRY/URINALYSIS
• In acute cases, CBC reveals reduced erythrocyte count and blood hemoglobin concentrations with normal erythrocyte morphology. Surviving animals quickly mount evidence of a regenerative response.
• Chronic haemonchosis results in depletion of iron, cobalt, and copper; hence microcytic, hypochromic anemia may occur.
• Serum protein concentrations are reduced, with reduced albumin/globulin ratio.

OTHER LABORATORY TESTS
• Fecal flotation using saline or sugar flotation media with a specific gravity of 1.18 or higher will float the eggs of *Haemonchus* and other nematodes. Fecal examination will reveal strongylid, thin-shelled segmented eggs. However, visualization of eggs is not diagnostic for *Haemonchus* since other genera of strongylids produce visually identical eggs.
• A quantitative test such as the modified McMaster method allows strongylid egg identification and enumeration. There is a somewhat linear relationship between egg count and the number of adult worms. Fecal egg counts of more than 4,000 eggs per gram of feces are associated with haemonchosis in small ruminants (though this depends upon the time of examination after infection).
• Measuring egg counts before and then 7–10 days after anthelmintic treatment (Fecal Egg Count Reduction Test) can be vital in determining the level of anthelmintic resistance on a specific property.

IMAGING
N/A

OTHER DIAGNOSTIC PROCEDURES
• Coproculture, the development of eggs to the infective L3 stage under laboratory conditions, enables specific identification of larvae but can take 10–14 days. This technique also has applicability in assessing anthelmintic resistance via *in vitro* larval development assays.
• A fluorescein-labeled peanut agglutinin test can provide rapid differentiation of *Haemonchus* eggs from those of other strongyles.
• PCR testing is being explored as a method of specifically identifying and quantitating *Haemonchus* infection, and for characterizing anthelmintic resistance in this parasite.

• FAMACHA© testing, the comparison of ocular mucus membrane color to a commercially available chart, allows evaluation of the severity of anemia in individuals. This facilitates selection for treatment of those animals with the highest worm burden to help protect pastures and reduces parasite selection for anthelmintic resistance.

PATHOLOGIC FINDINGS
• Gross postmortem examination identifies adult worms in the abomasum if performed within 24 hours of death. Adults are approximately 2 cm long; males are red and females have a characteristic "barber-pole" appearance arising from the combination of the blood-filled digestive tract against the white reproductive tract. Body cavities may contain transudate, and the abomasal mucosa may range from normal to markedly thickened and ulcerated. Intermandibular edema and pallor of mucus membranes is commonly evident. Feces may be normal, loose, or dark and dry. Bone marrow may appear red and hyperplastic.
• Histologic findings are associated with anemia, hypoxemia, hypoproteinemia, abomasitis, and bone marrow hyperplasia. There may be centrilobular hepatic necrosis, interstitial edema of organs, and infiltration of the abomasal mucosa with lymphocytes, eosinophils, and mast cells.

TREATMENT
THERAPEUTIC APPROACH
• Successful control of haemonchosis should rely on the use of multiple management strategies rather than sole dependence on the periodic administration of anthelmintics. Strategies can include pasture rotation, selective anthelmintic therapy based on fecal and clinical monitoring, and use of non-pharmaceutical control procedures such as administration of copper oxide wire particles, oral feeding of nematophagous fungi (*Duddingtonia flagrans*), and the feeding of condensed tannin forage sources such as *Sericea lespedeza*.
• Anthelmintic resistance in *Haemonchus* has occurred rapidly and is widespread in some areas. Selection by treatment rather than mutation appears to be the driving force in the establishment of resistance. Some of the features that contribute to the rise and spread of anthelmintic resistance include:
  ◦ Tolerant or resistant worms often accompany livestock being introduced into new areas.

  ◦ Underdosing of anthelmintic agents by underestimating body weight, dosing based on the average size of animals in a flock, and by dosing goats at recommendations for sheep (goats and cervids metabolize anthelmintics more quickly than do cattle or sheep).
  ◦ Providing anthelmintics via injectable form – as blood concentrations decline, parasites with some level of tolerance of the drug will be able to establish in the host.
  ◦ Use of cattle pour-on formulations in other species in which they are not as well absorbed.
• Techniques that might enhance the impact of anthelmintic therapy also exist:
  ◦ The effectiveness of benzimidazoles may be enhanced by dividing the dose over several days or by fasting the animals overnight in a dry lot.
  ◦ Combining anthelmintics by administration of two or more drugs from different classes simultaneously. Proprietary drugs using all three main families of anthelmintics are being used for *Haemonchus* resistance problems particularly in Australia and New Zealand.
  ◦ Selection of anthelmintics for individual properties based on those with the likely highest efficacy for that property.
  ◦ In regard to anthelmintic drug rotation, currently it is often suggested that rather than rotate products, a product should be used until it fails before switching to the use of a drug in another class.

SURGICAL CONSIDERATIONS AND TECHNIQUES
N/A

MEDICATIONS
DRUGS OF CHOICE
• *Haemonchus* in cattle and in small ruminants in cooler climates are currently still susceptible to some benzimidazoles, levamisole/morantel, or macrocyclic lactones if administered at an adequate dose via an appropriate route.
• Several new classes of anthelmintics are available in different geographic areas and include the aminoacetonitrile derivative Monepantel, the octadepsipeptide Emodepside, and a member of the Spiroindoles class, Derquantel.
• Drugs which are able to block the ability of *Haemonchus* to clear some anthelmintics are being evaluated.

CONTRAINDICATIONS
• Most of the currently available anthelmintics have a wide safety margin.

H

However, levamisole, especially when injected, can cause signs of nervous stimulation including salivation, lacrimation, urination, and defecation.
• Albendazole in early pregnancy can cause embryonic loss or teratogenic effects.

PRECAUTIONS
Appropriate milk and meat withdrawal times must be followed for all compounds administered to food-producing animals.

POSSIBLE INTERACTIONS
N/A

FOLLOW-UP

EXPECTED COURSE AND PROGNOSIS
Animals surviving acute disease and treated appropriately are expected to recover, though short-term consequences such as wool break and decreased production may be observed. Peracute and chronically diseased animals have a poor prognosis for survival or return to optimal production.

POSSIBLE COMPLICATIONS
Hypoxemia, recumbency, death

CLIENT EDUCATION
Should support periodic fecal analyses and herd health assessments, pasture management, animal selection, and judicious use of anthelmintic medications

PATIENT CARE
N/A

PREVENTION
• Prevention programs should be based on individualized practices that fit with the environment and management practices of the operation in question. The most effective control programs comprise integrated strategies using a number of different approaches simultaneously.
• Programs that recognize that some individuals are much more at risk than others, and which strive to ensure that the at-risk population is exposed to fewer worms or, if exposed, are treated differently, have a greater potential for success.
• Programs based on chemical control alone are likely to fail unless the season of transmission is very short or new anthelmintics with completely different modes of action are employed.
• Management strategies:
  ◦ In warm humid climates, rapid pasture rotation (where pastures are vacated for as few as 30 days) may be of value during the hottest time of the year in high rainfall areas or on irrigated pastures.
  ◦ Utilizing pastures that have been cropped, especially in the last half of the grazing season, insures that larvae deposited on the cropland will not survive until the next grazing.
  ◦ Alternate or co-grazing with other species or classes of livestock may harvest *Haemonchus* larvae from the pasture, reducing infection of ruminants; typically, *Haemonchus* of sheep and goats does not do well in cattle and vice versa. However, recent observations question this assumption as some populations of *H. contortus* may thrive in calves. Horses do not share *Haemonchus* and can be safely grazed in areas dangerous to ruminants, and older cattle may become infected but are highly resistant to the effects of the worm burden, and can be used to clear larvae from a pasture.
  ◦ Zero grazing for a period of time after an outbreak may enable animals to recover both in terms of reestablishing a protective immune response and replenishing erythrocytes and serum protein.
  ◦ Provision of copper oxide (typically as wire particles) is postulated to alter the reproductive capacity of *Haemonchus* females, reducing fecal egg counts and ultimately decreasing infective larvae on pasture.
• Nutritional strategies:
  ◦ Providing sufficient protein is vital to supporting infected individuals and to facilitating recovery.
  ◦ Provision of increased dietary protein during the periparturient period can reduce egg production by gastrointestinal nematodes.
• Biological control strategies:
  ◦ Pastures in which plants are high in condensed tannins are safer for hosts as ingested larvae are adversely affected.
  ◦ The physical structure of some plants can present a challenge to larvae to ascend the vegetation.
  ◦ Browsing reduces the chance of acquiring larvae as the distance from the ground increases. Most infective larvae are found within two inches (50 mm) of the soil surface.
  ◦ Nematophagous fungi can kill larvae on the pastures. One species, *Duddingtonia flagrans,* is able to traverse the digestive tract and is present in the feces when the larvae hatch. Feeding spores or incorporating them into ruminal boluses has the capacity to lower pasture contamination.
• Vaccination:
  ◦ A vaccine, Barbervax®, was recently made available for use in Australia, where it is reported to have 75–95% efficacy against *Haemonchus* infection in sheep. The vaccine is directed against specific intestinal antigens of the parasite, and is administered as 4–9 subcutaneous injections at approximately 6-week intervals.
• Genetics:
  ◦ Individual animals that display some innate resistance or the capacity to rebound from the effects of parasitism can be selected for breeding, as some of these selection traits may be heritable.
  ◦ Immunity to *Haemonchus* is slow to develop, and cannot overcome exposure to large numbers of larvae; however, there may be an allergic response to massive larval exposure known as "self-cure," during which adult worms are expelled and the larvae that triggered the response may eventually take their place or are also eliminated.

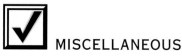

MISCELLANEOUS

ASSOCIATED CONDITIONS
Diarrhea may be observed in some infected individuals.

AGE-RELATED FACTORS
Young and recently weaned animals are at greater risk of clinical disease.

ZOONOTIC POTENTIAL
N/A

PREGNANCY
Pregnant animals are less resistant to infection and more susceptible to clinical disease.

BIOSECURITY
N/A

PRODUCTION MANAGEMENT
This is the most economically significant parasitic disease of pasture-based small ruminant systems, and results in stock losses, reduced production parameters, and expense associated with anthelmintic treatments and potentially vaccination.

SYNONYM
Barber's pole worm

ABBREVIATION
PCV = packed cell volume

SEE ALSO
• Anemia, Regenerative
• Copper Deficiency and Toxicity
• Sweet Clover Poisoning

Suggested Reading
Bassetto CC, Amarante AFT. Vaccination of sheep and cattle against haemonchosis. J Helminthol 2015, 89: 517–25.
Hein WR, Pernthaner A, Piedrafita D, et al. Immune mechanisms of resistance to

gastrointestinal nematode infections in sheep. Parasite Immunol 2010; 32: 541–8.

Hoste H, Torres-Acosta JFJ. Non chemical control of helminths in ruminants: Adapting solutions for changing worms in a changing world. Vet Parasitol 2011, 180: 144–54.

Larsen M. Biological control of helminths. Internat J Parasitol 1999, 29: 139–46.

Radostits OM, Gay CC, Hinchcliff KW, Constable PD. 2008. Veterinary Medicine: A Textbook of the Diseases of Cattle, Horses, Sheep, Pigs, and Goats, 10th ed. New York: Elsevier Saunders, 2008.

Sutherland IA, Leathwick DM. Anthelmintic resistance in nematode parasites of cattle: a global issue? Trends Parasitol 2011, 27: 176–81.

Van Wyk JA, Bath GF. The FAMACHA© system for managing haemonchosis in sheep and goats by clinically identifying individual animals for treatment. Vet Res 2002, 33: 509–29.

Authors Thomas Craig and Nicholas A. Robinson
Consulting Editor Erica C. McKenzie

H

HEARTWATER (COWDRIOSIS)

BASICS

OVERVIEW
• A tick-borne rickettsial disease of domestic and wild ruminants is caused by *Ehrlichia* (formerly *Cowdria*) *ruminantium*. This rickettsial agent is transmitted by ticks of the genus *Amblyomma*, particularly the tropical bont tick (*A. variegatum*).
• At least two *Amblyomma* species found in North America are potential vectors and this poses the threat of the disease introduction. Introduction of the vector is also possible through importation of wildlife from endemic areas.
• It is colloquially called "heartwater" due to the common finding of hydropericardium in infected cattle.

INCIDENCE/PREVALENCE
• In areas with the vector the disease is enzootic. The mortality rate in susceptible livestock is in the range <10%–90%, depending on the animal's species, breed, and previous exposures.
• Morbidity and mortality rates are normally higher in non-native than indigenous breeds, and sheep and goats are usually affected more severely than cattle.

GEOGRAPHIC DISTRIBUTION
The disease is enzootic throughout sub-Saharan Africa, Madagascar, and the Caribbean islands of Guadeloupe, Marie-Galante, and Antigua. The disease is exotic to the United States.

SYSTEMS AFFECTED
• Cardiovascular
• Nervous

PATHOPHYSIOLOGY
• Once in the host, the organisms may replicate first within the regional lymph nodes with subsequent dissemination via the bloodstream to invade endothelial cells of blood vessels elsewhere in the body. In domestic ruminants, there seems to be a predilection for endothelial cells of the brain.
• During the febrile stage, and for a short while thereafter, the blood of infected animals is infective to susceptible animals if subinoculated.
• Signs and lesions are associated with functional injury to the vascular endothelium, resulting in increased vascular permeability without recognizable histopathologic or even ultrastructural pathology.
• The concomitant fluid effusion into tissues and body cavities precipitates a fall in arterial pressure and general circulatory failure.
• The lesions in peracute and acute cases are hydrothorax, hydropericardium, edema and congestion of the lungs and brain, splenomegaly, petechiae and ecchymoses on mucosal and serosal surfaces, and occasionally hemorrhage into the GI tract, particularly the abomasum.
• The typically straw-colored effusions are high in large-molecular-weight proteins, including fibrinogen; hence, this fluid readily clots on exposure to air.

SIGNALMENT
• Most domestic ruminants are susceptible. Sheep and goats are more susceptible than other ruminants.
• Among wild ruminants, water buffalo and bison are highly susceptible. Infection has been observed in eland, wildebeest, blesbuck, and Cape buffalo.
• Age resistance, or a reduction in severity of clinical signs after infection, occurs in very young animals (calves <4 weeks of age, lambs and goat kids <1 week), and results in immunity to reinfection with the same strain and a carrier state.

GENETICS
• Among sheep breeds, Persian and Afrikaner are more tolerant than European breeds. Angora goats are highly susceptible.
• *Bos indicus* breeds are more tolerant than *Bos taurus* breeds.

PHYSICAL EXAMINATION FINDINGS
• Incubation period following bite from infected tick is 9–29 days in cattle, 5–35 days in sheep.
• Signs can be peracute, acute (most common), subacute, or subclinical.
• Peracute signs include rapid development of fever, hyperesthesia, lacrimation, convulsions, and sudden death. This form occurs in susceptible breeds introduced into endemic areas and is the rarest form.
• Acute signs include several days of high fever, anorexia, depression, exaggerated gait, excessive blinking, chewing movements, circling, aggression, and most animals die. This is the most common form.
• The subacute form is characterized by mild fever and mild nervous signs and occurs in animals with some natural resistance.
• The subclinical form has been reported in animals with natural resistance including neonates.
• Hydropericardium (hence the name heartwater) and hydrothorax are some of the pathologic findings observed on necropsy.

CAUSES AND RISK FACTORS
• Cowdriosis is caused by *Ehrlichia* (formerly *Cowdria*) *ruminantium*, a rickettsial agent transmitted by ticks of the genus *Amblyomma*.
• Important tick species that transmit the organism are *A. variegatum*, *A. habraeum*, and *A. pomposum*.
• Naïve animals introduced to endemic areas are highly susceptible. Introduction of vectors carrying *E. ruminantium* may also result in outbreaks.
• In endemic areas, reduced tick populations may lower herd immunity through less-frequent challenge and thereby put herds at greater risk for an epidemic of illness when tick populations rebound.
• In the United States, Gulf Coast states from Florida to Texas are at risk for introduction of the tropical bont tick, and possibly *E. ruminantium*, from the Caribbean.
• Zebu breeds of cattle appear more resistant to infection than European breeds.
• Animals 3–18 months are most susceptible, while young calves, lambs, and goat kids exhibit age resistance.

DIAGNOSIS

DIFFERENTIAL DIAGNOSES
• Differential diagnoses include diseases that cause sudden death (peracute form) or cortical signs. These include anthrax, lightning strike, polioencephalomalacia, salt poisoning, lead poisoning, and rabies.
• The acute form may resemble babesiosis, theileriosis, and trypanosomiasis, especially in endemic areas.
• Nervous system abnormalities may suggest other diseases such as rabies, hypomagnesemia, nervous ketosis, listeriosis, tetanus, meningitis or encephalitis, or poisoning by some toxins.

CBC/BIOCHEMISTRY/URINALYSIS
N/A

OTHER LABORATORY TESTS
• Serologic assays (e.g., ELISA) are available but suffer from cross-reactions with other rickettsia.
• PCR and LAMP can identify *E. ruminantium* in tissues at necropsy, or in the blood of live animals from just before the onset of the fever to a few days after recovery.
• Cowdriosis should be suspected when an animal is infested with *Amblyomma* ticks and develops fever and nervous signs and dies.
• In fatal cases, presence of characteristic gross lesions and demonstration of *E. ruminantium* colonies using Giemsa stain on endothelial cells of brain smears.

PATHOLOGIC FINDINGS.
Gross lesions include hydrothorax, hydropericardium, pulmonary edema, splenomegaly, petechiae, and ecchymoses on serosal surfaces.

TREATMENT

THERAPEUTIC APPROACH
• Tetracyclines are the treatment of choice but must be given early in the course of the disease.
• Chemoprophylaxis with tetracyclines has been suggested in animals introduced to endemic areas.

(CONTINUED)

• Short-acting formulations of oxytetracycline, 10–20 mg/kg body weight, given two times at 24-hour intervals

MEDICATIONS

DRUGS OF CHOICE
• Tetracyclines are the drug of choice (see "Therapeutic Approach")
• Corticosteroids have been used as supportive therapy (prednisolone 1 mg/kg, IM), although there is debate as to the effectiveness and rationale for their use.

CONTRAINDICATIONS
Appropriate milk and meat withdrawal times must be followed for all compounds administered to food-producing animals.

FOLLOW-UP

EXPECTED COURSE AND PROGNOSIS
• Animals with the neurologic form have a poor prognosis.
• Animals with the acute form of heartwater usually die within a week.
• Heartwater can also present as a subacute disease with milder signs such as a prolonged fever, coughing and mild incoordination. CNS signs are inconsistent in this form. Subacute cases are reported to be infrequent (although some cases might not be recognized if diagnostic testing is not done). In this form, the animal either recovers or dies within 1–2 weeks.

PATIENT CARE
Affected animals must be kept quiet in a cool area with soft bedding and be totally undisturbed; any stimulation can preempt a convulsive episode and subsequent death.

PREVENTION
• Various vaccines are available in endemic areas with varying success.
• Tick control is essential.
• Exposure of young animals may permit development of resistance.

MISCELLANEOUS

AGE-RELATED FACTORS
Young animals are more resistant to infection.

ZOONOTIC POTENTIAL
N/A

PREGNANCY
Heartwater has been associated infrequently with abortion in infected animals.

BIOSECURITY
Heartwater is a foreign animal disease in the United States. Contact appropriate animal health officials (e.g., USDA—APHIS Veterinary Services http://www.aphis.usda.gov/vs) for suspected cases.

PRODUCTION MANAGEMENT
N/A

SYNONYMS
• Cowdriosis
• Hidrocarditis Infecciosa
• Idropericardite dei Ruminanti
• Malkopsiekte
• Péricardite Exsudative Infectieuse

ABBREVIATIONS
• APHIS = Animal and Plant Health Inspection Service
• ELISA = enzyme-linked immunosorbent assay
• IM = intramuscular
• LAMP = loop-mediated isothermal amplification
• PCR = polymerase chain reaction
• USDA = United States Department of Agriculture

SEE ALSO
• Anthrax
• Babesiosis
• Grass Tetany/Hypomagnesemia
• Ketosis: Dairy Cattle
• Lead Toxicosis
• Lightning Strike
• Listeriosis
• Rabies
• Sodium Disorders: Hypernatremia
• Trypanosomiasis
• Vitamin B Deficiency

Suggested Reading
Heartwater. 2015. The Center for Food Security & Public Health, Iowa State University, accessed July 26, 2016. http://www.cfsph.iastate.edu/Factsheets/pdfs/heartwater.pdf
Mebus CA, Logan LL. Heartwater disease of domestic and wild ruminants. J Am Vet Med Assoc 1988, 192: 395–8.
Peter TF, Burridge MJ, Mahan SM. 2002. *Ehrlichia ruminantium* infection (heartwater) in wild animals. Trends Parasitol 2002, 18: 214–18.
Radostits OM, Gay CC, Blood DC, Hinchcliff KW. Veterinary Medicine, 10th ed. New York: Saunders, 2007, pp. 1462–4.
Shakespeare AS. Overview of heartwater. In: The Merck Veterinary Manual Online, 2014. Accessed July 26, 2016, http://www.merckvetmanual.com/mvm/generalized_conditions/heartwater/overview_of_heartwater.html
Wagner GG, Holman P, Waghela S. Babesiosis and heartwater: threats without boundaries. Vet Clin North Am Food Anim Pract 2002, 18: 417–30.
Author Munashe Chigerwe
Consulting Editor Christopher C.L. Chase

H

HEAT STRESS

BASICS

OVERVIEW
- Disease syndrome in ruminants secondary to exposure to conditions of excessively high ambient temperature or combinations of high ambient temperature and high humidity.
- The thermoneutral zone for cattle is between 41°F (5°C) and 77°F (25°C).
- The temperature humidity index is a good tool to determine risk. A THI ≥72 indicates some degree of risk.

INCIDENCE/PREVALENCE
N/A

GEOGRAPHIC DISTRIBUTION
Heat stress can occur in any part of the world where ambient temperature rises above 75°F (24°C), particularly with high humidity.

SYSTEMS AFFECTED
- Multisystemic

PATHOPHYSIOLOGY
- The preoptic area of the anterior hypothalamus receives and processes information from thermosensors throughout the body.
- Hyperthermia arises from thermoregulatory malfunction. In cases of heat stress, malfunction arises due to an elevated thermal burden that the body is incapable of handling.

HISTORICAL FINDINGS
Temperature rises above 75°F (24°C), particularly with high humidity ± increased stress

SIGNALMENT
Potentially all ruminant species. Disease is more severe in heavily fleeced animals.

PHYSICAL EXAMINATION FINDINGS
- Signs may vary due to the severity of the disease.
- Decreased fertility, decreased signs of estrus in females, increased number of abnormal spermatozoa in males, depressed libido in males, early embryonic death if early in gestation.
- Dullness, lethargy, increased respiratory and heart rates, open mouth breathing may all occur.
- Congested conjunctiva as well as pupil dilation or constriction depending on severity of disease may be present.
- Weak pulses and electrolyte and acid-base disturbances may occur as the disease progresses.

GENETICS
N/A

CAUSES AND RISK FACTORS
- Breakdown of thermoregulatory function due to exposure to periods of high heat ± high humidity

- Environmental factors
  - Temperature
  - Humidity
  - Air movement
  - High nighttime ambient temperatures
- Animal factors
  - Dehydration
  - Exercise
  - Dark coat color
  - Heavy fiber in sheep and fiber goats
  - Obesity
  - Stage of production—pregnant and lactating are at greater risk
  - Age—old and young are at greater risk
  - Current or recent illness
- Nutritional factors
  - Excess dietary protein—removing excess nitrogen requires energy and generates heat
  - Poor-quality hay—increases the heat of digestion
  - Selenium-deficient diets
  - Vitamin- and mineral-deficient diets
  - Salt-deficient diets
- Management factors
  - Availability of fresh drinking water—water consumption increases with ambient temperature.
  - Availability of shade.
  - Availability of cooling water.
  - Timing of stressful activity—early morning before the heat of the day is best. Evening is less preferable as animals are dissipating heat from the day at that time.
  - Timing of feeding—late day feeding will allow for the heat of digestion to be during cooler nighttime hours.

DIAGNOSIS

DIFFERENTIAL DIAGNOSES
- Infectious diseases that generate fever
- Pneumonia
- Rumen acidosis
- GI causes of colic
- Abomasal ulcers

CBC/BIOCHEMISTRY/URINALYSIS
- CBC often shows a mature neutrophilia with no left shift, platelet count may decrease with time.
- Biochemistry—abnormalities vary depending on organ systems involved. Increases can be seen in creatinine, urea nitrogen, AST, CK, bilirubin, and SDH. Hypoproteinemia may be present. Electrolytes (Na and Cl) may be decreased. Whole body potassium is often decreased, but serum levels may be increased in the presence of acidemia. Metabolic and respiratory acidosis also may be present.
- Urinalysis—initially increased specific gravity that may become isosthenuric if renal failure ensues, tubular casts may be present in individuals with severe disease, positive blood and protein also may be present.

OTHER LABORATORY TESTS
Clotting profiles—clotting times may be increased.

IMAGING
N/A

OTHER DIAGNOSTIC PROCEDURES
CSF—used to rule out other causes of neurologic disease

PATHOLOGIC FINDINGS
- Gross postmortem
  - Autolysis beyond what is expected for time of death
  - Hemorrhages and other signs consistent with DIC
  - Serous atrophy of fat
- Histologic changes
  - Renal necrosis
  - Hepatic necrosis
  - Coagulation necrosis of neurons
  - Vascular congestion in the lungs, liver, spleen, and myocardium

TREATMENT

THERAPEUTIC APPROACH
- Cooling to within a normal rectal temperature—care should be taken as affected animals may lack the ability to warm themselves if overcooled. Intact fleece in sheep will help insulate the animal even when wet, so cooling water must soak through to the skin.
- IV fluids—correction of dehydration, electrolyte disturbances, and acidosis. Intranasal oxygen therapy if indicated.
- Shearing (sheep)—if not already shorn, will increase area for heat loss.
- Limit activity as muscle activity increases heat production.

MEDICATIONS

DRUGS OF CHOICE
- Anti-inflammatory agents
  - Steroids—for shock
  - Dexamethasone—0.05–0.1 mg/kg, IV or SC, q48h for 2 treatments
  - Prednisolone sodium succinate—0.5–1.0 mg/kg IV or SC, q12–24h
  - Nonsteroidal anti-inflammatory agents—flunixin meglumine 1.1 mg/kg or meloxicam (0.5 mg/kg SC, IV, or PO). NSAIDs should be used cautiously as many heat-stressed animals may have severe renal compromise at presentation.
- Antimicrobial agents—for prevention of secondary infection. May not be necessary in all cases.
  - Oxytetracycline 200 mg/mL—18 mg/kg SC q72h. Use with caution in animals with renal compromise.

○ Ampicillin trihydrate—11 mg/kg IM q24h. Sodium ampicillin can be used q8h at the same dose.
○ Penicillin—22,000 IU/kg IM or SC q12h. Potassium penicillin can be used IV q6h at the same dose.
• Antioxidant agents
○ Vitamin E—immediate antioxidant activity: 1 mL/100 lb or 45 kg SC or IM (300 IU/mL)
○ Selenium—antioxidant activity will take 7–10 days for effect: Bo-Se® (1 mg/mL selenium and 50 mg/mL vitamin E)— 1 mL/50 lb; or 22 kg Mu-Se (5 mg/mL selenium and 50 mg/mL vitamin E)— 1 mL/200 lb or 90 kg.

CONTRAINDICATIONS
NSAIDs should be used with caution because severe renal compromise is often present at presentation.

PRECAUTIONS
Appropriate milk and meat withdrawal times must be followed for all compounds administered to food-producing animals.

POSSIBLE INTERACTIONS
N/A

FOLLOW-UP

EXPECTED COURSE AND PROGNOSIS
• Prognosis varies from good to grave depending on condition at the time of admission.
• Early heat stress with no systemic complications will often resolve with cooling and several days in a cooler environment.
• Individuals with organ failure and other serious manifestations may not survive despite aggressive therapy.

POSSIBLE COMPLICATIONS
• Severely affected animals are more predisposed in the future.
• Infertility:
○ Male—excessive heat is spermicidal to primary spermatocytes.
○ Female—ovarian activity will decrease in times of high heat.
• Pregnancy loss
• Congenital abnormalities in the fetus

PATIENT CARE
• Rectal temperature should be monitored regularly until stabilized, then several times daily.
• Serum biochemistry should initially be monitored depending on severity of disease to assess progress and provide a basis for alteration in fluid therapy.

PREVENTION
• Clients should be educated on risk factors and prevention techniques as well as early recognition of affected animals.
• Adequate access to clean drinking water.
• Adequate access to a mineral and salt supplement.
• Provide shade, fans, and other cooling mechanisms for animals during high heat and humidity.
• Observe animals and institute immediate treatment at signs of trouble.

MISCELLANEOUS

PREGNANCY
• Steroid use during pregnancy may induce abortion.

• Thermal damage to the developing fetus may result in congenital abnormalities, particularly of the CNS.

ABBREVIATIONS
• AST = aspartate aminotransferase
• CK = creatine kinase
• CNS = central nervous system
• CSF = cerebrospinal fluid
• DIC = disseminated intravascular coagulation
• GI = gastrointestinal
• IM = intramuscular
• IV = intravenous
• NSAIDs = nonsteroidal anti-inflammatory drugs
• SC = subcutaneous
• SDH = sorbitol dehydrogenase

SEE ALSO
Camelid: Heat Stress

Suggested Reading
Fidler, AP, Van Devender K. Heat stress in dairy cattle. Publication FSA3040. University of Arkansas Cooperative Extension Service Printing Services, 2014. Available at http://www.uaex.edu/publications/PDF/FSA-3040.pdf
Smith MC, Sherman DM. Goat Medicine, 2nd ed. Ames: Wiley-Blackwell, 2009.
Author Dusty W. Nagy
Consulting Editor Kaitlyn A. Lutz

H

HEAVY METAL TOXICOSIS

 BASICS

OVERVIEW

- The term "heavy metals" has been given a wide range of inconsistent meanings and has not been defined by any authoritative body such as IUPAC.
- Here "heavy metals" describes a group of metals and metalloids (semimetals), specifically arsenic (As), copper (Cu), lead (Pb), molybdenum (Mo), selenium (Se), and zinc (Zn), which have been associated with toxicity in ruminants under natural conditions.
- Toxicity arising from exposure (mostly by ingestion) to heavy metals.
- Injectable products containing minerals have the potential to contribute to toxicosis when not used according to the label.

INCIDENCE/PREVALENCE

- Incidence of heavy metal toxicosis is to some extent influenced by nutrition and other management factors, age, sex, and breed (see "Signalment").
- Arsenic toxicity is now less frequent because of reduced use of As-containing compounds as pesticides.
- Peak incidence of Cu toxicity occurs in the fall and winter while most cases of Pb toxicity are associated with seeding and harvesting activities.

GEOGRAPHIC DISTRIBUTION

- Heavy metal toxicoses can occur virtually anywhere.
- In the United States, Cu toxicosis is more common in western states.
- Mo is naturally high in soils in some US states (Florida, Oregon, California, Utah, Hawaii, Montana, Colorado, and Nevada) and in several areas of other countries around the world.

SYSTEMS AFFECTED

- As—digestive, nervous, respiratory, cardiovascular, multisystemic
- Cu—digestive, hemolymphatic, cardiovascular, multisystemic
- Pb—nervous, digestive, hemolymphatic, musculoskeletal, multisystemic
- Mo—digestive, hemolymphatic, musculoskeletal, nervous, cardiovascular, integument
- Se—integument, musculoskeletal, cardiovascular
- Zn—hemolymphatic, digestive, multisystemic

PATHOPHYSIOLOGY

- Arsenic (As)—exists in trivalent and pentavalent forms. Trivalent arsenicals bind to sulfhydryl (−SH) groups, leading to inactivation of enzymes and enzyme cofactors including those involved in cellular respiration (TCA cycle). They also impair capillary integrity resulting in plasma transudation into the GI tract. Pentavalent arsenicals uncouple oxidative phosphorylation, leading to cellular energy deficits.
- Copper (Cu)—acute exposure causes irritation and coagulative necrosis of GI mucosa. Chronic toxicity occurs when the capacity of the liver to regulate Cu (by sequestration and excretion) is exceeded. Excess Cu undergoes redox cycling (Cu$^+$ ⇔ Cu^{++}) and generates reactive oxygen species that cause membrane lipid peroxidation and necrosis of hepatocytes. Cu is then released from necrotic hepatocytes to blood circulation and damages RBC, causing intravascular hemolysis and release of hemoglobin. Damage to RBC causes anoxia, more centrilobular hepatic necrosis, and more release of Cu, which accumulates in and damages the kidney. Cu also inactivates proteins and enzymes by binding to −SH groups and may displace other essential trace metals (e.g., Zn) from their proteins.
- Lead (Pb)—binds to −SH groups and inactivates several enzymes including those involved in heme synthesis, impairs nerve and muscle transmission by competing with calcium (Ca), displaces Ca in bone and Ca-binding proteins (e.g., calmodulin), impairs membrane-bound enzymes (e.g., Na$^+$,K$^+$-ATPase) leading to RBC fragility and renal tubular injury, impairs vitamin D metabolism, and interferes with GABA production and activity in the CNS. Pb is also irritating (GI mucus membrane), toxic to germ cells (gametes), teratogenic, and immunosuppressive.
- Molybdenum (Mo)—interferes with Cu metabolism leading to Cu deficiency—Mo and sulfur (S) form insoluble thiomolybdates in the rumen, which bind and reduce absorption of Cu—and stimulate urinary loss of Cu. Some thiomolybdates increase hepatobiliary excretion of Cu, decrease blood Cu availability, and directly inhibit Cu-dependent enzymes. Mo may also alter Zn metabolism and impair myelin maintenance and function, leading to enzootic ataxia in lambs.
- Selenium (Se)—acts as an antioxidant, especially in conjunction with vitamin E. Necessary for glutathione peroxidase formation. Glutathione peroxidase catalyzes the reduction of hydrogen peroxide and lipid hydroperoxides, preventing oxidative damage to body tissues. A second selenium dependence enzyme is iodothyronine 5′-deiodinase. This enzyme catalyzes the deiodination of thyroxine (T4) to the more metabolically active triiodothyronine (T3) in tissues. Acute toxicity is associated with myocardial and secondary liver pathology. Chronic toxicity affects hooves and hair.
- Zinc (Zn)—exact pathophysiology of Zn toxicity in ruminants is unknown. However, Zn irritates the GI tract; antagonizes Ca, Cu, and iron (Fe) metabolism; and injures the pancreas and pancreatic ducts.

SIGNALMENT

- All ruminants are susceptible to heavy metal toxicosis.
- Sheep are very sensitive to Cu, while Pb most commonly poisons cattle.
- Ruminants are more sensitive than nonruminants to Mo.
- As, Pb, and Zn toxicities have no breed predilections.
- Cu—British breeds of sheep (e.g., Suffolk, Oxford, and Shropshire), Texel sheep, and Jersey cattle are more susceptible.
- Mo—Scottish Blackface and Finnish Landrace sheep are apparently more prone to develop swayback.
- Young and old animals are more susceptible to heavy metal toxicosis.

PHYSICAL EXAMINATION FINDINGS

- As—abdominal pain, weakness, staggering, ataxia, watery diarrhea, ruminal atony, weak rapid pulse and shock, oliguria, proteinuria, dehydration, uremia, and acidosis.
- Cu—*acute toxicity:* vomiting, anorexia, hypersalivation, abdominal pain, greenish diarrhea, dehydration, shock, collapse, and death. *Chronic:* sudden onset of hemolytic crisis with weakness, anorexia, thirst, depression, hyperventilation, trembling, anemia, hemoglobinemia, methemaglobinemia, hemoglobinuria (port wine urine), icterus, dyspnea, and death.
- Pb—depression, hyperesthesia, muscle tremors, convulsions, blindness, ataxia, seizures, incoordination, aggression, head pressing, spastic twitching of eyelids, bloat, tenesmus, diarrhea, teeth grinding, jaw champing, and death.
- Mo—sudden death, anorexia, severe diarrhea with gas bubbles, emaciation, reduced growth, anemia, lameness, ataxia, swayback in lambs, recumbency, protrusion of nictitating membrane, blindness, achromotrichia (depigmentation of hair/wool), rough hair coat, alopecia, deformity of limbs, muscular degeneration, decreased milk production, and decreased reproductive performance.
- Se—acute toxicosis causes anorexia, depression, abnormal posture, diarrhea, colic, increased pulse and respiration, frothy nasal discharge, moist rales, respiratory difficulty, weakness, dyspnea, garlicky odor to the breath, and sudden death in calves. Myocardial and hepatic pathology may be observed. Chronic toxicosis causes hoof deformation, hair loss, discoloration and general roughness of the coat.
- Zn—green-colored diarrhea, dehydration, anemia, jaundice, weakness, paresis, anorexia, reduced weight gain, decreased milk yield, subcutaneous edema, polydipsia, polyuria, polyphagia, depression, listlessness, chemosis, exophthalmia, convulsions, and death.

CAUSES AND RISK FACTORS

• As—grazing in areas around As mining and smelting sites, exposure to herbicides or old pesticides that have been improperly discarded or stored.

• Cu—excessive administration of Cu formulations or ingestion of improperly formulated rations, feeding sheep feeds formulated for other animals, consumption of vegetation or water contaminated with Cu (e.g., near mining/smelting operations or pastures amended with poultry or swine manure), consumption of forage/feeds low in Mo and S and grazing animals in areas containing hepatotoxic plants (e.g., plants containing pyrrolizidine alkaloids). Chronic toxicity is precipitated by stress (e.g., shipping, bad weather, deteriorating plane of nutrition, or lactation).

• Pb—consumption of forages contaminated by airborne emissions near Pb smelters or along roadsides, consumption of contaminated water or feed from Pb-lined pipes and drinking/feeding utensils, ingestion of Pb-containing products (automotive batteries, farm machinery grease or oil, paints, putties, and pesticides). In cattle, many cases are associated with seeding and harvesting activities when used oil and batteries are likely to be improperly disposed. Toxicity is exacerbated in animals deficient in Ca, Zn, iron (Fe), and vitamin D. The restricted use of leaded gasoline and oils has significantly reduced environmental Pb contamination.

• Mo—consumption of contaminated pastures (near mining or metal production plants) or forage grown with heavy application molybdic or phosphate fertilizers and lime. Low dietary Cu and high dietary S exacerbate the toxicity. High soil pH increases Mo absorption and decreases Cu absorption.

• Se—the only metal regulated by the Food and Drug Administration because of the low safety margin in feed. Only 0.3 ppm Se is allowed to be supplemented in the total diet. Injectable Se products may cause toxicosis if label directions are not followed. If two different types of injectable Se products are used there may be an overdose. Selenium-accumulating plants may also contribute to chronic selenium toxicosis. Elevated concentrations of organic or chelated Se sources may contribute to toxicosis. Injection of selenium at 0.2–0.5 mg/kg in young cattle and 1 mg/kg in mature cattle will cause acute toxicosis. Diets >50 ppm will cause acute toxicosis. Chronic toxicosis is observed when dietary concentration of Se is >20–50 ppm for >3 days.

• Zn—consumption of improperly formulated diets or zinc-contaminated forage (e.g., near galvanizing factories and mines), access to substances containing Zn, and careless use of Zn sulfate as a prophylactic and treatment of diseases (e.g., ovine foot rot, facial eczema, and lupinosis).

DIAGNOSIS

DIFFERENTIAL DIAGNOSES

• As—Pb toxicity, insecticide poisoning, selenium (Se) toxicity, Mo toxicity, Cu toxicity, bovine viral diarrhea.

• Cu—infectious gastroenteritis, leptospirosis, arsenic or selenium toxicoses, phenothiazine and other anthelmintic poisonings, bacillary hemoglobinuria, nitrate/nitrite poisoning, postparturient hemoglobinuria, babesiosis, *Corynebacterium renale* infection.

• Pb—other diseases with nervous signs including rabies, PEM, TEME, listeriosis, ammoniated feed toxicosis, hepatic encephalopathy, nervous coccidiosis, tetanus, hypovitaminosis A, thiamine deficiency, sodium (Na) ion toxicity, hypomagnesemic tetany, nervous acetonemia, As poisoning, brain abscess or neoplasia, *Haemophilus* meningoencephalitis.

• Se—acute toxicosis has to be differentiated from acute Se deficiency, anaphylaxis, ionophores, Japanese yew, gossypol, organophosphates and carbamates.

• Mo—primary Cu deficiency, enzootic ataxia, infectious gastroenteritis, internal parasitisms, leptospirosis, anthelmintic poisoning, As toxicosis, Se toxicosis.

• Zn—other causes of diarrhea or anemia, such as acute autoimmune hemolytic anemia.

CBC/BIOCHEMISTRY/URINALYSIS

• As—elevated hematocrit, BUN and urine specific gravity, and proteinuria.

• Cu—hemoglobinemia, methemoglobinemia, reduced blood glutathione, reduced PCV, increased WBC, AST, LDH, AP, GGT, SDH, and bilirubin.

• Pb—microcytic hypochromic to normocytic normochromic anemia, basophilic stippling, high nucleated RBC counts, mature leukocytosis, decreased myeloid/erythroid ratio, increased RBC fragility leading to anisocytosis, polychromasia, echinocytosis, poikilocytosis, and target cells. Also urinary ALA levels are elevated; RBC ALAD and porphyrin levels are reduced and elevated, respectively.

• Mo—microcytic hypochromic anemia, elevated AST, GGT, GDH, CK, SDH, bilirubin, creatinine, and Ca, and increased or decreased BUN (depending on the stage of the toxicosis).

• Se—with chronic Se toxicosis there may be increased PT, PTT, fibrinogen, GTH, ALT, AST, and ALP.

• Zn—anemia, neutrophilia, immature RBCs, uremia, reduced erythrocyte ALAD, elevated blood Na, glucose, LDH, GGT, AP, and SDH.

OTHER LABORATORY TESTS

• As—analyze for As concentration in liver, kidney, urine, GI contents, feces, and in suspected feeds.

• Cu—analyze for Cu concentration in serum, liver, kidneys, and in suspected feed.

• Pb—analyze for Pb concentration in whole blood (>0.6 ppm is diagnostic), kidney, and liver as well as urinary ALA.

• Mo—determine Mo concentration in blood, liver, and kidney. Blood levels that result in toxicity depend on dietary intake of Cu and S. Quantify Mo and Cu in feeds and forage.

• Se—analyze for Mn concentration in serum, whole blood or liver. Whole blood will reflect what the diet has been for the last 30 days.

• Zn—analyze for Zn concentration in serum and tissues (e.g., kidney, liver, pancreas) and urine. Special royal-blue top tubes are recommended for blood collection to avoid contamination.

PATHOLOGIC FINDINGS

• As—abomasum and intestines show redness and congestion of mucosa, submucosal edema, and epithelial necrosis.

• Cu—acute toxicity results in severe gastroenteritis with hemorrhage, edema, erosions, and ulcerations in the abomasum, faint-blue color of GI contents, generalized icterus, and swollen friable livers. In chronic toxicity, livers appear yellowish, swollen, and friable; kidneys are dark-red or bluish-black (gunmetal blue kidneys); and gall bladders are distended with greenish bile. Histopathology reveals centrilobular coagulative necrosis with fibrosis of portal areas and lymphocytic inflammation in liver, proliferation and apoptosis of bile ducts with bile stasis, necrosis of renal tubular and glomerular cells and hemoglobin in renal tubules, brown-black and enlarged spleen with numerous fragmented RBCs, and status spongiosus in the CNS white matter.

• Pb—emaciation, muscle wasting, and degenerative changes in the nervous system and kidney. Histopathology reveals laminar cortical cerebral necrosis, necrosis of renal tubules with high numbers of mitotic figures, and osteoporosis.

• Mo—emaciation, coarse and poorly pigmented hair/wool, osteoporosis and fractures, swollen friable livers, and swollen kidneys with perirenal edema. Histopathology shows hydropic hepatocellular degeneration and periacinar hemorrhagic necrosis, hydropic renal degeneration with tubular necrosis, lysis of cerebral white matter, and demyelination and degeneration of motor tracts in the spinal

H

H

cord and neurons (in lambs with swayback).
• Se—acute myocardial and/or secondary hepatic necrosis. Acute toxicosis causes pulmonary edema, pulmonary congestion, pulmonary hemorrhage, hepatic necrosis, myocardial necrosis, myocardial hemorrhage, and renal necrosis. Chronic toxicosis may cause hoof abnormalities, degeneration of the joint cartilage and bone, and reduced fertility.
• Zn—poor body condition, abomasitis and duodenitis with greenish mucosa, submucosal edema in the rumen and abomasum, catarrhal enteritis and congestion of small intestines, subcutaneous edema, hydrothorax, hydropericardium, and pancreatic atrophy. Cattle also show pulmonary emphysema, pale flabby myocardium, severe hepatic degeneration, and lesions in the pancreas. Histopathology reveals fibrosing pancreatitis, renal glomerular and tubular lesions, multifocal granulomas in the liver, and proliferation of neck cells of gastric glands.

TREATMENT

THERAPEUTIC APPROACH
Stabilize the patient, eliminate source of heavy metal, decontaminate (e.g., by physical removal through rumenotomy, washing off topically or by administration of cathartics), administer antidote (chelation therapy), enhance elimination, and provide symptomatic and supportive care.

MEDICATIONS

DRUGS OF CHOICE
• As—dimercaprol (BAL) 3 mg/kg IM q8h (before clinical signs) or 6 mg/kg IM q8h (after onset of clinical signs) for 3–5 days; sodium thiosulfate (30–60 g PO q6h for 3–4 days).
• Cu—ammonium molybdate (50–500 mg PO q24h per head) and sodium thiosulfate (300–1000 mg PO q24h per head) for 3 weeks (an aqueous mixture of the two salts can be sprayed on the feed to reduce labor); three treatments of ammonium tetrathiomolybdate (sheep, 1.7–3.4 mg/head IV or SC) on alternate days; D-penicillamine (52 mg/kg/day PO for 6 days), but it is expensive for treating on a flock basis.
• Pb—diazepam (0.55–1.5 mg/kg IM) for seizures; Ca-EDTA (73.3 mg/kg slow IV, divided q24h or q8h) for 3–5 days; BAL (3–6 mg/kg IM q8h for 3–5 days). Thiamine 250–1000 mg q12h is a useful adjunct to Ca-EDTA.

• Mo—copper glycinate (60 mg/calf and 120 mg/adult cattle SC); 1000 mg copper sulfate per adult cow; copper sulfate (1–5% depending on Mo levels in the feed) in salt-mineral mix.
• Se—primarily supportive therapy. Adding arsenic-containing compounds may be helpful in chronic toxicosis. Feeding rations containing 50–100 ppm of arsanilic acid may be helpful for calves. This may accelerate the excretion of Se.
• Zn—chelation therapy with Ca-EDTA as for Pb and supplementation of ration with Cu.

CONTRAINDICATIONS
• Ca-EDTA and BAL—use with extreme caution and adjust dose in patients with impaired renal function.
• Ca-EDTA and BAL should not be used in patients with anuria and impaired liver function, respectively.
• Exercise extra caution when using Cu compounds in sheep (very sensitive to Cu).
• Appropriate milk and meat withdrawal times must be followed for all compounds administered to food-producing animals.

POSSIBLE INTERACTIONS
• Ca-EDTA—use with caution with nephrotoxic drugs (e.g., aminoglycosides) and glucocorticoids.
• BAL—do not administer with Fe and Se salts (forms toxic complexes).
• Chelation therapy can cause depletion of essential minerals (e.g., Zn and Fe).

FOLLOW-UP

EXPECTED COURSE AND PROGNOSIS
• Generally favorable in animals with mild to moderate signs provided that the source of the heavy metal can be identified and removed from the animal's environment.
• Guarded to poor in animals with severe signs (e.g., hemolytic crisis, severe CNS signs).

PREVENTION
Prevent access to sources of heavy metals and ensure correct mineral nutrition and proper pasture management.

MISCELLANEOUS

ASSOCIATED CONDITIONS
As and Pb toxicities—none; Cu toxicity—Zn deficiency, possibly Mo deficiency; Mo and Zn toxicities—Cu deficiency

ZOONOTIC POTENTIAL
• None. However, organ meat may contain levels of heavy metals that pose a risk to humans (e.g., livers containing >500 mg/kg Cu are considered a risk to public health).
• Lead and Mo are secreted in milk and can present a risk to humans.

PREGNANCY
• Pb crosses placental barrier and is secreted in milk and thus can cause fetal and neonatal poisoning.
• Zn exposure in ewes can cause fetal and/or neonatal Cu deficiency.
• Pregnant ruminants are more susceptible to Zn toxicity.

PRODUCTION MANAGEMENT
• Nutrition—Ca, Zn, S, Fe, and vitamin D supplementation can reduce incidence of heavy metal toxicity. For example, the maintenance of correct Cu-to-Mo-to-S ratio in feeds is imperative to reduce incidence of Mo toxicity.
• Pasture management—use of some fertilizers may induce mineral imbalances in forage, hepatotoxic plants increase toxicity of Cu, and some plants may reduce bioavailability of essential heavy metals such as Cu.
• Cu : Zn ratio in the feed should be 1:4, Cu : Mn ratio in the feed should be 2:1.

SYNONYMS
As toxicity—arsenic toxicosis. Other names for As-containing compounds include arsenicals, arsenites, arsenates, arsine
Cu toxicity—enzootic icterus of sheep, copper toxicosis, copper poisoning, copper sulfate poisoning
Pb toxicity—plumbism, saturnism, lead intoxication, lead poisoning, lead toxicosis
Mo toxicity—molybdenosis, molybdenum toxicosis, teart disease, peat scours
Zn toxicity—zinc poisoning, new wire disease (in birds), zincalism (in humans)

ABBREVIATIONS
• ALA = δ-aminolevulinic acid
• ALAD = δ-aminolevulinic acid dehydratase
• AP = alkaline phosphatase
• AST = aspartate aminotransferase
• BAL = British anti-Lewisite
• CK = creatinine kinase
• EDTA = ethylenediaminetetraacetic acid
• GABA = gamma aminobutyric acid
• GDH = glutamate dehydrogenase
• GGT = gamma-glutamyl transferase
• GI = gastrointestinal
• IM = intramuscular
• IUPAC = International Union of Pure and Applied Chemistry
• LDH = lactate dehydrogenase

- Na^+, K^+-ATPase = sodium, potassium adenosine triphosphatase (sodium pump)
- PCV = packed cell volume
- PEM = polioencephalomalacia
- PO = per os (by mouth)
- SDH = sorbitol dehydrogenase
- RBC = red blood cell
- TCA = tricarboxylic cycle (Krebs cycle)
- TEME = thromboembolic meningoencephalitis
- WBC = white blood cell

SEE ALSO
See "Differential Diagnoses"

Suggested Reading
Beasley VR, Dorman DC, Fikes JD, Diana SG, Woshner V. A Systems Affected Approach to Veterinary Toxicology. Urbana: University of Illinois, 1999.
Duffus JH. "Heavy metals"—a meaningless term. Chemistry International 2001, 23(6).
Plumlee KH. Clinical Veterinary Toxicology. St. Louis: Mosby, 2004.

Author Steve Ensley
Consulting Editor Christopher C.L. Chase
Acknowledgment The author and book editors acknowledge the prior contribution of Collins N. Kamunde.

H

HEMORRHAGIC BOWEL SYNDROME

BASICS

OVERVIEW
• Hemorrhagic bowel syndrome (HBS) is a disease condition thought to be caused by *Clostridium perfringens* type A (or possibly other agents) and which leads to a necrohemorrhagic enteritis of one or more intestinal segments (usually jejunum).
• This condition can cause passage of very bloody diarrhea with blood clots in the feces or can cause an obstructive-type syndrome with production of scant or no manure and signs of colic.

INCIDENCE/PREVALENCE
• Sporadic, but occasionally occurs as an outbreak affecting up to 10% of a herd.
• Higher-producing herds have higher prevalence.
• Herds with higher rolling herd averages have higher prevalence.

GEOGRAPHIC DISTRIBUTION
• Worldwide
• Western states in the United States have a higher prevalence

SYSTEMS AFFECTED
• Digestive
• Cardiovascular
• Hemolymphatic

PATHOPHYSIOLOGY
The exact pathogenesis has not been established and attempts to replicate the disease in studies using specific pathogenic agents have not been successful. Postulated pathophysiologic mechanisms include the following:
• *C. perfringens* type A organisms are ubiquitous in environment but proliferate rapidly in the intestines under conditions of high carbohydrate or protein digestion, and liberate exotoxins that potentially play a pivotal role in disease.
• Hemorrhage occurs into the intestinal wall and lumen. Blood acts as a substrate for further proliferation of clostridial organisms.
• The fungus *A. fumigatus* has been proposed to incite tissue damage and releases immunosuppressive mycotoxins which can promote more rapid proliferation.
• Segmental intestinal necrosis develops in affected locations. Devitalized bowel provides a good environment for further proliferation of anaerobic bacteria and provokes the onset of peritonitis and shock.
• Intraluminal blood clots can act as an intraluminal foreign body, causing obstruction; hemorrhage can be severe enough to cause anemia and shock.
• Associated ileus also contributes to physiologic GI obstruction; fluid and gas distension of the bowel creates colic and potentially hypochloremic metabolic alkalosis.

HISTORICAL FINDINGS
Sudden decline in milk production with anorexia and diarrhea with clotted blood, progressing to scant or absent fecal passage in early lactation dairy cattle is a common complaint.

PHYSICAL EXAMINATION FINDINGS
• Thick, viscous, dark, tarry feces.
• Decreased to absent ruminations.
• Signs of hypovolemic and/or septic shock:
  ○ Tachycardia
  ○ Weak pulse
  ○ Dehydration
  ○ Pale/congested mucus membranes
  ○ Cold extremities
• Right abdominal distension ("papple" shaped).
• Succussable fluid in the right ventral abdomen.
• Colic.
• Intestinal distension on per rectum palpation. Per rectum examination may rarely identify an intestinal mass.
• Clinical signs generally worsen with duration of disease. Sudden death is also possible.

SIGNALMENT
• Usually affects dairy cows in second or higher lactation and within the first 100 days in milk.
• Brown Swiss cattle may be predisposed.
• Occasionally affects beef cows and bulls.

GENETICS
N/A

CAUSES AND RISK FACTORS
• Likely a multifactorial disorder arising from a combination of management factors (nutrition) and pathogen interaction.
• *Clostridium perfringens* type A is most commonly implicated, and the β2 toxin of this organism has been implicated. However, *C. perfringens* type A can be isolated from unaffected cows, and studies inoculating healthy cows with *C. perfringens* type A have failed to reproduce the syndrome.
• *Aspergillus fumigatus* has been hypothesized to play a role in some studies.
• A more recently proposed hypothesis is the combination of mycotoxic fungi in association with Shiga toxin–producing *E. coli*.
• Risk factors:
  ○ Brown Swiss cows were predisposed, in one study
  ○ High milk production
  ○ Early lactation: first 100 days in milk
  ○ Larger dairy herds (>100 cows)
  ○ Older cows (median parity = third lactation)
  ○ Dairies with higher rolling herd averages
  ○ Dietary risk factors are significant and include high energy and low fiber diets and feeding a total mixed ration.

DIAGNOSIS

DIFFERENTIAL DIAGNOSES
• Intussusception
• Intestinal incarceration
• Intestinal volvulus
• Salmonellosis
• Coccidiosis
• Winter dysentery
• Abomasal ulceration
• Vagal indigestion

CBC/BIOCHEMSTRY/URINALYSIS
• Mild inflammatory leukogram is common.
• Hematocrit can be normal early in the course of the disease or anemia can be apparent due to blood loss. As disease progresses the hematocrit may normalize as a result of combined anemia and hypovolemia.
• Hypochloremic, hyopokalemic, metabolic alkalosis can occur with proximal intestinal obstruction.

OTHER LABORATORY TESTS
N/A

IMAGING
Abdominal ultrasound (transabdominal or transrectal) can reveal small intestinal distension with hypomotility. Intraluminal blood clots may be apparent. The intestinal wall of devitalized segments can appear thickened and hyperechoic.

OTHER DIAGNOSTIC PROCEDURES
• Abdominocentesis—increased total nucleated cell count, total protein and lactate concentration combined with low glucose concentration of the peritoneal fluid suggests devitalization and secondary septic peritonitis.
• Exploratory laparotomy.

PATHOLOGIC FINDINGS
• Segmental necrohemorrhagic enteritis is apparent. The jejunum is most commonly affected but the ileum and duodenum can also be affected.
• Intramural hematomas and intraluminal blood clots.
• Mucosal ulceration and necrosis.
• Submucosal hemorrhage and edema.
• Neutrophilic infiltration.
• Fibrinous covering on serosal surfaces.
• Peritoneal effusion.

TREATMENT

THERAPEUTIC APPROACH
• Affected cows require supportive medical care with appropriate fluid treatment (preferably IV) to restore circulating volume and to reverse electrolyte and acid-base imbalances.

(CONTINUED)

HEMORRHAGIC BOWEL SYNDROME

• A combination of surgical and medical therapy is generally regarded as optimal; however, the prognosis is typically poor, regardless (<50% survival expected).

SURGICAL CONSIDERATIONS AND TECHNIQUES

• Right flank exploratory laparotomy is indicated.
  ◦ The lesion can usually be palpated but may be difficult to exteriorize.
  ◦ Affected bowel loops feel distended and turgid. If visualized, they may appear dark, congested, and necrotic.
• Extraluminal massage of affected segments allows fragmentation of intraluminal blood clots and is preferred if possible.
• Enterotomy can be performed to remove intraluminal hematomas, and resection and anastomosis of necrotic bowel segments might be necessary; both are associated with worse prognosis compared to extraluminal massage.

MEDICATIONS

DRUGS OF CHOICE

• Antimicrobial drugs are indicated, such as procaine penicillin G.
• NSAIDs, such as flunixin and ketoprofen, provide analgesia and anti-inflammatory effects.
• Prokinetic agents such as metoclopramide may help restore GI motility after surgery.
• Laxatives.
• Whole blood transfusion is indicated for cattle with severe anemia or signs of hemorrhagic shock.

CONTRAINDICATIONS

Prokinetic agents should not be given to animals with suspected GI obstruction.

PRECAUTIONS

Appropriate milk and meat withdrawal times must be followed for all compounds administered to food-producing animals.

POSSIBLE INTERACTIONS

N/A

FOLLOW-UP

EXPECTED COURSE AND PROGNOSIS

• The prognosis is guarded to poor with reported mortality rates varying from 55% to 100%.

• Recurrence is possible in cows that recover from clinical disease.
• Cows that undergo enterotomy or enterectomy have a worse prognosis than cows undergoing extraluminal massage of affected bowel segments.
• Cows undergoing surgical intervention may need to be reoperated if they fail to improve postoperatively.

POSSIBLE COMPLICATIONS

• Peritonitis
• Hemorrhagic or septic shock

CLIENT EDUCATION

Educate clients to closely monitor the most vulnerable group (high-producing mature cows in second or higher lactation and the first 100 days of milk).

PATIENT CARE

Transfaunation or supplemental nutrition may be required for cows with prolonged anorexia.

PREVENTION

• Improve feed management
• Increase fiber content in feed
• Administer *C. perfringens* type A toxoid (vaccine) to adult cows
• Addition of mycotoxin binding agents or probiotics to the ration

MISCELLANEOUS

ASSOCIATED CONDITIONS

Peritonitis

AGE-RELATED FACTORS

Older cows are predisposed: median parity of affected cows is third lactation.

ZOONOTIC POTENTIAL

None

PREGNANCY

N/A

BIOSECURITY

Not usually regarded as a contagious disorder

PRODUCTION MANAGEMENT

Although this is usually a sporadic disorder, economic losses can be severe due to reduced milk production, treatment and surgical expenses, and mortality.

SYNONYMS

• Jejunal hemorrhage syndrome
• Bloody gut
• Dead gut
• Hemorrhagic enteritis

ABBREVIATIONS

• GI = gastrointestinal
• HBS = hemorrhagic bowel syndrome
• NSAIDs = nonsteroidal anti-inflammatory drugs

SEE ALSO

Colic: Bovine

Suggested Reading

Dennison AC, VanMetre DC, Callan RJ, et al. Hemorrhagic bowel syndrome in dairy cattle: 22 cases (1997–2000). J Am Vet Med Assoc 2002, 221: 686–9.

Ewoldt JM, Anderson DE. Determination of the effect of single abomasal or jejunal inoculation of *Clostridium perfringens* type A in dairy cows. Can Vet J 2005, 46: 821–4.

Francoz D, Guard, CL. Obstructive intestinal diseases. In: Smith BP ed, Large Animal Internal Medicine, 5th ed. St. Louis: Elsevier, 2015, pp. 823–4.

Juhala P, Pyörälä S, Heinonen M. Hemorrhagic jejunitis in dairy cows: literature review with two case reports. Suomen Eläinlääkärilehti 2008, 114: 351–6.

Owaki S, Kawabuchi S, Ikemitsu K, Shono H, Furuoka H. Pathological findings of hemorrhagic bowel syndrome (HBS) in six dairy cattle cases. J Vet Med Sci 2015, 77: 879–81.

Peek SF, Santschi EM, Livesey MA, et al. Surgical findings and outcome for dairy cattle with jejunal hemorrhage syndrome: 31 cases (2000–2007). J Am Vet Med Assoc 2009, 234: 1308–12.

Van Metre DC. Hemorrhagic bowel syndrome. In: Anderson DE, Rings DM eds., Current Veterinary Therapy Food Animal Practice, 5th ed. St. Louis: Saunders, 2009, pp. 55–8.

Author Andrew J. Niehaus
Consulting Editor Erica C. McKenzie

Acknowledgment The author and book editors acknowledge the prior contribution of Kevin Washburn.

H

HEMOTROPIC MYCOPLASMAS (FORMERLY EPERYTHROZOONOSIS)

BASICS

OVERVIEW
• Epierythrocytic parasites (*Candidatus Mycoplasma* spp.) are often considered to be a subclinical disease of cattle, small ruminants, and camelids. However, it can be a significant cause of hemolytic anemia in immunologically naïve, immunosuppressed, or debilitated individuals.
• Current nomenclature recommendations are as follows: *Mycoplasma* (formerly *Eperythrozoon*) *wenyonii* in cattle, *Mycoplasma* (formerly *Eperythrozoon*) *ovis* in sheep, and *Mycoplasma haemolamae* in camelids. Collectively, these are often referred to as the hemoplasmas.

INCIDENCE/PREVALENCE
The disease is often subclinical, and widely used diagnostic methods (examination of blood smears or serology) are not sensitive enough to detect latent infection. Thus, it is difficult to actually determine the prevalence of the disease. The use of a recently developed and highly sensitive PCR assay has thus far detected latent infection in approximately 20% of New World camelids in the United States, Canada, and Australia. Recently, *Mycoplasma wenyonii* was found in 89% of cattle in Japan and was associated with lower milk yield.

GEOGRAPHIC DISTRIBUTION
Cases have been reported worldwide

SYSTEMS AFFECTED
• Cardiovascular
• Hemolymphatic
• Integument
• Reproductive

PATHOPHYSIOLOGY
• Hemoplasmas are contractible via inoculation of infected blood. Biting insects are considered vectors, though a specific insect has not been identified as the principal vector. *Mycoplasma wenyonii* has been detected by PCR in lice, flies, and mosquitoes. Transmission may also occur vertically and via blood-contaminated needles or instruments.
• Parasitemia develops within days of inoculation, but the rapid onset of an effective immune response curtails proliferation, halting further progression. Thus, latent infection can be common in endemic herds and the organism often coexists symbiotically within the host without causing clinical signs of anemia.
• The recent development of highly sensitive PCR assays have detected the organism in the blood of otherwise apparently healthy individuals.
• Debilitated, immunosuppressed, or immunologically naïve individuals are susceptible to uncontrolled parasitemia and

clinical signs of disease develop. The organism is found on the surface of erythrocytes, which are primarily removed from the circulation by the mononuclear phagocytes in the spleen and liver.
• Icterus without hemoglobinemia or hemoglobinuria is a cardinal clinical sign. In sheep, intravascular hemolysis may also occur. Anemia develops and, in severe cases, death from hypoxemia may ensue.

SIGNALMENT
• Cattle, small ruminants, camelids, mule deer, elk. Sheep and camelids appear to be most susceptible.
• Any age may be affected but younger immunosuppressed or immunologically naïve ruminants may be more susceptible.

HISTORICAL FINDINGS
Concurrent illness, progressive depression, weakness and lethargy, poor growth or chronic weight loss, poor coat quality, anorexia, and icterus.

PHYSICAL EXAMINATION FINDINGS
• Hemoplasmas rarely cause clinical signs of disease and their presence may be a coincidental finding. Severely debilitated or immunosuppressed individuals are more susceptible to clinical hemoplasmosis.
• The signs of the primary disease process that are responsible for immunosuppression often overshadow the clinical signs of hemoplasmosis.
• Clinical signs of disease infrequently occur in cattle and the presence of hemoplasma species may be a coincidental finding in some individuals.
• Immunosuppression from concurrent systemic disease may predispose individuals to hemoplasmosis; however, the primary disease process may conceal the signs of hemoplasmosis.
• Fever, weakness, and recumbency are expected if the condition progresses. In severe cases, tachycardia, tachypnea, pallor of the mucus membranes, lack of episcleral vessels, and icterus develop.
• Although hemolysis is primarily extravascular, intravascular hemolysis can occur in sheep and thus hemoglobinuria may be present.
• In chronic infection, signs of anemia or chronic ill thrift may be present without signs of active hemolysis (e.g., icterus). In cattle, mammary gland or scrotal and/or hindlimb edema, reduced fertility, reduced milk production, and lymphadenopathy may be the predominant signs.

CAUSES AND RISK FACTORS
• Hemoplasmosis is caused by a small (0.5 μm) coccoid prokaryotic organism that lacks a cell wall, is Gram-negative in staining, and cannot be cultivated. Although historically classified as a rickettsial organism, recent studies suggest that it is more closely related to mycoplasma.

• Current nomenclature recommendations are as follows: *Mycoplasma* (formerly *Eperythrozoon*) *wenyonii* in cattle, *Mycoplasma* (formerly *Eperythrozoon*) *ovis* in sheep, and *Mycoplasma haemolamae* in camelids.
• Hemoplasmosis is most commonly considered to be an opportunistic infection that infrequently results in clinical disease, unless an individual is severely immunosuppressed or systemically compromised.

DIAGNOSIS

DIFFERENTIAL DIAGNOSES
• Any cause of extravascular hemolysis in cattle would cause similar signs including anaplasmosis and autoimmune hemolytic anemia.
• The absence of hemoglobinemia and hemoglobinuria distinguishes hemoplasmosis from causes of intravascular hemolysis in cattle.
• With the occasional occurrence of intravascular hemolysis, leptospirosis and copper toxicity should be considered as differential diagnoses in sheep.

CBC/BIOCHEMISTRY/URINALYSIS
• Anemia: Regenerative anemia 5–7 days after onset (signs of regeneration include an increased MCV, anisocytosis, polychromasia, basophilic stippling, reticulocytes, Howell Jolly bodies, nucleated red blood cells); nonregenerative anemia may occur in chronic cases.
• Hemoglobinemia (pink plasma, MCH, and MCHC increased) and/or hemoglobinuria may occur in sheep.
• Hyperbilirubinemia (unconjugated) rarely occurs.
• Hypoglycemia.
• Acidosis.

OTHER LABORATORY TESTS
• Hemoplasma species may be seen in a routine Wright-stained peripheral blood smear on the surface of erythrocytes as a coccoid, rod, or ring-shaped organism. Smears should be made as soon as possible after blood is drawn as the organisms may detach from the red blood cells in vitro.
• Giemsa, Romanowsky, and acridine orange stains are particularly helpful to highlight the organisms. Parasitemia is often low, or affected cells are removed from the circulation by the mononuclear phagocytic system, therefore absence of visible hemoplasma species does not preclude the diagnosis.
• Complement fixation and indirect fluorescent antibody tests are positive within a few days of onset of clinical disease but, in some cases, may remain positive for only a short period of time. Unless paired serology is used, a single positive titer cannot distinguish

between recent infection and previous exposure.

• A PCR test has been developed to detect the organism in camelids and cattle and is more sensitive in detecting the organism than examination of blood smears.

• The evolution of an immune attack directed at the organism on the surface of red blood cells may lead to a positive Coomb's test.

PATHOLOGIC FINDINGS

Splenomegaly, edema, body cavity effusion, and widespread icterus

TREATMENT

THERAPEUTIC APPROACH

• Tetracyclines (see "Medications").

• If anemia is severe and clinical or laboratory evidence of hypoxemia is evident (intense lethargy or weakness, profound tachycardia or tachypnea, severe anemia, acidosis, increased anion gap), a whole blood transfusion is indicated.

• The normal total blood volume is approximately 8% of the body weight (i.e., 0.08 × body weight in kilograms equals the total blood volume in liters). Typically, transfusing one-fourth to one-third of the total blood volume is adequate.

MEDICATIONS

DRUGS OF CHOICE

Tetracycline (10 mg/kg IV q12–24h for 3–5 days in cattle or long-acting oxytetracycline 20 mg/kg SQ q72h for 2–5 treatments in camelids) is effective in controlling acute parasitemia, but it may be less effective in eliminating latency. Tylosin (5 mg/kg IM for 3 days) has also been reported to be effective in cattle.

CONTRAINDICATIONS

Appropriate milk and meat withdrawal times must be followed for all compounds administered to food-producing animals.

FOLLOW-UP

EXPECTED COURSE AND PROGNOSIS

The prognosis is good with treatment.

POSSIBLE COMPLICATIONS

Death from hypoxemia, poor wool quality, reduced fertility, chronic weight loss

PATIENT CARE

• Monitor heart rate, respiratory rate, attitude, appetite, PCV

• Limit activity by confining animal

PREVENTION

• Single use needles in infected herds to minimize transmission.

• Disinfect instruments between animals.

• Currently, there is no vaccine for hemoplasmosis.

MISCELLANEOUS

ZOONOTIC POTENTIAL

N/A

BIOSECURITY

In infected herds, since transmission may occur vertically and via blood-contaminated needles or instruments, use single use needles and disinfect instruments between animals.

SYNONYM

Eperythrozoonosis

ABBREVIATIONS

• MCH = mean corpuscular hemoglobin
• MCHC = mean corpuscular hemoglobin concentration
• MCV = mean corpuscular volume
• PCR = polymerase chain reaction

SEE ALSO

• Anaplasmosis
• Anemia, Regenerative
• Copper Deficiency and Toxicity
• Leptospirosis

Suggested Reading

Neimark H, Hoff B, Ganter M. 2004. *Mycoplasma ovis* comb. nov. (formerly *Eperythrozoon ovis*), an epierythrocytic agent of hemolytic anemia in sheep and goats. Intern J Systemic Evol Micro 54: 365–71.

Song Q, Wang L, Fang R, Khan MK, Zhou Y, Zhao J. Detection of Mycoplasma wenyonii in cattle and transmission vectors by the loop-mediated isothermal amplification (LAMP) assay. Trop Animal Health Prod 2013, 45: 247–50.

Strugnell B, McAuliffe L. *Mycoplasma wenyonii* infection in cattle. In Practice 2012, 34: 146–54. doi:10.1136/inp.e1550

Tagawa M, Yamakawa K, Aoki T, Matsumoto K, Ishii M, Inokuma H. Effect of chronic hemoplasma infection on cattle productivity. J Vet Med Sci 2013, 75: 1271–5.

Tornquist SJ, Boeder J, Rios-Phillips C, Alarcon V. Prevalence of *Mycoplasma haemolamae* infection in Peruvian and Chilean llamas and alpacas. J Vet Diagn Invest 2010, 22: 766–9.

Tornquist SJ, Boeder LJ, Cebra CK, Messick J. Use of a polymerase chain reaction assay to study response to oxytetracycline treatment in experimental *Candidatus Mycoplasma haemolamae* infection in alpacas. Am J Vet Res 2009, 70: 1102–7.

Tornquist SJ, Boeder LJ, Lubbers S, Cebra CK. Investigation of *Mycoplasma haemolamae* infection in crias born to infected dams. Vet Rec 2011, 168: 380. doi: 10.1136/vr.c6735

Author Michelle Henry Barton
Consulting Editor Christopher C.L. Chase

H

HEREDITARY CHONDRODYSPLASIA: OVINE

BASICS

Ovine hereditary chondrodysplasia (HC), also known as spider lamb syndrome (SLS).
• *Heritable* congenital defect that produces multiple, severe skeletal deformities in young lambs. "Spider" relates to severe valgus limb deformities that create a "spider-legged" appearance.
• *Genetic defect* disrupts normal ossification processes involving transformation of cartilage to bone resulting in skeletal overgrowth phenotype.
  ◦ Semilethal—affected lambs seldom survive past 6 months of age.
  ◦ Most common in black-faced breeds of sheep.
  ◦ First described in United States in 1980s in popular lines of Suffolk and Hampshire sheep.
  ◦ Documented in Suffolk, Hampshire, Shropshire, Oxford, Southdown, and associated crossbred sheep.
  ◦ Entered non-black-faced breeds (*ex: Southdown*) through crossbreeding programs.
  ◦ Prior to availability of DNA testing, *white* and *gray* pedigrees used to define carriers. *Gray* individuals—pedigrees linked to suspected carriers. *White* individuals—pedigrees with no apparent incidence of carriers. Pedigrees often inaccurate—now DNA testing a better option.
  ◦ Inheritance pattern—simple autosomal recessive. NN = normal; NS = carrier; SS = clinically affected lamb. Some researchers suggest codominant rather than simple autosomal recessive, with a single mutant (A) allele sufficient for long-bone growth enhancement.
• Inherited chondrodysplasia in crossbred Texel sheep
  ◦ Skeletal disease in Texel sheep characterized by disproportionate dwarfism, limb deformity, tracheal collapse.
  ◦ Inheritance pattern—recessive mode of inheritance in Texel sheep.

INCIDENCE/PREVALENCE

• In a German Suffolk mutation frequency study, 125 healthy, unrelated Suffolk rams were analyzed; 11 HC carriers were observed, indicating an FGFR3 allele mutation frequency of 4%.
• Another study found 97 of 336 (28.9%) carriers of A allele (HC-associated).
• During 5-year study of Texel sheep, 20 of 1,500 (1.3%) lambs per year were affected.

GEOGRAPHIC DISTRIBUTION

• United States and Canada as well as other countries where carrier sheep have been imported (Australia, New Zealand, Germany).

• Regions where black-faced breeds are common (Midwestern US).

SYSTEMS AFFECTED

• Musculoskeletal
• Respiratory (Texel sheep)

PATHOPHYSIOLOGY

Genetic defect linked to fibroblast growth factor receptor 3 (FGFR3) on sheep chromosome 6.
• Single-base change in tyrosine kinase II domain of the ovine FGFR3.
• FGFR3 normally downregulates chondrocyte growth in bone development process.
• Homozygous SS disrupts downregulation of process resulting in excessive and disorderly proliferation and transformation of chondrocytes to bone.
• Newly-recognized in the Texel breed.
• Recessively-inherited genetic disease with a defect in synthesis of glycosaminoglycans in cartilage matrix.

HISTORICAL FINDINGS

Two distinct clinical entities can confuse practitioners:
• *Affected lambs that appear grossly normal at birth.* While subtle deformities are present at birth, typical limb deformities and muscle atrophy associated with HC may not be readily apparent until the lamb is 4–6 weeks old.
• *Affected lambs with visible deformities at birth.* Severe skeletal deformities obvious at birth, may affect neonatal survival.

SIGNALMENT

• Ovine, primarily US black-faced Suffolk and Hampshire sheep, of both sexes.
• Larger-framed.
• Young (between 3 weeks and 9 months of age) or congenital disorder.
• Clinical signs as early as 1 week and as late as 2 years in Texel sheep.

PHYSICAL EXAMINATION FINDINGS

Clinical description of skeletal deformities observed in both groups include:
• Abnormally long, thin-boned legs with a long, fine neck (extreme type for breed).
• Small, rounded head (Roman nose) with occasional lateral deviation of the nose.
• Moderate-to-severe muscle atrophy—progresses with age.
• Scoliosis (usually) and/or kyphosis (less common) of the spine.
• Wide, flattened-appearing sternum with small palpable "dimple."
• Moderate-to-severe valgus deformities distal to the hock and/or carpus; severity increases with age and growth.

GENETICS

See "Pathophysiology"

CAUSES AND RISK FACTORS

• Breeds commonly associated with the problem

• Mating carrier sheep: NN × NN = 100% NN; (NS × NS = 25% SS + 50% NS + 25% NN

DIAGNOSIS

DIFFERENTIAL DIAGNOSES

• Inherited ovine arthrogryposis (IOA)
• AGH syndrome (arthrogryposis-hydranencephaly syndrome) and/or limb deformities
• Cache Valley Virus—joints feel "frozen," lack of articulation; die at birth
• Plant toxicities—*Veratrum californicum*, locoweed (*Astragalus or Oxytropis* spp.)
• Maternal manganese deficiency

CBC/BIOCHEMISTRY/URINALYSIS

Nondiagnostic: Slightly increased alkaline phosphatase activity associated with bone lesions

OTHER LABORATORY TESTS

• Blood or semen can be submitted for DNA testing to confirm genotype.
• Genetic test based on A > T polymorphism in exon 17 of ovine FGFR3.
• DNA isolated from blood or semen can identify NN, NS, or SS status.

IMAGING

• Radiographic findings—abnormal areas of ossification observed throughout skeleton.
• Live animal or postmortem: Flexed lateral of the elbow reveals multiple irregular "islands" of ossification in the olecranon.
• Postmortem: VD or DV view of the sternum (disarticulated from ribs) reveals multiple irregular islands of ossification instead of normal symmetrical bipartite pattern.

OTHER DIAGNOSTIC PROCEDURES

Clinical signs (suggestive), radiologic and necropsy findings (supportive)

PATHOLOGIC FINDINGS

• *Skull*: Rounding of dorsal silhouette (Roman nose appearance) with elongation and erosion of cartilage on the occipital condyles.
• *Sternum*: Sternebrae irregular shape and size, failure to fuse, malalignment and dorsal deviation of second-to-sixth sternebrae.
• *Vertebrae*: Consistent scoliosis, misshapen, excessive amounts and abnormal configuration to vertebral body cartilage.
• *Appendicular skeleton*: Excessive cartilage in olecranon and scapula, lateral "bowing" of distal radius and ulna, hindlimbs usually less severely affected, erosion of articular cartilage in most joints.

Texel Sheep

• Erosions of articular cartilage (femoral head).
• Exaggerated convex curvature of the ribs and costal cartilages, creating a "barrel-chested" appearance and a wide-based stance.

H

(CONTINUED)

HEREDITARY CHONDRODYSPLASIA: OVINE

• Gross and microscopic lesions in tracheal, articular, epiphyseal, and physeal cartilage.
• Affected sheep that survive to breeding age: prematurely developed DJD, especially in major weight-bearing joints (shoulder, hip, and stifle).

TREATMENT

None. Euthanasia suggested once diagnosis confirmed.

FOLLOW-UP

EXPECTED COURSE AND PROGNOSIS
• Semilethal in US black-faced Suffolk and Hampshire
• Lethal chondrodysplasia in Texel sheep

POSSIBLE COMPLICATIONS
N/A

CLIENT EDUCATION
Breeders should be informed about the DNA-based test for the detection of HC carriers.

PATIENT CARE
• Due to the ALD, may need to help lambs to stand so they can nurse.
• Avoid excessive exercise/stress (exercise intolerance) in Texel sheep (i.e., movement with sheepdogs).
• Euthanasia is justified upon diagnosis or with lameness/reluctance to walk.

PREVENTION
Where appropriate, DNA test and utilize only NN rams in the breeding program.

MISCELLANEOUS

AGE-RELATED FACTORS
Clinical signs noted upon birth, some noted at 1 week and some as late as 2 years.

PRODUCTION MANAGEMENT
The continued use of rams from the same breeder will, eventually, lead to carrier ewes in the commercial herd being bred to carrier rams.

SYNONYMS
• Congenital chondrodysplasia in sheep
• Ovine hereditary chondrodysplasia or hereditary chondrodysplasia
• Spider lamb syndrome
• Spider leg syndrome
• Spider syndrome
• Inherited chondrodysplasia in Texel sheep

ABBREVIATIONS
• ALD = angular limb deformity
• DJD = degenerative joint disease
• DV = dorsoventral
• FGFR3 = fibroblast growth factor receptor 3
• VD = ventrodorsal

SEE ALSO
• Arthrogryposis
• Cache Valley Virus
• Euthanasia and Disposal (Appendix 2)

Suggested Reading
Beever JE, Smit MA, Meyers SN, et al. A single-base change in the tyrosine kinase II domain of ovine FGFR3 causes hereditary chondrodysplasia in sheep. Anim Genet 2006, 37: 66–71.
Doherty ML, Kelley EP, Healy AM, et al. Congenital arthrogryposis: an inherited limb deformity in pedigree Suffolk lambs. Vet Rec 2000, 146: 748–53.
Drögemüller C, Wöhlke A, Distl O. Spider Lamb Syndrome (SLS) mutation frequency in German Suffolk sheep. Anim Genet 2005, 36: 511–42.
Rook JS, Trapp AL, Krehbiel J, et al. Diagnosis of hereditary chondrodysplasia (spider lamb syndrome) in sheep. J Am Vet Med Assoc 1988, 193: 713–18.
Thompson KG, Blair HT, Linney LE, West DM, Byrne T. Inherited chondrodysplasia in Texel sheep. N Z Vet J 2005, 53: 208–12.
Whittington RJ, Glastonbury JR, Plant JW, Barry MR. Congenital hydranencephaly and arthrogryposis of Corriedale sheep. Aust Vet J 1988, 65: 124–7.
Author Francisco C. Rodriguez
Consulting Editor Kaitlyn A. Lutz
Acknowledgment The author and book editors acknowledge the prior contribution of Joseph S. Rook.

H

HISTOPHILUS SOMNI COMPLEX

BASICS

OVERVIEW
• *Histophilus somni* is a small, pleomorphic, Gram-negative bacterium.
• An infection with *Histophilus somni* is often referred to as "Histophilosis," implying that the infection is systemic even though the clinical manifestation may be specific to an organ system. It was first identified in 1960 as the cause of infectious thromboembolic meningoencephalitis (ITEME) in feedlot cattle. It was later modified to thrombotic meningoencephalitis (TME) when it was recognized that embolism was not part of the pathogenesis.
• Historically this encephalitic form of the infection was recognized to be the main manifestation.
• More recently it has been shown to be an important cause of sporadic "sudden death" in groups of weaned, confined cattle and associated with diverse pathologic processes.
• Investigators have isolated the organism from the reproductive tract of both male and female cattle, but descriptions of overt disease are not common.

INCIDENCE/PREVALENCE
• Culture of normal animals and serologic evidence suggests infection is widespread. Clinical disease is less common.
• While histophilosis is probably a common infection of cattle in North America and elsewhere, the disease is often undiagnosed or misdiagnosed.

GEOGRAPHIC DISTRIBUTION
• In Canada and the northern United States, *H. somni* infection is considered to be a significant cause of morbidity and mortality in feedlot cattle.
• Commonly isolated in Canada, western and midwestern US. Rarely isolated in northeastern and southeastern US.
• Identified in South America, Europe, Australia, New Zealand, Russia, Israel, and Japan in both beef and dairy cattle.

SYSTEMS AFFECTED
• Respiratory
• Nervous
• Cardiovascular
• Musculoskeletal
• Ophthalmic
• Reproductive

PATHOPHYSIOLOGY
• The organism can survive in biologic fluids for several weeks in the environment. It has been established that pathogenic strains can survive within macrophages and neutrophils. Additionally, the mechanism by which this organism manages to evade antimicrobial sensitivity in vivo is not well described and it

has been suggested that the presence of biofilm formation, as well as the unique pathogenesis of the lesions, may explain the often reported nonresponse to treatment.
• *H. somni* can be isolated from respiratory and reproductive tracts of a healthy animal.
• Entry via the respiratory tract is the probable route of systemic exposure to the organism. *H. somni* initially colonizes mucus membranes and contributes to the etiology of routine undifferentiated respiratory disease in this fashion.
• The presence of the organism in the bloodstream or septicemia probably initiates all other manifestations of the disease, occasionally even causing an embolic pneumonia.
• Structurally the organism has the ability to adhere to the endothelium of vessels, especially veins, causing a thrombophlebitis. This adhesion initiates a pathologic cascade in the vessel wall and leads to a thrombus formation, which ultimately compromises the blood supply leading to that portion of the organ or organs.
• All subsequent pathologic processes associated with histophilosis can be attributed to destruction of viable tissue due to the interrupted blood supply (see Web Figures 1 and 2), referred to as an infarction.
• Clinical and pathologic observations have shown that some organ systems are more affected than others, indicating that different strains may have a varying predilection for specific organ tissues.
• Thus, historically, isolated strains were associated with encephalitic pathology; however, current isolates seem more predisposed to produce pathology in the myocardium, specifically, the papillary muscles of the left ventricle.
• The change in organ system preference of *H. somni* to produce the predominant pathology has been clinically but not microbiologically described.

SIGNALMENT
• Bovine—similar disease syndromes seen in sheep infected with *Haemophilus agni* and *Histophilus ovis*. These organisms are very similar to *H. somni* and the assigned nomenclature has and may change.
• Systemic disease is seen predominantly in beef cattle and only sporadically in dairy cattle.
• Reproductive disease can be seen in both beef and dairy cattle, predominantly in females although *H. somni* can easily be cultured from semen.
• Respiratory, neurologic, and cardiovascular disease are predominantly in feedlot cattle (6–12 months of age). *H. somni*-associated respiratory disease has also been anecdotally reported in beef calves as young as 2 months still sucking their dams on range.

PHYSICAL EXAMINATION FINDINGS
Septicemia/ Systemic Disease
• Sudden death is commonly the presentation in this form of the disease.
• Depression, reluctance to move (it may be difficult to differentiate between joint pain and depression) (see Web Figure 3).
• Febrile (e.g., >104.9°F, >40.5°C).

Meningoencephalitis
• Usually found "down." If not "down," affected animals usually become recumbent quite quickly, e.g., within 8–12 hours (see Web Figure 4). Occasionally cases will demonstrate signs of hyperesthesia, opisthotonus, nystagmus, and strabismus. Convulsions can occur, rarely.
• The animal acutely affected is febrile (often high).
• Extremely depressed.
• If treatment is initiated early, thereby sparing the progression of the disease, "head-pressing" may be reported by the stock attendants (see Web Figure 5).
• Blindness is often present but may be difficult to determine when depression is so profound.
• Hemorrhagic and/or fibrinous lesions may be visible in the fundus of the eyeball if an ocular examination is possible (see Web Figure 6).

Pleuritis
The thoracic space may fill with fluid and fibrin (see Web Figure 7) so rapidly that animals die without showing clinical signs.

Pneumonia
• Pneumonia caused by *H. somni* alone is impossible to differentiate clinically from pneumonia caused by other microorganisms, especially *Pasteurella multocida*.
• The acutely affected animal is febrile (often high).
• *H. somni* most often is part of the disease complex referred to as bovine respiratory disease complex (BDRC).

Myocarditis
• Animals affected with the myocardial form of histophilosis may also be found "down" and with no treatment history.
• If not, they will usually show exercise intolerance and when movement is initiated, extreme dyspnea may develop. They too, may collapse and die "in transit."
• The hypoxemia of cardiovascular malfunction or a thoracic space lesion may mean the animal presents with signs of ataxia or apparent lameness that may confuse the attending diagnostician.

Arthritis/Synovitis
• Currently, it is uncommon to make a diagnosis of arthritis or polyarthritis caused by *H. somni* alone, because the other manifestations of the infection predominate

clinically and quickly overwhelm what is usually a mild disease.
• The *infarctive* pathologic process, so typical of this disease, may also develop in the skeletal muscles, especially in the semimembranosus and semitendinosus muscles of the hindlimbs. Animals with these lesions will usually present with "knuckling over" from the fetlock of the affected limb, ataxia, stilted gait, or even recumbency.

Reproductive Disease
• Sporadic abortion with little or no clinical signs in the dam has been reported to occur. Additionally, the organism often can be cultured from the female reproductive tract in suspect cases of infertility.
• Reproductive disease is spread via respiratory or urinary tract routes, although venereal spread remains highly probable.

CAUSES AND RISK FACTORS
• *H. somni* is a Gram-negative, nonmotile, non spore-forming, nonencapsulated, pleomorphic coccobacillus. The original name of *Haemophilus* given to the genus derived from the fact that hemolysis occurred when cultured on blood agar within 24 hours.
• Recently weaned calves are at a higher risk of infection and disease. In western Canada a possible seasonal effect (historically demonstrated by increased diagnostic laboratory submissions during November, December, and January) occurs because 80% of calves are spring-born and therefore weaned and placed in the fall.
• Confined "high risk" (e.g., multiple-source, sorted and commingled via the sale barn) calves are exposed early in the feeding period.
• Method of transmission in confinement is assumed via respiratory secretions or urine.
• Titers to *H. somni* peak within first 3 weeks of confinement, suggesting early transmission of the organism, but immunologically naïve cattle experience higher morbidity and mortality following feedlot entry.
• *H. somni*-caused mortality commonly occurs 20–60 DOF, but pathologic sequelae to a previous infection may cause death sporadically at any time during the entire feeding period.
• *H. somni*-associated reproductive tract disorders such as mastitis, abortions, vaginitis, and metritis have been reported but were not duplicated in an infectious disease model.

DIAGNOSIS
DIFFERENTIAL DIAGNOSES
Sudden Death
• Animals can "suddenly die" but the primary differentiation must be between "sudden death" and "suddenly found dead" to enable the attending clinician to highlight the possibility of "selection failure" or "delayed detection" to the stock attendants.

Histophilosis cases in the form of bronchopneumonia, myocarditis, pleuritis, septicemia, and meningoencephalitis can all die acutely without any apparent premonitory signs.
• The exercise intolerance so characteristic of extensive *H. somni* pleuritis and myocarditis can be confused with severe viral interstitial pneumonia, overwhelming bronchopneumonia caused by *Mycoplasma bovis*, and monensin sodium toxicity.

Central Nervous System Disease
• *H. somni* meningoencephalitis must be differentiated from listeria meningoencephalitis, the nervous form of coccidiosis, hypovitaminosis A, polioencephalomalacia, including that caused by salt toxicity/water deprivation, and other toxicities (lead, nitrate, urea). Some systemic conditions, such as ruminal overload, may resemble CNS disease on first examination by the attending clinician.
• In North America, nonsuppurative encephalopathies in the bovine can also be caused by viruses such as rabies, malignant catarrhal fever virus, Astrovirus, and West Nile virus. In addition, the nervous system vasculitis caused by bovine virus diarrhea virus must be ruled out.
• Protozoal causes of bovine meningoencephalitis such as *Neosporum caninum* and *Sarcocystis*, as well as parasites such as *Baylisascaris procyonis*, should not be overlooked.
• Swollen joints caused by *H. somni* usually resolve with treatment. If not, the putative pathogen is more likely to be *Mycoplasma bovis* and treatment is more likely to be more unsuccessful.
• Animals with a "wild" disposition may present with apparent CNS disease from cranial or upper spinal trauma of varying degrees.

Reproductive
• An *H. somni* abortion must be differentiated from other bacterial causes of abortion: *Leptospira* spp., *Listeria monocytogenes*, *Brucella abortus*, and *Campylobacter* spp.
• Other routine causes of abortion must be considered and ruled out as well—protozoa such as *Neospora caninum*; viruses such as IBR, BVDV; toxicities such as mycoses, pine needle, nitrate; and the oft incriminated, but rarely defined, trauma.

CBC/BIOCHEMISTRY/URINALYSIS
No unique or specific changes. Nonspecific changes associated with inflammation may be seen—increased fibrinogen, leukocytosis, increased neutrophil : lymphocyte ratio, increased serum globulin.

OTHER LABORATORY TESTS
• The slow-growing nature of bacterial culture can lead to overgrowth of contaminants. Similarly, previous antibiotic treatment may decrease ability to isolate organism and

increase the use of molecular modalities such as polymerase chain reaction (PCR) or immunohistochemistry (IHC) to identify the organism in the lesion. Most current diagnoses of histophilosis are confirmed using IHC.
• Presence of bacteria, increased total protein, increased globulin, and a heavy concentration of neutrophils from a cerebrospinal fluid (CSF) tap at either the lumbar-sacral site or via the cisterna magna would confirm the diagnosis of meningoencephalitis.
• Similarly, isolation of the pathogen from blood, CSF, or urine of a febrile animal is much more likely if the sample is taken prior to antimicrobial treatment and confirms the diagnosis of histophilosis.
• Given the use of troponin I to confirm acute myocardial necrosis in other species in other applications, sampling of suspect histophilosis cases would help to determine the extent of clinical and subclinical myocardial disease.
• Serology—requires both acute and convalescent samples for accurate interpretation.

PATHOLOGIC FINDINGS
Sudden Death or Acute Cases
• Excessive petechiation and fibrinous synovitis is often associated with septicemia.
• Grossly visible hemorrhagic infarcts in the cerebrum are good presumptive evidence of encephalitis or TME.
• A finding of fibrinous pleuritis without pneumonia would support a tentative diagnosis of *H. somni* pleuritis.
• A gross pathologic finding of fibrinosuppurative bronchiolitis and bronchopneumonia would need further diagnostic support, such as culture and/or IHC, to definitively rule in a diagnosis of *H. somni* bronchopneumonia.
• The very common finding of extensive pulmonary edema or left-sided heart failure (LSHF) (see Web Figure 8) and focal myocardial necrosis confirms a diagnosis of *H. somni* myocarditis (see Web Figure 9). On occasion, field necropsy may demonstrate a more extensive peracute myocardial necrosis without LSHF referred to as pan-myocarditis (see Web Figure 10).
• When the synovial fluid of the major joints is cloudy and discolored with flecks of fibrin, portions of the joint capsule should be sampled and submitted for *H. somni* IHC to confirm a diagnosis of *H. somni* polyarthritis, recognizing that some diagnostic laboratories would still only use standard culture to identify the organism.
• Occasionally all organ systems or spaces lined by mucus or smooth membranes, e.g., joints, pericardium, inner ear (see Web Figure 11), mammary gland, thorax, and abdominal space, may be affected and *H. somni* polyserositis may be the most probable consideration.

• A diagnosis of *H. somni*-caused abortion is characterized by a necrotizing placentitis and nonspecific lesions in the usually semi-autolyzed fetus that must be confirmed by additional diagnostic support.

Chronic Cases
• Over time, the fibrinous pathologic process will be replaced by fibrosis, which may add to the repertoire of clinical signs, e.g., more free gas bloat and congestive heart failure. Thus, previous fibrinous pathologic processes will have become fibrotic adhesions.
• Necrotic foci in the lung and heart may sequestrate (see Web Figure 9), or an extensive fibrinous pleuritis may effectively eliminate the pleural space. The animal's demise is then caused by compression pulmonary atelectasis.

Musculoskeletal System
An *H. somni* septicemia may cause pale areas in the semimembranosus or semitendinosus muscles that are grossly visible muscle infarctions that can usually be confirmed with IHC examination of the sampled muscle tissue. Similarly, *H. somni* arthritis can usually be confirmed with IHC examination of the synovial membrane of an affected joint.

TREATMENT

THERAPEUTIC APPROACH
• For histophilosis in general, more important than the treatment of choice is the length of treatment and early detection. For example, atreatment protocol for animals in recumbency, animals losing weight, or animals whose lameness does not resolve, should be developed by the attending veterinarian with sound animal welfare, appropriate nursing care, and a definitive diagnosis in mind.
• Treatment for *H. somni* infection should be started as soon as signs are noted.

MEDICATIONS

DRUGS OF CHOICE
Respiratory Disease
• Treatment for pneumonia would resemble treatment for pneumonias of all other causes. Typically, affected animals are treated for undifferentiated BRDC with many antibiotics labeled for that treatment.
• Several antibiotics are specifically labeled for treatment of *H. somni*:
  ○ Ceftiofur (1.1–2.2 mg/kg SQ for 3–5 days)
  ○ Enrofloxacin (7.5–12.5 mg/kg SQ)
  ○ Florfenicol (40 mg/kg SQ).

Neurologic Disease
• Treatment for *H. somni* meningoencephalitis as well as the other manifestations of the infection should be started as soon as signs are noted. While common antimicrobials at labeled doses are all good choices, in Canada, florfenicol is recommended.
• However, no drugs are labeled for this use in the US. Extra-label use requires that the practitioner provide an appropriate drug withdrawal timetable.
• Common antibiotics that will cross the blood–brain barrier: Florfenicol and oxytetracycline should be considered.
• To limit or reduce the development of the cerebral edema that sometimes occurs with TME, the labeled dose of dexamethazone is indicated.

Herd Medication
• Mass medication with sustained-action oxytetracycline injections in the face of a histophilosis outbreak has not been shown to be an effective control of histophilosis; however, it was significant in controlling death loss due to undifferentiated BDRC.
• Medicating the feed with chlortetracycline or oxytetracycline at 5–6 g per head (~ 250 kg calf) per day has given equivocal results in controlling an outbreak of histophilosis.

PRECAUTIONS
Appropriate milk and meat withdrawal times should be followed for all compounds administered to food-producing animals.

FOLLOW-UP

EXPECTED COURSE AND PROGNOSIS
• Generally, cattle treated in the early stages of disease have a better chance of recovery than those with more advanced disease, regardless of the affected system.
• Cattle with advanced neurologic disease have a poor to grave prognosis even with aggressive treatment, and "other-than *H. somni* caused" CNS disease should be contemplated and ruled out.
• If the polyarthritis-like syndrome being treated has a poor response to therapy, leading to chronic lameness, it is unlikely to be *H. somni* disease, and the diagnosis should be re-evaluated.

PATIENT CARE
• Typically involves evaluation of improvement or deterioration of clinical signs (attitude, appetite, ambulation, rectal temperature, system-associated signs).
• Clinically affected animals should have constant access to fresh, palatable feedstuffs and clean water.
• Animals should be removed from their "home" pens and confined in a low-stress, low-competition environment; preferably sheltered from the ambient local climate.
• If affected individuals become laterally recumbent and are unable to rise, or if their condition has severely deteriorated, euthanasia is appropriate. Euthanasia is especially indicated if the patient is subject to a very cold ambient environment.

PREVENTION
• The risk of histophilosis could potentially be reduced by minimizing the amount of commingling that normally occurs when calves are weaned, sorted, mixed, and transported during the sale process.
• Post-arrival metaphylaxis with sustained-action injectable antibiotics or feed additives are commonly used when a high BRDC morbidity is expected, but have given equivocal results in preventing histophilosis.
• Appropriate *H. somni* immunization, requiring two doses at a 2- to 3-week interval, has been shown in challenge models to prevent the disease.
• Results of field trials to evaluate clinical efficacy have yielded conflicting results and often demonstrated significant vaccination failure.
• Vaccination failure in field trials may be explained because immunization and challenge likely occur spontaneously.

MISCELLANEOUS

AGE-RELATED FACTORS
• Systemic disease typically is seen in feedlot cattle (age 6–12 months).
• Reproductive disease is seen in breeding-age animals.

ZOONOTIC POTENTIAL
None

PREGNANCY
Organism can cause abortion.

BIOSECURITY
Biosecurity is difficult to attain in a feedlot setting due to movement of cattle from multiple sources onto the premises.

PRODUCTION MANAGEMENT
H. somni plays a role in BRDC, which is the most economically significant disease in the beef industry.

SYNONYMS
Neurologic disease "brainer," "sleeper", "downer"

ABBREVIATIONS
• BRDC = bovine respiratory disease complex
• BRSV = bovine respiratory syncytial virus
• BVDV = bovine viral diarrhea virus
• CNS = central nervous system
• CSF = cerebrospinal fluid
• DOF = days on feed
• IBR = infectious bovine rhinotracheitis (bovine herpesvirus-1)
• IHC = immunohistochemistry
• PCR = polymerase chain reaction

SEE ALSO

Suggested Reading

Corbeil LB. *Histophilus somni* host-parasite relationships. (Review). An Health Res Rev 2007, 82: 151–60.

Gagea MI, Bateman KG, van Dreumel T, et al. Diseases and pathogens associated with mortality in Ontario beef feedlots. J Vet Diagn Invest 2006, 18: 18–28.

Harris WH, Janzen ED. The *Haemophilus somnus* disease complex. Can Vet J 1989, 30: 816–22.

Howard MD, Cox AD, Weiser JN, Schurig CG, Inzana TJ. Antigenic diversity of *Haemophilus somnus* lipooligosaccharide: phase-variable accessibility of the phosphorylchlorine epitope. J Clin Microbiol 2000, 38: 4412–19.

Kwiecien JM, Little PB. *Haemophilus somnus* and reproductive disease in the cow: a review. Can Vet J 1991, 32: 595–601.

McDougall S. Gross abnormalities, bacteriology and histological lesions of uteri of dairy cows failing to conceive or maintain pregnancy. N Z Vet J 2005, 53: 253–6.

O'Connor A, Martin SW, Harland RJ, Shewen P, Menzies P. The relationship between the occurrence of undifferentiated bovine respiratory disease and titer changes to *Haemophilus somnus* and *Mannheimia hemolytica* at three Ontario feedlots. Can J Vet Res 2001, 65: 143–50.

Saunders JR, Janzen ED. *Haemophilus somnus* infections: II) A Canadian field trial of a commercial bacterin; clinical and serological results. Can Vet J 1980, 21: 219–24.

Van Donkersgoed J, Janzen ED, Harland RJ. Epidemiological features of calf mortality due to haemophilosis in a large feedlot. Can Vet J 1990, 31: 821–5.

Author Eugene Janzen

Consulting Editor Christopher C.L. Chase

H

HYDROMETRA

BASICS

OVERVIEW
• Hydrometra is an accumulation of aseptic fluid in the uterine lumen in absence of pregnancy and in the presence of a persistent corpus luteum (CL).
• Also known as pseudopregnancy, it can occur in all ruminants, but is most common in goats.
• It is one of the major causes of anestrus in goats during the breeding season.
• May also be referred to as "cloud burst."
• Hydrometra and mucometra may also be seen in animals with segmental aplasia of the tubular genitalia.

INCIDENCE/PREVALENCE
• Incidence of congenital abnormalities associated with hydrometra/mucometra is not known, but seems to be frequent in SAC.
• In goats, the reported incidence of hydrometra varies between 6.0% and 30%.
• Hydrometra is more prevalent in aged does.
• In a large study on 40,340 early pregnancy diagnoses in dairy goats, the mean incidence of hydrometra was 10.4% and varied from 0 to 66.6%. Incidence after breeding was higher in older goats (18.8%) than in yearlings (4.5%).

GEOGRAPHIC DISTRIBUTION
Worldwide

SYSTEMS AFFECTED
Reproductive

PATHOPHYSIOLOGY
• Hydrometra is an accumulation of fluid in the uterus resulting from an abnormality (segmental aplasia) or persistence of the CL.
• Fluid accumulation in the uterus may also be observed with cystic ovarian disease.
• The etiology and pathophysiology of hydrometra in cycling animals is poorly understood. Hydrometra was induced in goats following immunization against PGF2$_\alpha$.
• There is no correlation between prolactin concentration and development or persistence of the CL.
• The following have been suggested as contributing factors:
  ○ Mechanisms that decrease the production or release of PGF2$_\alpha$ from the endometrium.
  ○ Exposure to phytoestrogens.
  ○ Early fetal death with subsequent fetal resorption and a persistent CL; however, this condition has been identified in unmated females.
  ○ Out of season breeding.
  ○ Overuse of hormones for manipulation of the reproductive cycle.
  ○ Congenital malformations of the cervix and uterus.

GENETICS
• A genetic predisposition has been suggested for the incidence of pseudopregnancy.
• In a study on Dutch Saanen goats, there was a 16.3% repeatability of hydrometra, and daughters of does that experienced pseudopregnancy had a significant frequency compared to controls.

HISTORICAL FINDINGS
• Anestrus in absence of pregnancy
• Failure to deliver after mating and/or a positive pregnancy diagnosis
• History of synchronization

SIGNALMENT
• Adult female goat with bilateral abdominal distention.
• Occasionally found in other ruminant species.
• Occurs most commonly in pet and dairy goats who experience estrous cycles with no opportunity to be bred.

PHYSICAL EXAMINATION FINDINGS
• Early cases may be diagnosed during pregnancy diagnosis by ultrasonography.
• Advanced cases may show signs of pregnancy (abdominal enlargement), udder development.
• Signs of parturition and spontaneous evacuation of large amount of fluid from the vagina.
• Persistent anestrus with elevated progesterone levels.
• Purulent vaginal discharge when the accumulated uterine fluid is discharged either due to PGF2$_\alpha$ administration or the CL spontaneously lyses and the prolonged luteal phase comes to an end.

CAUSES AND RISK FACTORS
• Age, out-of-season breeding, overuse of hormonal manipulation on the reproductive cycle, and exposure to phytoestrogens are suspected predisposing factors in cyclic goats.
• Congenital abnormalities such as unperforated hymen and segmental aplasia of the tubular genitalia (vagina, cervix, uterus) result in accumulation of various amounts of fluid (mucometra or hydrometra).

DIAGNOSIS

DIFFERENTIAL DIAGNOSES
• Other causes of anestrus: Ovarian hypoplasia, mineral deficiencies, pituitary adenoma, pregnancy, fetal mummification.
• Other causes of fluid accumulation in the uterus: Mucometra, pyometra.
• Fluid accumulation in the uterus may be due to congenital (cervical aplasia, persistent hymen, vaginal aplasia) or acquired (cervical stenosis, vaginal adhesions) disorders.

CBC/BIOCHEMISTRY/URINALYSIS
N/A

OTHER LABORATORY TESTS
• Serum progesterone level will confirm the presence of a CL, but will not rule out a true pregnancy.
• Estrone sulfate (blood and urine) should only be present with a true pregnancy.
• Pregnancy-associated glycoproteins (PAGs) would be low in the case of hydrometra and would confirm absence of viable pregnancy.

IMAGING
• Transabdominal ultrasonography: Uterine enlargement with anechoic fluid in the lumen and no evidence of placentomes or a fetus.
• The character of fluid in the uterus varies from anechoic to echogenic with hyperechoic debris.

PATHOLOGIC FINDINGS
• The uterus is thin walled and contains thin, clear fluid.
• The amount of fluid varies from less than 250 mL to several liters (12 liters).
• The endometrium is thin and the glands are slightly dilated.
• The cervical glands and lumen are often filled with mucus.

TREATMENT

THERAPEUTIC APPROACH
• A single injection of PGF2$_\alpha$ is usually effective, but repeated doses may be necessary. In one study 59% of does responded to the first injection and 89.5% following two injections.
• In the case of congenital malformations of the cervix and uterus, consider culling the animal to prevent further complications in the future.

SURGICAL CONSIDERATIONS AND TECHNIQUES
Ovariectomy or ovariohysterectomy may be considered in pet or service animals with recurrent hydrometra.

MEDICATIONS

DRUGS OF CHOICE
• Dinoprost tromethamine (5–10 mg) or cloprostenol sodium (75–100 μg/45 kg of body weight).
• Oxytocin 50 IU q12h for 4 days results in luteolysis and evacuation of fluid but this treatment is not commonly used.

CONTRAINDICATIONS
Pregnant animals or animal with congenital defects

PRECAUTIONS
Confirm pregnancy status prior to treatment.

POSSIBLE INTERACTIONS
N/A

(CONTINUED)   **HYDROMETRA**

FOLLOW-UP

EXPECTED COURSE AND PROGNOSIS
• Some cases may resolve spontaneously.
• Animals treated with PGF2$_\alpha$ will experience luteolysis. The fluid is expelled following decreased progesterone level and cervical dilation. Various amount of clear or cloudy fluid may be observed. The hindquarters of the female may appear soiled or wet.
• Prognosis is fair to good for fertility. Some females may develop hydrometra again if not mated.
• Culling of affected goats is generally not indicated unless a congenital malformation is detected.

POSSIBLE COMPLICATIONS
Infertility

CLIENT EDUCATION
• Importance of pregnancy diagnosis
• Wellness examination for pet goats
• SAC should undergo prebreeding examination of the reproductive system because of the high incidence of congenital abnormalities

PATIENT CARE
Observe for return to estrus

PREVENTION
• Ovariectomy
• Since the etiology of hydrometra is poorly understood, the following are suggestions for possible modes of prevention:
  ◦ Limit exposure to phytoestrogens.
  ◦ Limit out-of-season breeding.
  ◦ Limit use of hormonal manipulation on the reproductive cycle.

MISCELLANEOUS

ASSOCIATED CONDITIONS
• Mucometra: These uterine conditions are only differentiated by the gross characteristics of the fluid present in the uterus.
• Infertility.
• Early pregnancy loss.
• In SAC, congenital defects may result in other clinical signs: Systemic disease in neonates with vulvar aplasia and urine accumulation in the uterus. Vaginal aplasia and unperforated/persistent hymen can result in tenesmus and rectal prolapse.

AGE-RELATED FACTORS
• Older does are overrepresented.
• Congenital defects are seen in neonates and nulliparous females.

ZOONOTIC POTENTIALL
N/A

PREGNANCY
The affected does are anestrous with elevated progesterone levels similar to those in pregnant ewes at 5 months' gestation.

BIOSECURITY
N/A

PRODUCTION MANAGEMENT
• Hydrometra is considered a very important pathologic condition because it represents one of the main causes of temporary infertility in goats.
• It is recommended to perform pregnancy examination via transabdominal ultrasonography at 35–45 days' gestation to verify the presence of a viable fetus and confirm pregnancy.

SYNONYM
Cloud burst

ABREVIATIONS
• PGF2$_\alpha$ = prostaglandin F2$_\alpha$
• CL = corpus luteum
• PAG = pregnancy-associated glycoprotein
• SAC = South American camelids

SEE ALSO
• Anestrus
• Congenital Defects: Camelid
• Pregnancy Diagnosis: Small Ruminant
• Reproductive Pharmacology
• Reproductive Ultrasonography: Small Ruminant (see www.fiveminutevet.com/ruminant)
• Uterine Anomalies

Suggested Reading
Batista M, Alamo D, Caballero MJ, et al. Segmental aplasia of the uterus associated with hydrometra in a goat. Vet Rec 2016, 159: 597–8.
Bretzlaff KN. Development of hydrometra in a ewe flock after ultrasonography of determination of pregnancy. J Am Vet Med Assoc 1993, 203: 122–5.
Hesselink JW. Incidence of hydrometra in dairy goats. Vet Rec 1993, 132: 110–12.

Hesselink JW. Hydrometra in dairy goats: reproductive performance after treatment with prostaglandins. Vet Rec 1993, 133: 186–7.
Kaulfuss KH. Scheinträchtigkeit bei Ziegen – Ursache, Diagnostik und wirtschaftliche Bedeutung. 5. Fachtagung für Ziegenhaltung. Management, Fütterung und Zucht von Milchziegen, Raumberg-Gumpenstein, Austria, 4 November 2011, pp. 3–6.
Kormalijnslijper JE, Bevers, MM, van Oord HA, Taverne MAM. Induction of hydrometra in goats by means of active immunization against prostaglandin F2α. Anim Reprod Sci 1997, 46: 109–22.
Pieterse MC, Taverne MAM. Hydrometra in goats: Diagnosis with real time ultrasound and treatment with prostaglandin or oxytocin. Theriogenology 1986, 26: 813–21.
Souza JMG, Mai ALRS, Brandao FZ, et al. Hormonal treatment of dairy goats affected by hydrometra associated or not with ovarian follicular cyst. Small Rumin Res 2013, 111: 104–9.
Taverne MAM, Hesselink JW, Bevers MM, Van Oord HA, Kornalijnslijper JE. Etiology and endocrinology of pseudopregnancy in the goat. Reprod Domest Anim 1995, 30: 228–30.
Wittek T, Erices J, Elze K. Histology of the endometrium, clinical-chemical parameters of the uterine fluid and blood plasma concentrations of progesterone, estradiol-17ß and prolactin during hydrometra in goats. Small Rumin Res 1998, 30: 105–12.

Author Clare M. Scully
Consulting Editor Ahmed Tibary

H

HYDROPS

BASICS

OVERVIEW
• Hydrops or dropsical condition ("dropsy") is a pregnancy disorder characterized by excessive fluid accumulation in either the allantoic or the amniotic cavity.
• Hydrallantois (hydrops allantois) is related primarily to placental dysfunction or insufficiency.
• Hydramnios (hydrops amnion) is attributable to congenital abnormalities of the fetus that contribute directly to fluid accumulation, such as impaired swallowing or renal dysgenesis/agenesis.

INCIDENCE/PREVALENCE
• Hydrallantois represents 85–90% of dropsical conditions in the bovine.
• Hydramnios is rare, accounting for only 5–10% of uterine dropsy cases.
• In the bovine, incidence of dropsical conditions is estimated at 1 in 7,500 pregnancies.
• Increased incidence (1 in 200 pregnancies) has been reported in pregnancies resulting from embryos produced by SCNT.
• Hydrops is relatively rare in sheep, goats, and camelids.

GEOGRAPHIC DISTRIBUTION
Worldwide

SYSTEMS AFFECTED
• Reproductive
• Musculoskeletal
• Multisystemic in advanced cases

PATHOPHYSIOLOGY
• Dysfunction of either the placenta or the fetus results in accumulation of excessive amounts of allantoic or amniotic fluid. The excessive weight from the rapid fluid accumulation is detrimental to the dam's health, leading to dyspnea, dehydration, and compromised GI function.
• The cause of hydrallantois is not certain. Adventitious placentation is commonly present and there may also be a deficient number of caruncles. This deficiency may be due to either a congenital lack of development or uterine disease acquired in later life.
• Hydramnios has been associated with a genetic (autosomal recessive) or congenitally defective fetus in which swallowing is impaired.
• Increased risk for hydrops in pregnancies obtained by nuclear transfer reconstructed embryos is due to errors in reprogramming of the donor genome.
• Hybrids produced by mating of an American bison bull with a domestic cow.
• Hydrops amnii in sheep may be associated with hydranencephaly due to Wesselsbron disease and Rift Valley fever.

HISTORICAL FINDINGS
• Rapid increase in abdominal girth during pregnancy
• Respiratory distress
• Reluctance or inability to stand

SIGNALMENT
• Reported in both dairy and beef cattle.
• Not as common but reported in sheep and goats usually after mid-gestation.
• Hydrallantois is seen in older cows that may lack caruncles due to prior uterine damage/trauma.

PHYSICAL EXAMINATION FINDINGS
• The major outward sign of hydrops is excessive abdominal distention during the last trimester that progressively worsens and can result in decreased appetite and difficulty in moving or rising.
• Hydrallantois: Affected cows show bilateral, rapid ventral distension of the abdomen. They are distressed, anorexic, and have no rumen activity due to compression. Dehydration and constipation follow and they eventually become recumbent. Transrectal palpation is difficult because of uterine distension and some cows may strain during the examination. The fetus and placentomes are generally not palpable. Rupture of the prepubic tendon may occur in advanced cases.
• Hydramnios: Due to the gradual nature of the increase in amniotic fluid, the cow does not show any overt clinical signs, except when viewed from the rear she shows a pear-shaped abdomen in the last 6 weeks of gestation.

GENETICS
• Hydrallantois: Pregnancies from cloned or transgenic embryos are more commonly affected by abnormal placentation and subsequently have a higher risk for hydrops allantois. Risk is also increased in pregnancies with multiple fetuses.
• Hydramnios has been associated with a genetic (autosomal recessive) mode of inheritance. Fetal abnormalities that cause this defect include bulldog calves (Dexter cattle), brachygnathic calves (Angus cattle), muscle contracture monsters (Red Danish cattle), pituitary hypoplasia/aplasia (Guernsey cattle), and hydrocephalic calves (Hereford cattle).
• Hydrops has been described in interspecies pregnancy (bison × cattle; sheep × goat).

CAUSES AND RISK FACTORS
• Pregnancy with multiple fetuses
• Mating of an American bison bull with a domestic cow
• Cloning (SCNT)
• Genetics: Certain breeds are overrepresented

DIAGNOSIS

DIFFERENTIAL DIAGNOSES
• Dropsical conditions should be differentiated from other conditions characterized by abdominal distention such as:
   ○ Ascites
   ○ Uroperitoneum due to bladder rupture
   ○ Abdominal masses
   ○ Gastrointestinal problems resulting in bloat (intestinal obstruction, vagal indigestion)
   ○ Uterine distension due to hydrometra, pyometra or multiple fetuses
• History (breeding, onset of symptoms), transrectal palpation, and transrectal and transabdominal ultrasonography are usually sufficient to make a diagnosis.

CBC/BIOCHEMSTRY/URINALYSIS
• Cases of hydrallantois may show hypoglycemia and/or hypocalcemia.
• Ketosis is a potential complication of significant abdominal distention.

OTHER LABORATORY TESTS
In an academic setting, differentiation between hydrallantois and hydramnios may be achieved by biochemical analysis of fetal fluids.

IMAGING
• Ultrasonography may help distinguish between hydrallantois and hydramnios (location and echogenicity of fluid). Also, placentome abnormalities may be detected. In hydramnios, the amnion may be thickened.
• Fetal abnormalities may be visualized.

OTHER DIAGNOSTIC PROCEDURES
Transrectal palpation: In cases of hydrallantois, the uterine wall is too tight and does not allow ballottement of the fetus or palpation of fetal parts and placentomes. In hydramnios, the fetus and placentomes can still be palpated.

PATHOLOGIC FINDINGS
• Hydrallantois:
• Fluid is watery, clear and may be amber in color.
• Presence of adventitious placentation.
• Fetus is normal but small.
• Hydramnios:
• Fluid is thick and viscous and may contain meconium.
• Placentation is normal.
• Fetal malformations may be present.

TREATMENT

THERAPEUTIC APPROACH
• Induction of parturition with dexamethasone and PGF2$_\alpha$. Overstretching of the myometrium due to excessive fluid accumulation may result in primary uterine inertia.
• Cervical relaxation may be enhanced by application of misoprostol.
• Supportive therapy to correct other abnormalities caused by the abdominal distention (hypoglycemia, hypocalcemia).

• Fluid replacement therapy is essential in management of hydrallantois.
• Extreme cases of hydrallantois should be humanely euthanized.

SURGICAL CONSIDERATIONS AND TECHNIQUES

Cesarean section may be considered. However, fluid must be removed and replaced slowly and simultaneously to avoid hypovolemic shock.

MEDICATIONS

DRUGS OF CHOICE
• Dexamethasone
• PGF2$_\alpha$ (dinoprost tromethamine) or cloprostenol.
• Misoprostol, a synthetic PGE1, topical application onto the cervix.
• Prophylactic antibiotics to treat the metritis and/or retained fetal membranes that occurs commonly with hydrallantois.

CONTRAINDICATIONS
• Misoprostol is not labeled for use in food-producing animals in some countries.
• Appropriate milk and meat withdrawal times must be followed.

PRECAUTIONS
Hypovolemic shock

POSSIBLE INTERACTIONS
N/A

FOLLOW-UP

EXPECTED COURSE AND PROGNOSIS
• Spontaneous abortion may occur in hydrallantois. The condition may recur in subsequent pregnancies. Prognosis for life and fertility is guarded to poor. The fetus is usually dead at birth or dies shortly after. Humane euthanasia is often the best approach in advanced cases.
• Cows may deliver normally in cases of hydramnios. The fetus is abnormal and, in most cases, nonviable. The prognosis for fertility is fair to good.

POSSIBLE COMPLICATIONS
• Prepubic tendon rupture
• Abortion
• Dystocia
• Retained placenta
• Metritis
• Infertility
• Metabolic, respiratory, and circulatory complications resulting in death

CLIENT EDUCATION
• Rare condition except when pregnancies are obtained from SCNT-produced embryos or with hybridization.
• Clients should be aware of risk factors and early signs.

PATIENT CARE
• Close monitoring and supportive care may be required following induction of parturition or abortion.
• Humane euthanasia may be the only option for some advanced cases.

PREVENTION
• Culling
• Do not rebreed to same sire

MISCELLANEOUS

ASSOCIATED CONDITIONS
• Adventitious placentation
• Fetal abnormalities
• Dystocia

AGE-RELATED FACTORS
Hydrallantois is seen in older cows that may lack caruncles due to prior uterine disease or damage.

ZOONOTIC POTENTIAL
N/A

PREGNANCY
• The affected animals (primarily bovine) show signs in mid to late gestation.
• Prognosis for viable offspring is grave for both conditions.

BIOSECURITY
N/A

PRODUCTION MANAGEMENT
• Cull affected animals
• Fetal and placental evaluation in high risk animals (pregnancies from SCNT produced embryos, hybrids)

ABBREVIATIONS
• GI = gastrointestinal
• PGE = prostaglandin E
• PGF = prostaglandin F
• SCNT = somatic cell nuclear transfer

SEE ALSO
• Dystocia: Bovine
• Induction of Parturition
• Reproductive Pharmacology

Suggested Reading

Drost, M. Dystocia and accidents of gestation. In: Hopper RM ed, Bovine Reproduction. Ames: Wiley Blackwell, 2014, pp. 409–15.

Farin PW, Piedrahita JA, Farin CE. Errors in development of fetuses and placentas from in vitro-produced bovine embryos. Theriogenology 2006, 65: 178–91.

Hanna WJB, Scott WD. An outbreak of placental hydrops in beefalo (bison X cattle) herd. Can Vet J 1989, 30: 597–8.

Hillman R, Gilbert RO. Diseases of the uterus. In: Divers TJ, Peek S eds, Rebhun's Diseases of Dairy Cattle. St. Louis: Elsevier, 2007.

Jones SL, Fecteau G. Hydrops uteri in a caprine doe pregnant with goat-sheep hybrid fetuses. J Am Vet Med Assoc 1995, 206: 1920–2.

MacDonald R. Hydrops in a heifer as a result of in-vitro fertilization. Can Vet J 2011, 52: 791–3.

Roberts SJ. Diseases and accidents during the gestation period. In: Roberts SJ, Veterinary Obstetrics and Genital Diseases. Ithaca, NY: Roberts, 1971, pp. 179–83.

Author Clare M. Scully
Consulting Editor Ahmed Tibary

H

HYPOCALCEMIA: BOVINE

BASICS

OVERVIEW
Hypocalcemia, also known as milk fever and postparturient paresis, is a metabolic disease affecting mostly dairy cows which occurs around parturition. It is characterized by low plasma calcium concentration and neuromuscular dysfunction.

INCIDENCE/PREVALENCE
Depending on prepartum feed management and other factors, the incidence of hypocalcemia is highly variable. Subclinical hypocalcemia may range from 25% in primiparous cows to over 53% in multiparous cows. Milk fever may range from 0.7% in primiparous cows to 5% or more in multiparous cows.

GEOGRAPHIC DISTRIBUTION
N/A

SYSTEM AFFECTED
• • Musculoskeletal
• • Digestive
• • Cardiovascular
• • Reproductive

PATHOPHYSIOLOGY
• Calcium is essential for neuromuscular physiology, primarily for the muscular contraction mechanism.
• Circulating concentrations of calcium and phosphorus are precisely regulated by parathyroid hormone (PTH) secreted by the parathyroid glands, calcitonin secreted by the C cells of the thyroid gland, and 1,25-dihydroxycholecalciferol (1,25-[OH]$_2$D; vitamin D) produced by the kidney. Phosphorus is less strictly controlled than is calcium. Both minerals are absorbed in the small intestine, with phosphorus being absorbed in the proximal small intestine.
• Hypocalcemia stimulates production of PTH, which in turn stimulates synthesis of vitamin D by the kidney. The efficiency of calcium absorption is increased by vitamin D. When excess calcium is present, calcitonin inhibits resorption of calcium by the kidney, leading to urinary loss.
• During the final days of gestation, the mammary gland extracts large amounts of calcium from blood for colostrum production. Normally, total plasma contains 3 g of calcium and colostrum contains 2 g of calcium per liter, or 30 g total (15 liters of colostrum). At the same time, fecal and urine losses may account for another 5–8 g of calcium. Additionally, feed intake is markedly depressed in periparturient cows. If a typical nonanionic diet (rich in potassium and sodium and low in chloride and sulfur) is fed to prepartum animals, parathyroid hormone and vitamin D activity are compromised; therefore, calcium absorption and its bioavailability is reduced. This is the result of a more alkaline blood (pH = 7.45) induced by high potassium levels or low content of dietary magnesium. As a result, a negative calcium balance is established with a decrease in the concentration of plasma calcium (<8.0 mg/dL). Signs will depend on the degree of hypocalcemia.

HISTORICAL FINDINGS
• This condition occurs mostly within the first 24–48 hours postpartum, although some high producing multiparous cows will develop clinical hypocalcemia just prior to signs of parturition. Signs will depend on the degree of hypocalcemia. A common history includes a postpartum animal becoming recumbent in the milking parlor just after completion of milking.
• A history of changes within the dry cow ration may precede an increased prevalence of clinical hypocalcemia within a herd. Subclinical hypocalcemia may be suspected in a herd with a high incidence of retained fetal membranes, displaced abomasum, and other postpartum disease.

SIGNALMENT
• Bovine (see separate chapter, Hypocalcemia: Small Ruminant)
• All dairy breeds but highest incidence in Jerseys
• Highest risk in multiparous cows 3rd lactation and greater

PHYSICAL EXAMINATION FINDINGS
• When examining a cow with suspected hypocalcemia, it is judicious to obtain a blood sample to hold for testing in the event she does not respond to calcium treatment.
• Subclinical hypocalcemia is present with blood calcium levels between 5.5 and 8.0 mg/dL. Animals will have decreased feed intake and be at increased risk of secondary diseases such as retained fetal membranes, uterine prolapse, and displaced abomasum.
• Hypocalcemia is considered clinical when neuromuscular signs develop and is generally broken down into three stages:
• Stage I (4.5–5 mg/dL) is short in duration and animals exhibit hypersensitivity, excitability, and muscle tremors. Head bobbing, ear twitching, and fine tremors over flank will be seen. Affected animals have a reduced appetite and most resist walking. If affected animals are willing to move, they tend to be ataxic and fall easily. Animals will proceed into stage II, if treatment is not instituted.
• Stage II (2–4.5 mg/dL) milk fever is characterized by sternal recumbency and the inability to rise. Many cows appear drowsy with a characteristic kink (S-curve) in their neck. The muzzle is dry, ears and other extremities are cold with a body temperature of 97–101°F (36.1–38.3°C), and pupils are dilated. Most affected cows have a faint pulse and the heart rate is increased (80 beats/min). Constipation and rumen stasis are common findings.
• Stage III milk fever is characterized by lateral recumbency and progression to a comatose state. Bloat may result due to an inability to eructate gas. Cardiac output decreases, the heart rate may reach 120 beats/min, and the pulse is nearly undetectable. If treatment is not instituted quickly, affected cows will die from cardiac arrest or respiratory failure within a few hours.

GENETICS
Jersey breed is the most susceptible.

CAUSES AND RISK FACTORS
• Prepartum diets rich in cations (mostly potassium) and low in magnesium, especially in high-producing animals that have had 3 or more parities.
• Management, breed, parity, milk production, nutrition or acid-base status around calving, season, herd size, geographic location.

DIAGNOSIS

DIFFERENTIAL DIAGNOSES
Downer cow syndrome, trauma, lymphosarcoma (spinal), hypomagnesemia, infectious diseases (rabies, listeriosis, BSE, TEME)

CBC/BIOCHEMISTRY/URINALYSIS
Plasma calcium levels for subclinical hypocalcemia are <8.0 mg/dL (<2.0 mmol/L) (see Table 1). In cases with neuromuscular signs, mostly recumbency, Ca levels are below 4.0 mg/dL (1.0 mmol/L). In recumbent animals it is common for CK and AST to be elevated in association with muscular damage.

OTHER LABORATORY TESTS
N/A

IMAGING
N/A

OTHER DIAGNOSTIC PROCEDURES
N/A

PATHOLOGIC FINDINGS
Variable. Muscular necrosis, gastrointestinal atony, and gas accumulation. Pericardial hemorrhages.

TREATMENT

THERAPEUTIC APPROACH
• Treatment efforts are aimed at returning serum calcium to within the normal range. The treatment should be administered as soon as possible to avoid muscular and nerve damage.
• Calcium borogluconate is commonly administered IV but can be administered via subcutaneous and intraperitoneal (IP) routes. Subcutaneous administration allows for slow

Table 1

Blood Serum Analysis of Normal Dairy Cows and Dairy Cows with Milk Fever			
	Mineral (mg/dL)		
Condition	*Calcium*	*Phosphorus*	*Magnesium*
Normal	8.4–10.2	4.6–7.4	1.9–2.6
Normal at parturition	6.8–8.6	3.2–5.5	2.5–3.5
Milk fever			
Stage I	6.2 ± 1.3	2.4 ± 1.4	3.2 ± 0.7
Stage II	5.5 ± 1.3	1.8 ± 1.2	3.1 ± 0.8
Stage III	4.6 ± 1.1	1.6 ± 1.0	3.3 ± 0.8

Note: Mean ± standard deviation.
Adapted from Church DC, The Ruminant Animal. Prospect Heights, IL: Waveland Press, 1993, table 24.1, p. 494.

H

calcium absorption, which may reduce the risk of cardiac arrest. Animals that relapse or fail to respond should be reexamined and treated in 8–12 hours.
• Calcium is directly cardiotoxic; any calcium-containing solution should be administered slowly (over about 10–20 min) during cardiac auscultation. Administration of calcium should be discontinued if dysrhythmias develop. To eradicate cardiac dysrhythmias associated with administration of calcium, atropine can be given intravenously. The cardioexcitatory consequences of intravenous calcium can be reduced by rapid administration of $MgSO_4$.
• In the case of mild parturient paresis, oral calcium can be administered. Oral calcium administration will decrease the risk of cardiotoxicity. The best combination of calcium preparation is calcium propionate in a propylene glycol gel. In order to achieve a 4 g rise in blood calcium levels, oral administration of 50 g of soluble calcium is required. Calcium propionate is a better alternative than calcium chloride.
• The administration of calcium chloride has a tendency to cause a slight metabolic acidosis.

Chronic Cases
• Any case that does not correct immediately with calcium administration should be safely moved to a clean, dry area with adequate bedding, mattresses, or pasture. Muscle and nerve damage from recumbency starts as early as 6 hours after the onset and may be irreversible; therefore, prevention with proper nursing care is imperative. Animals should be assisted to stand and rotated 3–4 times per day and kept on a soft surface.
• For the 15% of parturient paresis cows that do not react to calcium therapy, administer 1α- hydroxycholecalciferol, 1α-$(OH)_3$, a synthetic analog of vitamin D_3. It should be administered at 1 μg/kg of body weight, half IV and half IM.
• The advantages and disadvantages of vitamin D_3 in treating milk fever have been reported elsewhere.

• It is also judicious to test serum phosphorus, potassium and magnesium levels (see Table 1) to rule out concurrent deficiences as causes of recumbency.

SURGICAL CONSIDERATIONS AND TECHNIQUES
N/A

MEDICATIONS

DRUGS OF CHOICE

Injectable
Solutions of calcium salts supplying 10 g of Ca for intravenous application (Ca borogluconate, CMPK) in the case of clinical conditions (recumbency).

Oral
Calcium salts for oral supplementation (calcium propionate 510 g, calcium chloride 300 g) in the case of subclinical conditions. These salts may be accompanied with glucose precursors such as propylene glycol (250–400 mL). Oral calcium may be formulated as a dissolvable salt, gel, or bolus. More recently, fat-coated oral calcium boluses have gained popularity as they are less likely to cause chemical irritation in the esophagus. See "Precautions" regarding oral products.

CONTRAINDICATIONS
N/A

PRECAUTIONS
IV solutions must be applied slowly to avoid cardiac arrest. Some oral products may be irritants (calcium chloride), causing esophageal ulceration, and are therefore not recommended in recumbent animals whose ability to swallow may be impaired. Aspiration pneumonia must be considered as normal neuromuscular function of the oropharyngeal and esophageal regions will be impaired, especially in moderate to severe cases.

POSSIBLE INTERACTIONS
Phosphorus and magnesium metabolism.

FOLLOW-UP

POSSIBLE COMPLICATIONS
In clinical cases without treatment, death is very likely.

EXPECTED COURSE AND PROGNOSIS
Good prognosis when diagnosis and treatment are adequate.

PATIENT CARE
Nursing care and proper handling of the down animal are extremely important. After 30 minutes of IV treatment, recumbent animals should have experienced certain improvement. A second treatment might be recommended. See "Treatment."

PREVENTION
Proper prepartum nutritional management. Anionic salts to establish a cation-anion difference between −25 and −75 mEq/kg of dry matter. This diet will induce a mild metabolic acidosis with a consequent increase in calcium bioavailability. Monitor the anionic diet program by evaluating the urine pH of prepartum cows (~10–20% of the animals) on a weekly basis. Urine pH should be between 6.0 and 7.0, otherwise the diet should be modified. Alternatively, a low calcium diet can be fed prepartum when the forage profile allows.

MISCELLANEOUS

ASSOCIATED CONDITIONS
Gastrointestinal and reproductive conditions such as displacement of abomasums, retained fetal membranes, metritis, and mastitis.

HYPOCALCEMIA: BOVINE   (CONTINUED)

AGE-RELATED FACTORS
Parity 3 or older are more likely to develop this condition.

PRODUCTION MANAGEMENT
See "Prevention"

SYNONYMS
• Milk fever
• Postparturient paresis

ABBREVIATIONS
• BSE = bovine spongiform encephalitis
• IM = intramuscular
• IP = intraperitoneal
• IV = intravenous
• PTH = parathyroid hormone
• TEME = thromboembolic meningoencephalitis

SEE ALSO
• Dairy Nutrition: Ration Guidelines for Milking and Dry Cows (see www.fiveminutevet.com/ruminant)
• Transition Cow Management (see www.fiveminutevet.com/ruminant)

Suggested Reading
Goff P. Calcium and magnesium disorders. Vet Clin North Am Food Anim Pract 2014, 30: 359–81.
National Research Council. Nutrient Requirements of Dairy Cattle, 7th ed. Washington, DC: National Academy Press, 2001.

Author Pedro Melendez
Consulting Editor Kaitlyn A. Lutz
Acknowledgment The author and book editors acknowledge the prior contribution of Douglas C. Donovan.

H

BASICS

OVERVIEW
• Hypocalcemia in ewes and does is most common during the last 4–6 weeks of gestation. The developing ovine/caprine fetus has a relatively high demand for calcium.
• Hypocalcemia may occur during the first 6 weeks of lactation even in the face of relatively low milk yield.
• In dairy goats during lactation, hypocalcemia may occur and can be diagnosed several weeks into lactation.
• Stressful events may precipitate clinical hypocalcemia in sheep and goats.
• Plasma calcium tends to be higher during pregnancy and peaks at 5–7 weeks prepartum in cervidae. In these species, hypocalcemia can be observed 1–2 weeks postpartum.
• Nonparturient hypocalcemia makes up a higher proportion of cases in small ruminants.
• Prompt hypocalcemia therapy reduces the incidence of secondary complications.

INCIDENCE/PREVALENCE
• Typically <5% of animals in a herd or flock are affected, but rates of up to 20% have been documented.
• The incidence of hypocalcemia is increased in ewes or does carrying multiple fetuses during late lactation.
• In one study of the hypocalcemic cases that recovered, approximately 25% required more than one treatment. Ewes that developed hypocalcemia before lambing and that recovered, lost 22% of their lambs, the main reason probably being premature birth.

GEOGRAPHIC DISTRIBUTION
Worldwide

SYSTEMS AFFECTED
• Metabolic
• Musculoskeletal

PATHOPHYSIOLOGY
• Muscular contraction is impaired several ways by hypocalcemia: (1) loss of the membrane-stabilizing effect of calcium on peripheral nerves resulting in hyperesthesia and mild tetany, and (2) impaired role of calcium in the release of acetylcholine at the neuromuscular junction resulting in paralysis due to blockade of the transmission of nerve impulses to the muscle fibers.
• Increased disease susceptibility has been observed around the time of parturition. Low extracellular calcium in vitro decreases phagocytosis and intracellular killing in polymorphonuclear neutrophils.
• In contrast to most species, ruminants must secrete excess phosphate in the saliva and, to a lesser extent, in the urine. A fraction of phosphate excreted in saliva is resorbed in the small intestine while the remainder is eliminated from the body in the feces.

• Sheep with chronic hypomagnesemia also have profound alterations in calcium homeostasis. Hypomagnesemia prevents production or secretion of both PTH and 1,25-dihydroxyvitamin D_3.

HISTORICAL FINDINGS
• Periparturient most common
• History of stressful event (e.g., transport, group handling, adverse weather)

SIGNALMENT
• Potentially all small ruminant species.
• Predominantly female.
• The effect of age and parity is likely related to capacity for milk yield and the ability to mobilize calcium.
• In sheep and goats, the tendency to develop hypocalcemia increases with increasing age.

PHYSICAL EXAMINATION FINDINGS
• Early clinical signs
  ○ Hyperexcitability
  ○ Ataxia
  ○ Tetany
• Later signs
  ○ Dilated pupils with slow PLR
  ○ Mild depression
  ○ Bloat, rumen stasis, and no fecal passage
  ○ Rapid muffled heart sounds
  ○ Recumbency and coma
• Transit tetany may occur in pregnant ewes and lambs following the stress of transportation. Lambs will present with muscle tremors and tetany rather than flaccid paralysis.

GENETICS
N/A

CAUSES AND RISK FACTORS
• Inappropriate calcium homeostasis around the time of parturition.
• The developing fetuses have a high demand for calcium that may exceed dietary intake and availability.
• Excessive ingestion of plants that bind calcium such as oxalates (i.e., beet pulp, alfalfa leaves and sugar beet leaves).

DIAGNOSIS

DIFFERENTIAL DIAGNOSES
• Pregnancy toxemia
• Hypomagnesemia

CBC/BIOCHEMISTRY/URINALYSIS
• Decreased total (<6 mg/dL) or ionized calcium
• Magnesium levels variable but often low (<1.5 mg/dL)

OTHER LABORATORY TESTS
Hypocalcemia may be difficult to differentiate from pregnancy toxemia, so assessment of urine or blood for ketones may be helpful.

IMAGING
N/A

OTHER DIAGNOSTIC PROCEDURES
N/A

PATHOLOGIC FINDINGS
No significant pathologic findings at necropsy are directly attributable to hypocalcemia.

TREATMENT
See "Medications"

MEDICATIONS

DRUGS OF CHOICE
• Calcium: 1 g Ca/45 kg of BW intravenous, response to therapy should be rapid (within 5–10 minutes).
• Subcutaneous or oral calcium may be administered subsequently for a longer-acting effect in severe cases. Care must be taken to administer in small boluses (no more than 50 mL per site) using clean technique or to ensure oral calcium is administered carefully or directly into the rumen (avoid calcium chloride boluses due to esophageal irritation).

CONTRAINDICATIONS
• Subcutaneous calcium may rarely cause irritant reactions or skin sloughing subsequent to administration by this route.
• Steroids should not be used in pregnant animals.

PRECAUTIONS
• IV calcium solutions must be given slowly over 5–7 minutes to avoid cardiac arrhythmia/arrest.
• Appropriate milk and meat withdrawal times must be followed for all compounds administered to food-producing animals.

POSSIBLE INTERACTIONS
N/A

FOLLOW-UP

EXPECTED COURSE AND PROGNOSIS
Animals are expected to recover if treatment is instituted early in the course of disease.

POSSIBLE COMPLICATIONS
Recumbency progressing to death may occur if inadequately treated, or untreated.

CLIENT EDUCATION
Prevention of hypocalcemia through proper transition management should be the focus since clinical and subclinical hypocalcemia will lead to a cascade of negative health implications.

PATIENT CARE
• Response to therapy is suggestive of at least a temporary cure.

H

HYPOCALCEMIA: SMALL RUMINANT

• Recheck calcium +/− magnesium levels if unresponsive to treatment or if relapse occurs.
• Some animals will require multiple treatments, especially if dietary calcium has not been adequately managed.

PREVENTION
• Little work specific to small ruminants is available. Most recommendations are borrowed from prevention strategies in dairy cattle.
  ◦ A continuously increasing plane of nutrition during the last 6 weeks of gestation will increase calcium intake and prevent hypocalcemia and pregnancy toxemia in most cases.
  ◦ Alternatively, limiting calcium intake for 30 days before parturition can be helpful in prevention programs. Utilizing hay from cereal crops rather than alfalfa hay will lower the concentration of calcium in the diet, stimulating mobilization of calcium from bone which may reduce hypocalcemia.
• Avoid stressful events in late gestation.

 MISCELLANEOUS

ASSOCIATED CONDITIONS
• Pregnancy toxemia
• Hypomagnesemia
• Vaginal prolapse—some data would suggest no association

AGE-RELATED FACTORS
• The effect of age and parity is likely related to capacity for milk yield and mobilization of calcium.
• In sheep, the tendency to develop hypocalcemia increases with increasing age.

PREGNANCY
Commonly occurs in all small ruminant species in the last month of gestation.

PRODUCTION MANAGEMENT
This can occur as a herd problem if diet is inappropriate.

ABBREVIATION
• BW = body weight

SEE ALSO
• Body Condition Scoring (see www.fiveminutevet.com/ruminant)
• Ewe Flock Nutrition (see www.fiveminutevet.com/ruminant)
• Grass Tetany/Hypomagnesemia
• Nutrition and Metabolic Diseases: Small Ruminant

Suggested Reading
Brozos C, Mavrogianni VS, Fthenakis GC. Treatment and control of Peri-parturient metabolic diseases: pregnancy toxemia, hypocalcemia, hypomagnesemia. Vet Clin North Am Food Anim Pract 2011, 27: 105–13.

Cockcroft PD, Whiteley P. Hypocalcaemia in 23 ataxic/recumbent ewes: clinical signs and likelihood ratios. Vet Rec 1999, 144: 529–32.
Martens H, Schweigel M. Pathophysiology of grass tetany and other hypomagnesemias: Implications for clinical management. Vet Clin North Am Food Anim Pract 2000, 16: 339–68.
Nosdol G, Waage S. Hypocalcaemia in the ewe. Nord Vet Med 1981, 33: 310–26.
Sweeney HJ, Cuddeford D. An outbreak of hypocalcaemia in ewes associated with dietary mismanagement. Vet Rec 1987, 120: 114.
Author Dusty W. Nagy
Consulting Editor Kaitlyn A. Lutz

BASICS

OVERVIEW
• Simple indigestion is a form of gastrointestinal distress causing transient anorexia, usually with minimal signs of systemic illness.
• Defined as a less severe illness than other forms of rumen (vagal) indigestion.
• Results from an abrupt change in the feed regimen in regard to type, amount, and/or frequency.

INCIDENCE/PREVALENCE
• Simple indigestion is a common disorder of nongrazing animals and is the most common sequela to an abrupt change in ration.
• This condition may present as an individual animal problem, but more often affects several members of a herd.

GEOGRAPHIC DISTRIBUTION
Occurs in regions in which conditions or production systems limit grazing or feed availability.

SYSTEMS AFFECTED
Digestive

PATHOPHYSIOLOGY
• Animals are suddenly exposed to feedstuffs to which they are previously unaccustomed in either type or amount.
• This results in a change in the rumen environment, including pH, as a result of the presence of unusual substrates.
• The rumen microflora change in population as a result of change in feed substrate.
• Microflora then produce fermentation products which have deleterious effects on rumen motility, digestion, and nutrient absorption.
• Simple indigestion can also arise from the accumulation of relatively indigestible feedstuffs in the rumen that can physically impair rumen function.

HISTORICAL FINDINGS
• Change in feeding regimen.
• Acute onset of anorexia of 1–2 days duration, potentially with malodorous diarrhea or reduced fecal production 12–24 hours after signs commence, and decreased milk production in lactating animals.

SIGNALMENT
Any ruminant species of any age, breed or gender are susceptible. Young animals being intensively fed for growth, and adult dairy cattle being fed for production, are at greatest risk.

PHYSICAL EXAMINATION FINDINGS
• Signs are generally less severe and more transient than other rumen indigestion disorders such as grain overload.
• Generally there is minimal evidence of significant systemic illness.
• Rumen motility is typically reduced, reflected by decreased frequency and strength of contractions.
• Rumen fill is nearly normal, but contents are fluid and may slosh with succussion, or the rumen may feel full, firm or doughy on palpation/ballottement.
• Mild bloat may occur.
• Malodorous diarrhea may be noted.
• Vital signs (temperature, pulse, respiration) and demeanor are typically normal.

GENETICS
N/A

CAUSES AND RISK FACTORS
• Condition arises due to an abrupt change in feed type or amount, exposing rumen microflora to substrates to which they are not accustomed, or in greater quantities than those to which they are acclimated.
• This can occur when high-quality feeds are suddenly provided in large amounts or with a change in one or more components.
• Provision of compromised feeds such as those that are moldy or overheated; frosted forages; or incompletely fermented, spoiled, sour silage may also cause indigestion.
• Risk factors include minimal or complete lack of grazing time or hay availability, or accidental exposure to large amounts of novel feeds.

DIAGNOSIS

DIFFERENTIAL DIAGNOSES
• Traumatic reticuloperitonitis
• Left displaced abomasum
• Ketosis
• Lactic acidosis
• Rumen alkalosis
• Rumen putrefaction
• Vagal indigestion
• Peritonitis
• Any early systemic illness causing anorexia

CBC/BIOCHEMISTRY/URINALYSIS
May indicate mild dehydration and prerenal azotemia reflected by increases in serum total protein concentration, hematocrit, urea nitrogen, and creatinine.

OTHER LABORATORY TESTS
• Rumen fluid might display a decrease in size, numbers, and activity of protozoa under light microscopy.
• Rumen fluid pH may be slightly acidic (<6) or alkaline (>7), depending on the nature of the offending feedstuff and the duration of imbalance.
• Prolonged methylene blue reduction time might be evident in rumen fluid samples.

IMAGING
Radiographs or ultrasound might be indicated in some cases to rule out specific differential diagnoses such as traumatic reticuloperitonitis.

OTHER DIAGNOSTIC PROCEDURES
Abdominocentesis might be indicated to rule out peritonitis and other potential differential diagnoses.

PATHOLOGIC FINDINGS
Uncomplicated cases of simple indigestion are transient and rarely result in death.

TREATMENT

THERAPEUTIC APPROACH
• Supportive care (fluid and acid-base therapy, transfaunation) and dietary modifications are typically sufficient to manage uncomplicated cases of simple indigestion.
• Animals with simple indigestion may be treated as outpatients, though valuable animals may warrant hospitalization for monitoring of their condition and to facilitate intervention if their condition should deteriorate.
• Transfaunation with 8–16 L (2–4 gallons) of rumen fluid from a healthy cow can help reestablish normal rumen flora and function.
• The remainder of the herd should be closely monitored for additional incidence.

SURGICAL CONSIDERATIONS AND TECHNIQUES
In cases of simple indigestion, surgery (rumenotomy) is rarely required.

MEDICATIONS

DRUGS OF CHOICE
• If rumen pH alterations are confirmed, acidic pH may be addressed by providing magnesium hydroxide or magnesium oxide (450 g per adult cow) PO or by ororuminal tube; alkalotic pH can be managed by providing acetic acid (4–10 L) PO or by ororuminal tube.
• Administration of mineral oil (4–6 L) by ororuminal tube may reduce absorption and facilitate excretion of offending feedstuffs.
• Probiotic products are frequently used, but their utility is limited due to low volume and narrow spectrum of organisms provided.
• Ruminatorics including nux vomica, ginger and tartar can be used but are likely of limited use.
• Parasympathomimetic agents, such as neostigmine, are not useful in rumen atony, but may stimulate motility in cases where some motility remains.

CONTRAINDICATIONS
• Rumen pH should be confirmed before administering corrective substances. Magnesium hydroxide is contraindicated in absence of rumen acidosis, to avoid iatrogenic systemic alkalinization.

INDIGESTION

• Rumen motility agents are contraindicated if potential obstruction has not been ruled out.

PRECAUTIONS
• Rumen fluid for transfaunation should be obtained from healthy cows only, with regard to biosecurity concerns.
• Appropriate milk and meat withdrawal times must be followed for all compounds administered to food-producing animals.

POSSIBLE INTERACTIONS
N/A

 FOLLOW-UP

EXPECTED COURSE AND PROGNOSIS
• Typical course of anorexia is 1–2 days, with diarrhea occurring 12–24 hours after onset.
• If uncomplicated and managed by removal of offending feedstuffs, prognosis is good.
• Animals return to normal once rumen microflora and fermentation products achieve homeostasis and inhibitory products have been eliminated.
• Transfaunation encourages a more rapid return of a stable rumen environment.

POSSIBLE COMPLICATIONS
• Rumen environment may further deteriorate requiring more intensive therapy.

CLIENT EDUCATION
• Animals being fed for production should be introduced to concentrated feeds gradually and also provided quality forage.
• When new feedstuffs are incorporated into a production system, they should be incorporated prior to full depletion of previous feedstuffs, in order to allow gradual introduction.

• Feed should be inspected immediately prior to feeding for signs of damage or contamination.
• Silage and other stored feeds should be properly protected from environmental damage (moisture, oxygen, feces).

PATIENT CARE
• Oral or parenteral polyionic fluid therapy may be indicated depending on severity of dehydration and acid-base or electrolyte imbalances.
• Offending feedstuffs should be identified and removed.
• Animals should be provided unlimited access to good-quality grass hay or straw.
• Unless the offending feedstuff is inherently damaged (ie. moldy, spoiled, contaminated) it may be reintroduced in small, graduated amounts, along with good-quality hay or other forage source.
• Monitor closely for return to feed in 24–48 hours.

PREVENTION
• Any concentrate feeds should be gradually increased to the desired feeding rate over 10–14 days.
• Avoid rapid changes in feeding practices.
• Provide animals on feed with smaller volumes more frequently, to more closely mimic grazing.

 MISCELLANEOUS

ASSOCIATED CONDITIONS
• Lactic acidosis
• Rumen alkalosis

AGE-RELATED FACTORS
Young animals may be more inclined to overindulge in concentrated feeds.

ZOONOTIC POTENTIAL
N/A

PREGNANCY
Unlikely to be affected in mild disease.

BIOSECURITY
N/A

PRODUCTION MANAGEMENT
• Silage and other processed feeds should be properly prepared and stored to prevent spoilage.
• Animals should be gradually introduced to increasing amounts or different types of feeds.
• New feedstuffs should be ordered and introduced prior to depletion of previous feed to allow for mixing and gradual introduction.

SYNONYMS
N/A

ABBREVIATION
PO = per os

SEE ALSO
• Abomasal Impaction
• Bloat
• Rumen Dysfunction: Alkalosis
• Rumen Fluid Analysis (see www.fiveminutevet.com/ruminant)
• Rumen Transfaunation (see www.fiveminutevet.com/ruminant)
• Ruminal Acidosis

Suggested Reading
Leek BF. Clinical diseases of the rumen: a physiologist's view. Vet Rec 1983, 113: 10–14.
Nagaraja TG, Titgemeyer EC. Ruminal acidosis in beef cattle: the current microbiological and nutritional outlook 1,2. J Dairy Sci 2007, 90: E17–E38.
Author Meredyth L. Jones
Consulting Editor Erica C. McKenzie

BASICS

OVERVIEW
• Induction of parturition involves the pharmacologic initiation of parturition.
• Protocols to induce parturition in ruminants are aimed at mimicking the physiology of normal parturition by either inducing luteolysis to remove the luteal source of progesterone (goats and camelids), initiating hormonal cascades to remove placental progesterone (sheep), or both (cattle).
• Treatment used before term can terminate pregnancy and result in a nonviable fetus.

INCIDENCE/PREVALENCE
N/A

GEOGRAPHIC DISTRIBUTION
Worldwide

SYSTEMS AFFECTED
Reproductive

PATHOPHYSIOLOGY
• Parturition is initiated by fetal stress which leads to cortisol secretion from the fetal adrenal glands.
• Cortisol promotes the conversion of placental progesterone to estradiol, effectively removing placental progesterone and increasing uterine contractility.
• Fetal cortisol also initiates placental synthesis of $PGF2_\alpha$, which causes luteolysis and further decreases progesterone.
• Rising levels of $PGF2_\alpha$ and estradiol cause strong myometrial contractions that apply pressure upon the cervix to simulate oxytocin release (Ferguson's reflex), causing more uterine contractions and facilitating movement of the fetus through the birth canal.

HISTORICAL FINDINGS
• Management decision to synchronize parturitions and enable personnel to more closely attend to the dam and fetus during delivery or to ensure parturition coincides with peak pasture availability in seasonal grazing systems.
• Maternal compromise such as pregnancy toxemia, traumatic injury, or periods of prolonged recumbency.
• Prolonged pregnancy (to prevent dystocia due to fetal oversize) or other abnormalities of pregnancy.
• High risk pregnancies (SCNT embryo transfer).
• Breeding and accurate pregnancy diagnosis dates should be obtained.

SIGNALMENT
Induction of parturition is performed when indicated in all species of ruminants and camelids.

PHYSICAL EXAMINATION FINDINGS
• Normal pregnancy at stage compatible with extrauterine life.
• Mammary gland development and presence of colostrum.
• Findings vary depending on pregnancy disorder in compromised females.

GENETICS
N/A

CAUSES AND RISK FACTORS
Elective procedure or indicated in cases of compromised pregnancy

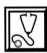

DIAGNOSIS

DIFFERENTIAL DIAGNOSES
N/A

CBC/BIOCHEMSTRY/URINALYSIS
Useful in cases of dam compromise

OTHER LABORATORY TESTS
N/A

IMAGING
Ultrasonography to determine viability of the fetus

OTHER DIAGNOSTIC PROCEDURES
N/A

PATHOLOGIC FINDINGS
Depends on reason for induction

TREATMENT

THERAPEUTIC APPROACH
Cattle
• Long- or short-acting corticosteroids, $PGF2_\alpha$, or a combination of $PGF2_\alpha$ and dexamethasone.
• Calf survival is optimal when parturition is induced no earlier than 2 weeks prior to gestational term.
• Induction of parturition with short-acting corticosteroids and/or prostaglandin results in a high rate (50–75%) of retained fetal membranes due to lack of placental maturation.

Sheep
• Normal gestation length in sheep is 145–150 days. Breeding dates should be accurate.
• CL functions as a source of progesterone only until 50–60 day gestation. At term, the placenta is the primary source of progesterone and prostaglandin alone is ineffective at inducing parturition.
• Induction can be achieved with dexamethasone after 137 days gestation. However, fetal viability is better if treatment is given after 142 days.

Goats
• Normal gestation length in goats is 147–155 days. Breeding dates should be accurate.
• Goats are CL-dependent throughout gestation and induction of parturition may be achieved with a luteolytic dose of $PGF2_\alpha$.
• In does suffering from pregnancy toxemia, treatment with dexamethasone (10–20 mg IM) prior to induction with $PGF2_\alpha$ may enhance maturation of fetal lungs and improve neonatal survival.
• Retained fetal membranes are rare in goats following induction of parturition.

Camelids
• Normal gestation length is highly variable. Induction of parturition should only be considered if there is sufficient mammary development and presence of colostrum.
• Camelids are CL-dependent throughout gestation. $PGF2_\alpha$ or analogs induce abortion or parturition reliably.

SURGICAL CONSIDERATIONS AND TECHNIQUES
Induction of parturition may be an initial step before planned cesarean section.

I

MEDICATIONS

DRUGS OF CHOICE
Cattle
• Long-acting corticosteroids should only be used when calf survival is not the primary goal of induction. Reported calf survival rates are around 64%. Fetal dysmaturity contributes to high calf mortality rates.
  ○ Dexamethasone trimethylacetate (25–30 mg IM) or triamcinolone acetonide (4–8 mg IM) can be administered 2–4 weeks prior to term. Timing of parturition after injection is variable, although most will calve within 10–14 days following induction (range = 3–30 days).
  ○ Calving occurs 48–72 hours after administration of $PGF2_\alpha$ (dinoprost tromethamine, 25 mg IM or SC) or cloprostenol sodium (500 μg IM) 9–14 days following induction with a long-acting corticosteroid.
• Short-acting corticosteroids, dexamethasone (20–30 mg IM), can be used to induce parturition within 2 weeks of gestational term with no increase in dystocia rates or neonatal mortality. Response rate to a single injection is 80–90% with cows calving 24–72 hours following administration.
• $PGF2_\alpha$ (dinoprost, 25 mg IM or SC) or cloprostenol sodium (500 μg IM) can be used for induction of parturition in the last 2 weeks of gestation. Parturition occurs within 24–72 hours in 80–90% of cows after a single injection.

INDUCTION OF PARTURITION

• The combination of corticosteroids and prostaglandin results in a more predictable time from administration to onset of parturition (25–42 hours) and a lower rate of induction failure.

Sheep
Dexamethasone (15–20 mg IM) will result in onset of parturition 36–48 hours following administration.

Goats
• Administration of PGF2$_\alpha$ (dinoprost, 15 mg IM) or cloprostenol sodium (75–100 µg IM) results in onset of parturition within 30–35 hours, on average.
• Although lower doses of prostaglandin (dinoprost, 2.5–5 mg) have been used successfully to induce parturition in goats, a higher dose of 15 mg results in a more reliable and predictable onset of parturition.

Camelids
• A luteolytic dose of PGF2$_\alpha$ (dinoprost, 5 mg IM) or analog (cloprostenol sodium, 250 µg IM) can be used to induce parturition.
• Parturition will occur, on average, 20 hours after prostaglandin injection with a range of 8–30 hours.
• Fetal viability may be assessed using transabdominal ultrasonography at 12 and 20 hours post-induction if parturition has not occurred. If fetal distress is suspected or parturition has not occurred by 24 hours post-induction, a C-section is indicated.

CONTRAINDICATIONS
• Appropriate milk and meat withdrawal times must be followed.
• Dexamethasone is contraindicated in induction of parturition in camelids due to an association with fetal death.
• In camelids, it is important to rule out uterine torsion and ensure that colostrum is present in the udder prior to induction of parturition. Viscous, sticky colostrum is most likely to result in adequate transfer of passive immunity to the neonate following parturition. In compromised females, synthetic analogs should be used for induction as natural prostaglandin (dinoprost) may cause respiratory distress or pulmonary edema and its use should be avoided.

PRECAUTIONS
Accuracy of breeding dates and viability of the fetus should be verified before induction.

POSSIBLE INTERACTIONS
Induction of parturition in compromised females may result in dystocia. Measures should be taken to proceed with cesarean section in case of complications.

FOLLOW-UP

EXPECTED COURSE AND PROGNOSIS
Response to induction of parturition treatment is very reliable if the prerequisite conditions are fulfilled.

POSSIBLE COMPLICATIONS
• Retained placenta is the major complication. Lower rates of retained placenta are observed with long-acting corticosteroids than with short-acting ones because they allow more time for placental maturation prior to parturition.
• Retained fetal membranes are uncommon in ewes following induction of parturition.
• Females with compromised health or abnormal pregnancies are at higher risk for dystocia.

CLIENT EDUCATION
• Natural parturition should be promoted whenever possible.
• Proper breeding record keeping.
• Welfare issues are raised in some countries.

PATIENT CARE
• Depends on reason for induction and complications.
• Monitor fetal viability, and emergency cesarean section should be planned if any complications arise.

PREVENTION
N/A

MISCELLANEOUS

ASSOCIATED CONDITIONS
Retained fetal membranes

AGE-RELATED FACTORS
N/A

ZOONOTIC POTENTIAL
N/A

PREGNANCY
N/A

BIOSECURITY
N/A

PRODUCTION MANAGEMENT
Farms practicing control measures for diseases that can be transmitted through colostrum, including mycoplasma and caprine arthritis and encephalitis virus, may elect to induce parturition to ensure the kidding can be attended and the kid can be removed from the doe prior to ingestion of colostrum.

SYNONYMS
N/A

ABBREVIATIONS
• CL = corpus luteum
• IM = intramuscular
• PGF2$_\alpha$ = prostaglandin F2$_\alpha$
• SC = subcutaneous

SEE ALSO
• Dystocia: Bovine
• Dystocia: Camelid
• Dystocia: Small Ruminant
• Hydrops
• Pregnancy Toxemia: Bovine
• Pregnancy Toxemia: Camelid
• Pregnancy Toxemia: Small Ruminant
• Prolonged Pregnancy
• Retained Placenta

Suggested Reading
Barth A. Inducing parturition or abortion in cattle. In: Hopper RM ed, Bovine Reproduction. Ames: Wiley, 2015.
Edmondson MA, Roberts JF, Baird AN, Bychawski S, Pugh DG. Theriogenology of sheep and goats. In: Pugh DG, Baird AN eds, Sheep and Goat Medicine. Maryland Heights, MO: Elsevier, 2012.
Rodriguez JS, Pearson LK, Tibary A. Parturition and obstetrics. In: Cebra C, Anderson DE, Tibary A, Van Saun RJ, Johnson LW eds, Llama and Alpaca Care. St. Louis: Elsevier, 2014.
Romano JE, Rodas E, Ferreira A. Timing of prostaglandin F$_{2\alpha}$ administration for induction of parturition in dairy goats. Small Rumin Res 2001, 42: 199–202.
Author Jennifer N. Roberts
Consulting Editor Ahmed Tibary

INFECTIOUS BOVINE RHINOTRACHEITIS

BASICS

OVERVIEW
• Infectious bovine rhinotracheitis (IBR) is a mild to severe upper respiratory disease in cattle caused by bovine herpesvirus 1 (BHV-1). This viral infection is one of the viral factors in bovine respiratory disease complex.
• BHV-1 can also cause conjunctivitis, reproductive disease, and abortion.
• Although of the same antigenic type, respiratory and genital strains can be differentiated by molecular methods and have been divided into subtypes BHV-1.1 (respiratory) and BHV-1.2 (genital). It is uncommon to see both strains circulating concurrently within the same herd.
• Bovine herpesvirus 5 (BHV-5), a cause of viral encephalitis, was previously classified as another variant of BHV-1 (BHV-1.3) but has since been given its own designation.

INCIDENCE/PREVALENCE
• BHV-1 is endemic in cattle.
• Symptoms in BHV-1 infected calves can vary from subclinical to severe disease with 100% morbidity and 10% mortality.
• Nonvaccinated pregnant cattle are highly susceptible to BHV-1 infection and up to 25% can abort (so-called "abortion storm").

GEOGRAPHIC DISTRIBUTION
Worldwide. Several European countries and regions within the European Union have achieved "IBR-free" status; however, sporadic outbreaks still occur in states contiguous with infected areas.

SYSTEMS AFFECTED
• Nervous
• Ophthalmic
• Respiratory
• Reproductive

PATHOPHYSIOLOGY
• BHV-1 is spread through nasal exudate, droplets, genital secretions, embryos, semen, and fetal fluids. BHV-1 multiplies in the nasal cavities and upper respiratory tract, resulting in rhinitis, laryngitis, and tracheitis.
• The virus spreads from the nasal cavity to the ocular system by the lacrimal gland. BHV-1 induces damage to the upper respiratory tract (URT) epithelium and conjunctiva of the eye (Figure 1).
• The damage to URT epithelium coupled with inflammatory changes increases the susceptibility of the lung to secondary bacterial infection.
• Conjunctivitis results from inflammation and edema of the conjunctiva.
• BHV-1 can induce late-term abortions in pregnant cattle by causing a viremia that results in BHV-1 infection of the ovary, placenta, and the corpus luteum (Figure 1).

Clinical Forms of IBR

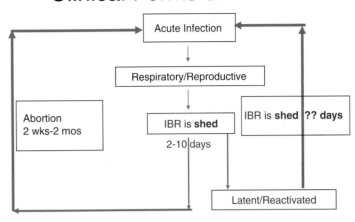

Figure 1.

Clinical Outcomes of IBR Infection.

The genital strain of BHV-1 is associated with genital tract infections of both the male [infectious pustular balanoposthitis (IPB)] and female [infectious pustular vulvovaginitis (IPV)].
• Once animals are infected with BHV-1, the virus spreads to the nervous system, becomes latently infected in the nervous and lymphoid system, and the animals are a lifelong source of infectious virus. The site of latent infection can vary depending on the initial tissue infected.

SIGNALMENT
• Bovine
• IBR is seldom seen in calves <6 months of age and is most prevalent and severe in animals between 6 and 18 months of age.
• Goats and buffalo can act as reservoirs for BHV-1.

PHYSICAL EXAMINATION FINDINGS
• Clinical signs of rhinotracheitis can occur within one or two days of infection and are characterized by a mucopurulent nasal discharge, sneezing, conjunctivitis, and ulcerative lesions in the nasal mucosa.
• An increased rectal temperature (104–108°F; 40–42°C) often occurs from 2 to 7 days following infection.
• Anorexia with depression occur early following infection. A cough may be observed later in the course.
• Secondary pneumonia with bacterial pathogens (*Mannheimia haemolytica, Pasteurella multicida, Histophilus somni*) or *Mycoplasma bovis* is a frequently sequela.
• Conjunctivitis can occur with respiratory disease or it may appear alone. Conjunctivitis originates from the corneoscleral line and is usually bilateral.
• Abortion usually occurs in the last trimester of gestation (range 4–8 months) in response to the respiratory strain (BHV-1.1) rather

than an extension of the genital strain (BHV-1.2) into the fetoplacental unit. Fetal death occurs within 48 hours of viral invasion of the reproductive tract but expulsion may take up to 7 days, resulting in pronounced fetal autolysis.

CAUSES AND RISK FACTORS
• BHV-1 is an enveloped double-stranded DNA virus in the subfamily alphaherpesvirus of the Herpesvirus family. The virus is easily inactivated by desiccation, heat, and disinfectants.
• Stress (weaning, shipping, etc.) will increase the risk. Maternal antibody will inhibit vaccine response. Dexamethasone administration has been shown to reactivate latent infections, resulting in viral shedding and potentially clinical disease.

DIAGNOSIS

DIFFERENTIAL DIAGNOSES
• Three other bovine viruses—bovine viral diarrhea virus, bovine respiratory syncytial virus (BRSV), and bovine parainfluenza-3 virus (PI-3)—commonly cause similar respiratory disease.
• BVDV is associated with oral ulcers, mucopurulent discharge and upper respiratory disease.
• BRSV is characterized by increasing harshness in respiratory sounds to severe distress with dyspnea, forced expiration, and open-mouth breathing. Spontaneous cough can be easily induced and can vary from dry and nonproductive to moist.
• PI-3 infection is usually a mild lower respiratory disease.
• Bovine coronavirus (BCV) has also been associated with respiratory disease. In younger

I

calves it is also seen with calves suffering from enteritis and diarrhea. BCV in 5- to 13-month-old cattle causes symptoms of dyspnea, nasal discharge, and increased respiratory rate.
• Abortion: The differential diagnosis would include BVDV, mycotic abortion, *Neospora caninum*, and leptospirosis.

CBC/BIOCHEMSTRY/URINALYSIS
N/A

OTHER LABORATORY TESTS
• BHV-1 is readily detected by virus isolation. Clinical specimens should be collected during the febrile, acute phase of infection. Respiratory and ocular specimens can be collected antemortem using swabs. Swabs can also be used for the detection of genital infections. On postmortem, virus isolation samples from IBR animals can be collected from the upper respiratory tract and trachea.
• From aborted fetuses, the liver, adrenal, kidney, and lung are the preferred tissues. However, the marked fetal autolysis that often accompanies abortion can make virus isolation more difficult in these tissues. In animals with encephalitis, several regions (olfactory lobes, midbrain, cortex, etc.) should be sampled.
• BHV-1 can also be detected using polymerase chain reaction (PCR).
• Other procedures that have proved useful in detection of BHV-1 are fluorescent antibody tests of fresh tissue and immunohistochemistry staining of cell cultures or formalin-fixed paraffin embedded tissues. Intranuclear inclusion bodies are often present in the liver of BHV-1 infected fetuses.
• A rise in serum neutralizing antibody titer also can be used to confirm BHV-1 infection. Paired serum samples collected 2–3 weeks apart are necessary; a single sample, even if it has a high titer, is of little value. It is not possible to detect a rising antibody titer in abortions, because infection generally occurs a considerable length of time before the abortion, and titers are already maximal. BHV-1 ELISA antibody detection tests are also available.
• The presence of characteristic venereal lesions is sufficient for a clinical diagnosis of the genital strain.

PATHOLOGIC FINDINGS
• Gross lesions of uncomplicated IBR are restricted to the upper respiratory tract and trachea. Petechial to ecchymotic hemorrhages with edema are found in the mucus membranes of the nasal cavity and the sinuses.
• There may be focal areas of necrosis in the nose, pharynx, larynx, and trachea that may coalesce to form plaques. The sinuses may be filled with a serous or serofibrinous exudate. As the disease progresses, the pharynx becomes covered with a serofibrinous exudate, and blood-tinged fluid may be found in the trachea.

• The pharyngeal and pulmonary lymph nodes may be acutely swollen and hemorrhagic. The tracheitis may extend into the bronchi and bronchioles; when this occurs, epithelium is sloughed in the airways. In animals with bacterial bronchopneumonia, the viral lesions are often masked. Aborted fetuses may have pale, focal, necrotic lesions in all tissues, which are especially visible in the liver, and serosanguinous fluid in the body cavities. Placental edema is sometimes seen.
• Histologic examination of IBR tissues reveals acute catarrhal inflammation of the mucosa with rare inclusion bodies.
• In encephalitic calves, histologic changes consisted of a widespread nonsuppurative meningoencephalitis, more severe in the anterior cerebrum, the dorsolateral cortex and, to a lesser extent, the posterior cerebrum and the midbrain. The lesions are characterized by gliosis, disruption of the neuropil and perivascular cuffing, consisting of macrophages, histiocytes, and lymphocytes.
• In aborted fetuses, intranuclear inclusion bodies are often present in the liver. Marked autolysis of aborted fetuses is common, which can complicate histologic examination.

TREATMENT
THERAPEUTIC APPROACH
The therapy for IBR is supportive. Severely diseased animals that are dehydrated may receive oral and/or intravenous fluids.

MEDICATIONS
DRUGS OF CHOICE
• Nonsteroidal anti-inflammatory drugs (NSAIDs) may have some benefit to lessen the severity of BHV-1 disease.
• Antimicrobial treatment is used to reduce secondary bacterial infections.

FOLLOW-UP
EXPECTED COURSE AND PROGNOSIS
• Uncomplicated BHV-1 respiratory infections will resolve in 5–7 days.
• Animals that have secondary infections usually will develop bronchopneumonia with varying levels of morbidity and mortality.

POSSIBLE COMPLICATIONS
• Intramuscular (IM) modified-live virus (MLV) BHV-1 vaccines may cause abortion in pregnant cattle.
• Maternal antibodies in calves interfere with development of an effective IBR immune response with parenterally administered MLV

vaccines. Maternal antibodies have no effect on intranasal (IN) MLV vaccines.

PATIENT CARE
• Respiratory characteristics along with rectal body temperature should be frequently monitored to assess IBR clinical progression and also the development of secondary bacterial infections that would result in bovine respiratory disease complex (BRDC).
• Minimize handling of animals and use preventive vaccines.

PREVENTION
• Vaccination is an important part of a BHV-1 control plan. Both MLV and inactivated virus BHV-1 vaccines are on the market. The MLV vaccines are available as either parenteral (IM or subcutaneous, SC) or intranasal (IN) vaccines.
• Use of MLV vaccines is not without risk due to persistence of the virus and its potential for reactivation.
• Eradication of the virus is possible by serologic testing and culling reactors. Eradication programs have been implemented in Europe. To aid in eradication, deletion mutant vaccines have been developed that permit antibody discrimination between BHV-1 vaccine and natural exposure. BHV-1 vaccines are cross-reactive and should be efficacious against BHV-5.

MISCELLANEOUS
ASSOCIATED CONDITIONS
BRDC is a frequent sequela to IBR. Retained placenta and metritis are possible sequelae to BHV-1 abortion.

AGE-RELATED FACTORS
A rare generalized disease may occur in neonatal calves <2 weeks of age. Most IBR disease is seen in animals >6 months of age.

ZOONOTIC POTENTIAL
N/A

PREGNANCY
BHV-1 infections result in late-term abortions that can occur as long as 100 days following infection.

BIOSECURITY
BHV-1 survives very poorly in the environment and is susceptible to UV light, desiccation, heat, and disinfectants. The virus will survive better in the winter. Animals exhibiting clinical signs of IBR should be isolated from other cattle as transmission of these viruses occurs by the oronasal route. Semen and embryos should be from BHV-1-free donors or prepared according to IETS guidelines for the control of infectious diseases.

(CONTINUED) **INFECTIOUS BOVINE RHINOTRACHEITIS**

PRODUCTION MANAGEMENT
In herds with a history of IBR or BHV-1 abortion, a BHV-1 vaccine program should be implemented

SYNONYMS
Rednose, IBR

ABBREVIATIONS
- BHV-1 = bovine herpesvirus 1
- ELISA = enzyme-linked immunosorbent assay
- IBR = infectious bovine rhinotracheitis
- IETS = International Embryo Technology Society
- IM = intramuscular
- IN = intranasal
- MLV = modified-live virus
- IPB = infectious pustular balanoposthitis
- IPV = infectious pustular vulvovaginitis
- PCR = polymerase chain reaction
- SC = subcutaneous
- UPT = upper respiratory tract

SEE ALSO
- Abortion: Viral, Fungal, and Nutritional
- Bovine Respiratory Syncytial Virus
- Bovine Viral Diarrhea Virus
- Coronavirus
- Leptospirosis
- Neosporosis
- Nonsteroidal Anti-inflammatory Drugs (NSAIDs) (see www.fiveminutevet.com/ruminant)

Suggested Reading
Fulton RW, Briggs RE, Payton ME, et al. Maternally derived humoral immunity to bovine viral diarrhea virus (BVDV) 1a, BVDV1b, BVDV2, bovine herpesvirus-1, parainfluenza-3 virus bovine respiratory syncytial virus, *Mannheimia haemolytica* and *Pasteurella multocida* in beef calves, antibody decline by half-life studies and effect on response to vaccination. Vaccine 2004, 22: 643–9.

Jones C. Herpes simplex virus type 1 and bovine herpesvirus 1 latency. Clin Microbiol Rev 2003, 16: 79–95.
Meyer G, Lemaire M, Ros C, et al. Comparative pathogenesis of acute and latent infections of calves with bovine herpesvirus types 1 and 5. Arch Virol 2001, 146: 633–52.
Zimmerman AD, Buterbaugh RE, Herbert JM, et al. Efficacy of bovine herpesvirus-1 inactivated vaccine against abortion and stillbirth in pregnant heifers. J Am Vet Med Assoc 2007, 231: 1386–9.

Author Christine M. Winslow
Consulting Editor Christopher C.L. Chase
Acknowledgment The author and book editors acknowledge the prior contribution of Christopher C.L. Chase and Sagar Goyal.

I

INFECTIOUS NECROTIC HEPATITIS

BASICS

OVERVIEW
Infectious necrotic hepatitis is a disease affecting mainly ruminant animals on pasture and causing sudden death. Rare cases have been reported in horses.

INCIDENCE/PREVALENCE
• Tends to be a seasonal disease related to the liver fluke life cycle, occurring in the warmer months when fluke transmission is active. Cases may, however, occur throughout the year. Occasionally, cases of necrotic hepatitis have been reported in animals without liver fluke.
• Incidence in affected sheep flocks is usually low, but the lethality of affected animals is close to 100%. Individual cases of the disease occur rarely in cattle and horses.

GEOGRAPHIC DISTRIBUTION
• Worldwide wherever liver flukes are present and occasionally in liver fluke-free areas.
• Important problem in Australia, New Zealand, and several South American countries; lesser importance in Europe, the United Kingdom, and the United States.

SYSTEMS AFFECTED
Multisystemic

PATHOPHYSIOLOGY
• *Clostridium novyi* type B is a Gram-positive spore-forming anaerobic bacterium, which may be found in soil, where the spores are very resistant to environmental conditions and can survive for long periods of time. The spores are more prevalent and resistant in poorly drained pastures with alkaline water pH. The spores are ingested by animals and absorbed through the intestinal mucosa into the bloodstream, reaching the liver via the portal circulation. In the liver, they are phagocytized by Kupffer cells, in the cytoplasm of which they can survive for several years.
• Liver damage, typically from larval migration of *Fasciola hepatica*, and occasionally from other liver parasites such as *Fascioloides magna*, *Dicrocoelium dendriticum* and *Cysticercus tenuicolis*, produces anaerobic conditions, allowing the clostridial spores to germinate and proliferate, producing exotoxins, mainly lethal and edema-inducing alpha-toxin and, to a lesser extent, the necrotizing and hemolytic beta-toxin, which cause coagulative necrosis in the liver. The exotoxins enter the general circulation, damaging vascular endothelium in multiple organs.

HISTORICAL FINDINGS
• Sudden death is the most common presentation.
• Presence of liver fluke in the flock is common.

SIGNALMENT
• Mainly sheep. Occasionally cattle.
• Mostly animals >1 year but can occasionally affect younger animals. Usually animals in good body condition.

PHYSICAL EXAMINATION FINDINGS
• Animals most often found dead, in ventral recumbency.
• When observed, clinical signs are nonspecific and include reluctance to move, weakness, anorexia, hyperthermia, tachypnea, tachycardia, and eventual recumbency. Affected animals tend to get separated from the flock. Jaundice and hemoglobinuria are not observed.

GENETICS
The so-called molecular Koch postulates have not been fulfilled for necrotic hepatitis and the definitive role of the toxins mentioned above in the virulence of *C. novyi* type B remains, therefore, unconfirmed.

CAUSES AND RISK FACTORS
• Causes: Toxins alpha and, to a lesser extent beta, produced by *Clostridium novyi* type B proliferating in liver tissue damaged by migrating liver flukes or, occasionally yet unidentified factors.
• Risk factors: *Fasciola hepatica*, other liver parasites or unidentified factors. Lack of or improper *C. novyi* type B vaccination.

DIAGNOSIS

DIFFERENTIAL DIAGNOSES
• Bacillary hemoglobinuria. Icterus and hemoglobinuria characteristic of bacillary hemoglobinuria is not usually seen in necrotic hepatitis.
• Other diseases causing sudden death: anthrax, toxic plants, others.

CBC/BIOCHEMISTRY/URINALYSIS
Neutrophilia with left shift, metabolic acidosis, azotemia, and increase in liver and muscle enzymes.

OTHER LABORATORY TESTS
• Anaerobic culture followed by PCR.
• PCR.
• Fluorescent antibody test.
• Gram-stain and microscopic inspection of an impression smear of the liver shows numerous large Gram-positive rods with central or subterminal spores.
• Histopathology and immunohistochemistry.

PATHOLOGIC FINDINGS
• Foci of coagulative necrosis in the liver, well delimited, usually small and multifocal.
• Migrating fluke lesions in the liver.
• Congested subcutaneous blood vessels giving a dark aspect to the carcass ("black disease").

• Blood-tinged fluid in all body cavities (urine appears normal in color; no hemoglobinuria).

TREATMENT

THERAPEUTIC APPROACH
• Rarely treated since the disease is usually acute and animals are frequently found dead.
• High doses of procaine penicillin and supportive care. Antibiotic effectiveness is usually poor due to the presence of toxins in tissues and bloodstream.

MEDICATIONS

DRUGS OF CHOICE
• Penicillin 20,000–40,000 IU/kg IV q6h.
• Clorsulon 7 mg/kg, PO.
• Mass medicate herd with long-acting penicillin or tetracycline when cases occur. Flukicide use (e.g., clorsulon).
• Vaccinate flock/herd.

CONTRAINDICATIONS
Appropriate milk and meat withdrawal times must be followed for all compounds administered to food-producing animals.

FOLLOW-UP

EXPECTED COURSE AND PROGNOSIS
• Prognosis is grave in animals showing clinical signs.
• Rapid clinical course in sheep, usually found dead before clinical signs noted.
• Short clinical course in cattle, with nonspecific clinical signs (depression, anorexia), occasionally seen just before death.

CLIENT EDUCATION
• Routine vaccination against clostridia, making sure *C. novyi* type B antigens are included in the vaccine used.
• Control of liver fluke infestation by pasture management, limiting access to streams and ponds, and strategic flukicide treatment.

PATIENT CARE
Restrict movement of animals being treated, since stress of physical exertion can precipitate sudden death.

PREVENTION
• Vaccination with clostridial toxoid with booster in 4–6 weeks and annual revaccination, preferably in early spring at least 1 month before expected fluke exposure.
• Use of flukicides in animals.
• The effectiveness of the use of molluskicides in streams and drainage of marshy areas is very limited.

MISCELLANEOUS

ASSOCIATED CONDITIONS
Fascioliasis

AGE-RELATED FACTORS
Typically adult animals 1 year and older

ZOONOTIC POTENTIAL
None known

BIOSECURITY
Carcasses should be deeply buried, burned, or removed from the premises to avoid spread of spores.

SYNONYM
Black disease

ABBREVIATIONS
• IV = intravenous
• PCR = polymerase chain reaction
• PO = per os, by mouth

SEE ALSO
• Anthrax
• Bacillary Hemoglobinuria
• Body Condition Scoring: Sheep (see www.fiveminutevet.com/ruminant)
• Liver Flukes
• Serology (see www.fiveminutevet.com/ruminant)

Suggested Reading
Bagadi HO, Sewell MM. An epidemiological survey of infectious necrotic hepatitis (black disease) of sheep in Southern Scotland. Res Vet Sci 1973, 15: 49–53.

Navarro M, Uzal FA. Infectious necrotic hepatitis. In: Uzal FA, Prescott J, Songer G, Popoff M eds, Clostridial Diseases of Animals. Ames: Wiley Blackwell, forthcoming.

Smith BP, ed. Large Animal Internal Medicine, 3rd ed. St. Louis: Mosby, 2002, pp. 796–8.

Uzal FA, Olaechea FV, VannelliSA. Un caso de hepatitis infecciosa necrosante en oveja sin *Fasciola hepatica*. Rev Med Vet 1996, 77: 377–9.

Whitfield LK, Cypher E, Gordon S, et al. Necrotic hepatitis associated with *Clostridium novyi* infection (black disease) in a horse in New Zealand. N Z Vet J 2015, 63: 177–9.

Author Francisco A. Uzal
Consulting Editor Christopher C.L. Chase

I

INFECTIOUS PUSTULAR VULVOVAGINITIS

BASICS

OVERVIEW
- Infectious pustular vulvovaginitis (IPV) is characterized by vulvitis and vaginitis and it is one of the granular venereal diseases.
- IPV is caused by alphaherpesvirus, bovine herpes virus (BoHV) type 1, subtype 2, of the Herpesviridae family.
- BoHV-1 is divided in two subtypes (BoHV-1.1 and BoHV-1.2) according to genetic differences and the systems that they affect.
- BoHV-1.1 affects the respiratory system causing infectious bovine rhinotracheitis (IBR), while BoHV-1.2 affects both the respiratory, causing IPV in females and infectious pustular balanoposthitis (IPB) in males.
- BoHV-5, which is responsible for the encephalitic form of the disease, was previously classified as BoHV-1.3.
- IPV and IBR rarely occur concurrently within the same herd.

INCIDENCE/PREVALENCE
- IPV was considered endemic in Europe during the 1960s and 1970s. Control measures (vaccination and elimination of serologically positive animals) have greatly reduced its prevalence and the disease has been completely eradicated in some countries.
- Seroprevalence surveys have indicated that 10–50% of cattle may be serologically positive for BoHV, but the prevalence depends on vaccination practices.

GEOGRAPHIC DISTRIBUTION
Bovine herpesvirus has been isolated in Africa, Asia, North America, Australia, New Zealand, and Europe.

PATHOPHYSIOLOGY
- The virus establishes latency in sacral spinal ganglia following genital infection and may reactivate, resulting in viremia and shedding.
- The incubation period for BoHV-1.2 is usually between 1 and 3 days.
- The virus produces an acute catarrhal inflammation with a neutrophilic infiltration of the mucosa and lymphocytic and plasmocytic infiltration of the submucosa.
- Experimental infection in heifers results in oophoritis, decreased luteal function, and early pregnancy loss. Cervicitis and endometritis have been reported. The inflammatory process may result in short cycles and, rarely, abortion.
- Insemination with virus-contaminated semen results in poor-quality embryos.

HISTORICAL FINDINGS
- Introduction of new animals or untested semen
- Poor reproductive performance (return to estrus after AI)

- Clinical signs: Frequent posturing for urination, constant tail twitching

SIGNALMENT
- Species affected include bovine, ovine, and wild ruminants.
- Animals of breeding age are more likely to be infected.
- Nonbred animals can also be affected.
- Bovine females infected with BoHV-1.2 usually develop IPV.
- Male infected with BoHV-1.2 develop IPB.

PHYSICAL EXAMINATION FINDINGS
- Vulvitis and vaginitis: Swelling of the vulva and hyperemic mucosa surface of the vestibular area.
- Mucopurulent vaginal secretion may develop secondary to bacterial infection.
- Lymphoid tissue develops pustules that become small ulcers (<3 mm) and may result in coalescing erosions. The vulvar mucosa in the latter stages of the disease presents small but numerous necrotic focal areas.

GENETICS
- Bovine herpesvirus 1 is the herpesvirus serologically related to IBR and IPV/IPB, and is divided in two main subtypes according to genetic differences (BoHV-1.1 and BoHV-1.2).
- The genetic differences may be responsible for the diverse epidemiologic and pathologic patterns of virus behavior. While BoHV-1.1 is related to IBR, the respiratory form of the disease, BoHV-1.2, is related to the genital form of the ailment (IPV/IPB).
- Bovine herpesvirus 1.2b is a different strain of the virus and it is usually related to the occurrence of IPV/IPB and outbreaks of low/medium virulence of IBR.
- Some specific genotypes of bovine animals are more resistant to challenges with BoHV-1, developing less severe disease. This is an indication that breeding programs that increase the occurrence of these specific genes may alter the sensitivity of populations to BoHV-1 infection.

CAUSES AND RISK FACTORS
- The causative agent in cattle is bovine herpesvirus type 1 subtype 2 (BoHV-1.2). A similar disease has been described in goats, caused by caprine herpesvirus 1 (CpHV-1).
- IPV is transmitted directly by coitus or artificial insemination.
- Mechanical means are also possibilities for the transmission of the causal agent.
- Transmission of BoHV-1.2 is rapid and can affect 60–90% of the herd.
- Reactivation of latent virus is observed following stress (parturition, transport, inclement weather).
- Dexamethasone administration can cause recrudescence of clinical disease and viral shedding.

DIAGNOSIS

DIFFERENTIAL DIAGNOSES
- Granular venereal disease caused by *mycoplasma*, *ureaplasma*, *Histophilus somni*, and *T. pyogenes*
- Transmissible fibropapilloma
- Granular vulvitis
- Necrotic vulvitis

CBC/BIOCHEMISTRY/URINALYSIS
N/A

OTHER LABORATORY TESTS
- Indirect: Serology—ELISA and virus neutralization test; skin test—delayed-type hypersensitivity (DTH) reaction
- Direct: Fluorescent microscope; polymerase chain reaction (PCR)

IMAGING
N/A

OTHER DIAGNOSTIC PROCEDURES
N/A

PATHOLOGIC FINDINGS
- Females develop mucopurulent secretion from the vagina and inflammation of the vulva and vagina.
- Lymphoid follicles present pustules that develop from small-sized ulcers to coalescing erosions.
- Male bovines infected with BoHV-1.2 that develop infectious pustular balanoposthitis (IPB) are reluctant to mate.
- The animals tend to recover within 10–30 days of the beginning of signs and remain transiently immune.

TREATMENT

THERAPEUTIC APPROACH
- Although lavage of the vagina with antiseptic solutions and emollients has been recommended, treatment is usually not required.
- Animals usually recover within 30 days of the initial infection.

SURGICAL CONSIDERATIONS AND TECHNIQUES
N/A

MEDICATIONS

DRUGS OF CHOICE
N/A

CONTRAINDICATIONS
N/A

PRECAUTIONS
N/A

(CONTINUED) | **INFECTIOUS PUSTULAR VULVOVAGINITIS**

POSSIBLE INTERACTIONS
N/A

FOLLOW-UP

EXPECTED COURSE AND PROGNOSIS
• Animals usually develop clinical signs of infection within 1–3 days after exposure.
• Spontaneous recovery occurs within 10–30 days of infection.
• Infectious pustular vulvovaginitis has a very good prognosis.
• The disease is notifiable in many countries.

POSSIBLE COMPLICATIONS
• Female bovids infected with BoHV-1.2 that develop IPV have an increased rate of return to estrus after insemination. This can have a major impact in the breeding programs and consequently to the profitability of dairy and beef operations.
• It is rare for IPV to be followed by abortion outbreaks.

CLIENT EDUCATION
Educate client on biosecurity measures.

PATIENT CARE
N/A

PREVENTION
• Vaccination can be of benefit. However, in the face of an outbreak, vaccination has little effect.
• Avoid mating among infected animals to decrease the risk of dissemination of the disease.
• The virus can be spread via fomites such as contaminated breeding equipment. Strong biosecurity protocols are essential.
• BoHV-1.2 can survive cryopreservation. Therefore, semen donors and semen should be tested and free of BoHV-1.2, and semen from these bulls should not be stored in the same tank as semen of unknown status.
• Eradication of the disease requires vaccination and often elimination of animals that are carriers of the genital form of BoHV.

MISCELLANEOUS

ASSOCIATED CONDITIONS
• During the initial phases of the disease, animals may present less-specific signs such as pyrexia and decreased milk production.
• Animals of breeding age infected with BoHV-1.2 may present increased rate of return to estrus.
• Conjunctivitis with serous discharge and bilateral nasal discharge are signs of BoHV-1.2 when the respiratory tract is affected.

AGE-RELATED FACTORS
Although breeding-age animals are more likely to develop the condition, unbred heifers can also be infected.

ZOONOTIC POTENTIAL
N/A

PREGNANCY
Infectious pustular vulvovaginitis is rarely related to abortion outbreaks.

BIOSECURITY
• Vaccination (vaccination is prohibited in countries that have eradicated the disease)
• Testing of bulls and frozen semen
• Avoid the use of shared hired bulls
• Proper sanitation of breeding and collection equipment

ABBREVIATIONS
• AI = artificial insemination
• BoHV = bovine herpesvirus
• DTH = delayed-type hypersensitivity
• ELISA = enzyme-linked immunosorbent assay
• IBR = infectious bovine rhinotracheitis
• IPB = infectious pustular balanoposthitis
• IPV = infectious pustular vulvovaginitis
• PCR = polymerase chain reaction

SEE ALSO
• *Histophilus somni* Complex
• Infectious Bovine Rhinotracheitis
• *Mycoplasma bovis* Associated Diseases

• Penile Disorders
• Ulcerative Posthitis and Vulvitis
• Ureaplasma
• Vaginitis
• Vulvitis

Suggested Reading
Ackermann M, Belak S, Bitsch V, et al. Round table on infectious bovine rhinotracheitis/infectious pustular vulvovaginitis virus infection diagnosis and control. Vet Microbiol 1990, 23: 361–3.
Miller JM, Van Der Maaten MJ, Whetstone CA. Effects of a bovine herpesvirus-1 isolate on reproductive function in heifers: classification as a type-2 (infectious pustular vulvovaginitis) virus by a restriction endonuclease analysis of viral DNA. Am J Vet Res 1988, 49: 1653–6.
Nandi S, Kumar M, Monohar M, Chauhan RS. Bovine herpes virus infections in cattle. Anim Health Res Rev 2009, 10: 85–98.
Piper KL, Fitzgerald CJ, Ficorilli N, Studdert MJ. Isolation of caprine herpesvirus 1 from a major outbreak of infectious pustular vulvovaginitis in goats. Austr Vet J 2008, 86: 136–8.
Pritchard G, Cook N, Banks M. Infectious pustular vulvovaginitis/infectious pustular balanoposthitis in cattle. Vet Rec 1997, 140: 587.
Tibary A. Infectious agents: infectious bovine rhinotracheitis. In. Hopper R ed, Bovine Reproduction. Hoboken, NJ: Wiley, 2014, pp. 541–2.
Whetstone CA, Miller JM, Bortner DM, Van Der Maaten MJ. Changes in the bovine herpesvirus 1 genome during acute infection, after reactivation from latency, and after superinfection in the host animal. Arch Virol 1989, 106: 261–79.
Author Christine M. Winslow
Consulting Editor Ahmed Tibary
Acknowledgment The author and book editors acknowledge the prior contribution of Ricardo Caronari Chebel.

I

INFERTILITY AND SUBFERTILITY ISSUES

BASICS

OVERVIEW
• Infertility is defined as the inability to produce young. Subfertility is a condition of less than normal or desired fertility, that is, a relative infertility. In common veterinary parlance, however, the terms are used interchangeably to describe less than optimal functioning of a reproductive system and we will make no distinction between them here.
• Sterility is a term generally reserved for cases of profound, permanent infertility in individual animals. It is important to keep in mind that while producing a single offspring defines a male or female animal as fertile, this level of performance is seldom satisfactory for livestock systems.
• Fecundity defines a livestock system that is functioning well from a reproductive point of view and infertility/subfertility (I/S) describes a system in need of improvement.

INCIDENCE/PREVALENCE
• Poor reproductive performance is one of the major areas in production medicine.
• Incidence is highly variable with local conditions and farm management.

GEOGRAPHIC DISTRIBUTION
Worldwide

SYSTEMS AFFECTED
Reproductive

PATHOPHYSIOLOGY
• The etiology and pathophysiology of I/S are highly complex. Investigation of fertility problems is a highly reductive process.
• Initial problem identification and refinement must account for all three elements of the fertility equation (the male animal; the female animal; and the human/management element) as well as the fundamental nature of the problem—usually expressed as either a failure to breed, a failure to become pregnant, or a failure to maintain pregnancy/stillbirth.
• Many approaches are used to further develop a diagnosis but expert systems tend to focus on cause (e.g., use of the DAMNIT system), timing of the problem within the reproductive life cycle, and anatomic localization. Further diagnostic tests are almost invariably necessary to make a specific diagnosis.
• Both the quality and the quantity of feed and water should be a major concern and subject of investigation in any herd-level problem with I/S in production animals.

HISTORICAL FINDINGS
• Vary with species, sex of the animal, and disease but can be broadly categorized as:
  ◦ A failure to copulate or express estrus
  ◦ A failure to conceive a pregnancy after copulation, insemination, or embryo implantation
  ◦ A failure to maintain a viable pregnancy to term, or fetal death within 48 hours of delivery (stillbirth)
  ◦ Disorders of lactation are not covered here.
• Herd infertility investigation may reveal a poor pregnancy rate, increased services per conception, or an elevated rate of abortion.

SIGNALMENT
Any intact animal at any stage of sexual development or the reproductive cycle

PHYSICAL EXAMINATION FINDINGS
• General physical examination may show underlying cause: Poor BCS, poor health
• Examination of the reproductive tract:
  ◦ Male—testicular or penile abnormalities
  ◦ Females—abnormal vaginal discharge, abnormal ovarian activity or uterine disorders

GENETICS
• Some I/S issues have a direct genetic causation (e.g., DUMPS, BLAD, CVM, and brachyspina in Holstein cattle), some have a less definitive genetic predisposition (e.g., the influence of offspring size on dystocia and subsequent stillbirth incidence), while others (e.g., infectious abortion, toxin ingestion) have little or no genetic influence.

CAUSES AND RISK FACTORS
• Suboptimal management, especially nutritional but including all aspects of reproductive program management
• Local infectious disease prevalence and virulence factors
• Trauma at mating or parturition
• Heredity

DIAGNOSIS

DIFFERENTIAL DIAGNOSES
• Establishing a differential list at the herd level requires a detailed epidemiological approach, including a review of records, management, nutrition and disease prevention programs as well as a careful evaluation of specific breeding practices.
• Individual animals need to undergo a complete breeding soundness examination (BSE).

CBC/BIOCHEMISTRY/URINALYSIS
N/A

OTHER LABORATORY TESTS
• Genomic testing where available
• Hormone analysis and response to stimulation tests
• Microbial culture and sensitivity
• Serology
• Virus isolation
• Molecular diagnostics
• Toxicology
• Feed/water analysis

IMAGING
• Ultrasonography has become the standard for imaging reproductive tissues in both male and female animals. Specific methods and applications will vary with species and suspected disease.
• While radiography is seldom indicated in ruminant I/S work-ups, contrast radiography can assist with diagnosis of penile disorders.

OTHER DIAGNOSTIC PROCEDURES
• A thorough reproductive examination of affected individuals (BSE).
• Diagnosis of herd-level I/S problems focuses on signalment, history, and records analysis and places a premium on local knowledge and professional acuity.
• Obtaining a specific diagnosis is complicated by the fact that the signs of reproductive disease are not specific or pathognomonic and there is often considerable time lag from the disease insult to the manifestation of the signs of disease.
• Diagnostic efforts are often delayed so that by the time a diagnostic investigation is begun, the trail may have gone cold.
• Palpation per rectum is a critical diagnostic skill for investigation of bovine I/S and is used variably in llamas and alpacas depending on size of the animal and the examiner.

PATHOLOGIC FINDINGS
• Vary with species and disease or disorders.
• Local or regional veterinary diagnostic laboratory should be contacted for advice on sample selection and handling.

TREATMENT

THERAPEUTIC APPROACH
• Depends on the specific disease condition responsible for the problem.
• Assisted reproductive technologies (e.g., ET, IVF and SCNT) are options for highly valuable animals with poor prognoses with more conventional breeding options.

SURGICAL CONSIDERATIONS AND TECHNIQUES
Surgical correction is possible for some specific disorders.

MEDICATIONS

DRUGS OF CHOICE
• Antibiotics are indicated for primary bacterial diseases. Culture and sensitivity testing are ideal but many cases are treated empirically, for economic reasons.
• Hormonal treatments can be used to stimulate and inhibit reproductive functions. Classes of hormones available for use in ruminants include GnRH, gonadotropins

(eCG and hCG), PGF, and the sex steroids or their agonist and antagonists.
• The choice of drug varies with the condition and regional availability.
• In general, prevention is a more economical approach to I/S management than is treatment.

CONTRAINDICATIONS
• Abortifacients and teratogenic agents should not be used in pregnant animals unless the life of the dam is the higher priority.

PRECAUTIONS
• Milk and meat withdrawal times should be observed.
• Extra-label drug use in food animals is not permitted in the United States in the absence of disease, and suboptimal reproductive function is not considered a disease.

POSSIBLE INTERACTIONS
N/A

FOLLOW-UP

EXPECTED COURSE AND PROGNOSIS
• Highly variable depending on the specific disorder and treatment options.
• Animals of minimal value (financial or genetic) may be culled quickly; more valuable animals may merit specific treatment or be given time to recover spontaneously.

POSSIBLE COMPLICATIONS
• The majority of I/S conditions are not life-threatening but some (e.g., dystocia) are both emergent and potentially serious if not fatal disorders.
• The greatest risk for animals experiencing I/S is that they will be involuntarily culled for economic reasons.
• Loss of genetic value of culled breeding animals.

CLIENT EDUCATION
• Record keeping
• Sound breeding management protocols
• Breeding soundness examination

PATIENT CARE
Individual animals and groups of animals should be monitored by appropriate physical examination and records to assess recovery.

PREVENTION
• Adequate biosecurity including pre-entry testing of new arrivals, adequate quarantine procedures and duration, and re-testing before entry to the herd.
• Biologically sound vaccination programs.
• Use semen and embryos that are certified to be free of diseases of concern. At the very least, be sure of the disease status of the facility where germplasm originates.
• Reproductive management protocols on the farm should include training, monitoring,

and establishing performance standards that will trigger rewards or remediation.

MISCELLANEOUS

ASSOCIATED CONDITIONS
N/A

AGE-RELATED FACTORS
Reproductive efficiency tends to increase for a period of years after puberty, followed by a plateau, and then a gradual decline with age. The inflection point will vary with species and management systems employed on each farm.

ZOONOTIC POTENTIAL
Many infectious reproductive diseases are capable of infecting humans. Special care should be taken when examining females that are aborting.

PREGNANCY
Pregnancy wastage is a common manifestation of reproductive disorders. Treatment and prevention programs often target pregnant animals and in such cases the potential for negative drug/vaccine effects on the fetus should be carefully considered before treatment is instituted.

BIOSECURITY
• Biosecurity is an obvious component of management for infectious disease control.
• The specific measures will vary with the cost and severity of the diseases one is trying to avoid. Tuberculosis and brucellosis are examples of diseases with an extremely high cost to ruminant production systems and grave zoonotic potential, so the tolerance for these diseases is essentially zero. The best approach to managing these diseases is a national disease eradication effort and continuous surveillance. Less serious diseases or those that do not affect humans as severely may be managed more economically by test and cull programs at the farm level. Others may respond well to vaccination or other disease prevention programs.
• Special attention should be paid to the disease status of semen, ova, and embryos used in ART programs.

PRODUCTION MANAGEMENT
• Adequate record systems that allow evaluation of reproductive efficiency and track disease occurrence. Computerized record systems are essential for large-scale operations.
• Local, regional and national recording and management systems are available that can help with interpretation of farm-level metrics. These systems can establish farm performance benchmarks and assist with setting goals for the future. They can also be useful in determining when interventions are necessary and assessing the performance of the interventions.

ABBREVIATIONS
• AI = artificial insemination
• ART = assisted reproductive technology
• BCS = body condition score
• BLAD = bovine leukocyte adhesion deficiency
• BSE = breeding soundness examination
• CVM = complex vertebral malformation
• DAMNIT = (D)egenerative, (A)utoimmune, (M)etabolic, (N)eoplastic, (I)nfectious/(I)atrogenic, (T)raumatic; an organizational system for developing a diagnosis, commonly expanded beyond this initial list
• DUMPS = deficiency of uridine monophosphate synthetase
• eCG = equine chorionic gonadotropin (primarily FSH activity)
• ET = embryo transfer
• GnRH = gonadotropin releasing hormone
• hCG = human chorionic gonadotropin
• I/S = infertility and subfertility
• IVF = in vitro fertilization
• PGF = prostaglandin F2α and its analogs
• SCNT = somatic cell nuclear transfer (cloning)

SEE ALSO
• Breeding Soundness Examination: Bull
• Breeding Soundness Examination: Camelid
• Breeding Soundness Examination: Small Ruminant
• Endometritis
• Heat Stress
• Orchitis and Epididymitis
• Penile Disorders
• Repeat Breeder Management
• Seminal Vesiculitis
• Testicular Disorders: Bovine
• Testicular Disorders: Camelid
• Testicular Disorders: Small Ruminant
• Uterine Anomalies

Suggested Reading
Edmondson MA, Roberts JF, Baird AN, et al. Theriogenology of sheep and goats. In: Pugh DG ed, Sheep and Goat Medicine, 2nd ed. Philadelphia: Saunders, 2012, pp. 150–230.
Hopper RM. Bovine Reproduction. Ames: Wiley Blackwell, 2015.
Pearson LK, Tibary A. Reproductive failure in female camelids. Clinical Theriogenology 2014, 6: 555–70.
Pearson LK, Tibary A. Reproductive failure in male camelids. Clinical Theriogenology 2014, 6: 571–7.
Youngquist RS, Threllfall WR. Large Animal Theriogenology, 2nd ed. St. Louis: Saunders, 2007.
Authors Harry Momont and Celina Checura
Consulting Editor Ahmed Tibary

INJECTION SITE LESIONS

BASICS

OVERVIEW
• Injection site lesions occur due to disruption of tissue constituents and architecture in response to physical or chemical trauma associated with the injection process or medications.
• Injection of any substance has the potential to result in immediate or delayed clinical symptoms and/or long-term changes in tissue structure.
• The term "injection site lesion," in ruminants, most commonly refers to the scar tissue found after almost any intramuscular injection, leading to the development of a tough, gristly area of meat.
• IM injection site lesions are of most significance in food-producing animals when located in the top sirloin, blade, and round cuts of meat as they cause economic losses due to trimming.
• Injection site lesions that occur after treatment of young animals persist into adulthood and can enlarge with time as the animal grows. They may be readily apparent in harvested carcasses.

INCIDENCE/PREVALENCE
• Unknown in many ruminant species, but substantial in cattle where injection sites include primary economic muscle groups.
• Investigators of a 3-year audit (1998–2000) reported frequencies of injection site lesions in outside round muscles from beef cow carcasses and dairy cow carcasses to be 26% and 49%, respectively. Higher frequencies in dairy cows are associated with greater injection frequencies linked to production management.
• A trend in declining frequencies is associated with educational programs and continued improvements in beef quality assurance practices among beef and dairy producers.

GEOGRAPHIC DISTRIBUTION
Worldwide

SYSTEMS AFFECTED
Musculoskeletal

PATHOPHYSIOLOGY
• Short-term and clinically evident effects of injections are uncommon but include local inflammation, hyperemia, hematoma formation, cellulitis, necrosis, and lymphadenitis.
• Most commonly, the long-term result of IM injections have no clinical consequence to the animal, but lesions are present and grossly identified at slaughter as a clear scar, woody callus, or cyst.
• A fibroproliferative process occurs subsequent to IM injection of a pharmacologic agent resulting in significant increases in total, soluble, and insoluble collagen concentrations at the lesion center,

which decrease in concentration as the radius from the lesion center increases.
• Histologically, lesions can be classified as clear, woody, nodular, metallic, or cystic.
• Clear and woody lesions are typical of injections given to animals in earlier stages of their life (as calves or during the time before weaning); metallic and nodular lesions are typical of pharmaceuticals administered to cattle in mid-to-late feeding phases; and cystic lesions are typical of injections given to cattle late in the finishing phase.
• IM injections significantly reduce the tenderness of affected tissues in an area up to 7.62 cm away from the lesion center.

HISTORICAL FINDINGS
Parenteral administration of pharmaceutical products

SIGNALMENT
Meat-producing livestock species: bovine, ovine, caprine, and camelids

PHYSICAL EXAMINATION FINDINGS
Palpation and/or observation of fibrous/cystic muscle tissue or a reduction in tenderness of muscle

GENETICS
N/A

CAUSES AND RISK FACTORS
• Administration of IM pharmaceuticals in regions of high value for meat processing
• Multiple use needles
• Injections >10 mL of any product at a single site and use of needles larger than 16 G
• IM injections in young animals that may enlarge with time
• Clostridial bacterin/toxoids, *Mycobacterium avium* subsp. *paratuberculosis* vaccination, oxytetracycline, vitamin A/D

DIAGNOSIS

DIFFERENTIAL DIAGNOSES
• Any disease or trauma causing a fibroproliferative tissue response
• Abscess
• Cyst
• Neoplasia

CBC/BIOCHEMISTRY/URINALYSIS
N/A

OTHER LABORATORY TESTS
N/A

IMAGING
Radiography and ultrasonography may reveal increased soft tissue density and mineralization of some lesions.

OTHER DIAGNOSTIC PROCEDURES
Biopsy, resection, or evaluation of tissue at time of meat processing

PATHOLOGIC FINDINGS
• Histologic section of lesions in affected cattle musculature have sheets of fibroblasts

with extensive collagen deposition at the core; a combination of dense fibrous connective tissue and mature adipose tissue progressing outwards; and a mixture of partially degenerated muscle fibers, mature connective tissue, and occasional adipose cells on the outside border.
• Tissue ossification and granulation may be identified.
• Alterations in relative proportions of muscle, connective tissue, and fat to a distance of 5.08 cm from the site of the lesion center may be present in beef cattle and confirm severe disruption of muscle tissue constituents and architecture.

TREATMENT

THERAPEUTIC APPROACH
• Surgical resection
• Trimming of affected tissue at meat processing

MEDICATIONS
N/A

FOLLOW-UP

PREVENTION
• All possible injections, especially those of potentially irritating animal health products, should be give via the SC route or by transdermal needleless injection.
• Use the "tent method" for SC injections to avoid injection into the muscle.
• SC injections in non-prime cut areas should start with baby calves and be practiced for the life of the animal.
• All injections should be given in the neck in front of the point of shoulder when possible.
• Choice of IM injection site should be based on minimal loss of retail product. Do not administer IM injections in the rear leg or hip areas. Administer IM injections in the neck area, but avoid the following landmarks: neck vertebrae, nuchal ligament, front edge of the scapula, the lymph node at the point of the shoulder.
• Inject in a clean and dry site.
• Select the needle gauge to fit animal size and liquid viscosity. Use the smallest practical size without risk of bending or breakage.
• If using multi-dose injectors, change needles when dull or damaged or in a manner consistent with disease transfer minimization.
• Use proper injection equipment, which is cleaned and functioning properly.
• Use a clean needle to fill syringes with drugs and vaccines.

(CONTINUED)   **INJECTION SITE LESIONS**

• Use products as labeled in their appropriate manner in consideration of route of administration and frequency.
• Use low dosage products, with a recommended space of 10 cm between injection sites, and do not exceed the recommended volume per injection site.

POSSIBLE COMPLICATIONS
Abscessation at injection site

EXPECTED COURSE AND PROGNOSIS
Injection site lesions rarely cause clinical problems for the affected animal but result in economic losses for the producer at time of slaughter.

 MISCELLANEOUS

ASSOCIATED CONDITIONS
N/A

AGE-RELATED FACTORS
IM injection site lesions in calves may enlarge with age, resulting in greater trim at slaughter.

ZOONOTIC POTENTIAL
N/A

PREGNANCY
N/A

BIOSECURITY
N/A

PRODUCTION MANAGEMENT
• Use strategies that do not compromise beef quality by reducing bruises, decreasing hide damage, preventing drug residues, and eliminating injection site lesions.
• Avoid giving medications close to slaughter that could cause injection site lesions and residue violations in meat.
• Use of products, where possible, that are approved for SC, IV, or oral administration.
• SC injections should be given in front of the shoulder.
• IM injections should be given in the neck region with no more than 10 mL administered in one site, using the smallest gauge needle possible.

ABBREVIATIONS
• IM= intramuscular
• IV = intravenous
• SC= subcutaneous

SEE ALSO
• Drug Hypersensitivities
• Food Animal Residue Avoidance Databank (FARAD) (see www.fiveminutevet.com/ruminant)
• Vaccination Programs
• Vaccinology (see www.fiveminutevet.com/ruminant)

Suggested Reading

George MH, Morgan JB, Glock RD, et al. Injection-site lesions: incidence, tissue histology, collagen concentration, and muscle tenderness in beef rounds. J Anim Sci 1995, 73: 3510–18.
Roeber DL, Cannell RC, Wailes WR, et al. Frequencies of injection-site lesions in muscles from rounds of dairy and beef cow carcasses. J Dairy Sci 2002, 85: 532–6.
Dairy Animal Care and Quality Assurance Manual. http://www.bqa.org/Media/BQA/Docs/dairybqamanual.pdf
Author Rachel H.H. Tan
Consulting Editor Kaitlyn A. Lutz
Acknowledgment The author and book editors acknowledge the prior contribution of Daniel Rule.

I

IODINE DEFICIENCY AND TOXICITY

BASICS

OVERVIEW
• Iodine is an essential micronutrient whose primary function is the synthesis of thyroxine (T4) and tri-iodothyronine (T3).
• Iodine cannot be synthesized by the body, thus diet is the primary source.
• Deficiency occurs when animals inhabit areas of iodine-deficient soil.
• Daily iodine requirement for cattle is 0.016 mg/kg body weight.
• Toxicity occurs through intake above the daily requirement either thru long-term consumption of diet with an excess, incorrect management of mineral feed mix, or chronic use of therapeutic iodine compounds.
• Toxic doses:
  ◦ Adult cattle prolonged administration at 0.12–1 mg/kg BW daily
  ◦ Calves prolonged administration at 0.4–2.2 mg/kg BW daily
  ◦ Sheep prolonged administration at 13.1 mg/kg BW daily
• Clinical signs associated with toxicity can be affected by the amount and length of administration, the type of compound administered, and the physiologic and metabolic status of the animal.

INCIDENCE/PREVALENCE
Since this is a nutritional issue, morbidity can vary greatly in a herd.

GEOGRAPHIC DISTRIBUTION
Iodine-deficient soil areas within the United States may include Texas, California, Pacific northwest, mountain states, North Dakota, and some of the Midwestern states.

SYSTEMS AFFECTED
• Hemolymphatic
• Reproductive

PATHOPHYSIOLOGY
• Iodine is an essential micronutrient whose primary function is the synthesis of thyroxine (T4) and tri-iodothyronine (T3). These hormones have a role in controlling metabolism, cell growth, and maturation as well as growth and development of tissues.
• Iodine additionally has a role in the immune system, especially in the functioning of leukocytes. Deficiency thus results in a depression of cellular and humoral immunity, leading to a decreased response to infectious agents.

HISTORICAL FINDINGS
• History of iodine-deficient diet, such as areas located with iodine-deficient soil without supplementation.
• Prolonged administration of iodine compounds such as EDDI (organic) or calcium or potassium iodate (inorganic) for therapeutic uses.

• Improper supplementation of iodine in the diet, potentially through improper mineral mix or diet concentrations.

SIGNALMENT
Cattle and sheep. The developing fetus is particularly susceptible to iodine deficiency.

PHYSICAL EXAMINATION FINDINGS
• Deficiency
  ◦ Goiter or thyroid enlargement especially in newborn calves and lambs
  ◦ Reproduction issues such as decreased conception rates and stillbirths
  ◦ Increased newborn mortality
  ◦ Ill-thrift in growing animals
• Toxicity
  ◦ Cattle
    ▪ Persistent cough
    ▪ Nasal discharge
    ▪ Lacrimation
    ▪ Salivation
    ▪ Hyperthermia
    ▪ Inappetence
    ▪ Depression
    ▪ Dermatitis (dry, scaly) and alopecia
    ▪ Infectious disease especially of the respiratory system
    ▪ Reduction in milk production
  ◦ Sheep
    ▪ Depression
    ▪ Anorexia
    ▪ Hyperthermia
    ▪ Changes in respiratory system

CAUSES AND RISK FACTORS
• Iodine is required for production of thyroid hormones
• Areas with iodine-deficient soils
• Feeding of goitrogenic feeds that interfere with the availability of iodine (brassica fodder crops—bok choy, kale, rape, sugar beet pulp, turnips—and vegetable crop residues of cauliflower and broccoli)
• Excess iodine supplementation

DIAGNOSIS

DIFFERENTIAL DIAGNOSES
Infectious respiratory disease

CBC/BIOCHEMISTRY/URINALYSIS
• Toxicity may result in leukopenia with neutrophilia and lymphopenia on full blood count
• Toxicity may result in:
  ◦ Increase in serum glucose, AST and BUN
  ◦ Decrease in serum cholesterol and urinary creatinine

OTHER LABORATORY TESTS
• Plasma inorganic iodine (PII) measures current daily iodine intake (short-term), and is thus susceptible to changes in feed intake.
• T4 levels reflect the thyroid and iodine status of the animal (>50 nmol/L, normal; <20 nmol/L, abnormal), and are useful in the diagnosis of deficiency. Care must be taken in

interpretation of T4 values, as there is natural variation according to stage of lactation (levels are much lower in early lactation), season, age of animal, etc.

OTHER DIAGNOSTIC PROCEDURES
Clinical signs

TREATMENT

THERAPEUTIC APPROACH
• Deficiency: Supplement as needed.
• Toxicity: Remove source and return diet to daily intake requirement levels.

MEDICATIONS

DRUGS OF CHOICE
• Oral dosing using potassium iodide is relatively short-acting and laborious. Intraruminal boluses provide slow release of iodine for 6 months. Painting 5% tincture of iodine onto the flank skinfold once a week in milking dairy cattle can work well, but is too labor-intensive in dry cows and beef animals. Free-access minerals, medication of water supplies, and pasture fertilizers can all be used to varying effect.
• For suckling lambs and calves with goiter, tincture of iodine can be applied to the teats for up to 2 weeks to treat iodine deficiency.

FOLLOW-UP

PREVENTION
• Iodine is frequently added to concentrate rations for feeding to cattle and sheep, for example using seaweed preparations. Rapeseed meals are usually treated to eliminate goitrogens prior to feeding, and newer "double-zero" oilseed rape varieties are lower in goitrogens.
• On the label of free-choice mineral mixes, iodine may be in the form of calcium iodate or ethylenediamine dihydroiodide, which are both quite stable and available. Additional supplementation of iodine in less stable forms (more susceptible to loss of iodine with exposure to light, heat, moisture, or other factors) includes potassium or sodium iodide, which are often used to fortify salt with iodine.
• If 25% or more of the diet is made up of feedstuffs associated with goitrogenic crops, then dietary iodine levels should increase to 1.0 ppm, especially for cows and ewes in late gestation or early lactation.
• Dosing ewes with iodine compounds in the fourth and fifth months of pregnancy prevents goiter in their lambs. The iodine compounds can be given directly or mixed

with worm drenches. Recommendations on the dosage and the compatibility of iodine compounds with various drenches can be obtained from your local veterinarian.

MISCELLANEOUS

PREGNANCY
Iodine deficiency results in abortion and stillbirths.

PRODUCTION MANAGEMENT
• Iodized salt is still a recommended source of supplemental iodine for all parts of the country, especially where origin of crops is unknown.
• If practical, avoid grazing pregnant livestock over "at risk" areas such as the sandier soil types, especially during the latter half of pregnancy.

• Sheep or cattle fed on brassica fodder crops such as bok choy, kale, rape, sugar beet pulp, turnips and vegetable crop residues of cauliflower and broccoli are likely to produce goiter in their progeny if access to these crops is prolonged. This is because brassicas contain goitrogens which interfere with the availability of iodine.

SYNONYM
Goiter

ABBREVIATIONS
• EEDI = ethylenediamine dihydroiodide
• T3 = tri-iodothyronine
• T4 = thyroxine

SEE ALSO
• *Brassica* spp. Toxicity
• Respiratory Disease: Bovine
• Respiratory Disease: Small Ruminant

Suggested Reading
Anderson PD, Dalir-Naghadeh B, Parkinson TJ. Proc N Z Soc Anim Prod 2007, 67: 248–54.
Grobbel J. Stillborn calves in Michigan linked to iodine deficiency. Beef Brief, Michigan State University, 2008, http://msue.anr.msu.edu/uploads/236/58572/Stillborn CalvesinMichiganLinkedtoIodine.pdf. Accessed July 27, 2016.
Gupta RC. Chromium, iodine and phosphorus. In: Gupta RC ed, Veterinary Toxicology: Basic and Clinical Principles. Massachusetts: Elsevier, 2012, p. 508.
Paulikova I, Kovac KJ, Paulik S, Seidel H, Nagy O. Iodine toxicity in ruminants. Vet Med Czech 2002, 47: 343–50.
Author Jennifer S. Taintor
Consulting Editor Christopher C.L. Chase
Acknowledgment The author and book editors acknowledge the prior contribution of Lauren Palmer.

I

JIMSONWEED TOXICITY (*DATURA STRAMONIUM*)

BASICS

OVERVIEW
• Caused by ingestion of jimsonweed (Jamestown weed, thorn apple, downy thornapple, devil's trumpet, angel's trumpet, mad apple, stink weed, tolguacha or *Datura stramonium*) and its toxic tropane alkaloids.
• All parts of the green or dried plant are toxic including the seeds. Plants become more toxic as they mature. Seeds are considered to be the most toxic part of the plant. • The green plant is generally unpalatable due to its strong odor. Thus, lack of other forage, drying of the plant in hay, or contamination of cereal grains or feed with the seeds are the primary routes of ingestion and toxicity. • Toxicity is often somewhat self-limiting as anorexia is induced early in the toxic process, limiting ingestion of further toxins. • Signs predominantly involve the neuromuscular, ophthalmic, and gastrointestinal systems.

INCIDENCE/PREVALENCE
Plant is unpalatable. Dried material in hay may be eaten inadvertently. This is particularly true for ruminants. Up to 1% of body weight per day of leaves or fruits fed to sheep or goats produced clinical signs after 2 or more days, but it was not lethal unless fed for several weeks or longer.

GEOGRAPHIC DISTRIBUTION
Jimsonweed is commonly found in fencerows, barnyards, and roadsides throughout much of the United States.

SYSTEMS AFFECTED
Nervous

PATHOPHYSIOLOGY
• Contain two tropane alkaloids: (1) L-hyoscyamine (atropine) and (2) scopalamine (L-hyoscine). • Tropane alkaloids act as a competitive antagonist of acetylcholine at muscarinic cholinergic receptors of the parasympathetic nervous system. • Clinical signs are attributable to this receptor blockade and are manifest as (1) blockage of contraction of the muscles of the iris and mydriasis, (2) decreased smooth muscle contraction of the gastrointestinal system, (3) decreased salivary secretions, and (4) increased vagal tone.

SIGNALMENT
• All ruminant species can be affected.
• Cattle appear to be more susceptible than other ruminants. • No sex, age, or breed predilection among animals consuming the plant.

SIGNS
• Mydriasis • Depression • Restlessness
• Anorexia • Sinus tachycardia • Weakness
• Photophobia • Dry mucus membranes
• Constipation/ileus • Rumen atony

CAUSES AND RISK FACTORS
Associated with ingestion of toxin-containing plant. Consumption of feed or cereal grains containing 1,000 seeds/kg can be toxic in cattle.

DIAGNOSIS

DIFFERENTIAL DIAGNOSES
• Other toxic plants with tropane alkaloids including moonflower, angel's trumpet, deadly nightshade, belladonna, black henbane, horse or bull nettle, Texas thistle, tropical soda apple, and ground cherries.
• Parenteral or topical atropine therapy.

CBC/BIOCHEMISTRY/URINALYSIS
No changes specific for jimsonweed toxicity

OTHER LABORATORY TESTS
• Urine and gastrointestinal contents can be tested for tropane alkaloids. • Test administration of parasympathomimetic drugs *may not* cause appreciable improvement.

OTHER DIAGNOSTIC PROCEDURES
• If acute consumption is suspected, a rumenotomy with confirmation of plant material or seeds in the ingesta would be diagnostic and may be indicated. • Urine from affected animal is said to induce mydriasis if applied topically to the eye of a test animal.

PATHOLOGIC FINDINGS
• Identification of seed or plant material in the rumen • No distinct lesions • May see hemorrhages of the liver or kidney or effusions of the pericardium

TREATMENT

THERAPEUTIC APPROACH
• Remove animals from source of toxin (plants or seed). • If acute ingestion of large volumes of toxin is suspected, rumenotomy with evacuation of the ingesta may be beneficial. • Often self-limiting due to anorexia, an early sign.

MEDICATIONS

DRUGS OF CHOICE
• Orogastric administration of mineral oil or activated charcoal may decrease absorption of the toxin. • Rarely administration of a cholinergic drug (such as physostigmine, pilocarpine, or arecoline) is used; however, no
clear benefit from the use of these drugs has been demonstrated.

CONTRAINDICATIONS
Atropine

FOLLOW-UP

EXPECTED COURSE AND PROGNOSIS
• Often self-limiting due to decreased ingestion of the toxin after initial signs of toxicity. • Most have a good prognosis with supportive care.

PATIENT CARE
Monitor for signs of continued ileus or intestinal obstruction secondary to ileus.

PREVENTION
Do not pasture animals on fields with jimsonweed or feed hay or grain containing the plant or seeds.

MISCELLANEOUS

ZOONOTIC POTENTIAL
N/A

PREGNANCY
• Some studies have demonstrated teratogenic properties of tropane alkaloids; however, more recent studies have not been able to clearly demonstrate a cause and effect relationship.
• Until further work is done, tropane alkaloids should be considered possible teratogens.

ABBREVIATIONS
N/A

SEE ALSO
Nightshade (*Solanum* spp.) Toxicosis

Suggested Reading
Burrows GE, Tyrl RJ, ed. Toxic Plants of North America. Ames: Iowa State University Press, 2001.
Burrows GE, Tyrl RJ. Datura. In: Burrows GE, Tyrl RJ eds, Toxic Plants of North America, 2nd ed. Ames: Wiley-Blackwell, 2013, Kindle Edition, pp. 1139–43.
Nelson PD, Mercer HD, Essig HW, Minyard JP. Jimson weed seed toxicity in cattle. Vet Hum Toxicol 1982, 24: 321–5.
Piva G, Piva A. Anti-nutritional factors of Datura in feedstuffs. Nat Toxins 1995, 3: 238–41; discussion 242.
Schulman ML, Bolton LA. Datura seed intoxication in two horses. J S Afr Vet Assoc 1998, 69: 27–9.
Author Paul J. Plummer
Consulting Editor Christopher C.L. Chase

J

BASICS

OVERVIEW
• Johne's disease (pronounced Yo-nees) is a serious disease of most ruminants that can cause significant economic loss if not controlled.
• Johne's disease is caused by the bacteria *Mycobacterium avium* subsp. *Paratuberculosis* (MAP).
• The primary source of infection is feces that contain MAP. Infected animals can produce large amounts of the bacteria and shed this organism in their feces.
• Most infected animals do not begin shedding the Johne's organism until they are adults.

INCIDENCE/PREVALENCE
It is estimated that >50% of the dairy and 20% of the beef cow-calf operations in the United States have at least one animal infected with Johne's disease. The prevalence is higher in larger dairy operations.

GEOGRAPHIC DISTRIBUTION
Worldwide

SYSTEMS AFFECTED
Digestive

PATHOPHYSIOLOGY
• The primary source of infection is feces that contain MAP. Infected animals can produce large amounts of the bacteria and shed this organism in their feces.
• After ingestion and uptake in the Peyer's patches of the lower small intestine, this intracellular pathogen infects macrophages in the GI tract and associated lymph nodes. It is possible that some animals may eliminate infection through a cell-mediated immune response that encourages microbiocidal activity in macrophages, but the frequency with which this occurs is unknown.
• In most cases, the organisms multiply and eventually provoke a chronic granulomatous enteritis that interferes with nutrient uptake and processing, leading to the cachexia typical of advanced infections.
• This may take months to years to develop and is usually paralleled by a decline in cell-mediated immunity, a rise in serum antibody, and bacteremia with dissemination of the infection beyond the GI tract.
• Fecal shedding begins before clinical signs are apparent, and animals in this "silent" stage of infection are important sources of transmission.

SIGNALMENT
• All breeds of cattle, sheep, and goats are susceptible to Johne's disease. Camelids are also susceptible.
• Newborn animals are most susceptible to infection with MAP. As they get older, risk of

infection decreases. In cattle, most infections likely occur in the first 6 months of life.
• Following a long incubation period of months to years, clinical disease typically occurs in an adult animal.

PHYSICAL EXAMINATION FINDINGS
• There is a long incubation period between infection with MAP and the appearance of clinical signs. In cattle, this period of time may range from 1 year to several years.
• Prior to the development of observable clinical signs, animals may be affected subclinically. Syndromes that have been associated with subclinical Johne's disease in cattle include reduced milk production, reduced reproductive performance, and increased disease susceptibility.
• The classical clinical sign of Johne's disease in cattle is chronic, watery diarrhea. This diarrhea may be intermittent at first, but eventually progresses to chronic and unrelenting. Diarrhea is not as evident in sheep and goats.
• The diarrhea has no distinguishing characteristics such as blood, mucus, or foul odor. It is often referred to as "pipe stream" in nature because of its watery and projectile appearance.
• Secondary to diarrhea, animals lose weight despite the maintenance of a good appetite. Weight loss is the primary clinical sign in sheep and goats.
• Depending on concurrent metabolic loads (milk production, pregnancy), weight loss may occur gradually over months or very rapidly over the course of a few weeks.
• In advanced cases, the development of submandibular edema may occur secondary to a decrease in total serum protein.

CAUSES AND RISK FACTORS
• Johne's disease is caused by the bacteria *Mycobacterium avium* subsp. *Paratuberculosis* (MAP).
• Animals <6 months of age are most susceptible to infection. Older animals are less susceptible to infection.
• Any method by which young stock become exposed to fecal material from adult animals may serve as a source of infection with MAP.
• This may include being born in a dirty maternity pen, nursing a dirty teat, being housed in direct contact with adult animals, using common feeding/manure handling equipment (skid-loader), or having manure run-off from mature cow areas going through the environments of young stock.
• Another important source of transmission is milk and colostrum. About one third of cows infected with MAP, whether they are showing clinical signs or not, will shed the bacteria in their colostrum or milk.
• Approximately 20% of cows with Johne's disease will pass MAP across their placenta to the developing fetus. The risk of this happening increases dramatically in cows with clinical signs of Johne's disease.

DIAGNOSIS

DIFFERENTIAL DIAGNOSES
• Parasitism
• Copper deficiency
• Bovine leukosis
• Salmonellosis
• Amyloidosis
• Chronic reticuloperitonitis/peritonitis

CBC/BIOCHEMISTRY/URINALYSIS
Hypoproteinemia, characterized by low serum albumin, may be present in advanced clinical cases of Johne's disease.

OTHER LABORATORY TESTS
• MAP can be cultured from feces using standard solid media culture methods, which require 10–16 weeks to complete, or new rapid liquid media culture methods that shorten the culture time to 7–10 weeks.
• PCR/DNA probe—organism detection assay used on feces or tissue.
• Antibody detection ELISA, agar gel immunodiffusion, and complement fixation assays on serum.
• The antibody ELISA assay can also be used on milk to screen individual animals or herds.
• Acid-fast stains can be used for direct visualization of organism in appropriate tissue samples such as ileum or ileal cecal lymph nodes.
• The specificity of all the assays for Johne's disease is high (>98%) whereas the sensitivity is generally low (30–50%).

PATHOLOGIC FINDINGS
• In cattle, gross lesions are primarily found in the distal jejunum, ileum, cecum, proximal colon, and associated lymph nodes.
• Thickening of the intestine three to four times normal thickness is characteristic.
• Affected mucosa takes on a corrugated appearance.
• The ileocecal valve is typically thickened and often reddened in color.
• In sheep, intestinal mucosa may be thickened, but it does not typically become corrugated.
• Mesenteric lymph nodes are enlarged and edematous in cattle. In sheep, they have areas of necrosis and calcification.
• Histologically, the earliest cellular changes are increased numbers of macrophages and lymphocytes.
• As the infection progresses, the mononuclear inflammatory infiltrate becomes pronounced and giant cells become more numerous. The inflammation is diffuse; the lesions are not walled off or circumscribed by fibrous connective tissue.
• Acid-fast bacteria will be present in areas of mononuclear inflammation.

J

TREATMENT

THERAPEUTIC APPROACH
There are no chemotherapeutic agents approved for use in food-producing animals for the treatment of MAP.

MEDICATIONS

DRUGS OF CHOICE
There are no approved drugs for the treatment of MAP. Use of antimycobacterial chemotherapeutic agents has largely been ineffective. Isoniazid, rifampin, clofazimine, dapsone, aminoglycosides, and ethambutol may result in transient reduction in clinical signs and slowing of disease progression, but response is inconsistent and they have failed to cure the disease.

PRECAUTIONS
Drug withdrawal times must be determined and maintained for food-producing animals.

FOLLOW-UP

EXPECTED COURSE AND PROGNOSIS
• Johne's is a chronic progressive disease.
• Progression of Johne's disease typically occurs over a 2–3-year period.
• Johne's disease progression can be divided into four stages. Stage 1 is the period of inapparent infection that occurs early in the disease progression. Stage 2 is a subclinical phase where shedding of the organism is intermittent. Stage 3 is characterized by consistent heavy shedding. Stage 4 is the clinical stage of the disease.
• Johne's disease is inevitably fatal if allowed to progress.

PREVENTION
• Stopping the transmission of MAP from infected cattle that are shedding the bacteria (generally adult animals) to susceptible animals (generally young animals) is key to controlling the disease.
• Specific recommendations include making sure newborns are born into and housed in a clean environment, reducing the chance of spread through colostrum and milk by not sharing colostrum and milk between multiple young stock or feeding only pasteurized sources of milk or milk replacers, making sure that weaned young stock are separated from adult animals.
• Feed and water sources for young stock should be protected from contamination with adult cow feces.
• Infected animals should be identified and either culled or managed so as to reduce the chances that they spread MAP to susceptible animals, primarily young stock.
• Calves born to known MAP-infected cattle should be considered at high risk for being infected with MAP, and managed accordingly.

MISCELLANEOUS

AGE-RELATED FACTORS
• Calves are most at risk for becoming infected with MAP. As cattle get older, infection becomes less likely.
• Because of the long incubation period, clinical signs of disease typically do not appear until adulthood.

ZOONOTIC POTENTIAL
There has been some association of MAP with Crohn's disease in humans, but no definitive link has been made.

PREGNANCY
MAP can cross the placenta and infect the fetus. This occurs about 20% of the time in Johne's-infected cows. The risk of fetal transmission in utero increases as the disease progresses in the dam.

BIOSECURITY
• The primary source of infection is feces that contain MAP. Infected animals can produce large amounts of the bacteria and shed this organism in their feces.
• The primary source of new infection into a herd is the acquisition of infected cattle.
• Studies have demonstrated that MAP can survive for months in the environment.
• Cleaning and disinfection is essential for MAP control.

SYNONYM
Paratuberculosis

ABBREVIATIONS
• ELISA = enzyme-linked immunosorbent assay
• PCR/DNA = polymerase chain reaction/deoxyribonucleic acid

SEE ALSO
• Bovine Leukemia Virus
• Copper Deficiency and Toxicity
• Parasite Control Programs: Bovine
• Salmonellosis
• Traumatic Reticuloperitonitis

Suggested Reading
Collins MT ed. Johne's Disease. Vet Clin North Am Food Anim Pract 2011, 27(3).
Collins MT, Gardner IA, Garry FB, Roussel AJ, Wells SJ. Consensus recommendations on diagnostic testing for the detection of paratuberculosis in cattle in the United States. J Am Vet Med Assoc 2006, 229: 1912–19.
Overview of Paratuberculosis. The Merck Veterinary Manual Online, 2013. Accessed July 28, 2016, http://www.merckvetmanual.com/mvm/generalized_conditions/paratuberculosis/overview_of_paratuberculosis.html

Author Daniel L. Grooms
Consulting Editor Christopher C.L. Chase

JUVENILE LLAMA IMMUNODEFICIENCY SYNDROME

BASICS

OVERVIEW
• Juvenile llama immunodeficiency syndrome (JLIDS) is a syndrome in young llamas characterized by failure to grow or gain weight as expected, and generalized ill thrift, which routinely progresses to multiple and/or chronic systemic infections and eventually to death.
• Research suggests an inherited impairment in B-cell development as a potential primary cause.

INCIDENCE/PREVALENCE
Not well established. Confirmed cases have greatly decreased since the late 1990s though this may be due to decreased intensive management of unthrifty llamas.

SYSTEMS AFFECTED
• Hemolymphatic
• Respiratory
• Digestive
• Musculoskeletal
• Urinary
• Reproductive
• Ophthalmic

PATHOPHYSIOLOGY
• Poorly understood.
• The specific immunodeficiency has not been determined, but an autosomal recessive defect in B-cell development has been proposed.
• Immunodeficiency leads to opportunistic or overwhelming systemic infections, and failure of the animal to respond to appropriate therapies, ultimately resulting in death.

SIGNALMENT
• Juvenile llamas, usually between the ages of 6 and 18 months, of either sex
• Not well documented in alpacas but occasionally suspected

GENETICS
An autosomal recessive inherited basis is suspected but not proven.

PHYSICAL EXAMINATION FINDINGS
• There are no pathognomonic signs—signs vary with the organ system(s) involved and the stage of the disease, including respiratory signs, lameness, dermatitis, ocular signs, or CNS signs/ataxia.
• Common reported complaints include:
  ○ Poor body condition and/or poor growth as compared to herdmates
  ○ Recurring infections or infections that fail to respond to treatment, particularly *Mycoplasma haemolamae*, ocular infections, and tooth root abscesses
  ○ Anemia, with pale mucus membranes, tachycardia, and mild heart murmur
  ○ Lethargy, depression
  ○ Occasionally, peracute infection may lead to rapid weight loss and death without prior signs.

CAUSES AND RISK FACTORS
• A hereditary component to the development of the clinical disease is likely, but a specific inheritance pattern has not been identified.
• No specific risk factors have been identified.

DIAGNOSIS

DIFFERENTIAL DIAGNOSES
Malnutrition, nutritional deficiency (copper, zinc, or selenium), iron deficiency, intestinal parasitism, and *Mycoplasma haemolamae*.

CBC/BIOCHEMISTRY/URINALYSIS
• Anemia—usually mild, normocytic, normochromic, and nonregenerative, though if the animal is infected with *M. haemolamae* the anemia can be severe and mildly regenerative.
• Hypoproteinemia with hypoalbuminemia and low to low-normal globulin levels, even in the face of infection.
• Low serum iron concentration with low to low-normal total iron binding capacity.

OTHER LABORATORY TESTS
• *Clostridium perfringens* C and D antibody ELISA: Paired serum samples are collected prior to and 2 weeks after vaccination with *C. perfringens* C and D toxoid, and antibody levels are measured. Healthy llamas show at least a twofold increase in titers, while JLIDS llamas have a low initial titer and fail to show any significant rise in titer after vaccination.
• Immunologic testing: Lymphocyte blastogenesis assays, serum protein electrophoresis, and flow cytometry can be used to characterize the specific immunodeficiency in an affected llama. Although these tests are still in the process of being validated for camelids, initial reports suggest consistent findings in JLIDS llamas including low levels of serum IgG and low numbers of B-lymphocytes.

IMAGING
Radiography may be indicated if clinical signs of lower respiratory tract disease and/or septic arthritis are present.

OTHER DIAGNOSTIC PROCEDURES
Lymph node biopsy: Affected llamas show regions of paracortical lymphocyte depletion.

PATHOLOGIC FINDINGS
• Gross lesions include muscle wasting, lack of body fat stores, and poor body condition.
• Since these animals usually have bacterial infections there is often evidence of bacterial septicemia or embolic bacterial spread in multiple organ systems. These appear as multiple foci of hemorrhage or inflammation within the parenchyma of various organs (kidney, spleen, and liver). Serosal surfaces of the thoracic and abdominal cavity and pericardium are usually reddened, with multifocal petechial hemorrhages and variable

amounts of adherent fibrin. Joint spaces may also be involved in a similar manner. Mild to moderate suppurative bronchopneumonia is often seen. Chronic dermatitis, embolic hepatitis, and both fibrinous and nonsuppurative leptomeningitis are other septicemia sequelae observed with JLIDS.
• Histologically, the major lesion is paracortical lymphocyte depletion. There is a lack of secondary follicles and germinal center formation. Ocular lesions including fibrinous anterior uveitis and neutrophilic choroiditis may also be seen.

TREATMENT

THERAPEUTIC APPROACH
• In the early stages, rule out intestinal parasitism as a cause for ill thrift with appropriate anthelmintic therapy.
• Lack of a functional immune system requires life-long antimicrobial intervention.

MEDICATIONS

DRUGS OF CHOICE
Antimicrobial therapy is indicated to treat systemic infections, with the caveat that infections in llamas with JLIDS routinely fail to respond to therapy and ultimately are fatal.

PRECAUTIONS
• Appropriate milk and meat withdrawal times must be followed for all compounds administered to food-producing animals, though withdrawal times are not established for camelids.

FOLLOW-UP

EXPECTED COURSE AND PROGNOSIS
This is a fatal disease. Animals diagnosed with this syndrome should be euthanized.

PREVENTION
Since this is likely a recessive genetic disorder, careful consideration should be taken in purchasing animals from herds with a history of JLIDS.

MISCELLANEOUS

ASSOCIATED CONDITIONS
• *Mycoplasma haemolamae* is prevalent in camelids in North America, but is rarely associated with clinical anemia except in animals with underlying disease.
• Secondary infections with typically nonpathogenic organisms, such as *Pneumocystis carinii*, *Bordetella* sp., or fungal

J

JUVENILE LLAMA IMMUNODEFICIENCY SYNDROME (CONTINUED)

organisms, are commonly associated with JLIDS.

AGE-RELATED FACTORS
Juvenile llamas (aged 6–18 months, typically)

PRODUCTION MANAGEMENT
• The specific immunodeficiency has not been determined, but an autosomal recessive defect in B-cell development has been proposed.
• Recent research suggests an inherited impairment in B-cell development as a potential primary cause.
• Cull/euthanize affected animals; evaluate parental records for possible genetic correlation.

SYNONYM
Failure to thrive

ABBREVIATIONS
• BCS = body condition score
• CNS = central nervous system
• ELISA = enzyme-linked immunosorbent assay
• JLIDS = juvenile llama immunodeficiency syndrome

SEE ALSO
• Anemia, Non-regenerative
• Body Condition Scoring: Alpacas and Llamas (see www.fiveminutevet.com/ruminant)
• Camelid Parasitology
• Copper Deficiency and Toxicity
• Nutrition and Metabolic Diseases: Camelid (see www.fiveminutevet.com/ruminant)
• Selenium/Vitamin E Deficiency
• Zinc Deficiency and Toxicity

Suggested Reading
Cebra C, Sisson D. Llama and Alpaca Care: Medicine, Surgery, Reproduction, Nutrition, and Herd Health. St. Louis: Elsevier, 2014, pp. 413–14.
Davis WC, Heirman LR, Hamilton MJ, et al. Flow cytometric analysis of an immunodeficiency affecting juvenile llamas. Vet Immunol Immunopathol 2000, 74: 103–20.
Hutchison JM, Garry F. Ill thrift and juvenile llama immunodeficiency syndrome. Update on Llama Medicine. Vet Clin North Am Food Anim Pract 1994, 10: 331–43.
Hutchison JM, Garry FB, Belknap EB, et al. Prospective characterization of the clinicopathologic and immunologic features of an immunodeficiency syndrome affecting juvenile llamas. Vet Immunol Immunopathol 1995, 49: 209–27.
Hutchison JM, Garry FB, Johnson LW, et al. Immunodeficiency syndrome associated with wasting and opportunistic infection in juvenile llamas: 12 cases (1988–1990). J Am Vet Med Assoc 1992, 201: 1070–6.

Author Kate O'Conor
Consulting Editor Christopher C.L. Chase
Acknowledgment The author and book editors acknowledge the prior contribution of Kelsey A. Hart.

KETOSIS: DAIRY CATTLE

BASICS

OVERVIEW

• Ketosis is a metabolic disorder characterized by high levels of ketone bodies affecting dairy cows mostly from parturition to 6 weeks postpartum. The ketone bodies, acetone, acetoacetate, and ß-hydroxybutyrate (BHB), are synthesized in the liver during oxidation of fatty acids. Acetone, a three-carbon compound, is produced in small quantities and is exhaled to the environment. Acetoacetate (four carbons) is either reversibly reduced to BHB in mitochondria, or is enzymatically or spontaneously decarboxylated to acetone. BHB is the most stable and important ketone body that can be tested in blood or milk.

• Historically, ketosis has been classified as primary or secondary, in which cows with primary ketosis have a decreased appetite and elevated serum, milk, urine, or breath ketones in the absence of another concurrent disease. Today, the words subclinical and clinical ketosis are more common terms for ketosis definition. Clinical ketosis is characterized by high levels of ketone bodies in blood, urine, or milk in combination with other signs, such as off-feed, severe body condition loss, depression, or altered behavior. Subclinical ketosis (SCK) is defined as an increase in blood, urine, or milk ketone bodies, above a threshold (e.g., 1.0–1.4 mmol/L of serum BHB) associated with lower milk yield, infertility and other conditions (e.g. displacement of the abomasum, metritis, mastitis) in the absence of noticeable clinical signs.

• Another classification for this metabolic disorder is type 1 and type 2 ketosis. Type 1 ketosis occurs when the cow experiences a sudden drop in energy intake. This is the case of underfeeding or poor cow comfort that prevents the cows from eating sufficient amounts of energy. Type 2 ketosis generally occurs around parturition when the cow is mobilizing excessive body fat in the form of nonesterified fatty acids (NEFA). Cows that are too fat at calving (BCS >3.75, scale 1–5) or cows that have been overfed during the dry period are at higher risk to develop this condition.

INCIDENCE/PREVALENCE

Incidence of SCK (≥1.2 mmol/L of BHB) can go between 15% and 60% of lactating dairy cows, while clinical ketosis may reach incidences between 2% and 15% of lactating dairy cows.

GEOGRAPHIC DISTRIBUTION

Worldwide, depending on production management. Ketosis has been diagnosed in both confined and grazing cattle.

SYSTEMS AFFECTED

Multisystemic

PATHOPHYSIOLOGY

• Every cow, starting around parturition, experiences a typical period of negative energy balance (NEB). Fat is mobilized from adipose tissue in the form of NEFA. This occurs because the activation of hormone-sensitive lipase (HSL) stimulates the breakdown of the ester link between NEFA and glycerol in the triglycerides (TAG).

• Once liberated, circulating NEFA is a significant energy precursor for several body tissues. In addition, it is a contributor to almost half of the milk fat produced in the mammary gland. NEFAs are also metabolized in the liver. Uptake of NEFA from plasma by the hepatocytes is proportional to the plasma concentration and the rate of blood flow. Consequently, when plasma NEFAs are extremely high, the uptake by the liver is also increased.

• Once taken up by the liver, NEFAs are oxidized to a number of molecules of acetyl-CoA (two carbon units) depending on the number of carbons present in the NEFA (16 or 18). Acetyl-CoA has four possible fates: complete oxidation through the Krebs cycle, incomplete oxidation through ketogenesis, TAG synthesis and packing as very low density lipoprotein (VLDL) for export from the liver, or TAG synthesis for storage in the liver. When oxaloacetate is depleted from the Krebs cycle, because of insufficient glucose availability, acetyl-CoA cannot continue its oxidation process and is accumulated and re-directed to form ketone bodies. This metabolic pathway is a normal secondary strategy to supply energy to the heart, brain, liver, and mammary tissue when the Krebs cycle is shut down. When excessive ketone bodies are built up, a negative impact on animal health, fertility, and productivity may occur.

• Simultaneously, accumulation of TAG in the liver may occur and it can be as high as 10% on wet weight basis during the peripartum period. Fatty liver is the result of a combination of increased fatty acid synthesis within the liver, decreased oxidation of hepatic fatty acids, and decreased export of hepatic TAG as VLDL.

• The evolution and extent of ketosis and hepatic lipidosis is finally the result of the level of adaptation from gestation to lactation.

HISTORICAL FINDINGS

For SCK, although there are no evident clinical signs, herd or individual animal history may indicate further investigation. Affected cows are at higher risk of developing several related conditions including displacement of the abomasum, metritis, mastitis, etc. In addition, cows with SCK are more likely to be culled during the first third of lactation, and less likely to conceive at first service than cows without SCK. Furthermore, cows with SCK produce less milk compared to cows without SCK.

SIGNALMENT

Female bovine, small ruminants, and camelids.

• Due to their high genetic merit for milk production, ketosis can be more prevalent in American Holsteins than other dairy breeds.

• Older cows are more prone to ketosis due to their greater potential milk yield.

PHYSICAL EXAMINATION FINDINGS

For clinical ketosis, the most common clinical signs are: drop in dry matter intake, constipation or loose feces, depression, gawking expression, evident losses in body condition, decreased milk production, odor due to ketones, neurologic signs such as circling, staggering, licking, chewing, bellowing, hyperesthesia, compulsive walking, and head pressing.

GENETICS

Ketosis has a certain genetic component. Heritability estimates for milk and plasma BHBA at different stages of early lactation have been determined to be between 0.10 and 0.29. Higher genetic merit for milk yield is associated with higher milk and plasma BHB concentrations.

CAUSES AND RISK FACTORS

• Risk factors for both clinical and SCK are over-conditioned animals at calving, development of other postpartum diseases, high milk production, poor cow comfort, stress, unbalanced diets, improper feed and nutritional management, and poor overall management. Ketosis may occur as either primary or secondary ketosis.

• Primary ketosis is caused either by a severe negative energy balance and/or obesity at parturition accompanied by a marked reduction in feed intake. In contrast, secondary ketosis occurs due to a decrease in feed intake, commonly due to a preexisting condition such as metritis, mastitis, lameness, traumatic reticulitis, or displacement of the abomasum.

DIAGNOSIS

DIFFERENTIAL DIAGNOSES

• Differential diagnoses for nervous ketosis include listeriosis, polioencephalomalacia, hypomagnesemia, and hypocalcemia.

• Differential diagnoses based on the nonspecific examination findings listed above and signalment should include postpartum diseases such as displaced abomasum, metritis, and mastitis.

CBC/BIOCHEMISTRY/URINALYSIS

• Biochemistry may show hypoglycemia.

• Urinalysis will show ketonuria in the vast majority of cases.

K

KETOSIS: DAIRY CATTLE   (CONTINUED)

OTHER LABORATORY TESTS

BHBA testing is routinely performed using a handheld glucometer/ketonometer (e.g., Precision Xtra) and 0.1 mL of whole blood. Levels above 1.2 mmol/L are considered to be abnormal.

IMAGING

N/A

OTHER DIAGNOSTIC PROCEDURES

N/A

PATHOLOGIC FINDINGS

N/A

TREATMENT

THERAPEUTIC APPROACH

• Several treatments have been recommended for ketosis in dairy cattle, with varying degrees of efficacy. However, in the scientific literature there is lack of well-designed clinical trials to answer this question.
• The only treatment of ketosis that has been scientifically shown to improve resolution of this metabolic disorder is oral propylene glycol (1,2 propanediol), in a dose of 300 g q24h. Although the duration of treatment may vary on a case-by-case basis, 5 days of treatment has yielded good response rates in numerous studies.
• The use of dextrose should be considered for animals with severe ketosis with concurrent hypoglycemia, especially in animals with nervous signs. The dose recommended is 250–500 mL 50% dextrose IV. Administration of IV dextrose leads to an immediate hyperglycemic state, lasting approximately 2 hours, and leading to excretion of excess dextrose in the urine. Dextrose for type 2 ketosis (related to insulin resistance) is not a recommended treatment, because glucose cannot enter the liver.
• Corticosteroids have long been used as an adjunctive therapy for ketosis based on their role in inducing hyperglycemia and catabolism of fat and protein stores. Few studies have evaluated the effect of corticosteroid use for ketosis in cattle and no significant benefit was found in the latest review in the *Veterinary Clinics of North America* in 2013. Due to the potential for immunosuppression secondary to corticosteroid use and the frequency of underlying postpartum disease in ketotic patients, corticosteroid use is not recommended as part of routine ketosis treatment.
• Insulin has been used in conjunction with dextrose and corticosteroid therapy due to its anabolic effects (decreases fat breakdown, increases ketone body utilization, increases fat synthesis). Benefits have been shown, albeit in limited studies. Insulin is best reserved for chronic cases that are refractory to the above

treatments or those where hepatic lipidosis is suspected. Note that the high cost and labile nature of insulin products may prohibit its use on farm.
• Vitamin B12 (cyanocobalamin) and phosphorus (butaphosphan) are often used in combination as a supportive therapy for ketosis since they are integral to the Krebs cycle. Their use in prevention of ketosis has been shown and preliminary studies show benefit as an adjunctive treatment for ketosis.

SURGICAL CONSIDERATIONS AND TECHNIQUES

N/A

MEDICATIONS

DRUGS OF CHOICE

See "Therapeutic Approach"

CONTRAINDICATIONS

Appropriate milk and meat withdrawal times must be followed for all compounds administered to food-producing animals.

PRECAUTIONS

• Corticosteroids should not be administered to pregnant animals.
• Use care when administering dextrose 50% IV as it causes severe tissue irritation and risk of abscessation when administered perivascularly.
• Do not use insulin without concurrent glucose support.

POSSIBLE INTERACTIONS

N/A

FOLLOW-UP

EXPECTED COURSE AND PROGNOSIS

With rapid diagnosis and treatment, as well as treatment of any underlying disease, the prognosis is good. If hepatic lipidosis has developed as a result of profound negative energy balance, the prognosis for return to productivity is worse.

POSSIBLE COMPLICATIONS

Ketosis will increase the risk of developing a displaced abomasum due to its effect on feed intake and gut motility. A study in 2012 found 95% of cows to be hyperketonemic prior to diagnosis of displaced abomasum.

CLIENT EDUCATION

See "Prevention"

PATIENT CARE

Insure that animals have easy access to fresh, palatable feed at all times to encourage increased feed intake. Optimize cow comfort and insure that the underlying cause of disease is being properly addressed in the case of secondary ketosis.

PREVENTION

• Ketosis must be prevented through rational feed management programs and adequate cow comfort. Diets should be properly balanced in energy, protein, vitamins, and minerals. Feeding programs should be designed to promote good body condition scores at calving (3.25–3.5). Avoid excess of energy during the dry period.
• Inclusion of gluconeogenic precursors that increase the energy density of the diet and plasma glucose concentrations during the entire transition period is recommended. Supplementation of glucose precursors should promote hepatic gluconeogenesis and increase circulating concentrations of insulin. This should decrease hepatic triglyceride accumulation and NEFA mobilization.
• Additives based on glycerol, calcium propionate, and/or propylene glycol have been used efficaciously. These products work better when they are top-dressed instead of mixed with the entire TMR.
• The use of sodium monensin (ionophore) either as a powder or as slow-release rumen bolus has also been demonstrated to be efficacious in controlling ketosis. Monensin stimulates the synthesis of rumen propionate. This effect spares oxaloacetate in the liver; consequently, the Krebs cycle continues in progress and ketogenesis is reduced.
• Another feed additive with secondary positive effects is niacin (6 g/day) incorporated into the ration for up to 10 weeks after calving.
• During recent years the use of rumen-protected choline (60 g/day), especially during the prepartum period, have been shown to be effective in the prevention of fatty liver and ketosis in dairy cattle, especially in obese animals.
• Propylene glycol administration protocols should be in place in dairy herds and should be based on herd ketosis incidence. If the herd incidence of ketosis is 15–50% then twice-weekly testing of cows 3–9 DIM is most economical. If incidence is above 50% then it is more economical to use blanket treatment for all cows starting at 5 DIM. The above management recommendations are integral to lowering the incidence of ketosis.

MISCELLANEOUS

SYNONYMS

N/A

ABBREVIATIONS

• BCS = body condition score
• BHB = beta hydroxybutyrate
• DIM = days in milk
• HSL = hormone-sensitive lipase
• NEB = negative energy balance
• NEFA = non-esterified fatty acids
• SCK = subclinical ketosis

K

- TAG = triglycerides
- TMR = total mixed ration
- VLDL = very low density lipoprotein

SEE ALSO
- Body Condition Scoring (see www.fiveminutevet.com/ruminant)
- Grass Tetany/Hypomagnesemia
- Hypocalcemia: Bovine
- Hypocalcemia: Small Ruminant
- Listeriosis
- Pregnancy Toxemia: Bovine
- Pregnancy Toxemia: Camelid
- Pregnancy Toxemia: Small Ruminant
- Transition Cow Management (see www.fiveminutevet.com/ruminant)
- Vitamin B Deficiency

Suggested Reading
Bobe G, Young JW, Beitz DC. Pathology, etiology, prevention, and treatment of fatty liver in dairy cows. J Dairy Sci 2004, 87: 3105–24.
Esposito G, Irons P, Webb E, Chapwanya A. Interactions between negative energy balance, metabolic diseases, uterine health and immune response in transition dairy cows. Anim Reprod Sci 2014, 144: 60–71.
Goff JP. Major advances in our understanding of nutritional influences on bovine health. J Dairy Sci 2006, 89: 1292–301.
Gordon JL, LeBlanc SJ, Duffield TF. Ketosis treatment in lactating dairy cattle. Vet Clin North Am Food Anim Pract 2013, 29: 433–45.
Grummer RR. Nutritional and management strategies for the prevention of fatty liver in dairy cattle. Vet J 2008, 176: 10–20.
LeBlanc SJ, Lissemore KD, Kelton DF, Duffield TF, Leslie KE. Major advances in disease prevention in dairy cattle. J Dairy Sci 2006, 89: 1267–79.
Ospina PA, McArt JA, Overton TR, Stokol T, Nydam DV. Using nonesterified fatty acids and β-hydroxybutyrate concentrations during the transition period for herd-level monitoring of increased risk of disease and decreased reproductive and milking performance. Vet Clin North Am Food Anim Pract 2013, 29: 387–412.

Author Pedro Melendez
Consulting Editor Kaitlyn A. Lutz
Acknowledgment The author and book editors acknowledge the prior contribution of Douglas C. Donovan.

K

LACTATION FAILURE (DYSGALACTIA, AGALACTIA, HYPOGALACTIA)

BASICS

OVERVIEW
- Agalactia is a clinical sign characterized by the absence of milk secretion, or the inability of a dam to lactate after parturition.
- Hypogalactia refers to an abrupt reduction in the normal amount of milk produced, and the term "dysgalactia" is sometimes used as a synonym.
- True agalactia can be present in situations of mammary gland aplasia or endocrinologic problems that compromise milk synthesis.
- Secondary agalactia is much more common and is present as one of the clinical signs of infectious diseases, intoxications, or neoplasia.
- Contagious agalactia (mycoplasma mastitis) of small ruminants is a syndrome that principally affects the mammary glands, joints, and eyes. The main causal agents are *Mycoplasma agalactiae* in sheep, and *M. agalactiae, M. mycoides* subsp. *mycoides* large colony type, and *M. capricolum* subsp. *capricolum* in goats. *M. putrefaciens* can produce a similar clinical picture, particularly in goats.
- In alpacas and llamas, agalactia may be seen in maiden females or in multiparous animals maintained on exogenous progesterone during pregnancy.

INCIDENCE/PREVALENCE
Will vary depending on etiology. With the small ruminant lentiviruses, CAEV and OPP (also known as Maedi-Visna), prevalence increases with age.

GEOGRAPHIC DISTRIBUTION
Contagious agalactia occurs worldwide and is often enzootic.

SYSTEMS AFFECTED
Mammary

PATHOPHYSIOLOGY
Will vary depending on etiology.

HISTORICAL FINDINGS
Will vary depending on etiology.

SIGNALMENT
Postparturient females are most commonly affected.

PHYSICAL EXAMINATION FINDINGS
In secondary agalactia or hypogalactia, some of the specific signs for the primary disease can be present, including:
- Depression
- Inappetence
- Fever
- Swollen or inflamed quarter(s)
- Conjunctivitis and arthritis (contagious agalactia of small ruminants)

GENETICS
Can be cause of mammary gland aplasia. Affected animals should be culled.

CAUSES AND RISK FACTORS
Common
- Mammarian aplasia, dysplasia
- Peracute toxigenic mastitis (agalactia)
- Clinical mastitis (hypogalactia)
- Contagious agalactia in small ruminants (mycoplasma mastitis)
- Lentiviruses (CAEV and OPP)
- Caseous lymphadenitis (caprine, ovine)
- Agalactia due to exogenous progesterone (camelids)

Less Common
- Leptospirosis (hypogalactia)
- Self-suckling or others suckling
- Water deprivation
- Endocrine dysfunction
- Intoxication (fungal toxins)
- Nutritional deficiency or imbalance (hypogalactia)
- Injury
- Neoplasia (lymphosarcoma, malignant melanoma, squamous cell carcinoma)
- Chapped teats, teat dip irritation
- Milk allergy
- Fescue toxicity
- Papillomatosis
- Anemia
- Severe toxicity

Risk Factors
- Cows affected by peracute toxigenic mastitis caused by *Staphylococcus aureus, Escherichia coli,* or *Klebsiella* spp. show signs of severe toxemia. Although not all quarters are usually affected, agalactia as a consequence of severe systemic illness can be present. The lactation curve is compromised and loss of the affected quarter is not uncommon. However, if treatment is successful, cows can reestablish milk production within 1–3 days.
- Contagious agalactia of sheep and goats is caused by *Mycoplasma agalactia* and can manifest in an acute, subacute, or chronic form. The udder shows signs of inflammation at the beginning of infection, milk secretion is watery and becomes purulent as the disease progresses, and agalactia is observed in the latter stages. Herd outbreaks may be accompanied by conjunctivitis and lameness.
- Dysgalactia and agalactia caused by leptospirosis outbreaks have been described in cow and sheep herds.
- Grazing of tall fescue (*Festuca arundinacea*) that is contaminated with an endophytic fungus (*Acremonium coenophialum*) has been shown to cause hypogalactia in cows. Feeding of grains contaminated with ergot (*Claviceps purpurea* in rye or *Claviceps africana* in sorghum) has produced clinical symptoms characterized by hypogalactia and eventual gangrene of extremities.
- In llamas and alpacas, exogenous progesterone may alter proper mammary development because of hormonal interactions, resulting in agalactia. Exogenous progesterone is used for treatment of luteal insufficiency in these species. Despite cessation of exogenous progesterone at 300 days of pregnancy, often these females do not develop adequate production of milk to meet their cria's needs.
- Risk factors for CAEV and OPP include feeding pooled colostrum, feeding virus-infected colostrum from a single dam to multiple kids or lambs, and addition of unscreened animals into herd.

DIAGNOSIS

DIFFERENTIAL DIAGNOSES
- Inability to secrete milk needs to be differentiated from inability to release milk from the alveolus or to pass it through the teat canal. Blockages need to be more fully examined.
- Primiparous females may have trouble adapting to the environment in the milking parlor and the administration of exogenous oxytocin (20 IU) may be necessary the first few days of lactation. This may need to be repeated for some days until the animal has adapted.
- Proliferative granulation tissue or fibrosis (pencil obstruction, "teat spider") after teat injury can cause partial or total obstruction of a teat canal. This is more common in one or two teats rather than the entire gland.
- Any systemic illness or stress may compromise lactation.

CBC/BIOCHEMISTRY/URINALYSIS
N/A

OTHER LABORATORY TESTS
- California Mastitis Test (CMT).
  - CMT is not useful in llamas and alpacas due to false negatives.
  - CMT may not be useful in goats due to false positives. Goats have a propensity for high milk somatic cell counts that may protect from mastitis.
- Culture and sensitivity of milk, including for mycoplasma.
- Bulk tank testing.
- CAEV AGID and ELISA.
- CAEV virus isolation (PCR).
- Microscopic examination of fescue for endophytic fungus.

IMAGING
- Ultrasound, using a 5–10 MHz linear probe. Can use contralateral teat as control.
- Radiology (contrast and double contrast).
- Teat endoscopy.

OTHER DIAGNOSTIC PROCEDURES
Diagnostics should be based on case history and specific laboratory analyses.

L

(CONTINUED)   LACTATION FAILURE (DYSGALACTIA, AGALACTIA, HYPOGALACTIA)

TREATMENT

Treatment should be directed against the underlying disease.

MEDICATIONS

DRUGS OF CHOICE
N/A

PRECAUTIONS
Appropriate milk and meat withdrawal times must be followed for all compounds administered to food-producing animals.

FOLLOW-UP

EXPECTED COURSE AND PROGNOSIS
Will vary depending on etiology.

POSSIBLE COMPLICATIONS
Culling may be indicated if production is not reestablished.

PREVENTION
See prevention strategies in appropriate chapter based on underlying disease.

MISCELLANEOUS

ASSOCIATED CONDITIONS
CAEV and OPP are lentiviruses that can manifest as "hard bag" (indurant mastitis).

AGE-RELATED FACTORS
Will vary depending on etiology. For example, prevalence of CAEV infection increases with age.

ZOONOTIC POTENTIAL
Certain strains of *Leptospira* and *Mycoplasma* are zoonotic.

PREGNANCY
Mycoplasma spp. and *Leptospira* spp. can cause abortions in ruminants.

BIOSECURITY
Will vary depending on etiology (e.g., screening new additions to herd with ELISA or milk culture).

PRODUCTION MANAGEMENT
• Will vary depending on etiology. Feeding heat-treated colostrum and isolation of kids at birth are control measures for both contagious agalactia and CAEV, for example.
• Mammary development in females often is minimal until immediately before or after parturition, although glandular development is palpable during late gestation and should be monitored.

ABBREVIATIONS
• AGID = agar gel immunodiffusion
• CAEV = caprine arthritis encephalitis virus
• CMT = California mastitis test
• ELISA = enzyme-linked immunosorbent assay
• OPP = ovine progressive pneumonia
• PCR = polymerase chain reaction

SEE ALSO
• Biosecurity (see www.fiveminutevet.com/ruminant)
• Caseous Lymphadenitis (CLA)
• Leptospirosis
• Maedi-Visna (Ovine Progressive Pneumonia)
• Mastitis: Coliform
• Mastitis: Mycoplasmal
• Mastitis: Pharmacology (see www.fiveminutevet.com/ruminant)
• Mastitis: Small Ruminant
• Reproductive Pharmacology
• Respiratory Disease: Small Ruminant

Suggested Reading
Bergonier D, Berthelot X, Poumarat F. Contagious agalactia of small ruminants: current knowledge concerning epidemiology, diagnosis and control. Rev Sci Tech 1997, 16: 848–73.
Blaney BJ, McKenzie RA, Walters JR, et al. Sorghum ergot (*Claviceps africana*) associated with agalactia and feed refusal in pigs and dairy cattle. Aust Vet J 2000, 78: 102–7.

Cebra C, Anderson DE, Tibary A. Llama and Alpaca Care. St. Louis: Elsevier, 2014.
Kautz FM. Use of a Staphylococcus vaccine to reduce prevalence of mastitis and lower somatic cell counts in a registered Saanen Dairy Goat Herd. Res Vet Sci 2014, 97: 18–19.
Kinde H, DaMassa AJ, Wakenell PS, Petty R. Mycoplasma infection in a commercial goat dairy caused by *Mycoplasma agalactiae* and *Mycoplasma mycoides* subsp. *mycoides* (caprine biotype). J Vet Diagn Invest 1994, 6: 423–7.
Madanat A, Zendulková D, Pospisil Z. Contagious agalactia of sheep and goats: a review. Acta Vet Brno 2001, 70: 403–12.
McKeown JD, Ellis WA. *Leptospira hardjo* agalactia in sheep. Vet Rec 1986, 118: 482.
Pugh DG, Baird AN. Sheep and Goat Medicine, 2nd ed. Maryland Heights: Elsevier Saunders, 2012.
Quinlan JF, McNicholl VJ. Agalactia and infertility due to *Leptospira interrogans* serovar *hardjo* infection in a vaccinated dairy herd. Irish Vet J 1993, 46: 97–8.
Smith BP. Causes of agalactia and hypogalactia in ruminants. In: Smith BP ed, Large Animal Internal Medicine, 5th ed. St. Louis: Elsevier Mosby, 2015.
Souza FN, Blagitz MG, Penna CFAM, et al. Somatic cell count in small ruminants: friend or foe? Small Rumin Res 2012, 107: 65–75.
Thomas DL. Effect of prepartum photoperiod on milk production and prolactin concentration of dairy ewes. Dairy Sheep Production Research at University of Wisconsin-Madison, A Review. J Anim Sci Biotech 2014, 5: 22.

Author Kyle G. Mathis
Consulting Editor Kaitlyn A. Lutz
Acknowledgment The author and book editors acknowledge the prior contribution of Sérgio O. Juchem.

L

LAMENESS: BOVINE

BASICS

OVERVIEW
• Lameness is a leading cause of culling and welfare problems in dairy cattle.
• Although less common in beef cattle, lameness remains an important welfare concern and can result in significant loss of productivity.
• In dairy cattle, 90% of lameness is associated with the foot, with 90% of that being associated with the hind foot lateral claw.
• In cow-calf operations the majority of lameness is associated with upper leg issues.
• In beef feedlots, approximately 70% of lameness is foot-associated with the remainder being related to lesions of the proximal limb.

INCIDENCE/PREVALENCE
• The incidence and prevalence varies widely between production systems and operations. Cattle confined on hard surfaces such as concrete tend to have more lameness compared with cattle housed on pasture.
• In many dairy operations the annual incidence of lameness varies between 15% and 30%. Lameness is the leading cause of culling in dairy operations and represents the most costly clinical disease process of dairy cattle, surpassing mastitis, when chronic lost production is considered.

GEOGRAPHIC DISTRIBUTION
Worldwide

SYSTEMS AFFECTED
• Musculoskeletal
• Integument

PATHOPHYSIOLOGY
• The majority of lameness in the foot is associated with uneven weight bearing between the claws. In the hind feet the normal posture of a cow results in increased weight bearing on the lateral claw. This results in compensatory overgrowth of horn on the lateral claw, which further exacerbates the disparity in weight bearing. In the front limb the medial claw bears the most weight.
• Bovine lameness can be subdivided into three major classifications:
  ○ Upper leg lameness—generally associated with trauma to the musculoskeletal system of the upper leg. This type of lameness is generally associated with a characteristic altered gait and a lack of sensitivity to hoof testers on the hoof capsule.
  ○ Claw horn lesions—generally associated with disease of the white line or a combination of mechanical and metabolic disease resulting in sole ulceration. The white line is the weakest portion of the claw horn capsule and in some cases allows foreign bodies to penetrate the white line and cause abscessation of the corium.
  ○ Infectious skin disease—most commonly associated with either bovine foot rot or bovine digital dermatitis. These diseases are bacterial in nature and result in infectious transmission between animals when environmental conditions are favorable.

HISTORICAL FINDINGS
• Upper leg lameness is often associated with a history of trauma, slipping or falling during movement, or calving.
• Housing in environments that keep the hoof moist and allow excessive buildup of mud or manure slurry are associated with an increased risk of infectious foot disease.
• Housing on concrete pads or confinement barns are associated with increased risk of lameness compared to housing on pasture. Housing cattle where they spend excessive periods of time standing due to a lack of comfortable areas on which to lie down is also associated with an increased risk of lameness.
• Introduction of cattle to an operation from outside operations is often identified as a source of new infectious disease, especially digital dermatitis.

SIGNALMENT
• Reported in all types of cattle.
• Disease is often most severe in mature heavier cattle compared to calves.
• Beef cows on grass most commonly present with upper leg lameness.
• Dairy cattle most commonly present with claw horn lesions or infectious skin disease.
• Feedlot cattle most commonly present with foot rot, digital dermatitis, or toe lesions.
• Particular causes of lameness may show breed predilections.
• Digital dermatitis is most often reported in Holstein dairy cattle, compared with other dairy and/or beef breeds.
• Lameness is more common in adults than in juveniles.

PHYSICAL EXAMINATION FINDINGS
• Lameness is generally recognized as unwillingness to place normal weight on one or more limbs.
• Lameness is best assessed by observation of animals walking on a solid surface (concrete) and evaluating gait for evidence of a shortened or inconsistent stride length, arched back while moving, head bob, and in severe cases a complete reluctance to place weight on a limb.
• Multiple schemes have been developed for classifying the severity of lameness; however, the easiest to apply is a three-point grading system. In this system animals are classified as normal, lame (one or more of the signs listed above but still willing to bear weight on the limb), or severely lame (unwillingness to bear weight on the limb).
• In cases of claw horn lesions, use of hoof testers applied to all areas of the sole will generally result in a withdrawal response associated with pain.
• In cases of infection involving the deep tissues of the foot or distal limb, a key clinical indicator is severe swelling in comparison to the contralateral foot. In foot rot, the swelling is most commonly symmetrical, while other infectious processes secondary to sole ulcers or white line disease often result in asymmetrical swelling confined to one claw of the foot.
• Careful examination of the interdigital skin, skin of the heel adjacent to the interdigital cleft, and the coronary band will be abnormal in cases of infectious foot disease. Lesions may vary from overt breaks in the skin with bovine foot rot to more ulcerative lesions or papillomatous lesions with bovine digital dermatitis.

GENETICS
N/A

CAUSES AND RISK FACTORS
• Upper leg lameness can occur from a variety of causes, the most common of which include fractures to the axial skeleton or pelvis, luxated or subluxated femorocoxial joint, ruptured cruciate ligaments and collateral ligaments of the stifle. In some cases, neurologic disease may induce clinical signs similar to lameness and should be ruled out.
• Hoof horn lesions
  ○ Sole ulcers are most commonly associated with ischemia and contusive effects damaging the corium between the flexor tuberosity of P3 and the floor or standing surface. As a consequence, these lesions are located beneath the anatomic location of the flexor tuberosity (located on the axial-caudal portion of the weight-bearing surface) and are typically located on the lateral hind claws or medial front claws because of greater weight bearing on these claws.
  ○ White line lesions typically form in the abaxial-caudal portion of the white line secondary to the penetration of foreign material from the environment. This area of the white line is vulnerable to penetration by foreign debris because of heel strike during locomotion. Laminitis predisposes to white line disease by further softening the white line and making it easier to penetrate. The foreign material results in formation of a deep anaerobic pocket that then migrates to the corium and causes an abscess.
• Infectious skin disease
  ○ Digital dermatitis is polybacterial in nature, meaning that there is no single bacterial organism that has been identified as an etiologic agent. Mature lesions are predominated by bacteria of the *Treponema* spp.; however, earlier lesions have small numbers and different treponemes, suggesting that this family is not exclusively causal for the disease.
  ○ Foot rot is caused by a deep infection of the soft tissue structures of the foot by *Fusobacterium necrophorum.*
• Once digital dermatitis is in the herd it is thought to spread through unsanitary conditions in the barn.

• Muddy or wet conditions and purchasing animals from off premises are the two most common risk factors for digital dermatitis.
• Poor freestall and bedding management will exacerbate lameness problems since cows will spend more time standing in the manure slurry, not allowing the feet to dry out periodically.

DIAGNOSIS

DIFFERENTIAL DIAGNOSES
• Neurologic disease
• Myositis

CBC/BIOCHEMISTRY/URINALYSIS
N/A

OTHER LABORATORY TESTS
N/A

IMAGING
In some cases of upper leg lameness or distal limb swelling, radiographs of the affected region may aid in diagnosis of fractures or infectious disease impacting the joints or bone.

OTHER DIAGNOSTIC PROCEDURES
• Observation of the animal in motion and the limb for swelling.
• Thorough evaluation of the lame foot with hoof testers, paying special attention to common areas of lesions (i.e., the abaxial white line for white line disease and the area of the flexor tuberosity of P3 for sole ulcers).
• Corrective hoof trimming and balancing of weight bearing will often identify underrun sole or loose tissue that will assist in identifying the lesion for claw horn lesions.
• Careful observation of the skin around the corium for evidence of breaks in the skin, ulceration, or abnormal appearances.
• In cases where it may be difficult to discern from the above procedures if the lesion is in the foot or proximal limb, intravenous regional anesthesia may be useful. If gait improves subsequent to anesthesia of the foot, the problem is likely in the foot.

PATHOLOGIC FINDINGS
Histopathology is typically unnecessary to identify the cause of lameness.

TREATMENT

THERAPEUTIC APPROACH
The treatment for lameness varies by cause and the reader is referenced to individual chapters in this text related to each condition, for more details.

SURGICAL CONSIDERATIONS AND TECHNIQUES
N/A

MEDICATIONS

DRUGS OF CHOICE
Readers are referred to the individual chapters related to each process for details on medications.

PRECAUTIONS
When using any antibiotics or anti-inflammatories for therapy, appropriate milk and meat withdrawal times should be followed for food-producing animals.

CONTRAINDICATIONS
N/A

POSSIBLE INTERACTIONS
N/A

FOLLOW-UP

EXPECTED COURSE AND PROGNOSIS
• Simple, uncomplicated white line abscesses typically resolve without complication in 4–6 weeks with corrective trimming and the application of a foot block to the healthy claw.
• Simple sole ulcers typically take longer to fully resolve but should heal within 2 months.
• The prognosis for infections that involve the deep structures of the claw or foot are always guarded. Since many of these cases typically present late in the disease course, the infection is well established and there is already significant pathology.
• Aggressive antibiotic therapy is warranted when deep structures of the hoof are involved, but it is rarely successful alone.
• Animals treated for digital dermatitis with topical antibiotics typically show increased discomfort immediately after treatment, but lameness should resolve almost fully within 48 hours.

POSSIBLE COMPLICATIONS
Some claw horn lesions will progress to deep-seated infectious arthritis cases.

CLIENT EDUCATION
Clients should be educated regarding diagnosis, risk factors, and treatment strategies. Importance should also be placed on prevention and degree of economic losses associated with lameness.

PATIENT CARE
• Lameness is a significant welfare issue and animals need to be treated promptly and given appropriate medication for pain control.
• Claw horn lesions treated with corrective trimming and having an orthopedic block applied to the opposite claw generally show significant improvement in lameness once weight bearing on the claw with the lesion has been removed. If the animal remains lame after trimming and placement of the block they should be promptly reevaluated for an alternate cause of lameness or incorrect block placement. They should be monitored regularly for evidence of increased lameness.
• Most cases of digital dermatitis treated with topical antibiotics will show rapid improvement in lameness. Animals that remain lame after 72 hours should be reexamined for an additional cause of lameness.
• Cows should be monitored for recurrence of all types of lameness and re-treated as necessary.

PREVENTION
• Providing housing conditions that promote the animals' lying and spending less time standing.
• Minimizing accumulation of excessive amounts of mud or manure and keeping standing areas dry.
• In cases of digital dermatitis, preventive foot bathing will assist in control.
• Routine foot trimming of cattle will assist in early detection of lesions and will improve equal weight bearing while minimizing lameness.

MISCELLANEOUS

ASSOCIATED CONDITIONS
• Decreased milk production, increased culling
• Recumbency
• Welfare

BIOSECURITY
• Introduction of digital dermatitis commonly occurs with purchase and introduction of new animals to a herd or feedlot. For this reason, it is prudent to inquire and evaluate potential animals for purchase for the presence of DD prior to introduction.
• Any individual involved in foot care should take great care to insure that equipment is suitably disinfected between farm visits.
• DD-free herds should avoid the purchase of replacements from off-site premises.

PRODUCTION MANAGEMENT
• Recommendations that pertain to cow comfort, including well-designed and bedded freestalls or open housing.
• Prompt and aggressive treatment of lameness will reduce suffering, losses in milk yield, and culling.

ABBREVIATION
• DD = digital dermatitis

SEE ALSO
• Bovine Digital Dermatitis
• Foot Rot: Bovine
• Sole Lesions in Dairy Cattle

Suggested Reading
Berry SL. Diseases of the digital soft tissues. Vet Clin North Am Food Anim Pract 2001, 17: 129–42.

L

LAMENESS: BOVINE

Demirkan I, Murray RD, Carter SD. Skin diseases of the bovine digit associated with lameness. Vet Bull 2000, 70: 149–71.

Hernandez J, Shearer JK, Webb DW. Effect of lameness on milk yield in dairy cows. J Am Vet Med Assoc 2002, 220: 640–4.

Krull AC, Shearer JK, Gorden PJ, Cooper VL, Phillips GJ, Plummer PJ. Deep sequencing analysis reveals the temporal microbiota changes associated with the development of bovine digital dermatitis. Infect Immun 2014, 82: 3359–73.

Krull A, Shearer J, Gorden P, Scott HM, Plummer PJ. Digital dermatitis: natural lesion progression and regression in Holstein dairy cattle over three years. J Dairy Sci 2016, 99: 3718–31.

Shearer JK, Plummer PJ, Schleining JA. Perspectives on the treatment of claw lesions in cattle. Vet Med Res Rep 2015, 6: 273–92.

Shearer JK, Elliott JB. Papillomatous digital dermatitis: treatment and control strategies—part I. Compend Cont Educ Pract Vet 1998, 20: S158–73.

Shearer JK, Hernandez J, Elliott JB. Papillomatous digital dermatitis: treatment and control strategies—part II. Compend Cont Educ Pract Vet 1998, 20: S213–23.

Trott DJ, Moeller MR, Zuerner RL, et al. Characterization of *Treponema phagedenis*-like spirochetes isolated from papillomatous digital dermatitis lesions in dairy cattle. J Clin Microbiol. 2003, 41: 2522–9.

van Amstel SR, Shearer JK, Palin FL. Moisture content, thickness, and lesions of sole horn associated with thin soles in dairy cattle. J Dairy Sci 2004, 87: 757–63.

Webster AJ. Effects of housing practices on the development of foot lesions in dairy heifers in early lactation. Vet Rec 2002, 151: 9–12.

Authors Paul J. Plummer and Jan K. Shearer

Consulting Editor Kaitlyn A. Lutz

L

BASICS

OVERVIEW
• Lameness is defined as an abnormality in the gait or posture of an animal. It may be related to pain or some other type of dysfunction in the locomotor system.
• Causes of lameness
  ○ Congenital lameness—defects in nerves, bones, muscles, or other associated soft tissue structures
  ○ Acquired lameness
    ▪ Traumatic soft tissue, bone, or neurologic injuries
    ▪ Bone or soft tissue infections
    ▪ Nutritional causes such as hypophosphatemic rickets and white muscle disease (WMD)
    ▪ Patellar luxation from abnormal skeletal growth due to early castration
    ▪ Arthritis in geriatric animals is common; animals have difficulty walking and rising; spend increased time recumbent
    ▪ Joint ill in neonates is not common in camelids, usually a single joint, non weight-bearing on affected limb with pain and swelling
    ▪ Meningeal worm infections (MW disease, MWD) resulting in spinal cord damage

INCIDENCE/PREVALENCE
One survey conducted for alpaca and llama farms in 18 different states in the United States, Canada, Australia, and New Zealand showed an incidence rate of 50% among farms surveyed and an overall prevalence of approximately 3% of the animals involved in the survey.

GEOGRAPHIC DISTRICUTION
• Worldwide
• MWD: Eastern US

SYSTEMS AFFECTED
• Musculoskeletal
• Nervous

PATHOPHYSIOLOGY
Varies depending on the nature of lameness and causes

HISTORICAL DATA
• Abnormal conformation
• Acute or chronic onset of abnormal gait
• Recent history of trauma on physical exertion
• Excessive recumbency

SIGNALMENT
• Any age and sex
• Lateral patellar luxation common in camelids castrated before 18 months of age
  ○ Due to growing taller with more upright conformation than animals castrated later
  ○ Leads to femoropatellar joint arthritis

PHYSICAL EXAMINATION FINDINGS
• Non-uniform gait (head nod, stilted gait) at the walk and faster.
• Decreased or lack of weight bearing on the affected limb or limbs.
• Kyphosis, excessive recumbency, and/or pain on palpation of physeal regions in crias with rickets; also may just appear to be lethargic.
• Swelling of limbs or muscles depending on etiology.

GENETICS
• Congenital defects resulting in lameness may have a hereditary basis.
• It is recommended that animals which produce offspring with congenital defects not be bred together again.

CAUSES AND RISK FACTORS
• Muscle infections and myositis
  ○ *Sarcocystis* spp.
    ▪ Camelids are intermediate hosts with carnivores such as dogs as the final host.
    ▪ Carnivores consume feces from infected, uncooked camelid muscles and shed sporocysts in the feces after 1–2 weeks for several months.
    ▪ Camelids are reinfected through consuming the sporocysts as they eat.
    ▪ More advanced stages of the protozoa cause damage to tissues such as muscles where they migrate.
    ▪ Eliminating contaminated meat intake by carnivores breaks the infection cycle.
  ○ *Clostridium septicum, C. chauvoei, C. sordellii,* and *C. novyi* can affect camelids depending on geographic prevalence of the species:
    ▪ Caused by exogenous introduction through wounds (such as snake envenomation) or localization in traumatized muscles from hematogenous origin.
    ▪ Death from toxemia may occur.
• Muscle and/or skeletal trauma from overcrowding and fighting among animals.
• White muscle disease (WMD) from deficiency of vitamin E and/or selenium in the diet.
  ○ No published reports in camelids but empirically diagnosed primarily in young animals.
  ○ Muscle weakness and excessive recumbency possible.
  ○ Sudden death possible if heart muscles affected.
• Skeletal dysfunction
  ○ Dietary causes
    ▪ Hypophosphatemic rickets in young growing animals between 3 and 7 months of age when exposed to low UV light conditions during rapid bone growth periods.
    ▪ Prevents activation of dietary vitamin D precursor to the active form of vitamin D3.
    ▪ Results in poor absorption and deposition of calcium and phosphorus in

bones, further resulting in growth plate abnormalities and signs such as leg deviations and pain in the physeal regions of bones.
    ▪ Excessive recumbency and poor body condition and growth may be the end result.
  ○ Traumatic causes
    ▪ Foot injuries are the most common cause of lameness: punctures, sole infections, fractured toenails, interdigital dermatitis from topical infections, space-occupying lesions (tumors)—bottom of foot, interdigital space
    ▪ Bone fractures
    ▪ Ligament, tendon, and joint injuries
    ▪ Back and neck injuries—fighting
    ▪ Congenital bone and ligament formation abnormalities: incomplete ossification of long bones—seen in the femur with no pain but abnormal gait in a neonate; arthrogryposis—unknown etiology but hereditary basis suspected
    ▪ Arthritis in mature animals may be progressive and accompanied by weight loss
  ○ Miscellaneous causes
    ▪ Joint ill in neonates from acquired systemic infections—umbilicus most likely the entrance point for environmental contaminants
    ▪ Angular limb deformities in premature crias—mildly affected animals will recover without treatment
    ▪ MWD from consumption of *Parelaphostrongylus tenuis* infectious larval stage where intermediate host (some species of terrestrial gastropods) and definitive host (Virginia white tailed deer) are present
    ▪ Lateral patellar luxation and associated arthropathy from early castration (before 18 months of age) in alpacas and llamas

DIAGNOSIS

DIFFERENTIAL DIAGNOSES
• Neurologic lameness—should observe weakness, ataxia, and/or proprioceptive deficits.
• Meningeal worm disease causing brain or spinal cord damage is seen as a lameness with abnormal locomotion, excessive recumbency, and/or inability to rise from the prone position.

CBC/BIOCHEMSTRY/URINALYSIS
Elevated muscle enzymes (CPK, LDH) from chronic time down; hypophophosphatemia with rickets, nonspecific elevations in enzymes associated with bone metabolism.

OTHER LABORATORY TESTS
• Whole blood selenium low for WMD

L

• Elevated eosinophilic white blood cells in cerebrospinal fluid tap for animals with MWD
• Muscle biopsies and cultures for infectious causes of lameness

IMAGING
• Radiography for bone lesions
• Ultrasonography for soft tissue lesions

OTHER DIAGNOSTIC PROCEDURES
Neurologic examination, posture and gait observation, palpation, withdrawal response to joint flexion or sole pressure

PATHOLOGIC FINDINGS
• Heat, swelling, pain on palpation, loss of function
• Possible osteomyelitis, bone sequestration, draining tracts
• Muscle biopsies with abnormal gross and/or microscopic findings
• Inflammatory tracts and/or larvae on histologic section of the spinal cord of camelids with MWD

TREATMENT
THERAPEUTIC APPROACH
• Confinement/rest
• Support wraps, casts, internal and/or external fixation as required
• Antibiotics for infections associated with wounds
• Nonsteroidal anti-inflammatory drugs for relief of pain and swelling
  ○ Flunixin meglumine at 0.5 mg/lb q24h by subcutaneous, intramuscular, or intravenous injection for 7–14 days
  ○ Phenylbutazone at 4 mg/lb orally q24h
  ○ Etodolac at 4.5 mg/lb orally q24h for 7 days, then decrease to q48h
  ○ Meloxicam @ 0.5 mg/lb orally q48h
• Joint-specific drugs to treat arthritis—Adequan IM (Luitpold Animal Health) @ 1.0 mg per lb body weight weekly by intramuscular injection for 3–4 weeks
• Physical therapy to restore range of motion and prevent pressure sores in recumbent animals
• Corticosteroids—drug choice and dose depends on clinician preference
• Acupuncture
• Chiropractic care
• Rickets treatment
  ○ Injectable vitamin D3 @ 1,000 IU/lb by subcutaneous injection
  ○ Repeat weekly as needed until serum phosphorus levels are raised to the normal range
• Angular limb deformities—periosteal stripping, growth plate screws and wires or staples depending on the severity and preferences of the surgeon
• Injectable selenium (bovine selenium product BoSe ®) for WMD in acute cases,

plus adequate dietary supplementation thereafter
• Lavage septic joints and use systemic antibacterial therapy for joint ill
• See chapter, Parasite Control Programs: Camelid, for treatment of MWD

CONTRAINDICATIONS
• Topical or systemic corticosteroid use in pregnant animals usually results in abortion.
• Appropriate milk and meat withdrawal times must be followed for all compounds administered to food-producing animals.

PRECAUTIONS
N/A

POSSIBLE INTERACTIONS
N/A

FOLLOW-UP
EXPECTED COURSE AND PROGNOSIS
• Good for most injuries including fractures.
• Clostridial myositis has a grave prognosis and may cause sudden death from effects of toxin.
• Rickets cases usually respond to medical treatment if discovered and treated early in the course.
• Joint ill may result in septicemia and death.
• MWD survivors are often left with abnormal locomotion—50% of cases die or require euthanasia.

POSSIBLE COMPLICATIONS
• Septicemia from infectious causes
• Chronic non-union fractures may necessitate amputation of a limb
• Chronic, progressive arthritis due to multiple causes
• Death—WMD, Clostridial infections, joint ill, *Sarcocystis* infections, MWD

CLIENT EDUCATION
Observe gait and behavior of the animal

PATIENT CARE
• Look for improvement in gait and/or less time recumbent
• Repeat radiographs to monitor bone healing
• Serial neurologic examinations
• Serial serum phosphorus levels to monitor improvement in hypophosphatemic rickets cases

PREVENTION
• Environmental cleanliness for neonates at birthing time helps prevent joint ill.
• Use of multivalent Clostridial vaccines depending on area risk.
• MWD prevention program in at-risk locations in the US (see chapter, Parasite Control Programs: Camelid).
• Avoid overcrowding to minimize traumatic injuries.
• Vitamin D3 injections for rickets prevention—1,000 IU/lb subcutaneously

every 2 months in October, December, and February in at-risk areas of the US.

MISCELLANEOUS
ASSOCIATED CONDITIONS
• Pressure sores from excessive recumbency
• Weight loss and poor growth from insufficient access to food
• Septicemia and death possible from infections

AGE-RELATED FACTORS
• Congenital incomplete ossification of femur seen rarely in crias
• Joint ill in neonates
• Angular limb deformities in premature crias
• Arthritis in mature animals may be progressive and accompanied by weight loss

ZOONOTIC POTENTIA
N/A

PREGNANCY
Increased weight as pregnancy progresses may increase lameness.

BIOSECURITY
N/A

PRODUCTION MANAGEMENT
• Separate animals into manageable group sizes to avoid injuries from overcrowding.
• Separate animals by body size to prevent injuries to smaller, young animals.
• Maintain a clean environment for birthing.
• Provide adequate diet for growth and maintenance.
• MWD prevention programs.

ABBREVIATIONS
• CPK = creatine phosphokinase
• LDH = lactate dehydrogenase
• MWD = meningeal worm disease
• WMD = white muscle disease

SEE ALSO
• Congenital Defects: Camelid
• Nutrition and Metabolic Diseases: Camelid (see www.fiveminutevet.com/ruminant)
• Physical Examination: Camelid (Appendix 5)
• Selenium/Vitamin E Deficiency
• Vitamin D Deficiency/Toxicosis

Suggested Reading
Harr B, Anderson, DE. Survey of Lameness in Alpacas and Llamas. The Ohio State University College of Veterinary Medicine, 2003.
Reed SK, Semevolos SA, Newman KD, Anderson DE. Musculoskeletal surgery. In: Cebra C et al. eds, Llama and Alpaca Care. Elsevier, 2014.
Van Saun RJ. Nutritional diseases of South American camelids. Small Rumin Res 2006, 61: 153–64.
Author Stephen R. Purdy
Consulting Editor Ahmed Tibary

L

LAMENESS: SMALL RUMINANT

BASICS

OVERVIEW
- Lameness is an important welfare and management problem of small ruminant operations.
- Most lameness observed in small ruminants is infectious in nature. Thus biosecurity is of paramount importance in limiting and managing lameness of small ruminants.
- In some jurisdictions (especially portions of Australia), active efforts to eradicate some forms of small ruminant lameness are under way and require specific reporting mechanisms with governmental oversight. No such systems are in place in the United States.
- Farms with active lameness issues should consider biosecurity implications of selling or moving animals from the farm.

INCIDENCE/PREVALENCE
- Varies greatly by disease process, season, and location.
- In severe cases of virulent foot rot, within-herd prevalence can exceed 50%.

GEOGRAPHIC DISTRIBUTION
- Varies by disease process.
- Ovine foot rot (benign and virulent) have a worldwide distribution. Efforts are under way to eradicate virulent foot rot in some regions of the world.
- Ovine contagious digital dermatitis and similar lesions in goats have been predominantly reported in Europe, although recently suggestive lesions have been identified in the US.
- White line disease, heel abscesses, and toe abscesses are reported worldwide.

SYSTEMS AFFECTED
Musculoskeletal

PATHOPHYSIOLOGY
- Most cases of small ruminant lameness are associated with an infectious agent.
- Penetration of the dermis or corium with infectious bacteria results in dermatitis or under-running of the sole and in some cases severe lameness.

HISTORICAL FINDINGS
Lameness scoring system
- Score 0 (SOUND) Bears weight evenly on all four feet and walks with an even rhythm.
- Score 1 (MILD) Steps are uneven but it is not clear which limb or limbs are affected.
- Score 2 (MODERATE) Steps are uneven and the stride may be shortened; the affected limb or limbs are identifiable.
- Score 3 (SEVERE) Mobility is severely compromised such that the sheep frequently stops walking or lies down due to obvious discomfort. The affected limb(s) are clearly identifiable and may be held off the ground.

SIGNALMENT
Sheep and goats. Any growing or mature animal is at risk.

PHYSICAL EXAMINATION FINDINGS
- Varies by disease process
- Interdigital dermatitis (also known as foot scald, benign foot rot, or grade 1–2 foot rot)
  - Erythema and inflammation of the interdigital space
  - Often multiple feet
- Virulent foot rot
  - Distinct odor often present when foot is lifted.
  - Erythematous and/or an erosive or ulcerative lesion affecting the interdigital space leading to hoof horn separation axially which may lead to necrosis of the sole and in very severe cases avulsion of the hoof capsule.
  - Severe and progressive separation of the soft and hard horn from the underlying corium. Starts as a portion of the sole (stage 3) and progresses.
  - Often involves the majority of the sole (stage 4) and extends up the outer wall in severe lesions (stage 5).
  - Usually involves both claws and often more than one foot.
  - Foot may be swollen or warm.
  - In chronic cases the claw may be severely misshapen.
- Contagious ovine digital dermatitis (CODD, contagious caprine digital dermatitis)
  - Ulcerative or chronic inflammatory lesion originating at the coronary band, which may extend dorsally and abaxially under the hoof wall and in many cases leads to avulsion of the hoof capsule.
  - The affected digit may be swollen and shortened.
- White line disease (shelly hoof, "hoof abscess")
  - Separation of the hard horn from the underlying corium without separation of the sole.
  - Confined to the region of the white line.
  - Pockets of manure and debris that can be cleaned out and do not have evidence of inflamed or hemorrhagic corium.
  - In severe cases it may extend to the coronary band and discharge purulent material.
- Strawberry foot rot
  - Ulcerative dermatitis affecting the skin of the legs from the coronet to as high as the knee or hock.
  - Scabs that when removed expose an ulcerative skin lesion with the appearance on the surface of a strawberry.
- Toe granuloma
  - Granulomatous mass of tissue originating from the corium at the toe end of the sole. The mass of tissue protrudes above the level of the surrounding sole and prevents normal formation of hoof horn.

CAUSES AND RISK FACTORS
- Wet environmental conditions predispose to all diseases due to softening of the hoof horn.
- Use of contaminated hoof trimming equipment is a significant risk factor.
- Purchase or housing of infected animals is the most common source of disease.
- Interdigital dermatitis: *Dichelobacter nodosus.*
- Virulent foot rot: *Dichelobacter nodosus.*
- Contagious ovine digital dermatitis: Polybacterial disease process that includes significant numbers of *Treponema* spp. organisms similar or identical to those seen in bovine digital dermatitis.
- White line disease
  - Packing of manure and debris into the normally softer white line.
  - Moist conditions that keep the hoof horn soft
- Strawberry foot rot: *Dermatophilus congolensis.*
- Toe granuloma: In most cases this is associated with overtrimming of the hoof. Less commonly it may be the sequela of a previous severe foot rot or undermined sole.

DIAGNOSIS

DIFFERENTIAL DIAGNOSES
- See "Causes and Risk Factors"

CBC/BIOCHEMISTRY/URINALYSIS
N/A

OTHER LABORATORY TESTS
N/A

IMAGING
Radiographs are helpful when trauma or osteoarthritis are suspected, or in chronic conditions with potential joint involvement.

OTHER DIAGNOSTIC PROCEDURES
N/A

PATHOLOGIC FINDINGS
N/A

TREATMENT

THERAPEUTIC APPROACH
- Segregate lame animals and do not sell.
- If possible keep lame animals in dry environment to allow hoof walls to harden.

Interdigital Dermatitis
- Preferred methods
  - Topical application of oxytetracycline as a spray to interdigital region.
  - Footbathing
  - Formalin—2–5%, although care should be taken as higher strengths can cause irritation to the skin. Start at 2–3% and increase only if needed. Does not require animals to stand in bath for long periods.

L

LAMENESS: SMALL RUMINANT

○ Zinc sulfate—typically 10% solution. Addition of a surfactant may benefit treatment success. Ideally have animals stand in bath for 2–20 minutes.

○ Copper sulfate—should be avoided due to risk of copper toxicosis in sheep.

• Injectable antibiotics are not necessary in flocks or herds with only interdigital dermatitis and no history of virulent foot rot.

Virulent Foot Rot

• Preferred method is injection of long-acting antibiotic:

○ Long-acting oxytetracycline

○ Long-acting macrolide

• Ancillary treatments

○ Topical application of oxytetracycline as a spray

○ Footbathing—same recommendations as for interdigital dermatitis

• While trimming of infected animals used to be recommended it has now been demonstrated to slow healing and to act as a means of transmission. Therefore, this is no longer recommended.

• Vaccination is available in some countries, with variable success. There is evidence to suggest that multivalent strain vaccines have limited efficacy due to antigenic competition. As a consequence, the most effective approach is culture of strains from infected farms and the development of single or double strain autogenous vaccines. Multiple studies demonstrate that farms and individual animals are often concurrently infected with multiple strains, complicating this approach. Cattle foot rot vaccines focused on *Fusobacterium* spp. are unlikely to provide significant protection.

• Some animals remain chronically infected despite repeated treatment and should be culled to minimize maintenance within the flock or herd.

Contagious Ovine Digital Dermatitis

• Relatively new disease process with minimal evidence-based medicine data to support the benefit of specific treatments.

• Anecdotal evidence supporting the use of injectable long-acting macrolides.

• Anecdotal response to topical lincomycin and spectinomycin soluble powder or tylosin soluble powder made up at 1 g per 2 L in water and applied repeatedly.

• Footbath recommendations as outlined above.

White Line Disease

• Remove the manure and soil packed in the wall and trim away the undermined wall.

• Do not disturb or trim away at the inner wall.

Strawberry Foot Rot

• Systemic therapy with penicillin may be beneficial.

• Topical therapy standard for dermatophylosis in other species.

SURGICAL CONSIDERATIONS AND TECHNIQUES

Toe granuloma—regional anesthesia of the limb (either ring block or IV regional) followed by placement of a tourniquet and surgical excision of the granuloma. Wrap to control hemorrhage.

MEDICATIONS

DRUGS OF CHOICE

See "Treatment"

CONTRAINDICATIONS

Foot trimming in cases of virulent foot rot is contraindicated.

PRECAUTIONS

• Be aware of human-health risks associated with formalin footbaths.

• Consideration of extra-label drug use and appropriate withdrawal times is necessary.

POSSIBLE INTERACTIONS

N/A

FOLLOW-UP

EXPECTED COURSE AND PROGNOSIS

Disease and severity dependent

POSSIBLE COMPLICATIONS

N/A

CLIENT EDUCATION

Biosecurity with infectious causes of lameness is of paramount importance.

PATIENT CARE

Lame animals should be examined and treated promptly.

PREVENTION

Keeping a closed herd and well-drained fields or dry indoor housing.

MISCELLANEOUS

BIOSECURITY

• Minimize new animals entering herd or flock.

• Separate lame animals promptly.

PRODUCTION MANAGEMENT

• Refer to recommendations in "Follow-Up"

ABBREVIATIONS

• CODD = contagious ovine digital dermatitis

• IV = intravenous

SEE ALSO

• Anesthesia: Local and Regional

• Foot Rot: Small Ruminant

Suggested Reading

Angell JW, Blundell R, Grove-White DH, Duncan JS. Clinical and radiographic features of contagious ovine digital dermatitis and a novel lesion grading system. Vet Rec 2015, 176: 544. doi: 10.1136/vr.102978.

Crosby-Durrani HE, Clegg SR, Singer E, et al. Severe foot lesions in dairy goats associated with digital dermatitis treponemes. J Comp Pathol 2016, 154: 283–96. doi: 10.1016/j.jcpa.2016.04.001.

Internet Resources

• http://www.nadis.org.uk/bulletins/lameness-control-in-sheep.aspx

• http://www.dpi.nsw.gov.au/__data/assets/pdf_file/0015/102381/Footrot-in-Sheep-and-Goats.pdf

Author Paul J. Plummer

Consulting Editor Kaitlyn A. Lutz

L

BASICS

OVERVIEW
Laminitis is a common, multifactorial disease causing lameness in cattle. Laminitis is very common in confined dairy cattle and beef cattle on high-concentrate diets. The pathology that occurs in the hoof is the result of systemic physiologic changes that affect the functionality of the keratinocytes that produce the horn of the hoof and compromise the integrity of the collagen connecting the third phalanx (P3) to the hoof capsule. These changes lead to abnormal horn production that is often manifested as a sole ulcer, white line disease, or misshapen hooves. Acute laminitis is uncommon. Subacute, subclinical, or chronic laminitis is much more common in both dairy and beef cattle.

INCIDENCE/PREVALENCE
Uncommon in pastured cattle. Variable incidence in cattle housed on concrete or fed diets containing grain with incidence ranging from 5% to 50%.

GEOGRAPHIC DISTRIBUTION
Worldwide

SYSTEMS AFFECTED
• Integument
• Musculoskeletal

PATHOPHYSIOLOGY
• The dermis, basement membrane, and epidermal keratinocytes are subject to physiologic and physical damage which can disrupt the production of normal hoof horn. The generally accepted mechanisms are disruption in blood flow and disruption in collagen attachment. The theories share the common endpoint of altering the function of germinal layers of the epidermis.
• Ruminal acidosis can cause laminitis. Vasoactive compounds such as histamine, released as a consequence of acidosis, are thought to decrease blood flow in the microvasculature of the hoof, either by vasoconstriction or arteriovenous shunting, which leads to local ischemia and edema. The compromise in blood flow disrupts nutrient supply to the epidermis. An increase in cytokines, specifically IL-1, has been documented to occur in the hoof following ruminal acidosis. IL-1 upregulates matrix metalloproteinases (MMP) which are involved in the turnover of collagen in the hoof. Upregulation of MMPs leads to loosening of the collagen attachment of P3 to the hoof capsule. Disruption of laminar corium attachment and support of P3 leads to damage to the corium through a combination of compressive and shearing forces.
• Dietary micronutrients such as zinc, copper, sulfur, biotin, and cysteine are critical to normal keratin production and horn formation. Deficiencies in these nutrients may contribute to the laminitis syndrome.
• Increased biomechanical load on the hoof from walking on concrete also contributes to the laminitis syndrome. Similarly, overgrowth of the hoof that causes abnormal weight bearing in the hoof will increase the risk for laminitis.
• The combination of changes in blood flow, inflammation, swelling, and loosening of attachments of P3 leads to cellular disruption in the corium which is manifested as some combination of sole ulcer, white line disease, and abnormal horn growth. It should be noted that the time from the physiologic insult until manifestation of changes in the hoof can be 2 months or more.

HISTORICAL FINDINGS
Recent feed or feeding management change can contribute to improper intakes and ruminal acidosis. Change in housing or recent bout of hot weather.

SIGNALMENT
Typically, adult dairy cows and feedlot cattle

PHYSICAL EXAMINATION FINDINGS
• Lameness.
• Overgrown hooves.
• Misshapen hooves with the hoof being broader and flatter, and dorsal wall furrowed and concave (slipper foot).
• On inspection of the hooves, sole hemorrhages, sole ulcer, or white line separation/abscess will likely be evident.
• Horizontal grooves are often evident on the dorsal aspect of the wall.
• The sole horn may be flaky or chalky.
• A double sole may be found.

GENETICS
The estimated heritability is 0.14–0.22.

CAUSES AND RISK FACTORS
• There is an interaction between diet and housing. Feeding high grain diets can cause SARA and predisposes cattle to laminitis. Housing cattle on concrete predisposes cattle to laminitis by increasing the biomechanical load on the corium. If the two conditions occur together, the risk increases substantially.
• In addition to diet, during hot weather, rumination time decreases and meal sizes increase which can exacerbate SARA.
• Also, overstocking and poorly designed stalls or resting surfaces will lead to increased standing time and thus increased biomechanical load on the foot.
• Overgrowth of hooves will change weight bearing, increase biomechanical load, and predispose to laminitis.

DIAGNOSIS

DIFFERENTIAL DIAGNOSES
Digital dermatitis, interdigital phlegmon, hoof overgrowth, thin soles

CBC/BIOCHEMISTRY/URINALYSIS
N/A

OTHER LABORATORY TESTS
N/A

IMAGING
N/A

OTHER DIAGNOSTIC PROCEDURES
Hoof trimming

PATHOLOGIC FINDINGS
Postmortem examination and biopsy are not necessary in clinical cases. Sinkage of P3, decreased fat content of the digital cushion, inflammation of the corium and epidermis.

TREATMENT

THERAPEUTIC APPROACH
• Functional hoof trimming should be performed to return all the claws to a normal conformation. Sole ulcers and white line abscesses should have the surrounding horn pared away until normal horn is seen well adhered to the corium. The sole surrounding the lesion should be sloped so as not to create a deep hole that will become filled with debris.
• A block (wood, rubber or plastic) should be glued to the sound claw to relieve weight bearing on the affected claw until healing can occur.

SURGICAL CONSIDERATIONS AND TECHNIQUES
N/A

MEDICATIONS

DRUGS OF CHOICE
Typically, medications are not necessary. For more severe lesions, NSAIDs can be used for pain relief. Flunixin meglumine (1.1–2.2 mg/kg once daily) or meloxicam (0.5 mg/kg PO once daily). Injectable meloxicam, ketoprofen, and carprofen are available in some countries.

PRECAUTIONS
Appropriate milk and meat withdrawal times must be followed for all compounds administered to food-producing animals.

FOLLOW-UP

EXPECTED COURSE AND PROGNOSIS
Most cases of laminitis that cause lameness can be treated by functional hoof trimming and treating the lesion and will have a good prognosis for recovery. Animals should be improved within 1 week of treatment, mostly sound within 2 weeks, and sound by 3 weeks after treatment. If improvement does not

L

LAMINITIS IN CATTLE   (CONTINUED)

proceed as expected, the animal should be re-evaluated. In some cases of chronic or severe laminitis, a shift in the position of P3 or scarring of the basement membrane may result in recurring problems with a poor prognosis for resolution.

POSSIBLE COMPLICATIONS
Granulation tissue may develop during the healing phase and, if it protrudes above the wound margin, must be removed. Sole ulcers or white line abscesses, if not treated early, can progress into deeper infections involving the bones, joints, and tendons of the foot. Deeper infections may require aggressive debridement and wound care or claw amputation as a salvage operation.

CLIENT EDUCATION
See "Prevention"

PATIENT CARE
Animals should be housed in a clean, dry area with a comfortable resting surface. They should be observed daily to ensure they are generally healthy and sufficiently mobile to access feed and water. If lameness worsens or swelling develops above the hoof, the animal should be re-evaluated promptly.

PREVENTION
• Nutrition and environmental management are the keys to preventing laminitis. The following comments are primarily for dairy cattle but can be adapted to other feeding situations. Diets should be formulated to provide adequate chemical and effective fiber and not exceed recommended maximum levels of starch or nonstructural carbohydrates. Diets should provide adequate physically effective fiber without promoting excessive sorting. Feeding diets to a low level of refusal, providing adequate bunk space, and providing heat abatement during warm

weather will promote the consumption of more moderate-size meals during the day and reduce the risk of SARA. Zinc methionine and biotin have been shown to decrease lesions associated with laminitis.
• For beef cattle, there must be a gradual transition from high roughage to concentrate feeding to avoid SARA and laminitis. The use of by-product feeds to replace corn can reduce the starch level in the diet without compromising performance.
• Reducing the biomechanical load on the feet is an important component in preventing laminitis. The housing environment should provide a comfortable resting place and be stocked such that animals can be reasonably expected to lie down at least 10 hours per day. The use of rubber mats in high traffic areas to provide a yielding walking surface with good traction has been shown to improve hoof health.
• Periodic locomotion scoring of cows will alert management when lameness incidence is increasing and allow corrective action to be taken in a timely manner.

 MISCELLANEOUS

ASSOCIATED CONDITIONS
SARA

PREGNANCY
Hormonal changes at parturition may affect the digital cushion and suspensory apparatus of the hoof, thus contributing to the risk for laminitis.

PRODUCTION MANAGEMENT
Lameness has significant economic consequences for all production sectors. There is also a significant animal welfare

concern with lameness. The sequelae to laminitis account for at least half of the cases of lameness that occur in dairy cattle. Controlling laminitis is critical to maintaining a healthy, profitable herd. Refer to the section "Prevention" for management considerations to control laminitis.

ABBREVIATIONS
• MMP = matrix metalloproteinase
• NSAID = nonsteroidal anti-inflammatory drug
• P3 = third phalanx
• PO = per os, by mouth
• SARA = subacute ruminal acidosis

SEE ALSO
• Lameness: Bovine
• Ruminal Acidosis

Suggested Reading
Bergsten C. Causes, risk factors, and prevention of laminitis and related claw lesions. Acta Vet Scand Suppl. 2003, 98: 157–66.
Greenough PR. Bovine laminitis and lameness. London: Saunders, 2007, pp. 8–69.
Hoblet KH, Weiss W. Metabolic hoof horn disease. Vet Clin North Am Food Anim Pract 2001, 17: 111–27.
Lischer CJ, Ossent P, Raber M, Geyer H. Suspensory structures and supporting tissues of the third phalanx of cows and their relevance to the development of typical sole ulcers (Rusterholz ulcers). Vet Rec 2002, 151: 694–98.

Author Edgar F. Garrett
Consulting Editor Kaitlyn A. Lutz
Acknowledgment The author and book editors acknowledge the prior contribution of Steven L. Berry.

LANTANA TOXICOSIS

BASICS

OVERVIEW
• Lantana is a perennial, branching herb or shrub. Both erect and creeping varieties exist, ranging between 0.5-2 meters tall.
• Lantana resides in the Verbenaceae, commonly known as the verbena or vervain family. Some 150–160 species exist, producing flowers in dense spikes from spring to fall.
• Simple leaves with serrated margins are ovate to lanceolate in shape and are arranged in opposite or whorled patterns. They emit an unpleasant odor when crushed.
• Fruits occur in clusters, initially green, then becoming dark purple to black when ripe. They are 5–7 mm in diameter. Stems are square (four-sided) and may be prickly with small hairs.
• The plants are often used as ornamentals because of their showy flowers that come in a wide variety of colors. Most lantana have flowers with two colors (yellow and orange, orange and red, purple and white), but single-colored varieties exist. "Ham and Eggs" is a common name for a variety with yellow and red flowers.
• Frequently planted as an ornamental, lantana has often escaped and become "wild."
• An uncommon cause of intoxication, lantana can be a significant cause of poisoning and death loss where it grows wild.
• Cattle are most frequently intoxicated by lantana and mortality is high in severe cases.

INCIDENCE/PREVALENCE
• Poisonings are most common in summer and fall, often due to clippings.
• The incidence is related to the availability of the plants.

GEOGRAPHIC DISTRIBUTION
• Lantana is widely spread throughout the tropical and subtropical regions of the world.
• It is primarily found in the southern portions of the United States as it is not cold tolerant.

SYSTEMS AFFECTED
• Multisystemic
• Hepatic
• Integument
• Digestive
• Urinary

PATHOPHYSIOLOGY
• Lantana produces lantadene A and B. These compounds are found in the leaves and are toxic to both the liver and gastrointestinal systems.
• Other plant parts including flowers, fruits and stems may contain other toxins.
• Toxicity varies considerably between different varieties of lantana. Those with red flowers are considered most toxic and purple/lavender flowered varieties least toxic.

• The amount of liver disease is directly related to the quantity of leaves ingested.
• As lantadenes are absorbed from the gastrointestinal tract, they cause direct irritation to the gastrointestinal mucosa.
• Lantadenes are transported to the liver, resulting in damage to hepatocytes.
• They cause inflammation of the bile ducts (cholangitis) as they are excreted and subsequently slow or stop the transport of bile (cholestasis).
• This causes phylloerythrin (a photodynamic agent from chlorophyll metabolism of plants) and bilirubin to accumulate in hepatocytes and capillary beds of the skin. When phylloerythrin is activated by sunlight, tissue damage occurs with resultant photosensitization.
• Time from ingestion to death may be several weeks.
• Death is likely due to hepatic disease and renal failure, while anorexia and metabolic acidosis contribute.

SIGNALMENT
• Although ruminants tend to be more commonly poisoned, most animal species, including sheep, goats, wildlife, and children are susceptible.
• Cattle are most frequently intoxicated during late summer and fall.
• There are no known breed, species, or sex predilections.

PHYSICAL EXAMINATION FINDINGS
• Intoxication and related clinical signs depend upon the quantity consumed and the time period of ingestion.
• Signs of acute intoxication may be seen within 24 hours post-consumption.
• Subacute poisoning over 1–2 days is more common than acute intoxication.
• Initial signs may include depression, weakness, anorexia, depressed ruminal motility, and constipation. Dehydration and electrolyte imbalances (metabolic acidosis) also play roles.
• Within 2–4 days, icterus, bloody diarrhea, skin changes associated with photosensitization, paralysis, and death can be seen.
• Chronic disease is characterized by oronasal ulcerations, keratitis, icterus and photosensitization progressing over days to weeks. Keratitis may vary from light sensitivity to complete blindness.

CAUSES AND RISK FACTORS
• Lantadenes are hepatotoxic triterpene acids. Lantadene A is considered the most toxic, while lantadene B is less toxic.
• Differing varieties exist, possessing varying amounts of lantadenes with differing levels of potency. Although flower colors are often indicative of the level of danger, it is best not to fully rely on this method for determining toxicity.

• Fresh or dry leaves are the primary source of lantadenes.
• Green fruits may possess other toxins.
• Ripened fruits and seeds are not toxic.
• Consumption of 5–10 g leaves will often produce fatal poisoning in livestock. Smaller doses, if consumed daily over several days, can be toxic as well.
• Lantadenes are absorbed primarily from the gastrointestinal tract.
• They are transformed in the liver and excreted in the bile, resulting in an obstructive cholangitis.
• The effects of lantadenes are cumulative as the hepatic and renal changes are permanent.

DIAGNOSIS

DIFFERENTIAL DIAGNOSES
• The signs of lantana intoxication are nonspecific. A number of hepatotoxic plants are listed:
  ◦ *Crotalaria* spp.—rattlebox
  ◦ *Helenium* spp. sneeze weed
  ◦ *Hymenoxys* spp.—rubber weed, bitterweed
  ◦ *Senecio* spp. and *Packera* spp.
• Oak poisoning may produce signs similar to acute lantana intoxication.
• St. John's wort—photosensitization
• Numerous other causes of liver disease
• Clinical signs, history of ingestion, finding plants in feed, hay, or rumen contents are supportive of a diagnosis.

CBC/BIOCHEMISTRY/URINALYSIS
• Serum bilirubin is elevated.
• With hepatocyte damage, serum hepatic enzymes are typically elevated, including AST, GGT and ALP.

OTHER LABORATORY TESTS
BSP clearance is decreased.

PATHOLOGIC FINDINGS
• Icteric tissues
• Skin lesions due to photosensitization
• Keratitis
• Enteritis/Abomasitis
• Obstructive cholangitis
• Enlarged green-tinted liver (bile staining)
• Enlarged gall bladder
• Enlarged kidneys with perirenal edema

TREATMENT

THERAPEUTIC APPROACH
• Remove affected animals from sunlight and provide shade for those affected by photosensitization.
• Prevent animals' access to lantana.
• Treat patients symptomatically, give supportive care, and maintain hydration and electrolyte balance with oral or intravenous fluids.

L

LANTANA TOXICOSIS

• Rumenotomy with evacuation of contents may be worthwhile if performed early.
• Broad-spectrum antibiotics to assist in preventing secondary bacterial infections of skin lesions associated with photosensitization.

MEDICATIONS

DRUGS OF CHOICE

• Activated charcoal—2–5 g/kg given orally to control absorption of toxins from the gastrointestinal tract (1 g charcoal per 5 mL water).
• Mineral oil administered orally to more rapidly transport plant materials from gastrointestinal tract.
• Generally, it is considered best to use either activated charcoal or mineral oil, but not both at the same time.
• Sodium thiosulfate may be beneficial.
• Systemic antibiotics are warranted in animals with photosensitization to assist in protecting them from secondary bacterial infections.

FOLLOW-UP

EXPECTED COURSE AND PROGNOSIS

• Variable, dependent upon the amount and rate of consumption.
• High mortality is expected with acute cases.
• Many animals will survive moderate cases of intoxication.

PREVENTION

• Providing a proper diet and adequate nutrition to animals will help to minimize the consumption of many toxic plants.
• Protective immunization has been studied and further research is needed.

MISCELLANEOUS

PREGNANCY
None

PRODUCTION MANAGEMENT
Removal/destruction of lantana—it is susceptible to 2,4-D and other broad-leaf herbicides.

ABBREVIATIONS
• AST = aspartate aminotransferase
• BSP = bromsulphalein
• GGT = gamma-glutamyl transpeptidase
• IV.= intravenous
• SDH = sorbitol dehydrogenase

SEE ALSO
• Oak (*Quercus* spp.) Toxicity
• St. John's Wort Toxicity

Suggested Reading
Burrows GE, Tyrl RJ. Toxic Plants of North America, Ames: Iowa State University Press, 2001.
Burrows GE, Tyrl RJ. Toxic Plants of North America, 2nd ed. Ames: Wiley-Blackwell, 2013.
Knight AP, Walter RG. A Guide to Plant Poisonings of Animals in North America. Jackson, WY: Teton New Media, 2001.
Poisonous Plants of the Southern United States. Agricultural Extension Service, University of Tennessee, 1980.
Toxic Plants of Texas. Texas AgriLife Extension Service, Texas A&M Press, 2003.
Author Matt G. Welborn
Consulting Editor Christopher C.L. Chase

L

LEAD TOXICOSIS

BASICS

OVERVIEW
• Among ruminants, most cases of lead poisoning occur in cattle.
• The vast majority of lead poisoning cases are the result of acute oral exposures; chronic exposures are rare in ruminants.
• Lead sources commonly encountered by ruminants include discarded auto batteries, discarded crankcase oil, paint, solder, greases, oil-well pipe dope, lead shot, roofing material, and burn piles.
• In acute toxicosis, the onset of clinical signs is rapid and typically includes signs associated with the gastrointestinal tract and central (and to a lesser extent, peripheral) nervous systems.
• Death with few to no premonitory signs may be observed in calves and young animals.
• Antemortem diagnosis relies on elevated blood lead levels and evidence of radiodense objects in the gastrointestinal tract (more common to find in the reticulum).
• Elevated liver and kidney lead levels, evidence of lead particles in the GIT (reticulum, rumen), and histologic evidence of laminar cortical necrosis provide postmortem evidence for a diagnosis of lead poisoning.
• Treatment, if possible and economically viable, includes administration of oral magnesium sulfate, thiamine, Ca-EDTA, along with supportive care targeted to observed clinical signs.
• Prognosis is generally poor in acute cases, and care must be taken in considering home or custom slaughter due to tissue residues.

INCIDENCE/PREVALENCE
Sporadic, unpredictable incidence but most cases occur in cattle in the spring, when they are turned out in pastures with access to lead-containing sources.

GEOGRAPHIC DISTRIBUTION
Worldwide

SYSTEMS AFFECTED
• Digestive
• Nervous
• Hemolymphatic
• Urinary
• Multisystemic
• Musculoskeletal
• Reproductive

PATHOPHYSIOLOGY
• Lead is relatively insoluble and poorly absorbed from the gastrointestinal tract. However, once absorbed, it is retained in the soft tissues initially and later the bone.
• In the blood, lead binds to surface proteins of red blood cells.
• Lead has a wide tissue distribution and long total body half-life, and ultimately forms deposits in bone where it resides (biologically inert) for years. Remodeling of bone can lead to its release.
• Lead is excreted primarily by the kidneys, crosses the placental barrier, and can be secreted into milk.
• Lead affects multiple systems, and the effects are varied depending on whether the exposure is acute or chronic.
• Lead interferes with sulfhydryl- and zinc-containing enzymes, leading to erythrocyte fragility, bone marrow suppression, and interference with heme synthesis (more common to see these changes with chronic exposures), along with interfering with various neurotransmitters in the CNS.
• Neurologic signs may be due to cerebral edema as a result of increased vascular permeability.
• Segmental demyelination of peripheral nerves (e.g., pharyngeal, buccal) may be seen.
• In young animals lead poisoning may result in suppression of bone growth.
• Lead interferes with calcium absorption from the gut, along with displacing calcium in multiple sites.

Toxic Dose
• The single acute lethal dose for cattle ranges from 400 to 800 mg/kg and daily intakes of 1–7 mg/kg/day can eventually result in toxicosis. These are from experimental exposures and differ from clinical cases where the amount and form of lead ingested is generally not known.
• Cattle—intakes of >6 mg/kg body weight can lead to chronic poisoning, and intakes >10 mg/kg BW may cause acute lead poisoning.
• Sheep—generally occurs in lambs; symptoms of poisoning appear at intakes >4.5 mg/kg BW.
• Goats—more resistant than sheep or cattle. Very minor signs of poisoning occur at intakes of 60 mg/kg BW. This is equal to blood concentrations of 130 µg/dL.

SIGNALMENT
• All ruminant species are at risk.
• Cattle more likely than other ruminants due to less-discriminating grazing.
• All ages are susceptible.
• Younger animals are at greater risk of intoxication due to increased capacity to absorb lead from the intestines.

PHYSICAL EXAMINATION FINDINGS
Signs appear to occur abruptly, though there may be a delay of several days (depending on the lead source) between the time of lead ingestion and the onset of signs.
• Blindness, circling, aimless wandering, head pressing
• Anorexia
• Grinding of the teeth
• Rhythmic twitching of the muscles, often involving the face (e.g., eyelids)
• Tucked and painful abdomen; rumen atony, constipation, or diarrhea may be present
• Salivation, due to pain or pharyngeal paralysis
• Excitement and/or seizures (depression may also be observed)
• Bradycardia and hypertension have both been observed in cattle

CAUSES AND RISK FACTORS
• Discarded broken batteries are by far the most common source of lead poisoning in ruminants. The interior lead plates often contain >90% lead.
• Other less common sources of lead include machinery grease, old used motor oil, paint, pesticides, caulk and putty, contamination from mines and smelters, water, and grazing pastures contaminated with lead shot.
• Burning batteries does not destroy lead; this practice only provides animals a more concentrated lead source in the remaining ash.

DIAGNOSIS

DIFFERENTIAL DIAGNOSES
• Polioencephalomalacia, salt poisoning and/or water deprivation, vitamin A deficiency, rabies, listeriosis, abscess, thromboembolic meningoencephalitis, nervous coccidiosis, rabies, nonprotein nitrogen poisoning, and hepatic encephalopathy.
• There are many differentials for "sudden" death in ruminants; these could include enterotoxemia, water hemlock (*Cicuta*), botulism, nonprotein nitrogen intoxication, cyanobacteria (blue-green algae), *Delphinium* (larkspur), *Zigadenus* (death camas), *Astragalus* (locoweed), and nitrate poisoning.

CBC/BIOCHEMISTRY/URINALYSIS
• Basophilic stippling is commonly mentioned as a potential alteration; however, its finding is inconsistent and may be mistaken for other disease processes.
• Anemia (subchronic to chronic lead toxicosis).
• Increased RBC fragility.

OTHER LABORATORY TESTS
• Definitive diagnosis requires detection of lead in appropriate clinical specimen.
• Diagnostic samples:
  ○ Whole blood: >0.35 ppm (35 µg/dL) lead with compatible clinical signs is diagnostic.
  ○ Kidneys: >10 ppm lead wet weight is diagnostic.
  ○ Liver: >10 ppm lead wet weight is diagnostic.
• Even though blood lead levels are diagnostic for confirming exposure, blood Pb levels sometimes do not correlate with clinical signs. For instance, one might see a blood lead level

L

of 0.30 ppm in a cow that is seizing; and one might see a blood lead level of 0.90 ppm in a cow that is not showing any clinical disease. Because of the variability, lead poisoning is diagnosed in an individual animal; remaining animals in the "exposed" group should be tested, regardless of whether they are showing signs.

IMAGING
Radiography carried out antemortem or postmortem may show radiographic densities in the GIT, most commonly in the reticulum.

OTHER DIAGNOSTIC PROCEDURES
Formalin-fixed tissue can still be used for lead analysis, retrospectively for diagnosis.

PATHOLOGIC FINDINGS
• No findings are pathognomonic for lead poisoning.
• Gross lesions include cerebral edema, flattened or yellow cerebral cortical gyri.
• Gastrointestinal inflammation, ulceration, and/or hemorrhages.
• Histologic lesions of the CNS include laminar cortical necrosis with swelling of the capillary endothelium within the brain.
• Kidney lesions include proximal renal tubule degeneration and necrosis. Lead inclusion bodies in the proximal renal tubules. Inclusions are described as intranuclear inclusions in the proximal tubules with periglomerular nephritis.
• Liver—centrilobular degeneration.

TREATMENT

THERAPEUTIC APPROACH
• Removal of the lead from the multicompartmental ruminant GIT is difficult.
• Treatment of lead intoxication may not be rewarding and deaths may occur prior to the initiation of therapy.
• The prolonged retention of lead may be due to continued release and absorption of lead from metal particles in the reticulum or rumen.
• Chelation therapy (enhances renal excretion)
  ○ Ca-EDTA—55–90 mg/kg body weight slowly IV or IM, q12h.
  ○ Treat for 3–5 days.
  ○ If additional treatment is indicated (clinical signs still present), wait for at least 2 days before administering another round of chelation therapy. Blood lead levels should be periodically monitored to evaluate the effectiveness of the chelation therapy.
• Symptomatic therapy—thiamine HCl—administer 250–1000 mg SC or IM, q12h. Treat for 5–10 days.
• Supportive therapy—mineral supplementation may be required if there is prolonged chelation therapy.

MEDICATIONS

DRUGS OF CHOICE
• Magnesium sulfate can be added to the diet to help bind lead within the gastrointestinal tract (one recommended dosage: 0.5 g/lb BW daily).
• Depending on the severity of clinical signs, symptomatic care may include diazepam or barbiturates for seizure control, IV fluid therapy to correct dehydration, monitoring for the development of electrolyte abnormalities, monitoring feed and caloric intake, and addressing deficiencies accordingly such as zinc supplementation (1.0 mg/kg/day).
• British anti-Lewisite (dimercaprol or BAL) penetrates into the brain, and can be a helpful chelator in animals showing severe neurologic signs. One suggested dosage is 3.0 mg/kg IM as a 5% solution in a 10% solution of benzyl benzoate in peanut oil q4h for 2 days, q6h on day 3, then q12h for the next 10 days. BAL is potentially nephrotoxic and is painful when injected. It can be difficult to obtain and expensive to use.

CONTRAINDICATIONS
• Ca-EDTA is potentially nephrotoxic, so monitoring renal parameters and maintaining adequate hydration status are recommended.
• Lead may interfere with copper, calcium, zinc, iron, and selenium metabolism.
• Appropriate milk and meat withdrawal times must be followed for all compounds administered to food-producing animals.

FOLLOW-UP

EXPECTED COURSE AND PROGNOSIS
• The more severely affected animals have a poor prognosis. It is often impossible to remove the lead from the gastrointestinal tract of ruminants, and patients showing severe neurologic signs often do not respond well to treatment.
• Mild or moderately affected animals may improve if one can remove the lead from the gastrointestinal tract, and enhance renal excretion through chelation therapy.

PATIENT CARE
• Blood lead levels should be monitored periodically to determine the efficacy of chelation therapy and to assist with decision making in regard to slaughter withdrawal times. Normal blood levels should be <0.10 ppm.
• Lead can be secreted into milk; milk should be tested and discarded if levels are too high.
• It is common for neurologic signs (e.g., blindness) to persist. Ill thrift may be present in "recovered" young.

PREVENTION
• Knowledge of the common sources of lead should help producers avoid this potentially devastating disease.
• Identify the source (through history, pasture examination, etc.) and remove it from the animal's environment; or remove the animals from the contaminated environment.
• Keep at-risk animals away from junk, burn, or "resource" piles located on the property.

MISCELLANEOUS

ASSOCIATED CONDITIONS
• The half-life of lead in an intoxicated animal depends on a number of factors including age and physiologic status.
• In some references, the half-life of lead in cattle is reported to be several weeks to >2 years.
• A study from Michigan examined the half-life of lead in poisoned animals and reported that lead tended to have a shortened half-life in pregnant or lactating cattle as compared to castrated bulls.

AGE-RELATED FACTORS
Younger animals are at greater risk of intoxication due to increased capacity to absorb lead from the intestines.

ZOONOTIC POTENTIAL
• Lead is immunosuppressive and carcinogenic in people. The developing fetus and young children are very susceptible to lead's toxic effect on the nervous system. Care should be taken when using meat or milk from lead exposed animals for human consumption.
• There is potential for lead exposure in others animals from the milk and meat of poisoned animals.
• In some states, there are restrictions on movement or marketing of cattle poisoned with lead.
• The veterinarian should consult the local diagnostic laboratory or department of public health for questions specific to their practice area.

PREGNANCY
• Lead poisoning is reported to cause infertility, abortions, and fetal resorption.
• Lead crosses the placental barrier and may exert a deleterious effect on the developing ruminant fetus.
• Pregnant ruminants that suffer from lead toxicosis may transfer significant amounts of lead to the developing fetus.

PRODUCTION MANAGEMENT
Restrict animals' access to lead sources (e.g., paint-cribbing, batteries, grease, etc.). Avoid access to junk piles in the pastures.

L

SYNONYMS
- Plumbism
- Saturnism

ABBREVIATIONS
- BAL = British anti-Lewisite
- Ca-EDTA = calcium disodium ethylenediaminetetraacetic acid
- CNS = central nervous system
- GIT = gastrointestinal tract
- IM = intramuscular
- IV = intravenous
- Pb = lead
- ppm = parts per million
- RBC = red blood cell
- SC = subcutaneous

SEE ALSO
- Blue-Green Algae Poisoning
- Clostridial Disease: Nervous System
- Coccidiosis
- Death Camas
- *Histophilus Somni* Complex
- Listeriosis
- Nitrate and Nitrite Toxicosis
- Rabies
- Sodium Disorders: Hypernatremia
- Urea Toxicity
- Vitamin A Deficiency/Toxicosis
- Vitamin B Deficiency
- Water Hemlock

Suggested Reading

Bischoff K, Higgins W, Thompson B, Ebel JG. Lead excretion in milk of accidentally exposed dairy cattle. Food Addit Contam Part A 2014, 31: 839–44.

Galey FD, Slenning BD, Anderson ML, et al. Lead concentrations in blood and milk from periparturient dairy heifers seven months after an episode of acute lead toxicosis. J Vet Diagn Invest 1990, 2: 222–6.

Gwaltney-Brant S. Lead. In: Plumlee KH ed, Clinical Veterinary Toxicology. St. Louis: Mosby, 2004.

Rumbeiha WK, Braselton WE, Donch D. A retrospective study on the disappearance of blood lead in cattle with accidental lead toxicosis. J Vet Diagn Invest 2001, 13: 373–8.

Waldner C, Checkley S, Blakley B, Pollock C, Mitchell B. Managing lead exposure and toxicity in cow-calf herds to minimize the potential for food residues. J Vet Diagn Invest 2002, 14: 481–6.

Authors Adrienne C. Bautista and Birgit Puschner
Consulting Editor Christopher C.L. Chase

Acknowledgment The authors and book editors acknowledge the prior contribution of Patricia Talcott and Joe Roder.

L

LEPTOSPIROSIS

BASICS

OVERVIEW
• Leptospirosis is a bacterial zoonotic disease of multiple animal species caused by *Leptospira* species.
• It is an acute febrile disease with clinical manifestations depending on the animal species and the serologic variant of *Leptospira*.
• The chronic form of leptospirosis causes septicemia, agalactia, hepatitis, nephritis, and abortion in domestic livestock and wildlife hosts.

INCIDENCE/PREVALENCE
• Mature cattle could develop into renal carriers of *Leptospira* with serovars *hardjo, pomona,* and *grippotyphosa*. *L. hardjo* cause endemic reproductive problems in cattle. *L. pomona* is common in calves.
• *L. grippotyphosa* and *L. pomona* are common in dogs. Raccoons are a reservoir of *Listeria* species. *L. pomona* is common in goats and sheep but are rarely infected. Sheep also harbor *L. hardjo*.
• High seroprevalence of various leptospira serovars (10–70%) has been reported in several species and countries.

GEOGRAPHICAL DISTRIBUTION
• Worldwide distribution favoring warm, wet climates and surviving in standing water for prolonged periods.
• Different serovars predominate in different regions.

SYSTEMS AFFECTED
• Urinary
• Multisystemic
• Cardiovascular
• Nervous
• Reproductive
• Mammary

PATHOPHYSIOLOGY
• Leptospires enters the body from the exposed mucus membranes or abraded skin. Venereal or transplacental routes of transmission have also been reported. Incubation period extends from 4 to 20 days.
• The bacteria replicate in the blood and are transmitted to the liver, lungs, kidney, GI tract, and CNS. Septicemia follows for 4–7 days resulting in systemic dispersion of bacterial toxins causing fever, capillary damage, hepatic necrosis, renal tubular damage, and agalactia.
• In calves, hemolysin toxin may cause intravascular hemolysis, hemolytic anemia, and hemoglobinuria.
• Humoral response increases serum antibody level, resolving the septicemia and fever. Bacteria localize in the liver and renal parenchyma, causing hepatitis and interstitial nephritis respectively, which resuls in persistent leptospiruria.

• Animals succumb due to acute septicemia, hemolytic anemia, and interstitial nephritis.
• Leptospires can cross the placental barrier. In the second half of gestation the bacteria invade the placenta and fetus during the septicemic phase, resulting in abortion several weeks later.
• Sheep and goats develop encephalitis/meningitis due to localization of the leptospires in the nervous system.
• Leptospires colonize the proximal renal tubules and are intermittently excreted in the urine of carrier animals.

HISTORICAL FINDINGS
• Ruminants: Infertility, early pregnancy loss, increased number of service per conception, prolonged calving interval, abortion, stillbirth, and weak offspring.
• Camelids: Early pregnancy loss, abortion, poor milk production.

SIGNALMENT
• Leptospirosis is common in dogs, cats, cattle, sheep, goats, pigs, camelids, wild ruminants, and water buffalo.
• *Leptospira* is isolated at higher rates from beef cattle than dairy cattle.
• Most wildlife are the maintenance host but dogs, pigs, and cattle may also be the maintenance host.
• The host-adapted serovars generally cause a mild or unapparent disease developing into a carrier state. For example:
  ◦ *Leptospira borgpetersenii* serovar *hardjo-bovis* is adapted to cattle.
  ◦ *Leptospira interrogans* serovar *hardjo-prajitno* is adapted to sheep.
• Animals, especially young animals, infected by a non-host-adapted serovar may develop acute, severe clinical disease; it also may cause abortion in pregnant animals. Examples are *Leptospira interrogans* serovars *pomona, grippotyphosa, canicola,* and *icterohaemorrhagiae* in cattle.
• Calves and lambs are more typically affected by the acute form; the subacute form predominatesin adult cattle; and the chronic form in sheep, goats, and adult cattle. It is acute in dogs <6 months of age and most of the dogs do not develop clinical symptoms and may develop into a carrier state.
• A survey isolating *Leptospira* from kidneys of cattle at slaughter in the United States reported higher isolation rates from bulls than cows.
• Males are often nonsymptomatic carriers that may excrete *Leptospira* in the urine and semen.

PHYSICAL EXAMINATION FINDINGS
Cattle
• A sudden drop in milk production (up to 50%) in lactating cows can be noticed, which lasts 7–14 days. Sometimes the milk is thick, yellow, and may contain clots.
• It can be an acute, systemic, often febrile illness characterized by renal and/or hepatic

damage depending upon the strain involved and recumbency lasting 1–7 days.
• Increased rate of abortion, retained fetal membranes, stillbirth, fetal infection, and birth of weak neonates.
• Infertility due to low conception rates or early pregnancy loss may be seen.
• Uveitis, pancreatitis, bleeding, hemolytic anemia, and respiratory disease may be noticed.

Sheep and Goats
• Sheep and goats rarely develop the clinical disease but in young stock: pyrexia, dyspnea, depression, anorexia, may be hemoglobinuria, pale or yellowish mucus membranes; death due to septicemia may occur within 12 hours.

Dogs
• Uveitis, pancreatitis.
• Fever and depression are the most common signs. Dogs feel cold, shivery, and stiff. They may carry their tummies tucked up due to pain. Some dogs may drool and vomit. They may drink excessively due to fever.
• Later in the course of disease, a few pets will develop uveitis, nervous system abnormalities, and red-tinged urine. As the disease progresses, the pet may become dehydrated due to the lack of interest in drinking. When body temperature drops to subnormal, the prognosis is very grave. Juvenile dogs may die suddenly before the clinical signs develop.
• When liver is involved the dog's skin may take on a yellowish tinge and show all the symptoms of hepatitis. When the kidneys have been severely damaged, they develop uremia.

GENETICS
N/A

CAUSES AND RISK FACTORS
• Pathogenic serovars of the *Leptospira* species.
• Pathogenic leptospires are classified as a single species, *Leptospira interrogans,* with >200 serovars in 23 serogroups.
• Direct transmission through contact with urine, vaginal discharge, post-abortion discharge, or the fetus of an infected host. Indirect transmission through contact with contaminated environment.
• Climatic conditions (high temperature and humidity) play an important role in maintenance of the bacteria in the environment and increase risk of contamination.

DIAGNOSIS

DIFFERENTIAL DIAGNOSES
• Uveitis, pancreatitis: Leptospirosis is confused with the other diseases that cause hematuria, abortion, and jaundice.
• The disease should be differentiated from water toxicosis in young calves, postparturient hemoglobinuria, anaplasmosis, babesiosis,

bacillary hemoglobinuria, enzootic hematuria, acute hepatitis, and cholangiohepatitis.
• Among the reproductive signs, it should be differentiated from anaplasmosis, bluetongue, bovine viral diarrhea mucosal disease, brucellosis, campylobacteriosis, trichomoniasis, infectious bovine rhinotracheitis (IBR), malnutrition, mycoplasma, and mycosis.

CBC/BIOCHEMISTRY/URINALYSIS
• CBC may show a hemolytic anemia and leukocytosis; there may be leukopenia.
• Urinalysis may reveal increased bilirubin, hemoglobin, and albumin. *Note:* Urine may be infectious.
• Biochemistry may show increased liver enzymes (AST and ALT), bilirubinemia, and azotemia.

OTHER LABORATORY TESTS
• Leptospirosis should be diagnosed on a herd level from several suspected animals.
• Microscopic agglutination test (MAT) on acute and convalescent (7–10 days later) serology is a commonly used test for leptospirosis. MAT titer >1:800 coinciding with clinical signs or by a four-fold rise in paired samples is diagnostic.
• In cases of abortion, MAT titer declines and identification of titer of >300 in several cows would be significant in an unvaccinated herd.
• Results of samples taken in early infection may show cross-reactivity to other serovars.
• Chronic carriers and animals that abort may be seronegative after several months of infection.
• Serologic titers due to vaccination cannot be distinguished from infection, although they tend to be lower and more transient.
• Isolation of bacteria in the kidneys from chronic carriers may not have diagnostic titer. Presence of spirochete in dark field microscopy is a tentative but not specific diagnosis.
• Diagnosis with immunofluorescence is rapid and confirmatory. Immunofluorescence detection in urine samples is fast and specific if samples arrive to the laboratory quickly and chilled. Formalin can be added to a final concentration of 0.8% to preserve the bacteria in the sample. As excretion in cattle is intermittent, a negative result does not preclude the disease. Detection of *Leptospira* in aborted fetal tissues by FA has also been reported with variable success.

IMAGING
N/A

PATHOLOGIC FINDINGS
• Calves present with fever, anorexia, depression, (with *L. hardjo*) hemolytic anemia, hemoglobinuria, icterus, and petechiae (with *L. pomona*.)
• Hemoglobinuria typically resolves within 72 hours; anemia begins to resolve at 4–5 days and is typically resolved 7–10 days later.

• Mortality rate in calves is higher than in adult cattle.
• Adult cattle present with abnormal milk (thick, yellow, blood tinged) without obvious inflammation of the mammary gland, or later with abortions.
• Aborted fetuses are usually autolyzed.
• In endemically affected herds, younger animals may have an increased incidence of abortions.

TREATMENT
THERAPEUTIC APPROACH
• Infected animals can be treated with any antibiotics to prevent irreversible liver and kidney damage, abortion, establishment of a carrier state, and hemolytic anemia. *Leptospira* are not found to be developing any antibiotic resistance. Antibiotics such as penicillin, tetracycline, and erythromycin are helpful. Doxycycline prevents dogs from becoming chronic carriers.
• Animals with acute disease may require blood transfusions, oral or intravenous fluid therapy, and other supportive nursing care.
• Treating lactating dairy cattle with agalactia may hasten return to near normal yields, but requires discarding the milk for the withdrawal period. Treatment at this time may also reduce the likelihood of abortion.
• Acute disease in calves should be treated aggressively both symptomatically and with antibiotics. Supportive care can be given through the use of antiemetics for vomiting, antidiarrheal for diarrhea, and fluid therapy usually with lactated Ringer's solution or normal saline.

SURGICAL CONSIDERATIONS AND TECHNIQUES
N/A

MEDICATIONS
DRUGS OF CHOICE
• Tetracycline, 10–15 mg/kg q12h for 3–5 days.
• Long-acting oxytetracycline, 20 mg/kg two doses at 10-day intervals.
• Long-acting amoxicillin, 15 mg/kg, two to three doses 48 hours apart.
• Tilmicosin, 10 mg/kg SQ.
• Ceftiofur sodium 2.2 or 5 mg/kg IM q24h for 5 days or 20 mg/kg IM q24h for 3 days.
• Streptomycin or dihydrostreptomycin, 12.5 mg/kg q12h for 3 days. A single dose of 25 mg/kg will usually clear the carrier state from *L. pomona* or other non-host-adapted serovars.

CONTRAINDICATIONS
N/A

PRECAUTIONS
• Appropriate meat and milk withdrawal times must be followed for all compounds administered to food-producing animals.
• Previously, streptomycin, dihydrostreptomycin, or dihydrostreptomycin-penicillin G was used for treatment, but is no longer available in certain countries for use in food-producing animals.

POSSIBLE INTERACTIONS
N/A

FOLLOW-UP
EXPECTED COURSE AND PROGNOSIS
• Prognosis is good if treated early.
• Animal may become a carrier and shed the bacteria.

POSSIBLE COMPLICATIONS
Abortion, early pregnancy loss

CLIENT EDUCATION
Awareness of risk factors: Purchase or comingling with infected animal, access to contaminated water source

PATIENT CARE
Supportive treatment during convalescence.

PREVENTION
• Minimizing access to wildlife, rodents, and contaminated water sources.
• Vaccination using multiple serovars generally confers protection against abortion and death and significantly reduces renal colonization.
• Selection of seronegative replacement stock will help prevent introduction into the herd.

MISCELLANEOUS
ASSOCIATED CONDITIONS
• Prompt vaccination and antimicrobial therapy for pregnant beef cows early in the epizoonosis can prevent further abortions.
• Leptospirosis is a zoonotic agent so appropriate hygiene and sanitary methods must be followed by practitioners and owners to prevent transmission.

AGE-RELATED FACTORS
• The acute form more typically affects calves and lambs, subacute form in adult cattle, and chronic form in sheep, goats, and occasionally adult cattle.

ZOONOTIC POTENTIAL
• Leptospirosis has zoonotic potential through direct contact with contaminated urine and the environment. People are also infected by aerosol.
• People working with infected cattle should take precautionary measures such as

L

LEPTOSPIROSIS

protective clothing, rubber boots, latex gloves, and protective eyeglasses or facemasks.

PREGNANCY
• In endemically affected herds, younger animals may have an increased incidence of sporadic abortions.
• Animals in the second half of gestation (>4 months) can suffer invasion of the placenta and fetus during the septicemic phase, resulting in abortion several weeks later.

SYNONYMS
N/A

ABBREVIATIONS
• ALT = alanine aminotransferase
• AST = aspartate transaminase
• FA = fluorescent antibody
• IBR = infectious bovine rhinotracheitis
• IM = intramuscular
• MAT = microscopic agglutination test
• PCR = polymerase chain reaction
• SQ = subcutaneous

SEE ALSO
• Abortion: Bacterial
• Abortion: Camelid

• Abortion: Small Ruminant
• Babesiosis
• Postparturient Hemoglobinuria
• Pyrrolizidine Alkaloids
• Snakebite

Suggested Reading

Bolin CA, Alt DP. Use of a monovalent leptospiral vaccine to prevent renal colonization and urinary shedding in cattle exposed to *Leptospira borgpetersenii* serovar *hardjo*. Am J Vet Res 2001, 62: 995–1000.

Esmaeli H, Moradi Geravand M, Hamedi M, Sharifi A, Kalateh Rahmani H. Outbreak of leptospirosis in cattle, sheep and goats of Hilla wetland in Bushehr in 2003. Vet J 2014.

Grooms DL. Infectious agents: Leptospirosis. In: Hopper RM ed, Bovine Reproduction. Hoboken: Wiley, 2014, pp. 529–32.

Levett PN. Leptospirosis. Clin Microbiol Rev 2001, 14: 296–326.

Llorente P, Leoni L, Martinez Vivot M. Leptospirosis en camélidos sudamericanos. Estudio de prevalencia serologica en distincas regiones de la Argentina. Archiv Med Vet 2002, 34: 59–68.

Martins G, Lilenbaum W. Leptospirosis in sheep and goats under tropical conditions. Trop Anim Health Prod 2014, 46: 11–17.

Rebhun WC. Diseases of dairy cattle. Philadelphia: Lippincott, Williams & Wilkins, 1995.

Rosardio AR, Véliz AA, Castillo DH, et al. Seroprevalencia a serovares de laptospiras patogenas en alpacas y vicunas de los departamentos de Huancavelica y Ayacucho, Peru. Rev Invest Vet Peru 2012, 23: 350–6.

Author Suvash Shiwakoti
Consulting Editor Ahmed Tibary
Acknowledgment The author and editors acknowledge the prior contribution of Noah Barka and Michael D. Bernstein.

 Client Education Handout available online

LEUKOCYTE RESPONSES IN CATTLE

BASICS

- Complete blood count (CBC) is indicated to evaluate cattle for the presence of inflammatory, infectious, or neoplastic disorders.
- CBC may improve diagnostic accuracy and treatment monitoring, ultimately helping clients make a more informed decision.
- CBC is a diagnostic test that should be performed based on historical and clinical findings and should never preclude a complete physical examination.
- Blood smear examination is a key component of the CBC because it allows clinicians to verify the white blood cell (WBC) count and the differential cell counts.
- Blood smear is also required to identify neutrophil precursors, neoplastic cells, blood parasites, and morphologic changes in neutrophils and lymphocytes.
- WBC count can be estimated from a blood smear using the following equation:
  - WBC (cells/μL) = 2,000 × mean number of WBCs per field at the 40× objective.
- Blood leukocytes can be classified as:
  - Granulocytes or polymorphonuclear cells: neutrophils, eosinophils, and basophils
  - Mononuclear cells: lymphocytes and monocytes.

Neutrophils
- Neutrophils develop from stem cells located in the bone marrow in about 6 days.
- Once the neutrophil storage pool in the bone marrow is depleted, precursors including band neutrophils, metamyelocytes, and myelocytes are released into the blood.
- Neutrophils usually circulate for 5–10 hours in the blood before entering tissues to phagocytose and kill invading microorganisms.
- Neutrophils migrate very rapidly to tissues and act as a first line of defense, but are incapable of repeated phagocytosis, unlike macrophages.
- Blood neutrophils are either free (circulating neutrophil pool) or temporarily adhered to the vascular endothelium (marginal neutrophil pool).

Eosinophils
- Eosinophils develop in the bone marrow, then circulate for few minutes before entering tissues.
- Eosinophils have a high tropism for tissues, and therefore blood eosinophil counts may not truly reflect tissue eosinophilia.
- Eosinophils play a major role in defense against parasites and modulation of inflammation, especially in allergic disorders.

Basophils
- Basophils develop in the bone marrow, then circulate for a few hours before entering tissues.
- Basophils play a major role in modulation of inflammation in allergic disorders.

Lymphocytes
- Blood lymphocytes include T-lymphocytes, B-lymphocytes, and natural killer cells.
- All lymphocytes arise from a common stem cell located in the bone marrow, then mature within primary lymphoid organs.
- T- and B-lymphocytes mature in the thymus and Peyer's patches, respectively.
- Mature lymphocytes leave the primary lymphoid organs to reside in secondary lymphoid organs including lymph nodes, spleen, bone marrow, and lymphoid tissues in the digestive, respiratory, and urogenital tracts.
- Lymphocytes are specialized in recognizing foreign antigens and mediate the humoral and cellular immunity.
- Blood lymphocytes are either free or adhered to endothelial cells.
- Lymphocytes are unique because these long-lived cells are able to recirculate from peripheral tissues to their lymphoid tissue of origin for several weeks to years.

Monocytes
- Monocytes develop from stem cells located in the bone marrow, then circulate for few days before entering tissues.
- Once in tissues, they may differentiate into different macrophage subtypes including Kupffer cells, alveolar macrophages, microglia, and Langerhans cells.
- Macrophages are specialized in phagocytosing and killing invading microorganisms.
- Macrophages also initiate tissue repair and act as antigen-presenting cells.

OVERVIEW

Leukogram Interpretation Principles
- Lymphocytes are the predominant blood leukocytes in adult cattle with a neutrophil to lymphocyte (N:L) ratio of about 1:2.
- Neonatal calves usually have a N:L ratio of about 1:1.
- Cattle have a limited ability to recruit bone marrow stem cells, and therefore WBC counts are typically lower in the face of acute inflammation than in other domestic animals.
- WBC counts greater than 20,000 cells/μL are considered markedly increased.
- It should be kept in mind that WBC counts vary naturally over time, both as a result of disease processes and biologic variation (age, diet, breed, pregnancy).

- CBC provides a snapshot of a dynamic process, and therefore does not reveal whether the situation is improving or deteriorating.

Reference Intervals
- Reference intervals (RIs) typically represent the central 95% of values of 60–120 healthy animals.
- 5% of healthy animals are expected to have a result outside of the RI for any single test, and therefore a single result outside of the RI should not be overinterpreted.
- Repeat testing is recommended when a test result does not fit the clinical context.
- Use of the term "normal range" is discouraged, because a test result can be within the RI and not be appropriate for the patient's condition.

Preanalytic and Analytic Variation
- Preanalytic variation is associated with patient preparation and handling, time of collection, and sample collection, storage, and handling.
- Analytic variation is associated with accuracy and precision of the hematology analyzer.
- Assessment of the analytic performance of in-clinic analyzers is recommended following instrument purchase and should be repeated annually.
- Standardization and control of preanalytic and analytic conditions may minimize intra- and inter-individual variation.
- Participation in an external quality assurance program is recommended to help ensure accuracy of results.

Sample Collection and Handling
- Blood collected in a tube containing EDTA is the sample of choice for a CBC.
- Blood tubes should be filled to completion to insure the proper blood-to-EDTA ratio and gently inverted several times immediately after filling.
- Blood should be analyzed within 30–60 minutes of collection or stored at refrigerator temperature (4°C) and analyzed within 24 hours.
- Delayed analysis may result in nuclear lobulation or cytoplasmic vacuolization of lymphocytes and marked cellular swelling.

INCIDENCE/PREVALENCE
N/A

GEOGRAPHIC DISTRIBUTION
N/A

PATHOPHYSIOLOGY
Neutrophilia
- Neutrophilia is usually caused by an increased production of neutrophils than an increased release from the bone marrow because cattle have a limited pool of neutrophils stored in the bone marrow.

L

LEUKOCYTE RESPONSES IN CATTLE (CONTINUED)

• Neutrophilia is usually due to acute or chronic inflammation caused by infectious agents, neoplasia, or tissue necrosis

• However, chronic or low-grade inflammation is not always associated with neutrophilia.

• Neutrophilia can also be due to changes in neutrophil kinetics caused by administration or endogenous release of catecholamines or glucocorticoids.

Neutropenia

• Neutropenia develops when margination or migration of neutrophils into tissues exceeds the release of neutrophils from the bone marrow.

• Neutropenia is common in the first 12–24 hours following an acute inflammatory stimulus because the pool of neutrophils stored in the bone marrow is limited.

• Persistent neutropenia is usually caused by severe acute inflammation and associated with degenerative left shift and toxic changes in neutrophils.

• Neutropenia can also be due to a shift from the circulating pool to the marginal pool caused by endotoxemia.

Left Shift

• The term "left shift" indicates the presence of neutrophil precursors in the peripheral blood including band neutrophils, metamyelocytes, and myelocytes.

• Left shift is usually due to severe, often acute, inflammation.

• Degenerative left shift is characterized by the presence of neutrophil precursors in the blood in numbers exceeding the mature neutrophils.

• It indicates an inappropriate production or release of neutrophils and is usually caused by endotoxemia or sepsis.

Right Shift

• The term "right shift" indicates an increased amount of hypersegmented neutrophils in the blood, which is usually caused by administration or endogenous release of glucocorticoids.

• Right shift has also been reported in cattle with bovine leukocyte adhesion deficiency (BLAD) and cobalt deficiency.

Toxic Neutrophils

• Toxic changes refer to morphologic abnormalities of neutrophils including cytoplasmic basophilia or vacuolization, toxic granules, Döhle bodies, and nuclear immaturity.

• It can be caused by any inflammatory disorder severe enough to stimulate neutrophil maturation.

Lymphocytosis

• Lymphocytosis is usually caused by an increased production of lymphocytes due to acute or chronic inflammation.

• Lymphocytosis can also result from neoplastic proliferation of lymphoid cells in lymph nodes, bone marrow, or other lymphoid tissues.

• Lymphoma associated with infection by bovine leukemia virus (BLV) is the most common lymphoproliferative disorder in cattle.

• BLV infection may also cause persistent lymphocytosis (7,000–15,000 cells/μL) without tumors.

• Lymphocytosis can also be due to changes in lymphocyte kinetics caused by administration or endogenous release of catecholamines.

Lymphopenia

• Lymphopenia is usually caused by an increased margination and migration of lymphocytes into tissues, increased movement of lymphocytes to lymphoid tissues, and decreased movement of lymphocytes from lymph nodes.

• Lymphopenia is usually due to changes in lymphocyte kinetics caused by administration or endogenous release of glucocorticoids.

• Lymphopenia can also be due to acute inflammation or bone marrow failure.

Reactive Lymphocytes

• Reactive changes refer to morphologic features of lymphocytes including fine cytoplasmic vacuoles, enhanced cytoplasmic basophilia, and nuclear changes.

• Reactive lymphocytes are seen in cattle with acute or chronic inflammation.

• Inflammation can cause marked lymphocyte atypia that can be very difficult to differentiate from neoplastic changes.

Monocytosis

• Monocytosis is usually caused by an increased production and release of monocytes due to acute or chronic inflammation.

• However, inflammation does not always cause monocytosis.

• Monocytosis can also be due to changes in lymphocyte kinetics caused by administration or endogenous release of glucocorticoids.

Eosinophilia and Basophilia

• Eosinophilia and basophilia are relatively rare but may be seen in cattle with parasitism or allergic disorders.

• Eosinophilia and basophilia are more commonly associated with tissue parasites than blood or gastrointestinal parasites.

• Chronic eosinophilia is usually caused by inflammation affecting mast cell-rich organs including skin, lung, and gastrointestinal tract.

Bovine Leukocyte Adhesion Deficiency

• BLAD is a hereditary disorder described in Holstein cattle.

• BLAD is caused by a single mutation in a gene that encodes an integrin controlling adherence, migration, and aggregation of leukocytes.

• Gene mutation causes neutrophils to lose their ability to adhere to vascular endothelium and migrate to tissues, leading their prolonged circulation in the blood.

• Affected cattle typically have marked neutrophilia and recurrent infections.

• PCR assays are commercially available to identify cattle with BLAD.

Chédiak-Higashi Syndrome

• Chédiak-Higashi Syndrome (CHS) is a hereditary disorder described in Hereford, Brangus, and Japanese Black cattle.

• CHS is caused by a mutation in a gene that controls lysosomal membrane fusion, leading to enlarged lysosomes in leukocytes and pigment cells.

• Presence of enlarged lysosomes in neutrophils, eosinophils, and monocytes is diagnostic.

• Affected cattle usually have a dilute coat color and light-colored irises (pseudoalbinism).

• Recurrent infections and/or excessive bleeding may be present because function of platelets, natural killer, and cytotoxic T-cells is usually altered.

SIGNALMENT
N/A

GENETICS

• BLAD is an autosomal recessive trait in Holstein cattle.

• CHS is an autosomal recessive trait in Hereford, Brangus, and Japanese Black cattle.

PHYSICAL EXAMINATION FINDINGS
N/A

CAUSES AND RISK FACTORS

Neutrophils
Causes of Neutrophilia
• Genetic disorders

- ○ Bovine leukocyte adhesion deficiency
- Increased production of neutrophils
  - ○ Acute or chronic inflammation
    - Common causes include pneumonia, peritonitis, deep digital sepsis, liver abscesses, paratuberculosis, and lymphoma
- Increased release from the bone marrow
  - ○ Acute or chronic inflammation
  - ○ Administration of glucocorticoids
  - ○ Endogenous release of glucocorticoids
    - Common causes include pain, circulatory shock, transportation, handling, and extreme temperatures
- Shift from the marginal pool to the circulating pool
  - ○ Administration or endogenous release of glucocorticoids
  - ○ Administration or endogenous release of catecholamines
    - Common causes include pain, circulatory shock, transportation, handling, and extreme temperatures

Causes of Neutropenia
- Decreased production
  - ○ Bone marrow failure
    - Common causes include bracken fern toxicosis, bovine neonatal pancytopenia, irradiation, myelofibrosis, and neoplasia
- Increased margination or migration into tissues
  - ○ Severe acute inflammation
- Shift from the circulating pool to the marginal pool
  - ○ Common causes of endotoxemia include coliform mastitis, puerperal metritis, and salmonellosis.

Lymphocytes
Causes of Lymphocytosis
- Increased production
  - ○ Chronic inflammation
- Neoplastic proliferation of lymphoid cells in lymph nodes or other tissues
  - ○ Lymphoma (BLV-associated or sporadic)
- Shift from the marginal pool to the circulating pool
  - ○ Administration or endogenous release of catecholamines

Causes of Lymphopenia
- Bone marrow failure
  - ○ Causes of bone marrow failure include bracken fern toxicosis, bovine neonatal pancytopenia, irradiation, myelofibrosis, and neoplasia.
- Shift from the marginal pool to the circulating pool
  - ○ Acute inflammation
  - ○ Administration or endogenous release of glucocorticoids

Monocytes
Causes of Monocytosis
- Increased production and release
  - ○ Acute or chronic inflammation
    - Common causes include pneumonia, peritonitis, deep digital sepsis, liver abscesses, paratuberculosis, and lymphoma
- Shift from the marginal pool to the circulating pool
  - ○ Administration or endogenous release of glucocorticoids

Eosinophils and Basophils
Causes of Eosinophilia and/or Basophilia
- Allergic disorders
  - ○ Common causes include dermatitis, eosinophilic enteritis, and milk allergy
- Parasitism
  - ○ External parasites
  - ○ Mites, lice fleas or ticks
  - ○ Internal parasites
    - Lungworms
    - Gastrointestinal strongyles
    - Sarcocystosis

DIAGNOSIS

DIFFERENTIAL DIAGNOSES
N/A

CBC/BIOCHEMISTRY/URINALYSIS
Common Leukogram Findings
- Severe acute inflammation is usually associated with neutropenia, degenerative left shift, toxic changes in neutrophils, and lymphopenia.
- Chronic inflammation is are usually associated with neutrophilia and lymphocytosis.
- Administration or endogenous release of glucocorticoids is usually associated with neutrophilia, lymphopenia, and monocytosis.
- Administration or endogenous release of catecholamines is usually associated with transient neutrophilia and lymphocytosis.

OTHER LABORATORY TESTS
- Determination of fibrinogen, haptoglobin, and serum amyloid A can be helpful when chronic or low-grade inflammation is suspected.

IMAGING
- Thoracic or abdominal radiography and ultrasonography may help identify inflammatory disorders including pneumonia, liver abscesses, traumatic reticuloperitonitis, urolithiasis, and lymphoma.

OTHER DIAGNOSTIC PROCEDURES
- Bone marrow examination is indicated when neutropenia persists for more than 3–4 days and/or atypical or unexplained immature cells are observed on the peripheral blood smear.

- Lymph node aspiration or biopsy is indicated in cattle with enlarged lymph node(s) and historical or clinical findings consistent with lymphoma.

PATHOLOGIC FINDINGS
N/A

TREATMENT
N/A

MEDICATIONS
N/A

FOLLOW-UP

EXPECTED COURSE AND PROGNOSIS
- Severe acute inflammation usually causes neutropenia with left shift followed by neutrophilia after 3–4 days.
- Resolution of degenerative left shift suggests a more favorable prognosis.
- Disappearance of toxic changes in neutrophils suggests resolution of inflammation.
- Persistent lymphopenia suggests ongoing inflammation.
- Marked persistent lymphocytosis is associated with a guarded prognosis until lymphoma can be excluded.

MISCELLANEOUS

AGE-RELATED FACTORS
- WBC and lymphocyte counts are usually higher in younger cattle and decrease with age.
- Neutrophil counts are usually higher in neonatal calves and decrease with age.
- Eosinophil counts are usually lower in younger cattle and increase with age.

PREGNANCY
- Parturition is usually associated with neutrophilia, lymphopenia, and variable monocytosis.

ABBREVIATIONS
- BLAD = bovine leukocyte adhesion deficiency
- BLV = bovine leukemia virus

L

LEUKOCYTE RESPONSES IN CATTLE

- CBC = complete blood count
- CHS = Chédiak-Higashi syndrome
- EDTA = ethylenediaminetetraacetic acid
- N:L = neutrophil to lymphocyte
- PCR = polymerase chain reaction
- RI = reference interval
- WBC = white blood cell

SEE ALSO
- Anemia, Nonregenerative
- Anemia, Regenerative
- Blood Chemistry (see www.fiveminutevet.com/ruminant)

Suggested Reading
Tornquist SJ, Rigas J. Interpretation of ruminant leukocyte responses. In: Weiss DJ, Wardrop KJ eds, Schalm's Veterinary Hematology, 6th ed. Ames: Blackwell, 2010, pp. 307–13.
Author Thibaud Kuca
Consulting Editor Christopher C.L. Chase

L

BASICS

OVERVIEW
• A discharge of electricity occurring in association with thunderstorms, damaged power lines, or faulty wiring that results in death or injury to one or more animals.
• Sudden death in groups of animals without signs of struggle are strongly suggestive of lightning strike.
• Lightning may cause death after **direct strike** (lightning strikes animals directly), **contact** (electrical charge passing through object (tree or fence) to animal(s)), **side flash** (jumps from one object to animal), **step voltage** (lightning strikes object which allows radiation of energy in all directions including where animal(s) are standing, thereby killing animals instantly), or **blunt trauma** (lightning strike injures animal by knocking it to ground or via falling objects).

INCIDENCE/PREVALENCE
Commonly observed in specific geographic locations during the spring, summer, and early autumn months of the year.

GEOGRAPHIC DISTRIBUTION
Where thunderstorms occur

SYSTEMS AFFECTED
• Multisystemic
• Integument

PATHOPHYSIOLOGY
The massive electrical current and voltage applied to animals by lightning most commonly results in subacute cardiac and respiratory arrest. Neurologic damage in animals can be observed in or around the 4th ventricle, leading to cardiac and respiratory arrest. Survivors may develop multiple organ system dysfunction including severe burns, vascular injury (subcutaneous hemorrhages to DIC), traumatic injury to limbs (falling, blunt trauma), or nerve excitation resulting in massive muscle contraction and thermal injury to muscle. This may result in myonecrosis that may progress to renal compromise in survivors. Renal damage associated with rhabdomyolysis and myoglobinuria can also result in hyperkalemia, hypocalcemia, hyperglycemia, and acidosis. Gastrointestinal effects may be due to direct effect of electrical injury on abdominal organs leading to hemorrhage or the result of blunt trauma secondary to falling or objects striking the animal.

HISTORICAL FINDINGS
• Careful evaluation of animal(s) and immediate environment (up to 40 meters in diameter), for signs of burns, burnt or damaged trees or other objects. Useful information may include number of animals affected, number in herd, specific management practices (feeding, watering, housing), recent medical history of animals, last observation of animal and time of death (if known). History of recent severe weather, although this may confuse some cases.
• Animal(s) found dead often after severe weather storms in areas where thunderstorms are frequent. Animals may be found dead where they were standing in various postures. Single or multiple animals may be found near large trees, against fences, or near watering holes and dead or unconscious. Feed (hay, grass) may be present within the oral cavity. Burn or singe marks on the animal and damage to the environment may be present in cases; however, animals that are electrocuted secondary to charged water or earth or objects (step voltage) may not have visible signs of electrocution (burns).

SIGNALMENT
Any animal. More commonly observed in pastured animals.

PHYSICAL EXAMINATION FINDINGS
• Death is often instantaneous with little visible indication of a struggle. Singe or burn marks on animals are most commonly observed and are commonly present on medial surface of limbs, jaw, neck, and shoulders. Often, singe marks are located at one end of tree (scorch lines). Peripheral blood vessels are often distended with blood that clots poorly. Capillary damage leading to subcutaneous hemorrhage and in some instances subcutaneous gas is noted. Ruminal distension may engorge venous structures with blood from abdomen to cranial aspect of animal. This is often accompanied by blood accumulation in muscle, lymph nodes, and subcutaneous tissues of the thorax, head, and neck. The lungs are generally not compressed as in cases of severe premortem bloat. Nasal mucosal and frontal sinus congestion is observed in some cases, and linear mucosal hemorrhages of the larynx, trachea, and bronchi are present in most cases of lightning-induced death. This may lead to blood-tinged frothy fluid or ropes of clotted blood draining from mouth and nares.
• Infrequently, animals rendered unconscious by lightning strike followed by recovery may manifest neurologic signs and evidence of struggling may be present. A recent report of ocular disease in dairy cows following lightning strike indicates that electrical or blunt trauma to eyes may occur, as is observed in human victims. Swine in outdoor pens struck by lightning manifested acute hindlimb paralysis. Lesions were limited to fractures of caudal lumbar and sacral vertebrae with dorsal displacement of sacral spine and transection of the spinal cord. Bilateral femur fractures were also observed in two calves associated with lightning strike.

GENETICS
N/A

CAUSES AND RISK FACTORS
A recent review demonstrated that season of the year (spring-summer), age of the animal (>1 year), presence of tree(s), water, ruminal distension with feed present in oral cavity were associated with greater odds of lightning-associated fatalities.

DIAGNOSIS

DIFFERENTIAL DIAGNOSES
Any cause of acute death in livestock. Anthrax (*Bacillus anthracis*), clostridial intoxications (*Clostridium hemolyticum, Cl. chauvoei, Cl. perfringens, Cl. botulinum*), *Mannheimia hemolytica, Histophilus somni* (previously haemophilus somnus), Listeria monocytogenes septicemia, organophosphate, carbamate, lead, ionophore, gossypol, toxic gases, blue-green algae intoxication, Japanese yew, nitrates, cyanogenic plants, salt poisoning, and other toxicants. Necropsy of potentially electrocuted animals is imperative.

CBC/BIOCHEMISTRY/URINALYSIS
N/A

OTHER LABORATORY TESTS
Feed or plants consumed may also be evaluated for pesticides, herbicides, and heavy metals.

IMAGING
N/A

OTHER DIAGNOSTIC PROCEDURES
N/A

PATHOLOGIC FINDINGS
Necropsy of animal(s) is highly recommended and therefore transport to local state diagnostic laboratory or field necropsy should be performed by a veterinarian. Samples to collect would include heart, lung, liver, spleen, kidneys, gut, lymph nodes, endocrine glands (thyroid, pancreas, adrenals), rumen content, skin and subcutaneous tissues, muscle (especially from limbs), paying particular attention to lesions or abnormalities observed. Samples should be saved for histopathology (10% buffered formalin), toxicology (frozen organs such as liver, kidney, rumen content, whole eyes or ocular fluid aspirates) and microbiology (blood, brain, liver spleen, lymph nodes, kidney, and muscle, thoracic or abdominal fluids, CSF, urine). Samples for microbiology should be collected in sterile containers and stored on ice but not frozen.

TREATMENT

THERAPEUTIC APPROACH
Treatment of survivors should focus on clinical signs. Neurologic sequelae are common, and nonsteroidal and steroidal anti-inflammatory agents, hyperosmolar

LIGHTNING STRIKE

agents (mannitol, 50% dextrose, hypertonic saline) to reduce inflammation and swelling in critical locations (CNS, muscle) are recommended. Local wound care for burns and systemic antimicrobial agents. Euthanasia for more severely affected animals may be appropriate.

SURGICAL CONSIDERATIONS AND TECHNIQUES
N/A

MEDICATIONS
See "Treatment"

FOLLOW-UP

EXPECTED COURSE AND PROGNOSIS
Normally sudden death occurs with lightning strike. The prognosis in cases of survival will vary.

POSSIBLE COMPLICATIONS
Neurologic signs, fractures, paralysis

CLIENT EDUCATION
N/A

PATIENT CARE
Euthanasia is recommended in survivors with severe traumatic injury.

PREVENTION
N/A

MISCELLANEOUS

PRODUCTION MANAGEMENT
N/A

ABBREVIATIONS
• CNS = central nervous system
• CSF = cerebrospinal fluid
• DIC = disseminated intravascular coagulation

SEE ALSO
• Burn Management
• Wound Management

Suggested Reading
Blackwell JG. Lightning incriminated in the sudden death of 18 steers. Vet Med Small Anim Clin 1976, 71: 1375–7.

Boeve MH, Huijben R, Grinwis G, Djajadiningrat-Laanen SC. Visual impairment after suspected lightning strike in a herd of Holstein-Friesian cattle. Vet Rec 2004, 154: 402–4.

Casteel SW, Turk JR. Collapse/sudden death. In: Smith BP ed, Large Animal Internal Medicine. St. Louis: Mosby, 2002, pp. 246–53.

Ramsey FK, Howard JR. Diagnosis of lightning strike. J Am Vet Med Assoc 1970, 156: 1472–4.

Van Alstine WG, Widmer WR. Lightning injury in an outdoor swine herd. J Vet Diagn Invest 2003, 15: 289–91.

Vanneste E, Weyens P, Poelman DR, Chiers K, Deprez P, Pardon B. Lightning related fatalities in livestock: Veterinary expertise and the added value of lightning location data. Vet J 2015, 203: 103–8.

Author Jeff Lakritz
Consulting Editor Kaitlyn A. Lutz

L

BASICS

OVERVIEW
- The genus *Listeria* contains five species: *L. monocytogenes, L. ivanovii, L. innocua, L. seeligeri,* and *L. welshimeri.*
- *L. monocytogenes* is the only significant pathogen in this group, causing septicemia, abortion, central nervous system infection, and mastitis in ruminants.
- In ruminants, listeriosis can manifest in several ways, including CNS infection, abortion, septicemia, and mastitis.

INCIDENCE/PREVALENCE
Clinically diseased animals in a group can reach 9% but rarely exceed 1–2%.

GEOGRAPHIC DISTRIBUTION
Worldwide, particularly temperate climates

SYSTEMS AFFECTED
- Reproductive
- Nervous
- Mammary
- Ophthalmic

PATHOPHYSIOLOGY
- Typically *Listeria* causes meningoencephalitis in adults and meningitis in the young after an incubation of 2–3 weeks.
- Infection is thought to occur following injury to mucus membranes of the oral and nasal cavities, conjunctiva, or through the dental pulp when animals are cutting or losing teeth.
- *L. monocytogenes* has been proposed to invade the trigeminal nerves (CN-V) and travels centripetally along the axons to the brain, proliferates in the pons and medulla and can spread elsewhere.
- The trigeminal nerve and its neighboring CN nuclei are subject to injury as a consequence of neuritis, encephalitis, and meningitis.
- *L. monocytogenes* can invade the fetoplacental unit with or without signs of encephalitis or septicemia, typically causing late gestation abortion with or without obvious clinical signs.
- *L. monocytogenes* can also produce septicemia and focal necrosis of the liver and spleen of neonates, after incubation as short as one day. The organism is thought to invade from the GI tract after consumption of colostrum or milk from infected dams.
- Mastitis can be subclinical to severe and suppurative in cattle. Sheep tend to develop chronic inflammatory mastitis, and goats, subclinical interstitial mastitis. The organism is thought to be contracted from feces and the dairy farm environment in these cases.

HISTORICAL FINDINGS
Typically acute to subacute onset of cranial nerve dysfunction (facial paralysis and vestibular signs) in juvenile or young adult ruminants.

SIGNALMENT
- CNS infection—juvenile and adult animals
- Septicemia—common in neonates
- Abortion—reported in adult cattle and sheep
- Mastitis—reported in cattle, sheep, and goats

PHYSICAL EXAMINATION FINDINGS
- Intracranial disease commences with depression, anorexia, decreased milk production, dehydration, and inconsistent fever.
- Neurologic signs are usually asymmetric with conscious proprioceptive deficits, head pressing, obtundation, compulsive circling, and cranial nerve deficits (CNs V through XII). Deficits are described in relation to the inciting lesion location:
  - CN–V—dropped jaw or asymmetric jaw closure, difficulty in prehension and mastication, facial analgesia and anesthesia.
  - CN–VI—ipsilateral medial strabismus.
  - CN–VIII—ptosis, loss of menace response, absent palpebral reflex, droopy ear, decreased lip tone, unilateral drooling, and exposure keratitis. In small ruminants deviation of the philtrum also occurs. Ipsilateral head tilt, nystagmus, and ataxia.
  - Basal ganglia—head pressing, compulsive circling.
  - CN IX and X—dysphagia, salivation, stertor.
  - CN XII—paresis or paralysis of the tongue.
  - Irritation of parasympathetic vagal neurons in the medulla—vomiting and bloat.
  - Spinal myelitis without brainstem disease can occur in lambs, with flaccid paralysis, hemiparesis, tetraparesis, tetraplegia, paraplegia, and recumbency.
- Animals with septicemia display fever, depression, and anorexia. Diarrhea commonly occurs in small ruminants. Neurologic signs are rare. Pregnant does and ewes can abort.
- Adult cattle can develop keratitis, conjunctivitis, or uveitis due to *L. monocytogenes* with no other clinical signs.
- Abortion related to *L. monocytogenes* usually occurs in the last 2 months of gestation in cattle and during the last month in ewes and does. Clinical signs of disease are uncommon in these cases; however, fever, depression, retention of fetal membranes, or endometritis can occur.

GENETICS
N/A

CAUSES AND RISK FACTORS
- *L. monocytogenes* is widely distributed in the environment, contained in soil, vegetation, water, and the feces of different mammals.
- Resistant and persistent in the environment, able to resist high salt concentrations, to grow over a wide pH range (5–9) and temperature range (0 to 45°C). These characteristics are related to some outbreaks.
- Poorly prepared silage does not achieve appropriate acidity (pH <4) and allows the organism to multiply.
- Improper ensiling, excessive dryness of the forage, lack of fermentation caused by trench ensiling, silage inoculants, and other factors such as long fiber length, inadequate packing of forage, use of bunker rather than tower silos, absence of silo covers, and relatively slow feeding, may prevent the silage from achieving a pH <5.
- Quality of fermentation of baled silage is generally less adequate.
- In sheep and goats, pasture contamination is the most likely source in outbreaks, but it can occur in winter and spring when animals are housed indoors.

DIAGNOSIS

DIFFERENTIAL DIAGNOSES
- CNS signs—rabies, otitis media/interna, cranial trauma, thromboembolic meningoencephalitis (cattle), aberrant parasite migration, brainstem abscesses.
- Abortion and mastitis—see relevant chapters.
- Septicemia—salmonellosis, yersiniosis, and enterotoxemia.

CBC/BIOCHEMISTRY/URINALYSIS
- Leukocytosis, neutrophilia, and monocytosis can occur, or leukopenia, neutropenia in the septicemic form.
- Decreased water and feed intake and excessive salivation can create hemoconcentration, hyperproteinemia, metabolic acidosis and hyponatremia, hypochloremia, hypokalemia, and hypocalcemia.
- Hyperketonemia in lactating cattle due to reduced feed intake.

OTHER LABORATORY TESTS
N/A

IMAGING
N/A

OTHER DIAGNOSTIC PROCEDURES
- Analysis of CSF—increased nucleated cell count (predominantly monocytes and lymphocytes), increased microprotein. Positive culture supports the diagnosis; however, negative CSF cultures are common.
- ELISA—detects specific antibodies in the milk of animals with mastitis.

PATHOLOGIC FINDINGS
- Minimal gross anomalies. Perivascular cuffing of mononuclear cells and multifocal

L

LISTERIOSIS

inflammatory foci (micro-abscesses) that contain mononuclear cells and predominantly neutrophils, are observed in the brainstem.
• In aborted fetuses—gray-white foci (2 mm) are seen in liver and cotyledons; abomasal erosion has been reported in aborted lambs.

TREATMENT

THERAPEUTIC APPROACH
• Fluid and electrolyte therapy is critical to correct dehydration and severe metabolic acidosis, and can be given orally or IV.
• Manage or prevent exposure keratitis.
• Well-bedded stall with good footing.
• Appropriate antimicrobials.

SURGICAL CONSIDERATIONS AND TECHNIQUES
Temporary rumenostomy can be considered to facilitate the administration of food, water and electrolytes to severely affected valuable animals.

MEDICATION

DRUGS OF CHOICE
• Penicillin: 20,000–40,000 IU/kg, IV, q6–8h for 7 days, then q24h for 14–21 more days.
• Oxytetracycline (100 mg/mL): 10 mg/kg, IV, q12h for 14 days.
• Treatment is usually recommended to continue for at least 1 week beyond apparent cure.

CONTRAINDICATIONS
N/A

PRECAUTIONS
• Isolation of *Listeria* spp. requires cold enrichment procedures and extended incubation times which limit timely diagnosis, and false-negative results are common.
• Appropriate milk and meat withdrawal times must be followed for all compounds administered to food-producing animals.

POSSIBLE INTERACTIONS
N/A

FOLLOW-UP

EXPECTED COURSE AND PROGNOSIS
• Prognosis improves if therapy is instituted early in the disease course.
• Sheep and goats respond poorly to treatment and have a higher case fatality rate than cattle.
• Recumbent or comatose animals rarely recover and have a guarded prognosis.
• Abortion usually has a transient effect on fertility and animals tend to resist reinfection.

POSSIBLE COMPLICATIONS
• Exposure keratitis
• Pneumonia
• Myopathy

CLIENT EDUCATION
Focus on prevention measures and the zoonotic potential of this disease.

PATIENT CARE
Consider euthanasia of animals with no improvement after 2–3 days of treatment.

PREVENTION
• Use high quality, low pH silage.
• Avoid contamination of silage with soil or manure.
• Use pasteurized colostrum or milk.
• Keep bulk tank temperatures low.
• Attenuated or killed vaccines have efficacy and are available in some countries (outside of the United States).

MISCELLANEOUS

ASSOCIATED CONDITIONS
• Exposure keratitis
• Aspiration pneumonia

AGE-RELATED FACTORS
N/A

ZOONOTIC POTENTIAL
• Listeriosis is a food-borne disease of humans, transmitted directly from contaminated meat and raw milk products, or indirectly by contaminated vegetables.

• Most commonly causes miscarriage in pregnant women; septicemia and meningitis can occur in immunodeficient adults.

PREGNANCY
Abortion can occur.

BIOSECURITY
• Aborted fetuses, placentas, and discharges must be handled wearing gloves and a facemask with proper disposal.
• During outbreaks, a high number of asymptomatic animals can shed the organism in their feces; this might have implications for animal transport or biosecurity protocols.

PRODUCTION MANAGEMENT
N/A

SYNONYMS
• Silage disease
• Circling disease

ABBREVIATIONS
• CN = cranial nerve
• CNS = central nervous system
• CSF = cerebrospinal fluid
• ELISA = enzyme-linked immunosorbent assay
• IV = intravenous

SEE ALSO
• Abortion: Bacterial
• Abortion: Small Ruminant
• Bacterial Meningitis
• Coenurosis
• Cranial Nerve Assessment and Dysfunction (see www.fiveminutevet.com/ruminant)
• *Histophilus somni* Complex
• Otitis Media/Interna

Suggested Reading
George LW. Listeriosis. In: Smith BP ed, Large Animal Internal Medicine, 5th ed. St. Louis: Elsevier, 2015, pp. 969–71.
Morin DE. Brainstem and cranial nerve abnormalities: listeriosis, otitis media/interna, and pituitary abscess syndrome. Vet Clin North Am Food Anim Pract 2004, 20: 243–73.
Author Diego Gomez-Nieto
Consulting Editor Erica C. McKenzie

L

LIVER ABSCESSES

BASICS

OVERVIEW
• Hepatic abscesses are a common sequela to ruminal acidosis in cattle fed highly fermentable diets.
• Neonatal calves are susceptible to ascending navel infections, which can occasionally result in hepatic abscesses.
• Foreign bodies can cause abscessation by penetrating the liver parenchyma.
• The most common bacterial species cultured from hepatic abscesses in cattle and sheep are predominantly *Fusobacterium necrophorum,* and also *Trueperella pyogenes* and *Streptococcus, Staphylococcus,* and *Bacteroides* spp.
• Liver abscesses represent a major economic loss to producers of feedlot cattle.
• Goats that have hepatic abscesses are usually older than 1 year of age and in poor body condition. The abscesses are usually secondary to a primary disorder and the most common bacterial species involved are *Corynebacterium pseudotuberculosis, E. coli* and other *Corynebacterium* spp.

INCIDENCE/PREVALENCE
• In general the incidence of liver abscesses is increased in ruminants fed diets high in carbohydrates and low in roughage.
• Holsteins are fed a consistently higher energy diet than beef cattle for longer periods; therefore, they have a higher incidence of liver abscesses.
• Feedlot steers have a somewhat higher incidence than heifers, believed to relate to greater feed intake.
• Cattle fed long-stem, dry, coarse hay are more prone to rumen wall penetration and abscess formation.
• Calves born into a dirty environment or that do not receive adequate colostrum are predisposed to ascending umbilical vein infections.
• Cattle in areas where liver flukes are endemic and not provided adequate prophylaxis can have abscesses form along the parasites' migratory tract.

GEOGRAPHIC DISTRIBUTION
Relates to distribution of specific management systems (feedlots) and parasites (flukes).

SYSTEMS AFFECTED
• Digestive
• Integument
• Respiratory

PATHOPHYSIOLOGY
• Liver abscessation in ruminants results from compromise to the integrity of the rumenal wall arising from ruminal acidosis and/or objects penetrating the rumen wall.

• *F. necrophorum* is isolated from 85% of liver abscesses. This organism is a commensal microbe of the rumen. Its primary energy substrate is lactate, allowing it to proliferate in an anaerobic environment that is using highly fermentable substrates to produce lactate.
• As bacteria colonize the ruminal wall, bacterial emboli shed into the vascular drainage of the rumen and enter the portal circulation. Bacteria and other foreign debris are phagocytized from the blood by Kupffer cells and leukocytes in the liver.
• The liver is highly vascular and well oxygenated. The causative anaerobic bacteria have virulence factors that allow them to establish an anaerobic microenvironment in which they can proliferate and produce an abscess.
• *F. necrophorum* has leukotoxin and endotoxic lipopolysaccharides that help defend against phagocytosis, and also promote intravascular coagulation, which results in infarcts in the parenchyma of the liver.
• As the abscess forms it becomes encapsulated with connective tissue. In time, fluid reabsorption and connective tissue infiltration result in scar tissue formation with net loss of hepatic parenchymal tissue.
• Occasionally an abscess may rupture into the venous circulation, resulting in anaphylaxis or showering of the lungs with bacterial emboli. Ruptured abscesses can also cause formation of a thrombus in the caudal vena cava, which can result in portal hypertension and lead to ascites. If an abscess continues to increase in size, it may occlude the common bile duct and prevent bile secretion into the gastrointestinal tract.
• Liver abscesses in neonates result from ascending umbilical vein infections. Neonates that have failure of passive transfer can also form liver abscesses independent of the nidus as they become bacteremic.
• Liver abscesses have also been reported in cattle infected with *Fasciola hepatica.*

HISTORICAL FINDINGS
• Weight loss.
• Reduction in feed intake.
• Decrease in feed efficiency.
• Dairy cows or dairy goats may have a decrease in milk production.

SIGNALMENT
• Liver abscesses have been identified in cows, sheep, and goats.
• In cattle and sheep abscesses are primarily associated with a highly fermentable, low roughage diet, provoking ruminal acidosis.
• Affected goats are usually older than one year and in poor body condition, with an accompanying pathologic disorder.

PHYSICAL EXAMINATION FINDINGS
• Affected animals may display fever, anorexia, stiff gait, diarrhea, and septic joints.
• Epistaxis and hemoptysis may be evident in animals with metastatic pneumonia.
• Most cases are subclinical and are not recognized until slaughter.

GENETICS
N/A

CAUSES AND RISK FACTORS
• Rumen acidosis
• Septicemia/bacteremia
• Ascending umbilical vein infection
• Liver flukes
• Highly fermentable feeds
• Long stem, dry, coarse hay
• Dirty environments (neonates)

DIAGNOSIS

DIFFERENTIAL DIAGNOSES
• Parasitism
• Malnutrition
• Poor quality feed
• Johne's disease
• Lymphosarcoma
• Traumatic reticuloperitonitis
• Hepatic lipidosis
• Polioencephalomalacia
• Septicemia

CBC/BIOCHEMISTRY/URINALYSIS
• In general, CBC and biochemistry analysis are not reliable indicators of hepatic abscessation. If alterations are observed, they usually support the diagnosis but are not specific.
• CBC may identify leukocytosis characterized by neutrophilia, and increased or decreased total protein. Anemia may be present due to chronic inflammation.
• Serum biochemistry may identify increases in liver enzyme activities (sorbitol dehydrogenase, gamma glutamyltransferase, and aspartate transaminase). If biliary obstruction occurs, direct (conjugated) bilirubin may increase in the serum and bilirubinuria might occur.

OTHER LABORATORY TESTS
Liver function tests are costly and can be challenging to interpret in ruminants.

IMAGING
• Ultrasonography is a useful tool for the diagnosis of liver abscesses, particularly in individual valuable animals. It may not be cost-effective in feedlot settings.
• Ultrasonography can also be used to evaluate the caudal vena cava and lungs of animals with hepatic abscesses.

L

LIVER ABSCESSES

• Radiology can be used to assess the thorax of valuable animals for accompanying pulmonary abscessation from septic emboli.

OTHER DIAGNOSTIC PROCEDURES
N/A

PATHOLOGIC FINDINGS
• Abscesses in the liver can appear as large single lesions or as multiple irregular, granular yellow lesions randomly distributed throughout (telangiectasis).
• Abscesses may have a thin capsule and a central area of necrosis and purulent material, or may have a thick fibrous capsule, with a central cavity and little to no purulent material evident. Central mineralization of these lesions may be evident.
• Histologically, abscesses that are a result of bacterial emboli have a central area of coagulative necrosis with numerous phagocytic cells. Bacteria may be present in the center, but more often are concentrated in the periphery of the necrotic core due to the length of time lesions have been present.
• Abscesses resulting from migration of hepatic parasites include focal and multifocal coalescences of eosinophils forming granulomatous inflammation.

TREATMENT

THERAPEUTIC APPROACH
• Treatment is often unrewarding due to the diffuse nature of abscesses and limited blood supply to the heavy capsular lining. However, antibiotic treatment can be combined with supportive therapy and may be effective in some cases.
• Anti-inflammatory agents can be administered to reduce damage from inflammatory factors and to provide pain management.

SURGICAL CONSIDERATIONS AND TECHNIQUES
If the abscess is in an area where it can be accessed surgically, it can be drained. This procedure is cost prohibitive and impractical in most food animal cases.

MEDICATIONS

DRUGS OF CHOICE
• Penicillins, ampicillin, and oxytetracycline are the drugs of choice to treat animals diagnosed with liver abscesses. The drugs are usually administered at very high doses for long periods of time, to facilitate penetration of the abscess capsular lining.

• Antimicrobials used as feed additives for the prevention of abscess formation include bacitracin, oxytetracycline, tylosin, tilmicosin, and virginiamycin.
• Monensin and lasalocid are ionophores that achieve the same purpose.

CONTRAINDICATIONS
N/A

PRECAUTIONS
• Antibiotics have the potential to alter normal ruminal microflora which alters feed efficiency.
• Administering high amounts of oxytetracyclines can cause hypocalcemia in cattle.
• Appropriate milk and meat withdrawal times must be followed for all compounds administered to food-producing animals.
• Antibiotics or drugs that require metabolism by the liver should be used with caution if there are indications that the majority of the liver is diseased.

POSSIBLE INTERACTIONS
N/A

FOLLOW-UP

EXPECTED COURSE AND PROGNOSIS
The vast majority of liver abscesses are not detected until slaughter, so this is primarily a subclinical disease with major economic impact in the cattle industry.

POSSIBLE COMPLICATIONS
Liver abscesses may result in caudal vena cava thrombosis syndrome.

CLIENT EDUCATION
• Educate clients how to introduce highly fermentable feeds into the diet.
• Feed a balanced ration with enough fiber and roughage.
• Proper neonatal management to prevent failure of passive transfer of immunity and septicemia.
• Ensure the client has an adequate parasite management program to avoid liver fluke infestation.

PATIENT CARE
N/A

PREVENTION
• Prevention of ruminal acidosis by feeding adequate amounts of appropriate roughage is a key factor in reducing the incidence of liver abscesses in animals being fed highly fermentable feeds.
• Roughage increases the amount of saliva produced to buffer VFAs in the rumen. Introducing highly fermentable feeds slowly

into the diets of ruminants allows adaptation of the microflora and improves absorptive capacity of the rumen, to prevent a build-up of acidic agents.
• A number of feed additives are used to decrease the incidence of ruminal acidosis and subsequently liver abscesses. These additives include ionophore antibiotics, which control the growth of Gram-positive bacteria in the rumen, and reduce the number of lactic acid producing bacteria.
• Tylosin can be added to feed to directly decrease the number of *F. necrophorum* and *T. pyogenes* bacteria in the rumen, and reduces the incidence of bacterial emboli formed in the ruminal wall that can travel to the liver.
• Regular preventive anthelmintic treatment may reduce the risk of liver flukes producing migratory tracts in the liver that can become infected and abscess.
• Proper environmental management, along with navel dipping and assuring ingestion of an adequate quantity of high-quality colostrum by neonates will help prevent ascending umbilical vein infections.

MISCELLANEOUS

ASSOCIATED CONDITIONS
• Rumen acidosis
• Bloat
• Caudal vena cava thrombosis
• Pulmonary arterial thromboembolism
• Laminitis
• Polioencephalomalacia

AGE-RELATED FACTORS
Hepatic abscesses in neonates generally relate to omphalophlebitis.

ZOONOTIC POTENTIAL
N/A

PREGNANCY
N/A

BIOSECURITY
N/A

PRODUCTION MANAGEMENT
• See "Prevention."
• Feed additives that contain antimicrobials help to decrease bacterial populations that can acidify the rumen. The United States Veterinary Feed Directive requires producers to obtain prescriptions from veterinarians in order to add antimicrobials into feed.

SYNONYMS
• Septic cholangiohepatitis
• Telangiectasis
• Sawdust liver

LIVER ABSCESSES

(CONTINUED)

ABBREVIATION
• VFAs = volatile fatty acids

SEE ALSO
• Caudal Vena Caval Thrombosis Syndrome
• Laminitis
• Liver Flukes
• Ruminal Acidosis
• Umbilical Disorders
• Vitamin B Deficiency

Suggested Reading
Brent BE. Relationship of acidosis to other feedlot ailments. J Anim Sci 1976, 43: 930–5.
Brink DR, Lowry RA, Parrott JC. Severity of liver abscesses and efficiency of feed utilization of feedlot cattle. J Anim Sci 1990, 68: 1201–7.
Johnson B. Nutritional and dietary interrelationships with diseases of feedlot cattle. Vet Clin North Am Food Anim Pract 1991, 7: 133–42.
Nagaraja TG, Lechtenberg KF. Liver abscesses in feedlot cattle. J Vet Clin Food Anim 2007, 23: 351–369.
O'Sullivan EN. Two-year study of bovine hepatic abscessation in 10 abattoirs in County Cork, Ireland. Vet Rec 1999, 145: 389–93.
Author Clemence Z. Chako
Consulting Editor Erica C. McKenzie
Acknowledgment The author and book editors acknowledge the prior contribution of Margo R. Machen.

L

LIVER FLUKES

BASICS

OVERVIEW

• Liver flukes are Platyhelminthes (flatworms) of the class Trematoda that mainly infect domestic and wild ruminants and camelids; these species typically serve as definitive hosts.

• Three species of liver fluke commonly infect livestock: *Fasciola hepatica* (common liver fluke), *Dicrocoelium dendriticum* (lancet liver fluke), and *Fascioloides magna* (giant liver fluke). *Fasciola gigantica* is significant to ruminants in Asia and Africa.

• Flukes have a relatively long, complex life cycle that requires a snail intermediate host and, for *D. dendriticum*, also an ant intermediate host. Livestock are infected by ingesting the encysted metacercariae stage of *Fasciola* and *Fascioloides* from vegetation, or by ingesting ants containing the metacercariae of *D. dendriticum*.

• Disease arises from parasite-associated inflammation and damage to the liver, and can be exacerbated by secondary infection of the liver with bacterial organisms, particularly *Clostridium*.

INCIDENCE/PREVALENCE

• The prevalence of fluke infestation varies substantially between geographic regions, depending on intermediate host distribution and climactic factors.

• *F. hepatica* tends to be endemic in regions with favorable climactic conditions; prevalence of infection in some regions can exceed 50%.

• *D. dendriticum* infection can achieve 100% in small ruminant flocks in many European and Eastern countries.

• *F. magna* infection can exceed 15% in cattle (a dead-end host) in areas in which the definitive deer hosts are prevalent, particularly the upper Midwestern United States.

GEOGRAPHIC DISTRIBUTION

• *F. hepatica* is found worldwide where intermediate hosts and climactic conditions facilitate the life cycle of this parasite. It has been identified on all continents except Antarctica, and in more than 50 countries.

• *D. dendriticum* is found throughout Europe, the Middle East, Asia, Africa; in North and South America, and in Australia.

• *F. magna* is native to the US, where it has been identified in at least 25 states, particularly the upper Midwest. It was introduced to Europe where it has regional distribution, and it is occasionally identified in imported stock in other countries.

• *F. gigantica* is significant in ruminants in Southern Asia, Southeast Asia, and Africa

SYSTEMS AFFECTED

Digestive

PATHOPHYSIOLOGY

• Adult *Fasciola* and *Fascioloides* flukes reside in the definitive host in either the bile ducts (*Fasciola*) or in thin-walled cysts which communicate with the bile ducts (*F. magna*), and produce operculated ova, which are passed in the feces.

• The most common definitive hosts of *F. hepatica* and *F. gigantica* are cattle and sheep, and species of wild cervidae are definitive hosts for *F. magna*. Fluke eggs release free-living miracidia, which seek out and invade the tissues of the snail intermediate host (often *Lymnaea* spp. or *Galba* spp.) where asexual replication occurs to produce motile cercariae.

• Cercariae escape the snail and attach to pasture and other vegetation, where they mature to encysted metacercariae.

• After ingestion by the definitive or aberrant host, the metacercariae excyst in the bowel and migrate through the intestinal wall, peritoneal cavity, and liver parenchyma, finally taking up residence in either the bile ducts or hepatic cysts to mature to adults.

• Infection with *Fasciola* can result in clinical disease due to blood and protein loss, irritation of the biliary tree, and occasional secondary infection of damaged parenchyma with bacteria, leading to formation of abscesses. Germination of the spores of specific species of *Clostridium* in anaerobic regions of damaged liver tissue can result in severe disease related to infectious necrotic hepatitis or bacillary hemoglobinuria.

• *F. magna* generally becomes encapsulated in infected cattle with no overt clinical signs. However, in sheep, goats, and camelids, *F. magna* tends to migrate continuously; hence, small numbers of these flukes can cause substantial hepatic damage and even death in these species.

• The life cycle of *D. dendriticum* exhibits substantial differences from that of *F. hepatica* and *F. magna*. The intermediate hosts include over 90 species of land snails with broad distribution. Cercariae that leave snails subsequently infect a second intermediate host (often *Formica* spp. ants) in which they mature to metacercariae. Ants are ingested by grazing herbivores and display distinct behavior changes after infection that greatly enhance their chances of being ingested, by migrating to the tips of vegetation and waiting there for extended periods (typically at night).

• Once ingested, excysted juvenile *Dicrocoelium* flukes migrate via the biliary tree versus the hepatic parenchyma, which reduces their potential for significant tissue destruction. However, heavy burdens in small ruminants can cause biliary irritation and inflammation.

HISTORICAL FINDINGS

N/A

SIGNALMENT

• *F. hepatica* affects a range of wild and domestic ruminants, including sheep, goats, and cattle, as well as some nonruminant species. Young animals are more susceptible to infection and more likely to demonstrate clinical disease, and small ruminants are most likely to develop clinical disease. Similarly, *F. gigantica* tends to affect cattle, buffalo, sheep, and goats, again with greater pathogenicity for small ruminants.

• *D. dendriticum* infects a range of domestic and wild ruminants including sheep, goats, cattle, buffaloes, some deer, and camels, and also some nonruminant species. Higher egg counts may be identified in younger animals of grazing age, versus older animals, and small ruminants are most likely to develop clinical disease with heavy burdens.

• The definitive hosts of *F. magna* in the US are white-tailed deer, caribou, and wapiti, and there are a variety of deer hosts in Europe. Domestic ruminants including cattle, sheep, and goats, as well as alpacas and llamas can become infected, but infection is not typically patent. Cattle rarely show clinical disease with infection, but this fluke is highly pathogenic in small ruminants.

PHYSICAL EXAMINATION FINDINGS

• In general, fluke infestation in cattle is typically asymptomatic, though significant burdens, particularly with *Fasciola*, can decrease productivity and may cause poor growth, reduced fertility, weight loss, and ill thrift. Calves with heavy infections may demonstrate anemia, submandibular edema, and ascites.

• Fluke infestation in small ruminants and camelids can also be asymptomatic with light infestations; signs of anemia, anorexia, weight loss, submandibular edema, ascites, and death can occur with moderate to heavy infections of *Fasciola*. However, only one or two migrating *F. magna* flukes can cause substantial damage and death in small ruminants.

• Acute disease resembling acute haemonchosis may occur in small ruminants experiencing heavy burdens of juvenile *Fasciola*, which can occur in outbreak fashion.

(CONTINUED)   **LIVER FLUKES**

• Infectious necrotic hepatitis (infection with *Clostridium novyi* type B) and bacillary hemoglobinuria (infection with *Clostridium haemolyticum*) can result in sudden death in affected ruminants, particularly sheep.
• In alpacas, thrombotic endocarditis inducing signs of cardiac failure including jugular distension, ventral edema, tachycardia, recumbency, and cavitary effusions has been linked to infection with *F. hepatica.*

GENETICS
N/A

CAUSES AND RISK FACTORS
• Presence of the definitive and intermediate hosts involved in the various life cycles influences the probability and prevalence of infection in domestic ruminants and camelids.
• Intermediate hosts of *F. hepatica* are typically amphibious, inhabiting shallow water sources in areas with neutral soils (pH 6–8) and poor drainage. Years with above-normal rainfall and mild temperatures (≥50°F, ≥10°C) promote increased risk of infection.
• Ruminants and camelids grazing low-lying wet pastures or pastures containing lakes or ponds in enzootic regions for *F. magna* are at increased risk.
• Calcareous or alkaline soils are most often associated with *D. dendriticum* infection, likely representing influence on the reproduction and survival of the intermediate hosts; moisture is much less of an influence for this fluke than for *Fasciola* and *Fascioloides.*
• Stress-inducing factors, such as transportation and confinement, can potentially increase egg production (*D. dendriticum*), suggesting that immunosuppression can be detrimental for these infections.
• Gender may present as a risk factor in some systems in which females are exposed to grazing at much higher rates than males or castrated males.

DIAGNOSIS

DIFFERENTIAL DIAGNOSES
• Gastrointestinal nematode infections, particularly *Haemonchus contortus.*
• *Taenia hydatigena* larvae in hepatic parenchyma may require distinguishing at necropsy.

CBC/BIOCHEMISTRY/URINALYSIS
• Anemia and hypoproteinemia (related to hypoalbuminemia) may be observed on CBC.
• Serum biochemistry can reveal elevations in hepatic enzyme activities, particularly GGT.

OTHER LABORATORY TESTS
• Fecal sedimentation is indicated for identification of *F. hepatica* ova, which will not float. The eggs are large, golden brown, and operculated (~140 × 80 μm in size) and should be distinguishable from the ova of the nonpathogenic rumen fluke, *Paramphistomum.* Repeated examinations can be necessary, particularly in subacute or chronic disease in cattle. A commercially available test, Flukefinder®, isolates ova by differential filtration, followed by differential sedimentation, and can identify low numbers of ova.
• Fecal flotation in solutions with a specific gravity of 1.30–1.45 is indicated for identification of the eggs of *D. dendriticum* which are small (~40 × 25 μm), thick-walled, yellowish-brown, and contain miracidium.
• The Flotac® technique is a dual chamber method gaining popularity for use as a diagnostic test to identify a wide range of parasite eggs (including trematodes) from fecal samples.
• A copro-antigen ELISA is available for the diagnosis of *F. hepatica* and an ELISA assay can detect serum antibodies to *D. dendriticum*; both of these tests can identify infection weeks before patency is established.
• PCR-based assays also exist to help distinguish *F. hepatica* from *F. gigantica.*

IMAGING
• Ultrasound can aid diagnosis after 9 weeks post-infection in sheep. Dilation of bile ducts is visible, and moving echogenic forms may be observed within the dilated bile ducts.
• In alpacas with thrombotic endocarditis, ultrasonography can detect echogenic material within the right ventricle and pleural and/or peritoneal effusion.

OTHER DIAGNOSTIC PROCEDURES
Necropsy can identify characteristic liver lesions and/or flukes, and is necessary for confirmation of *F. magna* infection in sheep, goats, and cattle which do not develop patent infections and therefore will not shed *F. magna* ova into the feces.

PATHOLOGIC FINDINGS
• Lesions of *F. hepatica* infestation often reflect chronic infection, resulting in proliferative cholangitis with bile duct dilation, thickening, and fibrosis. In cattle, calcification of bile ducts can occur ("pipe-stem" lesion). The liver may become fibrotic, firm and indurated, and adult flukes are evident within bile ducts.
• Acute disease related to exposure to large numbers of juvenile *Fasciola* can result in an enlarged liver with necrohemorrhagic tracts. The liver surface may be covered with

fibrinous exudate, and serosanguineous fluid may be present in the abdominal cavity.
• Thrombotic endocarditis in alpacas is reflected by accumulation of fibrinous material in cardiac chambers (typically the right ventricle); vegetative lesions may be present on cardiac valves with peripheral edema and cavitary effusions evident.
• Heavy burdens of *D. dendriticum* can result in anemia, edema, emaciation, and eventually cirrhosis of the liver with accompanying biliary distension. The small, semi-transparent adult flukes (~10 mm length, and 2 mm wide) may be evident in the biliary tract.
• *F. magna* infection in cattle results in the production of thick-walled cysts that encapsulate the adult flukes but which do not communicate with bile ducts. In small ruminants, severe damage to liver parenchyma can be evident as a result of uncontrolled migration, with necrohemorrhagic tracts in the liver containing black hematin pigmentation.

TREATMENT

THERAPEUTIC APPROACH
• The availability of various flukicidal drugs and their respective efficacy for adults versus juvenile flukes varies between different countries. In the US, available treatments are generally only effective for adult flukes.
• Timing of treatments should be based on local patterns of transmission and is particularly critical if drugs that only reliably affect adult flukes are used.
• In areas with extended transmission seasons for *F. hepatica*, two or even three treatments may be indicated, extending from late summer through spring, to ensure maximum fluke destruction is achieved.

SURGICAL CONSIDERATIONS AND TECHNIQUES
N/A

MEDICATIONS

DRUGS OF CHOICE
• Only two drugs are currently available to treat liver fluke infections in the US—clorsulon (a benzenesulphonamide), and albendazole (a benzimidazole).
• Outside of the US, other drugs available to treat fluke infestations in ruminants also include triclabendazole, netobimin, closantel, thiophanate, brotianide, rafoxanide, and

L

LIVER FLUKES

oxyclozanide. Drugs such as triclabendazole have efficacy against juvenile flukes <8 weeks of age.
• No drugs have FDA label approval for treatment of *F. magna*, but it has been suggested to use albendazole at twice the recommended label dose for 2 or 3 consecutive days. Outside of the US, triclabendazole is currently the recommended agent.
• There are no approved flukicidal drugs for alpacas or llamas.
• Clorsulon dosed at 7 mg/kg PO will apparently kill 99% of *F. hepatica* adults and over 85% of flukes >8–12 weeks old. When given subcutaneously at 2 mg/kg (usually in a combination product with ivermectin), or orally at 3.5 mg/kg, clorsulon will kill most adult *F. hepatica*.
• Albendazole dosed at 10 mg/kg PO will kill >70% of adult *F. hepatica*, in addition to other parasites; withholding feed for 24 hours prior to treatment will improve efficacy. Doses of 15 and 20 mg/kg PO have been reported for treatment of *D. dendriticum*.

CONTRAINDICATIONS
• Flukicidal drugs are typically not approved for use in lactating dairy cattle.
• Albendazole should be avoided in pregnant animals.

PRECAUTIONS
• Drug resistance has been reported in *F. hepatica,* including to albendazole, clorsulon, and triclabendazole.
• Appropriate milk and meat withdrawal times must be followed for all compounds administered to food-producing animals.

POSSIBLE INTERACTIONS
N/A

FOLLOW-UP

EXPECTED COURSE AND PROGNOSIS
• The prognosis for *Fasciola* or *Dicrocoelium* infection is expected to be good, particularly in cattle compared to small ruminants, with appropriate treatment. However, the prognosis is guarded for severe acute disease, particularly in calves and small ruminants.
• The prognosis for *F. magna* infection is excellent in cattle and poor to guarded in small ruminants.

POSSIBLE COMPLICATIONS
• Chronic liver failure
• Infectious necrotic hepatitis
• Bacillary hemoglobinuria

PATIENT CARE
N/A

PREVENTION
• A key management strategy can include preventing access to or proliferation of the intermediate host(s). This can include:
  ○ Improved pasture drainage (*Fasciola, Fascioloides*).
  ○ Fencing off natural water sources and marshy areas.
  ○ Moving animals off suboptimal pastures during high transmission periods.
  ○ Use of molluscicides – these can be toxic to the host species (copper-containing products in sheep) and are environmentally undesirable.
  ○ Introduction of turkeys, chickens, geese, and ducks into small pastures (about 50 birds per hectare) to consume snails and ants.
  ○ Avoiding grazing in the early morning or evenings to reduce the risk of infection with *Dicrocoelium*-infested ants.
• Strategic deworming in the spring or early summer may limit the degree to which snail populations become infected with immature stages of flukes and can limit amplification of infection.
• Deworming prior to introduction of livestock into low-lying pastures will have a long-term beneficial effect.

MISCELLANEOUS

ASSOCIATED CONDITIONS
• Concurrent infections with gastrointestinal nematodes is usually present in fluke-infected animals, which will exacerbate the impact of flukes on the host.
• Infectious necrotic hepatitis and bacillary hemoglobinuria can develop in affected hosts (particularly sheep) due to activation of dormant *Clostridium* spores in damaged liver tissue.

AGE-RELATED FACTORS
All ages are susceptible, but young animals are more likely to suffer severe disease.

ZOONOTIC POTENTIAL
• Metacercariae of *F. hepatica* are infective to humans, and present occasional risk through the consumption of contaminated produce such as watercress.
• Metacercariae of *D. dendriticum* are also infective to humans. The occurrence is rare and is usually the result of consumption of infected ants.
• There is no zoonotic transmission directly from animals to humans.

PREGNANCY
Albendazole is potentially teratogenic in early pregnancy.

BIOSECURITY
• *F. hepatica* can be spread between farms by infected rabbits and deer, making eradication almost impossible.
• Fencing of pastures (and ponds) with deerproof fencing should prevent *F. magna* infections in livestock in enzootic areas.

PRODUCTION MANAGEMENT
Flukes, particularly *F. hepatica*, are a significant cause of economic loss, due to morbidity and mortality, treatment expense, reduced productivity, and condemnation of affected livers at slaughter.

SYNONYMS
• *F. magna*: giant liver fluke, large American liver fluke, deer fluke
• *F. hepatica*: liver fluke, common liver fluke
• *D. dendriticum*: small liver fluke, lancet fluke, *D. lanceolatum*

ABBREVIATIONS
• FDA = Food and Drug Administration
• GGT = serum gamma glutamyltransferase activity

SEE ALSO
• Bacillary Hemoglobinuria
• Haemonchosis
• Infectious Necrotic Hepatitis

Suggested Reading
Aiello SE ed. The Merck Veterinary Manual, 2015. Retrieved from http://www.merckvetmanual.com/mvm/index.html
Cringoli G, Rinaldi L, Maurelli MP, Utzinger J. FLOTAC: new multivalent techniques for qualitative and quantitative copromicroscopic diagnosis of parasites in animals and humans. Nat Protoc 2010, 5: 503–15.
Duff JP, Maxwell AJ, Claxton JR. Chronic and fatal fascioliasis in llamas in the UK. Vet Rec 1999, 145: 315–16.
Fairweather I, Boray JC. Fasciolicides: efficacy, actions, resistance and its management. Vet J 1999, 2: 81–112.
Firshman AM, Wünschmann A, Cebra CK, et al. Thrombotic endocarditis in 10 alpacas. J Vet Intern Med 2008, 22: 456–61.
Kaplan RM. Liver flukes in cattle—control based on seasonal transmission dynamics. Compend Contin Edu Pract Vet 1994, 5: 687–94.
Kaplan RM. Liver flukes in cattle: a review of the economic impact and considerations for control. Vet Ther 2001, 1: 40–50.

Otranto D, Traversa D. A review of dicrocoeliosis of ruminants including recent advances in the diagnosis and treatment. Vet Parasitol 2002, 107: 317–35.

Loyacano AF, Williams JC, Gurie J, DeRosa AA. Effect of gastrointestinal nematode and liver fluke infections on weight gain and reproductive performance of beef heifers. Vet Parasitol 2002, 3: 227–34.

Radostits OM, Gay CC, Hinchcliff KW, Constable PD. Veterinary Medicine: A Textbook of the Diseases of Cattle, Horses, Sheep, Pigs, and Goats, 10th ed. New York: Elsevier Saunders, 2008.

Rokni MB, Mirhendi H, Mizani A, et al. Identification and differentiation of *Fasciola hepatica* and *Fasciola Gigantica* using a simple PCR-restriction enzyme method. Exp Parasit 2010, 124: 209–13.

Author Nicholas A. Robinson
Consulting Editor Erica C. McKenzie
Acknowledgment The author and book editors acknowledge the prior contribution of Ray M. Kaplan and Jeff W. Tyler.

L

LOW-FAT MILK SYNDROME

BASICS

OVERVIEW
• Milk fat depression (MFD) is a common nutritional/metabolic condition affecting modern dairy cattle. Sometimes drop in milk fat content is related to normal seasonal changes in lactation that occurs every year; however, occasionally, MFD may be related to nutritional problems. Fat is the most variable milk solid constituent in which several nutritional factors have been related to MFD. Yeast and molds, management, forages and fiber, starch and fats are the major nutritional factors that affect the risk of MFD. Too much fat in the diet of dairy cows is a classic cause of MFD. The amount of fat fed, especially the rumen polyunsaturated fatty acid load (C18:1 + C18:2 + C18:3) or PUFA is the most important risk factor.
• Milk fat depression is also related to low fiber diet content and rumen pH. Rumen pH below 6.0 induces an undesirable biohydrogenation pathway of excessive rumen PUFA to trans-10, cis-12 18:2 fatty acid. This isomer has been strongly associated with low milk fat synthesis at the level of mammary gland. When rumen pH is normal, rumen PUFA are biohydrogenated to different isomers, mostly cis-9, trans-11 18:2 fatty acid. These isomers are not involved in the low synthesis of milk fat.
• When rumen PUFA are > 3.5% of total dry matter content of the diet trans-10, cis-12 18:2 isomers increase dramatically in the rumen. When the only source of fiber is from corn silage, trans-10 fatty acids are also higher as compared with diets based on corn silage and alfalfa hay. In addition, free fatty acids increase the risk of MFD. Conservation processes such as silage rise the levels of free fatty acids from fresh forages. This is because plant lipases are released after cutting the grass. Corn silage contaminated with yeast and molds are also at higher risk for MFD, especially when yeast counts approach 1 million cfu/g.
• A well-balanced diet for a high producing dairy cow should contain no less than 30% of total NDF, no less than 17% of ADF, no more than 44% of nonfiber carbohydrates, no less than 20% of forage NDF, no less than 17.5% crude protein or 11.6% of metabolizable protein, and no more than 6% of fat.

PATHOPHYSIOLOGY
• Milk fat is constituted by short, medium and long chain fatty acids and minor lipids. They are formed by two mechanisms. The mammary gland synthesizes short and medium chain fatty acids (C4:0 to C14:0) and part of the palmitic acid (C16:0) from acetate and butyrate. The long chain fatty acids (> C16:0 and the rest of palmitic acid)

are incorporated into milk fat directly from dietary lipids and from the mobilization of adipose tissue (triglycerides) in the form of nonesterified fatty acids.
• Biohydrogenation process of RUFAL is modified in favor of trans-10, cis-12 linoleic acid (C18:2) under certain rumen environmental conditions. Risk factors for this alteration are high levels of rumen PUFA (> 3.5% of total DM), high levels of dietary starch, free fatty acids, silages, yeast and molds, low levels of effective fiber, and overall poor management.
• Trans-10, cis-12 linoleic acid is transported through the blood towards the mammary gland. At the level of parenchyma cells this isomer alters gene expression of key enzymes for the de novo fatty acid synthesis. The end result is low production of short and medium chain fatty acids with the consequent MFD.

SIGNALMENT
Holstein cows at or after peak lactation are at higher risk.

HISTORICAL FINDINGS
Fat may drop dramatically from 3.4% to 2.5%. In addition, the rumen acetate : propionate ratio may also drop from 3.1 to 1.7, but most likely due to high production of propionate and maintenance of levels of acetate.

CAUSES AND RISK FACTORS
Milk fat depression is a consequence of changes in dietary lipids as they pass through the rumen. Biohydrogenation of polyunsaturated fatty acids in the rumen leads to several isomers (18) of conjugated linoleic acid (CLA), trans-fatty acids, and saturated fatty acids. Under certain rumen negative conditions, three CLA isomers, especially trans-10, cis-12 CLA predominate over the rest. This isomer has an inhibitory effect on milk fat synthesis at the level of the mammary gland.

Risk Factors
• High dietary levels of polyunsaturated fatty acids (>3.5% of total dry matter).
• Type of oil. Fatty acids from canola oil are less dangerous than fatty acids from corn oil.
• Low-forage diets and excessive grain with large amount of rumen propionate.
• Small forage particle size (effective or forage NDF).
• Type of forages. Annual ryegrass is less likely than rye to decrease milk fat content.
• Conservation methods. Hay and silages are more harmful than fresh forages.
• Processing of grains. Overheated cotton seed is more likely to produce MFD than normal.
• High rates of starch degradability (>85%) in a 7-hour in vitro test.
• Moldy and spoiled feed and high count of yeast.
• Large amounts of dietary free-fatty acids.
• Use of ionophores.

DIAGNOSIS

DIFFERENTIAL DIAGNOSES
N/A

CBC/BIOCHEMISTRY/URINALYSIS
N/A

OTHER LABORATORY TESTS
N/A

IMAGING
N/A

OTHER DIAGNOSTIC PROCEDURES
Milk fat depression is diagnosed through milk plant fat determination and/or monthly milk fat test day records.

TREATMENT

THERAPEUTIC APPROACH
• MFD is a multifactorial problem. No single dietary factor is responsible for MFD. Interaction among various risk factors can increase the rumen production of milk fat inhibitory CLA isomers. Proper feed management and control of all risk factors should be the main objective.
• Some preventive or complementary strategies should be the addition of rumen buffers or replacement of dietary starch by rich-pectin by-products (e.g., almond hulls, whole cotton seed, soy hulls, beet or citrus pulp) to modulate rumen pH.

MEDICATIONS

DRUGS OF CHOICE
N/A

CONTRAINDICATIONS
N/A

POSSIBLE INTERACTIONS
N/A

PRECAUTIONS
Avoid risk factors. Polyunsaturated fatty acids (PUFA) should be no more than 3.5% of total dry matter.

FOLLOW-UP

EXPECTED COURSE AND PROGNOSIS
N/A

POSSIBLE COMPLICATIONS
See "Associated Conditions"

CLIENT EDUCATION
• Monitoring of feed management on a daily basis should be stressed to personnel
  ◦ Time of TMR mixing

L

(CONTINUED)

◦ Feeding frequency
◦ Quality of forages (mold contamination)

PATIENT CARE
N/A

PREVENTION
• Evaluation of diet composition should consider:
  ◦ Total NDF (no less than 30%)
  ◦ Forage NDF (no less than 20%)
  ◦ Non fiber carbohydrate (no more than 44%)
  ◦ Source and amount of starch in the diet (no more than 28%)
  ◦ Processing characteristics of grains
  ◦ Total fatty acid content, especially PUFA
  ◦ Type of fat supplement (vegetable oils, marine oils, oil seeds, protected fat, animal fat, etc.)

MISCELLANEOUS

ASSOCIATED CONDITIONS
The following can accompany a low milk fat test: subclinical or subacute ruminal acidosis (SARA), decreased feed intake, and higher incidence of laminitis-related claw lesions (sole ulcers, hemorrhages, soft horn tissue).

AGE-RELATED FACTORS
N/A

ZOONOTIC POTENTIAL
N/A

PREGNANCY
N/A

BIOSECURITY
N/A

PRODUCTION MANAGEMENT
• Major target: Maintenance of rumen health and low levels of milk fat inhibitory CLA isomers.
• All risks have to be considered with regard to the combination of factors at play in a given ration formulation and with regard to the limitations of management and physical or effective fiber (NDF).

SYNONYMS
N/A

ABBREVIATIONS
• CLA = conjugated linoleic acid
• DM = dry matter
• MFD = milk fat depression
• NDF = neutral detergent fiber
• NFC = nonfiber carbohydrate
• NRC = National Research Council
• PUFA = polyunsaturated fatty acids
• TMR = total mixed ration

SEE ALSO
• Body Condition Scoring: Dairy Cattle (see www.fiveminutevet.com/ruminant)
• Dairy Heifer Nutrition: Basics (see www.fiveminutevet.com/ruminant)
• Dairy Nutrition: Ration Guidelines for Milking and Dry Cows (see www.fiveminutevet.com/ruminant)
• Feeding for Milk Components (see www.fiveminutevet.com/ruminant)

Suggested Reading
Bauman DE, Griinari JK. Nutritional regulation of milk fat synthesis. Annu Rev Nutr 2003, 23: 203–27.
Jenkins TC, Harvatine KJ. Lipid feeding and milk fat depression. Vet Clin North Am Food Anim Pract. 2014, 30: 623–42.
National Research Council. Nutrient Requirements of Dairy Cattle, 7th ed. Washington, DC: National Academies of Science, 2001.
Author Pedro Melendez
Consulting Editor Kaitlyn A. Lutz
Acknowledgment The author and book editors acknowledge the prior contribution of Sergio O. Juchem.

L

LUMPY SKIN DISEASE

BASICS

OVERVIEW
• Lumpy skin disease (LSD) is a viral disease related to a capripoxvirus infection of cattle.
• Disease is characterized by deep dermal skin nodules that eventually undergo central necrosis.
• Affected animals also usually have a high fever and generalized lymphadenitis.

INCIDENCE/PREVALENCE
Depending on the susceptibility of the cattle
• Channel Island breeds:
  ◦ Most susceptible
  ◦ Morbility may range from 3% to 80%
  ◦ Mortality is very low (1-3%)

GEOGRAPHIC DISTRIBUTION
Endemic throughout most of Africa and Madagascar with occasional incursions into the Middle East.

SYSTEMS AFFECTED
• Integument
• Digestive

PATHOPHYSIOLOGY
• Disease arises from systemic capripoxvirus infection that affects primarily the skin and mucus membranes of cattle.
• Animals become viremic with systemic spread to epithelial tissues throughout the body.
• The incubation period varies between 7 and 28 days with most cases observed 10–12 days after exposure.

HISTORICAL FINDINGS
Formation of skin nodules over the body approximately 48 hours after onset of fever.

SIGNALMENT
Channel Island breeds are most susceptible; calves more so than adults.

PHYSICAL EXAMINATION FINDINGS
• Fever (104–107°F, 40–42°C) is the first clinical sign and may persist up to 4 weeks.
• 1–5 cm nodules develop under the skin, usually within two days of fever onset and primarily affect the neck, muzzle, nares, eyelids, dorsum, legs, scrotum, perineum, mammary gland, teats, and tail. The oral mucosa may also become involved.
• Nodules enlarge and involve the epidermis, dermis, and subcutaneous tissues, and can involve the superficial musculature. Nodules are often painful to the touch.
• Lesions can involve the mucus membranes of the mouth, esophagus, rumen, trachea, and lungs, which may result in dysphagia, respiratory distress, and pneumonia.
• Edematous nodules eventually become necrotic and collapse centrally, leaving an umbilicated lesion with a central necrotic core covered by a scab (sitfast). These lesions heal slowly and are often complicated by secondary bacterial infection.
• Necrotic lesions may take up to 5–6 weeks to heal and nodules may remain for some time.
• In severe infections, lameness may occur due to cutaneous nodules causing swelling and inflammation in the joints, tendon sheaths, and coronary bands.
• Lymph nodes draining infected regions may become large and swollen.
• Late-term abortions can occur in infected animals, believed to relate to high fever rather than fetal infection.
• Bulls may become sterile due to fever and mechanical damage to the skin and mucosa of the prepuce and penis, or from virus-induced orchitis.

GENETICS
The virus affects cattle (*Bos taurus* and *Bos indicus*) but experimental infection has been demonstrated in giraffe and impala. Many African wildlife species have seroconverted but have not been observed with lesions.

CAUSES AND RISK FACTORS
• Transmission of LSD is believed to be mechanical, by an arthropod vector.
• *Aedes aegypti* mosquitoes can infect susceptible cattle 2–6 days after feeding on infected/viremic cattle.
• Stable flies (*Stomoxys* sp.) have been shown to maintain live LSD virus after feeding on infected cattle but have not demonstrated transmission of the disease.
• Hard ticks might possibly also transmit the virus. *Rhipicephalus* (*Boophilus*) *decoloratus* ticks display transovarian and transstadial transmission of LSD virus; *Rhipicephalus appendiculatus* and *Amblyomma hebraeum* ticks display transstadial transmission.
• Outbreaks of LSD tend to occur most commonly during rainy seasons.
• Cattle are viremic for 2 weeks; all body secretions, blood, and nodules contain virus; viral DNA can be identified in semen for up to 5 months post-exposure.
• Contact with infected scabs and fomites can also spread disease to a lesser extent. Movement of contaminated raw hides have been implicated in some outbreaks.

DIAGNOSIS

DIFFERENTIAL DIAGNOSES
• Insect bites and associated urticaria.
• *Hypoderma bovis* infection.
• Photosensitization.
• Bovine papular stomatitis—usually affects the lips, muzzle, and oral and esophageal mucosa without fever or pain, and young animals are usually the only animals affected in the herd.
• Bovine herpes mammillitis (pseudo-LSD).
• Cowpox/pseudocowpox viruses—superficial pox-like lesions occur in the dermis of the teats and udder, and are not as deep or as extensive as in LSD.
• Dermatophilosis.

CBC/BIOCHEMISTRY/URINALYSIS
N/A

OTHER LABORATORY TESTS
N/A

IMAGING
N/A

OTHER DIAGNOSTIC PROCEDURES
• Biopsies of early lesions that have not scabbed can be used for virus isolation, histopathology, electron microscopy, PCR and ELISA testing.
• Aspirates of swollen lymph nodes should be placed in viral transport media and shipped on ice for virus isolation.
• Whole blood (heparinized or EDTA) can detect early viremia.
• Acute and convalescent sera should be obtained for serologic testing.

PATHOLOGIC FINDINGS
• Gross findings consist of generalized skin (dermal) nodules of 1–5 cm diameter composed of edema, hemorrhage, and necrotic debris. Older nodules have a central center of necrosis with a central scab present.
• Individual or coalescing pox lesions can be present in the oral cavity, nares, pharynx, esophagus, and trachea. These lesions reflect coalescing thickening of the mucosa and submucosa with some edema, hemorrhage, and necrosis.
• Lymph nodes are swollen and enlarged.
• Pox lesions may be present in the urinary bladder mucosa/submucosa and testicles.
• Fibrin may be present in joints and tendon sheaths.
• Histopathologically, early skin lesions consist of swelling of the dermis with edema and some hemorrhage.
• Variable numbers of lymphocytes, neutrophils, and macrophages are present in the dermis with some fibroblastic proliferation present. Older lesions have vasculitis and thrombosis of vessels with necrosis of the associated tissues.
• The epidermis is acanthotic with orthokeratotic and parakeratotic hyperkeratosis, ballooning degeneration of the stratum spinosum, and necrosis of keratinocytes.
• Eosinophilic intracytoplasmic inclusions are present in swollen keratinocytes in the epidermis and in macrophages, fibroblasts, and endothelial cells in the affected dermis and subcutis. In old infarcted lesions, inclusion bodies are usually absent.

L

(CONTINUED)

TREATMENT

THERAPEUTIC APPROACH
• LSD is a reportable disease in most areas of the world. Notification of state and/or federal veterinary authorities is important if there is suspicion of this disease.
• Treatment is supportive.

SURGICAL CONSIDERATIONS AND TECHNIQUES
N/A

MEDICATIONS

DRUGS OF CHOICE
• Antipyretic drugs (such as flunixin meglumine) can relieve fever and improve appetite.
• Antibiotics are indicated for severe secondary bacterial infections of the skin, mammary gland, joints, or tendon sheaths.

CONTRAINDICATIONS
N/A

PRECAUTIONS
• Antibiotic selection for treatment of bacterial complications should be based on antimicrobial sensitivity of the offending agent.
• Appropriate milk and meat withdrawal times must be followed for all compounds administered to food-producing animals.

POSSIBLE INTERACTIONS
N/A

FOLLOW-UP

EXPECTED COURSE AND PROGNOSIS
• In naïve animals, morbidity can reach 85–100% but mortality is usually low (<3%).
• In severe cases, lesions may persist for up to 6 months.
• Secondary bacterial infections are common.

POSSIBLE COMPLICATIONS
• Secondary bacterial infections of necrotic lesions.
• Bacterial infections of lesions of the mammary gland, joints, and penis can cause serious complications including loss of the mammary gland and loss of breeding capability in males.

CLIENT EDUCATION
Insuring that clients restrict movement of affected animals is key to preventing spread.

PATIENT CARE
• Sick animals should be monitored for secondary bacterial infections of the skin.
• Animals in regions in which old world screwworms are endemic should be kept under observation for wound myiasis.

PREVENTION
• In endemic areas, vaccination has been successful in controlling outbreaks; options include a live attenuated version of the sheeppox virus, or live attenuated Neethling virus.
• The control of insects has not proven effective at stopping spread.

MISCELLANEOUS

ASSOCIATED CONDITIONS
Bacterial infections of necrotic lesions are common.

AGE-RELATED FACTORS
Calves are more susceptible than adults.

ZOONOTIC POTENTIAL
N/A

PREGNANCY
Late-term abortions can occur related to fever.

BIOSECURITY
Affected animals should be quarantined and movement restricted.

PRODUCTION MANAGEMENT
Infection results in economic losses due to body condition loss, reductions of milk yield, and devaluation of hides.

SYNONYM
Neethling poxvirus

ABBREVIATIONS
• EDTA = ethylenediaminetetraacetic acid
• ELISA = enzyme-linked immunosorbent assay
• LSD = lumpy skin disease
• PCR = polymerase chain reaction

SEE ALSO
• Bovine Papular Stomatitis
• Cowpox
• Dermatophilosis
• Parasitic Skin Diseases: Bovine
• Pseudocowpox

Suggested Reading

Annandale CH, Holm DE, Ebersohn K, et al. Seminal transmission of lumpy skin disease virus in heifers. Transbound Emerg Dis 2014, 61: 443–8.

Hunter P, Wallace D. Lumpy skin disease in southern Africa: a review of the disease and aspects of control. J S Afr Vet Assoc 2001, 72: 68–71.

Kitching RP. Vaccines for lumpy skin disease, sheep pox and goat pox. Dev Biol Basel 2003, 114: 161–7.

Kitching P. Capripoxviruses. In: Brown C, Torres A eds, Foreign Animal Diseases, 7th ed. Boca Raton, FL: Committee on Foreign and Emerging Diseases of the United States Animal Health Association, 2008, pp. 377–82.

Rwetemanu M, Paskin R, Benkirane A, et al. Emerging diseases of Africa and the Middle East. Ann N Y Acad Sci 2000, 916: 61–70.

Tuppuraninen ESM, Oura CAL. Review. Lumpy skin disease: An emerging threat to Europe, the Middle-East, and Asia. Transbound Emerg Dis 2012, 59: 40–8.

World Organization for Animal Health. Lumpy skin disease. In: Fernandez PJ, White WR eds, Atlas of Transboundary Diseases. World Organization for Animal Health, 2010, pp. 150–7.

Author Robert B. Moeller Jr
Consulting Editor Erica C. McKenzie

L

LUPINE TOXICITY

BASICS

OVERVIEW
• Lupines (*Lupinus* spp.) cause two distinct forms of poisoning in livestock: lupine poisoning and lupinosis. Alkaloid-containing lupines are *Lupinus formosus* and *L. arbustus*.
• Lupine poisoning is a nervous syndrome caused by alkaloids present in bitter lupines.
• Lupinosis is a mycotic disease characterized by liver injury and jaundice.
• The genus *Lupinus* contains a large number of species. In some parts of the world they form a useful fodder crop.
• Lupines are found in climax and grassy habitats and are toxic even when dry.
• Many species of lupines contain quinolizidine or piperidine alkaloids known to be toxic or teratogenic to livestock.
• Defects caused by quinolizidine and piperidine teratogens include cleft palate and contracture-type skeletal defects such as arthrogryposis, scoliosis, torticollis, and kyphosis.
• Lupinosis affects sheep, and occasionally cattle. Horses and pigs are also susceptible.
• Cleft palate and minor front limb contractures are induced in calves by maternal ingestion of the piperidine alkaloid-containing lupines, *Lupinus formosus* and *L. arbustus*. Crooked calf disease, which includes an occasional cleft palate, is a congenital condition of widespread occurrence in cattle in the western United States and Canada. It is known to occur after maternal ingestion of certain species of *Lupinus* during specific gestational periods.

INCIDENCE/PREVALENCE
Like most toxic plants, incidence is variable. Crooked calf disease generally has been seen to affect <10% of a herd but incidence varies by year, area, and herd.

GEOGRAPHIC DISTRIBUTION
• *Lupinus* has two principal areas of distribution in the world: The first is the western North and South America, and second is the Mediterranean region.
• In North America, the genus is most abundant in the western half. Only a few species occur in the eastern half of the continent.

SYSTEMS AFFECTED
• Multisystemic
• Nervous
• Reproductive

PATHOPHYSIOLOGY
• The toxic and teratogenic effects from these plant species have distinct similarities including maternal muscular weakness and ataxia and fetal contracture-type skeletal defects and cleft palate.
• It is believed that the mechanism of action of the piperidine and quinolizidine

alkaloid-induced teratogenesis is the same; however, there are some differences in incidence, susceptible gestational periods, and severity between livestock species.
• Although many lupine species contain quinolizidine alkaloids including the teratogenic alkaloid anagyrine, *L. formosus* and *L. arbustus* produce piperidine alkaloids including the reported teratogen ammodendrine. In addition to ammodendrine, *L. formosus* contains both N-acetyl hystrine and N-methyl ammodendrine, whereas *L. arbustus* contains ammodendrine, trace amounts of N-methyl ammodendrine, and no N-acetyl hystrine.

SIGNALMENT
Most common in sheep and cattle

PHYSICAL EXAMINATION FINDINGS
Lupine Poisoning
• Inappetence and dyspnea, depression, ataxia, muscle twitching, labored breathing, violent struggles, convulsions, and hyper-excitability.
• Signs are most common in sheep but all ruminants are susceptible.
• Cattle will display excess salivation, protrusion of the nictitating membrane, weakness, recumbency, and death.
• Death is due to respiratory paralysis. It may be acute or take 2–3 days.
• There is no icterus.
• Defects caused by quinolizidine and piperidine teratogens include cleft palate and contracture-type skeletal defects such as arthrogryposis, scoliosis, torticollis, and kyphosis.

Lupinosis
• Early signs in sheep and cattle may include inappetence and listlessness, blisters, erythema, edema, reluctance to move, constipation, hemoglobinuria, hepatoencephalopathy (head pressing and wandering into fences); complete anorexia and jaundice follows, and ketosis is common.
• Cattle may show lacrimation and salivation.
• Ruminants may become photosensitive. In sheep with heavy fleece, lesions occur on head and coronary band, but in shorn sheep lesions can occur on the back. Sheep can also have extensive head edema. Onset of lesions may just take hours and initially include erythema and edema followed by blisters, exudation, necrosis, and sloughing of necrotic tissue. In cattle, lesions occur on areas of the body that are nonpigmented and on the teats, udder, perineum, and nose.
• In acute outbreaks, death occurs in 2–14 days.

CAUSES AND RISK FACTORS
Lupine Poisoning
• Acute poisoning occurs when a considerable amount of the plant is eaten in a short time.
• Lupins contain a number of alkaloids; D-lupanine is the most toxic and the most widely distributed.

• The concentration of alkaloid is greatest in the seeds, and the plants are most dangerous at the seeding stage.
• The alkaloids are not destroyed by drying.
• Lupine-induced "crooked calf disease": Crooked calf disease is characterized as skeletal contracture-type malformations and occasional cleft palate in calves after maternal ingestion of lupines containing the quinolizidine alkaloid anagyrine during gestation days 40–100.
• Toxic and teratogenic effects have been linked to structural aspects of these alkaloids, and the mechanism of action is believed to be associated with an alkaloid-induced inhibition of fetal movement during specific gestational periods.

Lupinosis
• The causal fungus is *Phomopsis leptostromiformis*, a phytopathogen causing phomopsis stem blight, especially in white and yellow lupines; blue varieties are very resistant.
• The fungus is also a saprophyte and under favorable conditions grows well on dead lupine material.
• The fungus produces hepatotoxic secondary metabolites. The main one is phomopsin A.

DIAGNOSIS

DIFFERENTIAL DIAGNOSES
Lupinosis
Acute aflatoxicosis

Photosensitization
• Chronic fluke damage
• Congenital porphyria
• Liver disease
• Phenothiazines
• St. John's wort
• Toxin absorption

Arthrogryposis
• BVD, IBR, bluetongue virus, akabane virus, and Cache Valley virus.
• Arthrogryposis-hydranencephaly syndrome (AHS) in lambs may be confused with spider lamb syndrome (SLS), in which there is characteristic hyperflexion of forelimbs, cranial overextension of hindlimbs, with a corkscrew deviation of the spine. In lambs with AHS, severe deformities result from primary abnormalities of the CNS and not of the skeleton. Hydranencephaly, micromyelia, hydrocephalus, and cerebellar hypoplasia are also seen with AHS.

CBC/BIOCHEMISTRY/URINALYSIS
Lupine poisoning: Elevated serum GGT, AST, LDH, and GDH concentrations

OTHER LABORATORY TESTS
N/A

IMAGING
N/A

PATHOLOGIC FINDINGS

Lupine Poisoning
• No icterus
• No characteristic postmortem lesions

Lupinosis
• In acute disease, icterus is marked. Livers are enlarged, orange-yellow, and fatty.
• Chronic disease shows bronze- or tan-colored livers that are firm, contracted in size and fibrosed, and often likened to a boxing glove.
• Copious transudate may be found in the abdominal and the pericardial sac.

Histopathologic Findings
Lupinosis: Diffuse scattered hepatocyte necrosis with a background of mitotic figures, often appearing to be arrested in metaphase. Later in the course of the disease, diffuse fibrosis and biliary hyperplasia predominate.

TREATMENT

THERAPEUTIC APPROACH

Lupine Poisoning
Remove animals from the source.

Lupinosis
• Frequent surveillance of sheep or cattle, and of lupine fodder material for characteristic black spot fungal infestation, especially after rain.
• The utilization of lupine cultivars, bred and developed for resistance to *P. leptostromiformis*, is advocated.

MEDICATIONS

DRUGS OF CHOICE

Lupine Poisoning
None

Lupinosis
Oral doses of zinc (0.5 g of zinc or more, per day) are useful in protection from phomopsin-induced liver injury in sheep.

PRECAUTIONS
Appropriate milk and meat withdrawal times must be followed for all compounds administered to food-producing animals.

FOLLOW-UP

EXPECTED COURSE AND PROGNOSIS
With acute lupine poisoning, if the animal survives it will likely make a full recovery, because the lupine alkaloid is readily excreted in the urine.

POSSIBLE COMPLICATIONS
Lupines have a marked teratogenic effect on cattle and give rise to crooked calf disease, characterized by arthrogryposis, scoliosis, torticollis, and cleft palate.

MISCELLANEOUS

ASSOCIATED CONDITIONS
• Liver failure, respiratory failure, cleft palate, and contracture-type skeletal defects such as arthrogryposis, scoliosis, torticollis, and kyphosis.
• Cleft palate and minor front limb contractures are induced in calves by maternal ingestion (crooked calf disease).

PREGNANCY
Crooked calf disease is characterized as skeletal contracture-type malformations and occasional cleft palate in calves after maternal ingestion of lupines containing the quinolizidine alkaloid, anagyrine, during gestation days 40–100.

PRODUCTION MANAGEMENT
• Producers should be aware of the association between certain toxic plants (e.g., lupines) and angular limb deformities such as CCD.
• To reduce the incidence of crooked calf syndrome, graze lupines during their least hazardous growth period and reduce exposure of pregnant cows. Lupines are most hazardous when either young or in the mature seed stage.
• Fence off heavily infested pasture areas and use intermittent, short-term grazing of lupine pastures.

SYNONYM
Crooked calf syndrome

ABBREVIATIONS
• AHS = arthrogryposis-hydranencephaly syndrome

• AST = aspartate aminotransferase
• BVD = bovine viral diarrhea
• CNS = central nervous system
• GDH = glutamate dehydrogenase
• GGT = gamma-glutamyl transferase
• IBR = infectious bovine rhinotracheitis
• LDH = lactate dehydrogenase
• SLS = spider lamb syndrome

SEE ALSO
• Akabane
• Arthrogryposis
• Bluetongue Virus
• Bovine Viral Diarrhea Virus
• Cache Valley Virus
• Infectious Bovine Rhinotracheitis
• Mycotoxins
• St. John's Wort Toxicity

Suggested Reading
Burrows GE, Tyrl RJ. Toxic Plants of North America, 2nd ed. Ames: Wiley-Blackwell, Kindle edition, 2013.
Panter KE, Gardner DR, Molyneux RJ. Teratogenic and fetotoxic effects of two piperidine alkaloid-containing lupines (*L. formosus* and *L. arbustus*) in cows. J Nat Toxins 1998, 7: 131–40.
Panter KE, James LF, Gardner DR. Lupines, poison-hemlock and *Nicotiana* spp. toxicity and teratogenicity in livestock. J Nat Toxins 1999, 8: 117–34.
Panter KE, Keeler RF. Quinolizidine and piperidine alkaloid teratogens from poisonous plants and their mechanism of action in animals. Vet Clin North Am Food Anim Pract 1993, 9: 33–40.
Panter KE, Keeler RF, Bunch TD, Callan RJ. Congenital skeletal malformations and cleft palate induced in goats by ingestion of *Lupinus, Conium* and *Nicotiana* species. Toxicon 1990, 28: 1377–85.

Author Troy E.C. Holder
Consulting Editor Christopher C.L. Chase

L

LYMPHOCYTOSIS

BASICS

OVERVIEW
• Absolute number of lymphocytes greater than the reference range—bovine >7,500/μL; ovine >9,000/μL; caprine >,9000/μL; camelids >7,000/μL.
• Absolute lymphocyte counts are greater in young animals than adults.

INCIDENCE/PREVALENCE
• Pathologic lymphocytosis is uncommon in ruminants except for cattle infected with bovine leukosis virus (BLV).
• Sporadic lymphosarcoma with concurrent lymphocytosis (also known as calf or juvenile form) is extremely rare and multiple cases within the same herd are even less common.

GEOGRAPHIC DISTRIBUTION
N/A

SYSTEMS AFFECTED
Hemolymphatic

PATHOPHYSIOLOGY
• Lymphocytes are produced in the bone marrow, lymph nodes, spleen, thymus, and Peyer's patches.
• Lymphocytes retain mitotic capability and can recirculate from the blood to lymphoid tissue. The number of lymphocytes in the blood represents a balance between cells leaving and entering circulation. Therefore, changes in peripheral lymphocyte counts may not necessarily indicate altered lymphopoiesis.
• Blood lymphocytes represent an assortment of lymphocyte subpopulations including B- and T-lymphocytes. B-cells are involved with humoral immunity and produce antibodies, while T-lymphocytes are responsible for cell-mediated immunity and cytokine responses involved in immune system regulation.
• Approximately 95% of all lymphocytes are B- and T-lymphocytes with T-cells predominating. The remaining lymphocytes make up a third group classified as "null" cells. Null cells consist of several subtypes including large granular lymphocytes and natural killer cells.
• In general, most lymphocyte subtypes cannot be identified on a blood film examination. However, large granular lymphocytes are occasionally observed in ruminant blood and can be recognized by the presence of small, red cytoplasmic granules.
• Infrequently, activated B-lymphocytes (i.e., immunoblasts) are identified on blood film evaluation by their large size, deep blue cytoplasm, and perinuclear clear zone.
• Ruminant lymphocytes generally have diameters equal to those of neutrophils, but can be quite irregular in size.
• Hepatosplenomegaly may occur as a result of hyperplasia or neoplasia; bone marrow may be hyperplastic; neoplastic populations of lymphocytes may rarely result in anemia and thrombocytopenia due to myelophthisis.

SIGNALMENT
• Reference values for absolute lymphocyte counts vary with ruminant species. Sheep and goats have higher mean absolute lymphocyte counts than cattle or camelids. However, alpacas and llamas generally have lower lymphocyte counts than camels.
• Sporadic lymphosarcoma (calf or juvenile form) generally affects calves 3–6 months of age, but may be observed in calves as young as 1 month or cattle as old as 3 years.
• Lymphocytic leukemia and BLV-associated lymphosarcoma affect adult ruminants >2 years of age.

PHYSICAL EXAMINATION FINDINGS
• If cause is physiologic (rare cause in ruminants), excited or fearful.
• If cause is persistent lymphocytosis associated with subclinical stage of BLV infection, affected cattle rarely exhibit clinical signs.
• If cause is pathologic (sporadic lymphosarcoma, lymphosarcoma, or lymphocytic leukemia), lymphadenopathy, anorexia, decreased milk production, poor body condition. Depending on the involvement of other organ systems, melena or diarrhea (intestinal tract), heart failure (myocardium), posterior paresis/paralysis (spinal canal), pelvic masses (uterus), and exophthalmia (retrobulbar tissue) may be observed. Anemia may result in pale mucus membranes, tachypnea, and tachycardia.

CAUSES AND RISK FACTORS

Physiologic
Epinephrine release due to excitement, pain, fear, restraint. The change occurs within minutes and usually lasts <30 minutes. Effect is usually observed in young healthy animals. Physiologic lymphocytosis is uncommon in most ruminants.

Antigenic Stimulation
Uncommon cause, but may occur occasionally with chronic viral or bacterial infections (e.g., caprine arthritis encephalitis virus, bacterial pneumonia) and within 10–14 days of vaccination.

Persistent Lymphocytosis
Subclinical BLV infection in cattle results in decreased B-cell turnover and an inverted B:T cell ratio. B cells in this condition are non-neoplastic.

Sporadic Lymphosarcoma
Cause is unknown.

Lymphosarcoma or Lymphocytic Leukemia
• Although reported in all ruminant species, lymphosarcoma with lymphocytosis and lymphocytic leukemia are rare except in cattle infected with BLV.
• Approximately 30% of BLV-infected cattle are leukemic. Lymphocytosis is primarily due to decreased cell death of B-cells.

DIAGNOSIS

DIFFERENTIAL DIAGNOSES
• Transient physiologic lymphocytosis typically occurs in young, healthy, and excitable animals.
• Persistent lymphocytosis (3-months duration) in cattle without clinical signs is associated with subclinical BLV infection.
• Ill cattle with absolute lymphocytosis—consider lymphosarcoma or lymphocytic leukemia; may be seropositive for BLV.

CBC/BIOCHEMISTRY/URINALYSIS
Physiologic Lymphocytosis
CBC
• Mild lymphocytosis
• Rarely, mild increases in RBC, Hgb, and PCV due to epinephrine-mediated splenic contraction
• Mild neutrophilia
• Plasma proteins typically normal
Serum Biochemistry/Urinalysis
No characteristic changes

Persistent Lymphocytosis of Cattle
CBC
• Mild to moderate lymphocytosis that persists over an interval of at least 3 months.
• Morphologically atypical and large lymphocytes may be present on blood film examination, but similar lymphocytes may occasionally be observed in normal cattle or cattle with various non-BLV-associated conditions.
Serum Biochemistry/Urinalysis
No characteristic changes

Lymphocytic Leukemia
CBC
• Marked to severe lymphocytosis with atypical lymphocytes observed in approximately 50% of the cases. (Approximately 5%–10% of BLV-infected cattle manifest with massive increases in circulating neoplastic lymphoblasts, but <2% develop lymphosarcoma.)
• Anemia (may be regenerative or nonregenerative depending on cause).
• Plasma proteins may be decreased if there is neoplastic involvement of gastrointestinal tract.
Serum Biochemistry/Urinalysis
No characteristic changes.

OTHER LABORATORY TESTS
• For cattle with persistent lymphocytosis—BLV antibody ELISA or AGID.
• Bone marrow evaluation in cases of lymphocytic leukemia often reveals a large population of infiltrating lymphoblasts.

IMAGING
Radiographic or ultrasonographic imaging may reveal evidence of hepatosplenomegaly.

OTHER DIAGNOSTIC PROCEDURES
• Fine-needle aspiration cytology and culture of enlarged lymph nodes is occasionally helpful in differentiating an abscess from lymphosarcoma.
• Histopathologic examination of tumor or lymph node biopsies may be more useful than cytology in confirming lymphosarcoma.

PATHOLOGIC FINDINGS
• No gross or histologic lesions with physiologic or persistent lymphocytosis.

TREATMENT

THERAPEUTIC APPROACH

Physiologic Lymphocytosis
Treatment is not warranted as lymphocyte counts typically return to normal within 30 minutes.

Lymphocytosis Due to Antigenic Stimulation
Treatment should be directed at the primary disease causing the lymphocytosis.

Lymphosarcoma and Lymphocytic Leukemia
No curative treatment for lymphosarcoma or lymphocytic leukemia exists in ruminants. Supportive or palliative therapy may be indicated to reduce discomfort.

MEDICATIONS

DRUGS OF CHOICE
• Chemotherapeutics: Case report data regarding chemotherapy are rare. A few reports summarizing unsuccessful attempts in treating lymphosarcoma and lymphocytic leukemia with dexamethasone and cylcophosphamide exist. Drug withdrawal periods must be determined and maintained.

• Fluid therapy: Rehydration with IV fluids appropriate for the primary cause (e.g., polyuric renal failure, diarrhea, etc.) and to correct any electrolyte and acid-base imbalances.

FOLLOW-UP

EXPECTED COURSE AND PROGNOSIS

Persistent Lymphocytosis of Cattle
Precedes the onset of lymphosarcoma in approximately 65% of cases, but <5% of cows with persistent lymphocytosis develop lymphosarcoma.

Sporadic Lymphosarcoma
Rapidly progressive and usually fatal within 2–8 weeks of onset.

Lymphosarcoma or Lymphocytic Leukemia
The prognosis for patients with lymphosarcoma or lymphocytic leukemia is poor, with median survival times following diagnosis of <2–3 months.

PATIENT CARE
Restrict activity

PREVENTION
See chapters Bovine Leukemia Virus, Leukocyte Responses in Cattle, and Lymphosarcoma for control suggestions.

MISCELLANEOUS

ASSOCIATED CONDITIONS
Persistent lymphocytosis of cattle is associated with BLV infection.

AGE-RELATED FACTORS
• Young animals—lymphocyte counts generally increase from birth to a maximum at approximately 11–12 months of age. Absolute lymphocyte counts begin to slowly decline in adult animals.
• Physiologic lymphocytosis occurs in young healthy animals.

• Sporadic lymphosarcoma occurs most commonly in 3- to 6-month-old calves.
• Lymphosarcoma and lymphocytic leukemia generally occur in adult animals >4 years.

ZOONOTIC POTENTIAL
N/A

SYNONYMS
• Bovine leukosis
• Bovine lymphoma
• Chronic lymphocytic leukemia
• Malignant lymphoma

ABBREVIATIONS
• AGID = agar gel immunodiffusion
• BLV = bovine leukemia virus
• ELISA = enzyme-linked immunosorbent assay
• Hgb = hemoglobin
• IV = intravenous
• PCV = packed cell volume
• RBC = red blood cells

SEE ALSO
• Bovine Leukemia Virus
• Leukocyte Responses in Cattle
• Lymphosarcoma

Suggested Reading
Ferrer JF, Marshak RR, Abt DA, Kenyon SJ. Persistent lymphocytosis in cattle: its cause, nature and relation to lymphosarcoma. Ann Rech Vet 1978, 9: 851–7.
Valentine BA, McDonough SP. B-cell leukemia in a sheep. Vet Path 2003, 40: 117–19.
Author Daniel L. Grooms
Consulting Editor Christopher C.L. Chase
Acknowledgment The author and book editors acknowledge the prior contribution of Frederic S. Almy.

L

LYMPHOSARCOMA

BASICS

OVERVIEW
• Lymphosarcoma is a lymphoid cancer caused by a single-stranded RNA retrovirus that integrates into the host cell genome.
• The cause of lymphosarcoma in cattle and sheep is believed to be bovine leukemia virus. Cattle are the natural host for BLV. However, only about 30% of BLV-positive cattle develop persistent lymphocytosis and only 5% of these develop lymphosarcoma.
• There are four forms of bovine leukemia: juvenile, thymic, cutaneous, and enzootic. The first three are considered sporadic because the animals are BLV negative for antibodies. The enzootic bovine leukemia animals are positive for BLV antibodies, have persistent lymphocytosis, and can develop lymphosarcoma.
• It can be hard to distinguish between the thymic form of BLV and lymphosarcoma.
• There are no indicators to predict which animals with persistent lymphocytosis will develop lymphosarcoma.
• BLV has not been associated with goats that develop lymphosarcoma.

INCIDENCE/PREVALENCE
• USDA NAHMS surveys estimate 39% and 89% of beef cow-calf and dairy herds, respectively, contain BLV-infected cattle.
• In the cattle industry, BLV-positive cattle are estimated to account for >285 million dollars in losses a year in the dairy industry. These losses are in the form of genetics, carcass condemnation, trade restrictions, and veterinary costs.
• Lymphosarcoma accounts for 13.5% of beef cow and 26.9% of dairy cattle condemnations at slaughter.

GEOGRAPHIC DISTRIBUTION
Widespread throughout the United States and the world

SYSTEMS AFFECTED
• Cardiovascular
• Musculoskeletal
• Digestive
• Hemolymphatic
• Ophthalmic
• Reproductive

PATHOPHYSIOLOGY
• In cattle and sheep, seroconversion occurs after exposure to the virus between 14 and 98 days. The wide temporal range of conversion is attributable to dose, route of infection, and immune status of the animal. Concurrent infection with a retro- or herpes virus may make the BLV infection more pathogenic.
• Currently it is believed that the virus is necessary only to initiate tumor development, but after initiation, the tumor self-replicates.
• Tumors can occur in every organ but primarily develop in lymph nodes.

SIGNALMENT
• Cattle are the natural host for BLV. Sheep are highly susceptible to forming lymphosarcoma once exposed to BLV. Goats tend to form tumors but do not seroconvert.
• Cattle and sheep have the highest incidence of tumor formation between the ages of 2 and 4. Goats >2 years of age tend to be identified with tumors.

GENETICS
Cattle that have been identified with the BoLA-A allele w8.1 are more resistant to BLV infections and therefore have a lower incidence of lymphosarcoma.

PHYSICAL EXAMINATION FINDINGS
• Depending on location of the developing tumor, animals will present with a wide variety of clinical signs.
• Cattle and sheep: Peripheral lymphadenopathy (prescapular, femoral, suprascapular, supramammary), weight loss, anorexia, decreased milk production, ketosis, diarrhea, ataxia, edema on ventral abdomen and udder due to blocked lymphatic drainage, exophthalmia, melena from gastrointestinal ulcers, dyspnea, cardiac dysrhythmia, pounding jugular pulse, masses in the reproductive tract, dog-sitting due to posterior paresis, and recumbent animals.
• Goats: Pyrexia, emaciation, diarrhea, and dyspnea.
• Masses may be visualized or palpated, typically associated with lymph nodes.

CAUSES AND RISK FACTORS
• Transmission of BLV occurs both horizontally and vertically.
• Horizontal transmission of BLV primarily occurs through fomites during normal cattle processing procedures. These include dehorning, rectal palpation, injections, tattoos, and surgeries. When instruments are not properly sterilized between procedures, contamination of naïve animals with the virus may occur. Body secretions from saliva, nasal discharge, broncho-alveolar fluids, and urine have all been demonstrated to seroconvert exposed ruminants. Insects have been hypothesized to be a transmitting vector, but to date, experimental infection has not been demonstrated between animals.
• Experimental vertical transmission of virus can occur through semen, ova, and embryos. It is not believed that these reproductive products are a significant source of infection. None of these products may be sold internationally if the animals are identified as having BLV. In utero, cell-free transmission of virus to offspring occurs through the placenta in 3–25% of infected dams after the third month of gestation. Colostrum and milk from BLV-positive cows are not believed capable of causing an infection in calves that ingest them if given after gut closure.

• Fomites contaminated with whole blood from an infected cow that are not cleaned and disinfected properly.
• Sheep that are comingled with infected cattle.
• Dairy cattle have more intense management and interaction than most beef cattle, which accounts for a higher incidence of transmission.

DIAGNOSIS

DIFFERENTIAL DIAGNOSES
• Lymphadenopathy due to systemic infection
• Fat necrosis
• Melanomas
• Carcinomas
• Internal abscesses
• Caseous lymphadenitis in goats and sheep

CBC/BIOCHEMISTRY/URINALYSIS
• Cattle
  ○ CBC may be normal
  ○ May see a lymphocytosis but rare
  ○ May be anemic, due to gastrointestinal bleeding (microcytic, hypochromic)
  ○ Can have an increase in liver enzymes if there is hepatic involvement
  ○ Hyperglobulinemia
  ○ Hypoalbuminemia
• Sheep and goats
  ○ Anemia that is nonregenerative
  ○ Hyperglobulinemia
  ○ Hypoalbuminemia

OTHER LABORATORY TESTS
• Tests for BLV antibodies:
  ○ *Agar gel immunodiffusion (AGID)*—this is the primary test used to screen cattle and the official test for export of cattle. Most labs that run this test are identifying antibodies to gp51 viral antigen, which appears to be more sensitive than testing for p24. Antibodies to gp51 can occur as early as 3 weeks post-exposure. A negative test indicates that the animal has not been exposed to BLV for 3–12 weeks prior to testing. A strong response to gp51 does not necessarily indicate that the animals will develop lymphosarcoma.
  ○ *Radioimmunoassay (RIA)*—this test is more sensitive than AGID and can detect smaller amounts of antibody within the first 2 weeks of infection. It has been developed for both the detection of p24 and gp51. Both serum and milk can be used for testing.
  ○ *Enzyme-linked immunosorbent assay (ELISA)*—sensitivity and specificity of this test are equal to RIA.
• A bone marrow aspirate and cytologic examination may reveal clonal expansion of lymphoid precursors.

IMAGING
Can see masses on survey radiographs in the cranial thorax in ruminants that could be heart-based tumors. Ultrasonography may be used to further characterize and differentiate masses.

OTHER DIAGNOSTIC PROCEDURES
• Physical examination revealing peripheral lymphadenopathy or other masses upon careful palpation.
• Fine-needle aspirate of the mass and cytologic examination. Examination of the aspirate may reveal a large number of lymphoblasts, but it may be hard to distinguish between lymphadenopathy and systemic infections.
• Lymph node biopsy during a laparotomy.

PATHOLOGIC FINDINGS
• Grossly, tumors appear to have a heavy fibrous capsular lining with cream-colored, friable inner contents and a necrotic, soft center.
• Tumor masses can occur in one or multiple organs and lymph nodes. The most common sites for development are:
  ◦ Cardiac tumors primarily occur in the myocardium and right atrium. They are very rarely seen in the left side of the heart.
  ◦ Gastrointestinal involvement of the pylorus is common and often will result in ulcers.
  ◦ Ocular masses develop in the retrobulbar region.
  ◦ Lymphatics in the area of the cranial udder.
  ◦ Uterine masses diffusely distributed throughout the tissues.
  ◦ Ventral spinal cord masses are readily palatable rectally.
  ◦ Liver diffusely.
  ◦ Lungs diffusely but rare to find.
  ◦ Spleen diffusely.
• Histologically, the masses have a large number of lymphoblast cells.

TREATMENT
THERAPEUTIC APPROACH
None

MEDICATIONS
DRUGS OF CHOICE
None

FOLLOW-UP
EXPECTED COURSE AND PROGNOSIS
• Animals are usually culled from the herd once they present with clinical signs and are diagnosed as having lymphosarcoma.
• Ruminants with lymphosarcoma may deteriorate within a week to 2 months after clinical signs and eventually need to be humanely euthanized.

CLIENT EDUCATION
• It is important to educate clients on the modes of horizontal transmission to prevent use of contaminated equipment on BLV-negative ruminants.
• It is important to discuss the economic impact of the disease on the production goals of the farm, to determine if testing and culling of infected animals are reasonable options.
• There are a number of international shipping restrictions that prevent the sale of breeding stock and their reproductive by-products if they are BLV positive.

PATIENT CARE
• Monitor patients as their health degenerates to ensure they are humanely treated.
• Some affected animals with high genetic value may need supportive care until they can have ova or semen harvested from them. Also, pregnant animals may need nursing care until they have their offspring.
• Depending on what the animals are presenting as clinical signs, nursing care could range from soft bedding if the animal is recumbent or ataxic to slinging animals to prevent pressure necrosis.
• Limit activity to prevent further injury if the animal is ataxic or recumbent and struggling.

PREVENTION
• Identify BLV-positive animals and keep them isolated from BLV-negative animals.
• Properly clean instruments that have whole blood contamination.
• Do not reuse needles.
• Test bulls that are used for natural service for BLV and do not use them if they are BLV-positive.
• Vector control—although to date experimental transmission of BLV by vectors has not been shown to be a primary infectious route.
• Cull BLV-positive animals from the herd and maintain strict testing and biosecurity when introducing new animals to the herd.
• If the owners have BLV-positive cows, they can harvest the ova, rinse them, and implant them into a BLV-negative recipient.

✓ MISCELLANEOUS
ASSOCIATED CONDITIONS
Ataxia, anemia, ascites, ventral edema, bloat, choke

AGE-RELATED FACTORS
Lymphosarcoma occurs in mature ruminants, usually over the age of 4 years.

ZOONOTIC POTENTIAL
None

PREGNANCY
There is cell-free transmission of the virus after 3 months of gestation through the placenta to the fetus.

BIOSECURITY
The optimal biosecurity measures would be to test and cull BLV-positive ruminants from the herd. Culling positive animals is cost-prohibitive for most producers, so reducing the rates of transmission is a practical approach to eliminating the disease from the herd. Testing and adding only BLV-negative animals to the herd and eliminating positive animals through natural attrition and preferential selection can accomplish reducing the number of infected ruminants.

PRODUCTION MANAGEMENT
• There are several approaches to eradicating BLV from the herd. The producer is going to have to determine if the cost benefit of eradication is greater or less than having the disease present.
• Eradicating or reducing BLV from the herd begins with testing all the animals in the herd. This primarily applies to cattle and sheep. All negative animals need to be retested in 12 weeks, and calves <6 months need to be retested at 6 months of age. Once producers have this information, they have three options:
  ◦ Culling all positive animals identified can eliminate BLV from the herd in a few months. However, the economic hardship is extreme if the herd has a high rate of infection. There is also the loss of genetic material from the herd when culling.
  ◦ Segregating infected animals from negative animals and slowly eliminating them from the herd and replacing with negative animals is another option. It takes longer to eliminate BLV from the herd this way, and requires more frequent serologic testing of the herd. Segregating positive from negative animals also requires essentially two separate facilities and equipment.

L

LYMPHOSARCOMA

○ Managerial practices can be altered to prevent the transmission of the disease and allow for natural attrition of infected animals. This takes a long time to eliminate BLV from the herd, and requires frequent serologic testing and a long-term commitment by the producer.

SYNONYMS
• Enzootic bovine leukosis
• Persistent lymphocytosis

ABBREVIATIONS
• AGID = agar gel immunodiffusion
• BLV = bovine leukemia virus
• ELISA = enzyme-linked immunosorbent assay
• NAHMS = National Animal Health Monitoring System
• RIA = radioimmunoassay
• USDA = United States Department of Agriculture

SEE ALSO
• Bovine Leukemia Virus
• Euthanasia and Disposal (Appendix 2)
• Serology (see www.fiveminutevet.com/ruminant)

Suggested Reading
Bartlett PC, Sordillo LM, Byrem TM, et al. Options for the control of bovine leukemia virus in dairy cattle. J Am Vet Med Assoc 2014, 244: 914–22.

Johnson R, Kaneene JB. Bovine leukemia virus. Part I. Descriptive epidemiology, clinical manifestations, and diagnostic tests. Compend Contin Educ Pract Vet 1991, 13: 315–24.

Johnson R, Kaneene JB. Bovine leukemia virus. Part III. Zoonotic potential, molecular epidemiology, and an animal model. Compend Contin Educ Pract Vet 1991, 13: 1631–9.

Author Daniel L. Grooms
Consulting Editor Christopher C.L. Chase
Acknowledgment The author and book editors acknowledge the prior contribution of M. R. Machen.

L

MAEDI-VISNA (OVINE PROGRESSIVE PNEUMONIA)

BASICS

OVERVIEW
• Maedi-visna (MV), known as ovine progressive pneumonia (OPP) in North America, is a multisystemic disease characterized by chronic inflammation of the lungs, mammary gland, joints, and central nervous system (CNS).
• Maedi-visna is caused by maedi-visna virus (MVV), also called ovine lentivirus (OvLV) or ovine progressive pneumonia virus (OPPV).
• Maedi-visna is an Icelandic name used for two clinical forms of the disease. Maedi (dyspnea) is a slow, nonfebrile, progressive interstitial pneumonia. Visna (wasting) is a slow progressive encephalitis of sheep.
• MVV is a member of the small ruminant lentiviruses group (SRLVs), which also includes caprine arthritis encephalitis virus (CAEV).
• SRLVs are related to other lentiviruses of domestic animals and humans.
• MVV and CAEV were considered species specific, but molecular studies show that sheep comingled with CAEV-infected goats can become infected with CAEV and vice versa.
• Susceptible animals may be infected early in life, but clinical signs manifest several years after infection.

INCIDENCE/PREVALENCE
• MV prevalence ranges from <5% to >60%. High prevalence is more common in intensively raised flocks, and in animals housed indoors.
• In the United States, the average seroprevalence is 26%, but there is a wide range between states and individual flocks. In west Texas, MVV seroprevalence is 0.5%. This difference is likely due to differences in management between regions. In Texas, most sheep are raised on open range conditions in a hot, dry climate, and lambing occurs on pasture.

GEOGRAPHIC DISTRIBUTION
MV has been reported in most sheep-producing countries with the exception of Iceland, where it was introduced but eradicated, and Australia and New Zealand.

SYSTEMS AFFECTED
• Respiratory
• Musculoskeletal
• Mammary
• Nervous
• Hemolymphatic

PATHOPHYSIOLOGY
• Maedi-visna virus is a Lentivirus in the family Retroviridae, subfamily Orthoretrovirinae.
• The genome of MVV is single-stranded RNA. After infection, the MVV genome is reverse transcribed into a double-stranded DNA copy that integrates into the host DNA.

Infected sheep remain infected for life, irrespective of the presence of neutralizing antibodies and cell-mediated immunity.
• Based on phylogenetic analyses, SRLV isolates are classified into five phylogenetic clusters. Genotypes A and B are distributed throughout the world, whereas C, D and E are geographically restricted.
• Genotype A includes MVV-like strains and genotype B comprises CAEV-like isolates originally isolated from sheep and goats from across the world, respectively.
• Genotype C includes isolates that were originally detected in Norway. Isolates from Switzerland and Spain are grouped in genotype D. Italian SRLVs isolated from the Roccaverano goat breed have been designated as genotype E.
• Groups A, B, and E are subdivided into subtypes.
• Group A is heterogeneous and contains fifteen subtypes (A1–A15). Group B is less complex and contains three subtypes (B1–B3). Group E contains two subtypes (E1 and E2) which have only been found in Italy.
• SRLVs from groups B–D and most group A subtypes (A1–A6, A9, A11–A13) infect both sheep and goats. Other SRLV groups and subtypes have so far only been described either in sheep (A15), or goats (A7, A8, A10, A14, E1 and E2). Co-infection with more than one SRLV strain may occur and can result in recombination to form new MVV-CAEV strains.
• Small ruminant lentiviruses quasi-species are continuously generated through mutation, recombination, and selection pressure by the immune system.
• Routes of transmission vary depending on factors, including production purposes (dairy versus meat or wool), management (intensive versus extensive operations), housing, breed, climate, virus strain, and host genetics.
• Transmission by close contact occurs more often during periods when infected and noninfected sheep are housed close together, such as during lambing or in winter, mainly when housed in poorly ventilated pens.
• During lambing and the postpartum period, transmission may occur by contact of newborns with contaminated birth products or aerosols.
• Ingestion of infected colostrum or milk is less important in MVV transmission, but may be significant in dairy sheep raised under intensive conditions and with a high prevalence of mastitis.
• Feeding MVV- or CAEV-contaminated colostrum or milk to sheep can result in infection.
• Vertical intrauterine transmission from infected ewes to fetuses occurs in 5–10% of cases.
• Venereal transmission of MVV has not been shown to occur, but sheep experimentally infected with MVV and co-infected with

Brucella ovis shed MVV in semen, and proviral DNA has been detected in semen.
• Seroconversion usually occurs between 2 and 8 weeks post-infection. Some sheep may remain seronegative for several months or longer in spite of being infected.

HISTORICAL FINDINGS
N/A

SIGNALMENT
• Sheep are the natural host of MVV infection.
• Phylogenetic analyses indicate that cross-species transmission of SRLVs (MVV and CAEV) occurs regularly.
• Several factors including virus strain, age, breed, genetics of the animal, route of exposure, secondary infections, and management conditions influence the outcome of MVV infection.
• There is no sex predilection.
• The percentage of seropositive sheep in a flock increases with age.
• Although MVV transmission may occur at an early age, clinical signs rarely arise before 2–3 years of age.
• Some breeds of sheep may be more susceptible to MVV infection.

PHYSICAL EXAMINATION FINDINGS
• The majority of sheep infected with MVV remain clinically healthy for life.
• In a proportion of sheep, MVV infection leads to cachexia and chronic inflammation in the lungs, lymph nodes, joints, mammary gland, and CNS.
• In North America, the most common manifestation of MV is chronic pneumonia with signs of afebrile, progressive respiratory failure in sheep 2–3 years or older. There is gradual emaciation and loss of body condition despite good appetite. Affected sheep remain behind the rest of the flock when driven and exhibit open-mouth breathing and dry cough.
• In later stages of disease, fever, purulent nasal discharge, and depression are common due to secondary bacterial infections.
• In ewes with mastitis, there is symmetrical bilateral enlargement and hardening of the udder (hardbag). Milk is normal in appearance but scant in quantity.
• Sheep with arthritis become lame and exhibit cachexia. There is weight loss and swelling of carpal and tarsal joints. Clinical signs of arthritis appear 2–3 years after infection.
• Neurologic manifestations of MV are seldom seen in the US, but are common in Europe. In this form, there is aberration of gait affecting primarily the hindquarters. There is gradual weakening, leading first to paraplegia and then quadriplegia. Affected animals lose weight, and jerking of the lips and facial muscles or blindness may be observed.
• The nervous form of MV has been diagnosed in Spain in lambs aged between 4

M

and 6 months, belonging to Assaf flocks that were managed intensively.

GENETICS
• MVV infections of sheep are influenced by host genetics and viral factors.
• Artificially produced identical twin lambs, one inoculated with a high pathogenicity MVV strain (85/34) and the co-twin inoculated with a low pathogenicity strain (84/28), developed the same degree of lymphoid interstitial pneumonia, indicating that host genetic factors are important in determining the degree of disease.
• Genetic variation in the ovine transmembrane 154 (*TMEM154*) gene associates with infection susceptibility. Distinct SRLV genetic subgroups infect sheep in association with their *TMEM154* diplotypes.

CAUSES AND RISK FACTORS
• Coexistence of chronic respiratory diseases in the flock, such as ovine pulmonary adenomatosis (Jaagsiekte) or lung parasites, seems to increase the risk of transmission.
• Larger flocks have an increased risk of infection.

DIAGNOSIS

DIFFERENTIAL DIAGNOSES
• Caseous lymphadenitis, paratuberculosis (Johne's disease), chronic parasitism, and malnutrition
• Chronic suppurative pneumonia, parasitic pneumonia, and ovine pulmonary adenomatosis (Jaagsiekte)
• Bacterial mastitis (bluebag)
• Bacterial arthritis (*Chlamydia* and *Mycoplasma*)
• Scrapie, rabies, brain abscesses, parasitic lesions, and trauma of the spinal cord

CBC/Biochemistry/Urinalysis
N/A

OTHER LABORATORY TESTS
N/A

IMAGING
N/A

OTHER DIAGNOSTIC PROCEDURES
• Serologic screening is done with enzyme-linked immunosorbent assay (ELISA) and agar gel immunodiffusion (AGID). Western blot can be used for confirmation.
• There are several commercially available ELISA and AGID kits for detection of MVV serum antibodies.
• Competitive ELISA has high sensitivity and specificity.
• Standard PCR and real-time PCR have been developed and used mostly for research; they are currently used by only a few diagnostic laboratories.

• The sensitivity and specify of serologic tests and PCR protocols are influenced by the MVV strains circulating in a flock or region.
• A combination of ELISA and real-time PCR increases the likelihood of detecting infected animals and becomes useful in control programs and export testing.
• Serologic tests or molecular techniques with high sensitivity and specificity in Europe may have lower sensitivity and specificity in other countries, due to antigenic and genetic variability of SRLV subtypes; developing subtype-specific diagnostic tests is imperative.

PATHOLOGIC FINDINGS
• Grossly, evidence of chronic pneumonia, arthritis, and/or mastitis might be present.
• Lungs of sheep with MVV-induced chronic interstitial pneumonia do not collapse fully and have a white or gray color. Rib impression lines can occur on the costal surface of the lungs. Lungs are heavier than normal and firm. One to 2 mm or larger, gray foci may be observed throughout the lung. Well-demarcated areas of consolidation without exudate in the airways may be found in the cranioventral lobes. Mediastinal and peribronchial lymph nodes may be five times larger than normal.
• The mammary gland in ewes affected with mastitis is symmetrically enlarged and firm.
• In sheep with arthritis, there is swelling of the carpal and tarsal joints. Other joints are less frequently affected. There is increased synovial fluid, discoloration and thickening of the synovial membrane, and erosion of the articular cartilage.
• Gross lesions are not observed in the CNS of sheep affected with the neurologic form.
• Microscopically, lymphoid interstitial pneumonia is the typical lesion in the lungs. There is thickening of the interalveolar septa due to infiltration of mononuclear cells, hyperplasia of smooth muscle, and fibrosis. Numerous lymphoid follicles with active germinal centers are found adjacent to bronchioles and small vessels.
• Ewes with mastitis have follicular lymphoid hyperplasia and interstitial infiltration of mononuclear cells.
• Joints exhibit severe infiltration with lymphocytes, plasma cells, and macrophages as well as villus proliferation of the synovium. There is degeneration of the articular cartilage, mineralization of the joint capsule, and periosteal replacement growth in more advanced cases.
• In the brain of sheep affected by the neurologic form, there is periventricular encephalitis characterized by ependymal necrosis, widespread demyelination, and prominent perivascular lymphocytic cuffing.

TREATMENT

THERAPEUTIC APPROACH
There are no treatments available.

SURGICAL CONSIDERATIONS AND TECHNIQUES
N/A

MEDICATIONS

DRUGS OF CHOICE
Wide-spectrum antibiotics may be used for secondary bacterial infections.

CONTRAINDICATIONS
Appropriate milk and meat withdrawal times must be followed for all compounds administered to food-producing animals.

PRECAUTIONS
N/A

POSSIBLE INTERACTIONS
N/A

FOLLOW-UP

EXPECTED COURSE AND PROGNOSIS
• Infected sheep remain infected for life.
• Sheep often die within 6–8 months after initial clinical signs.

POSSIBLE COMPLICATIONS
Secondary bacterial pneumonia/infections

CLIENT EDUCATION
Should focus on methods of preventing this disease within the flock

PATIENT CARE
N/A

PREVENTION
• There are no vaccines available.
• MV-free accreditation programs are in existence in some European countries.
• Serologic testing and segregation of positive reactors are used to reduce prevalence; in some cases eradication is performed.
• Retesting every 3–6 months and elimination of new positive reactors is necessary until 3–5 consecutive tests result in 100% of sheep being negative.
• Yearly testing and acquisition of replacements from MVV-free flocks are recommended.
• Reappearance of occasional positive reactors years after eradication has been documented.
• Reporting requirements for MV differ between countries.
• Lentiviruses are very susceptible to environmental factors and are destroyed by common disinfectants.

☑ **MISCELLANEOUS**

ASSOCIATED CONDITIONS
N/A

AGE-RELATED FACTORS
Clinical signs are seen more often in sheep 2–3 years of age or older.

ZOONOTIC POTENTIAL
N/A

PREGNANCY
N/A

BIOSECURITY
Acquire replacement animals from SRLVs-free herds.

PRODUCTION MANAGEMENT
N/A

SYNONYM
Visna-maedi

ABBREVIATIONS
- AGID = agar gel immunodiffusion test
- CAEV = caprine arthritis encephalitis virus
- ELISA = enzyme-linked immunosorbent assay
- MVV = maedi-visna virus
- OPP = ovine progressive pneumonia
- OvLV = ovine lentivirus
- PCR = polymerase chain reaction
- SRLVs = small ruminant lentiviruses

SEE ALSO
- Caprine Arthritis Encephalitis Virus
- Johne's Disease
- Ovine Pulmonary Adenocarcinoma
- Respiratory Disease: Small Ruminant

Suggested Reading
Cardinaux L, Zahno ML, Deubelbeiss M, Zanoni R, Vogt HR, Bertoni G. Virological and phylogenetic characterization of attenuated small ruminant lentivirus isolates eluding efficient serological detection. Vet Microbiol 2013, 162: 572–81.
Clawson ML, Redden R, Schuller G, et al. Genetic subgroup of small ruminant lentiviruses that infects sheep homozygous forTMEM154 frameshift deletion mutation $A4_{\Delta}53$. Vet Res 2015, 46: 22.
de la Concha-Bermejillo A. Maedi-Visna and ovine progressive pneumonia. Vet Clin North Am Food Anim Pract 1997, 13: 13–33.
de la Concha-Bermejillo A, Brodie SJ, Magnus-Corral S, Bowen RA, DeMartini JC. Pathologic and serologic responses of isogeneic twin lambs to phenotypically distinct lentiviruses. J Acquir Immune Defic Syndr Hum Retrovirol 1995, 8: 116–23.
Herrmann-Hoesing LM, White SN, Broughton-Neiswanger LE et al. Ovine progressive pneumonia virus is transmitted more effectively via aerosol nebulization than oral administration. Open J Vet Med 2012, 2: 113–19.
Minguijón E, Reina R, Pérez M, et al. Small ruminant lentivirus infections and diseases. Vet Microbiol 2015, 181: 75–89.

Author Andrés de la Concha-Bermejillo
Consulting Editor Erica C. McKenzie

M

MALIGNANT CATARRHAL FEVER

BASICS

OVERVIEW
Malignant catarrhal fever (MCF) is an often lethal, acute and rarely chronic, viral infection that affects many species or the order Artiodactyla, which is caused by different members of the genus Macavirus, subfamily Gammaherpesvirinae; Ovine herpesvirus 2 and Alcelaphine herpesvirus 1. It is characterized by lymphoproliferation and inflammation of mucosas and blood vessels.

INCIDENCE/PREVALENCE
Varies according to the species. Very low morbidity and high mortality (>90%) in cattle. Variable morbidity and high mortality in bison. High morbidity and mortality within cervidae.

GEOGRAPHIC DISTRIBUTION
Worldwide distribution. OvHV-2 is found in wild and domestic sheep and goats. AlHV-1 is found in Africa and is widely distributed in zoological and wildlife parks.

SYSTEMS AFFECTED
- Multisystemic
- Digestive
- Urinary
- Hemolymphatic
- Respiratory

PATHOPHYSIOLOGY
- At least six member of the MCFv subfamily are pathogenic in natural conditions, of which AlHV-1 and OvHV-2 are the most prevalent.
- OvHV-2 is found in sheep and goats; AlHV-1 is found in wildebeest, which are well-adapted species and are able to spread the disease.
- Susceptibility varies depending on the affected species.
- Well-adapted, nonclinically susceptible reservoir hosts are capable of replicating and shedding the virus in the environment to clinically susceptible, poorly adapted hosts, which neither replicate nor shed the virus, and are considered dead-end hosts.
- The virus is shed through feces and ocular and nasal secretions into the environment.
- Nasal, ocular, and fecal contamination is common, and the virus is cell associated.
- There is serologic evidence of the infection, which should be evaluated together with clinical signs and lesions.
- Serologic evidence supports the theory that deer and cattle may become subclinically infected and the disease can be precipitated following stress or concurrent infection.
- Transmission is primarily horizontal and through direct contact. In wildebeest, transmission is vertical and horizontal.
- Long-distance transmission has been described. Traditional recommendations for spatial separation between sheep/goats/wildebeest and susceptible species are difficult to apply.
- Incubation period ranges from weeks to months, which is associated with viral dose exposure.
- CD8+ T-lymphocytes are the predominant cell associated with vascular lesions and lymphoid hyperplasia.

HISTORICAL FINDINGS
Susceptible species (cattle, bison, wild ruminants) grazing with reservoir species (sheep, goats, wildebeest). Long-distance transmission of aerosolized OvHV-2 has been described.

SIGNALMENT
- Susceptibility varies depending on the affected species.
- Wildebeest, sheep, and goats act as asymptomatic carrier species.
- AlHV-1 affects cattle and deer; OvHV-1 affects cattle deer, bison, swine, and giraffes.
- Domestic cattle, Indian gaur, Javan banteng or Balinese cattle, swamp or water buffaloes, American bison, red deer, sika deer, white-tailed deer, mule deer, axis deer, Pere David's deer, red brocket deer, rusa deer, water deer, Chinese water deer, mooses and pigs, among others.
- Frequently in animals >1 year, occasionally in 6-month-old to 1-year-old, rare in younger animals.

PHYSICAL EXAMINATION FINDINGS
- Depression and fever (1–3 days), followed by a serous to purulent oculonasal discharge.
- In all species, ulceration of the coronet, interdigital skin, teats, vulva, and perineum may occur.
- Dyspnea, open-mouth breathing; keratitis with corneal opacity and hypopion resulting in photophobia and partial blindness; upper respiratory and oral ulcers, with erosions of the buccal papillae and profuse mucopurulent nasal and conjunctival discharge; severe dysentery and diarrhea; neurologic signs may occur, with hyperesthesia, muscle fasciculation, and aggressive behavior; generalized lymphadenopathy, fever, epithelial bleeding, and ulcers.
- In highly susceptible animals, depression, separation from the herd, hematuria, diarrhea, and blood in feces.
- Sudden death can be observed, without premonitory signs.
- Disseminated intravascular coagulation is observed in different species.
- Fever, nystagmus, weakness, tremors, paralysis, lameness, vasculitis, mucopurulent nasal and conjunctival discharge, dyspnea, dysentery and diarrhea, oral and upper respiratory ulcers, hypopion, sudden death, generalized lymphadenopathy, and muzzle encrustation.

CAUSES AND RISK FACTORS
- MCF is caused by two different members of the genus Macavirus, subfamily Gammaherpesvirinae; Ovine herpesvirus 2 and Alcelaphine herpesvirus 1.
- The virus is spread from sheep, goats, and wildebeest to cattle, bison, deer, and other wild ruminants through shared grazing contact. Dissemination though aerosolized virus has also been proposed.
- Most sick animals will succumb to the disease. Cattle surviving the disease may have proliferative arteriopathy in medium-sized arteries and corneal lesions, which may evolve to perforating ulcers.
- Nasal, ocular, and fecal contamination is common and is thought to be spread by fomites.
- Direct contact of susceptible species (cattle, bison, wild ruminants) with reservoir species (sheep, goat, wildebeest).

DIAGNOSIS

DIFFERENTIAL DIAGNOSES
Vesicular diseases, foot and mouth disease, rinderpest, vesicular stomatitis, BVD/mucosal disease, IBR, Bluetongue, epizootic hemorrhagic disease, East Coast tick fever (*Theileria parva*) encephalitis, shipping fever, arsenic toxicity, C naphthalene toxicity, rabies, yersiniosis, tick-borne diseases.

CBC/BIOCHEMISTRY/URINALYSIS
- CBC initially will show lymphocytosis with subsequent lymphopenia.
- When severe tissue damage is evident, neutrophilia occurs.

OTHER LABORATORY TESTS
- Polymerase chain reaction (PCR) on peripheral leukocytes in nonclotted blood samples.
- Serologic tests: Virus neutralization, immunoblotting, enzyme-linked immonosorbent assay (ELISA), competitive inhibition ELISA (current choice), immunofluorescence assay, immunoperoxidase test, and complement fixation test. Serologic results should be interpreted in context, considering the pathologic features of MCF.
- Buffy coat analysis for virus isolation.

OTHER DIAGNOSTIC PROCEDURES
- Clinical signs and typical lesions, combined with a recent history of exposure to a reservoir host, are sufficient to make a presumptive diagnosis of MCF.
- Gross and histopathologic findings.
- PCR is highly specific and is the best test for the determination of carriers in a clinically normal population, and for the postmortem diagnosis of the disease.
- Immunofluorescence is used in research settings.

PATHOLOGIC FINDINGS
- Gross findings: Corneal opacity and hypopion; muzzle crusting; mucopurulent

nasal and ocular discharge; reddening of oral and nasal mucosas; multifocal to coalescing ulcers in the oral cavity, esophagus, rumen, reticulum, omasum, abomasum; ulcerative enteritis/colitis, with bloody contents; lymphadenomegaly (not a prominent feature in bison); swollen kidneys with pale focal raised areas; hemorrhagic cystitis; enlarged liver; disseminated hemorrhages.
• Histopathology: In addition to ulcerative lesions, disseminated vasculitis with fibrinoid necrosis of the vascular wall and thrombosis is common, together with multisystemic lymphoplasmacytic infiltrates (portal areas in liver, renal interstitium, myocardium, lung, brain). Lymph nodes may be hyperplastic with prominent paracortical areas (not a prominent feature in bison).

TREATMENT

THERAPEUTIC APPROACH
• No treatment is available. Cattle can recover without treatment.
• No vaccine is available.

MEDICATIONS

DRUGS OF CHOICE
Vitamins, antibiotics, corticosteroids, and antivirals have been attempted. The role of these treatments in recovery is uncertain, as animal can recover without treatment.

FOLLOW-UP

EXPECTED COURSE AND PROGNOSIS
• Disease course is generally 3–7 days; sudden death may occur.
• Prognosis is grave.

• Low morbidity and high mortality. Outbreaks with high morbidity and mortality have been described in highly susceptible species (e.g., bison).

CLIENT EDUCATION
• Physically separate susceptible species from sheep, goats, and wildebeest in known infective areas.
• Wildlife population may also spread the disease, so ensuring separation is essential to prevent disease introduction.

PREVENTION
• In areas affected by MCF, do not graze sheep, goats, and wildebeest with cattle, deer, or bison.
• Elimination of fomites, especially those contaminated with postparturient fluids, is essential. Insect control is also indicated.

MISCELLANEOUS

ZOONOTIC POTENTIAL
None

PREGNANCY
Abortion may occur in sick animals.

SYNONYMS
• Catarrhal fever
• Gangrenous coryza
• Malignant head catarrh
• Snotsiekte

ABBREVIATIONS
• AlHV-1 = Alcelaphine herpesvirus 1.
• BDV/MD = bovine viral diarrhea/mucosal disease
• ELISA = enzyme-linked immunosorbent assay
• MCF: malignant catarrhal fever
• OvHV-2: Ovine herpesvirus 2
• PCR = polymerase chain reaction

SEE ALSO
• Arsenic Toxicosis
• Bluetongue Virus
• Bovine Viral Ddiarrhea Virus
• Foot and Mouth Disease
• Infectious Bovine Rhinotracheitis
• Rabies

Suggested Reading

Li H, Cunha CW, Taus NS, Knowles DP. Malignant catarrhal fever: Inching toward understanding. Annu Rev Anim Biosci 2014, 2: 209–33.

O'Toole D, Li H. The pathology of malignant catarrhal fever, with emphasis on Ovine Herpesvirus 2. Vet Pathol 2014, 51: 437–52.

Li H, Karney G, O'Toole D, Crawford TW. Long distance spread of malignant catarrhal fever virus from feedlot lambs to ranch bison. Can Vet J 2008, 49: 183–5.

O'Toole D, Li H, Miller D, Williams WR, TB Crawford. Chronic and recovered cases of sheep-associated malignant catarrhal fever in cattle. Vet Rec 1997, 140: 519–24.

Author Francisco R. Carvallo
Consulting Editor Christopher C.L. Chase
Acknowledgment The author and book editors acknowledge the prior contribution of Dan Grooms.

M

MANAGEMENT OF GUNSHOT WOUNDS

BASICS

OVERVIEW
• The pathology associated with gunshot wounds (GSWs) can vary dramatically with the anatomic location(s) of the injury, type of firearm, and the ballistics (shape, weight, stability in flight, and velocity) associated with the bullet.
• Radiographs or other imaging modalities are often indicated to assist in patient evaluation. GSWs may be minor and heal with little or no intervention, may require significant medical and/or surgical intervention, or may be fatal with or without treatment.
• The degree of tissue injury depends on bullet weight, velocity, and the affected tissues' expansile ability.
• Injuries from GSWs should be treated as though they are contaminated wounds.

INCIDENCE/PREVALENCE
Sporadic

GEOGRAPHIC DISTRIBUTION
Worldwide

SYSTEMS AFFECTED
Multisystemic

PATHOPHYSIOLOGY
• Varies with anatomic location of injury, type of firearm, and ballistics of the bullet.
• Hemothorax and pneumothorax may occur with penetrating thoracic GSWs.
• Penetrating abdominal wounds may result in septic peritonitis secondary to disruption of hollow viscera.

HISTORICAL FINDINGS
History of GSW may or may not be known.

SIGNALMENT
All ruminant species

PHYSICAL EXAMINATION FINDINGS
Clinical signs are variable and dependent upon anatomic location of GSWs. Some animals may not show clinical signs, and GSWs may be inapparent or difficult to detect during physical examination. Evidence of hemorrhage may or may not be visible. Clinical signs may include:
• Hemodynamic instability
• Dyspnea
• Hemoptysis
• Epistaxis
• Hematuria
• Hematochezia or melena
• Lameness
• Limb fracture
• Neurologic impairment
• Nonspecific signs consistent with pain, including lethargy, depression, hypo/anorexia, and/or vocalizing. Dorsoflexion may also indicate thoracic or abdominal pain.

GENETICS
N/A

CAUSES AND RISK FACTORS
Wound severity is a function of bullet or projectile size, shape, velocity, and tissue characteristics.

Bullet Velocity
• Velocity is the most important single factor responsible for wound damage.
• Impact velocity is the speed at which the bullet meets target tissue and is important to wound characteristics.
• When impact velocities are low (non-military-civilian bullets) wounds have less tissue damage and do not exhibit explosive effect. High-velocity injuries can exhibit explosive effects.
• High-impact velocity wounds reflect maximum tissue destruction with remote injury.

Bullet Mass
• Projectile kinetic energy varies directly with the mass of the bullet.

Ballistic Shape
• Bullets of different weights, shapes, and calibers do not pass through the air in similar patterns.

Bullet Composition
• Soft-point bullets will mushroom or expand upon impact.
• Hollow-point bullets behave similarly to soft-point jacketed bullets and will mushroom or expand upon impact.

Bullet Yaw
• Yaw results from inherent asymmetry of the bullet.
• Yaw in part explains the aberrant bullet wounds seen in veterinary practice. Yaw is magnified in animal tissues.

Tissue Reaction
• Tissue retentiveness to the passing bullet contributes to its severity. Wound extent is determined by the projectile's energy upon impact and tissue energy transfer. An entering bullet's kinetic energy is transferred to the surrounding tissue when producing the wound.
• Tissue elasticity, cohesiveness, and density properties tend to oppose the bullet's inertia and slow it down.

Tissue Elasticity
• Tissues of different densities variably alter the kinetic energy transfer.
• Tissue absorption of the kinetic energy is the determinant of wound severity.

Tissue Cohesiveness
• Penetrating wounds reflect sufficient tissue resistance to cause dissipation of the bullet's kinetic energy.
• Perforating wounds reflect the difference between energy at wound entry and that remaining at exit.

Tissue Density
• Damage to bone may result from the bullet striking the long bone directly. Effects depend on the type of bone structure, the physical characteristics of the bullet, and the periosteal supporting structures.
• "Indirect fracture" occurs when a high-velocity bullet passes near a bone but does not strike it directly.

DIAGNOSIS

DIFFERENTIAL DIAGNOSES
Vary with affected system(s)

CBC/BIOCHEMISTRY/URINALYSIS
• Full CBC and serum biochemistry panel may be helpful to determine extent of blood loss, presence of organ damage, and evidence of systemic infection in valuable animals.
• PCV/TP alone may be helpful to determine the extent of blood loss; serial PCV/TP may be required for monitoring of animals with uncontrolled internal or external hemorrhage.

OTHER LABORATORY TESTS
As needed

IMAGING
• Radiographs are recommended for all cases of GSW. Anatomic location of projectile(s) or fragments is important in formulating prognosis.
• Ultrasound may assist in identifying abnormal fluid accumulation(s) in cases with thoracic or abdominal cavity involvement.
• In very valuable animals, CT may also be helpful in assessing extent of internal organ involvement and bullet/pellet location.

OTHER DIAGNOSTIC PROCEDURES
History and thorough physical examination (entrance/exit wounds)

PATHOLOGIC FINDINGS
Variable and dependent upon anatomic location(s) of injury, type of firearm, and ballistics of projectile.

TREATMENT

THERAPEUTIC APPROACH
• Varies with anatomic location and extent of injury.
• Hemothorax and pneumothorax may be managed with medical treatment including thoracocentesis or thoracostomy tube, or may require surgical intervention. Ruminants with thoracic GSWs that are hemodynamically stable and eupneic generally do not require a thoracotomy.
• Penetrating abdominal wounds usually warrant exploratory laparotomy or celiotomy, to thoroughly evaluate and repair damaged viscera. GSWs to the abdomen carry a high risk of septic peritonitis.
• Antimicrobials are often indicated as GSWs are usually contaminated with dirt, hair, and skin fragments.

M

• Whole blood transfusion may be necessary in cases with severe or uncontrolled hemorrhage.
• Conservative treatment is often sufficient in limb wounds not associated with fractures. Wounds should be allowed to heal as open wounds, or repaired surgically after infection has been controlled.
• Extremity wounds could require tissue debridement. Thorough irrigation with physiologic saline to remove surface debris and contaminants is indicated. Excision of devitalized exposed skin, muscle, and fascia may be warranted. Foreign bodies should be removed. In severe cases, limb amputation may be warranted.
• Fracture treatment varies. Casts or splints may be sufficient in some cases, while other fractures could necessitate surgical intervention, limb amputation, or even euthanasia.
• Euthanasia may be indicated for animals with GSWs.

SURGICAL CONSIDERATIONS AND TECHNIQUES
See "Therapeutic Approach"

MEDICATION

DRUGS OF CHOICE
• Antimicrobial choice varies with location of GSW and affected species of animal. Consider drug regulations when making this selection.
• Analgesics and anti-inflammatories as needed.
• Aminocaproic acid may be helpful in controlling active hemorrhage. This drug is not labeled in food-producing animals in most countries and therefore no milk or meat withdrawal times have been established.
• Whole blood transfusions may be indicated in some animals.
• Fly repellent may be required with open wounds.

PRECAUTIONS
• Appropriate milk and meat withdrawal times must be followed for all medications administered to food-producing animals.

CONTRAINDICATIONS
N/A

POSSIBLE INTERACTIONS
N/A

FOLLOW-UP

EXPECTED COURSE AND PROGNOSIS
• Highly variable dependent on anatomic location of wound(s), severity of injury, type of treatment (medical vs. surgical), and degree of wound contamination.
• Limb wounds are rarely fatal.

POSSIBLE COMPLICATIONS
• Hemo- or pneumothorax from thoracic GSWs.
• Septic peritonitis from abdominal GSWs.
• Wound infection(s).
• In GSWs from a shotgun, pellets decelerate rapidly, resulting in severe damage over a wide area. Extensive devitalization of skin and/or musculature secondary to vascular disruption may occur.

CLIENT EDUCATION
N/A

PATIENT CARE
Dependent upon anatomic location of wound(s), severity of injury, and type of treatment (medical vs. surgical).

PREVENTION
Following rules regarding firearm safety may prevent accidental GSWs.

MISCELLANEOUS

ASSOCIATED CONDITIONS
• Lead toxicosis following GSWs is rare but has been reported in humans. Clinical signs could develop if one or more lead bullets or fragments remain in the animal.
• Ruminants with lead poisoning have a potentially long meat and/or milk withdrawal period; periodic blood lead testing is advisable in these cases prior to entering the food chain.

ABBREVIATIONS
• GSW = gunshot wound
• PCV = packed cell volume
• TP = total protein

SEE ALSO
• Anesthesia: Local and Regional
• Euthanasia and Disposal (Appendix 2)
• Extralabel Drug Use and Compounding (see www.fiveminutevet.com/ruminant)
• Pain Management (see www.fiveminutevet.com/ruminant)
• Wound Management

Suggested Reading
Bebchuk TN, Harari J. Gunshot injuries: pathophysiology and treatments. Vet Clin North Am Small Anim Pract 1995, 25: 1111–26.
Dicpinigaitis PA, Fay R, Egol KA, Wolinsky P, Tejwani N, Koval KJ. Gunshot wounds to the lower extremities. Am J Orthop 2002, 31: 282–93.
Doherty MA, Smith MM. Contamination and infection of fractures resulting from gunshot trauma in dogs: 20 cases (1987–1992). J Am Vet Med Assoc 1995, 206: 203–5.
Fullington RJ, Otto CM. Characteristics and management of gunshot wounds in dogs and cats: 84 cases (1986–1995). J Am Vet Med Assoc 1997, 210: 658–62.
Olsen LE, Streeter EM, DeCook RR. Review of gunshot injuries in cats and dogs and utility of a triage scoring system to predict short-term outcome: 37 cases (2003–2008). J Am Vet Med Assoc 2014, 245: 923–8.
Velmahos GC, Demetriades D, Cornwell EE 3rd. Transpelvic gunshot wounds: routine laparotomy or selective management? World J Surg 1998, 22: 1034–8.
Vincent J, DiMaia M. Gunshot Wounds: Practical Aspects of Firearms, Ballistics and Forensic Techniques. Boca Raton, FL: CRC Press, 1999.
Author Katharine M. Simpson
Consulting Editor Kaitlyn A. Lutz

M

MASTITIS: CAMELIDS

BASICS

OVERVIEW
• Mastitis occurs in camelids, with the dairy dromedary camel being most commonly affected.
• Different forms have been reported including clinical (severe gangrenous, acute, chronic) and subclinical.
• Various pathogens have been isolated with species, environment, housing, management, and regional differences.
• There is more focus on udder infection and raw milk quality as the camel dairy industry continues to develop as camel dairy products are sought out for health purposes.

INCIDENCE/PREVALENCE
• Low prevalence of mastitis in South American camelids. Isolated cases have been reported both in llamas and alpacas.
• In the dromedary, the prevalence of clinical mastitis ranges from 2 to 8%. The herd and quarter prevalence of subclinical mastitis in camels range from 5% to 40%. Higher prevalence of subclinical mastitis (>60%) is observed in traditionally managed dairy camels.

GEOGRAPHIC DISTRIBUTION
Worldwide, infectious agents vary depending on environment and management.

SYSTEMS AFFECTED
• Mammary
• Multisystemic

PATHOPHYSIOLOGY
• Mastitis is an inflammation of the mammary gland tissue, usually associated with a bacterial infection.
• Several Gram-positive and Gram-negative bacteria have been isolated from cases of clinical and subclinical mastitis.
• Infection is generally ascendant but may also result from hematogenous spread (*Corynebacterium pseudotuberculosis, Mycobacterium bovis*).
• Infection results in tissue damage, and decreased quality and quantity of milk production.
• Irreversible changes and loss of function may be observed with chronic infections.
• Rarely, severe acute inflammation of the mammary gland will result in systemic disease and endotoxemia.
• Mammary gland abscesses may develop in some infections (fungal infection, *C. pseudotuberculosis, M. bovis*).

HISTORICAL FINDINGS
• Poor production
• Ill-thrift or poor growth of the cria or calf
• Abnormal conformation or enlargement of the mammary gland
• Lameness or other systemic signs in acute cases

SIGNALMENT
• More common in camels (*Camelus dromedarius* and *C. bactrianus*), rarely seen in llamas and alpacas
• Camels used for traditional dairying

PHYSICAL EXAMINATION FINDINGS
• Clinical signs vary from absent to various degrees of visible changes depending on type of mastitis and etiological agent.
• Clinical mastitis: The mammary gland presents various degrees of swelling, redness, hardening, and pain upon palpation. Lameness may be seen in some cases. Severe toxic mastitis may be accompanied by fever, depression, and dehydration. The mammary gland secretions may be serous, hemorrhagic, or purulent.
• Chronic mastitis: Hardening of the gland, poor milk production, asymmetry of the quarter, abnormal shape of the gland and cisterns.
• Subclinical mastitis: There are no visible clinical signs but usually an alteration of milk color and consistency. Abscesses may be felt. Some glands may present as a blind (nonfunctional) teat or quarter.

GENETICS
Some breeds of dairy camel due to mammary gland conformation and high production

CAUSES AND RISK FACTORS

Major Pathogens
• Clinical mastitis: *Staphylococcus aureus,* coagulase-negative *Staphylococcus* spp., *E. coli, C. pseudotuberculosis, Streptococcus zooepidemicus* (alpacas and llamas).
• Subclinical mastitis: *Staphylococcus aureus,* coagulase-negative *Staphylococci, Streptococcus agalactiae, Streptococcus dysgalactiae, Bacillus* spp., *Proteus* spp., *E. coli.*
• Fungal mastitis (*Candida* spp., *Aspergillus* spp.) occurs sporadically in acute and chronic mastitis.
• *Corynebacterium pseudotuberculosis* causes mammary abscesses in camelids.
• *Mycobacterium tuberculosis, M. bovis* (camels, alpacas).
• *Klebsiella* spp. mastitis has been described in camels.
• Peracute, toxic mastitis due to *E. coli* has been described in camels.

Risk Factors
• Poor mammary gland conformation
• Increased risk with parity
• Early stages of lactation
• Poor milking hygiene
• Environmental: corral hygiene, animal density, bedding
• Tick infestation (camels)
• Association with other disease such as camel pox
• Use of soiled harness to prevent suckling by the calf (camels)

DIAGNOSIS

DIFFERENTIAL DIAGNOSES
• Sepsis or endotoxemia in cases of toxic mastitis
• Other causes of mammary gland swelling: adenocarcinoma or trauma (rare)

CBC/BIOCHEMISTRY/URINALYSIS
• CBC may show toxic changes in acute and peracute mastitis.
• Serum biochemistry shows electrolyte disturbances.
• Severely depressed animals may show signs of hepatic lipidosis.

OTHER LABORATORY TESTS
• Gross examination of secretions shows changes in color (bloody or purulent) and consistency.
• Cytologic examination of milk shows increased leukocytes and causative organisms.
• Milk pH may be increased.
• Subclinical mastitis may be diagnosed by CMT (70% sensitivity and 91% specificity in camels) or SCC. SCC interpretation is difficult. Camel milk contains a large proportion of anucleated cell fragments. The use of non-DNA-specific methods such as particle counters or methylene blue staining results in overestimation of cell count.

IMAGING
Ultrasonography may be helpful in identifying mammary gland tissue changes and abscesses.

OTHER DIAGNOSTIC PROCEDURES
N/A

PATHOLOGIC FINDINGS
• Clinical mastitis: Mammary gland tissue inflammation, focal necrosis, granulomas
• Subclinical mastitis: Damaged or sloughed alveolar epithelium

TREATMENT

THERAPEUTIC APPROACH
Dependent on type of mastitis. Acute or peracute mastitis may require intensive care and hospitalization.

SURGICAL CONSIDERATIONS AND TECHNIQUES
• Surgical drainage of abscesses may be indicated
• Mastectomy in cases of severe gangrenous or chronic suppurative mastitis

MEDICATIONS

DRUGS OF CHOICE
Treatment is indicated in cases of clinical mastitis according to the following guidelines:

M

• Milk stripping
• Proper systemic (IM or IV) antimicrobial therapy based on culture and sensitivity. IMM antibiotic therapy is not practical due to the anatomy of mammary gland in these species
• Anti-inflammatory drugs
• Fluid therapy in cases of endotoxemia

CONTRAINDICATIONS
N/A

PRECAUTIONS
• Some drugs (NSAIDs and aminoglycosides) are nephrotoxic in camelids.
• Camel milk is a major source of nutrition for people in several countries. Withdrawal times for milk and meat are lacking but should be taken into consideration

POSSIBLE INTERACTIONS
N/A

FOLLOW-UP

EXPECTED COURSE AND PROGNOSIS
• Prognosis is good in subclinical mastitis
• Prognosis is guarded for severe or chronic mastitis

POSSIBLE COMPLICATIONS
N/A

CLIENT EDUCATION
• Hygiene of milking (camels)

• Regular evaluation of the mammary gland particularly if neonate shows poor growth or signs of gastrointestinal disease (llamas and alpacas)

PATIENT CARE
N/A

PREVENTION
• Cull production animals with severe damage from known contagious agents
• Regular testing (CMT, SCC)
• Observe proper milking hygiene

MISCELLANEOUS

ZOONOTIC POTENTIAL
Many infectious agents can cause sickness also in humans, particularly with consumption of raw milk. Tuberculosis and brucellosis are major concerns.

BIOSECURITY
Testing of purchased lactating animals

ABBREVIATIONS
• CMT = California Mastitis Test
• IM = intramuscular
• IMM = intramammary
• IV = intravenous
• NSAIDs = nonsteroidal anti-inflammatory drugs
• SCC= somatic cell count

SEE ALSO
• Mastitis (by organism)
• Mastitis: Milking Procedures and Teat Disinfection (see www.fiveminutevet.com/ruminant)
• Mastitis: Pharmacology (see www.fiveminutevet.com/ruminant)

Suggested Reading
Al-Dughaym AM, Fadlelmula A. Prevalence, etiology and its seasonal prevalence of clinical and subclinical camel mastitis in Saudi Arabia. Br J Appl Sci Technol 2015, 9: 441–9.
Regassa A, Golicha G, Tesfaye D, Abunna F, Megersa B. Prevalence, risk factors, and major bacterial causes of camel mastitis in Borana zone, Oromia Regional state, Ethiopia. Trop Anim Health Prod 2013, 45: 1589–95.
Nagy P, Faye B, Marko O, Juhasz J. Microbiological quality ad somatic cell count in bulk milk of dromedary camels (*Camelus dromedarius*): Descriptive statistics, correlations, and factors of variation. J. Dairy Sci 2013, 96: 5625–40.
Rowan LL, Morin DE, Hurley WL, et al. Evaluation of udder health and mastitis in llamas. J Am Vet Med Assoc 1996, 209: 1457–63.
Author Ahmed Tibary
Consulting Editor Kaitlyn A. Lutz

M

MASTITIS: COLIFORM

BASICS

OVERVIEW
Acute coliform mastitis (ACM), the most common cause of mastitis in dairy herds, is of significant importance to farm economics and welfare. *Escherichia coli, Enterobacter aerogenes, Klebsiella pneumoniae,* and *Serratia marcesans* are four common coliform bacteria that cause mastitis. Coliform bacteria are normal inhabitants of the soil, digestive tract, and manure. They accumulate and multiply in contaminated bedding. Acute coliform mastitis occurs primarily during first trimester and less commonly during the dry period. Cow-to-cow transmission has minimal impact on disease transmission. The majority (60–80%) of coliform mastitis results in intramammary infection whereas only 15–23% results in acute systemic signs.

INCIDENCE/PREVALENCE
Herd susceptibility to infection is the greatest at 2 weeks after drying off and 2 weeks prior to parturition; however, the majority of the infection during the dry period does not lead to clinical cases but is persistent and leads into acute coliform mastitis immediately after parturition. Incidence of acute coliform mastitis during lactation varies with the herd, determined by various risk factors such as husbandry practices, stage of lactation, season, age, and previous exposure. A well-managed herd has as low as 1–2 clinical mastitis cases in 100 milking cows per month, and the incidence of acute coliform mastitis is 1 –2 cases in 100 lactating cows per year. Coliform-induced acute mastitis, on the other hand, has higher rate of death and agalactia-related culling which ranges from 30% to 40% of cases, compared with other forms of mastitis.

GEOGRAPHIC DISTRIBUTION
Spatial distribution of coliform mastitis has not been established yet but temperature and precipitation are the factors affecting the incidence rate. Coliform mastitis is more common in tropical areas with high precipitation than in temperate and dry areas.

SYSTEMS AFFECTED
Mammary

PATHOPHYSIOLOGY
Infection occurs when coliform bacteria invade the mammary gland through the teat canal, most commonly immediately after milking. Bacteria multiply rapidly in the mammary gland and release the potent toxin commonly called "endotoxin." Increased level of endotoxin in the mammary gland changes the vascular permeability, resulting in acute swelling of the gland. Extravasation (diapedesis) of neutrophils in the affected quarter follows within a few hours of infection. Neutropenia and leukopenia is the immunologic response to clear the bacteria. Tissue healing starts 24 hours after the action of immunologic cells. Acute release of endotoxin leads to systemic effects such as anorexia, fever, diarrhea, and death in some cases. Local effects include changes in the color and consistency of the milk. This may lead on into the chronic form of mastitis with agalactia.

HISTORICAL FINDINGS
Increases in coliform mastitis may be seen following wet weather, changes in milking routines, worsened housing hygiene, or changes in drying-off treatment.

SIGNALMENT
• Any species of large or small, domestic or wild ruminant.
• Most prevalent and clinically relevant in high-yielding dairy cattle and goats.
• Primarily lactating cows, immediately after drying-off and a few weeks before parturition.

PHYSICAL EXAMINATION FINDINGS
• Signs vary in severity from those involving only localized changes of the mammary gland and secretion, to those involving systemic signs of peracute septicemia with a death rate of 5–15%.
• Varying levels of heat, pain, swelling, and discoloration of the infected gland(s). The majority of cases of ACM (>70%) are localized to the udder and exhibit only mild, if any, systemic signs of disease. Affected glands may be warm, firm, and swollen, often with an abnormal secretion.
• Milk closely resembles serum. Additional manifestations can include the presence of flakes, clots, or blood.
• General systemic signs can include fever, anorexia, sunken eyes, ruminal stasis, diarrhea, dehydration, and recumbency.
• Signs of septicemia can include petechiation or scleral injection, injected mucus membranes with toxic ring at gingival margins, prolonged capillary refill time, hypothermia, tachycardia, and altered mentation (depression, coma).

CAUSES AND RISK FACTORS
• Poor sanitation and environmental hygiene
• Poor milking hygiene (milking wet udders, use of communal towels to dry teats, etc.)

DIAGNOSIS

DIFFERENTIAL DIAGNOSES
Acute mastitis characterized by swelling and pain can be caused by numerous organisms in addition to coliforms. A partial list includes *S. agalactiae, S. aureus, S. dysgalactiae, S. uberis, Clostridium* spp*., and Bacillus* spp. Common conditions that may be manifest by signs of septicemia (in addition to coliform mastitis) include metritis, peritonitis, and pneumonia.

CBC/BIOCHEMISTRY/URINALYSIS
• CBC is variable and may include hemoconcentration, leukocytosis with neutrophilia, left shift, and leukopenia with neutropenia. Toxic changes to neutrophils may also be observed (Doehle bodies, toxic granulation, cytoplasmic vacuolization, and basophilia).
• Hyperfibrinogenemia.
• Nonspecific changes in serum biochemical parameters may include hypocalcemia, hypokalemia, hypergammaglobulinemia, and hyper- or hypoglycemia.

OTHER LABORATORY TESTS
• Milk bacterial culture.
• Blood bacterial culture. *Note:* In cows suffering severe ACM, positive blood cultures may isolate coliform organisms originating from the mammary gland or noncoliform organisms (e.g., *Bacillus* spp*., Pasteurella* spp.), which presumably originate from other organ systems (e.g., respiratory, gastrointestinal).

IMAGING
N/A

OTHER DIAGNOSTIC PROCEDURES
California Mastitis Test (CMT): Useful in detecting increased somatic cell count (SCC) in cases of subclinical mastitis.

PATHOLOGIC FINDINGS
Gross and histologic postmortem findings either can be confined to local mammary changes associated with inflammation or may include signs of sepsis.

TREATMENT

THERAPEUTIC APPROACH
• ACM is likely to respond to conservative therapy including frequent stripping of the affected gland, administration of anti-inflammatory agents, and oral fluid therapy (e.g., 16–24 liters of water containing 8 oz NaCl, 2 oz KCl, and 12 oz calcium propionate).
• Use of systemic antimicrobials with intravenous fluid therapy is recommended in ACM when bacteremia is suspected. IV fluid therapy will aid in flushing of endotoxin, produced by both live and dead Gram-negative bacteria, which otherwise may cause significant and irreversible organ damage.
• In severely affected cows exhibiting marked systemic signs, fluid therapy is an important consideration. Since oral administration is generally ineffective in cows with marked gastrointestinal stasis, intravenous administration is preferred. The type and volume of fluid for intravenous administration should be based on abnormalities in blood parameters and clinical interpretation. Most cows with ACM are

(CONTINUED)

hypoglycemic, hypocalcemic, hypokalemic, and alkalotic.
• Administration of hypertonic saline (7.5% NaCl, 5 mL/kg or 1–2 L per adult cow) is a reasonable alternative to administration of large volume intravenous fluids. This must always be followed by adequate oral fluids (20–40 L per adult cow).

SURGICAL CONSIDERATIONS AND TECHNIQUES
N/A

 MEDICATIONS

DRUGS OF CHOICE
• Ceftiofur (1.1–2.2 mg/kg, IM, SC, q24h)
Note: IM administration is preferred in dehydrated patients (IV administration in cattle is prohibited in the USA based on current labeling).
• Oxytetracycline (6–10 mg/kg IV, IM, SC, q24h)
Note: IV administration is preferred in dehydrated patients. Administer slowly.
• Flunixin meglumine (1.1–2.2 mg/kg, IV, q12–24h)

CONTRAINDICATIONS
N/A

PRECAUTIONS
• Appropriate milk and meat withdrawal times must be followed for all compounds administered to food-producing animals.
• Flunixin meglumine and oxytetracycline both can cause renal toxicity in the compromised patient and therefore fluid therapy is essential when treating with these medications.

 FOLLOW-UP

EXPECTED COURSE AND PROGNOSIS
• The majority of cows diagnosed with ACM resolve within 5 days of treatment and return to production.
• Cows with marked systemic signs and prolonged disease have a guarded to poor prognosis.
• Cows with marked systemic signs and concurrent bacteremia have a poor to grave prognosis.

POSSIBLE COMPLICATIONS
Possibility of persistent infections

CLIENT EDUCATION
Awareness of the client about the good animal husbandry practices and maintaining the farm hygiene dramatically reduces the incidence of ACM. Clients should be aware of using milking machine only after the drying of the teats.

PATIENT CARE
Monitor local changes to mammary gland and secretion.

PREVENTION
• Insure proper environmental hygiene.
• Insure proper premilking and milking hygiene.
• Provide fresh, palatable feeds and management conditions to help insure that cows remain standing for approximately 30 minutes after milking to allow formation of the keratin plug prior to lying.

 MISCELLANEOUS

ASSOCIATED CONDITIONS
Apart from the involvement of the mammary gland, fever and shock leading to death are associated with severe coliform mastitis cases. Agalactia is also common in acute coliform mastitis.

AGE-RELATED FACTORS
Acute coliform mastitis is common in the first three lactation periods, but repeated exposure to the coliform bacteria reduces the chances of ACM at a later age.

ZOONOTIC POTENTIAL
Coliform agents can be zoonotic.

PREGNANCY
Bacteremia develops in a substantial proportion of cows with ACM concurrently showing systemic signs and possible abortion.

BIOSECURITY
• Isolation of the infected animal from the herd
• Immediate clean-up of areas that could be a source of bacteria
• Good husbandry practices by the workers on the farm

PRODUCTION MANAGEMENT
• Avoid using fine beddings such as sawdust for 3 weeks before and after calving.
• Provide adequate space per individual.
• Avoid wet milking using excessive water and no drying before milking time.
• Avoid excessive liner slippage at the end of milking from dirty and wet teats.

ABBREVIATIONS
• ACM = acute coliform mastitis
• CMT= California Mastitis Test
• IM = intramuscular
• IV = intravenous
• KCl = potassium chloride
• NaCl = sodium chloride
• SC = subcutaneous

SEE ALSO
• Fluid Therapy: Oral
• Mastitis (by species and etiology)

Suggested Reading
Cebra CK, Garry FB, Dinsmore RP. Naturally occurring acute coliform mastitis in Holstein cattle. J Vet Int Med 1996, 10: 252–7.
Gonzalez RN, Cullor JS, Jasper DE, et al. Prevention of clinical coliform mastitis in dairy cows by a mutant *Escherichia coli* vaccine. Can J Vet Res 1989, 53: 301.
Laven R. Treatment of *Escherichia coli* mastitis: are antibiotics needed? Livestock 2013, 18: 59–62.
Smith KL, Todhunter DA, P. S. Schoenberger PS. Environmental mastitis: cause, prevalence, prevention 1, 2. J Dairy Sci 1985, 68: 1531–53.
Tyler JW, Cullor JS. In: Smith BP ed, Large Animal Internal Medicine, 3rd ed. St. Louis: Mosby, 2002.
Wenz JR, Barrington GM, Garry FB, Dinsmore RP. Use of systemic disease signs to assess disease severity in dairy cows with acute coliform mastitis. J Am Vet Med Assoc 2001, 218: 567–72.
Wenz JR, Barrington GM, Garry FB, et al. Bacteremia associated with naturally occurring acute coliform mastitis in dairy cattle. J Am Vet Med Assoc 2001, 219: 976–81.
Author Suvash Shiwakoti
Consulting Editor Kaitlyn A. Lutz

M

MASTITIS: FUNGAL

BASICS

OVERVIEW
• Yeast and fungi are part of soil and water microflora, and opportunistic pathogens (if given the opportunity) will colonize the udder resulting in intramammary infection.
• Infections are usually sporadic, opportunistic, and limited to affected glands.
• Antimicrobials are suspected to depress host defense mechanisms and stimulate fungal growth.
• Most cases of fungal mastitis are mild and self-limiting; however, cases involving *Cryptococcus neoformans* can result in severe mastitis and permanent damage to the mammary gland.

INCIDENCE/PREVALENCE
Fungal mastitis is seen in ruminants, with low frequencies of occurrence; the true incidence is unknown.

GEOGRAPHIC DISTRIBUTION
Worldwide

SYSTEMS AFFECTED
• Mammary
• Hemolymphatic

PATHOPHYSIOLOGY
Opportunistic etiologic agents include *Candida* spp. (77% of cases), *Cryptococcus* spp., and *Prototheca* spp. algae. Rare genera include *Trichosporon, Aspergillus, Torulopsis, Saccharomyces, Rhodotorula, Pichia*, and *Hansenula*.

HISTORICAL FINDINGS
• Sharp drop in milk yield
• Anorexia
• Positive California Mastitis Test (CMT)
• Lack of positive response to antibiotic therapy
• Subclinical cases in herd mates are common.

SIGNALMENT
Potentially, females of all species used for milk production.
Lactating animals. The likelihood of infection increases with parity and is most often seen in the second month of lactation.

PHYSICAL EXAMINATION FINDINGS
• Abnormal mammary secretions (often watery secretions containing clots and flakes)
• Inflammation of the affected gland
• Fever (often spiking at 104–106°F, 40–41°C)

GENETICS
There is no evidence of genetic predisposition.

CAUSES AND RISK FACTORS
• Yeasts and fungi often gain entrance into the mammary gland through nonhygienic administration of intramammary antibiotics for treatment of bacterial mastitis.
• Injured or damaged regions of the mammary gland can provide the opportunity

for colonization by environmental yeast and fungi.
• Previous bacterial mastitis increases host susceptibility to fungal mastitis.
• Fungal mastitis is seen with milking machine malfunction and is associated with teat end damage.
• Inadequately sanitized milking units may act as fomites and result in epidemic infections.
• There is increased incidence and severity during warm, wet environmental conditions conducive to pathogen growth.
• The most common etiologic agents of fungal mastitis are *Cryptococcus neoformans* and *Candida albicans*. Others include:
  ◦ *Candida* spp.
  ◦ *Trichosporon beigelii*
  ◦ *Trichosporon cutaneum*
  ◦ *Rhodotorula* spp.
  ◦ *Hansenula holisti*
  ◦ *Hansenula polymorpha*
  ◦ *Hansenula anomala*

DIAGNOSIS

Diagnosis of fungal mastitis should be made based upon milk culture.

DIFFERENTIAL DIAGNOSES
Confusion and misidentification between prototexal mastitis and fungal mastitis is common based on colony morphology. Prototheca is an alga, which produce colonies similar to *Cryptococcus neoformans*.

CBC/BIOCHEMISTRY/URINALYSIS
• Leukocytosis and neutrophilia were found in experimental infections.
• Elevated urine ketones are possible with anorexia.

OTHER LABORATORY TESTS
Positive California Mastitis Test (CMT)

Microbiologic Laboratory Tests
• *Candida albicans:* Fermentation of various sugars
• *Cryptococcus neoformans:* Production of the enzyme urease and the assimilation of carbon substrates

Candida albicans
• *Germ tube test:* Rapid and reliable. This test utilizes media in which blastospores of *C. albicans* are suspended in serum and incubated at 37°C for 2–3 hours. The suspension must be examined between 2–3 hours for the presence of hyphal outgrowths.
• *Culture on cornmeal agar at 25°C:* Upon microscopic analysis, *C. albicans* will form chlamydospores, which are morphologically unique.

Cryptococcus neoformans
• *Direct culture:* *C. neoformans* is inhibited by cyclohexamide, but grows well on standard nonselective mycologic media. Identification is made on the presence of a capsule. Direct

culture is the definitive test for identifying *C. neoformans*.
• *India ink preparation:* Upon microscopic examination, *C. neoformans* appears as a budding yeast or single cell with a clear halo surrounding it due to the presence of a polysaccharide capsule.

IMAGING
N/A

OTHER DIAGNOSTIC PROCEDURES
• Direct microscopic examination of colonies or mammary secretions reveals yeast and fungi to be morphologically different from bacterial bacilli or cocci.
• The presence of hyphae or spores on direct microscopic examination of defatted milk smears renders a positive diagnosis.
• Predominant cultures on blood and/or Sabouraud's agar at 25°C or 37°C, respectively, are suggestive of a positive diagnosis.
• Both yeast and *Prototheca* are larger than bacteria, with yeast having buds and *Prototheca* being multinucleate.
• In the event of available histologic sections, Gomori methenamine silver (GMS) and periodic acid-Schiff (PAS) stains highlight morphology.
• Fluorescent antibody staining can be used with sections and cultures.

TREATMENT

THERAPEUTIC APPROACH
No effective and approved treatments are available for fungal mastitis (see "Medications"). Some general recommendations are as follows:
• Stop antibiotic therapy upon diagnosing fungal mastitis.
• Milking infected animals separately, sterilizing milking units between animals, and CMT testing may reduce spread to herd mates.
• Frequent milking/stripping of affected teat(s) increases the chances of a more favorable prognosis.

MEDICATIONS

DRUGS OF CHOICE
• Fungal mastitis is usually self limiting; however, clinically recovered cows may shed yeast/fungi for up to 8 months.
• Fungal mastitis is refractory to most drug treatments and there is little evidence to support such therapy in modifying the course of disease.
• Antipyretics (flunixin meglumine 1.1–2.2 mg/kg IV, q24h) are useful to help reduce high fevers and inflammation. Follow label

directions and abide by meat and milk withdrawal periods.
• Antimycotic drugs have been used; however, there exists no substantial evidence in regard to the efficacy of antimycotic drug therapy. There are no approved antimycotic treatments for fungal mastitis in milking animals in most countries. Prudent withdrawal times should be utilized.
• Intravenous sodium iodide (66 mg/kg body weight IV once per week) and oil-based intramammary iodine solutions have been reported to be of some value.
• While resistant to most antibiotics, experimental *Prototheca* infections have been treated with limited success using tertamisole hydrochloride or levamisole hydrochloride.

CONTRAINDICATIONS

Appropriate milk and meat withdrawal times must be followed for all compounds administered to food-producing animals.

FOLLOW-UP

EXPECTED COURSE AND PROGNOSIS
• Due to loss of production and persistent shedding, culling is a consideration.
• There is often irreversible tissue damage with near complete agalactia.
• Fungal mastitis does not respond well to antimicrobials.
• Tissue damage and infection are usually confined to the affected gland with rare systemic infections.

POSSIBLE COMPLICATIONS
There are rare incidences of systemic mycosis.

CLIENT EDUCATION
Unresolving cases of mastitis should be cultured rather than treated empirically.

PATIENT CARE
Monitoring temperature and milk secretions in addition to follow-up milk cultures are useful to gauge therapy effectiveness.

PREVENTION
• During the administration of antibiotics one should wear clean gloves, clean the teat end thoroughly prior to administration, and only use single-dose, sterile intramammary tubes in accordance to labeled instructions.
• Teat end hygiene is extremely important in preventing fungal contamination.
• Cull persistently infected animals.
• Use aseptic udder infusion techniques.
• Reduce environmental organic matter buildup.
• Practice aseptic milking hygiene.

MISCELLANEOUS

ASSOCIATED CONDITIONS
Bacterial and mycoplasmal mastitis

AGE-RELATED FACTORS
Incidence of fungal mastitis increases with parity.

PREGNANCY
Sodium iodide may lead to abortion.

PRODUCTION MANAGEMENT
• Yeasts and fungi compose part of the normal makeup of the soil and environmental microflora and, if given the opportunity, will colonize the udder resulting in intramammary infection.
• Injured or damaged teat or mammary gland can provide the opportunity for the colonization of environmental yeast and fungi.
• Affected cows should be culled from the herd.

ABBREVIATIONS
• CMT = California Mastitis Test
• GMS = Gomori methenamine silver
• IV = intravenous
• PAS = periodic acid-Schiff
• USDA/FDA = United States Department of Agriculture/Food and Drug Administration

SEE ALSO
• Mastitis: Involvement of Milking Equipment and Stray Voltage (see www.fiveminutevet.com/ruminant)
• Mastitis: Milking Procedures and Teat Disinfection (see www.fiveminutevet.com/ruminant)
• Mastitis: No Growth
• Mastitis: Pharmacology (see www. fiveminutevet.com/ruminant)

Suggested Reading
Casia dos Santos R, Marin JM. Isolation of Candida spp. from mastitic bovine milk in Brazil. Mycopathologia 2005, 159: 251–53.
Corbellini LG, Driemeier D, Cruz C, Dias MM, Ferreiro L. Bovine mastitis due to *Prototheca zopfii*: clinical epidemiological and pathological aspects in a Brazilian dairy herd. Trop Anim Health Prod 2001, 33: 463–70.
Erskine RJ, Kirk JH, Tyler JW, DeGraves FJ. Advances in the therapy for mastitis. Vet Clin North Am Food Anim Pract 1993, 9: 499–517.
Gonzalez RN. Prototheca, yeast, and Bacillus as a cause of mastitis. National Mastitis Council, www.nmconline.org/articles/prototheca.htm
Perez V, Corpa JM, Garcia Marin JF, Aduriz JJ, Jensen HE. Mammary and systemic aspergillosis in dairy sheep. Vet Pathol 1998, 35: 235–40.
Timony JF, Gillespie JH, Scott FW, Barlough JE. Hagen and Bruner's Microbiology and Infectious Diseases of Domestic Animls. 8th ed. Ithaca: Comstock Publishing Cornell University Press, 1988, pp. 407–19.
Watts JL. Etiological agents of bovine mastitis. Vet Microbiol 1988, 16: 41–66.
Author Michael Goedken
Consulting Editor Kaitlyn A. Lutz
Acknowledgment The author and book editors acknowledge the prior contribution of Gabriel J. Rensen.

M

MASTITIS: MINOR BACTERIA

BASICS

OVERVIEW
• The National Mastitis Council considers the primary minor bacterial mastitis pathogens to be *Corynebacterium bovis*, *Trueperella pyogenes* (formerly *Arcanobacterium pyogenes*) and *Nocardia* spp.
• Other uncommon bacterial causes of mastitis to be considered here are coagulase-negative *Staphylococcus* (CNS) spp., *Pseudomonas aeruginosa*, and *Serratia* spp.
• *Pseudomonas* spp. are found in organic bedding and water and can contaminate water sources, milking equipment, and rubber parts in hoses and the milking system.
• Sources of *Nocardia* spp. are soil, water, and udder skin.
• The reservoir for *Corynebacterium bovis* is normal teat skin and infected udders. Cases of *Corynebacterium bovis* mastitis are often associated with inadequate teat dipping or sanitizing.
• Purulent discharge from wounds, teat injuries, and abscesses are the major sources for *Trueperella pyogenes* infections.
• *Serratia* spp. are saprophytes and found in soil and plants.
• Most of the mastitis-causing CNS spp. are associated on teat skin.

INCIDENCE/PREVALENCE
Usually sporadic

GEOGRAPHIC DISTRIBUTION
Varies due to regional differences in housing, milking sanitation, intramammary treatments, teat dips, and use of pasture. "Summer mastitis" is seen with *Trueperella* infections of cows on pasture in Europe.

SYSTEMS AFFECTED
Mammary

PATHOPHYSIOLOGY
• Mastitis is inflammation of the mammary gland, usually as a result of bacterial infection. Pathogens gain entry into the gland either through ascending colonization of the streak canal (*Streptococcus* spp. and *Staphylococcus* spp.), by reverse-impaction during machine milking, or by contaminated intramammary treatments.
• Infection in the gland results in tissue damage either as the direct effect of infection in cells (e.g., *Staphylococcus* spp.) or from the immune response to the pathogen (e.g., Gram-negative bacteria).
• Inflammatory responses range from mild to severe, depending on the bacteria, the infectious dose, and the host immune function. Within the gland, the response can range from coagulation of milk or serum proteins (gargut), damage or destruction of

secretory tissue, blockage of ductules with necrotic debris and purulent material, endothelial leakage of serum and blood, fibrosis, abscess formation, granulomatous lesions to gangrene.
• Extravasation (diapodesis) of white blood cells, primarily neutrophils, into the gland results from chemotactic signals by macrophages (the primary leukocyte in healthy glands).
• The leukocyte response, or SCC, is a useful measure of inflammation in the mammary gland.
• Infections from CNS and *Corynebacterium* usually result in mild to moderate inflammation and the gland returns to normal after the infection is cleared.
• Infections from *Nocardia* spp., *Trueperella pyogenes*, *Pseudomonas aeruginosa*, and *Serratia* spp. often cause serious tissue damage and can become chronic with abscesses or granuloma formation (*Nocardia*).

SIGNALMENT
• Cattle; occasionally sheep and goats.
• Adults; *Corynebacterium bovis* can affect heifers prepartum.
• There are no breed predilections.

HISTORICAL FINDINGS
• Post-milking dipping of teats with non-iodine products is commonly associated with *Corynebacterium* and *Serratia* mastitis.
• Intramammary infusions with nonsterile products.

PHYSICAL EXAMINATION FINDINGS
• Palpation of the mammary gland reveals swelling, heat, firmness, or pain. The milk secretion may have small flakes or large pieces of gargut, actual pus (in the case of *Trueperella*), or may be watery from serum leakage into the gland (with *Serratia*).
• Abscesses or granulomas may be palpable (especially with *Nocardia*).
• Fever and tachycardia are usually present in acute infections but not in chronic mastitis.
• Decreased milk production.

GENETICS
N/A

CAUSES AND RISK FACTORS
• Contaminated intramammary infusions, bedding, or water used to sanitize teats or milking machines.
• Not employing post-milking teat dipping, improper teat dipping, or the use of ineffective teat dip preparations are associated with *Corynebacterium* and *Serratia* mastitis.
• Hyperkeratosis or damaged teat ends predispose for CNS mastitis.
• Maintaining cows with *Trueperella* or *Nocardia* mastitis with draining abscesses in the herd may also lead to infection.
• Using common medications for intramammary infusion rather than individual treatment tubes.

• Warm, moist organic bedding (*Pseudomonas* and *Serratia*).

DIAGNOSIS

DIFFERENTIAL DIAGNOSES
° Subclinical cases: *Streptococcus agalactia*, *Corynebacterium bovis*, and minor udder pathogens.
° Corynebacteria isolates from milk samples may represent teat streak canal colonization rather than infected glands.
° Clinical cases: Coliform bacteria, mycoplasma, or environmental streptococci.
° Gangrenous mastitis with bloody secretion: Trauma to the gland.
° Acute mastitis: A partial list includes *S. agalactiae*, *S. aureus*, *S. dysgalactiae*, *S. uberis*, *Clostridium* spp., and *Bacillus* spp.
° Common conditions that may be manifest by signs of septicemia (in addition to coliform mastitis) include metritis, peritonitis, and pneumonia.

CBC/BIOCHEMISTRY/URINALYSIS
N/A

OTHER LABORATORY TESTS
• SCC or CMT of milk from quarter or composite samples will indicate if excessive inflammation is present. SCC >200,000, CMT score of 2 or 3, or a log-linear score >4 indicates mastitis is present.
• Other indirect tests include the NAGase test (N-acetyl-β-D-glucosamidase) and electrical conductivity.
• Electrical conductivity is less sensitive due to normal variation of ions in milk.
• Microbiologic testing of an aseptically collected milk sample from the affected gland is the only way to determine the causative organism.
° Direct microbiology using suitable media is the most common method of determining the genus and often the species of bacteria involved in cases of mastitis.
° PCR techniques are becoming commercially available and are useful in determining species and subtypes of bacteria.

IMAGING
Ultrasound of the teat canal may be a helpful adjunct to diagnosis.

OTHER DIAGNOSTIC PROCEDURES
Finding inflammation in the mammary gland during physical examination or seeing abnormal milk secretion.

PATHOLOGIC FINDINGS
Gross pathology will show inflamed tissue in the affected glands, ranging from discoloration to fibrosis to severe tissue damage.

(CONTINUED) | **MASTITIS: MINOR BACTERIA**

TREATMENT

THERAPEUTIC APPROACH
• *Corynebacterium* and CNS spp. may self-cure but treatment with commercial intramammary antibiotics is advised.
• *Serratia* spp. and *Pseudomonas* mastitis usually respond poorly to antibiotic treatment.
• *Nocardia* and *Trueperella* mastitis is often refractory to treatment due to abscessation and purulent material.

MEDICATIONS

DRUGS OF CHOICE
Commercial mastitis preparations are advised for cases of *Corynebacterium* and CNS mastitis.

CONTRAINDICATIONS
N/A

PRECAUTIONS
Appropriate milk and meat withdrawal times must be followed for all compounds administered to food-producing animals.

POSSIBLE INTERACTIONS
N/A

FOLLOW-UP

EXPECTED COURSE AND PROGNOSIS
• Complete recovery of normal mammary tissue after treatment for cases of *Corynebacterium* and CNS spp. mastitis. *Corynebacterium* mastitis infections often are not associated with increased SCC.
• *Serratia*, *Nocardia*, and *Trueperella* mastitis usually become chronic.

POSSIBLE COMPLICATIONS
N/A

PATIENT CARE
Monitor for eating, drinking, reduction of inflammation in the gland, and return of normal milk secretion.

CLIENT EDUCATION
See "Causes and Risk Factors" and "Prevention"

PREVENTION
• Minimize risk factors.
• Vaccination with rough mutant Gram-negative vaccines (e.g., J-5) may reduce the severity and incidence of *Serratia* mastitis.

MISCELLANEOUS

ZOONOTIC POTENTIAL
Nocardia spp. infections are zoonotic and cultures should be considered dangerous. Colonies should be killed with formalin before opening the plates for examination.

SYNONYMS
• "Summer mastitis" for *Trueperella pyogenes* mastitis.
• "Environmental Staphylococcus" or "other Staphylococcus" for "CNS spp."

ABBREVIATIONS
• CMT = California Mastitis Test
• CNS = coagulase-negative *Staphylococcus*
• NAGase = N-acetyl-β-D-glucosamidase
• PCR = polymerase chain reaction
• SCC = somatic cell count

SEE ALSO
Mastitis (by species and etiology)

Suggested Reading
Barkema HW, Schukken YH, Lam TJ, Beiboer ML, Benedictus G, Brand A. Management practices associated with the incidence rate of clinical mastitis. J Dairy Sci 1999, 82: 1643–54.

Bexiga R, Pereira H, Pereira O, Leitão A, Carneiro C, Ellis KA, Vilela CL. Observed reduction in recovery of *Corynebacterium* spp. from bovine milk samples by use of a teat cannula. J Dairy Res 2011, 78: 9–14.
Gonçalves JL, Tomazi T, Barreiro JR, et al. Effects of bovine subclinical mastitis caused by *Corynebacterium* spp. on somatic cell count, milk yield and composition by comparing contralateral quarters. Vet J 2016, 209: 87–92.
Laboratory Handbook on Bovine Mastitis. National Mastitis Council, Inc. Madison, WI. 1999.
Levison LJ, Miller-Cushon EK, Tucker AL, et al. Incidence rate of pathogen-specific clinical mastitis on conventional and organic Canadian dairy farms. J Dairy Sci 2016, 99: 1341–50.
Radostits OM, Gay CC, Hinchcliff KW, Constable PD, eds. Veterinary Medicine: A Textbook of Diseases of Cattle, Sheep, Pigs, Goats and Horses, 10th Ed. London: Saunders, 2007.
Sargeant JM, Scott HM, Leslie KE, Ireland MJ, Bashiri A. Clinical mastitis in dairy cattle in Ontario: frequency of occurrence and bacteriological isolates. Can Vet J 1998, 39: 33–8.
Wilson DJ, Herer PS, Sears PM. N-acetyl-beta-D-glucosaminidase, etiologic agent, and duration of clinical signs for sequential episodes of chronic clinical mastitis in dairy cows. J Dairy Sci 1991, 74: 1539–43.

Author Jim P. Reynolds
Consulting Editor Kaitlyn A. Lutz

M

MASTITIS: MYCOPLASMAL

BASICS

OVERVIEW
• Inflammation of the mammary gland due to infection by various *Mycoplasma* spp.
• Mycoplasmas are contagious mastitis pathogens that can cause clinical, subclinical, and chronic intramammary infections (IMI).
• Spread primarily animal to animal at milking.
• *Mycoplasma bovis* is the most important agent of outbreaks of mycoplasmal mastitis in dairy cattle, but other species may cause mastitis outbreaks clinically indistinguishable from *M. bovis*.
• *M. agalactiae* is the primary etiologic agent of mycoplasmal mastitis in small ruminants and it is reportable in the United States. *M. mycoides* subsp. *mycoides* (large-colony type), *M. capricolum* subsp. *capricolum*, and *M. putrifaciens* are goat specific.
• Unresponsive to antibiotic therapy and has the potential to cause severe losses in milk production.
• This chapter will focus on mycoplasmal mastitis in cattle, with much of the information being applicable to small ruminants. See chapter, Mastitis: Small Ruminant, for more specific information on mycoplasma in small ruminants.

INCIDENCE/PREVALENCE
• The incidence/prevalence is variable among geographic regions and among herds in a region. There is a wide variation in quarter infection rates in herds. The condition is endemic in some areas.
• Based upon culture of a single bulk tank sample, prevalence estimates for mycoplasma mastitis in US dairy herds ranges from 1% to 10%.
• Most studies report a higher prevalence in large herds (>500 cows) compared to smaller herds.

GEOGRAPHIC DISTRIBUTION
Worldwide

SYSTEMS AFFECTED
Mammary

PATHOPHYSIOLOGY
• Mycoplasmas lack a cell wall and, therefore, are not affected by antimicrobials which act via an effect on the cell wall.
• The most common source of IMI due to mycoplasmas is the udder of infected cows.
• *Mycoplasma* spp. are commonly spread from infected cows to uninfected cows at milking via milking machines or milkers' hands.
• Mycoplasmal udder infections usually persist through the current lactation and into subsequent lactations.
• Mycoplasmas are present in the respiratory and urogenital tracts of healthy cattle and may serve as a source of IMI.

• Contaminated intramammary treatments or improper teat sanitation during or at the end of lactation are also means of new infections.
• Infection results in a purulent interstitial mastitis.
• Most damage in mycoplasmal mastitis is from the cow's immune response. However, metabolic by-products and toxins from mycoplasmas also contribute to tissue damage and reduction of milk production.
• Inflammatory cells accumulate in alveoli and ducts and reduce duct lumen space. Cells in alveoli regress and fluid accumulates, with an attendant drop in milk production. In the most severe reactions, fibrous tissue replaces alveoli and ducts, resulting in a permanent loss.
• Multiple abscesses, variable in size, can be found in cases of mastitis caused by *M. bovis*. These abscesses may contain *M. bovis*, which can cause long-term shedding.
• Mycoplasmas are sensitive to heat, sunlight, and environmental pressures but can survive on teat skin and in cool, moist, and protein-rich environments for variable periods.

HISTORICAL FINDINGS
• Classically, severe clinical mastitis in multiple quarters (often in multiple cows) without systemic involvement.
• Subclinical, clinical, and/or chronic mastitis.
• Lack of response to therapy.

SIGNALMENT
• *M. bovis* is highly adapted to the bovine species, with uncommon isolations reported from buffaloes and small ruminants.
• Mycoplasmal mastitis is a common cause of contagious mastitis in dairy sheep and goats.
• All ruminant species are potentially susceptible to mycoplasmal mastitis.
• No breed, age, or lactational stage predilections exist for mycoplasmal mastitis.

PHYSICAL EXAMINATION FINDINGS
• Sudden onset of swelling of the udder.
• Grossly abnormal milk. Appearance varies, ranging from normal to watery with clots, to tan or brown with flakes. However, the majority of milk samples positive for mycoplasmas are grossly normal.
• Sharp decrease in milk production, sometimes dramatic.
• Lack of systemic signs; maintenance of appetite and thirst.
• Mild fever is often present initially but is rarely observed in clinical cases.
• Agalactia/atrophy.
• Increased somatic cell count (SCC).
• Purulent mastitis (sometimes severe) without systemic signs.
• Supramammary lymph nodes may be enlarged.
• Acute arthritis with swollen joints and lameness.
• Multiple quarter involvement; sometimes all quarters are involved.

GENETICS
N/A

CAUSES AND RISK FACTORS
• Infection of the mammary gland with various species of mycoplasma. As few as 70 colony-forming units of *M. bovis* introduced via the teat canal can initiate mastitis.
• *M. bovis* is the most significant and common mycoplasmal agent of bovine mastitis although up to 11 species have been cultured from mastitis milk in the US including *M. alkalescens, M. arginini, M. bovigenitalium, M. bovirhinis, M. californicum, M. canadense, M. dispar,* and *M. capricolum*.
• Characteristics of mastitis produced by various *Mycoplasma* spp. are generally similar and cannot be distinguished clinically.
• *M. agalactiae* is the primary etiologic agent in dairy sheep and goats; *M. mycoides* subsp. *capri, M. capricolum* subsp. *Capricolum,* and *M. putrefaciens* are also commonly isolated.
• The purchase of replacement heifers and cows is frequently the origin of mycoplasmal mastitis outbreaks in previously *Mycoplasma*-free herds.
• Large herd size (>500 cows) is associated with an increased prevalence of positive mycoplasma cultures in bulk tank milk (BTM) samples.
• Outbreaks often originate in the hospital barn/string due to poor hygiene when performing intramammary treatments. Homemade mastitis treatments have also been associated with outbreaks of mycoplasmal mastitis.
• Cattle with the highest risk of infection are purchased cattle, fresh cows and heifers, and cattle that enter the treatment barn/string.
• Herds with and without mycoplasmal mastitis may contain both young and mature asymptomatic carriers.

DIAGNOSIS

DIFFERENTIAL DIAGNOSES
• *Staphylococcus aureus* mastitis
• Fungal mastitis
• Caprine arthritis and encephalitis virus infection in goats
• Other causes of chronic mastitis nonresponsive to antibiotic therapy

CBC/BIOCHEMISTRY/URINALYSIS
Marked leukopenia may be present in cases of acute infection.

OTHER LABORATORY TESTS
SCC numbers markedly increase in the milk. Often, secretions contain over 20 million cells/mL.

IMAGING
N/A

OTHER DIAGNOSTIC PROCEDURES
• Diagnosis is most commonly made using microbiologic procedures on aseptically

(CONTINUED)

MASTITIS: MYCOPLASMAL

collected quarter or composite milk samples or on culture of bulk tank milk samples.

• Isolation is most commonly attempted using direct inoculation onto plates containing modified Hayflick medium. Plates are incubated in moist 10% CO_2 at 35–37°C. They are observed for growth with a microscope at intervals after plating. Plates are not called negative for growth until incubated for 7–10 days. Intermittent shedding by carriers not demonstrating symptoms may make diagnosis difficult.

• Diagnosis of infection at the herd level is usually made by isolation of mycoplasmas from BTM samples.

• In large herds, culture of partial BTM samples collected after milking each production group or the use of string sampling or milk-line sampling may be used as a method to locate groups in which cows infected with mycoplasmas exist.

• Large numbers of mycoplasmas are usually present in milk samples from cows with clinical disease.

• False-negative diagnosis may occur in BTM because dilution could mask several low-level *Mycoplasma* shedders in the herd.

• Milk samples for culture of *Mycoplasma* must be collected aseptically, kept cool during transportation to the diagnostic laboratory or storage, and plated promptly to maximize isolation.

• If delay of more than 1 day is anticipated from collection to culturing, milk samples should be frozen at –30°C or below to assure viability, or stored in liquid nitrogen.

• Mycoplasmal colonies have a fried-egg appearance on solid medium because colonies have a dense, central core that grows down into the medium.

• The polymerase chain reaction (PCR) is a highly sensitive, specific, and rapid procedure for laboratory diagnosis, but several practical problems must be solved before full-scale adoption of this diagnostic procedure.

• Mycoplasmal shedding in milk will not impact the standard plate count (SPC), preliminary incubation count (PIC), or the laboratory pasteurized count (LPC).

PATHOLOGIC FINDINGS

• The pathology in mycoplasmal mastitis is most commonly described as a purulent interstitial mastitis.

• Widespread, scattered fibrosis and granulomatous changes with pus are found in the gland. Teat sinus and ductular linings are seen as thick and rough.

• Evidence of granulomatous mastitis is seen on histopathology.

TREATMENT

There is no known effective treatment.

MEDICATIONS

DRUGS OF CHOICE
N/A

CONTRAINDICATIONS
N/A

FOLLOW-UP

EXPECTED COURSE AND PROGNOSIS

• Cows diagnosed as positively infected should be considered positive for life.

• Some cows may become agalactic and/or develop complications (e.g., arthritis, etc.), may continue in production and produce normal-appearing milk with a high SCC, may be chronically infected with abnormal milk, or may return to production, go through a dry period, and calve again, still shedding mycoplasmas.

POSSIBLE COMPLICATIONS
N/A

CLIENT EDUCATION
See "Prevention" and "Production Management"

PATIENT CARE
N/A

PREVENTION

• Mycoplasmas survive for variable, but sometimes extensive, periods of time on teat skin and multiple environmental sites.

• Isolate or quarantine new additions.

• Culture new additions using procedures described under "Other Diagnostic Procedures."

• Investigate herd of origin of any animals brought into the herd.

• If milk from animals was not cultured at purchase, milk from these animals should be cultured as they calve.

• Culture all clinical cases of mastitis and all fresh cows for mycoplasma and screen bulk tank samples for mycoplasmas.

• Workers should practice strict hygienic milking and intramammary treatment procedures.

• Avoid any use of bulk intramammary treatment.

• Effective vaccines for mycoplasmal infections are not available.

Control

• There are divergent opinions and practices with respect to management and control of mycoplasmal mastitis.

• Due to the contagious nature of *Mycoplasma* spp. and its resistance to therapy, many owners elect to cull infected animals in order to limit new infections in the herd.

• Mode of handling will vary from dairy to dairy based on the owner's attitude, facilities,

number of infected animals, level of milk production, reproductive status of carrier animals, and the availability of replacements.

• Control of the disease, when present, is often based upon finding infected cows via culture of all lactating and dry cows in the herd, as well as all clinical cases and all animals at calving.

• An alternative approach is to use culture of bulk tank milk or string/group samples to identify infected groups. Alternative strategies have been proposed to deal with mycoplasmal mastitis.

Types of Approaches to Consider

If mycoplasma is diagnosed in a herd, there are two general types of approaches to be considered:

• Attempt to eliminate the organism from the herd:
  ° Culture all cows, identify infected animals, and cull those infected, (particularly if the number is limited).
  ° Culture milk from cows at dry-off, freshening, and from all clinical cases.
  ° Culture bulk tank milk at appropriate intervals to monitor new infections.
  ° Do not move cows between production groups until all cows have been cultured and classified as infected or uninfected (realizing limitations of a single culture).

• Limit spread of the disease:
  ° Separate mycoplasma-positive cows, and milk them last or with separate equipment.
  ° Cull cows with clinical mastitis or decreased production.
  ° Strict milking time hygiene—*M.* spp. is passed by fomites, such as the milking machine, hands, wash cloths.
  ° Culture milk for mycoplasmas—fresh cows, clinical mastitis cases, dry cows, bulk tanks.
  ° Either don't feed mastitic milk to calves or feed only after pasteurization or acidification following current recommendations.
  ° Back-flushing of the milking equipment.
  ° Strict teat dipping.

MISCELLANEOUS

ASSOCIATED CONDITIONS

• Enzootic pneumonia of calves: An infectious respiratory disease of young calves of multifactorial etiology. More common in housed dairy calves than beef calves. Feeding of unpasteurized waste milk from mastitic cows may allow transmission of *Mycoplasma* spp. to calves and result in respiratory disease characterized by dyspnea, anorexia, and depression. Mycoplasmal infections are often accompanied by head tilt secondary to otitis media/interna.

• Arthritis: The incidence of mycoplasmal arthritis is increased in herds experiencing

M

MASTITIS: MYCOPLASMAL   (CONTINUED)

outbreaks of pneumonia or mastitis due to *Mycoplasma* spp. Lameness due to polyarthritis and/or tenosynovitis. Affected joints are warm, distended, fluctuant, and may be painful. Concurrent mycoplasmal pneumonia or mastitis is common.

AGE-RELATED FACTORS
N/A

ZOONOTIC POTENTIAL
Very limited reports of human infections. Not considered a major zoonotic pathogen.

PREGNANCY
N/A

BIOSECURITY
• Since many infections are introduced into a herd by bringing replacements onto a farm, quarantine of newly introduced animals and milk culturing, as well as careful investigation into the status of the herd of origin of any introduced animals, will help limit this possibility.
• Practice strict milking time hygiene. Transmission is primarily at milking by fomites such as milking machines, milkers' hands, and wash cloths.
• The organism can also be spread when bulk mastitis treatments are administered from a contaminated vial, via a contaminated syringe, or with unsanitary treatment practices.
• Practice thorough teat dipping, iodine products preferred by some for mycoplasmal herds.
• Assure milking machine is functioning to standards.
• Use single-service towels for drying cows.
• Use gloves, disinfect between cows.
• Use single-service intramammary treatments.
• Either do not feed mastitic milk to calves or feed only after pasteurizing or acidifying using current recommendations.
• Monitor appropriate milk samples for mycoplasmas: bulk tanks, clinical mastitis cases, fresh cows, introduced cows, etc.

PRODUCTION MANAGEMENT
• Many, if not most, new mycoplasmal mastitis infections are introduced when animals are brought into a herd.
• Most cases are introduced through the teat canal but mastitis has also been proposed to occur following hematogenous spread of a respiratory infection to the mammary gland.

• Feeding of unpasteurized mastitic milk to young stock may predispose to mycoplasmal pneumonia and arthritis.
• Infected cows should be identified by culture of composite or quarter milk samples from all milking cows. Dry cows should be cultured upon calving.
• Cows diagnosed with *Mycoplasma* IMI should be considered positive for life.
• Any management plan for mycoplasmal mastitis following a whole herd culture should include segregation and/or removal of infected animals from the herd.
• Removal of infected animals from the herd to slaughter is advised when prevalence of infection is low and segregation is not practical.
• Segregation can be used when prevalence of mycoplasmal mastitis is high in the herd and culling is not economically feasible, but needs adequate facilities and management, and monitoring of the herd by repeated culturing of animals and BTM.
• Segregated cows should be milked last or with a separate milking unit from those used on uninfected cows to minimize the risk of infection for other cows.
• Mycoplasmal mastitis can be controlled with testing and discipline in the management of the disease, including the understanding by dairy personnel of the seriousness of the disease and their role to minimize its spread.
• Culture all replacements entering the herd, cows and heifers at calving, all mammary quarters with signs of clinical mastitis, cows with persistent high SCC, and BTM frequently.
• Use strict milking hygiene, including the wearing of nitrile or latex gloves by milkers, foremilking, pre- and post-milking teat disinfection with a high-quality product that covers almost the entire teat, and single use of paper or cloth towels.
• Clearly identify each infected animal by using a double identification system like leg bands and ear tags.
• Cows with blind quarters harboring mycoplasmas can spread the disease in the herd with uninformed or careless milkers and make isolation inconsistent from BTM samples.
• Avoid stresses, like the pressure effects of transportation, overcrowding, calving, and milking, particularly for the first calvers

because they can be important contributors to the disease.
• A dairy's hospital pen or treatment group is usually a key area for spreading the disease when treatments are administered without following aseptic procedures, including disinfection of gloved hands between treated cows.

ABBREVIATIONS
• BTM = bulk tank milk
• IMI = intramammary infections
• LPC = laboratory pasteurized count
• PCR = polymerase chain reaction
• PIC = preliminary incubation count
• SCC = somatic cell count
• SPC = standard plate count

SEE ALSO
• Caprine Arthritis Encephalitis Virus
• Cleaning and Disinfection (see www.fiveminutevet.com/ruminant)
• Enzootic Pneumonia of Calves
• Mastitis (by species and organism)

Suggested Reading
Bürki S, Frey J, Pilo P. Virulence, persistence and dissemination of *Mycoplasma bovis*. Vet Microbiol 2015, 179: 15–22.
Fox LK. Mycoplasma mastitis: causes, transmission, and control. Vet Clin North Am Food Anim Pract 2012, 28: 225–37.
Gómez-Martín A, Amores J, Paterna A, De la Fe C. Contagious agalactia due to *Mycoplasma* spp. in small dairy ruminants: epidemiology and prospects for diagnosis and control. Vet J 2013, 198: 48–56.
González RN, Wilson DJ. Mycoplasmal mastitis in dairy herds. Vet Clin North Am Food Anim Pract 2003, 19: 199–221.
Kumar A, Rahal A, Chakraborty S, Verma AK, Dhama K. *Mycoplasma agalactiae*, an etiological agent of contagious agalactia in small ruminants: a review. Vet Med Int 2014, doi: 10.1155/2014/286752.
Maunsell FP, Woolums AR, Francoz D, et al. *Mycoplasma bovis* infections in cattle. J Vet Intern Med 2011, 25: 772–83.
Author Benjamin W. Newcomer
Consulting Editor Kaitlyn A. Lutz
Acknowledgment The author and book editors acknowledge the prior contribution of Kevin L. Anderson and Ruben N. Gonzalez.

MASTITIS: NO GROWTH

BASICS

OVERVIEW
Mastitis yielding no bacterial growth on standard culture media.

INCIDENCE/PREVALENCE
Ten percent to 40% of clinical cases of mastitis yield no growth on culture.

GEOGRAPHIC DISTRIBUTION
Worldwide

SYSTEMS AFFECTED
Mammary

PATHOPHYSIOLOGY
• Varies depending on etiology. Most cases of no growth clinical mastitis are thought to be caused by bacteria; however, various other etiologies are possible.
• In this case, the offending organism has already been eliminated by the cow's immune system prior to sampling. Antigen-based studies indicate that Gram-negative bacteria may be a more likely cause than Gram-positive bacteria; yet there is good evidence for both occurring.

HISTORICAL FINDINGS
• Abnormal milk
• Previous treatment for mastitis

SIGNALMENT
Typically seen in lactating ruminants but also can occur during the dry period and in prepartum heifers.

PHYSICAL EXAMINATION FINDINGS
• Signs are almost always restricted to changes in the milk, such as clots or flakes.
• Systemic signs in the animal are quite rare in true no-growth cases of clinical mastitis.

GENETICS
N/A

CAUSES AND RISK FACTORS
• Bacteriologic factors: Phagocytized bacteria (within white blood cells but alive), L-forms of *Staphylococcus aureus*.
• Sample handling: Antibiotic inhibition if sample taken post-treatment, freezer kill (*Escherichia coli* tends to be more susceptible than Gram-positive organisms), inappropriate culture medium (i.e., *Mycoplasma* and *Trueperella pyogenes* do not grow on blood agar), numbers of bacteria are too low to be detected by the quantity of milk cultured.
• Interpretation: Inaccurate assessment of the significance of culture growth reported as no growth.
• Other infectious etiologies: Caprine arthritis encephalitis virus, ovine progressive pneumonia, and maedi-visna can cause an indurative viral mastitis which is characterized by hypogalactia or agalactia.
• Noninfectious etiologies: Trauma such as bruises or contusions from environmental hazards resulting in perforations into the gland or teat.
• Risk factors are the same as other forms of mastitis. The major risk factor for trauma with subsequent clinical mastitis is a pendulous udder.

DIAGNOSIS

DIFFERENTIAL DIAGNOSES
• Bacteria cleared by immune system
• Bacteria alive but phagocytized
• Bacteria numbers too low to detect by standard culture methods
• L-forms (*S. aureus*)
• Viral (sheep and goats)
• Organism does not grow on standard media (*Mycoplasma,* anaerobes)
• Trauma (noninfectious)
• Antibiotic or milk product inhibition
• Storage kill
• Inaccurate interpretation of culture result

CBC/BIOCHEMISTRY/URINALYSIS
N/A

OTHER LABORATORY TESTS
• No additional tests need to be performed routinely on the initial or sporadic case of clinical mastitis that yields no growth, especially in herds with no history of *Mycoplasma* mastitis. However, specialized media should be utilized when multiple cases of clinical mastitis in a single cow or in a group of cows yield no growth.
• Specifically, samples should be cultured for *Mycoplasma* spp.

IMAGING
N/A

OTHER DIAGNOSTIC PROCEDURES
Aseptic milk samples may be sent to a diagnostic laboratory for further testing to include *Mycoplasma* species and differentiation of other microorganisms other than bacteria (yeast etc.).

PATHOLOGIC FINDINGS
N/A

TREATMENT

THERAPEUTIC APPROACH
• No specific therapy is warranted for cows with clinical mastitis with no growth as the culture result.
• Cases are usually mild with clots or flakes in the milk with no swelling of the affected quarter(s) and no systemic effects on the cow.

SURGICAL CONSIDERATIONS AND TECHNIQUES
N/A

MEDICATIONS

DRUGS OF CHOICE
• It is difficult to justify the use of antimicrobial drugs for cases of no-growth clinical mastitis.
• If treatment must be given, oxytocin, to aid milk-out should do no harm. There are no studies that document the beneficial effects of oxytocin in the treatment of clinical mastitis.
• Intramammary antibiotic therapy of clinical mastitis will usually occur prior to knowledge of culture results. This treatment does not appear to affect time to cure.

CONTRAINDICATIONS
N/A

PRECAUTIONS
• Appropriate milk and meat withdrawal times must be followed.
• Long-term use of oxytocin may result in cows becoming dependent on oxytocin for milk letdown.

POSSIBLE INTERACTIONS
N/A

FOLLOW-UP

EXPECTED COURSE AND PROGNOSIS
• In one study, cows with clinical mastitis were cultured and evaluated once a day for 8 days, then once a week for 1 month, then monthly until completely cured.
• The geometric mean time to clinical cure of 21 no growth cases of clinical mastitis that were not treated with anything was 4.8 days (range 1–26 days) and time until the quarter somatic cell count (SCC) was <500,000 cells/mL was 10.5 days (range 1–66 days).
• In comparison, the geometric mean time to clinical cure of 19 no growth cases of clinical mastitis that were treated with intramammary cephapirin (by label) was 5.2 days (range 2–26 days) and time until the quarter SCC was <500,000 cells/mL was 10.7 days (range 1–111).
• Providing culture results remain negative and no *Mycoplasma* is cultured, the prognosis is good.

POSSIBLE COMPLICATIONS
N/A

CLIENT EDUCATION
Clients trained to obtain culture results prior to treatment should be able to reduce drug usage, thereby decreasing the chance of antibiotic residues in bulk tank milk. Proper sample handling is important in order to minimize inaccurate culture results.

PATIENT CARE
• Any cow with clinical mastitis, especially those that are not being treated, should be

M

MASTITIS: NO GROWTH   (CONTINUED)

evaluated on a daily basis to assess disease progression. Cows that have truly cleared the infection but are still showing clinical signs (abnormal milk) will show improvement.

• Any cow with repeated episodes of no growth clinical mastitis should be cultured for *Mycoplasma*. Cultures of cows with severe clinical mastitis that are reported as no growth should be held in suspicion.

• In one study where cows with clinical mastitis were cultured daily for 8 days, all cases of no growth were mild and did not progress to a more severe condition, whereas all cases of severe clinical mastitis yielded ample growth.

PREVENTION

• Standard mastitis control measures should always be used.

• Refer to other mastitis chapters or the National Mastitis Council's 10-point plan for a review of recommendations and a useful on-farm checklist (www.nmconline.org/docs/NMCchecklistNA.pdf).

 MISCELLANEOUS

ASSOCIATIED CONDITIONS

The vast majority of cases of clinical mastitis that result in no growth are largely thought to be due to bacteria.

AGE-RELATED FACTORS
N/A

ZOONOTIC POTENTIAL
N/A

PREGNANCY
N/A

BIOSECURITY
Closed herds decrease the chance of *Mycoplasma* spp. introduction.

PRODUCTION MANAGEMENT

• Any cow with clinical mastitis, especially those that are not being treated, should be evaluated on a daily basis to assess disease progression.

• Any cow with repeated episodes of no growth clinical mastitis should be cultured for *Mycoplasma* spp.

ABBREVIATIONS

• PCR = polymerase chain reaction
• SCC = somatic cell count

SEE ALSO

• Mastitis: Fungal
• Mastitis: Mycoplasma
• Mastitis: Pharmacology (see www.fiveminutevet.com/ruminant)
• Ultrasonography: Mammary

Suggested Reading

Beaudeau F, Fourichon C, Seegers H, Bareille N. Risk of clinical mastitis in dairy herds with a high proportion of low individual milk somatic-cell counts. Prev Vet Med 2002, 53: 43–54.

Sargeant JM, Scott HM, Leslie KE, Ireland MJ, Bashiri A. Clinical mastitis in dairy cattle in Ontario: frequency of occurrence and bacteriological isolates. Can Vet J 1998, 39: 33–8.

Schreiner DA, Ruegg PL. Relationship between udder and leg hygiene scores and subclinical mastitis. J Dairy Sci 2003, 86: 3460–5.

Smith MC, Sherman DM eds. Goat Medicine, 2nd ed. Ames: Wiley-Blackwell, 2009.

Suriyasathaporn W, Schukken YH, Nielen M, Brand A. Low somatic cell count: a risk factor for subsequent clinical mastitis in a dairy herd. J Dairy Sci 2000, 83: 1248–55.

Author Kaitlyn A. Lutz
Consulting Editor Ahmed Tibary
Acknowledgment The author and book editors acknowledge the prior contribution of Jerry R. Roberson.

M

BASICS

OVERVIEW
While the anatomy, normophysiology, and pathology of the small ruminant mammary gland is largely comparable to cattle, a number of significant species variations exist. The normal mammary gland consists of two functionally and anatomically distinct gland-teat complexes. More milk is stored in the gland cisterns than in cattle, decreasing dependence on hormonal milk letdown. Dairy goats are typically milked for a 305-day lactation and herds in the United States average ~1,500 pounds per doe annually. Dairy sheep have a 5-month lactation, producing 650–1,000 pounds per ewe per lactation. Milk fat (3.1–6.3% caprine, 7.62% ovine) and protein (2.7–4.4% caprine, 6.21% ovine) are similar to or higher than cattle. Cytoplasmic droplets from apocrine milk secretion are normal and may be mistakenly counted as somatic cells. Caprine SCC normally increases with parity, days in milk, and estrus, as well as in response to infection; increased ovine SCC is primarily related to infection.

INCIDENCE/PREVALANCE
• Mastitis is a very common problem on small ruminant operations, affecting more than 30% of US herds and almost 3% of lactating does annually.
• The majority of subclinical infections are caused by coagulase-negative *Staphylococcus* (CNS) (78% in ewes, 71% in does).
• *S. aureus* is the most common cause of acute clinical (11–65%) and peracute gangrenous (60%) mastitis and is a common cause of subclinical mastitis (4% in ewes, 8% in does).
• *Mannheimia* spp. are a major cause of acute clinical mastitis in nursing sheep.
• *Mycoplasma* spp. are major mastitis pathogens on a global basis. *M. agalactiae* is best known as the causative agent of contagious agalactia, an uncommon and reportable disease in the US. The term "contagious agalactia" is also used loosely to refer to any mycoplasma mastitis of small ruminants.
• Lentiviral infections affect 20–40% of US flocks, with a reported prevalence of as high as 25% on an overall basis.

GEOGRAPHIC DISTRIBUTION
Bacterial mastitis is widely distributed nationally and globally. *Mycoplasma* mastitis is relatively uncommon in the US but is widespread in the Mediterranean, Asia, and North Africa. Lentivirus seroprevalence varies across geographic regions.

PATHOPHYSIOLOGY
• Up to 90% of the late lactation increase in caprine SCC can be attributable to factors other than infections.

• Intramammary infections (IMIs) may present as subclinical, acute, peracute, or chronic conditions.
• Most small ruminant IMIs are caused by contagious bacteria which are spread during the milking process, via nursing offspring, or through other fomites.
• Signs of mastitis include increased SCC, decreased milk production, abnormal milk, and inflammation of the udder parenchyma.
• Subclinical and chronic infections, which are common with CNS, *S. aureus*, and mycoplasma IMIs, present a chronic exposure risk for herd mates.
• Peracute gangrenous presentations are associated with *S. aureus*, *Mannheimia*, and coliform infections. These severe infections cause systemic illness, septicemia, and death.
• *Mycoplasma*, *Mannheimia*, and lentiviral infections are associated with other disease syndromes such as pneumonia and polyarthritis.
• Resolved natural infections do not result in any effective degree of immunity.

SYSTEMS AFFECTED
• Mammary
• Other systems depending on etiology

HISTORICAL FINDINGS
See "Signalment"

SIGNALMENT
• Heavily milking does and ewes are most susceptible to IMI during the periparturient period and at dry-off/weaning. Mastitis may be observed in dry females and males.
• A strong correlation exists between CNS infection and increased days in milk and lactation number. Affected animals may have a history of decreasing milk production and increased individual SCC or the herd may have a history of increased bulk tank SCC or bacterial counts.
• Peracute gangrenous *S. aureus* mastitis typically occurs 10–15 days postpartum but may present just prior to parturition. Chronic *S. aureus* mastitis is more prevalent with increased days in milk or lactation number.
• *Mannheimia* mastitis is most common in sheep nursing lambs that have a rapid onset of glandular and systemic signs several weeks postpartum.
• Clinical *Mycoplasma* mastitis is more common in goats. It is characterized by increased bulk tank SCC and outbreaks of mastitis in early lactation, often in association with pneumonia, conjunctivitis, and polyarthritis in young stock.
• Lentiviral mastitis presents at parturition in sexually mature animals >2 years of age.

PHYSICAL EXAMINATION FINDINGS
• Over 90% of herds rely solely on clinical signs to diagnose clinical mastitis.
• Affected animals demonstrate elevated SCCs in the affected half; this may be the only signs with subclinical CNS and *S. aureus* infections.
• Milk production is decreased.

• Milk may be thin, watery, bloody, off-color, purulent, or contain visible flakes or clots.
• Udder may be asymmetrical, enlarged, inflamed, indurated, or abscessed.
• Signs of systemic illness, including depression, anorexia, pyrexia (or subnormal temperature), dehydration, altered gait, or acute death (<24 hours) with acute clinical presentations.
• Udder gangrene ("blue bag") is a particularly severe clinical syndrome associated with *S. aureus* or *Mannheimia* infection. The udder and teat may be erythematous to cyanotic, cool, and edematous. As the case progresses, a demarcation line can be observed on the udder surface, followed by sloughing of the affected tissues. Regional lymph nodes will be enlarged, and milk secretions are serum-like, bloody, and/or gassy.
• Chronic mastitis can cause udder induration.
• Palpable internal abscesses are common with chronic *S. aureus* infections.
• Lentiviral infection causes an indurative "hard bag" mastitis. The animal presents with agalactia and a full uniformly hard udder, but the overlying skin is loose, without edema, heat, or erythema. The milk appears normal but SCC will be elevated in affected goats.

GENETICS
Some association of breed with CAEV prevalence; highest in dairy breeds and least prevalent in Angora, Cashmere, and dwarf breeds but may be confounded by management.

CAUSES AND RISK FACTORS
• Small ruminant IMIs are commonly caused by bacterial and viral pathogens and rarely by fungi, prototheca, yeast, and *Bacillus* spp.
• *S. aureus* is arguably the most important major pathogen of the mammary gland in small ruminants.
• *Staphylococcus epidermidis*, *S. caprae*, *S. warneri*, *S. simulans*, and *S. xylosus*, and other species of CNS are significant pathogens of dairy sheep and goats.
• *Mannheimia haemolytica* and *M. glucosida* infection is associated with prior viral or physical trauma to the teat followed by introduction of the pathogen to the skin or teat duct. Risk factors include pre-existing orf or papilloma infection of the teat, physical trauma to the teat end, and cross-suckling.
• Contagious agalactia is specifically associated with *Mycoplasma agalactiae,* and loosely with other *Mycoplasma* species including *M. mycoides* subsp. *mycoides* (LC), *M. putrifaciens,* and *M. capricolum* subsp. *capricolum*. Specific risk factors include introduction of new animals; poor milking hygiene practices; and dam-raising of young stock.
• Lentiviral mastitis is caused by OPP and CAE. These retroviruses are easily transmitted through milk and colostrum.

M

MASTITIS: SMALL RUMINANT

DIAGNOSIS

DIFFERENTIAL DIAGNOSES
• Colostrum
• Edema
• Enlarged, nonfunctional gland from prior infection
• Internal teat sealant medications
• Normophysiologic elevations in SCC
• Nutritional agalactia or water deprivation
• Precocious udder
• Teat obstruction
• Trauma

CBC/BIOCHEMISTRY/URINALYSIS
Indicated when managing severe, systemically compromised cases, as a basis for fluid therapy interventions, or to evaluate for sepsis.

OTHER LABORATORY TESTS
• Milk culture: Ensure CNS growth is reported. *S. aureus* is associated with cyclic shedding and may require multiple cultures. Mycoplasma will not grow on routine culture.
• Serology is indicated to rule out lentiviral infections; both ELISA and AGID assays are readily available in the US. OPP antigen-based AGID test has reduced sensitivity for CAE. A mycoplasma ELISA has been developed but is not available in the US.
• PCR assays are available for mycoplasma and for OPP/CAE.

IMAGING
Ultrasound can be used to evaluate the udder parenchyma and teat for abnormalities (abscesses, teat spiders, and lactoliths) or to evaluate supranumary or bifid teats.

OTHER DIAGNOSTIC PROCEDURES
The California Mastitis Test is a pen-side screening tool that detects increased SCC and decreased milk pH. While colostrum and transitional milk specificity is poor, a negative result in the first few days of lactation is reliable. Both udder halves should be compared in goats to determine if a positive result is physiologic or due to infection.

PATHOLOGIC FINDINGS
• Intra- and extracellular Gram-positive cocci and elevated neutrophils are observed with staphylococcal infections. Peracute *S. aureus* causes connective tissue proliferation, venous thrombosis, tissue necrosis, and edematous/hemorrhagic supramammary lymph nodes. Internal macro- and micro-abscesses may be observed with chronic infections.
• *Mannheimia* are Gram-negative bipolar rods. Gross findings include an enlarged gland, subcutaneous edema, sanguineous parenchymal fluid exudates, and enlarged and edematous supramammary lymph nodes.
• *Mycoplasma* infections cause an interstitial mastitis, with fibrosis and parenchymal atrophy. Additional findings may include signs of septicemia, pneumonia, arthritis with periarticular edema, hyperemic synovial membranes, hemorrhagic joint fluid, and serous to mucopurulent conjunctivitis and keratitis. The mycoplasma organism can be identified through immunohistochemical or Giemsa staining of the affected tissue.
• Lentiviral infections cause an interstitial mastitis with generalized wasting and interstitial pneumonia. Affected tissues will be firm and noncollapsing.

TREATMENT

THERAPEUTIC APPROACH
• CNS: Therapeutic objective is to clear the infection in order to improve animal and herd production metrics and reduce transmission.
• *S. aureus*: The initial treatment priority for acute/gangrenous cases may be to save the animal and preserve milking capacity through early and aggressive therapy. The overall goal should be to eliminate this contagious organism from the herd. Chronic cases and some strains of *S. aureus* may be very resistant to treatment; multiple negative cultures and consistently low SCCs are required to declare an animal clear of infection.
• *Mannheimia*: Successful treatment of peracute cases is unlikely. Early and aggressive efforts should be directed first at saving the animal's life and then the gland.
• Lentivirus: No treatment is available for OPP/CAE. Herd goals may include managing endemic disease or obtaining and maintaining a disease-free status.
• Systemic antibiotics may be indicated in cases of *S. aureus* mastitis although research is inconsistent in showing a benefit. Antibiotic choice should be based on pharmacokinetic and pharmacodynamic properties which will affect activity within the mammary gland. Tylosin and penicillin G show some clinical efficacy with limited supportive research.
• Intramammary therapy is indicted for most Gram-positive infections when the animal is not showing signs of systemic illness. Splitting mastitis tubes between udder halves increases the risk of iatrogenic infection.
• Udder halves can be chemically killed by an intramammary infusion of chlorhexidine or povidine iodine along with adjunct anti-inflammatory therapy.
• Oral or intravenous fluid therapy may be required with severe and peracute gangrenous mastitis. Avoid alkalizing solutions and correct for hypocalcemia and hypokalemia as clinically indicated.

SURGICAL CONSIDERATIONS AND TECHNIQUES
• Teat amputation can be performed just distal to Furstenberg's ring under local anesthesia.
• Ligation of the external pudendal artery and vein can be performed under sedation when the animal is not a suitable surgical candidate for mastectomy.
• Radical mastectomy and removal of the associated supramammary lymph node under general anesthesia is well described in many texts.

MEDICATIONS

DRUGS OF CHOICE
• Adjust the initial antimicrobial selection based on the culture sensitivity results if available.
• CNS: Most cattle IMM antibiotics are effective at the label dosage, e.g., cephapirin (lactating) q12–24h for 2–3 doses and penicillin-dihydrostreptomycin once at dry-off. Florfenicol (20 mg/kg IM q24h, or SC once) may be used in nondairy animals.
• *S. aureus*: Extended lactating IMM therapy regimes (e.g., cephapirin or pirlimycin for 6–8 doses) and concurrent IMM and systemic drug administration are recommended in dairy cattle. Use a product approved for *S. aureus* at dry-off. Tilmicosin (10 mg/kg SQ once, **not for use in goats**) or florfenicol may be used in nondairy animals.
• *Mannheimia haemolytica* associated pneumonias are generally responsive to long-acting oxytetracycline, sulfonamides, ceftiofur, tulathromycin, and florfenicol. Lactating therapy protocols include cephapirin q12–24h for 2–3 doses. Tulathromycin (2.5 mg/kg SQ, once) or florfenicol may be used in nondairy animals.
• *Mycoplasma*: Antibiotic therapies are generally ineffective, subject to long milk withdrawals, and induce a carrier state.
• Anti-inflammatory therapy may include flunixin meglumine (1 mg/kg IV q12–24h, up to 3 days) or dexamethasone (0.44 mg/kg IM/SQ/IV, once).

CONTRAINDICATIONS
Tilmicosin is lethal in goats.

PRECAUTIONS
Very few drugs are approved for goats and no intramammary medications (IMM) are approved for small ruminants. Follow AMDUCA guidelines for extra-label drug use; US FARAD can assist with establishing appropriate withdrawal intervals.

FOLLOW-UP

EXPECTED COURSE AND PROGNOSIS
• As many as 60% of subclinical CNS cases will self-cure over the dry period; use of dry therapy will significantly increase the number of cures.
• Acute clinical cases of *S. aureus* may become chronic and refractory to therapy. New clinical cases are most likely to respond to an

extended treatment protocol while subclinical and chronic cases, or those that have survived a dry period, are unlikely to be cured.
• Untreated gangrenous mastitis has a 30–40% case fatality rate and permanent loss of the affected gland is common. Early, aggressive, effective intervention may increase recovery rates to >90%.
• A poor prognosis for survival is associated with *Mannheimia* mastitis.
• Mycoplasma morbidity in naïve flocks can reach 30–60% of the herd. Mortality in acute, untreated cases is generally ≤20%, but may reach as high as 40–70% especially in young stock that present with septicemia. In animals that survive the acute mastitis, milk production is significantly reduced in the current lactation but they may return to production in the next lactation. Carrier animals are common. Subclinical cases and chronic mastitis are more common in endemic herds.
• Lentiviral infections that lead to clinical disease are chronic, progressive, and invariably fatal as no treatment is available. In new cases, milk quantity may transiently improve over the course of a few weeks.

POSSIBLE COMPLICATIONS

Sepsis may develop with severe Gram-negative or *S. aureus* mastitis. Animals, especially goats, with lentiviral mastitis have higher rates of concurrent bacterial IMI due to the retrovirus's immunosuppressive effects.

PATIENT CARE

Monitor for worsening clinical presentation or onset of gangrenous signs.

CLIENT EDUCATION

Educate producers on the importance of herd and milking biosecurity, best milking practices, and control of conditions that impair the innate teat defenses.

PREVENTION

• Best milking practices from the cattle dairy industry can be used on small ruminant operations to improve udder health and decrease IMI transmission. Recommendations include milking primiparous and noninfected animals first, ensuring equipment is clean and well maintained, judicious application of dry therapy, and using gloves, individual towels, and teat dips.
• Control methods for *Mannheimia* mastitis include reducing orf and papilloma teat infections, teat chapping and trauma, cross-suckling (bum lambs), and respiratory spread of *Mannheimia* pneumonia in lambs; the cattle *Mannheimia* vaccine is not efficacious in small ruminants.

• The best defense against *Mycoplasma* is to maintain a clean herd and cull infected animals. Control measures include testing new herd additions, heat-treating colostrum, pasteurizing milk, and environmental hygiene. Request a mycoplasma culture if you repeatedly encounter culture-negative mastitis, or mastitis in conjunction with polyarthritis, conjunctivitis, and pneumonia in young stock.
• Test herd additions for OPP/CAE before purchase.

MISCELLANEOUS

ASSOCIATED CONDITIONS

• *S. aureus*: Diarrhea and pneumonia in nursing stock
• *Mannheimia*: Acute bronchopneumonia in 2-week to 2-month-old nursing stock
• *Mycoplasma*: Keratoconjunctivitis; polyarthritis and pneumonia in young stock
• Lentivirus: Chronic wasting, progressive interstitial pneumonia, arthritis, progressive inflammatory encephalomyelitis, and/or posterior paresis

AGE-RELATED FACTORS

• CNS mastitis is more common with increasing lactation number.
• Lentiviral mastitis typically presents at 2 years of age or older.

ZOONOTIC POTENTIAL

Staphylococci including *S. aureus* may present food safety or antimicrobial resistance concerns. Though less common, *E. coli* and *Salmonella* are documented causes of mastitis in small ruminants. Other pathogens such as *Listeria monocytogenes*, *Campylobacter* spp., and *Coxiella burnetii* may be shed in the milk of clinically normal animals.

PREGNANCY

Severe clinical mastitis during the pre-parturient period may cause abortion.

BIOSECURITY

Transmission of the most common and most severe mastitis organisms can be reduced through herd and milking biosecurity practices.

PRODUCTION MANAGEMENT

• Palpation of the udder at milking time is routinely performed to identify chronic cases of *S. aureus* mastitis that may otherwise serve as a source of infection for the herd.
• Follow recommended milking practices. Milk from affected animals should be pasteurized or acidified before it is fed to young stock.

• If monthly individual SCCs are available, the current month's SCC can be plotted against the previous month's SCC to monitor new, chronic, resolved, and cured IMIs.
• Bulk tank bacterial and SCCs can be rapidly reduced by selectively excluding the milk from the animals that are contributing the greatest **total** number of cells on a daily basis (cells/mL × production volume). These animals should be treated, dried off, or culled depending on the etiology.

ABBREVIATIONS

• AGID = agar gel immunodiffusion
• CAE = caprine arthritis encephalomyelitis
• CNS = coagulase-negative *Staphylococcus*
• ELISA = enzyme-linked immunosorbent assay
• IMI = intramammary infection
• IMM = intramammary medication
• OPP = ovine progressive pneumonia
• PCR = polymerase chain reaction
• SCC = somatic cell count

SEE ALSO

• Caprine Arthritis Encephalitis Virus
• Maedi-Visna (Ovine Progressive Pneumonia)
• Mastitis (by etiology)
• Precocious Udder

Suggested Reading
Bergonier D, de Crémoux R, Rupp R, et al. Mastitis of dairy small ruminants. Vet Res 2003, 34: 689–716.
Omaleki L, Browning GF, Allen JL, Barber SR. The role of Mannheimia species in ovine mastitis. Vet Microbiol 2011, 153: 67–72.
Paape MJ, Wiggans GR, Bannerman DD, et al. Monitoring goat and sheep milk somatic cell counts. Small Rumin Res 2007, 68: 114–25.
Plummer PJ, Plummer C. Diseases of the mammary gland. In: Pugh DG, Baird AN eds, Sheep and Goat Medicine, 2nd ed. Maryland Heights, MO: Saunders, 2012.
Rowan LL, Morin DE, Hurley WL, et al. Evaluation of udder health and mastitis in llamas. J Am Vet Med Assoc 1996, 209: 1457–63.
Smith MC, Sherman DM. Mammary gland and milk production. In: Smith MC, Sherman DM eds, Goat Medicine, 2nd ed. Ames: Wiley-Blackwell, 2009.
White E. The prevalence of mastitis in small ruminants and the effect of mastitis on small ruminant production. NMC Annual Meeting Proceedings, 2007.

Author Kelly M. Still Brooks
Consulting Editor Kaitlyn A. Lutz

M

MASTITIS: STAPHYLOCOCCAL

BASICS

OVERVIEW
• Mastitis is inflammation of the mammary gland. The majority of mastitis is caused by microorganisms, usually bacterial, that invade the mammary gland, multiply, and produce toxins harmful to the gland.
• Mastitis in dairy cattle and milk goats produces serious economic losses.
• Mastitis is the single most common disease in adult dairy cows.
• Staphylococci are Gram-positive bacteria.
• Staphylococci organisms that cause mastitis are usually identified as *S. aureus,* CNS (coagulase-negative *Staphylococcus*), or more generally as *Staphylococcus* species.

INCIDENCE/PREVALENCE
• *S. aureus:* The 2007 National Animal Health Monitoring Dairy Study found a herd-level prevalence of 40–45% in the USA.
• CNS: Most common cause of mastitis on farms where major contagious pathogens are controlled; between 7% and 30% of quarters infected during herd surveys.

SYSTEMS AFFECTED
Mammary

PATHOPHYSIOLOGY
• Establishment of infection and the inflammatory response is increased by adherence factors.
• Infection causes local destruction of alveolar tissue, involution of alveoli, and occlusion of ducts by tissue debris and clots.
• Each *S. aureus* strain possesses different virulence factors to aid in avoidance of the host's immune system, impacting the course of disease and treatability. These include surface proteins, presence of a capsule, and formation of a biofilm.
• Invasion of alveoli is followed by formation of micro-abscesses, fibrosis, and nonfunctional mammary tissue.
• Production of alpha-toxins may lead to gangrenous mastitis.

HISTORICAL FINDINGS
Loss of milk production and possibly local and systemic changes.

SIGNALMENT
Cows are most susceptible to clinical mastitis during early lactation.

PHYSICAL EXAMINATION FINDINGS
• Subclinical mastitis:
  ○ Lack of visible changes to the gland or the milk.
  ○ Elevation of somatic cell count of the infected gland.

• Clinical mastitis:
  ○ Changes in the gland, milk, and/or systemic signs.
  ○ Peracute clinical mastitis:
    ▪ Gland has swelling, heat, and pain.
    ▪ Secretion is abnormal and may contain clots, flakes, discolored serum, or sometimes blood.
    ▪ Signs of systemic illness are present. These include anorexia, depression, increased pulse rate, sunken eyes, and weakness.
    ▪ Onset is rapid and mortality may be high.
  ○ Acute, gangrenous clinical mastitis:
    ▪ Gangrenous form is due to *Staphylococcus* alpha-toxin.
    ▪ Acute systemic and local signs are due to toxemia.
    ▪ Starts with inflammation of the gland, then development of cold teats and bloody secretions.
    ▪ The gland has sharply delineated, blue discolorations.
    ▪ Mortality is generally high.
  ○ Acute clinical mastitis:
    ▪ Similar to peracute infections but systemic signs are less severe.
  ○ Subacute clinical mastitis:
    ▪ Mild to moderate alterations to the secretion and mammary gland.
    ▪ No systemic signs.

CAUSES AND RISK FACTORS
• *S. aureus:*
  ○ Primary source—infected udders.
  ○ Secondary sites include teat skin, udder skin, nose, lips, vagina, and other body sites.
  ○ Method of spread—via transfer of bacteria-laden milk from infected to noninfected glands. The milking process is a primary means of transfer, but nursing calves, flies, and milkers' hands can also transfer the organisms.
  ○ Often introduced into a herd by infected, purchased additions.
  ○ Flies have been associated with infection in prepartum heifers.
• CNS:
  ○ Normal inhabitants of bovine teat skin and can be free-living in the environment.
  ○ Infections are more common in first lactation cows.
  ○ Prevalence is high at parturition, then declines through the first month of lactation.
  ○ Primary source—commonly found on teat skin and in the streak canal.
  ○ Cow to cow spread is probably rare.
  ○ Most infections are transient but rarely become chronic.
  ○ May be associated with teat injuries or alteration of teat skin condition.

DIAGNOSIS

DIFFERENTIAL DIAGNOSES
• Subclinical cases: *Streptococcus agalactia, Corynebacterium bovis,* and minor udder pathogens.
• Clinical cases: Coliform bacteria, mycoplasma, and environmental streptococci.
• Gangrenous mastitis with bloody secretion: Trauma to the gland, and *Clostridium perfringens* type A mastitis.

CBC/BIOCHEMISTRY/URINALYSIS
Usually not performed.

OTHER LABORATORY TESTS
• Microbiological identification of the causative agent is essential:
  ○ Requires plating organisms to evaluate the colonial characteristics and hemolytic patterns on blood agar.
  ○ The catalase test is used to differentiate staphylococci from streptococci by mixing the colony with hydrogen peroxide.
    ▪ Staphylococci are catalase-positive (produces bubbles).
    ▪ Streptococci are catalase-negative (do not produce bubbles).
  ○ Colonies should be Gram stained.
    ▪ Gram-positive cocci that appear in clumps.
• *S. aureus*
  ○ Large colonies that are creamy, grayish-white, or yellowish.
  ○ Generally produce hemolysis, typically a double zone, around the colony.
  ○ Most are coagulase positive.
• CNS (*Staph.* species):
  ○ Large, creamy, grayish-white or yellowish.
  ○ Generally have no hemolysis.
  ○ Most are coagulase negative.

OTHER DIAGNOSTIC PROCEDURES
• Culture is the only method to identify the specific pathogen.
  ○ Culture and sensitivity results may be useful in determining methicillin-resistant strains of *S. aureus*; however, are not strongly correlated with in vivo treatment outcomes.
  ○ Strain typing for *S. aureus* is an excellent tool to determine virulence and transmissibility, both important when determining a herd-based treatment and control plan.

TREATMENT

THERAPEUTIC APPROACH
• Both intramammary and systemic therapy have been used.

M

• When possible, treatment should be influenced by culture and angiobiograms.
• Goal of treatment is to return the gland to production.
• Consider the economics of the treatment.
• Use only products approved for use in food-producing animals.
• Label instructions must be followed.
• Withholding times for milk and meat must be observed.
• Better response to treatment is attained during the dry period.

MEDICATIONS

DRUGS OF CHOICE
• Several commercial products for intramammary administration are available:
  ○ Pirlimycin
  ○ B-lactam antibiotics such as penicillin, hetacillin, and amoxicillin
  ○ Cephapirin
  ○ Ceftiofur HCl
  ○ Novobiocin
• No products are labeled for systemic therapy, but injectable ampicillin (3–5 mg/lb) and oxytetracycline (5 mg/lb) have been used in conjunction with intramammary therapy with variable results. These uses are considered extra-label, and the efficacy of combined intramammary and parenteral therapy has not been supported by research.
• Extended duration therapy can be used to improve efficacy of therapy. Approved intramammary antibiotics are administered for up to 8 days into infected quarters.
  ○ Pirsue® (pirlimycin) is labeled for treatment of clinical and subclinical mastitis associated with Staphylococcus species, including S. aureus.
  ○ Spectramast® (ceftiofur) is labeled for clinical and subclinical mastitis associated with coagulase-negative staphylococci.
• Prepartum antibiotic therapy has been demonstrated to be efficacious in reducing IMI with coagulase-negative staphylococci and S. aureus at calving. Most benefits have been demonstrated in herds with a high prevalence of staphylococci IMI.
• NSAIDs are used to control pain and fever.
• Fluid therapy is essential in systemically affected animals (gangrenous S. aureus) as hypovolemia will predispose to kidney damage from NSAIDs and certain antimicrobials.

PRECAUTIONS
Appropriate milk and meat withholding times must be followed for all compounds administered to food-producing animals.

FOLLOW-UP

EXPECTED COURSE AND PROGNOSIS
• Early treatment of S. aureus may be successful; success for chronic infections is poor.
• Response to therapy of S. aureus is poorer due to formation of L-forms, penicillinase production, and the formation of micro-abscesses within the udder parenchyma.
• CNS has a good prognosis but may become chronic in some cases.

POSSIBLE COMPLICATIONS
N/A

CLIENT EDUCATION
N/A

PATIENT CARE
• Infected quarters should be cultured 21–28 days after treatment to determine cure.
• In the case of S. aureus, three sequential cultures will significantly increase sensitivity due to cyclical shedding of the organism.

PREVENTION
• Maintain a closed herd and perform milk cultures on animals prior to purchase if this is necessary.
• See "Production Management" for prevention of transmission.

MISCELLANEOUS

AGE-RELATED FACTORS
First lactation animals have higher cure rates for S. aureus than multiparous animals.

ZOONOTIC POTENTIAL
S. aureus is an important zoonosis.

BIOSECURITY
Wear gloves while milking to prevent human-to-animal spread.

PRODUCTION MANAGEMENT
• Control of S. aureus:
  ○ Identify infected cows and isolate or milk last.
  ○ Cull chronically infected cows.
  ○ Treat all cows with appropriate, FDA-approved dry cow infusion products.
  ○ Apply an effective teat disinfectant to each teat following milking.
  ○ Backflushing systems have been used to reduce the bacterial load in the inflations.
  ○ Promote good milking hygiene and proper milking techniques to minimize teat end trauma.
  ○ Vaccines are available but of limited usefulness.

• Control of CNS:
  ○ Treat all cows with appropriate, approved dry cow infusion products.
  ○ Apply an effective teat disinfectant to each teat following milking.

ABBREVIATIONS
• CNS = coagulase-negative Staphylococcus
• FDA = (US) Food and Drug Administration
• NSAIDs = nonsteroidal anti-inflammatory drugs

SEE ALSO
• Mastitis: Bulk Tank Monitoring and Somatic Cell Counts (see www.fiveminutevet.com/ruminant)
• Mastitis (by pathogen)
• Mastitis: Milking Procedures and Teat Disinfection (see www.fiveminutevet.com/ruminant)
• Mastitis: Pharmacology (see www.fiveminutevet.com/ruminant)

Suggested Reading
Barkema HW, Schukken YH, Zadoks RN. Invited review: the role of cow, pathogen, and treatment regimen in the therapeutic success of bovine Staphylococcus aureus mastitis. J Dairy Sci 2006, 89: 1877–1895.
Current Concepts of Bovine Mastitis, 4th edition, 1996. National Mastitis Council, 421 S. Nine Mound Rd., Verona WI 53593 USA
Laboratory Handbook on Bovine Mastitis, revised edition, 1999. National Mastitis Council, 421 S. Nine Mound Rd., Verona WI 53593 USA
Prevalence of Contagious Mastitis Pathogens on US Dairy Operations, 2007. USDA APHIS, Veterinary Services, Center for Epidemiology and Animal Health. Accessed June 2016. https://www.aphis.usda.gov/nahms
Roy JP, Keefe G. Systematic review: what is the best antibiotic treatment for Staphylococcus aureus intramammary infection of lactating cows in North America. Vet Clin Food Anim 2012, 28: 39–50.
Ruegg P. Emerging Mastitis Threats on the Dairy. University of Wisconsin Dairy Quality Website. Accessed June 2016.

Author Richard W. Meiring
Consulting Editor Kaitlyn A. Lutz

M

MASTITIS: STREPTOCOCCAL

BASICS

OVERVIEW
• Streptococcal mastitis is among the most prevalent causes of intramammary infections (IMI) on dairy farms. These include contagious as well as environmental pathogens.
• *S. agalactiae* is a contagious, Gram-positive coccus that resides in the bovine mammary gland, generally not surviving for long outside of this environment. It tends to spread aggressively.
• *S. dysgalactiae* and *S. uberis* are Gram-positive cocci that are predominantly found within the environment.
• The latter two are often diagnosed as a group in mastitis and udder health programs.

INCIDENCE/PREVALENCE

S. agalactiae
• Fifteen percent of dairy herds in the northeast United States have *Streptococcus agalactiae* infections present at any given time, while 85% are free of this eradicable organism.
• Within infected herds, prevalence of *Streptococcus agalactia* varies considerably, ranging from 1% to 77% of the herd.
• Prevalence has declined dramatically in countries with robust extension programs but remains high in countries with developing dairy industries. For example, in Brazil and Colombia prevalence is 60% and 42%, respectively.
• Prevalence of *S. agalactiae* in camel herds ranges from 3% to 30%.
• Prevalence of *S. agalactiae* in buffaloes ranges from 15% to 30%.

Other Streptococcus spp.
• Of dairy herds in the US, 96% have *S. dysgalactiae* or *S. uberis* infecting at least one cow at any given time.
• Many laboratories and commercial dairy herd mastitis control programs do not distinguish between these two types of nonagalactiae streptococci, identifying them as *Strep* sp.
• Among cows, the prevalence of *Strep* sp. is 14–16% in reports from the US and other developed countries. One large study on dairy goats found a similar prevalence (16%) for *Strep* sp.
• In one study on camels, *S. dysgalactiae* and *S. uberis* were isolated in 22.2% and 7.6% of milk samples, respectively.
• In buffaloes, *S. dysgalactiae* and *S. uberis* were isolated in 30% and 73.5% of clinical mastitis milk samples, respectively.
• In goats, *Streptococcus* spp. are isolated in 11% of subclinical mastitis cases.
• In one study on sheep, *S. uberis* was isolated from 1.7% of clinical mastitis cases.

GEOGRAPHIC DISTRIBUTION
• Worldwide depending on bacterial species and environment.
• In dairy goats, *S. agalactiae* is seen in New Zealand, India, and Brazil but is uncommon in the US.

SYSTEMS AFFECTED
Mammary

PATHOPHYSIOLOGY
• The mammary gland is generally infected via ascendant route.
• Establishment of the infection and severity of the inflammation depends on the strain.
• The presence of inflammation results in an increase in SCC.

HISTORICAL FINDINGS
Increased bulk tank SCC

SIGNALMENT
Dairy cattle, dairy camels, and less frequently dairy goats

PHYSICAL EXAMINATION FINDINGS

S. agalactiae
• There is no one classical presentation of these pathogens within dairy herds; however, in most cases, *S. agalactiae* first becomes evident within months to 1 year following purchase of infected animals.
• Three percent of heifers have infections with *S. agalactiae* at first calving, and should not be assumed to be risk-free as herd additions.
• Ninety-six percent of *S. agalactiae* cases are subclinical.
• *S. agalctiae* results in bulk tank SCC usually >400,000/mL, with a geometric mean SCC for affected quarters of 857,000. The SCC often rises steadily once the increase begins.
• Sometimes associated with high bacterial counts in milk; can be >200,000/mL SPC.
• Often high (>10%/mo) new infection rate on DHIA (or other test service) monthly reports.
• May be high level (>10%/mo) of chronic infections as well.

Other Streptococcus spp.
• *Streptococcus* sp. can be major mastitis pathogens in any herd, including herds as described above.
• However, *Streptococcus* sp. are more likely to be at high levels when tank SCC >400,000/mL.
• *Streptococcus* sp. mastitis often is subclinical but may have severe clinical signs or LS >5.0.
• Often notice many new infections on DHIA among fresh cows <60 DIM.
• *Streptococcus* sp. mastitis increases from June through September in many herds in North America.

GENETICS
N/A

CAUSES AND RISK FACTORS
• Failure to employ standard milking time hygiene measures are risk factors for the spread of *S. agalactiae* IMI. Herds that do not use dry cow antibiotic therapy and herds that do not cull chronically high SCC cows would be at increased risk for *S. agalactiae*. There is also a suggestion that teat end hyperkeratosis increases the risk of *S. agalactiae*.
• Historically, the environmental streptococci (ES) are considered to be opportunist mastitis pathogens; however, the ES, especially *S. dysgalactiae*, may have some characteristics of contagious pathogens. A few studies have demonstrated a greater risk of ES IMI in cows with advancing age.
• Straw bedding increases the risk of cows to ES IMI. Deep-bedded straw packs tend to become contaminated with urine and feces and increase risk.
• Increased prevalence of ES was associated with poor sanitation, increased number of days dry, use of tie stalls, and lack of drying teats prior to milking. There is also a suggestion that the increased time associated with correcting liner slips increases the risk of ES IMI.

DIAGNOSIS

DIFFERENTIAL DIAGNOSES
• Streptococcal mastitis should be differentiated from other causes of mastitis based on epidemiology and culture

CBC/BIOCHEMISTRY/URINALYSIS
N/A

OTHER LABORATORY TESTS
• Bulk tank milk culture is a useful way to screen a herd or group for *S. agalactiae*.
• Sensitivity for a single bulk tank culture is 77% (across all ranges of prevalence). Three bulk tank milk culture samples should be collected approximately 3 days apart and cultured separately. This increases sensitivity to 99%.
• Bulk tank milk cultures are frequently positive for *Strep* sp., and have no practical value in monitoring for these infections.
• Culture of aseptic milk samples is the only definitive way to diagnose either type of mastitis in individual cows.
• Culture should be carried out on blood agar with incubation overnight at 37°C. Streptococci appear as small, somewhat transparent colonies with or without hemolysis at 18–24 hours.
• All mastitis-associated streptococci are catalase negative (no bubbling when a drop of hydrogen peroxide is added to a small amount of the colonies on a glass slide).
• Molecular diagnostic technique such as PCR may increase accuracy of detection and speciation.
• The three primary mastitis-associated streptococci can then be effectively differentiated from each other by a few simple tests (Table 1).

(CONTINUED)

Table 1

Streptococcus *spp.*	*Esculin*	*Camp*
agalactiae	–	+
dysgalactiae	–	–
uberis	+	+/–

IMAGING
N/A

OTHER DIAGNOSTIC PROCEDURES
N/A

PATHOLOGIC FINDINGS
N/A

TREATMENT

THERAPEUTIC APPROACH
• Spontaneous cure rate for streptococcal mastitis is low (<20%) and often results in chronically high SCC.
• Timely treatment with an appropriate antibiotic is essential and usually economical.

S. agalactiae
• IMM infusion of beta-lactam antibiotic in all four quarters for three milkings in a row should be done for all infected cows as soon as culture results are available. All infected cows should be treated at the same time.
• Cure rates are approximately 90% for *S. agalactiae* cases following any single course of IMM treatment.
• Individual cows may warrant two regimens of therapy before being considered nonresponsive; many animals will cure the second time. Cows that are positive on third culture after two rounds of therapy should be strongly considered for culling.
• Culture of entire lactating herd is usually necessary to eradicate *S. agalactiae*, with resampling of the herd 3 weeks after treatment is complete, repeated until eradication is accomplished.

Other *Streptococcus sp.*
• Teat dipping and other classical mastitis control measures are weakly associated with control of *Strep* sp.
• The definitive control program for *Strep* sp. has not been developed.
• Environmental sanitation is critical, including dry cow and replacement heifer housing.
• Bedding cultures are often useful. Counts <100,000 cfu/g are good.
• *Streptococcus* sp. >1,000,000 cfu/g in bedding (some are billions/g) is strongly associated with higher prevalence of the infection in cows.

• Bedding cultures often convince farm management that various types of housing and bedding really are in need of increased cleanliness efforts.
• *Streptococcus* sp. control programs including bedding, housing repair, and milking clean, dry teats must be developed with managers and employees of each farm.

SURGICAL CONSIDERATIONS AND TECHNIQUES
N/A

MEDICATIONS

DRUGS OF CHOICE
• Penicillin-based products are the IMM drugs of choice. Several studies have found that the streptococcal species are still quite susceptible to the penicillin products.
• The initial therapeutic protocol should be an approved IMM antibiotic used according to label directions. If this therapy is not successful, there are alternatives.
• Anecdotal evidence suggests that simply switching to a different class of approved IMM antibiotic used according to label is often sufficient to obtain a bacterial cure. Another option is to extend the IMM antibiotic therapy two to three times the labeled duration. Studies with pirlimycin and ceftiofur have demonstrated increasing bacterial cures with increasing duration of treatment. However, a study with extended amoxicillin did not demonstrate any benefit over the normal labeled dosage.
• One other option is to treat both IMM and systemically. In a recent study, increased bacterial cures were obtained by using intramuscular ampicillin with IMM amoxicillin.
• For herds with a high prevalence of *S. agalactiae*, blitz treatment during lactation should be considered as it is often effective (>80%) and often proves to be economical. *Enterococcus* species tend to be considerably more resistant to successful treatment than the other streptococci.
• Camelids should be treated systemically.

CONTRAINDICATIONS
N/A

PRECAUTIONS
Appropriate milk and meat withdrawal times must be followed for all compounds administered to food-producing animals. Note that extending treatment beyond that which is labeled may increase withdrawal times.

POSSIBLE INTERACTION
N/A

FOLLOW-UP

EXPECTED COURSE AND PROGNOSIS
• Spontaneous cure rate is around 20% for ES. The spontaneous cure rate for *S. agalactiae* is <10%.
• *S. agalactiae* remains highly susceptible to antimicrobials, with <5% of cases typically refractory to treatment.
• Extended IMM therapy has been shown to increase the bacterial cures up to 100% in some experimental studies.

PATIENT CARE
• Follow-up cultures are recommended on any treated streptococci cases.
• Recommended times to culture are 1–4 days after the milk antibiotic withdrawal (a negative culture at this time is most suggestive of the efficacy of the antibiotic) and at 28–30 days (helps to document that an actual bacterial cure did occur).
• Alternatively, a decrease in individual cow SCC to normal levels would be suggestive of a cure.

POSSIBLE COMPLICATIONS
Nonfunctional "blind" quarters in heifers

PREVENTION
• Although the significance of standard mastitis control procedures varies in importance among the streptococci, a complete mastitis control program is essential in control of the streptococci.
• Milking time hygiene will have the most effect on controlling *S. agalactiae* but will also help with control of the ES.
• Complete teat predipping with an effective germicide, which should be left in place for 30 seconds. Avoid water usage in the parlor. Teats should be dried completely with individual udder cloths or paper towels. Milking machines should be properly maintained. Avoid over- or undermilking. Quickly adjust milking units when liner slips occur. In the limited studies performed on backflushing, no benefit was found for the ES. At the end of milking, teats should be dipped up to the base of the udder with an effective germicide. Cows that have been treated and not cured should be retreated or culled to help remove the intramammary reservoir.
• The most reliable methods found to achieve a low SCC include annual milking system checks, establishing a consistent milking order, wearing gloves while milking, using automatic take-offs, and using an appropriate post-dip.
• Studies have shown that up to 50% of new streptococci infections occur during the dry period; therefore, the use of an internal teat sealant plus selective dry cow therapy is recommended. Blanket dry cow therapy is common and may be warranted based on herd dynamics.

M

MASTITIS: STREPTOCOCCAL   (CONTINUED)

• Proper nutrition, especially in regard to appropriate levels of vitamin E and selenium, is important for mammary immune function.
• Avoid the use of straw bedding when possible, and when not possible, proper maintenance of bedding areas is essential. Inorganic bedding is preferred; however, one study found ten times more ES on the teats of cows bedded on sand than on teats of cows bedded on sawdust. Even pasture areas may be heavily contaminated with ES (e.g., common shade area). These prevention measures are less effective against *S. uberis* possibly because of its ubiquitous nature on the dairy farm (shed in the feces). Vaccines are being studied and may be available in the future. However, several studies have found that *S. uberis* strains vary considerably among dairy herds and even within dairy herds, which becomes problematic in regard to an effective vaccine.
• Refer to the National Mastitis Council's 10-point plan for a review of recommendations and a useful on-farm checklist (www.nmconline.org/docs/NMCchecklistNA.pdf).

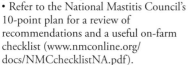

MISCELLANEOUS

ASSOCIATED CONDITIONS
Loss of milk production and increased culling rates

AGE-RELATED FACTORS
Three percent of heifers have infections with *S. agalactiae* at first calving, and should not be assumed to be risk-free as herd additions.

ZOONOTIC POTENTIAL
Although relatively rare, some streptococci of bovine origin have been identified in human infections. In particular, *S. agalactiae* is one of the leading causes of human neonatal infection. However, most studies have found that the *S. agalactiae* cultured from human infants is of a different strain than that found in bovine mastitis.

PREGNANCY
N/A

BIOSECURITY
See "Prevention"

PRODUCTION MANAGEMENT
See "Causes and Risk Factors" and "Prevention"

SYNONYMS
N/A

ABBREVIATIONS
• DHIA = Dairy Herd Improvement Association
• DIM = days in milk
• ES = environmental streptococci
• IMI = intramammary infection
• IMM = intramammary
• LS = linear score
• PCR = polymerase chain reaction
• SCC = somatic cell count
• SPC = standard plate count

SEE ALSO
• Environment and Mastitis (see www.fiveminutevet.com/ruminant)
• Manure Management and Environmental Planning (see www.fiveminutevet.com/ruminant)
• Mastitis (by etiology)
• Mastitis: Camelid
• Mastitis: Small Ruminant
• Microbiologic Sampling (see www.fiveminutevet.com/ruminant)

Suggested Reading

Al-Dughaym AM, Fadlelmula A. Prevalence. Etiology and its seasonal prevalence of clinical and subclinical camel mastitis in Saudi Arabia. Br J Appl Sci Technol 2015, 9: 441–9.

Charaya G, Sharma A, Kumar A, Singh M, Goel P. Pathogens isolated from clinical mastitis in Murrah buffaloes and their antibiogram. Veterinary World 2014, 7: 980–5.

Djabri, B, Bareille N, Beaudeau F, et al. Quarter milk somatic cell count in infected dairy cows: a meta-analysis. Vet Res 2002, 33: 335–7.

Elhaig MM, Selim A. Molecular and bacteriological investigation of subclinical mastitis caused by *Staphylococcus aureus* and *Streptococcus agalactiae* in domestic bovids

from Ismailia, Egypt. Trop Anim Health Prod 2015, 47: 271–6.

Gelasakis AI, Angelidis AS, Giannakou R, Filioussi G, Kalamaki MS, Arsenos G. Bacterial subclinical mastitis and its effect on milk yield in low-input dairy goat herds. J Dairy Sci 2016, 99: 3698–708.

Guerreiro O, Velez Z, Alvarenga N, Matos C, Duarte M. Molecular screening of ovine mastitis in different breeds. J Dairy Sci 2013, 96: 752–60.

Keefe GP. *Streptococcus agalactiae* mastitis: a review. Can Vet J 1997, 38: 429–37.

Keefe GP. Update on control of *Staphylococcus aureus* and *Streptococcus agalactiae* for management of mastitis. Vet Clin North Am Food Anim Pract 2012, 28: 203–16.

Leigh JA. *Streptococcus uberis*: a permanent barrier to the control of bovine mastitis? Vet J 1999, 157: 225–38.

Marogna G, Rolesu S, Lolai S, Tola S, Leori G. Clinical findings in sheep farms affected by recurrent bacterial mastitis. Small Rumin Res 2010, 88: 119–25.

Wahinya MM, Karuku KJ, Richard K, Muli MV, Younan M. Effect of subclinical mastitis caused by ss-haemolytic Streptococci on milk yields in Kenyan camels (*Camelus dromedarius*). Bull Anim Health Prod Afr 2014, 62: 267–74.

Wilson DJ, Gonzalez RN, Das HH. Bovine mastitis pathogens in New York and Pennsylvania: prevalence and effects on somatic cell count and milk production. J Dairy Sci 1997, 80: 2592–8.

Zdanowicz M, Shelford JA, Tucker CB, Weary DM, von Keyserlingk MA. Bacterial populations on teat ends of dairy cows housed in free stalls and bedded with either sand or sawdust. J Dairy Sci 2004, 87: 1694–701.

Zhao Y, Liu H, Zhao X, Gao Y, Zhang M, Chen D. Prevalence and pathogens of subclinical mastitis in dairy goats in China. Trop Anim Health Prod 2015, 47: 429–35.

Author Kaitlyn A. Lutz
Consulting Editor Ahmed Tibary
Acknowledgment The author and book editors acknowledge the prior contribution of David J. Wilson and Jerry R. Roberson.

BASICS

OVERVIEW
• Melioidosis, a disease caused by the bacterium *Burkholderia pseudomallei*, affects a wide variety of animal species.
• Disease is most commonly seen in sheep and goats.
• The disease causes caseous abscesses of the lungs, liver, and spleen.
• In disseminated forms, lameness, arthritis, mastitis, or encephalitis may also occur.

INCIDENCE/PREVALENCE
Outbreaks and cases typically occur in endemic areas during the wet season or after heavy rainfall or flooding in areas with high humidity or temperature.

GEOGRAPHIC DISTRIBUTION
• Endemic in tropical and subtropical regions, particularly southeast Asia, northern and central Australia, the Middle East, India, China, the Caribbean, and Central America.
• Most cases occur within 20° latitude of the equator.

SYSTEMS AFFECTED
• Respiratory
• Musculoskeletal
• Nervous
• Mammary
• Hemolymphatic

PATHOPHYSIOLOGY
• *B. pseudomallei* is an aerobic, Gram-negative, facultatively intracellular motile rod that is oxidase- and catalase-positive.
• *B. pseudomallei* measures approximately 0.8 μm × 1.5 μm and exhibits bipolar ("safety-pin appearance") staining.
• It is an opportunistic pathogen that produces exotoxins.
• Strain differences exist that affect virulence.
• The organism is found in soil and water in tropical and subtropical regions.
• Exposure occurs through ingestion, inhalation, contamination of wounds, or arthropod bites. Rare cases of transplacental transmission have been described.
• Disease can develop from the exotoxins produced by the organism (acute disease) or from the survival of the organism within phagocytic cells (latent or chronic disease).
• The incubation period can be days to years following exposure.

HISTORICAL FINDINGS
Residence within a geographic area where the disease is known to occur.

SIGNALMENT
• Sheep, goats, and Old World camelids are most commonly affected.
• Cattle, buffalo, New World camelids, and deer are rarely affected.

• Malnutrition and immunosuppression can predispose to disease.

SIGNS
• Incubation is variable ranging from a few days to many years.
• Many cases are subclinical, with lesions discovered at slaughter.
• Many seropositive animals never show clinical signs.
• *Sheep*
  ○ Acute form:
    ■ Fever, anorexia and generalized weakness
    ■ Respiratory distress/dyspnea
    ■ Coughing
    ■ Mucopurulent oculonasal discharge
    ■ Nasal plaques
    ■ Lameness with swollen joints
    ■ Neurologic signs may include circling, incoordination, nystagmus, recumbency, hyperesthesia and blindness
    ■ Death in 1–7 days
  ○ Chronic form (much less common)
    ■ Emaciation
    ■ Pneumonia
    ■ Orchitis and testicular abscesses
• *Goats*
  ○ Acute disease is rare.
  ○ Chronic form:
    ■ Lameness
    ■ Lymphadenopathy
    ■ Mastitis
    ■ Cough
    ■ Emaciation
    ■ Nasal discharge
    ■ Salivation
    ■ Fever
    ■ Hindlimb paresis
    ■ Abortion
    ■ Sudden death
• *Camelids*
  ○ Acute disease has been reported in an alpaca.
    ■ Anorexia
    ■ Dyspnea
    ■ Froth around the mouth
    ■ Lymphadenopathy/lymphadenitis
    ■ Death 2 days after first signs
  ○ Old World camelids tend toward chronic disease
    ■ Hacking cough
    ■ Nasal discharge
    ■ Dyspnea
    ■ Ataxia
    ■ Fever
    ■ Emaciation
• *Cattle*
  ○ Rarely show clinical disease
  ○ Fever
  ○ Dyspnea
  ○ Salivation
  ○ Staggering
  ○ Abscessation

GENETICS
N/A

CAUSES AND RISK FACTORS
• Transmission of *B. pseudomallei* is most commonly through contact with contaminated soil or water, via ingestion, inhalation, or by contamination of open wounds.
• Person-to-person and animal-to-person transmission can occur but is very rare.
• The primary risk factor for melioidosis is exposure to contaminated soil or water in endemic areas during the wet season or after periods of heavy rainfall in areas with high humidity and temperature.

DIAGNOSIS

DIFFERENTIAL DIAGNOSES
• Tuberculosis
• Caseous lymphadenitis (CLA)
• Actinobacillosis

CBC/BIOCHEMISTRY/URINALYSIS
No specific clinicopathologic changes have been noted.

OTHER LABORATORY TESTS
Submission of pus, nasal discharge, milk, or feces for culture should be considered.

IMAGING
• Pulmonary or mediastinal abscesses may be visible on radiographs.
• Ultrasound may be used to image abscesses for guided sampling of contents.
• Computed tomgraphy may be useful in valuable small ruminants.

OTHER DIAGNOSTIC PROCEDURES
• Culture of the organism from lesions confirms the diagnosis.
• Diagnosis of melioidosis is difficult but may be suspected at necropsy (see below).
• Although there are no pathognomonic lesions for the disease, isolation and identification of the organism should be attempted from swabs of nasal discharge and/or abscesses.
• Organisms may also be found in the feces or milk of infected animals.
• *B. pseudomallei* grows readily on blood agar, trypticase soy agar, chocolate agar, and MacConkey agar.
• Colonies are slow-growing, opaque brown, umbonate, and glistening. Beta hemolysis is evident on blood agar.
• The organism has a characteristic earthy or putrid odor that may be evident (although actual sniffing of plates is not recommended).
• Growth on MacConkey may be useful to distinguish *B. pseudomallei* from *B. mallei*, which will not grow on MacConkey.

M

- Suspect *B. pseudomallei* samples should be handled in a biosafety cabinet using BSL-3 precautions.
- Serologic tests (e.g., ELISA, indirect hemagglutination (IHA), and immunofluorescence) may also be used to assist diagnosis. IHA is recommended as a screening test for use in endemic areas, while CFT has been recommended for individual animal testing.
- Serology tests may cross-react with *B. mallei* (causative agent of glanders) and other related Gram-negative organisms.
- PCR tests have been developed to distinguish *B. pseudomallei* from *B. mallei* and other *Burkholderia* species.

PATHOLOGIC FINDINGS

- On necropsy, multiple abscesses may be found in any organ, but particularly the lungs, liver, spleen, internal and external lymph nodes, subcutis, and udder.
- Purulent material from the abscesses is green-tinged or gray, thick or caseous.
- Bronchopneumonia with abscesses.
- Nodular or plaque-like coalescing lesions of the nasal septum and turbinates in sheep and goats.
- Testicular or scrotal abscesses in sheep and goats.
- Aortic aneurysms in goats.
- Nodules around joints, arthritis, and/or osteomyelitis in sheep.
- Microscopic lesions in brainstem and spinal cord of sheep and goats.

TREATMENT

THERAPEUTIC APPROACH

- Treatment is seldom attempted due to the progressive nature of the disease.
- Treatment, if attempted, is often prolonged and unsuccessful once an animal is showing clinical signs.

SURGICAL CONSIDERATIONS AND TECHNIQUES

N/A

MEDICATIONS

DRUGS OF CHOICE

- In vitro susceptibility is noted to some 3rd-generation cephalosporins, tetracyclines, and potentiated beta-lactams (e.g., amoxicillin-clavulanate).
- Aminoglycoside resistance is well documented.

CONTRAINDICATIONS

N/A

PRECAUTIONS

No antimicrobial protocols have been evaluated in veterinary species.

POSSIBLE INTERACTIONS

N/A

FOLLOW-UP

EXPECTED COURSE AND PROGNOSIS

Clinically affected animals usually die despite treatment.

POSSIBLE COMPLICATIONS

Affected animals will contaminate the environment and place naïve animals at risk.

CLIENT EDUCATION

Focus on prevention (see "Prevention")

PATIENT CARE

N/A

PREVENTION

- No vaccine exists.
- Remove animals from any contaminated source; environmental testing may be useful.
- Use chlorinated water (2–6 mg/L) at a neutral pH.
- Ensure that water drains away from where animals are kept.
- Disposal of sewage/feces away from animal housing or forage cultivation.
- Pasteurization of milk.
- Rodent control.
- In nonendemic areas, affected animals should be culled.
- Risk factors for melioidosis include brush clearing around farms, multiple animal species present, and flooding or waterlogged conditions.

MISCELLANEOUS

ASSOCIATED CONDITIONS

- Malnutrition
- Immunosuppression

AGE-RELATED FACTORS

Young animals are more likely to suffer acute septicemic melioidosis.

ZOONOTIC POTENTIAL

- Melioidosis is considered a zoonosis, but transmission to humans from animals is considered very rare.
- Most cases acquired by humans are from environmental (contaminated soil or water) infection (i.e., aerosolization or direct contact with open wounds).
- Human clinical signs vary widely based on route of exposure and most human cases occur in conjunction with underlying diseases (diabetes, alcoholism, cystic fibrosis, etc.).
- Overall human mortality rate is 20%.

PREGNANCY

- Melioidosis has been reported to cause abortion in goats.

- Rare cases of transplacental transmission have been described in several species.

BIOSECURITY

- Isolation, quarantine, and testing of new stock entering the herd or flock.
- Cull infected animals if possible.
- Hypochlorite and cresol solutions have been recommended for disinfection of premises.
- *B. pseudomallei* can survive in 0.3% chlorhexidine.

PRODUCTION MANAGEMENT

- Cull positive cases if possible.
- Environmental management is important in preventing herd infection.

SYNONYMS

- Pseudoglanders
- Whitmore disease

ABBREVIATIONS

- CFT = complement fixation test
- ELISA = enzyme-linked immunosorbent assay
- IHA = indirect hemagglutination

SEE ALSO

- Actinobacillosis: Wooden Tongue
- Caseous Lymphadenitis (CLA)
- Tuberculosis: Bovine

Suggested Reading

Center for Food Security and Public Health, 2007. Melioidosis factsheet. Available at http://www.cfsph.iastate.edu/DiseaseInfo/factsheets.php accessed on February 22, 2016.

Dance DA. Ecology of *Burkholderia pseudomallei* and the interactions between environmental *Burkholderia* spp. and human-animal hosts. Acta Trop 2000, 74: 159–68.

Kahn CM, Line S eds. Merck Veterinary Manual, 10th ed. Whitehouse Station, NJ: Merck & Co., 2010.

Markey B, Leonard F, Archambault M, et al. *Pseudomonas, Burkholderia* and *Stenotrophomonas* species. In: Clinical Veterinary Microbiology, 2nd ed. New York: Mosby, 2013.

Musa HI, Hassan L, Shamsuddin ZH, et al. Case-control investigation on the risk factors of melioidosis in small ruminant farms in Peninsular Malaysia. J Appl Microbiol 2015, 119: 331–41.

Sprague LD, Neubauer H. Melioidosis in animals: a review on epizootiology, diagnosis and clinical presentation. J Vet Med B 2004, 51: 305–20.

Author Tamara Gull
Consulting Editor Erica C. McKenzie
Acknowledgment The author and book editors acknowledge the prior contribution of Glenda Dvorak.

METALDEHYDE TOXICOSIS

BASICS

OVERVIEW

• Metaldehyde is widely used for the control of slugs and snails in the United States. In some countries, metaldehyde is also used as a solid fuel in camping stoves and lamps.
• Available formulations include pellets, granules, liquids, or wettable powder. Baits may also contain other pesticides such as insecticides. The concentration of metaldehyde in baits sold in the US is generally between 1.5% and 5%.
• Metaldehyde poisoning is characterized by the abrupt onset of severe neurologic signs.
• Poisoning in ruminants is reported infrequently but has occurred in cattle, sheep, and goats.
• The onset of clinical effects may occur as soon as 30–60 minutes after ingestion, with death as soon as 1 hour.
• The poisoning is commonly referred to as the "shake and bake syndrome" due to the development of tremors and hyperthermia.
• The oral lethal dose of metaldehyde is estimated to be 300 mg/kg body weight in sheep and 200 mg/kg in cattle.

INCIDENCE/PREVALENCE

Usually results from accidental exposure to metaldehyde so mortality depends on amount consumed. Mortality rates of 10% or greater have been reported.

GEOGRAPHIC DISTRIBUTION

Occurs where metaldehyde is used

SYSTEMS AFFECTED

Nervous

PATHOPHYSIOLOGY

• Metaldehyde toxicity results in central nervous system stimulation as a result of disruption of the GABA-ergic system; may also involve other neurotransmitters.
• After ingestion, metaldehyde undergoes partial hydrolysis in the stomach to produce acetaldehyde. Both metaldehyde and acetaldehyde are readily absorbed from the GI tract. The nature of the stomach contents and the rate of gastric emptying influence the rate of absorption and the onset of the clinical syndrome.
• After absorption, metaldehyde is rapidly metabolized. Enterohepatic circulation may prolong retention of metaldehyde in the animal, but ultimately, both metaldehyde and acetaldehyde are excreted in the urine.
• Clinical manifestations are attributed primarily to metaldehyde, although acetaldehyde does play a role in the clinical syndrome. Metaldehyde exposure alters a variety of neurotransmitter concentrations and enzyme activities.
• Metaldehyde reduces concentrations of γ-aminobutyric acid, an inhibitory neurotransmitter that causes CNS excitation. Reduced concentrations of brain serotonin (5-hydroxytryptamine) and norepinephrine decrease the threshold for convulsions.
• Monoamine oxidase activity is increased after metaldehyde exposure. Increased muscle activity and the production of acidic metaldehyde metabolites cause severe electrolyte disturbances and metabolic acidosis (shake and bake).

SIGNALMENT

• All ruminant species are susceptible to metaldehyde including cattle, sheep, goats, deer, and camelids.
• Cases in cattle, sheep, and goats are reported infrequently. Most reported cases involve dogs.

PHYSICAL EXAMINATION FINDINGS

• Signs of poisoning generally begin within 30–60 minutes of exposure.
• Initial: Salivation, tremors of the fore and hind legs, staggering, and respiratory distress.
• This is quickly followed by weakness, ataxia, hyperventilation, hyperthermia, and convulsions. In severe cases, the animals become recumbent, unconscious, and show continuous convulsions with leg paddling.
• Disseminated intravascular coagulation may occur as a result of severe hyperthermia (body temperature may reach 110°F; 43°C).
• Death may occur within 60 minutes of exposure as a result of respiratory failure.

CAUSES AND RISK FACTORS

• Geographic areas with high slug and snail populations present a greater risk due to the increased use of metaldehyde baits.
• Bran or molasses is commonly added to the bait to increase its palatability. Some baits have chemicals added to make them less likely to be ingested by species other than slugs and snails.
• Wild ruminants with access to metaldehyde baits are at risk.

DIAGNOSIS

DIFFERENTIAL DIAGNOSES

• Cyanide toxicosis—initially bright cherry-red blood, history of exposure to cyanide-containing plants.
• Nitrate toxicosis—chocolate-brown discoloration of blood, history of exposure to nitrate-containing plants.
• Lead poisoning—determination of blood lead concentration.
• Organophosphorus or carbamate insecticide exposure—GI upset and neurologic signs, evaluation of cholinesterase activity, detection of pesticides in GI contents.
• Exposure to neurotoxic plants, such as poison hemlock, water hemlock, tree tobacco, lupine—history of presence of plants in the environment; identification of plant parts and chemical analysis for plant toxins in GI contents.
• Exposure to cardiotoxic plants, such as oleander, milkweed, and azalea—chemical analysis for plant toxins in GI contents, history of presence of plants in the environment.
• Nonprotein nitrogen toxicosis—history of NPN supplements in the feed ration, detection of toxic levels of ammonia in rumen content and blood.
• Strychnine toxicosis—history of exposure to strychnine-containing bait, detection of strychnine in GI contents or liver.
• 4-Aminopyridine—history of exposure to the avicide, detection of 4-aminopyridine in GI contents.
• Neurotoxic blue-green algae toxins—peracute onset, access to pond water, detection of anatoxin-A in GI contents.
• Seizures—nontoxic etiologies (e.g., trauma, neoplasia, infection, metabolic disorder).

CBC/BIOCHEMISTRY/URINALYSIS

• No specific clinical pathologic changes occur.
• Metabolic acidosis may be present.

OTHER LABORATORY TESTS

Detection of metaldehyde in serum, urine, rumen content, or liver. Confirmation of metaldehyde in suspect material.

PATHOLOGIC FINDINGS

• No clearly distinctive changes due to the rapidity of death.
• Generalized renal, hepatic, and pulmonary congestion.
• Petechial and ecchymotic hemorrhages in the heart, lung, and GI tract.
• Metaldehyde has a characteristic odor of formaldehyde; may be present in the rumen contents along with bait material.

TREATMENT

THERAPEUTIC APPROACH

• Rapid progression of metaldehyde poisoning necessitates immediate treatment.
• Control of CNS signs and hyperthermia is essential. Decontamination with activated charcoal should be considered after initial stabilization of the poisoned animal.
• Fluid therapy should be instituted to control acidosis and dehydration.

MEDICATIONS

DRUGS OF CHOICE

• No antidote available
• Pentobarbital at 20–30 mg/kg IV or diazepam at 0.5–1.5 mg/kg IV for control of seizures

M

METALDEHYDE TOXICOSIS (CONTINUED)

• Lactated Ringer's or sodium bicarbonate solutions IV
• Activated charcoal at 2 g/kg orally

CONTRAINDICATIONS
• Pentobarbital can cause respiratory depression.
• Appropriate milk and meat withdrawal times must be followed for all compounds administered to food-producing animals.

FOLLOW-UP

EXPECTED COURSE AND PROGNOSIS
• Animals poisoned with metaldehyde may be found dead.
• Poisoning progresses so rapidly that treatment is often too late. In most cases, the affected animals have a poor to grave prognosis.
• If treatment is initiated promptly after the onset of clinical signs, the prognosis is fair.

POSSIBLE COMPLICATIONS
Renal and hepatic disease may develop if poisoned animal survives the initial convulsive phase.

PATIENT CARE
Monitor progression of clinical signs.

PREVENTION
• Avoid metaldehyde-containing baits in areas accessible to livestock.

• Use bait according to label instructions.
• Consider the use of less-toxic alternatives to control slugs and snails.

MISCELLANEOUS

ASSOCIATED CONDITIONS
Concurrent toxicosis from other herbicides/pesticides that may be mixed in (most commonly carbamate insecticides).

PRODUCTION MANAGEMENT
Avoid metaldehyde-containing baits in areas accessible to livestock.

ABBREVIATIONS
• CNS = central nervous system
• GABA = gamma aminobutyric acid
• GI = gastrointestinal
• IV = intravenous
• NPN = nonprotein nitrogen

SEE ALSO
• Blue-Green Algae Poisoning
• Carbamate Toxicity
• Cardiotoxic Plants
• Cyanide Toxicosis
• Lead Toxicosis
• Lupin Toxicity
• Nitrate and Nitrite Toxicosis
• Organophosphate Toxicity
• Poison Hemlock (*Conium* spp.) Toxicity
• Pyrrolizidine Alkaloids

• Strychnine Poisonings
• Urea Toxicity
• Water Hemlock

Suggested Reading
Blakely BR. Overview of metaldehyde poisoning. The Merck Veterinary Manual Online, 2013. http://www.merckvet manual.com/mvm/toxicology/metaldehyde_ poisoning/overview_of_metaldehyde_ poisoning.html accessed July 30, 2016.
Booze TF, Oehme FW. Metaldehyde toxicity: a review. Vet Hum Toxicol 1985l 27: 11–19.
Brutlag AG, Puschner B. Metaldehyde. In: Peterson ME, Talcott PA eds, Small Animal Toxicology, 3rd ed. St. Louis: Saunders, 2013, pp. 635–42.
Dolder LK. Metaldehyde toxicosis. Vet Med 2003, 98: 213–15.
Gupta RC. Metaldehyde. In: Gupta RC ed, Veterinary Toxicology, Basic and Clinical Principles, 2nd ed. New York: Elsevier, 2012, pp. 624–8.
Talcott PA. Metaldehyde. In: Plumlee KH ed, Clinical Veterinary Toxicology. St. Louis: Mosby, 2004.
Valentine BA, Rumbeiha WK, Hensley TS, Halse RR. Arsenic and metaldehyde toxicosis in a beef herd. J Vet Diagn Invest 2007, 19: 212–15.
Author Marianne Polunas
Consulting Editor Christopher C.L. Chase
Acknowledgment The author and book editors acknowledge the prior contribution of Birgit Puschner.

M

BASICS

OVERVIEW
• Metritis is an inflammation of all layers (endometrium, myometrium, and serosa) of the uterus during the postpartum period, typically the first 7–14 days.
• Metritis is more commonly seen in dairy cattle but can affect all ruminant and camelid species.
• Affected cows have a fetid, watery, discolored genital discharge. Puerperal (toxic) metritis is distinguished by an elevation in body temperature and signs of systemic illness including anorexia, depression, and dehydration. In severe cases the condition can become septic and life threatening. In an effort to improve diagnostic, therapeutic, and prognostic precision, attempts have been made to distinguish metritic cows with and without systemic signs of disease. It should be noted that this distinction may be a temporal one as signs may have subsided at the time of the examination or they may occur later in the course of the disease. Cows with metritis are more likely to develop other postpartum disorders such as ketosis, displacement of the abomasum, endometritis, and pyometra.
• Cows with metritis usually have reduced feed intake, produce less milk, and experience a delay in days to first service, lower conception rates, and increased days open.

INCIDENCE/PREVALENCE
• The postpartum incidence of metritis varies among reports and with the definition criteria used for diagnosis.
• In North America, approximately 10–20% of dairy cows are affected with metritis. About one-half of the cows with an abnormal parturition (dystocia, RFM, twins) can be expected to develop metritis.

GEOGRAPHIC DISTRIBUTION
Worldwide; in hot climates the incidence of metritis may be higher due to the effect of heat stress.

SYSTEMS AFFECTED
• Multisystemic
• Reproductive

PATHOPHYSIOLOGY
• The vulva, vestibulovaginal sphincter, and cervix are mechanical barriers that protect the uterus from bacterial contamination. However, during parturition and shortly thereafter, these barriers break down and allow pathogenic and nonpathogenic bacteria to contaminate the uterus. Most of these bacteria are transient residents and are eliminated by the defense mechanisms of the uterus.

• The bacterial population is mixed and consists of both aerobic and anaerobic Gram-negative and Gram-positive organisms.
• Organisms frequently incriminated in bovine metritis include *Trueperella pyogenes*, *Escherichia coli*, and *Fusobacterium necrophorum*. Occasionally, *Clostridium* spp. infect the uterus and cause a gangrenous metritis. Depending on the species and location, a wide variety of pathogenic and opportunistic microorganisms have been isolated from cases of metritis.
• In cows with a normal parturition, the uterus resolves the bacterial infection by 4 weeks postpartum. However, in affected females the bacterial contamination becomes more severe and persistent.
• Unsanitary calving conditions and traumatic obstetric manipulation can also predispose the cow to uterine infections.
• Because of differences in husbandry practices and stress from lactation, postpartum metritis is more commonly seen in dairy cows than other ruminants.

GENETICS
Generally N/A; however, genomic testing has the potential to identify a genetic basis for many predisposing risk factors and possibly diseases themselves, including metritis.

HISTORICAL FINDINGS
Dystocia or RFM

SIGNALMENT
• More commonly seen in bovine than in caprine or ovine species.
• In camelid, metritis is observed after lengthy obstetric manipulation and in cases of fetal emphysema.
• Dairy cattle are more frequently affected than beef cattle.
• Reports are conflicting as to the effect of parity on incidence. However, most agree that the incidence is higher in primiparous than in multiparous animals.

PHYSICAL EXAMINATION FINDINGS
• Clinical signs of metritis are influenced by the virulence of the bacteria and predisposing risk factors.
• During the first few weeks postpartum, lochia is normally expelled from the reproductive tract. Normal lochia is red to brown in color.
• Metritis occurs more commonly in those cows that experienced an abnormal parturition and these cattle should be monitored carefully during the first 2 weeks postpartum.
• Fever (>103.0°F or 39.5°C).
• Partial or complete anorexia.
• Low milk production.
• Lethargy or depression.

• Fetid serosanguineous discharge from the reproductive tract.
• Enlarged, flaccid uterus.

CAUSES AND RISK FACTORS
• Risk factors associated with metritis have been studied mainly in dairy cattle and include: RFM, dystocia, delivery of a male calf, twinning, uterine prolapse, abortion or stillbirth, hypocalcemia.
• A variety of bacteria can establish an infection.

DIAGNOSIS

DIFFERENTIAL DIAGNOSES
• Normal discharge from the uterus or lochia
• Endometritis/vaginitis/cervicitis
• Parturient trauma (often iatrogenic)

CBC/BIOCHEMISTRY/URINALYSIS
• Neutropenia with or without a degenerative left shift
• Hypocalcemia
• Hypoglycemia
• Ketonemia

OTHER LABORATORY TESTS
Bacterial culture and sensitivity may be indicated for valuable individuals.

IMAGING
Ultrasonography and vaginoscopy may be used to verify the origin of the genital discharge but are generally not necessary in cattle. They may be of more use in small ruminants and camelidae.

OTHER DIAGNOSTIC PROCEDURES
• Palpation per rectum
• Vaginoscopy
• Ultrasonography

PATHOLOGIC FINDINGS
Necropsy findings in cows that die from toxic or septic metritis: peritonitis; friable, necrotic uterus.

TREATMENT

THERAPEUTIC APPROACH
• Because of the differences in diagnostic criteria and the lack of controlled studies, treatment of this condition remains controversial among clinicians.
• Therapy generally includes antibiotics (systemic or intrauterine). The efficacy of intrauterine antibiotic is questionable.
• Supportive treatment for clinical signs and associated conditions (e.g., hypocalcemia and ketosis).
• Fluid therapy and anti-inflammatory agents are indicated for animals with systemic signs of disease.

M

METRITIS   (CONTINUED)

• Camelidae are often treated in a manner similar to the mare. Typically this involves uterine lavage, systemic antibiotics, and supportive therapy.

SURGICAL CONSIDERATIONS AND TECHNIQUES
N/A

MEDICATIONS

DRUGS OF CHOICE
• Systemic administration of a broad-spectrum antibiotic is recommended for cows with metritis, particularly those that are pyretic. Follow label recommendations, maintain treatment records, and educate producers to avoid antibiotic residues in milk and meat.
   ○ Procaine penicillin G: 22,000 IU/kg IM q24h for 3–5 days
   ○ Ceftiofur: 2.2 mg/kg q24h IM or SubQ for 5 days
   ○ Ampicillin: 4.4–11 mg/kg IM for 3–7 days
   ○ Oxytetracycline: 6.6–11 mg/kg IM, SQ, or IV for up to 4 days
• Intrauterine penicillin and oxytetracycline are used by some clinicians but the efficacy is questionable.
• Sanitary procedures and avoidance of genital tract trauma are important considerations when intrauterine antibiotics are used.
• Estrogens and oxytocin have been advocated to increase uterine contractions and help evacuate uterine contents. Research is lacking that supports the use of these hormones for the treatment of metritis.
• Contractions induced by estrogen have been associated with flushing septic uterine contents into the uterine tubes, causing salpingitis or even peritonitis.
• Oxytocin causes contraction of the postpartum uterus if it is used within 6 days after calving. Doses of 20–40 IU repeated every 3–6 hours are generally used.

CONTRAINDICATIONS
• Systemic oxytetracycline is not recommended because of difficulty in reaching the minimal inhibitory concentration required for *T. pyogenes* in the uterine lumen.
• No antibiotic is approved for intrauterine use in the United States.
• Appropriate milk and meat withdrawal times must be followed.
• Veterinarians should be aware of local regulations that may restrict their choice of drugs or the method and frequency of administration.

PRECAUTIONS
N/A

POSSIBLE INTERACTIONS
N/A

FOLLOW-UP

EXPECTED COURSE AND PROGNOSIS
• Cows treated promptly can be expected to recover fully from metritis. However, milk production and reproductive performance are affected in the current lactation. In some cases, cows can develop uterine abscesses and pyometra.
• In camelids, prognosis for life is very good if metritis is treated promptly and adequately. Postpartum breeding should be delayed.

POSSIBLE COMPLICATIONS
• Septicemia
• Ketosis
• Displaced abomasum
• Mastitis
• Infertility
• Involuntary culling

CLIENT EDUCATION
• In dairy, clients should institute a postpartum monitoring program particular for high-risk cows.
• In camelids, females should be presented for postpartum evaluation and neonatal examination 24–36 hours after parturition.

PATIENT CARE
• In cattle, metritis patients should be monitored for development of ketosis, displaced abomasum, and mastitis.
• In camelids, metritis patients should be monitored for poor appetite and metabolic disorders. Neonates should be monitored to insure that they are getting enough milk.
• In addition, if the condition does not improve with 3 days of antibiotic treatment, an alternative antibiotic should be considered.

PREVENTION
• Effective transition cow management with special attention to adequate feed intake.
• Minimize dystocia incidence.
• Use of calving-ease bulls.
• Use of gender-enhanced semen (female) for heifers.
• Minimize abortion incidence.
• Biosecurity and quarantine procedures.
• Vaccination.
• Sanitary and atraumatic obstetric procedures.
• Sanitary maternity facilities.
• Postpartum health monitoring during the first 2 weeks postpartum should include milk production and attitude monitoring to help diagnose and treat the condition early.

MISCELLANEOUS

ASSOCIATED CONDITIONS
Ketosis, displaced abomasum, dystocia, RFM, endometritis, infertility

AGE-RELATED FACTORS
In general, incidence of metritis is greater in primiparous than in multiparous animals.

ZOONOTIC POTENTIAL
The common bacterial agents isolated from metritis cases are rarely a zoonotic concern for healthy, immunocompetent adults. However, metritis is frequently seen following abortion or stillbirth and these conditions in ruminants are often the result of potentially zoonotic diseases (e.g., leptospirosis, brucellosis, toxoplasmosis, and Q fever). Protective clothing, sleeves, and good hygienic practices are recommended.

PREGNANCY
Metritis occurs in postpartum animals.

BIOSECURITY
Prevention of infectious diseases that may cause abortion will reduce the incidence of metritis. Testing of new arrivals, quarantine, and vaccination programs are effective methods for limiting disease introduction.

PRODUCTION MANAGEMENT
Effective herd management can reduce the incidence of metritis as well as limit the financial impact of cases when they do occur.

ABBREVIATIONS
• IM = intramuscular
• IV = intravenous
• RFM = retained fetal membranes
• SQ = subcutaneous

SEE ALSO
• Displaced Abomasum
• Down Bovine
• Endometritis
• Hypocalcemia: Bovine
• Hypocalcemia: Small Ruminant
• Infertility and Subfertility Issues
• Ketosis: Dairy Cattle
• Mastitis
• Ovarian Hypoplasia, Bursal Disease, Salpingitis
• Postpartum Disorders
• Pyometra

Suggested Reading
Frazer GS. A rational basis for therapy in the sick postpartum cow. Vet Clin North Am Food Anim Pract 2005, 21: 523–68.
Machado VS, Bicalho ML, Meira Jr. EB, et al. Subcutaneous immunization with inactivated bacterial components and purified protein of *Escherichia coli*,

M

Fusobacterium necrophorum and *Trueperella pyogenes* prevents puerperal metritis in Hostein dairy cows. PLoS One 2014, PMID 24638139.

Risco CA, Youngquist RS, Shore MD. Postpartum uterine infections. In: Youngquist RS, Threlfall WR eds, Current Therapy in Large Animal Theriogenology,

2nd ed. Philadelphia: Saunders, 2007, pp. 339–44.

Sheldon IM, Lewis GS, LeBlanc S, Gilbert RO. Defining postpartum uterine disease in cattle. Theriogenology 2006, 65: 1516–30.

Tibary A. Breeding soundness evaluation and subfertility in female llamas and alpacas. In: Youngquist RS, Threlfall WR eds, Current

Therapy in Large Animal Theriogenology, 2nd ed. Philadelphia: Saunders, 2007, pp. 878–83.

Authors Harry Momont and Celina Checura
Consulting Editor Ahmed Tibary
Acknowledgment The author and book editors acknowledge the prior contribution of Carlos A. Risco.

M

MILK VEIN RUPTURE

BASICS

OVERVIEW
Hemorrhage from the caudal superficial epigastric vein (milk vein)

INCIDENCE/PREVALENCE
N/A

GEOGRAPHIC DISTRIBUTION
N/A

SYSTEMS AFFECTED
Cardiovascular

PATHOPHYSIOLOGY
• The milk vein is a common site for venipuncture by laypeople because it is very superficial cranial to the mammary gland on the ventral abdomen. It is an especially convenient vein for farmers and workers treating down cattle for conditions such as milk fever (hypocalcemia). The vessel is only thinly covered by skin and subcutaneous tissue.
• Perivascular hemorrhage or leakage of irritating products such as calcium, dextrose, or antimicrobials can cause small abscesses or fibrous tissue that weaken the covering over the milk vein, sometimes resulting in rupture.
• Hemorrhage also occurs due to direct trauma to the vein (e.g., lacerations, direct pressure from casting ropes).

SIGNALMENT
• Bovine species, usually adults after IV treatment.
• Predominant sex is females secondary to the propensity for hypocalcemia treatment.

HISTORICAL FINDINGS
• IV treatment in the milk vein some time prior to hemorrhage.
• Trauma.
• May see an increased incidence during times of biting flies and other insect activity due to bunching of cattle and increased leg kicking for fly avoidance.

PHYSICAL EXAMINATION FINDINGS
Bleeding from either of the caudal superficial epigastric veins.

GENETICS
N/A

CAUSES AND RISK FACTORS
• Weakened tissue superficial to the milk vein.
• Conditions requiring IV treatments, such as hypocalcemia, ketosis, or some mastitis treatments. Farmers treating cattle IV in milking parlors without adequate restraint tend to favor the milk vein. Reusing needles is associated with local sepsis and increased tissue damage due to dull or barbed needles.
• Infrastructure in milking parlors and barns, especially metal, with exposed sharp edges.

DIAGNOSIS

DIFFERENTIAL DIAGNOSES
N/A

CBC/BIOCHEMISTRY/URINALYSIS
PCV/TP can be monitored to evaluate level of whole blood loss; however, immediate on-farm treatment should be initiated based on clinical signs.

OTHER LABORATORY TESTS
N/A

IMAGING
N/A

OTHER DIAGNOSTIC PROCEDURES
N/A

PATHOLOGIC FINDINGS
Rupture in thin-walled area of milk vein.

TREATMENT

THERAPEUTIC APPROACH
• Suture ruptured area.
• Fluid therapy or blood transfusion may be required.

SURGICAL CONSIDERATIONS AND TECHNIQUES
Suturing may be complicated by friable tissue. Purse-string sutures surrounding the friable area are often required.

MEDICATIONS

DRUGS OF CHOICE
• Balanced electrolytes or whole blood transfusion if pale mucus membranes or low PCV.
• Broad-spectrum antibiotics are warranted in cases with significant contamination or cases occurring secondary to improper IV administration with surrounding cellulitis.

CONTRAINDICATIONS
N/A

PRECAUTIONS
• The rupture is often difficult to suture because of the friable tissue that resulted in the rupture.
• This is a medical emergency.

POSSIBLE INTERACTIONS
N/A

FOLLOW-UP

EXPECTED COURSE AND PROGNOSIS
Recovery if vein successfully sutured and hypovolemia is corrected.

POSSIBLE COMPLICATIONS
Hypovolemic shock and death

PATIENT CARE
Monitor for signs of hypovolemia and sepsis.

CLIENT EDUCATION
• Advise client not to utilize the milk vein for IV treatments.
• Train dairy personnel how to manage cases of milk vein rupture until the veterinarian arrives. This includes stopping hemorrhage with a tight belly-band (e.g., duct tape, elastikon) or clamp (e.g., hemostats, binder clips, locking plyers) and keeping the animal quiet.

PREVENTION
• Do not use milk vein for IV treatments. Do not reuse needles. Fly and insect control.
• Maintain facilities well, which includes frequent walk-throughs and prompt attention to damaged infrastructure.
• Use care when casting lactating cows using the double half-hitch method as the rope puts significant pressure over the superficial epigastric veins. The Burley/Flying-W method negates this risk.

MISCELLANEOUS

AGE-RELATED FACTORS
Usually adult dairy cows.

ABBREVIATIONS
• IV = intravenous
• PCV = packed cell volume
• TP = total protein

SEE ALSO
• Fluid Therapy: Intravenous
• Fluid Therapy: Oral

Suggested Reading
Davies RC. Rupture of the mammary vein in the cow. Vet Rec 1968, 83: 528.
Giles MB. Hematomas over the mammary veins in cows. Vet Rec 1968, 83: 333.
Swarbrick O. Hematoma over the mammary veins in cows. Vet Rec 1968, 83: 305–6.
Author Jim P. Reynolds
Consulting Editor Kaitlyn A. Lutz

MILKWEED (*ASCLEPIAS* SPP.) TOXICOSIS

BASICS

OVERVIEW
• Toxicity associated with ingestion of one of many *Asclepias* spp. (milkweed).
• Distribution of plants varies by species, however, there is at least one species present over most of North America.
• Two leaf types are present and vary in their expression of the relative amounts of toxins:
  ○ Wide leaf varieties (i.e., *A. speciosa* and *A. syriaca*) are more commonly associated with cardiac and gastrointestinal toxicity. Toxicity is less common as they are only eaten when no other feed choices are available.
  ○ Thin leaf (<1 cm wide) varieties (i.e., *A. fascicularis* and *A. subverticillata*), which contain higher levels of the neurotoxin and are consumed more commonly due to their more palatable nature and the animal's difficulty in selectively not consuming them in hay.
• Plants are most toxic during rapid growth but retain their toxicity even when dried in hay. Toxicity tends to decrease with maturity.
• Clinical signs develop with consumption of 0.05–2% of body weight depending on the species and toxin concentration in the plant.

INCIDENCE/PREVALENCE
Milkweed is considered to be one of the most toxic plants in North America and has been associated with mortality rates of >50% in sheep grazing milkweed for 24 hours or less.

GEOGRAPHIC DISTRIBUTION
There are over 100 species of *Asclepias* spp. growing naturally in North America and all are potentially toxic. There are few species in Canada. There are also a few species in other parts of the world.

SYSTEMS AFFECTED
• Cardiovascular
• Digestive
• Nervous

PATHOPHYSIOLOGY
• Two mechanisms of toxicity: (1) cardiovascular and gastrointestinal toxicity associated with cardenolides (cardiac glycosides) and (2) neuromuscular toxicity associated with neurotoxic pregnane glycosides.
• The cardenolides produced by the wide leaf varieties inhibit the function of the Na$^+$/K$^+$-ATPase pump and allow accumulation of Na and Ca inside the cell and depletion of intracellular K. This leads to abnormal membrane potentials and irregular action potential initiation. This results in cardiac arrhythmias and muscle weakness.
• The mechanism of action of the neurotoxin is not known.

SIGNALMENT
• Sheep are most commonly affected.
• Can occur in any ruminant species.
• Cattle require ingestion of twice as much toxin as sheep.
• Animals are consuming toxin-producing forages either green in the field or in hay.

PHYSICAL EXAMINATION FINDINGS
• Vary with the species of plant consumed (i.e., neurotoxin-producing thin leaf or cardiotoxin-producing wide leaf), amount consumed, and duration of toxicity.
• Acute death may be the only clinical sign.
• Signs generally develop within 12–18 hours of ingestion of cardiac glycosides and may be immediate or delayed (i.e., 12 hours) with ingestion of neurotoxic compounds.
• Cardiac glycoside (cardiac and gastrointestinal toxin) symptoms include depression, weakness, reluctance to stand, enteritis, bloat, labored respiration with grunt, and possibly cardiac arrhythmias.
• Neurotoxic symptoms include depression, mydriasis, ataxia, weakness, pelvic limb paresis, humped-up appearance, rabbit-like gait, seizures, opisthotonus, and death due to respiratory failure.

CAUSES AND RISK FACTORS
• Ingestion of toxin-containing *Asclepias* spp. in pastures or hay.
• Ingestion of neurotoxic compounds may be cumulative.
• Cattle on ionophore-containing diets may have an increased risk.

DIAGNOSIS

DIFFERENTIAL DIAGNOSES
• Other sources of cardiac glycosides, including dogbane, Indian hemp, lily of the valley, foxglove, and oleander.
• Other cardiotoxic plants including yew, rhododendron, and laurels.
• Other neurologic diseases including heavy metal toxicosis, buckeye toxicity, dallis grass toxicity, traumatic nerve damage (calving paralysis), spinal column lymphosarcoma, and rabies.
• Other causes of recumbency including fractures, hypocalcemia, hypomagnesemia, hypophosphatemia, and hypokalemia.
• Other causes of cardiac arrhythmias including traumatic reticulopericarditis, electrolyte disorder associated atrial fibrillation, cardiac neoplasia.

CBC/BIOCHEMISTRY/URINALYSIS
There may be an increase in serum creatinine kinase activity. However, this is not a specific indicator for milkweed toxicity.

OTHER LABORATORY TESTS
• Evaluation of the pasture or hay for evidence of milkweed contamination. Careful

examination for the narrow leaf varieties must be done, as they are often hard to identify due to their similarity to grasses even when contained in large quantities in hay.
• Analysis of urine, serum, tissue, and stomach contents for cardiac glycosides is available using high-performance liquid chromatography.

IMAGING
Echocardiography would be helpful in excluding other differential diagnoses. However, it is technically challenging and requires expensive equipment and thus is not routinely done.

PATHOLOGIC FINDINGS
• Depends on the toxin consumed.
• Cardiac glycoside toxicity is associated with a hyperemia with or without hemorrhage of the abomasum and small intestine, pulmonary congestion, acute ischemia-associated glomerulopathy and tubular necrosis, and in some cases mild nonsuppurative myocardial cellular degeneration. Hemorrhage may be present on the surface of the lung, kidney, and heart.
• Ingestion of the neurotoxic compound is more difficult to determine on necropsy, but there may be evidence of external trauma; hemorrhages in the trachea, heart, and lungs; and often an empty urinary bladder.

TREATMENT

THERAPEUTIC APPROACH
• If acute ingestion of large amounts of toxin is suspected, a rumenotomy to evacuate the ingesta may be beneficial.
• Other herd mates should be isolated from the source of the toxin (i.e., pasture or hay).

MEDICATIONS

DRUGS OF CHOICE
• Orogastric intubation with activated charcoal, cathartics, or mineral oil may decrease intestinal absorption of the toxins and increase rate of excretion in feces.
• Administering balanced polyionic fluids as needed to maintain hydration and for renal diuresis may minimize effects of ischemia-induced kidney damage.
• Sedative and/or anesthesia may be helpful in patients with severe convulsions associated with neurotoxin ingestion.
• Antiarrhythmic drugs such as procainamide, lidocaine, or atropine sulfate may be used in rare cases exhibiting arrhythmias. (Appropriate records for extra-label drug use must be maintained.)
• Appropriate drug withdrawal periods must be determined and maintained.

M

CONTRAINDICATIONS

Use of calcium-containing fluids is contraindicated as it may potentiate the effects of cardiac glycosides.

 FOLLOW-UP

EXPECTED COURSE AND PROGNOSIS

• Varies with amount of toxin ingested, duration of exposure, and response to treatment.
• Most animals will start developing signs within 12–18 hours of ingesting toxin.
• If symptoms are severe, animals will often die within 24 hours.
• If animal develops seizures and convulsions, the prognosis is grave.
• If animals survive the first 24–36 hours, they often will remain weak for a period of time before improving.

POSSIBLE COMPLICATIONS

If the animals survive, they may develop acute to chronic renal failure.

PATIENT CARE

• Evaluation of neurologic status and monitoring for seizure activity should be done frequently.

• Frequent auscultation of the heart should be performed to assess for development of cardiac arrhythmias.
• Monitoring of urinalysis and serum chemistry for azotemia is indicated in patients that survive the acute toxicosis.

PREVENTION

Prevent animals from grazing on pasture or eating hay containing milkweed.

 MISCELLANEOUS

PREGNANCY

N/A

ABBREVIATIONS

N/A

SEE ALSO

• Buckeye (*Aesculus* spp.) Toxicity
• Down Bovine
• Dystocia: Bovine
• Cardiotoxic Plants
• Fungal Tremorgens
• Grass Tetany/Hypomagnesemia
• Heavy Metal Toxicosis

• Hypocalcemia: Bovine
• Hypocalcemia: Small Ruminant
• Lymphosarcoma
• Oleander and Cardiotoxic Plant Toxicity
• Phosphorus Deficiency/Excess
• Rabies
• Traumatic Reticulopericarditis

Suggested Reading

Benson JM, Seiber JN, Bagley CV, Keeler RF, Johnson AE, Young S. Effects on sheep of the milkweeds *Asclepias eriocarpa* and *A. labriformis* and of cardiac glycoside-containing derivative material. Toxicon 1979, 17(2):155–65.

Burrows GE, Tyrl RJ ed. Toxic plants of North America. Ames: Iowa State University Press, 2001.

Burrows GE, Tyrl RJ. Toxic Plants of North America, 2nd ed. Ames: Wiley-Blackwell, 2013. Kindle edition.

Smith RA, Scharko P, Bolin D, Hong CB. Intoxication of sheep exposed to Ozark milkweed (*Asclepias viridis Walter*). Vet Hum Toxicol 2000, 42: 349–50.

Author Paul J. Plummer
Consulting Editor Christopher C.L. Chase

M

MOLYBDENUM TOXICITY

BASICS

OVERVIEW
• Molybdenum (Mb) is an essential micronutrient, which forms molybdenoenzymes. Dietary intake of excess Mb causes, in part, secondary hypocuprosis.
• The metabolism of copper, molybdenum, and inorganic sulfate is a complex interrelationship. Mb toxicity is directly associated with copper deficiency and has similar signs.
• Ruminants are especially susceptible to dietary molybdenum excess, leading to depressed growth, diarrhea, neurologic defects, and eventually death, if untreated.
• The ruminal interaction of molybdates and sulfides gives rise to thiomolybdates. At high levels, these compounds decrease the availability of dietary copper and, when absorbed, slow the metabolism of tissue copper and inhibit copper enzymes. This leads to signs of copper deficiency.
• Increased levels in the east and west coasts, increased in acidic, wet soil (peat bogs).
• Forage plants can accumulate Mb. Concentration is lowest in winter, increased in summer and fall.
• Seen in contamination of soils, industrial contamination, fertilizers, feeding of forages and grain. When Cu levels of feed or forages in the normal range of 8–11 ppm, cattle can be poisoned with Mb levels above 5–6 ppm and sheep on levels above 10–12 ppm.
• If Cu level is below 8–11 ppm, or sulfate level is high, even 1–2 ppm Mb may be toxic in cattle.
• High level of Cu in diet to 13–16 ppm can protect Mb poisoning up to 150 ppm dietary Mb.

INCIDENCE/PREVALENCE
Not unusual that large percentage of herd clinically affected.

GEOGRAPHIC DISTRIBUTION
Increased levels in the east and west coasts, increased in acidic, wet soil (peat bogs).

SYSTEMS AFFECTED
• Integument
• Musculoskeletal
• Nervous

PATHOPHYSIOLOGY
• In ruminants, various molybdates react with sulfides to produce thiomolybdate compounds, which react with copper to form an insoluble complex that is poorly absorbed.
• The reduced copper absorption impairs copper utilization and the synthesis of a variety of copper-dependent proteins. The reduced bioavailability of copper ultimately induces secondary copper deficiency. Causes cytochrome oxidase deficiency and limits heme synthesis.

• Excessive molybdenum intake also enhances the excretion of copper. Excessive molybdenum exposure may also impair a variety of enzymes involved in collagen and elastin maintenance and stability, which has been associated with cardiovascular disorders.
• Molybdenum exposure may reduce phospholipid synthesis in nervous tissue, resulting in demyelination and neurologic disorders clinically.

SIGNALMENT
• Ruminants tend to be more susceptible than nonruminants; cattle are more susceptible than sheep. Cattle and sheep are ~10-fold more susceptible than other species.
• Young animals have increased susceptibility.
• Calves can be poisoned by milk from cows on increased Mb.
• Lambs under 1 month of age, severely uncoordinated, ataxic, and usually blind.

PHYSICAL EXAMINATION FINDINGS
• Defects in pigmentation, keratinization, bone formation, myelination of the spinal cord, connective tissue formation, and pica.
• With chronic ingestion, osteoporosis, bone fractures, beaded ribs, and overgrowth of long bone ends are found.
• Emaciation, depressed growth.
• Liquid diarrhea full of gas bubbles, called peat scours, or teart.
• Swollen genitalia, impaired reproductive performance.
• Low-level toxicity linked to reduced fertility in cattle, result of binding to Cu.
• Anemia from decreased hematopoiesis.
• Achromotrichia (depigmentation) of the hair coat especially around the eyes, giving a "spectacled" appearance.
• In sheep, depigmentation of dark wool, loss of crimp and quality of the fine wool.
• In Australia, enzootic ataxia, in the United Kingdom "sway back" seen in the lysis of CNS white matter.
• Death is the result of starvation, exposure, or pneumonia.

CAUSES AND RISK FACTORS
The susceptibility of ruminants to a high intake of molybdenum depends on a number of factors:
• The copper contents and intake of the animal: The tolerance to molybdenum decreases as the content and intake of copper fall.
• The inorganic sulfate content of the diet: High dietary sulfate with low copper levels exacerbates the condition; low dietary sulfate causes high blood molybdenum levels due to decreased excretion.
• The chemical form of the molybdenum: Water-soluble in growing herbage is the most toxic, and curing decreases toxicity.
• The presence of certain sulfur-containing amino acids.
• The species of the animal: Cattle are less tolerant than sheep.

• The age: Young animals are more susceptible.
• The season of the year: Plants concentrate molybdenum beginning in the spring with the maximum level in the fall.
• The botanic composition of the pasture: Legumes take up more of the element than other plant species.
• In cattle forage a safe ratio of Cu : Mb is >2:1; when the ratio is <2:1, Mb poisoning occurs.

DIAGNOSIS
Made by clinical appearance, response to Cu treatment

DIFFERENTIAL DIAGNOSES
• Ca/phos/vit D metabolic imbalance
• Massive parasitism, GI parasites
• Johne's disease
• Demyelinating diseases of brain and spinal cord

CBC/BIOCHEMISTRY/URINALYSIS
• Decreased PCV, microcytic, hypochromic anemia
• Cu and Mb levels in forage and tissues
• Liver levels of Cu <10–30 ppm, Mb >5 ppm significant
• Whole blood Cu <0.6 ppm, Mb >0.1 ppm, significant
• Milk Mb up to 300 ppm significant

PATHOLOGIC FINDINGS
• Gross lesions include cardiovascular hemorrhage.
• Histologic lesions include lysis of white matter and degeneration of motor tracts of spinal cord.
• Microscopic to massive subcortical destruction.
• Neuronal degeneration and demyelination.

TREATMENT

THERAPEUTIC APPROACH
• Remove animal from feed source.
• Where Mb content of forage is <5 ppm, Cu sulfate in salt mineral mixture 1%. With higher Mb, use 2%.
• Repository Cu glycinate SQ and 60 mg for calves, 120 mg for mature cattle. May need to be repeated for a good response.
• Can use as top dressing in pasture, trace mineral mix free choice in feed.

MEDICATIONS

DRUGS OF CHOICE
Copper sulfate oral drench

MOLYBDENUM TOXICITY   (CONTINUED)

CONTRAINDICATIONS
• Sheep are highly susceptible to copper drench.
• Appropriate milk and meat withdrawal times must be followed for all compounds administered to food-producing animals.

 MISCELLANEOUS

ASSOCIATED CONDITIONS
N/A

AGE-RELATED FACTORS
• Young animals have increased susceptibility.
• Calves can be poisoned by milk from cows on increased Mb.
• Lambs <1 month of age, severely uncoordinated, ataxic, and usually blind.

PREGNANCY
Impaired reproductive performance

SYNONYMS
• Peat scours
• Teart

ABBREVIATIONS
• CNS = central nervous system
• Cu = copper
• GI = gastrointestinal
• Mb = molybdenum
• PCV = packed cell volume
• SQ = subcutaneous

SEE ALSO
• Coccidiosis
• Haemonchosis
• Hypocalcemia: Bovine
• Hypocalcemia: Small Ruminant
• Johne's Disease
• Ostertagiasis
• Phosphorus Deficiency/Excess
• Spinal Column and Cord Assessment and Dysfunction (see www.fiveminutevet.com/ruminant)
• Strongyloidiasis
• Vitamin D Deficiency/Toxicosis

Suggested Reading
Buck WB, Osweiler GD, Van Gelder GA. Clinical and Diagnostic Veterinary Toxicology, 2nd ed. Dubuque, IA: Kendall-Hunt Publishing Co, 1976.

Mason J. Thiomolybdates: mediators of molybdenum toxicity and enzyme inhibitors. Toxicology 1986, 42: 99–109.
Molybdenum Poisoning. In: Kahn CM ed, The Merck Veterinary Manual, 10th ed. Whitehouse Station, NJ: Merck & Co., 2010.
NADIS; National Animal Disease Information Service. Laven R. Molybdenum Toxicity. Accessed January 27, 2016. www.nadis.org.uk/bulletins/molybdenum-toxicity.aspx; http://www.thecattlesite.com/diseaseinfo/220/molybdenum-toxicity/
Roder JD. Veterinary toxicology. In: The Practical Veterinarian. Woburn, MA: Butterworth-Heinemann, 2001.
Ward GM. Molybdenum toxicity and hypocuprosis in ruminants: a review. J Anim Sci 1978, 46: 1078–85.

Author Marianne Polunas
Consulting Editor Christopher C.L. Chase
Acknowledgment The author and book editors acknowledge the prior contribution of Greg Stoner.

M

BASICS

OVERVIEW

• Monensin, a monovalent carboxylic ionophore antibiotic produced by the fungus *Streptomyces cinnamonensis,* is approved by the UnitedStates FDA for use as a feed additive in certain classes of ruminants.
• Commercially available as Rumensin and Coban, it is commonly added in feed to treat coccidiosis and to improve feed efficiency and growth by altering rumen microbial populations. It also spares dietary proteins in the rumen to prevent bloating and acidosis.
• Poisonings have been reported in cattle, sheep, goats, and camelids. Ingestion of toxic amounts of ionophores can cause effects to the cardiovascular, musculoskeletal, neuromuscular, hepatic, and renal systems.
• Toxicosis can result from overdosage and misuse. Mixing errors and ingestion of premix concentrates are the leading causes of such presentations.
• Clinical signs in affected animals may be acute, evident within a day, or subchronic, taking several weeks, depending on the concentration of monensin the animal was exposed to. Some effects may persist for months and lead to permanent damage.
• The following oral lethal doses have been reported for various ruminants on a body weight basis:
  ○ Cattle $LD_1 = 5.5$ mg/kg; $LD_{10} = 11$ mg/kg; $LD_{50} = 26.4$ mg/kg
  ○ Sheep $LD_0 = 4$ mg/kg; $LD_{50} = 10.7–13.1$ mg/kg
  ○ Goat $LD_{50} = 22.4–30.4$ mg/kg
  ○ Camelid $LD_{50} = 1–2$ mg/kg
• The FDA recommends 5.5–33 ppm monensin in the total diet of cattle and 22 ppm for goats.
  ○ 100 ppm, for about 1 year, had no effect on circulatory or reproductive functions of cattle.
  ○ 200–400 ppm monensin in feed for some days may lead to chronic toxicosis in cattle.
  ○ Goats consuming feed with 55 ppm monensin for 3 weeks may manifest hepatotoxicity. However, no such effect is seen in goats at 11 ppm for 3 weeks, or at 8 mg/kg BW × 5 days.
• Although not approved for sheep, monensin has been purposefully added to ovine feed at levels similar to that of cattle. In lambs <1 month of age, diffuse gastrointestinal hemorrhage has been reported. Single dose of monensin at 12 mg/kg resulted in no muscular abnormality. At 2–4 mg/kg × 4 days, listlessness and feed refusal were observed; and at concentrations ≥8 mg/kg × 2 days, toxicity was observed.

INCIDENCE/PREVALENCE
The incidences are sporadic and not very prevalent because of the awareness of monensin toxicity among producers.

GEOGRAPHIC DISTRIBUTION
N/A

SYSTEMS AFFECTED
• Cardiovascular
• Musculoskeletal
• Nervous
• Urinary
• Respiratory

PATHOPHYSIOLOGY
• Following ingestion, monensin is well absorbed from GIT, undergoes hepatic metabolism by P-450s and glutathione, and is excreted in the bile. O-demethylation and hydroxylation are the primary metabolic pathways. Urinary excretion is very low.
• Ionophores differ in their cation selectivity, forming dynamically reversible $Ca^{2+}/Mg^{2+}/Na^+/K^+$-lipid soluble complexes allowing ions to be transported across membranes, down the concentration gradient.
• Monensin shows preference for Na^+ ions, leading to increased intracellular sodium and loss of potassium from cells. Disruption of the normal cellular ionic gradient ensues, causing disturbances in cellular homeostasis (loss of osmotic pressure), metabolism (reduction in ATP production) and ion-mediated signaling events which can result in cell death.
• The loss of potential gradient across myocardial cells results in abnormal impulse transmission leading to cardiac arrhythmias and potentially congestive heart failure.
• In more chronic cases, reduction in ATP production leads to cell death or necrosis, followed by replacement with nonfunctional connective tissues such as fibroblasts.

SIGNALMENT
• Cattle, sheep, goats, and camelids have reportedly been affected. All ruminant species should be considered susceptible.
• Based on the LD_{50} values, among ruminants, the rank order of susceptibility to toxicosis is as follows: camelids > sheep > cattle = goats.
• No differentiation of toxicity on the basis of age, sex, or breed has been reported.

PHYSICAL EXAMINATION FINDINGS
Acute Effects
• Death
• Recumbency
• Arrhythmias
• Dyspnea
• Stiffness
• Ataxia and tremors due to alteration in normal impulse conduction
• Anorexia
• Edema of abdomen and legs

• Weakness
• Myoglobinuria, sometimes urinary bladder distension
• Diarrhea
Chronic Effects
• Anorexia
• Diarrhea
• Depression
• Dyspnea
• Arrhythmias
• Unthriftiness
• Exercise intolerance
• Death
• Decreased milk production
• Decreased weight gain

CAUSES AND RISK FACTORS
• Monensin toxicosis is generally a result of feeding of premix ration or other mixing errors.
• Exposure to other cardiotoxins and the absence of adequate amounts of selenium and vitamin E can result in aggravation of monensin toxicosis.

DIAGNOSIS

DIFFERENTIAL DIAGNOSES
• Selenium deficiency—evaluated by measuring selenium concentrations in blood, serum, or liver.
• Vitamin E deficiency—evaluated by measuring vitamin E in serum or liver.
• Cardiotoxic plants—identification of plant in feed, testing of rumen content for plant alkaloids.

CBC/BIOCHEMISTRY/URINALYSIS
• Hematologic parameters generally not affected; may see leukocytosis with increased PMN cells and decrease in lymphocytes.
• Muscle damage causing—increased AST, increased CPK.
• Diarrhea/rumenitis causing—hypokalemia, hyponatremia, and hypocalcemia.
• Myoglobinuria in severely affected animals.
• Myocardial damage causing—increased cardiac troponin I.

OTHER LABORATORY TESTS
• Analyze feed, GI contents, and molasses for identification and quantification of monensin. The analysis can be done using TLC, colorimetry, or the LC-MS method.
• Tissue samples (liver or heart) collected within 24 hours of intoxication can be used diagnostically for confirmation of exposure by LC-MS method.

IMAGING
Echocardiography may be used to determine the presence of myocardial damage in live, chronic cases. However, animals with acute

MONENSIN TOXICITY   (CONTINUED)

exposure cannot be diagnosed with this method, as the fibrosis is not present.

OTHER DIAGNOSTIC PROCEDURES
• Prolongation of Q-T interval and the QRS complex. Absence of P wave and increased amplitude of S and T waves have been observed.
• Atrial/ventricular fibrillation, ventricular tachycardia, and intermittent and premature ventricular contractions may be evident.
• ECG abnormalities are not consistent with severity of exposure or the amount of myocardial damage.

PATHOLOGIC FINDINGS
• Findings are similar to congestive heart failure.
• Animals with acute deaths may show no significant lesions.
• Enlarged heart with hydropericardium, epicardial hemorrhages, and a tigroid appearance.
• Permanent myocardial damage appears as diffusely pale and yellow myocardium with ventricular dilatation.
• Pulmonary congestion and edema.
• Hepatic congestion. Mottling of the liver along with hepatocellular necrosis have also been reported.
• Abomasal and SI mucosal congestion.
• Ecchymotic hemorrhages around subcutaneous layer and fascia of the neck and forelimbs.
• Subcutaneous edema.
• Yellow-to-gray necrotic streaks in skeletal muscles. Cattle have about equal predilection to develop heart and skeletal muscle lesions. In animals surviving an acute exposure, scarring and pallor of certain muscle groups may be noted.
• Cattle, histologic changes—mitochondrial swelling and vacuolar degeneration of cardiac myocytes. Pallor/pale streaking in ventricular walls and the septum. Centrilobular hepatic necrosis with vacuolar degeneration and focal degeneration of active skeletal muscles may be evident.
• Sheep, histologic changes—fibrosis and hyalinization with sarcoplasmic mineralization have been reported in ewes consuming 160 ppm monensin over a period of 70 days. Mononuclear infiltration was also observed. Unlike in cattle, the skeletal muscle lesions in sheep were more severe than the cardiac lesions.

TREATMENT

THERAPEUTIC APPROACH
• There is no specific antidote for monensin intoxication.

• Remove contaminated feed immediately.
• Monitor and correct the blood electrolyte imbalances, if any.
• Fluids can be administered to maintain hydration and enhance elimination or prevent renal casting by myoglobin.

SURGICAL CONSIDERATIONS AND TECHNIQUES
Apart from GIT decontamination and general supportive care, consider surgical evacuation of rumen contents in case of substantial exposure, followed by activated charcoal or mineral oil.

MEDICATIONS

DRUGS OF CHOICE
• No antidote
• AC/mineral oil/saline cathartics
• Vitamin E/Se to minimize secondary oxidative tissue damage

CONTRAINDICATIONS
IV fluids should not be administered in animals with cardiovascular problems.

POSSIBLE INTERACTIONS
Monensin toxicity may be potentiated by the concurrent use of tiamulin, oleandomycin, chloramphenicol, erythromycin, sulfonamides, furazolidone, and other cardiac glycosides.

FOLLOW-UP

EXPECTED COURSE AND PROGNOSIS
• Suspected animals may exhibit clinical signs within a few hours of exposure or, in some cases, may take months for the precipitation. Depending on the amount of exposure, the animals may manifest the acute or chronic effects (see "Physical Examination Findings").
• The prognosis is guarded to poor for any animal with suspected myocardial damage. These animals can be maintained, but their performance may be decreased.

POSSIBLE COMPLICATIONS
Myocardial damage may persist for a long period of time without noticeable clinical effects, predisposing the animal to succumb to factors resulting in an elevated heart rate or requiring an increase in cardiac output.

CLIENT EDUCATION
Animals surviving a toxic exposure may have permanent cardiac damage that can make the animal susceptible to sudden death following stress.

PATIENT CARE
• Stall rest and a nonstressful environment are essential to limit cardiac damage.
• A good plane of nutrition, ensuring adequate selenium and vitamin E intake.
• Restrict exercise and excitement.
• Serum chemistry, cardiac troponin I, ECGs, and echocardiography are helpful to monitor progress; however, they cannot predict the prognosis.

PREVENTION
• Proper storage of the premixes and concentrates.
• Maintain a proper feed management protocol to avoid mixing errors and possible miscalculations.
• Test feed to ensure monensin concentrations are within FDA recommended ranges (see "Overview").
• Keep animals at a good nutritional level, especially selenium and vitamin E.

MISCELLANEOUS

PREGNANCY
Ionophores have not been directly associated with reproductive problems. However, the compromised cardiovascular function may result in abortion.

BIOSECURITY
The tolerance level for monensin in edible tissues of cattle is 0.05 ppm.

PRODUCTION MANAGEMENT
• Do not feed to lactating dairy cows.
• Ensure proper mixing and final concentration within the FDA recommended ranges.

SYNONYMS
N/A

ABBREVIATIONS
• AC = activated charcoal
• AST = aspartate aminotransferase
• CPK = creatine phosphokinase
• ECG = electrocardiogram
• FDA = Food and Drug Administration
• GI = gastrointestinal
• GIT = gastrointestinal tract
• IV = intravenous
• LC-MS = liquid chromatography/mass spectrometry
• LD_0 = highest estimated dose at which none of the population is expected to die
• LD_1 = estimated dose at which 1% of the population is expected to die
• LD_{10} = estimated dose at which 10% of the population is expected to die
• LD_{50} = estimated dose at which 50% of the population is expected to die

- PMN = polymorphonuclear cells
- SDH = sorbitol dehydrogenase
- TLC = thin layer chromatography

SEE ALSO
- Cardiotoxic Plants
- Selenium/Vitamin E Deficiency

Suggested Reading

Anderson TD, Van Alstine WG, Ficken MD, Miskimins DW, Carson TL, Osweiler GD. Acute monensin toxicosis in sheep: Light and electron microscopic changes. Am J Vet Res 1984, 45: 1142–7.

Hall JO. Ionophore use and toxicosis in cattle. Vet Clin North Am Food Anim Pract 2000, 16: 497–509.

Langston VC, Galey F, Lovell R, Buck WB. Toxicity and therapeutics of moncnsin: a review. Vet Med 1985, 75–84.

Novilla MN. The veterinary importance of the toxic syndrome induced by ionophores. Vet Hum Toxicol 1992, 34: 66–70.

Potter EL, VanDuyn RL, Cooley CO. Monensin toxicity in cattle. J Anim Sci 1984, 58: 1499–511.

Authors Adrienne C. Bautista and Birgit Puschner

Consulting Editor Christopher C.L. Chase

Acknowledgment The author and book editors acknowledge the prior contribution of Asheesh K. Tiwary.

M

MYCOPLASMA BOVIS ASSOCIATED DISEASES

BASICS

OVERVIEW
• *Mycoplasma bovis* is a bacterial cause of mastitis, bronchopneumonia, otitis media, arthritis, and tenosynovitis in cattle and bison. Disease is common but sporadic; cattle and bison are the primary host, and infection is infrequent in other ruminants, which tend to host their own pathogenic species of *Mycoplasma*.
• Less commonly, *Mycoplasma bovis* has been associated with conjunctivitis and infection of the reproductive tract.

INCIDENCE/PREVALENCE
Mycoplasma bovis is the most pathogenic bovine mycoplasma in Europe and North America. It causes huge economic losses in cattle and milk production in both Europe and the United States. *M. bovis* is estimated to be responsible for at least a quarter or a third of losses caused by respiratory diseases in Europe. In the US, this organism causes a loss of $32 million per year as a result of the loss of weight gain and the diminished carcass value. The expenses due to *M. bovis* mastitis are estimated to be $108 million per year.

GEOGRAPHIC DISTRIBUTION
Worldwide

SYSTEMS AFFECTED
• Nervous
• Respiratory
• Reproductive
• Mammary
• Musculoskeletal
• Ophthalmic

PATHOPHYSIOLOGY
• *Mycoplasma bovis* can be found in both the upper respiratory (URT) and reproductive tracts in both young and old cattle.
• The URT mucosa and the mammary gland appear to be the most important sites of persistence and shedding of *M. bovis*. Although many cattle shed *M. bovis* for a few months or less, some cattle can shed *M. bovis* intermittently for many months or years. The factors responsible for intermittent shedding have not been determined. Cattle with clinical disease usually excrete especially large numbers of *M. bovis*. Stressful events such as transportation, comingling, entry into a feedlot, and cold stress are associated with increased rates of nasal shedding of *M. bovis* and increased clinical disease.
• *M. bovis* has characteristics that enable it to colonize and persist on mucosal surfaces, to invade tissues, and to persist at sites of disease despite an aggressive immune response. Molecules involved in adherence, antigenic variation, invasion, immunomodulation, biofilm formation, and production of toxic metabolites are likely to be important in

pathogenesis, but exactly how *M. bovis* interacts with the host is poorly understood.

SIGNALMENT
Cattle and bison; sheep can acquire *M. bovis* from infected cattle and may be a reservoir.

PHYSICAL EXAMINATION FINDINGS
• *Mycoplasma bovis* causes contagious mastitis in dairy cattle that can be enzootic or epizootic (outbreaks). Subclinical infection is common and contributes to persistent disease that can be difficult to eradicate.
• Cows with clinical mastitis do not usually develop severe systemic signs of disease. The mammary gland may be swollen but is not usually painful; milk may be discolored or purulent.
• *Mycoplasma bovis* is an important contributor to infectious bronchopneumonia in cattle (the "bovine respiratory disease complex" or BRDC). Co-infection with other bacterial or viral pathogens is common, though *Mycoplasma bovis* can be the sole pathogen isolated from pneumonic lungs. Experimental infections usually result in inapparent to mild signs of respiratory disease, but virulent strains have been identified that cause severe lung disease in calves.
• *Mycoplasma bovis* is a leading cause of otitis media in calves. Clinical signs include head tilt, loss of facial sensation, and loss of motor activity in the muscles of facial expression. Purulent drainage from the ear also is common. A large percentage (40–60%) of animals affected with otitis media also develop polyarthritis and tenosynovitis that causes severe chronic lameness.
• Septic arthritis and/or tenosynovitis may be caused by *Mycoplasma bovis,* with large joints in the proximal limb most often affected. Affected joints and tendon sheaths are enlarged and firm, leading to obvious lameness.
• It is common for cattle with otitis media and/or arthritis/tenosynovitis to have concurrent pneumonia due to *Mycoplasma bovis*.

CAUSES AND RISK FACTORS
• *Mycoplasma bovis* lacks a cell wall, and exposed membrane proteins form the primary interface with the host. These membrane proteins facilitate adherence to mucosal surfaces, although *M. bovis* adhesions are not yet well characterized. *M. bovis* has a large family of immunodominant variable surface lipoproteins that exhibit extensive strain variation in their coding sequences. These characteristics impart a vast capacity for antigenic variation in *M. bovis* populations that likely contributes to immune evasion and persistence and provides a challenge for vaccine development.
• Bacterial and/or viral co-infections are seen as an important co-factor for *M. bovis*-associated pneumonia and otitis media.

• The introduction of asymptomatically infected animals is thought to be the primary means by which *M. bovis*-free cattle and bison herds become infected. Transmission is delayed until, and if, shedding occurs; this delay can make it difficult to identify the source of infection and mycoplasma disease outbreaks occur in seemingly closed herds.

DIAGNOSIS

DIFFERENTIAL DIAGNOSES
• Bovine respiratory disease bacterial agents: *Histophilus somni, Mannheimia hemolytica, Pasteurella multocida*
• Bacterial mastitis: *Staph. aureus, Strep. uberis, Strep. agalactiae, E. coli*
• Bacterial otitis media: *P. multocida, Strep* spp., *M. hemolytica*
• Bacterial polyarthritis: navel ill, *H. somni*

CBC/BIOCHEMISTRY/URINALYSIS
N/A

OTHER LABORATORY TESTS
• Diagnosis is made by identification of *Mycoplasma bovis* from clinical specimens from animals with signs consistent with disease due to *Mycoplasma bovis*, or from materials collected at postmortem from typical lesions.
• *Mycoplasma* spp. are relatively difficult to isolate compared to other causes of mastitis or bronchopneumonia; thus diagnosis by culture requires that samples be kept cool but not frozen and submitted to the diagnostic laboratory as soon as possible. It will likely be necessary to specifically request that the laboratory carry out culture for mycoplasma, as special media and conditions are required.
• To confirm specific involvement of *Mycoplasma bovis* it will be necessary to also ask the diagnostic laboratory to identify the species of any mycoplasmas isolated; speciation is typically completed by immunofluorescence testing or PCR.
• It is possible to specifically identify *Mycoplasma bovis* by direct PCR testing of clinical materials. However, PCR alone may lack sensitivity for some samples.
• Diagnosis of mastitis at the herd level can be made by milk tank culture or PCR for *M. bovis*.

PATHOLOGIC FINDINGS
• Pneumonia, otitis media, and arthritis/tenosynovitis may be diagnosed by postmortem. In the lung, cranioventral consolidation typical of bronchopneumonia is seen, often with multiple small nodules that contain caseous material (caseous necrosis).
• Pleural effusion and/or fibrin deposition is not commonly seen in cattle with bronchopneumonia due to *Mycoplasma bovis*.
• Purulent or caseous material can be found in the tympanic bulla of animals with otitis

M

media, and in joint spaces or tendon sheaths in arthritis/tenosynovitis.

TREATMENT

THERAPEUTIC APPROACH

Mastitis

• Cows with mycoplasma mastitis respond poorly to treatment, and it appears that most if not all affected cows become permanent intermittent shedders even when clinical mastitis resolves. Thus it is recommended that cows with mycoplasma mastitis be culled from the herd.

• In herds with a high proportion of infected cows it may not be possible to cull all affected cattle; in such cases it may be advisable to maintain two milking strings, one of uninfected cows milked first, and a second string of infected cows milked second.

Bovine Respiratory Disease

• Antimicrobials most likely to be useful for treatment of bronchopneumonia due to *Mycoplasma bovis* include macrolides such as tulathromycin or gamithromycin, enrofloxacin, or florfenicol. Oxytetracycline or chlortetracycline have been used historically but resistance may be a problem; the same may be true for tilmicosin. Because mycoplasmas lack cell walls, beta-lactam antibiotics (penicillins and cephalosporins) will not be effective against these bacteria. Several antimicrobials are labeled for treatment of pneumonia due to *Mycoplasma bovis*.

Otitis and Arthritis

• Cases of otitis or arthritis/tenosynovitis are unlikely to respond to treatment with complete resolution unless treatment is initiated very early in the course of disease. Veterinarians should be attentive to the welfare of animals with chronic otitis or arthritis, and euthanasia may be the most appropriate course of action for severe, persistently infected cases.

MEDICATIONS

DRUGS OF CHOICE

Macrolides (tulathromycin or gamithromycin), enrofloxacin, or florfenicol

PRECAUTIONS

Although many drugs are labeled for treatment of pneumonia due to *Mycoplasma bovis,* cases in the field are commonly reported to respond poorly to treatment. This may be in part due the presence of lesions of caseous necrosis, which may require prolonged therapy for durations longer than indicated on the label. No evidence-based guidelines for duration of therapy for pneumonia due to *Mycoplasma bovis* are available.

FOLLOW-UP

EXPECTED COURSE AND PROGNOSIS

• When dealing with cattle with disease due to *Mycoplasma bovis*, producers will often report failure of disease to respond as expected to antibiotic therapy. In general *Mycoplasma bovis* infection in any organ is often manifested as disease that appears subacute to chronic, with resolution being difficult to effect.

PREVENTION

• Because disease due to *Mycoplasma bovis* can be difficult or impossible to treat, preventing disease in animals at risk should be a priority.

• Mastitis should be prevented by eliminating infected cows in herds where the disease is present, by practicing biocontainment to prevent transmission within infected herds, and by preventing the introduction of infected cows to herds that are free of disease.

• Because *Mycoplasma bovis* commonly causes bronchopneumonia in conjunction with other viral or bacterial pathogens, controlling other infectious causes of bronchopneumonia may also decrease rates of bronchopneumonia due to *Mycoplasma bovis*.

• Preconditioning beef calves prior to sale can help decrease bronchopneumonia due to any cause. Preconditioning includes castration and dehorning at birth or soon after, weaning at least 45 days before sale, and vaccination to protect against common respiratory pathogens well in advance of sale, in time to allow vaccinated calves to develop an adaptive immune response to vaccination.

• Vaccines exist for *Mycoplasma bovis*; unfortunately, at this time there are few scientific reports confirming their efficacy in the field.

• Septic arthritis and tenosynovitis likely occur secondary to bacteremia in cattle with bronchopneumonia; thus preventing bronchopneumonia should help prevent these conditions.

MISCELLANEOUS

ZOONOTIC POTENTIAL

None

BIOSECURITY

Cows from herds with a history of otitis or septic arthritis in calves should be avoided.

PRODUCTION MANAGEMENT

• Because *Mycoplasma bovis* is shed intermittently, it is not possible to reliably exclude an infected cow based on milk testing. The results of bulk tank testing from the herd of origin would ideally be evaluated if possible.

• Otitis in calves is associated with feeding calves infected milk; thus, otitis can be prevented or controlled by feeding calves pasteurized milk.

ABBREVIATIONS

• PCR = polymerase chain reaction
• URT = upper respiratory tract

SEE ALSO

• Enzootic Pneumonia of Calves
• Mastitis: Mycoplasmal
• Respiratory Disease: Bovine

Suggested Reading
Caswell JL, Archambault M. Mycoplasma bovis pneumonia in cattle. Anim Health Res Rev 2007; 161–86.
Caswell JL, Bateman KG, Cai HY, Castillo-Alcala F. Mycoplasma bovis in respiratory disease of feedlot cattle. Vet Clin North Am Food Anim Pract 2010; 365–79.
Maunsell FP, Donovan GA. Mycoplasma bovis infections in young calves. Vet Clin North Am Food Anim Pract 2009; 139–77.
Maunsell FP, Woolums AR, Francoz D, Rosenbusch RF, Step DL, Wilson DJ, Janzen ED. Mycoplasma bovis infections in cattle. J Vet Intern Med 2011; 772–83.

Author Amelia Woolums
Consulting Editor Christopher C.L. Chase
Acknowledgment The author and book editors acknowledge the prior contribution of Jeff W. Tyler.

M

MYCOTOXINS

BASICS

OVERVIEW
• Mycotoxins are naturally occurring compounds produced by a variety of fungi in grains, forages, and various foods/feeds/by-products. Their occurrence worldwide appears to be increasing with climatic events and better analytic techniques. This section is focused on the more common mycotoxins in North America.
• Typically, *Fusarium* and *Claviceps* fungi act as plant pathogens on cereal crops or grasses in the field. *F. verticilliodies* and *Aspergillus flavus* produce mycotoxins on drought-stressed or senescent plants, particularly corn in the field.
• *Aspergillus* and *Penicillium* fungi occur on developing crops in the field and later proliferate in storage, especially on ensiled cereals or baled forages under higher moisture conditions.
• Fungi have been associated with grass endophytes, such as *Neotyphodium coenophialum* in tall fescue.
• Functioning ruminants are often viewed as less sensitive to mycotoxins than monogastrics because of rumen microflora metabolism to less toxic compounds. However, ruminants occupy wide agricultural niches and are exposed to diverse toxins.
• Often the moldier and highly contaminated feeds end up in beef feedlots and, in poor crop years, beef cows are often fed poor-quality feedstuffs, exposing animals to a variety of mycotoxins and sometimes atypical rations for rumen microbes to digest.
• Dairy cows appear to be more sensitive to mycotoxins, perhaps due to greater stress and increased dry-matter intake, faster rumen turnover, and decreased rumen microbial degradation time.

INCIDENCE/PREVALENCE
Varying climatic conditions in the field (drought, wet, hail damage, insect damage, overwintered grain) and in storage and transport (higher stored moisture and temperatures which vary with the particular requirements of the feed).

Aflatoxins
Group of difuranocoumarin compounds produced by *Aspergillus flavus, A. parasiticus,* and *A. nomius* that can occur pre-harvest on starchy cereal crops, cottonseeds, and peanuts or post-harvest on stored commodities. Drought, hot weather, and insect damage favor fungal growth and production of aflatoxins, including aflatoxins B1, B2, G1, and G2, with aflatoxin B1 generally found in the highest concentration and considered the most toxic and carcinogenic. Aflatoxin M1 and M2 are hydroxylated metabolites of aflatoxin B1 and B2, respectively, and can occur in contaminated feed and more

importantly in tissue, milk, and dairy products. Young animals are more at risk. Ruminants fed rations with several hundred ppb aflatoxins may have reduced feed intake and growth. Sheep are considered to be the domesticated species most resistant to toxic effects of aflatoxins.

Ergot
Invasion by *Claviceps* spp. in the developing ovary of grasses and grain can cause a visible sclerotium or ergot body containing numerous ergot alkaloids. Cool, damp weather in the spring delaying pollination, no-till farming, shallow cultivation, and no crop rotation can increase ergot prevalence. Infection of tall fescue grass with an endophyte, *Neothyphodium coenophialum,* can result in production of ergot alkaloids, particularly ergopeptine alkaloids of which ergovaline predominates. Fescue toxicosis may produce syndromes of fescue foot (lameness and ischemic necrosis of hooves), summer slump (hyperthermia and ill thrift), and fat necrosis in cattle. Sheep can be affected also and develop tongue necrosis. Subacute to chronic exposures to concentrations of ergovaline at 200–600 ppb (0.2–0.6 ppm) in fescue grass pastures infected with the endophyte can result in fescue toxicosis. Extreme environmental conditions, at both cold and hot temperatures, can exacerbate thermoregulation in ergot-induced gangrene and summer slump (hyperthermia), respectively.

Fumonisins
Group of heat-stable, water-soluble mycotoxins occurring in white and yellow corn in the field produced by *Fusarium verticillioides* and *F. proliferatum.* Fumonisins can concentrate (3×) in co-products of corn ethanol production into the distiller's grains. A period of drought during the growing season followed by wet, warm conditions during pollination of corn favors development of fumonisins. Toxicity is associated with fumonisins B1 and B2, with fumonisin B2 usually occurring at about 30% of fumonisin B1 concentration. Ruminants are fairly resistant to fumonisins and generally high concentrations (>148 ppm) have been reported to depress feed intake. Dairy cows seem to be more susceptible to fumonisins, which is reflected in the FDA guidelines for feeding fumonisin-contaminated feed to ruminants (see "Follow-Up").

Ochratoxin A
Ochratoxins are potent nephrotoxins, immunosuppressants, and possible carcinogens (in humans) and teratogens produced by *Aspergillus alutaceus* var. *alutaceus* in tropical and subtropical areas and *Penicillium viridicatum* in temperate areas. These phenylalanine-dihydroisocoumarin compounds are generally produced in storage and occur on grains and various human

foods. The most toxic of the ochratoxins is ochratoxin A (OTA). A functioning rumen appears to metabolize ochratoxin A to the nearly nontoxic compound, ochratoxin α; and the elimination half-life for ochratoxin in ruminants is 17.3 hours, compared with 100 hours in pigs (a sensitive species). Therefore, functioning ruminants are less at risk for toxicity. Citrinin, another nephrotoxin mycotoxin, is produced by *Penicillium* spp. and *Monascus ruber* on cereal grains at high moisture. The US has no regulatory guidelines for ochratoxins; however, the EC guidelines are a maximum of 0.25 ppm OTA in feed materials fed to animals in a daily ration.

Tremorgens
Infection of perennial ryegrass (*Lolium perenne*) with the endophyte *Neotyphodium lolii* has been associated with grass staggers in sheep and cattle. Cattle consuming Bermudagrass (*Cynodon dactylon*) invaded by *Claviceps* or endophytes can develop periodic episodes of tremors that have been associated with paspalitrem-type indole alkaloids and perhaps ergot-type alkaloids *Penicillium* spp. can synthesize indole–diterpene tremorgenic mycotoxins including penitrem A and roquefortine that have been associated with staggers in ruminants. *Aspergillus* can produce tremorgenic mycotoxins, aflatrem and verruculogen.

Trichothecenes
Fusarium molds (*F. graminearum, F. culmorum, F. poae, F. sporotrichioides, F. equiseti, F. acuminatum* and others) can produce a variety of trichothecene mycotoxins, which are sesquiterpenoid compounds with an epoxy group at C12-13 that causes toxicity. Type A trichothecenes include the more toxic compounds such as T-2 toxin, its deacetylated metabolite Ht-2 toxin, and diacetoxyscirpenol (DAS). Type B trichothecenes are common field contaminants and include vomitoxin or deoxynivalenol (DON) and its acetylated derivatives 15- and 3-acetyl DON, nivalenol and fusarenone-X (4-acetylnivalenol). Generally, *Fusarium* grows on cereal grains during wet, warm conditions at pollination and during growth of plants in the field, but also in immature crops with warm days and cool nights, following hail damage, and in overwintered grains (esp. *F. sporotrichioides* and *F. poae*). *Fusarium* can invade forages and produce toxins, in some cases T-2 toxin, HT-2, DON, and zearalenone in grasses and hays. In bad scab years, DON contamination in wheat and barley straws can be significant (>50–100 ppm).
Trichothecene exposures are usually chronic to subchronic in nature with low dietary exposures to type B mycotoxins (e.g., DON) in ruminants associated with nutritional impairment and possible reduced production

and diminished immune responses. In general, beef cattle and sheep are more tolerant of higher DON concentration than are dairy cattle. See chapter, Vomitoxin, for further information.

Zearalenone

Zearalenone is a mycoestrogen produced by *Fusarium graminearum, F. culmorum,* and *F. equiseti* on cereal grains, ear corn, wet grasses, hay, and straw during wet conditions, with warmer days and cool nights. Zearalenone has low acute toxicity in most species.

GEOGRAPHIC DISTRIBUTION

Worldwide, with fungal growth dependent on climatic conditions, feed matrices, and production/storage practices.

SYSTEMS AFFECTED

• Cardiovascular
• Gastrointestinal
• Multisystemic
• Integument
• Hemolymphatic
• Nervous
• Reproductive
• Respiratory

PATHOPHYSIOLOGY

Aflatoxins

Aflatoxins are passively absorbed from the GIT, biotransformed into aflatoxin 8,9-epoxide, and can bind to DNA, RNA, and proteins causing disruption of cellular processes and organ function. The outcome is cellular necrosis, immune suppression, mutagenesis, neoplasms, possible abortions, and death.

Ergot

Ergot alkaloids are composed of ergoline alkaloids and ergopeptide alkaloids. The latter cause vasoconstriction through inhibition of the D1 dopaminergic receptor and partial agonism of the α1-adrenergic and serotonin receptors. Constriction of small arteries can lead to ischemia and necrosis of distal extremities and possibly uterine contractions in late pregnancy (evidence of abortions vague in ruminants). Ergopeptine stimulation of the D2-dopamine receptors can lead to decreased prolactin secretion by lactotropes in the anterior pituitary and low milk production and agalactia.

Fumonisins

Fumonisins, which are aliphatic hydrocarbons with a terminal amine group and tricarboxylic acid side chains and structurally similar to sphingolipids in cellular membranes, inhibit the ceramide synthase enzyme involved in converting sphinganine to sphingosine. Fumonisins can interfere with cellular growth and differentiation, resulting in toxicity and carcinogenicity. Liver toxicity is often involved across species.

Ochratoxin A

Ochratoxins inhibit protein synthesis and can deplete humoral factors, especially immunoglobulins and decrease natural killer cell activity. The most toxic of the ochratoxins is ochratoxin A (OTA). Citrinin, another nephrotoxin mycotoxin, is produced by *Pencillium* spp. and *Monascus ruber* on cereal grains at high moisture. Both toxins target the renal proximal tubule and can result in lowered milk production, diarrhea, ill thrift, polyuria/polydipsia, and immune suppression.

Tremorgens

Neurotoxic indole-diterpene tremogens, including lolitrems (esp. lolitrem B) are thought to interfere with excitatory amino acid neurotransmitter release mechanisms, especially inhibition of gamma aminobutyric acid (GABA) receptor function.

Trichothecenes

Trichothecenes exert several effects, including inhibition of protein, RNA and DNA synthesis, alteration of membrane structure and mitochondrial function, lipid peroxidation, induction of cell apoptosis, and activation of cytokines and chemokines. Significant metabolism of trichothecenes can occur in the rumen and GIT prior to absorption. Rumen microbes, particularly protozoa, appear to be active in the deacetylation of trichothecenes. The major rumen metabolite of DON is de-epoxydeoxynivalenol (DOM-1), which is much less toxic than DON.

Zearalenone

Zearalenone is a resorcyclic acid lactone that is fairly rapidly and extensively absorbed after oral exposure. Zearalenone can undergo rumen metabolism, with reduction to α-zearalenol (increased estrogenic activity) and to a lesser amount of β-zearalenol (lower estrogenic activity). Zearalenone has affinity for the 17β-estradiol receptor and can stimulate RNA and protein synthesis and clinical signs of estrogenism.

SIGNALMENT

• All ruminants are susceptible.
• Sheep are considered the most resistant domesticated species to toxic effects of aflatoxins.
• Ruminants are fairly resistant to fumonisins and generally high concentrations (>148 ppm) have been reported to depress feed intake.
• In general, beef cattle and sheep are more tolerant of higher DON concentration than are dairy cattle.

PHYSICAL EXAMINATION FINDINGS

Aflatoxins

• Young animals are more at risk.
• In acute outbreaks, deaths occur after a short period of inappetence; other acute signs

include vomiting, depression, hemorrhage, and icterus.
• Subacute outbreaks are more usual, with unthriftiness, weakness, anorexia, reduced growth and feed efficiency, and occasional sudden deaths.
• Ruminants fed rations with several hundred ppb aflatoxins may have reduced feed intake and growth.
• Chronic aflatoxicosis is associated with reduced appetite, feed efficiency, milk production, and icterus.

Ergot

• Fescue toxicosis may produce syndromes of fescue foot (lameness and ischemic necrosis of hooves), summer slump (hyperthermia and ill thrift), and fat necrosis in cattle. Symptoms include erythema and swelling of the coronary region occur, and cattle are alert but lose weight and may be seen "paddling" or weight-shifting. The back is slightly arched, and knuckling of a hind pastern may be an initial sign. There is progressive lameness, anorexia, depression, and later, dry gangrene of the distal limbs (hindlimbs first). Signs usually develop within 10–21 days after turnout into a fescue-contaminated pasture in fall. A period of frost tends to increase the incidence.
• Sheep can be affected also and develop tongue necrosis.
• Ergot alkaloids can produce gangrene of distal extremities, GIT changes, lowered milk production and feed intake.
• Extreme environmental conditions, at both cold and hot temperatures, can exacerbate thermoregulation in ergot induced gangrene and summer slump (hyperthermia), respectively.

Fumonisins

• Cattle and sheep tolerate fumonisin concentrations of 100 ppm with little effect. Dietary concentrations of 150–200 ppm cause inappetence, weight loss, and mild liver damage.
• Renal and hepatic damage have been reported in lambs fed high fumonisin diets (about 470 ppm). Dairy cows seem to be more susceptible to fumonisins,

Ochratoxin A

Citrinin, another nephrotoxin mycotoxin, is produced by *Pencillium* spp. and *Monascus ruber* on cereal grains at high moisture. Both toxins target the renal proximal tubule and can result in lowered milk production, diarrhea, ill thrift, polyuria/polydipsia, and immune suppression in cattle.

Tremorgens

• The clinical signs of perennial ryegrass staggers are ataxia, muscle rigidity, and convulsions.
• Cattle consuming Bermudagrass (*Cynodon dactylon*) invaded by *Claviceps* or endophytes can develop periodic episodes of tremors that

M

have been associated with paspalitrem-type indole alkaloids and perhaps ergot-type alkaloids. *Penicillium* spp. can synthesize indole–diterpene tremorgenic mycotoxins including penitrem A and roquefortine that have been associated with staggers in ruminants.
• *Aspergillus* can produce tremorgenic mycotoxins, aflatrem and verruculogen. The onset and duration of the "staggers" syndromes for these tremorgens can vary, but they are essentially identical to one another.

Trichothecenes
• The hallmark clinical sign of trichothecene toxicosis is feed refusal, and commonly diarrhea.
• Trichothecene exposures are usually chronic to subchronic in nature with low dietary exposures to type B mycotoxins (e.g., DON) in ruminants associated with nutritional impairment and possible reduced production and diminished immune responses. See chapter, Vomitoxin, for further information.
• Clinical effects of the more toxic type A trichothecenes include vomiting, feed refusal and weight loss, diarrhea, immunomodulation, coagulopathy, and hemorrhage.
• T-2 toxin can cross the placental barrier and cause abortions. Dairy cows appear to be more sensitive to trichothecene exposure.

Zearalenone
• Zearalenone has low acute toxicity in most species.
• Zearalenone has affinity for the 17β-estradiol receptor and can stimulate RNA and protein synthesis and clinical signs of estrogenism (swelling of vulva, increase in uterine size and sections, mammary gland hyperplasia and secretion, prolonged estrus, anestrus, pseudopregnancy, infertility, decreased libido, and secondary complications of rectal and vaginal prolapses).

CAUSES AND RISK FACTORS
Ingestion of moldy feedstuffs containing significant concentrations of a mycotoxin can lead to clinical effects. Pre-ruminants, immature animals which lack rumen microbial metabolism, and dairy cows, which are more highly stressed, are generally more at risk.

DIAGNOSIS

DIFFERENTIAL DIAGNOSES
• Aflatoxin liver damage: Plant pyrrolizidine alkaloids
• Type A trichothecenes: Radiomimetic poisoning, 4-ipomeanol pneumotoxin, *Perilla frutescens*
• Zearalenone hyperestrogenism: Phytoestrogens in alfalfa and clovers

CBC/BIOCHEMISTRY/URINALYSIS
• Aflatoxin can increase hepatic enzyme activity (ALP, AST, or ALT) and prothrombin time, and anemia can occur.
• Trichothecenes may cause leukopenia and anemia.
• Elevated BUN and creatinine levels due to ochratoxin A and citrinin.

OTHER LABORATORY TESTS
• Detection of mycotoxins in feed by liquid or gas chromatography-mass spectrometry, gas chromatography, and other reliable methods validated for the feed matrix.
• Laboratory analysis of feed for mycotoxins in tissues (milk and liver for aflatoxin M1) are the most practical assays.

PATHOLOGIC FINDINGS

Aflatoxin
• Aflatoxin-induced lesions include fatty degeneration of the liver, hepatic megalocytosis, fibrosis, necrosis, biliary hyperplasia, and possible veno-occlusive lesions and hemorrhages.
• In acute cases, there are widespread hemorrhages and icterus. The liver is the major target organ. Microscopically, the liver is enlarged and shows marked fatty accumulations and massive centrilobular necrosis and hemorrhage.
• In subacute cases, the hepatic changes are not so pronounced, but the liver is somewhat enlarged and firmer than usual. There may be edema of the gallbladder.
• Microscopically, the liver shows periportal inflammatory response and proliferation and fibrosis of the bile ductules; the hepatocytes and their nuclei (megalocytosis) are enlarged.
• The GI mucosa may show glandular atrophy and associated inflammation. Rarely, there may be tubular degeneration and regeneration in the kidneys.
• Prolonged feeding of low concentrations of aflatoxins may result in diffuse liver fibrosis (cirrhosis) and, rarely, carcinoma of the bile ducts or liver.

Ergot
• The most consistent lesions are in the skin and subcutaneous parts of the extremities. The skin is normal to the indented line, but beyond, it is cyanotic and hardened in advanced cases. Subcutaneous hemorrhage and some edema occur proximal to the necrotic area.
• In addition to gangrene of these extremities, the animals have a loss of body mass and a rough coat.

Ochratoxin
The lesions associated with ochratoxin are dilated renal tubules and fibrosis in the kidneys, thickened basement membranes, glomerular sclerosis, and fatty changes in the liver.

Trichothecenes
• Gross lesions including irritation of the skin and mucus membranes and gastroenteritis are typical signs of trichothecene toxicosis.
• Hemorrhagic diathesis can occur, and the radiomimetic injury (damage to dividing cells) is expressed as lymphopenia or pancytopenia.
• Because of the immunosuppressive action of trichothecenes, secondary bacterial, viral, or parasitic infections may mask the primary injury.
• The lymphatic organs are smaller than normal and may be difficult to find on necropsy.
• Type A trichothecenes histologic lesions include cellular necrosis of mitotically active tissues such as intestinal mucosa, skin, bone marrow, testis, and ovary.

TREATMENT

THERAPEUTIC APPROACH
• Stop feeding mycotoxin-contaminated feed or reduce exposure to concentrations associated with no clinical signs in ruminants when regulatory guidelines are available. Dilution with noncontaminated feedstuffs is one possibility, but this may not be acceptable on a regulatory basis.
• Cleaning to remove lightweight or broken grains will often substantially reduce mycotoxin concentration in remaining grain.
• Ammoniation reduces aflatoxin contamination in grain but is not currently approved by the FDA for use in food animals in the United States because of uncertainty about by-products produced.
• Provide clean feed and supportive fluids if necessary.

MEDICATIONS

DRUGS OF CHOICE
N/A

FOLLOW-UP

EXPECTED COURSE AND PROGNOSIS
• In many cases, low dose exposure to mycotoxins followed by a change to a clean ration will result in recovery within 3–6 weeks.
• Extensive organ damage (liver—aflatoxins, circulatory—ergot) can results in ill thrift or complications causing death.

PREVENTION
• Follow regulatory or action levels for aflatoxin in animal feed.

(CONTINUED)

• In the US, the Food and Drug Administration issued action levels for **aflatoxins in feed** for cattle:
  ○ 300 ppb for corn and peanut products intended for finishing (i.e., feedlot) beef cattle;
  ○ 300 ppb for cottonseed meal intended for beef cattle (regardless of age or breeding status);
  ○ 100 ppb for corn and peanut products intended for breeding beef cattle;
  ○ 20 ppb for corn, peanut products, and other animal feeds and feed ingredients, but excluding cottonseed meal, intended for immature animals;
  ○ 20 ppb for corn, peanut products, cottonseed meal and other animal feeds and feed ingredients intended for dairy animals, for animal species or uses not specified above, or when the intended use is not known.
  ○ 0.5 ppb for milk (aflatoxin M1).
• The FDA guidance levels for total **fumonisins in corn and corn by-products**:
  ○ 30 ppm (no more than 50% of diet, dry weight basis) for breeding ruminants;
  ○ 60 ppm (no more than 50% of diet, dry weight basis) for ruminants ≥3 months old being raised for slaughter;
  ○ 10 ppm (no more than 50% of diet) for other ruminants and immature ruminants.
• In the US, mycotoxin binders have not been approved by the Food and Drug Administration. The use of aluminosilicates and bentonite clays to bind aflatoxins is recognized as effective (based on in vivo and in vitro efficacy), but the use of other products to "bind" the varied mycotoxins in ruminants is equivocal.

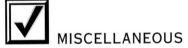 **MISCELLANEOUS**

AGE-RELATED FACTOR
Immature, pre-ruminants are generally more susceptible than older ruminants.

ZOONOTIC POTENTIAL
Aflatoxin M1 can be transferred to milk. The US FDA action level is 0.5 ppb in milk; the EC regulatory level is 0.05 ppb in milk. Note that all of these mycotoxins can occur in foods for human consumption.

PREGNANCY
Zearalenone can cause reproductive abnormalities, possibly anestrus and abortions. Aflatoxins, type A trichothecene mycotoxins (T-2, HT-2, DAS), and ergot can cause abortions.

BIOSECURITY
Avoid feeding moldy feedstuffs. Analyze suspect feed for vomitoxin prior to use and utilize appropriate guidelines. If possible, avoid feeding screenings that contain broken grains and possibly higher concentrations of mycotoxins.

PRODUCTION MANAGEMENT
Analyze moldy feedstuffs for mycotoxins prior to use. When available, follow regulatory guidelines (see "Prevention" and chapter, Vomitoxin).

ABBREVIATIONS
• AF = aflatoxins
• ALP = alkaline phosphatase
• ALT= alanine aminotransferase
• AST= aspartate aminotransferase
• BUN = blood urea nitrogen
• DAS = diacetoxyscirpenol
• DON = deoxynivalenol
• EC = European Community
• FDA = Food and Drug Administration
• GIT = gastrointestinal tract
• OTA = ochratoxin A
• ppb = parts per billion
• ppm = parts per million

SEE ALSO
• Plants Producing Acute Respiratory Distress Syndrome
• Pyrrolizidine Alkaloids
• Sweet Clover Poisoning
• Sweet Potato Poisoning
• Vomitoxin

Suggested Reading
Anon. Commission regulation (EC) No. 1881/2006 of 19 December 2006 setting maximum levels for certain contaminants in foodstuffs. 01.07.2010, p. 17. Official Journal European Union L364/5–24.
Anon. Commission recommendation on the presence of deoxynivalenol, zearalenone, ochratoxin A, T-2 and HT-2 and fumonisins in products intended for animal feeding. 17 August 2006. 2006/576/EC. Official Journal European Union 2006, 49, Part 229: 7–9.
Evans TJ. Diminished reproductive performance and selected toxicants in forages and grains. Vet Clin North Am Food Anim Pract 2011, 27: 345–71.
Evans TJ, Gupta RC. Tremorgenic mycotoxins. In: Gupta RC ed, Veterinary Toxicology. New York: Elsevier, 2007, pp. 1004–10.
Gallo A, Giubert G, Frisvad J, Bertuzzi T, Nielsen KF. Review on mycotoxin issues in ruminants: Occurrence in forages, effects of mycotoxin ingestion on health status and animal performance and practical strategies to counteract their negative effects. Toxins 2014, 7: 3057–111.
Mostrom MS, Jacobsen BJ. Ruminant mycotoxicosis. Vet Clin North Am Food Anim Pract 2011, 27: 315–44.
Internet Resources
• http://www.fda.gov/ICECI/Compliance Manuals/CompliancePolicyGuidance Manual/ucm074703.htm
• http://www.fda.gov/Food/Guidance Regulation/GuidanceDocumentsRegulatory Information/ChemicalContaminantsMetals NaturalToxinsPesticides/ucm109231.htm
Author Michelle Mostrom
Consulting Editor Christopher C.L. Chase
Acknowledgment The author and book editors acknowledge the prior contribution of Hussein S. Hussein.

M

NAIROBI SHEEP DISEASE

BASICS

OVERVIEW
• Nairobi sheep disease (NSD) is a noncontagious, highly pathogenic, tick-borne viral disease of sheep and goats with very high morbidity and mortality.
• It is a reportable disease in the United States and a notifiable disease of the International Office of Epizootics (OIE).

INCIDENCE/PREVALENCE
• Limited effect on animals bred in areas in which virus is endemic due to immunity from colostral antibodies.
• High mortality seen in naïve animals exposed to virus or in animals moved from dry to wet areas where ticks are abundant. Outbreaks are also seen in high rainfall when ticks expand their range.

GEOGRAPHIC DISTRIBUTION
• Mainly East Africa and Central Africa, may also be present in Botswana and Mozambique.
• The virus has been isolated in South Asia (India and Sri Lanka), and a novel strain identified in China, but no disease has been reported in these areas.

SYSTEMS AFFECTED
• Digestive
• Hemolymphatic
• Respiratory
• Reproductive

PATHOPHYSIOLOGY
• The virus causes a viral hemorrhagic fever; however, the virus is not contagious from animal to animal without a tick tick vector.
• Animals develop a viremia following the feeding of infected ticks.
• The virus increases the production of cellular factor, protein disulfide isomerase (PDI) that activates integrins at the surface of various uninfected cells, including endothelial cells and platelets, leading to increased vasodilatation and coagulopathy.
• Extracellular PDI activates tissue factor (TF), inducing intravascular coagulation, which may subsequently lead to disseminated intravascular coagulation (DIC) through depletion of platelets and clotting factors, resulting in hemorrhaging.
• Finally, since ERp57 another cell protein (and probably PDI) takes part in the folding of the major histocompatibility complex (MHC) class I and therefore assists in facilitating immune surveillance and elimination of virus-infected cells, viruses, which translocate these ER chaperones from the ER may avoid adaptive immune responses, although downregulation of MHC class I has not yet been described for nairovirus-infected cells.

GENETICS
• Animals in endemic areas are usually immune, and sheep are more susceptible than goats with mortality rates up to 75% in indigenous sheep breeds, e.g., East African hair sheep and Persian fat-tailed sheep.
• Few fatal cases of NSD have been reported in duikers, *Cephalophus monticola*, and experimental infection has been achieved in the African field rat, *Arvicathus abysinicus nubilans*.

SIGNALMENT
The virus affects small ruminants, particularly sheep; there is no age or sex predilection.

PHYSICAL EXAMINATION FINDINGS
• Incubation period is 1–15 days with most infections occurring in 2–6 days.
• Animals have sudden onset of fever (105.8–107.6°F; 41–42°C) that persists for up to 7 days; leukopenia and viremia coincide with the febrile stage and many animals die during this stage of the disease. This is often followed by rapid respiration, anorexia, and profound depression, followed by fetid diarrhea watery then hemorrhagic with straining and colic, and a concomitant drop in body temperature. Many animals die during the febrile stage of the disease.
• Palpable swollen prescapular and precrural lymph nodes.
• Bloodstained mucopurulent or serosanguinous nasal discharge.
• Abortion, ± conjunctivitis, death.

CAUSES AND RISK FACTORS
• NSD is caused by NSD virus, the prototype virus of the genus Nairovirus, family Bunyaviridae. Nairovirus is a negative sense, single-stranded RNA virus. The genus is divided into seven serogroups that include Crimean-Congo hemorrhagic fever. Ganjam virus is an Asian variant of the virus.
• The brown ear tick, *Rhipicephalus appendiculatus*, is the most common vector and transmission is both trans-ovarial and trans-stadial. The virus can persist in ticks for long periods and can be transmitted by unfed adult ticks for more than 2 years after infection. The virus can also be transmitted by *Amblyomma variegatum*, African bont tick, and has been isolated in South Asia (India and Sri Lanka) from ticks, *Haemaphysalis intermedia*, *H. wellingtoni*, and *R. haemaphysaloides*.
• A novel strain of NSD virus has been isolated in China with *H. longicornis* as the main vector but no disease has been reported in South Asia or China.
• Risk factors include movement of susceptible animals/naïve animals into endemic areas, expansion of tick vector range especially after high rainfall, and inadequate tick control measures.

DIAGNOSIS

DIFFERENTIAL DIAGNOSES
Heartwater, rinderpest, Rift Valley fever, anthrax, peste des petits ruminants, salmonellosis, coccidiosis, toxicosis (e.g., arsenic).

CBC/BIOCHEMISTRY/URINALYSIS
Leukopenia during the febrile stage

OTHER LABORATORY TESTS
• Detection of virus antigens during febrile stage of the disease using ELISA, virus isolation, indirect hemagglutination, IFAT.
• Serology: Indirect immunofluorescence antibody test (IFAT), agar gel immunodiffusion, complement fixation test, ELISA, and indirect hemagglutination. Fourfold or greater rise in antibody titers of paired sera samples.
• Virus isolation in BHK-21-C13 cells (baby kidney hamster cell line) from spleen and mesenteric lymph nodes.
• Inoculation of laboratory mice and sheep.

PATHOLOGIC FINDINGS
• Gross lesions include:
  ◦ Enlargement of superficial and mesenteric lymph nodes with congestion of most organs.
  ◦ Ecchymoses and petechiae on serosal surfaces of gastrointestinal tract, heart, spleen, liver, lungs, and kidney.
  ◦ Catarrhal mucoid or hemorrhagic gastroenteritis and dehydration; conjunctivitis.
  ◦ Ulceration and/or hemorrhages in abomasum, colon, cecum, distal ileum, and ileocecal valve; hemorrhages in mucosa of cecum and colon often appear as longitudinal striations (zebra striping). Hemorrhages are also present in genital tract of animals that have aborted.
  ◦ Swollen and hemorrhagic gallbladder.
  ◦ Edematous and hemorrhagic fetal membranes and hemorrhages throughout fetal organs.
• Histopathologic findings: Hyperplasia of lymphoid tissues, petechiae and ecchymoses in most organs, mucosal hemorrhages in gastrointestinal tract, myocardial degeneration, nephrosis, and coagulative necrosis of the gallbladder.

TREATMENT

THERAPEUTIC APPROACH
• No specific antivirals.
• Control of ticks by use of acaricides on unaffected animals.

N

(CONTINUED)

• Vaccination using either modified-live virus vaccine attenuated in mouse brain, or inactivated oil adjuvant vaccine before movement of naïve susceptible animals to an endemic area.

 MEDICATIONS

DRUGS OF CHOICE
N/A

 FOLLOW-UP

EXPECTED COURSE AND PROGNOSIS
• Prognosis is poor for naïve animals introduced into endemic areas.
• Goats are less susceptible than sheep and thus have a better prognosis.
• Animals that recover develop life-long immunity.

PREVENTION
• Avoid movement of naïve animals into endemic areas
• Vaccination
• Control of tick vector

 MISCELLANEOUS

AGE-RELATED FACTORS
Colostral antibodies confer immunity to young animals in endemic areas.

ZOONOTIC POTENTIAL
Febrile illness, headache, nausea, and vomiting

PREGNANCY
Abortion when infected

BIOSECURITY
Notifiable OIE disease and requires mandatory reporting

ABBREVIATIONS
• DIC = disseminated intravascular coagulation
• ELISA = enzyme labeled immunosorbent assay
• IFAT = indirect immunofluorescence antibody test
• MHC = major histocompatibility complex
• NSD = Nairobi sheep disease
• OIE = World Organization for Animal Health
• PDI = protein disulfide isomerase
• TF = tissue factor

SEE ALSO
• Anthrax
• Arsenic Toxicosis
• Coccidiosis
• Heartwater (Cowdriosis)
• Peste Des Petits Ruminants
• Rift Valley Fever
• Salmonellosis

Suggested Reading
Lasecka L, Baron MD. The nairovirus Nairobi sheep disease virus/ganjam virus induces the translocation of protein disulphide isomerase-like oxidoreductases from the endoplasmic reticulum to the cell surface and the extracellular space. PloS One 2014, 9: e94656. http://doi.org/10.1371/journal.pone.0094656
Marczinke BI, Nichol ST. Nairobi sheep disease virus, an important tick-borne pathogen of sheep and goats in Africa, is also present in Asia. Virology 2002, 303: 146–51.
Metwally SA. Overview of Nairobi sheep disease. In: Merck Veterinary Manual Online, 2015. Accessed July 30, 2016.
Radostits OM, Gay CC, Blood DC, Hinchcliff KW eds. Nairobi sheep disease. In: Diseases caused by viruses and Chlamydia. 1. Veterinary Medicine: A Textbook of the Diseases of Cattle Sheep, Pigs, Goats and Horses, 9th ed. London: Saunders, 2000, p. 1080.
Yadav PD, Vincent MJ, Khristova M, Kale C, Nichol ST, Mishra AC, Mourya DT. Genomic analysis reveals Nairobi sheep disease virus to be highly diverse and present in both Africa, and in India in the form of the Ganjam virus variant. Infect Genet Evol 2011, 11: 1111–20.

Author Akinyi Carol Nyaoke
Consulting Editor Christopher C.L. Chase
Acknowledgment The author and book editors acknowledge the prior contribution of Stacy M. Holzbauer.

N

NEMATODIROSIS

BASICS

OVERVIEW
• Nematodirosis related to infestation with the intestinal roundworm *Nematodirus* spp. is called nematodirosis.
• Disease can affect many ruminant species but is often most clinically relevant in sheep (lambs).

INCIDENCE/PREVALENCE
• Varies depending on management systems and climactic factors.
• Lamb mortality can reach 20% in untreated flocks in some regions (United Kingdom, New Zealand, Australia)

GEOGRAPHIC DISTRIBUTION
• Worldwide depending on species and environment
• UK, Europe, New Zealand, Australia, South Africa, North America

SYSTEMS AFFECTED
Digestive

PATHOPHYSIOLOGY
• Adult *Nematodirus* spp. reside in the anterior third of the small intestine of ruminants.
• Eggs are shed in the feces and, in the case of *N. spathiger* and *N. helvetianus*, development into the third stage larvae happens within the egg in 2–4 weeks. *N. battus* and *N. filicollis* have a delayed development and require conditioning by cold over winter. These infectious larvae (L3) remain within the egg until they are stimulated to hatch with rain and they can remain viable in the soil or on vegetation for many months. They are then ingested by the host during grazing and develop into mature adults in about 3 weeks.
• If the animal survives the effects of the parasite infestation, resistance to reinfection can develop.

HISTORICAL FINDINGS
• Pasturing in an enzootic area.
• A history of previous year's lambs, calves, or kids being infected and inhabiting the same premises.
• Infection is asymptomatic in resistant animals but acute illness can occur within 3 weeks of exposure in susceptible animals.
• Young animals are more likely to be affected.
• There is lack of an adequate anthelmintic program on the premises in question.

SIGNALMENT
• Potentially all ruminant species can be infected.
• Typically clinical disease occurs in lambs 6–12 weeks of age.

PHYSICAL EXAMINATION FINDINGS
• Sudden onset of diarrhea, anorexia, and loss of condition.
• Rapid dehydration and death (can be seen within 2–3 days of onset).

GENETICS
N/A

CAUSES AND RISK FACTORS
• *Nematodirus* spp.
  ○ Cattle—*N. helvetianus* primarily, also *N. spathiger*, *N. filicollis*, and *N. battus*.
  ○ Sheep and goats—*N. battus* primarily, also *N. spathiger*, *N. helvetianus*, *N. abnormalis*, *N. davitiani*, *N. filicollis*, and *N. lanceolatus*.
  ○ Bighorn sheep, deer, gemsbok—*N. spathiger*
  ○ Moufflon—*N. filicollis*
  ○ Bison—*Nematodirus* spp.
• Feeding on infested pasture, usually early in the grazing period
• Inadequate use of anthelmintics and preventive pasturing practices

DIAGNOSIS

DIFFERENTIAL DIAGNOSES
Infestation with other gastrointestinal parasites including *Trichostrongylus* spp., *Oesophagostomum* spp., and *Cooperia* spp.

CBC/BIOCHEMISTRY/URINALYSIS
CBC and biochemistry are indicated in severely affected animals, and may reveal changes consistent with systemic inflammation and protein loss.

OTHER LABORATORY TESTS
N/A

IMAGING
N/A

OTHER DIAGNOSTIC PROCEDURES
• Identification of eggs in feces; however, clinical signs often commence during the late pre-patent period prior to maturation of female parasites, which can complicate diagnosis early in flock outbreaks of disease.
• Eggs are distinctive and easily identified. They are large (180–230 μm × 90–170 μm), smooth and elongate, tapering at both ends. They are segmented (8 cells inside) when initially passed in the feces.

PATHOLOGIC FINDINGS
• Watery, dark-green diarrhea staining the escutcheon or breech.
• Dehydration, possibly cachexia.
• Fluid mucoid content of the upper small intestine and soft or fluid feces in the colon.
• Duodenal mucosa might show hyperemia with excess mucus, but is usually normal in appearance.
• Third stage larvae reside in the deeper layers of the mucosa and crypts. Fourth or fifth stage larvae reside coiled among the villi and, in high enough numbers, result in villous atrophy.
• Worm counts reveal tangled, cottony masses of elongate, lightly coiled nematodes in heavy infestations.

TREATMENT

THERAPEUTIC APPROACH
• All animals in an affected group should be treated with an appropriate anthelmintic product to reduce exposure level.
• If possible, prevent re-infestation by moving animals to a region or premises free of the parasite.

SURGICAL CONSIDERATIONS AND TECHNIQUES
N/A

MEDICATIONS

DRUGS OF CHOICE
• Ivermectin, moxidectin or doramectin given at 200 μg/kg body weight.
• Other anthelmintics that may be effective include levamisole (5 mg/kg), morantel and benzimidazoles (fenbendazole, oxfendazole and albendazole). Use as directed and observe withdrawal times.

CONTRAINDICATIONS
Do not treat animals that produce milk for human consumption with macrocyclic lactone drugs.

PRECAUTIONS
Appropriate milk and meat withdrawal times must be followed for all compounds administered to food-producing animals.

POSSIBLE INTERACTIONS
N/A

FOLLOW-UP

EXPECTED COURSE AND PROGNOSIS
Full recovery with resistance to re-infestation is expected if clinical disease is mild and treated early.

POSSIBLE COMPLICATIONS
Dehydration and death has been reported with high prevalence in affected lambs in the UK, New Zealand, and Australia.

CLIENT EDUCATION
Develop robust parasite prevention protocols appropriate for the specific region that rely heavily on management and monitoring techniques paired with judicious use of anthelmintic drugs.

PATIENT CARE
Supportive care, which includes adequate high-quality nutrition and ready access to fresh water.

(CONTINUED) **NEMATODIROSIS**

PREVENTION

• Anthelmintics can be given initially when young animals are put out to pasture in spring, and then again in 3–5 weeks.
• Repeated treatments may be needed depending on environmental conditions and the species of *Nematodirus* in the area. Single treatments can be used with a delayed spring turnout or if transfer to non-infested premises occurs.
• Protocols will vary with location, making the experience of local veterinarians essential.
• Avoid infested premises/pastures, and avoid lambing annually in the same area or pasture.
• Without re-infestation, premises should be relatively free of infective larvae or eggs after two seasons, so pasture rotation at that interval will decrease potential of exposure.
• Rotate pastures with different, nonsusceptible livestock species.
• If calves, lambs, or kids are put on the pasture, follow them with adults who are likely resistant.

 MISCELLANEOUS

ASSOCIATED CONDITIONS

• Other intestinal parasites
• Diarrhea, anorexia, dehydration

AGE-RELATED FACTORS

• Clinical disease occurs primarily in lambs, also calves and kids.
• Disease is most severe in young animals, but older nonresistant animals can also be affected.

ZOONOTIC POTENTIAL

N/A

PREGNANCY

N/A

BIOSECURITY

• Isolation and quarantine of new stock entering the herd or flock.
• Treat and/or cull new animals for disease conditions prior to herd introduction.
• If possible, prevent re-infestation by moving animals to premises free of the parasite.

PRODUCTION MANAGEMENT

• Avoid infested premises and pastures.
• Without re-infestation, premises should be relatively free of infective larvae or eggs after two seasons, so pasture rotation at that interval will decrease potential of exposure, and can involve different, nonsusceptible livestock species.

SYNONYMS

N/A

ABBREVIATIONS

N/A

SEE ALSO

• Anthelmic Resistence
• Diarrheal Diseases: Bovine
• Diarrheal Diseases: Small Ruminant
• Food Animal Residue Avoidance Databank (FARAD) (see www.fiveminutevet.com/ruminant)
• Haemonchosis
• Parasite Control Programs: Small Ruminant

Suggested Reading
Dorchies P, Jacquiet P, Bergeaud JP, et al. Efficacy of doramectin against *Oestrus ovis* and GI nematodes in sheep in the Southwest of France. Vet Parasitol 2001, 96:147–54.
Ivens VR, Mark DL, Levine ND. Principal Parasites of Domestic Animals in the United States. Special Publication 52, Colleges of Agriculture and Veterinary Medicine, University of Illinois at Urbana-Champaign, 2000.
Jubb KVF, Kennedy PC, Palmer N eds. Pathology of Domestic Animals, 4th ed, vol 3. San Diego: Academic Press, 1993.
Ranjan S, Trudeau C, Prichard RK, Daigneault J, Rew RS. Nematode reinfection following treatment of cattle with doramectin and ivermectin. Vet Parasitol 1997, 72: 25–31.
Rehbein S, Barth D, Visser M, Winter R, Langholff WK. Efficacy of ivermectin controlled release capsule against some rarer nematode parasites of sheep. Vet Parasitol 2000, 88: 293–8.
Vadlejch J, Kotrba, R, Cadkova, Z, Ruzickova, A, Langrova, I. Effects of age, sex, lactation and social dominance of faecal egg count patterns of gastrointestinal nematodes in farmed eland (*Taurotragus oryx*). Prev Vet Med 2015, 121: 265–72.
Internet Resource
• http://www.southeastsuffolks.co.uk/nadis1.htm
Author Saluna Pokhrel
Consulting Editor Erica C. McKenzie
Acknowledgment The authors and book editors acknowledge the prior contribution of Edward L. Powers.

N

NEONATAL DIARRHEA

BASICS

OVERVIEW
• Diarrhea is the most prevalent illness in ruminants during the first 28 days of life.
• The development of diarrhea in neonates can arise because of a lack of adequate passive transfer of protective maternal immunoglobulins, overwhelming exposure to enteric pathogens, environmental stressors, or a combination of these events.
• Most cases of diarrhea reflect mixed infections with more than one pathogen.
• Treatment centers on the correction of electrolyte and acid-base imbalances, and dehydration.
• Death occurs due to dehydration, metabolic derangements, and electrolyte imbalances, and occasionally sepsis.
• Prevention focuses on vaccination of dams with appropriate antigens prepartum, ensuring adequate colostrum intake by neonates, and providing a clean maternity area and neonatal environment.

INCIDENCE/PREVALENCE
• Incidence of disease is variable, influenced by management, and can be substantial when outbreak situations occur with infectious pathogens.
• Incidence is higher in neonates born to primiparous dams due to colostrum of lesser quality and volume.
• Incidence of disease is higher during conditions that favor increased pathogen survival, particularly when environmental conditions are cold and wet, resulting in neonatal stress.

GEOGRAPHIC DISTRIBUTION
Worldwide

SYSTEMS AFFECTED
• Digestive
• Cardiovascular

PATHOPHYSIOLOGY
• Diarrhea results from a variety of mechanisms occurring singly or in combination.
• Secretory diarrhea arises from stimulation of intestinal cells to secrete fluid into the lumen of the intestine. Although the absorptive capacity of the intestine may remain intact, the volume of fluid secretion overwhelms absorptive capacity, resulting in diarrhea.
• E. coli and Salmonella can produce entero- or exotoxins, which stimulate the intestinal epithelium to secrete sodium, chloride, bicarbonate, and potassium, along with fluid.
• The production of prostaglandins as a result of inflammatory processes also stimulates cellular secretions.
• Malabsorptive diarrhea results from injury to the absorptive epithelium of the intestinal tract. Viral agents, including coronavirus, rotavirus, and torovirus (Breda virus) as well

as parasitic agents (Cryptosporidium and Coccidia), are the main pathogenic agents that contribute to this mechanism of diarrhea.
• Injury to the intestinal epithelium results not only in the loss of absorptive capacity but also in the loss of the enzyme systems needed for the digestion of nutrients such as lactose and proteins, resulting in maldigestion.
• Osmotically active solutes result from incomplete digestion and subsequent bacterial fermentation of nondigested nutrients, and draw fluid into the intestine, overwhelming the absorptive capacity of the gut.
• Normal bacterial flora is disrupted and changed, which may contribute to the development of diarrhea.
• The severity of neonatal diarrhea is dependent on agent virulence factors as well as host factors. Some animals may remain bright and alert and only exhibit mild signs of diarrhea, while others may have profuse watery diarrhea and exhibit systemic disease, resulting in death.
• Clinical signs of disease most often relate to acid-base disturbances, electrolyte loss, and dehydration. Septic and hypovolemic shock can occur when the bowel is severely diseased or the pathogen invasive.
• Septicemia usually occurs in neonates with inadequate immunoglobulin status or that are infected with enteroinvasive E. coli or Salmonella spp.

HISTORICAL FINDINGS
• In a herd or flock situation, the number of diarrhea cases related to infectious disease typically increases with the duration of calving, lambing, or kidding season as the pathogen load builds over time.
• In systems in which neonates are hand reared, particular attention should be paid to feeding management in case of nutritional diarrhea or contagion as a result of feeding practices.

SIGNALMENT
• Neonatal diarrhea is common in cattle, kids, lambs, and crias.
• Enterotoxigenic E. coli usually causes disease within the first 4 days of life; this can extend to 2 weeks if viral or parasitic infections exist.
• Enteroinvasive E. coli tends to cause septicemic disease during the first week of life; joint infections may develop during the first 2 weeks of life.
• Enteropathogenic and enterohemorrhagic E. coli affect neonates typically in the second and third weeks of life (range 4–28 days).
• Salmonella can affect any age group, and tends to be very uncommon in camelids.
• Coronavirus typically creates disease in neonates 5–28 days of age.
• Rotavirus typically creates disease in neonates 5–14 days of age.
• Cryptosporidiosis afflicts animals 7–28 days of age.
• Coccidiosis usually causes clinical disease in animals 16 days of age and older.

PHYSICAL EXAMINATION FINDINGS
• Soiled perineal region and tail.
• Dehydration is suggested by increased skin tent time, sunken eyes, and tacky mucus membranes.
• Fever may be present. Body temperature may be subnormal in animals that are significantly dehydrated and in shock.
• Tachycardia is often present as a result of hypovolemia; however, bradycardia or irregular cardiac rhythm can occur due to hyperkalemia, hypothermia, and/or hypoglycemia.
• Respiratory rate can be elevated in animals with metabolic acidosis. Neonatal calves with diarrhea often have concurrent pneumonia which will influence respiratory rate and pattern.
• The abdomen may appear poorly filled if the animal is anorexic, or may appear distended, particularly on the right side, due to ileus and collection of fluid within the intestines.
• The umbilicus may be enlarged, suggesting omphalitis which is often associated with failure of passive transfer.
• Scleral injection and hypopyon may be observed in septicemic neonates.
• Animals may be recumbent and unable to rise as a result of severe hypovolemia, metabolic acidosis, hypoglycemia, septicemia, or severe electrolyte disturbances.

GENETICS
N/A

CAUSES AND RISK FACTORS
• A wide variety of viral, bacterial and parasitic agents can cause diarrhea in neonatal ruminants and camelids, as listed below (some species differences exist).
• Although infectious agents are by far the most frequent cause of neonatal diarrhea, other possible etiologies include nutritional mismanagement, toxicities, and nutritional deficiencies.
• Infectious agents:
  ○ Rotavirus
  ○ Enterotoxigenic E. coli
  ○ Cryptosporidium parvum, C. bovis, C. ryanae and C. andersoni
  ○ Coronavirus
  ○ Enteropathogenic and enterohemorrhagic E. coli
  ○ Enteroinvasive E. coli
  ○ Salmonella spp.
  ○ Clostridium perfringens type A, B, C, and D
  ○ Eimeria spp.
  ○ Bovine viral diarrhea virus (BVDV)
  ○ Bovine torovirus (Breda virus)
  ○ Calici virus
  ○ Astro virus
  ○ Parvovirus
  ○ Campylobacter coli and C. jejuni
• Inadequate passive transfer of immunoglobulins resulting in agammaglobulinemia or hypogammaglobulinemia is a major risk

factor in neonatal diarrhea, and can occur due to factors that influence the neonate's access to and intake of colostrum in an appropriate time window, or that adversely affect the quality of the dam's colostrum. These factors include dystocia, prematurity, dam health and parity, and separation of dam and neonate without adequate colostrum substitution.
• Maternity areas that are contaminated with fecal material containing pathogenic agents are also a risk, due to enhanced ingestion of pathogens by the neonate from dirty udders, overcrowded maternity areas, and where there is lack of adequate cleaning and replacement of dirty bedding between birthing dams.
• Inadequate or improper nutrition is a risk, including improper reconstitution of milk replacers, poor quality milk replacers, once daily feeding, provision of bacterially contaminated colostrum or milk from mastitic quarters, or milk/milk replacer containing antibiotics.
• Dirty and crowded neonatal housing increases the risk of high pathogen loads and transmission.
• Cold, wet, and/or drafty environments contribute to immunosuppression and enhance survival of some pathogens.

DIAGNOSIS

DIFFERENTIAL DIAGNOSES
• The gross characteristics of neonatal diarrheic feces are not diagnostic, although the presence of blood and mucus usually suggests large intestine involvement.
• Bloody diarrhea suggests *Salmonella*, coronavirus, enterohemorrhagic *E. coli*, BVDV, and *Coccidia*.
• Diarrhea with mucus can suggest *Salmonella*, coronavirus, enteropathogenic *E. coli*, enterohemorrhagic *E. coli*, and *Coccidia*.
• The presence of milk curds in the feces indicates a malabsorptive or maldigestive condition, often associated with viral agents.
• If fever is evident, *Salmonella*, enteropathogenic and enterohemorrhagic *E. coli*, and *Coccidia* should be considered.
• Tenesmus can also occur with coccidiosis in calves.
• Nutritional diarrhea.

CBC/BIOCHEMISTRY/URINALYSIS
• CBC can demonstrate hemoconcentration, with increased PCV and total protein concentrations. A left shift may be observed in animals in which the infectious agent invades the mucosa, produces toxins, or causes significant mucosal damage.
• Serum chemistry often reveals hypoglycemia, metabolic acidosis, and prerenal azotemia. Serum sodium and chloride might be low or normal. Hyperkalemia is often observed if metabolic

acidosis is present despite a whole body potassium deficit.

OTHER LABORATORY TESTS
• Determination of immunoglobulin status during the first five days of life can be performed by a variety of methods:
  ○ Plasma protein concentration determined by refractometry can provide an indirect measure; <5 mg/dL suggests of failure of passive transfer. However, the impact of dehydration and other plasma solutes on the plasma protein reading must be considered.
  ○ Zinc sulfate or sodium sulfite turbidity tests can be performed to estimate immunoglobulin status.
  ○ Single radial immmunodiffusion testing is accurately quantitative but takes 24 hours for results.
• Fecal floatation for observation of *Coccidia* and *Cryptosporidium* oocysts.
• Estimation of base deficit by evaluating serum or plasma total CO_2 concentration (which is 1–2 units higher than serum or plasma bicarbonate concentration).

IMAGING
N/A

OTHER DIAGNOSTIC PROCEDURES
• Necropsy
• Fecal culture
• Electron microscopy to detect viral agents

PATHOLOGIC FINDINGS
• At necropsy the intestines are filled with fluid and the mucosa may be congested, but gross lesions are often fairly minimal with most of the common causes of neonatal diarrhea.
• Hemorrhagic enteritis is associated with *Clostridium perfringens* type C infection.
• Fibrinonecrotic enteritis is associated with salmonellosis.
• Mucosal ulceration is associated with BVDV infection.
• Disruption of the mucosa and petechial hemorrhages may be observed in animals infected with *Salmonella* or *Coccidia*.
• Congestion of the lungs, liver, and spleen and petechial hemorrhages of the epicardium and serosal surfaces of organs are often observed in animals with septicemia resulting from *Salmonella* or enteroinvasive *E. coli* infection.
• Histopathologic findings vary. Colonization of the intestinal epithelium by enterotoxigenic *E. coli* may be evident, or adherence and effacement of epithelial cells by enteropathogenic and enterohemorrhagic *E. coli*.
• Developmental stages of *Cryptosporidium* and *Coccidia* can be observed within the small and large intestines.
• Desquamation of epithelial cells, villus shortening, and degrees of villus fusion are observed with viral infections.

TREATMENT

THERAPEUTIC APPROACH
• Fluid therapy is typically the foundation of treatment to correct dehydration, circulatory impairment, and electrolyte and acid-base imbalances. Fluid may be administered orally or intravenously depending on how severely diseased the neonate is.
• Commercial oral electrolyte solutions containing glucose and a nonbicarbonate alkalinizing agent are recommended if the neonate is still nursing.
• Neonates without a suckle response should receive IV fluids, such as physiologic saline with the addition of bicarbonate and glucose as needed. After establishment of rehydration, lactated Ringer's solution may be used for maintenance.
• With severe acidosis, isotonic sodium bicarbonate solution (1.3%, 13 g of sodium bicarbonate to 1 litre of distilled water) may be used.
• Dextrose solutions (2.5–5%) are indicated if hypoglycemia is present.
• With hypoglycemia and unknown electrolyte and acid-base status, a 2.5% dextrose and 0.45% saline solution has been recommended.
• Neonates with a suckle response should be left with the dam and allowed to nurse. Animals being artificially reared should remain on their diet or be switched to whole milk or colostrum. If the diarrhea becomes worse or the neonate becomes depressed, removal from the dam or milk is warranted for 24 hours.
• In hand-reared neonates that are depressed with no suckle, or neonates refusing to nurse the dam, a high-energy electrolyte solution can be administered at 10% of body weight (minimum) divided into a minimum of four feedings. Once neonates are suckling, feed milk at 5% of body weight divided into 4 feedings per day, increasing the amount per feeding gradually to full volume over 2–3 days.
• Neonates should not be denied milk for longer than 24 hours.
• Oral electrolytes containing an alkalinizing agent, other than acetate, should not be fed when neonates are receiving the dam's milk or whole milk, as milk digestion may be disrupted.

SURGICAL CONSIDERATIONS AND TECHNIQUES
N/A

N

NEONATAL DIARRHEA   (CONTINUED)

MEDICATIONS

DRUGS OF CHOICE
• Many causes of diarrhea in neonates are self-limiting and antibiotics are not indicated. However, approximately 30% of neonates with diarrhea will have bacteremia in which antimicrobial therapy may be beneficial.
  ○ Oral amoxicillin trihydrate (10 mg/kg PO q12h) for nonruminating calves.
  ○ Amoxicillin trihydrate-clavulanate potassium (12.5 mg combined drug/kg PO q12h for 3 days).
• Flunixin meglumine (1.1 mg/kg IV or 2.2 mg/kg IM) has been shown to decrease secretion induced by *E. coli* enterotoxins and to reduce days of morbidity in calves with fecal blood.
• Plasma transfusion is indicated in neonates with failure of passive transfer and sepsis if the value of the animal warrants the expense.

CONTRAINDICATIONS
Do not use kaolin and pectin in diarrheic neonates, as this may increase electrolyte loss.

PRECAUTIONS
Appropriate milk and meat withdrawal times must be followed for all compounds administered to food-producing animals.

POSSIBLE INTERACTIONS
N/A

FOLLOW-UP

EXPECTED COURSE AND PROGNOSIS
• Most cases of neonatal diarrhea are self-limiting and resolve over 2–3 days, depending on the cause.
• Diarrhea is more severe in animals in which multiple disease agents are present, such as viral diarrhea with secondary bacterial infection.
• Time to recovery is often proportional to the amount of mucosal damage the animal experiences.
• Prognosis is directly related to the ability of the animal to maintain hydration and its immunoglobulin status.
• Animals that are hypogammaglobulinemic or that are septicemic are at increased risk of mortality.

POSSIBLE COMPLICATIONS
• Sepsis
• Hypovolemic shock
• Septic arthritis

CLIENT EDUCATION
Focus on biosecurity measures and nutritional management

PATIENT CARE
• Monitor attitude, suckling response and appetite, fecal color and consistency, and hydration status.
• Monitor age cohorts for signs of diarrhea.

PREVENTION
• Ensure adequate colostrum quality through management and vaccination of dams, and monitoring of neonates for access and intake.
• Maternity areas should be kept clean and disinfected periodically as appropriate.
• Remove the dam and neonate from the birthing area into a clean environment as soon as safe and feasible.
• Dip neonatal navels in appropriate antiseptic agents.
• Eliminate access of neonates to areas of fecal buildup.
• Dams can be administered vaccines containing enterotoxigenic *E. coli*, rotavirus and coronavirus antigens, and autogenous *Salmonella* prepartum.
• Neonates should be kept dry and in a draft-free environment.
• Equipment used to treat or feed neonates should be cleaned and disinfected between animals.
• Diarrheic animals should be isolated from healthy animals since they are sources of a large numbers of pathogens.
• Caregivers should wash hands between animals and keep clothing free of fecal material.

MISCELLANEOUS

ASSOCIATED CONDITIONS
• Septic arthritis
• Omphalitis
• Meningitis

AGE-RELATED FACTORS
Diarrhea is a very common neonatal disease.

ZOONOTIC POTENTIAL
• All diarrheic animals should be handled as though zoonotic potential is present.
• *Salmonella*, *Cryptosporidium*, *Campylobacter*, and some *E. coli* are potentially transmissible and pathogenic to humans.

PREGNANCY
N/A

BIOSECURITY
• Equipment used to treat or feed neonates should be cleaned and disinfected between animals.
• Handle and feed the youngest animals first, then handle in order of increasing age.
• Diarrheic animals should be isolated from healthy animals as they are sources for large numbers of pathogens, and they should be fed and handled last.

• Caregivers should wash hands between animals and keep clothing free of fecal material.

PRODUCTION MANAGEMENT
Neonatal diarrhea is a significant cause of economic loss, and preventive measures are critical in controlling the incidence and prevalence within herds and flocks.

SYNONYM
Scours

ABBREVIATION
BVDV = bovine viral diarrhea virus

SEE ALSO
• Coronavirus
• Cryptosporidiosis
• Diarrheal Diseases: Bovine
• Diarrheal Diseases: Camelid
• Diarrheal Diseases: Small Ruminant
• *Escherichia coli*
• Rotavirus
• Salmonellosis

Suggested Reading
Barrington GM, Gay JM, Evermann JF. Biosecurity for neonatal gastrointestinal diseases. Vet Clin North Am Food Anim Pract 2002, 18: 7–34.
Gunn AA, Chuck G, McGuirk SA. Initial management and clinical investigation of neonatal disease. In: Smith BP ed, Large Animal Internal Medicine, 5th ed. St. Louis: Mosby, 2015, pp. 286–335.
Izzo M, Gunn AA, House JK. Neonatal diarrhea. In: Smith BP ed, Large Animal Internal Medicine, 5th ed. St. Louis: Elsevier Mosby, 2015, pp. 314–35.
Smith DR. Field disease diagnostic investigation of neonatal calf diarrhea. Vet Clin North Am Food Anim Pract 2012, 28: 465–81.
Smith GW, Berchtold, J. Fluid therapy in calves. Vet Clin North Am Food Anim Pract 2014, 30: 409–27.
Smith GW. Antimicrobial decision making for enteric diseases of cattle. Vet Clin North Am Food Anim Pract 2015, 31: 47–60.
Townsend HG. Environmental factors and calving management practices that affect neonatal mortality in the beef calf. Vet Clin North Am Food Anim Pract 1994, 10: 119–26.

Author Kevin D. Pelzer
Consulting Editor Erica C. McKenzie

N

NEONATAL SEPTIC ARTHRITIS

BASICS

OVERVIEW
• An inflammatory disease confined to the synovial membrane and articular surfaces as a result of sequestered bacteria.
• Route of infection is hematogenous as a result of bacteremia, which often originates from an umbilical infection or the GI tract.
• Often, this occurs in multiple joints ± physeal involvement.

INCIDENCE/PREVALENCE
• Incidence is not well described.
• Usually sporadic.
• Outbreaks in herds with endemic organisms or poor management.

GEOGRAPHIC DISTRIBUTION
N/A

SYSTEMS AFFECTED
• Musculoskeletal
• Nervous

PATHOPHYSIOLOGY
• Bacterial infections of newborn ruminants occur largely as a result of hypogammaglobulinemia (from FPT or depletion of immunoglobulins in the face of an overwhelming sepsis).
• Neonates become bacteremic or septicemic from an infection that often originates from the umbilical cord or via oral ingestion.
• Bacteria then sequester in the joint and cause inflammation of the synovial membrane.
• Multiple joints are often affected.
• Synovitis causes distention of the joint capsule with fluid.
• Arthritis may be suppurative or serofibrinous.
• Erosion of articular cartilage, infection of subchondral bone, and osteomyelitis can be sequelae.
• Synthesis of inflammatory mediators that can degrade cartilage.

HISTORICAL FINDINGS
• Unhygienic calving environment
• History of inadequate colostral intake
• Small, weak calves that remain recumbent for some hours
• Beef cows that reject their calves

SIGNALMENT
• All ruminants, but more common in dairy calves than beef calves
• Neonatal ruminants <4 weeks of age
• Usually evident within 2–3 days post-birth

PHYSICAL EXAMINATION FINDINGS
• Lameness is acute and severe.
• Joint effusion.
• Pain.
• Fever.
• Lethargy/Inappetence.
• Recumbency.
• Palpation and flexion of joint(s) reveal(s) heat and pain.
• Tachycardia and dehydration may be evident.
• Umbilicus may be moist and painful with purulent discharge.
• Nervous symptoms associated with meningitis may be present.

GENETICS
N/A

CAUSES AND RISK FACTORS
• Enterics are most common (Gram-negative)—*Trueperella pyogenes*, *Escherichia coli*, *Salmonella* spp.
• Skin commensals (Gram-positive cocci)—*Streptococcus dysgalactiae*, *Lactococcus lactis* (lambs)
• Respiratory tract commensals—*Histophilus somni*, *Mycoplasma bovis*
• *Chlamydia psittaci* (lambs)
• *Erysipelothrix rhusiopathiae* (lambs)
Risk factors include:
• Hypogammaglobulinemia as a result of inadequate colostral intake.
• Dystocia.
• Mismothering/abandonment.
• Hypothermia.
• Raw milk/fermented dairy products (source of Gram-positive pathogens).
• Poor-quality colostrums (source of Gram-positive pathogens).
• Environmental contamination—unhygienic or overcrowded calving area, fecal contamination of dam's hocks and tail (source of Gram-negative pathogens).
• Calves born to first-lactation cows tend to have lower immunoglobulin concentrations.

DIAGNOSIS

DIFFERENTIAL DIAGNOSES
• Primary infection arthritis: Penetration of joint by foreign body
• Extension of infection from surrounding tissues such as decubital lesions
• Idiopathic arthritis
• Myositis
• Degenerative myopathy
• Trauma
• Diseases of the nervous system that may cause recumbency or lameness
• Osteomyelitis
• Articular fracture
• Ligament injury
• Osteochondrosis

CBC/BIOCHEMISTRY/URINALYSIS
Elevated white blood cell counts

OTHER LABORATORY TESTS
• The neonate should be assessed for FPT.
• Blood culture improves the chance of finding bacteria in a febrile calf (use an ARD if the animal has received antibiotics prior to culture).
• Specific testing for *Mycoplasma* spp. (esp. if the umbilicus is normal and routine culture is negative).

IMAGING
• Radiology may only reveal soft tissue swelling in early stages, with destruction of articular cartilage and bone evident in advanced cases.
• Radiographic lesions more lytic with less new bone formation deposited at the joint periphery vs. older animals.
• Ultrasound joint (soft tissue swelling/effusion/fibrin) and umbilical structures.

OTHER DIAGNOSTIC PROCEDURES
• Joint aspiration may reveal purulent synovial fluid.
• Synovial fluid cytologic examination to evaluate TP and TNCC.
• Synovial fluid with TNCC >25,000 cells/µL, PMN count >20,000 cells/µL or >80% PMN cells should be considered septic.
• Total leukocyte counts range 50,000–100,000 cells/µL.
• Leukocytes are usually >90% neutrophils.
• Synovial fluid has elevated protein content (>4 g/dL).
• Joint culture is recommended, but is often unrewarding.

PATHOLOGIC FINDINGS
N/A

N

TREATMENT

THERAPEUTIC APPROACH
• Systemic antibiotic therapy should be initiated and maintained for 10 days to 3 weeks.
• Treatment of FPT should be considered (plasma/whole blood).
• Short-term analgesic therapy (24–48 hours) in the form of NSAIDs (flunixin meglumine, ketoprofen, or meloxicam) may be used to reduce pain.

SURGICAL CONSIDERATIONS AND TECHNIQUES
• Joint lavage using a "through-and-through" technique with two 18- to 14-gauge needles placed on either side of the joint (very effective in acute cases).
• Sterile, warmed isotonic fluid should be flushed through the joint to remove debris (1 liter if possible).
• A light dressing should be applied to the joint for 24–48 hours post-lavage.
• IA antibiotics provide concentrations above MIC for a long period of time.
• RLP (IV administration under tourniquet).
• Arthroscopy, arthrotomy, the use of AIPMMA, and arthrodesis are further options to consider if response to initial treatment is unsuccessful or the animal is highly valuable.

MEDICATIONS

DRUGS OF CHOICE
- Selection of antibiotic may be determined by results of joint culture and sensitivity.
- Empirically treat with broad-spectrum antibiotics while awaiting culture results. In neonates with septic arthritis, antimicrobials should also be effective against mycoplasma, especially if concurrent pneumonia or otitis.
- Florfenicol (reports of successful use in IA and RLP as well as systemically).
- Macrolides.
- Potentiated sulfonamides (trimethoprim sulfadiazine).
- Oxytetracycline (good joint penetration).
No mycoplasma coverage:
- Ampicillin/Penicillin (good joint penetration and do not cause chemical synovitis if IA).
- Ceftiofur (effective at increased dosage IV and in RLP; however now illegal to use extra-label in US).

CONTRAINDICATIONS
Do not use antibiotics not approved for food animals.

PRECAUTIONS
- If NSAID therapy is prolonged, neonates should be monitored/treated for abomasal/C3 ulcers.
- When treating via IA or RLP routes withdrawal times will differ, thus recommendations should be made based on available pharmacokinetic and pharmacodynamic data. FARAD is a useful resource for acquiring such information. All drugs are considered extra-label for the indication of septic arthritis in food animals in the US.

POSSIBLE INTERACTIONS
N/A

FOLLOW-UP

EXPECTED COURSE AND PROGNOSIS
- Prognosis is dependent on level of FPT and chronicity.
- Prognosis is poor if multiple joints or meningitis are evident.
- Rapid intervention after clinical signs increases the chance for recovery; delay in initial treatment will cause the prognosis to be poor.
- Cases involving a single joint that are treated early have a reasonably good prognosis (up to 80% of calves may recover).

POSSIBLE COMPLICATIONS
- Chronic arthritis may result in severe degenerative joint disease.
- Recurrence of infection may occur if source of infection is not eliminated.
- Osteomyelitis.
- Meningitis may occur in neonates with septicemia.

CLIENT EDUCATION
- Predisposing causes should be discussed and eliminated.
- Evaluate colostral management and calving area hygiene.
- Warn client of need for long-term antibiotics and guarded prognosis.
- Educate clients on the importance of hygiene in calf health as well as zoonoses prevention—wear gloves (assisting birth), clean animal and calving equipment when assisting delivery, promptly remove placentas, rebed maternity pen.

PATIENT CARE
- Calf may need to be assisted to stand and nurse if appropriate (beef cattle).
- Physiotherapy by gentle flexion and extension or regular exercise may improve return to function.

PREVENTION
- Insure adequate colostral intake
- Appropriate umbilical hygiene

MISCELLANEOUS

ASSOCIATED CONDITIONS
- Omphalophlebitis
- FPT
- Septicemia
- Meningitis

ZOONOTIC POTENTIAL
Salmonella spp., *E. coli* can have a zoonotic potential.

BIOSECURITY
Hygiene of calving area will aid in prevention.

SYNONYMS
- Joint ill
- Infectious arthritis
- Polyarthritis

ABBREVIATIONS
- AIPMMA = antibiotic-impregnated polymethylmethacrylate
- ARD = antimicrobial removal device
- C3 = compartment 3
- FARAD = Food Animal Residue Avoidance Databank
- FPT = failure of passive transfer
- GGT = gammaglutamyl transpeptidase
- IA = intra-articular
- IV = intravenous
- MIC = minimum inhibitory concentration
- NSAID = nonsteroidal anti-inflammatory drug
- PMN = polymorphonuclear
- RLP = regional limb perfusion
- TNCC = total nucleated cell count
- TP = total protein

SEE ALSO
- Enzootic Pneumonia of Calves
- Failure of Passive Transfer
- Neonatology (by species)
- Polyarthritis
- Umbilical Disorders

Suggested Reading
Desrochers A, Francoz D. Clinical management of septic arthritis in cattle. Vet Clin North Am Food Anim Pract 2014, 30: 177–203.
Haerdi-Landerer MC, Habermacher J, Wenger B, Suter MM, Steiner A. Slow release antibiotics for treatment of septic arthritis in large animals. Vet J 2010, 184: 14–20.
Jackson P. Treatment of septic arthritis in calves. Practice 1999, 21: 596–601.
Rohde C, Anderson DE, Desrochers A, et al. Synovial fluid analysis in cattle: A review of 130 cases. Vet Surg 2000, 29: 341–6.
Rutherford SJ, Rycroft AN, Ridler AL. Sources of *Streptococcus dysgalactiae* in English and Welsh sheep flocks affected by infectious arthritis (joint ill). Vet Rec 2014, 174: 579–82.
Weaver AD. Joint conditions. In: Greenough PR ed, Lameness in Cattle, 3rd ed. Philadelphia: Saunders, 1997.
Wichtel MEG, Fenwick SG, Hunter J, Stephenson A, Martin D, Wichtel JJ. Septicaemia and septic arthritis in a neonatal calf caused by *Lactococcus lactis*. Vet Rec 2003, 153: 22–3.

Author Francisco C. Rodriguez
Consulting Editor Kaitlyn A. Lutz
Acknowledgment The author and book editors acknowledge the prior contribution of John R. Campbell.

N

BASICS

OVERVIEW
• The neonatal period in cattle goes from 0 to 30 days of age.
• During the neonatal period the calf is subjected to physiologic and environmental changes and challenges that increase the risk of morbidity and mortality.

INCIDENCE/PREVALENCE
• Approximately 3% of anatomically normal beef calves can die in association with difficult calving (dystocia).
• Neonatal mortality in beef calves is in the range 4–10%, with approximately 50–70% of neonatal mortality occurring during the first 3 days after birth.

SYSTEMS AFFECTED
Multisystemic

HISTORICAL FINDINGS
• Failure in the transfer of passive immunity is the most common risk factor for morbidity and mortality in beef calves. Low IgG1 levels in calf's serum at 24–72 h after birth are significantly associated with higher morbidity and mortality rates and lower ADG in pre-weaned beef calves. Infectious diseases such as septicemia, diarrhea, and pneumonia are a common consequence of FPT in calves.
• Dystocia, premature delivery, inadequate colostral intake.
• Unable or no interest to stand and nurse/weakness.
• Depression.
• Diarrhea.

SIGNALMENT
Beef breed calves <4 weeks of age

PHYSICAL EXAMINATION FINDINGS
• Weakness/depression—hypoxic/ischemic encephalopathy leading to dummy calf syndrome; metabolic acidosis; hypoglycemia
• Dehydration
• Hypothermia
• Fever (may or may not be present)
• Nasal discharge of various types (serous to mucopurulent)
• Crackles and wheezes uni or bilaterally—meconium aspiration; inadequate surfactant in premature calves or those delivered via C section
• Heart murmurs—ventricular septal defect is the most common in cattle
• Enlarged joints—often seen with septic arthritis in septicemic calves
• Enlarged umbilical structures—umbilical hernias and abscesses
• Diarrhea—the most common disease manifestation in neonates
• Seizures—often associated with meningitis in septicemic calves
• Congenital abnormalities (e.g., cleft palate, arthrogryposis, hydrocephalus)

GENETICS
Some neonatal conditions are genetic (e.g., epitheliogenesis imperfecta in shorthorn and Angus; arthrogryposis multiplex in Angus).

CAUSES AND RISK FACTORS
Congenital
Numerous congenital defects that may affect calves linked to genetic, infectious, and toxic causes

Immune
Inadequate colostrum intake

Infectious
• Bacterial, viral, and fungal agents can cause infections in neonatal calves.
• Neonatal diarrhea and pneumonia are consistently the most common causes of beef calf morbidity and mortality in cow-calf operations.

Risk Factors
• Dystocia is one of the most important risk factors for beef calf morbidity and mortality.
• Calves born from a dystocic delivery have a higher risk of cerebral hypoxia and FPT.
• Calving first-calf heifers and adult cows in the same pasture/pen.
• FPT ranges from 9% to 32% in beef calves.
• Calves born in the winter months and calves from first-calf heifers.
• High infection pressure in the calving pasture/pen.
• Housing calves with adult cows and older calves.
• Poor quality nutrition and body condition score prepartum are associated with lower IgG1 levels in colostrum of beef cows.

DIAGNOSIS

DIFFERENTIAL DIAGNOSES
• Septicemia: *E. coli, Trueperella pyogenes, Staphylococcus aureus, Streptococcus* spp.
• Diarrhea: *E. coli*, Rotavirus, Coronavirus, *Cryptosporidium parvum, Salmonella* spp.
• Omphalitis: *Trueperella pyogenes, E. coli, Proteus, Enterococcus* spp.
• Pre-weaned calf pneumonia: *Pasteurella multocida, Mannheimia haemolytica* and *Mycoplasma* spp.
• Congenital defects
• Lameness: Septic arthritis, trauma (fracture)

CBC/BIOCHEMISTRY/URINALYSIS
• Leukocytosis/Leukopenia with left shift
• Hyperfibrinogenemia
• Hypoglycemia
• Hyponatremia
• Hyperkalemia/Hypokalemia
• Hypochloremia
• Metabolic acidosis
• Increased liver enzymes (SDH, AST, GGT)

OTHER LABORATORY TESTS
• FPT: Serum IgG or total protein at 24 hours of life <10 g/L or <5.5 g/dL, respectively

• Blood culture
• Fecal culture
• Fecal EM, ELISA or PCR for viral pathogens
• Fecal flotation

IMAGING
• Thoracic radiographs
• Ultrasonography of the heart and umbilical structures

PATHOLOGIC FINDINGS
Varies depending on disease condition

TREATMENT

Depends on specific disease or condition.

THERAPEUTIC APPROACH
• Maternal colostrum or colostrum replacers if within 24 hours of life.
• Plasma or whole blood transfusion (10–20 mL/kg).
• Fluid therapy to correct dehydration and metabolic acidosis. Oral solutions should contain 50–80 mmol/L of alkalinizing agent (acetate, lactate, citrate, gluconate, or bicarbonate), 90–120 mmol/L of sodium, and glucose. Acetate solutions provide best results for nursing calves.
• Supplemental oxygen.
• Antibiotic and anti-inflammatory medications as needed depending on condition.
• Keep recumbent neonates in sternal recumbency, if possible.
• Provide heat source to correct hypothermia.

SURGICAL CONSIDERATIONS AND TECHNIQUES
Infection of the umbilical structures or umbilical hernias may need surgical repair.

MEDICATIONS

DRUGS OF CHOICE
Varies depending on disease condition and antimicrobial susceptibility.

CONTRAINDICATIONS
N/A

PRECAUTIONS
• Prolonged use of antibiotics may alter intestinal microbiota and lead to diarrhea.
• Appropriate milk and meat withdrawal times must be followed for all compounds administered to food-producing animals.

FOLLOW-UP

PREVENTION
• Ensure nursing (colostrum intake) during the first 2 hours of life.

N

NEONATOLOGY: BEEF   (CONTINUED)

• Any calf that has not nursed during the first 6 hours of life should receive a colostrum replacer product or frozen colostrum from a dairy source.

• Minimal amount of total IgG mass present in colostrum replacers given to newborn beef calves should be 100 g or, ideally, 150 g.

• Calve first-calf heifers and adult cows separately. First-calf heifers should calve early in the season 3–4 weeks before adult cows.

• Clean, dry, and hygienic calving pastures and pens are essential (adequate drainage and low stocking density).

• Vaccinate cows against common enteric pathogens before the calving season with a final booster 2–3 weeks before the first calving.

 MISCELLANEOUS

ZOONOTIC POTENTIAL

Some neonatal diseases have zoonotic potential: *Salmonella, Cryptosporidium parvum, E. coli.*

BIOSECURITY

• Isolate pairs of sick calves and their dams to prevent disease spread.

• Maintain a closed herd and avoid introduction of pregnant cows/heifers or steers of unknown health status into the herd.

• If new animals are to be introduced into the herd, adequate quarantine and testing should be followed before introduction. Pregnant animals should be maintained isolated until calving and their offspring should be tested (persistent infection with BVDV) before herd introduction.

PRODUCTION MANAGEMENT

• Vaccination of cows during the prepartum will increase deposition of specific antibodies against common calf enteric and respiratory pathogens in colostrum and might decrease fecal shedding at calving as well as prevent clinical disease in neonatal calves.

• Adequate management of calving pasture/pen to decrease infection pressure to newborn calves is essential.

ABBREVIATIONS

• ADG = average daily gain
• AST = aspartate aminotransferase
• BVDV = bovine viral diarrhea virus
• ELISA = enzyme-linked immunosorbent assay
• EM = electron microscopy
• FPT = failure of transfer of passive immunity
• GGT = gamma glutamyltransferase
• IgG1 = immunoglobulin G
• PCR = polymerase chain reaction
• SDH = sorbitol dehydrogenase

SEE ALSO

• Colostrum and Milk Replacers (see www.fiveminutevet.com/ruminant)
• Congenital Defects: Bovine
• Neonatal Diarrhea
• Neonatal Septic Arthritis
• Neonatology: Dairy Cattle (see www.fiveminutevet.com/ruminant)

Suggested Reading

Bellows RA, Patterson DJ, Burfening PJ, Phelps DA. Occurrence of neonatal and postnatal mortality in range beef cattle. II. Factors contributing to calf death. Theriogenology 1987, 28: 573–86.

Dewell RD, Hungerford LL, Keen JE, et al. Association of neonatal serum immunoglobulin G1 concentration with health and performance in beef calves. J Am Vet Med Assoc 2006, 228: 914–21.

Larson RL, Tyler JW, Schultz LG, Tessman RK, Hostetler DE. Management strategies to decrease calf death losses in beef herds. J Am Vet Med Assoc 2004, 224: 42–8.

NAHMS. Beef Report. Calf Health and Management Practices, 1997, pp. 50–73.

Patterson DJ, Bellows RA, Burfening PJ, Carr JB. Occurrence of neonatal and postnatal mortality in range beef cattle. I. Calf loss incidence from birth to weaning, backward and breech presentations and effects of calf loss on subsequent pregnancy rate of dams. Theriogenology 1987, 28: 557–71.

Smith BP. Manifestation of disease in the neonate. In: Smith BP ed, Large Animal Internal Medicine, 5th ed. St. Louis: Mosby, 2014.

Townsend HGG. Environmental factors and calving management practices that affect neonatal mortality in the beef calf. Vet Clin North Am Food Anim Pract 1994, 10: 119–26.

Woolums AR, Berghaus RD, Smith DR, et al. Producer survey of herd-level risk factors for nursing beef calf respiratory disease. J Am Vet Med Assoc 2013, 243: 538–47.

Author Manuel F. Chamorro
Consulting Editor Kaitlyn A. Lutz
Acknowledgment The author and book editors acknowledge the prior contribution of Caroline Hammer.

N

BASICS

OVERVIEW
• Neonatal (<3 weeks of age) camelid problem management is more similar to the equine than to other ruminants.
• Camelid pregnancy and parturition physiology has unique features that affect camelid neonatology.
• Prematurity is a neonatal emergency.

INCIDENCE/PREVALENCE
• Neonatal losses are significant in camelid production systems.
• Losses may reach 50%.

GEOGRAPHIC DISTRIBUTION
Worldwide with a significant regional variation in incidence of specific disorders

SYSTEMS AFFECTED
Multisystemic

PATHOPHYSIOLOGY
• Transition to extrauterine life requires fetal maturity and excellent peripartum conditions.
• The rapid nature of parturition and the type of placentation predisposes to hypoxia.
• Camelids are born agammaglobulinemic. FPT is one of the major predisposing factors to septicemia.
• SAC are notorious for a high incidence of congenital abnormalities.

HISTORICAL FINDINGS
• Dystocia
• Premature birth
• Unattended birthing
• Prepartum conditions in the dam

SIGNALMENT
• Young less than 3 weeks of age.
• More than 50% are in the first week of life.

PHYSICAL EXAMINATION FINDINGS
• Assessment of the dam and placenta should be done first.
• Behavioral: Inactive, weak, recumbent, sleepy. "Wall baby"—unable to discern mother from physical environment or "dummy cria"—neonatal maladjustment syndrome; may be due to hypoxia. These crias can respond positively within a week or less with supportive care.
• Neurologic: Most crias will stand within 30 minutes after delivery and walk within 1 hour
• Ophthalmic: Cataracts, hyphema, hypopyon
• Cardiovascular
  ○ Normal neonate heart rate is 80–120 bpm immediately after birth and 60–100 bpm after several hours.
  ○ Perinatal murmurs are common and disappear after the first few days of life.
  ○ Congenital cardiac abnormalities are relatively common.
• Respiratory
  ○ The normal respiratory rate is 20–40 breaths per minute.

○ Choanal atresia can occur with subsequent open-mouth breathing with severe dyspnea when nursing.
• Gastrointestinal
  ○ Crias have brief and frequent suckle, this is not a sign of poor milk production.
  ○ Defection should be observed within the first 12 hours.
  ○ Colic, distension, straining, and gaunt are signs of GI disorders.
• Urogenital
  ○ Urination should be observed within the first 12 hours.
  ○ Lack of urination or straining warrant further evaluation.
• Prematurity: Low birth weight, silky hair coat, firmly attached epidermal membrane, floppy ears, tendon laxity, unerupted incisors, domed skull.
• Congenital defects: CA, atresia ani, atresia vulvi/fused labia, polydactyly, syndactyly, cleft palate, wry face.
• Medical emergency care is required if:
  ○ Hypothermia (temp <90°F, 32.2°C, normal temperature is 99–101°F, 37.2–38.3°C for cria)
  ○ Respiratory distress
  ○ Hypotension
  ○ Cyanosis
  ○ Blood loss
  ○ Blunt trauma to skull.

GENETICS
Several congenital defects are hereditary

CAUSES AND RISK FACTORS
Genetics, dystocia, abnormal gestation, parturition conditions, and FPT exposure to the environment contribute to neonatal diseases and loss.

DIAGNOSIS

DIFFERENTIAL DIAGNOSES
• Common neonatal problems
  ○ Failure of passive transfer (FPT) of immunoglobulins
  ○ Septicemia
  ○ Prematurity, hypoglycemic neonate
  ○ Hypoxia/hypothermia
  ○ Constipation: check for atresia ani, meconium impaction
  ○ Patent urachus and omphalitis/omphalophlebitis
  ○ Postpartum failure to stand and/or angular limb deformities
  ○ Aspiration distress and subsequent pneumonia
  ○ Choanal atresia
  ○ Cleft palate
  ○ Cataracts
  ○ Wry face/parrot jaw
• Neonatal concerns, first 24 hours
  ○ Premature neonate: hypothermia, acidosis, hypoglycemia, and hypoxia

○ Meconium retention: digital palpation and subsequent warm water enema
○ Dysuria: check for congenital problem or lack of nursing
○ Oral/nasal/respiratory complications: evaluation (manual or endoscopy) generally requires sedation with IV butorphanol at 0.05 mg/kg. CA can be diagnosed by passing of a small rubber catheter through the nostril. If CA exists, the catheter will not advance beyond the medial canthus of the eye. May be unilateral or bilateral
○ Blindness secondary to FPT
○ Umbilical hernia
• Neonatal concerns, after 24 hours
  ○ FPT/speticemia
  ○ Diarrhea: heavy milking dam, coliform bacteria, *Salmonella* spp., *Cryptosporidium* spp., rotaviral infection
  ○ Neonatal diseases are many times multisystemic in nature

CBC/BIOCHEMISTRY/URINALYSIS
Important in critically ill neonates. Abnormalities vary with condition.

OTHER LABORATORY TESTS
• IgG level evaluation
  ○ Evaluated after 15 hours post delivery
  ○ TSS in the field: <4.5 g/dL is evidence of FPT, 5–6 some transfer, >6 adequate.
  ○ Camelid specific immunoglobulin assay (serum radial immunodiffusion assay) is the gold standard: Inadequate <400 mg/dL; suspect 400–1,000 mg/dL; adequate >1,000 mg/dL. Healthy crias consuming good quality colostrum often have serum IgG >2,000 mg/dL at 24 hours of age.
• Parasitology, bacteriology (aerobic and anaerobic blood cultures).

IMAGING
Radiographs and ultrasonography

OTHER DIAGNOSTIC PROCEDURES
Depends on condition

PATHOLOGIC FINDINGS
Depends on condition

TREATMENT

THERAPEUTIC APPROACH
• Catheter placement: 18- to 20-gauge catheter in jugular vein.
• Failure of passive transfer: Plasma transfusion 15–25 mL/kg body weight IV or IP. Whole blood transfusions can be used if plasma is not available (>500 mL of whole blood in acid-citrate-dextrose administered over 2 hours).
• Fluid care and maintenance
  ○ Maintenance rate should begin at 2 mL/kg/h.
  ○ Hypoglycemia: 2.5% dextrose in half-strength saline IV. Regular monitoring of blood glucose is recommended.

- Thermal support: Maintain in sternal recumbency. Heating lamps, hot water units, and blankets (available commercially) all work well.
- Nutritional support
  ○ Tube or bottle-feed cria.
  ○ Parenteral nutrition if a poor suckle reflex.
  ○ It is important to monitor blood and urine glucose.
  ○ Repeated orogastric tube placement may be stressful to the cria. Indwelling nasogastric tubes may be better tolerated. Stallion catheters work well as orogastric tubes. The 18–22 French generally are the right size for smaller crias and 24–30 French stallion catheters should be used for larger crias.
- Respiratory support
  ○ Arterial blood gas from the medial saphenous artery.
  ○ Thoracic radiographs/ultrasonography may be indicated with compromised patients.
  ○ Hypoxemia is common in the critical neonate. Support with 100% humidified oxygen intranasally at a starting rate of 5 L/minute. Adjust according to the pO_2 and the oxygen tension should be at 80 mmHg.
- Pharmaceutical support
  ○ Antibiotic use should reflect culture and sensitivity results.
  ○ Commonly camelids have a Gram-negative or "mixed bag" culture and *Clostridium perfringens* A and C is not uncommon.
  ○ Ceftiofur is a good initial antibiotic choice in the cria while awaiting culture/sensitivity results.

SURGICAL CONSIDERATIONS AND TECHNIQUES
Surgery may be considered in some situations (umbilical hernia, angular limb deformities).

MEDICATIONS

DRUGS OF CHOICE
Antibiotics should be selected based on safety and sensitivity results.

CONTRAINDICATIONS
Aminoglycoside are nephrotoxic and should be avoided.

PRECAUTIONS
Many drugs are used off-label.

POSSIBLE INTERACTIONS
Drug interactions are not well-studied in camelids.

FOLLOW-UP

EXPECTED COURSE AND PROGNOSIS
- Prognosis is good for FPT and septicemia if diagnosis and implementation of critical care is early.
- Crias with severe congenital abnormalities should be humanely euthanized.

POSSIBLE COMPLICATIONS
Stunted growth, ill thrift

CLIENT EDUCATION
- Proper management of pregnant females and parturition.
- Recognize the normal newborn behavior and when to call the veterinarian.
- Prepare a source of colostrum replacement.

PATIENT CARE
- Prevent hypothermia and provide supportive (nutritional) care.

PREVENTION
- FPT can be prevented by providing an alternate colostrum source. Ovine or caprine colostrum is a good choice. Bovine colostrum is a last choice due to potential transmission of Johne's disease.
- For camels, a stock of good-quality camel colostrum is the best choice.
- Camelid plasma may also be administered orally if colostrum is unavailable.
- Colostrum requirements: 10% of the body weight fed q2h over 12 hours.

MISCELLANEOUS

ASSOCIATED CONDITIONS
- Berserk male syndrome can occur in camelids who form a human bond during the neonatal period.
- FPT may be associated with lactational problems (mastitis, agalactia, udder edema/mastitis, inadequate mothering behavior).

AGE-RELATED FACTORS
Neonates

ZOONOTIC POTENTIAL
Salmonella spp. and *Cryptosporidium* spp.

PREGNANCY
Proper nutrition and immunization during pregnancy insures colostral quality and good lactation.

BIOSECURITY
N/A

PRODUCTION MANAGEMENT
- Diet requirements throughout pregnancy
- Milk replacer: 6–8 ounces of goat milk replacer plus 2–3 ounces of live culture yogurt. It is essential that the milk/milk replacer contains no antibiotics as scours will result.

SYNONYMS
N/A

ABBREVIATIONS
- CA = choanal atresia
- FPT = failure of passive transfer
- IgG = immunoglobulin G
- IM = intramuscular
- IP = intraperitoneal
- IV = intravenous
- SAC = South American camelids
- TSS = total serum solids

SEE ALSO
- Body Condition Scoring: Alpacas and Llamas (see www.fiveminutevet.com/ruminant)
- Body Condition Scoring: Camels (see www.fiveminutevet.com/ruminant)
- Camelid: Reproduction
- Congenital Defects: Camelid
- Dystocia: Camelid
- Nutrition and Metabolic Diseases: Camelid (see www.fiveminutevet.com/ruminant)
- Parasite Control Programs: Camelid
- Vaccination Programs: Camelid

Selected Reading
Cebra CK, Anderson DE, Tibary A, Van Saun RJ, Johnson LW. Llama and Alpaca Care: Medicine, Surgery, Reproduction, Nutrition, and Herd Health. St. Louis: Elsevier, 2014.
Dolente BA, Lindborg S, Palmer JE, Wilkins PA. Culture-positive sepsis in neonatal camelids: 21 cases. J Vet Intern Med 2007, 21: 519–25.
Weaver DM, Tyler JW, Marion RS, Wallace LM, Nagy JK, Holle JM. Evaluation of assays for determination of passive transfer status in neonatal llamas and alpacas. J Am Vet Med Assoc 2000, 216: 559–63.
Weaver DM, Tyler JW, Scott MA, Wallace LM, Marion RS, Holle JM. Passive transfer of colostral immunoglobulin G in neonatal llamas and alpacas. Am J Vet Res 2000, 61: 738–41.

Author Kate O'Conor
Consulting Editor Ahmed Tibary
Acknowledgment The author and book editors acknowledge the prior contribution of Scott R. Haskell.

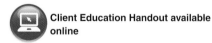
Client Education Handout available online

NEONATOLOGY: CAPRINE

BASICS

OVERVIEW
Common diseases found in goats from birth to 1 week of age. Management factors and environmental conditions play a very large part in the disease process of the neonate.

INCIDENCE/PREVALENCE
Dependent on specific disease process

GEOGRAPHIC DISTRIBUTION
N/A

SYSTEMS AFFECTED
Multisystemic

HISTORICAL FINDINGS
• Premature delivery
• Failure of passive transfer
• Diarrhea
• Anorexia

SIGNALMENT
Birth to 1 week of age

PHYSICAL EXAMINATION FINDINGS
• Congenital defects (e.g., cleft palate, contracted tendons, VSD)
• Dehydration
• Hypothermia
• Depression
• Weakness

GENETICS
Some conditions in neonates have a genetic predisposition.

CAUSES AND RISK FACTORS
Causes include:
• Congenital defects
• Failure of passive transfer
• Dehydration
• Hypothermia
• Hypoxia
• Hypoglycemia
• Nutritional deficiency in doe or kid
• Trauma
Risk factors include:
• Poor body condition or underlying disease in doe
• Failure of passive transfer
• Premature delivery
• Poor environmental conditions

DIAGNOSIS

DIFFERENTIAL DIAGNOSES
• Septicemia
• Floppy kid syndrome
• Hypothermia
• Starvation
• Meconium impaction
• Neuromusculoskeletal diseases: tetanus, white muscle disease, trauma
• Congenital defects
  ◦ Cleft palate

  ◦ Contracted tendons
  ◦ Umbilical hernia
  ◦ Patent urachus
  ◦ Cardiac (i.e., VSD)
• Diarrhea
  ◦ *E. coli*
  ◦ *Salmonella* spp.
  ◦ Adenovirus
  ◦ Coronavirus
  ◦ Rotavirus
  ◦ *Cryptosporidium* spp.
  ◦ *Giardia* spp.
  ◦ Clostridial enterotoxemia type B
• Respiratory disease: Aspiration pneumonia, *Mannheimia haemolytica*, rib fractures

CBC/BIOCHEMISTRY/URINALYSIS
• Hypoglycemia
• Hypoproteinemia
• Hyperfibrinogenemia
• Left shift in leukogram with neutropenia (toxic bands)
• Metabolic acidosis

OTHER LABORATORY TESTS
• IgG <400 mg/dL or TP <5.0 g/dL
• *Salmonella* positive on fecal culture
• Electron microscopy for viruses
• Fecal IFA for *Cryptosporidium* and *Giardia*
• Bacteremia on blood culture
• Hypoxemia on blood gas
• Decreased serum vitamin E
• Decreased EDTA or heparin whole blood selenium

IMAGING
Radiography if suspect fractures or aspiration pneumonia

OTHER DIAGNOSTIC PROCEDURES
N/A

PATHOLOGIC FINDINGS
N/A

TREATMENT

THERAPEUTIC APPROACH
Varies based on disease condition and the environment

SURGICAL CONSIDERATIONS AND TECHNIQUES
• Stabilize patient before beginning any surgical procedures.
• Congenital defects and/or traumatic injuries may need surgical correction.
• Neonates in many instances are not good surgical candidates.

MEDICATIONS

DRUGS OF CHOICE
• Antibiotics based on suspected problem and/or culture and sensitivity.

• NSAIDS may be indicated. Care should be used in selection and hydration status of the neonate. Some NSAIDs are contraindicated in the neonate.
• Intravenous plasma, oral plasma, or oral colostrum.
• Antidiarrheal medications.

CONTRAINDICATIONS
Avoid using drugs prohibited or not labeled for use in food-producing animals (e.g., aminoglycosides, metronidazole). Follow drug withdrawal periods for meat and milk.

PRECAUTIONS
Beware of drugs that may affect growing tissues.

POSSIBLE INTERACTIONS
N/A

ALTERNATIVE DRUGS
Probiotics may be indicated.

FOLLOW-UP

EXPECTED COURSE AND PROGNOSIS
Varies based on disease(s) encountered

POSSIBLE COMPLICATIONS
N/A

CLIENT EDUCATION
Correct any deficiencies in husbandry or breeding selection.

PATIENT CARE
• Warming neonate
• Oxygen supplementation
• Oral or intravenous fluids (correct electrolyte and acid-base disturbances)
• Meet caloric needs via PO or IV nutrition (i.e., oral sugar/syrup or IV dextrose for hypoglycemia)
• Enema for meconium impaction (warm soapy water)
• Activity
  ◦ Passive range of motion
  ◦ Rolling from side to side
  ◦ Maintain sternal recumbency
• Diet
  ◦ Proper nutrition of the prepartum doe
  ◦ Important to feed the kids a balanced diet that meets their caloric and nutritional requirements.

PREVENTION
• Correct management deficiencies.
• Avoid poor husbandry and/or breeding selection.
• Ensure colostral quality.
• Ensure adequate amount of colostrum is administered within the first 24 hours after birth.
• Adequate nutrition and vaccination of prepartum does.

N

✓ MISCELLANEOUS

ASSOCIATED CONDITIONS
N/A

AGE-RELATED FACTORS
N/A

ZOONOTIC POTENTIAL
Some diseases of small ruminants may have zoonotic potential (e.g., *Salmonella* spp., *E. coli*, *Campylobacter* spp., *Cryptosporidium* spp., *Giardia* spp.).

PREGNANCY
N/A

BIOSECURITY
• Biosecurity measures may help to decrease the severity and course of neonatal diseases and may improve the prognosis.
• Can decrease transmission among other neonates, adult goats, and humans.
• Isolation and quarantine of new stock entering the herd or flock.
• Treat and or cull new animals for disease conditions prior to herd introduction.

PRODUCTION MANAGEMENT
• A good environment is vital to neonatal health.
• Management of pregnant does is important to neonatal health and viability.
• Proper husbandry and breeding practices are crucial in selecting for healthy neonates.

Colostrum
• Does should be stripped after kidding to ensure functional teats and milk production.
• Kids should consume 2.5 ounces/lb (160 g/kg) BW of colostrum in the first 24 hours. Colostrum may be bottle fed or tubed using a red rubber catheter if the kid is weak or the dam will not allow nursing. The first feeding should take place within an hour after birth and subsequent volume should be given over four feedings. Stored colostrum should be refrigerated and re-warmed to 38–39°C (100–102°F) by immersing in warm water prior to feeding. Extra colostrum can be frozen and saved for instances of triplets or low production.
• If the farm tests and manages for Johne's, CAE and CL, kids should be given colostrum and milk from negative dams.

Umbilicus
The umbilicus should be dipped or thoroughly sprayed with 7% tincture of iodine immediately after birth. This may be repeated in 12–24 hours.

Housing
• Clean, dry bedding is essential to prevent infectious disease and aid in neonatal thermoregulation.
• Good ventilation is imperative to decrease risk of pneumonia and transfer of disease.
• Heat lamps may be used in particularly cold climates but caution should be observed as they present a fire hazard, especially with straw bedding. Kids must always have room to move away from the heat source to prevent hyperthermia.
• A creep feeding area should be set up to allow groups of kids a safe haven away from does as well as access to feed (grass hay and/or grain). Kids begin consumption of feed as early as 1 week of age and ruminal digestive function is complete by 2 months of age.

Disbudding
If clients plan on disbudding, arrangements should be made to perform by 1–2 weeks of age. If performed later, the procedure is much more difficult and stressful on the kid.

Vaccination
• Ideally, dams are vaccinated with CDT one month prior to kidding in order to enhance colostral antibody production. If adequate colostrum is consumed thereafter then kids will be adequately protected during the high-risk neonatal period.
• Vaccination with CDT (followed by booster vaccination according to label directions) should be administered by 30 days of age. If dams are unvaccinated or colostrum is not consumed, then earlier vaccination is warranted. Vaccine response may not be optimal due to developing immune system earlier than 1 month of age and therefore the above vaccination program may still be warranted.
• Other vaccinations (e.g., rabies) may be necessary based on location and herd management.

SYNONYMS
N/A

ABBREVIATIONS
• CDT = *Clostridium perfringens* type C & D plus tetanus vaccine
• CL = caseous lymphadenitis (CLA)
• EDTA = ethylene diamine tetraacetic acid
• IFA = immunofluorescence assay
• IgG = immunoglobulin G
• IM = intramuscular
• IV = intravenous
• NSAIDs = nonsteroidal anti-inflammatory drugs
• PO = per os, by mouth
• TP = total protein
• VSD = ventricular septal defect

SEE ALSO
• Congenital Defects: Small Ruminant
• Floppy Kid Syndrome
• Neonatal Diarrhea
• Respiratory Disease: Small Ruminant
• Starvation
• Vitamin E/Selenium Deficiency

Suggested Reading
Bulgin MS, Anderson BC. Salmonellosis in goats. J Am Vet Med Assoc 1981, 178: 720–3.
Foreyt WJ. Coccidiosis and cryptosporidiosis in sheep and goats. Vet Clin North Am Food Anim Pract 1990, 6: 655–70.
Smith MC, Sherman DM. Goat Medicine, 2nd ed. Ames: Wiley-Blackwell, 2009.
Van Der Lugt JJ, Randles JL. Systemic herpesvirus infection in neonatal goats. J S Afr Vet Assoc 1993, 64: 169–71.
Van Metre DC, Tyler JW, Stehman SM. Diagnosis of enteric disease in small ruminants. Vet Clin North Am Food Anim Pract 2000, 16: 87–115, vi.
Weese JS, Kenney DG, O'Connor A. Secondary lactose intolerance in a neonatal goat. J Am Vet Med Assoc 2000, 217: 340, 372–5.

Author Kate O'Conor
Consulting Editor Kaitlyn A. Lutz
Acknowledgment The author and book editors acknowledge the prior contribution of Jessica M. Dinham and Amanda S. Denisen.

BASICS

OVERVIEW
• *Neospora caninum,* an obligate intracellular coccidian parasite of ruminants, is the causative agent of late-term abortions or birth of congenitally infected, weak, or unthrifty calves in cattle.
• There are sporadic reports of abortion in sheep and goats due to infection with *Neospora caninum.*
• *N. caninum* has been reported as a cause of abortion in camelids.

INCIDENCE/PREVALENCE
• *Neospora caninum* infects 10–20% of all cattle worldwide and is incriminated in up to 20% of diagnosed bovine abortions.
• Seroprevalence studies have documented specific antibody responses in cattle, canids, and a multitude of likely intermediate hosts.
• Successful isolation of viable parasites has been limited to cattle, sheep, water buffalo, bison, white-tailed deer, and dogs.

GEOGRAPHIC DISTRIBUTION
• *Neospora caninum* infection has been detected in cattle populations and other ruminant and camelid species worldwide

SYSTEMS AFFECTED
• Reproductive
• Nervous

PATHOPHYSIOLOGY
• *N. caninum* has a heteroxenous life cycle highlighted by three infectious stages:
  ◦ Tachyzoites
  ◦ Tissue cysts
  ◦ Oocysts
• Dogs (*Canis familiaris*) and coyotes (*Canis latrans*) are the only recognized definitive hosts for *Neospora* sp.
• Cattle and a wide range of warm-blooded animals act as intermediate hosts.
• A sylvatic cycle including white-tailed deer and coyotes is important in maintaining a reservoir of infection.
• In cattle, *N. caninum* transmission may occur efficiently by both horizontal and vertical routes.
  ◦ Horizontal transmission occurs when cattle ingest sporulated *N. caninum* oocysts present due to fecal contamination from definitive hosts present in feed sources.
  ◦ Transplacental vertical transmission results in infection of a fetus carried by an acutely or persistently infected dam and can result in either abortion, birth of a weak, compromised neonate, or birth of a subclinically infected, apparently normal neonate.
• Abortions occur most commonly at 5–6 months of gestation, associated with chronic infection of the placenta and fetus.

• Abortion may be triggered either as a result of a recent primary maternal infection or following recrudescence of a persistent infection during pregnancy.
• Infected mature cows are asymptomatic but may abort or continually produce congenitally infected calves following transplacental transmission.
• A similar pathophysiology with abortion occurring in the second half of pregnancy has been reported in llamas and alpacas.
• Abortion, stillbirth, and neonatal mortality due to *N. caninum* infection has been reported in goats. Experimental infection at 40 days of pregnancy resulted in abortion. Infection at 90 days produced abortion and stillbirth while infection at 120 days of gestation resulted in birth of congenitally infected kids. Abortion occurred 17–21 days after infection. There were fewer placental lesions in small ruminants than in cattle.

HISTORICAL FINDINGS
• Abortion
• Birth of weak neonate with neurologic symptoms

SIGNALMENT
• Both beef and dairy cattle may be infected. Abortions due to *Neospora* are more common in dairy cattle.
• Both nulliparous and multiparous cattle may abort.
• Abortions are nonseasonal and may be seen in all months of the year.
• Bulls may be infected but there is no evidence that *N. caninum* is spread venereally or via artificial insemination.

PHYSICAL EXAMINATION FINDINGS
• Abortion is the main clinical manifestation of bovine neosporosis in dairy and beef cattle.
• Epidemic and endemic abortion outbreaks may occur.
• Fetuses dying in utero are generally expelled but mummification may occur.
• Postnatally infected cattle are unlikely to abort due to *Neospora* or to transmit the infection transplacentally more than once.
• 95% of congenitally infected calves appear normal at birth.
• Occasionally congenitally infected neonates exhibit neurologic deficits at birth or within the first 4 weeks of life. Neurologic signs include ataxia, weakness, decreased patellar reflexes, and loss of conscious proprioception.
• *Neospora* may occasionally cause birth defects of hydrocephalus, narrowing of the spinal cord, and arthrogryposis.
• Data on clinical and pathologic findings in sheep, goats, and camelids are scarce.

CAUSES AND RISK FACTORS
• *Neospora caninum*
• Presence of canids on farm

DIAGNOSIS

DIFFERENTIAL DIAGNOSES
• Any pathogen that may cause mid to late term abortion
• Protozoal: *Toxoplasma gondii* and *Sarcocystis cruzi*
• Viral: Bovine viral diarrhea virus, infectious bovine rhinotracheitis, bluetongue
• Bacterial: *Leptospira, Salmonella, Histophilus*
• Miscellaneous: Foothill abortion, mycotic abortion
• Causes of weak and unthrifty calves: Persistent infection with BVDV, selenium deficiency, iodine deficiency, congenital bluetongue virus, failure of passive transfer, or neonatal septicemia

CBC/BIOCHEMSTRY/URINALYSIS
Often unrewarding from cows that have aborted or congenitally affected calves, as results are unremarkable and nondiagnostic.

OTHER LABORATORY TESTS
• CSF obtained from neurologically abnormal congenitally infected neonates may demonstrate mild pleocytosis.
• Congenitally infected calves may be at increased risk of failure of passive transfer due to weakness.

IMAGING
N/A

OTHER DIAGNOSTIC PROCEDURES
• Laboratory submissions should include sera from aborting dams, fetal fluids, and tissues including placenta if available.
• Histopathology
  ◦ Gold standard for diagnosis of *Neospora.*
  ◦ Degenerative to inflammatory lesions may be found through fetal tissues but most commonly in central nervous system, heart, and liver.
  ◦ Tachyzoites in tissues are demonstrated with special stains.
• Gross pathology
  ◦ Aborted fetus, commonly autolyzed or mummified.
  ◦ Gross lesions, uncommon but may be present.
  ◦ Pale white foci may be observed in the heart or skeletal muscle.
  ◦ Very small, pale to dark necrotic foci may be observed in brain.
• Serology
  ◦ ELISA and IFAT serologic assays that detect specific antibodies allowing for confirmation of *Neospora* antibodies.
  ◦ Positive serology from an aborting cow is only indicative of exposure to *N. caninum* and diagnosis should be paired with histopathology.
  ◦ In contrast, a negative result on fetal submissions does not rule out *Neospora,* because of autolysis, immature fetal

N

NEOSPOROSIS

immunocompetence, or short interval between infection and death.
• Molecular techniques: PCR-based assays are available to detect *Neospora* in fetal tissues, amniotic fluid, milk, semen, or dog feces.

PATHOLOGIC FINDINGS
• Lesions most commonly observed in brain, spinal cord, heart, and liver, but may be present in other tissue.
• Most characteristic lesions are multifocal encephalitis, myocarditis, and periportal hepatitis associated with tachyzoites demonstrable by IHC.

TREATMENT

THERAPEUTIC APPROACH
• No pharmaceuticals are approved for treatment of bovine neosporosis.
• Experimental treatment of congenitally infected newborn calves with toltrazuril was shown to eliminate infection.

SURGICAL CONSIDERATIONS AND TECHNIQUES
N/A

MEDICATIONS

DRUGS OF CHOICE
There are no approved medications.

CONTRAINDICATIONS
N/A

PRECAUTIONS
N/A

POSSIBLE INTERACTIONS
N/A

FOLLOW-UP

EXPECTED COURSE AND PROGNOSIS
• Infected cows will often return to normal heath and conceive.

• There is an increased risk for abortion in subsequent pregnancies.

POSSIBLE COMPLICATIONS
• Milk production loss
• Other complications associated with abortion (retained fetal membranes, metritis, infertility)

CLIENT EDUCATION
• Role of canids in transmission
• Importance of biosecurity measures

PATIENT CARE
Farm biosecurity is important in controlling bovine neosporosis, with maintenance of a closed herd the best way to avoid introducing parasites.

PREVENTION
• Farm biosecurity is important in controlling bovine neosporosis, with maintenance of a closed herd the best way to avoid introducing parasites.
• Access of dogs and other canids to stored feeds should be minimized.
• No vaccine is currently commercially available.
• Determining the serostatus of each animal at birth and culling those congenitally infected.
• Embryo transfer to seronegative recipients can be used preserve the genetics of valuable seropositive animals.

MISCELLANEOUS

ASSOCIATED CONDITIONS
N/A

AGE-RELATED FACTORS
N/A

ZOOOTIC POTENTIAL
N/A

PREGANCY
Abortion

BIOSECURITY
See "Prevention"

PRODUCTION MANAGEMENT
• Serologic screening of new purchases may be considered, particularly for known negative herds.

• Consider presuckle serology of calves born to seropositive dams when attempting to reduce prevalence rate.
• Colostrum from seropositive dams does not appear to be a clinically significant means of vertical transmission.

SYNONYMS
N/A

ABBREVIATIONS
• BVDV = bovine viral diarrhea virus
• ELISA = enzyme-linked immunosorbent assay
• IFAT = indirect fluorescent antibody test
• IHC = immunohistochemistry
• PCR = polymerase chain reaction

SEE ALSO
• Abortion: Bovine
• Abortion: Camelid
• Abortion: Small Ruminant

Suggested Reading
Dubey JP, Schares G. Diagnosis of bovine neosporosis. Vet Parasitol 2006, 140: 1–34.
Dubey JP, Buxton D, Wouda W. Pathogenesis of bovine neosporosis. J Comp Pathol 2006, 134: 267–89.
Dubey JP. Neosporosis in cattle. Vet Clin North Am Food Anim Pract 2005, 21: 473–83.
Mazuz ML, Fish L, Reznikov D, et al. Neosporosis in naturally infected pregnant dairy cattle. Vet Parasitol 2014, 205: 85–91.
Noall D, Kasimanickam, Memon M, Gay J. Neosporosis in cattle. Clin Theriogenol 2013, 5: 109–17.
Porto WJN, Regidor-Cerillo J, Kim P, et al. Experimental caprine neosporosis: the influence of gestational stage on the outcome of infection. Vet Res 2016, 47: 29. doi 10.1186/s13567-016-0312-6.
Serrano-Martinez E, Collantes-Fernandez E, Chavez-Velasquez A, et al. Evaluation of *Neospora caninum* and *Toxoplasma gondii* infections in alpaca (*Vicugna pacos*) and llama (*Lama glama*) aborted foetuses from Peru. Vet Parasitol 2007, 150: 39–45.
Authors Jennifer H. Koziol and Herris Maxwell
Consulting Editor Ahmed Tibary
Acknowledgment The author and book editors acknowledge the prior contribution of Simon F. Peek.

NIGHTSHADE (*SOLANUM* SPP.) TOXICOSIS

BASICS

OVERVIEW
- Member of Solanaceae family; *Solanum* spp. (nightshade) has the largest number of species (>1,500 worldwide).
- Weeds, herbs, shrubs, small trees; erect stems or vines; annual or perennial; berry-like fruit.
- Present in pastures, gardens, waste areas, and cultivated crops.
- Common species of *Solanum* in North America include *S. nigrum* (black nightshade), *S. dulcamara* (bittersweet), *S. carolinense* (horse nettle), *S. elaeagnifolium* (silverleaf nightshade), *S. physalifolium* (hairy nightshade), *S. rostratum* (buffalo bur), *S. tuberosum* (potato), *S. ptychanthum* (eastern black nightshade).
- Related genera include *Lycopersicum* (tomato), *Datura* (jimsonweed or angel's trumpet), *Capsicum* (pepper), *Nicotiana* (tobacco).
- Depending on genera and species, gastrointestinal (GI) irritation, nervous system dysfunction, and teratogenicity are possible.

INCIDENCE/PREVALENCE
- Ruminants tend to be resistant, especially to the toxins solanine and solanidine
- Toxicosis with large ingestions

GEOGRAPHIC DISTRIBUTION
Worldwide

SYSTEMS AFFECTED
- Cardiovascular
- Digestive
- Nervous
- Reproductive

PATHOPHYSIOLOGY
- Toxins are concentrated in the green (unripe) fruits, leaves, sprouts, and green potato tubers.
- Steroidal alkaloids solanidine and solanine are primary toxins; many other toxins including solasonine, solamargine, chaconine; cause saponin-like effects with GI mucosal irritation and necrosis.
- Related genera contain tropane alkaloids (scopolamine, hyoscyamine, others), capsaicinoids, pyridine alkaloids (nicotine), other toxins; affects the autonomic nervous system. Activity of anticholinesterase is blocked, allowing accumulation of acetylcholine resulting in more severe GI, nervous, and cardiac effects.

SIGNALMENT
- All ruminant species can be affected
- All ages, both genders

PHYSICAL EXAMINATION FINDINGS
- Salivation, abdominal pain, vomiting, abdominal pain, diarrhea, or constipation from direct GI irritation.
- Decreased salivation, mydriasis, decreased GI motility, and increased heart rate may result from anticholinergic effects.
- Depression, incoordination, tremors, weakness, seizures.
- Rarely teratogenic effects.

CAUSES AND RISK FACTORS
- Lack of available food sources
- Season of year—consumed fresh in summer/fall; fed throughout the year in hay or silage

DIAGNOSIS

DIFFERENTIAL DIAGNOSES
Many other plants and chemicals produce similar signs of gastroenteritis or nervous dysfunction.

CBC/BIOCHEMISTRY/URINALYSIS
N/A

OTHER LABORATORY TESTS
N/A

OTHER DIAGNOSTIC PROCEDURES
- History of ingestion
- Clinical signs
- Presence of plant material in rumen or stomach

PATHOLOGIC FINDINGS
- Gastroenteritis, possibly severe with hemorrhage and necrosis
- Hyperemia of intestinal mucosa
- Increased peritoneal fluid, especially in calves
- Purkinje cell swelling and/or loss

TREATMENT

THERAPEUTIC APPROACH
- No antidote
- Symptomatic and supportive

SURGICAL CONSIDERATIONS AND TECHNIQUES
Rumenotomy and evacuation of contents may be useful early in the course of intoxication.

MEDICATIONS

DRUGS OF CHOICE
- Activated charcoal 1–5 g/kg PO as slurry; may repeat charcoal but add cathartic (magnesium or magnesium sulfate, sorbitol) × 1 dose only.
- Physostigmine 0.04–0.08 mg/kg IV (extra-label); use very cautiously and only if anticholinergic signs are severe.
- Atropine sulfate 0.1–0.5 mg/kg SC, IM, IV for severe cholinergic signs.

PRECAUTIONS
Appropriate milk and meat withdrawal times must be followed for all compounds administered to food-producing animals.

FOLLOW-UP

EXPECTED COURSE AND PROGNOSIS
- May have a latent period of hours to days before signs develop
- Variable, generally good with adequate treatment

PREVENTION
- Prevent further access to toxins
- Maintain good source of nutrition

MISCELLANEOUS

PREGNANCY
Teratogenic effects such as craniofacial malformations have been reported in laboratory animals.

ABBREVIATIONS
- GI = gastrointestinal
- IM = intramuscular
- IV = intravenous
- PO = by mouth
- SQ = subcutaneous

SEE ALSO
Jimsonweed (*Datura stramonium*) Toxicity

Suggested Reading
Bischoff K, Smith MC. Toxic plants of the Northeastern United States. Vet Clin North Am Food Anim Pract 2011, 27: 459–80.
Burrows GE, Tyrl RJ. In: Toxic Plants of North America, 2nd ed. Ames: Wiley-Blackwell, 2013, Kindle edition.
Jagatheeswari D. Black Night Shade *Solanum nigrum L*: An Updated Overview. Int J Pharm Biol 2013, 4(2).
Keeler RF, Baker DC, Gaffield W. Spirosolane-containing *Solanum* spp. and induction of congenital craniofacial malformations. Toxicon 1990; 28: 873–84.
Payne J, Murphy A. Plant poisoning in farm animals. In Practice 2014, 36: 455–65.
Qasem JR. Silverleaf nightshade (*Solanum elaeagnifolium*) in the Jordan Valley: Field survey and chemical control. J Hort Sci Biotech 2014, 89: 639–4.
Author Lynn R. Hovda
Consulting Editor Christopher C.L. Chase
Acknowledgment The author and book editors acknowledge the prior contribution of Matt G. Welborn.

N

NITRATE AND NITRITE TOXICOSIS

BASICS

OVERVIEW
• Toxicity most commonly results from ingestion of nitrate-accumulating forages or noxious weeds.
• Methemoglobin (MHb) formation gives the blood a chocolate-brown color and results in tissue hypoxia/anoxia giving rise to the observed clinical signs.
• Clinical signs develop acutely and include dyspnea, weakness, and sudden death.
• IV administration of methylene blue is the treatment of choice for affected animals.
• Many factors affect nitrate uptake by plants, and it is difficult to predict when problems may arise.

INCIDENCE/PREVALENCE
Generally unpredictable, but more likely to occur in times of drought and during the winter months.

GEOGRAPHIC DISTRIBUTION
Worldwide

SYSTEMS AFFECTED
• Cardiovascular
• Multisystemic

PATHOPHYSIOLOGY
• Nitrate (NO_3) is converted to nitrite (NO_2) by the rumen microflora.
• NO_2 is ten times more toxic than NO_3.
• NO_2, once absorbed systemically, converts hemoglobin (Fe^{2+}) to MHb (Fe^{3+}).
• MHb is incapable of oxygen transport and tissue anoxia results in the clinical signs observed.

SIGNALMENT
• All ruminant species can be affected.
• Adults are more susceptible due to conversion of NO_3 to NO_2 in the rumen. Functional ruminants are ten times more susceptible to toxicity than pre-ruminants.

PHYSICAL EXAMINATION FINDINGS
• Abrupt onset of dyspnea and weakness.
• Muscle tremors, stumbling, or recumbency.
• Salivation.
• Pale, cyanotic, or brown mucus membranes.
• MHb formation imparts a chocolate-brown color to the blood. This color will disappear within a few hours postmortem.
• Sudden death, with or without terminal convulsions.
• Abortion in pregnant animals follows acute signs by several days to a few weeks. The developing fetus is highly susceptible to anoxia, and abortion may occur in cattle with minimal signs of acute nitrate/nitrite toxicity.

CAUSES AND RISK FACTORS
• An acute oral lethal dose is approximately 0.5 g nitrate/kg body weight.
• Many forages and cereal grains have been associated with nitrate accumulation

including sorghum, alfalfa, oats, corn, barley, wheat and rye.
• Noxious weeds that are recognized as important accumulators of nitrate include pigweed (*Amaranthus* spp.), lambs quarter (*Chenopodium* spp.), Canada thistle (*Cirsium arvense*), and fireweed (*Kochia scoparia*) (See Table 1). Such plants may be consumed directly from pasture or can easily invade hay fields and be incorporated in dried harvested forages. This risk is especially true for the thistles that are likely to be sprayed with herbicides, some of which, for example, 2,4-D, cause the plants to accumulate higher levels of nitrates for a few days.
• Water can be the source of poisoning, but this is uncommon. Gross contamination of the water source and/or environment with nitrogen-containing fertilizers or use of tanks that once transported nitrogen-containing fertilizers as water troughs can be a risk. Nitrate levels <200 ppm are generally considered safe, and most animals can tolerate much higher levels (1,000–1,500 ppm).
• Animals that are more dominant, in an energy deficit, or debilitated with a pre-existing disease, may be more susceptible.
• Clinical signs in animals and death occur abruptly, despite feeding the same diet for days or weeks. This is not a cumulative or chronic problem. The sporadic nature of illness is directly related to the nonhomogeneous distribution of nitrate in the feed and lack of rumen adaptation.
• Once the animal's rumen has become "acclimated" to nitrate, the animal can tolerate much higher dietary levels.
• Any environmental stressors that limit photosynthesis but allow the plant to continue to take up nitrogen from the soil will result in increased nitrate accumulation. Examples of such stressors include frost, drought, pesticide application, and low light levels.
• Stunted plant growth results in nitrate accumulation in the lower part of the plant; this is clinically important when making silage from corn or other cereal grains.

DIAGNOSIS

DIFFERENTIAL DIAGNOSES
• Chlorate, copper, and *Mercurialis* toxicities are capable of causing methemoglobinemia.
• Other causes of "abrupt" onset of similar signs and death include anthrax, clostridial infection, cyanobacteria, lightning strike, and toxicities caused by *Cicuta* (water hemlock), *Taxus* (yew), *Zigadenus* (death camas), oleander, organophosphate and carbamate insecticides, ionophores, and nonprotein nitrogen.

CBC/BIOCHEMISTRY/URINALYSIS
No remarkable abnormalities are observed, other than the blood appearing "chocolate" brown.

OTHER DIAGNOSTIC PROCEDURES
• Muddy-colored mucus membranes, "chocolate brown" blood, and clinical signs suggestive of oxygen deprivation are consistent with nitrate/nitrite toxicosis.
• Due to the instability of MHb and the need for phosphate buffers for storage of blood samples, determination of MHb concentrations is rarely performed.
• Diphenylamine kits or nitrate/nitrite qualitative or semiquantitative strip tests can be used on feed and water to confirm high nitrate levels.
• Suspect forages can be tested using diphenylamine to semiquantitatively estimate the nitrate concentration, and ion chromatography can be used to quantitatively analyze for nitrate and nitrite in suspect forages and water.
• NO_3 concentrations can be measured in most biological fluids including refrigerated blood, serum or plasma, peritoneal, and pericardial fluids or urine along with feed or water using ion chromatography. Concentrations >15 ppm are suggestive, and concentrations >20–30 ppm are diagnostic of excessive exposure to nitrates; levels >50 ppm are consistent with NO_3 poisoning.
• Ocular fluid (aqueous humor) nitrate concentrations can be determined, using diphenylamine (semiquantitative) or ion chromatography (quantitative), for up to 72 hours postmortem or up to a week after death in refrigerated samples. Concentrations >10 ppm nitrate in ocular fluid are suggestive, and concentrations >20 ppm are diagnostic of exposure to excessive nitrates.
• Since neonatal calves normally have ocular fluid nitrate concentrations approximating 20 ppm during the first day of life, nitrate concentrations >30 ppm are generally more consistent with nitrate/nitrite toxicosis in these animals.
• Rumen contents are not useful diagnostically because of postmortem instability associated with the activity of microorganisms.

PATHOLOGIC FINDINGS
Postmortem changes are nonspecific. General vascular congestion may be observed. The blood is dark and may clot poorly.

TREATMENT
THERAPEUTIC APPROACH
• Stress associated with handling must be minimized in severely hypoxic animals.
• Exposure to the identified source of the excessive nitrates should be discontinued.

• Rumen lavage with cold water and oral penicillin may slow the continuous reduction of nitrate to nitrite in the rumen.
• Methylene blue is a specific antidote for nitrate/nitrite toxicosis. Administer 5–15 mg/kg body weight IV as a 1% solution in physiologic saline.
• Additional, lower doses of the antidote can be administered to animals still exhibiting signs.
• Mild to moderately affected animals may recover spontaneously if left untreated.

MEDICATIONS

DRUGS OF CHOICE
1% Methylene blue, 5–15 mg/kg IV, slow. Response should be immediate.

CONTRAINDICATIONS
The use of methylene blue is off-label. Consult FARAD for recommended withdrawal times.

FOLLOW-UP

EXPECTED COURSE AND PROGNOSIS
• The course of the disease is relatively short, generally lasting within one feeding period.
• The prognosis is heavily dependent on the exposure dose within a short time frame, and levels of methemoglobinemia (blood levels >80% are typically fatal).
• Pregnant animals may abort several days to a few weeks after the toxic insult, due to fetal hypoxia.

PATIENT CARE
No long-term problems have been documented other than abortions. Animals can completely recover, with or without treatment (depending on exposure dose), within a few hours.

PREVENTION
• Knowledge of the high-risk nitrate-accumulating plants and ability to recognize in the field or hay will minimize the risk.
• Knowledge of the risk factors predisposing high nitrates in the feed (e.g., fertilization, irrigation, soil conditions, environmental conditions) can lead one to be proactive in testing forages during the growing season and pre- and postharvest.
• Suspect forages or crops known to accumulate nitrate should be tested for nitrate concentrations prior to inclusion in the diet of ruminants, especially cattle.
• Forages containing <5,000 ppm nitrate are generally safe for consumption by ruminants.
• High-nitrate-containing forages can be diluted with low-nitrate-containing forages prior to feeding to ruminants, or suspect forages can be divided into two feedings to prevent rapid intake.

• Forages of high or questionable NO_3 content should not be fed to pregnant cattle; open cattle or growing calves may prove more resistant to toxicity.
• The harvest of forages or crops grown under conditions conducive to nitrate accumulation should be delayed until conditions improve to allow nitrate levels in stalks to drop.
• If the harvest of forages or crops grown under conditions conducive to nitrate accumulation cannot be delayed, then the harvesting cutter-bar should be raised to 18 inches to leave the lower portions of the stems or stalks in the field.
• Gradual adaptation of ruminants to high-nitrate-containing forages can be performed over a period of 7–10 days.
• Feeding readily fermentable carbohydrate sources in conjunction with high-nitrate-containing forages will promote a denitrifying environment within the rumen.

MISCELLANEOUS

AGE-RELATED FACTORS
• Younger animals with nonfunctional rumens are resistant to nitrate/nitrite toxicosis.
• The fetus has higher oxygen demands and is reported to be more susceptible to the adverse effects of methemoglobinemia.

PREGNANCY
• Abortions may occur several days to a few weeks after the initial toxic insult in those animals that survive.
• Abortion is a common sequela in pregnant cattle consuming forages containing excessive nitrates (>0.5% or 5,000 ppm).

Table 1

Genera and Species of Weeds that are Nitrate Accumulators	
Amaranthus spp.	pigweed
Ambrosia spp.	ragweeds
Carduus nutans	musk thistle
Chenopodium spp.	lambs quarter
Cirsium arvense	Canada thistle (to 4.8% NO_3)
Gnaphalium spp.	cudweeds
Helianthus annuus	annual sunflower
Heliomeris spp. (= *Viguiera*)	goldeneyes
Lygodesmia spp.	skeleton plants
Kochia scoparia	fireweed
Silybum marianum	milk thistle (to 10% NO_3)

Source: Adapted from Burrows, George E., Tyrl, Ronald J. Toxic Plants of North America (p. 151). Wiley. Kindle Edition.

PRODUCTION MANAGEMENT
Avoid feeding exceptionally weedy feeds, particularly avoiding those weeds that are well-recognized nitrate accumulators.

ABBREVIATIONS
• FARAD = Food Animal Residue Avoidance Databank
• IV = intravenous
• MHb = methemoglobin
• NO_3 = nitrate
• NO_2 = nitrite

SEE ALSO
• Abortion: Bovine
• Anthrax
• Blue-Green Algae Poisoning
• Carbamate Toxicity
• Clostridial Disease: Nervous System
• Death Camas
• Lightning Strike
• Monensin Toxicity
• Oleander and Cardiotoxic Plant Toxicity
• Organophosphate Toxicity
• Urea Toxicity
• Water Hemlock
• Yew Toxicity

Suggested Reading
Burrows GE, Tyrl RJ. Toxic Plants of North America, 2nd ed. Ames: Wiley-Blackwell, 2013.
Costagliola A, Roperto F, Benedetto D, et al. Outbreak of fatal nitrate toxicosis associated with consumption of fennels (*Foeniculum vulgare*) in cattle farmed in Campania region (southern Italy). Environ Sci Pollution Res Int 2014, 21: 6252–7.
McKenzie RA, Rayner AC, Thompson GK, Pidgeon GF, Burren BR. Nitrate-nitrite toxicity in cattle and sheep grazing *Dactyloctenium radulans* (button grass) in stockyards. Aust Vet J 2004, 82: 630–4.
Morgan SE. Water quality for cattle. Vet Clin North Am Food Anim Pract 2011, 27: 285–95.
Nitrate and nitrite poisoning. In: Radostits OM, Gay CC, Hinchcliff KW, Constable PD eds, Veterinary Medicine: A Textbook of the Diseases of Cattle, Horses, Sheep, Pigs, and Goats, 10th ed. Edinburgh: Saunders Elsevier, 2007, pp. 1855–8.
Osweiler, GD. Diagnostic guidelines for ruminant toxicoses. Vet Clin North Am Food Anim Pract 2011. 27: 247–54.
Villar D, Schwartz KJ, Carson TL, Kinker JA, Barker J. Acute poisoning of cattle by fertilizer contaminated water. Vet Hum Toxicol 2003, 45: 88–90.

Author Benjamin W. Newcomer
Consulting Editor Christopher C.L. Chase
Acknowledgment The author and book editors acknowledge the prior contribution of Patricia Talcott and Tim J. Evans.

N

NUTRITION AND METABOLIC DISEASES: BEEF

BASICS

OVERVIEW
• Nutrition and metabolism of the ruminant is a balance between meeting the nutrient needs of the host's microbial population and the host itself.
• Common diseases associated with nutrition and metabolism in beef cattle include bloat (ruminal tympany), ruminal acidosis, founder/laminitis, ketosis, atypical interstitial pneumonia, and numerous diseases associated with specific nutrient deficiencies, toxicities, and interactions (energy, protein, mineral, vitamin, water).
• Aberrations in ruminant nutrition and metabolism are frequently associated with nutrient excess, deficiency, or inappropriate timing for the needs of the microbial population and host.
• Proper nutrient analysis of feedstuffs, determining the nutrient requirements of the animal, and providing the right quantity, quality, and timing of nutrients are key areas of focus.
• Nutrient requirements of beef cattle vary based on factors such as body weight, stage of production, breed, and age.
• The nutrient quality and availability of feed can vary considerably over the course of a year and season, which can dramatically impact the nutrients available to the animal.
• Nutrient delivery, and subsequent nutrient intake, varies by production system; from feedlot systems where all nutrients are fed in a TMR to a grazing system where animals obtain nutrients provided by the environment.

INCIDENCE/PREVALENCE
• Feedlot Closeout digestive death loss prevalence can range from 0.1% to 0.5%, with bloat accounting for 20–40% of all feedlot mortalities. Digestive death loss in feedlot and backgrounded cattle occurs more commonly in the spring months in the northern hemisphere.
• Atypical interstitial pneumonia death loss prevalence ranges from 0.03% to 0.15%, with peak mortality occurring in the hottest and driest months of the year and more commonly in heifers.

GEOGRAPHIC DISTRIBUTION
• Worldwide
• Areas where cereal grains are fed to livestock are commonly associated with certain diseases
• Geographical areas with soil nutrient deficiencies or excesses which manifest in the feedstuffs

SYSTEMS AFFECTED
• Digestive
• Musculoskeletal
• Nervous
• Cardiovascular
• Reproductive
• Respiratory
• Integument

PATHOPHYSIOLOGY
• Abnormal ruminal fermentation can result in microbial metabolites that are harmful to the host (e.g., lactic acid, H_2S gas).
• Nutrients may be limited or in excess to a point where ruminal microbial populations experience an undergrowth or overgrowth. In either case, ruminal and postruminal nutrient metabolism are altered.

HISTORICAL FINDINGS
• Sudden death
• Poor growth
• Low body condition score
• Chronic morbidity

SIGNALMENT
N/A

PHYSICAL EXAMINATION FINDINGS
Dependent on specific nutritional and/or metabolic disease state

GENETICS
Genetic lines of cattle selected for greater growth and carcass traits are at a greater risk of certain nutrition and metabolic-related disease. This is primarily due to an increased nutrient requirement to meet maintenance and growth needs and a propensity for higher feed intake.

CAUSES AND RISK FACTORS
• Cattle with increased nutrient requirements based on stage of production (growth, lactation) may be at a greater risk.
• Seasonally or during abnormal weather patterns (e.g., drought) when feedstuff quality or quantity is altered.
• Abrupt changes to the diet resulting in unfavorable shifts in ruminal microbial population.
• Cereal grains that are rapidly fermentable; which is dependent on grain type, variety, and processing method utilized. More intensively processed grains increase surface area and starch availability, which can predispose cattle to metabolic diseases such as ruminal acidosis and bloat.

DIAGNOSIS

DIFFERENTIAL DIAGNOSES
Rule out infectious causes of lameness, gastrointestinal upset, pneumonia, and down animals.

CBC/BIOCHEMISTRY/URINALYSIS
Abnormalities dependent on underlying cause of disease—refer to specific chapters.

OTHER LABORATORY TESTS
• Ruminal fluid collection and analysis (pH and protozoal activity)
• Liver biopsy (assessment of trace mineral levels)
• Feed ingredient or pasture sampling and analysis (nutrient composition and processing efficacy, particle size, etc.)

IMAGING
N/A

OTHER DIAGNOSTIC PROCEDURES
Presumptive diagnosis based on collection of historical information, which includes feed records, ration composition, feed analysis, water analysis, and epidemiologic patterns.

PATHOLOGIC FINDINGS
• Gross necropsy should be performed on mortalities suspected from disease associated with nutritional and metabolic causes.
• Sample collection of primary organs and fluid (blood, rumen fluid, urine, cerebrospinal) can aid in diagnosis in more complicated cases lacking obvious gross necropsy signs.

TREATMENT
N/A

MEDICATIONS
N/A

FOLLOW-UP

EXPECTED COURSE AND PROGNOSIS
N/A

POSSIBLE COMPLICATIONS
Metabolic disease may result from a variety of nutritional issues including improper feed formulation, lack of available feed, decreased intake due to palatability or competition, or underlying disease processes inhibiting proper digestion and/or absorption (e.g., Johne's disease, subacute ruminal acidosis).

CLIENT EDUCATION
• The importance of proper nutrition throughout various life and production stages must be emphasized to all owners, managers, and workers. Nutritional requirements will vary depending on all of the factors described above and therefore unique feed formulation, delivery, and monitoring protocols will need to be developed with each client.
• Emphasis should also be placed on proper feed storage and pasture management in order to improve feed quality.

PATIENT CARE
N/A

PREVENTION
• For cattle provided nutrients solely as a TMR, diet formulation, mixing, delivery, and consumption are all areas to monitor closely.

N

(CONTINUED) | **NUTRITION AND METABOLIC DISEASES: BEEF**

Errors can happen in any of these steps, resulting in nutritional and metabolic disease.

• Diet changes should be as gradual as possible. Diet transition should consist of 2- to 3-week periods with multiple intermediate steps in diet composition progressing towards the final diet.

• Diet formulation should be adjusted when a change in feedstuff usage is expected, if feedstuff nutrient composition changes, or when the nutrient requirements change.

• Water testing should be conducted on an annual basis or when a change in water source occurs.

• Water consumption should be monitored closely, especially with cattle that are not familiar with certain water sources (e.g., automatic waterers). Floats can be set to overflow waterers and encourage consumption.

• Young calves may have difficulty reaching water tank heights designed for mature cattle.

• During the winter, if tank heaters are used, stray voltage is a possibility and water intake will be inhibited.

 MISCELLANEOUS

AGE-RELATED FACTORS
Young and old are likely more susceptible to nutritional and metabolic disturbances, especially around weaning and the periparturient period.

PREGNANCY
Pregnancy increases nutrient requirements and associated hormone changes can alter nutrient metabolism.

BIOSECURITY
Sound biosecurity practices will help rule out infectious causes of cattle disease and help maintain an overall low disease prevalence in the herd.

PRODUCTION MANAGEMENT
A production management plan that focuses on frequent cattle observation, routine feed and water sampling, and monitoring of cattle health and disease occurrence will minimize impacts of potential nutritional and metabolic diseases.

ABBREVIATION
• TMR = total mixed ration

SEE ALSO
• Atypical Interstitial Pneumonia
• Beef Herd Records (see www.fiveminutevet.com/ruminant)
• Bloat
• Feeding By-Products to the Beef Cow Herd (see www.fiveminutevet.com/ruminant)
• Ketosis: Dairy Cattle
• Laminitis in Cattle
• Ruminal Acidosis

Suggested Reading
Cheng KJ, McAllister TA, Popp JD, Hristov AN, Mir Z, Shin HT. A review of bloat in feedlot cattle. J Anim Sci 1998, 76: 299–308.

Nagaraja TG, Titgemeyer EC. Ruminal acidosis in beef cattle: The current microbiological and nutritional outlook. J Dairy Sci 2007, 90(E. Suppl.): E17–38.

National Research Council. Nutrient Requirements of Beef Cattle, 8th revised ed. Washington, DC: National Academy Press, 2016.

Smith BP, ed. Large Animal Internal Medicine, 5th ed. St. Louis: Mosby, 2015.

Vasconcelos KT, Galyean ML. ASAS Centennial Paper: Contributions in the Journal of Animal Science to understanding cattle metabolic and digestive disorders. J Anim Sci 2008, 86: 1711–21.

Vogel GJ, Bokenkroger CD, Rutten-Ramos SC, Bargen JL. A retrospective evaluation of animal mortality in US feedlots: rate, timing, and cause of death. Bov Pract 2015, 49: 113–23.

Author Nathan Meyer
Consulting Editor Kaitlyn A. Lutz

N

NUTRITION AND METABOLIC DISEASES: CERVIDAE

BASICS

OVERVIEW
• For deer of temperate origin, considerable seasonal fluctuations and variation in food availability result in observable changes in body weight, fatness, and food intake.
• Voluntary feed intake (VFI) in grazing cervid species is influenced by photoperiod, the feed value of the forage, and the stage of the reproductive cycle.
• Deer are generally considered to be "concentrate selectors" because of their tendency to choose the richest parts of consumed plant species, although some may be classified as intermediate.
• Optimizing pasture conditions and nutritional supplements can lead to improved growth rate in weanlings and improved reproductive performance in female cervids.
• Monitoring body condition score (BCS), especially during periods of nutritional stress, is the most effective way to monitor the status of a nutritional program and determine if any changes are necessary.

INCIDENCE/PREVALENCE
In one study on captive fallow deer, 28% of mortality was due to nutritional disease.

GEOGRAPHIC DISTRIBUTION
Worldwide where captive cervid are raised

SYSTEMS AFFECTED
Digestive

PATHOPHYSIOLOGY
• A basic understanding of the annual appetite cycle is crucial for making appropriate nutritional management decisions in captive populations.
• Cervid species of temperate origin undergo seasonal changes in body condition, with a large proportion of fat being stored during late summer to be later mobilized by males during autumnal rut or by females throughout the winter.
• Changes in body condition are modulated through variations in VFI, which is partially regulated by photoperiod.
• At mid-summer, VFI peaks and increased day length causes the hypothalamus to become resistant to leptin, enabling fat deposition.
• As day length decreases (autumn and winter), VFI declines (~20%) and the hypothalamus becomes more sensitive to leptin, allowing fat mobilization to occur.
• In autumn and winter, reduced appetite helps to avoid energy expenditure from unproductive searching for scarce or poor-quality food sources and is compensated for by improved efficiency of nutrient absorption, especially crude protein.
• Female cervids mobilize fat reserves gradually, allowing for maintenance of an appropriate body condition during the first

two trimesters of pregnancy in winter and early spring when nutritional resources are limited.
• Nutritional and/or mineral deprivation can negatively affect fetal development and mammary tissue development in most cervid species.
• In red deer, a variable gestation length has been reported, and it is speculated that this allows the fetus to obtain a critical mass before parturition can occur.
• Male cervids mobilize fat reserves rapidly during autumnal rut, devoting the majority of their energy expenditure to roaming and breeding.
• Weanlings (~3–4 months) also experience a decline in VFI in the autumn and winter months with maximal weight gain occurring in the following spring and summer months.
• If nutritional programs are poorly managed, malnourishment and premature depletion of fat stores may occur and result in clinical ketosis if animals must derive energy from stored fat and protein.

HISTORICAL FINDINGS
Poor BCS in the herd (especially outside of the breeding season), poor conception rates, and sudden death may be suggestive of malnourishment.

SIGNALMENT
All species and ages of cervidae

PHYSICAL EXAMINATION FINDINGS
• Seasonal variation in BCS should be considered.
• Dull/rough hair and sunken eyes might be noticeable.

GENETICS
N/A

CAUSES AND RISK FACTORS
• Males are most at risk for malnutrition during breeding season if summer nutrition was inadequate.
• Though rare in cervids, late-pregnant females may be at risk for pregnancy toxemia if overweight and carrying triplets/quadruplets.

DIAGNOSIS

DIFFERENTIAL DIAGNOSES
Debilitating disease (e.g., Johne's disease and chronic wasting disease) should be ruled out as a cause of poor BCS.

CBC/BIOCHEMSTRY/URINALYSIS
• Depend on the condition.
• Ketosis (urine/blood ketones) and hypoglycemia detectable in malnourished animals.

OTHER LABORATORY TESTS
N/A

IMAGING
N/A

OTHER DIAGNOSTIC PROCEDURES
N/A

PATHOLOGIC FINDINGS
Necropsy of malnourished animals may show lack of fat in subcutaneous, visceral, and bone marrow locations with diffuse muscular atrophy; GI organs may be empty/shrunken with rumen ulcerations.

TREATMENT

THERAPEUTIC APPROACH
• Supplemental feeding with pelleted formulated feeds may be required during high risk periods.
• Monitor BCS closely in the herd and make appropriate changes as needed.
• Animals diagnosed with severe ketosis may need to be managed with oral propylene glycol or IV fluids/dextrose if possible.

SURGICAL CONSIDERATION AND TECHNIQUES
N/A

FOLLOW-UP

EXPECTED COURSE AND PROGNOSIS
Good prognosis if appropriate changes to nutritional management programs are made.

POSSIBLE COMPLICATIONS
N/A

CLIENT EDUCATION
N/A

PATIENT CARE
N/A

PREVENTION
Pasture Considerations
• Cervids are considered "concentrate selectors" because of their behavioral tendency to select plants with better nutritive value when browsing.
• Most cervid feeding programs emphasize the feeding of good-quality legume/grass hay or pasture with grain (oats, corn, barley) as a supplemental energy source and a mineral supplement in deficient areas.
• Research has shown that grazing on red clover (*Trifolium pretense*) or chicory (*Chicorium intybus*) increased red deer weanling growth during autumn by 26–47% and during spring by 10–14% compared to traditional perennial ryegrass (*Lolium perenne*)/white clover (*Trifolium repens*) pasture (0.8/0.2). Additionally, pre-weaning growth during lactation was increased by ~20%.

• Grazing on the legume, sulla (*Hedysarum coronarium*), in autumn and spring has also been shown to improve growth rate of weanling deer by 33% and 10%, respectively, compared to other pasture-fed deer.

• Reduced parasitism has been reported in animals grazing chicory versus perennial ryegrass/white clover, likely due to the plant morphology and/or presence of secondary compounds (sesquiterpene lactones) which inhibit the motility of L1 and L3 lungworm and GI nematode larvae.

Energy and Protein Requirements

• Most grass hay feeding programs require additional protein, mineral, and vitamin supplementation. Commercial pellet supplements designed for cervids or sheep generally work quite well.

• Weanlings and stags feed ratio: 6:3:1, hay : concentrate : nutritional supplement.

• Pregnant females feed ratio: 8:1.5:0.5, hay : concentrate : nutritional supplement.

• Daily energy requirements can increase by as much as 2.5 times maintenance during the 3rd trimester of pregnancy and peak lactation.

• Dietary protein requirements vary by life stages:
  ○ Fawns (growth): 14–18%
  ○ Adults (maintenance): 6–10%
  ○ Females (late pregnancy): 11–15%
  ○ Females (lactation): 14–22%
  ○ Males (antler development): 15–16%

Trace Mineral Requirements

• General purpose mineral and trace element supplements should always be available.

• Copper (Cu) deficiency can have a significant impact on deer health and performance and usually manifests as clinical disease (enzootic ataxia and osteochondrosis).
  ○ Cu supplementation strategies can consist of Cu-EDTA injections, Cu oxide needles, or direct application of Cu to pasture.
  ○ Chicory contains higher concentrations of copper and cobalt than perennial ryegrass/white clover and may be included in mineral-deficient areas.

• Selenium and iodine deficiencies may also negatively impact reproductive performance if not managed appropriately.

MISCELLANEOUS

ASSOCIATED CONDITIONS

Ruminants on pasture or being supplemented with concentrates should always be monitored for bloat, though this is less common in cervids compared to other ruminants.

AGE-RELATED FACTORS

Feeding weanlings during the fall; it is imperative to prepare them for the winter feeding pattern. Required body weights, BCS, and gains are important early in the season.

ZOONOTIC POTENTIAL
N/A

PREGNANCY

• About 65% of a breeding hind's adult life is associated with pregnancy.

• The 3rd trimester of pregnancy, when the conceptus gains >70% of its ultimate mass, is when nutritional stress is most likely to occur, especially in years with prolonged winters. This can be overcome in captive herds with appropriate nutritional supplementation.

• Nutrition deprivation in the last trimester of pregnancy can hinder fetal development.

BIOSECURITY
N/A

PRODUCTION MANAGEMENT

• Flushing, the practice of heavy concentrate feeding immediately before the breeding season, has been found to induce an earlier first estrus and higher initial ovulation rates in the first cycle in cervids.

• The opportunity to increase live weight gain (LWG) in fawns/calves during late lactation can be improved by increasing metabolizable energy with dietary supplementation. LWG can be further maximized by feeding these supplements to the fawns/calves during weaning in early autumn.

• It is important to have multiple feeding supplementation stations. More aggressive animals can dominate a supplement program, leaving more submissive/subordinate animals without needed nutrients.

• Summer pastures should contain a mixture of grasses as well as legumes. These pastures should be tested annually for nutrient content and deficiencies supplemented on an as-needed basis.

• Concentrate or pelleted supplements may be fed to increase the diet's energy content, but they should not exceed 50% of the ration on an as-fed basis.

• Monitoring a nutrition management program requires regular live weight monitoring and body condition scoring. Setting individual animal and herd target weights allows nutritional and management program evaluation. Target weights should be evaluated on a per-farm basis.

SYNONYMS
N/A

ABBREVIATIONS

• BCS = body condition score
• LWG = live weight gain
• VFI = voluntary feed intake

SEE ALSO

• Body Condition Scoring: Cervidae (see www.fiveminutevet.com/ruminant)
• Cervidae: Captive Management
• Cervidae: Reproduction
• Vaccination Programs: Cervidae

Suggested Reading

Arnold W, Beiglböck C, Burmester M, et al. Contrary seasonal changes of rates of nutrient uptake, organ mass, and voluntary food intake in red deer (*Cervus elaphus*). Am J Physiol Regul Integr Comp Physiol 2015, 309: R277–85.

Asher GW, Mulley RC, O'Neill KT, Scott IC, Jopson NB, Littlejohn RP. Influence of level of nutrition during late pregnancy on reproductive productivity of red deer: I. Adult and primiparous hinds gestating red deer calves. Anim Reprod Sci 2005, 86: 261–83.

Barry TN, Hoskin SO, Wilson PR. Novel forages for growth and health in farmed deer. N Z Vet J 2002, 50: 244–51.

Huston JE, Rector BS, Ellis WC, Allen ML. Dynamics of digestion in cattle, sheep, goats and deer. J Anim Sci 1986, 62: 208–15.

Loudon ASI. Photoperiod and the regulation of annual and circannual cycles of food intake. Proc Nutri Soc 1994, 53: 495–507.

Mansell WD. Productivity of white-tailed deer on the Bruce Peninsula, Ontario. J Wildl Manage 1974, 38: 808–14.

Muller M, Weber A, Reith B, Kratzer R. Erkrankungen von Damwild aus nordbayerischen Gehegen Untersuchungsergebnisse von Sektionen im Zeitraum 1988 bis 2002. Tierärztliche Umschau 2003, 58: 476–81.

Mussa PP, Aceto P, Abba C, Sterpone L, Meineri G. Preliminary study on the feeding habits of roe deer (*Capreolus capreolus*) in the western Alps. J Anim Physiol Anim Nutr (Berl) 2003, 87: 105–8.

Pearse AJ, Drew KR. Ecologically sound management: aspects of modern sustainable deer farming systems. Acta Vet Hung 1998, 46: 315–28.

Scott IC, Asher GW, Barrell GK, Juan JV. Voluntary food intake of pregnant and non-pregnant red deer hinds. Liv Sci 2013, 158: 230–9.

Stevens DR, Webster JR, Corson ID. Effects of seasonality and feed quality on the feed requirements and live weight gain of young deer – a review. The nutrition and management of deer on grazing systems. Proc N Z Grassland Assoc Symp, Lincoln University, New Zealand, 2003.

Authors Jamie L. Stewart and Clifford F. Shipley
Consulting Editor Ahmed Tibary
Acknowledgment The authors and book editors acknowledge the prior contribution of Scott R. R. Haskell.

NUTRITION AND METABOLIC DISEASES: DAIRY

BASICS

OVERVIEW
Metabolic diseases are very important conditions affecting dairy cattle because they play a role in compromising milk production, fertility, and overall health. The majority of these diseases affecting milk production, fertility, and general health have a nutritional component, either as a primary cause or as a risk factor. The most significant metabolic diseases described in the dairy cow are hypocalcemia, hypomagnesemia, ketosis, and fatty liver.

INCIDENCE/PREVALENCE
See chapters on specific metabolic and nutritional disease.

GEOGRAPHIC DISTRIBUTION
Worldwide

SYSTEM AFFECTED:
• Mammary
• Musculoskeletal
• Digestive
• Nervous
• Multisystemic

PATHOPHYSIOLOGY
• In general, metabolic diseases are produced because an imbalance between inputs and outputs of a particular metabolite occurs within the body. Nutrition plays a key role in the pathophysiology of metabolic diseases by providing the necessary input to maintain balance of a metabolite within the body.
• Hypocalcemia arises because the entire Ca^{2+} homeostasis is altered during the transition period. Ca^{2+} intake is low around parturition and the output is high, because of lactational demands. In addition, Ca^{2+} intestinal absorption and Ca^{2+} bone resorption are depressed during this period.
• Hypomagnesemia primarily occurs in animals grazing lush pastures that are rich in potassium and nitrogen. For this reason, hypomagnesemia can often precipitate independent of a normal Mg^+ content within the pasture grasses. In this case, excessive amounts of nitrogen and potassium affect Mg^+ bioavailability by substantially decreasing the absorption of this mineral in the digestive tract.
• Ketosis and fatty liver are two metabolic diseases that are interrelated. In dairy cows, the energy demands for milk production after calving trigger the mobilization of nonesterified fatty acids (NEFA) from the adipose tissue. This mobilization is more severe in obese cows. The end result is the uptake of a large amount of NEFA by the liver. Inside the hepatocyte, NEFA are either oxidized or re-esterified to triglycerides. If NEFA are extremely high, the re-esterification

to triglycerides dominates over the normal mitochondrial oxidation process. This subsequently leads to pathologic fat accumulation (hepatic lipidosis). Often at the same time as NEFA mobilization, the blood glucose can become very low due to the high metabolic demands during lactation. In the case of the postpartum dairy cow, a temporary state of insulin resistance can even develop. Blood glucose concentrations determine the synthesis of oxaloacetate inside the hepatic mitochondria. A low blood glucose concentration reduces oxaloacetate production within the hepatic mitochondria and subsequently shuts down the Krebs cycle. As a result, acetyl-coA coming from the oxidation of NEFA cannot continue into the normal oxidative pathway of the tricarboxylic acid cycle; therefore, the acetyl-coA is redirected to the pathway of ketogenesis.

HISTORICAL FINDINGS
• The appearance of clinical signs related to metabolic disease are often correlated with a poor nutritional program and inadequate attention to cow comfort.
• In the case of hypocalcemia and hypomagnesemia, neuromuscular dysfunction is common.
• An increase in the incidence of other conditions such as retained fetal membranes, metritis, mastitis and displacement of the abomasum may also occur.

SIGNALMENT
• Bovine, dairy cows. Nutritional and feeding management related to dairy operations are essential.
• Older and high production animals are more likely to develop metabolic diseases. An efficient nutritional management strategy is required.

PHYSICAL EXAMINATION FINDINGS
Refer to individual chapters for unique physical examination findings.

GENETICS
• Some of these diseases may have a genetic component.
• High producing dairy cows (Holstein) are more likely to experience ketosis/fatty liver problems.
• The Jersey breed is more likely to develop hypocalcemia.

CAUSES AND RISK FACTORS
• Unbalanced diets which do not meet the requirements of the lactating dairy cow, overall poor feeding management such as improper mixing of the ingredients, insufficient bunk space, improper frequency of feeding, poor water quality, inadequate cow comfort, and poor environment management.
• Risk factors include genetic level, breed, days in milk, parity, milk production, environment, and nutrition.

DIAGNOSIS

DIFFERENTIAL DIAGNOSES
N/A

CBC/BIOCHEMISTRY/URINALYSIS
• CBC analysis is generally not indicated unless concurrent infectious disease is being investigated.
• Biochemistry panels can be useful to assess the mineral and protein profile within a herd, especially in herds with a high incidence of down cows and postpartum disease during the transition period.
• Urinalysis findings are very useful in the assessment and management of metabolic disease and transition cow rations specifically. Prepartum, urine pH should be assessed on a routine basis in herds managed on a DCAD system to control hypocalcemia (see chapter, Hypocalcemia: Bovine). Postpartum, blood or urine ketone assessment of cows between 4 and 11 DIM aids in ketosis detection and management (see chapter, Ketosis: Bovine).

OTHER LABORATORY TESTS
The Dairy Herd Improvement Association (DHIA) tests for milk production, SCC, milk solids, and MUN. This service offers invaluable information that can reflect changes in nutrition and metabolic status of the herd. Ration analysis is also important when investigating metabolic disease issues.

IMAGING
N/A

OTHER DIAGNOSTIC PROCEDURES
Liver biopsy will aid in diagnosis of mineral deficiencies (e.g., copper) and hepatic lipidosis.

PATHOLOGIC FINDINGS
N/A

TREATMENT

THERAPEUTIC APPROACH
Individual animal treatment should be instituted while the underlying cause of disease (i.e., management and nutritional factors) is determined and corrected.

SURGICAL CONSIDERATIONS AND TECHNIQUES
N/A

MEDICATIONS

DRUGS OF CHOICE
N/A

CONTRAINDICATIONS
N/A

N

PRECAUTIONS
N/A

POSSIBLE INTERACTIONS
N/A

FOLLOW-UP

EXPECTED COURSE AND PROGNOSIS
N/A

POSSIBLE COMPLICATIONS
N/A

PATIENT CARE
N/A

CLIENT EDUCATION
A proper nutrition and feeding management program, especially during the transition period, is fundamental to reach a low incidence of metabolic diseases and related disorders, maximize milk production, and achieve outstanding fertility. In order to accomplish these goals the following items must be addressed:
• Implement an efficient diet formulation.
• Optimize dry matter intake in all the steps of the production cycle.
• Feed balance diets in term of energy, protein, fiber, mineral, vitamins, and water.
• Maintain macromineral homeostasis, especially when considering the relationships between potassium, magnesium, calcium, and phosphorus.
• Consider animal grouping strategies to obtain a proper BCS and minimize the presence of excessively fat or thin cows (no more than 10% of the herd).
• Minimize stress and provide adequate cow comfort.
• Consider sufficient feed bunk and watering space.
• Minimize group changes and overcrowding.
• Institute an appropriate monitoring system to evaluate prepartum and postpartum health status and disease risk assessment.

PREVENTION
• Proper feed management and balanced diet
• Good overall management
• Health monitoring protocols

MISCELLANEOUS

AGE-RELATED FACTORS
Metabolic diseases are seen most commonly in lactating dairy cows and are uncommon in heifers.

PRODUCTION MANAGEMENT
Metabolic diseases continue to be a problem in the dairy cow that is managed and fed for high milk production standards. This trend is related to progressive genetic improvement for milk yields and solids. Consequently, dairy cows must adapt properly to the tremendous metabolic and physiologic changes that modern genetics imposes on them. Nutrition and feed management must evolve at the same level in order to succeed.

ABBREVIATIONS
• BCS = body condition score
• BHBA = beta-hydroxybutyrate
• DCAD = dietary cation anion difference
• DHIA = Dairy Herd Improvement Association
• DIM = days in milk
• MUN = milk urea nitrogen
• NEFA = nonesterified fatty acid
• SCC = somatic cell count

SEE ALSO
• Dairy Nutrition: Ration Guidelines for Milking and Dry Cows (see www.fiveminutevet.com/ruminant)
• Fatty Liver
• Hypocalcemia: Bovine
• Ketosis: Dairy Cattle
• Transition Cow Management (see www.fiveminutevet.com/ruminant)

Suggested Reading
Herdt TH. Metabolic diseases of dairy cattle. Vet Clin North Am Food Anim Pract 2013, 29: 267–468.
National Research Council. Nutrient Requirements of Dairy Cattle, 7th ed. Washington, DC: National Academy Press, 2001.
Van Saun RJ, Sniffen CJ. Transition cow nutrition and feeding management for disease prevention. Vet Clin North Am Food Anim Pract. 2014, 30: 689–719.
Author Pedro Melendez
Consulting Editor Kaitlyn A. Lutz

N

NUTRITION AND METABOLIC DISEASES: SMALL RUMINANT

BASICS

OVERVIEW
• Nutrition is a critical component of metabolic diseases of small ruminants.
• Key metabolic diseases in adult small ruminants include pregnancy toxemia, ketosis, milk fever, grass staggers, and transit tetany (low blood calcium and/or magnesium in transported small ruminants).
• The most important metabolic diseases in young small ruminants are drunken lamb and floppy kid syndromes, which are forms of acidosis without dehydration.

INCIDENCE/PREVALENCE
• Pregnancy toxemia has a low incidence (2–5%).
• Milk fever and grass tetany are less common in small ruminants than in cattle.
• Floppy kid and drunken lamb syndromes have been reported as affecting >10% of lamb/kid drops in the United Kingdom. Client education and earlier treatment with oral antacids have reduced recent incidence rates.

GEOGRAPHIC DISTRIBUTION
Worldwide

SYSTEMS AFFECTED
• Multisystemic

PATHOPHYSIOLOGY
• Stress is often a trigger for metabolic diseases (e.g., dog worry, extreme weather).
• In late pregnancy multiple fetuses drain energy from the dam. In addition, the fetuses take up abdominal space, limiting feed intake. This can be further restricted if there are large amounts of abdominal fat. Goats lay down fat internally, rather than subcutaneously.
• When blood glucose levels drop, fat reserves are utilized, ketone bodies are released, and the liver becomes fatty.
• Glucose is the main energy source needed for both the fetus and the brain. Nervous signs occur as the brain no longer has enough glucose to function properly.
• In milk fever, there is a sudden increase in calcium demands due to colostrum or milk production around parturition.
• Magnesium is absorbed in the rumen and reticulum but excreted in the saliva. Absorption is reduced if there are high potassium levels.

HISTORICAL FINDINGS
Dependent on underlying cause

SIGNALMENT
• Milking sheep and dairy goats
• Females of breeding age for adult metabolic diseases; drunken lamb syndrome, 1–4 weeks; floppy kid syndrome, 3–10 days

PHYSICAL EXAMINATION FINDINGS
• For pregnancy toxemia, ketosis, and milk fever, there is reduced appetite progressing to anorexia, depression, and swollen lower limbs (from fetlock down). There is often teeth grinding and inability to rise. In the terminal stages there can be additional nervous signs, e.g., blindness, twitching of facial muscles, or lack of response to stimuli. The affected ewes or does are generally emaciated or over-conditioned and in late gestation.
• Signs of milk fever include constipation, dragging foot/feet, ataxia, weak uterine contractions, trembling, and recumbency. Signs may be very subdued in goats.
• Signs of grass tetany vary according to whether acute (excited, tremors, facial twitching, convulsions, death), subacute (inappetence, reduced yield, apprehension), or chronic (dullness, poor milk production, poor growth rate of young).
• In lambs and kids the signs of metabolic acidosis syndromes are ataxia, recumbency, and lethargy.
• Lambs and kids with metabolic acidosis syndromes are not hypothermic nor dehydrated, yet have the above signs.

GENETICS
• Heavy milking lines and breeds with multiple young are more likely to be affected.

CAUSES AND RISK FACTORS
• Very low or high body condition scores in late pregnancy or early lactation.
• Does with 3 or more fetuses are 40 times more likely to get pregnancy toxemia than those with only 1 or 2.
• Small ruminants grazing lush heavily fertilized pastures and low-sodium pastures are at high risk for grass tetany.
• In drunken lamb syndrome, smaller lambs are more likely to be affected.

DIAGNOSIS

DIFFERENTIAL DIAGNOSES
• Any illness that causes anorexia can result in a secondary pregnancy toxemia.
• Ruminal acidosis is a differential diagnosis for milk fever.

CBC/BIOCHEMISTRY/URINALYSIS
• Low blood calcium levels for milk fever.
• In drunken lamb and floppy kid syndromes, the levels of D-lactate are very high and there is a severe acidosis (pH 7).

OTHER LABORATORY TESTS
• Animals with pregnancy toxemia would have ketones in the urine identified by urine test strips of values above 1.5 mmol/L as well as ketones in the blood. Blood glucose, serum 3-OH butyrate concentrations (>3 mmol/L) or blood β-hydroxybutyrate (>0.8 mmol/L) can be used for a diagnosis of pregnancy toxemia and ketosis.

• Handheld devices (as used in human medicine) can diagnose high levels of β-hydroxybutyrate and low glucose levels in ewes with pregnancy toxemia.

IMAGING
For pregnancy toxemia, ultrasound is useful to confirm if fetuses are still alive by observing movements.

OTHER DIAGNOSTIC PROCEDURES
Response to treatment will confirm a diagnosis of milk fever, grass tetany, or transit tetany.

PATHOLOGIC FINDINGS
• For pregnancy toxemia, ketosis, and milk fever, the main pathophysiology is a pale or yellow/orange, greasy and friable liver. Adrenal glands may be enlarged.
• Aqueous humor levels of 3-OH butyrate >2.5 mmol/L is also seen in the above diseases.

TREATMENT

THERAPEUTIC APPROACH
Dairy goats or ewes should not be milked for 24 hours after being treated for milk fever.

SURGICAL CONSIDERATIONS AND TECHNIQUES
An emergency cesarean may be necessary in advanced cases of pregnancy toxemia, where death of the ewe/doe is likely to occur before induction would take effect. If dam is unlikely to survive, use local blocks, recover the young, then euthanize the dam.

MEDICATIONS

DRUGS OF CHOICE
• Treatment for pregnancy toxemia involves drenching with an energy source, e.g., 60–200 mL propylene glycol (higher dose initially then reduce) or 60 mL of glycerin q12h plus NSAID such as flunixin meglumine (2.5 mg/kg).
• The best treatment for pregnancy toxemia is induction of parturition. If the due date is known, then dexamethasone can be given at day 143; parturition should occur in the next 48–96 hours. In the doe, where the corpus luteum is the sole source of progesterone, prostaglandin can be given after day 144 (when the kids' lungs would have matured enough to survive).
• Ketosis is treated with drenching with energy sources as per pregnancy toxemia plus an injection of dexamethasone (2–6 mg) to stimulate appetite and glucogenesis.
• Milk fever is treated with 80–100 mL 20% warm calcium borogluconate solution or ideally a commercial combined product with Ca, Mg, and P either slow IV or SC, or half

(CONTINUED) NUTRITION AND METABOLIC DISEASES: SMALL RUMINANT

IV and the rest SC. Grass tetany and transit tetany are treated with the combined commercial product given SC.
• Drunken lamb syndrome has been successfully treated with 50 mmol sodium bicarbonate as an 8.4% solution given orally plus parenteral antibiotics. Stomach tube as young cannot suckle and keep warm.

CONTRAINDICATIONS
N/A

PRECAUTIONS
Ca, Mg, and P solutions should be given slowly IV, while monitoring the heart, and SC doses spilt across 2 sites.

POSSIBLE INTERACTIONS
Sodium bicarbonate should not be added to fluids containing calcium.

 FOLLOW-UP

EXPECTED COURSE AND PROGNOSIS
• Pregnancy toxemia has a high mortality rate (80%) for both dam and offspring.
• Grass tetany cases can often relapse.

POSSIBLE COMPLICATIONS
Lower lactation yields

CLIENT EDUCATION
• Increase quality and quantity of feed in the last 6 weeks of gestation and first few weeks of lactation to meet animals' needs.
• Early oral treatment with antacids for metabolic acidosis of lambs and kids.

PATIENT CARE
Appropriate management of recumbent animals is essential and includes clean, dry bedding, shelter, and availability of feed and water.

PREVENTION
• Exercise may be useful for preventing dairy does and pet sheep from becoming over-conditioned, and in preventing pregnancy toxemia in general. Data loggers confirm that does that spend more time lying down are at higher risk for pregnancy toxemia or ketosis after kidding.
• Reducing calcium intake in the last few weeks before parturition, so that animals start using bone stores of calcium as recommended for cattle, is **not** recommended for small ruminants. Instead the cation/anion balance of the diet should be adjusted by adding more anionic salts to prevent milk fever. Magnesium levels should also be checked.
• High-quality fiber should be used in the periparturient period.
• Providing ½ oz/day of magnesium oxide has stopped outbreaks of grass tetany in ewes. It can be sprayed onto hay or grain as a suspension (can also add molasses to improve palatability). If strip grazing, dust pastures with 10-gram magnesium oxide per day per small ruminant. Alternatively add supplements to livestock water supplies, i.e., 500 g Epsom salts or 420 g magnesium chloride per 100 L water. Rumen boluses have been used. Salt and Mg licks are available but intakes by individuals are variable.

 MISCELLANEOUS

ASSOCIATED CONDITIONS
Ketoacidosis should be suspected in pregnancy toxemia cases with nervous signs, and sodium bicarbonate given.

PREGNANCY
Pregnancy toxemia occurs in the last weeks of gestation.

SYNONYMS
• Twin lamb disease or hyperketonemia for pregnancy toxemia
• Hypocalcaemia, parturient paresis, and lambing sickness for milk fever
• Hypomagnesemia and grass staggers for grass tetany
• Lamb D-lactic acidosis syndrome for drunken lamb syndrome

ABBREVIATIONS
• IV = intravenous
• NSAID = nonsteroidal anti-inflammatory drug
• SC = subcutaneous

SEE ALSO
• Grass Tetany/Hypomagnesemia
• Hypocalcemia: Small Ruminant
• Ketosis: Dairy Cattle
• Pregnancy Toxemia: Small Ruminant

Suggested Reading
Brozos C, Mavrogianni VS, Fthenakis GC. Treatment and control of peri-parturient metabolic diseases: pregnancy toxemia, hypocalcemia, hypomagnesemia. Vet Clin North Am Food Anim Pract 2011, 27: 105–11.
Matthews, John (2009) Diseases of the Goat, Third edition, Wiley-Blackwell.
Author Sandra Baxendell
Consulting Editor Kaitlyn A. Lutz

N

NUTRITION AND METABOLIC DISEASES: WATER BUFFALO

BASICS

OVERVIEW
• Buffalo need more feed and grasses than cattle on a body weight basis.
• Buffalo generally graze during the day time but, in high ambient temperatures, grazing takes place in the morning and afternoon and sometimes during the night.
• Newborn buffalo calves suckle their mothers within 2 hours of birth and start to nibble grass at 3–4 weeks of age.
• Natural weaning of calves usually takes place within a year or before its mother's next calving.
• Buffalo are more efficient in converting highly fibrous low-grade foods than domestic cattle.
• Buffalo have a larger gut with a slower passage of digesta and a higher rate of crude fiber digestion.
• The rumen in buffalo is well adapted to utilize cellulose material.
• They are better converters of nonprotein nitrogenous (NPN) compounds into protein than domestic cattle. This gives an opportunity to improve poor-quality roughage with various NPN compounds.
• Metabolic diseases are important for high-producing dairy water buffalo.
• Ketosis, milk fever, fatty cow syndrome, hypomagnesemia, and down cow syndrome are major metabolic diseases of water buffalo.
• Correcting the diet and proper management during pregnancy and the lactation period reduce the incidence of such diseases.

INCIDENCE/PREVALENCE
High among high-producing dairy water buffalo

GEOGRAPHIC DISTRIBUTION
Worldwide

SYSTEMS AFFECTED
• Digestive
• Musculoskeletal
• Reproductive

PATHOPHYSIOLOGY
The pathophysiology of metabolic disorders and nutritional deficiency syndromes is similar to that of cattle.

HISTORICAL FINDINGS
Depends on complaint.
Nutritional deficiencies result in a wide variation of presentation ranging from poor fertility to increased predisposition to disease.

SIGNALMENTS
• Nutritional disorders are mainly seen in growing animals.
• In adult animals, production and reproduction may suffer due to nutrition restrictions.

PHYSICAL EXAMINATION FINDINGS
• Varies depending on the complaint.
• Poor weight gain and poor body condition score.

GENETICS
N/A

CAUSES AND RISK FACTORS
• *Parturient paresis (milk fever)*—generally occurs in high-yielding dairy buffalo within 72 hours of calving due to decreased blood calcium level (<6 mg/dL), calcium borogluconate 400–800 mL IV is the preparation of choice to treat clinical cases. Dietary management during prepartum period, calcium gel containing calcium chloride dosing (24 hours before and 10–14 hours after calving), administration of vitamin D_3 and its metabolite can help prevent milk fever.
• *Ketosis*—blood glucose levels are decreased from the normal of 50 mg/dL to 20–40 mg/dL and increased ketone bodies in blood from normal (up to 10 mg/dL) to 10–100 mg/dL. Ketonuria and ketogalactia are the evidence of ketosis in buffalo.
• *Down cow syndrome*—generally occurs after milk fever cases, leg injuries, and other metabolic conditions. Creeper cow syndrome is the principal sign; animal is bright and alert but cannot rise. Injection of calcium, magnesium, phosphate salts, vitamin E and Se, proper bedding, frequent turning of buffalo side to side will be useful in such animals.
• *Hypomagnesemic tetany*—occurs due to decreased serum magnesium level, i.e., below 1 mg/dL compared with the normal level of about 1.7–3 mg/dL. For treatment calcium and magnesium preparation, e.g., 500 mL of solution containing 25% calcium borogluconate and 5% magnesium hypophosphite IV followed by SC injection of magnesium salt can be used. Similarly 200–300 mL of 20% magnesium sulfate solution may be injected intravenously.
• *Postparturient hemoglobinuria*—occurs after several weeks after calving in high-yielding dairy buffalo and cow. Low phosphorus diet and the feeding of cruciferous are considered the common cause of this disease. Transfusion of large quantity of whole blood (minimum 5 liters of blood for a 500 kg buffalo) and administration of 60 g of sodium acid phosphate in 300 mL distilled water SC repeated 24-hourly same dose SC will protect the severely affected animal.

DIAGNOSIS

DIFFERENTIAL DIAGNOSES
• Differential diagnoses of the cause of poor production or poor growth require a thorough evaluation of the feeding system, feed analysis, and ration calculation.
• Trace mineral deficiencies may present in various clinical forms. Laboratory analysis of feed and blood may help refine the diagnosis.
• Metabolic disorders are often the result of poor feeding management.

CBC/BIOCHEMESTRY/URINALYSIS
Alterations in CBC, serum biochemistry, and urinalysis are similar to those described for cattle for various metabolic disorders.

OTHER LABORATORY TESTS
N/A

IMAGING
N/A

OTHER DIAGNOSTIC PROCEDURES
N/A

PATHOLOGIC FINDINGS
Similar to those described for cattle

TREATMENT

THERAPEUTIC APPROACH
Therapeutic approach for the major metabolic disorders is similar to that used in cattle.

SURGICAL CONSIDERATIONS AND TECHNIQUES
N/A

MEDICATIONS

DRUGS OF CHOICE
Similar to cattle; dosage needs to be adjusted (see "Causes and Risk Factors")

CONTRAINDICATIONS
Appropriate milk and meat withdrawal times must be followed.

PRECAUTIONS
N/A

POSSIBLE INTERACTIONS
N/A

FOLLOW-UP

EXPECTED COURSE AND PROGNOSIS
The prognosis for malnutrition is relatively good if ration is corrected before onset of severe disorders.

POSSIBLE COMPLICATIONS
Poor conception rate, abortion birth of weak calves

CLIENT EDUCATION
Importance of nutrition and mineral supplementation, particularly in high-producing dairy animals.

(CONTINUED) NUTRITION AND METABOLIC DISEASES: WATER BUFFALO

PATIENT CARE
Varies depending on the disorder.

PREVENTION
Prevention of metabolic and nutritional disorders is based on a solid preventive (vaccination, parasite control) program as well as adequate ration formulation for different ages and stages of production.

 MISCELLANEOUS

ASSOCIATED CONDITIONS
Malnutrition can predispose animals to infertility, pregnancy loss, and poor immunity (increased risk for infectious diseases).

AGE RELATED FACTORS
Adult buffalos above 3–4 calvings are more susceptible to metabolic diseases.

ZOONOTIC POTENTIAL
N/A

PREGNANCY
Nutritional requirement should be adjusted based on stage of gestation.

BIOSECURITY
N/A

PRODUCTION MANAGEMENT
Feeding from Birth to Weaning
• Buffalo calves should take milk about 10% of their body weight.
• It is better to introduce a mash starter from 2 weeks of age and offer good-quality berseem leaves ad libitum after 3 week of age.
• Water buffalo are superior to cows in lignin turnover.
• TDN output/input ratio varied from 6% to 30% and protein output/input ratio from 5% to 40%, indicating that buffalo fed on straw and a grain-based diet were more efficient than cows.
• Maintenance and production requirements are higher in Murrah buffalo than in cows, indicating that cows are more efficient in utilizing ME for milk production than buffalo.
• To achieve ADG of 0.7–0.8 kg a highly palatable starter ration with 70–75% TDN and 15–17% DCP is essential for growing male calves.
• The concentrate to roughage ratio ranges between 50:60 and 60:40 on a DM basis, with good-quality berseem hay making up at least half of the roughage.
• A report in Egypt compared fattening from 200 kg to 350 kg over a short fattening period of about 4 months, and fattening from 250 kg to about 500 kg over a relatively longer period of 10–11 months; the first practice produces

relatively juicier meat but the second is popular because of its high dressing percentage. The overall ADG during fattening is usually 800 900 g/d, depending on the level of concentrates. ADG was 800–1,000 g when the concentrate fraction was 75% and when 1 kg concentrate was offered for each 50 kg body weight.

Feeding of Growing and Pregnant Heifers
• Raising a good buffalo heifer is a prerequisite for achieving a high-yielding buffalo cow. In Egypt a good buffalo heifer is characterized as weighing 350–370 kg at 16–18 months of age when the heifer reaches sexual maturity.
• From weaning to about 180 kg, heifers require the same special attention as described for feeding males.
• About 2 kg/100 kg body weight of the pellet starter is required to achieve about 700 g ADG.
• A typical ration during this growing phase (average weight 125 kg) is composed of 2.5 kg starter concentrate and 1 kg each of berseem hay and rice straw.
• Calculated intakes of nutrients in this ration are as follows: DM 4.1 kg, DM % of body weight 3.2, TDN 2.5 kg, DP 0.455 kg, ME 229 kcal/kg $W^{0.75}$.
• ME requirement for maintaining buffalo heifers as 188 kcal/kg $W^{0.75}$; others reported a value of 206 kcal/kg $W^{0.75}$ for maintenance and growth. Late-pregnant buffalo heifers need an extra 0.5 kg of corn per day.

Feeding Lactating Buffalo Cows
• A standard water buffalo cow weighing 500 kg, in her 3rd lactation, producing 7 kg/d milk for 300 days with average 7% fat requires 2 kg TDN and 400 g DCP for maintenance plus 750 g TDN and 80 g DP per kg milk produced.
• Common concentrates include cereal grains, cane molasses, cottonseed cake, wheat bran, rice (polish), horse bean, soybean meal, linseed meal, and sunflower seed.
• Common roughages include teosinte, sudan grass, bajra, berseem hay; rice, wheat and barley straw; wheat and rice brans; rice hulls and silage. The main green forages in winter are berseem (*Trifolium alexandrinum*), vetch, and oat.
• In practice, a mixture of concentrates (60% TDN, 14% DP) is prepared in a cube form and comprises yellow corn 23–25%, undecorticated cottonseed cakes 25–40%, wheat bran 10–15%, rice bran 10–15%, sugar cane molasses 3–6%, and common salt plus limestone 1.5–2.5%.
• In winter, the feeding system for dairy buffalo depends on green berseem and rice

straw for dry, nonpregnant, or early-pregnant buffalo cows.
• The level of roughage in rations for lactating buffalo has been generally accepted as 50% of total DM.
• Research on the use of cheaper sources of nitrogen indicated that urea can replace up to 50% of total nitrogen in rations for lactating buffalo with no adverse effect on milk or fat yield.
• Supplementary minerals and vitamins when required.

SYNONYMS
N/A

ABBREVIATIONS
• ADG = average daily gain
• DCP = digestible crude protein
• DM = dry matter
• DP = digestible protein
• IV = intravenous
• ME = metabolizable energy
• SC = subcutaneous
• TDN = total digestible nutrient
• $W^{0.75}$ = the power function of body weight

SEE ALSO
• Down Bovine
• Hypocalcemia: Bovine
• Ketosis: Dairy Cattle
• Nutrition and Metabolic Diseases: Beef
• Postparturient Hemoglobinuria

Suggested Reading

Chandra BS, Das N. Behaviour of Indian river buffaloes (*Bubalus bubalis*) during short-haul road transportation. Vet Rec 2001, 148: 314–15.
Devendra C. Forage supplements in feeding systems for buffaloes. Buffalo J 1987, 2: 93–113.
El-Ashry MA. Impact of feeding and management on maturity in buffalo. Proc II World Buffalo Congress, New Delhi, India, 1988. Vol II, Part II, pp. 548–55.
El-Ashry MA, Shehata O, Aboul-Selim IA, Saleh Youssef AS. The effect of level of concentrates in the ration on the efficiency of feed utilization for milk production in buffaloes. Agric Res Rev 1975, 53: 45–50.
El-Serafy AM, El-Ashry MA. The nutrition of Egyptian water buffaloes from birth to milk and meat production. Proc Int Symp on Constraints of Ruminant Production in the Dry Subtropics, Cairo, Egypt 5–7 November 1988. EAAP Pub. No. 38, 1989, pp. 230–43.
Jasiorowski HA. Perspective and prospective of buffalo breeding for milk and meat production in the world. Proc II World Buffalo Congress, New Delhi, India, 1988. Vol II, Part I, pp. 285–94.

N

NUTRITION AND METABOLIC DISEASES: WATER BUFFALO (CONTINUED)

Khattab HM, El-Ashry MA, El-Serafy AM, El-Shoubokshy AS. Effect of feeding different levels of urea on the production performance of milking buffaloes. Egypt J Anim Prod 1981, 21: 155–66.

Mudgal VO. Comparative efficiency for milk production of buffaloes and cattle in the tropics. Proce II World Buffalo Congress, New Delhi, India, 1988. Vol II, Part II, pp. 454–62.

National Research Council. Nutrient Requirements of Dairy Cattle, 5th revised ed. Washington, DC: National Research Council, 1978.

Radostits OM, Blood DC, Gay CC. Veterinary Medicine: A Textbook of the Diseases of Cattle, Sheep, Pigs, Goats and Horses, 8th revised ed. London: Bailliere Tindall, 1994.

Ranjhan SK, Pathak NN. Management and Feeding of Buffaloes, 2nd ed. New Delhi: Vikas, 1983, pp. 210–29.

Author Egendra Kumar Shrestha
Consulting Editor Ahmed Tibary

N

OAK (*QUERCUS* SPP.) TOXICITY

BASICS

OVERVIEW
• Renal damage and gastroenteritis can occur in ruminants following ingestion of leaves, buds, and acorns from oak trees.
• Cases involving other species such as horses, goats, sheep, and camelids are rare. Pigs and deer are resistant.
• Tannins are the toxic principle, and high concentrations are found in oak leaves, buds, and acorns. Tannins cause direct damage to epithelial cells in the GI tract, causing oral, esophageal, and ruminal ulceration. Protein-bound tannins can be refractory to ruminal hydrolysis and once they reach the abomasum are released, creating further GI ulceration in the abomasum and intestine.
• Animals that survive acute renal insults often develop chronic renal disease and demonstrate poor weight gains compared with their cohorts.

INCIDENCE/PREVALENCE
• Approximately 90 species of oak are found in North America, and while many are reported to be toxic, differences exist in the amount of toxin present.
• Case fatality rate is high, often >80%.

GEOGRAPHIC DISTRIBUTION
• Oak or acorn poisoning has been reported worldwide.
• Most oak species found in Europe and North America are considered toxic.

SYSTEMS AFFECTED
• Digestive
• Urinary

PATHOPHYSIOLOGY
• Tannins are the toxic principle, from which pyrogallol, gallotannins, polyhydroxyphenolic compounds, and other phenolic metabolites are produced by microbial hydrolysis in the rumen.
• Gallic acid and pyrogallols bind and precipitate proteins, which are extremely toxic to renal tubules, causing acute renal tubular necrosis. Acute tubular necrosis leads to severe azotemia, anuria, electrolyte imbalances, and uremia, which results in GI and renal dysfunction.
• Hydrolyzed tannins can also be absorbed and become bound to plasma proteins and endothelial proteins, which leads to hemorrhage and fluid loss from blood vessels resulting in edema.
• Severity of renal damage depends on the duration of exposure to oak and the amount ingested.

SIGNALMENT
• Cattle are the species most commonly affected. Young cattle often appear to be more severely affected than adult cattle.

• Oak poisoning has been reported in sheep, goats, and camelids.

HISTORICAL FINDINGS
A history of ingestion for 2–14 days (average of 1 week) usually precedes clinical signs; however, some reports describe disease occurring 21 days after removal from oak exposure.

PHYSICAL EXAMINATION FINDINGS
• Clinical signs usually occur within 3–7 days after consumption of green oak leaves or acorns.
• In peracute poisoning, cattle may be found dead. If observed closely, affected cattle may be recumbent, weak, and listless.
• Clinical signs include anorexia, depression, and ruminal stasis. Affected ruminants develop constipation, which is often followed by hemorrhagic diarrhea. Edema is observed in the ventral abdomen, perineum, vulva, submandibular area, and brisket, and can be severe.
• Anuria is present in peracute disease; however, polyuria and hematuria may also be observed.
• Secondary complications including bronchopneumonia and GI perforation with abscessation may occur.

CAUSE AND RISK FACTORS
• Immature leaves, stems, acorns, and buds are the most toxic and the most palatable.
• Oak poisoning is associated with ingestion of leaves and buds in the spring and with ingestion of acorns in the fall months.
• Toxicosis may occur when adequate forage is available but more commonly is associated with drought or other circumstances that lead to poor grazing.
• Cases may also be seen following wind or rain storms that drop leaves, acorns, or branches into pastures where cattle are grazing. Early spring snowstorms can cause oak branches containing oak buds and/or young leaves to break, making them accessible to grazing animals.
• Some animals develop a craving for acorns, occasionally to the exclusion of other available forage, and this may explain why individuals with the same access to oaks may remain unaffected.

DIAGNOSIS

DIFFERENTIAL DIAGNOSES
• Diagnosis of oak poisoning is made on history of exposure and characteristic clinical signs or necropsy findings.
• Primary differentials include diseases that cause sudden death, GI ulceration, and acute or chronic renal failure in ruminants.
• Pigweed (*Amaranthus retroflexus*) poisoning, obstructive urolithiasis, clostridial diseases, heavy metal poisoning, leptospirosis, and

renal injury due to nephrotoxic antibacterial drugs should be considered.
• Other differentials include diseases that cause GI ulceration: Infectious bovine rhinotracheitis, bovine viral diarrhea, foot and mouth disease, and bluetongue.

CBC/BIOCHEMISTRY/URINALYSIS
• Azotemia (elevated serum urea nitrogen and creatinine), hyponatremia, hyperkalemia, hyperphosphatemia, and/or hypocalcemia are present on serum biochemistry profiles. Mild metabolic acidosis with a high anion gap may be observed. Elevations in liver enzymes may also be observed.
• The animal may be anuric, or the urine may be isosthenuric with proteinuria, hematuria, and/or glucosuria.
• Granular or proteinaceous casts are often found on urinalysis.
• In chronic cases, elevated serum urea nitrogen, creatinine, and anion gap in addition to variable electrolyte imbalances may be seen.
• Elevated white blood cell counts usually indicate chronic GI ulceration or abscessation.
• Chronic inflammation may lead to a normocytic normochromic anemia. Serum protein levels may be abnormally low due to GI and renal losses.

OTHER LABORATORY TESTS
Serum and urine may be evaluated for concentrations of pyrogallol; however, detectable levels of pyrogallol in urine and serum usually precede clinical signs.

PATHOLOGIC FINDINGS
• Subcutaneous edema, ascites, hydrothorax, and hydropericardium are observed in peracute and acute cases.
• Tubular necrosis and perirenal edema are prominent. Grossly, the kidneys are pale, enlarged, and may contain multifocal hemorrhages.
• Multifocal ulcerative lesions are found in the mouth, esophagus and throughout the GI tract. Perforation and associated inflammation may be observed.
• Histopathologic examination reveals coagulation necrosis of the cortical tubular epithelium. Tubules are dilated and devoid of epithelium but with intact basement membranes. Many tubules contain granular, hyaline, or cellular casts. Necropsy findings after 3–6 weeks of disease may show GI abscessation associated with perforated ulcers, and secondary bacterial pneumonia. Some tubular regeneration may also be seen.

TREATMENT

THERAPEUTIC APPROACH
• Immediately remove affected and unaffected animals from oak trees and provide fresh hay and water.

O

OAK (*QUERCUS* SPP.) TOXICITY

• Intravenous fluid therapy to promote diuresis, establish urine production, and correct acid-base and electrolyte abnormalities is critical. Oral fluid therapy can be used in some cases, but is less effective.
• Antibiotic therapy should be initiated to treat secondary pneumonia and GI abscessation.
• Transfaunation is beneficial to restore rumen motility.
• Adding calcium hydroxide into feed as a 10% concentration has been shown to be effective in decreasing the incidence of intoxication and mortality rates.

MEDICATIONS

DRUGS OF CHOICE
• There is no specific antidote for oak poisoning.
• Calcium hydroxide, activated charcoal, ruminatorics, and purgatives (such as mineral oil [1 L/500 kg], sodium sulfate [1 kg/400 kg], or magnesium sulfate [450 g/400 kg]) may be effective antidotes if administered early in the course of disease.
• Polyethylene glycol (1 g/kg/day) administered in the feed or water will bind tannins and reduce tissue damage.

CONTRAINDICATIONS
Nephrotoxic antibiotics should be avoided.

PRECAUTIONS
Appropriate milk and meat withdrawal times must be followed for all compounds administered to food-producing animals.

FOLLOW-UP

EXPECTED COURSE AND PROGNOSIS
Clinical recovery usually occurs within 60 days but is rare if renal dysfunction is severe.

PATIENT CARE
Monitoring kidney function is essential for animals recovering from oak poisoning.

PREVENTION
• Improved range management to limit grazing in immature oak stands will prevent development of the syndrome.
• Consumption of a pelleted ration supplement (1 kg/head/day) containing 10–15% calcium hydroxide plus access to more palatable feeds may be used as a preventive measure if exposure to acorns or oak leaves cannot be avoided.

MISCELLANEOUS

PREGNANCY
Ingestion of large numbers of acorns in the second trimester of pregnancy can result in congenitally malformed calves. "Acorn calves" seem to be a result of poor nutrition and ingestion of acorns.

SYNONYMS
• Acorn calves
• Acorn toxicity

ABBREVIATION
• GI = gastrointestinal

SEE ALSO
• Acute Renal Failure
• Bluetongue Virus
• Bovine Viral Diarrhea Virus
• Clostridial Disease: Gastrointestinal
• Foot and Mouth Disease
• Heavy Metal Toxicosis
• Infectious Bovine Rhinotracheitis
• Leptospirosis
• Oxalate Toxicity
• Urolithiasis

Suggested Reading
Blakley BR. Overview of Quercus poisoning. In: The Merck Veterinary Manual Online, 2013. http://www.merckvetmanual.com/mvm/toxicology/quercus_poisoning/overview_of_quercus_poisoning.html, accessed July 31, 2016.
Blodgett DJ. Renal toxicants. In: Howard JL, Smith RA eds, Current Veterinary Therapy 4: Food Animal Practice. Philadelphia: Saunders, 1999.
Burrows GE, Tyrl RJ. Quercus. In: Burrows GE, Tyrl RJ eds, Toxic Plants of North America, 2nd ed. Ames: Wiley-Blackwell, 2013, Kindle edition, pp. 674–87.
Chamorro MF, Passler T, Joiner K, Poppenga RH, Bayne J, Walz PH. 2013. Acute renal failure in 2 adult llamas after exposure to Oak trees (*Quercus* spp.). Can Vet J 2013, 54: 61–4.
Doce RR, Belenguer A, Toral PG, Hervás G, Frutos P. Effect of the administration of young leaves of *Quercus pyrenaica* on rumen fermentation in relation to oak tannin toxicosis in cattle. J Anim Physiol Anim Nutr 2013, 97: 48–57.
Perez V, Doce RR, Garcia-Pariente C, et al. Oak leaf (*Quecus pyrenaica*) poisoning in cattle. Res Vet Sci 2011, 91: 269–77.
Smith BP. Oak (acorn) toxicosis. In: Smith BP ed, Large Animal Internal Medicine, 5th ed. St. Louis: Elsevier, 2015, pp. 827–9.
Spier SJ, Smith BP, Seawright AA, Norman BB, Ostrowski SR, Oliver MN. Oak toxicosis in cattle in northern California: clinical and pathologic findings. J Am Vet Med Assoc 1987, 191: 958–64.
Author Paul H. Walz
Consulting Editor Christopher C.L. Chase

BASICS

OVERVIEW
• Infestation of the nasal cavity and/or sinuses with larval stages (bots or maggots) of *Oestrus ovis*.
• Infestation can produce a chronic rhinitis and sinusitis, most commonly associated with a mucopurulent nasal discharge.

INCIDENCE/PREVALENCE
The incidence/prevalence is variable among geographic regions and within flocks in a given region. The condition is endemic in some areas.

GEOGRAPHIC DISTRIBUTION
The parasite is found worldwide. Various sources report it as widely distributed in Africa, Australia, Europe, countries of the Mediterranean basin, South Africa, some countries in South America, countries of the former USSR, and the United States.

SYSTEMS AFFECTED
• Respiratory
• Nervous

PATHOPHYSIOLOGY
• *Oestrus ovis* is a dipteran fly in the same family as the warble fly of cattle.
• The adult fly is dark gray and is approximately 1 cm long with rudimentary or vestigial mouthparts. It cannot feed.
• Female flies deposit larvae (larviposit or oviposit) in and around the nostrils of the ruminant host.
• Adult *Oestrus ovis* live 2–28 days and each female produces up to several hundred larvae.
• The parasite can "overwinter" as first-stage larvae in the nasal cavities of hosts and/or as pupae in the ground.
• The first-stage larvae, or instars, initially less than 2 mm long, enter the nasal cavity and feed upon mucus and exfoliated epithelial cells.
• The first-stage instars migrate in the nasal passages and undergo maturation to second-stage larvae in the frontal and maxillary sinuses. Further maturation leads to third-stage instars. After a total larval period of weeks to several months, the fully developed third-stage larvae migrate back to the nostrils, are sneezed out, and pupate in the ground.
• The pupal period is 3–9 weeks.
• Adult flies arise after a period of approximately 4 weeks in summer but require much longer in cooler weather.
• Mechanical damage and trauma occur to the nasal mucosa due in part to attachment by the oral hooks and cuticular spines of the larvae.
• Hypersensitivity has been proposed to play a role in the pathophysiology. In the sinuses, dead larvae may produce an allergic and inflammatory response.

• Larvae and/or their products may produce inflammatory reactions in the lung.

HISTORICAL FINDINGS
The female adult flies bother sheep, causing one or more of the following signs: head shaking, sneezing, rubbing the nose on the ground or on other sheep, foot stomping, circling with nose to the ground, blowing, and interference with grazing.

SIGNALMENT
• Most common in sheep, reported less commonly in goats.
• Has been reported in bighorn sheep (*Ovis canadensis*) and the European ibex (*Capra ibex*), some deer, elk, camels and camelids, dogs, and humans.
• All ages and breeds of sheep are affected.
• Larval burdens have been reported by some sources as being higher in younger animals.

PHYSICAL EXAMINATION FINDINGS
• Rhinitis with nasal discharge (initially clear and mucoid; later mucopurulent and often with blood), sneezing, and stertorous (snoring) respiration.
• Chronic sinusitis, secondary bacterial pneumonia is possible in some cases.
• Very uncommonly, larvae may enter the brain from the sinuses or there can be the spread of purulent inflammation from the sinuses to the brain.

CAUSES AND RISK FACTORS
Infestation of the nasal cavity/sinuses with larvae or bots of *O. ovis*.
• Environmental factors may play a major role in influencing the frequency of infestation.
• In North America, the adult fly is seen from spring to summer or autumn.
• The fly is particularly active in warm weather. In warm climates, the fly can be active over a greater portion of the year.

DIAGNOSIS

DIFFERENTIAL DIAGNOSES
• Foreign bodies (visualization of foreign body in nasal cavity), nasal adenocarcinoma (visualization of tissue and/or biopsy), pneumonia (characteristic clinical signs, evidence of pulmonary pathology), sinusitis (clinical signs, lack of evidence of oestrosis), trauma (history), and others depending upon specific symptoms.
• When the brain is involved (rare), signs of incoordination and a high-stepping gait may simulate signs of gid, a parasitic invasion of the CNS due to larval stages of a canine tapeworm (*Coenurus cerebralis*) and related species (*Taenia multiceps*).

CBC/BIOCHEMISTRY/URINALYSIS
N/A

OTHER LABORATORY TESTS
Serologic techniques such as an enzyme-linked immunosorbent assay (ELISA) test have been developed.

IMAGING
Techniques such as endoscopy may be used to visualize the parasite in the nasal cavity.

OTHER DIAGNOSTIC PROCEDURES
Diagnosis is usually based upon clinical signs; it can be confirmed by necropsy or visualization of the larvae in the sinuses (e.g., endoscopy) antemortem.

PATHOLOGIC FINDINGS
• Up to 20 or more larvae at different developmental stages may be found in the sinuses.
• Sinuses with live larvae may be seen as normal; sinuses with dead larvae may demonstrate edematous and thickened membranes and cavities with exudates.

TREATMENT

THERAPEUTIC APPROACH
• Treatment may be administered at various times during the year, based upon climatic factors and occurrence of infestations.
• In temperate climates, treatment in autumn has been recommended. The majority of larvae are small during this time period.

SURGICAL CONSIDERATIONS AND TECHNIQUES
N/A

MEDICATIONS

DRUGS OF CHOICE
These recommendations refer to treatment of the disease in the US in sheep.
• Some anthelmintics used in control/treatment programs for GI parasites may be effective in maintaining control of *O. ovis*.
• Ivermectin at 0.2 mg/kg (200 µg/kg) PO kills all instars and is reported as highly effective. A controlled-release form of ivermectin is available in some countries and has been shown to be effective over an extended period of time.
• It has been recommended in temperate zones to treat in autumn when the majority of larvae are small.
• Closantel, moxidectin, ruelene, rafoxanide, trichlorfon, and other systemic products have been reported in the literature.
• Some authors have recommended various treatments applied directly into the nostrils.

O

OESTRUS OVIS INFESTATION

CONTRAINDICATIONS
Ivermectin is not recommended for use in dairy animals due to its extended milk withdrawal time.

PRECAUTIONS
• Obtain current and complete information on any drugs used.
• Appropriate milk and meat withdrawal times must be followed for all compounds administered to food-producing animals.

POSSIBLE INTERACTIONS
Check drug label and follow all regulations within individual country.

 FOLLOW-UP

EXPECTED COURSE AND PROGNOSIS
Treatment at the appropriate life cycle stage with an effective drug should produce high cure rates.

POSSIBLE COMPLICATIONS
• Calcified or septic sinusitis with possible extension to the brain (rare) with presence of dead larvae
• Interstitial pneumonia and lung abscesses
• Killing mature larvae may result in marked reactions in the membranes of the sinuses.

CLIENT EDUCATION
Strategic treatment may interrupt life cycle before the parasite becomes widely established.

PREVENTION
Prevention is difficult. Attempts to minimize the effects of adult flies have been made by utilizing insecticides and by providing shelter or access to cool areas where flies are less active.

 MISCELLANEOUS

ASSOCIATED CONDITIONS
Chronic sinusitis and secondary bacterial pneumonia are possible.

AGE-RELATED FACTORS
Young animals may experience greater larval burdens.

ZOONOTIC POTENTIAL
• *Oestrus ovis* is a zoonosis.
• It most commonly causes ocular myiasis or ophthalmomyiasis, primarily among individuals with close contact with sheep or infested animals (e.g., shepherds).
• Affected individuals most commonly report the sensation of being struck in the eye by an insect or foreign body, followed by pain and inflammation in the ocular conjunctiva.

BIOSECURITY
Spread of the parasite may be promoted by importation of infested animals.

PRODUCTION MANAGEMENT
• Moderate numbers of larvae cause little harm; heavy infestations may produce effects such as decreased grazing and feeding times.
• Heavy infestations may interfere with feeding and lead to loss of condition and a significant decline in production of milk or a decrease in weight gains.

SYNONYMS
• Head bot/grub
• Nasal bots
• Nostril fly
• Oestrosis
• Sheep nasal fly
• False gid

ABBREVIATIONS
• CNS = central nervous system
• ELISA = enzyme-linked immunosorbent assay
• GI = gastrointestinal
• PO = per os
• USSR = Union of Soviet Socialist Republics

SEE ALSO
• Ovine Pulmonary Adenocarcinoma
• Parasite Control Programs: Small Ruminant
• Parasitic Pneumonia

Suggested Reading
Acha PN, Szyfres B. Zoonoses and communicable diseases common to man and animals. 3rd ed. Vol. III, Parasitoses. Scientific and Technical Publication No. 580. Washington, DC: Pan American Health Organization, 2003.
Dorchies P, Duranton C, Jacquiet P. Pathophysiology of *Oestrus ovis* infection in sheep and goats: a review. Vet Rec 1998, 142: 487–9.
Georgi JR, Georgi ME, Theodorides VJ. Parasitology for Veterinarians, 5th ed. Philadelphia: Saunders, 1990.
Horak IG, Snijders AJ. The effect of *Oestrus ovis* infestation on Merino lambs. Vet Rec 1974, 94: 12–16.
Kimberling CV. Jensen and Swift's Diseases of Sheep, 3rd ed. Philadelphia: Lea & Febiger, 1988.
Soulsby EJL. Helminths, arthropods and protozoa of domesticated animals. In: Monnig's Veterinary Helminthology and Entomology, 6th ed. Baltimore: Williams & Wilkins., 1968.
Tabouret G, Jacquiet P, Scholl P, Dorchies P. *Oestrus ovis* in sheep: relative third-instar populations, risks of infection, and parasite control. Vet Res 2001, 32: 525–31.

Author Kate O'Conor
Consulting Editor Kaitlyn A. Lutz
Acknowledgment The author and book editors acknowledge the prior contribution of Kevin L. Anderson.

O

OLEANDER AND CARDIOTOXIC PLANT TOXICITY

BASICS

OVERVIEW
• Toxicosis caused by exposure to cardiotoxic plants.
• Major toxins are cardiac glycosides, which are found in a number of unrelated plants, such as oleander (*Nerium oleander*), summer pheasant's eye (*Adonis aestivalis*), foxglove (*Digitalis purpurea*), lily-of-the-valley (*Convallaria majalis*), dogbane (*Apocynum* spp.), and some species of milkweed (*Asclepias* spp.).
• Oleander is cultivated widely in the southern United States and is most commonly associated with plant poisonings in livestock. Therefore, oleander is discussed in detail as a representative of plants containing cardiac glycosides.
• Other cardiotoxic plants that have resulted in poisoning of cattle include yew (*Taxus* spp.), grayanotoxin-containing plants, avocado (*Persea* spp.) and death camas (*Zigadenus* spp.)
• Sudden death is often the primary reported finding.
• In camelids, oleander poisoning may present as renal failure that develops several days post-exposure.

INCIDENCE/PREVALENCE
• Oleander poisoning is relatively common in camelids and cattle and is especially reported in California, Arizona, and Texas. Most cases of oleander poisoning are a result of ingestion of dried oleander clippings or oleander contamination in hay.
• Not all animals in a herd may be affected. Oleander contamination of hay may be uneven.
• Yew, death camas, and avocado poisoning are relatively uncommon in ruminants. Poisonings should be suspected if plants are identified in the environment of the animal or found in hay or burn piles (e.g., yew).
• Grayanotoxin poisoning is usually reported in goats due to browsing azaleas and rhododendrons.

GEOGRAPHIC DISTRIBUTION
• Cardiotoxic plants have specific distribution in the US.
• Oleander is commonly found across the southern US.
• Grayanotoxins are found in several members of the Ericaceae (Heath) family and are widely distributed in the US. They are often found along coastal regions as well as in mountain areas.
• Avocado is extensively cultivated in California and Florida, but can also be found as an ornamental in Gulf coast areas.
• Many species of death camas occur across the US and are seasonal with the greatest abundance being in the spring.

SYSTEMS AFFECTED
Cardiovascular

PATHOPHYSIOLOGY
• Oleander contains cardiac glycosides or cardenolide glycosides that are composed of a steroid core, an unsaturated lactone ring, and a sugar moiety. Cardiac glycosides such as oleandrin, digitoxin, and digoxin inhibit Na^+/K^+-ATPase with similar efficacy to their respective aglycones. The addition of sugar moieties to the steroid core is not essential for the Na^+/K^+-ATPase inhibition, but affects the pharmacodynamics and pharmacokinetics of cardenolide glycosides. Inhibition of the Na^+/K^+-ATPase on myocardial and other cells leads to intracellular retention of Na^+, followed by increased intracellular Ca^{2+} concentrations through the reverse operation of the Na^+-Ca^{2+} exchanger. Elevated intracellular Ca^{2+} concentrations promote inotropy. Other signaling pathways involving NF-κB, TNF-α, and Na^+-dependent amino acid transport have also been identified as targets of cardenolides. The toxic effects are primarily attributable to cardiac conduction alterations and other electrical activity changes. Atrioventricular block is one of the most common manifestations of toxicity, and death is typically due to ventricular fibrillation.
• Yews contain taxine alkaloids (major alkaloids are taxine A and taxine B) that are rapidly absorbed, metabolized, conjugated in the liver, and eliminated in urine as conjugated benzoic acid (hippuric acid). Taxine alkaloids can cause an increase in cytoplasmic calcium by interfering with both calcium and sodium ion channel conductance across myocardial cells. This results in depression of cardiac depolarization and conduction of the heart.
• Grayanotoxins are diterpenes that bind to sodium channels in excitable cell membranes, resulting in increased membrane permeability to sodium ions and maintaining excitable cells in a state of depolarization. Accumulation of intracellular sodium results in an exchange with extracellular calcium, and plays an important role in the control of transmitter release. The membrane effects caused by grayanotoxins account for the observed responses of skeletal and myocardial muscle, nerves, and central nervous system.
• The toxic compound of avocado is called persin. While the exact mechanism of action remains unclear, persin and its analogs arrest the cell cycle.
• Death camas contains steroidal alkaloids, such as zygacine and zygadenine. The alkaloids decrease blood pressure, slow the heart rate, and lead to respiratory depression.

SIGNALMENT
• All ruminant species are susceptible to oleander. Oleander poisoning has been reported in cattle, sheep, goats, and camelids.

• Goats are particularly sensitive to the mammary effects caused by avocados.
• No breed, age, or sex predilections.

PHYSICAL EXAMINATION FINDINGS
• Animals exposed to cardiotoxic plants are often found dead.
• Clinical signs of abdominal pain are often seen within hours of exposure.
• Progression of disease is rapid and animals develop weakness, tremors, excessive salivation, incoordination, dyspnea, and sometimes convulsions.
• In cardiac glycoside poisonings, animals often have an irregular fast pulse with tachycardia, ventricular arrhythmias, or gallop rhythms.
• Clinical signs of *Taxus* poisoning in cattle include incoordination, nervousness, difficulty in breathing, bradycardia, diarrhea, and convulsions, but sudden death is often all that is seen.
• Grayanotoxin poisoning can lead to depression, severe salivation, abdominal pain, and vomiting. In severe cases, animals may then become laterally recumbent, and develop seizures, tachycardia, tachypnea, and pyrexia.

CAUSES AND RISK FACTORS
• Cardiotoxic plants most commonly associated with acute poisoning are oleander and yew. The toxic principles are glycosidic cardenolides and/or cardiotoxic glycosides.
• All parts of oleander are extremely toxic, whether the plant is fresh or dried. Ingestion of dried oleander clippings is a common source of poisoning. Five medium-sized oleander leaves can cause illness and death in an adult cow or camelid.
• All parts of the yew, green or dried, with the exception of the red fleshy part surrounding the seed (aril portion), are toxic. Ingestion of yew clippings is most often the cause of poisonings. All species of *Taxus*, including *T. baccata* (English yew), *T. cuspidata* (Japanese yew) and *T. brevifolia* (Pacific or Western yew), are considered toxic.
• Grayanotoxin poisoning usually occurs when animals are offered plant trimmings or stray into wooded areas where little else is available to eat. The leaves of the plants are considered the greatest risk.
• Avocado leaves are especially toxic, but ingestion of fruit and seeds can also result in poisoning.
• Death camas leaves during the early stages of growth pose the greatest risk for poisoning. Seeds and fruits as well as the dried plant in hay are also toxic.
• Fresh plant material of cardiotoxic plants is often considered to be of low palatability, so animals are most likely to ingest dried plant material.
• Plant trimmings present the most common source for oleander and yew poisoning.
• Contamination of hay or hay cubes with oleander is of great risk.

O

OLEANDER AND CARDIOTOXIC PLANT TOXICITY   (CONTINUED)

• The Guatemalan strain of avocados and its hybrid ("Fuerte") are reportedly toxic, while the Mexican strain has low toxicity.
• Many species of death camas occur across the US and are seasonal with the greatest abundance being in the spring.

DIAGNOSIS

DIFFERENTIAL DIAGNOSES
• Ionophore antibiotics—history of ionophores (e.g., monensin) in the feed ration, detection of toxic concentrations of ionophores in the feed, histologic lesions.
• Cyanide poisoning—mucus membranes are initially bright cherry red, evidence of exposure to cyanogenic plants, chemical analysis for cyanide in gastrointestinal contents, liver or muscle.
• Organophosphorus or carbamate insecticide exposure—commonly associated with gastrointestinal irritation and neurologic signs, evaluation of cholinesterase activity, detection of pesticides in gastrointestinal contents.
• Exposure to neurotoxic plants, such as poison hemlock, water hemlock, tree tobacco, lupine—chemical analysis for plant toxins in gastrointestinal contents, history of presence of plants in the environment.
• Myocarditis—murmurs are usually present, differentiate echocardiographically.
• Endocarditis—fever, differentiate echocardiographically.

CBC/BIOCHEMISTRY/URINALYSIS
• Changes are limited in acute poisonings.
• BUN and CREA may be elevated in camelids several days after exposure.
• Myocardial damage may result in hyperkalemia, elevated LDH, CK and AST activities, and elevated cardiac troponin I.

OTHER LABORATORY TESTS
• Detection of oleandrin, gitoxin, digitoxin, grayanotoxins, strophanthidin, or other cardiac glycosides or aglycones in serum, stomach, cecal, or colon contents, and liver.
• Detection of taxine alkaloids in stomach contents.
• Visual and microscopic examination of stomach or intestinal contents for plant fragments. Direct microscopic examination of water and gastrointestinal contents.

OTHER DIAGNOSTIC PROCEDURES
ECG disturbances are supportive—atrioventricular conduction blocks and ventricular arrhythmias.

PATHOLOGIC FINDINGS
• In peracute cases, no lesions are found.
• Postmortem lesions are generally nonspecific in animals that died of exposure to cardiotoxic plants. Lesions include reddening of the mucosa of the gastrointestinal tract and congestion of organs.

• Ruminants with oleander poisoning have evidence of fluid in the pericardium and body cavities, endocardial hemorrhages, and multifocal myocardial degeneration and necrosis. Mural thrombi and hemorrhage under the epicardial surface may be seen.
• *Taxus* poisoning is associated with mild to moderate endocardial hemorrhages in both ventricles, acute multifocal contraction band necrosis of the ventricular wall and the papillary muscles, and occasional neutrophilic and lymphocytic infiltrates in the interstitium of the myocardium.
• There are no or very few lesions in cases of grayanotoxin and death camas poisoning.
• Avocado poisoning can result in fluid accumulation in the pericardial sac and in the thoracic and abdominal cavities. Edema of the gallbladder and perirenal tissues and a flabby, pale heart has been observed. In lactating animals, mammary glands are edematous and reddened.

TREATMENT

THERAPEUTIC APPROACH
• Treatment of animals exposed to cardiotoxic plants is primarily supportive and symptomatic. Supportive therapy should include administration of intravenous fluids, antiarrhythmics, and antibiotics if indicated.
• Prevention of further exposure to the cardiotoxic plant is essential.
• Adsorption of toxins with activated charcoal (AC) has been suggested. Multi-dose AC is beneficial in oleander intoxications.
• Any possible stress or trauma should be avoided.
• Atropine should be considered in cases of severe bradycardia.

SURGICAL CONSIDERATIONS AND TECHNIQUES
Rumenotomy or a rumen lavage may be considered in valuable animals.

MEDICATIONS

DRUGS OF CHOICE
• No antidote is available.
• Antiarrhythmics according to cardiac function (e.g., ECG).
• Atropine (0.01–0.02 mg/kg IV) to treat bradyarrhythmias.
• AC (2–5 g/kg PO in a watery slurry [1 g of AC in 5 mL of water]) via nasogastric tube
• Recommended IV fluid administration in oleander poisonings is 0.9% NaCl with 2.5% dextrose.
• Anticardiac glycoside Fab antibodies have been used in humans and small animals but their usefulness in the treatment of cardiac

glycoside-poisoned ruminants has not been evaluated.

CONTRAINDICATIONS
• Do not administer potassium in fluids if hyperkalemia is present.
• Avoid calcium-containing solutions and quinidine.

FOLLOW-UP

EXPECTED COURSE AND PROGNOSIS
• Animals poisoned with cardiotoxic plants are often found dead.
• Cardiotoxic plant exposure progresses so rapidly that treatment is often too late. In oleander and yew intoxications, the prognosis is poor.
• If treatment is initiated promptly after the onset of clinical signs, the prognosis is fair.
• Animals that survive the acute poisoning may suffer from myocardial damage and may be more prone to stress.
• Camelids that survive 24–72 hours after exposure may develop renal failure.

CLIENT EDUCATION
• Recognize cardiotoxic plants of concern in the geographic location and prevent access by ruminants.
• Provide adequate forage to limit ingestion of toxic plants.

PATIENT CARE
Monitor progression of clinical signs and evaluate ECG.

PREVENTION
• Ruminants should be denied access to landscaped yards and discarded clippings.
• Suspect forage should be inspected for the presence of cardiotoxic plants before allowing access.
• Hay should be inspected carefully for weeds, as many cardiotoxic plants remain toxic when dried (oleander, death camas, yew).

MISCELLANEOUS

PREGNANCY
None

ABBREVIATIONS
• AC = activated charcoal
• AST = aspartate aminotransferase
• BUN - blood urea nitrogen
• CK = creatine kinase
• CREA = creatinine
• ECG = electrocardiogram
• IV = intravenous
• LDH = lactate dehydrogenase
• PO = per os

SEE ALSO
• Carbamate Toxicity
• Cyanide Toxicosis

- Grass Tetany/Hypomagnesemia
- Lead Toxicosis
- Lupine Toxicity
- Nitrate and Nitrite Toxicosis
- Organophosphate Toxicity
- Poison Hemlock (*Conium* spp.) Toxicity
- Tobacco Toxicosis
- Water Hemlock

Suggested Reading
Burrows GE, Tyrl RJ. Lauraceae, Apocynaceae. In: Burrows GE, Tyrl RJ eds, Toxic Plants of North America, 2nd ed. Ames: Wiley-Blackwell, 2013.
Forero L, Nader G, Craigmill A, DiTomaso J, Puschner B, Maas J: Livestock-poisoning plants of California. Oakland, CA: Division of Agriculture and Natural Resources, 2010, Publication 8398. 44 pp. http://anrcatalog.ucdavis.edu/pdf/8398.pdf
Casteel SW. Taxine alkaloids. In: Plumlee KH ed, Clinical Veterinary Toxicology, 1st ed. St. Louis: Mosby, 2004, pp. 379–81.
Galey FG. Cardiac glycosides. In: Plumlee KH ed, Clinical Veterinary Toxicology, 1st ed. St. Louis: Mosby, 2004, pp. 386–8.
Kozikowski TA, Magdesian KG, Puschner B. Oleander intoxication in New World camelids: 12 cases (1995–2006). J Am Vet Med Assoc 2009, 235: 305–10.

Authors Birgit Puschner and Adrienne C. Bautista
Consulting Editor Christopher C.L. Chase
Acknowledgment The authors and book editors acknowledge the prior contribution of Asheesh K. Tiwary.

O

ORAL DISORDERS

 BASICS

OVERVIEW
• Disorders of the oral cavity and esophagus often provoke decreased feed intake, weight loss, and reduced production.
• The lips of cattle are relatively immobile and insensitive, which may contribute to indiscriminate eating habits.
• The lips of small ruminants and camelids are much more mobile and allow superior prehension compared with cattle. In cattle and goats, the upper lip is complete; sheep and camelids have a dividing philtrum, enhancing mobility.
• Dental formula of cattle, sheep, and goats
  ◦ Deciduous: 2 (incisors 0/4, premolars 3/3) = 20
  ◦ Permanent: 2 (incisors 0/4, premolars 3/3, molars 3/3) = 32
• Dental formula of camelids
  ◦ Deciduous: 2 (incisors 1–2/3, canine 1/1, premolars 2–3/1–2) = 18–22
  ◦ Permanent: 2 (incisors 1/3, canine 1/1, premolars 1–2/1–2, molars 3/3) = 30–32
  ◦ The upper incisor is caudal to the last lower incisor. Adult canine and upper incisor teeth are the "fighting teeth," which are larger in males.
• The parotid, mandibular, and sublingual glands are the three largest salivary glands.

INCIDENCE/PREVALENCE
Oral disorders are normally sporadic unless a contagious pathogen (typically viral) is involved.

GEOGRAPHIC DISTRIBUTION
Worldwide

SYSTEMS AFFECTED
Digestive

PATHOPHYSIOLOGY
• The lips and tongue of cattle are relatively insensitive, which contributes to oral trauma and ingestion of foreign bodies.
• Lip lesions are more often clinically significant in camelids and small ruminants; tongue lesions are more likely to adversely affect feeding of cattle.
• Grazing short grass and sandy soil can predispose to abnormal dental wear, dental injuries, decay, and dental loosening.
• The feeding of abrasive materials may predispose to the development of actinomycosis, actinobacillosis, and necrotic stomatitis through mucus membrane trauma.

HISTORICAL FINDINGS
• Anorexia or abnormal feeding activity, often accompanied by weight loss or reduced production, is common.

SIGNALMENT
N/A

PHYSICAL EXAMINATION FINDINGS
• Poor condition
• Fever (variable)
• Lesions on gums, dental pad, hard palate, or tongue
• Protruding tongue
• Abnormal odor
• Quidding
• Ptyalism
• Milk/feed from nostrils
• Swellings or tracts of maxilla or mandible
• Facial deformity
• Swelling of the throat or neck
• Extended head and neck
• Coughing
• Lymphadenopathy

GENETICS
N/A

CAUSES AND RISK FACTORS
• Causes of oral ulcers, erosions, or vesicles include trauma, foreign body penetration (e.g., foxtails), and viral infections—bluetongue, orf, bovine papular stomatitis, BVDV, VS, MCF, and FMD.
• Bacterial infections associated with erosions include *F. necrophorum* (necrotic stomatitis/laryngitis), and *Actinobacillus lignieresii* (wooden tongue). *Actinobacillus* spp. have been reported to cause stomatitis in camelids.
• Oral neoplasias include fibropapillomas (lip, mucosa, esophagus), squamous cell carcinoma, hemangioma, or hamartoma.
• Ptyalism or dysphagia can reflect retropharyngeal trauma/abscessation, foreign bodies, necrotic laryngitis, actinobacillosis, choke, megaesophagus, esophagitis, cleft palate, toxicity (slaframine, grayanotoxin, lead) and neurologic disorders (rabies, tetanus, botulism, listeriosis, and otitis media/interna).
• Mandibular/maxillary masses, swellings, or draining tracts can arise from tooth root abscesses, fractures, sequestrae, actinomycosis (lumpy jaw; *A. bovis*) sialocele, sialoadenitis, abscesses (*F. necrophorum*, *T. pyogenes*, *C. pseudotuberculosis*), cryptococcomas, or neoplasia (odontogenic, osteoma, fibroma, fibrosarcoma, lymphosarcoma).
• Quidding or abnormal regurgitation can reflect dental attrition, malocclusion, periodontal disease, retention of deciduous teeth, retropharyngeal trauma or infection, or choke, megaesophagus, and esophagitis.
• Respiratory distress can reflect retropharyngeal trauma/abscess, necrotic laryngitis, obstruction to the respiratory tract by feed material or masses, and aspiration pneumonia secondary to dysphagia.

DIAGNOSIS

DIFFERENTIAL DIAGNOSES
• Vary with signalment and clinical signs.

• Oral disorders can be associated with disease of other body systems, complicating diagnosis (e.g., concurrent respiratory signs, lameness).

CBC/BIOCHEMISTRY/URINALYSIS
• Hemoconcentration.
• Increased WBC count and fibrinogen with bacterial infection or inflammatory conditions.
• Lymphopenia reflects stress or viral infections.
• Metabolic acidosis may arise with ptyalism or dysphagia (salivary bicarbonate loss).

OTHER LABORATORY TESTS
• Bacterial culture
• Biopsy and histopathology assist confirmation of actinomycosis, actinobacillosis, neoplasia, cryptococcoma, and viral mucosal infections.
• Serology, PCR, or virus identification procedures are indicated to confirm the etiology of viral mucosal infections.

IMAGING
• Radiography: Mandibular or maxillary fractures, infections or neoplasia, sequestrae, tooth root abscesses, tooth fracture, retropharyngeal trauma, and metallic foreign bodies. Addition of contrast is useful for megaesophagus.
• Endoscopy: Cleft palate, necrotic laryngitis, retropharyngeal trauma, choke, megaesophagus, esophagitis, and neoplasms.
• Ultrasound: Retropharyngeal abscess, cellulitis, sialocele, sialoadenitis, and neoplasia.
• Computed tomography provides excellent imaging of the skull and dental structures; soft tissue anomalies are enhanced by IV contrast administration.

OTHER DIAGNOSTIC PROCEDURES
• Observe animals eating and swallowing different types of feeds.
• Complete oral examination requires physical restraint ± sedation, and an oral speculum used in concert with a good light source to visualize and palpate the oral cavity and pharynx if possible.

PATHOLOGIC FINDINGS
Vary with specific disorders.

TREATMENT

THERAPEUTIC APPROACH
• Medical management is often beneficial depending on the disorder.
• Antibiotics are indicated for bacterial infections or secondary complications such as pneumonia.
• For animals with severe and noncorrectable dental anomalies, a presoaked well-balanced pelleted diet may be fed as a mash.
• Abscessed teeth may require extraction and antimicrobials.

• Nutritional support may be necessary in animals that are dysphagic, via eosphagostomy, rumenostomy, ororuminal intubation, or parenteral nutrition.
• IV fluids may be necessary in dehydrated animals that cannot swallow and should target the animal's acid-base and electrolyte disturbances.

SURGICAL CONSIDERATIONS AND TECHNIQUES
• Emergency tracheostomy may be necessary in animals with respiratory distress related to upper airway obstructions.
• Retropharyngeal abscessation or other abscesses of the head and neck may require surgical drainage into the mouth or externally, and debridement of the affected areas.

MEDICATIONS

DRUGS OF CHOICE
• Antibiotic recommendations are made in chapters on specific conditions.
• NSAIDs are often indicated to assist pain and inflammation; flunixin meglumine is often used (1.1 mg/kg q12–24h).

CONTRAINDICATIONS
NSAIDs should not be used in dehydrated, azotemic animals.

PRECAUTIONS
Appropriate milk and meat withdrawal times must be followed for all compounds administered to food-producing animals.

POSSIBLE INTERACTIONS
N/A

FOLLOW-UP

EXPECTED COURSE AND PROGNOSIS
The prognosis is good in acute and transient infectious conditions such as orf, and guarded for severe and chronic diseases of soft tissue and bone such as actinomycosis.

POSSIBLE COMPLICATIONS
• Azotemia/renal insufficiency
• Aspiration pneumonia
• Secondary bacterial infections
• Dental loss

CLIENT EDUCATION
Focus on provision of high-quality, palatable feedstuffs and regular assessment of body condition score.

PATIENT CARE
• Response to treatments should be monitored closely, and treatment course modified accordingly.
• Monitor hydration status, electrolyte abnormalities, and acid-base status in patients that are anorexic and/or dysphagic.

PREVENTION
• Specific viral disorders can be prevented by vaccination.
• Dental care is commonly needed in aged small ruminants with dental attrition. Excessive enamel points that cause oral discomfort and ulceration, and hooks or wave mouths can be managed by floating the arcades.

MISCELLANEOUS

ASSOCIATED CONDITIONS
Aspiration pneumonia

AGE-RELATED FACTORS
Some disorders such as orf and necrotic stomatitis are much more common in young animals.

ZOONOTIC POTENTIAL
Contagious ecthyma can be transmitted to humans via contact with infected animals, fomites, or during vaccination procedures.

PREGNANCY
N/A

BIOSECURITY
• Viral mucosal diseases are contagious and appropriate biosecurity methods should be employed within herds and flocks diagnosed with one of those conditions.
• Mucosal diseases such as BVD, bluetongue, MCF, and VS require differentiation from foreign animal diseases (e.g., FMD) that threaten livestock in the United States. Consultation with regulatory veterinarians is imperative when these diseases are identified.

PRODUCTION MANAGEMENT
N/A

SYNONYMS
NA

ABBREVIATIONS
• BVDV = bovine viral diarrhea virus
• FMD = foot and mouth disease
• MCF = malignant catarrhal fever
• NSAIDs = nonsteroidal anti-inflammatory drugs
• PCR = polymerase chain reaction
• VS = vesicular stomatitis
• WBC = white blood cell

SEE ALSO
• Actinobacillosis: Wooden Tongue
• Actinomycosis: Lumpy Jaw
• Bluetongue Virus
• Calf Diphtheria/Necrotic Stomatitis
• Foot and Mouth Disease
• Orf (Contagious Ecthyma)
• Tongue Trauma
• Vesicular Stomatitis

Suggested Reading
Cebra C. Disorders of the digestive system. In: Cebra C, Anderson DE, Tibary A, Van Saun RJ, Johnson LW eds, Llama and Alpaca Care: Medicine, Surgery, Reproduction, Nutrition, and Herd Health, 1st ed. St. Louis: Elsevier, 2014, pp. 477–536.
Navarre CB, Lowder MQ, Pugh DG. Oral-esophageal diseases. In: Pugh DG ed, Sheep and Goat Medicine, 1st ed. Philadelphia: Saunders, 2002, pp. 61–8.
Smith BP. Ruminant alimentary disease. In: Smith BP ed, Large Animal Internal Medicine, 5th ed. St. Louis: Elsevier, 2015, pp. 739–67.
Van Metre DC, Tennant BC, Whitlock RH. Infectious diseases of the gastrointestinal tract. In: Divers TJ, Peek SF eds, Rebhun's Diseases of Dairy Cattle, 2nd ed. St. Louis: Saunders, 2008, pp. 200–94.
Author Marie-Eve Fecteau
Consulting Editor Erica C. McKenzie
Acknowledgment The author and book editors acknowledge the prior contribution of Jennifer M. Ivany Ewoldt and Dusty W. Nagy.

O

ORCHITIS AND EPIDIDYMITIS

BASICS

OVERVIEW
• Inflammation of the testes and epididymides may occur separately but often occur concurrently and frequently have the same etiology.
• The inflammation is most often the result of infection or trauma but can also have an autoimmune component.

INCIDENCE/PREVALENCE
• The incidence and prevalence are variable with local disease conditions. Where brucellosis and tuberculosis have been eradicated or controlled, the conditions are sporadic and relatively uncommon.
• Incidence of contagious epididymitis due to *Brucella ovis* in rams may be very high in some regions.

GEOGRAPHICAL DISTRIBUTION
Worldwide

SYSTEMS AFFECTED
Reproductive

PATHOPHYSIOLOGY
• Hematogenous spread of bacteria is the most common route of infection. Extension from other parts of the genitourinary tract is also an important route of infection.
• Periorchitis, an inflammation of the tunica vaginalis testis within the scrotum, may be directly related to orchitis or occur as an extension of peritonitis or penetrating trauma.
• Unilateral disease is more common but bilateral disease may also occur.
• In unilateral cases, local swelling and inflammation often disrupt scrotal thermoregulation, leading to problems with spermatogenesis and eventually degenerative changes in the unaffected testis.
• In most cases, epididymitis is the more common initial disease with either an extension of the infection to the testis (orchitis) or subsequent testicular degeneration.

HISTORICAL FINDINGS
• Male infertility
• Poor libido
• Observed testicular or epididymal swelling
• Incidental finding during BSE

SIGNALMENT
• All males at any age but especially those that are sexually mature.
• A form of contagious epididymitis has been described in ram lambs and may be caused by a variety of organisms including *Actinobacillus seminis*.

PHYSICAL EXAMINATION FINDINGS
• Warm, painful swelling of the entire testis or one or more segments of the epididymis is the most common sign of acute disease.

• Epididymitis most frequently involves the tail segment (cauda epididymis).
• Some cases of *Brucella ovis* epididymitis in rams are subclinical and cannot be detected by palpation alone.
• Painful animals may refuse to mate or may be reluctant to move. Frequently they walk with a stilted gait.
• Chronic disease of these organs may not be accompanied by either heat or pain. Swelling of the head, body, or tail of the epididymis may be the only clinical sign of chronic epididymitis.
• Transient testicular degeneration usually occurs subsequent to inflammation of either the testis or epididymis. Severe inflammation of one or both testes may lead to irreversible atrophy.
• Blood and/or pus may be seen in the ejaculate. In some cases, abscessation and liquefaction of the testicular parenchyma may occur with subsequent eruption and drainage through the scrotum. This is especially evident with cases of brucellosis in bulls and caseous lymphadenitis in goats.

GENETICS
N/A

CAUSES AND RISK FACTORS
Infectious
• *Brucella abortus* (bulls, camelids)
• *Brucella melitensis* (bucks, camelids)
• *Brucella ovis* (sexually mature rams)
• Epivag virus (bulls, only in Africa)
• Caseous lymphadenitis (CLA) (*Corynebacterium pseudotuberculosis*) (bucks, rams, camels)
• Tuberculosis (*Mycobacterium tuberculosis/bovis*) (bulls and camels, but scrotal lesions are uncommon)
• *Trueperella pyogenes* (bulls and rams)
• *Hemophilus* spp. (bulls, young rams)
• *Mycoplasma* spp. (ram)
• Herpesvirus III (IBR-IPV) (bulls)
• A variety of nonspecific bacteria, protozoa, and parasites have been isolated from or identified in sporadic cases of ruminant orchitis and epididymitis. Of special note are those that cause orchitis or epididymitis in rams and are differentials for *B. ovis* (i.e., *Actinobacillus seminis, Histophilus ovis, Haemophilus* spp., *Corynebacterium pseudotuberculosis ovis, Chlamydophila abortus*, and *B. melitensis*).

Traumatic
Management practices that predispose to male-male aggression can lead to problems with scrotal trauma.

DIAGNOSIS

DIFFERENTIAL DIAGNOSES
• Inguinal hernia
• Scrotal hydrocele or hematocele

• Sperm granulomas secondary to trauma or obstructive lesions
• Metastatic mesothelioma
• Lymphoma

CBC/BIOCHEMISTRY/URINALYSIS
Hematuria or pyuria

OTHER LABORATORY TESTS
• Hematospermia or pyospermia
• Immunologic or molecular-based tests for specific infectious agents (e.g., *B. ovis*)

IMAGING
• Ultrasonography may help differentiate hernia, hydrocele, etc. It will also localize the swelling to the epididymis or testis.
• Thermography may also localize inflammation.

OTHER DIAGNOSTIC PROCEDURES
• Scrotal palpation
• Semen collection and evaluation
• Semen culture
• Aseptic aspiration of scrotal fluid for culture/cytology
• Testicular fine-needle aspiration or biopsy
• *Brucella Brucellosis ovis* serologic test—complement fixation test

PATHOLOGIC FINDINGS
• Local infiltration of inflammatory cells, edema with disruption of normal histology
• Transient testicular degeneration
• Testicular atrophy
• Occluded seminiferous tubules, rete testes, vas deferens, or epididymis

TREATMENT

THERAPEUTIC APPROACH
• Unilateral castration can be effective in preserving fertility if the disease is unilateral.
• Systemic antibiotic therapy for 7–14 days or longer, combined with anti-inflammatory treatment, may resolve cases of acute bacterial orchitis. Culture and sensitivity of the organism is indicated if a bacterial etiology is suspected.
• Treatment is reportedly less effective for cases of epididymitis which is not unexpected given epididymal anatomy, as any significant occlusion of the duct can result in a spermatocele.
• Cool water hydrotherapy 30 minutes q12h for 7–10 days.
• Sexual rest.

SURGICAL CONSIDERATIONS AND TECHNIQUES
Unilateral castration should be considered if infection is not due to a contagious or reportable disease.

MEDICATIONS

DRUGS OF CHOICE
• Antibiotic selection based on culture and sensitivity testing
• Flunixin meglumine or meloxicam to reduce inflammation and for pain relief

CONTRAINDICATIONS
• Appropriate meat withdrawal times must be followed.
• Animals suspected or confirmed to have reportable or regulated diseases should not be treated with the intention of returning them to the breeding population.

PRECAUTIONS
N/A

POSSIBLE INTERACTIONS
N/A

FOLLOW-UP

EXPECTED COURSE AND PROGNOSIS
• Poor prognosis for return to fertility for the affected testis/epididymis.
• Good to guarded prognosis for normal fertility in cases where medical or surgical treatment is successful.

POSSIBLE COMPLICATIONS
Reduced fertility or sterility

CLIENT EDUCATION
• Report any detected testicular abnormalities to a veterinarian.
• Perform BSE on all males before the breeding season.

PATIENT CARE
• Frequent monitoring during therapy is recommended to evaluate the effectiveness. If no improvement is seen, unilateral castration should be considered along with a change in antibiotic.
• Re-evaluate the scrotum and testes for adhesions or atrophy 1 month after the end of therapy.
• Re-evaluate semen quality a minimum of 60 days after the end of the insult or removal of the affected testicle.

PREVENTION
• Vaccination (*Brucella ovis, Corynebacterium pseudotuberculosis*)
• Test and quarantine of herd or flock additions

MISCELLANEOUS

ASSOCIATED CONDITIONS
Seminal vesiculitis

AGE-RELATED FACTORS
N/A

ZOONOTIC POTENTIAL
Brucella abortus and *B. melitensis* are significant zoonotic concerns.

PREGNANCY
N/A

BIOSECURITY
• Report and appropriately dispose of animals infected with *Brucella* spp.
• Routine screening for scrotal disease is recommended for sheep flocks and affected animals should be tested and culled.

PRODUCTION MANAGEMENT
N/A

ABBREVIATION
• BSE = breeding soundness examination

SEE ALSO
• Breeding Soundness Examination: Bovine
• Breeding Soundness Examination: Camelid
• Breeding Soundness Examination: Small Ruminant
• Reproductive Ultrasonography: Bovine (see www.fiveminutevet.com/ruminant)
• Reproductive Ultrasonography: Camelid (see www.fiveminutevet.com/ruminant)
• Reproductive Ultrasonography: Small Ruminant (see www.fiveminutevet.com/ruminant)
• Testicular Disorders: Bovine
• Testicular Disorders: Camelid
• Testicular Disorders: Small Ruminant

Suggested Reading
Ivany JM, Anderson DE, Ayars WH, et al. Diagnosis, surgical treatment and performance after unilateral castration in breeding bulls: 21 cases (1989–1999). J Am Vet Med Assoc 2002, 220: 1198–202.
McEntee K. Reproductive Pathology of Domestic Animals. San Diego: Academic Press, 1990, pp. 263–70.
Authors Harry Momont and Celina Checura
Consulting Editor Ahmed Tibary
Acknowledgment The authors and book editors acknowledge the prior contribution of Steven D. Van Camp.

O

ORF (CONTAGIOUS ECTHYMA)

BASICS

OVERVIEW
• Orf is a highly contagious, zoonotic viral disease characterized by the development of ulcerative, pustulo-proliferative, or wart-like lesions of the skin of sheep, goats, camelids, and a variety of wild ruminants.
• Although rarely fatal, orf is an economically important disease that has resulted in severe economic losses due to international trade barriers.
• Orf can cause growth retardation and loss of body condition in young lambs and kids, and predisposes to secondary infections.

INCIDENCE/PREVALENCE
• Orf virus (ORFV) is a ubiquitous pathogen with high prevalence worldwide
• Morbidity often reaches 60–80% in a susceptible group; mortality rarely exceeds 1%.

GEOGRAPHIC DISTRIBUTION
• Worldwide in regions where sheep and goats are raised.

SYSTEMS AFFECTED
• Integument
• Digestive

PATHOPHYSIOLOGY
• Caused by the double-stranded DNA orf virus of the Parapoxvirus genus.
• ORFV can be transmitted by close contact between infected and susceptible animals, and through contact with contaminated fomites and dirt.
• ORFV does not cause latent infections; however, clinically healthy animals can act as mechanical carriers.
• ORFV is environmentally resistant and has been found to survive for up to 17 years in wool and contaminated material in dry climates.

HISTORICAL FINDINGS
Flocks or herds may be endemically affected, allowing the virus to infect vulnerable individuals; individual animals may be exposed during transport or with introduction of infected animals into groups.

SIGNALMENT
• Young kids and lambs are most often affected.
• Does and ewes may develop teat lesions while nursing affected offspring.

PHYSICAL EXAMINATION FINDINGS
• Skin lesions consist of macules, papules, vesicles, pustules, crusts, scabs, and papillomatous wart-like growths that usually start at the commissures of the lips and spread around the lip margins to the muzzle. Lesions can occasionally occur at earmarking or tail docking sites.

• In more severe cases, the skin of other areas, such as the eyes, feet, vulva, or udder may be affected.
• Occasionally, lesions may develop in the oral cavity and skin of the interdigital space, and animals may be reluctant to suckle, eat, or walk. Esophageal lesions can occur.
• A generalized persistent form of orf, characterized by severe, multifocal, proliferative dermatitis, occurs in sheep and goats. In these cases, secondary bacterial infections or maggot infestation of affected areas may occur.
• Animals that have recovered or that have been vaccinated can develop lesions that are usually less severe with a shorter clinical course.
• Outbreaks usually last 6–8 weeks.

GENETICS
N/A

CAUSES AND RISK FACTORS
Orf primarily affects young animals, and is enhanced by comingling and stress.

DIAGNOSIS

DIFFERENTIAL DIAGNOSES
Other ulcerative vesicular or proliferative dermatitis disorders, including capripox and sheep poxviruses, bluetongue virus, foot and mouth disease, or pearmouth (dermatitis of lips and muzzle caused by ingestion of prickly pear cactus).

CBC/BIOCHEMISTRY/URINALYSIS
N/A

OTHER LABORATORY TESTS
N/A

IMAGING
N/A

OTHER DIAGNOSTIC PROCEDURES
• Real-time PCR from scab material is replacing electron microscopy (EM). Unfixed scabs should be submitted at room temperature or refrigerated in a double container.
• EM relies on the identification of typical ovoid-shaped parapoxvirus virions. Other parapoxviruses, including bovine papular stomatitis virus and pseudocowpox virus, are indistinguishable by EM.
• Virus isolation is often unsuccessful but can be attempted using primary cell cultures.
• Serologic tests including serum neutralization, agar gel immunodiffusion, and complement fixation have limited diagnostic value.
• Demonstration of typical microscopic lesions (proliferative and erosive dermatitis with intracytoplasmic inclusions in keratinocytes) can aid in the diagnosis.

PATHOLOGIC FINDINGS
• Macroscopically lesions consist of ulcers, crusting, and papillomatous wart-like growths on the skin of the lips and muzzle, ranging from a few millimeters to several centimeters in size.
• Macules, papules, vesicles, and pustules can be observed. In the majority of cases, these lesions are transient and rapidly progress to crusting lesions. Within 3–4 weeks the scabs drop off, and the lesions heal.
• Orf lesions can occur in the oral cavity, and rarely extend to the esophagus and forestomachs.
• Lymph nodes draining affected areas of skin may be enlarged.
• Histologically orf lesions are characterized by papillated, hyperplastic dermatitis with a mixture of epidermal and dermal proliferation with hyperkeratosis and parakeratosis.
• Eosinophilic intracytoplasmic viral inclusions may be found in the stratum spongiosum. Subcorneal vesicles and pustules may be present throughout the epidermis.
• Ulcers covered by serocellular crust containing bacterial colonies or foreign debris can occur.

TREATMENT

THERAPEUTIC APPROACH
• No specific treatments in animals.
• When possible, affected animals should be isolated in shaded pens and provided with clean water and good-quality feed.

SURGICAL CONSIDERATIONS AND TECHNIQUES
N/A

MEDICATIONS

DRUGS OF CHOICE
Broad-spectrum antibiotics and topical insecticides should be used in animals with secondary bacterial infections or maggot infestation, respectively.

CONTRAINDICATIONS
N/A

PRECAUTIONS
• Appropriate milk and meat withdrawal times must be followed for all compounds administered to food-producing animals.
• Common zoonotic disease.

POSSIBLE INTERACTIONS
N/A

FOLLOW-UP

EXPECTED COURSE AND PROGNOSIS
• In the majority of cases, lesions heal spontaneously within 3–4 weeks.
• Disseminated persistent orf occurs in some animals. In these cases, lesions can be severe and can extend to other areas including the face, ears, feet, vulva, teats, and scrotum. In these cases, lesions can persist for weeks or months, with the risk of death from secondary bacterial infections.

POSSIBLE COMPLICATIONS
• Secondary bacterial infections or maggot infestation of ulcerated surfaces are common in animals with disseminated persistent orf.
• Foot lesions co-infected with *Dermatophilus congolensis* may result in "strawberry foot rot."
• Lesions on the udder can provoke abandonment of offspring by dams.

CLIENT EDUCATION
Ensure clients understand this is a zoonotic disease that can be contracted via handling of infected animals or the orf vaccine.

PATIENT CARE
N/A

PREVENTION
• Live ORFV vaccines, prepared by sheep skin passage or attenuated virus in cell culture, are commonly used to control the disease, but perpetuate the infection in the environment.
• The vaccine should not be used in locations where the disease has never been diagnosed.
• When animals in a flock/herd are vaccinated for the first time, all susceptible animals on the premises should be vaccinated to avoid vaccine-induced orf in nonvaccinated animals.
• On premises where orf is endemic, all lambs and goat kids should be vaccinated at 6–8 weeks of age. In subsequent years, only new lambs or kids and newly acquired animals need to be vaccinated.
• Vaccines contain live virus and can induce disease in naïve animals and humans.
• During vaccination, an area of the skin of the animal to be vaccinated is scarified, most commonly the medial aspect of the thigh, and the vaccine is brushed onto the site. The appearance of a localized lesion at the site 2–3 days later indicates successful vaccination.
• Vaccinated animals or those that recover from natural infection are susceptible to re-infection which tends to be milder and more transient.
• Sheep and goat ORFVs are essentially the same, but phylogenetic analyses have shown that ORFV has co-evolved with the species. A higher degree of protection is achieved in each species when vaccines are prepared with ORFV from the homologous species.
• Gloves should be worn during physical examination and vaccination of ruminants.
• Disinfection of surfaces and areas potentially contaminated with ORFV can be achieved using detergents, hypochlorite, alkalis, glutaraldehyde or multifaceted products (e.g., Virkon®).

 MISCELLANEOUS

ASSOCIATED CONDITIONS
N/A

AGE-RELATED FACTORS
Orf primarily affects young animals.

ZOONOTIC POTENTIAL
• Orf is more common among farmers, sheep shearers, and veterinarians due to exposure to small ruminants. Slaughterhouse workers, butchers, and meat handlers are sometimes infected from carcasses.
• Orf infection in humans manifests as one or several localized pustules and scabby lesions on the hands, face, or ears. The lesions form painful nodules that heal in 4–6 weeks.
• Multifocal, widespread skin lesions can occur in immunocompromised people.

PREGNANCY
N/A

BIOSECURITY
• New animals should be acquired from orf-free flocks or herds.
• The purchase of new animals from sale barns should be avoided.

• Visitors should wear clean boots and coveralls, and gloves if handling small ruminants.

PRODUCTION MANAGEMENT
N/A

SYNONYMS
• Contagious ecthyma
• Soremouth
• Cutaneous or contagious pustular dermatitis or stomatitis
• Infectious labial dermatitis
• Scabby mouth
• Ecthyma contagiosum

ABBREVIATIONS
• EM = electron microscopy
• ORFV = orf virus
• PCR = polymerase chain reaction

SEE ALSO
• Bluetongue Virus
• Foot and Mouth Disease
• Photosensitization
• Sheep and Goat Pox

Suggested Reading
de la Concha-Bermejill A, Guo J, Zhang Z, et al. Severe persistent orf in young goats. J Vet Diagn Invest 2003, 15: 423–31.
Guo J, Rasmussen J, Wünschmann A, et al. Genetic characterization of orf viruses isolated from various ruminant species of a zoo. Vet Microbiol 2004, 99: 73–82.
Guo J, Zhang Z, Edwards J, et al. Characterization of a North American orf virus isolated from a goat with persistent, proliferative dermatitis. Virus Res 2003, 93: 169–79.
Nandi S, De UK, Chowdhury S. Current status of contagious ecthyma or orf disease in goat and sheep: A global perspective. Small Rumin Res 2011, 96: 73–82.
Spyrou V, Valiakos G. Orf virus infection in sheep or goats. Vet Microbiol 2015, 181: 178–82.

Author Andrés de la Concha-Bermejillo
Consulting Editor Erica C. McKenzie

 Client Education Handout available online

O

ORGANOPHOSPHATE TOXICITY

BASICS

OVERVIEW
• Organophosphates are anticholinesterase agents commonly found in crop and animal insecticides.
• The binding of organophosphates is irreversible.

INCIDENCE/PREVALENCE
Unknown

GEOGRAPHIC DISTRIBUTION
Worldwide

SYSTEMS AFFECTED
• Nervous
• Digestive
• Respiratory
• Musculoskeletal
• Cardiovascular

PATHOPHYSIOLOGY
• Anticholinesterase insecticides bind with and inhibit acetylcholinesterase, the enzyme that breaks down the neurotransmitter acetylcholine.
• These compounds cause acetylcholine to accumulate at nerve junctions and cause excessive synaptic activity.
• The effects are in the parasympathetic nervous system and at neuromuscular sites. Nicotinic and muscarinic receptors are activated.

SIGNALMENT
Any species can be exposed to toxic levels of organophosphate insecticides.

PHYSICAL EXAMINATION FINDINGS
Muscarinic Symptoms
Result from stimulation of the parasympathetic nervous system and are described by the acronym SLUD:
• Salivation
• Lacrimation
• Urination
• Defecation

Other Possible Muscarinic Signs
• Vomiting
• Myosis
• Bradycardia
• Dyspnea
• Bloating
• Transient diarrhea

Nicotinic (Neuromuscular) Signs
• Muscle tremors
• Hyperthermia
• Ataxia
• Progressive paresis to paralysis

Central Nervous System (CNS) Signs
• Depression
• Seizures
• Behavioral changes

CAUSES AND RISK FACTORS
• Domestic animals are usually exposed to organophosphate insecticides due to accidental ingestion, or improper treatment by owners. Organophosphate insecticides are used primarily on crops and other plants but can be used as topical insecticides on animals. They were previously commonly used for ectoparasite control.
• Organophosphates are anticholinesterase agents commonly found in insecticides.
• Acute toxicity of organophosphates depends strongly on kinetics of absorption:
  ○ LD50 for parathion in mice is 5 mg/kg orally.
  ○ 10–40 mg/kg can be lethal in calves exposed to coumaphos.
  ○ A dermal dose of 8 mg/kg has caused death in sheep when using coumaphos.
  ○ Malathion causes clinical signs at 10–20 mg/kg in calves and 50–100 mg/kg in adult cattle when applied externally.
  ○ Toxic dose of malathion in sheep is 50–100 mg/kg dermally.

DIAGNOSIS

DIFFERENTIAL DIAGNOSES
• Gastrointestinal causes of diarrhea
• Metabolic disturbances such as nervous ketosis
• Nonprotein nitrogen toxicosis
• Pesticides including carbamates, rodenticides
• Plant toxicities that cause tremor or ataxia
• Rabies
• Toxins such as strychnine or lead

CBC/BIOCHEMISTRY/URINALYSIS
N/A

OTHER LABORATORY TESTS
N/A

OTHER DIAGNOSTIC PROCEDURES
• Diagnosis is often based on known exposure to organophosphate and response to treatment with atropine.
• Cholinesterase activity will be inhibited with exposure to an organophosphate.
• Cholinesterase activity in whole blood, retina, or brain that is 25–50% of normal for the species being tested indicates cholinesterase inhibitor toxicosis. If less than 25% of normal, clinical correlation of symptoms is required for diagnosis.
• Check with the laboratory before submitting blood samples because some testing methods may require serum instead of whole blood samples.
• Half of the brain should be submitted for homogenization, as cholinesterase activity varies in different brain regions.

PATHOLOGIC FINDINGS
None

TREATMENT

THERAPEUTIC APPROACH
• Provide supportive care for SLUD or secondary clinical signs such as dehydration.
• Wash the animal with soap and water if dermal exposure occurs, to decrease absorption. Clipping may be advisable in long-haired animals.
• Administer activated charcoal at a dose of 1–2 lb PO per 500 kg animal.
• Atropine should be given at a dose of 0.5–1.0 mg/kg to competitively bind acetylcholine. Give one-fourth of the initial dose IV (watch the pupils and see if they start to return to normal) and the rest subcutaneously or intramuscularly. Dosage can be repeated in 6 hours if clinical signs recur.

MEDICATIONS

DRUGS OF CHOICE
• Activated charcoal
• Atropine
• Oximes such as pralidoxime chloride (2-PAM) that are used to release the acetylcholinesterase-organophosphate bond can **not** be used due to the irreversible nature of organophosphate binding to acetylcholinesterase.

PRECAUTIONS
Appropriate milk and meat withdrawal times must be followed for all compounds administered to food-producing animals.

FOLLOW-UP

EXPECTED COURSE AND PROGNOSIS
Good prognosis if treated promptly

POSSIBLE COMPLICATIONS
Bloating, inhalation pneumonia

PATIENT CARE
• Heart rate
• Respiration
• Fluid and feed intake

PREVENTION
• Closely follow instructions for dilution and application found on organophosphate insecticide label.
• Premises should be washed and contaminated soil removed. Runoff can poison fish and aquatic animals.

• Avoid use of organophosphate insecticides for ectoparasite control, especially on sick or debilitated animals.

 MISCELLANEOUS

ZOONOTIC POTENTIAL
• Organophosphate toxicity is not a transmissible disease; however, humans are also susceptible to toxic exposures.
• Follow labeled instructions and precautions when handling organophosphate insecticides.
• Use caution when washing poisoned animals.

ABBREVIATIONS
• 2-PAM = pralidoxime chloride
• LD50 = estimated dose at which 50% of the population is expected to die
• SLUD = salivation, lacrimation, urination, defecation

SEE ALSO
• Ketosis: Dairy Cattle
• Lead Toxicosis

• Metaldehyde Toxicosis
• Rabies
• Rodenticide Toxicity
• Strychnine Poisoning

Suggested Reading
Aiello SE ed. Organophosphate insecticides. In: Merck Veterinary Manual, 8th ed. Whitehouse Station, NJ: Merck & Co., 1998.
Budavari S. The Merck Index, 12th ed. CD-ROM. Version 12:3a. Whitehouse Station, NJ: Chapman & Hall/CRCnetBASE, 2000.
Lewis RA: Lewis' Dictionary of Toxicology. Boca Raton, FL: Lewis Publishers, 1998.
Lloyd WE. Chemical detection techniques for diagnosing dairy herd health problems. J Dairy Sci 1978, 61: 676–8.
Meister RT. Farm Chemicals Handbook. Willoughby, OH: Meister Publishing Co., 2001.
Osweiler GD. Organophosphorus and organophosphate insecticides. In: Toxicology. Baltimore: Williams & Wilkins, 1996.
Pohanish RP. Sittig's Handbook of Toxic and Hazardous Chemicals and Carcinogens, 4th ed. Norwich, NY: Noyes Publications/William Andrew Publishing, 2002.
Smith BP ed. Toxicology of organic compounds. In: Large Animal Internal Medicine, 3rd ed. St. Louis: Mosby, 2002.
Tilley LP, Smith FWK Jr. ed. Organophosphate and carbamate toxicity. In: The 5-Minute Veterinary Consult—Canine and Feline, 3rd ed. Philadelphia: Lippincott, Williams & Wilkins, 2004.
Author Steve Ensley
Consulting Editor Christopher C.L. Chase

O

OSTEOCHONDROSIS

BASICS

OVERVIEW
Osteochondrosis (OCD) results from defective endochondral ossification. The defect may cause dissection cartilage flaps (osteochondrosis dessicans), subchondral bone cysts, or physitis. "Dyschondroplasia" and "chondrodysplasia" are other terms used for osteochondrosis.

INCIDENCE/PREVALENCE
True incidence is unknown. It appears most commonly among registered beef bulls and male and female show cattle of both beef and, to a lesser extent, dairy breeds because these animals are fed diets supporting maximum growth for extended periods of time. Among commercial beef and dairy replacements, the condition is rare because these animals are fed to support relatively slow growth. Although lesions are common in feedlot cattle, these animals rarely show clinical disease because they attain market weight before clinical signs become severe.

GEOGRAPHIC DISTRIBUTION
N/A

SYSTEMS AFFECTED
Musculoskeletal

PATHOPHYSIOLOGY
• In osteochondrosis, cartilage cells fail to differentiate normally and calcification fails to occur; however, the cartilage cells continue to grow, resulting in a zone of hypertrophied cartilage cells.
• Synovial fluid provides nutrition to the immature joint cartilage. A thicker zone of cartilage results in decreased nutrition to the basal layer of the cartilage cells. This results in degeneration and necrosis of the cartilage cells. The necrotic area can form the basis of a fissure that can lead to dissecting flaps, which present as osteochondrosis dissecans.
• Direct trauma has also been cited as a source of necrosis and eventual fragmentation.
• Subchondral bone cysts may result from thickened cartilage that infolds into subchondral bone of weight-bearing surfaces. Studies suggest that subchondral bone cysts may develop from defective connective tissue or cartilage rather than endochondral ossification. This theory suggests that the cartilage cracks following mechanical trauma, creates an opening, and synovial fluid pumps through the defect into subchondral bone during weight bearing.
• Physitis is associated with thickening and weakening of the growth plate cartilage.

HISTORICAL FINDINGS
Animals often have a post-legged conformation with abnormally straight stifle and tarsus joints.

SIGNALMENT
• There is no specific breed predilection in cattle, pigs, and goats. Hereditary dyschondroplasia ("spider lamb syndrome") in Suffolk and Suffolk crossbred lambs has been recognized.
• Reported in animals as young as 5–7 months, but overt clinical signs usually are observed in cattle between 12 and 24 months of age.
• More common in males and among males, bulls.

PHYSICAL EXAMINATION FINDINGS
• The primary clinical sign in cattle is lameness and joint effusion. Joint effusion is thought to be associated with joint capsule proliferation and synovial fluid production due to inflammation. The most commonly affected joints include stifle, tarsus, carpus, and shoulder, and multiple joint involvement is common.
• Affected cattle are usually reluctant to move and walk with a short-strided gait with minimal flexion of the stifle and hock.

GENETICS
May reflect the effects of genetic selection for rapid growth

CAUSES AND RISK FACTORS
• The exact cause of osteochondrosis is unknown.
• The most important risk factor for OCD is rapid weight gain during a young animal's period of cartilage maturation, prior to 2 years of age.
• High-energy and protein diets producing rapid growth have been implicated.
• The disease is more common among registered or valuable animals; however, this apparent predisposition probably reflects superimposed effects of genetic selection for rapid growth, diets composed to support maximum growth, and the increased likelihood of more definitive diagnostics in valuable animals.
• Mineral imbalances including calcium, phosphorus, copper, and zinc are thought to contribute to the development of osteochondrosis.
• Cattle raised on concrete floors with limited exercise are thought to be more predisposed.

DIAGNOSIS

DIFFERENTIAL DIAGNOSES
• Differential diagnoses include disease conditions causing either polyarthritis or multiple limb lameness. Thus, diseases such as mycoplasmosis, *Histophilus somni* infections, and bacterial endocarditis are likely differentials. Mycoplasmosis and *Histophilus* infection are usually associated with respiratory signs. *Histophilus* can also result in

encephalitis. Joint fluid analysis with both mycoplasmosis and *Histophilus somni* infections are associated with marked increase in white cell count and protein. PCR on joint fluid can be used to identify *Mycoplasma*. Signs of right-sided heart failure and presence of a systolic murmur are characteristic in endocarditis.
• Septic physitis, a common sequela to salmonellosis, may appear as a lameness involving multiple limbs and multiple swollen joints; however, joint distention is usually absent in this condition and examination will reveal that the swelling is localized to the physis, rather than joints.
• Laminitis should be considered as a differential. Cattle with chronic laminitis will have altered hoof growth. Laminitis will be confirmed by close examination and trimming of the hooves. Joint distention will be absent in cattle with laminitis.

OTHER LABORATORY TESTS
Joint fluid analysis reveals a nonseptic inflammation with mild to moderate increase in leukocyte count and protein.

IMAGING
Radiology
• Definitive diagnosis of osteochondrosis is confirmed by radiographic findings.
• Lesions are either the appearance of subchondral bone irregularity with bone fragmentation referred to as osteochondrosis dessicans or subchondral bone cysts characterized by periarticular focal areas of subchondral bone lucency.
• The stifle joint is the most commonly affected joint followed by the tarsal joint.
• Bilateral radiographs should be considered although clinical signs of bilateral disease might not occur.
• Osteochondrosis can lead to degenerative joint disease.

Arthroscopy
• Arthroscopy can be an effective technique for the diagnosis and treatment of osteochondrosis in cattle, sheep, goats, and camelids.
• Equipment costs and subsequent surgery may be prohibitive for most individuals.

TREATMENT

THERAPEUTIC APPROACH
• Conservative therapy includes stall rest for 1–3 months.
• Deep bedding and dirt-floored or pasture housing are recommended.
• Rations should be balanced with respect to mineral micronutrients. Energy content of the diet should be dramatically decreased to limit the patient's rate of gain.

• Nonsteroidal anti-inflammatory drugs may be considered for short-term palliative therapy.
• In feedlots, therapy should not be attempted and affected cattle should be marketed immediately.

SURGICAL CONSIDERATIONS AND TECHNIQUES

Surgical treatment involving removal of the osteochondral fragment and debridement of the fragment bed or debridement of the cyst in cases of subchondral bone cyst may be considered in valuable animals; however, no controlled clinical trials have examined the efficacy of these procedures in cattle.

MEDICATIONS

DRUGS OF CHOICE

• Meloxicam: 0.5 mg/kg SQ or IV, 1 mg/kg PO q24h (cattle), 2 mg/kg loading dose then 1mg/kg q24h (goats and sheep)
• Flunixin meglumine: 1.1–2.2 mg/kg IV q12–24h
• Ketoprofen: 2–4 mg/kg IV or IM q24h (cattle and sheep); 3 mg/kg IV or IM q24h (goats)
• Phenylbutazone: 10–20 mg/kg orally as loading dose then 5–10 mg/kg q48h. In the United States, use is discouraged in food-producing animals and prohibited for use in female dairy cattle 20 months of age or older.

PRECAUTIONS

Appropriate milk and meat withdrawal times must be followed for all compounds administered to food-producing animals.

FOLLOW-UP

EXPECTED COURSE AND PROGNOSIS

Cases with signs of lameness and secondary degenerative joint disease have a poor

prognosis. May improve with surgical intervention.

POSSIBLE COMPLICATIONS

• Degenerative joint disease
• Decreased production

CLIENT EDUCATION

Breeding stock with clinical disease will likely have a shortened productive lifespan due to the anticipated development of degenerative joint disease and culling should be considered.

PATIENT CARE

• Rations should be balanced with respect to mineral micronutrients. Energy content of the diet should be dramatically decreased and the patient's rate of gain limited.
• Activity should be restricted.

PREVENTION

• The diet and housing of herd mates of affected animals should be examined.
• Rations should be balanced with respect to mineral micronutrients. Energy content of the diet should be decreased to the level needed to support economically relevant rates of gain.

MISCELLANEOUS

ASSOCIATED CONDITIONS

Degenerative joint disease

AGE-RELATED FACTORS

Osteochondrosis has been reported in animals as young as 5–7 months, but overt clinical signs usually are observed in cattle 12–24 months of age.

PRODUCTION MANAGEMENT

See "Causes and Risk Factors"

SYNONYMS

• Chondrodysplasia
• Dyschondroplasia

ABBREVIATIONS

• OCD = osteochondrosis
• PCR = polymerase chain reaction

SEE ALSO

• Lameness (by species)
• Laminitis in Cattle
• Pain Management (see www.fiveminutevet.com/ruminant)

Suggested Reading

Davies IH, Munro, R. Osteochondrosis in bull beef cattle following lack of dietary mineral and vitamin supplementation. Vet Rec 1999, 145: 232–3.

Hill BD, Sutton RH, Thompson H. Investigation of osteochondrosis in grazing beef cattle. Aust Vet J 1998, 76: 171–5.

Lardé H, Nichols S. Arthroscopy in cattle: technique and normal anatomy. Vet Clin North Am Food Anim Pract 2014, 30: 225–45.

Nichols S, Lardé H. Noninfectious joint disease in cattle. Vet Clin North Am Food Anim Pract 2014, 30: 205–23.

Trostle SS, Nicoll RG, Forrest LJ, et al. Bovine osteochondrosis. Compend Contin Educ Pract Vet 1998, 20: 856–63.

Trostle SS, Nicoll RG, Forrest LJ, Markel MD. Clinical and radiographic findings, treatment, and outcome in cattle with osteochondrosis: 29 cases (1986–1996). J Am Vet Med Assoc 1997, 211: 1566–70.

Tryon KA, Farrow CS. Osteochondrosis in cattle. Vet Clin North Am Food Anim Pract 1999, 15: 265–74.

Author Munashe Chigerwe
Consulting Editor Kaitlyn A. Lutz

O

OSTERTAGIASIS

BASICS

OVERVIEW
• *Ostertagia* is a nematode parasite of the gastric glands and lumen of the abomasum of cattle.
• The subfamily Ostertaginae is divided into several morphologically distinguishable but biologically similar genera that are somewhat host specific.
• *Teladorsagia* and *Marshallagia* of sheep and goats, *Camelostrongylus* and other genera of ostertagids in cameloids, cervids, and antelope may cause a similar syndrome in their hosts.

INCIDENCE/PREVALENCE
• All animals in a pasture are exposed to infection but younger animals are more likely to show clinical signs of disease.
• Older cattle become resistant to the parasite but still may have economically important infection, presumably due to anorexia and decreased milk production.
• Clinical disease has decreased tremendously in the past 30–40 years but economic losses still appear to be prevalent where cattle are grazed in high rainfall or irrigated pastures.

GEOGRAPHIC DISTRIBUTION
• *Ostertagia ostertagi* is the most economically important nematode parasite of cattle in temperate regions and *Teladorsagia circumcincta* and *Marshallagia marshalli* are among the most important parasites of small ruminants in temperate and Mediterranean climates.
• Transmission occurs in cool temperate climates following the onset of spring grazing.
• Transmission in Mediterranean climates begins after the onset of rains and persists until the warm dry season.

SYSTEMS AFFECTED
• Digestive
• Cardiovascular

PATHOPHYSIOLOGY
• The disease is associated with the emergence of larvae from the gastric glands, causing cellular hyperplasia leading to increased abomasal pH, lowered serum protein, and anorexia. The number of larval worms emerging from gastric glands determines the severity of disease.
• Because of increased pH, pepsinogen is not converted into pepsin and protein is not denatured.
• Abomasal hyperplasia may be associated with leakage of fluid, leading to hypoproteinemia and diarrhea.
• Anorexia causing failure to gain weight and/or produce milk is the most common observation with this infection. The animals eat less and lie around more.
• The infection/disease may be manifest at different times of the year depending on the emergence of larvae from the gastric glands.
• *Ostertagia* causes a nonspecific suppression of immunity by the host.
• Hypersensivity reactions occur with infections, which may be deleterious to both host and parasite.

HISTORICAL FINDINGS
• Anorexia manifest by lying around rather than grazing is the reason for economic loss.
• Most cattle do not exhibit signs of disease but fail to gain weight at their genetic potential.

SIGNALMENT
• All ages may become infected but young are more at risk for disease.
• Stressed animals such as first calf heifers or those which have not been previously exposed to the parasite are more likely to show signs of disease.
• Breeds that evolved in cool moist environments are more likely to possess traits making them able to become resistant to infection.

PHYSICAL EXAMINATION FINDINGS
• Weight loss and diarrhea are the most common clinical signs.
• Hypoalbuminemia and dehydration may be seen in individual animals.
• The disease is seasonal and manifest in different ways depending on the epidemiology in a geographic region.
• Type I ostertagiasis occurs following exposure to larvae on pasture during the transmission season. Emergence from the glands begins approximately 2 weeks following infection.
• Pretype II infection occurs later in the transmission season as larvae acquired on pasture enter hypobiosis (arrest). No signs are observed.
• Type II ostertagiasis occurs when the previously arrested (hypobiotic) larvae resume development. This tends to occur near the onset of the transmission season. Because large numbers of larvae emerge simultaneously, there is a much higher likelihood of clinical signs.
• Watery diarrhea with the color depending on the forage consumed.
• Submandibular edema (bottle jaw), anemia, and dehydration with a dull hair coat may be seen.

GENETICS
Zebu cattle and zebu crosses are more likely to exhibit signs of disease than European breeds of cattle.

CAUSES AND RISK FACTORS
• Ostertagids are transmitted during cool, moist grazing conditions.
• Young animals and those in early lactation are at greatest risk.
• Heavily stocked and overgrazed pastures.
• Animals on low protein diets.
• Breeds that evolved in arid or moist tropical conditions.
• When animals are producing at their genetic maximum they are at greater risk of parasitic disease because they are immunologically and nutritionally challenged.
• Hypobiosis, or arrested development within the host's abomasum during the early 4th stage. These larvae are in a state of inactivity and are not affected by the host's immune system. They survive until conditions in the environment are more favorable for resuming their life cycle.

DIAGNOSIS

DIFFERENTIAL DIAGNOSES
• Malnutrition, especially a protein-deficient diet
• Diarrhea due to intestinal parasitism
• Hypoproteinemia due to haemonchosis or fasciolosis
• Enteric viral or bacterial diseases

CBC/BIOCHEMISTRY/URINALYSIS
• Anemia with low packed cell volume but not clinically apparent.
• Hypoproteinemia, especially low serum albumin levels.
• Elevated serum pepsinogen levels >3.0 IU tyrosine, cattle or >2.0 sheep.

OTHER LABORATORY TESTS
• Fecal flotation egg counts are usually elevated but the level may not be high as individual ostertagids do not produce as many eggs as some other nematodes, and there may be dilution due to diarrhea.
• Eggs are not diagnostic as other genera of gastrointestinal nematodes produce identical thin-shelled segmented eggs.
• Culturing larval nematodes to the infective L3 stage will enable a differential identification of worms at the generic level.
• Species-specific PCR will detect eggs in feces.

OTHER DIAGNOSTIC PROCEDURES
• History of grazing permanent cool season pastures
• Age and source of animals with clinical signs
• Weight loss, diarrhea, and no fever
• Elevated serum pepsinogen and low serum protein

PATHOLOGIC FINDINGS
Gross findings include
• Edematous roughened (Morocco leather) abomasal folds
• Enlarged regional lymph nodes
• Raised umbilicated nodules on surface of abomasum
• May be sloughing of mucosa
• Elevated abomasal pH

(CONTINUED)

• Adult worms (reddish brown and about 1 cm long) may be seen on surface of abomasum; easily overlooked if not fresh and moving.

Histopathologic findings include:
• Distended gastric glands containing developing worms.
• Cells lining glands are undifferentiated with a scarcity of acid-producing cells.
• Reactive regional lymph nodes.
• Edema and inflammatory cells in submucosa.

TREATMENT
See "Medications" and "Production Management"

MEDICATIONS
DRUGS OF CHOICE
• Broad-spectrum anthelmintics approved for use in food-producing animals are the primary means of treatment and control. Withholding periods (meat and milk) should be observed.
• Virtually all of the available anthelmintics should be effective against adult and metabolically active larvae.
• Benzimidazoles and macrocyclic lactones are effective against some populations of arrested larvae. Levamisole is only effective against adult worms.
• Macrocyclic lactones have a residual effect against incoming larvae, killing them before they can enter gastric glands. This residual period (weeks to months) varies with the chemical and carrier. Residual activity may be a selection mechanism for resistance or may eradicate the worm from the facility until reintroduced by infected cattle.
• Strategic deworming selects for anthelmintic-resistant worms but also has a greater impact on total worm populations, lowering numbers below the economic threshold for a longer time than other approaches.
• Not treating all the animals in a herd or flock will allow the parasites in the untreated population to survive and become the refugia (a population of worms not selected for resistance). Worms in the refugia will presumably mate with survivors of the treatment and preserve the usefulness of the anthelmintic used for a longer time.
• Schemes that recognize that some animals are much more at risk than others and strive to assure that the at-risk population is exposed to fewer worms or, if exposed, treated have a chance of success.
• Providing refugia by not treating all the animals in a population may preserve the value of anthelmintics longer than treating all

the animals in a herd. Treating bulls, first and second calf cows but not older cows or treating mother cows but not suckling calves may be approaches to provide refugia.

CONTRAINDICATIONS
• The currently available anthelmintics have a wide safety margin. However, levamisole, when injected, can cause nervous signs such as salivation, lacrimation, urination, and defecation.
• Albendazole in early pregnancy in small ruminants can cause loss of the embryo or act as a teratogen.

Enhancement of Anthelmintics
• The effectiveness of benzimidazoles may be enhanced by dividing the dose over several days or by fasting overnight in a dry lot prior to treatment.
• Drug choice for each individual farm should be based on what has the highest efficacy on that farm.
• Strategic treatment with a product effective against arrested larvae in the late autumn/winter in cool climates or spring/summer dosing in the warm climates when the pasture larvae die out.

Rotation of Anthelmintics
• Slow rotation (yearly) is thought to slow onset of resistance in comparison to continual rotation.
• See chapter, Anthelmintic Resistance.

PRECAUTIONS
• Anthelmintic resistance is common in some geographic areas in *Teladorsagia* in sheep and goats but rare in *Ostertagia* in cattle, probably due to the frequency with which anthelmintics are used in the livestock populations.
• See chapter, Anthelmintic Resistance.

FOLLOW-UP
EXPECTED COURSE AND PROGNOSIS
Good when appropriate management strategies and effective anthelmintics are used in combination.

POSSIBLE COMPLICATIONS
Economic loss due to decreased production (weight gains)

CLIENT EDUCATION
It is important to educate clients on the proper administration of anthelmintics and alternative management practices in order to decrease resistance.

PATIENT CARE
• Providing sufficient protein is vital with ostertagiasis. During the periparturient period, increased protein will lessen egg production by gastrointestinal nematodes.
• A high protein diet may mask some signs of disease and may also aid in the immune response of the host against the parasite.

PREVENTION
• See "Production Management."
• Vaccination is an approach likely to be successful. Commercial vaccines have not been produced although experimental vaccines have shown promise.

MISCELLANEOUS
AGE-RELATED FACTORS
• Livestock develop resistance to infection following repeated exposure to larvae. However, the resistance is not complete and parasites can occur in any age animal.
• Older cattle may become infected but are more resistant to effects of the worms and can be used to clear larvae from a pasture.

PRODUCTION MANAGEMENT
• Management systems that lower the exposure of hosts to parasites can be devised. These systems may not optimize the value of forages but they result in healthier livestock.
• Utilizing pastures that have been used for cropping, especially in the last half of the grazing season, results in grazing parasite-free pastures and by the following year any larvae deposited on the cropland will not survive until the next grazing.
• Alternate or co-grazing with other species or classes of livestock may harvest larvae from the pasture. The Ostertaginae in sheep and goats do not infect cattle, and vice versa. Horses do not share *Ostertagia* and can be safely grazed in areas dangerous to ruminants.
• Warm season transmission: Autumn/winter treatment and move young animals into barns or dry lots.
• Cool season transmission: Late spring/summer treatment and move young animals to pastures with low numbers of parasitic larvae.
• Pastures in which plants high in condensed tannins are grazed may be helpful as some of the incoming larvae are adversely affected.
• The physical structure of browse plants is a challenge for larvae to ascend, so the animals' chance of acquiring larvae diminishes as the distance from the ground increases.
• Predacious fungi have been evaluated as agents which kill larvae in pastures. One species, *Duddingtonia flagrans*, is able to traverse the digestive tract and is present in the fecal pat when the larvae hatch. Feeding spores or incorporating them in ruminal boluses has the capacity to lower pasture contamination.

SEE ALSO
• Anthelmintic Resistance
• Parasite Control Programs (by species)

Suggested Reading
Barger IA, Lewis RJ, Brown GF. Survival of infective larvae of nematode parasites of

O

cattle during drought. Vet Parasitol 1984, 14: 143–52.

Canals A, Zarlenga DS, Almeria S, Gasbarre LC. Cytokine profile induced by a primary infection with *Ostertagia ostertagi* in cattle. Vet Immunol Immunopathol 1997, 58: 63–75.

Charlier J, Demeler J, Hoglund J, et al. *Ostertagia ostertagi* in first-season grazing cattle in Belgium, Germany and Sweden: General levels of infection and related management practices. Vet Parasitol 2010, 171: 91–8.

Mihi B, Van Meulder F, Rinaldi M, et al. Analysis of cell hyperplasia and parietal cell dysfunction induced by *Ostertagia ostertagi* infection. Vet Res 2013, 44: 121–32.

Ploeger HW, Kloosterman A, Rietveld FW. Acquired immunity against *Cooperia* spp.

and *Ostertagia* spp. in calves: effect of level of exposure and timing of the midsummer increase. Vet Parasitol 1995, 58: 61–74.

Qu G, Fetterer R, Leng L, et al. *Ostertagia ostertagi* macrophage migration inhibitory factor is present in all development stages and may cross-regulate host functions through interaction with host receptor. Int J Parasitol 2014, 44: 355–67.

Suarez VH, Cabaret J. Similarities between species of the Ostertaginae (Nematoda: Trichostrongyloidea) in relation to host-specificity and climatic environment. Systemic Parasitol 1991, 20: 179–85.

Suarez VH, Busetti MR, Lorenzo RM. Comparative effects of nematode infection on *Bos taurus* and *Bos indicus* crossbred calves grazing on Argentina's Western Pampas. Vet Parasitol 1995, 58: 263–71.

Waghorn TS, Leathwick DM, Miler CM, Atkinson DS. Brave or gullible: Testing the concept that leaving susceptible parasites in refugia will slow the development of anthelmintic resistance. N Z Vet J 2008, 56: 158–63.

Williams JC, Knox JW, Marbury KS, et al. The epidemiology of *Ostertagia ostertagi* and other gastrointestinal nematodes of cattle in Louisiana. Parasitol 1987, 95: 135–53.

Yang C, Gibbs HC, Xiao L. Immunologic changes in *Ostertagia ostertagi*-infected calves treated strategically with an anthelmintic. Am J Vet Res 1993, 54: 1074–83.

Author Thomas M. Craig
Consulting Editor Kaitlyn A. Lutz

OTITIS MEDIA/INTERNA

BASICS

OVERVIEW
Inflammation of the middle ear (otitis media) or inner ear (otitis interna) usually associated with respiratory infections caused by viruses, bacteria, and *Mycoplasma* spp.

INCIDENCE/PREVALENCE
• True prevalence unknown but likely underestimated
• Incidence varies from year to year, even on the same premises
• More frequently encountered during the fall and winter months

GEOGRAPHIC DISTRUBTION
Worldwide

PATHOPHYSIOLOGY
• Otitis media/interna most commonly results from ascending viral or bacterial infection from the nasopharynx into the middle or inner ear via the eustachian tube.
• Progression from the external ear into the middle ear is uncommon but may occur secondary to ectoparasites or foreign bodies.

SYSTEMS AFFECTED
Nervous

SIGNALMENT
• All domestic ruminant species (cattle, sheep, goats, camelids).
• There is no apparent breed or sex predisposition.
• Animals of all ages are susceptible; however, pre- and post-weaned stock seem to be predisposed. Calves and lambs <1 month of age and calves 6–9 months of age are at greatest risk of disease.

PHYSICAL EXAMINATION FINDINGS
• The most common and prominent clinical signs are neurologic in origin and related to cranial nerve (CN) VII dysfunction. Drooping of the ear is often the first sign noted and occurs ipsilateral to the lesion. Ipsilateral ptosis and lip droop may be present in some cases. Deviation of the muzzle opposite the lesion may be seen in small ruminants and camelids but will not be detected in cattle.
• Signs consistent with dysfunction of CN VIII are also common and are usually manifested as head tilt and circling towards the lesion. Nystagmus and strabismus may occur but are generally uncommon.
• Concurrent bronchopneumonia is common and clinical signs consistent with respiratory disease (lethargy, anorexia, fever, increased respiratory rate and effort, nasal discharge, crackles) may also be seen.
• If associated with *Mycoplasma bovis,* polyarthritis and conjunctivitis may be encountered in affected animals or their herd mates.

GENETICS
N/A

CAUSES AND RISK FACTORS
• Progression from the external ear into the middle ear is uncommon but may occur secondary to infestation with ectoparasites (*Otobius megnini, Raillietia auris, Psoroptes cuniculi*) or damage from foreign bodies (e.g., foxtail awns).
• Feeding of contaminated waste milk has been implicated as a source of *Mycoplasma bovis* in outbreaks of otitis on dairies.
• Respiratory pathogens such as *Mannheimia haemolytica, Pasteurella multocida, Mycoplasma* spp., and *Histophilus somni* can frequently be isolated from animals with otitis. Of the aforementioned pathogens, *Mycoplasma* spp. is the organism most frequently associated with clinical disease and has the most impact on the design of treatment regimens.
• *Trueperella pyogenes* can be frequently isolated from animals with chronic otitis and isolation of this organism should not be considered significant.
• Numerous environmental organisms (*Bacillus* spp., *Staphylococcus* spp., *E. coli*) have been isolated from affected individuals.

Risk Factors
• Factors that increase the risk of respiratory disease within a population greatly increase the occurrence of otitis.
• Overcrowding, failure of passive transfer, co-mingling, long distance transport, excessive weight loss during transport (shrink), adverse environmental conditions, feeding of raw, unpasteurized waste milk, and poor herd health management programs are likely to contribute to the development of disease within both individual animals and populations.

DIAGNOSIS

DIFFERENTIAL DIAGNOSES
• Although signs of peripheral vestibular disease predominate in ruminants with otitis media/interna, differentiation from central vestibular disease is important to establish a list of differential diagnoses. With peripheral vestibular disease animals are bright, alert, and aware of their surroundings and have no evidence of conscious proprioceptive deficits. If nystagmus is detected in animals with peripheral disease, it is consistently horizontal. Animals affected with central vestibular disease are obtunded and show evidence of marked conscious proprioceptive deficits. If nystagmus is detected in animals with central vestibular disease it will vary in direction.
• Common differential diagnoses include listeriosis, brainstem abscesses, and thromboembolic meningoencephalitis (TEME) caused by *Histophilus somni.*

CBC/BIOCHEMISTRY/URINALYSIS
N/A

IMAGING
• Radiographs have been used to identify lesions in the tympanic bullae. Lateral and lateral oblique projections are needed to optimize diagnostic utility. With the advent of digital equipment the practicality of using radiographs as a diagnostic tool in a field setting is improved. Very specific but insensitive diagnostic modality.
• Ultrasound using a lateral approach caudal to the ramus of the mandible, and ventral to the base of the ear, provides visualization of the tympanic bullae and surrounding structures. Ultrasound is well tolerated by most ruminants and requires minimal restraint.
• Computed tomography (CT) is considered the gold standard in diagnosing otitis media. For many cattle producers, CT would not be an economically feasible option. However, for more valuable individuals, CT has the potential to increase the amount of information available to clinicians managing cases. Access to this form of diagnostic imaging would only be available at referral facilities and institutions.

OTHER DIAGNOSTIC PROCEDURES
Ancillary Diagnostic Tests
• Rarely needed to establish a specific diagnosis.
• A necropsy should be performed on all dead or moribund animals, especially when multiple animals in a group are affected.
• Analysis of cerebrospinal fluid (CSF) in calves with meningitis.
• Cultures of brain and lung tissue should be performed. When necropsy specimens are not available, specific efforts should be made to characterize the source and etiology of ongoing herd respiratory disease.
• Transtracheal wash or bronchoalveolar lavage cytology and culture may permit identification of the offending pathogens.
• *Mycoplasma* spp. are laborious and difficult to culture and some laboratories will use PCR to identify *Mycoplasma* spp.
• Cerebrospinal fluid analysis may be helpful in differentiating causes of asymmetric brainstem disease in feedlot cattle. Otitis will cause either a normal CSF composition, or alternatively, a CSF with increased concentrations of protein and neutrophils.
• Thromboembolic meningoencephalitis will typically result in a CSF which has a high cell count, a high protein concentration, a visible yellow color, and a preponderance of neutrophils.
• Listeriosis will generally cause milder increases in CSF cell counts and protein concentrations, with the predominant cell type being mononuclear cells. Likewise culture of the CSF may support specific

O

differential diagnoses; however, negative CSF cultures are common.

• In those animals with polyarthritis in concert with middle ear infections, arthrocentesis with culture and cytology may be useful in determination of the specific etiology.

• Septicemia and TEME tend to cause more dramatic changes in joint fluid composition and the predominant cell type is the neutrophil with both agents.

Herd Diagnostic Procedures

• In dairy herds, the recognition of otitis should encourage practitioners to re-evaluate the herd status with regard to *Mycoplasma bovis* mastitis, particularly if the herd has practiced feeding waste milk to calves.

• Bulk tank cultures performed on three sequential days are reasonable, low-cost strategies to screen herds for *Mycoplasma* spp. mastitis.

• When multiple cases of otitis are recognized in calves <1 month of age on a dairy, practitioners should establish the effectiveness of colostrum administration practices. Serum protein concentration should be determined on all calves <10 days of age. Calves with serum protein concentrations <5.2 g/dL should be classified as having inadequate passive transfer.

• If >20% of calves have less than adequate passive transfer status, immediately targeted intervention should be undertaken to correct deficiencies.

TREATMENT

THERAPEUTIC APPROACH

• Antimicrobials are usually used in affected animals. Unfortunately, no antimicrobials are labeled for the treatment of otitis media/interna in food-producing animals. Any antimicrobials used for treatment should follow extra-label guidelines, and those that are strictly prohibited should not be administered.

• Antimicrobial treatment designed to target pathogens associated with respiratory disease for calves that have concurrent infections should be considered.

• Due to the role that *Mycoplasma* spp. play in the disease process, antimicrobials with a spectrum of activity against this pathogen should be considered first-line agents.

SURGICAL CONSIDERATIONS AND TECHNIQUES

Tympanic bulla osteotomy is a surgical option to treat otitis media/interna in valuable individuals and has been used with some success in small ruminants and camelids.

MEDICATIONS

DRUGS OF CHOICE

• Reasonable antimicrobial choices include florfenicol, tulathromycin, and gamithromycin since they have documented efficacy against *Mycoplasma bovis*.

• In animals with respiratory disease, enrofloxacin would be a reasonable antimicrobial choice. However, extra-label use of fluoroquinolones in food-producing animals in the United States is strictly prohibited and their use in animals without respiratory disease is considered illegal.

• Anti-inflammatory drugs (flunixin meglumine 1.1–2.2 mg/kg IV q12–24h, meloxicam 1 mg/kg PO q24h) are indicated to provide pain relief.

CONTRAINDICATIONS

• No antimicrobials are currently labeled specifically for the treatment of food-producing animals with otitis media/interna. Guidelines for extra-label drug use as defined by the Animal Medicinal Drug Use Clarification Act (AMDUCA), or similar organization guidelines in other countries, should be followed.

• Appropriate milk and meat withdrawal times must be followed for all compounds administered to food-producing animals.

FOLLOW-UP

EXPECTED COURSE/PROGNOSIS

Prognosis for recovery is fair to good with long-term antimicrobial therapy, with 50–75% of treated animals demonstrating partial to complete improvement in clinical signs. Animals with chronic disease or meningitis have a poor prognosis.

POSSIBLE COMPLICATIONS

Extension of infection into the central nervous system and subsequent development of meningitis is possible, particularly in cases with a prolonged course.

PATIENT CARE

Affected animals should be examined regularly with examinations focused on evaluating improvement in clinical signs related to the vestibular system. In animals that fail to respond or that worsen, complicating factors should be considered. See "Possible Complications" and Expected Course and Prognosis."

PREVENTION

See "Age-Related Factors" and "Biosecurity."

MISCELLANEOUS

ASSOCIATED CONDITIONS

Pneumonia. See "Causes and Risk Factors."

AGE-RELATED FACTORS

• Among older calves 6–9 months of age, factors which increase the incidence of respiratory disease will likely increase the incidence of otitis media/interna. In neonatal calves, group housing, inadequate passive transfer of colostral immunoglobulins and feeding raw milk, particularly waste milk on dairies with endemic *Mycoplasma bovis* mastitis, are important additional risk factors.

• When multiple cases of otitis are recognized in calves <1 month of age on a dairy, practitioners should establish the effectiveness of colostrum administration practices.

ZOONOTIC POTENTIAL

N/A

PREGNANCY

N/A

BIOSECURITY

Avoid buying stock from co-mingled groupings (e.g., sale barns). Quarantine of newly arriving stock for a minimum of 3 weeks and testing each arrival for persistent infection with bovine viral diarrhea virus (BVDV) can be helpful in the diagnosis and prevention of the disease. Screen any purchased lactating animals for mastitis or test newly purchased heifers or dry cows upon initiation of lactation.

PRODUCTION MANAGEMENT

• Inadequate vaccination against respiratory disease, mixing animals from multiple sources, and inadequate preconditioning programs should all be considered risk factors.

• In a feedlot setting, adequate preconditioning programs including single sourcing of pen lots, immunization programs for respiratory viruses, and *M. haemolytica* and bunk adjustment are important factors.

• On dairy farms, efforts should focus on adequacy of passive transfer in calves, elimination of group housing for young calves (if disease present or at high risk), and avoiding feeding of unpasteurized or nonacidified waste milk.

SYNONYMS

N/A

ABBREVIATIONS

• AMDUCA = Animal Medicinal Drug Use Clarification Act
• BVDV = bovine viral diarrhea virus
• CN = cranial nerve

- CSF = cerebrospinal fluid
- CT = computed tomography
- PCR = polymerase chain reaction
- TEME = thromboembolic meningoencephalitis

SEE ALSO
- Cranial Nerve Assessment and Dysfunction (see www.fiveminutevet.com/ruminant)
- *Histophilus somni* Complex
- Listeriosis

Suggested Reading
Bernier VB, Francoz D, Babkine M, et al. A retrospective study of 29 cases of otitis media/interna in dairy calves. Can Vet J 2012, 53: 957–62.
Francoz D, Fecteau G, Desrochers A, et al. Otitis media in dairy calves: A retrospective study of 15 cases (1987–2002). Can Vet J 2004, 45: 661–6.

Van Biervliet J, Perkins GA, Woodie B, et al. Clinical signs, computed tomographic imaging, and management of chronic otitis media/interna in dairy calves. J Vet Intern Med 2004, 18: 907–10.
Villarroel A, Heller MC, Lane VM. Imaging study of myringotomy in dairy calves. Bov Pract 2006, 40: 14–17.

Author Brent C. Credille
Consulting Editor Kaitlyn A. Lutz

O

OVARIAN CYSTIC DEGENERATION

BASICS

OVERVIEW
• Ovarian cystic degeneration (OCD) is an anovular condition that occurs most commonly in dairy cattle and goats but can affect any ruminant species.
• Affected females may or may not display estrus. The core pathology is a failure of the dominant follicle to ovulate.
• Anovulatory follicles are a common finding in camelids that are not mated. It is sometimes referred to as cystic ovarian disease. However, it does not have the same physiopathology as OCD in cattle.

INCIDENCE/PREVALENCE
• Highly variable among herds and species.
• 10–20% in lactating dairy cows.
• The apparent incidence in dairy cattle is greatly influenced by the timing of postpartum examinations as many cows will develop OCD and then spontaneously recover before the end of the voluntary waiting period.
• Anovulatory follicles are common in camelids that are not mated (5–8% alpacas, 10–20% llamas, 30–40% camels).

GEOGRAPHIC DISTRIBUTION
Worldwide

SYSTEMS AFFECTED
Reproductive

PATHOPHYSIOLOGY
• Ovulation failure, associated with follicular growth to the point of deviation and beyond, appears to be related to inadequate LH pulses for follicular development or the absence of an LH surge sufficient to cause ovulation.
• Large follicular cysts (greater than normal ovulatory size) may represent a lack of a positive feedback effect of estrogen on the hypothalamic-pituitary axis, resulting in the absence of the LH surge necessary for ovulation and luteinization of the follicle.
• There are two types of cyst described. Follicular cysts are thin-walled structures that produce varying amounts of estradiol but they do not produce progesterone. Luteal cysts have a thicker wall and represent a degree of luteinization occurring without ovulation. Luteal cysts produce variable amounts of progesterone.
• Cysts are generally larger than normal follicular and luteal structures but this is not a necessary condition. OCD occurs when the cysts are steroidogenically active and interrupt normal ovulatory cycles. Cysts may occasionally be diagnosed in cycling or pregnant animals but these are presumed to be steroidogenically inactive and of no clinical consequence.
• In small ruminants, OCD diagnosis is complicated by seasonal factors (ewes and does).

• In camelids, in a large proportion of non-mated cycling females the follicle continues to grow, forming a large anovulatory follicle which loses its ability to ovulate after mating. These follicles may become hemorrhagic or even luteinize. They do not seem to affect follicular wave dynamics in all cases.

HISTORICAL FINDINGS
Complaint of anestrus or erratic estrus cycles

SIGNALMENT
• All ruminants but principally dairy cattle.
• Reported more commonly in Holstein cattle, related to the predominance of this breed throughout the world and affinity for high milk production.
• In dairy cattle, OCD is more common in the 2nd–5th lactations.

PHYSICAL EXAMINATION FINDINGS
• Anestrus is the common presenting complaint.
• Occasional animals may display erratic, prolonged, or persistent estrus behavior or even masculine behavior.

GENETICS
• A genetic predisposition has been implicated in dairy cows.
• In camelids, some females seem to be more predisposed to development of anovulatory hemorrhagic follicles in absence of mating.

CAUSES AND RISK FACTORS
• Genetic predisposition
• Dystocia
• Retained placenta and uterine infection (metritis/endometritis)
• High milk production, metabolic disease, and negative energy balance
• Stressful conditions (e.g., lameness, heat, severe overcrowding)
• Repeated MOET procedures in beef and dairy cattle
• Exogenous estrogen treatment and possibly phytoestrogens or estrogenic toxins in feed
• The causes and risk factors for anovulatory follicles in camelids are not known.

DIAGNOSIS

DIFFERENTIAL DIAGNOSES
• Normal ovarian structures: Preovulatory follicle, cystic corpus luteum
• Paraovarian cysts
• Ovarian abscess
• Ovarian tumors (especially GCT)

CBC/BIOCHEMISTRY/URINALYSIS
N/A

OTHER LABORATORY TESTS
Milk or blood progesterone concentration may help distinguish a luteal from a follicular cyst.

IMAGING
Use of ultrasonography to evaluate ovarian structures increases the diagnostic accuracy.

DIAGNOSTIC PROCEDURES
Palpation or ultrasonography per rectum to assess uterine character and ovarian structures is usually sufficient to make the diagnosis in the absence of a corpus luteum.

PATHOLOGIC FINDINGS
N/A

TREATMENT

THERAPEUTIC APPROACH
• Successful treatment of OCD is generally directed at re-establishment of normal ovulatory cycles rather than targeting the cystic structure. An exception is the use of ultrasound-guided aspiration or ablation of follicular cysts. The reported success of this approach, in contrast to the lack of success with manual rupture of cysts, must be interpreted with caution due to the lack of untreated controls.
• Prophylactic treatment with GnRH during the voluntary waiting period decreases the incidence of anovular conditions at the onset of the breeding period, as does exogenous progesterone therapy.
• Any significant predisposing disease or management condition should also be addressed.

SURGICAL CONSIDERATIONS AND TECHNQUES
N/A

MEDICATIONS

DRUGS OF CHOICE
• Gonadotropin releasing hormone (GnRH) (100 μg IM in cattle and camels; 10–50 μg IM in SAC and small ruminants) or hCG (human chorionic gonadotropin) (3,000–5,000 IU IV in cattle and camels; 500–1,000 IU IV in SAC and small ruminants) may luteinize a follicular cyst but more commonly causes the ovulation of a responsive follicle present on the ovary.
• $PGF2_\alpha$ at the luteolytic dose (cattle and camels 25 mg IM) or cloprostenol (cattle and camels 500 μg IM; 250 μg for SAC) is an effective treatment for luteal cysts as well as follicular cysts that have responded to GnRH with partial luteinization.
• Progesterone (PRID) for 7–14 days may initiate normal ovarian cyclic activity.
• Perhaps the most effective treatment for OCD in dairy cattle is an ovulation synchronization program as follows
  ○ Day 0, inject GnRH and insert a PRID.

○ Day 7, remove the PRID and inject PGF2$_\alpha$.

○ Inject GnRH again, 56 hours after PRID removal, and inseminate 16–20 hours later. It should be noted that this treatment regimen eliminates the need to distinguish between follicular cysts and luteal cysts as the basis for OCD.

CONTRAINDICATIONS
• Estrogenic compounds
• Appropriate milk and meat withdrawal times must be followed.
• PGF2$_\alpha$ should never be used in pregnant animals unless pregnancy termination is desired.

PRECAUTIONS
N/A

POSSIBLE INTERACTIONS
N/A

FOLLOW-UP

EXPECTED COURSE AND PROGNOSIS
• About 60% of cows with OCD early in the voluntary waiting period will spontaneously resume normal cycles by the time they enter the breeding period.
• Most cows affected with ovarian cystic degeneration respond favorably to treatment in terms of resumption of cyclicity; however, fertility may be compromised.

POSSIBLE COMPLICATIONS
• Animals with OCD have more days to first service, lower conception rates, longer days open, and a greater risk of being culled than do unaffected herd mates.

• Poor response to superovulation is observed in embryo donor camelids with anovulatory follicles.

PATIENT CARE
Careful observation for estrus is imperative following treatment in order to inseminate the cow in a timely manner or re-treat refractory cases as soon as possible.

PREVENTION
Reduce stressful condition on dairy farms.

MISCELLANEOUS

ASSOCIATED CONDITIONS
Anestrus

AGE-RELATED FACTORS
A higher incidence has been observed in multiparous cows.

ZOONOTIC POTENTIAL
N/A

PREGNANCY
• OCD will delay pregnancy and even prevent it in chronic, refractory cases.
• Pregnant cows will occasionally be diagnosed with follicular cysts. No treatment is necessary for these cows.
• IVF programs may offer a way to propagate valuable animals with chronic or refractory OCD.

BIOSECURITY
N/A

PRODUCTION MANAGEMENT
Sound nutrition, health, and reproductive management practices can minimize the economic impact of OCD.

ABBREVIATIONS
• GCT = granulosa cell tumor
• GnRH = gonadotropin releasing hormone
• hCG = human chorionic gonadotropin
• IM = intramuscular
• IV = intravenous
• IVF = in vitro fertilization
• LH = luteinizing hormone
• MOET = multiple ovulation and embryo transfer
• OCD = ovarian cystic degeneration
• PGF = prostaglandin F2$_\alpha$ and synthetic analogs
• PGF2$_\alpha$ = prostaglandin F2$_\alpha$
• PRID = progesterone-releasing intravaginal device
• SAC = South American camelids

SEE ALSO
• Anestrus
• Estrus Synchronization: Bovine
• Estrus Synchronization: Small Ruminant

Suggested Reading
Gaverick HA. Ovarian follicular cysts. In: Youngquist RS, Threlfall WR eds, Large Animal Theriogenology. 2nd ed. St. Louis: Saunders, 2007, p.379.
Peter AT. An update on cystic ovarian degeneration in cattle. Reprod Domest Anim 2004, 39: 1–7.
Smith JD. Cystic ovarian follicles. In: Hopper RM ed, Bovine Reproduction. Ames: Wiley Blackwell, 2015, p. 449.
Authors Celina Checura and Harry Momont
Consulting Editor Ahmed Tibary
Acknowledgment The authors and book editors acknowledge the prior contribution of Carlos A. Risco.

O

OVARIAN HYPOPLASIA, BURSAL DISEASE, SALPINGITIS

BASICS

OVERVIEW
- Ovarian hypoplasia: An incomplete development of the ovary characterized by lack of follicles; less severe than aplasia
- Bursal disease: Diseases associated with the ovarian bursa
- Salpingitis: Inflammation of the uterine tube (oviduct)

INCIDENCE/PREVALENCE
- Ovarian hypoplasia is rare in common breeds of cattle but was found in nearly 17% of infertile camelids at postmortem examination.
- A 10% incidence of bursal/oviductal disorders was reported in cattle with about one quarter being bilateral.
- Bursal disease and salpingitis may occur together.
- A high incidence of ovariobursal adhesions with hydrobursitis has been reported in infertile or subfertile camels.

GEOGRAPHIC DISTRIBUTION
Worldwide

SYSTEMS AFFECTED
Reproductive

PATHOPHYSIOLOGY
Ovarian Hypoplasia
- Occurs as an autosomal recessive trait in Swedish Highland cattle; the condition can be partial or complete, unilateral or bilateral.
- The condition is also associated with intersex conditions (e.g., freemartinism, XO monosomy, etc.) or may be acquired in cases of severe, chronic disease (e.g., tumor cachexia, lameness, starvation, etc.).
- In alpacas, ovarian hypoplasia has been associated with several chromosomal abnormalities (XX/XY, XO, XXX, minute chromosome).

Bursal Disease
- Causes include trauma, aggressive per-rectal palpation of the reproductive tract, developmental defects such as paraovarian cysts, and inflammation associated with metritis or perimetritis.
- Bursal adhesions and abscesses are a rare complication of transvaginal, ultrasound-guided oocyte aspiration (OPU) in bovine IVF programs.
- In camelids ovariobursal adhesions and hydrobursitis may be due to rupture of large hemorrhagic follicles. *Chlamydophila abortus* infection has been suspected to cause this condition.

Salpingitis
- Causes include ascending infection from the uterus, perimetritis, peritonitis, and ineffective treatments for retained fetal membranes and metritis.
- Inflammation may lead to adhesions and fluid accumulation (cysts) or in some cases abscess formation.
- A variety of bacterial and viral agents have been implicated.
- Factors that interfere with ova transport in the bursa and uterine tube or obstruct the uterotubal junction are a cause of repeat breeding.

HISTORICAL FINDINGS
Infertility, repeat breeding

SIGNALMENT
- Potentially all ruminant and camelid species may be affected.
- Ovarian hypoplasia: Swedish Highland cattle, shorthorn cattle.
- Ovarian hypoplasia is one of the most common congenital defects of the reproductive tract in alpacas.
- Salpingitis has been reported with a much higher incidence in water buffalo than in domestic cattle.

PHYSICAL EXAMINATION FINDINGS
Anestrus and infertility

GENETICS
- Ovarian hypoplasia has been attributed to a single recessive autosomal gene with incomplete penetration in some cattle breeds.
- Future expansion of genomic testing for economically important food and fiber species, coupled with careful disease definition and good record systems, will provide an opportunity to reduce or eliminate diseases with a heritable component.

CAUSES AND RISK FACTORS
- Causes and risk factors for ovarian hypoplasia include inheritance, female intersex conditions, and chronic, severe systemic disorders.
- For salpingitis and bursal disease, infectious conditions are most common and associated with a variety of nonspecific organisms (e.g., *Trueperella pyogenes, Streptococcus* spp., *Staphylococcus* spp., *Campylobacter* spp., *Mycoplasma* spp., *Histophilus somni,* and *Mycobacterium tuberculosis*) as well as specific genital infectious agents (e.g., *C. fetus* subsp. *venerealis*). Infectious agents usually ascend from the uterus and are often associated with abortion or metritis. Traumatic ovarian palpation or CL enucleation may cause inflammation and adhesions. Rarely, adhesions and abscesses may occur after OPU procedures in bovine IVF programs.
- The cause of the high incidence of ovariobursal adhesions with accumulation of fluid (hydrobursitis) in camels is not yet well understood.

DIAGNOSIS

DIFFERENTIAL DIAGNOSES
- Other causes of repeat breeding such as infectious diseases (endometritis) and deficiencies in reproductive management
- Other causes of anestrus:
  - Pregnancy
  - Inadequate estrus detection
  - Freemartinism
  - Heat stress
  - Ovarian cystic degeneration
  - Starvation
  - Lactational anestrus in beef cattle
  - Seasonal anestrus in ewes and does
  - Pyometra
  - Mummified fetus

CBC/BIOCHEMISTRY/URINALYSIS
N/A

OTHER LABORATORY TESTS
Culture and sensitivity may be helpful to rule out bacterial causes and select appropriate therapy.

IMAGING
Ultrasonographic imaging of the reproductive tract may help to increase diagnostic accuracy. Endoscopy is particularly useful for diagnosis of subtle lesions of the bursae and oviducts.

OTHER DIAGNOSTIC PROCEDURES
- Palpation per rectum and transrectal ultrasonography are most commonly employed for cattle and camelids.
- Endoscopy or laparoscopy are often required for antemortem diagnosis of small ruminants or more subtle lesions in all species.
- Oviductal blockage is most reliably confirmed by repeated failure to obtain embryos from animals that respond well to superstimulation protocols.

Ovarian Hypoplasia
Hypoplastic ovaries are small, thin, narrow, and firm. It may be difficult to find them by palpation or ultrasonography.

Bursal Disease
In cases of adhesion, the ovary is difficult to palpate per rectum. Fluid accumulation associated with bursal disease may develop due to adhesions of the fimbriae to the ovary.

Salpingitis
- *Tubo-ovarian cysts*—in cases of salpingitis, clear fluid accumulates in the proximal portion to reflux into the bursa. The cranial portions of the uterine tube distend in a cystic manner.
- Per-rectum palpation and ultrasonographic imaging of the reproductive tract are mandatory. The use of a dye test or embryo flush technique to diagnose the distended tube or oviductal blockage can be helpful. It allows differentiation of a unilateral or bilateral condition.

O

(CONTINUED) OVARIAN HYPOPLASIA, BURSAL DISEASE, SALPINGITIS

PATHOLOGIC FINDINGS

Ovarian Hypoplasia
• Hypoplastic ovaries are small, thin, narrow, and firm; the ovary may be so small that it is difficult to locate.
• In severe cases, only a cordlike thickening of the cranial border of the ovarian ligament may be evident. On palpation it may resemble a pea- or kidney-bean-like structure in partial hypoplasia or as a shrunken structure in total ovarian hypoplasia.

Bursal Disease
Pathologic lesions may range from mild adhesions of a few fibrous threads between the bursa and the ovary to extensive ovariobursal lesions. The lesions include narrow, shallow, or closed bursa, roughness of the internal wall of the bursa, and cysts of the bursa.

Salpingitis
• Hydrosalpinx—secondary to segmental aplasia or uterine/oviductal blockage due to adhesions distally, proximally, or at both ends of oviduct.
• Pyosalpinx—accumulation of pus in the oviduct following extensive uterine infection.
• The oviduct usually distends to a diameter of 0.5–2.0 cm (depending on species) containing clear mucus or pus; it is elongated, coiled, and thin-walled on palpation.

TREATMENT

THERAPEUTIC APPROACH
• There is no treatment for congenital ovarian hypoplasia.
• Medical treatment of acquired bursal and oviductal disorders is often unrewarding. Acute inflammatory disease may respond to antibiotics and anti-inflammatory drugs but these disorders are seldom diagnosed early. Elective culling is the most common outcome but extremely valuable animals may be candidates for IVF or even cloning.

SURGICAL CONSIDERATIONS AND TECHNIQUES
Ovariectomy may be justified for valuable animals with unilateral localized lesions.

MEDICATIONS

DRUGS OF CHOICE
If an acute infectious condition is suspected, appropriate antibiotic and anti-inflammatory treatment may be considered.

CONTRANDICATIONS
Appropriate milk and meat withholding times must be followed for all compounds administered to food-producing animals.

PRECAUTIONS
N/A

POSSIBLE INTERACTIONS
N/A

FOLLOW-UP

EXPECTED COURSE AND PROGNOSIS
Prognosis—guarded to poor, especially if bilaterally affected

POSSIBLE COMPLICATIONS
Infertility or sterility is the most common complication of these disorders. Peritonitis and gastrointestinal problems are rare.

CLIENT EDUCATION
• Importance of pre-breeding evaluation of maiden females, particularly in camelids
• Importance of submission of females that fail to become pregnant to examination
• Cost associated with examination procedures

PATIENT CARE
N/A

PREVENTION
• For heritable conditions, culling of the affected animal may help reduce the incidence.
• Measures to reduce the incidence of infectious diseases that may lead to bursal and oviductal problems include farm biosecurity, sound vaccination and nutrition programs, and hygienic and appropriate interventions for dystocia and postpartum uterine infections.

MISCELLANEOUS

ASSOCIATED CONDITIONS
• Infertility, repeat breeding
• Anestrus

AGE-RELATED FACTORS
N/A

ZOONOTIC POTENTIAL
Not a concern where tuberculosis and brucellosis are well-controlled or eradicated but should be considered in areas where this is not the case.

PREGNANCY
See "Differential Diagnoses" and "Pathophysiology."

BIOSECURITY
N/A

PRODUCTION MANAGEMENT
N/A

ABBREVIATIONS
• CL = corpus luteum
• IVF = in vitro fertilization
• OPU = ovum pick-up; a transvaginal ultrasound-guided oocyte aspiration procedure

SEE ALSO
• Anestrus
• Endometritis
• Repeat Breeder Management

Suggested Reading
Ali A, Al Sobayil FA, Hassanein KM, et al. Ovarian hydrobursitis in femal camels (*Camelus dromedarius*): the role of *Chlamydophila abortus* and a trial for medical treatment. Theriogenology 2011, 77: 1754–8.
Roberts SJ. Bovine Obstetrics and Genital Diseases (Theriogenology). Published by the author, 1986, p.535.
Smith KC, Long SE, Parkinson TJ. Abattoir survey of congenital reproductive abnormalities in ewes. Vet Rec 1998, 143: 679–85.
Tibary A. Breeding soundness evaluation and subfertility in female llamas and alpacas. In: Youngquist RS, Threlfall WR eds, Large Animal Theriogenology. St. Louis: Saunders/Elsevier, 2007, p. 880.

Authors Harry Momont and Celina Checura
Consulting Editor Ahmed Tibary
Acknowledgment The authors and book editors acknowledge the prior contribution of Ramanathan Kasimanickam.

O

OVINE ENCEPHALOMYELITIS (LOUPING ILL)

BASICS

OVERVIEW
• Louping ill refers to an acute, tick-transmitted encephalomyelitis that mainly affects sheep, but which can occur in other vertebrates including humans.
• Louping ill virus (LIV) is a single-stranded, neurotropic, RNA virus in the genus *Flavivirus* (family Flaviviridae). The virus has four subtypes and belongs to a subgroup of related viruses known as the tick-borne encephalitis complex.
• Small mammals and birds such as hares, red grouse, and ptarmigan can carry and amplify the virus.

INCIDENCE/PREVALENCE
• Yearling sheep are the most susceptible to clinical disease after waning of maternal protection occurs and they encounter ticks on pasture. Mortality rates in young sheep can reach 60%.
• Prevalence of infection may be as high as 60% in adult sheep, but the incidence of clinical disease is low unless the sheep are new to an endemic area; mortality rarely exceeds 15% in adults.
• The disease is most prevalent during spring, late summer, and fall during periods of heightened tick activity.

GEOGRAPHIC DISTRIBUTION
• Louping ill occurs in the British Isles and Norway, and has also been reported in sheep in Bulgaria, Turkey, and the Basque region of Spain.
• Outbreaks typically occur in swampy areas where dense populations of infected ticks overlap with wild animals.

SYSTEMS AFFECTED
• Nervous
• Respiratory
• Digestive

PATHOPHYSIOLOGY
• Louping ill is transmitted by a tick vector, *Ixodes ricinus*. Other tick species including *Rhipicephalus appendiculatus*, *Ixodes persulcatus*, and *Haemaphysalis anatolicum* can also carry the virus but appear less important.
• The larva, nymph, and adult tick contract the virus by feeding on a viremic host. Transmission between life stages of the tick appears to be transstadial, wherein the pathogen persists between life stages. The virus survives in the salivary glands of infected ticks.
• Infection can also occur via transmission on needles or in blood products. Ptarmigan may be infected by ingesting ticks.
• After susceptible sheep contract the virus, it migrates to regional lymph nodes and the spleen to replicate. Animals become viremic 6–20 days later. Those capable of generating a

rapid antibody response may recover with minimal clinical effects. In others, viral replication in the brain can induce nonsuppurative inflammation and cell death, resulting in neurologic disease.
• Concurrent infection with *Anaplasma phagocytophilum* (the agent of tick-borne fever) results in increased viremia and mortality of LIV infected sheep.
• LIV can be transmitted in unpasteurized sheep and goat milk. Lactating goats can shed significant amounts of virus creating fatal infection in neonatal kids.

HISTORICAL FINDINGS
Rapid onset of suggestive clinical signs in young sheep weeks or months after introduction to a pasture environment in a region in which louping ill is possible.

SIGNALMENT
Sheep, cattle, goats, and deer can be affected. Young animals are typically most vulnerable once maternal protection wanes.

PHYSICAL EXAMINATION FINDINGS
• Initial signs of infection include high fever (42°C, 107.6°F), lethargy, hypophagia, and generalized muscle tremors.
• As disease progresses with CNS invasion, affected animals develop gait abnormalities including ataxia, conscious proprioceptive deficits, and severe hypermetria. Some animals develop a characteristic bunny hopping gait, responsible for the name louping (leaping) ill.
• Head tremors, hyperexcitability, head pressing, opisthotonus, jaw champing, hyperesthesia, recumbency, and seizures can develop in advanced disease prior to death, which occurs after 3–12 days.

GENETICS
N/A

CAUSES AND RISK FACTORS
• Grazing pastures containing infected ticks is the most common way to acquire infection.
• Concurrent infection with *Anaplasma phagocytophilum*, spread by the same tick species, can exacerbate the clinical course of louping ill, possibly via immunosuppression.

DIAGNOSIS

DIFFERENTIAL DIAGNOSES
• In small ruminants, other infectious disorders should be considered (scrapie, maedi-visna, tetanus, listeriosis, rabies, and hydatid disease) as well as metabolic or nutritional disorders (pregnancy toxemia, polioencephalomalacia, hypocalcemia, copper deficiency); and toxic disorders (heavy metal toxicity, plant toxicities, strychnine poisoning).
• In cattle, consider other infectious disorders with similar signs (tetanus, malignant catarrhal fever, listeriosis, pseudorabies, rabies,

hydatid disease, and bovine spongiform encephalopathy); metabolic or nutritional disorders (hepatic lipidosis, hypomagnesemia, hypocalcemia); and toxic disorders (heavy metal toxicity, strychnine and plant toxicities).

CBC/BIOCHEMISTRY/URINALYSIS
N/A

OTHER LABORATORY TESTS
N/A

IMAGING
N/A

OTHER DIAGNOSTIC PROCEDURES
• Virus isolation from blood during the febrile stage prior to onset of neurologic signs, or from the brain or spinal cord of deceased animals. Sterile unfixed tissue should be placed in 50% glycerol and normal saline or frozen on dry ice.
• Virus isolation has been largely superseded by RT-PCR on brainstem tissue; immunohistochemistry (monoclonal antibody) can also be performed.
• Hemagglutination inhibition testing can detect specific serum IgM, which suggests recent infection (<10 days).
• Serum neutralization, ELISA, and complement fixation tests are also available. Cross-reaction with other flaviviruses is possible.

PATHOLOGIC FINDINGS
• Gross lesions are typically minimal; however, congested meningeal vessels and secondary pneumonia may be observed.
• Microscopically, there is nonsuppurative (mononuclear) polio- and meningoencephalomyelitis with gliosis, perivascular infiltration, and neuronal degeneration. Lesions are primarily located in the brainstem and cerebellum, as well as in the ventral horn of the spinal cord.

TREATMENT

THERAPEUTIC APPROACH
There are no specific treatments.

SURGICAL CONSIDERATIONS AND TECHNIQUES
N/A

MEDICATIONS

DRUGS OF CHOICE
N/A

CONTRAINDICATIONS
N/A

PRECAUTIONS
N/A

POSSIBLE INTERACTIONS
N/A

FOLLOW-UP

EXPECTED COURSE AND PROGNOSIS
• Approximately 50% of animals with clinical signs succumb after 1–12 days. Those that survive clinical disease typically have residual deficits.
• Animals infected with LIV are immune for life.

POSSIBLE COMPLICATIONS
Animals that survive clinical disease often have residual central nervous system deficits of variable severity.

CLIENT EDUCATION
• Educate clients about tick control and vaccination protocols to prevent infection.
• Inform clients this is a zoonotic disease which can be transmitted via skin wounds or unpasteurized milk.

PATIENT CARE
• Recovering animals should be provided with basic supportive care and sedation if needed to prevent convulsions stimulated by noise or touch. Cattle may fare well with basic nursing care, compared to sheep.
• Affected animals may require hand feeding for adequate nutrition.

PREVENTION
• An inactivated, tissue-culture-propagated vaccine is available for sheep, cattle, and goats. One subcutaneous injection will provide protection for >2 years. All animals kept for breeding should be vaccinated at 6–12 months of age, and pregnant ewes can be vaccinated in the last trimester to optimize maternal antibodies.
• Pour-on insecticides should be used to reduce tick exposure.

MISCELLANEOUS

ASSOCIATED CONDITIONS
N/A

AGE-RELATED FACTORS
Where the disease is endemic, it usually afflicts animals <2 years of age; adults are immune due to previous infection, and lambs are protected by maternal antibodies.

ZOONOTIC POTENTIAL
• LIV may infect humans through tick bites, skin wounds, and potentially aerosol exposure.
• Ingestion of unpasteurized sheep or goat's milk may also result in infection.
• Infected humans may develop an illness that resembles influenza, polio, biphasic encephalitis, or a hemorrhagic fever.

PREGNANCY
N/A

BIOSECURITY
Louping ill is exotic to the United States, but is listed as a reportable disease. Any suspicion of this disease should therefore be reported to state and federal authorities.

PRODUCTION MANAGEMENT
Appropriate herd vaccination procedures are indicated in areas where the disease is endemic.

SYNONYMS
• Infectious encephalomyelitis of sheep
• Trembling ill

ABBREVIATIONS
• CNS = central nervous system
• ELISA = enzyme-linked immunosorbent assay
• IgM = immunoglobulin M
• LIV = louping ill virus
• RT-PCR = reverse transcription-polymerase chain reaction

SEE ALSO
• Clostridial Disease: Nervous System
• Hypocalcemia: Bovine
• Hypocalcemia: Small Ruminant
• Listeriosis
• Maedi-Visna (Ovine Progressive Pneumonia)
• Pregnancy Toxemia: Bovine
• Pregnancy Toxemia: Small Ruminant
• Rabies
• Scrapie
• Tetanus

Suggested Reading
Callan RJ, Van Metre DC. Viral diseases of the ruminant nervous system. Vet Clin North Am Food Anim Pract 2004, 20: 327–62, vii.
Gritsun TS, Nuttall PA, Gould EA. Tick-borne flaviviruses. Adv Virus Res 2003, 61: 317–71.
Jeffries CL, Mansfield KL, Phipps LP, et al. Louping ill virus: an endemic tick-borne disease of Great Britain. J Gen Virol 2014, 95: 1005–14.
Laurenson MK, Norman R, Reid HW, Pow I, Newborn D, Hudson PJ. The role of lambs in louping-ill virus amplification. Parasitology 2000, 120(Pt 2): 97–104.
Sheahan BJ, Moore M, Atkins GJ. The pathogenicity of louping ill virus for mice and lambs. J Comp Pathol 2002, 126: 137–46.
Timoney PJ. Louping ill. In: Foreign Animal Diseases. Richmond, VA: United States Animal Health Association, 1998. http://www.vet.uga.edu/wpp/graybook/FAD.

Author Kate O'Conor
Consulting Editor Erica C. McKenzie
Acknowledgment The author and book editors acknowledge the prior contribution of Stacy M. Holzbauer.

O

OVINE PULMONARY ADENOCARCINOMA

BASICS

OVERVIEW
• A beta retrovirus called jaagsiekte sheep retrovirus (JSRV) causes a contagious disease characterized by the formation of pulmonary tumors in sheep.
• The disease is known as ovine pulmonary adenocarcinoma (OPA); however, it is also referred to as ovine pulmonary adenomatosis, jaagsiekte, and sheep pulmonary adenocarcinoma.

INCIDENCE/PREVALENCE
• Accurate information on the prevalence of OPA is difficult to obtain because OPA is not a notifiable disease and therefore very few countries collate data regarding the number of cases diagnosed.
• In the United Kingdom where JRSV is endemic, approximately 0.2–0.65% of sheep per year submitted to diagnostic laboratories for postmortem examination between 1975 and 2008 were diagnosed with OPA.

GEOGRAPHIC DISTRIBUTION
• OPA is found in sheep populations throughout the world; however, disease does not occur in Australia and New Zealand, and Iceland has successfully eradicated OPA.
• OPA is a significant problem in sheep-raising countries where it is enzootic. OPA is an economically important disease in Scotland, South Africa, and Peru; it is a minor disease in Canada and the United States.

SYSTEMS AFFECTED
• Hemolymphatic
• Respiratory

PATHOPHYSIOLOGY
• JSRV infection initiates OPA. The majority of tumor cells express markers of type II pneumocytes or Clara cells. However, the presence of undifferentiated cells makes likely that bronchioloalveolar stem cells (BASCs) are the also a target.
• Once JSRV has infected its target cell in the lung, it is able to promote neoplastic transformation of that cell. The JSRV Env glycoprotein functions as a viral oncoprotein to stimulate cellular transformation directly, in addition to its primary role in cellular entry.
• Following the initial activation of signaling pathways by JSRV Env, additional genetic mutations are needed for OPA to develop. This would be consistent with the long incubation period of natural OPA. Multiple events are generally required for other retrovirus-induced tumors such as the activation of additional cellular oncogenes or inactivation of tumor suppressors.
• JSRV has the ability to evade the immune system, allowing infection and tumors to progress.
• By the stage at which clinical OPA is apparent, a large proportion of the lung is commonly taken over by tumor and multiple lobes of the lung may be affected. Tumors may metastasize to thoracic lymph nodes and occasionally to other tissues.
• The reduction in functional lung parenchyma and the increased production of lung fluid cause respiratory difficulties, and the resultant coughing or spilling out of fluid via the nose promotes transmission of JSRV through aerosol production and contamination of the environment.
• Frequently, a bacterial infection appears to be the cause of death in the OPA-affected animal.

SIGNALMENT
• Sheep most susceptible.
• Goats: The disease has been experimentally transmitted from sheep to goats. Goats have a low susceptibility to infection. The disease appears to occur naturally at a low prevalence in goats.
• Some breeds appear to be more susceptible to OPA.
• The incubation period ranges from 3 weeks in lambs to several years in older animals.
• Average duration of clinical signs is 2 months (range of a few days to 6 months).
• The normal course of overt disease occurs in adult sheep 2–4 years of age; lambs are more susceptible to infection if exposed prior to 10 weeks of age.
• The peak incidence of OPA after natural infection is thought to be 3–4 years.

GENETICS
• There appears to be some breed predilection.
• There is some evidence that the presence of endogenous viral sequences in ovine genomes may increase the OPA susceptibility in sheep. Polymorphisms in MHC are linked to progression of disease.

PHYSICAL EXAMINATION FINDINGS
• Marked dyspnea, sporadic coughing, and copious watery nasal exudate
• Weight loss and increased secretion from the lungs

CAUSES AND RISK FACTORS
• Jaagsiekte sheep retrovirus (JSRV), a beta retrovirus, is the cause. It is in the same family as mouse mammary tumor virus but only distantly related to maedi-visna virus which is a retrovirus but a member of the lentivirus group.
• Transmission occurs by aerosol and, experimentally, by contact. OPA is highly contagious and susceptibility is age dependent.
• Detection of subclinical infection is difficult. Field diagnosis relies on identifying overt animals within a flock with typical clinical and postmortem symptoms.
• The presence of the disease may not be recognized in flocks containing a predominance of animals <4 years of age.
• When purchasing new stock, the infection status of individual animals depends on the disease status of the originating flock.

DIAGNOSIS

DIFFERENTIAL DIAGNOSES
• Epithelial hyperplasia, a sequela to chronic infections of sheep
• Maedi-visna virus
• Bacterial pneumonia
• Verminous pneumonia

CBC/BIOCHEMISTRY/URINALYSIS
N/A

OTHER LABORATORY TESTS
• Detection of infected sheep prior to development of clinical disease may be extremely difficult.
• Sheep do not develop detectable antibody responses to JRSV so standard serologic methods are not applicable.
• A blood PCR test for JSRV has been developed but is not commercially available. It is more accurate for herd-level diagnosis because it is not sensitive for infection at early stages.
• JSRV antigen can be detected in tumors and lung fluids using immunohistochemistry, PCR, immunoblotting, or interspecies competition radioimmunoassay. The JRSV 26-kD antigen cross-reacts with a primate-derived type D retrovirus.

IMAGING
Transthoracic ultrasound may be used to detect animals with overt tumors; however, a normal thoracic ultrasound does not rule out the potential for JSRV infection.

PATHOLOGIC FINDINGS
• On gross examination a large percentage of the lungs is taken over by the tumors and multiple lung lobes are involved. The tumor mass is frequently necrotic at the center.
• Metastases are found most commonly in the bronchial or mediastinal lymph nodes in 10–50% of cases.
• Histologically, pulmonary tissue pathologic changes occur as multiple, well-circumscribed nodules of transformed secretory epithelial cells, multifocal nodules of neoplastic cuboidal epithelial cells in acinar or papillary patterns, peribronchiolar and interstitial lymphoid hyperplasia, type II pneumocytes and nonciliated bronchiolar (Clara) cells, and fibromuscular proliferation.
• Virus replicates actively in the transformed epithelial cells of the lung, and viral DNA and RNA have been detected in lymphoid tissues.
• Electron microscopically, cells have microvilli, tight junctions, and cytoplasmic lamellar bodies reflecting alveolar type II cells.

(CONTINUED) **OVINE PULMONARY ADENOCARCINOMA**

TREATMENT

THERAPEUTIC APPROACH
Not effective. Humane euthanasia is indicated where infection is suspected.

MEDICATIONS

DRUGS OF CHOICE
None

FOLLOW-UP

EXPECTED COURSE AND PROGNOSIS
Grave; 95% of all clinical cases die. Surviving animals spread the disease.

PREVENTION
• Due to the long preclinical incubation period, OPA may disseminate widely in a flock prior to disease recognition.
• Lung fluids from affected sheep contain large numbers of virus particles and can survive in the environment for many days, so decontamination and rotation of grazing areas is recommended if clinical cases are identified.

MISCELLANEOUS

AGE-RELATED FACTORS
Adult sheep between 1 and 4 years of age with 4 years of age being the norm; lambs are more susceptible to infection if exposed prior to 10 weeks of age.

ZOONOTIC POTENTIAL
None

PREGNANCY
OPA has not been detected in embryos or uterine fluids. However, during the later stages of disease, exposure of embryos, ova, and semen to virus may be possible.

BIOSECURITY
• Restrict movement of sheep from known infected flocks.
• Purchase replacement stock from known disease-free farms and ranches.

PRODUCTION MANAGEMENT
Economic losses can arise from mortalities, the cost of eradication programs, and control measures.

SYNONYMS
• Jaagsiekte
• Jaagsiekte sheep retrovirus (JSRV)
• Ovine pulmonary carcinoma
• Ovine pulmonary adenomatosis
• Sheep pulmonary adenocarcinoma

ABBREVIATIONS
• BASCs = bronchioloalveolar stem cells
• JSRV = jaagsiekte sheep retrovirus
• MHC = major histocompatibility complex
• OPA = ovine pulmonary adenomatosis
• PCR = polymerase chain reaction

SEE ALSO
• Caprine Arthritis Encephalitis Virus
• Maedi-Visna (Ovine Progressive Pneumonia)
• Parasitic Pneumonia

Suggested Reading
Cousens C, Scott PR. Assessment of transthoracic ultrasound diagnosis of ovine pulmonary adenocarcinoma in adult sheep. Vet Rec 2015, 177: 366–42.

Demartini JC, Rosadio RH, Lairmore MD. The etiology and pathogenesis of ovine pulmonary carcinoma (sheep pulmonary adenomatosis). Vet Microbiol 1988, 17: 219–36.

Griffiths DJ, Martineau HM, Cousens C. Pathology and pathogenesis of ovine pulmonary adenocarcinoma. J Comp Pathol 2010, 142: 260–83.

Hecht SJ, Sharp JM, De Martini JC. Retroviral aetiopathogenesis of ovine pulmonary carcinoma: a critical appraisal. Br Vet J 1996, 152: 395–409.

Palmarini M, Sharp JM, de las Heras M, Fan H. OPA sheep retrovirus is necessary and sufficient to induce a contagious lung cancer in sheep. J Virol 1999, 73: 6964–72.

Parker BNJ, Wrathall AE, Saunders RW, et al. Prevention of transmission of sheep pulmonary adenomatosis by embryo transfer. Vet Rec 1998, 142: 687–9.

Peterhans E, Greenland T, Badiiola J, et al. Routes of transmission and consequences of small ruminant lentiviruses (SRLVs) infection and eradication schemes. Vet Res 2004, 35: 257–74.

Rosadio RH, Sharp JM, Lairmore MD, Dahlberg JE, De Martini JC. Lesions and retroviruses associated with naturally occurring ovine pulmonary carcinoma (sheep pulmonary adenomatosis). Vet Pathol 1988, 25: 58–66.

Scott P, Griffiths D, Cousens C. Diagnosis and control of ovine pulmonary adenocarcinoma (Jaagsiekte). In Practice 2013, 35: 382–97.

Author Kate O'Conor
Consulting Editor Christopher C.L. Chase
Acknowledgment The author and book editors acknowledge the prior contribution of Scott R.R. Haskell.

O

OXALATE TOXICITY

BASICS

OVERVIEW
• Due to ingestion of plants containing large amounts of soluble potassium and sodium oxalate salts that, when absorbed, form insoluble calcium and magnesium oxalate salts.
• Associated with ingestion of a number of different plant species; the most commonly seen include *Halogeton glomeratus* (halogeton), *Sarcobatus vermiculatus* (greaseweed, black greaseweed), and *Oxalis* (shamrock, soursob, sorrel).
• Many other plants contain oxalates but are less commonly associated with toxicity including, but not limited to, *Amaranthus* (red-pig root), *Chenopodium* (lamb's quarters), *Rheum rhaponticum* (rhubarb), *Panicum* spp. (elephant grass), and *Alocasia* (elephant's ear).
• Concentration of the oxalates depends on season, stage of plant growth, weather, soil, geographic area, and variation between plant species.
• Ruminants are able to detoxify oxalates in the rumen by bacterial degradation and this accounts for decreased toxicity in ruminants compared to some other species.
• Rapid absorption of oxalates and formation of insoluble calcium and magnesium salts yields a rapid decline in serum calcium and magnesium levels. Acutely, these animals may present with signs commonly seen with hypocalcemia due to impaired cellular membrane function.
• More chronic ingestion will yield formation of oxalate-containing urinary stones and oxalate nephrosis (due to precipitation of these salts in the tubules).
• Toxicity most commonly occurs when unadapted sheep or cattle are placed in or move through areas containing large stands of these plants.
• Local oxalate crystal formation in the rumen wall may induce a rumenitis or more severe gastroenteritis.

INCIDENCE/PREVALENCE
• Depends on season, stage of plant growth, weather, soil, geographic area, and variation between plant species.
• Host factors affecting the toxicity following ingestion include the amount and rate of ingestion, previous adaptation to the plant in allowing increased bacterial degradation (can occur over 2–3 days), and volume of other nontoxic plants in rumen.

GEOGRAPHIC DISTRIBUTION
• Worldwide
• These plants grow throughout continental North America; however, those most commonly associated with toxicity (halogeton

and greaseweed) are found mainly in the western areas of the continent.

SYSTEMS AFFECTED
• Digestive
• Nervous
• Urinary

PATHOPHYSIOLOGY
• When a ruminant consumes an oxalate-containing plant, the oxalate is metabolized in four possible ways. Three of the pathways render oxalate nontoxic to the animals.
• Only when Ca is low in the diet and/or large quantities of dietary oxalate is consumed, are the conditions right for oxalate toxicosis. Oxalate remains soluble in the liquid portion of the intestine contents and is readily absorbed from the intestine into the bloodstream.
• If the oxalate ion concentration becomes very high in the blood being filtered by the kidney, it may combine with Ca^{2+} or Mg^{2+} to form insoluble oxalate crystals that may block urine flow and cause kidney failure.
• The acute toxicosis is the result of low serum Ca^{2+}.

SIGNALMENT
• All ruminant species and swine can be affected, but the disease is seen more commonly in sheep.
• Acute exposure to the plant in unadapted animals is important in toxicity.

PHYSICAL EXAMINATION FINDINGS
• Acute toxicity present with signs of hypocalcemia.
• Signs occur within several hours and death can occur within 12 hours.
• First signs may include dullness, anorexia, belligerence (mainly cattle), stiffness, weakness, muscle tremors, tetany, and recumbency. As disease progresses without treatment, coma and death may occur.
• Rumenitis, rumen stasis, and gastroenteritis.
• If animal lives through acute stages, then azotemia and kidney failure ensue.
• Azotemia may be associated with increased depression, anorexia, and death.

CAUSES AND RISK FACTORS
• Ingestion of plants containing high levels of soluble oxalate salts.
• Most commonly halogeton or greaseweed.
• Ingestion of large amounts rapidly is a risk factor.
• Increased rumen fill by nontoxic forage is protective.
• Slow adaptation to oxalate plants over a period of 4 days can increase the rumen's ability to degrade the oxalates by up to 30%.
• Diets high in calcium may be protective due to formation of insoluble calcium oxalate salts in the GI tract.

DIAGNOSIS

DIFFERENTIAL DIAGNOSES
• Hypocalcemia of other causes, including lactational hypocalcemia (cattle) and gestational hypocalcemia (sheep and goats).
• Hypomagnesemia of other causes including grass tetany, lactation tetany, wheat pasture tetany, transport tetany, and grass staggers.
• Other causes of acute renal failure—ischemia, heavy metal toxicosis (arsenic, mercury, lead), drug-related nephropathies, *Quercus* (oak toxicity), pigment nephropathies (hemoglobin, myoglobin), and monensin toxicity.
• Other urinary tract disease—pyelonephritis, urolithiasis (struvite and silicates, calcium carbonate), and amyloidosis.
• History of exposure to oxalate-containing plants is helpful in differentiating oxalate toxicity from other processes.

CBC/BIOCHEMISTRY/URINALYSIS
• Oxalate crystals in urine (may not be present in acute cases).
• With chronic toxicity, an azotemia would be consistent with but not diagnostic of oxalate toxicity.

OTHER LABORATORY TESTS
Quantification of oxalate levels in suspect forage

IMAGING
Transabdominal or transrectal ultrasound of the kidneys may demonstrate perirenal edema (especially if pigweed is the plant involved) or cortical hyperechogenicity due to deposition of crystals in tissue.

PATHOLOGIC FINDINGS
• Depends on the severity, chronicity, and plant of oxalate origin.
• Ingestion of *Amaranthus* spp. (pigweed) often leads to perirenal edema in pig and cattle.
• Acute cases may have enlarged edematous, red kidneys, while more chronic cases may have smaller kidneys with histopathologic evidence of renal tubular nephrosis and oxalate crystal formation.
• Rumen wall may be hemorrhagic due to oxalates in the wall.
• Histopathology may demonstrate oxalate crystals in rumen wall.

TREATMENT

THERAPEUTIC APPROACH
• Evaluate rest of the herd for early evidence of disease.

(CONTINUED)
OXALATE TOXICITY

• Consider relocating rest of herd to a new area without plants or try to slowly introduce oxalate-containing forage and maintain intake with additional nontoxic forage to dilute the oxalates.
• Adaptation to oxalate forage should be done by cautiously allowing animals to graze for increasing periods of time over a minimum of 4 days.
• Add supplemental dicalcium phosphate to the diet to bind oxalates in the GI tract in the form of dicalcium phosphate–containing salts of alfalfa pellets.
• Hospitalization and fluid therapy to actively diurese the patient may slow down renal crystaluria and subsequent nephrosis.

MEDICATIONS

DRUGS OF CHOICE
• Hypocalcemic or hypomagnesemic patients should receive a slow IV infusion of 23% calcium gluconate or a commercially available mixture of calcium, magnesium, and glucose.
• IV fluid for diuresis is indicated.

PRECAUTIONS
• Infusion of IV calcium should be done slowly and the heart rate and rhythm monitored. Calcium infusion should be discontinued if any abnormalities are observed.
• Appropriate milk and meat withdrawal times must be followed for all compounds administered to food-producing animals.

FOLLOW-UP

EXPECTED COURSE AND PROGNOSIS
• Severely affected animals often succumb to renal failure if they survive the acute disease process.

• Early treatment of less severely affected cases may be successful.
• Aggressive fluid therapy and diuresis may improve the prognosis in animals with renal involvement.

POSSIBLE COMPLICATIONS
Chronic renal failure

PATIENT CARE
• Cases with renal involvement should have repeated serum chemistries and urinalysis to monitor renal function, evaluate efficacy of diuresis, and determine when fluids can be safely discontinued.
• Electrolytes, PCV, acid-base status, and albumin should be monitored in cases that survive severe renal compromise, as alterations in these values may continue after treatment.

PREVENTION
• If possible, avoid grazing oxalate-containing forages.
• Cautiously and slowly introduce oxalate forages over a period of 4 or more days.
• Increase calcium diphosphate in the diet (this may have an effect on DCAD balance and induce other metabolic syndromes if done long term).

MISCELLANEOUS

PREGNANCY
N/A

ABBREVIATIONS
• DCAD = dietary cation anion difference
• GI = gastrointestinal
• IV = intravenous
• PCV = packed cell volume

SEE ALSO
• Acute Renal Failure
• Arsenic Toxicosis
• Bacillary Hemoglobinuria
• Bracken Fern Toxicity
• *Brassica* spp. Toxicity
• Grass Tetany/Hypomagnesemia
• Heavy Metal Toxicosis
• Hypocalcemia: Bovine
• Hypocalcemia: Small Ruminant
• Lead Toxicosis
• Monensin Toxicity
• Oak (*Quercus* spp.) Toxicity
• Pyelonephritis
• Ryegrass Staggers (Annual Lolitrem B)
• Urolithiasis

Suggested Reading

Burrows GE, Tyrl RJ. Toxic Plants of North America, 2nd ed. Ames: Wiley-Blackwell, 2013, Kindle edition.
Knight AP, Walter RG. A Guide to Plant Poisoning of Animals in North America. Jackson, WY: Teton New Media, 2001.
Rahman MM, Abdullah RB, Wan Khadijah WE. A review of oxalate poisoning in domestic animals: tolerance and performance aspects. J Anim Phys Anim Nutr 2013, 97: 605–14. http://doi.org/10.1111/j.1439-0396.2012.01309.x
Author Paul J. Plummer
Consulting Editor Christopher C.L. Chase

O

PARAINFLUENZA-3 VIRUS

BASICS

OVERVIEW
• Parainfluenza-3 (PI-3) is an RNA virus in the Paramyxoviridae family.
• Infection is very common and found in cattle populations worldwide.
• Uncomplicated infections are generally associated with subclinical or mild disease.
• Viral infection can predispose to secondary bacterial infection and bovine respiratory disease complex (BRDC).

INCIDENCE/PREVALENCE
• Infection is considered nearly ubiquitous in cattle populations.
• Seroprevalence in sheep is also widespread; prevalence in goats is likely similar to rates seen in sheep.

GEOGRAPHIC DISTRIBUTION
• The virus is found worldwide.
• Large differences in geographic distribution of the three genotypes has been noted. Genotype A is found worldwide; genotype B is found primarily in Australia; and genotype C has been found primarily in Southeast Asia.
• Recent surveys have found the presence of all three genotypes in American livestock.

SYSTEMS AFFECTED
Respiratory

PATHOPHYSIOLOGY
• Virus spread is primarily through large droplet transmission.
• PI-3 is absorbed across the respiratory epithelium.
• Viral infection antagonizes innate immune responses, including interferon production and function of the mucociliary apparatus.
• PI-3 replicates readily in pulmonary alveolar macrophages, resulting in decreased phagocytic activity and bacterial killing.
• Depression of immune responses predisposes to secondary bacterial invasion.

SIGNALMENT
• Infection is considered widespread in all domestic ruminant species; exotic species are also susceptible to PI-3 infection.
• Infection seen most commonly in young animals following the waning of maternal immunity (2–6 months of age).

PHYSICAL EXAMINATION FINDINGS
• Most infections are subclinical with no detectable signs. Seroconversion follows infection.
• Mild fever develops 2–3 days following infection.
• Harsh coughing is often the first observed sign in outbreaks.
• Serous to mucopurulent discharge.
• Uncomplicated infections generally resolve within 7–10 days.

CAUSES AND RISK FACTORS
• Infection results from exposure of susceptible animals to the PI-3 virus.
• Aerosol and direct contact are the means of viral spread.
• Close contact, inadequate ventilation, and stress increase likelihood of spread.

DIAGNOSIS

DIFFERENTIAL DIAGNOSES
Other mild, uncomplicated viral respiratory infections:
• IBR
• BRSV
• BVDV
• Bovine adenovirus
• Bovine respiratory coronavirus

CBC/BIOCHEMISTRY/URINALYSIS
No specific changes observed.

OTHER LABORATORY TESTS
• Virus isolation
• Serology
• RT-PCR
• Positive results may not indicate the primary cause of disease since infection with PI-3 is very widespread. Testing for other viral respiratory pathogens should be performed concurrently.

OTHER DIAGNOSTIC PROCEDURES
• Nasal or laryngeal swabs are most commonly obtained for viral detection assays. A transtracheal wash could also be performed.
• Lung tissue or airway swabs can be obtained for postmortem testing.

PATHOLOGIC FINDINGS
• Gross lesions may be absent in uncomplicated cases.
• Rhinitis with mucopurulent nasal discharge.
• Atelectasis and consolidation of the anterior-ventral lung lobes.
• Thoracic lymphadenopathy.
• Histologic lesions include acute necrotizing bronchitis and bronchiolitis, infiltration by a mixed population of inflammatory cells, and intracytoplasmic eosinophilic inclusion bodies.

TREATMENT

THERAPEUTIC APPROACH
• Uncomplicated infections are generally mild and self-limiting.
• Treat as undifferentiated bovine respiratory disease.
• Broad-spectrum antibiotics may be warranted to prevent secondary bacterial infection.

MEDICATIONS

DRUGS OF CHOICE
Broad-spectrum antibiotics labeled for the control of BRDC

FOLLOW-UP

EXPECTED COURSE AND PROGNOSIS
• Spontaneous recovery following mild course of illness is likely in uncomplicated viral infection.
• Prognosis for bacterial pneumonia depends on the severity of clinical signs and progression of the disease before diagnosis and treatment.

POSSIBLE COMPLICATIONS
PI-3 infection can predispose to secondary bacterial pneumonia (BRDC).

PATIENT CARE
Worsening of clinical signs may indicate BRDC.

PREVENTION
• Vaccination
  ○ Both killed and modified live (MLV) parenteral vaccines are commercially available. Typically, PI-3 is included with other viral respiratory antigens in a multivalent vaccine.
  ○ A vaccine for intranasal administration containing temperature-sensitive, MLV strains of PI-3 and IBR is commercially available.
• Nonspecific prevention measures include adequate colostral intake, limiting nose-to-nose contact of housed dairy calves, and providing suitable ventilation for animals housed indoors.

MISCELLANEOUS

ASSOCIATED CONDITIONS
• BRDC may follow PI-3 infection.
• BRSV also belongs to the Paramyxoviridae family but is generally characterized by more severe respiratory disease.

AGE-RELATED FACTORS
• Infection is more common in young (age 2–6 months) animals.
• Maternal immunity is short-lived and disease is often seen shortly after weaning as passive immunity wanes.

ZOONOTIC POTENTIAL
None

P

(CONTINUED) | **PARAINFLUENZA-3 VIRUS**

BIOSECURITY
Virus is ubiquitous in most ruminant populations. Thus, specific biosecurity measures are often not employed.

PRODUCTION MANAGEMENT
Uncomplicated PI-3 infection is not a significant production concern. However, predisposition to BRDC is noteworthy. PI-3 infection should be addressed as part of the overall program to prevent and control BRDC.

ABBREVIATIONS
• BRDC = bovine respiratory disease complex
• BRSV = bovine respiratory syncytial virus
• BVDV = bovine viral diarrhea virus
• IBR = infectious bovine rhinotracheitis (bovine herpesvirus-1)
• MLV = modified live virus
• PI-3 = parainfluenza-3
• RT-PCR = reverse transcription-polymerase chain reaction

SEE ALSO
• Bovine Respiratory Syncytial Virus
• Bovine Viral Diarrhea Virus
• Infectious Bovine Rhinotracheitis
• Respiratory Disease: Bovine
• Respiratory Disease: Small Ruminant

Suggested Reading
Ellis, JA. Bovine parainfluenza-3 virus. Vet Clin North Am Food Anim Pract 2010, 26: 575–93.
Grissett GP, White BJ, Larson RL. Structured literature review of responses of cattle to viral and bacterial pathogens causing bovine respiratory disease complex. J Vet Intern Med 2015, 29: 770–80.
Neill JD, Ridpath JF, Valayudhan BT. Identification and genome characterization of genotype B and genotype C bovine parainfluenza type 3 viruses isolated in the United States. BMC Vet Res 2015, 11: 112.
Theurer ME, Larson RL, White BJ. Systematic review and meta-analysis of the effectiveness of commercially available vaccines against bovine herpesvirus, bovine viral diarrhea virus, bovine respiratory syncytial virus, and parainfluenza type 3 virus for mitigation of bovine respiratory disease complex in cattle. J Am Vet Med Assoc 2015, 246: 126–42.

Author Benjamin W. Newcomer
Consulting Editor Christopher C.L. Chase
Acknowledgment The author and book editors acknowledge the prior contribution of William R. DuBois.

P

PARASITE CONTROL PROGRAMS: BEEF

BASICS

OVERVIEW
• Parasite control programs are designed to limit clinical as well as subclinical disease within the beef herd. Effective programs incorporate appropriate management strategies to limit exposure along with tailored protocols to properly treat infected animals.
• The majority of internal parasites undergo part of their life cycle on grassland, making cow-calf and pastured stocker cattle at highest risk. Finishing animals and others within a drylot or feedlot system are more likely to perpetuate external parasites due to close proximity.
• Young cattle and immunosuppressed animals (e.g., pregnant) are at higher risk of internal parasitism due to lack of developed/effective immunity.
• Adults generally develop immunity to nematodes and coccidia if exposed over their lifetime; however, highly contaminated pastures and pens may still lead to clinical infection of adults.
• Subclinical losses due to parasitism may be greater than acknowledged and come in the form of decreased milk production leading to decreased average daily gain and weaning weights, delayed puberty, decreased fertility, and in general, reduced feed efficiency.

INCIDENCE/PREVALENCE
Nematode parasitism is common whenever cattle are pastured.

GEOGRAPHIC DISTRIBUTION
Worldwide, with parasitic species varying based on region.

SYSTEMS AFFECTED
• Integument
• Digestive
• Respiratory

SIGNALMENT
• Bovine species.
• Younger cattle are more susceptible to endoparasites, with the exception of liver flukes and *Neospora*.

CAUSES AND RISK FACTORS
• Nematodes infecting cattle include: *Haemonchus, Ostertagia, Trichostrongylus,* and *Nematodirus*. The nematode that has historically caused the greatest pathology and economic loss in cattle is *Ostertagia*; however, the NAHMS survey in 2008 found *Cooperia* spp. as the most prevalent nematode in beef cow-calf operations in the United States. This change is speculated to be due to the widespread use of avermectins, whose efficacy is questionable for *Cooperia* spp.
• The most common protozoa in cattle include *Isospora, Eimeria, Cryptosporidium parvum,* and *Neospora caninum*.

• The cattle liver fluke, *Fasciola hepatica,* thrives in wet environments and needs a snail intermediate host to complete the life cycle. Due to these requirements, flukes are regionally specific and at-risk animals can be determined based on herd of origin.
• The cattle lungworm is *Dictyocaulus viviparus,* which is found worldwide.
• Tapeworms affecting cattle most commonly are *Moniezia* spp. Their significance relating to production is not well documented.
• The most important ectoparasites of beef cattle include lice (sucking and biting) and various fly species.

Risk Factors
• Cattle grazing pasture are at risk of nematode infection, with management practices (i.e., stocking rate and pasture length) and climactic factors (i.e., rainfall, temperature, and season) greatly influencing the degree of risk.
• Calves 1–4 weeks of age are at highest risk for cryptosporidiosis.
• Young cattle >1 month of age and in a confinement system are at risk for coccidiosis. Poor sanitation is a major risk factor due to fecal-oral transmission.
• The definitive host for *N. caninum* is the canine and therefore free-roaming dogs defecating on pasture or in feed areas are a major risk factor.
• Liver fluke infestation depends on a wet environment and the presence of the snail intermediate host.
• *Moniezia* spp. require an intermediate host, the oribatid mite, which lives in soil and litter. Pastured animals are at highest risk.
• Lice infestations generally occur in the winter months, in closely confined animals with thick hair coats. Underlying immunosuppressive disease is also a risk factor.
• Flies are closely associated with environmental conditions and poor manure management.

DIAGNOSIS

DIFFERENTIAL DIAGNOSES
N/A

CBC/BIOCHEMISTRY/URINALYSIS
• Eosinophilia may exist in highly parasitized cattle.
• Anemia may be present with haemonchosis, heavy infestations of sucking lice and liver flukes, or any chronic parasitism (anemia of chronic disease).

OTHER LABORATORY TESTS
• Fecal egg counts are used to diagnose nematode infestation; however, sensitivity and specificity will vary based on technique and season. Hypobiotic larvae may present a large worm burden during very cold or very hot

weather, leading to underestimates of the true worm burden.
• Quantitative PCR is available in some areas to discern nematode species present in fecal samples. Eggs can also be speciated by culture and identification.
• Lungworms are diagnosed using the Baermann technique.
• Fecal sedimentation and ELISA serology (*F. hepatica*) can diagnose liver flukes.
• Coccidia can be seen on fecal flotation.
• Cryptosporidia are diagnosed by using acid-fast staining of fecal smears.
• Serology can be used to diagnose cows infected with *Neospora,* but confirmation of abortion requires either necropsy of the fetus or case control studies using serology.
• Lice can be easily identified as either sucking or biting types based on the shape of their head and mouthparts grossly or, more easily, under a microscope. Lice can be sampled directly from the hair coat of the affected animal.

OTHER DIAGNOSTIC PROCEDURES
Necropsy examination is the most definitive method of diagnosing internal parasites in cattle. Histochemistry can be used along with gross examination.

TREATMENT

THERAPEUTIC APPROACH
• Nematodes: Anthelmintic treatment should be targeted around times when worm burden is most significant. Specifically, the late winter/early spring when hypobiotic nematode larvae will start to become active again and grass growth, rainfall, and moderate temperatures will allow for reinfection. At this time, a class of drug effective against arrested larvae should be used, such as the macrocyclic lactones (MLs), which include the avermectins and moxidectin. Treatment is often repeated at the end of the grazing season (i.e., after the first frost of the late autumn/early winter) to "clean" animals and decrease the number of larvae that will overwinter within the GI tract. In warmer climates, larvae are arrested during the hot, dry summer months rather than during the winter.
• Lungworms: Various classes of anthelmintics are effective including MLs, benzomidazoles, and levamisole.
• Liver flukes: Clorsulon and albendazole are effective against adult liver flukes.
• Coccidiosis: Calves with clinical coccidiosis should be treated with sulfamethazine or amprolium. Amprolium is easily dosed in the water and is therefore convenient for large groups of calves.
• Cryptosporidiosis: Supportive care with oral or parenteral fluids and anti-inflammatories as

there is no specific treatment. Quarantine and good hygiene are important to prevent spread.
• Lice: Treatment is usually only necessary during the winter months and only in herds with clinically relevant lice infestation (pruritus and hair loss). MLs are effective against sucking lice (injectable or pour-on). Biting lice may be treated with pour-on MLs but efficacy may be higher with permethrin pour-on or dust treatments. Treatment should be repeated in 2 weeks.

MEDICATIONS

DRUGS OF CHOICE
• The appropriate anthelmintic to use should be primarily based on the parasite(s) being targeted and the season (see "Therapeutic Approach"). Other factors to consider include processing facilities, availability, and withdrawal times. The facilities may impact whether oral, injectable, or pour-on products are feasible. Oral products are less likely to perpetuate resistance whereas more resistance (or treatment failure) has been shown with the use of pour-on products. Pour-on products are generally considered less appropriate for calves since licking-behavior can decrease their efficacy.
• See "Therapeutic Approach."

CONTRAINDICATIONS
Anthelmintic classes showing resistance should not be used on that particular operation.

PRECAUTIONS
• Anthelmintic drugs should be used only as labeled and the labeled withholding periods must be followed for each drug.
• Average truck weights should not be used to determine dosing as this perpetuates underdosing of a percentage of cattle. It is safer to base dosage on the heaviest animal, taking into account the margin of safety for the product being used and the variability in the lot of cattle being processed.
• Amprolium may cause thiamine deficiency.

FOLLOW-UP

EXPECTED COURSE AND PROGNOSIS
N/A

POSSIBLE COMPLICATIONS
Anthelmintic resistance, significant production loss

CLIENT EDUCATION
• Clients should be advised that they must adhere to the parasite control program in order to achieve decreased pasture contamination.

• Education regarding the importance of judicious anthelmintic usage (i.e., storage, selection, dosage, administration) is imperative to avoid worsening of anthelmintic resistance.

PATIENT CARE
• On the herd level, fecal egg count reduction tests should be used to monitor the effectiveness of various anthelmintics on individual operations.
• On the individual level, severely parasitized animals should be dewormed using an anthelmintic known to be effective for the parasite in question. Supportive care includes a good-quality diet, hydration support, iron and vitamin B complex in the face of anemia and malabsorption, and appropriate shelter.

PREVENTION
• Maintain lowest possible stocking rates or employ pasture rotations.
• Good sanitary practices are necessary to prevent coccidia and cryptosporidia as both are transmitted by the fecal-oral route with the reservoir being adult cattle.
• If young stock are being intensively reared, such as drylot cow-calf operations, coccidiostats may be continuously fed to prevent coccidiosis.
• A vaccine is licensed in some countries to control *N. caninum* abortions.

MISCELLANEOUS

ASSOCIATED CONDITIONS
• General unthriftiness, poor performance, diarrhea, immunosuppression.
• Bacillary hemoglobinuria (*Clostridium haemolyticum*) may occur secondary to significant damage from liver fluke migration.

ZOONOTIC POTENTIAL
• *C. parvum* is a serious zoonotic pathogen.

PRODUCTION MANAGEMENT
• Good pasture management is imperative to a holistic parasite management program. The goal is to decrease the larval burden on grazing lands through various practices. These practices include:
  ○ *Pasture rotation:* Ideal rotation time will vary greatly based on climate.
  ○ *Mowing/hay making:* Mowing pastures for hay after cattle have been grazing and prior to the next rotation will allow for dessication of parasites.
  ○ *Pasture selection:* Place most susceptible animals (young stock) on pasture not grazed over winter (in mild climates) due to higher parasite burden on pasture.
• Targeted deworming
  ○ Deworm animals most at risk (i.e., dairy calves reared in a dry lot entering a feedlot

are unlikely to need treatment upon entry, whereas unthrifty, pastured stocker calves from the southeastern US are at high risk).
• All anthelmintic dosing equipment should be well maintained and calibrated to ensure proper doses are being administered. The use of scales to accurately weigh and dose animals is ideal.
• Anthelmintics must be stored properly and expiration dates should be observed as efficacy will decline accordingly.

ABBREVIATIONS
• ELISA = enzyme-linked immunosorbent assay
• MLs = macrocyclic lactones
• NAHMS = National Animal Health Monitoring Survey
• PCR = polymerase chain reaction

SEE ALSO
• Anthelmintic Resistance
• Coccidiosis
• Cryptosporidiosis
• Liver Flukes
• Ostertagiasis

Suggested Reading
Coles GC. Sustainable use of anthelmintics in grazing animals. Vet Rec 2002, 151: 165–9.
Gasbarre LC, Ballweber LR, Stromberg BE, Dargatz DA, Rodriguez JM, Kopral CA, Zarlenga DS. Effectiveness of current anthelmintic treatment programs on reducing fecal egg counts in United States cow-calf operations. Can J Vet Res 2015, 79: 296–302.
Gasbarre LC, Stout WL, Leighton EA. Gastrointestinal nematodes of cattle in the northeastern US: results of a producer survey. Vet Parasitol 2001, 101: 29–44.
Hansen J, Perry B. The Epidemiology, Diagnosis and Control of Helminth Parasites of Ruminants. Rome: International Laboratory for Research on Animal Diseases, 1994, pp. 3.1–3.8.
Irie T, Sakaguchi K, Ota-Tomita A, Tanida M, Hidaka K, Kirino Y, Nonaka N, Horii Y. Continuous *Moniezia benedeni* infection in confined cattle possibly maintained by an intermediate host on the farm. J Vet Med Sci 2013, 75: 1585–9.
Smith BP ed. Large Animal Internal Medicine, 5th ed. St. Louis: Mosby, 2015.
Yazwinski TA, Tucker CA, Powell J, Beck P, Wray E, Weingartz C. Current status of parasite control at the feed yard. Vet Clin North Am Food Anim Pract 2015, 31: 229–45.

Author Kaitlyn A. Lutz
Consulting Editor Kaitlyn A. Lutz

P

PARASITE CONTROL PROGRAMS: CAMELID

BASICS

OVERVIEW
• Camelids have a variety of gastrointestinal parasites, some of which can be transmitted to or from sheep, goats, and cattle.
• The most common GI parasites of camelids include:
  ◦ Nematodes (strongyles: *Haemonchus contortus*, *Ostertagia*, *Trichostrongylus*, and *Nematodirus*)
  ◦ Cestodes (*Moniezia*)
  ◦ Whipworms (*Trichuris*)
  ◦ Protozoa (*Eimeria macusaniensis* [large coccidia], *Eimeria* species [small coccidia], *Giardia*, and *Cryptosporidium*)
  ◦ Trematodes (liver flukes: *Fasciola*, *Fascioloides*, and *Dicrocoelium*)
  ◦ *Parelaphostrongylus tenuis* (meningeal worm) is an important cause of central nervous system disease in camelids, which serve as an aberrant host.
• Overcrowding and poor sanitation must be addressed to overcome parasite infestation and to minimize the potential for re-infection.
• Sound management practices, rather than anthelmintics alone, must be implemented to prevent clinical disease from endoparasites.

INCIDENCE/PREVALENCE
• Endoparasitism is common, especially in young, malnourished, and immunocompromised animals subject to overcrowded conditions which propagate re-infection.
• The incidence/prevalence of infection varies with seasonal/climactic factors, and management practices including anthelmintic administration and other methods of prevention and treatment.

GEOGRAPHIC DISTRIBUTION
• Worldwide, especially in temperate climates.
• Cold weather may allow for a break from infection with parasites that rely on pasture consumption (strongyles and cestodes), but not those primarily spread through environmental contamination (coccidia, whipworms, *Giardia,* and *Cryptosporidium*).
• The geographic distribution of specific parasite species also varies substantially with geographic region, climate, availability of hosts and vectors, and management practices.

SYSTEMS AFFECTED
• Digestive
• Nervous
• Multisystemic

PATHOPHYSIOLOGY
• Strongyle infections
  ◦ Include *Haemonchus contortus*, *Ostertagia*, *Trichostrongylus*
  ◦ These are typically the most common gastrointestinal parasites of camelids and small ruminants on farms.

◦ Eggs are passed in the feces and under the right conditions of temperature and moisture they hatch into infective larvae.
◦ The infective L3 stage is found primarily in the first two inches of pasture, and camelids are infected during consumption of contaminated pasture.
◦ Adults reside in the GI tract for months; eggs passed in feces hatch into larvae under favorable conditions of temperature and humidity.
◦ Larvae mature to the infective stage in the feces over at least one week (longer if cooler).
◦ Larvae dispersed by rain, traffic, etc. follow moisture films up and down grass blades and are consumed.
◦ Larvae die more rapidly in hot and dry conditions.
◦ *Haemonchus contortus* ("barber pole worm") is ingested from pasture as infective larvae, then adults reside in the C3 stomach compartment of camelids where blood-sucking behavior creates anemia, weakness, and potentially death.
◦ Disease can be severe and may be acute with onset in the warmer months and warmer climates since warm, humid weather favors development.
◦ *H. contortus* has a short life cycle of approximately 3 weeks from infection to egg-laying adults; adult females are prolific egg producers, releasing up to 5,000 eggs per day; 200 females release up to 1 million eggs per day.
◦ Mild winters extend transmission season.
◦ Other nematodes can contribute to disease and can cause diarrhea, including *Ostertagia* (brown stomach worm in C3); *Trichostrongylus* (C3 and small intestine); and *Nematodirus* (*N. battus* is considered particularly pathogenic and resides in the small intestine).
• *Trichuris* (whipworm)
  ◦ Life cycle is slightly different than other common GI nematodes; eggs are passed in feces, and infective larvae form inside the egg which is ingested by grazing camelids.
  ◦ Adult parasites reside in the large intestine and can cause diarrhea, severe anemia, and even colonic perforation.
• Tapeworm infection
  ◦ Primarily *Moniezia* species; infection occurs by consuming the intermediate hosts (orbatid mites) from pasture, and adult tapeworms subsequently reside in the small intestine.
  ◦ Not usually an important clinical problem; occasionally cause diarrhea and visible tapeworm segments on the manure pile.
  ◦ Infection occurs sporadically in specific locations, even on the same farm and usually in individual animals.
• Small coccidia (*Eimeria* species)
  ◦ Problematic under conditions of overcrowding, contamination, and re-infestation.

◦ Species-specific, with no cross-infection between sheep, goats, camelid, and bovine coccidia.
◦ Infective oocysts are consumed on pasture or in other feces-contaminated feed, with a pre-patent period of ~10 days.
◦ Usually infection is not a significant clinical problem in adults, and treatment is not required if asymptomatic.
◦ Young animals (usually <8 months old) can have diarrhea (occasionally bloody) and poor weight gain.
• *Eimeria macusaniensis (E. mac)*
  ◦ Can be very pathogenic, but oocysts are also commonly identified in animals with no clinical signs.
  ◦ Pre-patent period is approximately 32 days after ingestion of sporulated oocysts from pasture or other feces-contaminated feed.
  ◦ Endogenous development of the parasite in the small intestine of infected hosts gives rise to clinical signs of intestinal damage and the shedding of unsporulated oocysts in the feces.
  ◦ Clinical signs are most likely in compromised adults, or young animals; consisting of transient diarrhea, poor appetite, weakness, and rarely neurologic signs, accompanied by low blood protein (hypoalbuminemia) disproportionate to mild anemia.
  ◦ Severe thickening of the distal small intestine can occur in some cases.
• *Cryptosporidium* and *Giardia*
  ◦ Protozoan parasites spread via the fecal-oral route in feed and in water, as well as by fomites.
  ◦ Diarrhea is the main clinical sign, generated by disruption to the intestinal lining, particularly in the small intestine.
  ◦ Young animals are especially vulnerable to morbidity and mortality (especially crias <14 days old), as are immunocompromised adults which may present with ill thrift and not diarrhea.
  ◦ These are highly infectious pathogens among in-contact animal species, including humans.
• Liver flukes
  ◦ Primarily *Fasciola hepatica* in the high Andes, Pacific Northwest, northern Midwest, and Louisiana delta region of the US.
  ◦ Sporadic appearance of *Fasciola gigantica* and *Fascioloides magna* in US and South America.
  ◦ *Dicrocoelium dendriticum* in central Europe and northeastern US.
  ◦ Intermediate hosts are aquatic snails for larger flukes, and ants and terrestrial snails for *Dicrocelium*.
  ◦ Cattle, deer, and sheep are definitive hosts.
  ◦ Camelids are infected by ingesting larvae from pasture, which penetrate the duodenum and migrate to the liver, maturing in bile ducts.

P

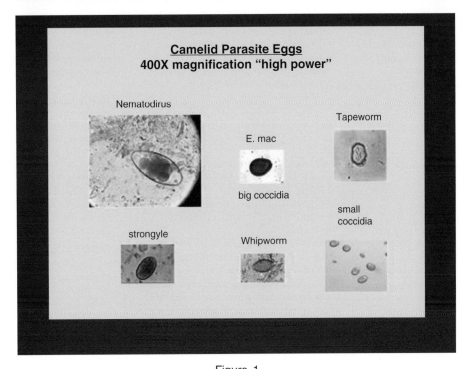

Figure 1.

Ova and oocysts of Common Gastrointestinal Parasites of Camelids

○ Liver damage occurs during migration and due to inflammation of the biliary tract; secondary bacterial hepatitis is also possible.
• *Parelaphostrongylus tenuis* (meningeal worm)
○ Camelids are exposed in regions where the definitive host, the white-tailed deer, exists (eastern US).
○ Camelids are infected by ingesting vegetation contaminated by infective L3 larvae in the slime trail from intermediate slug and snail hosts.
○ L3 migrates from the stomach to the spinal cord and brain of infected camelids, causing inflammation, damage, and neurologic signs.

HISTORICAL FINDINGS
• Relate to clinical signs associated with GI disease (poor growth, weight loss, diarrhea, anemia) or in the case of *P. tenuis*, onset of signs suggesting central nervous dysfunction.
• Historical findings might also reveal inadequate management or treatment practices relevant to parasite control.

SIGNALMENT
• Alpacas, llamas, vicunas, and guanacos
• No breed or sex predilection
• GI parasites primarily affect animals <2 years of age, although heavy environmental contamination can lead to older animals displaying clinical disease.

PHYSICAL EXAMINATION FINDINGS
• Thin body condition, evidence of diarrhea, pale mucus membranes, tachycardia,

tachypnea, submandibular edema, and dehydration depending on the severity and GI parasite involved.
• Meningeal worm disease can result in lameness, incoordination, weakness, inability to rise, circling or drifting gait, head tilt, depression, and/or blindness. Signs are often asymmetric.

GENETICS
• There is evidence that susceptibility to severe parasitism is related to certain blood lines, likely related to functional immunity.
• It is recommended that mature animals with repeated clinical disease not be used in breeding.

CAUSES AND RISK FACTORS
• Environmental exposure from eating contaminated feed and grazing on infected pastures.
• Malnutrition, overcrowding, and immunosuppression predispose.
• Short pasture lengths (overgrazing).
• Exposure to definitive and intermediate hosts of relevant parasites (white-tailed deer, gastropods).
• Warm and humid climates.
• Access to natural water sources.
• Physiologic status (young or old age, pregnancy, lactation).

DIAGNOSIS
DIFFERENTIAL DIAGNOSES
• Bacterial or viral enteritis

• Hepatic lipidosis (liver flukes)
• Neoplasia
• Trauma, encephalitis, meningitis (recumbent animals)

CBC/BIOCHEMISTRY/URINALYSIS
• No specific findings: inflammation, anemia, and hypoalbuminemia possible.
• Anemia can be profound in severe *H. contortus* infections (PCV <10%).
• Anemia, hypoproteinemia, and elevated liver enzymes can occur with liver flukes.

OTHER LABORATORY TESTS
Serum ELISA exists for early liver fluke infection before patency.

IMAGING
Not typically utilized; however, ultrasonographic examination can reveal ascites, abnormalities of the liver (flukes), or thickening of small intestine (*E. mac*) in severe infestations.

OTHER DIAGNOSTIC PROCEDURES
• Fecal testing for visual identification of ova, oocysts, and protozoa (see Figure 1) can include Modified Wisconsin test with concentrated sugar solution (SG 1.33); McMasters Slide using concentrated sugar solution; fecal sample centrifugation in water then examine sediment; or Flukefinder® for fluke eggs (also for *Giardia*).
• Individual animals with weight loss, poor body condition, poor growth rate, or diarrhea

P

PARASITE CONTROL PROGRAMS: CAMELID (CONTINUED)

can be tested, or herd test 25% of animals in each housing group.
• Strongyle eggs are not readily differentiated, hence nematode larval cultures can be used for identification of genus and species to differentiate *Haemonchus* from other trichostrongyles.
• Fluorescein-labeled peanut agglutinin assay can differentiate *Haemonchus* ova from those of other trichostrongyles.
• Immunologic fecal testing for *Cryptosporidium* and *Giardia* (ImmunoCard STAT!® enzyme immunoassay® from Meridian Bioscience, Inc.) or examination of fecal smears.
• Fecal egg count reduction test is used to determine anthelmintic resistance; compare quantitative fecal ova results before and 10–14 days after treatment; count should decrease by 90–95% or drug resistance is present and alternative therapy should be selected.
• FAMACHA-Scoring: Ocular mucosa is compared to a color chart to estimate anemia and the need for active treatment in suspected *Haemonchus* infestation.
• Cerebrospinal fluid can be obtained to evaluate *P. tenuis* infection (eosinophilic pleocytosis).
• Nested PCR assay described for *E. mac* infection.

PATHOLOGIC FINDINGS
Consistent with anemia, cachexia, hypoproteinemia, diarrhea, hepatic fluke migration, or aberrant CNS larval migration depending on the parasite species in question.

TREATMENT
THERAPEUTIC APPROACH
• Successful control of parasitism requires the use of multiple management strategies versus sole reliance on periodic medication with anthelmintics.
• Pasture rotation minimizes exposure to infective parasite stages and avoids re-infection; it can include interspecies grazing with horses.
• Medical treatment should be provided judiciously, to animals with clinical disease, and on the basis of fecal testing to identify at-risk groups.
• Drug resistance is a major concern for GI parasites and describes a change in the gene frequency of a population that is produced by drug selection, whereby more drug is required to exert its effect than was required prior to selection. Drugs lose efficacy because of selection pressure for parasites that have some means of resisting that drug's effects.
• Management practices which hasten development of drug resistance and which should be avoided include:
   ◦ Frequent drug treatments.
   ◦ Treating all animals at once.

   ◦ Underdosing animals.
   ◦ Treating and moving to clean pastures.
   ◦ Treating when there are not many worms on pasture (drought, end of winter).
   ◦ Buying resistant worms within animals.
• All of the above decrease the refugia, which are important to maintain.
   ◦ Refugia = the proportion of the worm population that is not selected by drug treatment and are therefore in "refuge" from drugs.
   ◦ Provides pool of sensitive genes for cross-breeding with other parasites.
   ◦ Dilutes resistant genes.
   ◦ Considered the most important factor in preventing the development of drug resistance.
• Treatment should also be based on the nature of identified parasites; those that are minimally pathogenic, such as tapeworms and small coccidia, do not necessitate treatment.
• Serial fecal examinations may be indicated to detect infection with parasites with long pre-patent periods (*E. mac*) or intermittent shedding (*Trichuris*), and treatment can be appropriate in the face of clinical signs even with a negative fecal result if these parasites are suspected to be causing disease.
• Ideally focus on emphasizing cleanliness in the herd to prevent re-infection; monitor individuals for fecal abnormalities, growth rate, and body condition; and analyze periodic fecal samples to determine which animals might require treatment and to evaluate the effectiveness of the control program.

SURGICAL CONSIDERATIONS AND TECHNIQUES
N/A

MEDICATIONS
DRUGS OF CHOICE
• See Table 1, best applied for treatment rather than prevention.
• Nematodes can respond to benzimidazoles (albendazole, fenbendazole [strongyles and whipworms], mebendazole, and thiabendazole); macrocyclic lactones (ivermectin, moxidectin, and doramectin); tetrahydropyramidine (pyrantel pamoate); imidazothiazole (levamisole); and quinolones. Aminoacetonitrile anthelmintics (monepantel) represent a new class of drug available in some countries but not the US (used in Australia and New Zealand at 7.5 mg/kg PO against *Haemonchus*).
• Cestodes—praziquantel and pyrantel pamoate
• Liver flukes—benzenesulfonamide (clorsulon) and albendazole. Limited efficacy since damage is most profound during migration of immature fluke stages unaffected by these drugs. Triclabendazole (10–15 mg/kg PO) can be used in some countries outside of

the US and has efficacy against migrating flukes.
• *Giardia*—fenbendazole.
• *Cryptosporidium*—no efficacious drugs available, supportive treatment often required while management steps are taken (feces removal) to avoid autoinfection or re-infection.
• *P. tenuis*—early, aggressive treatment maximizes success and can include ivermectin (on days 1, 3, and 5 @ 4 mL/100 lb body weight, SC) plus fenbendazole (5 days at 10–50 mg/kg, PO), dimethylsulfoxide (DMSO) solution (diluted with 3 parts water, on days 1, 3, and 5 at 0.5 mL DMSO per lb body weight, PO) and flunixin meglumine (5 days at 1 mL/100 lb, IM or IV).

CONTRAINDICATIONS
• Albendazole has caused abortion in pregnant camelids and severe neutropenia in overdosed crias.
• Macrocyclic lactones are considered environmental contaminants—the effect of composting on drugs is under investigation.

PRECAUTIONS
Polioencephalomalacia can develop in camelids treated with amprolium; therefore treatment with thiamine (10 mg/kg SC) may be provided at the beginning and/or end of treatment.

POSSIBLE INTERACTIONS
N/A

FOLLOW-UP
EXPECTED COURSE AND PROGNOSIS
• Animals should respond to management changes and/or treatment unless repeated or continuous exposure to parasite infection occurs.
• Neurologic signs are expected to improve within 5 days of treatment of *P. tenuis* infestation.

POSSIBLE COMPLICATIONS
• Severe infestations can result in farm quarantine, especially for *Cryptosporidium*.
• Death/euthanasia from liver failure (flukes), severe anemia (*H. contortus*), severe GI disease (nematodes, protozoa), or severe neurologic deficits (*P. tenuis*).

CLIENT EDUCATION
Focus on encouraging periodic fecal analyses and herd health assessments, pasture management, animal selection, and judicious use of anthelmintic medications.

PATIENT CARE
• Evaluate improvement in clinical signs ± fecal ova/oocyst scores after treatment.
• Repeat fecal examinations periodically.
• Monitor body condition score.
• Monitor FAMACHA score when *H. contortus* is a concern.

P

Table 1

Anthelmintics and Coccidiostats used in Llamas and Alpacas		
Drug	*Dose/Route*	*Spectrum of Activity*
Ivermectin	0.2 – 0.6 mg/kg SC	Nematodes
Moxidectin	Not advised unless resistant nematodes are documented, then 0.2–0.4 mg/kg PO	Nematodes
Doramectin	0.2 mg/kg SC	Nematodes
Albendazole	10 mg/kg PO (may result in abortion)	*Fasciola hepatica, Moniezia,* nematodes
Fenbendazole	10–20 mg/kg PO (high dose for 3 days for *Trichuris*)	Nematodes, whipworms, *Giardia*
	20 mg/kg PO, 5 days	*Nematodirus*
	50 mg/kg PO, 5 days	*Moniezia* and *P. tenuis* (clinical)
Mebendazole	22 mg/kg PO, 3 days	Nematodes
Pyrantel pamoate	8.5 mg/kg PO	Nematodes
	18 mg/kg PO, 3 days	Cestodes
Levamisole	5–8 mg/kg PO or 6 mg/kg SC (not in lactating animals)	Nematodes
Clorsulon	7 mg/kg PO	*Fasciola hepatica*
Praziquantel	50 mg/kg PO	*Dicrocoelium dendriticum*
	2.5–10 mg/kg	Cestodes
Ponazuril	20 mg/kg PO	*E. macusaniensis*
Amprolium	10 mg/kg PO for 5–10 days	Small coccidia (5 days) and *E. mac* (10 days)

PREVENTION
• Avoid overcrowding and exposure of resident herd to new animals.
• Quarantine new herd additions and check their feces after 4–6 days; treat as needed before moving into the resident herd.
• Keep pastures from being overgrazed to decrease infection rate.
• Fence off natural water sources.
• In geographic regions with *P. tenuis*, prevention often involves the administration of injectable ivermectin monthly during snail and slug season (April to January in the northeastern US), which can contribute to anthelmintic resistance and can be detrimental to beneficial soil arthropods and nematodes.
• Deerproof fences, fowl, and gravel paths around camelid enclosures will limit exposure to *P. tenuis*.

MISCELLANEOUS
ASSOCIATED CONDITIONS
• Infectious necrotic hepatitis (*Clostridium novyi*) can occur with liver flukes.
• Rhabdomyolysis and heat stress may occur in animals recumbent with severe cachexia or *P. tenuis* infection.
• Renal failure can result from severe diarrhea and dehydration.
• Hepatic lipidosis can arise due to systemic compromise and anorexia.

AGE-RELATED FACTORS
Young animals and immunocompromised adults are the most susceptible to infection and clinical disease.

ZOONOTIC POTENTIAL
Cryptosporidium and *Giardia* have high potential for zoonotic transmission to animal caretakers or children via fecal-oral contamination.

PREGNANCY
Severe infestations can result in abortion due to metabolic stress, anemia, and cachexia, or inappropriate albendazole administration.

BIOSECURITY
• Avoid infection and spread from outside animals introduced into the resident herd.
• Protective clothing for animal caretakers avoids infection with *Cryptosporidium* and *Giardia*.

PRODUCTION MANAGEMENT
• Avoid overcrowding and check body condition score of all animals periodically.
• Examine manure piles for abnormalities of fecal consistency or presence of tapeworm segments.
• Manure should be removed twice daily to limit pasture contamination.
• Limit exposure of camelids to swamps, ponds, streams and other areas frequented by snail and slug intermediate hosts to reduce exposure to infective larvae of *P. tenuis*.

SYNONYMS
N/A

ABBREVIATIONS
• ELISA = enzyme-linked immunosorbent assay
• GI = gastrointestinal
• L1 = first larval stage
• L3 = third larval stage
• PO = per os
• SC = subcutaneous

SEE ALSO
• Cryptosporidiosis
• Haemonchosis
• Liver Flukes
• Nematodirosis
• Ostertagiasis

Suggested Reading
Ballweber L. Endoparasite control. In: Cebra C, et al. eds, Llama and Alpaca Care: Medicine, Surgery, Reproduction, Nutrition, and Herd Health, 1st ed. St. Louis: Elsevier, 2014.
Cebra C. Hepatic, pancreatic and metabolic disorders. In: Cebra C, et al. eds, Llama and Alpaca Care: Medicine, Surgery, Reproduction, Nutrition, and Herd Health, 1st ed. St. Louis: Elsevier, 2014.
Franz S, Wittek T, Joachim A, et al. Llamas and alpacas in Europe: Endoparasites of the digestive tract and their pharmacotherapeutic control. Vet J 2015, 204: 255–62.

Author Stephen R. Purdy
Consulting Editor Erica C. McKenzie

P

PARASITE CONTROL PROGRAMS: DAIRY

BASICS

OVERVIEW

• Parasite control programs on dairy farms are aimed at decreasing clinical and subclinical disease. This is achieved by decreasing the exposure to parasites and by strategic treatment of exposed or infested animals.

• Because most internal parasites of cattle require pasture or grasslands in their life cycles, cattle in drylot or confinement dairies are at small or no risk for disease from the nematode parasites.

• Dairy cattle or replacements that are pastured are at risk and parasite control programs should be considered.

• Young cattle are at risk of coccidiosis from oral-fecal contamination when they are raised in groups. Young cattle and cattle in their first year on pasture require parasite control.

• Adult cattle tend to develop immunity to nematodes and coccidia with exposure and may not benefit from anthelmintic treatment. Cattle on highly infected pastures will benefit from treatment.

INCIDENCE/PREVALENCE

• Nematode parasitism is common whenever cattle are pastured. Confined cattle are not at risk of nematode parasitism owing to the life cycle of the parasites.

• The reservoirs for coccidiosis and cryptosporidiosis are primarily the calves in a population, although older cattle can be a source of coccidia and cryptosporidia on a farm.

• *Neospora* is very common in dairy cattle in North America.

GEOGRAPHIC DISTRIBUTION

Worldwide

SYSTEMS AFFECTED

• Digestive,
• Respiratory
• Multisystemic

PATHOPHYSIOLOGY

N/A

SIGNALMENT

• Bovine species.

• Because cattle develop immunity to most parasites with exposure, younger cattle are most susceptible. Exceptions are liver flukes and *Neospora*.

• Mean age and range of clinical disease and infection for cryptosporidia is from 5 days to 3 months and for coccidia from 21 days to 12 months.

GENETICS

N/A

CAUSES AND RISK FACTORS

• The nematode that causes the greatest pathology and economic loss in cattle is *Ostergia*.

• Other nematodes that infect cattle include *Cooperia, Haemonchus, Trichostrongylus,* and *Nematodirus.* Lungworms (*Dictyocaulus*) also parasitize cattle.

• Protozoal parasitism in dairy cattle includes coccidiosis from *Isospora* and *Eimeria,* cryptosporidiosis from *C. parvum* and sometimes *C. muris,* and neosporosis from *Neospora caninum.*

• Coccidiosis is mainly a disease of young confined animals and risk increases with poor sanitation, especially in the feed area, because the route of transmission is fecal-oral.

• Cryptosporidia have a short prepatent period (5 days), a low infectious dose, and often infect young calves.

• *Neospora* infection in dairy cattle is common and the main route of transmission is vertical from dam to calf. Cattle are a secondary host for the parasite and are infected for life. *Neospora* can be a cause of second trimester abortions.

Risk Factors

• Cattle grazing on pasture.

• Young cattle are at risk for coccidiosis and cryptosporidiosis.

• Neosporosis has been associated with canine species interactions (the definitive host) but actual initial infection in a cow or herd has not been documented. Once infected, cattle remain infected and tachyzoites cross the placenta and infect the fetus (vertical transmission).

DIAGNOSIS

DIFFERENTIAL DIAGNOSES

N/A

CBC/BIOCHEMISTRY/URINALYSIS

Parasitized cattle may have eosinophilia.

OTHER LABORATORY TESTS

• Fecal egg counts can be used to detect nematode parasitism, but the technique is not specific or sensitive for disease.

• Fecal sedimentation can diagnose liver flukes.

• Coccidia can be visualized on fecal flotation.

• Cryptosporidia can be diagnosed by using acid-fast stains on fecal smears.

• Serology can be used to diagnose cows infected with *Neospora,* but confirmation of abortion requires either necropsy of the fetus with detection of *Neospora* lesions associated with mortality or case control studies using serology.

IMAGING

N/A

OTHER DIAGNOSTIC PROCEDURES

Necropsy examination with histochemistry is the most sensitive and specific way to diagnose parasitism in cattle.

TREATMENT

THERAPEUTIC APPROACH

• Nematode and lungworm parasite control programs based on avermectins or moxidectin should be used when dairy cattle are grazing.

• A common program is to treat cattle twice early in the grazing season, approximately 6–8 weeks apart. Another approach is to treat at the beginning of the pasture season and again at the end. Heavily infested pastures may require treating every 3 weeks with non-ivermectin drugs or every 5 weeks with ivermectin. Fecal egg counts can be used to monitor the program and estimate the level of infestation of the pasture.

• Coccidiosis: Calves with clinical coccidiosis should be treated with sulfamethazine (110 mg/kg for 5 days).

• Cryptosporidiosis: There are no documented effective drugs available for prevention or treatment of cryptosporidiosis in cattle in the United States. In many countries, Halocur® (Halofuginone lactate) is labeled for treatment and prevention of Cryptosporidiosis in calves.

SURGICAL CONSIDERATIONS AND TECHNIQUES

N/A

MEDICATIONS

DRUGS OF CHOICE

• The appropriate anthelmintic to use should be primarily based on the primary parasite being targeted and the season (whether hypobiotic stages of larvae must be targeted). Other factors to consider include available processing facilities and withdrawal times. The facilities may impact whether oral, injectable, or pour-on products are feasible. Oral products are less likely to perpetuate resistance. Pour-on products are generally considered less appropriate for calves since licking behavior can decrease their efficacy.

• Numerous products with zero milk withdrawal time are available in the US (eprinomectin, fenbendazole, morantel, moxidectin). Ivermectin is not approved for dairy cattle of breeding age in the US. Product approval and withdrawal times will vary by country.

CONTRAINDICATIONS

• Anthelmintics should not be administered on dairy operations in which resistance has been shown.

PRECAUTIONS

• Anthelmintic drugs should be used only as labeled and the labeled withholding periods must be followed for each drug.

(CONTINUED) **PARASITE CONTROL PROGRAMS: DAIRY**

• Overestimation of weight is preferable to underestimation since underdosing anthelmintics perpetuates resistance.

POSSIBLE INTERACTIONS
N/A

 FOLLOW-UP

EXPECTED COURSE AND PROGNOSIS
N/A

POSSIBLE COMPLICATIONS
Animals should not be treated with avermectin drugs when the larval migration of *Hypoderma* spp. is near CNS tissue. See chapter, Parasitic Skin Diseases: Bovine, for information regarding *Hypoderma* infestation.

CLIENT EDUCATION
Clients should be advised that they must adhere to the parasite control program in order to achieve decreased parasite loads in the pastures.

PATIENT CARE
Fecal egg counts and reductions can be used to monitor parasitism in cattle and the effectiveness of the program.

PREVENTION
• Contagious disease control procedures such as improved sanitation and strict adherence to working only from young to old animals during feeding and treatment should be employed in calf housing systems.

• Do not overcrowd pastures.
• Coccidia and cryptosporidia require fecal-oral contamination for transmission and sanitation is the primary management factor associated with disease from either organism. The reservoir for all of the parasites is older cattle.
• The coccidiostats lasalocid or monensin (1 mg/kg continuously) in the feed in group housing prevents clinical disease. Breakthroughs do occasionally occur due to improper mixing at the feed mill, inadequate intakes, etc. Individually housed calves and adult cattle do not require coccidiostats due to low exposure and increased immunity, respectively.
• A vaccine is licensed in the US to control abortions from *Neospora*.

 MISCELLANEOUS

ASSOCIATED CONDITIONS
Anemia, weakness, decreased growth, diarrhea, decreased immune response.

ZOONOTIC POTENTIAL
Cryptosporidia are a serious zoonotic pathogen.

ABBREVIATIONS
• CNS= central nervous system

SEE ALSO
• Anthelmintic Resistance
• Coccidiosis
• Cryptosporidiosis
• Liver Flukes
• Ostertagia
• Parasitic Skin Diseases: Bovine

Suggested Reading
Barger I. Control by management. Vet Parasitol 1997, 72: 493–500; discussion 500–6.
Coles GC. Sustainable use of anthelmintics in grazing animals. Vet Rec 2002, 151: 165–9.
Gasbarre LC, Stout WL, Leighton EA. Gastrointestinal nematodes of cattle in the northeastern US: results of a producer survey. Vet Parasitol 2001, 101: 29–44.
Smith BP ed. Large Animal Internal Medicine, 5th ed. St. Louis: Mosby, 2015, pp. 314–45, 1503–1517.
Stromberg BE, Averbeck GA. The role of parasite epidemiology in the management of grazing cattle. Int J Parasitol 1999, 29: 33–9; discussion 49–50.
Stromberg BE, Gasbarre LC. Gastrointestinal nematode control programs with an emphasis on cattle. Vet Clin North Am Food Anim Pract 2006, 3: 543–65.
Williams JC. Anthelmintic treatment strategies: current status and future. Vet Parasitol 1997, 72: 461–70; discussion 470–7.
Author Jim P. Reynolds
Consulting Editor Kaitlyn A. Lutz

P

PARASITE CONTROL PROGRAMS: SMALL RUMINANT

BASICS

OVERVIEW
• In most of North America, *Haemonchus contortus* is the most important nematode pathogen of small ruminants and *Trichostrongylus colubriformis* is the next most common. *Teladorsagia (Ostertagia) circumcincta* is an important pathogen in cool climates. Other species such as *Trichostrongylus axei, Cooperia* spp., *Oesophagostomum, Trichuris ovis, Strongyloides papillosus, Nematodirus* spp., *Coccidia* spp. and *Bunostomum* are less common and by themselves, or in small loads, usually do not cause important levels of disease. *Parelaphostrongylus tenuis* and *Dictyocaulus filaria* are less common. The proportions of each of these nematodes in small ruminant populations vary according to geographic location.
• The number of approved drugs available for use in the treatment of parasites in small ruminants is severely limited.
• Extra-label anthelmintic drug use is a standard practice in small ruminants, but this is an exclusive privilege of the veterinary profession and is only permitted when a bona fide veterinarian-client-patient relationship exists and an appropriate medical diagnosis has been made.
• Anthelmintic resistance is extremely prevalent in gastrointestinal nematodes (GIN) of small ruminants and camelids and must be calculated into all treatment decisions.
• Multiple-drug-resistant parasites are becoming quite prevalent; now and in the future, anthelmintics must be thought of as extremely valuable and limited resources that must be preserved.
• Anthelmintic therapy needs to follow "smart drenching" principles and a medically based selective approach to treatment should be implemented wherever possible.
• Goats metabolize drugs more rapidly than do other ruminants and therefore should receive a dose one and a half to two times greater than is required for sheep and cattle.

GEOGRAPHIC DISTRIBUTION
Climate will greatly affect parasite load and seasonality and therefore programs must be adjusted accordingly.

SYSTEMS AFFECTED
• Digestive
• Respiratory
• Nervous

HISTORICAL FINDINGS
Dependent on parasite species. See "Physical Examination Findings."

SIGNALMENT
• Ruminants and pseudo-ruminants of all ages.

• Young, recently weaned and periparturient animals are at greatest risk for severe diseases.

PHYSICAL EXAMINATION FINDINGS
• Gastrointestinal nematodes
  ° Anemia, hypoproteinemia (more common with *Haemonchus contortus* infestation), weakness, weight loss, poor hair coat, diarrhea, death
• Meningeal worm: *Parelaphostrongylus tenuis*
  ° Hind leg paresis or paralysis extending to forelimbs, poor anal tone, poor tail tone, alertness, anuria or inability to defecate
• Lungworm: *Dictyocaulus filaria*
  ° Moderate to severe coughing, tachypnea, respiratory distress, neck extension, drooling saliva, weight loss

CAUSES AND RISK FACTORS
• Young, recently weaned animals are more susceptible
• Overstocking of pasture
• Poor nutrition
• Periparturient immune suppression
• Drug-resistant parasites
• Over-administration of anthelmintic
• Poor pasture management

DIAGNOSIS

• Clinical examination of the animal affected and recognition of signs of parasitosis.
• Parasite egg identification with fecal flotation-sedimentation and fecal egg count or PCR.
• *Note*: Several methods of fecal flotation exist with sensitivity varying for different parasite species based on method.

PATHOLOGIC FINDINGS
Postmortem visualization of the parasite in the abomasum, small intestine, trachea, spinal cord indicates the causative agent.

TREATMENT

THERAPEUTIC APPROACH
• See Table 1.
• Administration of single anthelmintic class, oral or injectable. Multiple classes of anthelmintics may be used together to increase efficacy (see "Production Management").
• Increasing the dosing frequency at 12 hours apart when using short-acting anthelmintics (fenbendazole).
• Restricting feed intake for 24 hours before treatment slows ingesta flow, increases drug availability and efficacy, and may increase efficacy of benzimidazoles. Ivermectin or levamisole are not affected by fasting.

MEDICATIONS

DRUGS OF CHOICE
CONTRAINDICATIONS
• Most anthelmintics used in small ruminants are administered in an extra-label fashion; therefore appropriate withdrawal times will not be listed on the product label, and it is the responsibility of the veterinarian to ensure that appropriate meat and milk withdrawal times are known by the client. When in doubt, contact the Food Animal Residue Avoidance Databank (FARAD).

PRECAUTIONS
• Appropriate meat and milk withdrawal times must be followed for all anthelmintics administered to food-producing animals.

FOLLOW-UP

EXPECTED COURSE AND PROGNOSIS
N/A

POSSIBLE COMPLICATIONS
If the herd shows signs of parasite resistance, perform a herd investigation to test efficacy of drugs:
• *Fecal egg count reduction test:* Using the modified McMaster technique to determine pre- and post-anthelmintic treatment fecal egg counts. Reduction of 95% in parasite load after deworming is considered optimal.
• *Egg hatch assays larval development tests:* Eggs from feces are incubated with concentrations of the anthelmintic to be tested, and the eggs are allowed to hatch.
• If resistance is noted, consider change in anthelmintic class.
• It is advisable to use the same anthelmintic until the drug is no longer effective. Alternating anthelmintic is not advisable and may cause resistance to multiple drug classes.
• Please refer to chapter, Anthelmintic Resistance, for more information.

CLIENT EDUCATION
Educating small ruminant owners on proper management and anthelmintic usage is extremely important. Most anthelmintics are available over-the-counter and without veterinary advice their inappropriate use will lead to poor efficacy and perpetuate resistance. Ensure that goat owners know about increasing the dose to one and a half to two times the labeled dose when using oral anthelmintics in goats.

PREVENTION
See "Production Management"

P

Table 1

		Commonly Used Anthelmintics and Coccidiostatic/Coccidiocidal Drugs in Sheep and Goats					

Drug	Class	Approved Sheep	Approved Goats	Dosage (mg/kg)	How Supplied	Prevalence of Resistance[a]	Meat WDT	Milk WDT for Goats
Ivermectin	AM	Yes	No	Sheep: 0.2 Goats: 0.4	Sheep: oral drench	High	Sheep: 11 days Goats: 14 days	Not approved 8 days
Remarks: Injectable formulation not recommended								
Doramectin	AM	No	No	Sheep: 0.2 Goats: 0.4	Injectable	High	ND	NE
Remarks: Not recommended because residual activity promotes resistance								
Moxidectin	AM	Yes	No	Sheep: 0.2 Goats: 0.4	Cattle Pour-on	Moderate	Sheep: 14 days Goats: 23 days	NE
Remarks: Only use pour-on product orally. Use sparingly to preserve efficacy. Kills avermectin-resistant *Haemonchus*, but when used in this fashion, resistance to moxidectin may develop rapidly.								
Levamisole	I/T	Yes	No	Sheep: 8.0 Goats: 12.0	Soluble drench powder	Low	Sheep: 3 days Goats: ND	NE
Remarks: Toxic side effects = salivation, restlessness, muscle fasciculations. Recommend weighing goats before treatment.								
Morantel	TETR	No	Yes	10	Feed premix	Moderate to high	30 days	0 days
Remarks: Approved for use in lactating goats								
Fenbendazole	BZ	No[b]	Yes	Sheep:5.0 Goats: 10.0[c]	Paste Suspension feed block, mineral pellets	High	Goats: 6 days[d] (suspension only)	Not approved 0 days[d]
Albendazole	BZ	Yes	No	Sheep: 7.5 Goats: 15–20	Paste Suspension	High	Sheep: 7 days Goats: 7 days	Not approved
Remarks: Do not use within 30 days of conception.								
Lasalocid	ION	Yes	No	Sheep 20–30 g/ton feed 15–70 mg/head/day	Powder feed additive	Moderate	Sheep: 0 days Goats: not approved	Not approved
Monensin	ION	No	Yes	20 gr/ton feed	Powder feed additive	Moderate	Sheep: not approved Goats: 0 days	Not required
Remarks: Monensin can be toxic to equine and dogs								
Decoquinate	QUI	Yes	Yes	13.6 gr/ton feed	Powder feed additive	Moderate	Sheep: 0 days	NE
Amprolium	THIA	No	No	10–50 or 4 oz/ 50 gal. of water-	Suspension	Moderate	1 day	NE
Remarks: Thiamine supplementation may be necessary during treatment with amprolium.								
Sulfadimethoxine	SULF	No	No	55 loading dose- 27.5 subsequent days	Suspension	Moderate	21 days	NE
Toltrazuril	ST	No	No	20–25	Suspension Paste	Moderate	Not approved	Not approved
Remarks: Coccidiostats and coccidiocidals used for control of coccidiosis in lambs and kids								

Note: AM = avermectin/milbemycin; BZ = benzimidazole; I/T = imidazothiazole TETR = tetrahydropyrimidine; ION = ionophore; QUI = quinolones; THIA = thiamine analogs; SULF = sulfonamide antibiotics; ST = symmetrical thiazinetrione; WDT = withdrawal time, consult with FARAD for WDTs in small ruminants; NE = milk WDT has not been established in goats; product should not be used in lactating dairy goats; ND = meat withdrawal time has not been established in goats. To be safe, it is probably best to double sheep WDT.

[a]In the southern United States. Prevalence of resistance has not been established elsewhere.

[b]Approved in big-horned sheep and wildlife.

[c]Label dose is 5.0 mg/kg but 10–15 mg/kg is recommended.

[d]Listed WDTs are for the 5 mg/kg dose. If used at the 10 mg/kg level, these WDTs should be extended.

PARASITE CONTROL PROGRAMS: SMALL RUMINANT   (CONTINUED)

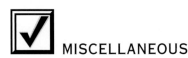

MISCELLANEOUS

AGE-RELATED FACTORS
Young, recently weaned, and periparturient animals are at the greatest risk for severe disease.

PREGNANCY
Periparturient ewes and does from approximately 2 weeks before to 8 weeks after parturition have a clinically significant suppression in immunity to GI nematodes.

BIOSECURITY
See "Production Management"

PRODUCTION MANAGEMENT

Smart Drenching
Smart drenching is an approach whereby we use the current state of knowledge regarding host physiology, anthelmintic pharmacokinetics, parasite biology, dynamics of the genetic selection process for resistance, and the resistance status of worms on the farm to develop strategies that maximize the effectiveness of treatments while also decreasing selection for drug resistance. A smart drenching approach requires that a medically based program be used for parasite control, rather than adherence to some calendar-based recipe. The following are the components to a smart drenching program.

Famacha—Selective Rather Than Whole-Herd Treatment
• Famacha is a color-based chart that evaluates sheep ocular mucus membrane color for the detection of anemia. It can be used only where *Haemonchus contortus* is the primary parasite. This approach should only be applied to adult animals.
• For pregnant ewes, lambs, and kids fecal egg count and PCV/TP is more reliable. Lambs and kids have comparatively small blood volume and anemia can progress rapidly from moderate to severe. Ewes and does can have periparturient rise in gastrointestinal nematodes.

Know the Resistance Status of the Worms Infecting the Herd
• With the prevalence of resistance so high, it is critical that anthelmintic efficacy be determined on each farm and be monitored every 2–3 years.
• There are two methods for determining resistance on a farm: (1) perform an on-farm fecal egg count (FEC) reduction test; (2) send in a fecal sample to a laboratory offering the DrenchRite larval development assay.

"In Refugia" Population: Keep Some Animals Untreated
In refugia refers to the subpopulation of parasites that has not been exposed to anthelmintics. Maintaining a percentage of animals untreated on farm secures presence of susceptible parasites, which helps dilute the frequency of resistant genes in the parasite pool on farm. Selection of animals that can be excluded from treatment can be based on fecal egg count results, Famacha score and clinical examination. It is advisable to avoid treating animals with low fecal egg counts, high Famacha scores, with no clinical signs of diarrhea and weight loss. The larger the in refugia population the slower resistance to anthelmintics is formed.

Keep Resistant Worms Off the Farm
• Anthelmintic-resistant worms can come from only two sources: either they are home-grown by selection with drug treatment or they are purchased.
• All new additions to the herd or flock should be quarantined in a dry lot (without any grass) or on concrete and aggressively dewormed upon arrival.
• Recommended protocol: withhold feed for 24 hours (free choice water), and then deworm sequentially with moxidectin, levamisole, and albendazole at recommended individual-drug dosage. 14 days after the last treatment, FEC should be performed and the animal should be allowed to enter the herd only if the fecal test is negative. Simultaneous treatment with different drug families is recommended only for quarantine animals.
• After receiving this treatment, animals should be placed on a contaminated pasture. Never should an animal be placed onto a clean pasture after a triple anthelmintic class treatment regimen is administered, because any surviving worms will be triple resistant and there will be no "in refugia" on pasture to dilute the future transmission of any eggs that are shed.

Vaccination
Successful vaccines have been developed for lungworms in cattle and tapeworms in sheep.

Administer the Proper Dose
• Underdosing exposes worms to sublethal concentrations of drug, which increases the selection for resistance, and several studies have demonstrated that sheep/goat producers often underestimate the weight of their animals.
• Animals should be weighed individually or dosed according to the heaviest animals in the group (except when treating with levamisole in goats where overdosing can be risky).
• Check accuracy of dosing equipment on a regular basis.
• Anthelminthic administration with a drenching gun, syringe, or drench adapter is recommended.

Utilize Host Physiology to Maximize Drug Availability and Efficacy
• All oral anthelmintics should be delivered into the rumen. This helps put ingesta in contact with the drug, therefore inducing slow release as feed particles pass down the digestive tract. This is accomplished by delivering drugs over the back of the tongue using a properly designed drenching apparatus. Presenting a drench to the buccal cavity, rather than into the pharynx/esophagus, can stimulate closure of the esophageal groove with significant drench bypassing the rumen.
• Once in the rumen, the duration of drug availability, as it is absorbed from the rumen and flows to more distal sites of absorption, is largely dependent on the flow rate of the digesta. Restricting feed intake for 24 hours prior to treatment decreases digesta transit flow rate, thereby increasing drug availability and efficacy. This recommendation is most useful for BZ and AM drugs. It is not useful for levamisole.
• Similar increases in efficacy can be achieved by repeating the dose in 12 hours. For levamisole, treatment should be repeated after 24 hours.
• Pour-on formulations designed for cattle are poorly absorbed in small ruminants. If used, these products should only be administered orally.

Drug Selection and Rotation
• Instead of a calendar-based rotation, drug choice should be made after considering many factors, the most important of which are the number of drugs that remain effective on that farm (and level of effectiveness) and the degree of parasite-induced illness in the animals being treated.
• Rotation of anthelmintics is an overblown concept that gives farmers and veterinarians a false sense that they are actually doing something worthwhile in terms of resistance prevention. Rotation actually does very little to prevent the development of anthelmintic resistance, and is not a replacement for proper resistance prevention measures.
• Two different anthelmintics (from different drug classes) given together will produce a synergistic effect, which may significantly increase the efficacy of treatment compared to the individual drugs. This synergistic effect is most pronounced when the level of resistance is low, but once high-level resistance to both drugs is present, the synergistic effect will be lost.
• Since the available drug arsenal is limited, a suggested approach is to use one drug until not effective anymore. This will allow easier monitoring of resistance development on farm.
• Prophylactic treatment against migrating larvae of *Parelaphostrongylus tenuis* in alpaca may induce problems of anthelmintic resistance in other populations of parasites normally infecting susceptible species. Use of long-acting anthelmintics is suggested to reduce frequency of treatments.

Pasture Management
• Good pasture management can significantly reduce the impact of parasitism and dependence on dewormers.

P

• To prevent the rapid development of drug resistance, it is important that animals are not treated immediately before moving to safe pasture unless a significant proportion of animals is left untreated.

• Treating animals and leaving them on a confined area for 24–48 hours before moving them to a clean pasture is advisable. In this period animals should be fed from elevated feed bunks to reduce ingestion of parasite eggs. Fecal material passed in the 24–48 hours after treatment should be removed and not applied to pastures that will be grazed by sheep and goats. Dispose of fecal material by incineration or by application to ground that will be grazed by cows.

• Managing pastures so that safe grazing areas (low larval contamination) are available will permit movement of animals to a safe area, reducing the number of treatments that are needed.

• Few parasites are acquired when animals browse forage high off the ground; therefore browse areas should be utilized as much as possible.

• Reducing stocking rates will greatly decrease the number of parasites that sheep and goats are exposed to and also will improve the quality and quantity of forage available to the animals (suggested 6–10 sheep/acre). Overstocking can often make control of *H. contortus* nearly impossible. Co-grazing sheep and cattle (not goats) can reduce density of host and therefore reduce pasture contamination of parasite.

• Alpacas and goats should not graze on the same pastures as white-tailed deer. Molluscicides, together with drainage of standing water or reducing access to swampy areas, may be considered to destroy or reduce contact with snails and slugs, which serve as intermediate hosts for meningeal worm spread.

Alternative Control Methods
• Copper wire particles may have some anthelmintic activity against abomasal worms, but not other gastrointestinal worms. Copper use should be limited in sheep due to toxicity. 1 g or 2 g of copper wire particles may remove substantial numbers of *H. contortus* in lambs and ewes, respectively. Similar doses may apply in goats but have not been tested adequately.

• Other methods such as tannin-containing forages and nematode-trapping fungi have shown positive effect at reducing intestinal parasite load.

Prevention of Coccidiosis
• Coccidia are the most common parasite causing diarrhea in young small ruminants.

• Prevention is key and involves both management and therapeutics. Cleaning barns before lambing and kidding, maintenance of dry and clean bedding, feeding at elevated bunks reduces environmental loads.

• Several coccidiostatic drugs are labeled for sheep or goats and are incorporated with feeding. Since kids and lambs do not eat enough feed in the first days of life to secure coccidia control, treatment of ewes and does in late gestation may be more beneficial.

ABBREVIATIONS
• AM = avermectin/milbemycins
• BZ = benzimidazoles
• FARAD = Food Animal Residue Avoidance Databank
• FEC = fecal egg count
• GIN = gastrointestinal nematodes
• PCR = polymerase chain reaction
• PCV/TP = packed cell volume/total protein

SEE ALSO
• Anthelmintic Resistance
• Food Animal Residue Avoidance Databank (FARAD) (see www.fiveminutevet.com/ruminant)
• Haemonchosis
• Ostertagia
• Parasitic Pneumonia
• Parasitic Skin Diseases: Small Ruminant
• Parasitology chapters
• *Parelaphostrongylus tenuis* (Meningeal Worm)

Suggested Reading
Fleming SA, Craig T, Kaplan RM, Miller JE, Navarre C, Rings M. Anthelmintic Resistance of Gastrointestinal Parasites in Small Ruminants. ACVIM Consensus Statements 2006, 20: 435–44.

Van Wyk JA, Bath GF. The FAMACHA(c) system for managing haemonchosis in sheep and goats by clinically identifying individual animals for treatment. Vet Res 2002, 5: 509–29.

Young G, Alley ML, Foster DM, Smith GW. Efficacy of amprolium for the treatment of pathogenic *Eimeria* species in Boer goat kids. Vet Parasitol 2011, 178: 346–9.

Internet Resource
SCOPS. Sustainable control of parasites in sheep. www.scops.org.uk

Author Eleonora Po
Consulting Editor Kaitlyn A. Lutz

P

PARASITIC PNEUMONIA

BASICS

DEFINITION
Alveolar and interstitial pneumonia in ruminants can be caused by the lungworm *Dictyocaulus viviparus* and aberrant migration of *Ascaris suum* larvae in cattle, and the lungworms *Dictyocaulus filaria*, *Protostrongylus rufescens*, and *Muellerius capillaris* in sheep and goats.

INCIDENCE/PREVALENCE
• Mainly areas with mild climate, high rainfall, intense irrigation, in late summer through fall.
• In southern United States, season of maximum *D. viviparus* infection in calves may be from December to March.
• Typically occurs in groups of animals on pasture.

GEOGRAPHIC DISTRIBUTION
Worldwide, mainly northern temperate climates

SYSTEMS AFFECTED
Respiratory

PATHOPHYSIOLOGY
• Generally, lungworms have a prepatent phase when larvae are migrating and adults are not present in large airways, and a patent phase when adults are present in large airways. *D. viviparus* and *D. filaria* have direct life cycles.
• Adults live in the trachea and bronchi, lay eggs, and hatch quickly. First larval stage L1 are coughed up, swallowed, passed in feces, then develop in environment. Third larval stage L3 migrate onto grass and are ingested, penetrate intestine, and are taken by lymphatic drainage to mesenteric lymph nodes. Fourth larval stage L4 travel through blood and lymphatics to lungs, lodge in pulmonary capillaries of caudoventral lung lobes, enter alveoli, and molt to adults in bronchioles.
• *P. rufescens* and *M. capillaris* have indirect life cycles.
• Adults live in trachea and bronchi, lay eggs, and hatch quickly. L1 are coughed up, swallowed, passed in feces. They enter snail or slug intermediate host, develop to L3. Intermediate host and L3 migrate onto grass and are ingested, penetrate intestine, and are taken by lymphatic drainage to mesenteric lymph nodes. L4 travel through blood and lymphatics to lungs, lodge in pulmonary capillaries of caudoventral lung lobes, enter alveoli, and molt to adults in bronchioles.
• *A. suum* can infect cattle exposed to large amounts of eggs in pens heavily contaminated by swine. Cattle are typically affected about 10 days after exposure, with signs due to allergic reaction to the larvae migrating through the lungs. Larvae in the alveoli initiate allergic reaction, with eosinophilic

exudate being produced, causing coughing and tachypnea. More larvae tend to be aspirated into the caudoventral lung lobes, with consolidation developing there and in the interstitium as larvae migrate.
• Adult worms in the trachea and bronchi cause inflammation. Generally, larvae in the alveoli cause inflammatory reaction with eosinophilic exudate blocking bronchioles and causing coughing and tachypnea.
• Adult worms in larger airways cause marked inflammatory response with consolidation of caudoventral lung lobes.

HISTORICAL FINDINGS
Areas of high rainfall or intense irrigation, young animals turned out onto infected pasture, older animals moved from nonendemic to endemic areas.

SIGNALMENT
• All ruminant species.
• Beef cattle tend to be less affected by *D. viviparus* since management is more extensive, therefore infective larvae are not as concentrated.
• Mainly a disease of dairy calves.
• *D. viviparus* infection tends to occur in cattle <1 year old, or previously unexposed adults, turned out onto infected pasture.
• Infection also occurs in older cattle, previously infected and considered immune, re-infected when they are moved from nonendemic to endemic areas.

PHYSICAL EXAMINATION FINDINGS
Marked coughing (inconsistent finding in sheep and goats), tachypnea, dyspnea, fever (high fever in *A. suum* larval migration), anorexia, weight loss, harsh breath sounds, and widespread crackles and wheezes on lung auscultation (crackles over dorsal half of lungs in *D. viviparus* infection in cattle).

CAUSES AND RISK FACTORS
• Cattle—*D. viviparus*, aberrant migration of *A. suum*.
• Sheep and goats—*D. filaria*, adults in trachea and bronchi, most pathogenic. *P. rufescens*, adults in bronchioles, lesions smaller, less pathogenic. *M. capillaris*, adults in lung parenchyma, which become encysted so relatively benign; most common but least pathogenic lungworm of sheep and goats; more pathogenic in goats than in sheep; causes a more diffuse inflammation and interstitial pneumonia in goats.
• Exposure to vector (snail or slug) habitat (i.e., marshy land, wet muddy areas around waterholes, areas of high rainfall, intense irrigation).

DIAGNOSIS

DIFFERENTIAL DIAGNOSES
• Acute bovine pulmonary emphysema and edema or ABPEE (atypical interstitial

pneumonia, fog fever)—cattle >2 years old suddenly switched from sparse dry forage to lush green pasture.
• Bacterial/viral bronchopneumonia.

CBC/BIOCHEMISTRY/URINALYSIS
May see increase in eosinophils 2–6 weeks after infection.

OTHER LABORATORY TESTS
Baermann sedimentation technique on feces or fluid from transtracheal aspirate to look for lungworm larvae; need to check several animals in herd.

IMAGING
• Radiography—may see consolidation of caudoventral lung lobes.
• Endoscopy—may see adult lungworms in large airways.

OTHER DIAGNOSTIC PROCEDURES
N/A

PATHOLOGIC FINDINGS
• Prepatent phase—lungs grossly normal, few atelectic lobules in caudoventral lung lobes. May see larvae in microscopic smears of bronchial exudate, and eosinophilic infiltration.
• Patent phase—bilaterally symmetrical caudoventral lung consolidation. See adult worms in trachea and bronchi, with hemorrhage and fluid exudate.
• *D. filaria*—adult worms mainly in caudodorsal diaphragmatic lung lobes.
• *M. capillaris*—adult worms mainly in lung parenchyma, form grayish nodules 2–3 mm in diameter in subpleural tissue of sheep.

TREATMENT

THERAPEUTIC APPROACH
N/A

SURGICAL CONSIDERATIONS AND TECHNIQUES
N/A

MEDICATIONS

DRUGS OF CHOICE
• Ivermectin 0.2 mg/kg SC.
• Fenbendazole 5 mg/kg PO, approved for dairy cattle of breeding age in the US.
• Fenbendazole, levamisole, ivermectin, and moxidectin are effective in sheep and goats. See chapter, Parasite Control Programs: Small Ruminant, for dosing information for sheep and goats.

CONTRAINDICATIONS
N/A

PRECAUTIONS
• Appropriate milk and meat withdrawal times must be followed for all compounds administered to food-producing animals.

• Move animals to fresh pasture after treatment to avoid re-infection.

POSSIBLE INTERACTIONS
N/A

FOLLOW-UP

EXPECTED COURSE AND PROGNOSIS
• Good prognosis if animal only has cough and tachypnea.
• Guarded prognosis if animal also has dyspnea, fever, or anorexia.

POSSIBLE COMPLICATIONS
N/A

CLIENT EDUCATION
• Avoid infected pastures
• Vector control (e.g., molluscicides)

PATIENT CARE
N/A

PREVENTION
• Avoid infected pastures.
• Vector control (e.g., molluscicides).
• Strategic deworming (e.g., ivermectin at 3, 8, and 13 weeks after turning out on new pasture).

MISCELLANEOUS

ASSOCIATED CONDITIONS
N/A

AGE-RELATED FACTORS
Acute infection in young animals or previously unexposed adults turned out onto infected pasture, or re-infection in older animals previously infected and considered immune and moved from nonendemic to endemic areas.

ZOONOTIC POTENTIAL
N/A

PREGNANCY
Benzimidazoles (e.g., albendazole) may be teratogenic in first trimester of pregnancy; use with caution.

BIOSECURITY
N/A

PRODUCTION MANAGEMENT
Control of vectors and implementation of proper parasite control programs in affected herds are important to minimize production losses and improve animal health.

SYNONYMS
• Husk
• Parasitic bronchitis
• Parasitic pneumonitis
• Verminous bronchitis
• Verminous pneumonia

ABBREVIATIONS
• ABPEE = acute bovine pulmonary emphysema and edema
• FARAD = Food Animal Residue Avoidance Databank

SEE ALSO
• Atypical Interstitial Pneumonia
• Food Animal Residue Avoidance Databank (FARAD) (see www.fiveminutevet.com/ruminant)
• Parasite Control Programs (by species)
• Respiratory Disease (by species)
• Respiratory Disease: Pharmacology (see www.fiveminutevet.com/ruminant)

Suggested Reading
Pugh DG, Baird N, eds. Sheep and Goat Medicine. Philadelphia: Saunders, 2012.
Radostits OM, Gay CC, Hinchcliff KW, Constable PD, eds. Veterinary Medicine, 10th ed. London: Saunders, 2007.
Smith BP ed. Large Animal Internal Medicine, 5th ed. St. Louis: Mosby, 2015.
Author Kate O'Conor
Consulting Editor Kaitlyn A. Lutz
Acknowledgment The author and book editors acknowledge the prior contribution of David McKenzie.

PARASITIC SKIN DISEASES: BOVINE

BASICS

OVERVIEW
- Cattle can be affected by a wide range of parasitic skin diseases which can cause significant production losses and compromised animal welfare.
- External parasites feed on body tissues such as blood, skin and hair, and can cause skin irritation, self-trauma, and secondary infections.
- External parasites also serve as vectors for transmission of many important infectious diseases.

INCIDENCE/PREVALENCE
N/A

GEOGRAPHIC DISTRIBUTION
Worldwide; influenced by distribution of specific causative species and cattle management systems

SYSTEMS AFFECTED
- Integument
- Ophthalmic

PATHOPHYSIOLOGY
- Warble flies include *Hypoderma bovis*, *H. lineatum*, and *H. sinense*.
  - Adult flies attach eggs to hair in spring to late summer; larvae penetrate skin and migrate in the tissues of the esophagus (*H. lineatum*) or spinal canal (*H. bovis*); they then move to subdermal tissue along the back and emerge from a breathing hole they create, fall to the ground to pupate, and emerge as adult flies.
  - Infection can create focal swellings of the dorsum, poor growth and production, and damage to hides and carcasses. Migration of larvae in the spinal cord can occasionally cause posterior paralysis.
- Pediculosis or louse infestation is common in cattle due to host-specific biting (chewing) lice (*Damalinia bovis*) or sucking lice (*Linognathus vituli, Solenopotes capillatus, Haematopinus eurystemus*, and *H. quadripertusus*). Infestation causes irritation, rubbing, skin damage, decreased milk production, and sometimes anemia.
- Ticks are much less host-specific than lice, and can act as vectors of important blood-borne diseases in addition to reducing production and potentially causing anemia and paralysis.
  - There are two main types of tick that affect cattle: *Argasidae* (soft ticks) for which important examples in North America include *Otobius megnini* and *Ornithodoros coriaceus*; and *Ixodidae* (hard ticks) for which important examples in North America include the genera *Dermacentor, Ixodes, Amblyomma*, and *Rhipicephalus* (*Boophilus*).

- Ticks tend to be fairly long-lived and environmentally resistant, living away from their hosts for extended periods of time.
  - Tick feeding can result in hide damage, otitis, secondary bacterial infections, and transmission of important diseases including babesiosis and heartwater. Some species are also capable of causing paralysis as a result of the neurotoxins they inject into their hosts during feeding.
- Cutaneous myiasis (infestation with fly larvae or maggots) usually relates to *Calliphoridae* flies. "Blowfly strike" tends to be most problematic in sheep infested with *Lucillia cuprina* or *L. sericata*. Cattle can be significantly affected by screwworms, *Cochliomyia hominovorax* (in the New World) and *Chrysomyia bezziana* (in southern Europe, Africa, and Asia); larvae initially hatch into and feed on damaged skin, but then continue to invade living tissues causing severe damage, inflammation, secondary infection, and toxemia.
- A large variety of other fly species also affect cattle which can cause distress, pain, behavioral changes, reduced feed intake, and reduced productivity. In addition, flies may act as vectors for a variety of parasitic and infectious diseases.
  - Stable flies (*Stomoxys calcitrans*) are present in most countries and are small and gray. They are most significant to confined livestock in North America because they attack cattle to feed on blood. They can serve as mechanical vectors for anthrax and BVDV.
  - Horse and deer flies (*Tabanidae*) are large, robust, blood-feeding flies that are widespread in temperate and tropical regions. Only female flies take blood meals; bites are severe and distressing. These flies can act as mechanical vectors of bovine leukosis, vesicular stomatitis, and anthrax. These flies attack principally the legs and ventral abdomen; attacks lead to bunching of animals which can promote overheating and sometimes stampeding behavior.
  - Horn flies (*Haematobia* spp.) are small gray flies. *H. irritans exigua* occurs in Australia and Southeast Asia, *H. irritans irritans* in Europe, North and South America, and Hawaii, and *H. minuta* in Africa. Both sexes are obligate blood feeders and attack pastured cattle. They can act as a vector for *Stephanofilaria stilesi* spp. which can cause skin lesions on the ventral abdomen of cattle.
  - Biting midges are very tiny flies (1–3 mm long) that belong to the family *Ceratopogonidae; Culicoides* is the most important genus. These are also blood feeders that cause irritation and distress and which can transmit bluetongue and ephemeral fever, and act as an intermediate host for *Onchocerca*.

- Black and sand flies are small gray to black flies that belong to the family *Simuliidae*. Some important species include *Cnephia pecuarum* (southern US), *Simulium arcticum* (northern Canada), *Austrosimulium pestilens* and *A. bancrofti* (Australia), and *Simulium ornatum* (Great Britain). Female flies are active blood feeders in summer and cause distress, skin wheals and papules, and sometimes blood loss, and can transmit *Onchocerca* spp.
  - Face flies (*Musca autumnalis*) are slightly larger than house flies and gather on the faces of cattle to feed on nasal and lacrimal secretions and saliva. This can cause stress and ocular irritation, and this species can act as vectors for eyeworms (*Thelazia* spp.) and enhance transmission of *Moraxella bovis* (the primary agent of bovine infectious keratoconjunctivitis).
  - Head flies (*Hydrotea irritans*) are similar to house flies but have an olive abdomen and yellow wing bases. They are found mainly in Europe and do not bite, but create irritation, head shaking, rubbing, and scratching which may result in trauma and secondary myiasis. They can aid transmission of summer mastitis.
  - Tsetse flies (*Glossina* spp.) in Africa are blood feeders and critical vectors of trypanosome diseases including Nagana (a complex of disease associated in cattle with *Trypanosoma brucei* infection).
- Several species of mites affect cattle, including *Demodex bovis, Sarcoptes scabei, Psoroptes ovis*, and *Chorioptes bovis*.
  - Demodectic mange (follicular mange) can cause significant damage to the hide. This mite spends its entire life on the host, and spreads between animals by contact. Mites invade the hair follicles and sebaceous glands, creating chronic inflammation and alopecia. Affected animals have small nodules and pustules, general hair loss, and thickening of the skin without pruritus. Lesions occur most commonly on the brisket, lower neck, forearm, and shoulders.
  - Sarcoptic mange (barn itch) related to *Sarcoptes scabiei* var *bovis* infection is usually seen in cattle in overcrowded situations with poor feeding and poor husbandry. *Sarcoptes* is mainly transmitted by direct contact between hosts and it is a zoonotic and notifiable disease in most countries. Affected cattle have small red papules and general erythema, severe pruritus, hair loss and thick scabs distributed over the inner surface of the thighs, the neck, brisket, and tail base.
  - Psoroptic mange (body mange, ear mange) can also affect cattle and is caused by *Psoroptes ovis*. Infection can spread rapidly among animals and cause serious losses. Typical lesions are intensely itchy and appear first on the withers, neck, and around the root of the tail, eventually hair

loss, thickened skin, scabs, and papules occur.

° Chorioptic mange (tail mange, leg mange, scrotal mange) is the most common form of mange in cattle, caused by *Chorioptes bovis*. Again, transmission is mainly by direct contact and infection creates allergic, exudative dermatitis affecting the rump, tail, perineum, thighs, caudal udder, and scrotum with erythema, papules, crusts, alopecia, and pruritus.

° Psorergatic mange is caused by *Psorobia bos* (itch mite) which is usually an asymptomatic infestation; however, some cattle may display mild pruritus and alopecia.

HISTORICAL FINDINGS
• Vary with the underlying etiology but defining the history of skin disease within the herd, and any relevant treatment or management procedures, is important.
• A description of skin lesion appearance and duration, number of animals affected, and the presence or absence of pruritis are important historical factors.

SIGNALMENT
Generally, any age and breed of cattle are susceptible to parasitic skin diseases; however, *P. ovis* is very common in some breeds of beef cattle, whereas some dairy cattle breeds such as Holstein Friesians are considered resistant.

PHYSICAL EXAMINATION FINDINGS
• Ticks and lice are often readily visible on close examination of the skin.
• Skin should be closely evaluated for characteristics that include pruritis, alopecia, excoriations, lumps, perforations, and other anomalies.
• Signs of anemia or related infectious diseases may be observed.

GENETICS
N/A

CAUSES AND RISK FACTORS
• The presence of specific parasitic agents in the region
• Overcrowding and poor nutrition
• Lack of control and treatment procedures for external parasitism

 DIAGNOSIS

DIFFERENTIAL DIAGNOSES
• Dermatophilosis
• Lymphosarcoma
• Dermatophytosis
• Photosensitization
• *Staphylococcus* spp. dermatitis
• Tuberculosis
• Foot and mouth disease
• Poxvirus
• Pemphigus
• Contact dermatitis

• Trombiculidiasis
• Nutrient deficiency (selenium, zinc, vitamins A, D, or E)
• Pseudorabies
• Chemical burns

CBC/BIOCHEMISTRY/URINALYSIS
N/A

OTHER LABORATORY TESTS
Bacterial culture and sensitivity might be relevant in secondary infections of the skin or ear canals

IMAGING
N/A

OTHER DIAGNOSTIC PROCEDURES
• Skin scrapings can provide positive diagnosis and clarification of mite-related mange conditions
• Skin biopsy

PATHOLOGIC FINDINGS
• Mites are evident in deep scrapings or biopsies, and the species responsible can be differentiated by morphologic identification.
• Other findings are dependent on the causative etiology.

 TREATMENT

THERAPEUTIC APPROACH
• Specific conditions respond very well to topical or parenteral treatment with insecticides provided via ear tags, residual livestock sprays, pour-on formulations, dust bags, back rubbers, oilers, or wipe-ons.
• Animals should be supported via good management, adequate nutrition, and where relevant, good hygiene procedures.
• For reportable conditions, contact appropriate state/provincial/government bodies to determine specific quarantine requirements and treatments.

SURGICAL CONSIDERATIONS AND TECHNIQUES
• Skin biopsy is a quick and relatively painless procedure that can be achieved using a 6 mm skin biopsy punch with no preceding preparation of the skin or local anesthesia to avoid lesion disruption and artifact.
• Biopsy sites can be left to heal by granulation but should be protected from invasion by external parasites.

 MEDICATIONS

DRUGS OF CHOICE
• Warble flies respond to macrocyclic lactone products (doramectin, ivermectin, eprinomectin, moxidectin). If systemic insecticides are not allowed, tetrachlorvinphos dust can be applied to the dorsum.

• Mange mites are typically also responsive to macrocyclic lactone endectocides.
• Lice respond to treatment with topical pyrethroid insecticides which are effective against chewing and sucking lice, whereas macrocyclic lactone products mainly affect sucking lice.
• Ticks can respond to diazinon, pyrethroids, carbaryl and macrocyclic lactone drugs which can be provided via dipping, pour-on preparations, or injection.
• Flies can be managed through pour-on products, insecticide-impregnated ear tags, oral larvicides, and insect growth regulators to kill fly larvae developing in manure.

CONTRAINDICATIONS
Topical ectoparasiticides that fall under the jurisdiction of the EPA rather than the FDA in the US cannot be applied in an extra-label manner.

PRECAUTIONS
• Appropriate milk and meat withdrawal times must be followed for all compounds administered to food-producing animals.
• Crushing or damaging warble fly larvae during treatment procedures can induce acute anaphylaxis in host cattle.

POSSIBLE INTERACTIONS
N/A

 FOLLOW-UP

EXPECTED COURSE AND PROGNOSIS
• Depends upon the causative agent; the prognosis for *Demodex* infestation is guarded, but for other mites is fair to good with adequate diagnosis and subsequent treatment.
• Most parasitic conditions of the integument cause anxiety and production loss as the main concern.

POSSIBLE COMPLICATIONS
• Secondary bacterial infection and toxemia
• Cutaneous myiasis

CLIENT EDUCATION
Focus on methods of control and prevention to reduce ectoparasite-related distress and disease

PATIENT CARE
N/A

PREVENTION
• Quarantine new animals before introduction into the herd, with close inspection for skin lesions.
• Lice can live for a limited time off the host (varies with species); therefore, leaving facilities dormant for 1–4 weeks (depending on the species involved) before re-introducing treated animals can help break the life cycle.
• Remove wet, rotting organic matter to reduce habitat for fly larvae; dragging pastures

P

to break up and dry manure masses is also helpful.
• Sterile male fly release programs have been very successful at controlling screwworm flies.
• Fly traps can be useful additions to the listed treatment methods which also often work in prevention.

MISCELLANEOUS

ASSOCIATED CONDITIONS
• Secondary infection
• Cutaneous myiasis

AGE-RELATED FACTORS
N/A

ZOONOTIC POTENTIAL
Sarcoptes scabiei is zoonotic and can cross between species.

PREGNANCY
N/A

BIOSECURITY
• Quarantine new animals before introducing into the herd.
• Isolate affected herd members or whole herds during testing and treatment.

• Contact regulatory bodies if notifiable conditions are suspected.

PRODUCTION MANAGEMENT
Ectoparasites are a significant cause of economic loss due to reduced production including lower weaning weights, hide damage, secondary disease, and treatment expenses.

SYNONYMS
• Hypoderma—cattle grubs, warble fly, heel fly, gad fly
• Stable flies—biting house fly
• Demodectic mange—follicular mange
• Sarcoptic mange—barn itch
• Psoroptic mange—body mange, ear mange
• Chorioptic mange—tail mange, leg mange, scrotal mange

ABBREVIATIONS
• BVDV = bovine viral diarrhea virus
• EPA = Environmental Protection Agency
• FDA = Food and Drug Administration

SEE ALSO
• Dermatophilosis
• Dermatophytosis
• Food Animal Residue Avoidance Databank (FARAD) (see www.fiveminutevet.com/ruminant)

• Foot and Mouth Disease
• Lymphosarcoma
• Photosensitization
• Tuberculosis: Bovine

Suggested Reading
Cortinas R, Jones CJ. Ectoparasites of cattle and small ruminants. Vet Clin North Am Food Anim Pract 2006, 22: 673–93.
Radostitis OM, Gay CC, Hinchcliff KW, et al. Diseases associated with arthropod parasites. In: Radostitis OM, Gay CC, Hinchcliff KW, et al. eds, Veterinary Medicine: A Textbook of the Diseases of Cattle, Horses, Sheep, Pigs and Goats, 10th ed. Philadelphia: Saunders, 2007, pp. 1585–612.
Scott DW. Color Atlas of Farm Animal Dermatology, 1st ed. Ames: Blackwell, 2007.

Author Sameeh M. Abutarbush
Consulting Editor Erica C. McKenzie
Acknowledgment The author and book editors acknowledge the prior contribution of Melissa Carr.

P

BASICS

OVERVIEW
• A variety of parasitic agents cause skin disease in camelids including mites, ticks, lice, fleas and flies.
• External parasites can feed on blood, skin, tissue, and hair, and can cause irritation, self-trauma, and secondary infection.
• External parasites can also facilitate transmission of infectious diseases.

INCIDENCE/PREVALENCE
Varies depending on the parasite and relevant management factors; contagious disorders can achieve high prevalence in herds.

GEOGRAPHIC DISTRIBUTION
Worldwide; variation in distribution of specific agents

SYSTEMS AFFECTED
Integument

PATHOPHYSIOLOGY
• *Mite* infestation is common in camelids.
  ○ *Chorioptes bovis* is not host specific and lives on the skin surface, feeding on organic material (epidermal scaling, hair, and dandruff). It is the most common mange mite in North America and Europe and is transmitted by direct contact.
  ○ *Sarcoptes* spp. has incomplete host specificity. It is highly contagious and a serious disease of dromedaries (*Sarcoptes scabiei* var. *camelis*). *Sarcoptes scabiei* var *auchinae* affects new world camelids (NWC). The mite burrows in the stratum corneum layer until reaching living cells in the stratum granulosum and stratum spinosum. Transmission is by direct/indirect contact and mites may survive off host for several days if climate is moist/cool. Mites are transmitted by direct contact and fomites.
  ○ *Psoroptes* sp. is also not host specific and lives on the skin surface, feeding superficially on lipid emulsion of skin cells, bacteria, and lymph. It is transmitted by direct contact.
  ○ *Demodex* sp. is a commensal organism with transmission believed to occur from dam to offspring via nursing. The mites burrow in hair follicles/sebaceous glands and destroy the inner root sheath of hair, causing it to fall out. Lesions represent nodules containing developmental stages, inflammatory products, and detritus. *Demodex* has been isolated from camels in Iran and Africa, llamas and alpacas in Bolivia, llamas imported to South Korea and Germany, and alpacas imported to New Zealand.

  ○ Miscellaneous mites include *Trombicula* spp. (chiggers) which may be seen on the skin surface. *Ornithonyssus sylviarum* (northern fowl mite) and *Dermanyssus gallinae* (red poultry mite) are reported as occasional skin irritants of camelids housed with poultry.
• *Ticks* are potential vectors of bacterial, protozoal, rickettsial, and viral diseases. They tend to be more problematic in old world camelids (OWC) than in NWC.
  ○ Ticks live on hosts for a short time. Some ticks are able to adapt to climates by altering their life cycles using multiple hosts depending on environmental conditions.
  ○ Camel host-specific hard ticks: *Hyalomma* spp. most important. *H. dromedarii* is the most common. *H. asiaticum* is the most common tick in Asia (affecting Bactrian camels in Mongolia).
  ○ Others found in camels include *Amblyomma* spp., *Rhipicephalus* spp., and *Dermacentor* spp.; *Boophilus* spp. reported on dromedaries in Australia and India.
  ○ Few hard body ticks affect NWC. *Amblyomma* spp. and *Haemaphysalis* spp. have been reported in South America; *Dermacentor* spp. and *Ixodes holocyclus* in llamas in western US, and *Amblyomma* spp. have been reported in vicuñas.
  ○ Larvae of *H. dromedarii* are implicated in tick paralysis of dromedaries. Other *Hyalomma* spp. and *Rhipicephalus* spp. also reported. The disorder can cause high calf mortality. *Dermacentor* spp. was reported in two llamas in Washington State. A salivary neurotoxin produced by female *Dermacentor* spp. ticks is injected during the blood meal. Ataxia/generalized muscle flaccidity resolves 2–12 hours after tick removal. Death is due to ascending paralysis if untreated. *I. holocyclus* produced serious tick paralysis in one llama in Australia. Animals may not recover after tick removal. Specific tick anti-serum may be administered to save the animal.
  ○ Soft ticks: *Ornithodoros* spp. live in sandy soils, cracks and crevices, seeking shade from hot arid deserts. Large numbers may be seen in the sand in marketplaces or holding pens where animals co-mingle. *Otobius megnini* (NWC): Adults do not feed. Nymphs molt twice in the ear, fall to ground and molt to an adult. Habitat off host is around outbuildings, feed bunks, wooden fences, or rough-barked trees. Animals in open pastures/rangelands are less commonly affected.
• *Lice* are host specific, and can be seen with the naked eye; sucking lice (spindle-shaped head) are smaller than biting lice (broad blunt head).

  ○ The life cycle is completed on one host. Females lay eggs (nits) on fiber and secure them there. Lice molt for growth.
  ○ Transmission occurs by direct contact between animals, or indirectly via contact with equipment, blankets, scratching posts, feed bunks, or dust bath areas.
  ○ Lice populations increase during colder months.
  ○ Shearing, exposure to sunlight, and fluctuating temperatures reduce lice populations.
  ○ Sucking lice: *Microthoracius cameli* (OWC), *M. mazzai*, *M. minor*. *M. praelongiceps* (NWC). Occur more often in temperate regions where animals have long winter hair. Sucking lice cause more significant disease than biting lice as they suck blood and lymph from host.
  ○ Biting lice: *Bovicola breviceps* (NWC). Llamas more often affected than alpacas. Seen in Chile and also on animals imported to New Zealand, Australia and the United Kingdom. Feed on dandruff, lipids, and bacteria.
• *Fleas* are not host specific and spend time on hosts for a blood meal. Eggs are laid in the environment.
  ○ Fleas can serve as vectors/intermediate hosts of disease pathogens. They are not reported in NWC.
  ○ *Vermipsylla* spp. and *Dorcardia ioffi* (Bactrian camels in Mongolia) affect OWC. Infestation by the cat flea *Ctenocephalides felis felis* has been reported.
• *Flies* distract animals from feeding and result in decreased productivity. They can also transmit infectious disease agents.
  ○ Myiasis (infestation with fly larvae) is caused by many fly species.
    ■ Flesh flies: *Wohlfahrtia magnifica*, *W. nuba*, and *Sarcophaga dux* (OWC in India). *W. magnifica* is an important cause of myiasis in the Mediterranean basin, southern Russia, Turkey, Iran, the Far East, Spain, and Mongolia. Flies deposit eggs/larvae near wounds.
    ■ Blow flies: *Lucilia cuprina*, *Chrysomya bezziana* (OWC), *Cochliomyia hominivorax* (OWC/NWC), and *Calliphora* spp., *Phaenicia* spp., *Phormia* spp. (NWC).
      □ *C. bezziana* (old world screwworm) affects camels in Africa and Southern Asia. Eggs are deposited at wound edges. Skin trauma from surgery, branding, scalding from dips, tick bites, and injection sites attract flies.
      □ *L. cuprina*: Australia, Middle East, India, and Africa. Eggs deposited in carcasses, infected/necrotic wounds, soiled/matted fiber around infected lesions, and on rotting vegetation.

P

PARASITIC SKIN DISEASES: CAMELID   (CONTINUED)

Larvae feed on epidermal cells, lymph, and necrotic tissue.
- □ *C. hominivorax* (new world screwworm) invades fresh wounds and can penetrate healthy tissue, exacerbating lesions.
○ Biting and nonbiting flies: *Musca domestica*, *M. autumnalis*, *Stomoxys calcitrans*, *Hydrotea* spp., *Haematobia* spp. are vectors/intermediate hosts for some bacterial, viral, helminth, and protozoal disease-causing organisms.
- ■ *M. domestica* deposits eggs in feces and decaying organic matter.
- ■ *M. autumnalis* lays eggs in fresh cattle feces. Camelids housed with cattle are affected.
- ■ *S. calcitrans* lays eggs in feces and decaying organic matter.
○ *Glossinia* spp.: Important intermediate host for *Trypanosoma* in OWC in tropical Africa.
○ *Tabanus* spp., *Haematopota* spp., *Chrysops* spp.
- ■ *Tabanus* spp. and *Haematopota* spp. are vectors of *Trypanosoma* for OWC in Africa and Asia and potentially NWC in South America; and aid in the transmission of other pathogens. Eggs are deposited in damp soil/organic matter near water sources. Larvae and pupae overwinter in mud.
- ■ Tabanids (horse flies, deer flies) are found throughout the world and are diurnal. They are attracted to animals by sight, odor, and body heat. Animals dislodge the feeding flies, which then move from animal to animal to complete feeding. Several blood meals expose multiple animals to potential disease transmission.
○ *Midges*: Small, biting flies. Transmit viruses, protozoa, and helminthes.
- ■ Simuliidae: Related to mosquitoes. Found in warm climates worldwide. Eggs are deposited in running water on the surface, or on submerged stones/twigs/vegetation. Eggs remain there for months (overwintering) or may hatch in a few days. The flies take blood meals from hosts. Swarms are annoying and lead to reduced feed intake by the host. Bites are similar to fleas/mosquitoes.

HISTORICAL FINDINGS
- Vary with the underlying etiology but defining the history of skin disease within the herd, and any relevant treatment or management procedures, is important.
- A description of skin lesion appearance and duration, number of animals affected, and the presence or absence of pruritis are important historical factors.

SIGNALMENT
Any age, species and breed of camelid is susceptible to ectoparasitism; however, some parasites are host-specific.

PHYSICAL EXAMINATION FINDINGS
Mites
- *Sarcoptes* spp.
  ○ Severe pruritus leading to excoriation, erythema, cracked/bleeding skin, skin thickening/wrinkling, or alopecia.
  ○ Affects nostrils, lips, orbit, chest, interdigital clefts, knee/hock joints, medial thighs, ventral abdomen, axillae, tail, perineum, and prepuce.
  ○ May become generalized.
- *Psoroptes* spp.
  ○ Pruritus less severe than *Sarcoptes* spp.
  ○ Ear canal lesions in NWC. Otitis externa, crusting/alopecia of pinnae, and dry flakes in ear canals. Animal may shake head or appear uncoordinated.
  ○ May be generalized without ears being affected. Nares, shoulders, neck, axillae, chest, back, sides, groin, legs, tail head, and perineum.
  ○ Erythema, crusting, papules, serum exudate, alopecia.
- *Chorioptes* spp.
  ○ Pruritus less severe than *Sarcoptes* spp. or *Psoroptes* spp.
  ○ Alopecia and scaling of distal limbs/feet, ventral abdomen, medial aspect of limbs base of tail; forehead, ears, trunk and perineum in severe cases.
  ○ Animals may be asymptomatic.
- *Demodex* spp.
  ○ Nonpruritic to mildly pruritic papular or nodular alopecic lesions on face, neck, axillary/inguinal regions (may extend to medial upper limbs). May be found in ears without concurrent otitis.
  ○ Secondary infections lead to excoriation, erythema, and crusting.
- Trombiculidae: Pruritic dermatitis of distal extremities.

Ticks
- Ticks may be identified in the perineal, inguinal and axillary regions, lips, ears, eyes, nostrils, between toes, and on udder.
- Cause direct/indirect irritation of the skin. Secondary bacterial infection/pyoderma may develop. Chronically skin may become thickened/scarred. Sores may be observed at mucocutaneous junction of nose, lips, vulva.
- *Otobius megnini* larvae/nymphs prefer the ears, causing excess wax production, purulent exudate in ears, and severe inflammation in the outer ear canals. Affected animals shake their heads and may appear uncoordinated. May cause anemia.

Lice
- Movement of lice causes pruritus and restlessness.

- Biting lice affect dorsal midline, base of tail, sides of neck/body. Cause matting of fiber, lackluster coat, ragged coat, and alopecia. Llamas more often affected than alpacas.
- Sucking lice affect flanks, head, neck, and withers causing alopecia. Alpacas more often affected than llamas. May cause anemia. Anemic animals are susceptible to cold stress and secondary infections.
- Lice may be observed if the hair is parted down to the skin which is examined with a light or magnifying glass, or nits may be visible attached to fiber. Sucking lice may be seen on fibers close to skin or embedded in the skin surface.

Fleas/Flies
- Distract animals from feeding, resulting in decreased productivity.
- Fleas: Deposit saliva when biting host, causing an allergic response which varies from mild irritation to marked pruritus. Bites may lead to anemia and death.
- Flesh flies: Ulcerative, oozing lesions.
- *Lucilia cuprina*: Prefer skin folds, especially in the perineal region, neonatal umbilicus, and decubital ulcers. Animals may rub or bite affected areas.
- *S. calcitrans*: Constant irritation may result in decreased production and conjunctivitis.
- *Tabanus* spp.: Prefers ventral abdomen, legs, and inguinal region. Bite wounds may be erythematous and swollen, attracting other flies. Bites are so intensely painful that reduced productivity occurs.

GENETICS
N/A

CAUSES AND RISK FACTORS
- The presence of specific parasites in a region
- Lice and mites tend to be more problematic in the cooler months
- Overcrowding and poor nutrition
- Lack of control procedures for external parasitism

 DIAGNOSIS

DIFFERENTIAL DIAGNOSES
- Camel pox
- Contagious ecthyma
- Dermatophytosis
- Endocrine disorders of the skin
- Foot and mouth disease
- Hyperkeratotic skin disease
- Irritant/Contact dermatitis
- Lymphosarcoma
- Nutrient deficiency (selenium, zinc, vitamins A, D, E)
- Pemphigus
- Photosensitization
- Poxvirus
- Pruritic skin disease

- Pseudotuberculosis
- Scrapie
- Tuberculosis

CBC/BIOCHEMISTRY/URINALYSIS
CBC may show anemia or inflammatory leukogram.

OTHER LABORATORY TESTS
Fecal analysis may yield dead mites as a result of pruritis and mite ingestion.

IMAGING
N/A

OTHER DIAGNOSTIC PROCEDURES
- Deep skin scrapings from lesion edges are indicated for *Sarcoptes* and *Demodex* spp. Adding warmed 10% potassium hydroxide to the scraping debris may allow for better visualization.
- Multiple superficial skin scrapings between toes or axillae, or by skin biopsy identifies *Chorioptes* sp.
- Examine swabs or ear exudates for *Psoroptes* sp. or *Otobius megnini*.
- Bacterial culture and sensitivity are relevant for infections.

PATHOLOGIC FINDINGS
- Mites are evident in scrapings or biopsies, and the species responsible can be differentiated by morphologic identification.
- Other findings are dependent on causative etiology.

TREATMENT
THERAPEUTIC APPROACH
- Follow adequate nutrition, management, and hygiene practices.
- Differentiate demodectic nodules from those of tuberculosis. Mites may not always be found and a treatment trial may be warranted using systemic or topical agents.
- Quarantine new animals before introduction to the herd.
- Treat all affected animals and all animals in the herd since they can be asymptomatic carriers. This includes animals in close contact, such as cattle or poultry.
- Multiple treatments are often necessary.
- Traditional topical treatment method (using products made from plants, oils, other) are used frequently by producers throughout the world. These generally require lengthy preparation time and can be laborious to apply.
- Treat secondary bacterial infections and otitis appropriately.
- *Cochliomyia hominivorax*: Treatment is aimed at reducing irritation of the lesion and cleansing of the wound. Remove larvae manually or by insecticides. Topical

application of hydrogen peroxide, ether, or chloroform drives larvae out of wounds.

SURGICAL CONSIDERATIONS AND TECHNIQUES
N/A

MEDICATIONS
DRUGS OF CHOICE
- Ivermectin at 0.2 mg/kg SC (repeated at 2-week intervals) is effective against many mites, ticks (nymphs/larvae), sucking lice, and some flies. Not effective for biting lice or *Chorioptes* due to their superficial feeding habits. Clients should be informed of extra-label use.
- Topical and systemic therapies are often utilized concurrently to improve treatment success.
- Topical acaricides must reach the skin layer to be effective. Clean affected areas with keratinolytic solution/soap to loosen and remove scabs. Brush away debris before application. Repeat at 7–14 day intervals.
- NWC fiber does not contain lanolin, reducing efficacy of topical products. Poor penetration of the product into damaged skin also limits efficacy. Many dusts, rinses, dips, sprays, powders containing pyrethroids, amitraz, spinosad, fipronil, avermectins and lime sulfur are safer alternatives to organophosphates/carbamates.
- Fipronil spray and ivermectin have been used in the ear after cleaning to improve efficacy against psoroptic mites. Not recommended if tympanic membrane is ruptured.

CONTRAINDICATIONS
- Corticosteroids are contraindicated in the treatment of mange.
- Corticosteroids should not be administered to pregnant animals.

PRECAUTIONS
- Appropriate milk and meat withdrawal times must be followed for all compounds administered to food-producing animals.
- Use caution when treating young crias with pyrethroids—of toxicity are possible.

POSSIBLE INTERACTIONS
N/A

FOLLOW-UP
EXPECTED COURSE AND PROGNOSIS
- Prognosis for demodectic mange is guarded, for other mites is fair to good with adequate diagnosis and subsequent treatment.

POSSIBLE COMPLICATIONS
Secondary bacterial infection.

CLIENT EDUCATION
Focus on methods of control and prevention to reduce ectoparasite-related distress and disease.

PATIENT CARE
- Monitor clinical signs and/or repeat skin scrapings.
- Observe animals for re-infestation.

PREVENTION
- Consider arthropod life cycles and length of treatment, as some animals may not show clinical signs.
- Implement scheduled anti-parasite programs (treatment, prevention, control).
- Free-ranging guineafowl or chickens decrease numbers of mites, ticks, and fleas in the environment.
- Management of environment to decrease breeding habitat of flies and mosquitoes. Fly traps/sticks, fly predators, and mosquito repellents may also be used.

MISCELLANEOUS
ASSOCIATED CONDITIONS
- Arthropod borne diseases
- Lymphadenopathy

AGE-RELATED FACTORS
N/A

ZOONOTIC POTENTIAL
Sarcoptes scabiei is zoonotic.

PREGNANCY
N/A

BIOSECURITY
- Quarantine new animals before introduction into herd.
- Isolate affected herd members or whole herds.
- Contact state/provincial/government veterinarian for reportable diseases.
- *Sarcoptes* spp. and *Psoroptes* spp. are reportable in the US and other countries.
- New world screwworm and old world screwworm are reportable. New world screwworm has been eradicated from the US, however, recent infestations in wild and domestic animals were reported in Florida in 2016 and 2017.

PRODUCTION MANAGEMENT
Parasites affecting the skin cause significant economic loss as a result of poor growth, reduced milk/meat production, hide damage, poor fiber quality, and death.

SYNONYMS
- Demodectic mange—follicular mange
- Sarcoptic mange—barn itch

P

• Psoroptic mange—body mange, ear mange, sheep scab
• Chorioptic mange—tail mange, leg mange, scrotal mange

ABBREVIATIONS

• FARAD = Food Animal Residue Avoidance Databank
• NWC = New World camelids
• OWC = Old World camelids

SEE ALSO

• Parasitic Skin Diseases: Small Ruminant

Suggested Reading

Bornstein S. Important ectoparasites of alpaca (*Vicugna pacos*). Acta Vet Scand 2010, 52(Suppl 1): S17.

El-Bannna HA, Elzorba H, El Baby MM. Efficacy of ivermectin and closantel combination on camel parasites. In: Proceedings of the 4th Conference of the International Society of Camelid Research and Development, 2015, pp. 244–6.

Fowler ME. Medicine and Surgery of Camelids, 3rd ed. Ames: Wiley-Blackwell, 2010, pp. 231–69.

Köhler-Rollefson I, Mundy P, Mathias E. A Field Manual of Camel Diseases: Traditional and Modern Health Care for the Dromedary. London: ITDG Publishing, 2001, pp. 69–98.

Merino O, Alberdi P, Pérez de la Lastra JM, de la Fuente J. Tick vaccines and the control of tick-borne pathogens. Front Cellular Infect Microbiol 2013, 3: 30.

Sisson D, Cebra C. Disorders of the skin. In: Cebra C ed, Llama and Alpaca Care. St. Louis: Elsevier Saunders, 2014, pp. 379–92.

Stitch, RW. Ectoparaciticides used in large animals. The Merck Veterinary Manual, 2015. http://merckvetmanual.com/mvm/pharmacology/ectoparasiticides/ectoparasiticides_used_in_large_animals.html

Wernery U, Kaaden O-R. Infestations with ectoparasites. In: Infectious Diseases in Camelids, 2nd ed. Berlin-Vienna: Blackwell-Science, 2002, pp. 312–46.

Wernery U, Kinne J, Schuster RK. Arthropod infections. In: Camelid Infectious Disorders. World Organisation for Animal Health. Paris: OIE, 2014, pp. 431–64.

Author Keely A. Smith
Consulting Editor Erica C. McKenzie

PARASITIC SKIN DISEASES: SMALL RUMINANT

BASICS

OVERVIEW
• Small ruminants are affected by a range of parasitic skin diseases which can cause significant economic loss and compromise animal welfare.
• External parasites can feed on blood, skin, tissue, and hair, and can cause irritation, self-trauma, and secondary infection.
• External parasites can also facilitate transmission of infectious diseases.

INCIDENCE/PREVALENCE
Varies depending on the parasite and management factors; contagious disorders can achieve high prevalence in herds.

GEOGRAPHIC DISTRIBUTION
• Lice affect sheep and goats worldwide.
• Chorioptic mange is present worldwide and is common in goats in North America and Europe.
• Psoroptic mange is not present in North America. It was eradicated in the United Kingdom but is now present and widespread. It is eradicated from Australia and New Zealand.
• Sarcoptic mange is not present in the United States and is a reportable disease. It is present in Southern European countries.
• Demodectic mange occurs worldwide.
• Myiasis is common worldwide, particularly in warmer climates.

SYSTEMS AFFECTED
Integument

PATHOPHYSIOLOGY
• Pediculosis (louse infestation) is related to lice from order Mallophaga (biting or chewing lice) and order Anoplura (sucking lice).
  ◦ Common species in sheep are *Damalinia (Bovicola) ovis* (biting body louse), *Linognathus ovillus* (sucking face louse) and *L. pedalis* (sucking foot louse).
  ◦ Common species in goats are *D. caprae, D. crassipes,* and *D. limbata* (biting) and *L. stenopsis* and *L. africanus* (sucking).
  ◦ Lice maintain their life cycle on the animal, living off the host for usually very brief periods, with transmission by direct or indirect contact.
• Mites can live off their hosts for more extended periods and transmission occurs by direct contact and indirect contact with fomites.
  ◦ Chorioptic mange: *Chorioptes ovis or C. bovis* in sheep; *C. caprae* in goats.
  ◦ Psoroptic mange: *Psoroptes ovis* in sheep, rare in goats. *P. cuniculi* is an ear mite of sheep and goats that can also affect the face and body.
  ◦ Sarcoptic mange: *Sarcoptes scabei* var *ovis* (sheep) and *S. scabei* var *caprae* (goats).
  ◦ Demodectic mange (demodecosis) generally affects goats. *Demodex caprae*

mites live in the hair follicles and can be transmitted from dam to kid; infection is associated with nodular lesions and is usually nonpruritic.
• Cutaneous myiasis (fly strike) is typically caused by blow flies or bottle flies; including *Lucilia* spp., *Phormia* spp., and *Calliphora* spp. Flies are attracted to warm, moist wool, hair, or skin, and to organic matter to lay their eggs. Soiled wool or wounds are particularly attractive. Eggs develop into larvae (maggots) which ingest skin and tissue.
• Screwworm fly (*Cochliomyia hominivorax*) occurs in Central and South America. It has been eradicated from North America and is reportable. Transient re-emergence was documented in Florida in 2016 and 2017. Adult females deposit eggs near wounds and larvae cause severe damage by feeding on body fluids and living tissue. Several other species of fly act in a similar manner.

HISTORICAL FINDINGS
• Vary with the underlying etiology, but defining the history of skin disease within the herd, and any relevant treatment or management procedures, is important.
• A description of skin lesion appearance and duration, number of animals affected, and the presence or absence of pruritis are important historical factors.

SIGNALMENT
Any age, species, and breed of small ruminant is susceptible to ectoparasitism; however, some parasites are host-specific. Demodectic mange tends to affect goats, and *Damalinia limbata* and *D. crassipes* lice are more common in Angora goats.

PHYSICAL EXAMINATION FINDINGS
• Mites typically cause pruritus. Chronic mange can result in hyperkeratinization and lichenification of skin, weight loss, decreased productivity (meat, wool, and milk), infertility, and even death from emaciation.
• Ear mites may cause head shaking and scratching with secondary aural hematomas and scarring of the pinnae.
• Lice tend to cause pruritis in sheep with accompanying wool damage, and are less often pruritic in goats. Large infestations of sucking lice can cause signs of anemia in neonates.
• Demodectic mange is typically nonpruritic, with formation of papules and nodules with a normal appearing coat. Lesions can be found on the face, neck, and shoulders of goats but may be extensive.
• Chorioptic mange can create erythema, papules, crusts, and scaling, usually localized to the lower legs (hind > fore), scrotum, and udder.
• Psoroptic mange lesions start as vesicles and papules resulting in yellow crusts and inflammation. Wool becomes stained and is lost due to pruritus. Lesions typically localize

on the dorsal midline progressing to the whole body, or occasionally localize to the ears.
• Sarcoptic mange affects non-wooled areas of the face, ears, neck, scrotum, and legs. Chronically, lesions may become generalized and the skin thickened. Peripheral lymphadenopathy may occur.
• Myiasis usually tends to affect wounds, the breech, and sometimes body areas, and occasionally the tail, poll, genitalia, prepuce, and foot.

GENETICS
N/A

CAUSES AND RISK FACTORS
• The presence of specific parasites in a region.
• Lice and mites tend to be more problematic in the cooler months.
• Angora goats are more at risk of infestation with some species of *Damalinia* lice.
• Overcrowding and poor nutrition.
• Lack of control procedures for external parasitism.

DIAGNOSIS

DIFFERENTIAL DIAGNOSES
Differential diagnoses for skin lesions in small ruminants besides ectoparasites include zinc-responsive dermatosis, bacterial skin disease (including dermatophilosis), fungal skin disease, and pyoderma.

CBC/BIOCHEMISTRY/URINALYSIS
N/A

OTHER LABORATORY TESTS
Bacterial culture and sensitivity might be relevant in secondary infections of the skin or ear canals.

IMAGING
N/A

OTHER DIAGNOSTIC PROCEDURES
• Lice are visible to the naked eye. Close examination of the hairs, or use of a flea comb, can yield lice which can be viewed under magnification for further identification. Sucking lice have longer, narrow mouthpieces compared to the flatter, wider mouthpiece of chewing lice.
• Mites are not easily visible to the naked eye. Identification requires sampling via skin scraping (superficial and deep) or skin biopsy. Acute lesions typically yield more mites than chronic lesions, and scraping at the edges of lesions is most helpful. Caseous material expressed from nodules can reveal *Demodex* mites in cases of demodecosis.
• For filarial dermatitis (elaeophoriasis or sorehead), a skin biopsy of the lesion is macerated in isotonic saline solution and rested for ≥6 h at room temperature. Tissue is strained off and the fluid examined for microfilariae.

P

PATHOLOGIC FINDINGS
• Mites are evident in scrapings or biopsies, and the species responsible can be differentiated by morphologic identification.
• Other findings are dependent on causative etiology.

TREATMENT

THERAPEUTIC APPROACH
• Specific conditions respond to topical or parenteral insecticides/pesticides.
• Animals should be supported via good management, adequate nutrition, and where relevant, hygiene procedures.
• For reportable conditions, contact appropriate state/provincial/government bodies to determine specific quarantine requirements and treatments.

SURGICAL CONSIDERATIONS
• Skin biopsy is a quick and relatively painless procedure that can be achieved using a 6 mm skin biopsy punch with no preceding preparation of the skin or local anesthesia to avoid lesion disruption and artifact.
• Biopsy sites can be left to heal by granulation but should be protected from invasion by external parasites.

MEDICATIONS

DRUGS OF CHOICE
• For mites, organophosphate compounds (OPs) (e.g., diazinon and propetamphos) and systemic pyrethroids (e.g., flumethrin and cypermethrin) have been used in plunge dipping, showers, and jetting. Both have significant health implications for operators and the environment, and resistance is widespread. Injectable macrocylic lactones (ivermectin, doramectin, moxidectin) are effective and labeled for use in some countries. Repeated use has implications for development of nematode resistance. In flocks affected with *Psoroptes ovis*, all animals should be treated with injectable macrocyclic lactones twice, 7–10 days apart (treatment may be less effective for chorioptic mange). Topical lime sulfur can be effective if repeated every 7 days for prolonged periods. A shampoo that loosens crusts can make topical treatment more effective in chronic cases. Topical amitraz may also be effective for *Demodex*.
• Lice are killed by many topically administered drugs including OPs, and synthetic pyrethroids and pyrethrins. Care must be taken for the product to have contact with the skin for full effect. Treatment should be applied 2–4 weeks after shearing for full effectiveness. Resistance to all drugs has been reported. The louse eggs (nits) are not responsive to these treatments, which should

therefore be repeated in 10–14 days. Injectable macrocyclic lactones are effective against sucking lice but not biting/chewing lice.
• Cutaneous myiasis is addressed after removing surrounding wool or hair from the affected area. Severe myiasis may result in shock, dehydration, and secondary bacterial infections which should be treated appropriately. Permethrins can be applied to kill maggots, selecting products that can be applied to open wounds.

CONTRAINDICATIONS
Topical pesticides that fall under the jurisdiction of the EPA rather than the FDA in the US cannot be applied in an extra-label manner.

PRECAUTIONS
Appropriate milk and meat withdrawal times must be followed for all compounds administered to food-producing animals.

POSSIBLE INTERACTIONS
N/A

FOLLOW-UP

EXPECTED COURSE AND PROGNOSIS
• Depends upon the causative agent; the prognosis for *Demodex* infestation is guarded, but for other mites is fair to good with adequate diagnosis and subsequent treatment.
• Most parasitic conditions of the integument cause anxiety and production loss as the main concern.

POSSIBLE COMPLICATIONS
Secondary bacterial infection

CLIENT EDUCATION
Focus on methods of control and prevention to reduce ectoparasite-related distress and disease

PATIENT CARE
N/A

PREVENTION
• Psoroptes, lice, and keds (wingless flies) can be eradicated from a flock with appropriate treatment and control.
• Prevention of myiasis in sheep can be achieved by decreasing fecal and urine contamination of the fleece by controlling causes of diarrhea (e.g., parasites); shearing the breech region; the mulesing procedure in Merinos; tail docking; use of fly traps; and genetic selection for fewer skin folds (Merinos).
• Drugs used in prevention and control of fly strike include synthetic pyrethroids (e.g., deltamethrin, cypermethrin), insect growth regulators (IGRs) (e.g., cyromazine, dicyclanil), OPs (e.g., diazinon) and permethrins. Use may be restricted depending on location. Dipping, showers, dusting, spray

races, and hand jetting have all been used to apply drugs to sheep. There is reported resistance to OPs and IGRs.
• Remove wet, rotting organic matter to reduce habitat for fly larvae; dragging pastures to break up and dry manure masses is also helpful.
• Quarantine new animals before introduction into the herd, with close inspection for skin lesions.
• Lice can live for a limited time off the host (varies with species); therefore, leaving facilities dormant for 1–4 weeks (depending on the species involved) before re-introducing treated animals can help break the life cycle.

✓ MISCELLANEOUS

ASSOCIATED CONDITIONS
• Keds (*Melophagus ovinus*) are wingless flies that can cause pruritis and wool staining in sheep. They are visible to the naked eye and the entire life cycle is spent on the animals; hence they can be eradicated through simple control procedures.
• Blackflies (Simuliidae), *Culicoides* gnats, mosquitoes, and biting flies (*Stomoxys* spp. and Tabanidae) may cause insect hypersensitivity and irritation in small ruminants.
• Ticks exist worldwide, are not particularly host-specific and in addition to skin lesions, anemia and reduced production, can facilitate disease including tick paralysis, babesiosis, heartwater, theileriasis, and anaplasmosis.
• Free-living pasture mites (*Trombiculidae* sp.) can cause hypersensitivity and dermatitis.
• *Strongyloides papillosus* larvae penetrate skin and migrate to the lungs. Repeated exposures may cause dermatitis. Similarly, *Pelodera* (*Rhabditis*) *strongyloides* is a soil-living nematode that may cause dermatitis in animals housed in dirty conditions.
• Psorergatic mange (*Psorobia ovis*, itch mite) is often asymptomatic but can cause pruritis and wool damage in some infested sheep and occurs in Australia, New Zealand, Africa, and South America.
• Elaeophoriasis (sore head) is related to infestation with *Elaeophora schneideri*, a deer parasite in western and southwestern US. Transmitted to sheep and goats by Tabanid flies, infection can cause severe neurologic disease and prominent microfilarial dermatitis of the poll, forehead, or face.

AGE-RELATED FACTORS
N/A

ZOONOTIC POTENTIAL
Sarcoptes mites are zoonotic.

PREGNANCY
N/A

P

(CONTINUED) PARASITIC SKIN DISEASES: SMALL RUMINANT

BIOSECURITY
• Prevent introduction of ectoparasites by quarantine and examination of new arrivals and effective treatment.
• Isolate affected herd members or whole flocks during testing and treatment.
• Contact regulatory bodies if reportable conditions are suspected.

PRODUCTION MANAGEMENT
• Ectoparasites are a significant cause of economic loss due to reduced production (milk, meat, wool), secondary disease, and expenses related to control and treatment.
• Psoroptic mange has significant welfare and economic implications in areas of the world where is it not eradicated.

SYNONYMS
• Demodectic mange—follicular mange
• Sarcoptic mange—barn itch

• Psoroptic mange—body mange, ear mange, sheep scab
• Chorioptic mange—tail mange, leg mange, scrotal mange
• Psorergatic mange—Australian mange
• Elaeophoriasis—sore head, filarial dermatosis, "clear-eyed" blindness

ABBREVIATIONS
• EPA = Environmental Protection Agency of the USA
• FDA = Food and Drug Administration of the USA
• IGRs = insect growth regulators
• OPs = organophosphates

SEE ALSO
• Dermatophytosis
• Dermatophilosis
• Wool Rot

Suggested Reading
McNair CM. Ectoparasites of medical and veterinary: drug resistance and the need for alternative control methods. J Pharm Pharmacol 2015, 67: 351–63.
Plant JW, Lewis CL. Treatment and control of ectoparasites in sheep. Vet Clin North Am Food Anim Pract 2011, 27: 203–12.
Scott DW. Color Atlas of Farm Animal Dermatology, 1st ed. Ames: Blackwell Scientific Publishing, 2007, chs 2.3, 3.3.
Smith MC, Sherman DM. Goat Medicine, 2nd ed. Ames: Blackwell Publishing, 2009, pp. 38–45.
Taylor MA. Emerging parasitic diseases of sheep. Vet Parasitol 2012, 189: 2–7.
Author Philippa Gibbons
Consulting Editor Erica C. McKenzie
Acknowledgment The author and book editors acknowledge the prior contribution of Melissa Carr.

P

PARELAPHOSTRONGYLUS TENUIS (MENINGEAL WORM)

BASICS

OVERVIEW
• Aberrant migration of the larvae of *Parelaphostrongylus tenuis* into the central nervous system of small ruminants, camelids, and specific cervidae including red deer and moose, causes mild to severe neurologic signs.
• White-tailed deer (WTD) are the definitive host and typically show no clinical signs.

INCIDENCE/PREVALENCE
P. tenuis does not affect camelids in regions that do not contain infected WTD; however, in some regions >50% of deer are infested, and there is evidence that the range of infection is expanding.

GEOGRAPHIC DISTRIBUTION
• Reflects the range of the WTD, which includes southern Canada and the continental United States typically east of the Mississippi river.
• Animals co-mingled in artificial habitats (zoos) may be affected outside of this geographic range.

SYSTEMS AFFECTED
Nervous

PATHOPHYSIOLOGY
• The natural host for *P. tenuis* is the white-tailed deer (*Odocoileus virginianus*). Clinical signs or pathologic findings associated with *P. tenuis* infestation in this species are rare.
• Adult worms reside in the subarachnoid space of WTD. Eggs leave the CNS through the venous sinuses and embryonate into first stage larvae which migrate up the trachea, and are swallowed and passed in the feces.
• Larvae penetrate into a snail or slug and mature for 3–4 weeks. Larvae can overwinter in the intermediate host. During the grazing season infected slugs and snails are ingested by WTD. Alternatively, the L3 stage may leave the gastropod and deer ingest them in slime trails on vegetation.
• Ingested larvae penetrate the abomasal wall, migrate through the body to the dorsal gray columns of the spinal cord, and become adults in 20–30 days. They then migrate along the dorsal nerve rootlets to the subarachnoid space.
• The prepatent period is approximately 90 days, and the life cycle is complete in 4 months.
• When aberrant hosts such as sheep, goats, and camelids ingest infected gastropods or slime, the larvae are released in the abomasum and after variable periods of time eventually reach the spinal cord and/or brain, where aberrant migration causes inflammation and disease. Larvae rarely reach maturity in the aberrant host.
• Self-cure has been reported in sheep, and goats.

HISTORICAL FINDINGS
Acute or chronic onset of neurologic signs that commence in the hindlimbs and progress cranially, in an area where *P. tenuis* is known or possible, and in animals not subject to frequent preventive treatment.

SIGNALMENT
The disease is most common in adult camelids ≥2 years of age. Goats, sheep, moose, elk, antelope, and reindeer can be affected.

PHYSICAL EXAMINATION FINDINGS
• Clinical signs vary based on the number and location of migrating larvae.
• Most commonly signs indicate focal, asymmetric disease of the spinal cord, reflected by gait abnormalities (lameness, spasticity, ataxia) and proprioceptive deficits. Paresis, or paralysis, may also be present and animals may present recumbent.
• Cortex and brainstem involvement may cause cranial nerve deficits, blindness, head tilt, circling, scoliosis, altered mentation, and seizures.

GENETICS
N/A

CAUSES AND RISK FACTORS
• The major cause for cerebrospinal nematodiasis in North America is *P. tenuis*. Other parasites such as *Oestrus ovis*, *Coenurus cerebralis*, and *Baylisascaris procyonis* can also cause disease.
• The major risk factor for infestation is grazing low-lying, damp treed pastures in the late summer and fall that are cohabited by WTD. After a killing frost, the risk for infestation is greatly decreased.

DIAGNOSIS

DIFFERENTIAL DIAGNOSES
• Differentials for recumbency and possible spinal cord disease include heat stress, rabies, spinal trauma, abscessation, neoplasia, listeriosis, tick paralysis, and nutritional deficiencies, especially in juveniles (copper, vitamin E/selenium, vitamin D).
• Differentials for signs suggestive of intracranial disease can include rabies, listeriosis, otitis interna, polioencephalomalacia, neoplasia, trauma, cerebral abscessation, and toxicity (lead, salt, plants). In sheep and goats, scrapie, louping ill, and lentivirus infection should be considered.

CBC/BIOCHEMISTRY/URINALYSIS
There are no specific tests for diagnosis of *P. tenuis*. Complete blood count, serum chemistry analysis, and urinalysis may be useful to investigate differentials.

OTHER LABORATORY TESTS
N/A

IMAGING
• Diagnostic imaging (radiographs, CT, MRI) is not specific for *P. tenuis*, but may help rule out differentials.
• Computed tomography with intravenous contrast may reveal subtle multifocal lesions in the brain of animals with intracranial signs.

OTHER DIAGNOSTIC PROCEDURES
CSF cytology—detection of an eosinophilic pleocytosis is highly suggestive for cerebrospinal nematodiasis. A mononuclear pleocytosis may also be observed which is less specific for parasite migration. CSF can be obtained readily from the lumbosacral space of camelids just caudal to the dorsal spinous process of the 7th lumbar vertebra.

PATHOLOGIC FINDINGS
Definitive diagnosis requires histopathologic identification of the parasite within the brain or spinal cord. In cases where the parasites are not definitively identified, microcavitation and spongiosis with multifocal areas of malacia, necrosis, and degenerating axons are often present, suggestive of aberrant parasite migration.

TREATMENT

THERAPEUTIC APPROACH
• Animals that remain standing with relatively mild signs should be separated or housed with a few gentle companions, in an area that is well bedded with a nonslip floor.
• Food and water should be readily accessible. Encouraging mild to moderate exercise is important to promote muscle strength and function.
• Animals with severe signs, such as paralysis of the forelimbs, hindlimbs, or both, require intensive nursing care. This may include use of a sling or a water flotation tank to support the animal and the provision of physical therapy. Food and water need to be immediately accessible.
• Animals that have signs associated with brain lesions present the greatest challenge since they are often recumbent and inappetent. Besides physical therapy, enteral feeding via stomach tube or temporary rumen fistula may be required. Parenteral (intravenous) nutrition may be required for severely affected animals.

SURGICAL CONSIDERATIONS AND TECHNIQUES
N/A

MEDICATIONS

DRUGS OF CHOICE
• Anthelmintics

(CONTINUED) *PARELAPHOSTRONGYLUS TENUIS* (MENINGEAL WORM)

○ Fenbendazole: 20–50 mg/kg, PO q24h for 5 days ±
○ Diethylcarbamazine: 50 mg/kg, PO q24h for 7 days
• Anti-inflammatory agents
○ Dexamethasone: 0.05–0.1 mg/kg, IV or SC, q48h for 2 treatments
○ Prednisolone sodium succinate: 0.5–1.0 mg/kg IV or SC, q12–24h
○ Flunixin meglumine: 0.5–1 mg/kg IV, q12h for 2–3 days
• Antioxidant agents
○ Vitamin E—immediate antioxidant activity: 1 mL/100 lb SC or IM (300 IU/mL)
○ Selenium—antioxidant activity will take 7–10 days for effect (Bo-Se®—1 mL/50 lb)

CONTRAINDICATIONS
• Dexamethasone will cause abortion in pregnant camelids, and possibly in small ruminants.
• Ivermectin is suggested to be contraindicated in *P. tenuis* treatment, to reduce the chance of exacerbating damage by crossing a compromised blood-brain barrier.

PRECAUTIONS
Appropriate milk and meat withdrawal times must be followed for all compounds administered to food-producing animals.

POSSIBLE INTERACTIONS
N/A

FOLLOW-UP

EXPECTED COURSE AND PROGNOSIS
Damaged nervous tissue may take 6 months or longer to heal, or for an animal to develop compensatory skills. The more severe the neurologic damage, the poorer the prognosis. Recovery may be incomplete and may require prolonged, intensive nursing care.

POSSIBLE COMPLICATIONS
Recumbency may create the risk of heat stress in warmer months, or promote muscle damage if prolonged without intervention.

CLIENT EDUCATION
Promote non-anthelmintic methods of control where feasible to reduce the contribution of frequent preventive treatments to anthelmintic resistance.

PATIENT CARE
Focuses on supportive nursing, provision of nutrition, and providing a safe environment during recovery.

PREVENTION
• Minimize exposure of susceptible animals to infected snails by using fowl, having vegetation-free zones around pastures, and preventing access to low-lying, snail- and deer-infested pastures during cooler, moist periods until after the first killing frost.
• Strategic anthelmintic treatment typically involves periodic treatment with an avermectin product every 30–60 days. Prior to reaching the CNS, *P. tenuis* is susceptible to multiple products using dosages recommended for treatment of gastrointestinal parasites.
• Livestock guard dogs can be used to repel deer, since fencing is typically of limited effectiveness.

 MISCELLANEOUS

ASSOCIATED CONDITIONS
N/A

AGE-RELATED FACTORS
Because of the *P. tenuis* life cycle, disease is typically confined to animals of grazing age.

ZOONOTIC POTENTIAL
N/A

PREGNANCY
See "Contraindications"

BIOSECURITY
N/A

PRODUCTION MANAGEMENT
See "Prevention"

SYNONYMS
• Brain worm
• Deer worm
• Meningeal deer worm

ABBREVIATIONS
• CNS = central nervous system
• CSF = cerebrospinal fluid
• CT = computed tomography
• MRI = magnetic resonance imaging
• WTD = white-tailed deer

SEE ALSO
Parasite Control Programs (by species)

Suggested Reading
Cebra C, Anderson D.E., Tibary A, Van Saun R.J., and Johnson L. 2014. Llama and alpaca care. 1st ed. St. Louis: Elsevier
Fowler, M. E. 2010. Medicine and surgery of Camelids. 3rd ed. Ames: Wiley-Blackwell.
Nagy D.W. 2004. *Parelaphostrongylus tenuis* and other diseases of the ruminant nervous system. Vet Clin Food Anim 20:393
Smith, M. C., Sherman, D. M. 2009. Goat medicine. 2nd ed. Ames: Wiley-Blackwell.
Author Dusty W. Nagy
Consulting Editor Erica C. McKenzie
Acknowledgment The author and book editors acknowledge the prior contribution of Michelle Kopcha.

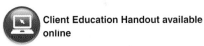 **Client Education Handout available online**

P

PARENTERAL NUTRITION

BASICS

OVERVIEW
• Parenteral nutrition (PN) refers to the intravenous administration of nutrients.
• Total PN (TPN) provides all daily nutrient requirements while partial PN (PPN) only provides part of daily nutrient requirements.
• PN is indicated when enteral nutrition is either contraindicated (dysphagia, regurgitation, malabsorption, maldigestion, or ileus) or impossible (esophageal obstruction or rupture).
• PN can also be useful in ruminants that have a history of prolonged anorexia and are not voluntarily ingesting enough to meet 75% of their daily maintenance requirements.
• PN can be beneficial and life-saving and should be considered as important as other medications in the management of critically ill ruminants.
• PN solutions usually include dextrose and lipids as energy sources and amino acids (AA) as protein sources.

INCIDENCE/PREVALENCE
N/A

GEOGRAPHIC DISTRIBUTION
N/A

SYSTEMS AFFECTED
N/A

PATHOPHYSIOLOGY
Maintenance Nutrient Requirements
• Daily maintenance energy requirements (MER) can be calculated as follows:
  ∘ MER (kcal) = $140 \times BW^{0.75}$ (kg) in cattle [1]
  ∘ MER (kcal) = $130 \times BW^{0.75}$ (kg) in small ruminants [1]
  ∘ MER (kcal) = $70 \times BW^{0.75}$ (kg) in camelids [1]
• Daily maintenance protein requirements (MPR) can be calculated as follows:
  ∘ MPR (g) = $3.5 \times BW^{0.75}$ (kg) in adults [2]
  ∘ MPR (g) = $4 \times BW^{0.75}$ (kg) in neonates [2]
• For example, a 50-kg calf should receive about 2,600 kcal and 75 g of protein per day.

HISTORICAL FINDINGS
• Prolonged anorexia
  ∘ 1–2 days in neonates
  ∘ 5–7 days in adults
• Weight loss

SIGNALMENT
N/A

PHYSICAL EXAMINATION FINDINGS
• Evidence of dysphagia or choke
  ∘ Dropping feed from the mouth
  ∘ Ptyalism
  ∘ Feed coming from the nares
  ∘ Neck swelling or pain
  ∘ Free-gas bloat
  ∘ Abnormal jaw or tongue tone
• Evidence of malabsorption or maldigestion
  ∘ Chronic diarrhea
  ∘ Weight loss or cachexia
• Anorexia is common in ruminants with
  ∘ Altered mentation
  ∘ Chronic renal failure
  ∘ Gastrointestinal obstruction or stasis
  ∘ Severe anemia
  ∘ Severe dyspnea

GENETICS
N/A

CAUSES AND RISK FACTORS
• Any disease causing prolonged anorexia, dysphagia, malabsorption, maldigestion, or gastrointestinal obstruction.

DIAGNOSIS

DIFFERENTIAL DIAGNOSES
N/A

CBC/BIOCHEMISTRY/URINALYSIS
• Sepsis, hyperglycemia, hyperlipidemia, hypokalemia, hypophosphatemia, and hypomagnesemia can develop in ruminants treated with PN.

OTHER LABORATORY TESTS
N/A

IMAGING
N/A

OTHER DIAGNOSTIC PROCEDURES
N/A

PATHOLOGIC FINDINGS
N/A

TREATMENT

THERAPEUTIC APPROACH
Composition Determination
• First, volume of AA solution required to provide 100% of MPR should be calculated.
• 8.5–10% AA solutions provide 0.085–0.1 gram of protein per mL, respectively.
• Volume of AA solution can be calculated as follows:
  ∘ Volume (mL) = [2] / 0.1 with 10% AA solution [3]
  ∘ Volume (mL) = [2] / 0.085 with 8.5% AA solution [3']
• A 50-kg calf should receive 750 mL of 10% AA solution or 900 mL of 8.5% AA solution per day to provide 100% of MPR.
• Each gram of AA provides 4 kcal and energy provided by AA solution can thus be calculated as follows:
  ∘ Energy (kcal) = [3] $\times$ 0.1 $\times$ 4 with 10% AA solution [4]
  ∘ Energy (kcal) = [3'] $\times$ 0.085 $\times$ 4 with 8.5% AA solution [4]

• For example, 750 mL of 10% AA solution or 900 mL of 8.5% AA solution provide 300 kcal.
• Second, volume of lipid solution required to provide 25% of MER should be calculated.
• 10–20% lipid solutions provide 1.1 and 2 kcal per mL, respectively
• Volume of lipid solution can thus be calculated as follows:
  ∘ Volume (mL) = (0.25 $\times$ [1]) / 2 with 20% lipid solution [5]
  ∘ Volume (mL) = (0.25 $\times$ [1]) / 1.1 with 10% lipid solution [5']
• A 50-kg calf should receive 330 mL of 20% lipid solution or 600 mL of 10% lipid solution per day to provide 25% of MER.
• Energy provided by lipid solution can be calculated as follows:
  ∘ Energy (kcal) = [5] $\times$ 2 with 20% lipid solution [6]
  ∘ Energy (kcal) = [5'] $\times$ 1.1 with 10% lipid solution [6]
• Third, volume of dextrose solution required to provide the remainder of the MER should be calculated
• Each gram of dextrose provides 3.4 kcal and 50% dextrose solution contains 0.5 g of dextrose per ml
• Volume of dextrose solution can thus be calculated as follows:
  ∘ Volume (mL) = ([1] − [4] − [6]) / (3.4 $\times$ 0.5) with 50% dextrose solution [7]
• A 50-kg calf should receive 1,000 mL of 50% dextrose solution per day to provide the remainder of the MER.
• Energy provided by dextrose solution can be calculated as follows:
  ∘ Energy (kcal) = [7] $\times$ 0.5 $\times$ 3.4 with 50% dextrose solution [8]
• Lipids can sometimes be omitted to reduce the cost of PN.
• Lipids should be avoided in ruminants with liver dysfunction or hypertriglyceridemia.
• If lipids are not used, volume of dextrose solution should be calculated as follows:
  ∘ Volume (mL) = ([1] − [4]) / (3.4 $\times$ 0.5) with 50% dextrose solution [7']
• A 50-kg calf should receive 1,400 mL of 50% dextrose solution should be administered per day if lipids are omitted.
• Nonprotein calories from dextrose and lipid solutions should be provided at a ratio between 100 and 300 kcal per gram of nitrogen to promote the use of AA for tissue maintenance and repair.
• Each gram of AA provides 0.16 g of nitrogen and amount of nitrogen provided from AA solution can thus be calculated as follows:
  ∘ Nitrogen (g) = [3] $\times$ 0.1 $\times$ 0.16 with 10% AA solution [9]
  ∘ Nitrogen (g) = [3'] $\times$ 0.085 $\times$ 0.16 with 8.5% AA solution [9]
• For example, 750 mL of 10% AA solution or 900 mL of 8.5% AA solution provide 12 g of nitrogen.

(CONTINUED)

- Nonprotein calorie to nitrogen ratio (NPC:N) can be calculated as follows:
  - NPC:N = ([6] + [8]) / [9]
- For example, a PN solution containing 750 mL of 10% AA solution, 330 mL of 20% lipid solution, and 1,000 mL of 50% dextrose solution, has a NPC:N of 190:1.
- Finally, the osmolarity of the PN solution should be calculated.
  - Osmolarity of AA solution (mOsm/L) = [3] × 938 or [3′] × 920 = [10]
  - Osmolarity of lipid solution (mOsm/L) = [5] or [5′] × 268 = [11]
  - Osmolarity of dextrose solution (mOsm/L) = [7] or [7′] × 2525 = [12]
- Osmolarity (mOsm/L) of the PN solution can be calculated as follows:
  - Osmolarity = ([10] + [11] + [12]) / ([3] or [3′] + [5] or [5′] + [7] or [7′])
  - Osmolarity should not exceed 1,400 mOsm/L to limit the risk of thrombophlebitis.
- PN solution containing 750 mL of 10% AA solution, 330 mL of 20% lipid solution, and 1,000 mL of 50% dextrose solution has an osmolarity of 1600 mOsm/L.
- Therefore, crystalloid fluids should be added to this PN solution prior to administration.

Preparation
- PN solution should be prepared aseptically, preferably under a laminar hood.
- AA, dextrose, and lipid solutions can be added to an empty 3-in-1 mixing bag.
- Crystalloid fluids are usually added to decrease the osmolarity of the PN solution.
- Lipid solution should be added last because lipid destruction droplets can occur if lipids are mixed directly with dextrose solution.
- Lipids can also be administered through a separate line to allow intermittent discontinuation if hyperlipidemia develops.

Administration
- Jugular catheter should be placed aseptically.
- Central venous catheter should ideally be placed.
- PN solution should be administered through a separate catheter to reduce the risks of sepsis and drug incompatibility.
- PN solution should be protected from light as much as possible.
- PN should be initiated gradually
- 50% of maintenance nutrient requirements are usually administered on the first day
- It is important to adjust fluid therapy to maintain hydration in the meantime
- Administration rate is then gradually increased to provide 100% of maintenance requirements on the second or third day.
- Similarly, PN should be gradually decreased before discontinuing PN.
- Administration rate should be decreased if hyperglycemia develops.
- Lipids should be discontinued temporarily if hyperlipidemia develops.

- Amount of AA solution should be reduced in ruminants with liver or renal dysfunction.
- Enteral nutrition should be reintroduced as early as possible.
- Enteral nutrition via rumen fistula is a practical and economical alternative to PN in ruminants with dysphagia or choke.

MEDICATIONS
DRUGS OF CHOICE
- Example of PN solution for a 50-kg calf
  - 1,900 mL of crystalloid fluids
  - 750 mL of 10% AA solution
  - 1,400 mL of 50% dextrose
- Administered at a maintenance rate (3.3 mL/kg/h), this solution provides 100% of maintenance requirements with a NPC:N of 190:1 and an osmolarity of 1,200 mOsm/L.
- Example of PN solution for an 80-kg alpaca
  - 3,000 mL of crystalloid fluids
  - 950 mL of 10% AA solution
  - 900 mL of 50% dextrose
- Administered at a maintenance rate (2.5 mL/kg/h), this solution provides 100% of maintenance requirements with a NPC:N of 100:1 and an osmolarity of 830 mOsm/L.
- Example of PN solution for a 40-kg goat
  - 800 mL of polyionic isotonic fluids
  - 550 mL of 10% AA solution
  - 1,100 mL of 50% dextrose
- Administered at a maintenance rate (2.5 mL/kg/h), this solution provides 100% of maintenance requirements with a NPC:N of 210:1 and an osmolarity of 1,400 mOsm/L.

Other Medications
- B vitamins can be administered every 2–3 days.
- Potassium supplementation (20–40 mEq/L) is indicated in ruminants with hypokalemia.
- Long-acting insulin (0.2–0.4 IU/kg SC) is indicated in camelids with severe prolonged hyperglycemia.
- Minerals, micronutrients, and vitamins should be added to the PN solution if administered for > 7 days.

CONTRAINDICATIONS
- Lipids should be avoided in ruminants with liver dysfunction or hypertriglyceridemia.

PRECAUTIONS
- Careful case selection is necessary because inappropriate use of PN may result in a higher incidence of complications and may worsen the outcome of the patient.

POSSIBLE INTERACTIONS
- Intravenous medications should be administered through a separate catheter and should not be added to the PN solution to reduce the risk of drug incompatibility.

FOLLOW-UP
EXPECTED COURSE AND PROGNOSIS
N/A

POSSIBLE COMPLICATIONS
- Sepsis, hyperglycemia, hyperlipidemia, hypokalemia, hypophosphatemia, and hypomagnesemia can develop in ruminants treated with PN.
- PN solutions are hypertonic and their use has been associated with thrombophlebitis.

CLIENT EDUCATION
- Due to the high cost of PN, this therapy should be considered in the light of the animal's value and prognosis.

PATIENT CARE
- Animals should be monitored closely for evidence of thrombophlebitis.
- Animals should be monitored closely for evidence of sepsis including
  - Tachycardia or tachypnea
  - Hyperthermia or hypothermia
  - Leukocytosis or leukopenia
  - >10% band neutrophils.
- Vitals and blood glucose should be monitored q8–12h.
- Urine output and urine specific gravity can be used to monitor hydration and renal function.
- PCV and total solids can be used to monitor hydration and prevent fluid overload, especially in calves, small ruminants, and camelids.
- Plasma should be evaluated daily for evidence of lipemia.
- Blood electrolytes and liver and renal enzymes should be monitored daily initially.

PREVENTION
N/A

MISCELLANEOUS
ABBREVIATIONS
- AA = amino acid
- BW = body weight
- K$^+$ = potassium
- MER = maintenance energy requirements
- MPR = maintenance protein requirements
- NPC:N = nonprotein calorie to nitrogen ratio
- PCV = packed cell volume
- PN = parenteral nutrition
- PPN = partial parenteral nutrition
- TPN = total parenteral nutrition

P

SEE ALSO
• Fluid Therapy: Oral
• Rumen Transfaunation (see
www.fiveminutevet.com/ruminant)

Suggested Reading
Chan DL, Freeman LM. Parenteral nutrition. In: DiBartola SP ed, Fluid, Electrolyte, and Acid-Base Disorders in Small Animal Practice, 4th ed. St. Louis: Saunders, 2012, pp. 605–22.
Sweeney RW, Divers TJ. The use of parenteral nutrition in calves. Vet Clin North Am Food Anim Pract 1990, 6: 125–31.
Van Saun RJ, Cebra C. Nutritional support. In: Cebra, C, Anderson DE, Tibary A, Van Saun RJ, Johnson LW eds, Llama and Alpaca Care, 1st ed. St. Louis: Saunders, 2014, pp. 357–65.
Author Thibaud Kuca
Consulting Editor Kaitlyn A. Lutz

P

BASICS

OVERVIEW
• Penile disorders in ruminants and camelids are often identified following breeding accidents or as part of a routine breeding soundness examination.
• These disorders affect the male's ability to service females in varying degrees and can lead to decreases in breeding efficiency.
• Penile disorders may be congenital, infectious, or traumatic in origin.
• Males with congenital disorders should be culled from breeding unless used as terminal sires. The most common congenital disorders are
  ○ Persistent frenulum
  ○ Short penis
  ○ Hypospadias
  ○ Penile deviations
• The most common acquired penile disorders are:
  ○ Rupture of the tunica albuginea: Mainly seen in bulls
  ○ Specific or nonspecific balanitis (all species)
  ○ Penile fibropapilloma (bulls)
  ○ Acquired peno-preputial adhesion or abscesses
  ○ Urethral fistulas

INCIDENCE/PREVALENCE
• Persistent frenulum is commonly found in bulls and camelids.
• Ruptured tunica albuginea (broken penis) is expected sporadically in breeding bulls. It is more commonly encountered early in the breeding season when libido would be expected to be at its highest.
• The prevalence of penile fibropapillomas is highly variable within populations but its incidence is higher in populations of young bulls housed together. It has been reported in 60–70% of bulls in a group.

GEOGRAPHIC DISTRIBUTION
Worldwide

SYSTEMS AFFECTED
Reproductive

PATHOPHYSIOLOGY
• Congenital defects
  ○ *Persistent frenulum:* Normally around the time of puberty the penis separates from its attachment to the prepuce. The process of separation is under the influence of testosterone. Complete separation should have occurred by 12 months of age in bulls and by 6–8 months in small ruminants. In SAC, peno-preputial adhesions may persist until 3 years of age, however >70% have separated by 2 years of age. Failure of separation results in incomplete

exteriorization of the penis during mating. Incomplete separation in bulls results in a persistent frenulum and causes varying degrees of ventral deviation of the distal penis during erection and breeding. This ventral deviation can potentially lead to breeding failure if the condition limits or prevents penetration during coitus.
  ○ *Short penis:* Described in bulls and camelids, abnormal development of the penile shaft or abnormalities of the sigmoid flexure result in shortness of the penis and inability to complete mating. Some bulls may be able to breed in their first breeding season, then lose this ability as they grow.
  ○ *Penile deviations:* Penile deviations are observed during erection in bulls and can be spiral, ventral, or S-shaped. It is not clear whether these deviations are congenital or may be acquired. Spiral deviation is the most common; it occurs normally within the vagina during peak erection and ejaculation. It hinders vaginal intromission if it occurs early and may predispose to penile hematoma.
  ○ *Hypospadias:* This is a failure of the embryonic urethral groove to close along its entire length or at its distal part.
  ○ *Vascular shunts:* These are abnormal vascular anastomoses between the erectile tissue and surrounding structures, leading to anomalies of erection.
  ○ *Diphalia:* Duplication of parts of the free portion of the penis have been reported in bulls.
• Infectious disorders
  ○ *Penile fibropapilloma or "penile warts":* A common condition affecting young or juvenile bulls, characterized by pedunculated growths on the distal penis. It is caused by the neoplastic growth of fibroblasts in animals carrying the bovine papillomavirus. This virus is common in young bulls and is easily spread from animal to animal via riding activity within groups of bulls. Abrasions on the penile epithelium appear to be the source of entry for the virus.
  ○ *Specific balanitis:* Infectious balanitis is caused by BoHV1-2 in bulls, caprine herpesvirus in bucks.
  ○ *Nonspecific balanitis* often observed in camelids.
  ○ *Abscesses and peno-preputial adhesions:* Usually develop as a complication of preputial lesions or penile hematomas. In camelids, penile adhesions are relatively common in males that frequently masturbate (breed objects or sand).
• Traumatic disorders
  ○ *Ruptured tunica albuginea:* This condition is reported primarily in bulls and results from an acute bend in the penis against the perineum. The resulting excessively high

pressure in the corpus cavernosum of the penis (CCP) causes a rent to occur in the tunica albuginea on the dorsal aspect of the penis at the distal sigmoid flexure. Blood escapes from the CCP forming a hematoma just cranial to the neck of the scrotum.
  ○ *Urethral fistulas:* Urethral fistulas may occur as a result of trauma, surgical removal of a mass or urethral calculi. This compromises potential semen deposition during mating.
  ○ *Penile lacerations* are not uncommon in range bulls.

HISTORICAL FINDINGS
• Incidental finding of the lesions during BSE.
• Inability to complete mating: Lack of exteriorization of the penis or abnormal erection.
• Observed abnormality of the external genitalia such as a mass in front of the spermatic cord (hematoma), bloody or purulent discharge from the prepuce, or preputial prolapse.

SIGNALMENT
• Congenital abnormalities are often seen in young virgin males submitted for BSE.
• Acquired disorders are seen in breeding age animals generally early in the breeding season.
• Penile fibropapilloma is more likely to occur in bulls housed with other young bulls.

PHYSICAL EXAMINATION FINDINGS
• Bulls are generally healthy at presentation. The only clinical sign may be an abnormality of the external genitalia.
• Congenital abnormalities of the penis are often discovered at the time of semen collection by electroejaculation.
• Ruptured tunica albuginea: Affected bulls present with a history of an acute onset of swelling at the location of the distal sigmoid flexure. It is also common for bulls to have a concurrent preputial prolapse with this condition.
• Penile fibropapilloma: Scant preputial discharge or bleeding from the prepuce may be observed. Phimosis and in more severe cases paraphimosis can be seen with this condition, depending on the location, number, and severity of the masses.
• Lacerations of the penis due to bites occur in camelid males housed together (fighting injuries).

GENETICS
• Persistent frenulum is considered heritable in bulls.
• Ruptured tunica albuginea is reputedly more common in the Hereford breed.

CAUSES AND RISK FACTORS
• Although several developmental abnormalities of the penis have been described, the causes and risk factors have not been elucidated.

P

PENILE DISORDERS

• Ruptured tunica albuginea: There are no known causes for this condition but there have been risk factors proposed. Young bulls with high libido (early in the breeding season) and bulls who may have lost condition or who have become clumsy in their breeding attempts (late in the breeding season) may be at increased risk for this condition.

• Penile fibropapilloma: The causative agent is bovine papillomavirus (BPV) which is spread among naïve animals through breeding behavior. The primary risk factors include bulls of young age and exposure to other bulls where transmission can occur.

• Balanitis may be caused by specific agents (BoHV1-2 and *Ureaplasma diversum* in cattle, CpHV-1 in goat, OHV-2 in sheep). In sheep balanitis may be a complication of ulcerative posthitis (pizzle rot due to *Corynebacterium renale*) or local infection with other organisms (*Histophilus ovis*, *Streptococcus pyogenes*, *Mycoplasma bovigenitalum*). In camelids, balanitis is often a result of infections of abrasions caused by masturbation against objects or sand.

DIAGNOSIS

DIFFERENTIAL DIAGNOSES

• Ruptured tunica albuginea should be differentiated from other masses. Ruptured urethra, retropreputial abscess would be two primary rule-outs for this condition. Retropreputial abscesses are generally further distal and are more closely associated with the shaft of the penis. Urethral rupture typically involves the ventral aspect of the penis, and urine escaping into the area leads to large areas of swelling typically associated with the ventrum of the bull.

• Persistent frenulum is easily diagnosed during routine breeding soundness examination. The band of tissue connecting the ventral aspect of the penis with the prepuce can vary in size from several millimeters to several centimeters in diameter. Also some persistent bands are flat in their orientation. During erection the band of tissue will restrict the penis's ability to fully extend. This condition should be differentiated from traumatic adhesions.

• Diagnosis of congenital defects is often very straightforward.

CBC/BIOCHEMISTRY/URINALYSIS
N/A

OTHER LABORATORY TESTS
Virology for viral causes of balanitis

IMAGING
Ultrasonography may aid in differentiating between a hematoma in the case of ruptured tunica albuginea and other masses (abscess or urine accumulation).

OTHER DIAGNOSTIC PROCEDURES
Radiography (cavernosogram) may be useful for the diagnosis of CCP vascular shunts.

PATHOLOGIC FINDINGS
• Penile papilloma can be submitted for confirmation of the diagnosis with histopathology; however, this is rarely indicated in most cases due to the consistent presentation and clinical signs associated with this condition.

• Viral balanitis is characterized by the presence of pustular lesions on the surface of the penis.

TREATMENT

THERAPEUTIC APPROACH
• Treatment of penile disorders is only indicated in valuable bulls. Bulls with congenital lesions should be discarded from breeding.

• Ruptured tunica albuginea: Conservative treatment involves sexual rest for a minimum of 60 days with antibiotic coverage for the first 1–2 weeks following injury.

• Penile papilloma: Warts involving the penis of bulls are best treated by surgical removal.

• Balanitis: Nonspecific balanitis may be managed by sexual rest and local antimicrobials. Viral balanitis is usually self-limiting.

SURGICAL CONSIDERATIONS AND TECHNIQUES
• Surgical treatment of ruptured tunica albuginea should be referred to a facility where there is expertise in the procedure. Bulls selected for surgery should preferably be not more than 10 days post-trauma as the associated fibrosis with older injuries makes a successful surgery and outcome less likely.

• Wart excision may be performed after local anesthesia with 1–2% lidocaine. The mass is excised with a scalpel, an electrosurgical unit, or a CO_2 laser. Large vessels associated with the mass are ligated and closed with 3-0 suture in routine fashion. Some large warts may not be easy to remove completely but can be successfully managed by debulking the mass with attention to adequate hemostasis. Special attention should be made to avoid damage to the urethra during removal. There are anecdotal reports of the benefits of immunostimulants such as Immunoboost (Bioniche Animal Health, USA) in managing large outbreaks. Both commercial and autogenous vaccines have been used with varying results and may help reduce recurrence when large numbers of bulls are affected.

• Persistent frenulum: A small bleb of 2% lidocaine can be injected into each end of the frenulum and a ligature should be tied at each

end. The band can then be easily transected. Very small frenulums can be broken down manually but there may be some minor hemorrhage noted.

MEDICATIONS

DRUGS OF CHOICE
Depending on the condition, a combination of local ointment, systemic antibiotics, and anti-inflammatories may be indicated.

CONTRAINDICATIONS
Appropriate meat withdrawal times must be followed for all compounds administered to food-producing animals.

PRECAUTIONS
N/A

POSSIBLE INTERACTIONS
N/A

FOLLOW-UP

EXPECTED COURSE AND PROGNOSIS
• Most bulls with severe penile disorders will be classified as unsatisfactory and culled from breeding.

• Prognosis is good for bulls with persistent penile frenulum but they should only be used as terminal sires.

• Prognosis is good for penile fibropapilloma if there are no complications.

• Penile hematoma: With proper patient selection 50% of bulls treated conservatively and 75% of bulls treated surgically are able to return to breeding soundness.

POSSIBLE COMPLICATIONS
Extensive fibrosis may limit the bull's ability to extend the penis during coitus without pain.

CLIENT EDUCATION
• All males should be submitted to BSE prior to breeding.

• Males should be closely monitored for any abnormality and submitted for examination by a practitioner immediately.

• Serving capacity is not part of the BSE. Client should observe male activity once joined with the females.

PATIENT CARE
• Sexual rest for a minimum of 60 days is recommended in cases of ruptured tunica albuginea.

• All bulls treated for penile fibropapilloma should be evaluated for complete healing and absence of any regrowth 4–6 weeks following surgery.

PREVENTION
N/A

MISCELLANEOUS

ASSOCIATED CONDITIONS
Infertility

AGE-RELATED FACTORS
Congenital defects are often discovered during examination of young virgin males.

ZOONOTIC POTENTIAL
N/A

PREGNANCY
N/A

BIOSECURITY
• Introduction of new breeding males into an operation is one of the most frequent causes of introduction of diseases.
• All males should be procured from a reputable source and examined prior to use for breeding.

PRODUCTION MANAGEMENT
Management of a group of males should take into account aggressive behavior which may result in serious injuries.

SYNONYMS
N/A

ABBREVIATIONS
• BoHV = bovine herpesvirus
• BPV = bovine papillomavirus
• BSE = breeding soundness examination
• CCP = corpus cavernosum of penis
• CpHV = caprine herpesvirus
• OHV = ovine herpesvirus

SEE ALSO
• Beef Bull Management (see www.fiveminutevet.com/ruminant)
• Breeding Soundness Examination: Bovine
• Breeding Soundness Examination: Camelid
• Breeding Soundness Examination: Cervidae
• Breeding Soundness Examination: Small Ruminant
• Infectious Pustular Vulvovaginitis
• Penile Hematoma

Suggested Reading
Maxwell H. Inability to breed due to injury or abnormality of the external genitalia of bulls. In: Hopper R ed, Bovine Reproduction. Ames: Wiley, 2015, pp. 113–27.
Pritchard GC, Scholes SFE, Foster AP, et al. Ulcerative vulvitis and balanitis in sheep flocks. Vet Rec 2009, 163: 86–9.
Tibary A, Pearson LK. Reproductive emergencies in camelids. Clin Theriogenol 2015, 6: 579–92.

Author Jack D. Smith
Consulting Editor Ahmed Tibary

P

PENILE HEMATOMA

BASICS

OVERVIEW AND PATHOPHYSIOLOGY
• Hematoma of the penis is probably the most common injury of the penis and is often referred to as a broken or fractured penis.
• Even observant owners/caretakers may not notice this condition for 2–3 days.

INCIDENCE/PREVALENCE
Frequent

GEOGRAPHIC DISTRIBUTION
N/A

SYSTEM AFFECTED
Reproductive

PATHOPHYSIOLOGY
• A bull typically has a fully engorged penis as he mounts in preparation for breeding. After two or three searching motions of the penis near the vulva, he normally makes one very forceful thrust, followed by intromission.
• Thus injury occurs when the penis misses the intended target, hits the cow's perineum, and bends.
• The hematoma results from rupture of the tunica albuginea and the subsequent hemorrhage from the corpus cavernosum. This rupture is typically a 2–7.5 cm tear.
• The initial volume of blood escaping is <250 mL but the size of the resultant hematoma varies as each subsequent erection results in further hemorrhage.
• Therefore the hematoma may range in size from 15 cm to 30 cm.
• The resultant swelling occurs in the sheath over and cranial to the rudimentary teats.

HISTORICAL FINDINGS
Observed lesion

SIGNALMENT
• Although it usually occurs in young inexperienced bulls, it can also occur in the older bull, which due to orthopedic injury or pain has altered his approach during mounting.
• Aggressive, high libido bulls, most commonly 2–4 years old.
• A previous history of this condition places an individual at risk for recurrence regardless of treatment, although surgical repair has been associated with a lower recurrence rate.

PHYSICAL FINDINGS
• A large symmetrical swelling cranial to the scrotum.
• In some instances the prepuce will be prolapsed.

GENETICS
Herefords are predisposed. Charolais are over-represented compared to other breeds.

CAUSES AND RISK FACTORS
• Sudden angulation of the penis during erection caused by misalignment during breeding may result in rupture of the tunica albuginea and hematoma formation.
• Aggressive (high libido) breeding bulls, awkward breeding attempts of novice bulls, over-fit bulls, older bulls with orthopedic problems.

DIAGNOSIS

DIFFERENTIAL DIAGNOSES
• Urethral rupture—swelling is ventral to the sigmoid flexure and more symmetric.
• Retropreputial abscess—this swelling is typically located along the more distal aspects of the penis.

CBC/BIOCHEMSTRY/URIANALYSIS
N/A

OTHER LABORATORY TESTS
N/A

IMAGING
Ultrasonography is helpful in differentiating a hematoma from an abscess.

OTHER DIAGNOSTIC PROCEDURES
• Physical examination:
  ○ Presence of a large swelling immediately cranial to the scrotum.
  ○ Bruising of the skin over the hematoma occurs but is only apparent in light-skinned bulls.
  ○ Secondary preputial prolapse secondary to a penile hematoma; this in fact may be the owner's reason for seeking help.
• Do not attempt to aspirate the swelling as inadvertent introduction of bacteria can convert a hematoma to an abscess.
• Do not attempt to manually extend the penis as this may further damage peri-penile elastic tissue.

PATHOLOGIC FINDINGS
N/A

TREATMENT

THERAPEUTIC APPROACH
• Systemic antibiotic treatment for 7–10 days
• Hydrotherapy
• Sexual rest for 60–90 days

SURGICAL CONSIDERATIONS AND TECHNIQUES
• Optimal time for surgery: 5–7 days post occurrence.
• Given that the owner or attendant typically may not notice this problem for 2–3 days and that the patient should be fasted for 36–48 hours prior to surgery, surgery must be scheduled immediately in an attempt to avoid clot organization and fibrosis that begins to occur 10 days post-injury.
• Surgery may again be attempted after 21 days post occurrence.

• Preparation: Antibiotics, fast for 36–48 hours, and withhold water overnight.
• General anesthesia can be utilized or regional anesthesia with heavy sedation.
• Surgery consists of clot removal and repair of the rent in the tunica albuginea.
• Antibiotic coverage should extend for 7 days.
• The bull should have 60–90 days of sexual rest following surgery.
• Seroma formation occurs often enough that it probably should not be considered a true complication.

MEDICATIONS

DRUGS OF CHOICE
Procaine penicillin: 44,000 IU/kg, IM, q12h

CONTRAINDICATIONS
Meat withdrawal time should be followed.

PRECAUTIONS
N/A

POSSIBLE INTERACTIONS
N/A

FOLLOW-UP

EXPECTED COURSE AND PROGNOSIS
• The success rate for medically managed cases is around 60–70% for hematomas measuring <20 cm across and 30% for larger hematomas.
• The surgical success rate is 70–80% regardless of the size.

POSSIBLE COMPLICATIONS
• Abscessation
• Suture dehiscence
• Permanent analgesia to the penis (i.e., loss of sensation, likely results from damage to the dorsal nerve of the penis occurring from the initial injury)
• Reoccurrence

CLIENT EDUCATION
Owner/caretakers should observe bulls daily during the breeding season.

PATIENT CARE
Bulls can be returned to a pasture environment with little oversight as long as they are away from cows.

PREVENTION
N/A

MISCELLANEOUS

ASSOCIATED CONDITIONS
N/A

AGE-RELATED FACTORS
N/A

P

(CONTINUED)   **PENILE HEMATOMA**

ZOONOTIC POTENTIAL
N/A

PREGNANCY
N/A

BIOSECURITY
N/A

PRODUCTION MANAGEMENT
N/A

SYNONYMS
N/A

ABBREVIATIONS
N/A

SEE ALSO
• Beef Bull Management (see
www.fiveminutevet.com/ruminant)
• Breeding Soundness Examination: Bovine
• Penile Disorders

Suggested Reading
Hopper RM. Management of male
reproductive tract injuries and disease. Vet
Clin North Am Food Anim Pract 2016, 32:
497–510.

Wolfe DF. Restorative surgery of the penis.
In: Hopper RM ed, Bovine Reproduction.
Ames: Wiley, 2014.
Author Richard M. Hopper
Consulting Editor Ahmed Tibary
Acknowledgment The author and book
editors acknowledge the prior contribution of
M.S. Gill.

P

PERICARDITIS

BASICS

OVERVIEW
• Inflammation of the pericardium with accumulation of fluid or exudate within the pericardial sac.
• In cattle, it most often relates to traumatic reticuloperitonitis (TRP) in which fibrinous septic pericarditis develops following perforation of the pericardial sac by a contaminated, metallic foreign body originating from the reticulum.
• Septic pericarditis can also arise from hematogenous infection or direct extension of infection from pleuropneumonia, pleuritis, or myocarditis.
• Other causes include viral infections, neoplasia, and idiopathic disease.
• Pericarditis can be effusive with accumulation of nonseptic fluid within the pericardial sac; or fibrinous (typically septic in nature), with accumulation of fibrin ± fluid in the pericardial sac which over time can lead to constrictive pericarditis with fibrosis and thickening of the pericardial sac.

INCIDENCE/PREVALENCE
Uncommon; septic pericarditis has high mortality.

GEOGRAPHIC DISTRIBUTION
Worldwide

SYSTEMS AFFECTED
• Cardiovascular
• Respiratory
• Digestive
• Integument

PATHOPHYSIOLOGY
• Can result from bacterial or viral inflammation, cardiac neoplasia, or is idiopathic.
• Initially, inflammation of the pericardium with hyperemia, fibrin deposition, and small amounts of exudate can cause pain and an audible friction rub due to the pericardium and epicardium interacting during cardiac motion.
• As fluid accumulates in the pericardial sac, friction sounds decrease, heart sounds become muffled, and tachycardia progresses.
• Gas can accumulate in the pericardial space if specific bacteria are present, resulting in more profoundly abnormal cardiac sounds.
• Heart chambers become compressed due to pericardial fluid ± fibrin, leading to cardiac tamponade. Inhibition of venous return may interfere with ventricular filling during diastole, resulting in decreased end-diastolic volume, stroke volume, and cardiac output, leading to congestive heart failure.

• With chronicity, fluid is resorbed and adhesions may form between the pericardium and epicardium, which over time can result in constrictive pericarditis and cardiac failure.

HISTORICAL FINDINGS
• Usually limited to the onset of clinical signs of disease.
• A history of previous cases of TRP is common on poorly managed establishments.
• Exercise intolerance and increased recumbency are common historical complaints in other ruminants and camelids.

SIGNALMENT
• Mature cattle; typically dairy cattle
• Uncommon in small ruminants
• Juvenile and pregnant camelids (*Streptococcus zooepidemicus* infection)

PHYSICAL EXAMINATION FINDINGS
• Early signs in cattle with traumatic reticuloperitonitis include reduced appetite, intermittent fever, tachypnea, tachycardia, elbow abduction, an arched back, and respiratory grunt. There may be pain on palpation of the thoracic wall over the cardiac region, and a "friction rub" evident on auscultation of the heart. Pinching of the withers or upward pressure on the xiphoid region may elicit a grunt on expiration.
• As disease progresses, signs of increased venous pressure/right-sided heart failure can occur, including peripheral edema, bilateral jugular distention ± abnormal pulsation, and abdominal and thoracic cavity fluid accumulation which may decrease lung sounds over the ventral thorax and contribute to dyspnea. A "splashing" or "washing machine murmur" may be apparent if gas is present in the pericardium.
• Diarrhea, dehydration, decreased milk production, decreased GI motility, and signs of toxemia and death can occur.
• In nonseptic pericarditis or in other species with pericarditis, the main findings are peripheral edema, jugular venous distention and pulsation, tachypnea, or dyspnea ± fever.
• Heart sounds are muffled, with an expanded area of cardiac dullness, decreased palpability of the apex beat, and weakened peripheral pulses. Reduced audibility of ventral lung sounds is common.

GENETICS
N/A

CAUSES AND RISK FACTORS
• Ingestion of metallic foreign bodies
• Extension from another focus of infection (e.g., pleuropneumonia)
• Secondary to lymphoma or other neoplasms
• Polyserositis (e.g., *S. zooepidemicus* in camelids)
• Mycoplasmosis in goats

DIAGNOSIS

DIFFERENTIAL DIAGNOSES
• Other causes of cranial abdominal pain and thoracic pain such as perforating abomasal ulcer, hepatic abscesses and pleuritis
• Infectious endocarditis
• Pasteurellosis or mycoplasmosis (cattle, sheep, and goats)
• *Histophilus somni* infection
• Cor pulmonale
• Cardiac lymphoma
• Idiopathic hemorrhagic pericardial effusion of cows
• Heartwater/cowdriosis (Africa and Caribbean)
• Other causes of vagal indigestion

CBC/BIOCHEMISTRY/URINALYSIS
• CBC: Leukocytosis ± left shift, elevated total protein, and hyperfibrinogenemia.
• Biochemistry can reflect heart failure, dehydration, anorexia, and rumen stasis, with azotemia, hypochloremic metabolic alkalosis, hypokalemia, hypocalcemia, increased AST and GGT, and increased CK if recumbent.

OTHER LABORATORY TESTS
• Cardiac troponin I
• Bovine leukemia virus: AGID, ELISA, or PCR

IMAGING
• Ultrasonography
  ○ Abdominal and thoracic ultrasound assist in ruling out other differentials.
  ○ Echocardiography determines the presence, amount, and character of pericardial effusion and fibrin, and the integrity of cardiac valves or presence of other anomalies (tumors).
  ○ Cardiac chamber collapse can be assessed; usually progresses in the order of right atrium, right ventricle, then left side chambers as fluid accumulation increases.
  ○ Pericardial effusion is imaged between the pericardium and epicardium, around both ventricles.
  ○ Clear anechoic effusion is most consistent with a transudate, and more echogenic fluid with fibrin is typical of septic or traumatic pericarditis.
  ○ Evaluating the cranial abdominal region can identify reticular abscesses and adhesions, abnormal reticular contour or wall, and abnormal reticular motility. Rarely, causative foreign bodies might be identified.
• Radiography
  ○ Main utility is in the detection of metallic foreign bodies and their position within the abdomen, thorax, or reticulum.

P

○ Thoracic radiographs may be obscured by pleural effusion or may display cardiomegaly, obscured cardiac silhouette, and gas fluid interfaces within the pericardium or near the reticulum.

OTHER DIAGNOSTIC PROCEDURES
• Pericardiocentesis
○ Can be performed standing in cattle, and in laterally recumbent goats, preferably using ultrasound guidance. Pneumothorax, cardiac puncture, arrhythmias, hemorrhage, and cardiac tamponade are all risks of this procedure
○ Aseptically prepare skin over the 5th intercostal space (ICS), then inject local anesthetic over the dorsal and cranial aspect of the 6th rib, blocking skin, subcutaneous tissue, and parietal pleura.
○ An 18-G spinal needle, or, after a small skin incision, a 4–8 inch intravenous catheter or small chest tube, is advanced through the left 5th ICS just dorsal to the elbow at the anterior aspect of the 6th rib.
○ For goats, use the right 4th ICS low on the chest wall to avoid lung and coronary arteries.
○ Fluid can be drained and submitted for analysis (cytology, and protein, lactate and glucose evaluation) and for bacterial/mycoplasma culture and sensitivity.
○ Traumatic pericarditis tends to produce fluid with a high protein concentration (>3.5 g/dL), high lactate and low glucose concentration, and an elevated cell count (>5,000/μL) composed primarily of neutrophils. The fluid may be discolored, with a foul odor. A mixed population of Gram-positive and Gram-negative aerobic and anaerobic bacteria (GI flora) are usually present.
○ Cardiac lymphoma is intermittently identified on cytologic evaluation of pericardial effusion.
• Electrocardiogram reveals diminished amplitude of QRS complexes, potentially cardiac arrhythmias, and electrical alternans in animals with significant pericardial effusion.
• Abdominocentesis provides fluid with increased protein concentration (>3 g/dL), cell count (>10,000 cells/μL), and presence of toxic or degenerate cells if suppurative peritonitis is present; however, normal results do not exclude disease or may reflect ascites.

PATHOLOGIC FINDINGS
• Pericardial effusion
• Fibrin tags on pericardial and epicardial surfaces
• Thickening of epicardium and pericardium, which may be adhered to each other
• Lesions of congestive heart failure
• Evidence of reticular penetration and peritonitis in TRP cases
• If present, cardiac lymphoma is typically identified invading the right atrium.

TREATMENT
THERAPEUTIC APPROACH
• Particularly in septic pericarditis, treatment is long-term, costly, and often unsuccessful, so culling is typically recommended. Treatment is not recommended in cardiac lymphoma.
• Broad-spectrum, parenteral, bactericidal antibiotics are preferred, and when possible selected based on cytology, culture, and sensitivity results from pericardial fluid.
• Analgesic and anti-inflammatory drugs as needed.
• If significant effusion is present, the pericardial sac can be drained and lavaged with isotonic, nonirritating fluid followed by installation of an antimicrobial drug. This is of limited use in constrictive pericarditis or neoplasia.
• Diuretics and restriction of dietary salt can be practiced if congestive heart failure is present.
• Idiopathic effusive pericarditis cases can benefit from drainage and provision of corticosteroids or nonsteroidal anti-inflammatory drugs.

SURGICAL CONSIDERATIONS AND TECHNIQUES
• Rumenotomy should be considered to remove definitively identified penetrating foreign bodies.
• If unresponsive to medical therapy, thoracotomy and pericardectomy or pericardiostomy can provide drainage or allow marsupialization of pericardium to body wall in valuable animals with septic pericarditis.

MEDICATIONS
DRUGS OF CHOICE
• Penicillin: 22,000 IU/kg q12h, IM (procaine) or q6h, IV (aqueous potassium penicillin)
• Amoxicillin: 10 mg/kg IM q12h
• Flunixin meglumine: 1.1 mg/kg q24h or 0.5 mg/kg q12h
• Aspirin: 30–100 mg/kg PO q12–24h
• Furosemide: 0.5–1.0 mg/kg IV q12–24h
• Potassium supplement (50–200 g/day PO) if on potassium-wasting diuretics

CONTRAINDICATIONS
N/A

PRECAUTIONS
• Extra-label use of antibiotics often occurs during treatment of septic pericarditis because few are labeled for such long-term therapy.
• Early withdrawal of therapy may result in relapse.
• Appropriate milk and meat withdrawal times must be followed for all compounds administered to food-producing animals.

POSSIBLE INTERACTIONS
N/A

FOLLOW-UP
EXPECTED COURSE AND PROGNOSIS
• Complete recovery is uncommon with septic pericarditis, with a prognosis likely <30%.
• Prognosis declines with chronicity.
• Idiopathic hemorrhagic pericarditis cases can recover completely.

POSSIBLE COMPLICATIONS
• Chronic disease may result in constrictive pericarditis and cardiac failure.
• Survivors may have myocarditis and arrhythmias.

CLIENT EDUCATION
Focus on maintaining a safe feed supply, particularly avoiding incidental inclusion of metallic foreign bodies in chopped rations.

PATIENT CARE
• Supportive care to maintain hydration, nutritional status, and electrolyte and acid–base balance.
• Appropriate treatment of secondary organ disease or dysfunction.

PREVENTION
• Relies on preventing exposure to metal objects in feed; large magnets can be placed on feed handling equipment.
• Prophylactic administration of forestomach magnets into the rumen at 6–8 months of age to confine ingested metallic objects.
• Protocols to reduce bovine leukemia infection within cattle herds.

MISCELLANEOUS
ASSOCIATED CONDITIONS
• Traumatic reticuloperitonitis
• Congestive heart failure
• Myocardial disease
• Bovine leukemia virus

AGE-RELATED FACTORS
A disease of mature cattle

ZOONOTIC POTENTIAL
N/A

PREGNANCY
Gravid uterus has been hypothesized to enhance migration of foreign bodies from the reticulum.

BIOSECURITY
N/A

PRODUCTION MANAGEMENT
Employ strategies to prevent exposure to metal objects; provide prophylactic forestomach magnet; control for bovine leukemia infection.

P

PERICARDITIS (CONTINUED)

SYNONYM
Hardware disease

ABBREVIATIONS
• AGID = agar gel immunodiffusion
• AST = aspartate transaminase
• CK = creatine kinase
• ELISA = enzyme-linked immunosorbent assay
• GGT = gamma glutamyl transferase
• GI = gastrointestinal
• ICS = intercostal space
• PCR = polymerase chain reaction
• TRP = traumatic reticuloperitonitis

SEE ALSO
• Bovine Leukemia Virus
• Cardiac Failure
• Heartwater (Cowdriosis)
• Respiratory Disease: Bovine
• Respiratory Disease: Camelid
• Respiratory Disease: Small Ruminant
• Traumatic Reticuloperitonitis

Suggested Reading
Firshman AM, Sage AM, Valberg SJ, et al. Idiopathic hemorrhagic pericardial effusion in cows. J Vet Intern Med 2006, 20: 1499–502.
Jones S, Smith B. Diseases of the alimentary tract. In: Smith BP ed, Large Animal Internal Medicine, 5th ed. St. Louis: Mosby, 2015.
Radostits OM, Gay CC, Blood DC, Hinchcliff KW. Diseases of the heart. In: Veterinary Medicine: A Textbook of Diseases of Cattle, Sheep, Pigs, Goats and Horses, 9th ed. New York: Saunders, 1999, pp. 389–91.
Reef VB, McGuirk S. Diseases of the cardiovascular system. In: Smith BP ed, Large Animal Internal Medicine, 5th ed. St. Louis: Mosby, 2015.
Smith MC, Sherman DM. Goat Medicine. Philadelphia: Lea & Febiger, 1994, pp. 233–236.
Sojka JE, White MR, Widmer WR, VanAlstine WG. An unusual case of traumatic pericarditis in a cow. J Vet Diagn Invest 1990, 2: 139–42.

Author Anna M. Firshman
Consulting Editor Erica C. McKenzie
Acknowledgment The author and book editors acknowledge the prior contribution of Susan Semrad and Sheila McGuirk.

P

PERINATAL LAMB MORTALITY

BASICS

OVERVIEW
- Mortality in lambs can be high and can significantly limit sheep production.
- Although it is easy to limit mortality in lambs, and essential if rearing sheep is to be profitable, it is often overlooked.
- Perinatal survival is influenced by late-term lamb development, uncomplicated parturition, appropriate udder development, and close monitoring of the ewe-lamb bond.

INCIDENCE/PREVALENCE
- Majority of losses occur during the first week of life (Figure 1a), particularly during the first 72 hours (Figure 1b).
- Mortality in lambs occurs during the last 3 weeks of gestation (15%), during parturition (20%), and the majority in the postpartum period (65%).
- Prevalence is recorded from various countries to be between 9% and 20%; <5% is regarded as good.

GEOGRAPHIC DISTRIBUTION
Worldwide distribution, although causes and timing of losses will vary.

SYSTEMS AFFECTED
Multisystemic

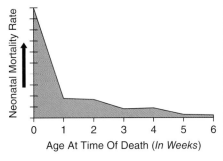

Figure 1a.

Most Neonatal Mortality Occurs During the First Week of Life

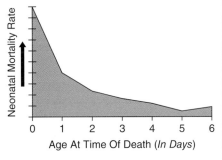

Figure 1b.

Mortality Rates are Highest During Days 1, 2, & 3 Following Birth

PATHOPHYSIOLOGY
- Caused by poor flock management.
- Majority of the losses are caused by (1) starvation, hypothermia, and exposure; (2) stillbirth (including dystocia); (3) pneumonia; and (4) abortion.

HISTORICAL FINDINGS
Critical illness leading to death or found dead.

SIGNALMENT
Majority of deaths occur in utero or during the first week after birth.

PHYSICAL EXAMINATION FINDINGS
Dependent on etiology

GENETICS
Some evidence of genetic components within breeds (e.g., Suffolks and spider lamb syndrome). In addition, selective breeding strategies to optimize production in certain breeds will likely reduce mortality.

CAUSES AND RISK FACTORS
There are ten top causes of perinatal lamb mortality.

1. Stillbirth
Usually the cause of mortality in 3–5% of lambs.

2. Death Secondary to Dystocia
- These lambs will often be meconium stained.
- May have rib fractures, ruptured liver, umbilical or abdominal herniation.

3. Hypothermia/Starvation Complex
- Simple hypothermia will be seen in lambs <6 hours old who are wet in predisposing environmental conditions.
- Hypothermia secondary to starvation (50% of lambs in the first week) will be seen in lambs >6 hours old who are usually dry.

4. Pneumonia
- These lambs are usually >4 hours of age.
- Cranioventral lobes affected, abscesses may be visible.
- When pneumonia is secondary to sepsis, lesions will be more extensive.

5. Abortion
- Independent of cause, most abortions are seen in the last month of gestation.
- Individual farms—may see 5–25%.
- Normal rate considered 1–2%.
- Oral transmission route.
- Campylobacteriosis
  - Abortion (132 days), stillbirths, and weak lambs that die shortly after birth.
  - Ewe not sick.
  - Lamb largely normal (immature lung—poor or no inflation).
  - History of ewes added to the flock.
- Toxoplasmosis
  - Abortion, stillbirth, mummified fetuses, weak lambs, open ewes.
  - Mummification of fetuses is common.
  - Fetal thoracic fluid useful to obtain a *Toxoplasma* antibody titer.
- *Chlamydia* (enzootic abortion in ewes)

- Abortion, stillbirth, and weak lambs.
- Sick ewes.
- Often seen in successive years.
- *Coxiella burnetii* (Q fever)
  - Abortion secondary to necrotizing placentitis.
  - Ewes may be well or sick.
  - Can become persistent carriers so low-grade problems remain in herd.
- Schmallenberg virus
  - Orthobunyavirus—transmitted via insects.
  - Caused significant lamb mortality in Europe since 2011—20–70% loss on affected farms.
  - Abortions, stillbirths due to congenital musculoskeletal malformations, weak lambs.
  - Ewes generally not ill.

6. Trauma, Particularly Fractured Ribs
Often secondary to hypothermia and starvation, dystocia, or farm movement procedures.

7. Diarrhea
- *Escherichia coli*
  - Usually causes disease in the first week of life.
  - Particularly seen to cause disease during days 2–4 secondary to poor immunity/failure of passive transfer.
  - Affected lambs will often be found dead within 24–48 hours of developing clinical signs.
  - Usually evident which lambs have diarrhea as they will have a wet, stained tail and rump area.
  - This is often an individual flock problem and may be seen at certain times of year when the weather changes.
- Coccidiosis
  - Seen in lambs 4–6 weeks old.
  - In addition to diarrhea, these animals will strain.
  - Blood in feces is rare.
  - Often an individual flock problem and may be seen at times of year when the weather is changing.

8. Sequelae to Sepsis—Umbilical and Joint Infection
- Seen in lambs 10–30 days (particularly those 2–3 weeks old).
- Due to foci of infection, lambs with be thin with weight loss or poor weight gain.
- Lambs will be lame, often in more than one limb, with distended joints.
- May have a swollen or discharging umbilicus.
- Secondary pneumonia common.
- Will often be seen following changes in weather.

9. Intestinal Obstruction
- History of abdominal pain preceding collapse and death.
- Distended abdomen.

P

• Causes include intestinal torsion, volvulus, or intussusception.
• Can be seen secondary to diarrhea, but also common in lambs reared on milk replacer.
• Can be misdiagnosed as overeating disease.

10. Clostridium perfringens Types C and D
• *Clostridium perfringens* type C
  ◦ Present with sudden death in 1- to 3-day-old lambs.
  ◦ Affected lambs collapse, and die within 24–48 hours.
  ◦ Diarrhea rare.
  ◦ More common in unvaccinated flocks and in lambs with failure of passive transfer.
• *Clostridium perfringens* type D
  ◦ Lambs >4 weeks of age found dead.
  ◦ Common in creep-fed and feedlot lambs, but is also seen in orphan lambs raised on milk replacer.

Risk Factors
The following risk factors influence perinatal or postnatal mortality:
• Highest stillbirth rates on smallest and largest farms and those with unaided and unsupervised parturition
• Intensive rearing systems, although housing sheep for parturition reduced losses
• Low lamb birthweight
• Triplets and quadruplets
• Fostering a large number of lambs
• Poor lambing pen hygiene
• Poor ewe condition at breeding and poor ewe nutrition
• Poor mothering leading to failure of passive transfer
• Relationship between losses and low ambient environmental temperatures

DIAGNOSIS
DIFFERENTIAL DIAGNOSES
See "Causes and Risk Factors," but these will fall into the following categories:
• Environmental factors
• Management effects
• Genetic factors
• Hygiene and infectious causes

CBC/BIOCHEMISTRY/URINALYSIS
N/A

OTHER LABORATORY TESTS
N/A

IMAGING
N/A

OTHER DIAGNOSTIC PROCEDURES
• Gross postmortem examination of all dead lambs is of great value.
• Economical means of confirming cause
  ◦ Examine all dead lambs to document flock trends
  ◦ Try to discern whether the lamb has breathed, nursed and the extent of fat coverage.

• Use caution (especially women of childbearing age) when handling dead lambs and placentas, especially if abortion is a problem.
• Use a diagnostic laboratory for persistent or undiagnosed problems.
• Educational tool for producers.
• Focus control programs by classifying into four to six basic categories.

PATHOLOGIC FINDINGS
1. Stillbirth
Necropsy reveals non-aerated lung.

2. Death Secondary to Dystocia
Necropsy reveals meconium staining; and rib fractures, ruptured liver, umbilical or abdominal herniation may be present.

3. Hypothermia/Starvation Complex
• Hypothermia. Minimal findings, but no fat depletion is present and milk may or may not be present in the abomasum.
• Hypothermia/starvation complex. Abomasum usually empty and there is marked fat depletion throughout, particularly evident surrounding the kidney and coronary groove.

4. Pneumonia
Consolidated lung lesions on necropsy will usually be clearly demarcated, may be in the cranioventral lobes, and abscesses may be visible. When pneumonia is secondary to sepsis, there may be evidence of adhesions, where the whole lung is edematous with evidence of epicardial hemorrhage and pericardial effusion.

5. Abortion
• Campylobacteriosis. Placenta normal in appearance; lamb largely normal (immature lung—poor or no inflation).
• Toxoplasmosis.
  ◦ Mummification of fetuses is common
  ◦ White, focal (1–2mm) lesions on cotyledons, but no intercotyledonary lesions
  ◦ Fetal thoracic fluid useful to obtain a Toxoplasma antibody titer
• *Chlamydia* (enzootic abortion in ewes). Placental examination shows necrotic cotyledons and thickened intercotyledonary areas.
• *Coxiella burnetii* (Q fever). Necrotic placental lesions.
• Schmallenberg virus
  ◦ Stillborn lambs with congenital musculoskeletal malformations.
  ◦ Minimal placental changes.

6. Trauma, Particularly Fractured Ribs
Necropsy reveals hemothorax, punctures to the lungs, ruptured liver or spleen leading to hemoperitoneum.

7. Diarrhea
• *Escherichia coli*
  ◦ Wet, stained tail and rump area
  ◦ Necropsy reveals signs consistent with sepsis to include petechial hemorrhages on the epicardium

◦ The intestines will have a thin, discolored wall and will be distended and fluid filled
◦ There may be intestinal perforation with adhesions and secondary peritonitis
◦ May see secondary lesions consistent with the hypothermia/ starvation complex
• Coccidiosis. At necropsy, the intestines will be thin and distended with fluid, but little blood with intestinal contents.

8. Sequelae to Sepsis—Umbilical and Joint Infection
Necropsy will often reveal thin carcasses with minimal fat, lung changes consistent with pneumonia spread hematogenously (changes throughout lungs), liver abscessation due to extension of infection from the umbilical vein; secondary peritonitis; thickened, fibrous umbilicus that may contain purulent, necrotic material; and distended joints with a thickened joint capsule containing thickened, purulent material.

9. Intestinal Obstruction
Necropsy reveals purple discoloration to the affected section of bowel. Changes secondary to sepsis (petechiae) may be present on other organs (epicardium; serosal surface of adjacent pieces of intestine) and peritonitis may also be present.

10. Clostridium perfringens Types C and D
• *Clostridium perfringens* type C. Necropsy reveals increased pericardial fluid, epicardial hemorrhage with or without fibrin. The abomasum often engorged with milk and hemorrhagic abomasitis. Minimal excessive fluid within the intestines.
• *Clostridium perfringens* type D. Necropsy often reveals minimal changes, but will include petechial hemorrhages on organ surfaces and necrotic intestine.

TREATMENT
THERAPEUTIC APPROACH
N/A

SURGICAL CONSIDERATIONS AND TECHNIQUES
N/A

MEDICATIONS
DRUGS OF CHOICE
Identification of infectious causes of abortion and mortality of lambs may allow an appropriate vaccination strategy to be of value.

CONTRAINDICATIONS
N/A

PRECAUTIONS
N/A

POSSIBLE INTERACTIONS

N/A

 FOLLOW-UP

EXPECTED COURSE AND PROGNOSIS

NA

POSSIBLE COMPLICATIONS

N/A

CLIENT EDUCATION

• Clients must appreciate financial losses with this condition.
• Need to appreciate the value of necropsy evaluation of all lambs in order to find causes and then solutions on all farms where losses are >5%.
• Need to evaluate aspects of rearing likely problematic:
  ◦ Ewe nutrition
  ◦ Hygiene
  ◦ Lamb-ewe bond affecting transfer of immunity
  ◦ Disease control when causes of mortality known.

PATIENT CARE

Good supportive care (i.e., thermal support, fluid therapy, etc.) and biosecurity (i.e., separating sick animals) are imperative to decrease mortality.

PREVENTION

See "Production Management"

 MISCELLANEOUS

ZOONOTIC POTENTIAL

Use caution (especially women of childbearing age) when handling dead lambs and placentas, especially if investigating an abortion problem.

PREGNANCY

• Appropriate ewe nutrition and identification of ewes with multiple fetuses will help prevent the birth of weak, small lambs.
• In flocks with sheep breeds producing >2 lambs, have management practices in place to ensure effective provision of colostrum and nutrition.

BIOSECURITY

Buying in ewes can predispose to certain infectious causes of abortion (see "Causes and Risk Factors").

PRODUCTION MANAGEMENT

• Often cannot truly assess or affect losses during the lambing season.
• Losses are seen with individual flock patterns that require assessment over time—losses and causes in one year may not reflect overall problems.
• Information on the cause or causes of mortality allows disease control and management changes to be made in a timely fashion.
• The major management areas to address include:
  ◦ Minimizing effects of the environment and weather
  ◦ Forage resources
  ◦ Ewe nutrition
  ◦ Genetic selection
  ◦ Monitoring of newborn lambs and minimization of mismothering
  ◦ Hygiene and disease control
  ◦ Appropriate use of labor and facilities.
• Lamb mortality should ideally be <5%, but is challenging to achieve; 5–10% is a more realistic goal.

SYNONYMS

• Lamb mortality
• Neonatal mortality
• Postmortem examination
• Preweaning losses

SEE ALSO

• Abortion: Small Ruminant
• Campylobacter
• Clostridial Disease: Gastrointestinal
• Neonatal Diarrhea
• Neonatal Septic Arthritis
• Neonatology: Ovine (see www.fiveminutevet.com/ruminant)

Suggested Reading

Binns SH. Cox IJ, Rizvi S, Green LE. Risk Factors for lamb mortality on UK sheep farms Prev Vet Med 2002, 52: 287–303.

Dutra F, Banchero G. Polworth and Texel ewe parturition duration and its association with lamb birth asphyxia. J Anim Sci 2011, 89: 3069–78.

Holmay IH, Waage S. Time trends and epidemiological patterns of perinatal lamb mortality in Norway. Acta Vet Scand 2015, 57: 65–76.

Miller DR, Jackson RB, Blache D, Roche JR. Metabolic maturity at birth and neonate lamb survival and growth: the effects of maternal low-dose dexamethasone treatment. J Anim Sci 2009, 87: 3167–78.

Riggio V, Finocchiaro R, Bishop SC. Genetic parameters for early lamb survival and growth in Scottish Blackface sheep. J Anim Sci 2008, 86: 1758–64.

Rook JS, Scholman G, Wing-Proctor S, Shea M. Diagnosis and control of neonatal losses in sheep. Vet Clin North Am Food Anim Pract 1990, 6: 531–63.

Author Gayle Hallowell
Consulting Editor Kaitlyn A. Lutz
Acknowledgment The author and book editors acknowledge the prior contribution of Joseph S. Rook.

P

PESTE DES PETITS RUMINANTS

BASICS

OVERVIEW
Peste des petits ruminants (PPR), also known as goat plague, contagious pustular stomatitis, kata, pneumoenteritis syndrome, and pseudo-rinderpest of small ruminants, is an acute viral disease of small ruminants. PPR is a significant threat to food security and sustainable small ruminant production in much of the eastern hemisphere. It is a listed and reportable disease in accordance with the OIE *Terrestrial Animal Health Code* and is a joint OIE/FAO target for eradication by 2030.

INCIDENCE/PREVALENCE
• Significant portions of the world are free of PPRV. The OIE WAHIS interface provides current information on disease status by country.
• Seroprevalence in endemic regions varies greatly by location, with reports ranging from 30% to over 90%. Apparent clinical prevalence may be low.
• Epizootics occur when a susceptible population is exposed. Morbidity rates may approach 100% with case fatality rates approaching 90%.

GEOGRAPHIC DISTRIBUTION
PRRV is widespread across major sections of Africa, the Arabian peninsula, and Asia.

SYSTEMS AFFECTED
• Digestive
• Hemolymphatic
• Respiratory

PATHOPHYSIOLOGY
• Transmission occurs through close contact with infected animals, their infectious ocular, nasal, oral, and fecal secretions, or inhalation of droplet aerosols.
• There is no true carrier state. Incubatory carriers shed virus prior to clinical disease. Affected animals shed virus for 3 weeks post-infection.
• Clinical signs typically appear 4–6 days post-infection and last 2 weeks in survivors. The *peste des petit ruminants* virus (PPRV) replicates in the host cells' cytoplasm, with an affinity for tonsillar, lymphoid, and epithelial tissues.
• PPRV is highly immunosuppressive, causing a profound leukopenia and CD4+ T-cell suppression. Secondary infections are common.
• Extremely high morbidity and case fatality rates occur in naïve herds. Goats and young stock are most severely affected. A peracute form has been observed in goats, causing high fevers, severe depression, and death before the onset of classical lesions. Subclinical infections may occur in enzootic settings.
• Infection with PPRV provokes both cellular and humoral immune responses, primarily

targeted against the H, F, and N viral protein antigens. Surviving affected animals are immune for life. Maternal antibodies are capable of virus neutralization for the first 3–4 months of life.

SIGNALMENT
• Goats, sheep, camels, and Indian buffalo.
• Some breed differences have been reported in goats. The West African Dwarf and Alpine breeds are considered highly susceptible; Saanens are reportedly more resistant.
• Young stock >4 months of age, up to about 18–24 months, are at greatest risk.

PHYSICAL EXAMINATION FINDINGS
• Cases observed only in the small ruminant population; co-located cattle are not affected.
• Nonspecific signs of depression, anorexia, and a dull, staring hair coat.
• Pyrexia 104–106°F (40–41°C).
• Profuse serous oculonasal discharge that becomes mucopurulent with chronicity resulting in matted eyes and crusting nasal occlusion.
• Hyperemic nasal and oral mucosa with necrotizing erosions and fibrinous pseudo-membranes on the nares, gingiva, dental pad, hard palate, buccal surfaces, and tongue; a putrid oral odor may be observed.
• Profuse diarrhea.
• Coughing, dyspnea, and other signs of pneumonia.
• Abortion.
• Dehydration.
• Emaciation.
• Death.

CAUSES AND RISK FACTORS
• PPR is caused by the *peste des petits ruminants* virus (PPRV), a paramyxovirus of the genus Morbillivirus. It is a single-stranded negative-sense RNA virus that is antigenically similar to the rinderpest virus.
• Circulating strains of PPRV can be organized into four distinct lineages. Lineages I–III have been associated with African outbreaks while lineage IV was originally found in the Middle East and Asia but is now present across all PPR enzootic regions.
• Major epizootics occur when the virus is introduced to a naïve susceptible population.
• Risk factors include co-mingling at animal centers, movement of transhumant populations, and waning passive immunity in the young stock. Poor nutritional status, stress, and concurrent infections may enhance the severity of disease.

DIAGNOSIS

DIFFERENTIAL DIAGNOSES
• Rinderpest
• Foot and mouth disease
• Bluetongue
• Contagious ecthyma

• Contagious caprine pleuropneumonia
• Respiratory pasteurellosis
• Nairobi sheep disease
• Heartwater
• Coccidiosis
• Plant or mineral poisoning

CBC/BIOCHEMISTRY/URINALYSIS
Leukopenia

OTHER LABORATORY TESTS
• Gold standard is virus isolation: Sample during the acute phase from clear oronasal secretions, buccal or rectal mucosa, anticoagulant whole blood, or erosion debris.
• Antigen and RNA-based diagnostics include immunochromatographic lateral flow, RT-PCR or QRT-PCR, immunohistochemistry, and immunocapture ELISA.
• Diagnostic serology includes serum cELISA, virus neutralization, AGID, and counter immunoelectrophoresis. Paired acute and convalescent serum samples will show a fourfold or greater rise in antibody titer. Cannot currently distinguish vaccinates from natural infections.

OTHER DIAGNOSTIC PROCEDURES
• Postmortem target tissues for virus isolation, antigen and RNA-based diagnostics include tonsils, lymph nodes (retropharyngeal, bronchial, and mesenteric), lung parenchyma, spleen, and intestinal mucosa (ileum and large intestine).
• Fresh tissues should be chilled (not frozen) and delivered cold to the laboratory within 12 hours of collection.
• 10% neutral buffered formalin fixed tissues should be submitted for histopathology.

PATHOLOGIC FINDINGS
• External: Severe emaciation and dehydration, conjunctivitis, and crusting of outer lips and nares.
• Gastrointestinal tract: Necro-erosive lesions from the oral cavity to the rumeno-reticular junction, abomasum, and small intestine. Severe ulceration and necrosis of Peyer's patches. Congestion and/or erosive and hemorrhagic enteritis around the ileocecal valve and ceco-colic junction. Linear congestion of the mucosal folds in the colon and rectum ("zebra stripes").
• Respiratory tract: Small erosions and petechial hemorrhages of the nasal mucosa, turbinates, larynx, and trachea. Severe interstitial bronchopneumonia, consolidation, and atelectasis, often compounded by signs of a secondary bacterial pneumonia. Lung histopathology may identify multinucleated giant cells with inclusions.
• Urogenital tract: Mucosal erosions.
• Hemic/lymphatic/immune: Enlarged and congested spleen and liver. Lymphadenopathy with syncytia and empty germinal centers on histopathology.

P

(CONTINUED)

TREATMENT

THERAPEUTIC APPROACH
• No specific treatment is available for individual animals, but in vitro RNA interference trials are promising.
• Access to veterinary care is limited in most enzootic areas, and individual animal care may not be feasible. Supportive supplementation may be indicated.
• Control for secondary infections.

MEDICATIONS

DRUGS OF CHOICE
• Use antimicrobials for control of secondary bacterial infections.
• Parenteral anti-inflammatory and B-complex vitamin supplementation may be indicated.

FOLLOW-UP

EXPECTED COURSE AND PROGNOSIS
• The severity and outcome of disease is correlated with the extent of oral pathology.
• Lesions that resolve in 2–3 days have a better prognosis while halitosis or respiratory signs indicate a grave prognosis.

POSSIBLE COMPLICATIONS
• Secondary bacterial pneumonia, specifically with *Mannheimia haemolytica*, is a frequent complication.
• Immunosuppression may permit secondary parasitemia or recrudescence of other infectious disease processes.

CLIENT EDUCATION
Educate producers on the importance of vaccination to prevent infection in countries where it is approved for use.

PATIENT CARE
• Monitor for respiratory distress due to blocked nasal passages or secondary infections.
• Fluid therapy to resolve fluid deficits and restore electrolyte and acid-base balance.
• Limit handling, stress, and movement to prevent respiratory embarrassment and limit spread of disease.
• Provide a nutritionally appropriate palatable and easily masticated feed.

PREVENTION
• PPR-free countries should prohibit import of animals or animal products from affected locations.
• Sheep and goats in enzootic areas should be vaccinated once maternal immunity has waned (3–4 months of age) and a booster administered every 3 years. In some countries, administration of the vaccine may be restricted to government personnel.
• Four live-attenuated vaccines are currently available. The Nigeria 75/1 (lineage II) and Sungri 96 (lineage IV) are the most widely used products, while Arasur 87 and Coimbatore 97 are sheep and goat origin lineage IV isolates licensed in India. Modifications have been made to make these vaccines more thermostable and decrease reliance on a cold chain.
• Effective live-attenuated vaccines must be administered several days prior to exposure to stimulate an effective immune response.
• New vaccines are in development that focus on recombinant H or F antigen subunit technology and DIVA capabilities.

MISCELLANEOUS

ASSOCIATED CONDITIONS
Secondary bacterial and parasitic infections

AGE-RELATED FACTORS
Young animals, 4–8 months of age, often have worse clinical disease than adult animals.

ZOONOTIC POTENTIAL
None

PREGNANCY
Abortions may occur.

BIOSECURITY
PPRV survives in the environment or on fomites for up to 72 hours in shaded conditions, but is otherwise sensitive to heat, UV radiation, and pH <5.5 or >10.

PRODUCTION MANAGEMENT
Goats and sheep in enzootic areas should be vaccinated by 3–4 months of age and then every 3 years with an attenuated isolate of PPR. Vaccinate ahead of the risk season (e.g., cool, dry season in Africa) or before known periods of mass herd movement.

ABBREVIATIONS
• AGID = agar gel immunodiffusion test
• cELISA = competitive enzyme-linked immunosorbent assay
• DIVA = differentiation of infected from vaccinated animals
• ELISA = enzyme-linked immunosorbent assay
• FAO = Food and Agriculture Organization of the United Nations
• OID = World Organization for Animal Health
• PCR = polymerase chain reaction
• PPR = peste des petits ruminants
• PPRV = peste des petits ruminants virus
• QRT = quantitative reverse transcription-polymerase chain reaction
• RT-PCR = reverse transcription-polymerase chain reaction

SEE ALSO
• Bluetongue Virus
• Coccidiosis
• Contagious Caprine Pleuropneumonia
• Foot and Mouth Disease
• Heartwater (Cowdriosis)
• Nairobi Sheep Disease
• Orf (Contagious Ecthyma)
• Respiratory Disease: Small Ruminant
• Rinderpest (see www.fiveminutevet.com/ruminant)

Suggested Reading
Albina E, Kwiatek O, Minet C, et al. Peste des petits ruminants, the next eradicated animal disease? Vet Microbiol 2013, 165: 38–44.
OIE World Animal Health Information System. At www.oie.int/wahis_2/public/wahid.php/Wahidhome/Home
OIE. Manual of Diagnostic Tests and Vaccines for Terrestrial Animals, 6th ed. Paris: Office International des Epizooties, 2008. At www.oie.int/manual-of-diagnostic-tests-and-vaccines-for-terrestrial-animals/
Parida S, Muniraju M, Mahapatra M, et al. Peste des petits ruminants. Vet Microbiol 2015, 181: 90–106.
Roeder PL, Obi TU. Recognizing Peste des Petits Ruminants: A Field Manual. Rome: FAO EMPRES (Livestock), 1999. At www.fao.org/docrep/003/x1703e/x1703e00.HTM#Acknowledgements
Spickler AR. Peste des Petits Ruminants. 2008 (Last Updated). At www.cfsph.iastated.edu/DiseaseInfo/factsheets.php
Author Kelly M. Still Brooks
Consulting Editor Christopher C.L. Chase
Acknowledgment The author and book editors acknowledge the prior contribution of Stacy M. Holzbauer.

P

PETROLEUM PRODUCT POISONING

BASICS

OVERVIEW
Ingestion, inhalation, or topical administration of petroleum products and their chemical constituents or waste products, resulting in morbidity and mortality.

INCIDENCE/PREVALENCE
- Dependent on access to petroleum products.
- Multiple animals are usually affected and may be found dead.

GEOGRAPHIC DISTRIBUTION
- Common in areas where grazing animals and petroleum production, transport, storage or land application of drilling waste or wastewater occurs.
- State regulations may vary on how special wastes and produced water from the petroleum industry are handled.
- Application of salty wastewater to melt road ice may create exposure distant from the source through melt and runoff.
- Dependent on access to petroleum products.

SYSTEMS AFFECTED
- Cardiovascular
- Digestive
- Integument
- Mammary
- Musculoskeletal
- Nervous
- Reproductive
- Respiratory
- Urinary

PATHOPHYSIOLOGY.
- Products with highly volatile hydrocarbon fractions or volatile organic compounds are more likely to result in inhalation or aspiration after ingestion compared to compounds of low volatility or high viscosity.
- Inhalation of volatile petroleum products or emissions from operations target the lungs. Hypoxia, chemical pneumonia, and cerebral anoxia are common.
- Ingestion of petroleum products also targets the lungs through eructation and inhalation, aspiration, or hematogenous exposure. A high salt content in petroleum muds and wastewater may contribute to morbidity and mortality. Expansion of hydrocarbon in the rumen results in bloat and rumen stasis. Petroleum products and associated chemical additives are caustic to gastrointestinal mucosa, resulting in gastroenteritis, colitis, mucosal edema, and hemorrhage.
- Dermal lesions occur when petroleum products are applied topically or used as a vehicle for insecticide sprays or dips resulting in contact dermatitis.

SIGNALMENT
All species and ages are susceptible to exposure, younger animals may be at higher risk due to curiosity and inquisitive nature.

PHYSICAL EXAMINATION FINDINGS
Clinical signs vary, often developing within 24 hours of exposure.
- Pyrexia, dehydration, tachycardia, bradycardia, arrhythmia, cardiac arrest
- Oily nasal discharge, petroleum odor on breath and feces
- Dyspnea, tachypnea, aspiration pneumonia, coughing
- Milk tainted with fuel odor, decreased milk production
- Dry integument with blisters, cracking, unthrifty
- Decreased rumen motility, bloat, displaced abomasum, anorexia, salivation, vomiting, oil in feces and rumen contents, diarrhea or constipation
- Reluctance to move, ataxia, recumbency, paddling, shivering, CNS signs (head tremors, decreased menace response and palpebral reflex, opisthotonus), blindness, coma, death
- Sudden death—multiple animals are usually affected and may be found dead.

CAUSES AND RISK FACTORS
Environmental Factors
- Contamination of feed, soil, or water supply by petroleum products resulting from broken pipes, leaking valves or storage tanks, spills, application of drilling muds or wastewater to grazing land, runoff from application of salty wastewater to melt ice, or road-oil used for dust control.
- Rainfall or flooding may mobilize petroleum products long after a spill occurs. Some components such as BTEX (benzene, toluene, ethylbenzene, and xylene) are highly soluble.
- Ambient temperature and wind factors increase volatility and dispersion.
- Poor-quality pasture may contribute to ingestion.

Animal Factors
- Age, preexisting health, hydration, and nutritional status, duration of exposure, duration of time to treatment.
- Direct application of petroleum product either topically or by drench may result in toxicosis.
- Ruminants willingly ingest petroleum-tainted soil, forage, or water. Petroleum products and waste fluids may have a high salt content that promotes consumption.

Petroleum Factors
- Amount of petroleum product consumed; viscosity, volatility, toxicity of chemical constituents, presence of heavy metals, and concentration of salt.

- The exact composition of proprietary mixtures of drilling compounds and nondisclosure agreements may make the product composition difficult to determine.

DIAGNOSIS

Opportunity for exposure and petroleum odor on breath, skin, or in feces is supportive of the diagnosis.

DIFFERENTIAL DIAGNOSES
Lead or other heavy metal exposure, other chemicals used in petroleum extraction, organophosphate ester poisoning, salt toxicity, nutritional deficiencies, other infectious diseases.

CBC/BIOCHEMISTRY/URINALYSIS
Results vary with exposure and chemical composition.
- Increased PCV, Hgb, Fib, TPP, leukopenia initially followed by leukocytosis
- Elevated AST, GGT, BUN, creatinine, LDH, CPK, cholesterol
- Decreased potassium, calcium, glucose
- Elevated Na^+Cl^-

OTHER LABORATORY TESTS
- Gas chromatography or "fingerprinting" of rumen contents, liver, lung, or kidney tissue, and the suspected source of poisoning.
- Heavy metal analysis of liver, GI contents, kidney, and brain to rule out other causes or as components of petroleum product composition.
- Test suspected soil, vegetation and water sources for salts, total petroleum hydrocarbons, heavy metals.
- Acetylcholinesterase level in blood and brain tissue to rule out organophosphate toxicity.

IMAGING
Thoracic radiography in smaller ruminants has prognostic value.

OTHER DIAGNOSTIC PROCEDURES
Tracheal wash and culture

PATHOLOGIC FINDINGS
Respiratory Tract
- Gross lesions: Cranial and middle lung lobe most often affected; consolidation, congested, dark red to purple, mottled, abscesses, and lesions are usually bilateral, serofibrinous exudate, pleural adhesions, and tracheitis
- Histologic: Lung—necrotizing bronchopneumonia, edema

Gastrointestinal
- Gross lesions: Esophagitis, bloat, enteritis, colitis, fuel odor to GI tract, petechial hemorrhages of GI tract, bloody intestinal contents

P

• Histologic: GI tract—mucosal and submucosal congestion and mucosal and serosal hemorrhage

Other Histologic Findings
• Brain—meningeal hyperemia, meningeal/choroid edema, parenchymal hemorrhage, malacia
• Heart—myocardial degeneration and necrosis, hemorrhage, edema, mineralization, congested myocardial and epicardial blood vessels, infiltrations of lymphocytes, macrophages, and neutrophils
• Kidney—renal tubular degeneration, interstitial nephritis, granular eosinophilic casts mixed with inflammatory cell infiltrates, renal vessel thrombi
• Liver—periacinar fatty degeneration and periportal infiltration of lymphocytes and plasma cells, bile duct hyperplasia

TREATMENT

THERAPEUTIC APPROACH
• Remove from source; use stomach tube to relieve bloat (use of a trocar increases risk of peritonitis); administer saline laxative.
• Intravenous fluids, supportive care by system.
• Euthanasia may need to be considered.

SURGICAL CONSIDERATIONS AND TECHNIQUES
Rumenotomy and transfaunation may be indicated.

MEDICATIONS

DRUGS OF CHOICE
Broad-spectrum antibiotics, IV or IM, until clinical signs abate.

CONTRAINDICATIONS
Rumen lavage via orogastric or nasogastric tube increases risk of aspiration.

FOLLOW-UP

EXPECTED COURSE AND PROGNOSIS
• Highly variable depending on type of compound and severity of exposure.

• Some animals survive the initial exposure with few clinical signs while others do poorly for weeks to months, requiring culling.
• Animals with aspiration pneumonia have a guarded to poor prognosis.

POSSIBLE COMPLICATIONS
Chronic wasting or neoplasia. Some chemical compounds are known carcinogens.

PATIENT CARE
• Physical examination and routine blood work as warranted by clinical findings.
• Restrict activity.
• Modifications to diet will depend on rumen motility. Some animals will continue to eat while others will be anorectic for days to weeks.

PREVENTION
• Fence off areas to keep animals away from potential sources.
• Locate petroleum storage tanks and pits away from well or surface water.
• Inspect tanks, pipes, valves, pits, and ponds associated with petroleum extraction and storage for leakage.
• Do not reuse petroleum storage containers for feed or water.
• If constituent chemicals are known, estimate potential risks of soil and water exposure using risk-based screening levels (RBSLs) or toxicity reference levels (TRLs).

MISCELLANEOUS

ASSOCIATED CONDITIONS
• Salt toxicity
• Many compounds associated with petroleum products are known carcinogens.

ZOONOTIC POTENTIAL
Inhalation of petroleum vapors is potentially toxic.

PREGNANCY
Abortions or stillbirths have been attributed to petroleum exposure.

PRODUCTION MANAGEMENT
• Fence off areas to keep animals away from potential sources.
• Quarantine of animals after natural gas exposure has been reported.

• Appropriate milk and meat withdrawal times must be followed for all compounds administered to food-producing animals.

ABBREVIATIONS
• AST = aspartate aminotransferase
• BUN = blood urea nitrogen
• CNS = central nervous system
• CPK = creatine phosphokinase
• Fib = fibrinogen
• GGT = gamma-glutamyl transferase
• GI = gastrointestinal
• Hgb = hemoglobin
• IM = intramuscular
• IV = intravenous
• LDH = lactate dehydrogenase
• PCV = packed cell volume
• RBSLs = risk-based screening levels
• TPP = total plasma protein
• TRLs = toxicity reference levels

SEE ALSO
• Agricultural Chemical Toxicities
• Gaseous Toxicities (see www.fiveminutevet.com/ruminant)
• Heavy Metal Toxicosis
• Lead Toxicosis
• Organophosphate Toxicity
• Toxicology: Herd Outbreaks

Suggested Reading
Bamberger M, Oswald RE. Impacts of gas drilling on human and animal health. New Solutions 2012, 22: 51–77.
Batista JS, Camara ACL, Almeida RD, Olinda RG, Silva TMF, Soto-Blanco B. Poisoning by crude oil in sheep and goats. Revue Med Vet 2013, 164: 517–20.
Coppock RW, Mostrom MS, Khan AA, Semalulu SS. Toxicology of oil field pollutants in cattle: a review. Vet Hum Toxicol 1995, 37: 569–75.
Edwards WC. Livestock poisoning from oil field drilling fluids, muds and additives. Vet Hum Toxicol 1991, 33: 502–4.
Edwards WC, Coppock RW, Zinn LL. Toxicosis related to the petroleum industry. Vet Hum Toxicol 1979, 21: 328–37.
Author Lauren Palmer
Consulting Editor Christopher C.L. Chase

P

PHENOXYL TOXICITY

BASICS

OVERVIEW

• Chlorophenoxylic herbicide compounds, such as 2,4-dichlorophenoxy acetic acid (also known as 2,4-D) and methylchlorophenoxy acetic acid (MCPA), are used to control weeds and aquatic plants, to increase fruit durability in storage, and to prevent premature fruit dropping. Animals' exposure is from accidental ingestion of concentrates or sprays, occasionally from chronic ingestion of treated forages. These herbicides are relatively nontoxic unless ingested in a concentrated form.

• Several hundred commercial products contain chlorophenoxy compounds in various forms, concentrations, and combinations.

• Repeated and massive doses are needed to cause poisoning in ruminants.

• These agents can cause liver and kidney failure, hypotension, and increased cancer risk; also there may be hemolysis.

• Chlorophenoxy compounds have been shown to demyelinate peripheral nerves, depress ribonuclease synthesis, uncouple oxidative phosphorylation, and increase hepatic peroxisomes.

• Examples—2,4-D; 2,4-dichlorophenyl; 2,2-dichloropropionic acid (Dalapon); 4-chloro-2-methylphenoxy acetic acid (MCPA); 2,4,5-trichlorophenoxy acetic acid (Sivex).

• The advent of commercial farming prompted the development of selective weed control chemicals. These organic herbicides are plant growth regulators altering the metabolism of plants and are associated with potential teratogenicity.

• A side effect of the compound's use is the increased levels of nitrates or cyanide in plants that can cause secondary poisoning to ruminants prior to the plant's death.

• Some toxic weeds, such as jimsonweed and nightshade, become more palatable after treatment with this type of herbicide.

• Essentially, usage has been stopped because of the toxic contaminants of dioxins (TCDD, HCDD).

INCIDENCE/PREVALENCE

These herbicides are relatively nontoxic unless ingested in a concentrated form.

GEOGRAPHIC DISTRIBUTION

Worldwide

SYSTEMS AFFECTED

Musculoskeletal
Nervous
Urinary

PATHOPHYSIOLOGY

Causes kidney and muscle damage, as the herbicide increases not only serum UA, TP, and CR levels but also CK activity. Reported effects include muscle weakness in cases of myopathy, as well as degeneration of skeletal muscle fibers and increased serum CK activity in cattle.

SIGNALMENT

• Potentially, all ruminant species are affected.

• 10 days of exposure may be required to produce poisoning. However, calves have been poisoned by a single oral dose of 200 mg/kg body weight.

• Oral administration of up to 125 mg/kg body weight to adult dogs did not result in lethality.

• Chronic administration of up to 500 ppm of 2,4-D in the diet for 2 years did not result in any adverse effects.

PHYSICAL EXAMINATION FINDINGS

• Clinical signs are only seen following massive and repeated exposures.

• Anorexia, depression, rumen atony, muscle weakness, especially in hindlimbs.

• Diarrhea, ulceration of oral mucosa, bloating.

• Animals progressively become emaciated and moribund.

CAUSES AND RISK FACTORS

• Feeding up to 2000 ppm herbicide in the diet amounted to 1 ppm in liver and kidneys and <0.05 ppm in the muscle and fat.

• Herbicide residues are not likely to be at >300 ppm in or on forage immediately after treatment at recommended rates for brush and weed control. Residues decline rapidly. Half-life in forage is 1–2 weeks.

• Meat residues occur only with extremely high exposure during continuous ingestion of freshly treated vegetation.

• Withdrawal of animals from treated forages for 1–2 weeks prior to slaughter should decrease any residues.

• Herbicide-treated forages do not seem to affect rumen microbial functions or development in the rumen; they are not readily degraded by ruminal microorganisms.

DIAGNOSIS

DIFFERENTIAL DIAGNOSES

• Severe parasitism

• Diseases causing anorexia, depression, rumen atony, muscle weakness, especially of hindlimbs

• Diseases causing diarrhea, ulceration of oral mucosa, bloating
  ◦ Abomasal torsion
  ◦ Acidosis/grain overload
  ◦ Bovine viral diarrhea virus (BVDV)
  ◦ Cathartic/laxatives
  ◦ Coccidiosis
  ◦ Colitis/typhlitis
  ◦ Displaced abomasum
  ◦ Enteritis
  ◦ Heart failure
  ◦ Indigestion
  ◦ Intussusception
  ◦ Jejunal hemorrhage syndrome
  ◦ Johne's disease
  ◦ Liver failure
  ◦ Malignant catarrhal fever
  ◦ Molybdenum toxicity/copper deficiency
  ◦ Parasitism
  ◦ Parasympathomimetic drugs
  ◦ Peritonitis
  ◦ Poisonous plants: Acorn (oak), *Brassica* spp., fungal toxicity, mushroom, oleander, pokeweed, pyrrolizidine alkaloids, rattlebox, selenium accumulators, *Solanum* spp., St. John's wort
  ◦ Salmonellosis
  ◦ Sepsis/toxemia/enterotoxemia
  ◦ Toxins: Aflatoxin, arsenic, chlorpyrifos (Dursban), copper, herbicides, levamisole, lincomycin, monensin, nicotine, phosphorus fertilizers, propylene glycol, sodium bicarbonate, sulfur, trichothecene, zinc
  ◦ Uremia/renal failure
  ◦ Winter dysentery
  ◦ Xylazine, large doses

• Diseases causing weight loss and emaciation

CBC/BIOCHEMISTRY/URINALYSIS

• Major elimination by the kidneys.

• CBC/biochemistry/urinalysis is indicated to monitor parameters for treatment.

• No parent compounds or metabolites found in milk from orally dosed cattle.

OTHER LABORATORY TESTS

• High levels of compound in kidney and liver, decreased levels in fat and muscle.

• Phenoxy acid esters and salts are primarily metabolized by acid hydrolysis, and a minor amount is conjugated.

OTHER DIAGNOSTIC PROCEDURES

Feed analysis, chemical analysis for the chlorophenoxylic herbicide compounds

PATHOLOGIC FINDINGS

• Epicardial hemorrhage

• Hydropericardium

• Bright green, undigested feed from ruminal stasis

• Liver swollen, friable

• Kidneys congested

• Hyperemia, enlargement of lymph nodes and mesenteric vessels

• High levels in liver and kidney, decreased levels in fat and muscle

TREATMENT

THERAPEUTIC APPROACH

• Activated charcoal, alkaline diuresis

• Control seizures; diazepam, phenobarbital

• Cathartic: Administer a dose of a saline or sorbitol cathartic such as magnesium or sodium sulfate (sodium sulfate dose is 1 gram/kilogram). If access to these agents is

(CONTINUED)   **PHENOXYL TOXICITY**

limited, give 5–15 mL magnesium oxide (Milk of Magnesia) per os for dilution.

MEDICATIONS

DRUGS OF CHOICE
Control seizures—diazepam, phenobarbital

PRECAUTIONS
• Appropriate milk and meat withdrawal times must be followed for all compounds administered to food-producing animals.
• Keep toxic chemicals away from livestock. Do not apply toxic chemicals to fields or crops on which animals may feed.
• Consult manufacturer and FARAD if accidental exposure occurs.

POSSIBLE INTERACTIONS
N/A

FOLLOW-UP

EXPECTED COURSE AND PROGNOSIS
Depends on quantity ingested; fair to poor depending on treatment and amount of agent consumed.

PREVENTION
• Withdrawal of animals from treated forages for 1–2 weeks prior to slaughter would decrease any residues.
• Keep toxic chemicals away from livestock. Do not apply toxic chemicals to fields or crops on which animals may feed.

• Meat residues occur only with extremely high exposure during continuous ingestion of freshly treated vegetation.

MISCELLANEOUS

ASSOCIATED CONDITIONS
• A side effect is the increased levels of nitrates or cyanide in plants that can cause secondary poisoning before the plant dies.
• Some toxic weeds, such as jimsonweed and nightshade, become more palatable after treatment.

PREGNANCY
N/A

PRODUCTION MANAGEMENT
Keep all chemicals and sprays away from feeding ruminants.

ABBREVIATIONS
• BVDV = bovine viral diarrhea virus
• CK = creatine kinase
• CR = creatinine
• FARAD = Food Animal Residue Avoidance Databank
• HCDD = dioxone; 1,2,3,4,5,6,7,8-HCDD
• TCDD = the most toxic member of the dioxin and furan family—2,3,7,8-TCDD; 2,3,7,8-tetrachlorodibenzo-p-dioxin
• TP = total protein
• UA = urine albumin

SEE ALSO
• Bovine Viral Diarrhea Virus
• Coronavirus

• Heavy Metal Toxicosis
• Johne's Disease
• Malignant Catarrhal Fever
• Molybdenum Toxicity
• Monensin Toxicity
• Mycotoxins
• Nightshade (*Solanum* spp.) Toxicosis
• Oak (*Quercus* spp.) Toxicity
• Oleander and Cardiotoxic Plant Toxicity
• Pyrrolizidine Alkaloids
• Salmonellosis

Suggested Reading
Clark DE, Palmer JS. Residual aspects of 2,4,5-T and an ester in sheep and cattle with observations on concomitant toxicological effects. J Agric Food Chem 1971, 19: 761–4.
Paulino CA, Oliveira GH, Palermo-Neto J. Acute 2,4-dichlorophenoxyacetic acid intoxication in cattle. Vet Hum Toxicol 1994, 36: 433–6.
Paulino CA, Palermo-Neto J. Effects of acute 2,4-dichlorophenoxyacetic acid on cattle serum components and enzyme activities. Vet Hum Toxicol 1995, 37: 329–32.
Rowe VK, Hymas TA. Summary of toxicological information on 2,4-D and 2,4,5-T type herbicides and an evaluation of the hazards to livestock associated with their use. Am J Vet Res 1954, 15: 622–9.
Author Steve Ensley
Consulting Editor Christopher C.L. Chase
Acknowledgment The author and book editors acknowledge the prior contribution of Greg Stoner.

P

PHOSPHORUS DEFICIENCY/EXCESS

BASICS

OVERVIEW
- Essential macromineral.
- Roles: Bone, teeth and cell membrane structure, regulation of metabolism, energy storage, and buffering.
- Elemental phosphorus is highly reactive → in the body phosphorus is present as phosphate (P), in both organic and inorganic (P_i) forms. Methods of determining [P] in body fluids specifically measures [Pi].
- *P deficiency* may manifest as rickets (RK), osteomalacia (OM), pregnancy toxemia (PT), hypophosphatemic down cow syndrome (HDCS), and postparturient hemoglobinuria (PPH).
- *P excess* may manifest as yellow (white) phosphorus toxicity (YPT), osteodystrophy fibrosa (OF), urolithiasis, and sodium phosphate toxicity (SPT).

INCIDENCE/PREVALENCE
- PPH: sporadic and low incidence
- Chronic P excess: uncommon

GEOGRAPHIC DISTRIBUTION
- OM/RK
  ○ Regional soil deficient in P: Africa, Australia, New Zealand, and arid or tropical regions
  ○ Reduced sunlight hours in southern and northern latitudes
- PPH: North America, New Zealand
- HDCS: Northern United States and Canada

SYSTEMS AFFECTED
P Deficiency
- Musculoskeletal
- Hematologic
- Cardiovascular

P Excess
- Nervous
- Musculoskeletal
- Urinary
- Digestive

PATHOPHYSIOLOGY
Compartments
- 85% hydroxyapatite (bones and teeth)
- 14–15% intracellular
- <1% extracellular

Homeostasis
- Losses (600 kg dairy cow)
  ○ Bone and muscle growth
  ○ Saliva and fecal loss (20–40 g/d)
    ■ ~80% saliva [P] is recovered by intestinal absorption
  ○ Urinary loss (<1 g/d)
  ○ Milk production (20–55 g/d)
  ○ Late gestation fetal skeletal development (2–6 g/d)

- Uptake
  ○ Intestinal absorption
    ■ Primary site: small intestines
    ■ Ruminal microbes are able to digest phytic acid → phytate-bound P (up to 70% of P in plants), is available for absorption in ruminants.
- PTH: Increases renal and salivary excretion of P but also increases osteoclast activity and increases renal production of 1,25-DHCC.
  ○ PTH is secreted primarily in response to hypocalcemia rather than P imbalance.
  ○ Renal tubular cells and bovine salivary gland cells become unresponsive to PTH in states of severe P depletion.
- 1,25-DHCC
  ○ Enhances intestinal P absorption.
  ○ Negative feedback to PTH secretion.
- Calcitonin: Decreases renal tubular P reabsorption.
- Phosphatonins: Modulate renal tubular reabsorption of P and inhibit activation of 1,25-DHCC.

P Deficiency
- Chronic P depletion primarily manifests as anorexia and bone demineralization.
  ○ RK: The cartilaginous matrix at the growth plate and the osteoid matrix formed during bone remodeling fail to mineralize.
  ○ OM: Failure of osteoid matrix to mineralize.
  ○ Soils deficient in P are often energy deficient, which when combined with anorexia results in weight loss, impaired fertility, and decreased milk production.
- PT: Fetal growth removes substantial amounts of P from the maternal circulation.
- HDCS: Recumbent hypophosphatemic periparturient cows unresponsive to Ca treatment.
  ○ Debated whether the P imbalance is a cause (losses in milk) or consequence (anorexia and decreased GIT motility) of recumbency.
  ○ Negative effects of P depletion on muscle function are well established in human medicine but the mechanisms have not been identified.
- PPH: Intravascular hemolysis during the first 6 weeks of lactation presumably due to intracellular ATP depletion → increased osmotic fragility.
- Refeeding syndrome (RFS): Potentially fatal shifts in fluids and electrolytes in malnourished animals receiving a high carbohydrate diet (particularly artificial enteral or parenteral feeding).
  ○ Refeeding → insulin release → increased glycogen, fat and protein synthesis, processes that require P, Mg, K, and thiamine → intracellular shift of these electrolytes and water and thiamine depletion

○ Total body P depletion → ATP and 2,3-DPG rapidly depleted → cellular dysfunction and inadequate oxygen delivery

P Excess
- Chronic P excess
  ○ Inhibits formation of 1,25-DHCC → downregulate P and Ca intestinal absorption
  ○ Reduced intestinal Mg absorption → hypomagnesemia decreases PTH binding affinity → hypocalcemia. Dry cow rations with a dietary P content >0.5% increase the risk of clinical hypocalcemia
  ○ PTH release → widespread osteoclastic resorption of bone and its replacement by fibrous tissue = OF
  ○ Dystrophic mineralization
  ○ Increased urinary [P] → urolithiasis
- Yellow (white) phosphorus toxicity (YPT)
  ○ Local irritant to the GIT
  ○ Distributes to all tissues → ~day 3: cardiac, hepatic, renal and multiorgan failure
- Sodium phosphate toxicity (SPT) (Iatrogenic MSP IV or P enema)
  ○ P is rapidly absorbed through the mucosa of the colon
  ○ P enema doses above recommended amounts or concurrent renal or GIT disease might result in toxicosis
    ■ >11 kg BW: 120 mL (human adult size)
    ■ <11 kg BW: 60 mL (human pediatric size)
  ○ Lethal dose in pigs: 20 mL/kg per rectum
  ○ Hypernatremia → hyperosmolar syndrome
  ○ Hypocalcemia: PTH-induced losses, intracellular shift, and hypernatremia-induced calciuresis
  ○ Hypokalemia: increased urinary K excretion
  ○ Metabolic acidosis
    ■ Hypertonicity of enema causes fluid influx into the colon (or body cavity if perforation occurs during administration) → dehydration and elevation in lactate
    ■ Hyperphosphatemia increases the nonvolatile weak acid pool.

HISTORICAL FINDINGS
N/A

SIGNALMENT
P Deficiency
- Cattle > sheep and goats
- RK: Young growing animals
- PT: Beef cows and ewes in late gestation
- HDCS: Postpartum dairy cows
- PPH: Mature, multiparous, high-yielding dairy cows

P Excess
OF: Goats > cattle and sheep

(CONTINUED) | **PHOSPHORUS DEFICIENCY/EXCESS**

PHYSICAL EXAMINATION FINDINGS

P Deficiency
• General: Anorexia, pica, unthriftiness, weight loss, reduced milk production, reduced reproductive performance
• OM: Shifting lameness, kyphosis, lordosis, spontaneous nonhealing fractures
• RK: Stiffness, lameness, joint enlargement, kyphosis, angular limb deformity
• PT/HDCS: Weakness, recumbency
• PPH: Weakness, marked decrease in milk production, red-brown urine, pallor of mucus membranes, tachycardia, tachypnea, and jaundice
• RFS: Neurologic disorders, seizures, rhabdomyolysis, cardiac arrhythmias, cardiac failure, and death

P Excess
• OF: Stiffness, shifting lameness, facial and physeal enlargement, multiple fractures
• YPT: Diarrhea, abdominal pain, garlic-like breath odor, jaundice, coagulopathies, convulsions, tachycardia, and torsades de pointes
• SP toxicosis: Prosencephalic neurologic signs (dullness, seizures, coma), cardiac arrhythmias, hypocalcemia (tetanic convulsions, weakness), hypokalemia (weakness) and dehydration. Incorrect enema administration → rectal or vaginal trauma

GENETICS
N/A

CAUSES AND RISK FACTORS

P Deficiency
• OM/RK
  ◦ Chronic PO_4 deficiency
    ▪ Diet deficient in P: green cereal crops, mature forages or crop residues; poor P content of soil: regional, heavy rains, continuous removal of crops
    ▪ P binding agents: Diet high in Ca, Al, Mg, and fat
    ▪ Hypovitaminosis D: lack of sunshine; bile duct aplasia
    ▪ Intestinal malabsorption disease
• PT
  ◦ Late gestation
  ◦ P-deficient diet
  ◦ Late winter
  ◦ Usually complicated by concurrent deficiency in Ca, Mg, and energy
• HDCS
  ◦ Initiation of lactation
  ◦ Acidogenic diet increases urinary P excretion
  ◦ Concurrent hypocalcemia → PTH → increased urinary and salivary loss of P
  ◦ Decreased feed intake
  ◦ Not associated with low P diets
• PPH
  ◦ P-deficient diet
  ◦ P deficiency is likely only a contributing factor
  ◦ Cows that have been treated for ketosis

  ◦ Concurrent Se, Cu, and energy deficiencies
• RFS
  ◦ Chronically undernourished animals
  ◦ Little or no energy intake for 10 days

P Excess
• Chronic
  ◦ Diet high in P, low in Ca: bran, grains, oxalates
  ◦ Excessive supplementation of feed with P
  ◦ Hypervitaminosis D: Cholecalciferol rodenticides, *Solanum* spp., *Cestrum diurnum*
• YPT: Rodenticides, fertilizer
• SP: Iatrogenic overdose or incorrect administration
  ◦ Inadvertent transvaginal administration of P enema reported in crias

 DIAGNOSIS

DIFFERENTIAL DIAGNOSES
• OM/RK
  ◦ Fluorosis arthritis
  ◦ Cu deficiency
  ◦ Physitis
• PPH
  ◦ Babesiosis
  ◦ Theileriosis
  ◦ Bacillary hemoglobinuria
  ◦ Water intoxication
  ◦ Increased oxidative stress: onions, bassicas, Se deficiency
  ◦ Saponins: sugar beet, alfalfa
• SP toxicity: Obstructive urolithiasis, ruptured bladder, renal failure

CBC/BIOCHEMISTRY/URINALYSIS
Serum [Pi] or plasma [Pi]: most commonly used tool to assess P
• Correlates well with short-term dietary P supply
• Chronic P deficiency might be masked by mobilization of P reserves from bone
• Altered acutely by multiple factors, particularly transcellular shifts
• Shift from ECF to ICF
  ◦ Hyperinsulinism: insulin injections, insulin-secreting neoplasm, or response to carbohydrate load (dextrose infusion in cattle can lower plasma [Pi] within minutes by >30% and remain below baseline for 90 minutes)
  ◦ Respiratory alkalosis
  ◦ Catecholamine and cortisol release
  ◦ Sepsis
• Shift from ICF to ECF
  ◦ Myopathies
  ◦ Sick cell syndrome
  ◦ Acute tumor lysis syndrome
  ◦ Acidemia and metabolic acidosis
• Dehydration
  ◦ Hyperphosphatemia is a common finding in cattle with right displaced abomasums or

abomasal volvulus and is associated with the degree of dehydration.
• Young, growing animals: Increased growth hormone → increases renal tubular resorption of P.
• Spurious decrease [Pi] by increased conjugated bilirubin; spurious increase with hyperbilirubinemia, monoclonal gammopathy, in vitro hemolysis or delayed harvesting of serum or plasma.

Reference Ranges
• Cattle:
  ◦ Adults 1.4–2.6 mmol/L (4–8 mg/dL)
  ◦ Growing 1.9–2.6 mmol/L (6–8 mg/dL)
• Sheep 1.6–2.4 mmol/L (5–7.3 mg/dL)
• Goats: 1.3–3 mmol/L (4.2–9.1 mg/dL)

Laboratory Findings for P-Associated Diseases
• OM/RK
  ◦ ± hypophosphatemia
  ◦ ± hypocalcemia
• PT
  ◦ Recumbent animals serum [Pi] often <1 mg/dL
  ◦ Herd average serum [Pi] 2–3 mg/dL
• PPH
  ◦ Moderate to marked anemia, polychromasia, and basophilic stippling of RBC, nucleated RBC, anisocytosis
  ◦ Hypophosphatemia common (<1.5 mg/dL)
  ◦ Increased indirect bilirubin
  ◦ Hemoglobinuria, bilirubinuria, and proteinuria
• OF
  ◦ ± hyperphosphatemia
  ◦ ± hypocalcemia
  ◦ Increased fractional excretion of P
• SP toxicosis
  ◦ Hyperphosphatemia
  ◦ Hypernatremia
  ◦ Hypocalcemia
  ◦ Hypokalemia
  ◦ Metabolic acidosis

OTHER LABORATORY TESTS
N/A

IMAGING
Radiographic changes:
• OM: Thin cortices, reduced bone density, noncalloused bone fractures
• RK: Clublike thickening of metaphysis, wide physes, bowed long bones
• OF: Reduced bone density, subperiosteal bone resorption, loss of dura dentes

OTHER DIAGNOSTIC PROCEDURES
• OM, RK, OF: Bone ash : organic ratio 1.2–1.3 (normal 3:2)
• Analysis of dietary P and Ca

PATHOLOGIC FINDINGS
• OM: Soft and brittle bones, thin cortices with large marrow cavities, noncalloused fractures. Accumulation of excess unmineralized osteoid on trabecular bone surfaces.

P

- RK: Bowed long bones, domed cranium, prominent costochondral junctions, rachitic metaphysis, retarded mandibular growth. Failure of osteoid and cartilaginous matrix to mineralize, overgrowth of fibrous tissue in metaphyses, persistent cartilage and irregular physes.
- PPH: Thin watery blood, jaundice of soft tissue, distended gall bladder, pigmenturia, nutmeg liver. Central lobular coagulative hepatic necrosis, bile and hemosiderin pigment in renal tubular epithelial cells and hemoglobin in tubules.
- OF: Thickening of flat bones particularly the calvarium, maxilla and mandible, soft bones, noncalloused fractures. Extensive erosion of periosteal and cortical bone by numerous osteoclasts, compact bone replaced by fibrocellular tissue, herniation of articular cartilage into the epiphysis.
- YPT: Severe icterus and fatty liver with periportal necrosis.

TREATMENT

THERAPEUTIC APPROACH

P Deficiency

Chronic
- Correct any dietary deficiency in P, Ca, or vitamin D
  ○ Ideal dietary ratio of Ca:P is 2:1
    ▪ Cattle: 150–300 kg body weight require 9–18 g/d of P
    ▪ Sheep: 10–100 kg body weight require 1.9–4.8 g/d of P
- OM/ RK
  ○ Adequate sunlight
  ○ Injectable vitamin D: 10,000–30,000 IU/kg

Acute
- Oral drench: 50 g of P (200 g MSP)
  ○ Duration: 8–12 hours
  ○ Rumen motility important
- IV: 6 g of P (23 g MSP) or 120 mL phosphate enema (19 g MSP + 7 g DSP) dissolved in 1 L sterile deionized water
  ○ Administer over several hours to avoid precipitation with Ca, and increased renal P excretion
  ○ Do not use with Ca- or Mg-containing solutions—precipitation

○ Ca-containing solutions used for milk fever often contain phosphorus but in the form of phosphite or phosphinic acid—remain soluble but are biologically inactive so should not be used with the intent of restoring plasma [Pi].
- RFS
  ○ Supplementation of P, K, and Mg orally, or IV if severe
  ○ Thiamine
  ○ Reduce energy intake → gradually increase over 4 days

P Excess
- Chronic: Reduce dietary P content + supplement Ca during adjustment period
- YPT: No antidote, supportive therapy
- SP toxicosis
  ○ Correct hypocalcemia only to level that controls clinical symptoms as extra Ca stimulates soft tissue mineralization
  ○ Correct hypernatremia
    ▪ IV fluids containing relatively lower [Na]
    ▪ Calculate amount Na required using Adrogue formula
    ▪ Acute (24 h): 2–3 mEq/L/h and then slow rate (max total, 12 mEq/L/24h)
    ▪ Chronic (>24h): max 0.5 mEq/L/h (max total of 8–10 mEq/L/24h)
    ▪ Do not allow free access to water if severely hypernatremic.
  ○ Correct acidosis and dehydration.

MEDICATIONS

See "Therapeutic Approach"

FOLLOW-UP

EXPECTED COURSE AND PROGNOSIS
- OM/RK/OF: Good with appropriate treatment
- PPH: Grave (death in 2–5 days)
- YPT: Grave

POSSIBLE COMPLICATIONS
N/A

PATIENT CARE
- SP toxicosis
  ○ ECG monitoring during calcium administration
  ○ Serial monitoring of serum [Na]

- RFS: Monitor serum electrolytes and for signs of fluid overload

PREVENTION
- HDCS: Avoid hypocalcemia.
- P enema toxicosis: Only use in cases refractory to soapy water enemas and aqueous lubricants.

MISCELLANEOUS

ABBREVIATIONS
- 1,25-DHCC = 1,25-dihydroxycholecalciferol
- DSP = disodium phosphate
- HDCS = hyperphosphatemic down cow syndrome
- MSP = monosodium phosphate
- OF = osteodystrophy fibrosa
- OM = osteomalacia
- P = phosphate
- P_i = inorganic phosphorus
- PPH = postparturient hemoglobinuria
- PT = pregnancy toxemia
- PTH = parathyroid hormone
- RFS = refeeding syndrome
- RK = rickets
- SP = sodium phosphate
- SPT = sodium phosphate toxicity
- YPT = yellow phosphorus toxicity

SEE ALSO
- Hypocalcemia: Bovine
- Hypocalcemia: Small Ruminant

Suggested Reading
Goff JP. Pathophysiology of calcium and phosphorus disorders. Vet Clin North Am Food Anim Pract 2000;16: 319–37.
Grünberg W. Treatment of phosphorus balance disorders. Vet Clin North Am Food Anim Pract 2014, 30: 383–408.
Mehanna HM, Moledina J, Travis J. Refeeding syndrome: what it is, and how to prevent and treat it. BMJ 2008, 336:1495–8.
Schropp DM, Kovacic J. Phosphorus and phosphate metabolism in veterinary patients. J Vet Emerg Crit Care 2007, 17: 127–34.
Author Laura Johnstone
Consulting Editor Kaitlyn A. Lutz
Acknowledgment The author and book editors acknowledge the prior contribution of Kurt L. Zimmerman and Daniel C. Rule.

P

PHOTOSENSITIZATION

BASICS

OVERVIEW
- Photosensitization is an abnormal reaction of the skin to sunlight due to the presence of a photodynamic agent in the dermis. Photodynamic agents absorb certain wavelengths of ultraviolet (UV) light, producing free radicals, which react with proteins in the dermal tissue, causing damage.
- Photosensitization can be divided into four categories: Type I (primary photosensitization), type II (photosensitization due to aberrant pigment synthesis), type III (secondary or hepatogenous photosensitization), and type IV (idiopathic).

INCIDENCE/PREVALENCE
Late spring, summer, and early fall are most common, but if photosensitizing plants are baled into hay, signs may be seen year round.

GEOGRAPHIC DISTRIBUTION
Worldwide

SYSTEMS AFFECTED
- Integument
- Multisystemic

PATHOPHYSIOLOGY
- In type I photosensitization, the photodynamic agents are absorbed into the blood from the gastrointestinal tract (GI) and react with UV light at the skin surface. Type I reactions may also occur with direct contact to the photodynamic agent (plant, chemical). Once in the dermis, the photodynamic agent absorbs the energy of a light photon and forms free radicals. The oxygen free radical reacts with amino acids, nucleic acids, and membrane lipids in the capillary endothelium and surrounding tissues, causing tissue destruction.
- Type II photosensitization is due to a genetic defect in the individual. The photodynamic agent is a pigment that is produced endogenously by an aberrant metabolic process.
- Type III photosensitization is secondary to liver damage. Chlorophyll is metabolized by microbes in the GI tract, forming phylloerythrin. Phylloerythrin, a photodynamic metabolite of chlorophyll, is absorbed into the bloodstream. Normally phylloerythrin is removed from the blood by the liver, and excreted in bile. With liver damage or biliary obstruction, phylloerythrin cannot be excreted, and thus enters the general circulation. Liver damage can occur from toxins, bacteria, viruses, or neoplasia. Secondary photosensitization is intensified when the consumption of chlorophyll from green plants is high.
- Type IV photosensitization is where the pathogenesis is unknown or the photodynamic agent is not identified.

HISTORICAL FINDINGS
- With plant ingestion, signs may appear from 24 hours to several months after the first ingestion.
- With drug eruptions, cutaneous lesions are noted 24–48 hours after drug administration, although there may occasionally be a longer interval.

SIGNALMENT
- All ruminant species
- White- or light-colored breeds
- Affects all ages, but young may be more susceptible
- Affects both sexes equally

GENETICS
- White- or light-skinned breeds are at higher risk for type I or type III photosensitivity. Black-skinned animals are rarely affected with photosensitization of any type.
- Type II photosensitization has been reported to occur as an inherited autosomal recessive congenital disease in Holstein, Ayrshire, and Shorthorn cattle and Southdown and Corriedale sheep.
- In bovine erythropoietic porphyria ("pink tooth"), affected cattle are deficient in uroporphyrin III cosynthetase, an enzyme needed for proper formation of hemoglobin. Uroporphyrin and coproporphyrin accumulate in the bones, teeth, skin, and urine, as well as other tissues and secretions. Accumulations of porphyrin metabolites in the skin predispose the animals to photosensitization.
- Southdown lambs may have a congenital defect that can cause hyperbilirubinemia and results in hepatogenous photosensitization. Corriedale lambs can have a similar condition, which is characterized by a failure to excrete phylloerythrin and conjugated bilirubin that also results in hepatogenous photosensitization.

PHYSICAL EXAMINATION FINDINGS
- Photosensitization occurs most frequently in hairless and white-skinned areas of the body. Eyelids, lips, ears, nose, white blazes, coronary bands, and other white areas are most commonly involved.
- Signs may be more severe in areas of the body that receive more sunlight (head, neck, back).
- In contact photosensitization, only areas of contact with the photodynamic agent are affected. The affected area first becomes erythematous, edematous, and painful. Honey-colored serum begins to seep from the thickened skin, and extensive scabs can form after 1–2 days. Secondary bacterial infections of the skin can occur.
- Animals tend to be very pruritic in the early stages. As signs progress, they resist handling and may not want to eat due to the discomfort. Occasionally, the eyes will be affected and these animals may become blind. Death is due to starvation or misadventure.

Table 1

Plants That Cause Type I (Primary) Photosensitization		
Latin Name	Common Name	Toxin
Hypericum spp.	St. John's wort	Conjugated quinone (hypericin)
Fagopyrum esculentum	Buckwheat	Conjugated quinone (fagopyrin)
Heracleum mantegazzianum	Giant hogweed	Furocoumarins
Ammi majus	St. Anne's lace	
Cymopterus spp.	Spring parsley	
Thamnosma texana	Dutchman's breeches	

- Signs consistent with hepatic encephalopathy (e.g., ceaseless walking, head pressing, behavior changes, etc.) are seen with secondary photosensitization.
- Animals may be restless and pruritic with reddened and swollen eyelids, muzzle, and lips. Affected animals may also exhibit tachypnea, tachycardia, hyperthermia, diarrhea, salivation, and jaundice (if type III or IV).

CAUSES AND RISK FACTORS
Plants
See Tables 1 and 2

Pharmaceuticals
- Antibiotics (penicillin, sulfas, tetracycline)
- Anticonvulsants
- Local anesthetics
- Nonsteroidal anti-inflammatory agents (NSAIDs), antipyretics (aspirin, phenylbutazone)
- Phenothiazines
- Thiazides

Chemicals
- Carbon tetrachloride
- Copper
- Methylene blue
- Phenanthridium
- Phosphorus

Fungal
- *Pithomyces chartarum*, *Aspergillus* spp., and *Fusarium* spp. can all produce hepatotoxic mycotoxins and cause secondary photosensitization.

Neoplasia
- Any neoplasia that affects hepatic function can cause secondary photosensitization. A major risk factor is any underlying liver disorder or genetic defect that decreases excretion of phylloerythrin.

P

PHOTOSENSITIZATION   (CONTINUED)

Table 2

	Plants That Cause Type III (Secondary) Photosensitization		
Latin Name	*Common Name*	*Toxin*	*Mechanism of Action*
Senecio spp. Crotalaria spp. Amsinckia intermedia Echium spp. Heliotropium spp. Symphytum spp. Cynoglossum officinale	Ragwort, groundsel, senecio Crotalaria, rattlebox Fiddleneck Blueweed, viper's bugloss Heliotrope Comfrey Hound's tongue	Pyrrolizidine Alkaloids (PA)	PAs are metabolized by the liver and the activated pyrrole form alkylates DNA in the hepatocyte, which impairs cell division. This prevents the hepatocyte from undergoing binary fission to regenerate hepatocytes, resulting in hepatocytomegaly and karyomegaly. When large numbers of hepatocytes die, the necrosis triggers a regenerative response accompanied by bile duct proliferation.
Microcystis Anabaena Oscillatoria Nodularia spumigena	Blue green algae	Microcystins	Microcystins cause disruption of the actin filaments of the hepatic cytoskeleton, leading to cellular collapse.
Lantana spp. Lippia spp.	Lantana, shrub verbena, yellow sage White brush	Triterpenoid compounds	Triterpenoids affect hepatocytes by inhibiting secretory function and decreasing bile canaliculi ATPase activity resulting in cholestasis and jaundice.
Helenium spp. Hymenoxys spp.	Sneezeweed Rubberweed, bitterweed	Sesquiterpene lactones	Sesquiterpene lactones bind to sulfhydryl groups and other nucleophilic components, inhibiting numerous aerobin and anaerobin enzymes.
Tetradymia and Artemisia spp.	Horsebrush Black sagebrush	Furanosesquiterpenens Sesquiterpene lactones	Tetradymol metabolites uncouple oxidative phosphorylation in electron transport. Phylloerythrin from other plants must be eaten to result in the development of photosensitization.
Panicum spp. Tribulus terrestris Nolina spp. Agave lecheguilla	Panicum, Kleingrass Puncture vine, goathead Sacahuiste, bunchgrass Agave, lecheguilla	Disogenin	Lithogenic steroidal saponins (disogenins) are responsible for formation of crystals in the bile ducts resulting in hepatogenous photosensitization.
Kochia scoparia	Kochia	Unknown, possibly saponins	Secondary photosensitization
Trifolium hybridum	Alsike clover	Unknown	Primary photosensitization has been seen with ingestion and possibly contact. Secondary photosensitization has been seen with long-term ingestions.
Phyllanthus abnormis Descurainia pinnata D. sophia	Abnormal-leaf Flower Tansymustard Flixweed	Unknown	Secondary photosensitization
Brassica rapa B. napus B. oleracea	Turnip Rape Kale	Nitriles?	Unknown photosensitization
Lotus corniculatus Trifolium incarnatum T. subterraneum T. pretense Medicago denticulate (polymorpha) M. sativa M. lupulina M. minima Avena sativa Sorghum Triticum Chamaesyce (Euphorbia) maculata	Bird's-foot trefoil Crimson clover Subterranean clover Red clover Burclover Alfalfa Black medic Small burclover Oats Sorghum Wheat Spotted spurge	Unknown	Unknown photosensitization

P

(CONTINUED)

DIAGNOSIS

DIFFERENTIAL DIAGNOSES
- Pemphigus foliaceus
- Irritant dermatitis
- Allergic dermatitis
- Folliculitis/furunculosis
- Dermatophytosis
- Chemical burns
- Thermal burns
- Malignant catarrhal fever
- Pediculosis
- Demodectic mange

CBC/BIOCHEMISTRY/URINALYSIS
- Elevations in GGT, AST, and ALP (most common)
- Elevations in SDH, GLDH, LDH (early in syndrome)
- Hyperbilirubinemia
- Inflammatory leukogram may be present.

OTHER LABORATORY TESTS
- Elevated bile acids
- Prolonged BSP clearance time
- Plasma phylloerythrin (>10 µg/dL is diagnostic) if available

OTHER DIAGNOSTIC PROCEDURES
Skin or liver biopsies can be performed.

PATHOLOGIC FINDINGS
- Dermal lesions vary from minimal reddening to urticarial lesions with erythema and swelling, to skin necrosis. The skin may have a gelatinous appearance extending down into the deeper corium. Microscopically, edema will be accompanied by necrosis and a polymorphonuclear infiltrate in the deeper corium. Both the epidermis and the superficial dermal vasculature may be damaged.
- Animals with secondary photosensitization will have hepatic and other systemic lesions. Bright yellow fat, hepatomegaly, liver cirrhosis, hepatic necrosis, and ascites are common. Depending on the extent of the liver damage, bruising and hemorrhage may be seen.
- If toxicosis is due to PAs, then hepatocytomegaly (always present), fibrosis, and bile duct proliferation may be seen.
- With certain plants, birefringent crystals may be evident in the bile ducts (small ducts may be obstructed), skin, kidney, adrenal gland, and heart.

TREATMENT

THERAPEUTIC APPROACH
- Therapy involves removing the animal from sunlight and preventing reexposure to the photodynamic agent.

- All drugs being administered when photosensitization occurred should be stopped.
- If the liver is involved, appropriate therapy for liver disease must be given.

MEDICATIONS

DRUGS OF CHOICE
- Pain relief with NSAIDs (e.g., flunixin 1.1–2.2 mg/kg PO or IV q6–12h; 72-hour milk withdrawal, 10-day meat withdrawal) if hepatopathy is not involved.
- Antibiotics if pyoderma is present (e.g., ceftiofur 1.1–2.2 mg/kg IM q24h; no milk or meat withdrawal).
- Liver protectants and blood transfusions may be attempted to prolong life in valuable animals.

CONTRAINDICATIONS
- If signs are due to a drug reaction, avoid using any related medications in the treatment of clinical signs.
- Appropriate milk and meat withdrawal times must be followed for all compounds administered to food-producing animals.

PRECAUTIONS
If secondary photosensitization, use caution when using drugs that must be metabolized by the liver.

FOLLOW-UP

EXPECTED COURSE AND PROGNOSIS
- Type I has a good prognosis. Type III has a poor prognosis due to liver involvement.
- The skin eruptions usually subside within 24–48 hours after exposure ceases, although lesions may persist up to 6 months.

POSSIBLE COMPLICATIONS
Prolonged grazing of *Echium* and *Heliotropium* may result in chronic copper poisoning of sheep.

CLIENT EDUCATION
Clients need to inspect hay and pastures for any phototoxic plants.

PATIENT CARE
- As many affected animals stop eating and drinking, supplemental feeding and fluid therapy are important.
- Mortality primarily occurs in lambs because the ewe's udders are so painful that lambs are not permitted to nurse. Cows also refuse to let calves nurse, but calf losses are usually low.
- Soothing skin medication or other pain relief can hasten healing.
- Prevent animal exposure to UV light. Let out on dry pasture only at night.
- Avoid any additional photosensitizing plants.

- Monitor until dermal lesions have resolved or until liver values return to normal.

PREVENTION
- Avoid future exposures to any implicated compounds and related substances.
- Avoid grain and hay contaminated by species of plants known to cause photosensitization.
- Control photosensitizing plants by spraying pastures and crop land with herbicides. Plants along trails and in shipping areas should be removed.
- Less-valuable animals or more resistant species may be used to "pregraze" pastures (e.g., sheep/goats may be used to graze groundsel before cattle).
- Provide supplemental feeding with more nutritious and palatable forage with contaminated pastures and follow a range management program that prevents overgrazing.
- Avoid exposure to blue-green algae by fencing off contaminated ponds.
- Facial eczema can be prevented by breeding animals for resistance, oral dosing with zinc, and spraying pastures with fungicides.

MISCELLANEOUS

ASSOCIATED CONDITIONS
Pyoderma

AGE-RELATED FACTORS
Affects animals of all ages, but increased mortality in young animals.

ZOONOTIC POTENTIAL
PA metabolites are secreted in milk.

PREGNANCY
PAs cross the placenta and can affect the fetus, leading to increased calf losses, even with clinically normal dams.

SYNONYMS
- Bighead = *Tribulus terrestris*, *Chamaesyce maculata*
- Facial eczema = *Pithymyces chartarum*
- Fagopyrism = *Fagopyrum esculentum*
- Geeldikkop = *Tribulus terrestris*
- Hard liver disease = chronic *Amsinkia intermedia toxicosis*
- Seneciosis, Pictou disease, sleepy staggers = chronic *Senecio* spp. intoxication
- Trifoliosis, dew poisoning, big liver disease = *Trifolium hybridum* intoxication

ABBREVIATIONS
- ALP = alkaline phosphatase
- AST = aspartate aminotransferase
- BSP = bromosulfophthalein
- GGT = gamma-glutamyltransferase
- GI = gastrointestinal
- GLDH = glutamate dehydrogenase
- LDH = lactate dehydrogenase
- NSAIDs = nonsteroidal anti-inflammatory drugs

P

PHOTOSENSITIZATION

- PA = pyrrolizidine alkaloids
- SDH = sorbitol dehydrogenase
- UV = ultraviolet

SEE ALSO
- Dermatophytosis
- Malignant Catarrhal Fever
- Parasitic Skin Diseases: Bovine
- Parasitic Skin Diseases: Camelid
- Parasitic Skin Diseases: Small Ruminant

Suggested Reading
Burrows GE, Tyrl RJ. Toxic plants of North America. Ames: Iowa State University Press, 2001.
Burrows GE, Tyrl RJ. Toxic Plants of North America, 2nd ed. Ames: Wiley-Blackwell, 2013, Kindle edition.
Cheeke PR, Shull LR. Natural Toxicants in Feeds and Poisonous Plants. Westport, CT: AVI Publishing Co, 1985.
Flaoyen A. Do steroidal saponins have a role in hepatogenous photosensitization diseases of sheep? Adv Exp Med Biol 1996, 405: 395–403.
Scruggs DW, Blue GK. Toxic hepatopathy and photosensitization in cattle fed moldy alfalfa hay. J Am Vet Med Assoc 1994, 204: 264–6.
Author Steve Ensley
Consulting Editor Christopher C.L. Chase

P

PINE NEEDLE TOXICITY

BASICS

OVERVIEW
• Ingestion of pine needles and bark from several north American pine species can induce abortion in cattle and bison and less frequently, systemic toxicity in cattle and sheep.
• Economic impact due to cattle abortions and death loss were estimated between $4.5 million and $20 million annually in the United States.
• Toxic pine trees are found in Western Canada, the US, and Northern Mexico.
• Toxicity has been reported with consumption of Ponderosa pine (*Pinus ponderosa*), Monterey pine (*Pinus radiata*), lodgepole pine (*Pinus contorta*), Monterey cypress (*Cupressus macrocarpa*), common juniper (*Juniperus communis*), Formosan juniper (*Juniperus formosana*), Utah juniper (*Juniperus osteosperma*), Rocky Mountain juniper (*Juniperus scopulorum*), Engelmann spruce (*Picea engelmannii*), Pinyon pine (*Pinus edulis*), single leaf pinyon (*Pinus monophylla*), and Jeffrey pine (*Pinus jeffreyi*).

INCIDENCE/PREVALENCE
Unknown

GEOGRAPHIC DISTRIBUTION
• *P. ponderosa* (Ponderosa or Western yellow pine) is the most widespread found across much of western North America, from southern Canada into Mexico and from Nebraska and Oklahoma to the Pacific Coast.
• *P. contorta* (lodgepole or limber pine) is found in western North America, from Alaska to Mexico and east to South Dakota.
• *P. radiata* (Monterey pine) is found around Monterey, California and cultivated in New Zealand and Australia.

SYSTEMS AFFECTED
• Nervous
• Reproductive
• Respiratory
• Urinary

PATHOPHYSIOLOGY
• The toxic and abortive actions are exerted by acids contained in pine needles and barks.
• Abortifacient effect is induced by pine diterpene labdane acids such as isocupressic acid (ICA). Pine resins compounds such as abietane acid have also neurotoxic and nephrotoxic effects.
• The induction of abortion is dependent on dosage of ICA ingested and on the stage of pregnancy.
• After consumption of pine needles, ICA is absorbed by the rumen into the systemic circulation and metabolized by the liver into agathic acid (AA), dihydroagathic acid (DHAA), and tetrahydroagathic acid (THAA).

• The mechanism of action for the abortion is not completely understood. The metabolites appear to modify hormonal changes, inducing increase in caruncular arterial tone and decrease in uterine caruncular blood flow. An effect on progesterone concentration inducing termination of pregnancy was also proposed.
• Clinical signs of toxicity happen from 24 hours to several days post-exposure.
• Abortifacient effects most often occur with ingestion of 1 kg needles/day for several days or higher amounts for 2–3 days. 100 mg ICA/kg body weight twice daily is required to initiate abortions in cattle. Ingestion of 62–78 mg ICA/kg BW of *Pinus contorta* induced abortion in 8–10 days. Ingestion of 190–245 mg ICA/BW of *Juniperus communis* induced abortion in 3–4 days.

SIGNALMENT
• Affects mainly bison and cattle.
• Sheep generally do not abort but increased incidence of dead lamb is noticed with pine needle consumption.
• Goats, elk, mule deer, and white-tailed deer are tolerant.

PHYSICAL EXAMINATION FINDINGS
Reproductive
• Abortion is more common than toxicity signs.
• Abortion or stillbirth happens in cattle in the second or third trimester of pregnancy, usually 3–4 days after ingestion. Early pregnancies do not seem to be affected. Increased incidence of abortion is noticed as pregnancy progresses.
• Early parturition with signs of depression, mucoid vulvar discharge (often bloody), weak uterine contractions, incomplete cervical dilation, uterine hemorrhage, dystocia, birth of dead or small weak calf. Alive calves are generally weak but stillbirth is also common.
• Maternal complications include retained placenta, septic metritis, agalactia, anorexia, rumen stasis, and death (if untreated).
• While significant exposure does not cause abortion in sheep, the number of dead lambs born at term may increase.

Systemic
• Intoxication and related clinical signs depend upon the amount consumed and the rate of ingestion.
• Initial clinical signs are depression, weakness, anorexia, lethargy, rumen atony, followed by hindlimb paresis and paralysis.

CAUSES AND RISK FACTORS
• Ingestion of pine needles, especially when green.
• Consumption of conifer foliage increases when limited forage is available, during snow cover, inclement weather, and reduced grazing time.
• Cattle with low body condition scores are induced to consume more pine needles compared to those with high body condition score.

• Cattle fed a low protein, high energy diet are induced to consume more pine needles.

DIAGNOSIS

DIFFERENTIAL DIAGNOSES
Abortion caused by BVD or IBR viruses, neosporosis, leptospirosis, brucellosis, campylobacteriosis, selenium deficiency, or foothill abortion (EBA).

CBC/BIOCHEMISTRY/URINALYSIS
• Systemic toxicity: Azotemia, hypercreatinemia, hyperbilirubinemia
• Increase in AST, CPK, LDH
• Proteinuria with hyaline and granular casts

OTHER DIAGNOSTIC PROCEDURES
• Investigating access to pine needles, presence of risk factors, and clinical signs.
• Collection of fetal thoracic fluid or stomach content for detection of THAA.

PATHOLOGIC FINDINGS
• Reproductive—dams that die exhibit heavy uterine exudate with necrotic placental tissue, edema, and focal ulceration of endometrium and necrosis in the caruncles. Stillborn calves may show malacia of white brain (cerebral leukomalacia) matter or may appear normal.
• Systemic—nephrosis, vacuolation of basal ganglia neutrophils, perivascular and myelinic edema, patchy neuronal degeneration, ischemic myonecrosis of rear leg muscles.

TREATMENT

THERAPEUTIC APPROACH
• Remove source of pine needles from affected animals.
• Bind metabolites and reduce their absorption from digestive system.
• Support patient, treat symptomatically, maintain hydration and electrolytes.
• Treat retained placenta and endometritis.
• Supportive care for calf.

SURGICAL CONSIDERATIONS AND TECHNIQUES
Rumenotomy with evacuation of contents may be worthwhile if performed early.

MEDICATIONS

DRUGS OF CHOICE
• Activated charcoal orally to control absorption of toxins from the GI tract. 2–5 g/kg in a water slurry given orally (1 g charcoal per 5 mL water).
• Na thiosulfate—0.5g/kg BW IV.
• Broad-spectrum antibiotics to treat uterine and/or systemic bacterial infection.

P

PINE NEEDLE TOXICITY   (CONTINUED)

PRECAUTIONS

Appropriate milk and meat withdrawal times must be followed for all compounds administered to food-producing animals.

FOLLOW-UP

EXPECTED COURSE AND PROGNOSIS

• Dams usually recover with treatment but death has been reported.
• Calf prognosis is dependent on stage of development at birth and supportive treatment for premature birth.
• Incidence of abortion: High abortive rate is expected in acute cases.

POSSIBLE COMPLICATIONS

Dams: Retained placenta, septic metritis, agalactia, anorexia, rumen stasis, and death (if untreated).

PREVENTION

• Prevent animal access to pine needles.
• Providing a proper diet and adequate nutrition to animals will minimize the intake of many toxic plants.
• Feeding 25% or more corn silage has shown to reduce pine intake.
• Increase protein content of diet if diet is composed of high energy and low protein.
• Conditioning cattle with pine needles has been proposed to reduce incidence of abortion but no data is supportive of its efficacy. The dose suggested for conditioning is 66 mg ICA/kg BW.

MISCELLANEOUS

ASSOCIATED CONDITIONS

Nutritional deficiency

PREGNANCY

Reproductive toxicity in last trimester of pregnancy

PRODUCTION MANAGEMENT

• Fence pregnant cows in the last trimester away from pines and provide supplemental feed.
• Reduce animal density at feeding and assure appropriate access to feeders.
• Remove young stands of pines where appropriate.

ABBREVIATIONS

• AA = agathic acid
• AST = aspartate aminotransferase
• BVD = bovine viral diarrhea
• CPK = creatinine phosphokinase
• DHAA = dihydroagathic acid
• EBA = epizootic bovine abortion
• IBR = infectious bovine rhinotracheitis
• ICA = isocupressic acid
• LDH = lactic acid dehydrogenase
• THAA = tetrahydroagathic acid

SEE ALSO

• Abortion: Bacterial
• Bovine Viral Diarrhea Virus
• Brucellosis
• Infectious Bovine Rhinotracheitis
• Leptospirosis
• Neosporosis
• Selenium/Vitamin E Deficiency

Suggested Reading

Burrows GE, Tyrl RJ, ed. Toxic plants of North America. Ames: Iowa State University Press, 2001.

Burrows GE, Tyrl RJ, ed. Toxic plants of North America. Ames: Wiley-Blackwell, 2013, Kindle edition.

Short RE, Ford SP, Grings EE, Kronberg SL. Abortifacient response and plasma vasoconstrictive activity after feeding needles from Ponderosa pine trees to cattle and sheep. J Anim Sci 1995, 73: 2102–4.

Snider DB, Gardner DR, Janke BH, Ensley SM. Pine needle abortion biomarker detected in bovine fetal fluids. J Vet Diagn Invest 2015, 27: 74–9.

Stegelmeier BL, Gardner DR, James LF, Panter KE, Molyneux RJ. The toxic and abortifacient effects of Ponderosa pine. Vet Pathol 1995, 33: 22–8.

Wang S, Panter KE, Gardner DR, Evans RC, Bunch TD. Effects of the pine needle abortifacient, isocupressic acid, on bovine oocyte maturation and preimplantation embryo development. Anim Reprod Sci 2004, 81: 237–44.

Welch KD, Gardner DR, Pfister JA, Panter KE, Zieglar J, Hall JO. A comparison of the metabolism of the abortifacient compounds from Ponderosa pine needles in conditioned versus naïve cattle. J Anim Sci 2012, 90: 4611–17.

Author Eleonora Po
Consulting Editor Christopher C.L. Chase

PLANTS PRODUCING ACUTE RESPIRATORY DISTRESS SYNDROME

BASICS

OVERVIEW
• An afebrile pneumonia-like disease of cattle but occasionally observed in other ruminants. Often called acute respiratory disease syndrome (ARDS). Also called acute bovine pulmonary emphysema and edema (ABPEE).
• Rapid death may result.
• Several etiologies exist for the disease including rapidly changing animals from poor to lush pasture, and the plant *Perilla frutescens* (purple mint, perilla mint). Moldy sweet potatoes, rape, kale, turnips, and moldy pink half-runner beans are also associated with the disease.
• Many lush grasses are associated with ARDS including Bermuda, fescue, alfalfa, and Kleingrass. In the southeastern United States, *Perilla frutescens,* or purple mint, is often associated with ARDS. *Perilla* is an annual weed that grows to a height of 1–2 meters. *Perilla* is readily identified by its square stem and is common along wood lines and waste areas. The plant has small terminal white flowers and a characteristic minty fragrance.
• Lush pasture of many grasses contains high quantities of L-tryptophan. Dry, nonsucculent pastures contain lower quantities of L-tryptophan.
• Perilla mint contains 3-substituted furans (perilla ketone, egomaketone, and isoegomaketone).
• L-tryptophan in high quantities can lead to atypical interstitial pneumonia (AIP).
• Ingestion of moldy sweet potatoes that contain *Fusarium solani* can develop AIP in ruminants.
• *Fusarium solani* produces 4-ipomeanol which is a pneumotoxin.
• 3-substituted furans can be pneumotoxic by their direct affects on the lung.
• The condition is often referred to as bovine asthma, or AIP, in the US and fog fever in the United Kingdom.

INCIDENCE/PREVALENCE
• Usually observed in the fall when cattle are moved from summer pasture to lush fall growth, it has been observed in spring when cattle are turned out on lush pasture after being fed hay over the winter.
• Outbreak usually occur on pastures. The morbidity rate is usually low but occasionally may exceed 50%. The case fatality rate is typically 25–50%.
• ARDS cases in Mexico have involved a variety of irrigated grasses.

GEOGRAPHIC DISTRIBUTION
Worldwide

SYSTEMS AFFECTED
Respiratory

PATHOPHYSIOLOGY
• The toxin can vary depending on the substrate but the pathogenesis is similar among the plants producing ARDS toxicants including *Brassica* spp. (kale, turnips), moldy sweet potatoes, and purple mint.
• Bioactivation of a pneumotoxin, primarily in Clara cells and macrophages of the lung rather than in cells in the liver, results in formation of reactive metabolite intermediates such as 3-methylindole (3-MI).
• These reactive metabolites bind to proteins in the lungs and cause tissue destruction, especially of type 1 pneumocytes and epithelial cells. Under the stimulus of factors released by macrophages, type 2 pneumocytes proliferate to replace lost type I cells and in the process cause formation of foci with massive increase in cellularity.
• During this period of proliferation, the ability of type II cells to synthesize and secrete functional surface-active phospholipids (surfactants) is decreased. Surfactant produced no longer effectively lowers surface tension. This compromises lung function.

SIGNALMENT
All ruminants, but cattle primarily

PHYSICAL EXAMINATION FINDINGS
• The clinical course is rapid and cattle may be found dead in 12–24 hours, especially if stressed.
• Animals are observed with very rapid and shallow open-mouth breathing. Foam is evident around their mouth. An expiratory grunt is very audible from 100 feet or more. Animals may be extremely cyanotic and die quickly if stressed.

CAUSES AND RISK FACTORS
• Animals are susceptible whenever moved from dry nonsucculent pasture to lush pasture. Signs may appear within 1 week following the transfer.
• L-tryptophan is metabolized by rumen microorganisms to indoleacetic acid, which is subsequently decarboxylated by *Lactobacillus* spp. to 3-methylindole (3-MI). The 3-methylindole is absorbed and metabolized by the lung mixed-function oxidase system to produce pneumotoxicosis.
• Usually observed in the fall when cattle are moved from summer pasture to lush fall growth, it has been observed in spring when cattle are turned out on lush pasture after being fed hay over the winter.
• If caused by *Perilla frutescens,* usually observed from August through October when this plant reaches maturity. The seed heads are the most toxic. Has been observed in cattle eating hay containing purple mint.
• Consumption of moldy sweet potatoes containing 4-IP can occur year round.
• There have been reports of acute respiratory disease associated with feed wet distiller's grains. There may be a pneumotoxin similar to 4-IP in this feed. Can occur year round but most reports are in the fall.

DIAGNOSIS

DIFFERENTIAL DIAGNOSES
• Other causes of pneumonia such as viruses, mycoplasma, and bacteria
• Hardware disease in cattle due to the pronounced expiratory grunt

CBC/BIOCHEMISTRY/URINALYSIS
N/A

IMAGING
• Thoracic radiography.
• Pulmonary emphysema and edema are common.
• Emphysematous bullae may be observed on the lung surface.

OTHER DIAGNOSTIC PROCEDURES
These are used to rule out viral and bacterial causes for the pneumonia.

PATHOLOGIC FINDINGS
• Lungs are enlarged and heavy due to edema, cellular proliferation, and congestion. Foam fills many airways.
• Interlobular edema and emphysema are commonly observed. Emphysematous bullae are often observed on the lung surface.
• Emphysema may extend into the mediastinum and subcutaneous cervical and thoracic areas.
• Microscopically, alveolar epithelial hyperplasia of type 2 pneumocytes is common along with interstitial emphysema, edema, and hyaline membranes.

TREATMENT

THERAPEUTIC APPROACH
• No specific treatment.
• Keeping animals as calm as possible is important.
• If stressed, animals often become anoxic and die.
• Remove animals from etiology (e.g., purple mint, moldy sweet potatoes, or lush pasture). Place on dry feed.

MEDICATIONS

DRUGS OF CHOICE
• No specific drugs are effective.
• Symptomatic treatment such as corticosteroids, atropine, diuretics, antihistamines, and antibiotics.
• Avoid stress (if possible) when treating.
• Weigh the value of therapeutic pharmacology versus the stress involved with handling and treatment.

P

PLANTS PRODUCING ACUTE RESPIRATORY DISTRESS SYNDROME   (CONTINUED)

PRECAUTIONS
• Appropriate milk and meat withdrawal times must be followed for all compounds administered to food-producing animals.
• Steroids should not be used in pregnant animals.

FOLLOW-UP

EXPECTED COURSE AND PROGNOSIS
• Depending on the amount of lung damage, very guarded early prognosis as death may occur within 12–24 hours.
• Clinical course may last 2–3 weeks.
• If animals survive 2 or 3 days and are not stressed, prognosis improves.
• Even severely affected animals may return to normal in 2–3 weeks when the type 2 pneumocytes resolve to type 1.

PREVENTION
• Gradually introduce cattle to lush pasture after feeding on nonsucculent, if possible.
• Inhibit certain ruminal microflora that reduce L-tryptophan to 3-MI with monensin or lasalocid.
• Avoid exposure to perilla mint.
• Supply ample good pasture as perilla is usually consumed only when other better forage is lacking.

MISCELLANEOUS

ASSOCIATED CONDITIONS
N/A

AGE-RELATED FACTORS
Calves fed the flowering perilla plant develop the toxic syndrome, while those fed earlier plants (collected before seed stage) and late plants (collected after frost) remain asymptomatic. Cases in cattle have been reported year round.

PRODUCTION MANAGEMENT
The time of year when *Perilla* reaches the seed stage often corresponds to periods when pasture grass is scarce, forcing cattle to consume plants not normally eaten when ample desirable forage is available.

SYNONYMS
• Atypical interstation pneumonia (AIP)
• Bovine asthma
• Fog fever

ABBREVIATIONS
• ABPEE = acute bovine pulmonary emphysema and edema
• AIP = atypical interstitial pneumonia
• ARDS = acute respiratory distress syndrome
• 3-MI = 3-methylindole
• 4-IP = 4 ipomeanol

SEE ALSO
• Aspiration Pneumonia
• Atypical Interstitial Pneumonia
• Bovine Respiratory Syncytial Virus
• *Brassica* spp. Toxicity
• Contagious Bovine Pleuropneumonia
• Enzootic Pneumonia of Calves
• Organophosphate Toxicity
• Parasitic Pneumonia
• Pericarditis
• Respiratory Disease: Bovine
• Sweet Potato Poisoning
• Toxicology: Herd Outbreaks

Suggested Reading
Apley MD, Fajt V. Feedlot therapeutics. Vet Clin North Am Food Anim Pract 1998, 14: 291–313.
Burrows GE, Tyrl RJ. Toxic Plants of North America. Ames: Wiley, 2013. Kindle edition.
Doster AR, Mitchell FE, Farrell RL, Wilson BJ. Effects of 4-ipomeanol, a product from mold-damaged sweet potatoes, on bovine lung. Vet Pathol 1978, 15: 367–75.
Kerr LA, Johnson BJ, Burrows GE. Intoxication of cattle by *Perilla frutescens* (purple mint). Vet Hum Toxicol 1986, 28: 412–16.
Kerr LA, Linnabary RD. Review of interstitial pneumonia in cattle. Vet Hum Toxicol 1989, 31: 247–54.
Loneragan GH, Morley PS, Wagner JJ, et al. Time-dependent changes in plasma concentrations of 3-methylindole and blood concentrations of 3-methyleneindolenine-adduct in feedlot cattle. Am J Vet Res 2002, 63: 591–7.
Pearson EG, Andreasen CB, Blythe LL, Craig AM. Atypical pneumonia associated with ryegrass staggers in calves. J Am Vet Med Assoc 1996, 209: 1137–42.

Author Steve Ensley
Consulting Editor Christopher C.L. Chase
Acknowledgment The author and book editors acknowledge the prior contribution of Larry A. Kerr.

P

POISON HEMLOCK (*CONIUM* SPP.) TOXICITY

BASICS

OVERVIEW
• Poison hemlock (*Conium maculatum*) toxicity in ruminants is an uncommon occurrence.
• Poison hemlock is a member of the Apiaceae family. It is a biennial. The first-year seedling plant contains leaves that are fernlike in appearance—three to four times pinnately divided, and the leaflets are 1/4 in. long and segmented. The foliage has a strong odor like mouse urine, or a parsnip-like odor.
• The mature plant is erect, 3–8 feet tall, with a stout hollow stem (except at the nodes) that is smooth and often purple splotched. The plant has a long white/yellow taproot, which resembles a carrot or parsnip.
• Small, white flowers are arranged in umbrella-shaped clusters at the tips of the uppermost stems.
• It is a commonly encountered weed throughout North America, sometimes forming heavy dense stands that are difficult to control.
• Two types of clinical conditions can be encountered—acute toxicities (nicotinic effects) and malformations in young exposed in utero ("crooked calf disease").
• Treatment is nonspecific in nature, and emphasis should be placed on identification of the plant and preventing access to it.

INCIDENCE/PREVALENCE
Not very common; the plant is not generally considered palatable (particularly the mature plant) and animals do not readily graze it unless forced to do so. Animals may acquire a taste for the plant.

GEOGRAPHIC DISTRIBUTION
Throughout North America

SYSTEMS AFFECTED
• Nervous
• Musculoskeletal

PATHOPHYSIOLOGY
• The piperidine alkaloids have nicotinic-like effects—stimulate, then paralyze the nicotinic receptors. Large exposures cause neuromuscular block, hypotension, and bradycardia.
• Gamma-coniceine is thought to be the agent responsible for the malformations; inhibits fetal movement. Both coniine and gamma coniceine are considered teratogenic in various animals.

SIGNALMENT
• All ruminants, particularly cattle (considered more susceptible).
• Cattle, sheep, and goats appear to be susceptible.

PHYSICAL EXAMINATION FINDINGS
• Abrupt onset (within a few hours of ingestion) of muscle tremors, ataxia, muscle weakness, weakened heartbeat, excessive salivation and lacrimation, mydriasis, and frequent urination and defecation.
• This can progress to recumbency, depression, abdominal pain, respiratory distress, and death from respiratory arrest.
• Skeletal deformations observed when pregnant animals are exposed include arthrogryposis, cleft palate, microphthalmia, and spinal column deformities.

CAUSES AND RISK FACTORS
• Concentrations of the toxic alkaloids vary between parts of the plant and stage of maturity.
• All parts of the plant are potentially toxic, and toxicity is thought to increase as the plant matures.
• Approximate toxic and lethal dose for poison hemlock—cattle >1.0 g fresh plant/kg body weight; sheep >5.4 g fresh plant/kg BW; goats >7.8 g fresh plant/kg BW.
• Some toxicity is lost in drying; but there have been cases where cattle have been poisoned as a result of ingesting contaminated hay.
• Grain that is contaminated by the seeds can be a problem as well. Concentration of the alkaloids is highest in the seeds.

DIAGNOSIS

DIFFERENTIAL DIAGNOSES
• Organophosphate or carbamate poisoning, poisoning with *Lupinus* or *Nicotiana* spp.
• Nitrate
• Cyanide
• Nonprotein nitrogen

CBC/BIOCHEMISTRY/URINALYSIS
No specific diagnostic changes have been reported.

OTHER DIAGNOSTIC PROCEDURES
• One can attempt to confirm exposure through feed microscopy of the rumen contents.
• Piperidine alkaloids can be detected in the rumen contents or urine, also in liver, kidney, and blood.

PATHOLOGIC FINDINGS
• Renal tubule necrosis and skeletal muscle degeneration has been reported in fatal cases involving people.
• A mouse urine or parsnip odor can be detected from the freshly open rumen.
• Skeletal malformations include cleft palate, arthrogryposis, scoliosis, kyphosis, and torticollis.

TREATMENT

THERAPEUTIC APPROACH
• Symptomatic and supportive in nature. Decontaminate the gastrointestinal tract with activated charcoal and saline cathartic.
• Providing adequate respiratory support would be next to impossible in the field.

MEDICATIONS

DRUGS OF CHOICE
Atropine should be used with caution.

PRECAUTIONS
Appropriate milk and meat withdrawal times must be followed for all compounds administered to food-producing animals.

FOLLOW-UP

EXPECTED COURSE AND PROGNOSIS
Highly dependent on the exposure dose or the severity of the malformations.

PATIENT CARE
Monitor respiratory function.

PREVENTION
• Avoid access to the plant.
• Control chemically with appropriate herbicides.

MISCELLANEOUS

ASSOCIATED CONDITIONS
• Depression, abdominal pain, respiratory distress, and death from respiratory arrest.
• Skeletal deformations observed when pregnant animals are exposed include arthrogryposis, cleft palate, microphthalmia, and spinal column deformities.

PREGNANCY
Attempts should be made to prevent pregnant animals' access to the plant during susceptible periods (cattle—days 40–100 of gestation; sheep and goats—30–60 days of gestation).

PRODUCTION MANAGEMENT
• Prevent animals from accessing the plant.
• Some toxicity is lost in drying; but there have been cases where cattle have been poisoned as a result of ingesting contaminated hay.
• Grain contaminated by the seeds can be a problem as well.

P

POISON HEMLOCK (*CONIUM* SPP.) TOXICITY   (CONTINUED)

SYNONYMS
- Fool's parsley
- Poison carrot
- Poison parsley
- Spotted hemlock
- St. Bennett's weed
- Stinkweed

ABBREVIATION
BW = body weight

SEE ALSO
- Arthrogryposis
- Carbamate Toxicity
- Lupine Toxicity
- Organophosphate Toxicity
- Tobacco Toxicosis

Suggested Reading
Burrows GE, Tyrl RJ. Conium. In: Burrows GE, Tyrl RJ eds, Toxic Plants of North America. Ames: Iowa State University Press, 2001.
Burrows GE, Tyrl RJ. Chapter 8 Apiaceae Lindl. In: Burrows GE, Tyrl RJ eds, Toxic Plants of North America, 2nd ed. Ames: Wiley-Blackwell, 2013, Kindle edition.
Galey FD, Holstege DM, Fisher EG. Toxicosis in dairy cattle exposed to poison hemlock (*Conium maculatum*) in hay: isolation of Conium alkaloids in plants, hay, and urine. J Vet Diagn Invest 1992, 4: 60–4.
Keeler RF. Coniine, a teratogenic principle from *Conium maculatum*, producing congenital malformations in calves. Clin Toxicol 1974, 7: 195–206.
Keeler RF, Ball LD. Teratogenic effects in cattle of *Conium maculatum*, producing congenital malformations in calves. Clin Toxicol 1978, 12: 49–64.
Lopez TA, Cid MS, Bianchini ML. Biochemistry of hemlock (*Conium maculatum L.*) alkaloids and their acute and chronic toxicity in livestock. A review. Toxicon 1999, 37: 841–65.
Panter KE. Piperidine alklaloids. In: Plumlee KH ed, Clinical Veterinary Toxicology. St. Louis: Mosby, 2004.
Panter KE, Keeler RF, Backer DC. Toxicosis in livestock from the hemlocks (*Conium* and *Cicuta* spp.). J Anim Sci 1988, 66: 2407–13.
Vetter J. Poison hemlock (*Conium maculatum L.*). Food Chem Toxicol 2004, 42: 1373–82.

Author Steve Ensley
Consulting Editor Christopher C.L. Chase
Acknowledgment The author and editors acknowledge the prior contribution of Patricia Talcott.

P

POLYARTHRITIS

BASICS

OVERVIEW
Inflammation of multiple joints resulting in persistent lameness

INCIDENCE/PREVALENCE
Varies based on etiology

GEOGRAPHIC DISTRIBUTION
N/A

SYSTEMS AFFECTED
Musculoskeletal

PATHOPHYSIOLOGY
Inflammation is a component of all joint disease, regardless of etiology, to varying degrees. The synthesis of inflammatory mediators results in degradation of synovial tissue. A common cause of polyarthritis, septic arthritis, results from the hematogenous seeding of bacteria or, less commonly, viral pathogens from a primary site of entry (e.g., omphalophlebitis, pneumonia). Direct trauma and congenital disorders can also cause polyarthritis, although often seen in a solitary joint. See chapters on each specific etiology for more detailed pathophysiology.

HISTORICAL FINDINGS
• The clinical signs typically observed in animals with polyarthritis include shifting limb lameness, stilted gait, and unwillingness to move. Close examination usually reveals multiple visibly-swollen and distended joints.
• Herd health history is important to narrow down underlying cause.

SIGNALMENT
This varies with the specific syndrome and etiology. All ruminant species can become affected.

PHYSICAL EXAMINATION FINDINGS
• A complete physical examination is important to determine underlying cause of disease.
• Joint capsules are palpably distended and pressure on the joint will cause increased distention of the joint at an alternate site. Warmth and pain upon palpation and flexion of joints may be observed.
• Look for signs of trauma over joints (e.g., puncture wounds, chronic decubital ulceration). Penetrating wounds should be cleaned and probed.
• Systemic signs include any of lameness, fever, lethargy, and inappetence.

CAUSES AND RISK FACTORS
Clinical syndromes presenting with multiple distended and/or painful joints:
• *Mycoplasma* spp. arthritis—fibrinosuppurative and necrotizing arthritis + tenosynovitis in calves and feedlot bison
• *Histophilus somni* arthritis
• Chlamydial arthritis

• Caprine arthritis encephalitis virus (CAEV)
• Polyarthritis secondary to septicemia
• Polyarthritis secondary to bacterial endocarditis
• Osteochondrosis—inheritance and gender are contributing factors
• Septic physitis secondary to salmonellosis
• Traumatic
• OA (DJD)—elbow joints in domestic sheep; cartilage lesions in the patellar groove lesions in bulls; temporomandibular joint in free-living Soay sheep on St. Kilda (geriatric females, predominantly)
• Mineral deficiency
• Osteomalacia
• Hock lesions (tarsal periarthritis) strongly associated with time spent lying on abrasive surfaces, prolonged high local pressure/friction of the hock on hard surfaces, and collisions of hock with cubicle fittings.

DIAGNOSIS

DIFFERENTIAL DIAGNOSES
See "Causes and Risk Factors." Make sure to rule out other extra-articular causes of lameness including infectious and noninfectious hoof lesions, some of which will cause swelling around the joints of the distal limb.

Diagnosis Criteria
• Herd histories of preceding or concurrent outbreaks of respiratory disease will greatly increase the likelihood of mycoplasmal, *Histophilus somni,* or chlamydial disease.
• Polyarthritis secondary to septicemia is seen almost exclusively in neonates <1 month of age. Most will have additional diagnoses of clinical signs strongly supportive of septicemia including omphalophlebitis, hypopion, fever, and scleral injection.
• Age of onset will vary among the common causes of polyarthritis. Polyarthritis secondary to septicemia is diagnosed in very young animals. Chlamydial arthritis is most common preweaning. *Mycoplasma* and *Histophilus* polyarthritis are most common in recently weaned calves. Osteochondrosis is most common in cattle between 1 and 2 years of age. Polyarthritis secondary to endocarditis is typically seen in adult cattle.

CBC/BIOCHEMISTRY/URINALYSIS
N/A

OTHER LABORATORY TESTS
• Microbiologic culture procedures or polymerase chain reaction (PCR) assays may be useful in the identification of the offending pathogens. However, it should be noted that negative results are common and should not exclude the possibility of a diagnosis.
• Serologic tests are available for chlamydia and CAEV.

IMAGING
• Radiography is a useful adjunct to the diagnosis of polyarthritis. Osteochondrosis with or without degenerative joint disease and septic physitis can readily be confirmed or ruled out by radiographic examination.
• Acute stages on radiographs will reveal only nonspecific soft tissue swelling and subchondral bone lysis does not appear until 14 days.
• Septic arthritis on radiographs can have narrowing or widening of the joint space, subchondral bone lysis and periarticular bone proliferation.
• Ultrasound is a reliable method for confirming tentative diagnosis (distention of joint pouch).

OTHER DIAGNOSTIC PROCEDURES
• Arthrocentesis and analysis of joint fluid is the single most useful test in most animals with polyarthritis. Cattle with polyarthritis caused by *H. somni* or endocarditis will generally have joint fluid with a profound increase in leukocytes, the predominant cell type being the neutrophil. Synovial fluid with at least 10,000 nucleated cells/µL and >90% neutrophils is indicative of purulent arthritis. Fluid is grossly cloudy with decreased viscosity compared to normal synovial fluid.
• Joint fluid in cattle with *Mycoplasma* spp. infection has a less dramatic increase in cell numbers and the predominant cell type is mononuclear cells.
• Cattle with either osteochondrosis or septic physitis secondary to salmonellosis will generally have near normal joint fluid composition.
• Fibrinous arthritis cannot always be diagnosed by arthrocentesis.
• Elevations in MMPs (gelatinase enzymes in CT involved in cartilage degradation) (MMP-9 = septic; MMP-2 = aseptic).

TREATMENT

THERAPEUTIC APPROACH
• Varies with the specific syndrome and etiology. See specific chapters for details.
• NSAIDs are indicated for pain management.

MEDICATIONS
Varies with the specific syndrome and etiology. See specific chapters for details.

FOLLOW-UP
Varies with the specific syndrome and etiology. See specific chapters for details.

P

POLYARTHRITIS

MISCELLANEOUS

ASSOCIATED CONDITIONS
N/A

AGE-RELATED FACTORS
• Chlamydial arthritis is most common preweaning.
• *Mycoplasma* and *Histophilus* polyarthritis are most common in recently weaned calves.
• Osteochondrosis is most common in cattle between 1 and 2 years of age.
• Polyarthritis secondary to endocarditis is typically seen in adult cattle.
• Polyarthritis secondary to septicemia is seen almost exclusively in neonates <1 month of age.

ZOONOTIC POTENTIAL
Chlamydia spp. and *Salmonella* spp. should be considered zoonotic agents and care should be used in sample collection.

PREGNANCY
Chlamydia spp. and *Salmonella* spp. can cause abortion in herds or flocks.

BIOSECURITY
Recommendations dependent on etiologic agent.

PRODUCTION MANAGEMENT
Recommendations dependent on etiologic agent. When polyarthritis is a result of improper housing conditions, animal husbandry and comfort must be addressed. See chapter, Dairy Cow Comfort (see www.fiveminutevet.com/ruminant), for recommendations.

ABBREVIATIONS
• CAEV = caprine arthritis and encephalitis virus

• CT = connective tissue
• DJD = degenerative joint disease
• MMP = matrix metalloprotease
• NSAIDs = nonsteroidal anti-inflammatory drugs
• OA = osteoarthritis
• PCR = polymerase chain reaction

SEE ALSO
• Bacterial Endocarditis
• Caprine Arthritis Encephalitis Virus
• *Histophilus somni* Complex
• Lameness (by species)
• *Mycoplasma bovis* Associated Diseases
• Neonatal Septic Arthritis
• Nonsteroidal Anti-inflammatory Drugs (NSAIDs) (see www.fiveminutevet.com/ruminant)
• Osteochondrosis
• Pain Management (see www.fiveminutevet.com/ruminant)
• Salmonellosis

Suggested Reading
Arican M, Coughlan AR, Clegg PD, Carter SD. Matrix metalloproteinases 2 and 9 activity in bovine synovial fluids. J Vet Med A 2000, 47: 449–56.

Arthur C, Watt K, Nussey DH, et al. Osteoarthritis of the temporo-mandibular joint in free-living Soay sheep on St. Kilda. Vet J 2015, 203: 120–5.

Dyer N, Hansen-Lardy L, Krogh D, Schaan L, Schamber E. An outbreak of chronic pneumonia and polyarthritis syndrome caused by *Mycoplasma bovis* in feedlot bison (*Bison bison*). J Vet Diagn Invest 2008, 20: 369–71.

Gagea MI, Bateman KG, Shanahan RA, et al. Naturally occurring *Mycoplasma bovis*-associated pneumonia and polyarthritis in feedlot beef calves. J Vet Diagn Invest 2006, 18: 29–40.

Heinola T, Sukura A, Virkki LM, Sillat T, Lekszycki T, Konttinen YT. Osteoarthritic cartilage lesions in the bovine patellar groove: A macroscopic, histological and immunohistological analysis. Vet J 2014, 200: 88–95.

Heppelmann M, Rehage J, Kofler J, Starke A. Ultrasonographic diagnosis of septic arthritis in cattle. Vet J 2009,179: 407–16.

Hill BD, Sutton RH, Thompson H. Investigation of osteochondrosis in grazing beef cattle. Aust Vet J 1998, 76: 171–5.

Hughes KL, Edwards MJ, Hartley WJ, Murphy S. Polyarthritis in calves caused by *Mycoplasma* spp. Vet Rec 1966, 78: 276–81.

Kester E, Holzhauer M, Frankena K. A descriptive review of the prevalence and risk factors of hock lesions in dairy cows. Vet J 2014, 200: 222–8.

Smith BP, Biberstein EL. Septicemia and meningoencephalitis in pastured cattle caused by a *Haemophilus*-like organism (*Haemophilus somnus*). Cornell Vet 1977, 67: 300–5.

Storz J, Shupe JL, Smart RA, Thornley RW. Polyarthritis in calves: isolation of psittacosis agents from affected joints. Am J Vet Res 1966, 27: 633–41.

Van Pelt RW, Langham RF. Nonspecific polyarthritis secondary to primary systemic infection in calves. J Am Vet Med Assoc 1966, 149: 505–11.

Author Francisco C. Rodriguez
Consulting Editor Kaitlyn A. Lutz
Acknowledgment The author and book editors acknowledge the prior contribution of Jeff W. Tyler.

POSTPARTUM DISORDERS

BASICS

OVERVIEW
• Postpartum disorders are common production diseases which often stem from a problem during the transition period (21 days before expected parturition to 21 days postpartum).
• These disorders may be exacerbated by calving conditions. Calving accidents are a separate entity that is not discussed here.
• The most important postpartum disorders are hypocalcemia, retained fetal membranes (RFM), metritis, displacement of abomasums (DA), ketosis, fatty liver, and udder edema.
• Other conditions such as lameness and mastitis are also related to the transition period but they may occur at any time during the production cycle.
• In beef cattle, prepartum nutrition and trace mineral supplementation affect colostrum quality and calf survival.

INCIDENCE/PREVALENCE
• Incidence of postpartum disorders is extremely variable and depends on factors such as season, geographic location, breed, type of housing and environment, management, herd, etc.
• Dairy cattle are more at risk than beef cattle.
• Reported incidence of various disorders in dairy cattle is
  ◦ Clinical hypocalcemia: 0.2–2%
  ◦ Retained fetal membranes: 8–14%
  ◦ Metritis: 6–12%
  ◦ Clinical ketosis: 2–6%
  ◦ Subclinical ketosis: 10–20%
  ◦ Displacement of abomasum: 0.5–6%.

GEOGRAPHIC DISTRIBUTION
Worldwide

SYSTEMS AFFECTED
• Reproductive
• Musculoskeletal
• Digestive
• Mammary
• Multisystemic

PATHOPHYSIOLOGY
• The transition period is a very dynamic stage. The fetus grows exponentially and cows start to decrease dry matter intake (DMI), especially during the last week of gestation. As a response, cows start to mobilize fat from adipose tissue. The result is an increase of nonesterified fatty acids (NEFA) in blood, especially in obese cows, which may develop fatty liver.
• Parturition is a stressful process involving metabolic and hormonal changes that contribute to immunosuppression and decrease of host resistance to diseases.
• Mammary gland removes high amounts of calcium from blood; therefore, there is a more intense negative calcium balance with development of hypocalcemia.

• If calving is complicated, hypocalcemia worsens, affecting uterine and gastrointestinal motility. This in turns contributes to increased risks for RFM with consequent metritis and displaced abomasum.
• When lactation advances, energy requirements increase dramatically and DMI recovers slowly. This causes a typical negative energy balance during the first weeks of lactation. In addition, mammary gland extracts large amounts of glucose from blood for lactose synthesis. Therefore, hypoglycemia may develop and ketosis may be established. In addition, a transient stage of insulin resistance may occur during the early postpartum period to promote glucose uptake by the mammary gland (insulin independent organ) and to block glucose uptake by other tissues. This stage of insulin resistance makes NEFA release more abundant, with a progressive likelihood of hepatic lipidosis. Finally, the catabolic stage of fat depots increases immunosuppression because adipocytes are very proactive inflammatory cells producing several cytokines and immunomodulatory responses, negatively affecting white blood cells.

HISTORICAL FINDINGS
• Herd with high rate of RFM, poor production, and increased rate of metabolic disorders
• Individual cows: Dystocia, twinning

SIGNALMENT
• Periparturient dairy cows
• Breed predisposition for some postpartum disorders (Jersey, hypocalcemia)

PHYSICAL EXAMINATION FINDINGS
• Clinical signs of postpartum disorders vary but can be monitored on farm by daily rectal temperature and demeanor and appetite of the cow. Infectious processes are often accompanied by fever, depression, increased heart and respiratory rate, and dehydration. Severe disorders may lead to a down cow syndrome.
• Retained fetal membranes: Visible membranes 24 hours postpartum.
• Metritis: Fever, foul-smelling discharge.
• Hypocalcemia: Musculoskeletal compromise.
• Ketosis: Decrease in milk yield, high ketones in blood, urine or milk.
• Displacement of abomasum (high-pitched "ping" sound at auscultation on left flank, last two rib spaces).

GENETICS
Some calving-related disorders have a hereditary component (ketosis and somatic cell count).

CAUSES AND RISK FACTORS
• Inadequate management of the prepartum, calving, and postpartum period. Improper nutrition, poor environment, and lack of cow comfort.

• Breed, genetic potential, season, herd size, geographic location, parity, and facilities.

DIAGNOSIS

DIFFERENTIAL DIAGNOSES
• Diagnosis of the specific condition is based on thorough physical examination of the animal.
• On herd basis, record analysis shows increased incidence of several postpartum disorders which are associated one to another.

CBC/BIOCHEMISTRY/URINALYSIS
• Ketosis (ketones in urine, blood, or milk)
• Hypocalcemia (plasma)
• Fatty liver (plasma NEFA or liver biopsy).

OTHER LABORATORY TESTS
Liver biopsy

IMAGING
N/A

OTHER DIAGNOSTIC PROCEDURES
N/A

PATHOLOGIC FINDINGS
N/A

TREATMENT

THERAPEUTIC APPROACH
Individual animals require appropriate therapy for the specific disorders. This may include antimicrobials, anti-inflammatory drugs, and fluid therapy to correct dehydration and electrolyte imbalances. Hypocalcemia should be addressed immediately.

SURGICAL CONSIDERATIONS AND TECHNIQUES
Surgical correction of DA

MEDICATIONS

DRUGS OF CHOICE
• Drugs should be selected based on the specific diagnosis.
• Broad-spectrum antibiotic therapy.
• NSAIDs.
• Corticosteroid in cases of endotoxemia.
• Fluids: Oral fluids are sufficient in mild cases, IV fluids are important in severe clinical cases. Hypertonic fluid for severely dehydrated animals.
• Feed additives to improve energy and mineral balance such as propylene glycol, niacin, protected choline, calcium propionate, glycerol, vitamin E, selenium, yeasts, and probiotics.

P

POSTPARTUM DISORDERS   (CONTINUED)

CONTRAINDICATIONS
PRECAUTIONS
Appropriate milk and meat withdrawal times must be followed for all compounds administered to food-producing animals.

POSSIBLE INTERACTIONS
N/A

 FOLLOW-UP

EXPECTED COURSE AND PROGNOSIS
• Most cases can be treated successfully if diagnosed early. However, there will be an effect on reproductive and production performance and increased risk for culling.
• Down cows present a peculiar challenge in its management. Welfare issues should be considered and humane euthanasia is required in severe cases.

POSSIBLE COMPLICATIONS
Postpartum disorders are often associated and it is not uncommon to see cows developing a succession of problems during the same lactation.

CLIENT EDUCATION
• Importance of transition cow management (proper nutrition, calving management).
• Train calving team to recognize dystocia and properly manage it.
• Importance of postpartum monitoring program.
• Importance of cow comfort and welfare issues.

PATIENT CARE
• Monitor response to treatment: Rectal temperature, appetite, manure quality.
• Provide a comfortable area.
• Transfaunation may be necessary in some cases.

PREVENTION
• Proper general and nutritional management.
• Monitoring of body condition score during dry period. Cows should not lose condition or gain excessive weight during the transition period.

• Urine pH should be monitored to evaluate anionic salts during prepartum period for the prevention of hypocalcemia. Urine pH should be between 6.0 and 7.0.
• Proper transition diet. Moderate energy (not more than 16 Mcal/day NE for lactation) and protein levels (not more than 1,200 g/day of metabolizable protein). Prepartum diet with a negative cation-anion difference between −25 and 75 mEq/kg DM. Fiber in sufficient quantity and of appropriate particle size.
• Prepare cows for calving ease.

 MISCELLANEOUS

ASSOCIATED CONDITIONS
• Calving-related disorders are intimately related to each other. Cows with hypocalcemia are more likely to develop RFM. Cows with RFM are more likely to develop metritis. Cows with metritis are more likely to develop ketosis, and cows with ketosis are more likely to develop displacement of abomasum.
• Delayed resumption of ovarian activity in beef cattle.

AGE-RELATED FACTORS
Older cows are more likely to develop clinical hypocalcemia, ketosis, and displacement of abomasum.

ZOONOTIC POTENTIAL
N/A

PREGNANCY
Prepartum management is critical for prevention of calving-related disorders. Enough feed bunk space, adequate shade, and comfortable environment are essential for prepartum dairy cows.

BIOSECURITY
N/A

PRODUCTION MANAGEMENT
• Nutrition and feeding management
• Housing management

SYNONYM
Periparturient disorders

ABBREVIATIONS
• DA = displaced abomasum
• DMI = dry matter intake
• NE = net energy
• NEFA = nonesterified fatty acids
• RFM = retained fetal membranes

SEE ALSO
• Displaced Abomasum
• Down Bovine
• Fatty Liver
• Hypocalcemia: Bovine
• Ketosis: Dairy Cattle
• Metritis
• Nutrition and Metabolic Diseases: Beef
• Nutritional and Metabolic Diseases: Dairy
• Postparturient Paresis (Hypocalcemia
• Retained Placenta

Suggested Reading

Mass J. Diagnostic considerations for evaluating nutritional problems in cattle. Vet Clin North Am Food Anim Pract 2007, 23: 527–39.

Melendez P, Risco CA. Management of transition cows to optimize reproductive efficiency in dairy herds. Vet Clin North Am Food Anim Pract 2005, 21: 485–501.

National Research Council. Nutrient Requirements of Dairy Cattle, 7th ed. Washington, DC: National Academy Press, 2001.

Risco CA, Melendez P. Periparturient disorders. In: Fuquay JW, Fox PF, McSweeney PLH eds, Encyclopedia of Dairy Sciences, 2nd ed. Amsterdam, Elsevier, 2011, pp. 514–19.

Risco C, Melendez P eds. Dairy Production Medicine, 1st ed. Ames, Wiley-Blackwell, 2011.

Author Pedro Melendez
Consulting Editor Ahmed Tibary

P

POSTPARTURIENT HEMOGLOBINURIA

BASICS

OVERVIEW
• This uncommon and sporadic condition causes intravascular hemolysis in cattle shortly after parturition, resulting in anemia and hemoglobinuria.

INCIDENCE/PREVALENCE
Although the condition is sporadic and the incidence is low, the mortality rate is high.

GEOGRAPHIC DISTRIBUTION
• Cases have been reported worldwide.
• In the United States, disease is more common in the winter months in northern states.

SYSTEMS AFFECTED
• Hemolymphatic
• Cardiovascular
• Urinary

PATHOPHYSIOLOGY
• The exact etiology of this disease is not entirely known; however, inadequate dietary phosphorus leading to hypophosphatemia is often detected in affected cows. Although hypophosphatemia is associated with postparturient hemoglobinuria, most cattle with hypophosphatemia do not experience intravascular hemolysis, suggesting that there are other causative aspects of the disease.
• Hypophosphatemia alters erythrocyte metabolism and membrane permeability, thus rendering the cells more susceptible to intravascular hemolysis.
• Hypocupremia may also be a predisposing factor. Hypocupremia predisposes erythrocytes to oxidative damage and Heinz body formation, also leading to fragility of the red blood cell membrane and intravascular hemolysis.

HISTORICAL FINDINGS
Recent calving, progressive depression, weakness and lethargy, anorexia, decreased milk production, red to brown discolored urine.

SIGNALMENT
• Cattle, most common in dairy breeds
• Multiparous cows within the first month of calving

PHYSICAL EXAMINATION FINDINGS
• The clinical signs depend on the severity and rate at which hemolysis occurs.
• Weakness and recumbency are expected as the condition progresses. In severe cases, signs of hypovolemic shock may be present, including tachycardia, tachypnea, pallor of the mucus membranes, lack of episcleral vessels, and cool extremities.
• A low-grade fever may be present. A grade I to III/VI systolic murmur may be audible over the heart base as blood viscosity decreases with advancing anemia.

• When the plasma hemoglobin concentration exceeds the renal threshold, hemoglobinuria will occur. Within 1–2 days, icterus of the mucus membranes and sclera will develop.

GENETICS
High-producing dairy cattle appear to be most susceptible.

CAUSES AND RISK FACTORS
• Low dietary phosphorus.
• Low dietary copper.
• Parturition.
• Ingestion of alfalfa hay or sugar beet that may contain saponins.
• Copper deficiency.
• High-producing multiparous dairy cow consuming diets low in phosphorus are at greatest risk of disease.
• Drought conditions, grazing phosphorus-deficient soil, prolonged housing, and exposure to extremely cold weather may also predispose to the disease.
• Consumption of rape, turnips, or other cruciferous plants, and large amounts of beet pulp or cold water are associated with the disease. In New Zealand, low blood and liver copper levels and grazing copper-deficient pastures are additional risk factors.

DIAGNOSIS

DIFFERENTIAL DIAGNOSES
Any cause of intravascular hemolysis in the cow would cause similar signs: babesiosis, bacillary hemoglobinuria, leptospirosis, onion, rape, or kale plant toxicity, copper toxicity, and autoimmune hemolytic anemia.

CBC/BIOCHEMISTRY/URINALYSIS
• Anemia
• Regenerative anemia 5–7 days after onset (signs of regeneration include an increased MCV, anisocytosis, polychromasia, basophilic stippling, reticulocytes)
• Hemoglobinemia (pink plasma, MCV, and MCHC increased)
• Hemoglobinuria
• Hyperbilirubinemia (unconjugated)
• Azotemia
• Acidosis
• Ketonuria

OTHER LABORATORY TESTS
• Decreased serum phosphorus concentrations are evident.
• In New Zealand cases, decreased blood copper concentration and Heinz bodies in erythrocytes have been noted.

IMAGING
N/A

OTHER DIAGNOSTIC PROCEDURES
N/A

PATHOLOGIC FINDINGS
Hemoglobinuria and widespread icterus

TREATMENT

THERAPEUTIC APPROACH
• Emergency inpatient or outpatient care.
• Intravenous fluid therapy with polyionic isotonic fluids is indicated.
• When anemia is severe and clinical or laboratory evidence of hypoxemia is evident (intense lethargy or weakness, profound tachycardia or tachypnea, severe anemia, acidosis, increased anion gap), a whole blood transfusion is indicated.
• The normal total blood volume is approximately 8% of the body weight (i.e., 0.08 × body weight in kilograms equals the total blood volume in liters). Typically, transfusing 1/4 to 1/3 of the total blood volume is adequate.

SURGICAL CONSIDERATIONS
N/A

MEDICATIONS

DRUGS OF CHOICE
• The current recommendation for intravenous treatment for hypophosphatemic cattle is the administration of either 30 g of anhydrous NaH_2PO_4 dissolved in 300 mL of sterile deionized water or 36 g of anhydrous Na_2HPO_4 (or 90 g of $Na_2HPO_4.12\ H_2O$) dissolved in 500 mL of sterile deionized water and administered as slow intravenous infusion. Because products approved for the use in cattle are frequently not available, this treatment would have to be administered in an extra-label manner.
• Human enema formulations that contain a mixture of monobasic sodium phosphate monohydrate and dibasic sodium phosphate heptahydrate in a buffered solution also have been administered to hypophosphatemic cattle orally (preferred) or intravenously but must be diluted with at least 4 mL of water for every 1 mL of enema solution if given intravenously.
• In experimentally phosphorus-depleted lactating Holstein-Friesian cows, 302 g NaH_2PO_4 dihydrate dissolved in 1.5 L warm water (38°C) and 263 g KH_2PO_4 dissolved in 1.5 L warm water administered by orogastric tube were equally effective in raising serum phosphorus concentration within 90 minutes and sustained for at least 24 hours.

CONTRAINDICATIONS
Appropriate milk and meat withdrawal times must be followed for all compounds administered to food-producing animals.

PRECAUTIONS
Avoid concurrent use of potentially nephrotoxic drugs.

P

POSTPARTURIENT HEMOGLOBINURIA   (CONTINUED)

POSSIBLE INTERACTIONS
N/A

 FOLLOW-UP

EXPECTED COURSE AND PROGNOSIS
• The prognosis is guarded to poor, even with appropriate treatment.
• The clinical course is acute, progressing to recumbency in 3–5 days. In severe cases, death can occur within hours.
• Surviving cows may need a 4-week period of convalescence.

POSSIBLE COMPLICATIONS
• Renal disease from hemoglobinuria
• Ketosis
• Death from hypoxemia

PATIENT CARE
• Monitor heart rate, respiratory rate, attitude, appetite, PCV, serum phosphorus and copper concentrations, creatinine.
• Keep confined.
• Increase dietary phosphorus intake.

CLIENT EDUCATION
Increase dietary phosphorus intake in unaffected herd mates.

PREVENTION
Ensure adequate dietary phosphorus and copper intake in the early postpartum period.

 MISCELLANEOUS

ASSOCIATED CONDITIONS
Ingestion of feeds that contain saponins may predispose to hemolysis.

AGE-RELATED FACTORS
Multiparous cows within the first month of calving

ZOONOTIC POTENTIAL
N/A

PREGNANCY
N/A

BIOSECURITY
N/A

PRODUCTION MANAGEMENT
• The dietary phosphorus and copper intake of the herd should be evaluated.
• Drought conditions, grazing phosphorus-deficient soil, prolonged housing, and exposure to extremely cold weather may also predispose to the disease.
• Consumption of rape, turnips, or other cruciferous plants, and large amounts of beet pulp or cold water are associated with the disease.

SYNONYMS
N/A

ABBREVIATIONS
• MCHC = mean corpuscular hemoglobin concentration
• MCV = mean corpuscular volume
• PCV = packed cell volume

SEE ALSO
• Anemia, Regenerative
• Babesiosis
• Copper Deficiency and Toxicity
• Leptospirosis
• Phosphorus Deficiency/Excess

Suggested Reading
Carlson GP. Postparturient hemoglobinuria. In Smith BP ed, Large Animal Internal Medicine, 5th edition. St. Louis: Elsevier Mosby, 2015, p. 1064.
Idink MJ, Grünberg W. Enteral administration of monosodium phosphate, monopotassium phosphate and monocalcium phosphate for the treatment of hypophosphatacmia in lactating dairy cattle. Vet Rec 2015, 176: 494. doi:10.1136/vr.102847
Grünberg W. Treatment of phosphorous balance disorders. Vet Clin North Am Food Anim Pract 2014, 30: 383–408.
Singh R, Rana YS, Beniwal BS, Tehlan M. Osmotic fragility of buffalo red blood cells in post-parturient haemoglobinuria. Haryana Vet 2007, 46: 96–8.
Cheng YH, Goff JP, Horst RL. Restoring normal blood phosphorus concentrations in hypophosphatemic cattle with sodium phosphate. Vet Med 1998, 93: 383–8.
MacWilliams PS, Searcy GP, Bellamy JEC. Bovine postparturient hemoglobinuria: a review of the literature. Can Vet J 1982, 23: 311–14.

Author Michelle Henry Barton
Consulting Editor Ahmed Tibary

P

POSTPARTURIENT PARESIS (HYPOCALCEMIA)

BASICS

OVERVIEW
• Increased calcium (Ca) demand with a delay in adaptation of Ca metabolism in dairy cows within the first 72 h postpartum leads to hypocalcemia.
• Hypocalcemia ultimately results in flaccid paralysis and inability to rise.
• The disorder is most easily prevented by altering dietary cation-anion difference (DCAD), which is the balance between absorbable cations and anions in the dry cow ration.

INCIDENCE/PREVALENCE
• Clinical disease in 5–6% of all dairy cows
• Up to 50% of older periparturient dairy cows have subclinical hypocalcemia
• Rare in first-calf heifers

GEOGRAPHIC DISTRIBUTION
Worldwide depending on production factors

SYSTEMS AFFECTED
• Musculoskeletal
• Nervous

PATHOPHYSIOLOGY
• Parathyroid hormone (PTH) controls plasma concentrations and urinary excretion of Ca and phosphorus (to a lesser extent, magnesium)
• PTH is released primarily in response to decreases in serum ionized Ca, and promotes mobilization of Ca from bone, resorption of Ca and magnesium in the renal tubules, and increases urinary phosphorus excretion.
• PTH also stimulates renal production of active 1,25 dihydroxyvitamin D_3, which stimulates active absorption of Ca from the GI tract.
• Rations with a higher ratio of cations (K^+, Na^+, Ca^{2+}, and Mg^{2+}) to anions (Cl^-, SO_4^{2-}, PO_4^{3-}) induce nutritional metabolic alkalosis, creating pseudohypoparathyroidism:
  ○ Altered conformation of the PTH receptor reduces sensitivity of tissue receptors to PTH
  ○ Subsequently there is reduced release of Ca from bone and reduced absorption of Ca in the GI tract
• Hypocalcemia impairs muscular contraction by delaying release of acetylcholine at neuromuscular junctions, causing flaccid paralysis.
• Hypomagnesemia prevents production and secretion of PTH and 1,25-dihydroxyvitamin D_3.

HISTORICAL FINDINGS
Recent parturition in mature cows receiving diets with inappropriate DCAD

SIGNALMENT
Female cows of Channel Island and Swedish Red breeds are predisposed, in their third or later lactation.

PHYSICAL EXAMINATION FINDINGS
○ *Stage I*
  ■ Early signs are subtle and transient; animals appear excitable, nervous, or weak without recumbency.
  ■ Shifting weight frequently, shuffling hind feet, may have fine tremors.
○ *Stage II*
  ■ Sternal recumbency, with low body temperature and poor anal tone
  ■ Tachycardia and decreased intensity of cardiac sounds
  ■ Moderate to severe depression and partial paralysis
  ■ S-shaped curve to the neck
○ *Stage III*
  ■ Lateral recumbency, paralysis and bloat
  ■ Severely depressed (coma)
  ■ Tachycardia and weak peripheral pulses

GENETICS
N/A

CAUSES AND RISK FACTORS
• High producing dairy cows in third or later lactation
• Inappropriate DCAD
• Increased dietary phosphorus (blocks renal production of 1,25 dihydroxyvitamin D_3)

DIAGNOSIS

DIFFERENTIAL DIAGNOSES
• Grass tetany
• Traumatic reticuloperitonitis
• Coxofemoral luxation
• Obturator paralysis
• Lymphosarcoma
• Musculoskeletal or spinal trauma
• Toxemia (mastitis, metritis, pneumonia)

CBC/BIOCHEMISTRY/URINALYSIS
• Serum Ca^{2+} declines from 8.5–10 mg/dL to <7.5 mg/dL (see Table 1).
• Hypophosphatemia, hypo- or hypermagnesemia, and hyperglycemia.
• Neutrophilia, lymphopenia, and eosinopenia with moderately increased serum

Table 1

Serum Concentrations (mg/dL) of Ca^{2+}, P, and Mg^{2+} in Cows in Different Stages of Postparturient Paresis		
	Calcium	*Phosphorus*	*Magnesium*
Stage 1	6.2 ± 1.3	2.4 ± 1.4	3.2 ± 0.7
Stage 2	5.5 ± 1.3	1.8 ± 1.2	3.1 ± 0.8
Stage 3	4.6 ± 1.1	1.6 ± 1.0	3.3 ± 0.8

*Adapted from Church DC, The Ruminant Animal. Prospect Heights, IL: Waveland Press, 1993, table 24.1, p. 494.

creatine kinase activity (CK) related to recumbency.

OTHER LABORATORY TESTS
Serum or urine ketone measurement

IMAGING
Applicable to animals with suspected musculoskeletal or spinal trauma

OTHER DIAGNOSTIC PROCEDURES
Ration analysis to determine DCAD

PATHOLOGIC FINDINGS
No gross findings; or evidence of intercurrent diseases (metritis, retained membranes, pneumonia) may be present.

TREATMENT

THERAPEUTIC APPROACH
• Cows with clinical signs require prompt recognition and treatment with Ca to prevent progression and death.
  ○ Oral Ca supplementation may be adequate in mild cases and reduces risk of cardiotoxicity.
  ○ Achieving a 4 g rise of calcium in the blood requires oral administration of ~50 g of soluble Ca (Ca chloride or Ca propionate ± propylene glycol).
• Relapses are common (25–30% of cows that initially respond) and may require additional therapy within 24–48 hours.
• Intercurrent diseases should be identified and treated.

SURGICAL CONSIDERATIONS AND TECHNIQUES
N/A

MEDICATIONS

DRUGS OF CHOICE
• Calcium gluconate
  ○ Can be administered via subcutaneous and intraperitoneal routes, but is most effective IV
  ○ IV solutions supply 8.5–11.5 g Ca/500 mL; effective IV Ca doses are about 2 g Ca/100 kg BW and may elevate blood Ca above normal for about 4 h.
  ○ Solutions should be administered over 10–20 min (~1 gram Ca/min) with concurrent auscultation for dysrhythmias.
  ○ Cows relapsing or failing to respond can be treated again at 8–12 h.
  ○ Cardioexcitatory consequences of IV Ca can be reduced by administration of magnesium.
• 1α-hydroxycholecalciferol is a synthetic analog of vitamin D_3, which can be given to cattle not responding to IV Ca (~15% cases). Administer at 1 μg/kg BW, half IV and half IM.

P

POSTPARTURIENT PARESIS (HYPOCALCEMIA) (CONTINUED)

CONTRAINDICATIONS
• Do not give Ca solutions containing formaldehyde or with >25 g dextrose/500 mL SC, and do not give >1–1.5 g Ca (~50–75 mL) at a single SC site.
• Do not use SC route as sole therapy in case of poor peripheral perfusion.

PRECAUTIONS
• Calcium-containing solutions are cardiotoxic and can cause death if given rapidly IV.
• Large doses of oral Ca (250 g soluble Ca) can also cause death.
• Calcium chloride is caustic to oral and pharyngeal mucosa and should not be given repeatedly.
• Cows with stupor and recumbency should not be medicated orally, to avoid aspiration.
• Appropriate milk and meat withdrawal times must be followed for all compounds administered to food-producing animals.

POSSIBLE INTERACTIONS
N/A

 FOLLOW-UP

EXPECTED COURSE AND PROGNOSIS
• Typically cows with hypocalcemia show rapid improvement and 75% should be standing within 2 hours.
• Severe hypocalcemia or intercurrent disease creates a poorer prognosis, especially with delayed treatment, and these animals can die within hours.

POSSIBLE COMPLICATIONS
• Low palatability of anionic salts and overacidification may reduce DM intake.
• Dystocia, uterine prolapse, retained fetal membranes, metritis, abomasal displacement, mastitis, and rhabdomyolysis may occur in cattle with hypocalcemia.

CLIENT EDUCATION
Focus on preventive measures; this is largely a disease of management.

PATIENT CARE
See "Precautions"

PREVENTION
• Reduce the content of potassium in prepartum diets.
• Formulate dry cow ration with a DCAD of –10 to –15 mEq/100 g DM; DCAD can be calculated as $(Na^+ + K^+) - (Cl^- + S^{2-})$.

• DCAD diet should be commenced no further out than 3 weeks from calving, and at least 4–5 days before.
• Measure urine pH during the last week of gestation by collecting midstream samples 6–9 h postprandially:
  ◦ Ideal value for Holstein cows is pH 6.2–6.8 for Jersey cows 5.8–6.3
  ◦ Urine pH of 5.0–5.5 suggests excessive anion supplementation which will reduce DM intake.
• Synthetic bovine PTH given IV 60 h before calving, or IM 6 days before calving.
• Supplement dry cow diet with 20,000–30,000 IU vitamin D/day.
• Minerals in prepartum diet (% DM) should be as follows:
  ◦ Na^+: 0.12%
  ◦ K^+: 1.0%
  ◦ Cl^-: 0.5% less than K^+ in the diet
  ◦ Ca^{2+}: 0.85–1.0%
  ◦ Mg^{2+}: 0.35–0.4%
  ◦ P: 0.35–0.4%
  ◦ S: >0.22% to ensure adequate substrate for rumen microbial amino acid synthesis but no more than 0.4% to prevent sulfur toxicity.
• Prophylactic use of vitamin D preparations or analogs is not ideal but has been used in high-risk cases; performed by feeding or injecting large doses 1–2 weeks prepartum, with the risk of renal damage and metastatic calcification.

 MISCELLANEOUS

ASSOCIATED CONDITIONS
• Dystocia, retained placenta, ketosis, left displaced abomasum, mastitis, and metritis.
• Rhabdomyolysis (crush syndrome): weight of a down cow can cause ischemic damage to muscles and nerves in as little as 4 h.

AGE-RELATED FACTORS
Incidence increases with age due to higher milk output and reduced number of vitamin D receptors in the intestine.

ZOONOTIC POTENTIAL
N/A

PREGNANCY
This is a disease established in late pregnancy and occurring soon after parturition; colostrum has 8–10 times the amount of Ca^{2+} as milk.

BIOSECURITY
N/A

PRODUCTION MANAGEMENT
See "Prevention"

SYNONYMS
• Hypocalcemia
• Milk fever

ABBREVIATIONS
• CK = creatine kinase
• DCAD = dietary cation anion difference
• DM = dry matter
• IM = intramuscular
• IV = intravenous
• PTH = parathyroid hormone
• SC = subcutaneous

SEE ALSO
• Dairy Nutrition: Ration Guidelines for Milking and Dry Cows (see www.fiveminutevet.com/ruminant)

Suggested Reading
Goff JP. Calcium and magnesium disorders. Vet Clin North Am Food Anim Pract 2014, 30: 359–81.
Goff JP. The monitoring, prevention, and treatment of milk fever and subclinical hypocalcemia in dairy cows. Vet J 2008, 176: 50–7.
Goff JP, Liesegang A, Horst RL. Diet-induced pseudohypoparathyroidism: A hypocalcemia and milk fever risk. J Dairy Sci 2014, 97: 1520–8.
Goff JP, Ruiz R, Horst RL. Relative acidifying activity of anionic salts commonly used to prevent milk fever. J Dairy Sci 2004, 87: 1245–55.
Lean IJ, DeGaris PJ, McNeil DM, Block E. Hypocalcemia in dairy cows: meta-analysis and dietary cation anion difference theory revisited. J Dairy Sci 2006, 89: 669–84.
Martin-Tereso J, Martens H. Calcium and magnesium physiology and nutrition in relation to the prevention of milk fever and tetany (dietary management of macrominerals in preventing disease). Vet Clin North Am Food Anim Pract 2014, 30: 643–70.
Author Douglas C. Donovan
Consulting Editor Erica C. McKenzie

P

BASICS

OVERVIEW
• The mammary gland increases in size during puberty in the female due to growth of connective tissue and fat deposition.
• Significant increase in size of mammary gland is observed during late pregnancy.
• A precocious udder is a mammary gland that is more developed than usual at a given age or stage of lactation. It is also called inappropriate lactation or galactorrhea.
• Gynecomastia, enlargement of male mammary tissue, in male goats can occur (e.g., Alpine and Saanen breeds) especially during the summer months.

INCIDENCE/PREVALENCE
Sporadic

GEOGRAPHIC DISTRIBUTION
N/A

SYSTEMS AFFECTED
• Reproductive
• Mammary
• Integument

PATHOPHYSIOLOGY
• Estrous periods stimulate the development of secretory and duct tissues. Growth of lactation tissue is dependent on two hormones: Estrogen from developing follicles and progesterone from the CL.
• Cyclic secretion of estrogen stimulates duct development of the mammary gland.
• Progesterone secretion is cyclic in nonpregnant animals, and nearly continuous in pregnant animals, and causes secretory tissue development.
• Milk secretion is activated by withdrawal of progesterone and increase in cortisol and prolactin at parturition.
• Precocious udder development is associated with many risk factors (see "Causes and Risk Factors") that affect the normal secretion of estrogen, progesterone, or prolactin.

HISTORICAL FINDINGS
• Early development of the mammary gland in the absence of pregnancy is the most common sign of precocious udder.
• Goat kids may be born with significant udders containing milk (witch's milk).

SIGNALMENT
• Precocious udders are most commonly seen in young milking breeds of goats such as the Saanen, Alpine, Toggenburg, LaMancha, and Nubian.
• Young kids may develop precocious udders more frequently during springtime.
• In adult bucks (Saanen and crossbreed) gynecomastia and galactorrhea has been reported unilateral or bilateral, not associated with other sexual organ abnormality, producing almost normal milk, and high testosterone but no changes in estrogen or prolactin.
• It has also been described in cattle and sheep much less commonly.

PHYSICAL EXAMINATION FINDINGS
Enlarged mammary gland with no signs of pregnancy or mastitis.

CAUSES AND RISK FACTORS
• Prolonged progesterone production of false pregnancy
• Estrogen, prolactin, GH, and IGF seem to be involved
• Exposure to high levels of estrogen
• Artificial lactation-induction programs
• Spring season (increased levels of prolactin)
• High estrogen levels in feed (e.g., clover, moldy corn)
• Suckling by herd mates (usually affects a single gland)
• Adrenal adenomas (producing estradiol)
• Ovarian neoplasms

DIAGNOSIS

DIFFERENTIAL DIAGNOSES
• Mastitis
• Intersex
• Neoplasia
• Fatty udder due to overconditioning

CBC/CHEMISTRY/URINALYSIS
N/A

OTHER LABORATORY TESTS
N/A

IMAGING
Imaging (ultrasound) may be useful to rule out neoplasia.

OTHER DIAGNOSTIC PROCEDURES
• The udder should be symmetric, firm to soft tissue consistency, and free of irregular lumps.
• Rule out mastitis by evaluating any secretions that are present for signs of inflammation.
• If abnormalities are found on palpation, especially in older lactation animals, imaging or biopsy of the mass is warranted to rule out neoplasia.

PATHOLOGIC FINDINGS
N/A

TREATMENT

THERAPEUTIC APPROACH
• No treatment is an accepted option since it may stop spontaneously.
• Once mastitis is ruled out, separate the animal from others, especially from young stock that may try to nurse.
• Hydrotherapy.
• If the milk production is persistent, the teats leak, or the animal is very uncomfortable and/or painful, it might be necessary to initiate milking. It should be noted that if milking is instituted, an increased risk of mastitis can be seen.
• The effect of milking on the lifetime production of the animal has not been documented.
• Infusion of iodine, chlorhexidine, and hypertonic solution has been mentioned but not tested. Refer to information in cattle where using these protocols to cause cessation of lactation is commonplace. Be aware that these procedures are not without risk as they cause significant acute inflammation in the mammary gland.
• Feeding management to dry off the animal (e.g., increase the level of poor-quality hay in the diet and eliminate grain).
• With gynecomastia in male goats, reduce energy and protein intake levels during spring and summer months.

SURGICAL CONSIDERATIONS AND TECHNIQUES
• In pet goats with large udders, amputation may be necessary.
• Although not tested, an ovariectomy may prevent this problem in pet goats.

MEDICATIONS

DRUGS OF CHOICE
• PGF2$_\alpha$ (5 mg IM has been utilized with persistent CL).
• NSAIDs if painful (flunixin meglumine 1–2 mg/kg IV).
• Diuretics and steroid treatment may be helpful (furosemide 2–10 mg/kg IM, dexamethasone (0.1–1.0 mg/kg IM).

CONTRAINDICATIONS
N/A

PRECAUTIONS
Appropriate milk and meat withdrawal times must be followed for all compounds administered to food-producing animals.

POSSIBLE INTERACTIONS
N/A

FOLLOW-UP
N/A

MISCELLANEOUS

ASSOCIATED CONDITIONS
Mastitis may be a sequela.

SYNONYMS
Galactorrhea

P

PRECOCIOUS UDDER

ABBREVIATIONS
- CL = corpus luteum
- GH = growth hormone
- IGF = insulin growth factor
- IM = intramuscular
- IV = intravenous
- NSAIDs = nonsteroidal anti-inflammatory drugs
- $PGF2_\alpha$ = prostaglandin $F2_\alpha$

SEE ALSO
Mastitis: Small Ruminant

Suggested Reading
Ambrose DJ, Emmanuel DGV. Precocious mammary development in an 8-month-old Holstein heifer. Can Vet J 2008, 49: 803–5.

Bchini O, Andres AC, Schubaur B, et al. Precocious mammary gland development and milk protein synthesis in transgenic mice ubiquitously expressing human growth hormone. Endocrinology 1991, 128: 539–46.

Dwyer CM. Behavioural development in the neonatal lamb: effect of maternal and birth-related factors. Theriogenology 2003, 59: 1027–50.

Haenlein GFW, Caccese R. The Goat Handbook. 1992. Available at: http://www.inform.umd.edu/EdRes/Topic/AgrEnv/ndd/goat/

Pilo C, Cannas EA, Coghe F, Dore S, Liciardi MA. Gynaecomastia and galactorrhea in goat buck: report in two subjects raised in the countryside of Sassari. Large Anim Rev 2011, 17: 23–6.

Author Julián A. Bartolomé
Consulting Editor Kaitlyn A. Lutz
Acknowledgment The author and book editors acknowledge the prior contribution of Angela M. Daniels.

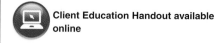

Client Education Handout available online

PREGNANCY DIAGNOSIS: BOVINE

BASICS

OVERVIEW
• Accurate early diagnosis of pregnancy in cattle is essential for optimization of reproductive performance, particularly in dairy cattle.
• The producer's primary economic incentive for pregnancy diagnosis is to accurately identify cattle that are not pregnant so they may be inseminated again as quickly as possible.
• Direct methods are based on clinical or laboratory findings that are only present during pregnancy. They are often more invasive and require slightly more time after breeding before they are effective. The overall accuracy of these methods tends to be very high.
• Indirect methods for pregnancy diagnosis are based on clinical or laboratory techniques to detect open cows. They are generally less invasive and are often applicable earlier in gestation. They tend to have a high negative predictive value but a low positive predictive value.

INCIDENCE/PREVALENCE
Common

GEOGRAPHIC DISTRIBUTION
Worldwide

PATHOPHYSIOLOGY
N/A

SYSTEMS AFFECTED
Reproductive

HISTORICAL FINDINGS
• Non-return to estrus after artificial insemination or natural mating dates
• Anestrus

SIGNALMENT
Bovine postpubertal female

PHYSICAL EXAMINATION FINDINGS
• See "Diagnosis"

GENETICS
• Age at puberty
• Conception rate (sire/daughter) and calving ease

CAUSES AND RISK FACTORS
• Pregnancy diagnosis is a routine activity in herd management.
• Indicated if there is suspicion of accidental breeding in young stock.

DIAGNOSIS

General Recommendations for Pregnancy Diagnosis
• Early pregnancy diagnosis techniques should focus on accurate identification of nonpregnant cows. In dairy cattle, pregnancy diagnosis should be scheduled no later than 35 days post-breeding.
• The appropriate diagnostic technique to be used in a herd will depend on several factors (heat detection efficiency, method of breeding, cost of labor, cost of the technique, pregnancy rate, size of the herd, etc.). An efficient system should be designed in collaboration between the attending veterinarian and the herd manager.
• Regardless of the method used for pregnancy diagnosis, dairy cows should be reexamined after 45 days of gestation and again after 90 days in order to manage the relatively high rate of pregnancy loss (15% between 30 and 60 days of gestation).
• Transrectal palpation and/or ultrasonography offer the advantage of an immediate result and the ability to diagnose pathology of the reproductive tract.

Observation for Estrus
• Return to estrus is considered a strong indication that a cow is not pregnant; however, up to 5% of pregnant females may display some signs of estrus.
• Nonreturn to estrus can be an indication of pregnancy; however, females that have a persistent CL (e.g., pyometra) or are anestrous contribute to increase in false positive diagnoses.
• Problems with estrus detection accuracy and efficiency on many dairy operations limit the utility of this method.

Clinical Diagnosis
Transrectal Palpation
• Per-rectum palpation of the uterus and its contents is the most commonly used technique for diagnosis and staging of pregnancy.
• Palpation of a CL in conjunction with an enlarged, fluid-filled uterus is suggestive of pregnancy but a positive diagnosis of pregnancy is only established if one of the following is identified:
  ○ Presence of fetal membrane slip, palpable as early as 30 days but more reliable after 35 days.
  ○ Palpation of the amniotic vesicle as early as 28 days. Useful for aging gestation between 30 and 60 days and confirming twins.
  ○ Palpation of placentomes after 75 days. Useful for aging gestation.
  ○ Palpation of the fetus after 60–65 days as the amniotic vesicle becomes less turgid.
• This technique is very accurate with moderate degree of expertise after 35 days. However, early pregnancy loss (5–12%) should be taken into account.
• Very safe when performed by a skilled practitioner.

DIFFERENTIAL DIAGNOSES
• Early pregnancy: Anestrus, mummification, pyometra, persistent CL, and poor estrus detection.

• Late gestation: Mummification, pyometra, hydropic conditions, and obesity.

CBC/BIOCHEMISTRY/URINALYSIS
N/A

OTHER LABORATORY TESTS
Progesterone Assay
• In absence of maternal recognition of pregnancy, luteolysis occurs and progesterone falls below 1 ng/mL approximately 18–24 days after breeding.
• Milk or serum progesterone concentration >2 ng/mL, 18–24 days after breeding, suggests maintenance of CL activity and possible pregnancy.
• Low milk or serum concentration (<1 ng/mL) is very accurate for diagnosis of nonpregnancy.
• In-line milk progesterone testing is available; cow-side tests are intermittently marketed.
• This technique suffers from the same problems with low specificity and positive predictive value as observation for estrus.

Pregnancy-Associated Glycoproteins
• PAGs is a group of specific proteins produced by the trophoblastic binucleate cells from the early ruminant conceptus.
• PAGs testing is available for serum and milk from a number of commercial laboratories.
• The assay is most accurate around 30 days after breeding. PAG concentrations in serum and milk decline between 6 and 10 weeks of gestation and testing at this time may result in more diagnostic errors.
• Sensitivity and specificity of bPSPB increases from 75% and 85% at 26–27 days to 100% and 85% by days 37–45, respectively.
• Most laboratories recommend testing begin 28–30 days after breeding with as much as a 7-day delay for embryo recipients. For both postpartum and post-breeding intervals, always follow the specific recommendations of the testing laboratory. Single-use needles and syringes are required to avoid cross-contamination of samples and errant results.
• PAG may remain elevated for a variable period of time after pregnancy loss.
• A significant limitation of this method is that results are not immediately available and therefore interventions for open cows are delayed.
• Pregnancy confirmation at a later date is still advised, to detect any early embryonic death/pregnancy loss.
• Because no clinical examination is conducted, uterine and ovarian pathologies may go unnoticed for a long time.

IMAGING
• Transrectal ultrasonography with a linear 5 MHz transducer.
• Timing: From 25 days in heifers and 27 days in cows.
• Accuracy: Increases with gestational age and sensitivity, and the specificity of the technique approaches 100% at 32 days. It is considered

P

the gold standard for evaluating pregnancy diagnostic tests.
• Specificity: Increases if the operator uses presence of fetal heartbeat as a sign of pregnancy rather than just fetal fluid. This is easily accomplished at 29 days but requires increased examination time.
• Other advantages
  ◦ Increased accuracy of diagnosis of twins and early pregnancy loss.
  ◦ Estimate gestational age (amniotic vesicle diameter, fetal biparietal diameter, abdominal diameter, fetal crown–rump length).
  ◦ Determination of fetal gender by identification of the position of the genital tubercle at 65 ± 10 days of gestation.

OTHER DIAGNOSTIC PROCEDURES
• Early conception factor (ECF), an immunosuppressive hormone, is elevated as early as 48 hours post-conception. Currently there is no reliable commercial assay for this substance.
• Interferon-tau is the initial signal for pregnancy recognition in ruminants. It is secreted by fetal trophectoderm and inhibits corpus luteum regression by suppressing the pulsatile release of $PGF2_\alpha$ from the endometrium. It is also responsible for upregulation of specific genes expressed on maternal leukocytes. It peaks in maternal serum about 17–21 days after estrus in pregnant cattle. No commercial assay is available.

PATHOLOGIC FINDINGS
N/A

TREATMENT
THERAPEUTIC APPROACH
N/A

SURGICAL CONSIDERATIONS AND TECHNIQUES
N/A

MEDICATIONS
DRUGS OF CHOICE
CONTRAINDICATIONS
$PGF2_\alpha$ is commonly used to manage re-breeding in cattle that are diagnosed not pregnant. Pregnancy diagnostic tests with a low sensitivity and/or low negative predictive value will increase risk of inducing abortion in cow <5 months pregnant.

PRECAUTIONS
N/A

POSSIBLE INTERACTIONS
N/A

FOLLOW-UP
EXPECTED COURSE AND PROGNOSIS
N/A

POSSIBLE COMPLICATIONS
N/A

CLIENT EDUCATION
• Importance of pregnancy diagnosis
• Accuracy of various methods and implications for management

PATIENT CARE
N/A

PREVENTION
N/A

MISCELLANEOUS
ASSOCIATED CONDITIONS
Infertility, abortion, retained fetuses, dystocia

AGE-RELATED FACTORS
N/A

ZOONOTIC POTENTIAL
Cattle may shed zoonotic organisms in their feces or genital discharges (e.g., *Salmonella* spp., *C. burnetii, B. abortus*).

PREGNANCY
See "General Recommendations for Pregnancy Diagnosis."

BIOSECURITY
Pregnant animals should be vaccinated as appropriate and isolated from transient animals, wildlife disease reservoirs, and disease fomites.

PRODUCTION MANAGEMENT
Efficient production of pregnant heifers and cows is a critical component of farm profitability.

SYNONYMS
N/A

ABBREVIATIONS
• bPSPB = pregnancy-specific protein B
• CL = corpus luteum
• ECF = early conception factor
• PAG = pregnancy associated glycoprotein
• $PGF2_\alpha$ = prostaglandin $F2_\alpha$

SEE ALSO
• Abortion: Bovine
• Artificial Insemination: Bovine
• Dairy Reproduction (see www.fiveminutevet.com/ruminant)
• Reproductive Ultrasonography: Bovine (see www.fiveminutevet.com/ruminant)

Suggested Reading
Cain AJ, Christiansen D. Biochemical pregnancy diagnosis. In: Hopper RM ed, Bovine Reproduction. Ames. Wiley-Blackwell, 2015, p. 320.
Colloton J. Reproductive ultrasound of female cattle. In: Hopper RM ed, Bovine Reproduction. Ames: Wiley-Blackwell, 2015, p. 326.
Ricci A, Carvalho PD, Amundson RH, Fourdraine RH, Vincenti L, Fricke PM. Factors associated with pregnancy-associated glycoprotein (PAG) levels in plasma and milk of Holstein cows during early pregnancy and their effect on the accuracy of pregnancy diagnosis. J Dairy Sci 2015, 98: 2502–14.
Romano JE, Kelsey B, Roney S, Ramos JV, Pinedo P. Effect of early pregnancy diagnosis by per rectum amniotic sac palpation on pregnancy loss, calving rates, and abnormalities in newborn dairy calves. Theriogenology 2016, 85: 419–27.

Internet Resource
• iPhone and iPad apps to assist with pregnancy diagnosis in cattle: http://www.vetmed.wisc.e.du/dms/fapm/apps.htm

Authors Harry Momont and Celina Checura
Consulting Editor Ahmed Tibary
Acknowledgment The author and book editors acknowledge the prior contribution of Ahmed Tibary.

P

BASICS

OVERVIEW
• Timely and precise pregnancy diagnosis is an important aspect of breeding management.
• The diagnosis of pregnancy is based on history, physical examination (sexual behavior), laboratory evaluation, and ultrasonography.
• Depending on the method used, pregnancy diagnosis can be performed as early as 14 days after mating. However, it is important to recognize that pregnancy loss occurs in 10–50% of females before 60 days of gestation.
• Additional examinations may be warranted in high-risk pregnancies or if a female has a history of recurrent pregnancy loss.
• Early pregnancy diagnosis is beneficial for detecting problems of infertility in either the female or the male.
• Females that are not pregnant after three matings with a proven male should be submitted for a complete breeding soundness examination.
• Evaluation of any pregnant female is warranted if she displays receptivity to the male after a positive pregnancy diagnosis.

INCIDENCE/PREVALENCE
Common procedure

GEOGRAPHIC DISTRIBUTION
Worldwide

PATHOPHYSIOLOGY
N/A

SYSTEMS AFFECTED
Reproductive

GENETICS
N/A

HISTORICAL FINDINGS
• Owners/breeders will often tease mated females to determine if they have ovulated (at 7 days post-mating) and if they are potentially pregnant (at 12 days post-mating).
• If a female does not become pregnant following mating she will be receptive to the male 12–14 days post-mating and can be mated again.

SIGNALMENT
Any postpubertal female that has been mated

PHYSICAL EXAMINATION FINDINGS
• A complete physical examination should be performed on any female presenting for pregnancy diagnosis.
• General health and nutritional status (BCS) is extremely important for pregnancy maintenance and fetal viability.

• Clinical evaluation for pregnancy in camelids is based primarily on two techniques: behavioral changes and transrectal palpation findings.

Behavioral Signs of Pregnancy
• Pregnant camelid females display specific behavior of non-receptivity to male sexual advances starting 14 days after mating.
• In SAC, this behavior is characterized by spitting and running away from the male.
• In camels, the female assumes a characteristic body stance with the head held high and the tail curled upward (tail cocking or tail curling).
• Accuracy of pregnancy diagnosis based on behavior is 83–95%.
• False positive diagnoses (5–30%) are due to other causes for maintenance of elevated progesterone (i.e., exogenous administration of progesterone, luteinized anovulatory follicles, persistent CL, early embryo loss) or abnormal behavior (e.g., dominant or inexperienced females, painful conditions).
• False negative diagnoses are rare (<5%) and mostly due to an overtly aggressive male or a submissive female.
• The major drawback of behavioral testing is the inability to determine the number of embryos and fetal development.

Transrectal Palpation
• Appropriate physical and/or chemical restraint and proper technique are important to prevent complications.
• Size of the hand, pelvic anatomy, and size of the female may limit the veterinarian's ability to perform transrectal palpation in SAC and young camels.
• Pregnancy evaluation by transrectal palpation is possible from 30–35 days post-mating.
• There is no membrane slip in camelids. Diagnosis is based solely on size of the left uterine horn (where almost all fetuses are carried), presence of fluid, and palpation of the fetus.
• The accuracy of pregnancy diagnosis by transrectal palpation increases with gestational age until 160 days, then decreases thereafter when the enlarging uterus is displaced cranially and ventrally and the fetus becomes out of reach.

Transabdominal Fetal Ballottement
Possible after 9 months of gestation

CAUSES AND RISK FACTORS
• Accidental mating may occur if young animals are housed with males. Alpacas and llamas may reach puberty as early as 6 months of age and become pregnant.
• Early pregnancy loss is relatively common in maiden and aged females. Pregnancy should be confirmed several times during pregnancy.

DIAGNOSIS

DIFFERENTIAL DIAGNOSES
Other causes of uterine enlargement: Pyometra/mucometra, mummification, maceration, uterine neoplasia

CBC/BIOCHEMISTRY/URINALYSIS
N/A

OTHER LABORATORY TESTS
Progesterone
• Luteal progesterone is required throughout gestation in camelids.
• Serum progesterone concentration >2 ng/mL 14 days post-mating is suggestive of pregnancy.
• Serum progesterone concentrations <1.5 ng/mL are not consistent with maintenance of pregnancy.

Estrone Sulfate
• Estrone sulfate concentrations may be measured in plasma or urine.
• This test is not commonly used in practice.

IMAGING
• Real-time B-mode ultrasonography is the gold standard for pregnancy diagnosis and evaluation of the fetus and placenta.
• Ultrasonography provides the earliest accurate diagnosis along with assessment of embryonic/fetal number, development, and wellbeing.
• Transrectal ultrasonography is performed prior to 35 days of gestation with 5–8 MHz linear transducer. The transducer is mounted on a rigid extension to allow external manipulation in alpacas and small llamas.
• It is recommended to perform pregnancy diagnosis and follow-up pregnancy confirmation/evaluation at 14, 25, and 35 days and between 46 and 60 days. Additional pregnancy evaluations may be recommended in mid- to late-gestation.
• The embryonic vesicle may be visualized as early as 9–10 days post-mating; however, accuracy is greatly increased if pregnancy diagnosis is performed >14 days post-mating.
• Presence, size, and number of CLs should be evaluated at the first pregnancy diagnosis examination. Double ovulations are not rare and increase the risk for twinning.
• The embryo proper is first visualized at 20–22 days as a small echogenic structure within the vesicle. The heartbeat becomes detectable at 22–25 days.
• Transabdominal ultrasonography is performed using a 3.5 MHz curvilinear transducer.
• High accuracy for pregnancy diagnosis using transabdominal ultrasonography can be

P

achieved by scanning the right inguinal area between 35 and 120 days of pregnancy.
• Pregnancy evaluation at later stage requires scanning the ventral abdomen all the way to the xiphoid.
• Gestational age may be estimated with measurements of fetal structures (biparietal diameter, thoracic height, aortic diameter, crown–rump length, etc.).

OTHER DIAGNOSTIC PROCEDURES
N/A

PATHOLOGIC FINDINGS
• Abnormal uterine content: Pyometra, mucometra
• Abnormal pregnancies: Early embryo loss, collapsed echogenic embryonic vesicle, placentitis, placental detachment, compromised fetus (tachycardia >130 bpm or bradycardia <50 bpm), fetal death (absence of cardiac activity).

TREATMENT

THERAPEUTIC APPROACH
• Sedation and/or epidural analgesia may be required for transrectal palpation, particularly if uterine torsion is suspected.
• Intra-rectal administration of lubricant containing 2% lidocaine may facilitate transrectal palpation.

SURGICAL CONSIDERATIONS
N/A

MEDICATIONS

DRUGS OF CHOICE
Sedation: Butorphanol 0.05 mg/kg IM

CONTRAINDICATIONS
N/A

PRECAUTIONS
See "Possible Complications"

POSSIBLE INTERACTIONS
N/A

FOLLOW-UP

EXPECTED COURSE AND PROGNOSIS
• Early embryo loss varies between 5% and 30%.
• Pregnancy confirmation should always be performed in the first trimester and whenever a female is showing signs of receptivity.

POSSIBLE COMPLICATIONS
Potential complications of transrectal palpation or ultrasonography include rectal irritation, colonic or rectal perforation, or prolapse.

CLIENT EDUCATION
Emphasize the importance of timely and accurate pregnancy diagnosis for management of breeding females.

PATIENT CARE
• Pregnant females should be monitored for appropriate BCS.
• Nutrition should be adjusted for stage of pregnancy.

PREVENTION
N/A

MISCELLANEOUS

ASSOCIATED CONDITIONS
Pregnancy loss, twinning

AGE-RELATED FACTORS
Early pregnancy loss is more common in maiden and aged females.

ZOONOTIC POTENTIAL
N/A

PREGNANCY
Pregnancy diagnosis should be part of the physical examination.

BIOSECURITY
N/A

PRODUCTION MANAGEMENT
• Early and accurate pregnancy diagnosis is critical for effective breeding management.
• Fertility disorders in males and females can be detected early.
• Accurate pregnancy diagnosis is important to modify management and nutritional plans for females based on their reproductive status.

SYNONYMS
N/A

ABBREVIATIONS
• BCS = body condition score
• CL = corpus luteum
• MHz = megahertz
• SAC = South American camelids

SEE ALSO
• Abortion: Camelid
• Camelid: Reproduction
• Nutrition and Metabolic Diseases: Camelid (see www.fiveminutevet.com/ruminant)
• Pregnancy Toxemia: Camelids
• Reproductive Ultrasonography: Camelid (see www.fiveminutevet.com/ruminant)
• Vaccination Programs: Camelid

Suggested Reading
Campbell A, Pearson LK, Spencer TE, Tibary A. Double ovulation and occurrence of twinning in alpacas (*Vicugna pacos*). Theriogenology 2015, 84: 421–4.
Ferrer MS. Diagnosis of pregnancy and evaluation of high risk pregnancy. In Cebra CK et al. eds, Llama and Alpaca Care: Medicine, Surgery, Reproduction, Nutrition, and Herd Health. St. Louis: Elsevier, 2014, pp. 250–6.
Ferrer MS, Jones M, Anderson DE, Larson R. Ultrasonographic parameters of fetal well-being and development in alpacas. Theriogenology 2013, 79: 1236–46.
Tibary, A., Anouassi, A. Breeding soundness examination of the female camelidae. In: Tibary A ed, Theriogenology in Camelidae: Anatomy, Physiology, BSE, Pathology and Artificial Breeding: Actes Editions. Institut Agronomique et Veterinaire Hassan II, 1997, pp. 243–310.
Volkery J, Gottschalk J, Sobiraj A, et al. Progesterone, pregnanediol-3-glucuronide, relaxin and oestrone sulphate concentrations in saliva, milk and urine of female alpacas (*Vicugna pacos*) and their applications in pregnancy diagnosis. Vet Rec 2012, 171: 195.

Author Alexis Campbell
Consulting Editor Ahmed Tibary
Acknowledgment The author and book editors acknowledge the prior contribution of Ahmed Tibary.

P

PREGNANCY DIAGNOSIS: SMALL RUMINANT

BASICS

OVERVIEW
• Pregnancy diagnosis in sheep and goats provides valuable management information to the livestock producer. It allows timely re-breeding or culling of nonpregnant animals and facilitates supervision at parturition and production planning for dairy operations.
• Diagnostic systems that count fetal numbers allow for separation and selective feeding of females carrying multiple fetuses.
• This chapter will focus on practical, clinically relevant methods of pregnancy diagnosis in sheep and goats.

INCIDENCE/PREVALENCE
• The prevalence of pregnancy in a herd or flock is highly dependent on the fertility of the male and female animals but also depends on the competence of the livestock management system.
• In a well-managed flock or herd, during the breeding season and with natural service, the pregnancy rate should be >95% in mature females and >75% in maiden females.
• It should be noted that the performance of diagnostic tests is not independent of the prevalence of the condition being tested.

GEOGRAPHICAL DISTRIBUTION
Worldwide

SYSTEMS AFFECTED
Reproductive

PATHOPHYSIOLOGY
N/A

HISTORICAL FINDINGS
• Historical findings depends on the primary reason for pregnancy diagnosis.
• In herds or flocks using AI followed by natural mating, producers may want to stage the pregnancies and determine which females are pregnant to AI and which are pregnant to natural service.
• Most flocks or herds will have a marking system to record breeding dates. However, in absence of such a system the dates of introduction and removal of the male should be known.
• Staging of pregnancy is desirable for adequate management of lambing or kidding.
• Pregnancy diagnosis may be sought after suspicion of an accidental mating.
• Pregnancy diagnosis is an essential part of any embryo transfer program.

SIGNALMENT
Postpubertal ewes and does

PHYSICAL EXAMINATION FINDINGS
The principal signs of pregnancy in ewes and does are the absence of estrus followed by abdominal distention and udder development later in gestation.

GENETICS
• Most sheep and goat breeds have been highly selected for fertility so seasonal pregnancy rates should be high, usually above 90–95%.
• Prolificacy (number of fetuses or newborns per pregnancy) is genetically determined and is an important measure of overall reproductive efficiency.

CAUSES AND RISK FACTORS
N/A

DIAGNOSIS

• Practical diagnostic tests for pregnancy in sheep and goats may be either direct or indirect.
• Direct diagnostic tests rely on the detection of physical evidence of pregnancy. They generally involve palpation, imaging, or laboratory detection of pregnancy-specific substances.
• Indirect tests rely primarily on behavior (return to estrus in nonpregnant females).

DIFFERENTIAL DIAGNOSES
• Hydrometra or related uterine pathologies
• Anestrus

CBC/BIOCHEMISTRY/URINALYSIS
N/A

OTHER LABORATORY TESTS
• Measurement of serum progesterone concentration is an indirect laboratory test for pregnancy in sheep and goats. It requires either frequent, repeated testing—which is generally not practical—or carefully timed sampling roughly one estrus cycle length after mating. Females with high progesterone concentration at this time are presumably pregnant (~80% diagnostic accuracy); those with low progesterone are almost certainly not pregnant (~95–100% diagnostic accuracy).
• Measurement of pregnancy-associated glycoproteins (PAGs) is a direct laboratory test for pregnancy. These substances are pregnancy specific; however, they will remain elevated in serum for up to a week after fetal death so false positives are a concern. Commercial tests are available and advertise 99% accuracy for open diagnoses 30 or more days after breeding.
• Historically, conjugated estrogen concentrations in serum or milk have been used to diagnose pregnancy. Since estrone sulfate is a product of placental metabolism, its measurement is considered a direct test for pregnancy. Goats may be tested as early as 50 days while sheep are usually tested after 70 days of gestation.

IMAGING
• Real-time B-mode ultrasonography is the gold standard for pregnancy diagnosis in most veterinary species, including sheep and goats.

• Transrectal ultrasonography will provide an earlier diagnosis but is not practical outside of research settings.
  ○ Use linear transducers with 5–8 MHz frequency mounted on an extension handle.
  ○ Embryonic vesicles (anechoic) are visible starting at 20 days.
  ○ Placentomes (echogenic) are visible starting at 21 or 22 days.
  ○ Embryos are readily visible within the vesicle starting at 25 days.
  ○ Accuracy is low before 30 days.
  ○ Up to 16% of pregnancies diagnosed at 30 days may be lost by 60 days.
• Transabdominal ultrasonography is the most commonly used technique in practice.
  ○ Scanning is done using a sector or curvilinear transducer with 3.5 MHz frequency. Female are scanned in the lower right flank, just above the base of the udder. This region is naturally devoid of fleece in most sheep but goats may need to be clipped to provide good acoustic coupling. The use of rubbing alcohol or coupling gel on the skin is necessary to obtain an image.
  ○ Pregnancy fluid may be detected as early as 25 days post-mating but accuracy is better at 35 days and continues to improve until about 60 days of gestation. At this early stage of gestation it is important to direct the transducers dorsally and caudally the area of the pelvic inlet. As gestation advances, the fetuses move cranially and ventral in the abdomen. The accuracy decreases after 100 days unless the ventral abdomen is clipped to provide better visualization.
  ○ The optimal time for fetal number determination is 45–85 days.
  ○ Sensitivity and specificity of this technique for pregnancy diagnosis are 99% and 100%, respectively.
  ○ Sensitivity and specificity of fetal number determination are 91% and 100%, respectively.
• Fetal age can be determined by measuring the embryonic vesicle (days 24–40), crown–rump length (days 24–40), and fetal thoracic diameter and parietal diameter (from day 41).
• Fetal gender determination is possible between 60 and 69 days. Accuracy is higher for single fetuses and males.

OTHER DIAGNOSTIC PROCEDURES
Ballotement of the fetus is possible late in gestation but provides limited economic return.

PATHOLOGIC FINDINGS
• A major advantage of diagnostic imaging, ultrasonography in particular, is the ability to detect reproductive pathology. This will allow for timelier, effective treatment interventions or a decision to cull the abnormal animal.
• Abnormal pregnancies: early embryonic loss, mummifications, fetal death.

P

PREGNANCY DIAGNOSIS: SMALL RUMINANT (CONTINUED)

TREATMENT

N/A

MEDICATIONS

N/A

FOLLOW-UP

EXPECED COURSE AND PROGNOSIS
• Early pregnancy losses are minimal after 45 days and any loss of pregnancy is generally visible.
• In absence of any abortion-causing etiology the lambing/kidding rate should be close to pregnancy rate.

POSSIBLE COMPLICATIONS
• Transrectal ultrasonography requires some expertise and may cause injury to the female if not done properly.
• Early pregnancy diagnosis is associated with both a reduced diagnostic accuracy and a higher rate of spontaneous loss of the pregnancy.
• While the tests described above are generally regarded as safe, testing of herds or flocks for pregnancy should always be done in a manner and in facilities that minimize stress on the animals.

CLIENT EDUCATION
Importance of pregnancy diagnosis in fertility investigation, management of pregnant females, and planning for lambing/kidding.

PATIENT CARE
While earlier pregnancy diagnosis may provide the greatest economic return to producers, the reality is that pregnancy loss rates are much higher in early gestation. Pregnancy diagnosis performed in ruminants before 40–45 days of gestation should always be accompanied by a recommendation to reconfirm pregnancy status sometime after 60 days.

PREVENTION
N/A

MISCELLANEOUS

ASSOCIATED CONDITIONS
• Hydrometra
• Fetal mummification

AGE-RELATED FACTORS
N/A

ZOONOTIC POTENTIAL
Diseases that cause abortion in sheep and goats are often zoonotic. Appropriate precautions should be taken when working with these species.

BIOSECURITY
• Equipment used on multiple sites should be sanitized between locations.
• When blood testing for pregnancy, a new syringe and needle must be used for each animal.

PRODUCTION MANAGEMENT
N/A

SYNONYMS
N/A

ABBREVIATIONS
N/A

SEE ALSO
• Anestrus
• Artificial Insemination: Small Ruminant
• Embryo Transfer: Small Ruminant
• Hydrometra
• Pregnancy Toxemia: Small Ruminant
• Reproductive Ultrasonography: Small Ruminant (see www.fiveminutevet.com/ruminant)
• Uterine Anomalies

Suggested Reading
Vinoles-Gil C, Gonzalez-Bulnes A, Martin GB, et al. Sheep and goats. In: DesCoteaux L, Colloton J, Gnemmii G eds, Practical Atlas of Ruminant and Camelid Reproductive Ultrasonography. Ames: Wiley- Blackwell, 2010, pp. 181–210.
Author Harry Momont
Consulting Editor Ahmed Tibary

P

PREGNANCY TOXEMIA: BOVINE

BASICS

OVERVIEW
• Pregnancy toxemia is an uncommon metabolic disease in cattle that results from the inability of the dam to maintain glucose homeostasis in the face of increasing energy demands during late gestation.

INCIDENCE/PREVALENCE
• Varies widely between herds and production styles.
• Individual variation may result in sporadic occurrence.
• Mortality rate in affected animals may reach 90% or more.

GEOGRAPHIC DISTRIBUTION
Worldwide

SYSTEMS AFFECTED
• Nervous
• Musculoskeletal
• Digestive
• Reproductive

PATHOPHYSIOLOGY
• Pregnancy toxemia is characterized by low glucose concentrations and high ketone body concentrations. Insufficient energy use rather than complete lack of energy supply may be a contributing factor.
• The fetoplacental unit requires glucose for energy and may consume up to 40% of the maternal glucose production during late gestation.
• In ruminants, absorption of dietary glucose is limited because of fermentation by the ruminal flora. Serum glucose concentrations are largely maintained by gluconeogenesis, 85% of which occurs in the liver.
• If the dam is unable to maintain glucose homeostasis a state of negative energy balance (NEB) occurs resulting in a metabolic state with a decreased ratio of insulin to glucagon and development of insulin resistance.
  ◦ NEB is defined as insufficient consumption of calories necessary to meet metabolic requirements for late prepartum or early postpartum cows.
  ◦ In cows, particularly dairy cows, the development of NEB and ketosis is more commonly associated with peak lactation.
• Insulin function is critical to glucose uptake by the cells, is an important factor in glucose homeostasis, and ultimately plays a role in the susceptibility of individual animals to development of pregnancy toxemia.
• Development of periparturient ketosis has been attributed to insulin resistance and impaired glucose utilization as a result of overfeeding dairy cattle during the dry period.
• In a state of NEB, NEFAs are mobilized and converted to glucose with production of ketone bodies (acetone, acetoacetate, and BHB) and development of metabolic acidosis.

• Reduced disposal of ketones during late gestation along with an increased rate of hepatic ketogenesis promotes hyperketonemia, facilitating development of pregnancy toxemia.
• Hyperketonemia depresses hepatic glucose production, resulting in a sustained hypoglycemia, and contributes to the pathogenesis of the disease.

HISTORICAL FINDINGS
• Late gestation (often carrying twins); typically 7–10 days prior to calving.
• Inadequate nutrition: overfeeding during the dry period (dairy cattle; BCS > 3.75/5), or obesity followed by limited feed quantity/quality.
• Initial clinical signs are vague: Rough appearance, off feed, obtunded, isolation from remainder of herd.
• Advancement to weakness, decreased rumen motility (firm, dry feces), mental dullness, neurologic signs (generally 10% of affected cows will develop neurologic signs; abnormal licking, head pressing, circling, blindness, tremors, tetany, etc.), recumbency, and eventually death without treatment.
• Even with aggressive therapy, death and culling rates are greatly increased among clinically affected cows.

SIGNALMENT
Mature cows in late gestation are primarily affected.

PHYSICAL EXAMINATION FINDINGS
• Physical examination findings dependent on duration and progression of the disease (vital signs are typically normal).
• Anorexia, weakness, incoordination, mental dullness, decreased rumen fill, firm/scant/dry feces, sweet acetone breath, recumbency, neurologic signs, death.

GENETICS
N/A

CAUSES AND RISK FACTORS
• Pregnancy toxemia is caused by an inability of the dam to maintain glucose homeostasis in the face of increased demand from the fetoplacental unit in late gestation (last 4–6 weeks).
• Primary pregnancy toxemia results from a combination of poor nutrition and a sharp increase in energy needs during late gestation (extreme lack of feed and poor feed quality).
• Pregnancy toxemia can be classified as primary pregnancy toxemia or fat cow pregnancy toxemia (type II ketosis).
• Overconditioning of the dam (body condition score > 4/5) resulting in compromise of gluconeogenic capacity with increased fatty infiltration ultimately leading to reduced glucose availability and increased ketogenesis, development of hepatic lipidosis.
• Cows with twins, having improper, declining, or interrupted nutritional inputs (especially in cows that were overconditioned

and then experience a sharp decline in nutrition). Cows with excessive parasite burden, poor dentition, lameness, or those experiencing stress such as sudden cold/wet weather, processing, or hauling may be more susceptible.

DIAGNOSIS

DIFFERENTIAL DIAGNOSES
• Hypocalcemia
• Listeriosis
• Polioencephalomalacia
• Impending abortion
• Copper toxicity
• Ruminal acidosis
• Hypomagnesemia
• Trauma
• Parasitism

CBC/BIOCHEMISTRY/URINALYSIS
• CBS is generally nonspecific but marked neutrophilia may be present.
• Hypoglycemia or normoglycemia, hypocalcemia, and in some cases elevated liver enzymes and hypocholesterolemia. Samples for blood glucose should be processed as soon as possible.
• Serum concentrations of both NEFAs (>0.4 mEq/L) and BHB (subclinical/moderate ketosis >15 mg/dL; clinical ketosis >25 mg/dL) are increased.
• Hypoproteinemia (hypoalbuminemia and hypoglobulinemia) can be observed in clinical cases of pregnancy toxemia and could potentially be attributed to hepatic and/or renal failure.
• In later stages of pregnancy toxemia hyperglycemia (often associated with fetal death), hypokalemia, elevated creatinine, and elevated BUN may be evident.
• Elevated ketones on urinalysis; ketonuria is present and usually detected before ketonemia.

OTHER LABORATORY TESTS
• Cow-side diagnostic tests available for estimation of ketone bodies concentration in milk.

IMAGING
N/A

OTHER DIAGNOSTIC PROCEDURES
N/A

OTHER PATHOLOGIC FINDINGS
• Gross necropsy findings vary with body condition and initiating causes.
• Twins or a large single fetus present and, depending on when fetal death occurred, autolysis may be present. Some cows will abort or calve prematurely before death.
• The carcass is either emaciated or overconditioned with large quantities of intra-abdominal and subcutaneous fat.
• Variable degrees of fatty liver infiltration with the liver potentially enlarged, pale, and

P

friable; however, the severity of these changes may be difficult to evaluate grossly.
• Histologic lesions include hepatic lipidosis and neuronal necrosis and astrocytosis.
• Aqueous humor concentrations of BHB can correspond to antemortem serum concentrations.

TREATMENT

THERAPEUTIC APPROACH
• Treatment protocols are based on two general principles: Administration of energy sources and removal of factors that increase energy requirements.
• Treatment costs and prognosis should be considered before any treatment is recommended. Individual animals should be segregated from the herd for treatment and monitoring purposes.
• If the cow is in early stages of the disease (prior to anorexia and recumbency), dietary modification and supplementation with glucogenic precursors may be sufficient.
• Without intensive care, cows with pregnancy toxemia are unlikely to recover.
• Propylene glycol, glycerol, calcium propionate, sodium propionate, or liquid molasses are routinely used as glucose precursors.
• Oral propylene glycol and electrolytes are useful to treat mild cases.
• In more advanced stages of the disease, more aggressive supportive therapy is necessary and the prognosis more guarded.
• Acid-base status, degree of dehydration, associated electrolyte abnormalities, and renal function should be evaluated and appropriate treatment and fluid therapy provided.
• To reduce the effects of the negative energy balance and improve the potential response to therapy, cesarean section or induction of parturition/termination of pregnancy to remove the fetus(es) is often recommended in affected females.
• Induction of parturition in cows can be accomplished with the administration of dexamethasone and/or prostaglandin F2$_\alpha$ with parturition generally occurring 24–72 hours following administration.
• In cases where the female is severely compromised, euthanasia may be indicated for welfare reasons.

SURGICAL CONSIDERATIONS AND TECHNIQUES
• If induction of parturition or termination of pregnancy does not result in delivery of the fetus(es) within 72 hours, or the animal is severely compromised, a cesarean section should be performed to reduce demands on glucose.
• Often the fetus(es) are nonviable and the procedure is used to save the cow.

MEDICATIONS

DRUGS OF CHOICE
• There are no specific drugs of choice; however, several drugs are occasionally used in individual cases of pregnancy toxemia in combination with glucose administration and fluid therapy.
• Administration of B-complex vitamins to stimulate appetite.
• Dexamethasone (25–30 mg IM) with parturition generally occurring 24–72 hours following administration.
• Prostaglandin F2α or an analog (25 mg dinoprost tromethamine IM; 500 μg cloprostenol IM) with parturition generally occurring 24–72 hours following administration.
• Females that are managed with induction of parturition or cesarean section should be treated with broad-spectrum antimicrobials, a nonsteroidal anti-inflammatory, and oxytocin to facilitate placenta delivery and prevent metritis.

CONTRAINDICATIONS
Appropriate milk and meat withdrawal times must be followed for all compounds administered to food-producing animals.

PRECAUTIONS
N/A

POSSIBLE INTERACTIONS
N/A

FOLLOW-UP

EXPECTED COURSE AND PROGNOSIS
• Treatment is often unrewarding and often noneconomic in commercial herds.
• The prognosis is usually poor for recovery if recumbency is prolonged.
• Induction of parturition/termination of the pregnancy or cesarean section is unpredictable for survival of the fetus(es), and if delayed, for the cow as well.

POSSIBLE COMPLICATIONS
Dystocia, retained placenta, and metabolic complications during early lactation are common in dams that survive to the induced or natural initiation of parturition.

CLIENT EDUCATION
• Repeated and prolonged treatments will be needed.
• The owner will need to evaluate the economics of therapy versus probable outcomes.
• Development of pregnancy toxemia in one cow may indicate other cows in the herd at risk; provision of energy supplement is an essential part of treatment on a herd basis.

PATIENT CARE
• Feed intake is a critical factor in monitoring for treatment success. If the animal is recumbent for a prolonged period, the odds of recovery are substantially reduced.
• The goal of therapy in pregnancy toxemia is to restore glucose homeostasis as soon as possible.
• Multiple electrolyte, acid-base, and fluid imbalances in addition to low blood glucose levels will need to be considered in any potential treatment plan.
• The affected cow should be isolated to reduce expenditures of energy and limit competition for feed resources.
• Considerations for management of recumbent cows.
• High-quality forages and concentrates should be offered in an attempt to stimulate intake.
• Transfaunation could be considered if a source of rumen fluid is available.

PREVENTION
• Prevention of future cases of pregnancy toxemia is best accomplished by evaluation of nutritional and management practices within the herd.
• Designing nutritional programs that meet the females' requirements based on the stage of production and relevant environmental and management conditions can prevent most cases of pregnancy toxemia.
• Cows should have an ideal body condition at the beginning of the breeding season through to the end of gestation.
• Appropriate dry and close-up rations in dairy cows.
• Where possible blood samples should be collected to evaluate BHB or NEFA levels. Females with elevated BHB or NEFA levels should be separated and monitored closely.

MISCELLANEOUS

ASSOCIATED CONDITIONS
Correction or treatment of concurrent disease is necessary.

AGE-RELATED FACTORS
More common in older cows

ZOONOTIC POTENTIAL
N/A

PREGNANCY
Pregnancy toxemia is present in cows in late gestation (generally the last 4–6 weeks).

BIOSECURITY
N/A

PRODUCTION MANAGEMENT
• Best managed as a production disease with primary emphasis placed on prevention of future cases.

• Nutritional and management factors must be addressed to minimize the impact within a population.

SYNONYMS
• Pregnancy ketosis
• Periparturient ketosis
• Type II ketosis
• Fatty liver syndrome
• Twinning disease

ABBREVIATIONS
• BCS = body condition score
• BHB = beta-hydroxybutyrate
• BUN = blood urea nitrogen
• IM = intramuscular
• IV = intravenous
• NEB = negative energy balance
• NEFA = nonesterified fatty acid
• SC = subcutaneous

SEE ALSO
• Cesarean Section: Bovine
• Grass Tetany/Hypomagnesemia
• Hypocalcemia: Bovine
• Induction of Parturition
• Ketosis: Dairy Cattle
• Listeriosis
• Nutrition and Metabolic Diseases: Beef
• Nutrition and Metabolic Diseases: Dairy
• Reproductive Pharmacology

Suggested Reading
Brozos C, Mavrogianni VS, Fthenakis GC. Treatment and control of peri-parturient metabolic diseases: pregnancy toxemia, hypocalcemia, hypomagnesemia. Vet Clin North Am Food Anim Pract 2011, 27: 105–13.

Holtenius P, Holtenius K. New aspects of ketone bodies in energy metabolism in dairy cows: a review. J Vet Med A 1997; 43: 579–87.
Rook JS. Pregnancy toxemia of ewes, does, and beef cows. Vet Clin North Am Food Anim Pract 2000, 16: 293–317.
Van Saun RJ. Metabolic and nutritional diseases of the puerperal period. In: Youngquist RS, Threlfall WR eds, Current Therapy in Large Animal Theriogenology, 2nd ed. St. Louis: Saunders; 2007, pp. 355–78.
Author Alexis Campbell
Consulting Editor Ahmed Tibary

P

PREGNANCY TOXEMIA: CAMELID

BASICS

OVERVIEW
• Metabolic disease resulting from a disruption in maternal glucose homeostasis associated with increased metabolic demands from the term fetus.
• The syndrome may also affect females during lactation.

PATHOPHYSIOLOGY
• Negative energy balance may occur due to inadequate nutrition to supply fetal metabolic demands, parasitism, or anorexia secondary to systemic disease or stress.
• In the face of negative energy balance, fat is mobilized from peripheral stores as an alternative energy source, causing hyperlipemia.
• Free fatty acids are metabolized into ketone bodies in the liver, resulting in ketosis.
• Bicarbonate conversion and loss leads to metabolic acidosis.
• Excessive accumulation of lipids in hepatocytes (hepatic lipidosis) results in loss of function.
• Osmotic diuresis can contribute to serum hyperosmolarity and dehydration.
• In severe cases with hepatic lipidosis, hepatic metabolism of ammonia into urea is altered, resulting in accumulation of ammonia in blood and hepatic encephalopathy.

INCIDENCE/PREVALENCE
Sporadic

GEOGRAPHIC DISTRIBUTION
Worldwide

SYSTEMS AFFECTED
• Reproductive
• Nervous
• Digestive

GENETICS
N/A

HISTORICAL FINDINGS
• Recent illness or uterine torsion
• Recent social or environmental (heat) stress
• Recent changes in management
• Acute (2 days) or progressive (weeks), severe weight loss

SIGNALMENT
• Reported in llamas and alpacas with variable BCS (overweight, normal or thin).
• Pregnant female in the last 2 months of gestation.
• Signs progress over 3–7 days.

PHYSICAL EXAMINATION FINDINGS
• Anorexia
• Depression
• Recumbency
• Weight loss
• Weakness
• Ataxia
• Mental dullness
• Head pressing
• Abortion
• Death
• Tachycardia
• Tachypnea
• Normothermia
• Reduced gastrointestinal sounds
• Normal to poor body condition

CAUSES AND RISK FACTORS
• Failure to increase the nutritional plane to meet the energy demands of the growing fetus.
• Transient feed deprivation or change in eating behavior associated with stress or disease.
• Concurrent disease affecting appetite and energy utilization.
• Inappropriate nutritional management.
• Obese animals or late pregnant females are at high risk.
• Improper or interrupted energy intake.

DIAGNOSIS

DIFFERENTIAL DIAGNOSES
• Cerebral edema
• Polioencephalomalacia
• Meningitis
• Meningeal worm
• Listeriosis
• Trauma
• Tick paralysis
• Hypomagnesemia
• Peripheral nerve damage

CBC/BIOCHEMISTRY/URINALYSIS
• Hyperglycemia.
• Increased liver enzymes and bile acids.
• Hyperlipemia; late pregnant females should have NEFA concentrations <400 µmol/L. NEFA concentration >800 µmol/L is life threatening.
• Metabolic acidosis.
• Hypokalemia.
• Hypocalcemia.
• Hypophosphatemia.
• Azotemia.
• Ketonuria.
• Glucosuria.

OTHER LABORATORY TESTS
Liver biopsy

IMAGING
• Transabdominal ultrasonography to evaluate fetal wellbeing: Fetal heart rate is particularly important in detection of fetal stress. Fetal heart rate constantly >130 bpm or constantly <50 bpm suggests fetal stress.
• Ultrasonographic evaluation of the liver: Mottled appearance and enlargement.

OTHER DIAGNOSTIC PROCEDURES
N/A

PATHOLOGIC FINDINGS
Hepatic lipidosis in advanced stages

TREATMENT

THERAPEUTIC APPROACH
• Correct or treat underlying problem.
• Correct hydration, electrolyte imbalances, and acidosis.
• Restore glucose homeostasis.
• Stimulate feed intake.
• Induce parturition with a term fetus.
• Potentially remove the fetus.

SURGICAL CONSIDERATIONS
• Cesarean section is indicated if the fetus is already dead or if the female is debilitated.
• Uterine inertia may result in dystocia and indication for cesarean section after induction of parturition.

MEDICATIONS

DRUGS OF CHOICE
• Insulin: 0.4 IU/kg SC q4–8h (regular crystalline) or q24h (long-acting).
• Vitamin B complex or diazepam (0.05 mg/kg IV) to stimulate appetite.
• Cloprostenol 250 µg IM for induction of abortion or parturition
• Anabolic steroid is an alternative to stimulate appetite and liver function

CONTRAINDICATIONS
Appropriate milk and meat withdrawal times must be followed for all compounds administered to food-producing animals.

PRECAUTIONS
• Fluid therapy should be performed carefully in compromised pregnant female to avoid pulmonary edema and fetal stress.
• Induction of abortion or cesarean section may result in further stress and exacerbate the problem.

POSSIBLE INTERACTIONS
N/A

FOLLOW-UP

EXPECTED COURSE AND PROGNOSIS
• Prognosis for life of the dam is guarded to poor. Development of hepatic lipidosis worsens the prognosis.
• Prognosis for pregnancy maintenance is guarded to poor and for neonatal survival is guarded to poor depending on the maturational stage of the fetus.

POSSIBLE COMPLICATIONS
• Maternal death
• Pregnancy loss
• Dystocia
• Retained fetal membranes
• Metritis

- Agalactia or hypogalactia
- Neonatal morbidity and mortality
- Hepatic injury and liver failure
- Neuropathy

CLIENT EDUCATION

- Contact a veterinarian promptly if illness, lack of appetite, or depression develops in a pregnant camelid.
- Work with your veterinarian to provide appropriate nutrition, management, and parasite control in pregnant females.
- Avoid stress in pregnant females.

PATIENT CARE

- Animal should be in stall rest in comfortable environment.
- Monitor blood glucose, electrolytes, and acid-base status q4h during treatment.
- Monitor feed intake.
- Monitor fetal wellbeing.
- Monitor for fetal expulsion within 30 h of treatment with cloprostenol.
- Transfaunation with bovine ruminal fluid (0.5–1.0 L via orogastric tube).
- Total parenteral nutrition if appetite is not restored.
- Reduce stress and avoid stressful procedures.
- Provide good-quality hay and feed (alfalfa cubes or pellets, sugar beet pulp, fresh grass cuts).

PREVENTION

- Provide appropriate nutritional management.
- Provide appropriate parasite control strategies.
- Avoid stress in pregnant females.

MISCELLANEOUS

ASSOCIATED CONDITIONS

- Heat stress
- High parasite load
- Septicemia

AGE-RELATED FACTORS

N/A

ZOONOTIC POTENTIAL

N/A

PREGNANCY

Pregnancy toxemia develops in late pregnant females and may lead to pregnancy loss.

BIOSECURITY

N/A

PRODUCTION MANAGEMENT

- Routine body condition scoring.
- Appropriate feeding management. Understand the unique metabolic processes of camelids, ensuring both adequate protein and energy intake.

SYNONYMS

- Ketosis, ketoacidosis
- Fatty liver disease

ABBREVIATIONS

- BCS = body condition score
- IM = intramuscular
- IV = intravenous
- NEFA = non-esterified fatty acids
- SC = subcutaneous

SEE ALSO

- Body Condition Scoring: Alpacas and Llamas (see www.fiveminutevet.com/ruminant)
- Body Condition Scoring: Camels (see www.fiveminutevet.com/ruminant)
- Induction of Parturition
- Nutrition and Metabolic Diseases: Camelid (see www.fiveminutevet.com/ruminant)

Suggested Reading

Anderson DE, Constable PD, Yvorchuk KE, Anderson NV, St-Jean G, Rock L. Hyperlipemia and ketonuria in an alpaca and a llama. J Vet Intern Med 1994, 8: 207–11.

Cebra CK. Disorders of carbohydrate or lipid metabolism in Camelids. Vet Clin North Am Food Anim Pract 2009, 25: 339–52.

Ferrer MS, Jones M, Anderson DE, Larson R. Ultrasonographic parameters of fetal well-being and development in alpacas. Theriogenology 2013, 79: 1236–46.

Paxson JA, Bedenice D. Severe acid-base and neurological derangements in pregnancy toxemia. Livestock 2015, 20: 102–6.

Tornquist SJ, Van Saun RJ, Smith BB, Cebra CK, Snyder SP. Hepatic lipidosis in llamas and alpacas: 31 cases (1991–1997). J Am Vet Med Assoc 1999, 214; 1368–72.

Van Saun RJ. Nutritional diseases of llamas and alpacas. Vet Clin North Am Food Anim Pract 2009, 25: 797–810.

Van Saun RJ. Nutritional diseases of South American camelids. Small Ruminant Res 2006, 61: 153–4.

Author Maria Soledad Ferrer
Consulting Editor Ahmed Tibary

P

PREGNANCY TOXEMIA: SMALL RUMINANT

BASICS

OVERVIEW
• Pregnancy toxemia is a common metabolic disease in sheep and goats that results from the inability of the dam to maintain glucose homeostasis in the face of increasing energy demands from multiple fetuses during late gestation.

INCIDENCE/PREVALENCE
• Varies widely between flocks/herds and production systems.
• Isolated cases in well-managed flocks; individual variation may result in sporadic occurrence and low morbidity (<3%).
• In contrast, flocks or herds with improper nutritional management could experience outbreaks with morbidity rates exceeding 10% of the ewes or does.
• Insulin resistance during late gestation has been evaluated as a potential predisposing factor to the development of pregnancy toxemia.

GEOGRAPHIC DISTRIBUTION
Worldwide

SYSTEMS AFFECTED
• Nervous
• Musculoskeletal
• Digestive
• Reproductive

PATHOPHYSIOLOGY
• Pregnancy toxemia is caused by a negative energy balance due to increasing energy demand of rapid fetal growth during late gestation (generally the last 4–6 weeks of gestation) combined with insufficient energy intake.
• Pregnancy toxemia is characterized by low glucose concentrations and high ketone body concentrations.
• The fetoplacental unit requires glucose for energy and may consume up to 40% of the maternal glucose production during the rapid growth that occurs during late gestation.
• In ruminants, limited dietary glucose is absorbed because the ruminal flora is proficient at fermenting glucose. Serum glucose concentrations are largely maintained by gluconeogenesis, 85% of which occurs in the liver.
• Excess glucose is stored in the liver as glycogen but these stores are inadequate to supply the dam's needs in late gestation.
• While it has long been demonstrated that a lack of energy supply is responsible for the development of pregnancy toxemia, it is not likely the only major factor.
• Insufficient energy utilization rather than complete lack of energy supply may be a contributing factor.
• If the dam is unable to maintain glucose homeostasis a state of negative energy balance occurs, resulting in a metabolic state with a

decreased ratio of insulin to glucagon and development of insulin resistance may result. It has been demonstrated that insulin plasma concentrations are reduced in ewes carrying more than three fetuses.
• Insulin function is critical to glucose uptake by the cells, is an important factor in glucose homeostasis, in part regulates ketogenesis, and ultimately plays a role in the susceptibility of individual animals to development of pregnancy toxemia.
• In a state of negative energy balance body fat stores in the form of nonesterified fatty acids (NEFAs) will be converted to glucose with the undesirable production of ketone bodies (acetone, acetoacetate, and BHB) and development of metabolic acidosis.
• Reduced disposal of ketones during late gestation along with an increased rate of hepatic ketogenesis promotes hyperketonemia, facilitating development of pregnancy toxemia.
• Hyperketonemia depresses hepatic glucose production, resulting in a sustained hypoglycemia, and contributes to the pathogenesis of the disease.
• It has been suggested that cell-mediated and humoral immunity are altered in subclinical and clinical cases of pregnancy toxemia.

HISTORICAL FINDINGS
• Late gestation ewes or does carrying multiple fetuses.
• Recently sheared, hauled, or fasted for a period of time.
• Initial clinical signs are vague: Isolation from the remainder of the flock or herd, off feed, depressed.
• Advancement to weakness, mental dullness, blindness, disoriented, head pressing, teeth grinding, recumbency, and eventually death within 3 or 4 days without treatment.
• Progression of clinical signs ranges from 12 hours to 7 days.

SIGNALMENT
• The disease occurs more frequently in ewes than in does.
• Prolific breeds may be at greater risk for nutritional mismanagement.
• Breeds consistently delivering >2 offspring per litter are more predisposed.
• Mature ewes and does primarily affected, rare in maiden females.
• Obese or severely underconditioned females.

PHYSICAL EXAMINATION FINDINGS
• Physical examination findings dependent on duration and progression of the disease.
• Anorexia, weakness, incoordination, mental dullness, impaired vision/lack of menace response, hyperesthetic to tactile or auditory stimuli, head pressing, circling, muscle tremors, ataxia, teeth grinding, recumbency, convulsions, death.

GENETICS
• Variation in clinical incidence within flocks and between flocks suggests that some

animals may be genetically susceptible to development of pregnancy toxemia.
• Individual variation appears to be related to hepatic metabolic efficiency and ability to maintain functional insulin concentrations and maternal tissue responses, with some breeds more predisposed to the condition.
• Some highly prolific breeds, such as Finnish Landrace and Booroola Merino sheep, do not experience an increased incidence of pregnancy toxemia.

CAUSES AND RISK FACTORS
• Pregnancy toxemia is caused by an inability of the dam to maintain glucose homeostasis in the face of increased demand from the fetoplacental unit in late gestation.
• Dams with multiple fetuses, late gestation, having improper, declining, or interrupted nutritional inputs.
• Pregnancy toxemia can be classified into one of the following general categories:
  ○ Primary pregnancy toxemia
    ■ Results from a combination of poor nutrition and a sharp increase in energy needs during late gestation
    ■ Factors that might predispose to the development of primary pregnancy toxemia: lack of feed availability, decreased feed quality, sudden feed changes, transportation during late pregnancy, shearing, vaccinating, and heat or cold stress.
  ○ Fat ewe pregnancy toxemia
    ■ Overconditioning of the dam (body condition score > 4/5) during early gestation, resulting in increased abdominal fat and reduced rumen capacity, possible hepatic lipidosis that also impairs glucose metabolism.
• Secondary pregnancy toxemia
  ○ Concurrent disease in affected ewes or does; examples would include lameness, pneumonia, water deprivation, heavy parasite infestation, vaginal prolapse.

DIAGNOSIS

DIFFERENTIAL DIAGNOSES
• Hypocalcemia
• Listeriosis
• Polioencephalomalacia
• Impending abortion
• Copper toxicity
• Ruminal acidosis
• Hypomagnesemia
• Trauma
• Parasitism

CBC/BIOCHEMISTRY/URINALYSIS
• CBC is usually nonspecific but potential marked neutrophilia.
• Hypoglycemia, hypocalcemia, and in some cases elevated liver enzymes and hypocholesterolemia; samples for blood

glucose should be processed as soon as possible.
• Serum concentrations of both NEFAs (>0.4 mEq/L) and BHB (subclinical/moderate ketosis >15 mg/dL; clinical ketosis >25 mg/dL) are increased.
• Hypoproteinemia (hypoalbuminemia and hypoglobulinemia) can be observed in clinical cases of pregnancy toxemia and could potentially be attributed to hepatic and/or renal failure.
• In later stages of pregnancy toxemia, hyperglycemia (often associated with fetal death), hypokalemia, elevated creatinine, and elevated BUN may be evident.
• Elevated ketones on urinalysis; ketonuria is present and usually detected before ketonemia.

OTHER LABORATORY TESTS
Impaired intravenous glucose tolerance test, not practical in clinical practice.

IMAGING
Transabdominal ultrasonography to determine the viability of fetuses in clinical pregnancy toxemia to better determine clinical management strategies.

OTHER DIAGNOSTIC PROCEDURES
N/A

PATHOLOGIC FINDINGS
• Gross necropsy findings vary with body condition and initiating causes.
• Multiple fetuses are present and, depending on when fetal death occurred, autolysis may be present.
• The carcass is either emaciated or in good condition with large quantities of intra-abdominal and subcutaneous fat.
• Variable degrees of fatty liver infiltration with the liver potentially enlarged, pale, and friable; however, the severity of these changes may be difficult to evaluate grossly.
• Histologic lesions include hepatic lipidosis, neuronal necrosis, and astrocytosis.
• Aqueous humor concentrations of BHB can correspond to antemortem serum concentrations.
• Complete postmortem examinations are rarely performed.

TREATMENT
THERAPEUTIC APPROACH
• Treatment protocols based on two general principles: Administration of energy sources and removal of factors that increase energy requirements.
• Treatment costs and prognosis should be considered before any treatment is recommended. Individual animals should be segregated from the flock for treatment and monitoring purposes.
• If the ewe or doe is in early stages of the disease, dietary modification and

supplementation with glucogenic precursors may be sufficient.
• Propylene glycol (60–200 mL PO q12h for 6 days), glycerol, calcium propionate, sodium propionate, or liquid molasses are routinely used as glucose precursors. Precautions should be taken when administering propylene glycol, as excessive amounts may lead to acidosis and/or cause diarrhea.
• Calf electrolytes for neonatal diarrhea (PO q12h for 1–2 days) can combat acidosis and dehydration.
• In more advanced stages of the disease, more aggressive supportive therapy is necessary and the prognosis more guarded.
• Acid-base status, degree of dehydration, associated electrolyte abnormalities, and renal function should be evaluated and appropriate treatment and fluid therapy provided.
• Glucose levels should be evaluated before initiation of treatment. Severe hypoglycemia should be treated by administration of 250–500 mL of 10–20% glucose solution IV followed by slower infusion of a 5–10% glucose solution. In combination with glucose treatment, insulin therapy should be initiated and monitored closely.
• To reduce the effects of the negative energy balance and improve the potential response to therapy, cesarean section or induction of parturition/termination of pregnancy to remove the fetuses is often recommended in affected females.
• Induction of parturition in ewes is usually accomplished with the administration of dexamethasone (10–20 mg IM) with parturition generally occurring 36–48 hours following administration. However, it is only successful if the fetuses are alive.
• Induction of parturition in does is usually accomplished with the administration of prostaglandin F2α or an analog (2.5–15 mg dinoprost tromethamine IM; 75–125 μg cloprostenol IM) with parturition generally occurring 30–48 hours following administration.
• In cases where the female is severely compromised, euthanasia may be indicated for welfare reasons.

SURGICAL CONSIDERATIONS
• Emergency cesarean section may be elected if the dam is severely compromised.
• If induction of parturition or termination of pregnancy does not result in delivery of the fetuses within 72 hours, or the animal is severely compromised, a cesarean section should be performed.

MEDICATIONS
DRUGS OF CHOICE
• Several drugs are occasionally used in individual cases of pregnancy toxemia in

combination with glucose administration and fluid therapy.
• Administration of B-complex vitamins to stimulate appetite.
• Protamine zinc insulin (20–40 units IM q48h) in combination with glucose and fluid therapy.
• Recombinant bovine somatotropin (0.15 mg/kg q24h SC or single injection of 160 mg of slow-release formulation SC) may increase efficiency of glucose and ketone usage. (Not currently approved for use in small ruminants in the US.)
• Dexamethasone (10–20 mg IM) with parturition in ewes generally occurring 36–48 hours following administration.
• Females that are managed with induction of parturition or cesarean section should be treated with broad-spectrum antimicrobials, a nonsteroidal anti-inflammatory, and oxytocin to facilitate placental passage and prevent metritis.

CONTRAINDICATIONS
Appropriate milk and meat withdrawal times must be followed for all compounds administered to food-producing animals.

PRECAUTIONS
N/A

POSSIBLE INTERACTIONS
N/A

FOLLOW-UP
EXPECTED COURSE AND PROGNOSIS
• Prognosis for dam survival and delivery of live offspring is good if the condition is diagnosed and treated early.
• The prognosis is usually poor if recumbency is prolonged.
• Induction of parturition/termination of the pregnancy or cesarean section is unpredictable for survival of the fetuses, and if delayed, for the dam as well.

POSSIBLE COMPLICATIONS
• Fetal death and septicemia
• Dystocia and retained placenta are common complications in dams that survive to the induced or natural parturition.

CLIENT EDUCATION
• The owner will need to evaluate the economics of therapy versus probable outcomes.
• Awareness of factors contributing to pregnancy toxemia and their avoidance.

PATIENT CARE
• Feed intake is a critical factor in monitoring for treatment success. If the animal is recumbent for a prolonged period, the odds of recovery are substantially reduced.
• The goal of therapy in pregnancy toxemia is to restore glucose homeostasis as soon as possible.

P

• Multiple electrolyte, acid-base, and fluid imbalances in addition to low blood glucose levels will need to be considered in any potential treatment plan.
• The affected dam should be isolated to reduce expenditures of energy and limit competition for feed resources.
• High-quality forages and concentrates should be offered in an attempt to stimulate intake.
• Transfaunation could be considered if a source of rumen fluid is available.

PREVENTION
• Prevention of future cases of pregnancy toxemia is best accomplished by evaluation of nutritional and management practices within the flock.
• Designing nutritional programs that meet the females' requirements based on the stage of production and relevant environmental and management conditions can prevent most cases of pregnancy toxemia.
• Ewes and does should have a BCS of 3 or 3.5/5 at the beginning of the breeding season and a BCS of 2.5–3.5/5 one month prior to parturition.
• Transabdominal ultrasonography performed in early gestation (day 40–70) can be useful for determination of fetal numbers and thus to adjust nutrition in the last trimester of pregnancy to meet the demands of twins and triplets.
• Close observation of ewes and does carrying multiple fetuses in the last 6 weeks of pregnancy.
• Avoid stress (transport, shearing) during the last month of pregnancy.
• Where possible blood samples should be collected to evaluate BHB levels. Females with elevated BHB levels should be separated and monitored closely.

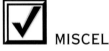 **MISCELLANEOUS**

ASSOCIATED CONDITIONS
Dystocia, retained placenta, respiratory disease

AGE-RELATED FACTORS
• More common in older ewes or does, not generally associated with maiden females.

ZOONOTIC POTENTIAL
• N/A

PREGNANCY
Pregnancy toxemia is present in dams in late gestation (generally the last 4–6 weeks).

BIOSECURITY
N/A

PRODUCTION MANAGEMENT
• Best managed as a production disease with primary emphasis placed on prevention of future cases.
• Nutritional and management factors must be addressed to minimize the impact within a population.

SYNONYMS
• Pregnancy ketosis
• Lambing ketosis
• Fatty liver syndrome
• Lambing paralysis
• Lambing sickness
• Pregnancy disease
• Twinning disease

ABBREVIATIONS
• BCS = body condition score
• BHB = beta-hydroxybutyrate
• BUN = blood urea nitrogen
• IM = intramuscular
• IV = intravenous
• NEFA = nonesterified fatty acid
• PO = per os
• SC = subcutaneous

SEE ALSO
• Cesarean Section: Small Ruminant
• Ewe Flock Nutrition (see www.fiveminutevet.com/ruminant)
• Goat Nutrition (see www.fiveminutevet.com/ruminant)
• Hypocalcemia: Small Ruminant
• Induction of Parturition
• Listeriosis
• Nutrition and Metabolic Diseases: Small Ruminant
• Reproductive Pharmacology
• Vitamin B Deficiency

Suggested Reading
Andrews A. Pregnancy toxaemia in the ewe. In Practice 1997, 19: 306–12.
Balikci E, Yildiz A, Gurdogan F. Investigation on some biochemical and clinical parameters for pregnancy toxemia in Akkaraman ewes. J Anim Vet Adv 2009, 8: 1268–73.
Brozos C, Mavrogianni VS, Fthenakis GC. Treatment and control of peri-parturient metabolic diseases: pregnancy toxemia, hypocalcemia, hypomagnesemia. Vet Clin North Am Food Anim Pract 2011, 27: 105–13.
Bulgin M. Diseases of the periparturient ewe. In: Youngquist RS, Threlfall WR eds, Current Therapy in Large Animal Theriogenology, 2nd ed. St. Louis: Saunders, 2007, pp. 695–700.
Campbell AJ, Pearson LK, Tibary A. Pregnancy toxemia in small ruminants: A review. Clin Theriogenol 2015, 7: 407–18.
Duehlmeier R, Fluegge I, Schwert B, et al. Insulin sensitivity during late gestation in ewes affected by pregnancy toxemia and in ewes with high and low susceptibility to this disorder. J Vet Intern Med 2013, 27: 359–66.
Duehlmeier R, Fluegge I, Schwert B, et al. Post-glucose load changes of plasma key metabolite and insulin concentrations during pregnancy and lactation in ewes with different susceptibility to pregnancy toxaemia. J Anim Physiol Anim Nutr 2013, 97: 971–85.
Duehlmeier R, Fluegge I, Schwert B, et al. Metabolic adaptations to pregnancy and lactation in German Blackheaded Mutton and Finn sheep ewes with different susceptibilities to pregnancy toxaemia. Small Rumin Res 2011, 96: 178–84.
Lacetera N, Bernabucci U, Ronchi B, et al. Effects of subclinical pregnancy toxemia on immune responses in sheep. Am J Vet Res 2001, 62: 1020–4.
Moallem U, Rozov A, Gootwine E, et al. Plasma concentrations of key metabolites and insulin in late-pregnant ewes carrying 1 to 5 fetuses. J Anim Sci 2012, 90: 318–24.
Rook JS. Pregnancy toxemia of ewes, does, and beef cows. Vet Clin North Am Food Anim Pract 2000, 16: 293–317.
Schlumbohm C, Harmeyer J. Twin-pregnancy increases susceptibility of ewes to hypoglycaemic stress and pregnancy toxaemia. Res Vet Sci 2008, 84: 286–99.
Van Saun RJ. Puerperal nutrition and metabolic diseases. In: Youngquist RS, Threlfall WR eds, Current Therapy in Large Animal Theriogenology, 2nd ed. St. Louis: Saunders, 2007, pp. 562–72.

Author Alexis Campbell
Consulting Editor Ahmed Tibary

BASICS

OVERVIEW
• A functional fetal hypothalamic-pituitary-adrenal (HPA) axis is required for onset of parturition in ruminants.
• Prolonged gestation is a rare occurrence resulting from alterations in the HPA axis that render the fetus incapable of secreting cortisol to initiate parturition.
• Prolonged gestation is that which extends beyond the expected mean for the species; 284 ± 10 days in the bovine and 148 ± 7 days in sheep.

INCIDENCE/PREVALENCE
Unknown; sporadic cases have been reported in various breeds of cattle and sheep.

GEOGRAPHIC DISTRIBUTION
N/A

SYSTEMS AFFECTED
Reproductive

PATHOPHYSIOLOGY
• Parturition involves a cascade of endocrine and biochemical events triggered by the fetal HPA.
• Briefly, under oxygenation limitation in late pregnancy the stressed fetus responds by an increase of ACTH. The fetal pituitary stimulates secretion of adrenal corticoids from the fetal adrenal cortex. Fetal cortisol promotes an enzymatic pathway to convert progesterone to estradiol and causes placental synthesis of $PGF2_\alpha$. These events promote luteolysis and stimulation of myometrial contractions and initiation of parturition.
• Prolonged gestation is primarily due to absence of this HPA cascade.
• In camelids, pregnancy length is extremely variable. Prolonged gestation may be due to placental insufficiency. Fescue toxicosis has been suspected but there is no scientific evidence as of yet.

HISTORICAL FINDINGS
• Overdue female based on breeding date.
• Failure of onset of parturition after expected date of parturition.
• In flocks of sheep where the breeding date is not known, ewes may go beyond the window of lambing based on joining period.

SIGNALMENT
• Prolonged pregnancy complaint is reported in cattle, sheep, and quite commonly in camelids.
• Some breeds of cattle are over-represented due to the implication of an autosomal recessive gene: Ayrshire, Belgian Blue, Guernsey, Holstein-Friesian, and Swedish Red.
• Reported gestation lengths in cases of prolonged gestation in cattle are in the range 305–526 days.

• In sheep, gestation lengths up to and exceeding 230 days have been reported.

PHYSICAL EXAMINATION FINDINGS
Lack of mammary development, vulvar edema, or relaxation of the sacro-sciatic ligaments of the dam.

CAUSES AND RISK FACTORS
• In cattle the condition is associated with some fetal abnormalities, genetics, and intoxication.
• In sheep, the condition has been associated with craniofacial deformities of the fetus induced by viral pathogens or teratogens.
• In camelids, prolonged pregnancy has been associated with severe nutritional restriction, harsh environmental conditions, and placental insufficiency.

GENETICS
Autosomal recessive type of prolonged gestation described in some breeds of cattle.

DIAGNOSIS

• First step in diagnosis is determining that insemination and calculated due dates are accurate and that no bull exposure occurred subsequent to recorded natural or artificial breeding.
• Transrectal palpation will reveal a fluid-filled uterus. A fetus may be palpable and its characteristics may differentiate prolonged gestation from fetal mummification or maceration.
• Transrectal ultrasonography may allow visualization of the fetus and placentomes.
• In some cases, prolonged gestation may be accompanied by abnormal fluid accumulation in the uterus resulting in hydrops amnii or hydrops allantois.
• Serial examinations may be necessary to definitively rule out inaccurate breeding dates.

DIFFERENTIAL DIAGNOSES
• Inaccuracies in record keeping due to human error include inaccurate insemination records, incorrect calculations of expected date of parturition, or undocumented natural or artificial breeding following initial insemination.
• Viral causes of hydrancephaly, anencephaly, porencephaly, microencephaly that may interfere with normal pituitary gland development such as Border disease, bovine viral diarrhea virus, Akabane virus, bluetongue virus, or Cache Valley virus.
• Abnormal development of the pituitary gland due to craniofacial deformities induced by ingestion of *Veratrum californicum* or *Veratrum album* during early gestation.
• Fetal death during gestation resulting in mummification or maceration of the fetus and apparently prolonged gestation due to a nonviable fetus.

CBC/BIOCHEMISTRY/URINALYSIS
N/A

OTHER LABORATORY TESTS
N/A

IMAGING
• Transrectal ultrasonography to identify structures associated with pregnancy such as placentomes and fetus.
• Transabdominal ultrasonography findings have not been reported to be different from healthy, nonstressed fetuses and would not differentiate prolonged gestation from a normal pregnancy.

OTHER DIAGNOSTIC PROCEDURES
N/A

PATHOLOGIC FINDINGS
• In some cases of prolonged gestation, the fetus continues to grow in utero and may weigh >90 kg at birth. Dystocia often results due to fetomaternal disproportion. These fetuses may also have hirsutism, long hooves, and delayed skeletal ossification.
• Alternately, fetal growth may cease during late gestation and the fetus remains in utero in a vegetative state. These fetuses are smaller in size, weighing 20–30 kg at birth. Affected fetuses may also have hypotrichosis, craniofacial deformities, or developmental arrest of the incisors and molars.
• Hypoplasia or aplasia of the adenohypophysis or adrenal cortex may be present on histologic examination of fetal tissues.
• Placentitis has also been reported in some cases of prolonged gestation.

TREATMENT

THERAPEUTIC APPROACH
• Induction of parturition is indicated upon determination of prolonged gestation.
• Induction in cattle may be achieved by administering a single dose of natural prostaglandin $F_{2\alpha}$ or analog (cloprostenol) or dexamethasone.
• Parturition should occur 24–72 hours following induction with either prostaglandin $F_{2\alpha}$ or dexamethasone. Induction failures may occur in 10–20% of cases.
• Induction in cattle with a combination of prostaglandin $F_{2\alpha}$ and dexamethasone allows for more predictable onset of parturition (25–42 hours in one study) and fewer induction failures.
• Since the ewe only relies on luteal progesterone through day 50 of gestation, prostaglandin $F_{2\alpha}$ alone is unlikely to be effective in inducing parturition in the case of prolonged gestation. Induction in sheep requires administration of dexamethasone (15–20 mg IM) to induce enzymes responsible for converting placental

P

PROLONGED PREGNANCY (CONTINUED)

progesterone to estradiol and initiate the parturition cascade.
• Induction of parturition in camelids should not be attempted unless the health of the dam is compromised.

SURGICAL CONSIDERATIONS AND TECHNIQUES
• In the case of induction failure or extreme fetal oversize due to prolonged gestation, cesarean section or fetotomy may be required.

MEDICATIONS

DRUGS OF CHOICE

Cattle
• PGF2$_\alpha$ (dinoprost tromethamine, 25 mg IM) or cloprostenol (500 mg, IM)
• Dexamethasone (20–30 mg, IM)

Sheep
• Dexamethasone (15–20 mg IM)

Goats
• PGF2$_\alpha$ (dinoprost, 15 mg IM) or cloprostenol sodium (75–100 µg IM)

CONTRAINDICATIONS
Appropriate milk and meat withdrawal times must be followed for all compounds administered to food-producing animals.

PRECAUTIONS
N/A

POSSIBLE INTERACTIONS
N/A

FOLLOW-UP

EXPECTED COURSE AND PROGNOSIS
• Animals should be monitored for dystocia, retained placenta, and metritis following induction of parturition.
• Camelids with prolonged pregnancy and no signs of distress should be monitored until

natural delivery. Neonates delivered after a prolonged pregnancy (>370 days in alpacas) should be examined for dysmaturity. Examination of the placenta may reveal lesions consistent with placental insufficiency.

POSSIBLE COMPLICATIONS
• Dystocia, retained placenta, metritis
• Neonatal maladjustment or death

CLIENT EDUCATION
Accurate record keeping for breeding and early pregnancy diagnosis

PATIENT CARE
Depends on decision for induction of parturition and follow-up.

PREVENTION
N/A

MISCELLANEOUS

ASSOCIATED CONDITIONS
Hydrops

AGE-RELATED FACTORS
N/A

ZOONOTIC POTENTIAL
N/A

PREGNANCY
• There is no data on recurrence of the problem in subsequent pregnancies, but animals should be monitored closely if rebred.

BIOSECURITY
N/A

PRODUCTION MANAGEMENT
Production animals with prolonged pregnancy and postpartum complications are usually culled from breeding.

ABBREVIATIONS
• ACTH = adrenal corticotropic hormone
• CL = corpus luteum
• HPA = hypothalamic pituitary adrenal

• IM = intramuscular
• PGF2$_\alpha$ = prostaglandin F2$_\alpha$
• SC = subcutaneous

SEE ALSO
• Camelid: Reproduction
• Hydrops
• Induction of Parturition
• Teratogens

Suggested Reading
Buczinski S, Belanger AM, Fecteau G, Roy JP. Prolonged gestation in two Holstein cows: Transabdominal ultrasonographic findings in late pregnancy and pathologic findings in the fetuses. J Vet Med A Physiol Pathol Clin Med 2007, 54: 624–6.
Cornellie P, Van Den Broeck W, Simoens P. Prolonged gestation in two Belgian Blue cows due to inherited adenohypophyseal hypoplasia in the fetuses. Vet Rec 2007, 161: 388–91.
Holm LW, Short RV. Progesterone in the peripheral blood of Guernsey and Friesian cows during prolonged gestation. J Reprod Fertil 1962, 4: 137–41.
Jackson PGG. Prolonged gestation in cattle and sheep. In: Kahn MA ed, The Merck Veterinary Manual, 9th ed. Whitehouse Station, Merck & Co., 2005.
McEntee K, Roberts SJ, Sears RM. Prolonged gestation in two Guernsey cows. Cornell Vet 1952, 42: 355–9.
Pearson LK, Rodrigues JS, Tibary A. Disorders and diseases of pregnancy. In: Cebra C, Anderson DE, Tibary A, et al. eds, Llama and Alpaca Care: Medicine, Surgery, Reproduction, Nutrition and Herd Health. St.Louis: Elsevier, 2014, pp. 256–73.
Van Kampen KR, Ellis LC. Prolonged gestation in ewes ingesting *Veratrum californicum*: Morphological changes and steroid biosynthesis in the endocrine organs of cyclopic lambs. J Endocr 1972, 52: 549–60.

Author Jennifer N. Roberts
Consulting Editor Ahmed Tibary

BASICS

OVERVIEW
• Proteins are nitrogen-containing compounds that occur in plants and animals, which are composed of amino acid (AA) chains of medium to large molecular weight. They are essential nutrients that serve as one of the building blocks of all tissues and can also serve as an energy source.
• In most if not all animal husbandry and production operations, adequate provision of protein represents the single highest cost in the diet, both through expenses associated with supplementation, as well as with production and preservation of forages.
• In animals, proteins function in structure, metabolism, transport, the endocrine system, and the immune system. Muscle, hormones and their receptors, enzymes and many blood constituents such as albumin are protein in nature.
• Prevention of protein-energy malnutrition (PEM) requires intake of essential AA.
• Accurately predicting AA requirements in ruminants poses the challenge of balancing for essential and limiting AA, not only for adequate nutrition, growth and maintenance functions, but also to support an adequate and efficient level of production.

INCIDENCE/PREVALENCE
N/A

GEOGRAPHIC DISTRIBUTION
N/A

SYSTEMS AFFECTED
Multisystemic

PATHOPHYSIOLOGY
• PEM results from a limited availability of protein, energy sources, or both. It can be primary, due to limited dietary content, or secondary, due to chronic, debilitating conditions.
• Though essential AA deficiency is rare in ruminants, low dietary AA, increased production demands, or chronic loss of protein lead to a catabolic state.

HISTORICAL FINDINGS
History of limited availability of food sources or presence of chronic wasting conditions.

SIGNALMENT
All ruminant species can be affected, without breed, age, or sex predilection.

PHYSICAL EXAMINATION FINDINGS
• Loss of body condition and in advanced cases cachexia, stunted growth, generalized weakness, decreased feed intake, marked loss of muscle mass, diarrhea, edema, impaired wound healing and immunity, and generalized impairment of all functions.
• Early changes in a herd or flock include decreased production, reproductive failure with delayed estrus, increased pregnancy losses, decreased conception rates, and low birthweights.

GENETICS
N/A

CAUSES AND RISK FACTORS
• Inadequate food availability or decreased intake
• Poor dietary formulation with low protein content
• Chronic, debilitating diseases

DIAGNOSIS

DIFFERENTIAL DIAGNOSES
All causes of chronic wasting disease.

CBC/BIOCHEMISTRY/URINALYSIS
None specific. Hypoalbuminemia in advanced stages with or without low urea/BUN.

OTHER LABORATORY TESTS
N/A

IMAGING
N/A

OTHER DIAGNOSTIC PROCEDURES
Diet analysis

PATHOLOGIC FINDINGS
Grossly, a cachectic carcass with complete fat depletion is observed.

TREATMENT

THERAPEUTIC APPROACH
The treatment of PEM is based on correction of dietary deficiencies to guarantee adequate provision of AA (particularly essential and limiting AA) to meet maintenance requirements and to support all production demands.

MEDICATIONS

DRUGS OF CHOICE
• Supplementary sources of enteral or parenteral AA can be used in addition to adequate dietary availability.
• If available and financially feasible, total parenteral nutrition may be used for initial rapid correction of the catabolic status of the patient.

PRECAUTIONS
N/A

CONTRAINDICTATIONS
Administration of partial or total parenteral nutrition is contraindicated in the presence of an active infection.

POSSIBLE INTERACTIONS
Many medications interact negatively with parenteral nutrition formulations.

FOLLOW-UP

EXPECTED COURSE AND PROGNOSIS
• If treated promptly and with provision of dietary sources of essential and limiting AA, the prognosis is good. A gradual weight gain, growth in young animals, and a return to production can be expected.
• Advanced cases of cachexia and debilitation secondary to PEM carry a poor prognosis and are unlikely to thrive.

POSSIBLE COMPLICATIONS
N/A

CLIENT EDUCATION
See "Production Management"

PATIENT CARE
Severely affected, cachectic animals should be sold if suitable for human consumption, or euthanized.

PREVENTION
Adequate access to a well-formulated diet and supplementation (variable for different species and production units)

MISCELLANEOUS

ASSOCIATED CONDITIONS
• Protein-losing nephropathy or enteropathy, neoplasia, and cachexia.
• Protein deficiency will result in partial anorexia, weight loss, stunted growth, delayed estrus, or decreased milk yield.

PREGNANCY
Appropriate protein nutrition is required for optimal fetal development and for normal reproductive function and lactation.

PRODUCTION MANAGEMENT
• Protein requirements vary between and within species. Within species, type and level of production, as well as stage of growth, affect protein requirements.
• Protein intake and essential AA balance is important to all animals.
• Primary methods of harvesting and preserving forage crops include silage making, hay making, green chopping, and pasturing. Each of these methods has benefits and limitations.
• Direct assessment of feed quality by appraisal, such as visual appearance, smell, and feel, are important tools for evaluating forages. Color, leaf content, stem texture, maturity, contamination from weeds, molds or soil, and observations on palatability are examples of useful visual determinations. Though useful, there are distinct limitations

P

PROTEIN NUTRITION

for measuring feed quality in this way only, therefore laboratory assessment is advised.

Protein Nutrition

• Adequate protein nutrition is required for optimal growth, reproduction, and maintenance in all animals, as well as for milk, meat, and wool production.
• Animals produce proteins from AA. Some AA can be synthesized and some, the essential AA, must be available in the diet and are required in the production of virtually all proteins.
• In ruminants, essential AA can be supplied by ruminal protozoa and bacteria. However, for optimal production, supplemental essential AA are usually incorporated into the diet.
• Sources of soluble nitrogen and carbon are required to synthesize bacterial proteins. Soluble dietary proteins are referred to as degradable intake proteins (e.g., soybean meal), whereas ruminal undegradable intake proteins (e.g., blood meal or feather meal) do not provide the ruminal bacteria with AA but must be digested in the abomasum and small intestine to obtain essential AA.
• An adequate balance of degradable and undegradable intake protein is essential for optimal ruminal health.
• Therefore, proper protein dietary formulations are absolutely essential for ruminant production.

Protein Sources and Analysis

• Protein is an important nutrient supplied by forages, and protein analysis assesses the quantity and quality of the protein present in the forage.
• A basic understanding of this analysis is essential for protein nutrition:
  ○ When a laboratory uses wet chemistry, crude protein will most likely be measured by the standard Kjeldahl procedure, which measures total nitrogen. The crude protein value includes both true protein and nonprotein nitrogen compounds.
  ○ The true protein derived from various plantstuffs is roughly 70% of the protein in

fresh forages, 60% in hay forage, and <60% in fermented forages.
  ○ Laboratories also frequently report a digestible protein value. This is an estimate of protein digestibility only, having limited value in ration formulation.
• Management and storage conditions of feedstuffs can also affect the nutritional quality and should be considered when assessing dietary protein content of forages:
  ○ When excessive heating of a forage occurs, a portion of the crude protein may be unavailable. If heat damage is suspected, an analysis for bound protein (acid detergent fiber crude protein, unavailable, insoluble protein) should be requested.
  ○ If bound or insoluble protein represents >12% of the crude protein content, enough heating to reduce protein digestibility has occurred.
• For ration formulation it is the amount of bound protein that is usually taken into account when determining protein requirements for animals:
  ○ Some laboratories report percent ACP as crude protein minus bound protein. Technically, this is incorrect as it does not account for the normal amount of bound protein in the forage.

ABBREVIATIONS

• AA = amino acids
• ACP = available crude protein
• BUN = blood urea nitrogen
• PEM = protein energy malnutrition

SEE ALSO

• Dairy Heifer Nutrition: Basics (see www.fiveminutevet.com/ruminant)
• Dairy Nutrition: Ration Guidelines for Milking and Dry Cows (see www.fiveminutevet.com/ruminant)
• Ewe Flock Nutrition (see www.fiveminutevet.com/ruminant)
• Goat Nutrition (see www.fiveminutevet.com/ruminant)
• Milk Cow Nutrition Monitoring (see www.fiveminutevet.com/ruminant)

• Nutritional Assessment (see www.fiveminutevet.com/ruminant)
• Starvation
• Urea Toxicity

Suggested Reading

Armstrong DG, Gong JG, Webb R. Interactions between nutrition and ovarian activity in cattle: physiological, cellular and molecular mechanisms. Reprod Suppl. 2003, 61: 403–14.

Britt JS, Thomas RC, Speer NC, Hall MB. Efficiency of converting nutrient dry matter to milk in Holstein herds. J Dairy Sci 2003, 86: 3796–801.

Cole NA, Todd RW. Opportunities to enhance performance and efficiency through nutrient synchrony in concentrate-fed ruminants. J Anim Sci 2008, 86(14 Suppl): E318–33.

Dunford LJ, Sinclair KD, Kwong WY, et al. Maternal protein-energy malnutrition during early pregnancy in sheep impacts the fetal ornithine cycle to reduce fetal kidney microvascular development. FASEB J 2014, 28: 4880–92.

Hersom MJ. Opportunities to enhance performance and efficiency through nutrient synchrony in forage-fed ruminants. J Anim Sci 2008, 86(14 Suppl): E306–17.

Lloyd LJ, Foster T, Rhodes P, Rhind SM, Gardner DS. Protein-energy malnutrition during early gestation in sheep blunts fetal renal vascular and nephron development and compromises adult renal function. J Physiol 2012, 590: 377–93.

Richardson JM, Wilkinson RG, Sinclair LA. Synchrony of nutrient supply to the rumen and dietary energy source and their effects on the growth and metabolism of lambs. J Anim Sci 2003, 81: 1332–47.

Author Carlos E. Medina-Torres
Consulting Editor Kaitlyn A. Lutz
Acknowledgment The author and book editors acknowledge the prior contribution of Daniel C. Rule.

P

BASICS

OVERVIEW
Pseudocowpox is a parapoxvirus that is closely related to contagious ovine ecthyma in sheep and bovine papular stomatitis in cattle.

INCIDENCE/PREVALENCE
Common disease of dairy cattle, less common in beef breeds

GEOGRAPHICAL DISTRIBUTION
Worldwide; common in North America

PATHOPHYSIOLOGY
• Virus spreads locally in the skin.
• The lesions are small, 2–5 mm erythematous macules and papules that develop on the teats, udder, and perineum.
• These lesions eventually rupture and crust over.

SIGNALMENT
• Most cases involve adult milking cows and tend to occur in cyclic infections with the introduction of new naïve animals and the waning of immunity in previously exposed older animals.
• The disease tends not to affect dry cows, heifers, and bulls.
• Calves suckling infected teats can develop oral lesions. Cutaneous lesions on the muzzle and lips of nonsuckling juvenile calves have also been observed.
• In camels, the disease forms proliferative lesions on the lips, muzzle, and eyelids.

PHYSICAL EXAMINATION FINDINGS
• Animals rarely develop fevers but there may be a drop in milk production due to teat irritation.
• Lesions begin as small macules and papules 2–5 mm in diameter, on the teat, udder, and perineum, which slowly expand to round reddened raised lesions 1–2 cm in diameter with an overlying ring-shaped scab or crust.
• Lesion does not usually form a central umbilicated pustule that is commonly observed in most poxvirus infections.
• In nursing calves, the lesions may be located in the oral cavity with raised, umbilicated, circular ulcers on the tongue or palate and can look similar to bovine papular stomatitis.

CAUSES AND RISK FACTORS
• Pseudocowpox, a parapox virus, is the causative agent.
• It is believed that there are no rodent or other animal vectors for pseudocowpox virus.
• Since cattle are the primary source of infection; exposure to virally contaminated milking equipment or udder cleaning supplies are the most common source of infection in adult cattle.
• The drinking of virally contaminated milk or drinking from contaminated bottles are a source of infection for calves.

DIAGNOSIS

DIFFERENTIAL DIAGNOSES
• Herpesvirus mammillitis (Allerton virus, bovine herpesvirus-2): This usually begins as small 2–3 mm vesicles or pustules that rupture, forming small slow-healing ulcers. These can coalesce into larger lesions that are slow to heal.
• Bovine papular stomatitis: This usually occurs in suckling calves but can occasionally be seen on the teats and udder of infected cattle. Lesions are often umbilicated with a central scab.
• Bovine papillomavirus: May cause fibropapillomas on the teats. Often the lesions are verrucous or plaque-like which may scab over due to trauma.
• Cowpox: This is a disease primarily of Europe with lesion having an umbilicated appearance on the udder and teat, which may have a central scab over the umbilicated region.
• Foot and mouth disease (FMD): Vesicles which ulcerate can be observed on teats and udder. Usually the oral vesicles and vesicles in the interdigital space are commonly seen associated with teat lesions, which would make it easy to differentiate from pseudocowpox.
• Vesicular stomatitis virus: Vesicles and ulcers can be seen on teats; however, most vesicles are usually associated with lesions in the mouth and occasionally on feet.
• Buffalo-pox virus (India/Pakistan region): Vaccina-virus with a disease similar to pseudocowpox virus. There are pox-like lesions on teats and udders of domesticated water buffalo and occasionally cattle.
• Brazilian vaccinia viruses: Endemic vaccinia-virus disease in Brazil with papules that develop into painful ulcers on the teats and udder of cattle.

CBC/BIOCHEMISTY/URINALYSIS
N/A

OTHER LABORATORY TESTS
• Virus isolation from infected scabs can assist in the identification of the virus.
• PCR testing of scab and other associated material.
• Electron microscopic evaluation of the scab will identify parapoxvirus particles.

PATHOLOGIC FINDINGS
• Gross findings: Small 2–5 mm erythematous macules and papules develop on the teats, udder, and perineum that rupture and crust over.
• As the lesions progress, the lesions enlarge to 1–2 cm in diameter with an erythematous outer rim and a peripheral ring-shaped scab present.
• If the scab is removed, there remains an ulcerated lesion that slowly heals.

• This differs from cowpox in that the lesion is not umbilicated.
• Histologically, the lesion is primarily epithelial with the epidermis undergoing vacuolar (ballooning) degeneration and vesicle formation. Older lesions have neutrophils filling the vesicle.
• Eosinophilic intracytoplasmic inclusions are present in the vacuolated epithelium.

TREATMENT

THERAPEUTIC APPROACH
• The lesions of pseudocowpox are usually self limiting and require little care other than keeping the lesion free of debris and preventing secondary bacterial infections of the open sore.
• In outbreaks, sanitation of the milking parlor equiptment and cleaning supplies is critical in lessening the spread of the disease.

MEDICATIONS

DRUGS OF CHOICE
If lesions become infected by secondary bacterial agents, systemic or topical antibiotics may be appropriate for treatment.

FOLLOW-UP

EXPECTED COURSE AND PROGNOSIS
Most animals recover without any problems.

POSSIBLE COMPLICATIONS
Secondary bacterial mastitis or dermatitis can occur in lesions.

PREVENTION
• Little immunity is present after infections.
• Animals probably transmit the disease during milking.

MISCELLANEOUS

AGE-RELATED FACTORS
Calves may become infected with the virus and have lesions in the mouth from suckling on infected teats.

ZOONOTIC POTENTIAL
• This disease can be transmitted to herdsmen working on infected animals.
• Lesions develop on the hands, fingers, and face.
• These lesions are usually discrete, round, slow healing ulcers.

ABBREVIATIONS
• FMD = foot and mouth disease
• PCR = polymerase chain reaction

P

SEE ALSO
- Bovine Papular Stomatitis
- Foot and Mouth Disease
- Teat Lesions
- Vesicular Stomatitis

Suggested Readings

Abubakr MI, Abu-Elzein EME, Housawi FMT, et al. Pseudocowpox virus: The etiological agent of contagious ecthyma (Auzdyk) in camels (*Camelus dromedarius*) in the Arabian peninsula. Vector Borne Zoonotic Dis 2007, 7: 257–60.

Cargnelutti JF, Flores MM, Teixeira FR, Weiblen R, Flores EF. An outbreak of pseudocowpox in fattening calves in southern Brazil. J Vet Diagn Invest 2012, 24: 437–41.

Gibbs EP. Viral diseases of the skin of the bovine teat and udder. Vet Clin North Am Large Anim Pract 1984, 6: 187–202.

Oguzoglu TC, Koc BT, Kirdeci A, Tan MT. Evidence of zoonotic pseudocowpox virus infection from a cattle in Turkey. Virusdisease 2014, 25: 381–4.

Wellenberg GJ, van der Poel WH, Van Oirschot JT. Viral infections and bovine mastitis: a review. Vet Microbiol 2002, 88: 27–45.

Author Robert B. Moeller Jr.

Consulting Editor Christopher C.L. Chase

P

PSEUDORABIES

BASICS

OVERVIEW
• Pseudorabies is a reportable disease caused by the alphaherpesvirus, Suid herpesvirus-1.
• The name is derived from the clinical similarities to rabies.

INCIDENCE/PREVALENCE
• Common herpesvirus virus of domestic swine; United States is free of the virus in domesticated swine. However, the virus is still identified in wild domestic swine.
• Rare occurrence in ruminants, usually history of cattle, sheep, or goats housed with infected swine.

GEOGRAPHIC DISTRIBUTION
Worldwide

SYSTEMS AFFECTED
Nervous

PATHOPHYSIOLOGY
• The primary host are domestic swine with aberrant infections in ruminants causing an encephalitis.
• Ruminants infected by exposure to the virus from infected swine (saliva or nasal secretions) through pig bites, open wounds, or contact with mucus membranes.
• Virus travels centripetally to the spinal cord and brain via peripheral nerves, resulting in a devastating progressive encephalitis/myelitis.

SIGNALMENT
• Swine are the primary host.
• Infections can occur primarily in sheep, goats, and cattle exposed to oral or nasal secretions from infected swine.
• Affected ruminants usually do not transmit the disease to other animals.

PHYSICAL EXAMINATION FINDINGS
• Duration of illness ranges from 2 hours to 3 days.
• Many animals die suddenly without clinical signs of illness.
• Ruminants often develop an intense local pruritus (mad itch) at the point of dermal contact with the pathogen. Sites of pruritus are often the head, shoulder, flank, limbs, and perineum. Head and neck region most commonly affected.
• Animals begin licking at the area, then scratch the skin against inanimate objects.
• This may progress until the animal becomes frenzied, resulting in hair loss, abrasions, or ulceration.
• Goats do not usually exhibit intense pruritus. Signs usually include restlessness, screaming, and profuse sweating.
• Animals progress to ataxia, depression or becomes excited with manic or aggressive behavior (rare). Head pressing, grinding of teeth, unusual bellowing, and convulsions may occur. Pharyngeal paralysis with excessive salivation and loss of tongue tone may occur.

• Elevated rectal temperatures up to 107°F (41.5°C) often are observed.
• Signs progress to lateral recumbency, paralysis, and death.
• Calves often develop oral and esophageal ulcers without pruritus, and clinical signs of an encephalitis in 6–48 hours. Pruritus is often absent.

CAUSES AND RISK FACTORS
• It is caused by a pseudorabies virus (Suid herpesvirus 1), an alphaherpesvirus.
• Close contact with infected swine is the primary source of infection for sheep, goats, and cattle.
• Swine that have recovered from infection are asymptomatic but continue to shed virus intermittently due to infection of the trigeminal ganglia. Viral shedding usually occurs when the pig is stressed.
• In ruminants, viral latency is not common, with these animals being a dead-end host.
• Infection can occur after exposure to the virus by intranasal, oral, intradermal, or subcutaneous routes. Virus spreads by retrograde axoplasmic transport to the CNS.
• Virus may be present in the ruminant's nasal mucosa, secretions, and saliva during acute infection.
• Ruminant and other animals infected (dog, cat, and rat) have a short transient infective period which may (highly unlikely) act as a source of infection.

DIAGNOSIS

DIFFERENTIAL DIAGNOSES
• Rabies
• Malignant catarrhal fever
• Bovine herpesvirus-1 and 5 (IBR)
• Ovine lentiviral encephalitis
• Bornavirus
• Ovine encephalomyelitis (louping ills, tick-borne encephalitis)
• Bovine spongiform encephalitis/scrapie
• Polioencephalomalacia
• Bacterial meningitis (*Listeria*, *Histophilus somni*, other septic bacterial pathogens)
• Hypomagnesemia/Hypocalcemia
• Toxicity—organophosphate, carbamate, lead, arsenic, salt poisoning, hepatotoxins
• Enterotoxemia (*Clostridium perfringens* type D)
• Pituitary abscess

CBC/BIOCHEMISTRY/URINALYSIS
Usually normal

OTHER LABORATORY TESTS
• CSF findings are consistent with encephalitis. Pleocytosis with increased mononuclear cells (50–200 cells/dL) and increased protein concentration (100–200 mg/dL).
• Virus isolation via cell culture or inoculation of rabbits with infected nervous tissues.

Sensory segments of the spinal cord serving the pruritic sites contain high concentrations of the virus.
• Immunofluorescent antibody, immunohistochemistry, or PCR testing on brain tissue may be useful to confirm the diagnosis.
• Serologic testing for rising antibodies is not useful in ruminants or other acutely infected animals.

PATHOLOGIC FINDINGS
• Gross lesions—alopecia, edema, dermal abrasions occur at the pruritic site with the possible presence of secondary bacterial pathogens.
• There is possible swelling or edema of regional lymph nodes.
• Histologic lesions—nonsuppurative meningoencephalitis with mononuclear perivascular cuffing and neuronal degeneration and necrosis observed in the brain.
• Eosinophilic intranuclear (Cowdry type A) inclusion bodies are often identified in neurons and glial cells.

TREATMENT

THERAPEUTIC APPROACH
• No effective treatment in ruminants.
• Supportive therapy and prevent self-injury due to pruritus if possible.
• Humane euthanasia may be the only source of relief if animal continues to deteriorate.

MEDICATIONS

DRUGS OF CHOICE
None

CONTRAINDICATIONS
• Do not vaccinate ruminants with modified-live virus vaccines targeted for use in swine.
• There have been reports of sheep infected by use of syringes contaminated with the MLV vaccine for swine.

FOLLOW-UP

EXPECTED COURSE AND PROGNOSIS
The majority of affected ruminants die within 2–3 days of the onset of clinical signs.

PREVENTION
• Prevent exposure of ruminants to swine or direct contact with any fomites that may transmit the virus from pigs to susceptible animals.

P

• Recovered swine should be culled as natural infections can result in the typical herpesvirus latency and a carrier state.
• Environmental inactivation of the virus can be achieved by drying, 6 hours of contact time with ultraviolet light, and high temperature (37°C).
• Contaminated pens and other surfaces can be disinfected with 10% bleach solution, quaternary ammonium compounds, iodine compounds, or phenolic compounds. At least 5 minutes of contact time is required before rinsing.
• Be sure to thoroughly clean all surfaces of organic matter before applying a disinfectant.

 MISCELLANEOUS

ASSOCIATED CONDITIONS
Infectious bovine rhinotracheitis (IBR) virus shares common antigens with the pseudorabies virus. Serologic tests can be affected by heterospecific antibodies to the IBR virus cross-neutralizing pseudorabies virus antibodies.

ZOONOTIC POTENTIAL
Humans are generally resistant to pseudorabies virus. There have been reports of pruritus when skin wounds came into direct contact with infected tissues. Use caution when working with infected swine or other animals.

BIOSECURITY
Do not allow swine direct contact with ruminants.

SYNONYMS
• Aujeszky's disease
• Infectious bulbar paralysis
• Mad itch

ABBREVIATIONS
• CNS = central nervous system
• CSF = cerebral spinal fluid
• IBR = infectious bovine rhinotracheitis
• MLV = modified-live virus
• PCR = polymerase chain reaction

SEE ALSO
• Arsenic Toxicosis
• Bovine Spongiform Encephalopathy
• Caprine Arthritis Encephalitis Virus
• Carbamate Toxicity
• Clostridial Disease: Gastrointestinal Down Bovine
• Clostridial Disease: Nervous System
• Grass Tetany/Hypomagnesemia
• *Histophilus somni* Complex
• Hypocalcemia: Bovine
• Hypocalcemia: Small Ruminant
• Infectious Bovine Rhinotracheitis
• Lead Toxicosis
• Listeriosis
• Maedi-Visna (Ovine Progressive Pneumonia)
• Organophosphate Toxicity
• Ovine Encephalomyelitis (Louping Ill)
• Rabies

• Scrapie
• Sodium Disorders: Hypernatremia
• Spinal Column and Cord Assessment and Dysfunction (see www.fiveminutevet.com/ruminant)
• Vitamin B Deficiency

Suggested Reading
Callan RJ, Van Metre DC. Viral diseases of the ruminant nervous system. Vet Clin North Am Food Anim Pract 2004, 20: 327–62.
Kahn CM, Line S ed. Pseudorabies. In: Merck Veterinary Manual, 10th ed. Whitehouse Station, NJ: Merck & Co., 2010.
Jones TC, Hunt RD, King NW ed. Pseudorabies (infectious bulbar paralysis, Aujeszky's disease, mad itch). In: Veterinary Pathology, 6th ed. Baltimore, MD: Williams & Wilkins, 1997.
Smith BP ed. Pseudorabies (mad itch; Aujeszky's disease). In: Large Animal Internal Medicine, 5th ed. St. Louis: Elsevier Mosby, 2015.
Timoney JF, Gillespie JH, Scott FW, Barlough JE ed. Pseudorabies. In: Hagan and Bruner's Microbiology and Infectious Diseases of Domestic Animals, 8th ed. Ithaca, NY: Comstock Publishing Associates, a division of Cornell University Press, 1992.
Author Robert B. Moeller Jr.
Consulting Editor Christopher C.L. Chase
Acknowledgment The author and book editors acknowledge the prior contribution of Lisa Nashold.

P

BASICS

OVERVIEW
• Pyelonephritis refers to bacterial infection of the kidney(s) that typically results from ascending infection of the lower urinary tract.
• In cattle, *E. coli* is the most common causal agent followed closely by *Corynebacterium renale* and other *Corynebacterium* species (*C. cystitidis* and *C. pilosum*). Whereas *E. coli* is an opportunistic pathogen of environmental origin, *C. renale* is a normal inhabitant of the ruminant genitourinary tract.
• Cattle subclinically infected with *C. renale* become carriers and can shed the organism in urine. The organism is capable of surviving in the environment for weeks.
• Other organisms associated with pyelonephritis in cattle include *Trueperella pyogenes*, alpha-hemolytic *Streptococcus* spp., *Proteus* spp., *Pseudomonas aeruginosa*, *Klebsiella* spp., and *Oligella urethralis*; some of these organisms establish infection via a hematogenous route (suppurative embolic nephritis).
• In small ruminants, *C. pseudotuberculosis* has been cultured from some renal infections.
• Both kidneys can be affected but pyelonephritis is usually unilateral, and can be acute or chronic in nature.

INCIDENCE/PREVALENCE
• Herd prevalence of pyelonephritis in one study ranged from 0.3% to 2.7%.
• 73% of cases of clinical disease developed within the first 90 days after calving.

GEOGRAPHIC DISTRIBUTION
Worldwide

SYSTEMS AFFECTED
Urinary

PATHOPHYSIOLOGY
• Irritation or damage of the caudal genitourinary tract from trauma (dystocia, obstetric manipulation, urolithiasis, bladder catheterization, etc.) provides ideal conditions for bacteria to attach and proliferate in the genitourinary mucosa.
• *C. renale* possesses pili that facilitate attachment to and colonization of the urinary tract mucosa. The organism can be contracted at breeding, from iatrogenic transmission, or through urine splashing and contact from carrier cows.
• Ascending infection to the bladder can result in signs of cystitis, and further ascension via the ureters to the kidneys results in inflammation, necrosis, and abscess formation within renal tissue.
• Fecal contamination of the caudal reproductive tract favors ascending infection with *E. coli*.
• Occasionally congenital disorders (ectopic ureters, abnormalities of the umbilicus/urachus) contribute to the development of pyelonephritis in juvenile ruminants.

HISTORICAL FINDINGS
• Many cases have a recent history of calving or urogenital procedures.
• Acute cases often have a history of sudden anorexia, fever, and reduced milk yield; chronically diseased animals may have a history of weight loss, wasting, diarrhea, and reduced milk production.

SIGNALMENT
Females, particularly adult postparturient dairy cows are most commonly affected.

PHYSICAL EXAMINATION FINDINGS
• Acute pyelonephritis is often represented by fever 103.5–105.5°F (39.7–40.8°C), anorexia, depression, tachycardia, and dehydration (reflected by enophthalmos).
• Some cows exhibit signs of colic such as treading, restlessness, kicking, tail swishing, and arched stance.
• Dysuria, stranguria, polyuria, hematuria, and pyuria can occur.

GENETICS
N/A

CAUSES AND RISK FACTORS
• Trauma to the caudal genitourinary tract associated with dystocia, obstetric manipulation, urolithiasis, bladder catheterization, etc.
• Urine stagnation (bladder paralysis, urolithiasis)
• Abnormal perineal/vulvar conformation
• Rectovaginal fistula
• Pneumovagina/metritis
• Presence of subclinical carriers of *C. renale* in the herd
• Venereal transmission
• Pregnancy

DIAGNOSIS

DIFFERENTIAL DIAGNOSES
• Enzootic hematuria
• Urolithiasis
• Vaginitis/cervicitis/metritis
• Perivaginal abscess
• Gastrointestinal disorders creating colic

CBC/BIOCHEMISTRY/URINALYSIS
• CBC can display neutrophilic leukocytosis and hyperfibrinogenemia. Anemia may be observed in chronic disease.
• Urine contains increased numbers of RBCs, WBCs; often substantially increased protein, and the presence of bacteria (perform Gram stain).
• Serum chemistry may demonstrate increased globulin and reduced albumin, particularly in chronic cases. Increases in BUN and creatinine can be prerenal (dehydration), renal (bilateral pyelonephritis with renal failure), or postrenal (obstruction of the ureters or urethra by blood clots or fibrin) in origin.
• The presence of azotemia in conjunction with non-concentrated urine specific gravity (<1.020) is suggestive of bilateral kidney involvement and probable renal insufficiency.

OTHER LABORATORY TESTS
Urine should be submitted for bacterial culture and antimicrobial sensitivity testing, preferably after collection by sterile catheterization to avoid sample contamination with skin organisms and reproductive discharge.

IMAGING
• Ultrasound examination may reveal dilation of renal calyces, presence of echogenic flocculent material within renal pelves, and renal enlargement.
• Thickening of the bladder wall might also be appreciated.
• The right kidney can be evaluated percutaneously; the left kidney may be obscured by the rumen in many animals and can be evaluated using per rectum ultrasonography.

OTHER DIAGNOSTIC PROCEDURES
• Per rectum examination may reveal loss of lobulations, increased size, and pain on palpation of the left kidney.
• Per vaginam examination may permit palpation of enlarged ureter(s) through the ventral vaginal wall.
• Cystoscopy allows evaluation of urine quality from each ureteral opening, and sampling of urine from each individual kidney. The bladder may appear inflamed, thickened, or ulcerated when visualized.

PATHOLOGIC FINDINGS
• Gross distortion of renal size and shape.
• Cross-section of affected kidney(s) may detect gray, viscous, odorless exudate in the renal pelvis with extension into the medulla and cortex.
• Renal abscesses may be present.
• Hemorrhage, ulceration, and fibrin deposition may be present on the mucosa of the bladder and urethra.
• Ureteral enlargement may be evident with purulent debris occluding the ureteral lumen.

TREATMENT

THERAPEUTIC APPROACH
• Antimicrobial selection is ideally based on the results of urine bacterial culture and sensitivity, and the ability of the drug to achieve high concentrations in the urine without nephrotoxic effects.
• Long-term (≥3 weeks) of antimicrobial therapy is crucial to treatment success.
• Intravenous or oral fluid therapy promotes diuresis and flushes the urinary tract, which is of value in acute disease.

P

PYELONEPHRITIS

• Acidification of urine to prevent adhesion of *C. renale* and other organisms may be of value.

SURGICAL CONSIDERATIONS AND TECHNIQUES

In cases of severe or nonresponsive unilateral pyelonephritis, nephrectomy may be indicated.

MEDICATIONS

DRUGS OF CHOICE

• Sodium, potassium, or procaine penicillin (22,000–44,000 IU/kg, q6–12h depending on formulation and severity of disease) is the usual drug of choice since *C. renale* is considered uniformly sensitive to penicillin; *E. coli* (despite being a Gram-negative organism) is often sensitive because of the very high concentrations of penicillin achieved in urine.
• Ampicillin trihydrate (11 mg/kg IM, q12h).
• Ammonium chloride (200 mg/kg PO, q24h).

CONTRAINDICATIONS

Nephrotoxic drugs should be avoided in azotemic animals.

PRECAUTIONS

• Appropriate milk and meat withdrawal times must be followed for all compounds administered to food-producing animals.
• Recommendations for specific drugs, including penicillin, involve extra-label administration.

POSSIBLE INTERACTIONS

N/A

FOLLOW-UP

EXPECTED COURSE AND PROGNOSIS

• Case fatality rate and cull rate due to pyelonephritis in cattle are approximately 18% and 33%, respectively.

• Bilateral pyelonephritis and pyelonephritis secondary to bladder paralysis, rectovaginal fistula, or other functional problems have a poorer prognosis.
• Chronic pyelonephritis and animals with azotemia are also associated with a lesser prognosis due to loss of renal function and lower likelihood of therapeutic response.

POSSIBLE COMPLICATIONS

• Renal insufficiency
• Renal abscessation

CLIENT EDUCATION

N/A

PATIENT CARE

Urinalysis and urine culture should be assessed one week after treatment is ceased, to ensure resolution; relapse rate can approach 10%.

PREVENTION

• Isolate affected animals to prevent shedding and environmental contamination.
• Practice aseptic technique when performing urogenital and obstetric procedures and thoroughly clean and disinfect equipment.
• Artificial insemination can help control venereal transmission in endemically affected herds.

MISCELLANEOUS

ASSOCIATED CONDITIONS

Renal failure

AGE-RELATED FACTORS

Usually a disease of mature females

ZOONOTIC POTENTIAL

N/A

PREGNANCY

Is a risk factor for this disorder

BIOSECURITY

N/A

PRODUCTION MANAGEMENT

Economic losses are associated with decreased production, culling, and treatment expense.

SYNONYMS

N/A

ABBREVIATIONS

• BUN = blood urea nitrogen
• RBCs = red blood cells
• WBCs = white blood cells

SEE ALSO

• Endometritis
• Postpartum Disorders
• Urolithiasis

Suggested Reading

Braun U, Nuss K, Wehbrink D, Rauch S, Pospischil A. Clinical and ultrasonographic findings, diagnosis and treatment of pyelonephritis in 17 cows. Vet J 2008, 175: 240–8.

Dominguez BJ. Urinary tract infection. In: Smith BP ed, Large Animal Internal Medicine, 5th ed. St. Louis: Elsevier Mosby, 2015, pp. 906–8.

Rebhun WC. Diseases of Dairy Cattle, 2nd ed. Philadelphia: Lippincott, Williams & Wilkins, 2008.

Rebhun WC, Dill SG, Perdrizet JA, Hatfield CE. Pyelonephritis in cows: 15 cases (1982–1986). J Am Vet Med Assoc 1989, 194: 953–5.

Rosenbaum A, Guard CL, Njaa BL, et al. Slaughterhouse survey of pyelonephritis in dairy cows. Vet Rec 2005, 157: 652–5.

Yeruham I, Elad D, Avidar Y, Goshen T. A herd level analysis of urinary tract infection in dairy cattle. Vet J 2006, 171: 172–6.

Author M.F. Chamorro
Consulting Editor Erica C. McKenzie
Acknowledgment The author and book editors acknowledge the prior contribution of M.S. Gill.

P

BASICS

OVERVIEW
• Pyometra is an intrauterine accumulation of pus associated with a persistent luteal state.
• It typically affects animals with existing uterine infections during the late postpartum period after the resumption of ovarian activity.
• As seasonal breeders, ewes and does generally deliver their young during the anovulatory season and are at very low risk for developing pyometra.
• Pyometra is described in camelidae but it is rarely associated with CL retention. In these species, pyometra is often the result of severe cervical or vaginal adhesions.

INCIDENCE/PREVALENCE
• Postpartum pyometra is relatively common in dairy cattle.
• Incidence of pyometra is in the range 5–15% in herds experiencing an outbreak of trichomoniasis.
• Pyometra is rare in camelids.

GEOGRAPHIC DISTRIBUTION
Worldwide

SYSTEMS AFFECTED
Reproductive

PATHOPHYSIOLOGY
• Pyometra develops when ovulation and CL formation occur in the presence of uterine infection, most commonly chronic endometritis.
• Failure of $PGF2_\alpha$ release from the endometrium results in luteal retention and maintenance of elevated serum progesterone which perpetuate the condition by keeping the cervix closed and inhibiting uterine contractions.
• In cattle, pyometra often develops following an infection with *Tritrichomonas foetus* and early pregnancy loss.
• The volume of purulent material in the uterus ranges from a few milliliters to several liters.
• In cows with preexisting uterine infections, exogenous GnRH treatment early in the postpartum period can result in an iatrogenic pyometra.
• In camelidae, pyometra has been linked to postpartum metritis, cervical or vaginal adhesions, and prolonged progesterone therapy.

HISTORICAL FINDINGS
• History of dystocia or postpartum complications
• Cattle herds using untested bulls for natural mating

SIGNALMENT
• Sexually mature female animals
• Lactating dairy cows in the postovulatory phase of the postpartum period
• Cycling beef or dairy cattle exposed to bulls infected with *Tritrichomonas foetus*

PHYSICAL EXAMINATION FINDINGS
• Systemic signs of disease are usually absent.
• Anestrus.
• Purulent or mucopurulent genital discharge may be present in some cases.

GENETICS
N/A

CAUSES AND RISK FACTORS
• Animals with retained fetal membranes with or without dystocia.
• Postpartum uterine infection.
• Animals that resume ovulatory cyclicity early in the postpartum and have concurrent endometritis.
• Ewes and does that cycle year-round may have a greater risk of developing pyometra as a sequela to postpartum metritis or endometritis.
• Birthing trauma and cervical adhesions, especially in camelids.
• Natural service with *Tritrichomonas fetus*–infected bulls may result in a post-breeding (as opposed to postpartum) pyometra.
• Although the initial insult is a microbial infection (*Fusobacterium necrophorum* and *Trueperella pyogenes* are most often incriminated), determining the specific etiologic agent is necessary only if *T. foetus* is suspected. Successful treatment of pyometra does not generally require identification of a specific etiologic agent, and newer diagnostic methods suggest that the microbiota of postpartum uterine disease may be vastly more complicated and dynamic than indicated by traditional culture techniques.

DIAGNOSIS

DIFFERENTIAL DIAGNOSES
• Mucometra or hydrometra
• Pregnancy
• Macerated fetus
• Anestrus

CBC/BIOCHEMISTRY/URINALYSIS
N/A

OTHER LABORATORY TESTS
Culture and sensitivity testing as well as cytologic evaluation of the uterine contents are rarely performed. Most affected animals are treated on the basis of physical diagnosis.

IMAGING
Transrectal or transabdominal ultrasonography

OTHER DIAGNOSTIC PROCEDURES
• Palpation per rectum (cattle, camelids)
  ○ Enlarged uterus with palpable fluid distention, the tone may or may not mimic normal pregnancy
  ○ Absence of positive signs of pregnancy (fetal membrane slip, amniotic vesicle, fetus, and placentomes in cattle, fetus in camelids)
• Ultrasonography (all species)
  ○ Transrectal (cattle, camelids) or transabdominal (sheep, goats) ultrasonography provides a definitive diagnosis.
• Vaginoscopy may reveal the presence of purulent material in the cranial vagina. In camelids, vaginal or cervical adhesions may be evident.

PATHOLOGIC FINDINGS
N/A

TREATMENT

THERAPEUTIC APPROACH
• In ruminants, treatment is directed at terminating what is essentially a pseudopregnancy. $PGF2_\alpha$ treatment is usually sufficient in cattle, sheep, and goats.
• Camelids may benefit from physical removal of the uterine contents by flushing or lavage followed by local or systemic broad-spectrum antibiotic therapy for 5–7 days. This is only possible if there are no vaginal or cervical adhesions.

SURGICAL CONSIDERATIONS AND TECHNIQUES
Ovariohysterectomy may be considered in companion animals.

MEDICATIONS

DRUGS OF CHOICE
• $PGF2_\alpha$ IM (dinoprost, cattle: 25 mg; small ruminants; 5–10 mg) or (cloprostenol, cattle: 500 µg, small ruminants, 75–250 µg) repeated at 11- to 14-day intervals until the uterus is emptied and normal cycles resume.
• Camelids should be treated IM with cloprostenol if a CL is detected by ultrasonography (100 µg for alpacas, 250 µg for llamas, 500 µg for camels).
• Antibiotic therapy is not indicated for pyometra in cattle, but sheep, goats, and camelids may benefit from a 5- to 7-day course of systemic therapy. Intrauterine antibiotic therapy may be used in camelids.

CONTRAINDICATIONS
Appropriate milk and meat withdrawal times should be followed for all compounds administered to food-producing animals.

PRECAUTIONS
N/A

POSSIBLE INTERACTIONS
N/A

P

PYOMETRA

FOLLOW-UP

EXPECTED COURSE AND PROGNOSIS
• Prognosis for fertility is good to fair in dairy cattle responding to the treatment. Most cattle (90%) will respond to PGF2$_\alpha$ treatments by evacuating the uterus. Normal fertility can be expected at the second or third estrus after resolution.
• Cattle with confirmed diagnosis of trichomoniasis should be culled.
• In camelids, prognosis for fertility depends on the cause. Prognosis is poor if there are cervical or vaginal adhesions.

POSSIBLE COMPLICATIONS
• Infertility due to failure to resolve the pyometra is the most frequent complication and may result in a decision to cull the female.
• Salpingitis, ovarian bursitis, and peritonitis may occur if uterine contents are expressed in a retrograde manner.

CLIENT EDUCATION
• Owners should submit anestrus females for reproductive evaluation.
• Trichomoniasis should be ruled out in bull bred herds.
• Use proper procedures during obstetric manipulations.

PATIENT CARE
• Treated animals should be monitored every 1–2 weeks to confirm that the uterine contents have been evacuated and estrous cycles have resumed.
• Most affected ruminants will respond after 1 or 2 treatments but rarely as many as 4 or 5 treatment cycles may be necessary.
• Camelids with vaginal or cervical adhesions should be removed from breeding and monitored for any complication.

PREVENTION
• Management of the peripartum animal to minimize the incidence of dystocia and postpartum uterine disease.
• Pre-breeding examinations.
• Incorporating PGF2$_\alpha$ presynchronization into ovulation synchronization programs for breeding dairy cows will prevent most cases of pyometra from developing.

MISCELLANEOUS

ASSOCIATED CONDITIONS
• Hydrometra
• Infertility and subfertility
• Metritis
• Endometritis
• Dystocia
• Retained fetal membranes

AGE-RELATED FACTORS
N/A

ZOONOTIC POTENTIAL
N/A

PREGNANCY
• Care should be taken to rule out normal pregnancy before initiating treatment as PGF2$_\alpha$ is abortigenic throughout pregnancy in goats and camelids and will terminate early pregnancy in sheep and cows.

BIOSECURITY
Measures to prevent the introduction of trichomoniasis

PRODUCTION MANAGEMENT
N/A

SYNONYMS
N/A

ABBREVIATIONS
• CL = corpus luteum
• GnRH = gonadotropin releasing hormone
• IM = intramuscular
• PGF2$_\alpha$ = prostaglandin F2$_\alpha$ and its synthetic analogs

SEE ALSO
• Congenital Defects: Camelid
• Dystocia: Bovine
• Dystocia: Camelid
• Dystocia: Small Ruminant
• Endometritis
• Hydrometra
• Infertility and Subfertility Issues
• Metritis
• Retained Placenta
• Uterine Anomalies

Suggested Reading
Knudsen LR, Karstrup CC, Pedersen HG, Agerholm JS, Jensen TK, Klitgaard K. Revisiting bovine pyometra–new insights into the disease using a culture-independent deep sequencing approach. Vet Microbiol 2015, 175: 319–24.
Palmer C. Postpartum uterine infection. In: Hopper RM ed, Bovine Reproduction. Ames: Wiley Blackwell, 2015, p. 440.
Tibary A. Breeding soundness evaluation and subfertility in female llamas and alpacas. In: Youngquist RS, Threlfall WR eds, Current Therapy in Large Animal Theriogenology, 2nd ed. Philadelphia: Saunders, 2007, pp. 878–83.
Authors Harry Momont and Celina Checura
Consulting Editor Ahmed Tibary
Acknowledgment The authors and book editors acknowledge the prior contribution of Carlos A. Risco.

P

PYRROLIZIDINE ALKALOIDS

BASICS

OVERVIEW
• Among ruminants, most cases of pyrrolizidine alkaloid (PA) poisoning occur in cattle.
• Sheep and goats are relatively resistant to PA intoxication.
• Llamas and alpacas appear to be similar to sheep and goats when it comes to susceptibility.
• The three plant families Compositae, Leguminosae, and Boraginaceae contain the majority of PA-containing plants.
• The genera *Senecio* (*S. vulgaris*, common groundsel; *S. jacobaea*, tansy ragwort; *S. riddelli*, Riddell's groundsel; *S. flaccidus*, threadleaf groundsel) and *Cynoglossum officinale* (houndstongue) have been implicated in most of the animal poisonings in the United States.
• Plants in the genera *Amsinckia*, *Crotalaria*, *Heliotropium*, and *Echium* less commonly cause poisonings either because they are not palatable or do not grow in dense enough stands to pose a significant risk.
• Poisonings generally occur as a result of cattle grazing heavily-contaminated pastures (rare—most of these plants are not palatable) or consuming contaminated hay (most common route). Exposures are typically over several weeks to months duration.
• The alkaloid content can vary tremendously among plants; concentrations vary with respect to age and stage of maturity of the plant, and soil and weather conditions.
• Poisonings are most commonly chronic in nature; acute exposures are rare.
• This is generally a herd problem, although individual animals may be selected.
• The clinical signs can be slow and insidious, with general debilitation and weight loss a common complaint. Some affected animals show abrupt onset of signs associated with hepatoencephalopathy.
• The liver is the primary target; kidney, lung, and heart tissue are less commonly affected.
• Megalocytosis, biliary hyperplasia, and fibrosis are commonly reported histologic findings on postmortem examination of the liver.
• Prognosis is guarded to grave for affected animals.

INCIDENCE/PREVALENCE
• Unpredictable and uncommon; however, it is one of the more common causes of plant intoxication in some areas of the US.
• Poisonings can occur all year round through grazing contaminated pastures or ingesting heavily contaminated hay.

GEOGRAPHIC DISTRIBUTION
Worldwide

SYSTEMS AFFECTED
• Multisystemic
• Respiratory
• Urinary

PATHOPHYSIOLOGY
• PAs are rapidly absorbed from the gastrointestinal tract.
• They undergo extensive metabolism in the liver. Some PAs are detoxified to harmless metabolites, but some are converted to highly toxic pyrroles.
• It is these pyrroles that alkylate DNA, leading to inhibition of cell mitosis and the ultimate histologic change of megalocytosis. As these megalocytes die, they are replaced by fibrous connective tissue.
• Though the liver is the primary target, lung, kidney, and heart tissue may be affected as well.

SIGNALMENT
• Cattle are most susceptible.
• Sheep, goats, llamas, and alpacas are relatively resistant.
• Resistance appears to be partly due to differences in rumen metabolism.
• Young animals appear to be more sensitive.

PHYSICAL EXAMINATION FINDINGS
• Some animals suffer chronic weight loss and debilitation associated with chronic liver insufficiency.
• Weakness and sluggishness.
• Secondary photosensitivity and icterus.
• Some animals exhibit an abrupt onset of signs associated with hepatic encephalopathy—mania, derangement, aimless walking, head pressing, blindness, and ataxia.
• Less commonly observed signs include inspiratory dyspnea (reported in horses), GI impactions, ascites, and diarrhea.

CAUSES AND RISK FACTORS
• A minimum of 2–4 weeks, up to several months, of exposure to these plants is generally required in order to induce toxicity.
• Acute exposures can occur if animals ingest 5–10% of their body weight of plant material within a few days to a few weeks (rare).
• It is more common to see poisonings in animals that ingest 25–50% of their body weight in plant material over a period of several months.
• Signs can occur suddenly in animals where the exposure to PA-containing plants ceased weeks or months previously.
• Approximate chronic toxic dose (for tansy ragwort) for an adult cow is 0.4 kg dry plant or 1.7 kg fresh plant per day for several weeks.
• For Riddell's groundsel, approximately 33 g dry or 176 g fresh plant daily for 3 weeks could be toxic to an adult cow.
• An approximate toxic dose of threadleaf groundsel in adult cows is 150 g dry or 750 g fresh plant daily for 2 weeks.

• A daily dose of 136 g dry or 680 g fresh houndstongue daily could be toxic to cattle over a period of a few weeks.

DIAGNOSIS

DIFFERENTIAL DIAGNOSES
Acute hepatitis or cholangiohepatitis, liver abscess, viral or bacterial encephalitis, aflatoxicosis, exposure to nitrosamines, hepatotoxic cyanobacteria.

CBC/BIOCHEMISTRY/URINALYSIS
• Inflammatory leukogram can be observed.
• Hyperbilirubinemia.
• Elevations in gamma-glutamyl transpeptidase, alkaline phosphatase, aspartate aminotransferase, and sorbitol dehydrogenase may also be elevated.
• Hypoalbuminemia, hypoproteinemia, and low blood urea nitrogen are less consistent abnormalities.

OTHER LABORATORY TESTS
• Severely elevated bile acids
• Characteristic histologic lesions of a liver biopsy

IMAGING
Ultrasound may reveal a small liver.

OTHER DIAGNOSTIC PROCEDURES
• One should examine the diet for the presence of PA-containing plants.
• Pyrrole testing of blood or hepatic tissue has been done, but it is not commonly performed at diagnostic laboratories. The analysis is not quantitative nor sensitive, particularly in the late stages of the disease.

PATHOLOGIC FINDINGS
• Poor body condition.
• Jaundice.
• Ascites and generalized edema.
• Small, pale, firm liver with mottled cut service may be visualized on necropsy.
• Characteristic lesions of hepatic megalocytosis with piecemeal necrosis, biliary hyperplasia, and generalized fibrosis.
• Kidney changes may include megalocytosis of the proximal convoluted tubules, glomerular atrophy, and tubular necrosis,
• Other less commonly recognized lesions include myocardial necrosis, gastrointestinal edema and hemorrhage, adrenal cortical hypertrophy, pulmonary edema, interstitial pneumonia, and status spongiosus of brain tissue (not all reported in ruminants).

TREATMENT

THERAPEUTIC APPROACH
• Find and remove the suspect source or remove animals from the contaminated environment.

P

• Most animals respond poorly to treatment, because by the time the disease is diagnosed, adequate regeneration of the liver is not possible.
• No specific treatment regime has been shown to be effective in treating these animals.
• Dietary changes could include switching to one that is highly digestible, high in calories, and low in protein.
• Treatment is typically not an economically viable option for most producers.

MEDICATIONS

DRUGS OF CHOICE
None

FOLLOW-UP

EXPECTED COURSE AND PROGNOSIS
• The more severely affected animals have a poor prognosis. Many are euthanized due to debilitation and poor response to therapy, or because of financial constraints.
• Patients showing severe neurologic signs often do not respond well to treatment.
• Some patients may survive after several months of intensive supportive care, but often are not able to regain their former activity or production level.

POSSIBLE COMPLICATIONS
• Avoid using medications that require extensive hepatic metabolism.
• Pneumonia and chronic wasting.

PATIENT CARE
• Monitor appetite, weight, and serum chemistries to evaluate liver enzymes, albumin, and protein.
• Serum chemistry panels should be run periodically to evaluate liver function.

PREVENTION
• Be able to recognize PA-containing plants either in the pasture or in hay.
• Avoid feeding "weedy" hay.
• Appropriate herbicide use can control the growth of these plants in the field.
• Sheep and goats can perhaps be used to control stands of these plants through rotational grazing.

MISCELLANEOUS

AGE-RELATED FACTORS
Young animals appear to be more susceptible.

PREGNANCY
PAs have been shown to cross the placenta and some are secreted into the milk. The risk of these routes having a significant impact on the developing fetus or nursing young is extremely low.

PRODUCTION MANAGEMENT
Avoid feeding "weedy" PA-containing hay. Be able to recognize these plants in pastures or hay.

SYNONYMS
• Seneciosis
• Venoocclusive disease

ABBREVIATIONS
• GI = gastrointestinal tract
• PA = pyrrolizidine alkaloid

SEE ALSO
• Mycotoxins
• Blue-Green Algae Poisoning
• Liver Abscesses

Suggested Reading
Burrows GE, Tyrl RJ. Zigadenus. In: Burrows GE, Tyrl RJ eds, Toxic Plants of North America. Ames: Iowa State University Press, 2013.
Cheeke P. Natural Toxicants in Feeds, Forages, and Poisonous Plants. Danville, IL: Interstate Publishers, 1998.
Molyneux RJ, Johnson AE, Olsen JD, Baker DC. Toxicity of pyrrolizidine alkaloids from Riddell groundsel (*Senecio riddellii*) to cattle. Am J Vet Res 1991, 52: 146–51.
Skaanild MT, Friis C, Brimer L. Interplant alkaloid variation and *Senecio vernalis* toxicity in cattle. Vet Hum Toxicol 2001, 43: 147–51.
Stegelmeier B. Pyrrolizidine alkaloids. In: Plumlee KH ed, Clinical Veterinary Toxicology. St. Louis: Mosby, 2004.

Author Steve Ensley
Consulting Editor Christopher C.L. Chase
Acknowledgment The author and book editors acknowledge the prior contribution of Patricia Talcott.

P

Q FEVER (COXIELLOSIS)

 BASICS

OVERVIEW
• Q (Query) fever is a highly infectious zoonotic disease caused by the intracellular bacterium *Coxiella burnetii* that primarily affects goats, sheep, cattle, and humans. Other species less commonly affected include dogs, cats, rabbits, a variety of wild and domestic mammals, and birds.
• The majority of *C. burnetii* infections in ruminants are subclinical, but abortion and infertility are common manifestations when naïve groups are exposed to the organism.
• Asymptomatic animals can shed *C. burnetii* for long periods of time in reproductive secretions, milk, urine, and feces.
• Epidemiologic studies indicate that Q fever is a public health problem in many countries.
• In humans, Q fever is considered an occupational hazard with the majority of infections occurring in livestock workers, veterinarians, and personnel of animal research facilities.
• In the United States, *C. burnetii* is classified as a category B potential aerosolized biological weapon.

INCIDENCE/PREVALENCE
• Information on the prevalence of Q fever in animal species is limited. Worldwide prevalence of serum antibodies from animal-based or farm-based surveys varies from 0% to 48% and from 0% to 100%, respectively.
• Q fever can be endemic in areas where reservoir animals are found.

GEOGRAPHIC DISTRIBUTION
Q fever is a zoonosis with a worldwide distribution with the exception of New Zealand.

SYSTEMS AFFECTED
Reproductive

PATHOPHYSIOLOGY
• *C. burnetii* is an obligate, intracellular, Gram-negative bacterium that replicates within the phagolysosome of infected cells.
• Among ruminants, *C. burnetii* is transmitted mainly through inhalation of contaminated dust or droplets and by ingestion of contaminated feed or water.
• After experimental inoculation of pregnant goats, the chorioallantoid membrane is the primary target for *C. burnetii*. The organism also localizes in the mammary gland, supramammary lymph nodes, and uterus in domestic ruminants.
• As with other infections, the initial antibody response is mediated by IgM, subsequently switching to a predominately IgG reaction.
• A characteristic of *C. burnetii* is its phase variation due to partial loss of polysaccharide that results in antigenic drift. During the acute phase of infection, ELISA can detect predominately IgM antibodies against phase II antigens. Later, IgG, IgA, and to a lesser extent IgM antibodies against phase I antigens appear. Studies to characterize the cellular immune response against phase I and II *C. burnetii* antigens in domestic animals are lacking.
• After inoculation, *C. burnetii* phase II specific antibodies, both IgM and IgG, can be detected 2 weeks post-infection and remain increased for up to 13 weeks. Antibodies directed against *C. burnetii* phase I increase as well, but about 4 weeks later compared to the phase II antibodies. Serum antibodies in infected animals can be detected for several months up to years.
• The organism can be shed in milk, urine, feces, placenta, and parturient discharges during subsequent pregnancies and lactations.
• In chronically infected animals, *C. burnetii* is also shed in the feces and urine.
• *C. burnetii* is highly resistant to heat, desiccation, and many common disinfectants, and can survive in the environment for long periods of time.
• Ingestion and inhalation of contaminated aerosols from amniotic fluid or placenta of infected animals are considered the main avenues of transmission.
• Contaminated hides and wool, and dust from barns, can be a source of infection for people and other animals either by direct contact or by inhalation of airborne particles.
• Consumption of raw milk contaminated with *C. burnetii* can be a risk factor for Q fever infection in humans and animals.
• *C. burnetii* has been found in the semen of bulls and rams, but the likelihood of this route of transmission is not well documented.
• Over 40 tick species can be naturally infected with *C. burnetii* and a sylvatic cycle based on *C. burnetii* tick-borne transmission has been proposed. However, the recent discovery of many tick-borne *Coxiella*-like bacteria with cross-reactivity to *C. burnetii* suggests that tick transmission may not be important.
• Dogs and cats may be infected by consumption of placentas or milk from infected ruminants, and by the aerosol route.

HISTORICAL FINDINGS
N/A

SIGNALMENT
• Sheep, goats, cattle, and ticks (ixodid and argasid) are considered the primary reservoirs. In general, goats are considered more susceptible than sheep.
• Humans and other animal species, including dogs, cats, rabbits, horses, pigs, rodents, pigeons, and other fowl, may also get infected with *C. burnetii*.
• Infection causes the greatest mortality in fetal or newborn animals. Adult animals are usually asymptomatic.

PHYSICAL EXAMINATION FINDINGS
• In domestic animals, Q fever is mostly associated with abortion outbreaks in small ruminants and sporadic abortions in cattle. The incubation period of Q fever is variable.
• Affected adult ruminants are usually asymptomatic; when clinical disease occurs, reproductive failure is usually the only signs. This can manifest as abortions, stillbirths, retained placentas, infertility; or the birth of weak neonates.
• Late-term abortions are typical and occur over a 2- to 4-week period. Between 5% and 50% and in some cases up to 90% of pregnant ewes or goats in a group may abort, with no previous clinical signs.
• An increased incidence of postpartum metritis has been observed in dairy goats that experience abortions caused by *C. burnetii*.
• Some infected animals can become carriers and the infection may be reactivated in subsequent pregnancies, resulting in shedding of the organism even though pregnancy may result in normal, viable offspring.
• In cattle, infertility, sporadic abortion, and low birthweights are seen.

GENETICS
N/A

CAUSES AND RISK FACTORS
• Parturient materials containing *C. burnetii* are highly infective and can contain large numbers of the organism.
• *C. burnetii* is extremely stable in the environment and can be transmitted to other animals via aerosol (airborne droplets or contaminated dust) and direct contact with placental tissues and parturient fluids, feces, or urine of infected animals.
• Fomites (e.g., wool, bedding, clothing), ingestion of parturient material, contaminated water or raw milk, or arthropods may also play a role in transmission.
• The infective dose of *C. burnetii* is very low, and it is considered that one to ten organisms can initiate an infection. In addition, due to the highly resistant nature of the organism to adverse environmental conditions, particles carrying *C. burnetii* can remain infectious for months and be transported long distances by wind currents.
• Young naïve pregnant small ruminants are very susceptible and abortion storms are common.
• The risk of animals in a herd or flock being infected increases in geographic areas with high wind speed, open landscape, high environmental temperature, low precipitation, and high animal densities.

 DIAGNOSIS

DIFFERENTIAL DIAGNOSES
Differentials include other causes of abortion and infertility, such as brucellosis,

Q

leptospirosis, campylobacteriosis, salmonellosis, listeriosis, chlamydiosis, mycotic abortion, toxoplasmosis, BVD, and IBR.

CBC/BIOCHEMISTRY/URINALYSIS
N/A

OTHER LABORATORY TESTS
N/A

IMAGING
N/A

OTHER DIAGNOSTIC PROCEDURES
• Currently, the preferred method to establish the diagnosis of Q fever in aborted fetuses is the demonstration of *C. burnetii* DNA within the affected placenta or other tissues, using several polymerase chain reaction (PCR) formats including conventional PCR, real-time PCR (RT-PCR), multiplex PCR, and nested PCR.
• Samples for PCR diagnosis include placenta, vaginal discharges, and liver, lung or stomach contents of aborted fetuses. However, performing necropsies of aborted fetuses of small ruminants in a veterinary clinic setting or farm facilities is discouraged due to the high risk of contaminating the premises. The entire placenta and fetus should be submitted overnight to the diagnostic laboratory, double bagged with refrigerant (gel coolants), and sealed in a leakproof insulating container.
• *C. burnetii* real-time PCR also has been used to detect the organism in vaginal swabs, milk, and colostrum of dams that have aborted.
• In general, the sensitivity of real-time PCRs based on multicopy genes (e.g., IS1111) is higher than those based on single copy genes.
• Loop mediated isothermal amplification (LAMP) assays have been developed with reportedly reliable results, but are not available in veterinary diagnostic laboratories.
• The demonstration of *C. burnetii*-specific antibodies in the serum of adult animals is the most practical indirect method to establish a diagnosis of Q fever. In domestic animals ELISA and complement fixation (CF) test are most often used.
• Testing of bulk tank milk samples by ELISA or real-time PCR has been used infrequently in sheep and goats.
• Currently, microagglutination and immunofluorescence assay (IFA) are less frequently used. Phase II antibodies dominate the humoral immune response in the acute phase of the infection, whereas phase I antibodies are prominent in the chronic phase. IFA is no longer available in most veterinary diagnostic laboratories.
• The sensitivity and specificity of ELISA and CF test vary depending on the tests used. When the sensitivity and specificity of two commercially available ELISA kits and the CF were compared, the sensitivity of the ELISA was in the range 97–100% and the specificity was in the range 95–100%. The sensitivity

and specificity of the CF test was 89% and 82%, respectively.
• Serologic tests are good indicators of previous exposure but provide no information on the infectious status of individual animals.
• *C. burnetii* does not grow on artificial media, but can be isolated in cell culture, embryonated chicken eggs, and some laboratory animals, such as mice and guinea pigs. *C. burnetii* can be detected from vaginal discharges, the placenta, placental fluids, aborted fetuses, as well as milk, urine, and feces. However, cultivation of *C. burnetii* is not recommended for routine diagnosis because the process is difficult, time-consuming, and dangerous; culture requires a biosafety level 3 (BSL-3) laboratory practice because the organism is highly infective and represents a health hazard for laboratory workers.
• *C. burnetii* does not stain well with the traditional Gram technique, but takes a magenta color with the Gimenez, modified Ziehl-Neelsen, or Macchiavello stains and stains purple with Giemsa stain.
• Confirmation of the diagnosis in formalin fixed tissues can be achieved by immunohistochemical staining.
• *C. burnetii* is a BSL-3 zoonotic agent; therefore, personal protective measures should be taken.
• Due to the recent identification of many *Coxiella*-like bacteria, future research about potential cross-reactivity between *C. burnetii* and *Coxiella*-like bacteria is necessary to better evaluate the current specificity of diagnostic methods and screening tools used in vertebrates.

PATHOLOGIC FINDINGS
• Macroscopically, the placenta (chorioallantoic membrane) is often affected and is the preferred sample for confirmation of the diagnosis.
• Grossly, the intercotyledonary areas are thickened, with a leathery appearance, and are covered with white-yellow or brownish-red exudate. Cotyledons are swollen and exhibit a yellow or brownish-red discoloration.
• In the majority of cases, Q fever-aborted fetuses do not show gross lesions, are generally fresh, and less often autolytic.
• Microscopically, the characteristic lesions consist of necrotic placentitis. The chorionic epithelium exhibits necrosis and accumulation of cell debris and leukocytes on the surface. The stroma of the intercotyledonary areas shows severe infiltration of leukocytes.
• Often, chorionic trophoblast cells are filled with large numbers of small intracytoplasmic coccobacilli that are visible in hematoxylin and eosin-stained sections. The organisms are Gram-negative and stain a magenta color with Gimenez stain.
• The organism cannot be differentiated by microscopic examination of tissues from other Gram-negative intracellular bacteria, such as

Brucella or *Campylobacter*, hence confirmation of the diagnosis requires ancillary tests.
• In the majority of cases, affected fetuses do not show microscopic lesions. Some fetuses may be found to have bronchopneumonia or mild granulomatous hepatitis.

TREATMENT
THERAPEUTIC APPROACH
Because *C. burnetii* replicates in phagolysosomes of infected cells, the effectiveness of antibiotics is theoretically limited by their ability to penetrate these organelles and remain active at the low pH that prevails in this environment.

SURGICAL CONSIDERATIONS AND TECHNIQUES
N/A

MEDICATIONS
DRUGS OF CHOICE
• Two successive injections of long-acting oxytetracycline (20 mg/kg SC) during the last month of pregnancy is often used in females that are still pregnant once an outbreak starts. However, the beneficial effect of antibiotic treatment in reducing *C. burnetii*-induced abortions and shedding is not well documented.
• Humans require long-term therapy with drugs including doxycycline and hydroxychloroquine.

CONTRAINDICATIONS
N/A

PRECAUTIONS
Appropriate milk and meat withdrawal times must be followed for all compounds administered to food-producing animals.

POSSIBLE INTERACTIONS
N/A

FOLLOW-UP
EXPECTED COURSE AND PROGNOSIS
N/A

POSSIBLE COMPLICATIONS
• Stillbirth or abortion in pregnant ruminants and humans.
• Chronically infected humans can develop endocarditis.

CLIENT EDUCATION
Education should focus on potential sources of infection and ways to reduce environmental contamination from infected placental membranes and aborted materials, and to avoid consumption of raw milk.

Q

(CONTINUED) **Q FEVER (COXIELLOSIS)**

PATIENT CARE
N/A

PREVENTION
• In the United States, there are no vaccines available for the prevention of Q fever in ruminants.
• Q fever vaccines for humans and animals are available in other countries. Vaccination of noninfected small ruminants before their first mating with a phase I vaccine leads to significant reduction of abortion rates and subsequent shedding of bacteria.
• Since the start of a compulsory vaccination campaign of all dairy sheep and dairy goats in the Netherlands in 2010, no abortions caused by *C. burnetii* have been reported. On average, it took 2–7 years to eradicate Q fever from a herd with preventive vaccination after this outbreak in the Netherlands.
• In addition to vaccination, sound biosecurity and management practices should be established in ruminant herds. Replacement animals should be obtained from Q fever-free flocks and herds.
• Aborted fetuses and placentas should be collected quickly and submitted to the laboratory for diagnosis or disposed of by incineration or deep burial.
• Lambing areas should be cleaned and disinfected with Lysol, bleach, or hydrogen peroxide.
• *C. burnetii* is highly resistant to physical and chemical agents. Variable susceptibility has been reported for hypochlorite, formalin, and phenolic disinfectants; a 0.05% hypochlorite, 5% peroxide, or 1:100 solution of Lysol® (benzalkonium chloride) may be effective.
• High-temperature pasteurization destroys the organism.

 MISCELLANEOUS

ASSOCIATED CONDITIONS
N/A

AGE-RELATED FACTORS
N/A

ZOONOTIC POTENTIAL
• Q fever in humans has different epidemiologic patterns. Often, it may consist of sporadic cases that are problematic to diagnose because clinical signs of acute infection are nonspecific and easily confused with those of other diseases.
• In some Mediterranean countries, such as France, Spain, and Israel, where Q fever is endemic, the disease is more frequently diagnosed in humans and animals.
• Epidemic outbreaks affecting large numbers of non-occupation related people and animals

occur sporadically, as was the case in the Netherlands where more than 4,000 human cases were diagnosed and 50,000 goats were euthanized between 2007 and 2010.
• In the US, approximately 50–60 cases of Q fever in humans are reported each year, but it is believed that they are underdiagnosed and underreported and that these numbers do not reflect the true incidence of disease.
• Humans are highly susceptible to Q fever by exposure to aerosols when assisting infected animals during parturition, when handling infected placental tissues, by performing necropsies on aborted fetuses, during slaughter or laboratory procedures, and by drinking raw, unpasteurized milk from infected animals.
• In the acute phase, Q fever in humans can manifest as fever, chills, retrobulbar headache, myalgia, chest pain, dyspnea, productive cough, and liver failure; however, in the majority of cases infection is asymptomatic.
• In a small proportion of infected individuals the infection may progress to a chronic phase characterized by chronic heart failure due to valvular endocarditis, vasculitis, granulomatous hepatitis, osteomyelitis, or by chronic inflammation in several other organs. At this stage, the infection is often life threatening and complicated by the fact that antibiotic therapy is generally not effective.
• Q fever occurring during pregnancy in humans is associated with a risk of miscarriage.
• Q fever clinical disease is more frequent among HIV-infected patients and other immunocompromised individuals.
• Several studies have shown that living in the proximity of a small ruminant farm with a history of *C. burnetii* abortions is a risk factor for Q fever in humans.

PREGNANCY
Abortion and pregnancy loss

BIOSECURITY
• Biosecurity consists of management practices to prevent the introduction and spread of infectious diseases in a herd.
• Unless other farms or animals have equal health status, do not loan or share bucks, do not breed does for other producers, and do not mix animals with other producers' animals.
• Do not share equipment unless it is disinfected after each use.
• Limit access by visitors to the farm and to the animals.
• Control cat, dog, bird, rodent, and insect populations as much as possible.

PRODUCTION MANAGEMENT
N/A

SYNONYMS
Query fever

ABBREVIATIONS
• BSL-3 = biosafety level 3
• BVD = bovine viral diarrhea
• CF = complement fixation
• ELISA = enzyme-linked immunosorbent assay
• IBR = infectious bovine rhinotracheitis
• IFA = immunofluorescence assay
• IgA = immunoglobulin A
• IgG = immunoglobulin G
• IgM = immunoglobulin M
• PCR = polymerase chain reaction
• RT-PCR = reverse transcription-polymerase chain reaction

SEE ALSO
• Abortion: Bacterial
• Abortion: Bovine
• Abortion: Small Ruminant
• Brucellosis
• Campylobacter
• Chlamydiosis
• Listeriosis

Suggested Reading
Angelakis E, Raoult D. Q Fever. Vet. Microbiol 2010, 140: 297–309.
Duron D, Sidi-Boumedine K, Rousset E, Moutailler S, Jourdain E. The importance of ticks in Q fever transmission: What has (and has not) been demonstrated? Trends Parasitol 2015, 31: 536–52.
Emery MP, Ostlund EN, Schmitt BJ. Comparison of Q fever serology methods in cattle, goats and sheep. J Vet Diagn Invest 2012, 24: 379–82.
Million M, Raoult D. Recent advances in the study of Q fever epidemiology, diagnosis and management. J Infect 2015, 71: Suppl.1, S2–S9.
Nusinovici S, Frössling J, Widgreen S, Beaudeau F, Lindberg A. Q fever infection in dairy cattle herds: increased risk with high wind speed and low precipitation. Epidemiol Infect 2015, 18: 1–11.
Tissot-Dupont H, Amadei MA, Nezri M, Raoult D. Wind in November, Q fever in December. Emerg Infect Dis 2004, 10: 1264–9.
van den Brom R, van Engelen E, Roest HIJ, van der Hoek W, Vellema P. *Coxiella burnetii* infections in sheep and goats: an opinionated review. Vet Microbiol 2015, 181: 119–20.

Author Andrés de la Concha-Bermejillo
Consulting Editor Erica C. McKenzie
Acknowledgment The author and book editors acknowledge the prior contribution of Glenda Dvorak and Richard Ermel.

Q

RABIES

BASICS

OVERVIEW
• Rabies is a disease caused by an RNA virus. Rabies virus is an important cause of acute viral encephalomyelitis in ruminants, with public health implications.
• Once clinical signs appear, the disease is consistently fatal.
• Exposure most commonly occurs subsequent to a bite, usually from an infected feral or wild animal. After infection in CNS neurons, the virus travels to the salivary gland, from where it may be transmitted to other mammals.
• Prevention and control of the disease involves vaccination; however, vaccination is not commonly performed in livestock.
• Humans risk exposure by reaching into the mouth of an infected ruminant when a foreign body is suspected due to inability to swallow or hypersalivation.

INCIDENCE/PREVALENCE
• Cattle are most frequent domestic ruminant in which cases of rabies are reported.
• In the report on rabies surveillance in the United States during 2013, 49 states and the District of Columbia and Puerto Rico reported 5,865 cases of rabies in nonhuman animals and 3 cases in human beings to the Centers for Disease Control and Prevention, a decrease of 4.8% from the 6,162 cases in nonhuman animals and 1 case in a human being reported in 2012. Hawaii was the only reporting jurisdiction in the US where no confirmed cases of rabies were reported. The majority of cases (92.0%; 5,398 cases) were in wild animals, whereas 8.0% (467 cases) were in domestic species.
• Rabies cases in cattle are usually <100 cases per year in the US (approximately 1.0% of all rabies cases), although a spike in rabies cases in cattle was reported in 2012 (115 cases, 1.87% of all rabies cases).
• Rabies cases among sheep and goats in the US average <0.25% of all cases, and numbers of cases have ranged between 6 and 13 individual cases each year during 2009–2013.
• The relative contributions of the major groups of animals reported to have rabies in 2013 were: raccoons (32.3%, 1,898 cases), bats (27.2%, 1,598), skunks (24.7%, 1,447), foxes (5.9%, 344), cats (4.2%, 247), dogs (1.5%, 89), and cattle (1.5%, 86).

GEOGRAPHIC DISTRIBUTION
Worldwide

SYSTEMS AFFECTED
Nervous

PATHOPHYSIOLOGY
Exposure most commonly occurs subsequent to a bite by an infected animal. After an animal is bitten, the rabies virus replicates locally. The virus travels by retrograde axonal transport to the brain. After infection in CNS, virus travels by antegrade axonal transport to the salivary gland and nasal epithelium. Shedding of the virus in saliva and nasal secretions may precede clinical signs.

SIGNALMENT
All ruminants

PHYSICAL EXAMINATION FINDINGS
• Early clinical signs are nonspecific and highly variable between individuals.
• In cattle, disease may manifest as different forms (furious or paralytic), although clinical signs associated with each form are not mutually exclusive. Oropharyngeal paralysis is considered one of the most common clinical signs of cattle, and rabid cattle can present with clinical signs indistinguishable from choke (esophageal obstruction).

Furious Form
• Restlessness, expression of anxiety, dilated pupils.
• Exaggerated response to auditory or tactile stimuli; aggression with minimal provocation.
• Animals may charge through stall doors or gates and roam extensively.
• Other signs can include bloat, convulsions, pruritis, pica, or tenesmus.
• Affected animals become progressively ataxic and eventually develop paresis.
• Death usually occurs within 10 days of onset of clinical signs.

Paralytic or "Dumb" Form
• Initial signs often include anorexia, depression, ataxia, shifting leg lameness, and fever.
• Paralysis of the masseter muscles.
• Laryngeal and pharyngeal paralysis.
• Cattle may bellow incessantly with altered phonation.
• Profuse salivation and inability to swallow.
• Abrupt cessation of lactation in dairy cattle.
• Flaccidity of the tongue, tail, anus, and urinary bladder. Some animals exhibit long periods of tenesmus.
• If able to stand, animals have a wide-base stance. Knuckling of the hind fetlock joints may occur.
• Paresis progresses rapidly to paralysis of all parts of the body.
• Death within 10 days of onset of clinical signs.

CAUSES AND RISK FACTORS
• Rabies is a disease caused by RNA viruses in the genus *Lyssavirus* (family Rhabdoviridae).
• Different variants of the rabies virus are endemic to a specific host population within a given geographic region. In the US, raccoons are the primary host species along the eastern seaboard, skunks in the north central and south central states, and the fox in Texas. Various species of bat also carry different strains of the rabies virus.
• Skunks and bats can become asymptomatic carriers serving as reservoirs.
• Antigenic variations in the rabies virus result in different reservoir species depending on geographic area, although extension to other species is common.

DIAGNOSIS

DIFFERENTIAL DIAGNOSES
• Behavioral aggression unrelated to disease.
• Oral or esophageal foreign body.
• Grass tetany, polioencephalomalacia, milk fever, nervous ketosis, nervous coccidiosis, hypoxemia (anaplasmosis), bacterial encephalitis (thromboembolic meningoencephalitis).
• Transmissible spongiform encephalopathy: Scrapie, bovine spongiform encephalopathy, or chronic wasting disease in elk and deer.
• Neurotoxins such as carbamates or organophosphates.
• Other viral encephalitis diseases in ruminants include bovine herpesvirus encephalomyelitis, pseudorabies, malignant catarrhal fever, ovine and caprine lentiviral encephalitis, West Nile virus encephalitis, Borna disease, paramyxoviral sporadic bovine encephalomyelitis, and ovine encephalomyelitis (louping ill).

CBC/BIOCHEMISTRY/URINALYSIS
N/A

OTHER LABORATORY TESTS
CSF may be normal or have increased protein, mononuclear cells, neutrophils, eosinophils, or xanthochromia. Remember to handle CSF with extreme caution, as the virus may be present in this cytologic specimen.

IMAGING
N/A

OTHER DIAGNOSTIC PROCEDURES
In ruminants, rabies is diagnosed using a direct fluorescent antibody test conducted on fresh CNS tissues (preferably brainstem and cerebellum).

PATHOLOGIC FINDINGS
• There are no gross findings specific to rabies infection.
• On histology, Negri bodies, cytoplasmic inclusion bodies containing rabies viral antigen, may be found in the hippocampus, cerebellum, or medulla oblongata. These cytoplasmic inclusion bodies are considered diagnostic for rabies but may not be present in up to 30% of cases.
• Diffuse encephalitis can be seen with perivascular cuffing and neuronal necrosis.

TREATMENT

THERAPEUTIC APPROACH
• No effective treatment.

• Any animal suspected of being exposed to rabies must be securely quarantined as required by state public health department regulations.

MEDICATIONS

DRUGS OF CHOICE
N/A

FOLLOW-UP

EXPECTED COURSE AND PROGNOSIS
• Incubation period varies from a few weeks to a year. The average incubation period is 2–6 months. Animals bitten near the head have shorter incubation periods than those bitten on an extremity or on the trunk.
• Death usually occurs within 10 days of the first symptoms.

PATIENT CARE
• Animals suspected to have rabies must be securely quarantined.
• Monitor for changes in behavior and attitude, or clinical signs suggestive of rabies.
• Check state regulations on specific requirements. Rabies is a reportable zoonosis.

PREVENTION
• Inactivated vaccines are the only licensed product for prevention of rabies in livestock in the US. The modified-live vaccines that are available for use in domestic dogs and cats may potentially produce fatal allergic or viral encephalitis when injected in ruminants.
• Due to the extreme public health concerns, state, provincial, and local regulations have been put in place and must be followed completely.

• The Compendium of Animal Rabies Control is compiled and updated annually by the National Association of State Public Health Veterinarians (NASPHV) and summarizes the most current recommendations for the US and lists all USDA-licensed rabies vaccines.
• Environmental disinfection can be accomplished with household bleach in a 1:32 dilution (4 ounces per gallon).

MISCELLANEOUS

ZOONOTIC POTENTIAL
• Extreme risk. Observe strict quarantine of animals suspected to have rabies.
• Humans risk exposure by reaching into the mouth of an infected animal when a foreign body is suspected due to inability to swallow or hypersalivation.

ABBREVIATIONS
• CNS = central nervous system
• CSF = cerebrospinal fluid
• NASPHV = National Association of State Public Health Veterinarians
• USDA = United States Department of Agriculture

SEE ALSO
• Bacterial Meningitis
• Bloat
• Borna Disease
• Bovine Spongiform Encephalopathy
• Caprine Arthritis Encephalitis Virus
• Carbamate Toxicity
• Cervidae: Chronic Wasting Disease
• Clostridial Disease: Nervous System
• *Histophilus somni* Complex
• Infectious Bovine Rhinotracheitis
• Ketosis: Dairy Cattle

• Malignant Catarrhal Fever
• *Oestrus ovis* Infestation
• Organophosphate Toxicity
• Ovine Encephalomyelitis (Louping Ill)
• Postparturient Paresis (Hypocalcemia)
• Pseudorabies
• Ruminal Acidosis
• Scrapie
• Tick Paralysis
• Urea Toxicity
• Vitamin B Deficiency

Suggested Reading
Callan RJ, Van Metre DC. Viral diseases of the ruminant nervous system. Vet Clin North Am Food Anim Pract 2004, 20: 327–62.
Chipman RB, Cozzens TW, Shwiff SA, et al. Costs of raccoon rabies incidents in cattle herds in Hampshire County, West Virginia, and Guernsey County, Ohio. J Am Vet Med Assoc 2013, 243: 1561–7.
Dyer JL, Wallace R, Orciari L, Hightower D, Yager P, Blanton JD. Rabies surveillance in the United States during 2012. J Am Vet Med Assoc 2013, 243: 805–15.
Dyer JL, Yager P, Orciari L, et al. Rabies surveillance in the United States during 2013. J Am Vet Med Assoc 2014, 245: 1111–23.
Bowen RA. Rhabdoviridae. In: MacLachlan NJ, Dubovi EJ eds, Fenner's Veterinary Virology, 4th ed. San Diego: Academic Press, 2011.
Author Paul H. Walz
Consulting Editor Christopher C.L. Chase
Acknowledgment The author and book editors acknowledge the prior contribution of Lisa Nashold.

Client Education Handout available online

R

RECTAL PROLAPSE

BASICS

OVERVIEW
Prolapse or eversion of the rectum through the anus

INCIDENCE/PREVALENCE
• Cattle: 0.1–1.5% within a population. • Sheep (lambs): 7.8%, 4% and 1.8% with respectively short, medium and long tail docking.

GEOGRAPHIC DISTRIBUTION
Feedlot lambs have higher incidence than grazing lambs.

SYSTEMS AFFECTED
Digestive

PATHOPHYSIOLOGY
• Increase in pressure gradient in the abdominal and pelvic cavities • Exposure of rectum from anus • Straining • Reduced blood circulation, with secondary vascular congestion, edema, and necrosis • Secondary tissue trauma is common

HISTORICAL FINDINGS
May be predisposed by:
• Increased abdominal fill
• Tenesmus • Coughing • Feed changes

SIGNALMENT
• Cattle aged 6–24 months, sheep aged 6–12 months.
• No breed or sex predilection.

PHYSICAL EXAMINATION FINDINGS
Grading system: • Grade 1 mucosal prolapse, small or intermittent • Grade 2 prolapse of all layers from mucosa to serosa, variable length • Grade 3 prolapse of the large colon • Grade 4 intussusception of rectum and colon through anus

GENETICS
• Inherited anal sphincter laxity may play a role. • Genetic analysis of rectal prolapse using half siblings indicated a low heritability factor.

CAUSES AND RISK FACTORS
• Increased abdominal fill • Growth implant administration • Obesity with excessive pelvic fat deposition • Parasitosis • Bloat • Dystocia • Retained fetus • Uterine torsion • Vaginal or uterine prolapse • Increased number of fetuses • Diarrhea • Enteritis or colitis • Urinary obstruction • Decreased perianal and anal tone (may be secondary to short tail docking) • Neuropathy secondary to trauma or breeding injury • Mounting during estrus • Spinal lymphoma • Epidural alcohol blocks • Diet: Clover, high estrogenic compound feedstuff (soybeans) • Toxins • Respiratory disease • Chronic coughing

DIAGNOSIS
Diagnosis is straightforward and based on physical examination. Underlying disease diagnosis is fundamental.

TREATMENT
Transport before rectal prolapse correction is contraindicated if prolapse is very large.

THERAPEUTIC APPROACH
• Perform epidural block • In case of extensive straining, perform mild standing sedation. • Clean prolapsed rectum with warm and clean water. • Identify any area of laceration or necrosis. • Suture lacerated areas. • Apply osmotic agents to reduce rectal edema (hypertonic saline, dextrose, or glycerol). • Gently reduce the prolapse manually with the aid of lubricant. • When replaced, gently invert rectum in the pelvis. • Perform purse-string suturing through the skin 2–4 cm from the anus, maintaining some patency for defecation. • Individuate and treat the primary cause of the prolapse.

SURGICAL CONSIDERATIONS AND TECHNIQUES
• Severely traumatized or necrotic rectal tissue may necessitate amputation. • Perform only if severe damage to the rectum is present. • Perform mucosal resection and anastomosis if only the mucosa is damaged. • If more severely compromised, a prolapse ring can be applied. • A commercial prolapse ring or open-ended tube (PVC pipe) is inserted into the rectum. • Application of prolapse ring or elastrator band is used to stop blood supply to the area. • The necrotic area and ring will slough off in 7–10 days.

MEDICATIONS

DRUGS OF CHOICE
• Broad-spectrum antibiotic therapy • NSAIDs (flunixin meglumine) • Osmotic agents (hypertonic saline or dextrose) • Lubricating agents

CONTRAINDICATIONS
N/A

PRECAUTIONS
Appropriate milk and meat withdrawal times must be followed for all compounds administered to food-producing animals.

POSSIBLE INTERACTIONS
N/A

FOLLOW-UP

EXPECTED COURSE AND PROGNOSIS
• Prognosis is guarded with tendency for recurrence unless causative agents are controlled.

POSSIBLE COMPLICATIONS
• Bleeding from rectal laceration or due to surgical amputation • Recurrence • Skin suture dehiscence or abscessation • Constipation • Bladder retroversion • Eventration of small intestine • Rectal stricture • Septic peritonitis • Death

CLIENT EDUCATION
• Animal's value should be discussed when deciding on treatment options. • Educate clients on controllable risk factors such as appropriate tail docking, parasite control programs, prompt treatment of respiratory disease, nutrition and body condition monitoring, and avoidance of estrogenic plants.

PATIENT CARE
• Restriction of activity is indicated. • Maintenance of soft feces can help risk of constipation post-suture placement (e.g., legume diet, mineral oil, cathartics such as magnesium hydroxide). • Remove purse-string sutures in 7–10 days.

PREVENTION
Proper management practices such as feeding to control body condition, long tail docking, and prompt attention to reproductive, gastrointestinal, and respiratory disease can reduce the risk of prolapse.

MISCELLANEOUS

ASSOCIATED CONDITIONS
• Enteritis • Vaginal or uterine prolapse • Bloat • Urolithiasis

PREGNANCY
May be more common in animals carrying multiple fetuses or very large fetus.

PRODUCTION MANAGEMENT
Market value and intended use of animal will determine treatment option

ABBREVIATION
• PVC = polyvinyl chloride

SEE ALSO
• Reproductive Prolapse • Uterine Prolapse

Suggested Reading
Anderson DE, Miesner MD. Rectal prolapse. Vet Clin North Am Food Anim Pract 2008, 24: 403–8.
Steiner A. Surgery of the colon. In: Fubini SL, Ducharme NG eds, Farm Animal Surgery. St. Louis: Saunders, 2004, pp. 257–62.
Thomas DL, Waldron DF, Lowe GD, et al. Length of docked tail and the incidence of rectal prolapse in lambs. J Anim Sci 2003, 81: 2725–32.
Author Eleonora Po
Consulting Editor Kaitlyn A. Lutz
Acknowledgment The author and book editors acknowledge the prior contribution of John R. Campbell.

R

REINDEER MANAGEMENT: OVERVIEW

BASICS

OVERVIEW
• Historically, more than 25 indigenous ethnic groups residing in the Eurasian circumpolar regions have participated in reindeer herding.
• Currently, the reindeer industry is a primary focus of the Koryak, Chukchi, Komi, Nenet, Yakut, Enets, Even, Evenk, Nganasan, Dolgan, and Sami (see map at https://en.wikipedia.org/wiki/Reindeer#Reindeer_husbandry).
• There are approximately 1.5 million domesticated reindeer in Russia, 200,000 in Finland, 250,000 in Sweden, and 200,000 in Norway.
• Although <1% of the total meat consumed in Fennoscandia is reindeer, its production is a vital source of income to remote regions of this subarctic region.
• Reindeer also plays a central role in the traditions of the circumpolar indigenous herding groups which are the few remaining groups that have maintained a traditional lifestyle.

INCIDENCE/PREVALENCE
N/A

GEOGRAPHIC DISTRIBUTION
Russia, Finland, Sweden, Norway, Greenland, Canada, and Alaska

SYSTEMS AFFECTED
Multisystemic

PATHOPHYSIOLOGY
N/A

HISTORICAL FINDINGS
N/A

SIGNALMENT
Species
• *Rangifer tarandus* is a circumpolar species consisting of seven subspecies formed through the isolation of populations during the ice age.
• North American subspecies of *Rangifer tarandus* are called caribou, while Eurasian subspecies are called reindeer.
• Peary caribou (*R.t. pearyi*) and Svalbard reindeer (*R.t. platyrhyncus*) inhabit the high Arctic.
• Alaskan caribou (*R.t. granti*), barren ground caribou (*R.t. groenlandicus*), and Eurasian reindeer (*R.t. tarandus*) inhabit the taiga; woodland caribou (*R.t. caribou*) and woodland reindeer (*R.t. fennicus*) inhabit the boreal forests.
• *Rangifer tarandus* are polygamous and sexually dimorphic with males being approximately twice the size of females.
• North American caribou are all wild.
• Eurasian reindeer: Both wild and domesticated herds exist.
• Domesticated reindeer are highly gregarious and form large herds, particularly during migration and periods of insect harassment.

Breed Predilections
• Eurasian reindeer are smaller than caribou.
• Females reach maximum body size at the age of 4–5 years, and senescence starts at the age of 7–10 years.
• Females are ~60 kg and males 120 kg at their prime. Body weights vary markedly depending on range conditions.
• Calves are born in April–June (one calf per year).
• Females with poor nutritional status have reduced fecundity and delayed calving.
• Birthweight is ~5 kg (males are 0.5 kg heavier) and is positively associated with neonatal survival.
• Weaning ends in September/October (i.e., when the rut starts), but the calf may follow its mother for a year.
• Calves following their mothers have easier access to food and are more likely to survive the winter. Males are less likely to follow their mothers and have higher mortality rates.
• Age of maturity is 1–3 years in females and 2–5 years in males. Poor nutritional conditions during early development may delay maturity. Conversely, good conditions may result in early maturity (age 1) in females, and this premature reproduction effort can permanently stunt somatic growth.

GENETICS
N/A

CAUSES AND RISK FACTORS
N/A

DIAGNOSIS

DIFFERENTIAL DIAGNOSES
N/A

CBC/BIOCHEMISTRY/URINALYSIS
N/A

OTHER LABORATORY TESTS
N/A

IMAGING
N/A

OTHER DIAGNOSTIC PROCEDURES
N/A

PATHOLOGIC FINDINGS
N/A

TREATMENT

THERAPEUTIC APPROACH
• The most important food during winter is lichens (*Cladina* spp.).
• During summer, the diet is more variable, and includes vascular plants, grasses (graminoids), herbs, shrubs such as willow (salicaceae), heathlike shrubs (ericoids), trees, and fungi.

• Inadequate harvesting and subsequent population growth exceeding the carrying capacity of the ranges have led to degradation of the winter pastures in many areas.
• Supplementation with hay and commercial feed pellets during winter is practiced (in Finland hay is subsidized by the European Union).

SURGICAL CONSIDERATIONS AND TECHNIQUES
N/A

MEDICATIONS
N/A

DRUGS OF CHOICE
N/A

CONTRAINDICATIONS
N/A

PRECAUTIONS
N/A

POSSIBLE INTERACTIONS
N/A

FOLLOW-UP

EXPECTED COURSE AND PROGNOSIS
N/A

POSSIBLE COMPLICATIONS
N/A

CLIENT EDUCATION
N/A

PATIENT CARE
N/A

PREVENTION
N/A

MISCELLANEOUS

ASSOCIATED CONDITIONS
N/A

AGE-RELATED FACTORS
N/A

ZOONOTIC POTENTIAL
Several reindeer diseases are zoonotic. Care must be taken in the collection of laboratory samples and the diagnosis and treatment of affected animals.

PREGNANCY
N/A

BIOSECURITY
• Isolation and quarantine of new stock entering the herd.
• Treat and or cull new animals for disease conditions prior to herd introduction.

R

REINDEER MANAGEMENT: OVERVIEW

PRODUCTION MANAGEMENT

Herding Systems

• Reindeer management has been recently introduced into Siberia and regions (Inuit in Alaska and Canada, and the Greenland Eskimos).

• The most intensive and modernized management of domesticated reindeer is found among the Sámi people in Fennoscandia. There, herding is a cooperative operation based on year-round free range with seasonally defined ranges and migration routes, intensive use of mechanical transportation for herding (motorcycles, snow mobiles, helicopters), and supplemental feeding during poor range conditions.

• Reindeer are in general individually owned in most regions of Fennoscandia, but reindeer cooperatives with joint ownership are common in Finland, southern Norway, and most of Siberia.

• Reindeer husbandry requires access to extensive land areas (34% of the land area in Finland, 50% in Sweden, and 40% in Norway).

• When available, coastal regions, with their moist climates, nutrient-rich grazing, and a relatively low intensity of flying, biting insects are used for summer range. Drier continental ranges with dense lichen beds, less snow, and stable cold conditions during the winter months are used for winter range.

• Historically, reindeer herders in Russia, Finland, Sweden, and Norway migrated freely across national borders.

• Governmental restrictions regarding crossing geopolitical boundaries have tended to break up traditional, ecologically determined migration patterns and seasonal ranges.

• During the nineteenth century, the Russian and Finnish borders were closed, and today severe restrictions exist on the movement of reindeer between pastures in Norway and Sweden. This has led to reduced availability of appropriate summer and winter pastures.

• Many Norwegian reindeer herds are forced to survive on winter pastures along the coast where heavy snowfall and ice prevent efficient foraging. This has been remedied to some extent by supplemental feeding during some of the winter months.

• Finnish and Swedish reindeer lack access to nutrient-rich pastures along the coast during the summer and experience a very high burden of parasites (nasal bot flies, *Cephenomyia trompe* Modeer and warble fly, *Hypoderma tarandi* L.).

Economic Considerations

• Historically, reindeer were used for clothing, milk production, transportation (sled and draft animals), and meat production.

• Today, meat production is the primary goal in reindeer husbandry. Reindeer meat is considered a delicacy and an organically, free-range-raised meat, and commands a high price in European markets.

• More recently, with incorporation of modern technology into the husbandry techniques, it became necessary to produce adequate revenue to support the increased mechanization (e.g., snow mobiles, modern dwellings).

• The length of time domesticated reindeer are in close contact with humans varies greatly among different management practices, from only a few times a year when the calves are marked in the summer or early fall, and in the fall when animals are slaughtered, to almost year-round with prolonged periods of round-the-clock surveillance.

• Herders follow the reindeer on their migration between the winter and summer pastures.

• Calves are marked to signal ownership by cutting away small parts of the ear (see https://merker.reindrift.no/sok.aspx) in complex patterns of markings. These marks are passed down from generation to generation.

• Families, or family groups, often share pastures and herd their reindeer together in cooperative style management operations.

Predation

• Wolverine (*Gulo gulo*), lynx (*Lynx lynx*), and golden eagle (*Aquila chrysaetos*) are important predators of reindeer.

• In some regions, bears can be significant predators.

• Wolf (*Canis lupus*) may be an important predator, but has effectively been removed by humans from most reindeer-herding areas.

• Red fox (*Vulpes vulpes*) may be an important predator on neonates.

• Neonates are particularly vulnerable to predators.

• Food limitation increases risk of predation.

SYNONYMS
N/A

ABBREVIATIONS
N/A

SEE ALSO

• Biosecurity: Cervidae (see www.fiveminutevet.com/ruminant)
• Cervidae: Captive Management
• Reindeer Management: Population Dynamics
• Vaccination Programs: Cervidae

Suggested Reading

Barboza PS, Hartbauer DW, Hauer WE, Blake JE. Polygynous mating impairs body condition and homeostasis in male reindeer (*Rangifer tarandus tarandus*). J Comp Physiol B 2004, 174: 309–17.

Gjostein H, Holand O, Weladji RB. Milk production and composition in reindeer (*Rangifer tarandus*): effect of lactational stage. Comp Biochem Physiol A 2004, 137: 649–56.

Jentoft S ed. Commons in a Cold Climate. Coastal fisheries and reindeer pastoralism in north Norway: the co-management approach. Paris: UNESCO, 1998.

Moen J, Danell O. Reindeer in the Swedish mountains: an assessment of grazing impacts. Ambio 2003, 32: 397–402.

Norsk Polarinstitutt. Proceedings of the human role in reindeer/caribou systems workshop. Polar Res 2000, 19(1), 1–142.

Tveraa T, Stien A, Brøseth H, Yoccoz NG. The role of predation and food limitation on claims for compensation, reindeer demography and population dynamics. - Journal of Applied Ecology 2014, 10.1111/1365-2664.12322.

Weladji, R. B., Holand, O. 2003, Jul. Global climate change and reindeer: effects of winter weather on the autumn weight and growth of calves. Oecologia 136(2): 317–23. Epub 2003, Apr 18.

Author Torkild Tveraa, Adun Stien and Andrew Karter

Consulting Editor Ahmed Tibary

R

REINDEER MANAGEMENT: POPULATION DYNAMICS

BASICS

OVERVIEW
• High-density herds (populations exceeding carrying capacity) have reduced fecundity and calf growth, and are more vulnerable to density-independent factors (e.g., climatic events). Particularly calves, yearlings, mature bulls (weakened by the rut), and old (>10 years) females with worn teeth, are at risk of starvation.
• In the absence of overgrazing, excessive mortality, or heavy animal harvesting, reindeer herds grow until their populations exceed carrying capacity and crash or move to new feeding regions.
• Reindeer in poor nutritional condition are more susceptible to parasites, disease, and metabolic deficiencies, which can increase winter losses of meat, hides, and antlers.
• Basic range management plans can prevent overgrazing and subsequent starvation of overpopulated reindeer herds.

INCIDENCE/PREVALENCE
N/A

GEOGRAPHIC DISTRIBUTION
Russia, Finland, Sweden, Norway, Greenland, Canada, and Alaska

SYSTEMS AFFECTED
Multisystemic

PATHOPHYSIOLOGY
N/A

HISTORICAL FINDINGS
N/A

SIGNALMENT
See chapter, Reindeer Management: Overview

PHYSICAL EXAMINATION FINDINGS
N/A

GENETICS
N/A

CAUSES AND RISK FACTORS
N/A

DIAGNOSIS

DIFFERENTIAL DIAGNOSES
N/A

CBC/BIOCHEMSTRY/URINALYSIS
N/A

OTHER LABORATORY TESTS
N/A

IMAGING
N/A

OTHER DIAGOSTIC PROCEDURES
N/A

PATHOLOGIC FINDINGS
N/A

TREATMENT

THERAPEUTIC APPROACH
N/A

SURGICAL CONSIDERATIONS AND TECHNIQUES
N/A

MEDICATIONS

DRUGS OF CHOICE
• Broad-spectrum anthelmintics (e.g., ivermectin MSD—Ivomec 1%, Merck-Sharp & Dohme), i.e., GABA (γ-amino butyric acid) inhibitors, are frequently used to combat nematodes and arthropods in reindeer.

CONTRAINDICATIONS
Appropriate milk and meat withdrawal times must be followed for compounds administered to food-producing animals.

PRECAUTIONS
N/A

POSSIBLE INTERACTIONS
N/A

FOLLOW-UP

EXPECTED COURSE AND PROGNOSIS
N/A

POSSIBLE COMPLICATIONS
N/A

CLIENT EDUCATION
N/A

PATIENT CARE
N/A

PREVENTION
• Semi-domesticated reindeer, like all free-ranging animals, are exposed to a wide variety of parasite species and infectious diseases. However, only a few species have substantive economic impact.
• Parasite burdens are to a large extent determined by density-dependent factors; herds exceeding carrying capacity, or that do not migrate seasonally to new ranges, may experience high transmission pressure and high parasite burdens. In addition, climate and weather play an important role (e.g., weather conditions influence the ability of flying parasites to breed and infect their hosts).
• Elaphostrongylus rangiferi Mitskevich (Nematoda: Metastrongylidae) causes cerebrospinal and muscular nematodiasis and mortality in the reindeer of the Palearctic.

• E. rangiferi likely has the greatest economic impact; epizootics have resulted in up to 25% mortality in a single year in select herds of northern Norway.
• The oestrids, Hypoderma tarandi L. (warble fly) and Cephenomyia trompe Modeer (nasal bot fly), cause substantial harassment during the warmer summer months, resulting in reduced feeding time and body mass growth.
• Finnish and Swedish reindeer lack access to nutrient-rich pastures along the coast during the summer and experience a very high burden of flying parasites such as nasal bot flies (Cephenomyia trompe Modeer) and warble fly (Hypoderma tarandi L.).
• Gastrointestinal nematodes (Trichostronglyus, Ostertagia, Nematodirus, Marshallagia, Trichuris, Skrjabinema species) have a detrimental impact on weight gain and somatic growth, but usually not a direct impact on survival.
• In North America and Siberia, brucellosis outbreaks in reindeer herds have caused serious morbidity,d mortality, and economic consequences.
• Brucellosis is a contagious, infectious, and communicable disease caused by bacteria of the genus Brucella.
• Because brucellosis is zoonotic (causing undulant fever in humans), eradication through a vaccination program has been a major veterinary medicine focus in recent years.

MISCELLANEOUS

ASSOCIATED CONDITIONS
N/A

AGE-RELATED FACTORS
N/A

ZOONOTIC POTENTIAL
• Several reindeer diseases are zoonotic. Care must be taken in the collection of laboratory samples and the diagnosis and treatment of affected animals.
• In North America and Siberia, brucellosis is a contagious, infectious, and communicable disease caused by bacteria of the genus Brucella.
• Because brucellosis is zoonotic (causing undulant fever in humans), eradication through a vaccination program has been a major veterinary medicine focus in recent years.

PREGNANCY
N/A

BIOSECURITY
• Isolation and quarantine of new stock entering the herd.
• Treat and or cull new animals for disease conditions prior to herd introduction.

R

REINDEER MANAGEMENT: POPULATION DYNAMICS   (CONTINUED)

PRODUCTION MANAGEMENT

Population Dynamics

• Sex ratio in domesticated herds is highly skewed toward females (i.e., 1:10–20) due to selective harvest.

• A skewed sex ratio increases growth and productivity due to the higher growth efficiency (per unit feed) of younger animals.

• Large variations in regional climate and management strategies, including harvest intensities, have led to profound variation in reindeer densities, size, and productivity.

• As a rule of thumb, summer range conditions are most important determinants for somatic growth, while winter range conditions are most critical for survival and population growth rates.

• Populations with access to winter pastures with little precipitation (snow) and stable (cold) continental conditions have good access to food in winter and higher survival rates.

• Intensive harvesting is needed to regulate such populations to sustainable levels that are appropriate for the winter range.

• Populations with winter pastures in coastal areas are exposed to high precipitation levels, bringing deep snow alternating with rain and ice. Resultant ice crystals embedded in the lichen beds reduce access and palatability, causing reindeer to wander constantly rather than graze with stability.

• High-density herds (populations exceeding carrying capacity) have reduced fecundity and calf growth and are more vulnerable to poor environmental conditions such as periods of poor winter weather. Particularly calves, yearlings, and mature bulls (weakened by the rut) and old (>10 years) females with worn teeth, are at risk of starvation.

Future Challenges

• Closing of national borders led to suboptimal use of pastures for reindeer in Fennoscandia, and international range-sharing agreements could lead to improved productivity.

• Increased pressure on reindeer pastures due to development of infrastructure for other activities such as mining, oil drilling, and power plants may permanently reduce the sustainability of reindeer herding activities.

• The recovery of predator populations, such as wolverine and lynx, has increased predation on reindeer in Fennoscandia.

• Reindeer densities are in many regions above sustainable levels. In such areas increased reindeer management plans, that increase harvest, are needed to match population densities to the food resources on the available pastures.

SYNONYMS

N/A

ABBREVIATION

GABA = γ-amino butyric acid

SEE ALSO

• Biosecurity: Cervidae (see www.fiveminutevet.com/ruminant)

• Reindeer Management: Overview

Suggested Reading

Aschfalk A, Josefsen TD, Steingass H, Muller W, Goethe R. Crowding and winter emergency feeding as predisposing factors for kerato-conjunctivitis in semi-domesticated reindeer in Norway. Dtsch Tierarztl Wochenschr 2003, 110: 295–8.

Aschfalk A, Thorisson SG. Seroprevalence of *Salmonella* spp. in wild reindeer (*Rangifer*

tarandus tarandus) in Iceland. Vet Res Commun 2004, 28: 191–5.

Laaksonen S, Pusenius J, Kumpula J, et al. Climate change promotes the emergence of serious disease outbreaks of filarioid nematodes. Ecohealth 2010, 7: 7–13.

Kutz SJ, Hoberg EP, Nagy J, Polley L, Elkin B. "Emerging" parasitic infections in arctic ungulates. Integr Comp Biol 2004, 44: 109–18.

Palmer MV, Stoffregen WC, Rogers DG, et al. West Nile virus infection in reindeer (*Rangifer tarandus*). J Vet Diagn Invest 2004, 16: 219–22.

Tikkanen MK, McInnes CJ, Mercer AA, et al. Recent isolates of parapoxvirus of Finnish reindeer (*Rangifer tarandus tarandus*) are closely related to bovine pseudocowpox virus. J Gen Virol 2004, 85: 1413–18.

Tveraa T, Stien A, Brøseth H, Yoccoz NG. The role of predation and food limitation on claims for compensation, reindeer demography and population dynamics. J Appl Ecol 2014, 51: 2164–72.

Vahtiala S, Sakkinen H, Dahl E, Eloranta E, Beckers JF, Ropstad E. Ultrasonography in early pregnancy diagnosis and measurements of fetal size in reindeer (*Rangifer tarandus tarandus*). Theriogenology 2004, 61: 785–95.

Vikoren T, Tharaldsen J, Fredriksen B, Handeland K. Prevalence of *Toxoplasma gondii* antibodies in wild red deer, roe deer, moose, and reindeer from Norway. Vet Parasitol 2004, 120: 159–69.

Author Torkild Tveraa, Adun Stien and Andrew Karter

Consulting Editor Ahmed Tibary

R

REPEAT BREEDER MANAGEMENT

 BASICS

OVERVIEW

• "Repeat breeding" (RB) is defined as a failure of conception following three or more services or artificial inseminations in the absence of obvious abnormalities
• RB is associated with considerable economic loss due to decreased productivity, veterinary expenses, replacement cost, loss of genetic gain, semen cost, and involuntary culling.
• RB is a common complaint in dairy cattle and camelids.

INCIDENCE/PREVALENCE

Incidence varies from 5% to 20% and is affected by herd size, age of the cows, season, and production.

GEOGRAPHIC DISTRIBUTION

Worldwide

SYSTEMS AFFECTED

Reproductive

PATHOPHYSIOLOGY

• RB is due to fertilization failure or embryonic death before maternal recognition of pregnancy.
• Fertilization failure may result from poor insemination protocol (e.g., heat detection inaccuracy, improper timing, handling or placement of semen). Semen factors (post-thaw quality and intrinsic fertility of the male) may play a role.
• Failure of fertilization or increased early embryonic death (EED) may be due to:
  ○ Poor oocyte quality due to age, metabolic disorders, and heat stress
  ○ Poor survival of the gametes or embryo due to poor uterine (i.e., endometritis) and endocrine environment (luteal insufficiency in high-producing cows).
• Derangement in synthesis of estrogen, progesterone, and luteinizing hormones is implicated in RB through impairment of oocyte competence and development.
• Failure of ovulation is a common cause of repeat breeding in camelids.

HISTORICAL FINDINGS

• Herd records show increased services per conception, increased calving interval, and increased interval from calving to conception.
• Increased rates of dystocia, postpartum disorders, metabolic disorders.
• High milk production.
• In individual females, history of infertility.

SIGNALMENT

Reproductively mature, parous females

PHYSICAL EXAMINATION FINDINGS

Most animals appear healthy.

GENETICS

N/A

CAUSES AND RISK FACTORS

• Dystocia and postpartum disorders
• Metabolic disorders (negative energy balance)
• Heat stress
• Poor breeding management

 DIAGNOSIS

DIFFERENTIAL DIAGNOSES

Rule Out Management/Human Factors

• History and analysis of conception rate by inseminator and method of heat detection
• Evaluation and retraining of inseminators

Rule Out Semen Factors

• Analysis of conception rate by bull and semen/tank batches
• Evaluation of semen tank management and semen handling
• Evaluation of a semen sample
• Breeding soundness evaluation of males if natural mating

Rule Out Fertilization Failure

Failure of fertilization may be due to:
• Defective oocytes: Estimated as a cause in 3–8% of RB. Aged oocytes may be implicated in repeat breeding of individual animals. In herd situations, poor oocyte quality is the result of poor timing of insemination (too late), heat stress, and negative energy balance.
• Oviductal anomalies: Estimated as a cause in 6–15% of RB. Bilateral congenital (segmental aplasia, hydrosalpinx) or acquired (salpingitis, pyosalpinx, perisalpingitis) conditions of the uterine tube or bursa (hydrobursitis, ovario-bursal adhesions) will interfere with gamete transport and prevent fertilization. Diagnosis requires detailed examination of the reproductive tract.
• Abnormalities of the uterus: The most common cause of fertilization failure is endometritis, which compromises sperm viability. Diagnosis of endometritis requires careful examination during estrus; uterine cytology and culture may help in diagnosis of endometritis. Immunologic reaction against semen may be a significant factor in some cases.
• Abnormalities of the cervix: Double cervix, cervical adhesion, double cervix or double external os of the cervix, cervicitis and pericervical adhesions/abscesses may be a cause of fertilization failure in individual cases but rarely as a herd problem. In some breeds (e.g., Santa Gertrudis), cervical morphology may be an important factor in poor conception rate. These disorders present as a difficulty to bypass the cervix and deposit semen into the uterus.
• Hormonal imbalances: Synchronization using MGA results in poor fertility of the induced heat. Improper timing or dosage of estrogens and GnRH used in some synchronization protocols. In dairy heifers, repeat breeding has been associated with prolonged duration of estrus, delayed LH

peak, prolonged lifespan of preovulatory follicle, late postovulatory rise in plasma progesterone, and the tendency for suprabasal periovulatory progesterone levels. Recent studies have shown that hormonal imbalance may also affect expression of epidermal growth factors in the uterus, which are important for embryonic development.

Rule Out EED

• Females experiencing EED before embryo-uterine signaling (day 16 of the cycle in cattle, day 9 in camelids) will have a normal cycle length and would manifest as a repeat breeder syndrome.
• In dairy cattle, EED before day 16 is estimated at 40–50% of all conceptions.
• EED can result from poor quality embryos originating from poorly timed insemination (aged oocytes), heat stress, aging, poor oviductal or uterine environment due to inflammation or hormonal imbalances, and genetics.
• In dairy herds, one of the most important causes of EED is heat stress.

Infectious Disease

• Infectious diseases may be implicated in increased RB in a herd.
• Most of these agents predispose to RB due to inflammatory changes to the ovaries, ovarian bursa (viruses), and/or the uterus, cervix and vagina. These include *Brucella abortus, Mycobacterium tuberculosis, BVDV, IBR, Ureaplasma diversum, Mycoplasma bovigenitalium, Histophilus somni, Leptospira harjo bovis, Tritrichomonas foetus,* and *Campylobacter fetus* ssp. *Venerealis.*

CBC/BIOCHEMSTRY/URINALYSIS

N/A

OTHER LABORATORY TESTS

• Semen evaluation
• Serum progesterone determination
• Serology and bacteriology for specific pathogens

IMAGING

N/A

OTHER DIAGNOSTIC PROCEDURES

• Endometrial cytology for diagnosis of endometritis
• Embryo collection and evaluation

PATHOLOGIC FINDINGS

Endometritis, cervicitis, salpingitis

 TREATMENT

THERAPEUTIC APPROACH

• Treatment of RB focuses on improving environmental conditions and addressing deficiencies in heat detection and insemination procedures.
• Intrauterine administration of antimicrobials is used in cows suspected to have endometritis, but this treatment is not

R

REPEAT BREEDER MANAGEMENT

approved in some countries (e.g. United States).

SURGICAL CONSIDERATIONS AND TECHNIQUES

Unilateral ovariectomy in the case of uterine tube abnormalities

MEDICATIONS

DRUGS OF CHOICE

Depends on diagnosis

CONTRAINDICATIONS

• Appropriate milk and meat withdrawal times must be followed for all compounds administered to food-producing animals.

PRECAUTIONS

N/A

POSSIBLE INTERACTIONS

N/A

FOLLOW-UP

EXPECTED COURSE AND PROGNOSIS

• Pregnancy may be achieved if predisposing factors are addressed. However, delayed conception may lead to decision for culling.
• Embryo collection and transfer may be considered in valuable animals.

POSSIBLE COMPLICATIONS

N/A

CLIENT EDUCTION

• Work with the veterinarian to set up a herd health monitoring program.
• Consider appropriate methods to combat heat stress.
• Emphasize the importance of parturition management and postpartum protocols.

PATIENT CARE

N/A

MISCELLANEOUS

ASSOCIATED CONDITIONS

Dystocia, postpartum disorders, metabolic disorders, heat stress

AGE-RELATED FACTORS

N/A

ZOONOTIC POTENTIAL

• Brucella abortus
• *Mycobacterium tuberculosis*

PREGNANCY

Progesterone supplementation has been shown to help in some cases.

BIOSECURITY

N/A

PRODUCTION MANAGEMENT

• Address human/management factors
  ◦ Improve heat detection efficiency and accuracy.
  ◦ Use fixed-time insemination.
  ◦ Periodic retraining of inseminators.
• Address female factors
  ◦ Cull cows with congenital or acquired nontreatable conditions.
  ◦ Determine causes of uterine infection and setup protocol for prevention (parturition management, retained placenta, nutrition, vaccination protocols).
  ◦ Early identification and treatment of uterine infection.
  ◦ Reduce ovulation failure/ovulation problems by the implementation of an ovulation synchronization protocol or systematic injections of GnRH at the time of insemination in RB cows.
  ◦ Improve embryo survival by administration of hCG or GnRH to create accessory corpora lutea and supplemental progesterone (CIDR) 6 days after insemination.
  ◦ Administration of 500 mg BST has been shown to improve embryo survival.
• Semen/Male factors
  ◦ Use semen from high fertility males.
  ◦ Use a double insemination regime.
  ◦ Use deep horn insemination (if technician is well trained).
  ◦ Perform breeding soundness evaluation on males.
  ◦ Use clean-up bulls only on cows that are known not to have an infectious cause of infertility.
• Address environmental factors
  ◦ Use cooling system during summer.
  ◦ Decrease incidence of uterine infection by improving calving conditions.
  ◦ Improve heat detection by addressing problems such as crowding and floor-surface issues.

SYNONYMS

N/A

ABBREVIATIONS

• BST = bovine somatotropin
• BVDV = bovine diarrheal virus
• CIDR = controlled internal drug release
• EED = early embryonic death
• GnRH = gonadotropin releasing hormone
• hCG = human chorionic gonadotropin
• IBR = infectious bovine rhinotracheitis
• LH = luteinizing hormone
• MGA = megestrol acetate
• RB = repeat breeder

SEE ALSO

• Artificial Insemination: Bovine
• Bovine Viral Diarrhea Virus
• Breeding Soundness Examination: Bovine
• Breeding Soundness Examination: Camelid
• Endometritis
• Infectious Bovine Rhinotracheitis
• Infertility and Subfertility Issues
• Ovarian Hypoplasia, Bursal Disease, Salpingitis
• Trichomoniasis

Suggested Reading

Bonneville-Hébert A, Bouchard E, Du Tremblay D, et al. Effect of reproductive disorders and parity on repeat breeder status and culling of dairy cows in Quebec. Can J Vet Res 2011, 75: 147–51.

Kendall NR, Flint APF, Mann GE. Incidence and treatment of inadequate postovulatory progesterone concentration in repeat breeder cows. Vet J 2009, 181: 158–62.

Sood P, Zachut M, Dube H, Moallem U. Behavioral and hormonal pattern of repeat breeder cows around estrus. Reproduction 2015, 149: 545–54.

Walsh SW, Williams EJ, Evans ACO. A review of the causes of poor fertility in high milk producing dairy cows. Anim Reprod Sci 2011, 123: 127–38.

Author Ahmed Tibary
Consulting Editor Ahmed Tibary

R

BASICS

OVERVIEW
• Reproductive pharmacology includes the indications for usage, dosage, and efficacy of different drugs in the treatment of reproductive disorders or for manipulation of reproductive functions.
• Reproductive disorders can be of inflammatory, infectious, or hormonal origin.
• Pharmacologic agents used to treat or prevent these problems include antimicrobials, antiseptics, hormones, and enzymes as well as other compounds.

INCIDENCE/PREVALENCE
Common

GEOGRAPHIC DISTRIBUTION
Worldwide

SYSTEMS AFFECTED
Reproductive

PATHOPHYSIOLOGY
• Reproductive disorders may originate from inflammatory or infectious processes or endocrine dysfunction.
• The most common treatable inflammatory/infectious disorders in the female are endometritis and metritis. These disorders often result from contamination during parturition or breeding. In the male ruminant, the most common inflammatory disorder treated is seminal vesiculitis.
• Among the treatable hormonal disorders is cystic ovarian disease.

HISTORICAL FINDINGS
Depend on the condition treated

SIGNALMENT
• All ruminant species and camelids may be concerned. However, in production medicine, individual treatment of endometritis is often limited because of cost and regulations.
• In camelids, a wide variety of pharmacologic substances are used in countries which do not consider these species as food-producing animals.

PHYSICAL EXAMINATION FINDINGS
Depends on the condition treated

GENETICS
N/A

CAUSES AND RISK FACTORS
Causes and risk factors are discussed in various chapters (see "See Also").

DIAGNOSIS

DIFFERENTIAL DIAGNOSES
N/A

CBC/BIOCHEMISTRY/URINALYSIS
N/A

OTHER LABORATORY TESTS
N/A

IMAGING
N/A

OTHER DIAGNOSTIC PROCEDURES
N/A

PATHOLOGIC FINDINGS
N/A

TREATMENT

THERAPEUTIC APPROACH
Antimicrobials
• Antimicrobials are used for the treatment of reproductive infections and in outbreaks of specific bacterial abortion agents in small ruminants.
• Efficacy of antimicrobials depends on several factors:
  ○ Sensitivity of the causative organism
  ○ Achievable concentration (minimum inhibitory concentration) in the tissue or site of infection
  ○ Physiologic properties of the target organ (lipid content, blood flow)
  ○ Dose, route of administration, and duration of treatment.
• In ruminants, antimicrobials are primarily administered systemically whereas in camelids, systemic or intrauterine administration is often used.
• Regulations restrict the in utero use of antimicrobials in food-producing animals in some countries.
• Residues are found in milk following intrauterine administration of antimicrobials but there are no guidelines for withdrawal time determination.
• Intrauterine delivery of an antimicrobial is only effective if the uterus is small and the milieu is compatible with drug activity (pH, pKa, and lack of debris).
• The antibiotic carrier is very important, as some antibiotics are inactivated by saline solutions.
Systemic Antibiotic Therapy
• Systemic antibiotic therapy is used to treat uterine infections or as part of perioperative management (cesarean section, castration).
• In the face of bacterial abortion storms of small ruminants, systemic antibiotics are often used as a first line of defense.
• In males, systemic antibiotics are often used to treat reproductive tract infections (e.g., seminal vesiculitis), although efficacy of this treatment is often poor.
• Antimicrobial selection
  ○ Legal use of an antibiotic is dictated by the FDA (or equivalent agency).
  ○ Antimicrobial culture and sensitivity patterns are generally not performed in production animals, and most practitioners

will select a drug based on the most common isolates.
  ○ For treatment of seminal vesiculitis:
    ▪ Most antibiotics do not reach the glands at high concentration.
    ▪ Tulathromycin and tilmicosin have had success in treating some bulls infected with *T. pyogenes* and *H. somni*.
Intrauterine Antimicrobial Therapy
• Indicated for the treatment of endometritis.
• In cattle, penicillins and cephalosporins (e.g., ceftiofur) are the drugs of choice if culture is not possible. Tetracyclines are not recommended because of negative effects on sperm and the endometrium. Ozone infusions have been shown to have antimicrobial action. The volume of the infusion solution depends on the size of the uterus (25–100 mL).
• In camelids, treatment of endometritis should be preceded by culture and sensitivity. Uterine lavage prior to infusion is recommended to remove any inflammatory debris.
  ○ Ceftiofur: 0.5 g/infusion
  ○ Penicillin: 1×10^6–3×10^6 IU/infusion
  ○ Oxytetracycline (povidone based): 0.5–1 g/infusion
  ○ Ticarcillin: 0.5–3 g/infusion
  ○ Infusions should be performed daily for 3–5 days. Indwelling catheters are highly discouraged.

Antiseptics
• Antiseptics have been used traditionally to treat uterine infections in cattle. These compounds, at higher concentrations, can result in uterine inflammation and intraluminal adhesions.
• Selection of an agent:
  ○ Povidone iodine solution or foam:
    ▪ Cattle: 0.5%–2% solution
    ▪ Camelids: 0.1% solution
    ▪ Iodine is an irritant with bactericidal and fungicidal properties.
  ○ Chlorhexidine solution: 1%–2% of the stock solution
  ○ Hydrogen peroxide diluted in saline at a ratio of 1:4
Uterine Lavage
• Uterine lavage is commonly practiced following dystocia and in cases of metritis.
• Uterine lavage should only be performed when uterine wall integrity is maintained.
• Large quantities of warm fluids (tap water for bovine and ovine or lactated Ringer's solution for camelids and goats) are used until the efflux, collected by gravity, is clear.
• The addition of a small volume of povidone iodine solution may be helpful.
• Excessive uterine lavage may prolong involution and inhibit the immunologic function of the uterus.

Hormonal Therapy
Gonadotropin Releasing Hormone (GnRH)
GnRH is a decapeptide produced in the hypothalamus. It stimulates the release of

R

REPRODUCTIVE PHARMACOLOGY   (CONTINUED)

FSH and LH. It is used for the induction of ovulation, induction of accessory corpora lutea in cattle, synchronization of ovulation, and treatment of follicular ovarian cysts (not all cysts are responsive to this treatment as some may lack receptors for LH).

Follicle Stimulating Hormone (FSH) and Equine Chorionic Gonadotropin (eCG)
• FSH is a glycoprotein secreted by the anterior lobe of the pituitary.
• eCG is a glycoprotein secreted by the endometrial cups of pregnant mares.
• Target tissues include granulosa cells of the ovary where it promotes follicular development, and Sertoli cells of the testis where it promotes Sertoli cell function and seminiferous tubule activity.
• In females these hormones are used for ovarian superstimulation or treatment of some forms of anestrus.

Luteinizing Hormone (LH) and Human Chorionic Gonadotropin (hCG)
• LH is a glycoprotein secreted by the gonadotropic cells of the anterior lobe of the pituitary.
• Human chorionic gonadotropin is a glycoprotein with LH activity secreted by the trophoblast of human blastocysts.
• Target tissues are the theca interna of the ovary, which when stimulated results in luteinization or ovulation, and Leydig cells of the testis, which when stimulated results in increased testosterone secretion.
• Indications:
  ○ In the female:
    ▪ Induction of ovulation
    ▪ Treatment of ovarian follicular cysts
    ▪ Development of accessory corpora lutea. In cattle, hCG given 5 days after insemination will luteinize large follicle(s) to help maintain pregnancy.
  ○ In the male:
    ▪ Increased testicular function (requires combination with FSH)
    ▪ Diagnostic testing for cryptorchidism (hCG stimulation test).

PGF2$_\alpha$ and Analogs
• Prostaglandin F2$_\alpha$ (PGF2$_\alpha$) is a C-20 fatty acid which is derived from arachidonic acid. It is secreted by the endometrium. It has a very short half-life and is eliminated by the respiratory system. Target tissues include the corpus luteum and smooth muscle, particularly the myometrium (female) and epididymis (male) where it causes contractions. PGF2$_\alpha$ and analogs are most effective to induce luteolysis at least 5 days after ovulation.
• Indications:
  ○ Luteolysis as a treatment for:
    ▪ Induction of abortion
    ▪ Estrus synchronization
    ▪ Endometritis
    ▪ Pyometra

▪ Mucometra/Hydrometra in goats
▪ Induction of estrus following treatment for cystic ovarian disease
  ○ Elimination of fetal mummies
  ○ Induction of parturition (alone for camelids and goats or in combination with dexamethasone in cattle and sheep)

Oxytocin
• Oxytocin is an octapeptide synthesized by the hypothalamus and released by the posterior lobe of the pituitary.
• It is also synthesized by the corpus luteum of ruminants and potentiates the activity of PGF2$_\alpha$.
• Target tissues in the female include the myometrium and myoepithelial cells of the mammary gland.
• Indications and dosage:
  ○ To enhance uterine contraction
  ○ To promote placental detachment in the first 24 hours postpartum, after obstetric manipulation or cesarean section
  ○ Milk letdown

Progesterone and Progestagens
• Steroids produced by the corpus luteum and placenta.
• Target tissue: Hypothalamus, uterus, mammary gland.
• Several natural and synthetic progestagens are available for use as injectable or oral formulations, or as vaginal pessaries.
• Indications
  ○ Estrus synchronization
  ○ Maintenance of pregnancy in camelids with a history of recurrent pregnancy loss due to low progesterone
    ▪ Can increase risk of failure of cervical dilation
    ▪ Altrenogest is not orally bioavailable
  ○ Induction of lactation (use not approved in several countries)

Estrogens
• Steroids produced by granulosa cells, placenta.
• Target tissues: Hypothalamus, uterus, cervix and ovaries, mammary gland.
• Effects: Luteolysis, induction of estrus behavior, stimulation of ovulation, stimulation of cervical mucus production, induction of mammary gland development, induction of uterine contraction.
• Common preparations: Estradiol benzoate (EB), estradiol cypionate (ECP). Their use is not approved in food-producing animals in several countries.
• Indications: Estrogens are used in estrus synchronization programs in countries which allow them.

Testosterone
• Steroid produced by Leydig cells and theca cells.
• Target tissues: Accessory sex glands, seminiferous tubules, skeletal muscle.
• Effects: Development of male characteristics, male behavior, and anabolic growth.

• Indications:
  ○ For preparation of teaser animals (cows or steers):
    ▪ Testosterone enanthate 500 mg IM + 1.5 g SC followed by 500–750 mg every 2 weeks.
    ▪ Testosterone propionate 200 mg IM on day 1, 4–9; 1,000 mg IM on day 10, and every 10–14 days thereafter.
    ▪ Wethers treated with lower doses of testosterone can be used for heat detection in sheep and goats.
  ○ For its anabolic steroid effect in feedlot animals.

Steroid Combination Implants
• These products are implants which contain androgens and estrogens (primarily synthetic) and are placed subcutaneously in the ear.
• These hormones increase rate of gain and feed efficiency in feedlot animals.
• Not approved in many countries.

Other Drugs Used in Reproductive Medicine
Anti-Inflammatory Agents
• Nonsteroidal anti-inflammatory drugs (NSAIDs):
  ○ Flunixin meglumine; Meloxicam
Ionophores
Decoquinate (2 mg/kg BW/day) or monensin (15–30 mg/animal/day) have been used for the prevention of abortion due to toxoplasmosis in sheep and goats.
Enzymes
• Collagenase administered directly into the umbilical arteries will result in faster detachment of placental membranes in cows.
• Its use may not be permitted in all countries.
Domperidone
May be used to treatment agalactia in camelids.

MEDICATIONS
DRUGS OF CHOICE
Antibiotics
• Penicillin or one of its synthetic analogs (20,000–30,000 IU/kg q12h): Active against most organisms that cause postpartum metritis.
• Ceftiofur (1–2 mg/kg q12h): Broad-spectrum antimicrobial action.
• Oxytetracycline: Not a good choice because minimal inhibitory concentration required for *T. pyogenes* is not reached in the uterine lumen.
• For the treatment of some bacterial abortion in small ruminants: Tetracycline can be used in the feed (200–300 mg/animal/day). Higher doses (300–500 mg) for leptospirosis infections. Long-acting tetracycline (20 mg/kg q48h). Tylosin (10 mg/kg IM daily for up to 5 days) can be used for tetracycline-resistant *Campylobacter* and *Chlamydophila* isolates.

R

(CONTINUED)   REPRODUCTIVE PHARMACOLOGY

Hormones

• GnRH IM or IV: Gonadorelin hydrochloride or gonadorelin diacetate tetrahydrate (natural GnRH, cattle and camels: 100 µg; sheep, goats, alpacas, and llamas: 50 µg); buserelin (synthetic GnRH with longer half-life, cattle and camels 8 µg, sheep, goats, alpacas, and llamas, 4 µg).
• eCG IM. Not approved for use in food animals in some countries. Animals may become refractory to eCG if it is used often. eCG is used generally in a single (long half-life) IM injection following a course of progesterone treatment.
  ◦ Ovarian superstimulation (cattle: 1,500–3,000 IU, sheep and goats 800–1,500 IU, alpacas and llamas: 750–1,000 IU, camels: 1,500–6,000 IU).
  ◦ Smaller doses are used in anestrous cows (500 IU) and out-of-season synchronization in small ruminants (250–500 IU).
• FSH (porcine and ovine FSH, IM) is most commonly used for ovarian superstimulation (see chapters, Embryo Transfer).
• hCG is administered IV and can cause anaphylaxis
  ◦ Cattle: 3,000–10,000 IU IV
  ◦ Sheep and goats: 500–1,000 IU IV
  ◦ Alpacas and llamas: 500–1,000 IU IV
  ◦ Camels: 1,000–1,500 IU IV
• PGF2$_\alpha$ IM, dinoprost tromethamine (cattle and camels: 25 mg, sheep 10 mg, goats 2.5 mg, alpacas and llamas: 5 mg) or cloprostenol (synthetic, cattle and camels: 500 µg, sheep: 125–250 µg, goats: 50–100 µg, alpacas and llamas: 250 µg).
• Oxytocin (IM or IV) (cattle: 20–40 IU; sheep and goats: 5–10 IU; alpacas and llamas: 5–10 IU; camels: 30 IU).

CONTRAINDICATIONS

Appropriate milk and meat withdrawal times must be followed for all compounds administered to food-producing animals.

PRECAUTIONS

Dinoprost has been shown to cause respiratory distress in a few llamas.

POSSIBLE INTERACTIONS

N/A

FOLLOW-UP

EXPECTED COURSE AND PROGNOSIS
N/A

POSSIBLE COMPLICATIONS
N/A

CLIENT EDUCATION
• Treatment should only be used after consultation with a veterinarian.
• Care in handling of hormones and other potentially harmful drugs.

PATIENT CARE
Depends on diagnosis

PREVENTION
N/A

MISCELLANEOUS

ASSOCIATED CONDITIONS
See "Therapeutic Approach"

AGE-RELATED FACTORS
N/A

ZOONOTIC POTENTIAL
N/A

PREGNANCY
See "Therapeutic Approach"

BIOSECURITY
N/A

PRODUCTION MANAGEMENT
See "Therapeutic Approach"

SYNONYMS
N/A

ABBREVIATIONS
• EB = estradiol benzoate
• eCG = equine chorionic gonadotropin
• ECP = estradiol cypionate
• FDA = Food and Drug Administration
• FSH = follicle stimulating hormone
• GnRH = gonadotropin releasing hormone
• hCG = human chorionic gonadotropin
• IM = intramuscular
• IV = intravenous
• LH = luteinizing hormone
• NSAIDs = nonsteroidal anti-inflammatory drugs
• PGF2$_\alpha$ = prostaglandin F2$_\alpha$
• PO = per os, by mouth
• SC = subcutaneous

SEE ALSO
• Abortion: Small Ruminant
• Artificial Insemination: Bovine
• Artificial Insemination: Small Ruminant
• Embryo Transfer: Bovine
• Embryo Transfer: Camelid
• Embryo Transfer: Small Ruminant
• Estrus Synchronization: Bovine
• Estrus Synchronization: Small Ruminant
• Induction of Parturition
• Metritis
• Retained Placenta
• Seminal Vesiculitis

Suggested Reading
Abecia JA, Forcada F, Gonzalez-Bulnes A. Hormonal control of reproduction in small ruminants. Anim Reprod Sci 2012, 130: 173–9.
Beagley JC, Whitman KJ, Baptiste KE, et al. Physiology and treatment of retained fetal membranes in cattle. J Vet Intern Med 2010, 24: 261–8.
Brodzki P, Bochniarz M, Brodzki A, et al. *Trueperella pyogenes* and *Escherichia coli* as an etiological factor of endometritis in cows and the susceptibility of these bacteria to selected antibiotics. Polish J Vet Sci 2014, 17: 657–64.
Duricic D, Valpotic H, Samardzija M. Prophylaxis and therapeutic potential of ozone in buiatrics: Current knowledge. Anim Reprod Sci 2015, 159: 1–7.
Lima FS, Vieira-Neto A, Vasconcellos GSFM, et al. Efficacy of ampicillin trihydrate or ceftiofur hydrochloride for treatment of metritis and subsequent fertility in dairy cows. J Dairy Sci 2014, 97: 5401–14.
Author Lisa Pearson
Consulting Editor Ahmed Tibary
Acknowledgment The author and book editors acknowledge the prior contribution of Ahmed Tibary.

R

REPRODUCTIVE PROLAPSE

BASICS

OVERVIEW
• A prolapse is a falling down or sinking of an anatomic structure from its normal position.
• Reproductive prolapses involve the uterus, cervix, and vagina in the female and the prepuce in the male. Uterine prolapse is covered separately; see chapter, Uterine Prolapse.

INCIDENCE/PREVALENCE
• Highly variable with calving management and genetic selection programs.
• Prepartum vaginal prolapse is relatively common in sheep (1–10% of ewes are affected in production flocks annually).

GEOGRAPHIC DISTRIBUTION
Worldwide

SYSTEMS AFFECTED
Reproductive

PATHOPHYSIOLOGY
• Vaginal prolapse occurs commonly in the later part of the pregnancy and is often the result of a combination of processes including the physiologic relaxation of the tissues (pelvic ligament) supporting the vagina and factors increasing the abdominal pressure.
  ○ In sheep, increased abdominal pressure can be due to presence of large multiple fetuses, tenesmus or straining due to other pathologic processes (lungworm, diarrhea), or obesity. In this species, a genetic component is suspected.
  ○ In cattle, late term vaginal prolapse is observed in older, generally thin, large frame cows.
  ○ In camelids, vaginal prolapse is observed in older females.
  ○ In all species, prepartum or postpartum vaginal prolapse may also result from traumatic disruption of the perineal body and the vestibulovaginal sphincter following excessive, forceful obstetric assistance.
• Prolapse of the cervical folds into the cranial vagina is relatively common in multiparous cattle and is assumed to be secondary to calving trauma. In Bos indicus cows, this may progress to the point of cervical eversion through the vulva.
• Preputial prolapse in males is often secondary to trauma. Preputial prolapse in bulls should not be confused with the intermittent eversion of the prepuce commonly seen in polled bulls. Preputial prolapse is commonly seen in camelids that have the tendency to masturbate against objects or the ground.

HISTORICAL FINDINGS
Cases are reported by owner after observing the abnormality.

SIGNALMENT
• Sexually mature ruminants or camelids.

• Vaginal prolapse is most common in late gestation and occurs more frequently in cattle, camelids, and sheep.
• Preputial prolapse is common in bulls and camelids.

PHYSICAL EXAMINATION FINDINGS
• Prolapse of the vagina and prepuce are generally visually obvious.
• Local tissue irritation and pain may lead to straining.
• Some affected animals may strain to urinate.

GENETICS
• Vaginal prolapse is often hereditary in beef cattle and sheep, so a standard recommendation is to cull the affected animal after weaning and avoid using female offspring as replacements.
• Preputial prolapse is more common in Bos indicus cattle and their crosses (e.g., Santa Gertrudis).

CAUSES AND RISK FACTORS
• Vaginal prolapse should be assumed to be a hereditary defect in beef cattle unless another cause can be established. Trauma and repeated superovulation treatment can also cause the condition.
• The hormonal milieu and abdominal fill of late gestation predispose to prolapse of the vagina.
• Excessive body condition can also predispose to vaginal prolapse.
• In dairy cattle, postpartum vaginal prolapse often occurs secondary to premature or excessive obstetric interventions, especially in heifers.
• Breeding injuries to the prepuce (e.g., preputial laceration) or penis (e.g., penile hematoma) can result in prolapse of the prepuce.

DIAGNOSIS

DIFFERENTIAL DIAGNOSES
• Eversion of the bladder
• Retained placenta
• Tumors

CBC/BIOCHEMISTRY/URINALYSIS
N/A

OTHER LABORATORY TESTS
N/A

IMAGING
Ultrasonography can assist with locating the bladder or diagnosis of abscessation in chronic cases.

OTHER DIAGNOSTIC PROCEDURES
• Visual inspection and manual palpation are usually sufficient to make the diagnosis.
• Vaginal prolapse can be graded as to severity.
  ○ Grade 1: Intermittent protrusion of vaginal tissue during recumbency
  ○ Grade 2: Continuous prolapse of vaginal tissue

  ○ Grade 3: Continuous prolapse of the vagina, cervix, and bladder
  ○ Grade 4: A chronic case resulting in tissue compromise that will result in fetal death and possibly peritonitis.

PATHOLOGIC FINDINGS
N/A

TREATMENT

THERAPEUTIC APPROACH
• See "Surgical Considerations and Techniques"

SURGICAL CONSIDERATIONS AND TECHNIQUES

Vaginal Prolapse
• Treatment of vaginal prolapse depends on the value of the animal, the stage of gestation, and the severity of the condition. An epidural anesthetic is administered before beginning. The prolapsed tissue is cleaned and replaced and the bladder emptied.
• In cattle, options for retaining the tissue include:
  ○ A Caslick's suture may suffice for grade 1 prolapse if no straining occurs. This is often the case with postpartum vaginal prolapse due to calving trauma, as frequently observed in Holstein dairy cattle.
  ○ A Buhner suture is an effective treatment for more severe grades but must be closely monitored to allow timely removal before delivery. Variations on this purse-string approach include a bootlace technique and placement of horizontal mattress sutures across the vulvar opening. With the Buhner and horizontal mattress sutures, leave about a 3 cm opening (access for two fingers) ventrally to allow for urination.
  ○ More complicated surgical options that allow for unobserved calving include the Minchev vaginopexy and the Winkler cervicopexy.
• In the ewe, especially if many animals are affected, a commercially available retaining device can be used. The device is tied to the body to maintain the vagina in place.
• In camels, options similar to those used in cattle are appropriate for camels. In SAC, a bootlace technique is preferable.

Preputial Prolapse
• The primary objective of treatment for preputial prolapse is to replace the swollen tissue and avoid surgery. The prolapsed tissue is cleaned and covered with a lubricating ointment.
• In bulls, a drainage tube is placed into the preputial cavity to allow urine to drain. The exposed tissue is covered with a stockinette and then bandaged from the distal end with an elastic tape that is applied with enough tension to reduce the swelling. The tape encircles the prepuce and is anchored to the

R

hair of the skin at the preputial opening. The bandage is changed as needed, usually daily or every other day, until the prepuce can be returned to the preputial cavity. A sling may be needed if the sheath is especially pendulous. The sling should be of porous material so that urine is not trapped. Once the prepuce is in place, it should be held in place with another bandage, changed as before and continued until it remains in place. Allow at least 60 days of sexual rest and then evaluate for normal penile erection and extension.
• In camelids, the prolapsed tissue is cleaned and covered with a lubricating ointment, replaced within the prepuce, and held in place with a purse-string suture on the preputial orifice. An antibiotic ointment is applied daily into the prepuce. Sutures are removed after 7–10 days.

MEDICATIONS

DRUGS OF CHOICE
• Systemic, broad-spectrum antibiotic therapy is indicated for chronic cases or when cellulitis is suspected.
• Flunixin meglumine or meloxicam can be used to reduce inflammation and for pain relief.

CONTRAINDICATIONS
Appropriate meat and milk withdrawal times must be followed for all compounds administered to food-producing animals.

PRECAUTIONS
N/A

POSSIBLE INTERACTIONS
N/A

FOLLOW-UP

EXPECTED COURSE AND PROGNOSIS
• Vaginal prolapse: Good prognosis for fetal survival after normal delivery if detected and managed early, poor otherwise.

• Preputial prolapse: Guarded prognosis for normal fertility in cases where surgical treatment is necessary.
• In camelids, if the male returns to masturbation against objects, preputial prolapse will recur with increased severity of tissue damage and adhesion formation and a poor prognosis.

POSSIBLE COMPLICATIONS
• Cellulitis, abscessation, and scarring with phimosis may occur after preputial prolapse.
• Abortion, dystocia, and peritonitis may complicate cases of chronic vaginal prolapse. In postpartum cattle, chronic vaginal prolapse may cause infertility.

CLIENT EDUCATION
Cull females with recurrent vaginal prolapse.

PATIENT CARE
• Vaginal prolapse: Frequent monitoring is required for the remainder of gestation in pregnant animals to assure normal delivery.
• Preputial prolapse: Daily monitoring is required during treatment to assure urine passage and absence of straining.

PREVENTION
• Sound genetic selection program for herd or flock replacements.
• Avoid unnecessary, premature, or excessive obstetric assistance.
• Select bulls with good sheath conformation.

MISCELLANEOUS

ASSOCIATED CONDITIONS
• Penile hematoma
• Preputial laceration

AGE-RELATED FACTORS
N/A

ZOONOTIC POTENTIAL
N/A

PREGNANCY
Vaginal prolapse usually occurs in late gestation.

BIOSECURITY
N/A

PRODUCTION MANAGEMENT
N/A

SYNONYMS
N/A

ABBREVIATION
SAC = South American camelids

SEE ALSO
• Penile Disorders
• Penile Hematoma
• Uterine Prolapse

Suggested Reading
Ennen S, Floss S, Scheiner-Bobis G, et al. Histological, hormonal and biomolecular analysis of the pathogenesis of ovine *Prolapsus vaginae ante partum*. Theriogneology 2011, 75: 212–19.
Jackson R, Hilson RPN, Roe AR, et al. Epidemiology of vaginal prolapse in mixed-age ewes in New Zealand. N Z Vet J 2014, 62: 328–37.
McEntee K. Reproductive Pathology of Domestic Animals. San Diego: Academic Press, 1990, pp. 207–8.
Peter AT. Vaginal, cervical and uterine prolapse. In: Hopper RM ed, Bovine Reproduction. Ames: Wiley Blackwell, 2015, pp. 383–95.
Tibary A, Pearson LK. Reproductive emergencies in camelids. Clin Theriogenol 2014, 6: 579–92.

Authors Harry Momont and Celina Checura
Consulting Editor Ahmed Tibary
Acknowledgment The authors and book editors acknowledge the prior contribution of Steven D. Van Camp.

R

REPRODUCTIVE TUMORS

BASICS

OVERVIEW
Tumors can arise in several locations of the female and male reproductive tract. In females, the ovary, uterus, cervix, vagina, and vulva can be affected. In the male, the testis and penis are the most common locations. Clinical signs are dependent on the tumor type, location, severity, and possible metastasis.

PATHOPHYSIOLOGY
• Tumors of the reproductive tract are highly variable in nature, depending on the tissue of origin, chronicity, malignancy, and location. In some cases, neoplasia of other tissues can metastasize to the reproductive tract.
• Females with ovarian tumors may present for infertility, anestrus, nymphomania, or male-like behavior, depending on the hormonal output of the tumor.
• Females with uterine, cervical, vaginal, or vulvar tumors may present for observation of a mass on examination or transrectal palpation, hemorrhagic discharge from the vulva, or abnormalities identified during artificial insemination.
• Reproductive tract tumors may have a metastatic component, depending on the tissue of origin and malignancy. Affected animals should be examined for metastasis to the lungs, liver, and kidneys. Metastasis may result in chronic weight loss, respiratory dysfunction, and dysuria.
• Males with testicular tumors may present for nonpainful, chronic enlargement of the scrotum.
• Males with penile tumors may have reduced libido, lower pregnancy rates in co-mingled females, and observation of hemorrhagic discharge from the prepuce.

SYSTEMS AFFECTED
Reproductive

GENETICS
N/A

INCIDENCE/PREVALENCE
Unknown

GEOGRAPHIC DISTRIBUTION
Worldwide

HISTORICAL FINDINGS
• In females, the history may include irregular estrous cycles, including persistent estrus or anestrus, male-like behavior, and a history of infertility. Vaginal discharge may be a complaint.
• In males, the history may include progressive enlargement of the scrotum, or discharge from the penis or prepuce. Decreased libido may also be reported.

SIGNALMENT
• Cows, sheep, goats, camelids.

• Although tumors are most often recognized in adult breeding animals, granulosa-theca cell tumors (GTCT) have been diagnosed in calves and nulliparous heifers.

PHYSICAL EXAMINATION FINDINGS
• Reproductive tumors in the female should be suspected if any or a combination of the following are observed:
  ◦ Abnormal or palpable masses in or around the ovaries, uterus, or cervix
  ◦ Hemorrhagic vaginal discharge
  ◦ Irregular estrus cycles (including anestrus, nymphomania, or male-like behavior)
  ◦ Mammary gland development and lactation in nonpregnant young animals
  ◦ Stranguria, dysuria, straining
  ◦ Abnormal ultrasonographic appearance of the ovaries, uterus, or cervix
  ◦ History of infertility
• Reproductive tumors in the male should be suspected if any or a combination of the following are observed:
  ◦ Deterioration of semen quality in the absence of detectable inflammatory, traumatic, degenerative, or environmental causes
  ◦ Chronic progressive, nonpainful enlargement of the testis
  ◦ Hemorrhagic discharge from the penis
  ◦ Observation of proliferative lesions on the penis
• The general physical examination may reveal nonspecific signs such as weight loss, vaginal or preputial discharge, or behavior changes.
• Specific examination should include palpation per rectum in large species, or palpation/ballottement of the abdomen or scrotum. Ultrasonography should be performed on any suspicious masses.
• The animal should be examined for metastasis, which can include imaging of the lung fields and liver.

CAUSES AND RISK FACTORS
Specific Tumor Types in Females
• Ovary
  ◦ Ovarian tumors are classified as epithelial, germ cell, sex cord, or mesenchymal in origin.
  ◦ Epithelial tumors
    ▪ Includes papillary adenoma or carcinoma, cystadenoma, cystadenocarcinoma, and adenocarcinoma.
    ▪ Papillary adenoma or adenocarcinoma are very rare and arise from the surface epithelium, subsurface epithelial structures, or rete ovarii.
    ▪ Cystadenomas, large single-cavity cystic structures, arise from the epoophoron and/or rete ovarii.
    ▪ A cystadenocarcinoma was reported in a cow, with metastasis to the peritoneum and iliac lymph nodes, kidney, and other organs.

    ▪ Adenocanthoma, carcinoma with squamous metaplasia, has been reported in a cow.
  ◦ Germ cell tumors
    ▪ Dysgerminoma has been reported in the cow as a firm, spherical, red-gray mass, 15 cm in size, which can metastasize. Hyperplasia of the endometrium can occur secondary to hyperestrogenism.
    ▪ Teratomas arise from all three germinal layers, with tissue representing any organ except ovary or testis. Teratomas of different sizes and content (cartilage, hair, bone, teeth, etc.) have been reported in sheep, cows, goats, and camelids.
    ▪ Dermoid cysts, or cystic ovarian teratomas, have been reported in Zebu cattle and water buffalo and vary in size and weight from 5.7 to 45 kg. Metastasis has been reported.
  ◦ Sex cord tumors
    ▪ GTCT dominate this category of tumor. Others include thecoma (theca cell tumor, a firm white/yellow/orange tumor), and luteoma (an interstitial cell tumor which is smooth, slightly lobulated, orange, and produces progesterone).
    ▪ GTCT can result in anestrus, nymphomania, or male-like behavior and development of male secondary sex characteristics (particularly of the head and neck). Mammary enlargement may be observed.
    ▪ GTCT have been reported in cows, sheep, goats, and camelids. They can occur in adults as well as newborn or prepubertal females.
    ▪ Typically the affected ovary is enlarged and the contralateral ovary small and inactive, due to effects of inhibin produced by the tumor. The tumor is generally benign.
    ▪ Serum endocrinology typically shows high anti-mullerian hormone, testosterone, estrogen, and inhibin.
  ◦ Mesenchymal tumors: This category includes hemangioma, leiomyoma, fibroma, and lymphoma (lymphosarcoma).
• Uterus
  ◦ Epithelial tumors
    ▪ Adenoma: Polyps of the endometrium are considered hyperplastic and rare.
    ▪ Adenocarcinomas have been reported in cows, goats, sheep, and camelids. Clinical signs include infertility, bloody vaginal discharge, palpable mass(es), depression, respiratory disease, and stranguria. Metastasis to the lungs, peritoneum, lymph nodes, and other organs can occur. Lesions from the endometrium may invade the myometrium.
  ◦ Mesenchymal tumors
    ▪ Fibromas are rare, hard, white, spherical tumors of the uterine wall.
    ▪ Fibrosarcomas are very rare.

■ Leiomyomas are benign, firm, tan, nodular tumors which generally affect the myometrium.

■ Leiomyosarcomas are very rare.

■ Uterine lymphosarcoma is common in cattle, associated with infection with bovine leukosis virus. Masses may be multiple, irregular shaped, and soft.

• Cervix

○ Cervical neoplasia is typically epithelial in origin, including adenocarcinoma and squamous cell carcinoma.

○ Cervical adenocarcinomas are relatively common in older goats and should be differentiated from cervical hyperplasia. Metastasis of adenocarcinoma is possible.

○ Mesenchymal tumors such as leiomyomas are typically associated with the uterus or vagina.

• Vagina and vulva

○ Papillomas and squamous cell carcinomas have been reported in cows, sheep, and goats.

○ Risk factors for squamous cell carcinoma include surgical resection of perineal skin folds to reduce myiasis, tail-docking of ewes, and pink vulvas of certain breeds.

○ Lesions may become ulcerated, necrotic, and covered by exudate and blood.

○ Fibropapillomas are firm, elevated, white or pink masses, smooth or cauliflower-like in texture, and are transmissible tumors in heifers.

Specific Tumor Types in Males

• Testes

○ The most common neoplasia of the testis is seminoma, followed by sustentacular cell tumors (Sertoli cell tumor, tubular adenoma, tubular adenocarcinoma), and interstitial cell tumors (Leydig cell tumors).

○ Seminomas have been reported in male cattle, sheep, goats, and camelids. The affected testis is usually enlarged, with variable effects on semen quality.

○ Sertoli cell tumors have been reported in bulls and rams, and an intersex goat. The affected testis is usually enlarged, with normal or decreased semen quality. The tumor is pale gray and firm with an irregular surface when sectioned.

○ Leydig cell tumors are often characterized by poor semen quality, large ejaculate volume with low motility, and low concentration of spermatozoa.

○ All testicular tumors are treated by hemilateral castration of the affected testis. Semen quality should be monitored postoperatively. The animal should be examined for metastasis.

• Penis

○ The most common penile tumor is the fibropapilloma, a result of the fibropapilloma virus. It is most often diagnosed in young bulls.

○ Treatment is by surgical excision.

○ The tumor can be prevented by use of autovaccines.

DIAGNOSIS

• Diagnosis in the female with suspected neoplasia is based on:

○ Transrectal (cow) or transabdominal (sheep and goat) palpation and ultrasonography of an enlarged ovary, uterus, or cervix. Transrectal ultrasonography may be performed in small ruminants and camelids with the transducer mounted on an extension rod.

○ Biopsy or *en bloc* excision of the mass via laparoscopy (sheep, goats, camelids) or laparotomy (cows). A fine needle aspirate may be performed for vaginal or vulvar masses.

○ Serum endocrinology: Elevations of anti-mullerian hormone are diagnostic for GTCT. Sex steroid hormones and inhibin are often assessed in conjunction.

• Diagnosis in the male with suspected neoplasia is based on:

○ Semen evaluation

○ Testicular measurements, palpation, and ultrasonography

○ Testicular biopsy (may be ultrasound-guided)

○ Exteriorization and examination of the penis

DIFFERENTIAL DIAGNOSES

• For females:

○ Other causes of ovarian enlargement (adhesions, large cysts)

○ Other causes of uterine masses (uteroperitoneal adhesions, mummified or macerated fetus, tuberculosis)

○ Other causes of cervical masses (cervicitis, abnormal cervical conformation, double cervix)

• For males:

○ Other causes of scrotal or testicular enlargement (testicular hematoma, abscess, orchitis, inguinal hernia)

○ Other causes of preputial hemorrhage or phimosis (preputial or penile laceration, preputial abscess or adhesions)

CBC/BIOCHEMISTRY/URINALYSIS

N/A

OTHER LABORATORY TESTS

Assay of serum anti-mullerian hormone concentrations can aid in the diagnosis of GTCT preoperatively.

IMAGING

• Ultrasonography is invaluable in the diagnostic evaluation of reproductive tract neoplasia. Transrectal and transabdominal ultrasonography can be performed in females, and ultrasonography of the scrotal contents in males.

• Radiography of the lungs can be useful in the diagnosis of metastasis.

OTHER DIAGNOSTIC PROCEDURES

• Biopsy of the mass is often performed to obtain a diagnosis prior to surgical excision; however, it is not required. Often the mass (or ovary or testis) is excised *en bloc* and submitted for histopathology.

• Penile fibropapillomas can be submitted for histopathology after removal.

PATHOLOGIC FIDINGS

On histopathology, each tumor type will demonstrate specific findings.

TREATMENT

THERAPEUTIC APPROACH

Animals which undergo surgical treatment should be treated with appropriate antibiotics, anti-inflammatories, and tetanus toxoid. Appropriate milk and meat withdrawal times must be followed for all compounds administered to food-producing animals.

SURGICAL CONSIDERATIONS AND TECHNIQUES

• In females, ovarian neoplasms are treated by ovariectomy. Ovariectomy is performed using a standing paralumbar flank approach in cattle and camels. In small ruminants and camelids a midline laparotomy or laparoscopy-assisted approach is preferred.

• Uterine and cervical masses require hysterectomy or partial hysterectomy. These techniques may be considered for companion goats or SAC. A midline laparotomy approach under general anesthesia is the best approach.

• Vulvar masses may be excised.

• In males, testicular neoplasms are treated by orchiectomy. Penile fibropapillomas are surgically excised, often with electrocautery.

• Animals submitted for surgery have the usual postoperative considerations of infection, incisional dehiscence, hemorrhage, and seroma formation.

• Surgical treatment may not be appropriate for animals with metastasis, or metastasis may need to be addressed after removal of the primary tumor.

MEDICATIONS

DRUGS OF CHOICE

• Depends on the surgical approach selected.

• General anesthesia is required for ovariectomy, hysterectomy, and ovariohysterectomy in small ruminants and camelids. Induction with xylazine, butorphanol, and ketamine is followed by maintenance with isoflurane in oxygen.

R

REPRODUCTIVE TUMORS

• Paralumbar flank approach for ovariectomy in cattle and camels: Sedation, paralumbar or inverted "L" block.
• Hemicastration in breeding bulls can be performed under heavy sedation.
• Hemicastration in small ruminants and camelids should be performed under general anesthesia.

CONTRAINDICATIONS
Appropriate milk and meat withdrawal times must be followed.

PRECAUTIONS
N/A

POSSIBLE INTERACTIONS
N/A

FOLLOW-UP

EXPECTED COURSE AND PROGNOSIS
• Highly dependent on the tumor type, location, malignancy, progression of disease, and metastasis.
• Breeding males can retain good fertility if no complications occur after unilateral castration of the affected testicle.
• Prognosis for fertility is fair to good after unilateral ovariectomy.

POSSIBLE COMPLICATIONS
• Metastasis to lungs, liver, and other organs is possible, particularly in cases of adenocarcinomas.
• Mastitis in subsequent pregnancies may be a complication of GTCT in young animals with premature udder development.
• Surgical complications for ovariectomy and ovariohysterectomy: Adhesions, peritonitis (infertility and recurrent pregnancy loss for unilateral ovariectomy).
• Surgical complications after castration: Hemorrhage, infertility in cases of hemicastration (compromise of spermatogenesis in the remaining testicle due to inflammation).

CLIENT EDUCATION
• Emphasize regular breeding soundness examinations in valuable breeding males.
• Seek veterinary consultation if behavioral abnormalities are observed.

PATIENT CARE
• Patients should be monitored for any surgical complication in the immediate period following surgery.
• Animals should be monitored for evidence of metastasis or recurrence of the tumor, particular at the vulva if excision was elected.
• Animals which undergo surgical treatment should be fasted appropriately prior to anesthesia to prevent regurgitation and aspiration as well as to reduce intestinal contents to increase visibility and handling of the ovaries and/or uterus, in females.

PREVENTION
N/A

MISCELLANEOUS

ASSOCIATED CONDITIONS
• Infertility
• Abnormal behavior
• Weight loss

AGE-RELATED FACTORS
• Diagnosis of adenocarcinoma tends to be in older females.
• GTCT have been reported in adult as well as neonatal and prepubertal females.

ZOONOTIC POTENTIAL
N/A

PREGNANCY
N/A

BIOSECURITY
N/A

PRODUCTION MANAGEMENT
N/A

SYNONYMS
N/A

ABBREVIATIONS
• GTCT = granulosa-theca cell tumor
• SAC = South American camelids

SEE ALSO
• Lymphosarcoma
• Reproductive Ultrasonography: Bovine (see www.fiveminutevet.com/ruminant)
• Reproductive Ultrasonography: Camelid (see www.fiveminutevet.com/ruminant)
• Reproductive Ultrasonography: Small Ruminant (see www.fiveminutevet.com/ruminant)
• Squamous Cell Carcinoma
• Testicular Disorders: Bovine
• Testicular Disorders: Camelid
• Testicular Disorders: Small Ruminant
• Uterine Anomalies

Suggested Reading
Ali HE, Kitahara G, Nibe K, et al. Plasma anti-Mullerian hormone as a biomarker for bovine granulomas-theca cell tumors: comparison with immunoreactive inhibin and ovarian steroid concentrations. Theriogenology 2013, 80: 940–9.
Buergelt CD. Color Atlas of Reproductive Pathology of Domestic Animals. Philadelphia: Mosby, 1997.
McEntee K. Reproductive Pathology of Domestic Mammals. New York: Academic Press, 1990.
Tibary A, Pearson LK, Van Metre DC, et al. Surgery of the sheep and goat reproductive system and urinary tract. In: Fubini SL, Ducharme N eds, Farm Animal Surgery, 2nd ed. Philadelphia: Saunders, 2016, pp. 571–95.
Author Lisa Pearson
Consulting Editor Ahmed Tibary
Acknowledgment The author and book editors acknowledge the prior contribution of Ahmed Tibary.

R

RESPIRATORY DISEASE: BOVINE

BASICS

OVERVIEW
- Bovine respiratory disease (BRD) or the BRD complex refers to the general development of respiratory disease in cattle. BRD most commonly occurs in weaned beef cattle as they move through the production cycle from weaned calves to the feedlot.
- BRD can also affect adult dairy animals with vaccine failure, immunosuppression caused by a primary microbial infection, transition from dry to lactation status, or transport.
- BRD is commonly called "shipping fever," or in preweaned calves, enzootic calf pneumonia.
- The etiology of BRD is often multifactorial, and may include viruses, bacteria, parasites, nutrition, environmental stressors, and host susceptibility. Many bacterial pathogens isolated from the lower airway are normal flora of the upper respiratory tract. The severity of BRD outbreaks is often influenced by the relative combination of these factors, and timing of disease is most often associated with transport.

INCIDENCE/PREVALENCE
BRD is the most prevalent and economically significant disease of the beef industry.

GEOGRAPHIC DISTRIBUTION
Worldwide; distribution influenced by management systems

SYSTEMS AFFECTED
Respiratory

PATHOPHYSIOLOGY
Stress (immunosuppression) + viral or *Mycoplasma bovis* infection + bacterial overgrowth = BRD (Figure 1).

HISTORICAL FINDINGS
Clinical signs become apparent 6–10 days after cattle are stressed or exposed to new animals.

SIGNALMENT
Younger animals under stressful conditions are most at risk.

PHYSICAL EXAMINATION FINDINGS
- Fever.
- Reduced appetite.
- Mild depression and separation from herd mates.
- Lowered head, drooped ears, and oculonasal discharge.
- Inducible or spontaneous cough.
- Reluctance to rise, exercise intolerance.
- Severely affected cattle may have dyspnea, extend the head and neck, and protrude the tongue.
- Thoracic auscultation may identify moist or dry crackles and harsh bronchovesicular sounds in the cranioventral thorax.

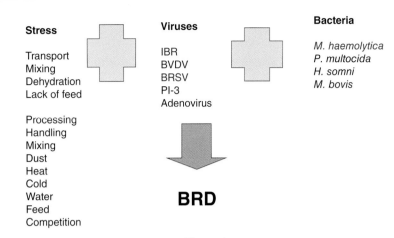

Stress	Viruses	Bacteria
Transport	IBR	*M. haemolytica*
Mixing	BVDV	*P. multocida*
Dehydration	BRSV	*H. somni*
Lack of feed	PI-3	*M. bovis*
	Adenovirus	
Processing		
Handling		
Mixing		
Dust		
Heat		
Cold		
Water		
Feed		
Competition		

BRD

Figure 1.

Bovine Respiratory Disease is Multifactorial

- Consolidated areas of lung associated with bronchopneumonia (or large abscesses) are silent due to lack of air motion.

GENETICS
N/A

CAUSES AND RISK FACTORS
- Viruses commonly incriminated in BRD include BHV-1, BVDV, BRSV, parainfluenza-3, BRCV, and adenoviruses.
- Bacteria commonly involved in BRD include *Mannheimia, Pasteurella multocida, M. bovis, Histophilus somni, Bibersteinia trehalosi,* and *Trueperella pyogenes.*
- Environmental stressors increase the risk of BRD and include poor sanitation, poor ventilation, and overcrowding.
- Weaning, transport, co-mingling of cattle from multiple sources and other stressors.
- Lack of preconditioning (vaccination, dehorning, castration, deworming) of animals prior to movement.

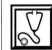

DIAGNOSIS

DIFFERENTIAL DIAGNOSES
- Interstitial pneumonia
- Aspiration pneumonia
- Pulmonary edema
- Pulmonary fibrosis
- Verminous pneumonia

CBC/BIOCHEMISTRY/URINALYSIS
- CBC may indicate acute and/or chronic inflammation with neutrophilia and hyperfibrinogenemia.
- Biochemistry may indicate chronic inflammation with hyperglobulinemia and hypoalbuminemia, and systemic illness with azotemia and electrolyte anomalies.

OTHER LABORATORY TESTS
Culture and antimicrobial sensitivity or PCR can be performed on nasopharyngeal swabs, lung tissue, transtracheal aspirate, or bronchoalveolar lavage fluid.

IMAGING
- Ultrasonography permits visualization of pulmonary consolidation and can be performed with a 5.5 MHz linear rectal probe with standard scoring systems available.
- Radiography is useful to define the extent and distribution of disease in valuable animals.

OTHER DIAGNOSTIC PROCEDURES
- Clinical scoring systems for respiratory disease are popular but accuracy relies on consistent and trained personnel. Automated systems have been assessed to identify affected cattle, but human observation remains the most sensitive detection method.
- Bacterial culture of nasal swabs are not diagnostic for several BRD bacterial pathogens that are normal flora of the upper respiratory tract, but can determine antimicrobial sensitivity patterns and the presence of *Mycoplasma* spp.
- PCR for bacterial pathogens may be helpful to identify presence of *Mannheimia* and *Histophilus*, which can be difficult to culture and are easily overgrown by other bacteria such as *Pasteurella*.
- Bacterial culture and/or PCR of transtracheal wash and bronchoalveolar lavage fluid can definitively identify pathogens.
- Necropsy provides useful information regarding etiologic agents and pathologic processes. Perform necropsy early in the course of the disease and prior to antibiotic therapy for the best results.

PATHOLOGIC FINDINGS
- Gross lesions depend on pathologic agents and chronicity.
- Necrotizing lesions of the upper respiratory tract and trachea most commonly represent viral pathogens.
- *M. bovis* associated otitis and otitis media are common with purulent debris in the

R

RESPIRATORY DISEASE: BOVINE   (CONTINUED)

external ear canal, fluid or purulent material in the tympanic bullae, and bony changes in the walls of the bullae.
- Pneumonic lesions are typically bilateral and cranioventral, often with a sharp line of demarcation between normal and abnormal, consolidated lung.
- Varying degrees of pleural adhesion between lung lobes and to the chest wall.
- Diseased lung parenchyma typically has a lobulated pattern that imparts a marbled appearance on both the pleural and cut surface.
- Affected parenchyma is firm and ranges in color (pink, tan, red, red-black) depending on the amount of necrosis.
- Necrotic tissue may progress to abscessation.
- Histology is consistent with consolidating bronchopneumonia due to secondary bacterial pathogens. Samples submitted from cattle early in the disease process may show interstitial changes.

TREATMENT

THERAPEUTIC APPROACH
- Antimicrobials should be selected for efficacy against common BRD bacteria, and should provide coverage for a minimum of 7–10 days.
- Supportive care for individual animals may include NSAIDs, nutritional support, and fluid therapy.
- Moving sick cattle to separate pens reduces the stress of competing for food with healthy cattle.

SURGICAL CONSIDERATIONS AND TECHNIQUES
N/A

MEDICATIONS

DRUGS OF CHOICE
- Common classes of antibiotics used in BRD include beta-lactams, tetracyclines, macrolides, and fluoroquinolones.
- Ancillary treatments such as NSAIDs, corticosteroids, antihistamines, and vitamin injections may be of value on an individual basis.

CONTRAINDICATIONS
Some antibiotics with a respiratory disease label are illegal for use off-label. AMDUCA does not apply in these cases.

PRECAUTIONS
- Appropriate milk and meat withdrawal times must be followed for all compounds administered to food-producing animals.
- Some macrolide antibiotics are cardiotoxic to humans if injected by mistake. Read the label for precautionary warnings.

POSSIBLE INTERACTIONS
N/A

FOLLOW-UP

EXPECTED COURSE AND PROGNOSIS
- Prognosis is generally favorable if intervention occurs early and the selection and time course of antimicrobial therapy is appropriate.
- If intervention is started early, most cattle respond to treatment in 24–72 hours but require extended antimicrobial coverage to decrease risk of treatment failure and recrudescence of clinical signs.
- Failure to respond to multiple treatments or development of complications generally indicates advanced disease and the prognosis is then guarded.
- Weight gain is associated with a good prognosis; continued weight loss is a poor sign.

POSSIBLE COMPLICATIONS
- Pericarditis
- Endocarditis
- Pleuritis
- Peripheral vestibular disease (*M. bovis* associated otitis media)
- Polyarthritis (*M. bovis* and *H. somni* pneumonia)
- Thromboembolic meningoencephalitis (TEME) and endocarditis can occur with *H. somni* pneumonia.

CLIENT EDUCATION
Management factors play a key role in influencing respiratory disease.

PATIENT CARE
- Daily observation of attitude and appetite will provide a good indication of treatment success. Available clinical scoring schemes aid in daily monitoring.
- Reduction of rectal temperature in 24–48 hours post-treatment suggests a good prognosis.
- Development of head tilt or ear droop is a negative prognostic indicator.

PREVENTION
- Ensure successful passive transfer of maternally derived antibodies via colostrum.
- Parenteral immunization against common BRD pathogens at 4–6 weeks prior to movement or stressful events.
- Intranasal immunization 2 weeks prior to movement or stressful change.
- Preconditioning (dehorning, deworming, castration) 2–4 weeks prior to movement or stressful change.
- Minimizing stressful events, e.g., direct sale of cattle to avoid sale barns and co-mingling from multiple sourced animals.
- Maintaining well-ventilated and sanitary environments with plenty of bunk space and water availability.

MISCELLANEOUS

ASSOCIATED CONDITIONS
- Arthritis
- Pericarditis
- Meningoencephalitis
- Otitis

AGE-RELATED FACTORS
Weaned calves are at high risk due to waning maternal antibodies and stress from weaning and transport for sale.

ZOONOTIC POTENTIAL
N/A

PREGNANCY
N/A

BIOSECURITY
N/A

PRODUCTION MANAGEMENT
It is estimated that more than 3 billion dollars are spent annually on prevention, treatment, and production losses related to BRD in the US fed cattle industry.

SYNONYMS
Shipping fever

ABBREVIATIONS
- BHV-1 = bovine herpes virus 1
- BRCV = bovine respiratory corona virus
- BRD = bovine respiratory disease
- BRSV = bovine respiratory syncytial virus
- BVDV = bovine viral diarrhea virus

SEE ALSO
- Bovine Respiratory Syncytial Virus
- Bovine Viral Diarrhea Virus
- Infectious Bovine Rhinotracheitis

Suggested Reading
Caswell JL, Hewson J, Slavic D, Delay J, Batemen K. Laboratory and postmortem diagnosis of bovine respiratory disease. Vet Clin North Am Food Anim Pract 2012, 28: 419–41.
DeDonder KD, Apley MD. A review of the expected effects of antimicrobials in bovine respiratory disease treatment and control using outcomes from published randomized clinical trials with negative controls. Vet Clin North Am Food Anim Pract 2015, 31: 97–111.
Hilton WM. BRD in 2014: Where have we been, where are we now, and where do we want to go? Anim Health Res Rev 2014, 15:120–2.
Mosier D. Review of BRD pathogenesis: the old and the new. Anim Health Res Rev 2014, 15: 166–8.
Author Keith P. Poulsen
Consulting Editor Erica C. McKenzie
Acknowledgment The author and book editors acknowledge the prior contribution of Daniel L. Grooms.

R

RESPIRATORY DISEASE: CAMELID

BASICS

OVERVIEW
• Respiratory disease in camelids most commonly reflects upper airway disorders, primary lung disease, or diaphragmatic paralysis.
• Diagnostic evaluation can be challenging, since llamas and alpacas may display subtle clinical signs despite progressive or severe respiratory disease.

INCIDENCE/PREVALENCE
Typically sporadic unless a contagious disorder is involved.

GEOGRAPHIC DISTRIBUTION
Worldwide

SYSTEMS AFFECTED
Respiratory

PATHOPHYSIOLOGY
• Upper airway dysfunction can arise from choanal atresia in which failure in embryologic development of the nasopharyngeal opening creates unilateral or bilateral, membranous or osseous, and complete or partial obstruction of nasal air flow in species that are obligate nasal breathers. Allergic rhinitis, nasopharyngeal feed impaction, neoplasia, sinusitis, and *Oestris ovis* infestation can cause upper airway disease in older animals.
• Lower airway disease can arise from infectious broncho- or pleuropneumonia, aspiration of medication, feed, or milk (neonates), and from neoplasia. Hematogenous pulmonary infection can occur in association with bacterial sepsis in neonatal crias (*E. coli, Enterococcus* spp., *Listeria monocytogenes,* and *Citrobacter* spp.). Secondary suppurative bronchopneumonia is documented in persistently BVDV infected crias.
• The etiologic diagnosis of diaphragmatic paralysis is unknown; genetic, metabolic (oxidative stress), infectious (aberrant parasite migration, EHV-1), traumatic, nutritional (vitamin E deficiency), and toxicologic causes have been proposed.

HISTORICAL FINDINGS
Dependent on the underlying etiology. While viral infections can present as a herd concern, neoplastic, fungal, and protozoal disease will generally affect individual animals.

SIGNALMENT
Choanal atresia is usually reported in crias with respiratory distress since birth.

PHYSICAL EXAMINATION FINDINGS
• Tachypnea, increased respiratory effort, open-mouth breathing, nostril flare, and asynchronous breathing may occur.
• Thoraco-abdominal asynchrony most commonly accompanies upper airway obstruction, phrenic nerve dysfunction, diaphragmatic or intercostal muscle paralysis, and diaphragmatic fatigue due to chronic airway disease.
• Changes in respiratory characteristics may also reflect nonrespiratory disorders including metabolic derangements (e.g., severe acidosis), pain, abdominal crisis, fever, high environmental temperatures, and excitement. Clinical signs of pulmonary disease can be nonspecific and difficult to differentiate by physical examination alone in camelids.
• Complete choanal atresia often presents with congenital respiratory distress and lack of air flow through the nares, while partial choanal atresia can be difficult to diagnose due to subtle or absent clinical signs.

GENETICS
Choanal atresia is considered a heritable disorder with a complex mode of inheritance.

CAUSES AND RISK FACTORS
• Bacterial pneumonia: Tuberculosis, nocardiosis, *Rhodococcus equi*-associated lymphadenitis
• Viral pneumonia: Coronavirus, adenovirus-associated pneumonia, bovine herpesvirus type 1, enterovirus
• Pulmonary neoplasia: Adenocarcinoma, squamous cell carcinoma, lymphosarcoma
• Fungal pneumonia: Pulmonary aspergillosis, pulmonary histoplasmosis, coccidioidomycosis, cryptococcosis
• Protozoal pneumonia: *Pneumocystis jiroveci*
• Pleuritis: *S. zooepidemicus,* penetrating thoracic wounds
• Lipoid pneumonia (endogenous or from oil aspiration)
• Diaphragmatic paralysis
• Risk factors include exposure to environmental pathogens, temperature extremes, poor ventilation, dust, overcrowding, stress, and transportation. Dysphagia can relate to structural abnormalities of the upper airways (cleft palate, malformation, cyst, or mass), central nervous system or cranial nerve disorders, and marked laryngeal inflammation.
• Risk factors specifically for crias include dystocia (meconium aspiration), failure of passive transfer (leads to lack of specific antibody protection as well as impaired neutrophilic function in neonates), prematurity or immaturity (lung immaturity, immature immune system), and neonatal

weakness (neonatal encephalopathy, sepsis, vitamin E or selenium deficiency).
• Iatrogenic risk factors include bottle feeding in the absence of a strong suckle reflex, and administration of mineral oil, rumen fluid, or medications.

DIAGNOSIS

DIFFERENTIAL DIAGNOSES
• Nonpulmonary causes of altered respiratory function include anemia, hypovolemia, cardiac disease, acidosis, hypoglycemia, botulism, nutritional myodegeneration, pain, fever, hyperthermia, and birth asphyxia.
• Developmental or noninfectious respiratory diseases in neonates include respiratory distress syndrome (hyaline membrane disease), diaphragmatic hernia, pulmonary hypoplasia, and persistent pulmonary hypertension.
• Differentials related to trauma include pneumothorax, rib fracture, and traumatic airway obstruction.

CBC/BIOCHEMISTRY/URINALYSIS
• Complete blood count changes include neutrophilic leukocytosis and hyperfibrinogenemia in bacterial infections.
• Neutropenia is often observed in neonatal crias with sepsis and in patients with viral diseases.
• Significant lymphopenia may be found in acute viral diseases, and in sepsis.

OTHER LABORATORY TESTS
• Arterial blood gas (ABG) analysis: Samples are best obtained from the medial saphenous artery (medial hindlimb above the stifle). The following ABG results (mean ± 95% confidence interval) have been documented in 14 healthy adult, male and nonpregnant female alpacas (mean age and weight: 4.5 years; 62 kg) and in 12 healthy neonatal alpaca crias (2–7 days old, 7.8 kg mean weight):
  ◦ pH = 7.47 (7.46–7.48)
  ◦ Bicarbonate (mEq/L) = 20.4 (19.6–21.3)
  ◦ PaO_2 (mmHg, adults) = 104.6 (100.7–108.4)
  ◦ Neonatal PaO_2 = 92 (87.7–96.4)
  ◦ $PaCO_2$ (mmHg, adults) = 27.7 (26.4–28.9)
  ◦ Neonatal $PaCO_2$ = 30.5 (27.2–33.8)
• Pleural fluid analysis: The preferred site of pleurocentesis is the 6th or 7th intercostal space, 10–15 cm dorsal to the midline ventrum or 2–4 cm dorsal to the costochondral junction of the ribs. The reported total nucleated cell count of pleural

RESPIRATORY DISEASE: CAMELID   (CONTINUED)

fluid from 17 healthy llamas was in the range of 200–1500 cells/μL (mean: 576 ± 361 cells/μL); with small lymphocyte, mononuclear cell, and neutrophil percentages representing 80–100%, 0–20%, and 0–10% of cells, respectively. Pleural fluid total protein concentrations were in the range <2.5–3.5 g/dL.
• Transtracheal aspirate fluid in clinically healthy adult llamas contained primarily vacuolated macrophages (60–100%), with 0–40% neutrophils, and fewer lymphocytes (0–2%), eosinophils (0–3%), and ciliated respiratory epithelial cells (0–10%).
• Bronchoalveolar lavage fluid from healthy alpacas contained 59 ± 12% alveolar macrophages, 31 ± 14% lymphocytes, 11 ± 9% neutrophils, 0% mast cells, and several ciliated epithelial cells.

IMAGING
• Thoracic radiographs are generally limited to lateral views in adult camelids.
• Thoracic ultrasonography can be useful to detect pulmonary consolidation, pleural effusion, abscesses, penetrating thoracic wounds, and rib fractures. However, lesions that do not involve the periphery of the lung or the pleural cavity cannot be imaged by this means.
• Upper airway endoscopy is useful to assess nasal and tracheal patency, and laryngeal and pharyngeal function, and to permit tracheal wash.
• Positive contrast rhinography, nasal catheter placement, endoscopy, and computed tomography (CT) have all been used to diagnose choanal atresia in camelids.

OTHER DIAGNOSTIC PROCEDURES
Noninvasive pulmonary function testing, including respiratory inductive plethysmography and pneumotachography, forced oscillatory mechanics, and assessment of functional residual capacity, have been described in camelids.

PATHOLOGIC FINDINGS
Vary depending on the underlying disease

TREATMENT
THERAPEUTIC APPROACH
• Antimicrobial therapy if indicated, preferably based on bacterial culture and sensitivity testing.
• Supportive care might include fluid therapy, enteral or parenteral nutrition, bronchodilators, gastroprotectants, and NSAIDs.
• Provision of oxygen via mask, nasal catheter, or potentially mechanical ventilation of neonates to address hypoxemia.

SURGICAL CONSIDERATIONS AND TECHNIQUES
Surgical intervention (with balloon dilation) may be beneficial in the membranous forms of choanal atresia, although the prognosis remains poor.

MEDICATIONS
DRUGS OF CHOICE
Camelid-specific pharmacokinetic data is available for the following antimicrobials:
• Ceftiofur (Naxcel®): 2.2 mg/kg IM q12h in alpacas will maintain plasma concentrations > 0.25 μg/mL. Naxcel® is usually dosed at higher amounts in the clinical setting (4.4–6.6 mg/kg SC q12h) to target more resistant bacteria. A long-acting ceftiofur crystalline-free acid (CCFA) formulation (Excede®) will also maintain plasma concentrations >0.25 μg/mL for 5–6 days if dosed at 6.6 mg/kg (effective for *Streptococcus* spp.)
• Enrofloxacin: 5–10 mg/kg, q24h SC or IV. Enrofloxacin will not target streptococcal, enterococcal, or anaerobic infections and is commonly used in combination with ceftiofur or penicillin.
• Florfenicol (Nuflor Gold®): 40 mg/kg SC q48h. Monitor serum protein concentrations during long-term use.
• Florfenicol (Nuflor®): 20 mg/kg IM q24h or 20 mg/kg SC q36–48h (use only for highly susceptible pathogens with an MIC ≤0.5 μg/mL). Monitor serum protein concentrations during long-term use.
• Ampicillin: 12 mg/kg IV q6–12h in llamas. Efficacy is expected against ampicillin-sensitive bacteria (with an MIC of 1–3 μg/mL).
• Gentamicin/amikacin: Use with caution while monitoring renal function.
• Penicillin-G (targets Gram-positive and some anaerobic infections): 22,000 IU/kg SC q12h.
• Long-acting tetracycline (200 mg/mL): 20 mg/kg SC q48h.
• Gastric protectant (C3): Pantoprazole 1 mg/kg IV or 2 mg/kg SC q24h.

CONTRAINDICATIONS
• Fluroquinolones should be avoided in neonatal crias.
• Avoid aminoglycosides in dehydrated animals.

PRECAUTIONS
Appropriate milk and meat withdrawal times must be followed for all compounds administered to food-producing animals.

POSSIBLE INTERACTIONS
N/A

FOLLOW-UP
EXPECTED COURSE AND PROGNOSIS
• Pulmonary disease is associated with a higher mortality in neonatal crias. Early diagnosis is essential for successful treatment.
• State and federal regulations impact management of animals with reportable disease.

POSSIBLE COMPLICATIONS
C3 ulceration

CLIENT EDUCATION
N/A

PATIENT CARE
• Serial chest radiographs are useful in monitoring the progress of lower respiratory tract conditions. Radiographic changes may, however, either follow or precede the onset of clinical signs and persist after their resolution.
• Repeated laboratory and clinical evaluation.

PREVENTION
Appropriate biosecurity for incoming animals (new members to the herds, animals returning from shows, breeding, etc.).

MISCELLANEOUS
ASSOCIATED CONDITIONS
• Sepsis
• Concurrent congenital defects in neonatal crias

AGE-RELATED FACTORS
Congenital conditions are most commonly observed in neonatal camelids.

ZOONOTIC POTENTIAL
Tuberculosis

PREGNANCY
Severe hypoxemia, as well as certain infectious diseases (e.g., BVDV and coronavirus infection), may be associated with reproductive losses.

BIOSECURITY
Relevant for individual contagious diseases including tuberculosis and coronavirus.

PRODUCTION MANAGEMENT
N/A

SYNONYMS
N/A

R

ABBREVIATIONS
- BVDV = bovine viral diarrhea virus
- C3 = third compartment of the camelid GI tract
- CT = computed tomography
- NSAIDs = nonsteroidal anti-inflammatory drugs
- $PaCO_2$ = partial pressure of carbon dioxide in arterial blood
- PaO_2 = partial pressure of oxygen in arterial blood

Suggested Reading
Byers S, Barrington G, Nelson D, et al. Neurological causes of diaphragmatic paralysis in 11 alpacas (*Vicugna pacos*). J Vet Intern Med 2011, 25: 380–5.
Crossley BM, Barr BC, Magdesian KG, et al. Identification of a novel coronavirus possibly associated with acute respiratory syndrome in alpacas (*Vicugna pacos*) in California, 2007. J Vet Diagn Invest 2010, 22: 94–7.
Pacheco AP, Bedenice D, Mazan MR, et al. Respiratory mechanics and results of cytologic examination of bronchoalveolar lavage fluid in healthy adult alpacas. Am J Vet Res 2012, 73: 146–52.

Author Daniela Bedenice
Consulting Editor Erica C. McKenzie

R

RESPIRATORY DISEASE: SMALL RUMINANT

BASICS

OVERVIEW
• A variety of upper and lower respiratory tract problems affect small ruminants.
• It is important to differentiate between upper and lower respiratory tract problems.
• Pathologic sounds may be referred from the upper airway and audible in the thorax.
• Auscultation has limitations in all species. Imaging modalities including ultrasound improve the accuracy of respiratory disease diagnosis.
• Lung sounds are typically easier to hear in small ruminants, which normally have fairly harsh inspiratory sounds.

INCIDENCE/PREVALENCE
• Variable; contagious disorders can achieve a high prevalence.
• Prevalence often influenced by herd or flock management.

GEOGRAPHIC DISTRIBUTION
• Variable depending on disorder.
• Pasteurellosis occurs worldwide.
• Contagious caprine pleuropneumonia is absent from the United States, but reported in other countries.

SYSTEMS AFFECTED
Respiratory

PATHOPHYSIOLOGY
• Often involves a primary infectious organism with secondary bacterial invasion creating or enhancing respiratory system injury.
• Upper airway disorders include neoplasia, pharyngeal trauma, *Corynebacterium pseudotuberculosis* infection, sinusitis, and *Oestrus ovis* infestation.
• Lower airway disease can arise from bacterial infections (*Pasteurella, Mannheimia Mycoplasma, Corynebacterium*), parasite infestation (*Dictyocaulus, Muellerius, Protostrongylus*), viral infections (OPP, OPA, CAE), aspiration of medication, feed, or milk (neonates), and from neoplasia.

HISTORICAL FINDINGS
Dependent on the underlying etiology. While viral infections can present as a herd concern, neoplastic, fungal, and protozoal disease will generally affect individual animals.

SIGNALMENT
Any breed or age of sheep and goats; respiratory disease may be more common in younger animals under stressful conditions.

PHYSICAL EXAMINATION FINDINGS
• Stridor or stertor, hyporexia inspiratory difficulty, limited air flow through the nostrils, facial asymmetry, and nasal discharge (especially unilateral) can indicate upper airway disease.
• Tachypnea, expiratory effort, exercise intolerance, fever, hyporexia, and coughing can indicate lower airway disease.
• Poor body condition suggests chronicity.

GENETICS
N/A

CAUSES AND RISK FACTORS
• A predisposing agent and/or stress (transport, poor nutrition, extreme weather, poor ventilation, overstocking, parasitism, weaning, and general husbandry procedures) may collaborate to overwhelm host immunity, allowing an opportunistic pathogen to invade the lower respiratory tract.
• Predisposing agents may be viral or bacterial and may include parainfluenza-3, respiratory syncytial virus, *Mycoplasma ovipneumoniae*, *Bordetella parapertussis*, adenovirus type 6, and *Chlamydia*.
• Pasteurellosis is one of the most important infectious bacterial diseases in sheep and goats, causing acute bacterial pneumonia. The condition is primarily associated with *M. haemolytica*, though *P. multocida* has been implicated. These are normal inhabitants of the upper respiratory system and opportunistic invaders of the lower respiratory system. *Bibersteinia trehalosi* (formerly *P. trehalosi*) results in systemic pasteurellosis and septicemia.
• Progressive pneumonia can result from viral infections, OPP, OPA, or from progressive interstitial retroviral pneumonia (PIRP) associated with CAE in goats. These are chronic disorders that progress over time, with weight loss and respiratory distress in afebrile animals as common signs.
• Mycoplasma pneumonia is also called atypical pneumonia, enzootic pneumonia, and chronic nonprogressive pneumonia. *M. ovipneumoniae* is thought to be the primary causative organism with secondary invading organisms.
• The *Mycoplasma mycoides* cluster is the most important group for goat mycoplasma pneumonia. *M. capricolum* ssp. *capripneumoniae* is the cause of contagious caprine pleuropneumonia (CCPP). This is very contagious with morbidity approaching 100% and mortality 60–100%. This is an exotic disorder in the US.
• *Mycoplasma mycoides* ssp. *capri* and *M. mycoides* ssp. *mycoides* large colony type are a common cause of arthritis and pneumonia in goats.
• Parasitic infestations of the respiratory tract can cause dyspnea, coughing, tachypnea, and weight loss particularly in young, pastured animals.

DIAGNOSIS

DIFFERENTIAL DIAGNOSES
• Ovine progressive pneumonia
• Bacterial pneumonia
• Caprine arthritis encephalitis
• Verminous pneumonia
• Causes of upper airway disease
• Other causes of weight loss and bacterial infection

CBC/BIOCHEMISTRY/URINALYSIS
A CBC may show inflammatory leukogram, a left shift, and increased fibrinogen and total protein concentrations.

OTHER LABORATORY TESTS
• Transtracheal aspiration or tracheal wash are superior for bacteriology.
• Bronchoalveolar lavage is superior for cytology.
• Baermann test on fresh feces is appropriate to detect verminous pneumonia.

IMAGING
• Ultrasonography with a 5–7.5 MHz probe allows visualization of the pleural cavity, pleural surface, and lung parenchyma (if consolidated at the pleural surface).
• Radiographs are useful for upper and lower respiratory tract lesions.
• Computed tomography under sedation provides excellent visualization of the upper and lower respiratory tract, particularly with intravenous contrast administration.

OTHER DIAGNOSTIC PROCEDURES
• Necropsy of affected representative individuals for flock/herd benefit
• Culture or PCR of tracheal wash and lung sections

PATHOLOGIC FINDINGS
• Fibrinopurulent pleuropneumonia
• Excess pleural and peritoneal fluid
• Lung abscessation and lung consolidation
• Verminous infestation

TREATMENT

THERAPEUTIC APPROACH
• Early detection and treatment with antibiotics is beneficial in bacterial disorders.
• Supportive therapy as needed.
• Vitamin C and E may be of additional benefit.
• Progressive pneumonias are terminal.

SURGICAL CONSIDERATIONS AND TECHNIQUES
N/A

(CONTINUED)

RESPIRATORY DISEASE: SMALL RUMINANT

MEDICATIONS

DRUGS OF CHOICE
• Common antibiotics include oxytetracycline (200 mg/ml at 20 mg/kg q72h), penicillin (22,000–44,000 U/kg q12–24h), ceftiofur (1.1–2.2 mg/kg q24h), florfenicol (20 mg/kg q48h, or 40 mg/kg once), tylosin (10–20 mg/kg q12–24h), tilmicosin at 10–20 mg/kg once in sheep only, and tulathromycin at 2.5 mg/kg once.
• Antibiotic selection may be based on drug cost, dose interval, culture and sensitivity results, and past effectiveness on each property.
• Oxytetracycline is commonly prescribed due to spectrum and cost effectiveness.
• Tylosin, tetracycline, and macrolides are appropriate for mycoplasma infections.
• Nonsteroidal anti-inflammatory drugs may benefit an individual animal for control of fever or to provide analgesia and to improve appetite.
• Anthelmintics are indicated for *Oestrus ovis* infestation and verminous pneumonia.

CONTRAINDICATIONS
• Tilmicosin is toxic to goats.
• Fluoroquinolones are illegal or prohibited from extra-label use in some countries.

PRECAUTIONS
• Appropriate milk and meat withdrawal times must be followed for all compounds administered to food-producing animals.
• Notifiable diseases must be reported to the appropriate regulatory bodies.

POSSIBLE INTERACTIONS
N/A

FOLLOW-UP

EXPECTED COURSE AND PROGNOSIS
• Progressive pneumonia is terminal; euthanasia and flock/herd implications need to be considered.
• For chronic pneumonias a prolonged course of therapy can achieve fair to good results.
• With mycoplasma infections, the hosts often remain carriers of the pathogens even with clinical recovery.

POSSIBLE COMPLICATIONS
• Polyarthritis
• Mastitis
• Otitis interna
• Septicemia

CLIENT EDUCATION
Management factors play a key role in respiratory disease. Depending on the causative agent, clients should be educated in regard to what management changes they can make to reduce the likelihood of additional cases.

PATIENT CARE
• Once to twice daily monitoring of attitude and appetite is a good indirect indication of therapy success.
• Imaging repetition can aid in disease monitoring.
• Normothermia within 48 hours of treatment is a good prognostic indicator in bacterial infections.

PREVENTION
• Isolate affected animals.
• Treat affected animals with antibiotics if definitively indicated.
• Reduce stress factors such as overcrowding and unnecessary handling.
• Divide up animal groups by age and production purpose.
• Consider vaccination for diseases such as caseous lymphadenitis and pasteurellosis.
• Purchase goat kids from herds with negative bulk tank culture for *Mycoplasma* and no history of kid deaths from arthritis and pneumonia.
• Isolate newcomers and culture milk before mixing goats with the rest of the herd.
• Provide neonates with heat-treated colostrum and milk.
• Practice good milking hygiene; teat dips, individual cloths for udder preparation.

MISCELLANEOUS

ASSOCIATED CONDITIONS
• Polyarthritis
• Leukoencephalomyelitis (goat kids with CAEV)
• Indurative mastitis (CAEV, OPP)
• Secondary bacterial pneumonia

AGE-RELATED FACTORS
Some conditions are more common in younger animals, such as septicemic pasteurellosis.

ZOONOTIC POTENTIAL
N/A

PREGNANCY
N/A

BIOSECURITY
• Quarantine new animals for 30–45 days.
• Visitors should wear clean clothes and footwear and wash their hands.

PRODUCTION MANAGEMENT
Minimize stress and biosecurity breaches.

SYNONYMS
• Ovine progressive pneumonia = maedi-visna
• Ovine pulmonary adenocarcinoma = sheep pulmonary adenomatosis, Jaagsiekte

ABBREVIATIONS
• CAEV = caprine arthritis encephalitis virus
• CCPP = contagious caprine pleuropneumonia
• OPA = ovine pulmonary adenocarcinoma
• OPP = ovine progressive pneumonia
• PCR = polymerase chain reaction
• PIRP = progressive interstitial retroviral pneumonia

SEE ALSO
• Caprine Arthritis Encephalitis Virus
• Contagious Caprine Pleuropneumonia
• *Oestrus ovis* Infestation
• Maedi-Visna (Ovine Progressive Pneumonia)
• Respiratory Disease: Pharmacology (see www.fiveminutevet.com/ruminant)

Suggested Reading
Plummer PJ, Plummer CL, Still KM. Diseases of the respiratory system. In: Pugh DG, Baird AN eds, Sheep and Goat Medicine, 2nd ed. Philadelphia: Saunders, 2012, pp. 126–49.
Scott PR. Cardiorespiratory system, Part 1: Thorax. In: Scott PR, Sheep Medicine. London: Manson Publishing Ltd, 2007, pp. 137–60.
Smith MC, Sherman DM. Respiratory system. In: Smith MC, Sherman DM, Goat Medicine. Ames: Wiley-Blackwell, 2009, pp. 339–76.

Author Brandon Fraser
Consulting Editor Erica C. McKenzie

R

RETAINED PLACENTA

BASICS

OVERVIEW
• Retained placenta (RP) or retained fetal membranes (RFM) is failure to expel the placenta (fetal membranes) within 12 hours after parturition in cattle and small ruminants and within 6 hours in camelids.
• Various authors define RP at 6, 12, or 24 h. Among cows that expelled the placenta within 24 h, 77% occurred within 6 h and 94% occurred within 12 h after calving. The 24 h definition may be most practical for monitoring in the field.

INCIDENCE/PREVALENCE
• The median lactational incidence risk was 8.6%, with a range of 1.3–39.2% of lactations affected in dairy cows in the United States.
• RFM is more common in sheep than in goats.
• RFM is rare in alpacas and llamas.

GEOGRAPHIC DISTRIBUTION
Worldwide

SYSTEMS AFFECTED
Reproductive

PATHOPHYSIOLOGY
• Ruminant placentation is classified as synepitheliochorial cotyledonary nondeciduate. Cotyledonary refers to the presence of localized areas of proliferated trophectoderm that constitute the fetal portion of the placentome. The placentome is formed by chorionic villi from the cotyledons that grow and interdigitate with corresponding maternal caruncular crypts, providing a finger-in-glove arrangement. Domestic ruminants have 75–125 placentomes.
• Placentation in camelids is epitheliochorial microcotyledonary diffuse nondeciduate. The placenta is delivered rapidly. RP is likely to results from uterine atony.
• The exact mechanism of placental detachment is not completely understood. Placental maturation along with appropriate structural, endocrinologic, and immunologic changes result in the separation and expulsion of the placenta. Critical biochemical, vascular, contractile, and involution changes occurring at the uterine-placental interface before and during parturition assist in separation and expulsion of the placenta.
• After expulsion of the fetus and loss of fetal circulation to the cotyledons, capillaries within the villi collapse, resulting in a decrease in size. Uterine contractions result in flattening of the caruncles and shrinkage of the caruncular stock, further enhancing the separation of the allantochorion.
• RFM results from the failure of detachment of the fetal-maternal interface following parturition.

• The increased incidence of RP after induced parturition or abortion supports the observation that placentome immaturity may be a contributing factor in ruminants.
• In a mature placenta, maternal immunologic recognition of fetal MHC class I proteins triggers immune and inflammatory responses that contribute to the detachment of the cotyledonary portion of the allantochorion at parturition. MHC compatibility has significant molecular consequences and can result in an increased incidence of RP. Given that immune function is critical to normal placental detachment, it is likely that molecular genetics has a role in RP.
• Production of neutrophil-activated factors and the chemotactic activity to neutrophils are important for successful immune-assisted detachment of the cotyledonary portion of the allantochorion. Prepartum immunosuppression, specifically impairment of neutrophil function, is a critical factor in RP. The function of peripheral leukocytes may be reduced in cases of RP, with decreased neutrophil function occurring 1–2 weeks before calving in cows that develop RP.
• Failure of proteolysis of the cotyledon and, in particular, a failure of collagenolysis to release the cotyledon from the caruncle also plays a role in RP. Injection of collagenase into the umbilical artery within the uterus (after RP occurs) or into the uterine artery during cesarean section is associated with detachment of the placenta within hours.
• In RP, detachment occurs around day 6–10 following parturition due to necrosis of the caruncle and liquefaction of the cotyledonary villi. While the RP is present in the uterus, partial necrosis contributes to bacterial growth, which along with ongoing metabolic activity by the placental tissue results in inflammation of the uterus, which may progress to clinical metritis.

GENETICS
RFM is more common in dairy cattle and camels.

HISTORICAL FINDINGS
• Recent parturition
• Dystocia
• Failure to find an expelled placenta

SIGNALMENT
• Bovine—more common in dairy cattle than in beef cattle
• Small ruminants—occurs uncommonly
• Camelids—rare

PHYSICAL EXAMINATION FINDINGS
• Presence of all or part of the placenta in the uterus >12–24 hours after parturition; commonly observed on inspection from a distance, with part of the placenta hanging downward from the vulva.
• Within 1–3 days a fetid odor and/or fetid red-brown discharge from the vulva are likely to be present.

• Other clinical signs or physical examination findings that might be observed include pyrexia, decreased milk yield, obtundation, tachycardia, loss of body condition, and marked systemic illness. These clinical signs are often associated with development of either clinical endometritis or metritis.
• In some cases, inspection or palpation per vagina is necessary to confirm the presence of placental tissue and rule out an RP.

CAUSES AND RISK FACTORS
• Failure of detachment of the fetal cotyledon from the maternal caruncle at the time of parturition in ruminants.
• In camelids, RFM is often due to failure of uterine contraction.
• Abortion, twins, fetal gigantism, induced parturition, dystocia, cesarean section, stillbirth, intensive heat stress, negative energy balance, trace mineral and vitamin deficiency (suboptimal availability of selenium, vitamin E, etc.), and milk fever (hypocalcemia) are all associated with an increased risk of RP.
• Cows with elevated serum NEFAs (>0.5 mEq/L) and/or suboptimal vitamin E status in the last week prepartum (serum α-tocopherol : cholesterol ratio <2.5×10^{-3}) are more likely to develop RP. Lower prepartum serum cholesterol concentration has also been associated with increased risk of RP.

DIAGNOSIS

DIFFERENTIAL DIAGNOSES
• Diagnosis is straightforward.
• If pyrexia (temperature >39.5°C) is present together with RP (in the absence of other causes), it is important to consider development of clinical/toxic metritis, particularly if dullness, decreased milk production, loss of appetite, anorexia, or signs of toxemia (dehydration, tachycardia, diarrhea, weakness, cold extremities) are also present.

CBC/BIOCHEMISTRY/URINALYSIS
May be indicated if signs of systemic illness are present.

OTHER LABORATORY TESTS
Potentially haptoglobin and serum amyloid A concentrations could potentially be used to identify cows at risk for RP.

IMAGING
Transrectal (cattle) and transabdominal ultrasonography (small ruminants and SAC) may be helpful in confirming RP in cases where the cervix may be closed making digital vaginal examination impossible.

OTHER DIAGNOSTIC PROCEDURES
Transrectal palpation or digital vaginal examination may be needed to confirm the diagnosis of RP.

R

PATHOLOGIC FINDINGS

Animals with RP have necrotic placental tissue attached at the caruncles, abundant mixed bacterial growth in the uterine lumen, and variable severity of inflammation of the layers of the uterus.

TREATMENT

THERAPEUTIC APPROACH

• The basic goals of any therapeutic plan should be to return the cow to reproductive usefulness as soon as possible and prevent complications that can lead to economic losses.
• Uncomplicated ruminant cases require no treatment. Treatment is often initiated early in the case of camelids.
• Manual removal should be attempted only if the placenta is detached and easy to remove.
• In camelids, oxytocin therapy with or without systemic antibiotic is considered the standard of care.
• In ruminants, intrauterine antibiotic treatment is generally not recommended. In cases when antibiotic treatment is necessary, systemic administration is recommended. Absorption of systemic antibiotics is not impaired as in local treatments; antibiotic concentrations attained in the uterine tissue are similar in blood concentrations.
• In ruminants, if the RP persists for >48 hours and the animal develops pyrexia or other clinical signs it should receive immediate attention and a treatment plan be developed. Therefore it is imperative that cows in the postpartum period are evaluated daily for attitude, appetite, and rectal temperature, with closer monitoring initiated in instances where an RP is identified.
  ◦ Several studies have demonstrated that approximately 50% of cows with untreated RP will have a temperature >39.5°C on at least 1 day. It is not clear if all of these cases require systemic antibiotic treatment. At a minimum, it establishes that approximately 50% of cows that develop RP do not require antibiotic treatment because they never become febrile. Therefore, automatic treatment of all cows having an RP with antibiotics is questionable.
  ◦ Limited published data evaluating conservative management (no antibiotic treatment) of cows developing a fever following an RP leaves an unclear picture as to the health or economic benefits of treating all cows with an RP, or even all febrile cows with an RP, with systemic antibiotics.
• Uterine lavage may be considered in cases where development of metritis or other secondary clinical signs are observed.

• Other agents that have been considered for intrauterine use include chlorhexidine, hydrogen peroxide, and more recently ozone.
• The use of ecbolic drugs has been suggested as a way to improve uterine and myometrial contractions to aid in the separation and expulsion of the placenta.
  ◦ Although there are some reports of benefits of $PGF2_\alpha$ or oxytocin, especially within 1 hour after calving, the data are limited and contradictory. There are persistent anecdotes in circulation, and some controversy in the scientific literature, but these arguments are not based on data from field studies of naturally occurring cases. There is no strong evidence that any of the suggested treatments hasten the passage of the RP, reduce the risk of displaced abomasum (DA), or improve subsequent reproductive performance.
• Estradiol compounds have been advocated as an adjunct treatment option to aid in the restoration of the endometrium and prevent metritis; however, lack of conclusive scientific evidence and lack of availability in some parts of the world due to regulatory measures precludes its use in many circumstances.
  ◦ Estradiol cypionate (ECP) in cows with RP did not reduce the incidence of fever with fetid discharge within 7–30 DIM, but significantly prolonged the time to pregnancy relative to no treatment in cows with RP.
  ◦ Similarly, in two other studies, ECP administration failed to reduce the incidence of fetid discharge (with or without fever).

SURGICAL CONSIDERATIONS AND TECHNIQUES
N/A

MEDICATIONS

DRUGS OF CHOICE

• Ceftiofur (Na- or -HCl): 1–2.2 mg/kg IM q24h for 3 days; up to maximum of 5 days if clinically improving but not resolved (WD = 0 milk, 3 d meat) – Labeled for use in cattle with metritis.
• Ceftiofur crystalline free acid: 6.6 mg/kg SC q4d (administration of 2 doses) (WD = 0 milk, 13 d meat). Labeled for use in cattle with metritis.
• Procaine penicillin G: 21,000 IU/kg IM q12–24h for 3–5 days (WD = 4–5 d milk; 10–30 d meat).
• Oxytocin IM administration q4h in the first 24 hours postpartum may be helpful (cattle and camels 20 IU, small ruminants and SAC 5–10 IU). Oxytocin administration is more helpful in the management of RFM in camelids.

CONTRAINDICATIONS

• Appropriate milk and meat withdrawal times must be followed for all compounds administered to food-producing animals.
• Manual removal is contraindicated in ruminants. There is some evidence that manual removal can exacerbate damage to the endometrium, increasing the risk of toxemia, and may delay return to cyclicity.
• Use of estrogen in food-producing animals is not legal in some countries.

PRECAUTIONS
N/A

POSSIBLE INTERACTIONS
N/A

FOLLOW-UP

EXPECTED COURSE AND PROGNOSIS

• The expected impact of RP depends on complications, which range from none (other than an esthetically unappealing condition for 1 week) to impaired reproductive performance, or progression to severe metritis and toxemia. The course of this disorder depends on immune function of the animal.
• The ability of the uterine immune system to respond to RP, inflammation, and increased bacterial challenge determines whether the animal will go on to suffer metritis or impaired reproductive performance.
• RP is a risk factor for metritis and endometritis. It is also a risk factor for DA in cattle. Conversely, many animals with RP do not have any clinical complications, even if untreated.
• In cattle, although many studies report negative impacts of RP on reproductive outcomes, the results are variable. The best analyses estimate that affected cows become pregnant approximately 15% more slowly (i.e., hazard ratio for pregnancy = 0.85) than unaffected cows (e.g., reduction in 21-day pregnancy rate from 15% to 12.8%).
• It is not clear whether impaired reproductive performance is directly attributable to RP, or (more likely) only if metritis or clinical and/or subclinical endometritis result.
• There are some reports of short-term reductions in milk yield associated with RP, but meaningful loss of production appears to be confined to those individuals that progress to clinical metritis. Likewise, RP itself appears not to increase culling risk.

POSSIBLE COMPLICATIONS

Metritis, endometritis, ketosis, DA, mastitis, increased time to pregnancy (days open), decreased probability of pregnancy, increased risk of culling.

R

RETAINED PLACENTA　(CONTINUED)

CLIENT EDUCATION
See "Prevention"

PATIENT MONITORING
• In camelids, aggressive treatment is usually instituted quickly to reduce the chance of complications.
• Ruminants with RP should be inspected daily until the placenta is expelled, to detect progression to metritis. Observation of the cow's attitude, appetite (if possible), and daily milk production is likely a useful screening test.
• Measurement of rectal temperature is indicated in animals that are dull, inappetent, producing less milk than expected, or declining in milk production. Some authors advocate daily monitoring of rectal temperature in all cows with RP for 10 days postpartum. More large-scale field studies are needed to determine if this approach results in early detection and mitigation of metritis, avoidance of other related diseases (e.g., displaced abomasum), and/or improved reproductive performance, or if this approach leads to medically or economically unnecessary treatment.
• It is recommended that all cows affected with RP be examined 20–30 days after expulsion of the placenta to determine the progress of uterine involution.
• Animals with RP will plausibly benefit from extra effort to provide easy access to feed and bedding space, as well as unrestricted access to water and heat abatement measures. It is important to recognize, however, that all transition cows may benefit from such measures.

PREVENTION
• In cattle, because the cause of RP is multifactorial, it is important to recognize that no one preventive measure will be universally effective. The principle for prevention is to optimize peripartum immune function.
• In general, best management and nutritional practices (i.e., transition diet to meet National Research Council [2001] requirements for >3 weeks prepartum with average DIM >12 kg/cow/day, >60 cm manger space/cow, calving at body condition score of 3.5 out of 5, lack of crowding, heat abatement measures above 27°C, free access to clean water) will plausibly help prevent RP.
• In particular, the prepartum diet should include 0.3 ppm selenium and 1,000–2,000 IU/cow/day of vitamin E. Among animals with suboptimum circulating vitamin E in the last week prepartum (serum

α-tocopherol : cholesterol ratio $<2.5 \times 10^{-3}$), injection of 3,000 IU α-tocopherol SC or IM 1 week before expected calving reduced the risk of RP. Unfortunately, there is no simple way to identify individuals or herds that may benefit from this treatment. In two studies, peripartum oral administration of calcium (one to three treatments of 60 g Ca within a 24 h period around calving) did not reduce the incidence of RP.
• One economic analysis estimated that at a herd incidence of 7% the economic loss was minimal. Therefore, decisions about preventive interventions should consider the magnitude of the problem as well as the evidence for the expected costs and benefits of proposed measures.
• In camelids, animals at risk of having RFM (i.e., following dystocia or C-section) are systematically treated with oxytocin and systemic antibiotics.

MISCELLANEOUS

ASSOCIATED CONDITIONS
• Abortion, twins, dystocia, metritis, endometritis
• In SAC, RFM and peritonitis has been reported following uterine rupture

AGE-RELATED FACTORS
N/A

ZOONOTIC POTENTIAL
Retained placenta is common following abortion due to zoonotic bacteria (brucellosis, Q fever, chlamydiosis).

PREGNANCY
N/A

BIOSECURITY
N/A

PRODUCTION MANAGEMENT
Record keeping of all instances of RFM helps monitor trends in postpartum complications and detection of problems in transition cow and calving management.

SYNONYMS
• Retained afterbirth
• Retained fetal membranes

ABBREVIATIONS
• DA = displaced abomasum
• DIM = days in milk (days postpartum)
• ECP = estradiol cypionate
• IM = intramuscular
• MHC = major histocompatibility complex
• NEFA = nonesterified fatty acid

• PGF2$_\alpha$ = prostaglandin F2$_\alpha$
• RFM = retained fetal membranes
• RP = retained placenta
• SAC = South American camelids
• SC = subcutaneous
• WD = withdraw

SEE ALSO
• Dystocia: Bovine
• Endometritis
• Ketosis
• Metritis
• Postpartum Disorders
• Postparturient Paresis (Hypocalcemia)

Suggested Reading
Beagley J, Whitman K, Baptiste K, Scherzer J. Physiology and treatment of retained fetal membranes in cattle. J Vet Intern Med 2010, 24: 261–8.
Davies C, Hill J, Edwards J, et al. Major histocompatibility antigen expression on the bovine placenta: its relationship to abnormal pregnancies and retained placenta. Anim Reprod Sci 2004, 82–83: 267–80.
Đuričić D, Valpotić H, Samardžija, M The intrauterine treatment of the retained foetal membrane in dairy goats by ozone: novel alternative to antibiotic therapy. Reprod Domest Anim 2015, 50: 236–9.
Đuričić D, Valpotić H, Žura Žaja I, Samardžija, M. Comparison of intrauterine antibiotics versus ozone medical use in sheep with retained placenta and following obstetric assistance. Reprod Domest Anim 2016, 51: 538–40.
Fathi E, Hamali H, Kaleibar MT, et al. Application of acute phase proteins as indicators of retained placenta and their relation to energy metabolites in postcalving dairy cows. Comp Clin Pathol 2015, 24: 47–51.
Frazer G. A rational basis for therapy in the sick postpartum cow. Vet Clin North Am Food Anim Pract 2005, 21: 523–68.
Fthenakis GC. Effects of retention of fetal membranes on subsequent reproductive performance of dairy ewes. Theriogenology 2004, 61: 129–35.
Zobel R, Tkalčić S. Efficacy of ozone and other treatment modalities for retained placenta in dairy cows. Reprod Domestic Anim 2013, 48: 121–5.

Author Alexis Campbell
Consulting Editor Ahmed Tibary
Acknowledgment The author and book editors acknowledge the prior contribution of Stephen LeBlanc.

R

BASICS

OVERVIEW

Rift Valley fever (RVF) is an acute febrile viral disease affecting cattle, sheep, goats, and camelids. It causes high mortality in neonates, necrotizing hepatitis, and abortion. It is reportable in the United States and a notifiable disease of the International Office of Epizootics (OIE).

INCIDENCE/PREVALENCE

- Sheep are most susceptible to infection, and mortality is influenced by age. Newborn lambs are highly susceptible, with a mortality rate >90% in lambs <1 week old, associated with acute necrotic hepatitis.
- Mortality rate in adult ruminants is 10–30%; the abortion rate can range between 40% and 100%.

GEOGRAPHIC DISTRIBUTION

- Endemic throughout much of the African continent. Epidemics occur every 5–10 years in eastern Africa.
- The virus has emerged in the Middle East, northern Egypt and the Comoros archipelago.
- The geographic range is likely to expand due to presence of appropriate vectors over a much larger geographic range

SYSTEMS AFFECTED

- Reproductive
- Digestive

PATHOPHYSIOLOGY

- RVF is caused by a mosquito-borne phlebovirus, family Bunyaviridae. It is a single-stranded RNA virus with a single serotype but with strains of variable virulence.
- The virus is transmitted mainly by *Aedes* mosquitoes, which are also a reservoir, but >20 species of mosquito can transmit RVF including *Culex, Anopheles,* and *Mansonia*; transovarial transmission occurs in *Aedes* spp.
- The virus circulates between wild ruminants and mosquitoes in endemic areas without causing disease.
- Viral replication occurs mainly in the liver and spleen of infected animals, although the brain may be affected; lesions arise mainly due to the lytic effects of the virus.
- Generalized infection in the mosquito is necessary for effective transmission, and movement of virus from the insect gut is facilitated by the presence of microfilariae in ingested blood.
- Cattle, sheep, and goats are considered the primary amplifying hosts.
- Virus is carried to the placenta and fetus during viremia with the liver as the target organ for multiplication.

- Peracute, acute, subacute, chronic, and convalescent forms of disease can occur in mature sheep and cattle.

HISTORICAL FINDINGS

Abortion or sudden neonatal death may be reported.

SIGNALMENT

- Most commonly infects cattle, goats, and sheep which are amplifiers of the virus, but RVF has been reported in other species including camelids, wild ruminants, African monkeys, and domestic carnivores.
- Lambs, kids, and calves are the most likely to show clinical disease.
- Pregnant females very commonly display abortion with infection.

PHYSICAL EXAMINATION FINDINGS

- The incubation period is approximately 12–36 hours, and viremia typically lasts for 1–3 days (up to 10 days).
- The mortality rate in infected newborn lambs is 95–100%, with death within two days. Affected lambs display high fever, which may be biphasic, loss of appetite, decreased activity, and prostration about 12–18 h prior to death. Salivation, diarrhea, and colic may occur.
- Adult sheep and cattle are often asymptomatic, though fever, bloody nasal discharge, and bloody diarrhea can occur, as can sudden death.
- Abortion occurs in the vast majority of pregnant animals.

GENETICS

N/A

CAUSES AND RISK FACTORS

- Heavy rainfall and flooding often precede outbreaks.
- Irrigation and dam building can promote RVF in a region.
- Exposure of pregnant animals to competent arthropod vectors presents great risk.
- Biting midges and ticks are also implicated in transmission.

DIAGNOSIS

DIFFERENTIAL DIAGNOSES

- Include other causes of abortion such as toxoplasmosis, brucellosis, trichomoniasis, ovine enzootic abortion, Q fever and campylobacterioisis.
- Additional differentials include ephemeral fever, Wesselsbron disease, enterotoxemia (sheep), peste des petits ruminants, toxic plant ingestion, pasteurellosis, heartwater (*Ehrlichia ruminantium* infection), and anthrax.

CBC/BIOCHEMISTRY/URINALYSIS

N/A

OTHER LABORATORY TESTS

N/A

IMAGING

N/A

OTHER DIAGNOSTIC PROCEDURES

- Virus isolation from whole blood or serum during the febrile stage, and from brain, liver, spleen, and fetal membranes of aborted fetuses via ELISA, serum neutralization, complement fixation, RT-PCR, agar gel diffusion, and immunohistochemistry
- Tests can be supplemented by virus isolation from inoculated rodents or cell cultures
- Cross-reactivity can be an issue between RVF virus and other phleboviruses in tests identifying serum antibodies to RVF; virus neutralization tests are the most specific. An IgM ELISA exists by which recent infection can be determined from a single serum sample.

PATHOLOGIC FINDINGS

- Gross findings include hepatomegaly with patchy congestion; petechial, ecchymotic to suffusive hemorrhages in skin, parietal and visceral serosal surfaces; enlarged and hemorrhagic lymph nodes; and hemorrhagic abomasitis and cholecystitis are often evident. Fetal malformations (arthrogryposis, brain defects) may occur.
- Histopathology identifies multifocal to massive coagulative or lytic hepatic necrosis often preserving portal areas; eosinophilic rod-shaped, round or oval intranuclear inclusions are evident in hepatocytes in 50% of affected ovine fetuses. Necrosis of the villi of the distal jejunum and ileum may occur; lymphoid depletion in spleen and lymph nodes; placentitis; and degenerative lesions in heart and renal tubules.

TREATMENT

THERAPEUTIC APPROACH

N/A

SURGICAL CONSIDERATIONS AND TECHNIQUES

N/A

MEDICATIONS

DRUGS OF CHOICE

N/A

CONTRAINDICATIONS

N/A

PRECAUTIONS

N/A

R

RIFT VALLEY FEVER

POSSIBLE INTERACTIONS
N/A

 FOLLOW-UP

EXPECTED COURSE AND PROGNOSIS
• Symptomatic adult animals are likely to recover quickly from abortion and other clinical signs in most cases.
• Severe illness and rapid death is expected in infected neonatal ruminants.

POSSIBLE COMPLICATIONS
Abortion is the most likely complication of infection in the pregnant female.

CLIENT EDUCATION
• Ensure clients understand that RVF is a zoonotic disease that can be readily transmitted to humans via inhalation or direct contact with body fluids from infected animals (some of which may be asymptomatic).
• All animal products should be pasteurized or cooked prior to consumption.

PATIENT CARE
N/A

PREVENTION
• Both live and killed vaccines exist for ruminants, including the live Smithburn strain which induces good immunity within a week after vaccination, and a naturally attenuated avirulent isolate (clone 13).
• Vaccination is not recommended during outbreaks due to the risk of inadvertently amplifying outbreaks through the use of multidose vaccine vials and reuse of needles.
• It is also not recommended to use live attenuated vaccines in areas where RVF is not endemic.

• Lambs can be vaccinated at 6 months old, and pregnant ewes and cows can be vaccinated (twice in 3 months) with the formalin inactivated vaccine to provide protection to the fetus and colostral immunity.
• Vector control should be practiced.
• Quarantine may be appropriate for preventing infection or reducing spread in outbreak situations.

 MISCELLANEOUS

ASSOCIATED CONDITIONS
N/A

AGE-RELATED FACTORS
• Greatest mortality occurs in fetuses and neonates of cattle, sheep, and goats.
• Decreased susceptibility to disease with age.

ZOONOTIC POTENTIAL
• Human infections can arise from mosquito bites, or through exposure to infected animals or animal tissues, since infected animals (sheep in particular) can display high titer viremia.
• Generally humans are asymptomatic or experience a short febrile illness with infection, sometimes with recurring fever and headaches for up to 10 days followed by 2 weeks of weakness before recovery.
• Some humans may develop severe disease with acute hepatitis, jaundice, encephalitis, renal failure, and hemorrhagic complications.

PREGNANCY
• RVF causes abortion, neonatal death, and fetal malformations in sheep, cattle, and goats.
• The live vaccines should not be administered to pregnant animals due to the risk of abortion or fetal defects.

BIOSECURITY
Notifiable OIE disease and requires mandatory reporting.

PRODUCTION MANAGEMENT
• Vector control
• Movement of animals to higher elevations
• Vaccination prior to breeding season
• Quarantine

SYNONYM
Enzootic hepatitis

ABBREVIATIONS
• ELISA = enzyme-linked immunosorbent assay
• IgM = immunoglobulin M
• OIE = International Office of Epizootics
• RT-PCR = reverse transcription-polymerase chain reaction
• RVF = Rift Valley fever

SEE ALSO
• Abortion: Bacterial
• Abortion: Viral, Fungal, and Nutritional

Suggested Reading
Ikegami T, Makino S. The pathogenesis of Rift Valley fever. Viruses 2011, 3: 493–519.
Mansfield KL, Banyard AC, McElhinney L, Johnson N, Horton DL, Hernández-Triana LM, Fooks AR. Rift Valley fever virus: A review of diagnosis and vaccination, and implications for emergence in Europe. Vaccine 2015, 33: 5520–31.
Author Akinyi Carol Nyaoke
Consulting Editor Erica C. McKenzie
Acknowledgment The author and book editors acknowledge the prior contribution of Glenda Dvorak.

BASICS

OVERVIEW
• Nondilation of the cervix that results in prolonged lambing (kidding), weak-born or dead lambs (kids), and cervical trauma or secondary infections in the ewe (doe).
• Mortality is often high in dam and offspring, even with veterinary intervention.

INCIDENCE/PREVALENCE
Incidence is usually higher in maiden dams; however, older animals may also present with ringwomb. The number of cases within a given flock or herd can vary dramatically from year to year. Predisposing factors are not well established.

GEOGRAPHIC DISTRIBUTION
Ringwomb is apparently common in most regions of the world, although complete data on distribution with emphasis on individual species have not been reported.

SYSTEMS AFFECTED
Reproductive

PATHOPHYSIOLOGY
• Complex interactions between fetal and maternal neural, endocrine, and paracrine systems lead to the efficient delivery of normal lambs or kids.
• Increased levels of fetal plasma cortisol result in an increase in estrogen and a decrease in progesterone in maternal plasma and an increase in maternal uterine prostaglandin production. These changes lead to the induction of normal delivery including efficient and coordinated myometrial contractions, dilation of the cervix, delivery of the fetus, and expulsion of the placenta.
• The exact mechanism by which estrogen and other hormonal factors regulate cervical ripening and dilation is not completely known.
• Failure of the cervix to dilate is referred to as ringwomb. (For a complete review of endocrine and paracrine regulation of preterm and birth processes, see Challis et al. (2000) in "Suggested Reading").

HISTORICAL FINDINGS
• Dystocia: Failure to progress through the second stage of parturition
• Depressed or down female
• Overdue ewe or doe

SIGNALMENT
• Commonly ewes and does in labor.
• Less commonly, cattle and camelid may present with failure of cervical dilation.
• In sheep and goats, all ages are affected; first or second parity dams are most commonly affected.

PHYSICAL EXAMINATION FINDINGS
• Affected ewes and does may go undetected until the fetuses have died from hypoxia, and the ewe is suffering systemic effects from uterine toxemia.
• Often the first indication of ringwomb is the presentation of fetal membrane through the vagina without concurrent evidence of active labor. The ewe may act restless or appear normal.
• Similar signs are observed in does, although vocalization may be more prominent.
• The cervix is not sufficiently dilated to allow expulsion of the fetus. Often, only a finger may be inserted through the cervical os on vaginal examination.
• Status of the fetus should be determined by stimulating fetal movement if possible. Oftentimes the presence of a malodorous discharge will confirm the demise of the lamb and impending metritis and septicemia in the ewe.

GENETICS
A clear genetic linkage has not been determined; however, there is anecdotal evidence that suggests that certain bloodlines within a particular breed may have an increased incidence of ringwomb.

CAUSES AND RISK FACTORS
• Nondilation of the cervix.
• Risk factors are not well understood.
• There is limited evidence of unknown genetic factors that may predispose to ringwomb.
• Infectious causes including *Chlamydophila ovis* have been implicated; however, many flocks have problems with enzootic abortion and report no significant problems with ringwomb.
• Factors that have been considered in the past but are not supported scientifically include trace mineral deficiencies, exogenous estrogen in feedstuffs, or simple malpresentation of the fetus.

DIAGNOSIS

DIFFERENTIAL DIAGNOSES
• Dystocia
• Uterine torsion
• Early dilation syndrome

CBC/BIOCHEMISTRY/URINALYSIS
N/A

OTHER LABORATORY TESTS
N/A

IMAGING
Transabdominal ultrasonography to determine fetal viability and integrity of the uterine wall.

OTHER DIAGNOSTIC PROCEDURES
Vaginal examination readily confirms nondilation of the cervix.

PATHOLOGIC FINDINGS
Often, postmortem examinations are not performed. If performed, gross examination reveals term or near-term fetuses that are fresh or variably autolyzed. The cervix is usually only slightly dilated to allow expulsion of minimal fetal membranes.

TREATMENT

THERAPEUTIC APPROACH
• Hormonal therapy (estrogen or application of misoprostol) may help dilate the cervix, although the response is variable and often delayed. In addition, neither product is approved in food animals in many countries.
• Oxytocin may stimulate uterine contractions but, if the cervix is not dilated, contractions will not be productive and will result in uterine tearing.
• Producers will often attempt to manually dilate the cervix with digital pressure. If care is taken, and the cervix is slowly dilated (30 minutes or more) with minimal tearing, live lambs or kids may deliver. More often, this procedure results in delayed delivery with dead fetuses and trauma to the dam's cervix that results in the need to treat aggressively for secondary bacterial infection of the cervix and uterus.

SURGICAL CONSIDERATIONS AND TECHNIQUES
If fetuses are alive, a cesarean section is the most reliable way to achieve a positive outcome for the dam and offspring.

MEDICATIONS

DRUGS OF CHOICE
• Broad-spectrum antibiotics are usually needed as follow-up therapy after manual dilation.
• Estrogen products have been recommended to assist in cervical dilation; however, the effects are minimal and the response is often delayed.
• Oxytocin administered IM, will stimulate uterine contractions; however, the cervix is usually not dilated and the uterus may tear or rupture.
• Calcium preparations have been administered as a preventive approach if hypocalcemia is suspected; however, a link between low blood calcium and ringwomb has not been established.

CONTRAINDICATIONS
• Appropriate milk and meat withdrawal times must be followed for all compounds administered to food-producing animals.
• Goats are extremely sensitive to the effects of lidocaine.

PRECAUTIONS
N/A

R

RINGWOMB

POSSIBLE INTERACTIONS
N/A

 FOLLOW-UP

EXPECTED COURSE AND PROGNOSIS
• Affected dams will usually recover if trauma to the cervix is minimized. However, all ewes experiencing ringwomb will need to be culled from production.
• Secondary infection is usually responsive to antibiotics.
• If trauma to the cervix is severe or the dam is toxic and the fetuses are dead at the time of presentation, the prognosis is poor.

POSSIBLE COMPLICATIONS
• Fetal death and toxemia
• Uterine rupture
• Post-surgical complications (retained placenta, peritonitis, surgical incision infection)

CLIENT EDUCATION
• All the risk factors for ringwomb are not known.
• If manual dilation is attempted, the ewe will need to be culled from production. If the producer has examined the dam prior to veterinary intervention, it is an appropriate time to provide education on the zoonotic risks associated with lambing ewes.

PATIENT CARE
Standard care following cesarean section: Monitor female for appetite, fever, and demeanor.

PREVENTION
N/A

 MISCELLANEOUS

ASSOCIATED CONDITIONS
N/A

AGE-RELATED FACTORS
All ages are affected; first or second parity dams are most commonly affected.

ZOONOTIC POTENTIAL
Any assisted delivery in the ewe and doe has the potential to transmit several zoonotic pathogens including *Chlamydophila abortus*, *Campylobacter jejuni*, and *Coxiella burnetii*. Appropriate safety precautions should be observed.

PREGNANCY
Ringwomb is a condition of parturition. If unresolved quickly, the fetal survival is compromised.

BIOSECURITY
N/A

PRODUCTION MANAGEMENT
Cull females which survive from breeding.

SYNONYM
Nondilation of the cervix

SEE ALSO
• Cesarean Section: Bovine
• Cesarean Section: Camelid
• Cesarean Section: Small Ruminant
• Dystocia: Bovine
• Dystocia: Camelid
• Dystocia: Small Ruminant

ABBREVIATIONS
• IM = intramuscular
• NSAIDs = nonsteroidal anti-inflammatory drugs

Suggested Reading
Braun W. Parturition and dystocia in the goat. In: Youngquist RS ed, Current Therapy in Large Animal Theriogenology. Philadelphia: Saunders, 1997.
Challis JRG, Matthews SD, Gibb W, Lye SJ. Endocrine and paracrine regulation of birth at term and preterm. Endocr Rev 2000, 21: 514–50.
Hindson JC, Winter AC. Manual of Sheep Diseases, 2nd ed. Oxford: Blackwell Science, 2002.
Menzies PI, Baily D. Lambing management and care. In: Youngquist RS ed, Current Therapy in Large Animal Theriogenology. Philadelphia: Saunders, 1997.
Author Larry D. Holler
Consulting Editor Ahmed Tibary

R

RODENTICIDE TOXICITY

BASICS

OVERVIEW
• A variety of rodenticides can be used around feedstuffs and buildings used for livestock or could be maliciously fed to animals. The livestock owner needs to monitor use of rodenticides in an operation and prevent access of animals to the chemicals.
• The US Environmental Protection Agency recently cancelled the registrations of a variety of second-generation anticoagulant rodenticide formulations. Products containing second-generation anticoagulants must be sold in large bait containers for use in professional applications or for use in or near agricultural structures. The use of over-the-counter rodenticide small package use has shifted away from anticoagulants to bromethalin and cholecalciferol.
• Much of the specific toxicity data and treatments for rodenticides is focused on small animals, and ruminant information is lacking.
• In some cases, the time between rodenticide ingestion and clinical signs is prolonged and the opportunity to use GIT decontaminants is no longer a viable option. Often, specific antidotes are not an option and treatment is supportive and symptomatic.

INCIDENCE/PREVALENCE
Anticoagulants
• Anticoagulant rodenticides were developed after investigations of moldy sweet clover (dicumarol) toxicosis in dairy cattle. Warfarin, a first-generation anticoagulant rodenticide, was synthesized during these investigations.
• Because of warfarin resistance in rodents, second-generation anticoagulants were developed with greater toxicity. The second-generation anticoagulants include brodifacoum, bromodiolone, chlorophacinone, coumafuryl, difenacoum, difethialone, and difacinone. These second-generation anticoagulants are more potent and longer acting, can poison with one exposure, and require longer treatment with vitamin K1 as an antidote.
• The anticoagulant rodenticides are well absorbed with oral exposure and are highly bound to plasma proteins. Anticoagulants can be dislodged from binding by drugs, including sulfonamides, phenylbutazone, phenobarbital, and adrenocorticosteroids; check veterinary drug handbooks for potential interactions.
• The anticoagulants are metabolized in the liver and some can undergo enterohepatic recirculation. The half-life of anticoagulants varies greatly with the compound and the species. The duration of action of anticoagulants in large animals is about 14 days for warfarin, 21 days for bromadiolone, and 30 days for brodifacoum.

Bromethalin
• Bromethalin is a substituted diphenylamine developed as a neurotoxin rodenticide for commercial use. Bromethalin is commercially available as 0.01% bait pellets, bars, and or place packs. It is marketed under a variety of trade names, including Assault®, Gladiator®, Trounce®, Fastrac®, and Tomcat®. Bromethalin can be sold to commercial pest control operators in bulk and in concentrated (2–10%) liquid or solid form.
• The toxic dose for ruminants has not been determined, but for other species appears to range from approximately 1–15 mg/kg body weight for an acute, single dose oral LD50.

Cholecalciferol
• Vitamin D or cholecalciferol toxicosis can occur after ingestion of rodenticides containing cholecalciferol, including the following products: Rampage Rat and Mouse Bait, Quintox Rat and Mouse Bait, Ceva True Grit Rampage, Mouse-B-Gone. These products can be manufactured as flakes, granules, cakes, briquettes, etc. containing 0.075% cholecalciferol (vitamin D3).
• Clinical signs can be seen in companion animals at 0.5 mg/kg body weight. Any dose causing clinical signs in an animal should be considered serious.
• Cholecalciferol and its metabolites have high lipid solubility and are slowly eliminated from the body; the terminal half-life of cholecalciferol is weeks to months.

Sodium Monofluoroacetate (Compound 1080)
• Monofluoroacetate naturally occurs in many plants in Africa, Australia, and South America and causes death in livestock. These plants belong to the Fabaceae, Rubiaceae, Bignoniaceae, Maliipighiaceae, and Dichapetalaceae families.
• Sodium monofluoroacetate or Compound 1080 has been used as a rodenticide since the 1940s in the United States. Currently, it is a restricted use rodenticide in the US with use in livestock protection collars in sheep and goat flocks throughout several western states. These livestock protection collars contain 30 mL with 1% active ingredient (300 mg of fluoroacetate).
• Monofluoroacetate is used for vertebrate pest control in New Zealand and other countries. Sodium monofluoroacetate also appears to be available over the counter in the US in foreign rodenticide products or herbal pesticides.
• Monofluoroacetate is a colorless, water-soluble salt, which is similar in appearance to flour or powdered sugar. The oral lethal dose for cattle is 0.15–0.62 mg/kg body weight, for goats is 0.3–0.7 mg/kg body weight, and for sheep is 0.25–0.5 mg/kg body weight.

Strychnine
• Strychnine baits are composed of red or green colored grains mixed with 0.5–1%

strychnine alkaloid. Some formulations may contain higher strychnine concentrations. Most baits are used to control rodent populations with below-ground use of these products.
• The lethal oral dose of strychnine for cattle is reported as 0.5 mg/kg body weight. Strychnine is rapidly absorbed from the GIT and metabolized by hepatic enzymes. Strychnine is widely distributed in the body with a small portion excreted unchanged into the urine.

Zinc Phosphide
• Zinc phosphide is a metallophosphide that is a dull, gray-black crystal with a faint, pungent odor. It is available as a paste, tracking powder, or grain-based pellet in concentration ranges 0.5–10%.
• The primary use of zinc phosphide is control of gophers and moles. The average lifetime of the bait when placed on wet soils is approximately 20 days, although the bait may retain some toxicity for several months in the field.
• In acid environments, zinc phosphide hydrolyzes to release phosphine gas, a dangerous systemic poison; the odor of phosphine gas is similar to rotten fish or acetylene. The lethal dose of zinc phosphide in ruminants is approximately 60 mg/kg body weight.

GEOGRAPHIC DISTRIBUTION
Worldwide, wherever there are rodenticides

SYSTEMS AFFECTED
Anticoagulants
Hemolymphatic

Bromethalin
Nervous

Cholecalciferol
• Musculoskeletal
• Digestive
• Urinary

Sodium Monofluoroacetate (Compound 1080)
• Cardiovascular
• Nervous

Strychnine
Nervous

Zinc Phosphide
• Gastrointestinal
• Nervous

PATHOPHYSIOLOGY
Anticoagulants
• Clinical toxicology is caused by a coagulopathy occurring because of reduction of the activatable forms of clotting factors II, VII, IX, and X. The reduction occurs due to insufficient amounts of vitamin K1 at sites of post-translation modification of these clotting factors.
• The lag time between ingestion of an anticoagulant bait and the onset of clinical signs is normally 3–5 days.

R

RODENTICIDE TOXICITY   (CONTINUED)

• The vitamin K1-dependent clotting factors are involved with one-stage prothrombin time, activated partial thromboplastin time, and activated clotting time that become prolonged.
• After depletion of clotting factors, hemorrhage can occur from any site.

Bromethalin
Post-ingestion, bromethalin is rapidly absorbed and metabolized by the liver to desmethylbromethalin (DMB), the active metabolite that uncouples mitochondrial oxidative phosphorylation leading to decreased cellular ATP production and disruption of sodium-potassium ATPase pumps.

Cholecalciferol
• Cholecalciferol is rapidly absorbed following oral ingestion.
• Cholecalciferol and its metabolites are tightly bound to vitamin D-binding protein, an α2-globulin; the primary circulating metabolite is 25-hydroxycholecalciferol. The liver converts cholecalciferol to 25-hydroxycholecalciferol, which can become activated in the kidneys to 1,25-dihydroxycholecalciferol.
• Clinical effects occur within 48 hours and include altered cell membrane permeability, altered calcium pump activity, decreased cellular energy production, and cellular necrosis.
• The vitamin D3 metabolites increase plasma calcium and phosphorus, stimulate calcium and phosphorus transfer from bone to plasma, and increase renal calcium reabsorption.

Sodium Monofluoroacetate (Compound 1080)
• Monofluoroacetate is readily absorbed from the GIT, but is slowly absorbed through intact skin. It is metabolized to monofluoroacetic acid, and reacts with coenzyme A to form fluoroacetyl CoA and then fluorocitrate.
• Fluorocitrate inhibits aconitase in the Krebs or tricarboxylic acid cycle resulting in energy depletion, citrate and lactate accumulation, and a decrease in blood pH.
• In general, monofluoroacetate causes cardiotoxic effects.

Strychnine
• Strychnine acts by blocking both inhibitory actions of glycine on the anterior horn of the cells in the spinal cord and that of the endogenous transmitter released from Renshaw cells.
• The inhibition leads to excessive neuronal activity and mild to severe muscle spasms and hyperextension of the limbs and body. Convulsions can occur.

Zinc Phosphide
• Phosphine gas can block cytochrome C oxidase, resulting in disruption of oxidative phosphorylation in mitochondria. The blockage of energy pathways leads to cell death and multi-organ failure.

• Brain, heart, liver, and kidney are most affected due to high metabolic rates and high demands for oxygen.
• Because of the higher pH of the rumen, ruminants should be more resistant to phosphide toxicants as compared with monogastric animals.

SIGNALMENT
All ruminants can be affected. See "Incidence/Prevalence.".

PHYSICAL EXAMINATION FINDINGS
Anticoagulants
• Hemorrhage can occur from any site, including hemorrhage into lungs, GIT, urine, joints, epidural and subdural spaces, and major body cavities.
• Animals can also exhibit pain, dyspnea, abdominal distention, collapse, seizures, abortions, and death.

Bromethalin
• Clinical signs of intoxication involve the central nervous system (CNS), including muscle tremors, hyperthermia, hyperexcitability, hyperesthesia, and focal to generalized seizures that appear to be stimulated by light or noise, and death.
• Clinical signs develop within 2–24 hours after ingesting near lethal doses.
• Animals ingesting sublethal doses have a more delayed onset of signs that develop within several days of exposure and can include lethargy, hind leg ataxia, and paralysis.

Cholecalciferol
• Clinical signs in companion animals occur within 12–36 hours after ingestion and include GIT damage and possible diarrhea, anorexia, depression, and polyuria/polydipsia.
• Acute renal failure and death can occur within 24–48 hours; animals that survive can have loss of renal function and musculoskeletal function, and cardiac abnormalities.

Sodium Monofluoroacetate (Compound 1080)
• Clinical signs can appear 30 minutes to 2 hours post-ingestion.
• Sheep tend to show a combination of cardiac and CNS responses, including restlessness, frequent urination, muscular tremors, polypnea, and tachycardia.
• Cattle ingesting lethal quantities of monofluoroacetate can stagger, tremble, sweat, and show GIT signs. In general, herbivores develop cardiotoxic effects.

Strychnine
• Clinical signs can occur 10 minutes to several hours post-ingestion.
• Initial signs can involve nervousness, increased respiratory rate, and excessive salivation.
• Subsequently, muscle spasms, stiffness, and generalized convulsions that are tonic extensor in nature develop. These convulsions

can be stimulated by loud noise, bright lights, and touch.
• Death results from impaired respiration and hypoxia.

Zinc Phosphide
• Clinical signs can occur 15 minutes to 4 hours or sometimes are delayed for as long as 12–18 hours post-ingestion. Animals ingesting lethal doses rarely survive longer than 48 hours.
• Clinical signs in ruminants are ruminal tympany and bloat, followed by ataxia, weakness, recumbency, hypoxia, dyspnea, and struggling. Some animals exhibit convulsions.
• Zinc phosphide tends to induce vomiting in animals that can vomit; this protective action prevents the conversion of zinc phosphide to phosphine gas and subsequent clinical signs.

CAUSES AND RISK FACTORS
See "Incidence/Prevalence" and "Pathophysiology"

DIAGNOSIS
DIFFERENTIAL DIAGNOSES
• Anticoagulants: Dicumarol, trauma.
• CNS signs: Organophosphorus/carbamate/chlorinated hydrocarbons, trauma, botulism, metaldehyde or lead toxicosis, tremorgenic mycotoxins, sodium ion toxicity, *Clostridium tetani*
• Cholecalciferol: Hypercalcemic diseases, renal failure, granulomatous diseases
• 1080: Cardiotoxic plants

CBC/BIOCHEMISTRY/URINALYSIS
• **Anticoagulants** Can cause prolonged one-stage prothrombin time, activated partial thromboplastin time, and activated clotting time.
• **Bromethalin** Changes in serum electrolytes are generally unremarkable.
• **Cholecalciferol** Can affect serum calcium, phosphorus, BUN, and creatinine.
• **Sodium monofluoroacetate (1080)** Can cause hyperglycemia and increased serum citrate, hypocalcemia (ionized), and acidosis.
• **Strychnine** No specific serum or blood chemistry changes occur following strychnine ingestion.
• **Zinc Phosphide** No specific clinical pathology or histopathology is reported in zinc phosphide toxicosis.

IMAGING
Cholecalciferol Calcification of tissues can be observed in radiology/ultrasound/histopathology.

OTHER DIAGNOSTIC PROCEDURES
• **Anticoagulants** Analytical methods can identify specific anticoagulant rodenticides in blood, serum, plasma, liver, GIT contents, and bait; some anticoagulants can be detected in plasma for over 3 weeks.

• **Bromethalin** Diagnosis is based on the history of exposure to a toxicant and clinical signs observed. DMB can be detected in tissues, such as liver, brain, and adipose tissue. Detection of DMB in adipose tissue provides a possible antemortem confirmation of exposure. Methods using mass spectrometry or liquid chromatography-mass spectrometry have been developed for detection of DMB in tissues; check with veterinary diagnostic laboratories for availability of this analysis.

• **Sodium monofluoroacetate (compound 1080)** A diagnosis is based on clinical signs, history of exposure, and detection of monofluoroacetate in GIT contents, kidney, liver, or bait; contact a veterinary diagnostic laboratory for available testing. Sodium monofluoroacetate can be detected in tissues using a gas chromatography-mass spectrometry method; detection limit is 10 μg/kg in tissues.

• **Strychnine** The diagnosis of strychnine can be confirmed by identification of strychnine in GIT contents, bait, liver, kidney, or urine.

• **Zinc Phosphide** Because zinc phosphide quickly hydrolyzes to phosphine gas, samples of GIT contents, liver, or kidney should be frozen in airtight containers prior to sending to a veterinary diagnostic laboratory for analysis. The detection of zinc phosphide is difficult.

PATHOLOGIC FINDINGS

• **Anticoagulant** After depletion of clotting factors, hemorrhage can occur from any site, including hemorrhage into lungs, GIT, urine, joints, epidural and subdural spaces, and major body cavities.

• **Bromethalin** A postmortem of DMB diagnosis is indicated by diffuse white matter vacuolization in the CNS (intramyelenic edema) and spongiosus.

• **Cholecalciferol** Lesions can include mineral crystal deposition in cortical tubule basement membranes and Bowman capsules. GIT lesions can include mucosal necrosis, sloughing, and hemorrhage. Cardiac lesions include necrotic, disrupted, and mineralized myocytes.

• **Sodium monofluoroacetate (compound 1080)** Postmortem lesions are generally nonspecific. Sheep and cattle can develop endocardial and epicardial petechiae and brain edema.

• **Strychnine** No specific lesions are noted; although, necrosis of the cerebral cortex and brainstem have been reported in strychnine poisoned humans.

• **Zinc Phosphide** The kidneys and liver can show congestion. Histologically, renal tubular degeneration and necrosis can be observed and congestion of the liver and kidneys.

TREATMENT
THERAPEUTIC APPROACH

Anticoagulant
• Treatment includes GIT decontamination shortly after ingestion.
• The use of vitamin K1 as an antidote may depend on presence or absence of coagulation abnormalities.
• If vitamin K1 therapy is not initiated, a clotting parameter can be checked periodically at 36 and 96 hours post-exposure for evaluation.
• If clotting times are prolonged, vitamin K1 treatment and whole blood (plasma) transfusions may be required. The use of vitamin K1 treatment may need to be prolonged (3 weeks or longer if necessary) with exposures to second-generation anticoagulants.
• Additional supportive treatment, oxygen therapy, IV fluid therapy, antibiotics, and stall rest to minimize trauma, may be needed.

Bromethalin
• Treatment immediately post-exposure includes the use of repeated doses of activated charcoal to stop absorption and prevent enterohepatic recirculation of bromethalin.
• It is very important to control cerebral edema and elevated intracranial pressure in a toxicosis. The use of mannitol and dexamethasone have been implemented in small animal cases, with varied success.
• Additionally, maintenance of animal hydration is important along with symptomatic and supportive care.

Cholecalciferol
• In general, treatment consists of GIT decontamination (activated charcoal at 1–4 g/kg PO as a slurry and saline cathartic) shortly after exposure, reduction of hypercalcemia and hyperphosphatemia, restriction of dietary calcium and phosphorus, and supportive therapy (such as 0.9% saline) to maintain adequate hydration, tissue perfusion, and urine flow.
• Corticosteroids have been used to suppress bone resorption and reduce intestinal calcium absorption.
• In small animals, calcitonin has been used for treatment of vitamin D hypercalcemia.

Sodium Monofluoroacetate (Compound 1080)
There is no antidote for monofluoroacetate toxicosis, and the rapid onset of clinical signs can prevent effective decontamination of the GIT with activated charcoal.

Strychnine
• Treatment initially involves GIT decontamination (activated charcoal) if appropriate and supportive and symptomatic care to reverse the hyperthermia and hypoxia.

• More importantly, the convulsions and muscle tremors have to be controlled and respiratory activity needs to be monitored.

Zinc Phosphide
• Treatment includes quick GIT decontamination following ingestion.
• The use of oral aluminum or magnesium hydroxide to slow the hydrolysis of zinc phosphide to phosphine gas is suggested.
• Gastric/rumen lavage with 5% sodium bicarbonate mixture is also recommended to slow the hydrolysis of zinc phosphide to phosphine gas.
• No specific antidote is available for zinc phosphide or phosphine gas.
• Therapy may also be directed towards treating respiratory difficulties (oxygen), treating shock, and supporting animals with liver failure.
• Additional symptomatic and supportive care may be required.

MEDICATIONS
DRUGS OF CHOICE

• **Anticoagulant** A dose of Vitamin K1 in large animals is 0.5–2.5 mg/kg body weight, either IM or SC.
• **Bromethalin** None
• **Cholecalciferol** None
• **Sodium monofluoroacetate (compound 1080)** None
• **Strychnine** None
• **Zinc phosphide** None

FOLLOW-UP
EXPECTED COURSE AND PROGNOSIS

• **Anticoagulant** Depending on the severity of hemorrhage, the prognosis can be guarded. Analytic methods can identify specific anticoagulant rodenticides in blood, serum, plasma, liver, GIT contents, and bait; some anticoagulants can be detected in plasma for over 3 weeks.
• **Bromethalin** Mild poisoning cases may recover; however, the prognosis is usually poor for recovery.
• **Cholecalciferol** Animals with progressive azotemia and elevated serum calcium and phosphorus values have a guarded prognosis.
• **Sodium monofluoroacetate (compound 1080)** Severely affected animals generally die within days of exposure. The prognosis is generally poor. No long-term effects on health or reproductive performance were reported in ewes that survived experimental dosing with a single near-lethal dose of 1080.
• **Strychnine** Because of the difficulty in treating large animals with convulsions, the prognosis is poor.

R

RODENTICIDE TOXICITY

• **Zinc phosphide** The prognosis for animals with clinical signs is poor. Animals ingesting lethal doses rarely survive longer than 48 hours.

PATIENT CARE

• **Anticoagulants** Animals can develop mild to severe anemia, thrombocytopenia, hypoproteinemia, and prolonged clotting factors.

• **Cholecalciferol** Serum calcium, phosphorus, BUN, and creatinine should be monitored. If these values stay in the normal range for 96 hours and the animal remains asymptomatic, no further monitoring is necessary.

PREVENTION

Keep rodenticides away from livestock.

 MISCELLANEOUS

PREGNANCY

Anticoagulant rodenticides can potentially cause early embryonic death and abortions.

BIOSECURITY

Monitor all use of rodenticides around feedstuffs. Keep rodenticides away from livestock.

PRODUCTION MANAGEMENT

Keep rodenticides away from livestock and facilities.

ABBREVIATIONS

• BUN = blood urea nitrogen
• CNS = central nervous system
• DMB = desmethylbromethalin
• GIT = gastrointestinal tract
• IM = intramuscular
• LD50 = lethal dose killing 50% of population
• SC = subcutaneous

SEE ALSO

• Bracken Fern Toxicity
• Cardiotoxic Plants
• Clostridial Disease: Nervous System
• Mycotoxins
• Oleander and Cardiotoxic Plant Toxicity
• Sodium Disorders: Hypernatremia
• Sweet Clover Poisoning
• Tobacco Toxicosis
• Vitamin D Deficiency/Toxicosis
• Water Hemlock
• Yew Toxicity

Suggested Reading

Dorman DC. Bromethalin. In: Peterson ME, Talcott PA eds, Small Animal Toxicology, 3rd ed. St. Louis: Elsevier, 2013, pp. 471–8.

Eason C. Sodium monofluoroacetate (1080) risk assessment and risk communication. Toxicology 2002, 181–182: 523–30.

Eason CT, Gooneratne R, Fitzgerald H, Wright G, Frampton C. Persistence of sodium monofluoroacetate in livestock animals and risk to humans. Hum Exp Toxicol 1994, 13: 119–22.

Filigenzi MS, Bautista AC, Aston LS, Poppenga RH. Method for the detection of desmethylbromethalin in animal tissue samples for the determination of bromethalin exposure. J Agric Food Chem 2015, 63: 5146–51.

Giannitti F, Anderson M, Caspe SG, et al. An outbreak of sodium fluoroacetate (1080) intoxication in selenium- and copper-deficient sheep in California. Vet Pathol 2013, 50: 1022–7.

Gooneratne SR, Eason DT, Milne L, Arthur DR, Cook E, Wiskstrom M. Acute and long-term effects of exposure to sodium monofluoroacetate (1080) in sheep. Onderstepoort J Vet Res 2008, 75: 127–39.

Lee ST, Cook D, Pfister JG, Colegate SM, Riet-Correa F, Taylor CM. Monofluoroacetate-containing plants that are potentially toxic to livestock. J Agric Food Chem 2014, 62: 7345–54.

Mostrom M. Pesticides and rodenticides. In: Smith BP ed, Large Animal Internal Medicine, 5th ed. St. Louis: Elsevier, 2015, pp. 1611–16.

Murphy MJ, Talcott PA. Anticoagulant rodenticides. In: Peterson ME, Talcott PA eds, Small Animal Toxicology, 3rd ed. St. Louis: Elsevier, 2013, pp. 435–45.

Author Michelle Mostrom

Consulting Editor Christopher C.L. Chase

BASICS

OVERVIEW
- Most common cause of neonatal ruminant diarrhea.
- Causative agent, a rotavirus.
- There are several serogroups of rotaviruses A, B, and C affecting ruminants: Serogroup A being the more common in calves and B (pararotavirus) being the more common in kids and lambs.
- Pathogenicity is related to serogroup and load of exposure, level of immunity to the virus, concurrent infection with other neonatal pathogens, and stress.
- Most infections are concurrent with other neonatal pathogens.
- Virus may survive for 9 months in the environment.
- Virus is ubiquitous with seroprevalence in the adult herd of 80–90%.

INCIDENCE/PREVALENCE
- Prevalence of rotavirus infections range from 50% to 100% with a large variation in mortality.
- Depending on immunity, calves may appear normal except for a mild voluminous diarrhea. Farmers often report that this "normal" diarrhea is due to the cow producing too much milk, "milk scours."

GEOGRAPHIC DISTRIBUTION
Worldwide

SYSTEMS AFFECTED
Gastrointestinal

PATHOPHYSIOLOGY
- The virus is acquired through the ingestion of fecal contaminated material.
- Absorptive epithelial cells lining the distal portions of the villi are infected, starting in the proximal portion and moving distally to the middle and distal portions of the small intestine.
- Infected cells contain large numbers of virus particles and are desquamated into the lumen.
- The villi become shortened due to exfoliation of the epithelial cells, resulting in the loss of digestive enzymes contained within the glycocalyx and decreased absorptive capacity of the villi.
- The virus produces an enterotoxin, NSP4, and also stimulates neurotransmitters which increases intestinal secretions.
- The loss of epithelial cells results in a maldigestive as well as a malabsorptive type diarrhea. Undigested carbohydrates undergo bacterial fermentation resulting in an increase in osmotic pressure and water being drawn into the intestinal lumen. Maldigestion and malabsorption alter bacterial flora which may contribute to the diarrhea.

- Diarrhea results due to increased osmotic pressure and decreased absorption.
- The physical loss of epithelial cells results in increased susceptibility to other pathogens due to loss of villous integrity and decreased secretion of lactoferrin and lysozymes.
- Epithelial damage predisposes attachment of ETEC and attaching and effacing *E. coli* to the intestinal villi.
- The loss of electrolytes, bicarbonate, and water leads to dehydration and metabolic acidosis.

HISTORICAL FINDINGS
- Sudden onset of diarrhea that spreads rapidly through the neonatal population.
- Initially a few cases are noted but the frequency of cases increases as the calving season progresses due to increased viral load in the environment.
- An increase in the number of cases is frequently observed following periods of stress such as a snowstorm or cold wet weather.
- Individuals within a specific population may develop diarrhea at the same day of age.

SIGNALMENT
- Bovine, caprine, and ovine.
- Most infections occur between 7 and 14 days of age.
- Range 1 day to 8 weeks.

PHYSICAL EXAMINATION FINDINGS
- Clinical signs will vary from mild to severe diarrhea. In uncomplicated disease, diarrhea may exist for 1–2 days.
- Secondary bacterial infection may result in diarrhea for 3–5 days.
- Mild to severe watery white diarrhea, often with large amounts of mucus; color, consistency, and composition vary with coexisting infections.
- Dehydration and depression with degrees of inappetance or reluctance to nurse.
- Some animals may be weak to the point of recumbency.

CAUSES AND RISK FACTORS
- Rotavirus serogroup A most common in calves.
- Rotavirus serogroup B, pararotavirus in small ruminants.
- Inadequate colostral transfer of immunoglobulins resulting in agammaglobulinemia or hypogammaglobulinemia.
- Lack of local colostral immunity in the case of neonates fed milk replacers.
- Lack of specific antibodies against the infective serogroup or type of rotavirus in colostrum.
- Birthing areas and neonatal housing contaminated with virus resulting from a build-up of manure or inadequate cleaning and disinfection.
- Neonates housed or maintained in a cold wet environment.

DIAGNOSIS

DIFFERENTIAL DIAGNOSES
- *E. coli*, coronavirus, cryptosporidia, *Salmonella* spp., and *Clostridium perfringens* type C are disease agents commonly cause diarrhea during the first 3 weeks of life.
- Nutritional causes of diarrhea may be differentiated from rotaviral diarrhea if history contains a dietary change or identification of nutritional deficiencies or excesses.

CBC/BIOCHEMISTRY/URINALYSIS
- CBC: Hemoconcentration, increased plasma proteins.
- Serum chemistry: Metabolic acidosis with low plasma bicarbonate. Glucose and electrolyte values may be low depending on severity of diarrhea.

OTHER LABORATORY TESTS
- Feces should be collected as soon as diarrhea is noted, within 48 hours of onset, because exfoliation of virus-laden enterocytes is short-lived and occurs early in the disease process.
- Bovine rotavirus (BRV) real-time PCR detects at least 30% more cases of group A rotaviruses in feces and intestinal tissues than antigenic detection methods.
- Feces can be submitted for electron microscopy and identification of virus. A few drops of formalin can be added to 10 mL of feces for preservation.
- Feces can be submitted for ELISA and latex agglutination tests for detection of viral antigens.
- Fresh sections of the small intestine, preferably mid ileum, tied at the cut ends to contain intestinal contents can be submitted on ice for fluorescent antibody testing.

PATHOLOGIC FINDINGS
- No gross lesions except for increased fluid contents throughout the intestinal tract.
- Histopathology: Intestinal villi are shortened.

TREATMENT

THERAPEUTIC APPROACH
- Fluid therapy is needed to correct dehydration, circulatory impairment, and electrolyte and metabolic imbalances.
- Fluid deficit should be calculated as well as maintenance requirement, 80–100 mL/kg, and fluid loss in the diarrhea to determine volume of fluids needed during a 24-hour period.
- Fluids may be administered orally or intravenously. Commercial oral electrolyte solutions containing glucose and a

R

non-bicarbonate alkalinizing agent are recommended if the neonate is still nursing. Although oral electrolytes are less likely to be absorbed due to enterocyte pathology, not all enterocytes are affected so some absorption does occur.

• Neonates without a suckle response need IV fluids. IV administration of isotonic 1.3% sodium bicarbonate solution initially (2 L) followed by lactated Ringer's solution.

• Dextrose solutions (2.5–5%) are indicated in cases of hypoglycemia. With hypoglycemia and after correcting acid-base status, a 2.5% dextrose and 0.45% saline solution has been recommended.

• Although not specific for rotaviral infections, in cases of failure of passive transfer and depending on value of the animal, plasma transfusion may be warranted.

MEDICATIONS

DRUGS OF CHOICE

• Broad-spectrum antibiotics may be considered because of the potential for mixed infections as well as the loss of mucosal integrity.

• Oral amoxicillin trihydrate 10 mg/kg PO q12h for nonruminating calves, 20-day slaughter withdrawal (extra-label in small ruminants). Amoxicillin trihydrate-clavulanate potassium 12.5 mg combined drug/kg PO q12h for 3 days (extra-label usage).

• Parenteral ceftiofur 2.2 mg/kg IM q24h for 3 days (extra-label usage).

• Drug withdrawal times must be determined and maintained in the treated animal.

CONTRAINDICATIONS

Do not use kaolin and pectin as may increase electrolyte loss.

PRECAUTIONS

Appropriate milk and meat withdrawal times must be followed for all compounds administered to food-producing animals.

FOLLOW-UP

EXPECTED COURSE AND PROGNOSIS

• In uncomplicated infections, diarrhea is present for 1–2 days.

• Prognosis is good, as this infection tends to be self-limiting and generally requires minor supportive care.

• Duration of diarrhea may be 3–5 days with secondary bacterial infections.

• Prognosis is dependent on the degree of pathology produced by the secondary bacteria.

• Prognosis is good to fair with supportive care.

POSSIBLE COMPLICATIONS

• Hypovolemic shock
• Secondary bacterial infections

CLIENT EDUCATION

• Neonates should be kept dry and in a draft-free environment.

• Animals should be moved and fed in such a way as to reduce the build-up of mud and fecal material in the neonate's environment.

• Diarrheic animals should be isolated from healthy neonates as they are sources for large numbers of pathogens.

PATIENT CARE

• Monitor attitude, suckling response and appetite, fecal color and consistency, and hydration status every 6–12 hours.

• Monitor age cohorts for signs of diarrhea.

• Neonates with a suckle response should be left with the dam and allowed to nurse.

• Animals being reared artificially should remain on their diet or switched to whole milk or colostrum. If the diarrhea becomes worse or the calf becomes depressed, removal from the dam or milk is warranted. In case of hand-fed neonates that are depressed and not interested in sucking, or neonates not nursing the dam, neonates should receive daily a high-energy electrolyte solution at a rate of 10% of body weight divided into a minimum of 4 feedings.

• Once neonates are suckling, feed milk at a rate of 5% of body weight in 4 feedings a day, increasing the amount per feeding gradually so calf is back on full feed within 2 days.

• Calves should also receive 5% of their body weight in electrolyte solutions spacing 2 hours before or after milk feedings. Milk should not be withheld longer than 24 hours and can be given via an esophageal feeder. No more than 1 liter should be tubed at a time.

• Oral electrolytes containing bicarbonate should not be fed when calves are receiving milk as milk digestion may be disrupted.

PREVENTION

• Reduce viral exposure, by calving in clean maternity areas and moving to a clean area after birth.

• Diarrheic animals should be isolated from healthy neonates as they are sources for large numbers of pathogens.

• Feed youngest animals first and oldest animals last.

• Those handling sick neonates should practice biosecurity measures to reduce exposure to healthy neonates, wash hands and disinfect boots, maintain clothes free of fecal material.

• Vaccination of dams prepartum according to manufacturers' recommendations with a rotaviral vaccine may increase colostral

antibody. Effectiveness will be dependent on field virus serogroup and type and that contained in the vaccine.

• Oral vaccination of neonate with a modified-live oral vaccine will produce IgA and IgM. This vaccine is cumbersome for management as it is to be given prior to colostrum consumption and colostrum must be withheld for several hours after vaccination. This may increase the opportunity for bacterial infections and failure of passive transfer.

• In the case of dairy animals, feed neonates colostrum for 30 days if rotavirus is an endemic problem.

• Eliminate areas of fecal build-up.

• Keep environment dry and draft free.

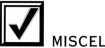

MISCELLANEOUS

AGE RELATED FACTORS

• Most cases between 7 and 21 days of age.
• Range 1 day to 8 weeks.

ZOONOTIC POTENTIAL

• Isolates from neonatal ruminants have not been infective to humans.

• Some human isolates have been found to be infective for calves.

BIOSECURITY

• Diarrheic animals should be isolated from healthy neonates as they are sources for large numbers of pathogens.

• Feed youngest animals first and oldest animals last.

• Those handling sick neonates should practice biosecurity measures to reduce exposure to healthy neonates, wash hands and disinfect boots, maintain clothes free of fecal material.

• Disinfect with bleach, or phenolic or peroxymonosulfate compounds. Surface must be free of organic material and surface contact is a minimum of 10 minutes.

ABBREVIATIONS

• BRV = bovine rotavirus
• ELISA = enzyme-linked immunosorbent assay
• ETEC = enterotoxigenic *E. coli*
• IM = intramuscular
• IV = intravenous
• PCR = polymerase chain reaction
• PO = per os, by mouth
• SC = subcutaneous

SEE ALSO

• Clostridial Disease: Gastrointestinal
• Coronavirus
• Cryptosporidiosis
• *Escherichia coli*
• Salmonellosis

R

Suggested Reading

Barrington GM, Gay JM, Evermann JF. Biosecurity for neonatal gastrointestinal diseases. Vet Clin North Am Food Anim Pract 2002, 18: 7–34.

Bendali F, Sanaa M, Bichet H, Schelcher F. Risk factors associated with diarrhoea in newborn calves. Vet Res 1999, 30: 509–22.

Cho Yong-il, Yoon Kyoung-Jin. An overview of calf diarrhea – infectious etiology, diagnosis, and intervention. J Vet Sci 2014,15: 1–17.

Izzo M, Gunn AA, House JK. Neonatal diarrhea. In: Smith BP ed, Large Animal Internal Medicine, 5th ed. St. Louis: Elsevier Mosby, 2015, pp. 314–35.

MacLachlan NJ, Dubovi EJ eds. Fenner's Veterinary Virology, 4th ed. San Diego: Elsevier, 2011, pp. 288–90.

Smith GW, Berchtold, J. Fluid therapy in calves. Vet Clin North Am Food Anim Pract 2014, 30: 409–27.

Smith GW. Antimicrobial decision making for enteric diseases of cattle. Vet Clin North Am Food Anim Pract 2015, 31: 47–60.

Townsend HG. Environmental factors and calving management practices that affect neonatal mortality in the beef calf. Vet Clin North Am Food Anim Pract 1994, 10: 119–26.

Author Kevin D. Pelzer

Consulting Editor Christopher C.L. Chase

R

RUMEN DYSFUNCTION: ALKALOSIS

BASICS

OVERVIEW
Indigestion resulting from rumen inactivity or toxins that promote alkaline rumen pH and dysfunction.

INCIDENCE/PREVALENCE
N/A

GEOGRAPHIC DISTRIBUTION
N/A

SYSTEMS AFFECTED
Digestive

PATHOPHYSIOLOGY
• Usually relates to continued production and swallowing of alkaline saliva during periods of reduced microbial fermentation that produce insufficient acid to neutralize saliva.
• Continued absorption of VFAs, especially acetate, across the rumen wall also contributes to alkalinity because of bicarbonate generation in the rumen fluid. • Rumen alkalosis can occur due to excessive ammonia production related to overfeeding of NPN sources or toxin ingestion.

HISTORICAL FINDINGS
Reduced feed intake or dietary accidents may be reported.

SIGNALMENT
Functional ruminants of any age can be affected.

PHYSICAL EXAMINATION FINDINGS
• Forestomach dysfunction
  ○ Decreased appetite ○ Rumen hypomotility
  ○ Bloat ○ Abnormal regurgitation
  ○ Abdominal pain
• Signs of urea toxicosis
  ○ Diarrhea ○ Muscle tremors ○ Incoordination
  ○ Weakness ○ Tachypnea ○ CNS excitation
  ○ Rapid deterioration and death

GENETICS
N/A

CAUSES AND RISK FACTORS
• Mild alkalosis (rumen pH 7.0–7.5) can result from prolonged anorexia, microflora inactivity, ingestion of poorly digestible roughage, and some cases of simple indigestion. • Severe alkalosis (rumen pH >7.5) usually relates to excessive ingestion of NPN sources such as urea, biuret, ammonium phosphate, and ammonium salt containing fertilizers.

DIAGNOSIS

DIFFERENTIAL DIAGNOSES
• Rumen acidosis • Simple indigestion • Vagal indigestion • Other systemic or primary diseases causing anorexia

CBC/BIOCHEMISTRY/URINALYSIS
• Dehydration is reflected by increased hematocrit, BUN, creatinine, and total protein. • Leukocytosis (stress) may occur.
• Hypokalemia and hypocalcemia. • Alkalemia.

OTHER LABORATORY TESTS
N/A

IMAGING
N/A

OTHER DIAGNOSTIC PROCEDURES
• Ruminocentesis/ororuminal tubing for rumen fluid analysis • Rumen fluid pH 7.5–8.5 • Strong odor of ammonia
  ○ Poor microbial activity under light microscopy ○ Exposure of tube to oral cavity during ororuminal tubing can falsely elevate pH due to exposure of tube to alkaline saliva.

PATHOLOGIC FINDINGS
• In acute cases, the rumen fluid pH is 7.5–8.5 and may smell of ammonia if NPN ingestion is the cause. • Histopathologic examination might show rumen epithelial exfoliation and, in cases of urea toxicity, lesions in other organs have included lymphocytic abomasitis, necrotic enteritis, follicular cholecystitis, and meningoencephalitis.

TREATMENT

THERAPEUTIC APPROACH
• Identify and manage primary disease.
• Correct acid-base and electrolyte aberrations with appropriate fluid therapy. • Establish normal rumen volume as relevant.
  ○ Increase volume with 8–16 L of rumen fluid and balanced oral electrolytes.
  ○ Decrease volume by removing abnormal rumen contents by siphon or rumenotomy.
  ○ Resolve rumen impaction.
• Can provide acetic acid 4–10 L in cold water orally to correct rumen pH and diminish systemic ammonia absorption from the rumen.

SURGICAL CONSIDERATIONS AND TECHNIQUES
Surgical evacuation of the rumen via rumenotomy may be relevant in cases of acute intoxication.

MEDICATIONS

DRUGS OF CHOICE
• Medications as indicated by primary disease.
• B vitamin supplementation since B vitamin production will be diminished during rumen dysfunction.

CONTRAINDICATIONS
Do not administer magnesium hydroxide if rumen alkalosis is present.

PRECAUTIONS
Appropriate milk and meat withdrawal times must be followed for all compounds administered to food-producing animals.

FOLLOW-UP

EXPECTED COURSE AND PROGNOSIS
• Mild cases are often easily corrected with transfaunation and gradual provision of good-quality feeds. • Severe alkalosis caused by intoxication may require rumen evacuation, along with rumen fluid replacement and supportive care, and the prognosis is poor.

POSSIBLE COMPLICATIONS
Rumen putrefaction can occur: high rumen pH and inoculation with bacteria such as coliforms and *Proteus* spp. from spoiled or fecal-contaminated feeds leads to putrefactive decomposition.

CLIENT EDUCATION
See "Prevention"

PATIENT CARE
• Monitor patient for return to appetite and normal rumen motility • Some cases may require repeat transfaunation

PREVENTION
• Good feed management • Provision of quality digestible feedstuffs • Proper administration of NPN sources • Securing fertilizers

MISCELLANEOUS

ASSOCIATED CONDITIONS
Rumen putrefaction

PRODUCTION MANAGEMENT
Prevention requires good management of feedstuffs and good security of fertilizer storage.

ABBREVIATIONS
• BUN = blood urea nitrogen • CNS = central nervous system • NPN = non-protein nitrogen • VFA = volatile fatty acids

SEE ALSO
Ruminal Acidosis

Suggested Reading
Gartley C, Ogilvie TH, Butler DG. Magnesium oxide contraindicated as a cathartic for cattle in the absence of rumen acidosis. Bovine Proc 1981, 13: 17–19.
Randhawa SS, Dhaliwal PS, Gupta PP, et al. Studies of clinic-biochemical and pathological changes in the urea-induced acute rumen alkalosis in buffalo calves. Acta Vet Brno 1989, 58: 225–43.
Author Meredyth L. Jones
Consulting Editor Erica C. McKenzie

R

BASICS

OVERVIEW
• Acute ruminal acidosis is the most dramatic form of indigestion in ruminants and, in some cases, can lead to death in <24 hours.
• Subacute ruminal acidosis (SARA) results from chronic indigestion leading to short- or long-term production inefficiencies.
• In camelids, the disease is known as forestomach acidosis. Similar to cattle and sheep, the clinical presentation can be acute or chronic.
• Ruminal acidosis results from ingestion of excessive quantities of rapidly fermentable carbohydrates (RFC). Therefore, it represents a major challenge for ruminants on high-concentrate diets (e.g., feedlot cattle).
• Rumen pH of 4.5–5.0 and 5.2–5.5 are used as benchmarks for acute and chronic ruminal acidosis, respectively.

INCIDENCE/PREVALENCE
N/A

GEOGRAPHIC DISTRIBUTION
Worldwide

SYSTEMS AFFECTED
• Digestive
• Multisystemic

PATHOPHYSIOLOGY
Acute Ruminal Acidosis
• Excessive consumption of RFC leads to a rapid fermentation with production of short-chain fatty acids and both D- and L-lactic acid. This causes a decrease in ruminal pH to physiologically inappropriate levels.
• Decreased rumen pH causes significant changes in the ruminal microbiome, especially rapid proliferation of the amylolytic or sugar-utilizing bacteria such as *Streptococcus bovis*.
• Under low pH conditions, lactate-producing bacteria (e.g., *Lactobacillus* spp.) also grow faster, increase in number, and produce excessive amounts of D- and L-lactate.
• The rumen's ability to use lactate is exceeded when large amounts of lactate are produced, resulting in its accumulation.
• If sufficient substrate is available, production of lactate by *S. bovis* continues, leading to a profound reduction in ruminal fluid pH (4.5–5.5) and a severe increase in ruminal osmolality.
• Low pH and high ruminal fluid osmolality kill or inhibit small protozoa which normally limit the production of lactate by using small sugars, and lactate-utilizing bacterial species (e.g., *Megasphaera elsdenii, Propionibacterium shermanii,* and *Selenomonas ruminantium*).

• Under these low pH conditions (pH ~ 4.5), lactate-producing bacterial species outnumber lactate-utilizing species (the number of *S. bovis* is decreased and the number of *Lactobacillus* species is increased) leading to a further lactic acid accumulation.
• Rapid increase of ruminal osmolality and accumulation of lactic acid draws fluid into the rumen producing dehydration, third space fluid sequestration, ruminal distension, and, in severe cases, circulatory shock.
• Lactic acid and increased ruminal fluid osmolality cause damage to the ruminal epithelium and vascular bed that can result in loss of albumin, absorption of enteric toxins or translocation of bacteria with subsequent toxemia, septicemia/bacteremia, SIRS and MODS associated hypovolemic and septic shock.
• Thiamine deficiency can be triggered by thiaminases produced by rumen bacteria under low pH conditions, causing poliocncephalomalacia and neurologic signs.

SARA
• Similar to acute ruminal lactic acidosis, SARA has been associated with feeding starch-rich diets.
• Unlike ruminal acidosis, SARA results from continued ingestion of these feeds over a prolonged period of time rather than sudden exposure without adequate adaptation.
• Upon induction of SARA, an increased concentration of toxin (LPS) is observed within several compartments of the rumen.
• Chronic ruminal wall lesions allow penetration of bacteria and endotoxin with dissemination to the bloodstream, predisposing the cow to a chronic systemic inflammatory response and laminitis.
• Translocation of bacteria frequently results in liver abscess.

SIGNALMENT
• Potentially all ruminant species.
• Sheep appear to be more susceptible to acidosis than other ruminants.

PHYSICAL EXAMINATION FINDINGS
Acute Ruminal Acidosis
• Anorexia
• Marked decreased milk production
• Diarrhea or loose feces
• Dehydration, circulatory shock, and death
• Tachycardia and tachypnea
• Laminitis or founder
• Vomiting
• Totally static rumen
• Polioencephalomalacia

Acute Forestomach Acidosis in Camelids
• Depression
• Weakness

• Ataxia
• Head arched over the back
• Abdominal distension
• Diarrhea

SARA
• *Herd:* Increased incidence of abomasal diseases, lameness (due to laminitis), indigestion
• Decreased milk production and milk fat content
• Reduced metabolic efficiency and overall performance

Chronic Forestomach Acidosis in Camelids
• Ill-thrift
• Cycles of weight gain and loss
• Intermittent diarrhea

CAUSES AND RISK FACTORS
• Feedlot cattle during the period of adaptation to high-concentrate diets.
• Feedlot cattle adapted to high-concentrate diets that suddenly ingest large quantities of RFC.
• Acute and chronic ruminal acidosis can occur in grazing cattle when large amounts of high-starch supplements are fed.
• Dairy cattle during the early postpartum period due to the introduction of high-concentrate diets containing more RFC than those fed during the dry period.
• Sources of RFC include immature/rapidly growing forages (i.e., high in intracellular carbohydrates), tubers/root crops (i.e., high in sugars), and cereal grains (i.e., high in starch).
• Cereal grains are considered the most important source of RFC (wheat is more fermentable than corn or milo).
• Cold weather as it promotes consumption of large amounts of feed, predisposing feedlot cattle to acidosis.
• Accidental ingestion of large quantities of grain by gaining access to the grain room (cattle and camelids).
• Improper mixing of total mixed rations.

DIAGNOSIS

DIFFERENTIAL DIAGNOSES
• *Acute ruminal acidosis*—Causes of acute abdomen in cattle and small ruminants.
• *SARA*—Causes of reduced metabolic efficiency and overall performance.
• *Chronic forestomach acidosis in camelids*—Causes of weight loss and chronic diarrhea. See chapter, Diarrheal Diseases: Camelid, for details.

CBC/BIOCHEMISTRY/URINALYSIS
Acute Ruminal and Forestomach Acidosis
• Hemoconcentration—dehydration

R

RUMINAL ACIDOSIS

• Neutropenia with left shift—septicemia/bacteremia
• Metabolic acidosis—increased D- and L-lactate and anion gap
• Hypocalcemia and hypomagnesemia
• Increased liver enzymes—dehydration, hypovolemic and septic shock
• Aciduria
• Azotemia—dehydration and shock
• Hyperglycemia—camelids
SARA
• Chronic inflammatory response (i.e., cattle with liver abscessation)
• Hypocalcemia
• Decreased milk fat content

OTHER LABORATORY TESTS
Analysis of Ruminal Fluid
Acute Ruminal Acidosis
• Acidic odor.
• Rumen pH of 4.5–5.0 (normal 6.0–7.0 on roughage and 5.5–6.5 on grain).
• Sedimentation and reduction-oxidation times are prolonged.
• Protozoa—reduced numbers.
• Bacteria—predominance of Gram-positive cocci and rods.
• Rumen osmolality—increased >300 mOsm due to accumulation of solutes such as VFA, lactate, glucose, and minerals.
Acute Forestomach Acidosis in Camelids
Ruminal fluid pH drops to 40–4.5 (normal 6.4–6.8).
SARA
• Rumen pH drops daily to <5.5 for a given period of time. This has negative effects on fermentation and the subsequent utilization of nutrients.
Chronic Forestomach Acidosis in Camelids
• Ruminal fluid pH drops to 5.5 (normal 6.4–6.8).
• Ruminal fluid pH below 6 is suspicious.

OTHER DIAGNOSTIC PROCEDURES
Acute Ruminal Acidosis
• History of feeding in the herd, physical examination, analysis of ruminal fluid.
• Biochemical profile, acid-base and electrolytes abnormalities.
SARA
• Made at the herd level rather than individual animals.
• Determination of ruminal pH.
• Ruminocentesis is preferred to oro-ruminal collection to avoid contamination with saliva.
• Collection should be performed 4–8 h post-feeding.
• A pH <5.5 in 40% or more of the cows from a sample of 12 animals from the herd has been suggested for diagnosis of SARA.

PATHOLOGIC FINDINGS
• Rumenitis, reticulitis, and inflammation of the small intestine.
• Liver abscesses (especially in chronic cases).

TREATMENT
THERAPEUTIC APPROACH
Acute Ruminal Acidosis
• Clinicians must decide whether surgical treatment is required or medical therapy will be sufficient.
• Rumen can be evacuated via rumenotomy or, in less severe cases, ruminal lavage can be performed using a Kingman tube or a large oro-ruminal tube.
• Rumen contents must be evacuated and the rumen washed with water several times.
• Magnesium hydroxide (500 g/450 kg body weight) can be administered once the rumen has been evacuated.
• Administration of good-quality hay (via rumenotomy)
• Rumen transfaunation may help to restore the ruminal microbiome.
• Determine fluid requirements—replacement, maintenance, and ongoing losses.
• Animals estimated to be more than 8% dehydrated: Rehydrate IV initially, and then may be maintained with IV or oral fluid therapy.
• Oral fluid therapy: Large volumes of water and rehydration solutions can be administered.
• The volume (L) of fluids to replace the deficit can be calculated as: Volume (L) = body weight (kg) × % *dehydration*. Lactated Ringer's solution or isotonic 0.9% saline at 20 mL/kg/h (highest rate reached through a 14-gauge catheter) is recommended for fluid replacement.
• Maintenance fluid rate: Recommended 2–4 mL/kg/h of lactated Ringer's solutions or isotonic 0.9% saline.
• Cows with mild acidemia (base deficits <10 mmol/L): Administer lactated Ringer's solution supplemented with potassium chloride and calcium.
• Cows with more severe acidemia (base deficits <10 mmol/L): Administer isotonic sodium bicarbonate (156 mmol/L).
• Bicarbonate requirements—calculate from values of base deficit (BD) obtained from the blood gas measurement. Bicarbonate (mmol) = body weight (kg) × base deficit (mmol/L) × 0.3.
• If blood gas is not available, BD can be calculated from values of TCO_2 provided in biochemical profiles. $BD = 25 - TCO_2$.
• Calcium, magnesium, and phosphates should be supplement to correct deficits.
• See chapter, Diarrheal Diseases: Camelid and chapter, Diarrheal Diseases: Small Ruminant, for fluid therapy recommendation in those species.
• Remove the RFC source from the diet.

SARA
Increasing buffer input from the diet and/or through salivation by increasing forage levels in the diet, especially long hay to stimulate rumination.

MEDICATIONS
DRUGS OF CHOICE
• Analgesic and anti-inflammatory drugs—flunixin meglumine or meloxicam to decrease the effects of the systemic inflammatory response.
• Antimicrobials—oxytetracycline and penicillin (ceftiofur in camelids) can be administered to prevent or treat bacteremia and liver abscess development.
• Broad-spectrum antimicrobial therapy can predispose to mycotic rumenitis.
• Prevention of polioencephalomalacia: Administer thiamine HCl (10 mg/kg, IM or IV q4h).

CONTRAINDICATIONS
• Appropriate milk and meat withdrawal times must be followed for all compounds administered to food-producing animals.
• Broad-spectrum antimicrobial therapy can predispose to mycotic rumenitis.

PRECAUTIONS
N/A

POSSIBLE INTERACTIONS
N/A

FOLLOW-UP
EXPECTED COURSE AND PROGNOSIS
N/A

POSSIBLE COMPLICATIONS
N/A

CLIENT EDUCATION
N/A

PATIENT CARE
N/A

PREVENTION
• Gradual adaptation of animals to high-concentrate diets. A 4-week adaptation period may provide the time necessary for adjustment to a new diet.
• Feeding long forages or by-products containing high fiber at 10–15% of dry matter will promote rumination and stimulate salivation (increase the quantities of buffers in the rumen).
• Decrease the amount of cereal grains. Wheat can increase the risk of ruminal acidosis.
• Management and close monitoring of feeding processed grains such as steam-flaked corn. The gelatinization of starch during

(CONTINUED)

steam flaking increases its rate of fermentation.
• Close monitoring of daily intake of diets containing high RFC levels.
• High protein and 6% fat in the diets.
• Oral administration of buffers such as sodium bicarbonate at 1% or 2% of dry matter to increase the buffering capacity of the rumen.
• Allow access to fresh feed and water at all times.
• Administration of ionophores including monensin and lasalocid—to alter rumen fermentation, allow adjustment to high-starch diets by inhibiting lactate-producing bacterial species.

 MISCELLANEOUS

ASSOCIATED CONDITIONS
• Diarrhea, frequently seen in small ruminants and camelids
• Laminitis
• Decreased rate of body weight gain
• Decreased milk production
• Polioencephalomalacia
• Rumen atony
• Liver abscess

PRODUCTION MANAGEMENT
• Ruminal acidosis has high economic significance because a large number of cattle and sheep are finished on high-concentrate diets.
• Economic losses include death and decreased performance of animals.

ABBREVIATIONS
• BD = base deficit
• LPS = lipopolysaccharides
• MODS = multiple organ dysfunction syndrome
• RFC = readily fermentable carbohydrates
• SARA = subacute ruminal acidosis
• SIRS = systemic inflammatory response syndrome
• TCO$_2$ = total carbon dioxide
• VFA = volatile fatty acids

SEE ALSO
• Dairy Nutrition: Ration Guidelines for Milking and Dry Cows (see www.fiveminutevet.com/ruminant)
• Ewe Flock Nutrition (see www.fiveminutevet.com/ruminant)
• Goat Nutrition (see www.fiveminutevet.com/ruminant)
• Milk Cow Nutrition Monitoring (see www.fiveminutevet.com/ruminant)
• Nutrition and Metabolic Diseases: Beef
• Nutrition and Metabolic Diseases: Camelid (see www.fiveminutevet.com/ruminant)
• Nutrition and Metabolic Diseases: Dairy
• Nutrition and Metabolic Diseases: Small Ruminant
• Nutritional Assessment (see www.fiveminutevet.com/ruminant)
• Rumen Dysfunction: Alkalosis
• Rumen Fluid Analysis (see www.fiveminutevet.com/ruminant)
• Rumen Transfaunation (see www.fiveminutevet.com/ruminant)
• Vitamin B Deficiency

Suggested Reading
Cebra C. Diseases of the digestive system. In: Cebra C, Anderson DE, Tibary A, Van Saun RJ, Johnson LW eds, Llama and Alpaca Care: Medicine, Surgery, Reproduction, Nutrition and Herd Health. St. Louis: Elsevier, 2014, pp. 477–537.
Crichlow EC, Chaplin RK. Ruminal lactic acidosis: Relationship of forestomach motility to nondissociated volatile fatty acid levels. Am J Vet Res 1985, 46: 1908–11.
Li S, Khafipour E, Krause DO, et al. Effects of subacute ruminal acidosis challenges on fermentation and endotoxins in the rumen and hindgut of dairy cows. J Dairy Sci 2012, 95: 294–303.
Nocek JE. Bovine acidosis: implications on laminitis. J Dairy Sci 1997, 80: 1005–28.
Owens FN, Secrist DS, Hill WJ, Gill DR. Acidosis in cattle: a review. J Anim Sci 1998, 76: 275–86.
Rodríguez-Lecompte JC, Kroeker AD, Ceballos-Márquez A, Li S, Plaizier JC, Gomez DE. Evaluation of the systemic innate immune response and metabolic alterations of nonlactating cows with diet-induced subacute ruminal acidosis. J Dairy Sci 2014, 97: 7777–87.
Zebeli Q, Metzler-Zebeli BU. Interplay between rumen digestive disorders and diet-induced inflammation in dairy cattle. Res Vet Sci 2012, 93: 1099–108.
Author Diego Gomez-Nieto
Consulting Editor Christopher C.L. Chase
Acknowledgment The author and book editors acknowledge the prior contribution of Hussein S. Hussein.

R

RYEGRASS STAGGERS (PERENNIAL, LOLITREM B)

BASICS

OVERVIEW
Infection of perennial ryegrass (*Lolium perenne*) with endophyte fungus *Neotyphodium lolii*.
- Consistent problem in Australia and New Zealand and occasional problem in the United States (north coast of California).
- Different from annual ryegrass (*Lolium rigidum*) staggers which is a much deadlier disease.
- Summer and fall during hot and dry weather.
- Same disease as bermudagrass staggers and paspalum staggers.

INCIDENCE/PREVALENCE
- In outbreaks, morbidity may reach 80–90%, but mortality is low (0–5%).
- Deaths are usually accidental, often by drowning when drinking from ponds or streams, or due to the inability to forage for food and water.

GEOGRAPHIC DISTRIBUTION
- US (California)
- Australia
- New Zealand

SYSTEMS AFFECTED
Nervous

PATHOPHYSIOLOGY
- Lolitrem B, produced by the endophyte, is a neurotoxic indole-diperpenoid.
- Currently it is thought that lolitrem B impairs or inhibits potassium channels.
- Caused by interference with neuronal transmission in the cerebellum.

HISTORICAL FINDINGS
Occurring mainly in the summer and fall during hot, dry weather, the disease has become quite common in certain areas.

SIGNALMENT
- Bovine, ovine
- Any age that grazes pastures

GENETICS
Within flocks and herds, individual susceptibility varies greatly, and this trait is heritable.

PHYSICAL EXAMINATION FINDINGS
- At rest, animals may exhibit only a fine tremor of the head or neck.
- When forced to move they move with a stiff, stilted, uncoordinated gait and may collapse.
- When in recumbency animals exhibit opisthotonus, nystagmus, and flailing of stiffly extended limbs.
- In less severe cases, the attack soon subsides, and the animal regains its feet within minutes.
- Reduced milk yield in cows has been recorded in New Zealand and Australia.

CAUSES AND RISK FACTORS
- Tremorgenic toxin
- Exposure to endophyte-infected plant

DIAGNOSIS

DIFFERENTIAL DIAGNOSES
- Fungal tremegons
- Grass tetany
- Mycotoxins
- Polioencephalomalacia
- Oxalate toxicity

CBC/BIOCHEMISTRY/URINALYSIS
No characteristic changes

OTHER DIAGNOSTIC PROCEDURES
- Analysis of grass for *Neotyphodium lolii*
- History of exposure to the endophyte infected plant
- Clinical signs

PATHOLOGIC FINDINGS
No specific gross or histologic lesions are recognized.

TREATMENT

THERAPEUTIC APPROACH
- Remove from source.
- Because movement and handling of animals exacerbates signs, individual treatment is generally impractical.
- Recovery is spontaneous in 1–2 weeks if animals are moved to nontoxic pastures or crops.

MEDICATIONS

DRUGS OF CHOICE
None

FOLLOW-UP

EXPECTED COURSE AND PROGNOSIS
- Full recovery when removed from source.
- Recovery is usually complete within a few days to a week. Occasionally, tremors are elicited in cattle several weeks later when they are handled.
- Death is rare.

PATIENT CARE
Avoid stressing the animals. If the animal is forced to run, the episode is repeated. Signs are most severe when the animal is heat stressed.

PREVENTION
- Control by grazing management can help reduce or prevent the disease.
- Lolitrems and ergovaline are concentrated in the leaf sheath and inflorescences. If pastures are not overgrazed down into the leaf sheath zone or grazed when the plants are flowering, then animals should be relatively safe even when a high proportion of the ryegrass plants are infected with endophytes.
- Encouragement of growth of other grass species and legumes in established swards also reduces the intake of toxic grass.

MISCELLANEOUS

PRODUCTION MANAGEMENT
- Good pasture management is essential.
- New pastures can be established using ryegrass seed with little or no endophyte infection. However, the presence of endophyte in grasses makes the plants resistant to attack from many insects; thus, infected pastures are more persistent than endophyte-free pastures.
- Cultivars of ryegrass artificially infected with a strain of endophyte that does not produce lolitrem B or ergovaline are available in New Zealand.

SYNONYMS
- Bermudagrass staggers
- Perennial ryegrass staggers
- Paspalum staggers

SEE ALSO
- Fungal Tremogens
- Grass Tetany/Hypomagnesemia
- Mycotoxins
- Ovine Encephalomyelitis (Louping Ill)
- Oxalate Toxicity

Suggested Reading

Burrows GE. Poaceae. In: Burrows GE, Tyrl RJ eds, Toxic Plants of North America. Ames: Iowa State University Press, 2001, pp. 908–11.

Burrows GE, Tyrl RJ. Toxic Plants of North America, 2nd ed. Ames: Wiley-Blackwell, 2013, pp. 919–21. Kindle edition.

Imlach WL, Finch SC, Dunlop JD, Meredith AL, Aldrich RW, Dalziel JE. The molecular mechanism of "Ryegrass Staggers" a neurologic disorder of K+ channels. J Pharmacol Exp Ther 2008, 327: 657–64.

Simpson W. Perennial Ryegrass Staggers. In: The Merck Veterinary Manual Online, 2013. http://www.merckvetmanual.com/mvm/toxicology/ryegrass_toxicity/perennial_ryegrass_staggers.html accessed August 4, 2016.

Author Jennifer S. Taintor
Consulting Editor Christopher C.L. Chase
Acknowledgment The author and book editors acknowledge the prior contribution of Heidi Coker.

R

SALMONELLOSIS

BASICS

OVERVIEW
• *Salmonella* infections are the second most economically important bacterial disease affecting the gastrointestinal system in ruminants.
• The severity of the disease is dependent on the virulence of the serovar, dose of organisms, the immune status of the animal, and environmental stressors.
• Infections in young animals are associated with contaminated environments and immune status.
• Outbreaks in adults are associated with stress and exposure to a virulent serovar.

INCIDENCE/PREVALENCE
• As farm size and concentration of animals has increased, so has the incidence of disease.
• Once an outbreak has occurred on a farm, the environmental prevalence of the organisms may be high, but the incidence of clinical disease is usually low.
• The farm prevalence of *Salmonella* was determined to be 9.2% for cow calf operations and 30% for dairy operations, based on the US National Animal Health Monitoring System Beef 07-08 study and Dairy 2002 study.

GEOGRAPHIC DISTRIBUTION
Worldwide

SYSTEMS AFFECTED
• Cardiovascular
• Digestive
• Musculoskeletal
• Nervous
• Respiratory
• Urinary
• Multisystem

PATHOPHYSIOLOGY
• *Salmonella* organisms are most commonly acquired through the fecal-oral route or consumption of contaminated feeds.
• Carrier cows may secrete organisms directly into milk, especially *S. Dublin*.
• Young calves are susceptible to infection because the organism easily passes through the rumen and the abomasum. There are no volatile fatty acids in the rumen nor is the abomasal pH low enough to kill the organism. Likewise, calves lack colonization resistance within the intestines.
• The organism attaches, via adhesins, to mucosal cells of the ileum, cecum, and colon invading epithelial cells, moving through the mucosa, resulting in an inflammatory response with macrophage uptake and entrance into lymphoid tissue and the bloodstream.
• Various virulence and host factors determine the extent of damage and invasiveness of the organism.

• The organism secretes exotoxins that stimulate fluid secretions and damage host cells. In addition, lipopolysaccharide (LPS) is released during bacterial replication and death. These LPSs stimulate the inflammatory cascade leading to tissue damage, cardiovascular changes, and signs of toxemia.
• Diarrhea results from increased cellular secretions, malabsorption, and maldigestion due to mucosal damage and the inflammatory response.
• Pneumonia results from septicemia.
• Dry gangrene results from cold agglutinins.

HISTORICAL FINDINGS
• Salmonellosis in animals >3 months of age is often associated with the introduction of a carrier animal into the herd as well as recent exposure to new water or feed sources.
• Periods of stress such as grouping of animals, late pregnancy, parturition, early lactation, transport, feed or water deprivation, surgery, or antibiotic usage are often associated with cases or outbreaks.

SIGNALMENT
• Bovine, caprine, and ovine.
• In calves, infections occur from 14 days to 2 months of age.
• All animals, regardless of age, are at risk of developing salmonellosis.

PHYSICAL EXAMINATION FINDINGS
• The disease may have three different presentations, including peracute, acute, and chronic.
• Acute infections may result in a chronic state.
• Depending on the virulence of the specific serotype and immune status of the host, the organism may be contained within the intestinal tract or invade the circulatory system resulting in multiple organ pathology.
• Clinical signs are often associated with the release of endotoxins and the development of endotoxemia.
• Animals infected with non-host adapted *Salmonella* may be convalescent carriers up to 6 months.

Peracute Infections
• May observe anorexia, depression, right-sided abdominal distension, and dehydration prior to sudden death, in cattle >6 months of age.
• Signs of overwhelming septicemia, meningitis, opisthotonus, and convulsions may be observed in animals <6 months.
• Signs of diarrhea and colic are not common consistent findings.

Acute Infections
• Most frequently encountered state.
• Animals exhibit enteritis, fever, anorexia, depression, and dehydration.
• Feces initially are watery in nature, becoming voluminous with a foul odor and may contain shreds of mucosa, fibrin casts, and frank blood.

• Animals are severely dehydrated, have sunken eyes, and may be too weak to stand.
• Body temperature initially is elevated but decreases and may be subnormal in the terminal stages of the disease.
• Calves infected with *S. Dublin* are unthrifty in appearance, weak, anorectic, and die acutely.
• Many calves will develop meningoencephalitis, polyarthritis, osteomyelitis, and pneumonia. Some calves, especially if infected with *S. Dublin*, may develop dry gangrene of the distal extremities, ears, and tail.
• Calves may have concurrent pneumonia due to septicemia.
• Adult animals exhibit fever; anorexia, diarrhea, dehydration; and pregnant animals may abort. Heat stress exacerbates clinical signs.

Chronic Infections
• Occur in animals >1 month of age; *S. Dublin* occurs in animals >8 weeks of age.
• These animals fail to thrive; stools may be pudding-like to diarrheic.
• The animals' body temperature may be normal to slightly elevated; animals have poor hair coats and are undersized.

CAUSES AND RISK FACTORS
• Gram-negative facultative intracellular organism.
• *Salmonella enterica* subsp. *enterica* containing 2,500 serovars.
• *Salmonella* Dublin is host adapted to cattle and *S. Arizonae* and *S. Abortusovis* (uncommon in North America) to sheep.
• The most frequently isolated serotypes from cattle include *Salmonella enteric* subsp. *enterica* serovars Typhimurium, Montevideo, Dublin, Newport, and Cerro.
• *Salmonella enterica* subsp. *enterica* serovars Typhimurium, Dublin, and Arizonae are frequently isolated serotypes of sheep and goats.
• Inadequate colostral transfer of immunoglobulins resulting in agammaglobulinemia or hypogammaglobulinemia.
• Birthing areas contaminated with fecal material containing *Salmonella* spp.
• Crowding and poor sanitation increases pathogen concentration and decreases host immunity.
• Use of common feeding and treatment equipment without proper cleaning and disinfection between uses.
• Late gestation, parturition, and induction of lactation are physiologic stressors.
• Factors which reduce immunity or cause alterations in microbial gut flora—transportation, concurrent disease, anesthesia, surgery, feed changes, antimicrobial therapy, and withholding food and water.

S

SALMONELLOSIS

• Herd introductions, especially from multiple sources.

• Wild birds having access to feed and water supplies, especially water fowl.

• Feeding high protein supplements, by-pass proteins and calcium-phosphorus supplements from animal sources as these are often contaminated with the organism.

DIAGNOSIS

DIFFERENTIAL DIAGNOSES

• Diarrhea may be caused by a variety of infectious agents as well as nutritional causes.

• *Clostridium perfringens* type C and *E. coli* occur during the first week of life.

• Cryptosporidia, rotavirus, and coronavirus are disease agents that cause diarrhea during the first 4 weeks of life.

• Coccidiosis occurs after 3 weeks of age and often associated with tenesmus.

• Salmonellosis develops after 2 weeks of age (generally) and is usually associated with a fever while the other agents generally are not associated with a fever.

• Pasteurellosis and mycoplasmosis in animals exhibiting pneumonia.

• Differential diagnoses in animals >1 month of age include dietary changes, indigestion, lactic acidosis, toxicosis, BVDV, and winter dysentery.

CBC/BIOCHEMISTRY/URINALYSIS

• CBC: Hemoconcentration, a slight anemia may exist but is masked by dehydration. A degenerative left shift with neutropenia and band neutrophilia is commonly observed. Plasma proteins are increased initially due to dehydration; however, plasma protein levels decrease due to decreased albumin levels as a result of malnutrition and protein losing enteropathy.

• Serum chemistry: Metabolic acidosis with low plasma bicarbonate. Cattle with nonfatal diarrhea do not develop significant acidosis. Electrolyte values will be low depending on severity of diarrhea and may appear normal but are deficient on a whole-body basis. BUN and creatinine levels are increased due to prerenal azotemia and acute nephrosis due to septicemia and endotoxemia.

• Urinalysis: Depending on state of dehydration, urine will be concentrated, resulting in an increased specific gravity.

OTHER LABORATORY TESTS

• Isolation of the organism from feces in live animals and tissues, bone marrow, and lymph nodes in dead animals along with clinical signs consistent with salmonellosis is confirmatory.

• Samples for bacterial culture should be collected and placed in Cary Blair Transport Media for shipment to the laboratory.

• Fecal PCR can be performed.

PATHOLOGIC FINDINGS

Peracute Infections

• Result in nonspecific gross lesions.

• Petechial hemorrhages on the serosal surfaces of the intestine and in epicardium.

• The lungs are congested.

• Intestines are distended with fluid. The presence of mucosal hemorrhage and necrosis in the intestines is variable.

Acute Infections

• May result in the following gross changes. The abdominal cavity contains increased peritoneal fluid and fibrin tags; the intestines are congested and distended with fluid containing a mixture of mucus and fluid feces along with frank blood, blood clots, pieces of sloughed mucosa, fibrin and mucosal casts; the spleen is enlarged and the liver swollen; lymph nodes are edematous and hemorrhagic; lungs may be congested with evidence of pneumonia.

Chronic Infections

• Result in thickened intestines with evidence of catarrhal enteritis in the distal small intestine, cecum, and colon.

• The mesenteric lymph nodes are hyperplastic and the gall bladder may be thickened containing fibrin.

• Chronic infections associated with *Salmonella* Dublin are exhibited by arthritis, osteomyelitis, and meningitis along with pneumonia.

TREATMENT

THERAPEUTIC APPROACH

• Fluid therapy is needed to correct dehydration, circulatory impairment, and electrolyte and metabolic imbalances. Fluid deficit should be calculated as well as maintenance requirement, 80–100 mL/kg body weight, and estimated fluid loss to determine volume of fluids needed during a 24-hour period.

• Fluid may be administered orally or intravenously. Commercial oral electrolyte solutions containing glucose and an alkalinizing agent (acetate if on whole milk) are recommended for neonates capable of nursing.

• Oral electrolytes are approximately 60% absorbed due to enterocyte pathology and absorption capacity. Neonates without a suckle response need IV fluids. IV administration of 0.9% NaCl is adequate if animals are not severely acidotic.

• With severe acidosis, isotonic sodium bicarbonate solution (1.3%, 13 of sodium bicarbonate to 1 litre of distilled water) may be used. Dextrose solutions (2.5–5%) are indicated in cases of hypoglycemia.

• With hypoglycemia and an unknown electrolyte and acid-base status, a 2.5%

dextrose and 0.45% saline solution has been recommended.

MEDICATIONS

DRUGS OF CHOICE

• Florfenicol 20 mg/kg IM q48h (extra-label usage).

• Ceftiofur 2.2 mg/kg IM/SC q12h for 4–7 days (extra-label usage).

• Flunixin meglumine 0.5 mg/kg IV q12h first day, then q24h (extra-label usage).

CONTRAINDICATIONS

• Do not use kaolin and pectin as use may increase electrolyte loss.

• Do not use hypertonic saline.

• Do not use flunixin if renal disease is evident.

PRECAUTIONS

Meat and milk withdrawal times must be followed for all compounds administered to food-producing animals.

FOLLOW-UP

EXPECTED COURSE AND PROGNOSIS

• Prognosis is dependent on the virulence of the serovar and the host's immune status.

• Animals will have diarrhea or loose stools for approximately 7–10 days.

• Poor weight gains can be expected for 2–3 weeks after clinical signs resolve.

• Some acute infections will become chronic infections.

• Animals may shed the organism in feces for up to 6 months post-recovery.

• Because the organism can survive for months in the environment, outbreaks may recur during periods of animal stress.

• Most outbreaks last 2 weeks, unless the infection becomes endemic, in which case, animals brought into the environment may develop signs over an extended time period.

POSSIBLE COMPLICATIONS

• Endotoxic shock and death.

• Pneumonia and dry gangrene of the distal extremities in calves.

• Retained placenta and metritis in animals that abort.

PATIENT CARE

• Monitor attitude, suckling response and/or appetite, fecal color and consistency, and hydration status.

• Neonates with a suckle response should be left with the dam and allowed to nurse.

• Animals being reared artificially should remain on their diet or switched to whole milk or colostrum. If the diarrhea becomes worse or the calf becomes depressed, removal from the dam or milk is warranted. In the case of hand-fed neonates that are depressed

(CONTINUED)

SALMONELLOSIS

and not interested in sucking, or neonates not nursing the dam, neonates should receive a high-energy electrolyte solution at a rate of 10% of body weight divided into a minimum of 4 feedings.
• Calves should also receive 5% of their body weight in electrolyte solutions spacing 2 hours before or after milk feedings. Milk should not be withheld longer than 24 hours and can be given via an esophageal feeder. No more than 1 liter should be tubed at a time.
• Milk and electrolyte solutions can be altered as described previously with a minimum of 10% body weight of fluid per day.
• Oral electrolytes containing bicarbonate should not be fed when calves are receiving milk as milk digestion may be disrupted.
• Ruminating animals should be provided a forage-based diet.
• Force feeding alfalfa meal and electrolytes in a water solution to inappetant animals is helpful.

PREVENTION
• Cleanliness is the basis of prevention. Clean and disinfect animal holding facilities between groups of animals.
• Do not overcrowd animals.
• Equipment should be cleaned and disinfected with iodine, chlorine, or phenolic compounds. Drying and exposure to sunlight increases pathogen die-off.
• Reduce manure build-up.
• Control bird and rodent populations as both may carry *Salmonella* organisms.
• Avoid run-off ponds as water sources.
• Vaccination with a LPS core antigen vaccine will not prevent infection but will reduce clinical signs.
• Sanitary storage and delivery of feedstuffs; keep feeding equipment free of manure.
• Quarantine new additions for 30 days.
• Those handling sick animals should practice biosecurity measures to reduce exposure to healthy animals, wash hands and disinfect boots, maintain clothes free of fecal material.

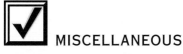 MISCELLANEOUS

ASSOCIATED CONDITIONS
• Acute infections may result in a chronic state.

• Depending on the virulence of the specific serotype and immune status of the host, the organism may be contained within the intestinal tract or invade the circulatory system resulting in multiple organ pathology.
• Clinical signs are often associated with the release of endotoxins and the development of endotoxemia.

AGE-RELATED FACTORS
• Most cases are 2 weeks to 2 months of age.
• All ages are susceptible.
• Infections in young animals are most often a result of contaminated environments.
• Outbreaks in adults are associated with stress and exposure to a virulent serovar.

ZOONOTIC POTENTIAL
• During outbreaks within animal populations, it is not uncommon for animal caregivers to become infected and develop clinical signs.

PREGNANCY
Abortions are common

BIOSECURITY
• Clients should be made aware of the potential for fecal shedding of *Salmonella* organisms by both clinically ill as well as convalescent animals into the environment.
• Isolation and biosecurity procedures to keep organisms from spreading throughout the environment should be developed and instituted.
• Potential for zoonotic spread should be addressed.

PRODUCTION MANAGEMENT
Avoid risk factors by implementing appropriate management and disinfectant procedures.

ABBREVIATIONS
• BUN = blood urea nitrogen
• BVDV = bovine viral diarrhea virus
• IM = intramuscular
• IV = intravenous
• LPS = lipopolysaccharide
• PCR = polymerase chain reaction
• SC = subcutaneous

SEE ALSO
• Bovine Viral Diarrhea Virus
• Clostridial Disease: Gastrointestinal
• Coronavirus
• Cryptosporidiosis

• *Escherichia coli*
• Johne's Disease
• Lymphosarcoma
• Malignant Catarrhal Fever
• Rotavirus
• Winter Dysentery

Suggested Reading
Aarestrup FM, Hasman H. Susceptibility of different bacterial species isolated from food animals to copper sulphate, zinc chloride and antimicrobial substances used for disinfection. Vet Microbiol 2004, 100: 83–9.
Bywater RJ. Veterinary use of antimicrobials and emergence of resistance in zoonotic and sentinel bacteria in the EU. J Vet Med B Infect Dis Vet Public Health 2004, 51: 361–3.
Hirsh DC, Zee YC. Veterinary Microbiology. Malden, MA: Blackwell Science, 1999.
Moxley R. Salmonella. In: McVey DS, Kennedy M, Chengappa MM eds, Veterinary Microbiology, 3rd ed. Hoboken: Wiley-Blackwell, 2013, pp. 74–85.
Nielsen LR, Schukken YH, Grohn YT, Ersboll AK. *Salmonella* Dublin infection in dairy cattle: risk factors for becoming a carrier. Prev Vet Med 2004, 65(1–2): 47–62.
Peek SE, Hartmann FA, Thomas CB, Nordlund KV. Isolation of *Salmonella* spp from the environment of dairies without any history of clinical salmonellosis. J Am Vet Med Assoc 2004, 225: 574–7.

Author Kevin D. Pelzer
Consulting Editor Christopher C.L. Chase

S

SARCOCYSTOSIS

 BASICS

OVERVIEW
Sarcocystosis is a zoonotic disease caused by an intracellular protozoan parasite, *Sarcocystis* spp.

INCIDENCE/PREVALENCE
• In humans, worldwide incidence of intestinal infection is estimated to be 6–10%.
• Ruminants are very prone to sarcocystosis, with an estimated prevalence of 10–100%.

GEOGRAPHIC DISTRIBUTION
Distribution is worldwide. Particular species vary with specific geographic locations.

SYSTEMS AFFECTED
• Hemolymphatic
• Musculoskeletal
• Cardiovascular
• Nervous
• Reproductive

PATHOPHYSIOLOGY
• *Sarcocystis* spp. Have a two-host life cycle involving humans and multiple species of animal. The definitive host is usually a predator or scavenger which is infected through its respective prey, the intermediate host.
• The definitive host is infected after ingesting muscle tissue infected with sarcocysts. The cysts develop into microgametes and macrogametes to an unsporulated oocyst and finally to sporulated oocysts which, after one week, are shed in feces for several months.
• The intermediate host ingests sporocysts during grazing or drinking and they release several sporozoites. The parasite invades the arteries and develops to a first-generation schizont into merozoites I, second-generation schizonts into merozoites II, and finally to third-generation schizonts which are then released in the bloodstream. Schizonts are then circulated to the intermediate host's muscle and nerve cells and form cysts. Infective zooites develop within the sarcocysts in 2–3 months.
• Clinical disease in the intermediate host may occur at two stages in the developmental cycle.
• The first stage occurs at 3–5 weeks after the initial infection and can last for 6–8 weeks. This stage corresponds with the formation of endothelial schizonts with fever, petechiation of mucus membranes, edema, icterus, and macrocytic hypochromic anemia.
• The second stage corresponds to the entry of schizonts into muscle tissue where extensive fiber degeneration and enzyme release can occur. The enlargement of the cysts in massive infestations can cause muscle pain and lameness. After about 100 days, maturation of the cysts occurs, and tissue reactions subside along with clinical signs.
• This recovery from clinical disease may explain the past impression that sarcocystosis was an innocuous condition. In cattle, *S. cruzi* seems to be the only species capable of causing significant clinical disease. In sheep, *S. tenella* can be very pathogenic to lambs.

HISTORICAL FINDINGS
N/A

SIGNALMENT
• Dogs, cats, mammalian wildlife, birds, reptiles, and humans are definitive hosts.
• Intermediate hosts include cattle, sheep, goats, and buffalo in addition to many nonruminant species (pigs, horses, poultry, birds, dogs, cats, rodents, rabbits).

PHYSICAL EXAMINATION FINDINGS
• Usually infection is asymptomatic.
• In ruminants infection can cause fever, anorexia, wasting, weakness, muscle spasms, decreased milk production, diarrhea, pneumonia, sloughing of the tip of the tail, hemorrhages, anemia, icterus, prostration, CNS signs, and death. Pregnant cows may abort.

GENETICS
N/A

CAUSES AND RISK FACTORS
• *Sarcocystis* spp.
• Dogs, cats, humans, and other carnivores are infected by consuming uncooked tissues of infected animals.
• Ruminants become infected with sporocysts shed in the feces of definitive hosts while grazing on contaminated pastures.

 DIAGNOSIS

DIFFERENTIAL DIAGNOSES
• Gastrointestinal parasitism
• Toxicity
• Brucellosis
• Leptospirosis
• Enzootic bovine abortion
• White muscle disease
• CNS diseases: rabies, spongiform encephalopathy, scrapie

CBC/BIOCHEMISTRY/URINALYSIS
• Hypergammaglobulinemia
• Elevations of muscle enzyme activities (creatine kinase, aspartate aminotransferase) and beta and gamma globulin concentrations.

OTHER LABORATORY TESTS
• Immunofluorescent antibody (IFA) test
• PCR-RFLP resolved by agarose gel electrophoresis
• Definitive (final) hosts – visualization of sporocysts in feces.
• Intermediate hosts – gross or microscopic visualization of cysts in muscle tissue (skeletal, cardiac, and esophageal).

IMAGING
N/A

OTHER DIAGNOSTIC PROCEDURES
Sarcocysts are evident in stained sections of relevant muscle tissue.

PATHOLOGIC FINDINGS
• Visible cysts of *S. gigantea* are found in sheep tissue and microscopic cysts are detected in the esophagus, diaphragm, heart, and other muscle. However, *S. gigantea* are mildly pathogenic.
• Massive infestation of *S. cruzi* in cattle forms visible lesions leading to carcass condemnation at slaughter.
• Severely affected animals may appear cachectic, or have hemorrhage of the visceral and myocardial serosa.

TREATMENT

THERAPEUTIC APPROACH
Therapeutic treatment is ineffective.

S

Table 1

Different *Sarcocystis* species		
Species	Definitive (final) hosts	Intermediate hosts
S. hominis, S. suihominis	Humans, primates	Cattle
S. cruzi	Dogs, wolves, coyotes, racoons, foxes, hyenas	Cattle
S. hirsuta	Cats	Cattle
S. medusiformis, S. moulei, S. gigantea	Cats	Goats
S. hircicanis, S. capracanis, S. tenella	Cats	Sheep
S. fusiformis, S. buffalonis	Cats	Water buffalo
S. fayeri, S. bertrami	Dogs	Horses
S. leporuum, S. cuniculi	Cats	Rabbits
S. muris, S. cymruensis	Cats	Rodents

(CONTINUED)   **SARCOCYSTOSIS**

SURGICAL CONSIDERATIONS AND TECHNIQUES
N/A

MEDICATIONS

DRUGS OF CHOICE
• Pharmacologic treatment is not generally practiced. Experimentally, amprolium administered at 100 mg/kg body weight per os once daily prophylactically for 30 days seemed to reduce the severity of illness in exposed sheep and calves. Except for calves, this is extra-label use.
• Anti-inflammatory medications or vitamin E and immunomodulators may be used as supportive therapy.

CONTRAINDICATIONS
• Do not use amprolium in animals producing milk for human consumption. Do not use in calves to be processed for veal.

PRECAUTIONS
• Amprolium can promote signs of thiamine deficiency (polioencephalomalacia) in ruminants, particularly if overdosed.
• Appropriate milk and meat withdrawal times must be followed for all compounds administered to food-producing animals.

POSSIBLE INTERACTIONS
N/A

FOLLOW-UP

EXPECTED COURSE AND PROGNOSIS
• In cattle, only *S. cruzi* has the potential to cause significant clinical disease, which can range from muscle pain, to abortions, to death. Full recovery is seen after 100 days when cysts mature. Sarcocysts will remain in the muscle and can result in carcass condemnation at slaughter.
• *S. tenella* has been associated with high morbidity and mortality in lambs.

POSSIBLE COMPLICATIONS
N/A

CLIENT EDUCATION
See "Prevention"

PATIENT CARE
N/A

PREVENTION
• Keep definitive carnivore hosts off pasture by means of fencing and other deterrents.
• Ionophore and coccidiostat drugs may help reduce incidence.

MISCELLANEOUS

ASSOCIATED CONDITIONS
• Other intestinal parasites
• Meningoencephalitis or encephalitis, hepatitis, and generalized coccidiosis

AGE-RELATED FACTORS
Clinical disease is seen primarily in calves, lambs, and kids.

ZOONOTIC POTENTIAL
• *S. bovihominis*: Humans are the primary host, and generally no clinically significant disease has been documented in humans or cattle in natural infections.
• In experimental infections, some humans experienced transient abdominal pain and diarrhea 10–14 days after exposure, and shed sporocysts in their feces for 5–12 days.
• Other *Sarcocystis* spp. have created rare cases of muscular weakness and pain, periarteritis and subcutaneous tumefaction, indicating humans can potentially serve as intermediate hosts as well. But a causal association has not been established. Immunosuppressed individuals may be at increased risk of clinical disease. It is thought that nearly half of the muscular cysts worldwide in bovines and swine are caused by *S. bovihominis* and *S. suihominis*.

BIOSECURITY
N/A

PRODUCTION MANAGEMENT
N/A

SYNONYMS
• Beef measles
• Sarcosporidiosis

ABBREVIATIONS
• IFA = immunofluorescent antibody
• PCR-RFLP = polymerase chain reaction-restriction fragment length polymorphism

SEE ALSO
• Abortion: Bovine
• Bovine Spongiform Encephalopathy
• Brucellosis

• Leptospirosis
• Rabies
• Scrapie
• Selenium/Vitamin E Deficiency

Suggested Reading
Fayer R. *Sarcocystis* spp. in human infections. Clin Microbiol Rev 2004, 17: 894–902, table of contents.
Fayer R, Esposito DH, Dubey JP. Human infections with *Sarcocystosis* species. Clin Microbiol Rev 2015, 28: 295–311.
Gunning RF, Jones JR, Jeffrey M, Higgins RJ, Williamson AG. Sarcocystis encephalomyelitis in cattle. Vet Rec 2000, 146(11): 328.
Harris VC, VanVugt M, deBree GJ, Stijnis C, Goorhuis A, Grobusch MP. Human extraintestinal sarcocystosis: What we know, and what we don't know. Curr Infect Dis Rep 2015, 17(8): 495.
Leek RG, Fayer R. Amprolium for prophylaxis of ovine sarcocystosis. J Parasitol 1980, 66: 100–6.
Ogunremi O, MacDonald G, Geerts S, Brandt J. Diagnosis of *Taenia saginata* cysticercosis by immunohistochemical test on formalin-fixed and paraffin-embedded bovine lesions. J Vet Diagn Invest 2004, 16: 438–41.
Oryan A, Moghaddar N, Gaur SN. The distribution pattern of *Sarcocystis* species, their transmission and pathogenesis in sheep in Fars Province of Iran. Vet Res Commun 1996, 20: 243–53.
Villar D, Kramer M, Howard L, Hammond E, Cray C, Latimer K. Clinical presentation and pathology of sarcocystosis in psittaciform birds: 11 cases. Avian Dis 2008, 52: 187–94.
Yang ZQ, Li QQ, Zuo YX, et al. Characterization of *Sarcocystis* species in domestic animals using a PCR-RFLP analysis of variation in the 18S rRNA gene: a cost-effective and simple technique for routine species identification. Exp Parasitol 2002, 102: 212–17.

Internet Resource
http://www.cfsph.iastate.edu/Factsheets/pdfs/sarcocystosis.pdf
Authors Edward L. Powers and Saluna Pokhrel
Consulting Editor Erica C. McKenzie

S

SCHMALLENBERG VIRUS

BASICS

OVERVIEW
- Schmallenberg virus (SBV) is a Bunyaviridae that causes malformations in newborn ruminants in Europe.
- It was first detected in Germany and other parts of Europe during the autumn of 2011.
- SBV infections are often asymptomatic; acute signs included a drop of milk yield, diarrhea, and fever.
- In pregnant animals, thee were abortions and congenital malformations in the parturition period. Besides cattle, sheep and goats, SBV infection was detected in a bison and in alpacas.

INCIDENCE/PREVALENCE
- Seroprevalence in naïve herds varies from 71% to 90%.
- The incidence of reproductive disease (abortion and congenital defects) morbidity and mortality is <3%.

GEOGRAPHIC DISTRIBUTION
- SBV infection was found in numerous European countries including Germany, the Netherlands, Belgium, United Kingdom, Italy, France, Spain, Luxembourg, Denmark, Ireland, Northern Ireland, and Switzerland and antibodies to SBV were detected in animals originating from Austria, Poland, Sweden, Finland, and Norway.
- SBV was discovered by metagenomic analysis of blood samples of cows from a farm in North Rhine-Westphalia in Germany. SBV belongs to a group of teratogenic arthropod-borne viruses, including Akabane virus (AKV).
- The virus infects primarily sheep, goats, and cattle and is supposed to be transmitted by *Culicoides* biting midges including *Culicoides obsoletus* complex, *C. dewulfi*, *C. scoticus*, and *C. chiopterus*.

SYSTEMS AFFECTED
- Reproductive
- Nervous
- Musculoskeletal

PATHOPHYSIOLOGY
- Arthropod transmission results in viremia.
- Neurons in the brain seem to be the major target for viral replication in the developing fetus. Sheep fetuses seem to be susceptible to SBV infection at 28–50 days of gestation which coincides with the development of the blood brain barrier (BBB). In sheep the BBB starts to develop between days 50 and 60 of gestation and reaches full development by day 123. Thus, the virus may gain easy access to the brain of the fetus during a short period of time: from day 28 of gestation when the placentomes develop until day 50 when the BBB starts to develop. This would explain why disease in adult animals, that have an intact BBB, is mild with no apparent

development of lesions in the CNS. SBV inhibits the interferon beta (INF-β) innate immune response of host. The lack of production of IFN-b transcripts, which in cells infected with wild type SBV indicating that the inhibition of IFN production occurred at the level of transcription. The SBV NSs protein is able to modulate at least indirectly the host innate immune response. Thus, the NSs protein of SBV acts as a virulence factor. Importantly, we also found SBV to replicate in neurons of in utero infected calves and lambs.
- In fetal sheep, SBV infection can result in cavitation of the white matter of the cerebrum, cerebellar hypoplasia, mild lymphohistiocytic perivascular encephalitis, and small glial nodules scattered throughout the brain. Thus, the cavitary lesions observed in naturally SBV infected lambs and calves appear to be the natural progression of vacuolar changes within the white matter.
- The malformations and deformities observed in SBV-infected lambs and calves are accompanied by muscle hypoplasia and demyelination. SBV infect the neurons of the gray matter of the spinal cord, which would suggest that muscular hypoplasia and muscular defects observed in SBV infected lambs and calves are mostly secondary to damage of the central nervous system (CNS).

HISTORICAL FINDINGS
Outbreak of aborted, stillborn, and malformed newborns.

SIGNALMENT
Aborting cattle, sheep (most susceptible), and goats

PHYSICAL EXAMINATION FINDINGS
- Mild transient disease can occur in adult ruminants.
- Severe fetal malformation, abortion, and stillbirth.
- The teratogenic effects due to SBV are mostly reported to affect the musculoskeletal system; arthrogryposis, hydranencephaly, brachygnathia, scoliosis, kyphosis, or lordosis were malformations frequently reported during the epidemic.
- Morphologically normal SBV infected animals may present central nervous system alterations, mostly porencephaly.

CAUSES AND RISK FACTORS
- SBV is an enveloped, negative-sense, segmented, single-stranded RNA virus. The three-segmented genome of Bunyaviridae creates a potential for reassortment, which may lead to emergence of new virus strains. Reassortment is a form of genetic recombination in RNA viruses. As with RNA recombination, reassortment requires that a cell be infected with more than one virus. Phylogenetic analysis indicated that Schmallenberg virus might be a reassortant, with segments from Sathuperi virus and Shamonda virus.

- SBV is transmitted by *Culicoides* spp.
- SBV has also been detected in semen of bulls naturally infected with SBV.

DIAGNOSIS

DIFFERENTIAL DIAGNOSES
- Acute symptoms (high fever, diarrhoea, milk reduction and abortion)
  - Bluetongue virus
  - Epizootic hemorrhagic disease virus of deer (EHD)
  - Foot and mouth disease (FMD)
  - Bovine viral diarrhea (BVD)
  - Border disease virus
  - Bovine herpesvirus 1
  - Rift Valley fever
  - Bovine ephemeral fever
- Congenital symptoms
  - Bovine viral diarrhea virus
  - Akabane virus
  - Bluetongue virus
  - Cache Valley virus
  - Nairobi sheep virus
  - Rift Valley Fever virus
  - Other orthobunyaviruses

CBC/BIOCHEMISTRY/URINALYSIS
N/A

OTHER LABORATORY TESTS
ELISA, indirect immunofluorescence and virus neutralization tests are available to detect SBV antibodies.

IMAGING
N/A

OTHER DIAGNOSTIC PROCEDURES
Real-time quantitative reverse transcription PCR (RT-qPCR) test for rapid detection of Schmallenberg virus.

PATHOLOGIC FINDINGS
- Gross lesions: The most common gross lesions were arthrogryposis, vertebral malformations, brachygnathia inferior, and malformations of the central nervous system, including hydranencephaly, porencephaly, hydrocephalus, cerebellar hypoplasia, and micromyelia.
- Histologic lesions: The most common histologic lesions are lymphohistiocytic meningoencephalomyelitis in some cases, glial nodules mainly in the mesencephalon and hippocampus of lambs and goats, and neuronal degeneration and necrosis mainly in the brainstem of calves. Micromyelia was characterized by a loss of gray and white matter, with few neurons remaining in the ventral horn in calves. The skeletal muscles had myofibrillar hypoplasia in lambs and calves. The lesions of SBV-associated abortion and perinatal death are similar to those attributed to Akabane virus and other viruses in the Simbu group of bunyaviruses. In fetal sheep, SBV infection can result in cavitation of the white matter of the cerebrum,

cerebellar hypoplasia, mild lymphohistiocytic perivascular encephalitis, and small glial nodules scattered throughout the brain.

TREATMENT
N/A

MEDICATIONS
N/A

FOLLOW-UP

EXPECTED COURSE AND PROGNOSIS
• In cattle, the disease is usually acute in form with visible clinical manifestations of fever, reduced milk yield, and diarrhea that subsides, with the animal recovering in 2–3 weeks.
• In sheep and goats, SBV infection is almost asymptomatic with transplacental transmission to fetuses in pregnant animals, causing abortions, stillbirths, and a variety of congenital malformations.

POSSIBLE COMPLICATIONS
N/A

CLIENT EDUCATION
Report any increase in abortion or neonatal abnormalities.

PATIENT MONITORING
Animals with congenital defects will have permanent neurologic deficits.

PREVENTION
• Control the *Culicoides* vectors by employing methods such as the application of insecticides and pathogens to habitats where larvae develop; environmental interventions to remove larval breeding sites; controlling adult midges by treating either resting sites such as animal housing or host animals with insecticides; housing livestock in screened buildings; and using repellents or host kairomones to lure and kill adult midges.
• The treatment of livestock and animal housing with pyrethroid insecticide combined with the use of midge-proofed housing for viremic or high-value animals and reduction of local breeding sites are the best options currently available. However, application of pour-on insecticides has been unsuccessful, with no noticeable reduction in the density of biting midges in highly challenged areas.
• There is an inactivated vaccine available in Europe.

MISCELLANEOUS

ASSOCIATED CONDITIONS
The other orthobunyaviruses have similar clinical outcomes but can be differentiated by serology.

AGE-RELATED FACTORS
Fetus is the most susceptible.

ZOONOTIC POTENTIAL
N/A

PREGNANCY
In pregnant animals, abortions and congenital malformations in the following parturition period occur in <3% of cases.

BIOSECURITY
Midge-proofed housing for viremic or high-value animals and reduction of local breeding sites are the best options currently available.

PRODUCTION MANAGEMENT
The timings of breeding or insemination of female animals can be selected such that the vulnerable stage of pregnancy (analogously to Akabane virus: 4–8 weeks in sheep and approximately 8–14 weeks in cattle) does not lie within the vector active area.

ABBREVIATIONS
• AKV = Akabane virus
• BBB = the blood brain barrier
• BDV = Border disease virus
• BVDV = bovine viral diarrhea virus
• CNS = central nervous system
• EHDV = epizootic hemorrhagic disease virus of deer
• INF-β = interferon-beta
• PCR = polymerase chain reaction
• RT-qPCR = real-time quantitative reverse transcription PCR
• SBV = Schmallenberg virus

SEE ALSO
• Abortion: Small Ruminant Teratogens
• Abortion: Viral, Fungal, and Nutritional
• Akabane
• Border Disease
• Bovine Viral Diarrhea Virus

Suggested Reading
Doceul V, Lara E, Sailleau C, et al. Epidemiology, molecular virology and diagnostics of Schmallenberg virus, an emerging orthobunyavirus in Europe. Vet Res 2013, 44: 31. http://doi.org/10.1186/1297-9716-44-31
Lievaart-Peterson K, Luttikholt S, Peperkamp K, Van den Brom R, Vellema P. Schmallenberg disease in sheep or goats: Past, present and future. Vet Microbiol 2015, 181: 147–53. http://doi.org/10.1016/j.vetmic.2015.08.005
Pawaiya R, Gupta VK. A review on Schmallenberg virus infection: a newly emerging disease of cattle, sheep and goats. Veterinarni Medicina 2013, 58: 516–26.
Poskin A, Martinelle L, Mostin L, et al. Dose-dependent effect of experimental Schmallenberg virus infection in sheep. Vet J 2014, 201: 419–22. http://doi.org/10.1016/j.tvjl.2014.05.031
Poskin A, Théron L, Hanon J-B, et al. Reconstruction of the Schmallenberg virus epidemic in Belgium: Complementary use of disease surveillance approaches. Vet Microbiol 2016, 183: 50–61. http://doi.org/10.1016/j.vetmic.2015.11.036
Varela M, Schnettler E, Caporale M, et al. Schmallenberg virus pathogenesis, tropism and interaction with the innate immune system of the host. PLoS Pathogens 2013, 9: e1003133. http://doi.org/10.1371/journal.ppat.1003133
Wernike K, Holsteg M, Saßerath M, Beer M. Schmallenberg virus antibody development and decline in a naturally infected dairy cattle herd in Germany, 2011–2014. Vet Microbiol 2015, 181: 294–7. http://doi.org/10.1016/j.vetmic.2015.10.014

Author Christopher C.L. Chase
Consulting Editor Ahmed Tibary

S

SCRAPIE

BASICS

OVERVIEW
- Scrapie is a nonfebrile, progressive neurodegenerative disease of sheep and goats that costs the sheep industry in the United States an estimated $20 million a year in lost productivity and potential export markets.
- Also referred to as "classical scrapie," scrapie is the oldest known agent in the family of transmissible spongiform encephalopathies (TSEs). Other examples of TSEs include chronic wasting disease (CWD) in cervids, bovine spongiform encephalopathy (BSE), and Creutzfeldt-Jakob disease (CJD) in humans.
- Contamination of the environment and oral exposure to placenta shed from infected dams are major sources for horizontal transmission.
- Transmission via the milk, colostrum, blood, and saliva has also been demonstrated.
- Scrapie has a long incubation period, clinical signs most common between 2–5 years of age.
- Clinical signs vary but can include altered behavior, incessant scratching, weight loss despite normal appetite, ataxia, and ultimately death.
- Scrapie is a reportable disease in the US and is subject to the National Scrapie Eradication Program (NSEP).
- Gold standard diagnosis is by immunohistochemistry (IHC) on formalin-fixed tissues. Biopsy of the rectoanal mucosa or nictitating membrane of the third eyelid are approved antemortem samples, whereas samples of the obex, retropharyngeal lymph node, and tonsil are preferred for postmortem testing.
- Relative genetic scrapie susceptibility testing, especially of prion protein codons 136 and 171, is an effective tool for controlling risk of infection in sheep.
- Scrapie has never been linked to disease in humans who consume sheep muscle.

INCIDENCE/PREVALENCE
- Scrapie was first diagnosed in the US in 1947 in a flock of Suffolk sheep in Michigan. The first US case of scrapie in a goat was reported in 2002.
- For the period April 2003 until February 2017, the Regulatory Scrapie Slaughter Surveillance (RSSS) program has tested just over one-half million culled small ruminants and confirmed 471 cases of classical scrapie (including 41 goats) and 9 cases of Nor98-like scrapie in US sheep.
- In the US, scrapie is most commonly diagnosed in black-faced sheep of which the Suffolk breed predominates. The annual

incidence of scrapie in black-faced cull sheep tested at slaughter has steadily dropped from approximately 0.15% in 2003 to 0.004% in 2015, a 98% decrease.

GEOGRAPHIC DISTRIBUTION
Scrapie has been diagnosed in all regions of the continental US and is endemic in many regions of the world. Current and historical infection status and monitoring efforts of each country is tracked and reported by the World Animal Health Organization (OIE).

SYSTEMS AFFECTED
Nervous

PATHOPHYSIOLOGY
- The infectious agent of scrapie is termed a prion and is thought to be primarily comprised of misfolded isoforms of the prion protein (PrP).
- Encoded by the host's prion protein gene (*PRNP*), the normal "cellular" form (PrP^C) is expressed as a glycoprotein linked to the surface membrane of many types of host cells, especially those of the nervous and lymphoreticular systems. PrP^C is rich in alpha helixes and is susceptible to degradation by proteases.
- In association with scrapie infection, PrP^C becomes misfolded to isoforms (PrP^{Sc}) with increased beta sheet content that renders PrP^{Sc} partially resistant to protease degradation and prone to self-aggregation and formation of characteristic scrapie-associated fibrils (SAFs).
- PrP^{Sc} slowly accumulates in the nervous system and typically also in lymphoid follicles and placental cotyledons. While accumulation in peripheral tissues does not cause significant dysfunction, accumulation of PrP^{Sc} in the central nervous system causes neurologic dysfunction and spongiform degeneration.
- Strains of prions are thought to arise from subtle differences in the conformation and aggregation of PrP^{Sc}. Typical or "classical" forms of scrapie are naturally transmissible between genetically susceptible small ruminants and are the primary focus of this chapter. Atypical forms include Nor98 (discovered 1998 in Norway) and Nor98-like scrapie strains, which may be sporadic forms of small ruminant TSE given the evidence to date suggesting poor or no transmission under natural conditions.

SIGNALMENT
- Sheep and goats.
- Most breeds of domestic sheep are affected but in the US, black-faced sheep, especially Suffolk, have been more likely to test positive for scrapie than white- or mottle-faced sheep.
- Diagnosis is much less common in goats but includes both meat and dairy type breeds.

- Scrapie is commonly diagnosed in animals 2–5 years of age, whereas Nor98-like strains are more common in sheep 5 years of age and older.
- No sex predilection.

GENETICS
- Major determinants of susceptibility and disease phenotype are the amino acid sequence of the host's PrP^C and the strain of scrapie present.
- Relative genetic scrapie susceptibility testing has been effectively utilized to control infection risk in sheep; research to identify susceptibility genotypes in goats continues. No *PRNP* genotype has been identified that is completely resistant to all prion strains.
- *PRNP* codon 171: Amino acid changes at codon 171 have a large effect on scrapie susceptibility. Virtually no sheep homozygous for arginine (171RR) have been identified with scrapie. (*Note:* 171RR sheep are not protected from developing atypical disease associated with Nor98 and Nor98-like strains. Fortunately, transmission of these atypical strains appears to be inefficient and not likely to occur under natural conditions.)
- *PRNP* codon 136: While sheep homozygous for alanine at codon 136 (136AA) are more resistant than are sheep homozygous for valine (136VV) or heterozygous (136AV), all three genotypes are considered susceptible to scrapie infection for regulatory purposes.

PHYSICAL EXAMINATION FINDINGS
- Incubation period is prolonged and >1 year.
- Signs vary among individuals but often develop insidiously and progress slowly over weeks to months.
- Signs may be singular or multiple and include abnormal behavior (confusion, separation from the group, somnolence, or hyperexcitability), weight loss despite normal appetite, pruritus (incessant scraping which may induce lip smacking behavior), fine head and neck tremors, limb ataxia (commonly symmetric), or general weakness progressing to recumbency.
- In addition, goats may be more likely to nibble at feet and limbs or trunk, removing hair in more-or-less vertical and sometimes bilaterally symmetric patterns.
- Infection is ultimately fatal. Occasionally death may occur without observation of clinical signs or coincident with stressful events such as shearing.

CAUSES AND RISK FACTORS
- Newborn lambs and kids are the most susceptible to infection. The mostly likely modes of transmission are spread from infected dams to offspring and to other lambs and kids through contact with the placenta

and placental fluids, but also may occur via ingestion of infected colostrum or milk and exposure to a contaminated environment.
• Transmission risk is lower from infected sires to dams and offspring, from infected adult to other adult small ruminants, and from a contaminated environment to adult small ruminants.
• There is a risk of iatrogenic transmission through injection of contaminated materials (e.g., blood components).

DIAGNOSIS

DIFFERENTIAL DIAGNOSES

Neurologic Signs: Sheep
• Brain abscess (caseous lymphadenitis—CLA/*Actinobacillus*)
• *Clostridium perfringens* type C
• Cobalt deficiency
• Copper deficiency
• Hypocalcemia
• Hypomagnesemia
• Inner ear infection
• Listeriosis
• Louping ill
• Mycotoxins
• *Parelaphostrongylus* (meningeal worm migration)
• Polioencephalomalacia/thiamine deficiency
• Pregnancy toxemia
• Rabies
• Swayback
• Tetanus
• Tick paralysis
• Uremia
• Vitamin A deficiency

Neurologic Signs: Goats
• Bacterial: Botulism, brain abscess, inner ear infection, *Listeria* infection, meningoencephalitis, tetanus
• Congenital: Hydranencephaly, hydrocephalus, progressive paresis
• Nutritional/metabolic: Cobalt deficiency, enzootic ataxia/swayback/copper deficiency, hypovitaminosis A, polioencephalomalacia/thiamine deficiency, pregnancy toxemia, uremia
• Parasitic: *Parelaphostrongylus tenuis*, tick paralysis
• Toxic ingestion
• Pyrethrin/organophosphates
• Salt toxicity
• Trauma
• Viral: Border disease, Borna disease, caprine arthritis encephalitis virus (CAE), louping ill, maedi-visna, pseudorabies, rabies

CBC/BIOCHEMISTRY/URINALYSIS
N/A

OTHER LABORATORY TESTS
• Diagnostic application of common serologic methods is not possible since an immune response to PrP^Sc is not a feature of scrapie.
• Development of a blood- or secretion-based antemortem test utilizing novel detection methodologies continues to be an active area of research.

OTHER DIAGNOSTIC PROCEDURES
• Conclusive diagnosis of scrapie is by detection of accumulated PrP^Sc by immunohistochemistry (IHC) staining of the obex, retropharyngeal lymph nodes, and tonsils of sacrificed sheep and goats.
• Antemortem testing is possible utilizing biopsy samples of the lymphoid follicles associated with the rectoanal mucosa or nictitating membrane of the third eyelid.

PATHOLOGIC FINDINGS
While immunohistochemical detection of PrP^Sc in brain or lymphoid tissues is the gold standard of diagnosis, central neuropathologic lesions may include bilaterally symmetric neuronal vacuolation, microcystic vacuolation (spongiform change) of the gray matter neuropil, astrocytosis, cerebral amyloidosis (rare), and the presence of scrapie-associated fibrils (SAF) as identified by negative-stain EM.

TREATMENT

There is no known treatment for scrapie.

MEDICATIONS

There is no treatment for scrapie.

FOLLOW-UP

EXPECTED COURSE AND PROGNOSIS
• Scrapie is a reportable disease. Clinical suspect animals >12 months of age should be reported to state or federal regulatory officials.
• A slowly progressive but ultimately fatal clinical course.

PREVENTION
• The National Scrapie Eradication Program (NSEP) is a joint state, federal, and industry supported program that employs both passive and active surveillance, animal identification, case management, and education measures in an effort to eradicate scrapie in the US.
• Participation in the Scrapie Flock Certification Program (SFCP): A voluntary program aimed at helping owners significantly reduce the risk of introducing scrapie into flocks.
• Breeding for genetic resistance in sheep.
• Lambing and kidding in a clean environment. Removing fetal membranes and contaminated bedding to prevent additional exposure.

MISCELLANEOUS

AGE-RELATED FACTORS
• Susceptibility to infection is greatest in neonates.
• Clinical signs are commonly observed in small ruminants between 2 and 5 years of age but rarely in animals <18 months of age.

ZOONOTIC POTENTIAL
Scrapie has never been linked to disease in humans who consume sheep muscle.

PREGNANCY
N/A

BIOSECURITY
• Lambing in a clean environment and removing fetal membranes and contaminated bedding to prevent additional exposure will also reduce exposure and disease risk.
• Scrapie prions have also been detected in milk and colostrum, and components of the blood.

PRODUCTION MANAGEMENT
See "Genetics"

ABBREVIATIONS
• BSE = bovine spongiform encephalopathy
• CAE = caprine arthritis encephalitis virus
• CJD = Creutzfeldt-Jakob disease
• CLA = caseous lymphadenitis
• CWD = chronic wasting disease
• EM = electron microscopy
• IHC = immunohistochemistry
• PrP = protease resistant prion
• SAFs = scrapie associated fibrils
• TSEs = transmissible spongiform encephalopathies

SEE ALSO
• Actinobacillosis (Wooden Tongue)
• Brain Assessment and Dysfunction (see www.fiveminutevet.com/ruminant)
• Caseous Lymphadenitis (CLA)
• Clostridial Disease: Nervous System
• Listeriosis
• Mycotoxins
• Ovine Encephalomyelitis (Louping Ill)
• *Parelaphostrongylus tenuis* (Meningeal Worm)
• Pregnancy Toxemia (by species)
• Rabies
• Tick Paralysis

S

- Vitamin B Deficiency
- Vitamin D Deficiency/Toxicosis

Suggested Reading
Baylis M, Goldmann W. The genetics of scrapie in sheep and goats. Curr Mol Med 2004, 4: 385–96.
Prusiner SB. Prions. Proc Natl Acad Sci 1998, 95: 13363–83.
USDA. Phase II: Scrapie: ovine slaughter surveillance study 2002–2003. Fort Collins, CO: National Animal Health Monitoring System, 2003. #N419.0104.
Vaccari G, Panagiotidis CH, Acin C, et al. State-of-the-art review of goat TSE in the European Union, with special emphasis on PRNP genetics and epidemiology. Vet Res 2009, 40(5): 48.
White S, Herrmann-Hoesing L, O'Rourke K, Waldron D, Rowe J, Alverson J. Prion gene (PRNP) haplotype variation in United States goat breeds. Genet Sel Evol 2008, 40: 553–61.
Windl O, Dawson M. Animal prion diseases. Subcell Biochem 2012, 65: 497–516.
Wineland NE, Detwiler LA, Salman MD. Epidemiologic analysis of reported scrapie in sheep in the United States: 1,117 cases (1947–1992). J Am Vet Med Assoc 1998, 212: 713.

Author David A. Schneider
Consulting Editor Christopher C.L. Chase
Acknowledgment The author and book editors acknowledge the prior contribution of Chris D. Calloway and Jeremy Schefers.

S

SEGMENTAL APLASIA OF THE REPRODUCTIVE TRACT

 BASICS

OVERVIEW
• Segmental aplasia refers to lack of development of part of one or more of the structures that are derived from the embryonic mesonephric (Wolffian) or paramesonephric (Müllerian) duct systems.
• In males, the mesonephric duct system differentiates into the epididymis, vas deferens, and accessory sex organs. The epididymis and vas deferens are the most commonly affected.
• In females, the paramesonephric duct system differentiates into the uterine tube, uterus, cervix, and vagina. All these structures may be affected by segmental aplasia.

INCIDENCE/PREVALENCE
• The prevalence in ruminants is very low.
• Relatively frequent in SAC.

GEOGRAPHIC DISTRIBUTION
Worldwide

SYSTEMS AFFECTED
Reproductive

PATHOPHYSIOLOGY
• Segmental aplasia conditions are congenital and represent a developmental error.
• The specific mechanisms have not been elucidated but a hereditary basis is often suspected.
• Segmental aplasia is often unilateral but both sides may be affected.
• Complete aplasia is rare and may represent a separate pathologic process.
• In males, the right side seems to be more frequently affected than the left side. Occlusion of the body or head of the epididymis results in testicular swelling and subsequent degeneration due to fluid backpressure.
• In females, the tubular genitalia may be affected at any level along its anatomy but the most commonly reported conditions are:
    ○ Uterus unicornis (absence of one uterine horn).
    ○ Segmental aplasia of a uterine horn resulting in an isolated distal segment.
    ○ Segmental vaginal aplasia or a persistent hymen.
• Cervical aplasia is possible but rare.

HISTORICAL FINDINGS
• Infertility is the most common presenting complaint.
• In unilateral cases, males are usually fertile.
• In females, unilateral affection may present as infertility, failure to accept the male, or recurrent pregnancy loss. Some cases may present for anestrus.

SIGNALMENT
• Although segmental aplasia can occur in all species, it is particularly well described in cattle and SAC.
• Historically, white Shorthorn cattle were considered at greater risk for paramesonephric disorders (hence, white heifer disease), but up-to-date breed prevalence data is lacking.

PHYSICAL EXAMINATION FINDINGS
• In most cases there are no outwards clinical signs.
• Vaginal aplasia and persistent imperforated hymen may be accompanied by variable degrees of vaginal prolapse, dysuria, and intermittent straining.

GENETICS
• Numerical chromosomal aberrations (e.g., XXY) have been identified as a risk factor.
• A hereditary basis is suspected in some cases.

CAUSES AND RISK FACTORS
Chromosomal abnormalities and specific genes have been implicated.

 DIAGNOSIS

DIFFERENTIAL DIAGNOSES
• In males:
    ○ Small cystic structures derived from either embryonic duct system can occur adjacent to the ampullae, vas deferentia, and head of the epididymis. These generally have no clinical significance.
    ○ Spermiostasis, sperm granuloma, epididymitis, epididymal neoplasia testicular degeneration.
    ○ Orchitis and epididymitis.
• In females:
    ○ Normal pregnancy
    ○ Pyometra and mucometra
    ○ Hydrometra in the doe

CBC/BIOCHEMISTRY/URINALYSIS
N/A

OTHER LABORATORY TESTS
N/A

IMAGING
• In the male, the head and tail of the epididymis as well as the pelvic accessory sex organs are readily assessed by ultrasonography. The complete absence of any expected structure provides a presumptive diagnosis of segmental aplasia.
    ○ In the bull, the rete testis is a narrow (5–6 mm) and hyperechoic (white) linear structure located in the center of the testis parenchyma. In cases of segmental aplasia in postpubertal bulls, the rete is often distended with hypoechoic (dark) fluid.
• In the female, transrectal ultrasonography shows fluid accumulation in the segment of the tubular tract distal to the aplastic area. This may lead to a mistaken diagnosis of pregnancy but the absence of a fetus and placenta is readily determined by ultrasonography. Transabdominal ultrasonography may be used in small ruminants and SAC.

• Vaginoscopy is used to diagnose aplasia caudal to the cervix.

OTHER DIAGNOSTIC PROCEDURES
• Palpation of a very small or absent epididymal tail is suggestive of the condition. The epididymal head may be enlarged due to distension with semen. If the defect is located in the vas deferens, the epididymal tail may be enlarged.
• Semen collection and evaluations: Bilaterally affected males (epididymal segmental aplasia) are azoospermic.
• Palpation per rectum is a common diagnostic procedure in the cow. Absence of a positive sign of pregnancy leads to a diagnosis of pathologic fluid accumulation. Segmental aplasia is confirmed by identifying a missing portion of the uterine horn.
• Exploratory laparotomy or laparoscopy confirms the diagnosis of segmental aplasia of the uterus.

 TREATMENT

THERAPEUTIC APPROACH
• No treatment is recommended for affected animals.
• Unilaterally affected females may be fertile. Females with uterus unicornis continue to cycle and may become pregnant and deliver normally if ovulation occurs on the ovary ipsilateral to the normal side.

SURGICAL CONSIDERATIONS AND TECHNIQUES
• Unilateral ovariectomy (affected side) or partial hysterectomy for cows with segmental aplasia of the uterus. Removal of the ovary on the affected side at the same time will solve the problem with infertile ovulation.
• Segmental aplasia of the vagina can be easily corrected if the aplastic segment is very short (<1 cm). This is especially true when fluid accumulates in the cranial vagina, resulting in a caudal bulging of the aplastic area.
• Nonetheless, the standing recommendation should be to cull all affected animals. Veterinarians should consider the ethical implications of surgically altering breeding animals, especially when those animals or their progeny may be sold without full disclosure.

 MEDICATIONS
N/A

 FOLLOW-UP
N/A

S

MISCELLANEOUS

ASSOCIATED CONDITIONS
N/A

AGE-RELATED FACTORS
Often diagnosed in maiden infertile females

ZOONOTIC POTENTIAL
N/A

PREGNANCY
N/A

BIOSECURITY
N/A

PRODUCTION MANAGEMENT
N/A

SYNONYMS
N/A

ABBREVIATION
SAC = South American camelids

SEE ALSO
• Breeding Soundness Examination: Bull
• Breeding Soundness Examination: Camelid
• Breeding Soundness Examination: Small
Ruminant
• Congenital Defects: Bovine
• Congenital Defects: Camelid
• Congenital Defects: Small Ruminant
• Orchitis and Epididymitis
• Testicular Disorders: Bovine
• Testicular Disorders: Camelid
• Testicular Disorders: Small Ruminant
• Uterine Anomalies

Suggested Reading
Anderson M, Alanko M. Ultrasonography
revealing the accumulation of rete testis
fluid in bull testicles. Andrologia 1991, 23:
75–8.

Blom E. Aplasia of the ductuli efferentes—a
new sterilizing congenital syndrome in the
bull. Nord Vet Med 1982, 34: 431–34.
Momont H, Checura C. Ultrasound
evaluation of the reproductive tract of the
bull. In: Hopper RM ed, Bovine
Reproduction. Ames: Wiley Blackwell,
2015, pp. 79–91.
Riley CB, Kuli K, Crane M, et al.
Management of infertility due to unilateral
segmental aplasia of the paramesonephric
(Mullerian) duct in Holstein Friesian cattle-
A case-based review and update. Bov Pract
2007, 41: 24–31.

Authors Harry Momont and Celina Checura
Consulting Editor Ahmed Tibary
Acknowledgment The authors and book
editors acknowledge the prior contribution of
Peter Chenoweth.

S

SELENIUM TOXICITY

BASICS

OVERVIEW
- Selenium (Se), an essential trace element, plays a vital role in various physiologic processes including immunity, reproduction, and productivity.
- It has a narrow margin of safety but is required in the diet to prevent deficiencies as seen with white muscle disease.
- Selenium is the only essential nutrient that does not have a GRAS (generally regarded as safe) status and so the FDA regulates Se supplementation in animals as if it were a drug.
- Selenium toxicosis can occur naturally, by the consumption of selenium-accumulating plants, or by human errors from over-supplementation of selenium in the diet and/or accidental overdosing (parenteral/oral).
- Organic forms of selenium such as selenomethionine and Se-methyl selenocysteine are the major selenium-containing compounds found in plants, whereas inorganic forms of selenium such as sodium selenite are the common supplemental/dosing form.
- Acute selenosis may occur at oral doses ≥2.2 mg Se/kg body weight.
- Chronic selenosis has been reported to occur in animals fed >5–40 ppm Se in feed.
- The toxic effects of the organic and inorganic forms of selenium are similar but, in most cases, the toxic dose of the inorganic form is greater than the organic form.
- Clinical signs involve the respiratory, cardiovascular, hematologic, and gastrointestinal systems.
- The fetus can concentrate Se in the liver at concentrations up to three times higher than the dam.
- Chronic selenosis or "alkali disease" causes hoof deformities and hair loss. The term "blind staggers" is a misnomer for selenium toxicosis.

INCIDENCE/PREVALENCE
- Seleniferous areas with alkaline soil
- Sporadic incidences resulting from accidental overdoses

GEOGRAPHIC DISTRIBUTION
N/A

SYSTEMS AFFECTED
- Cardiovascular
- Digestive
- Hemolymphatic
- Musculoskeletal
- Nervous
- Urinary
- Reproductive
- Respiratory
- Integument

PATHOPHYSIOLOGY
- Selenium replaces sulfur in amino acids leading to loss of disulfide bridges which results in weakening of keratin and disruption of hair, hoof, and horn integrity. Se also causes abnormal maturation of keratinocytes in the stratum spinosum which may give rise to degeneration and necrosis. Alopecia results from atrophy of primary hair follicles.
- In the hoof, cells on the coronary papillae produce dyskeratotic debris that accumulates in the horn tubules and distorts the normal architecture of the hoof wall.
- Cytotoxic effects of Se are the result of denaturation of critical protein thiols. Selenite and SeCys react with tissue thiols to produce ROS.
- Selenium has been reported to decrease erythrocytic volume by reducing hemoglobin synthesis, which may result in anemia.

HISTORICAL FINDINGS
- Recent administration of parenteral or oral selenium products.
- History of dietary changes with over-supplementation of selenium or grazing of selenium-accumulating plants when feed is limited.

SIGNALMENT
- Young animals are more susceptible to selenosis as a result of an underdeveloped rumen. Rumen microflora can reduce bioavailable forms of selenium to unavailable, elemental forms.
- No breed or sex predilections have been described in the literature.

PHYSICAL EXAMINATION FINDINGS
Acute Effects
- In some cases, there is acute death with few clinical signs.
- Generally, clinical signs include anorexia, depression, reluctance to move, and respiratory distress. Grinding of teeth, diarrhea, bloat, and abdominal pain may also be present.
- Elevated heart rate and respiratory rate and a weak pulse may be evident. Fever, polyuria, and hemolytic anemia have been reported in some cases.
- Death usually occurs within 12–48 hours of acute exposure, otherwise the animal usually recovers.
- Once clinical signs such as dyspnea and ataxia appear, animals generally succumb within the hour.
- A garlicky smell to the breath may be present, especially during the first 16 hours post-exposure.

Chronic Effects (Alkali Disease/Bobtail Disease)
- Clinical signs associated with chronic selenosis include depression, weakness, emaciation, anemia, bilateral alopecia (neck and tail), swelling of the coronary band, and hoof deformities that may result in separation and sloughing of the hoof wall.

- Reproductive performance may be reduced at concentrations ranging from 5–10 ppm Se in the total diet, although no outward clinical signs are present; may be the result of the interference with absorption and retention of copper.
- Blind staggers has been described in cattle and sheep but its causal link with selenium intoxication is questioned.
- Bovine—even in the absence of clinical alkali disease in cattle, elevated Se concentrations may adversely affect both pregnancy and immune response. Se administered as sodium selenite at 25 ppm (0.6–1 mg Se/kg BW) for 1 month or 15 ppm (0.4–0.6 mg Se/kg BW) for 6 months caused chronic selenosis.
- Sheep—chronic selenosis may result in death—without observing clinical signs. Unlike other ruminant species, wool loss and hoof lesions are not commonly identified, although wool production is known to decrease. Sheep fed diets containing 0.5–1 mg Se/kg BW (about 17–33 ppm in the diet) reportedly was lethal when exposed for 2.5–6 months. See Table 1.

GENETICS
N/A

CAUSES AND RISK FACTORS
- Vitamin E-deficient animals are more susceptible to acute selenosis.
- Se toxicosis has been reported to increase with concomitant cobalt deficiency.
- Signs of Se deficiency resemble those of selenium toxicosis.
- Primary (obligate) selenium accumulators such as *Astragalus, Machaeranthera, Xylorhiza,* and *Haplopappus* spp. can contain >1000 ppm selenium. Secondary (facultative) accumulators such as *Aster, Atriplex, Grindelia, Gutierrezia,* and *Castilleja* spp. can also contain toxic amounts of selenium. Most of the plants that have the ability to accumulate large amounts of selenium are unpalatable and are only eaten by animals when there is nothing else to eat.

DIAGNOSIS

DIFFERENTIAL DIAGNOSES
Pneumonia, cardiotoxic plant exposure, ionophore overdose, thallium toxicosis, vitamin E and selenium deficiency, and endotoxemia

CBC/BIOCHEMISTRY/URINALYSIS
- Usually unremarkable in acute cases.
- In chronic exposure, the liver enzymes may be elevated as a result of liver damage.

OTHER LABORATORY TESTS
N/A

IMAGING
N/A

S

SELENIUM TOXICITY　　(CONTINUED)

Table 1

	Comparative Selenium Toxicosis in Cattle and Sheep	
	Se as sodium selenite (inorganic) (orally)	*Se as selenomethionine (organic) (orally)*
Cattle	• 7 mg Se/kg BW—no effect • 10.1 mg Se/kg BW—anorexia and low milk production for 5 days • 9–11 mg Se/kg BW—anorexia, dyspnea, garlicky breath, followed by death within 2 days • Oral MLD at 9.9–11 mg Se/kg BW • 15 ppm Se in diet for 231 days—decreased weight gain, sore foot, cracked hooves, excitability in 1 of 5 heifers	• 2.2 mg Se/kg/day (*A. pectinatus*) for 6–16 days caused blind staggers in steers. • 3.4 mg Se/kg/day (*A. bisulcatus*) for 7 days caused blind staggers in steers. • 25 ppm Se (*Astragalus hay*) for 46 days caused joint stiffening and cracking of hooves in 4 weeks. By the end of 4 months, sloughing of the hoof started. • 9 out of 11 bullocks showed stiffness and lameness in all four legs, pale mucosa, and slow but gradual sloughing of the hoof. Mean concentrations of Se in the herbage was 37 ppm.
Sheep	• 1.7 mg Se/kg BW—35% mortality within 12–16 h • 2.2 mg Se/kg BW—35% mortality within 12–48 h • 6.4 mg Se/kg BW—pulmonary cong., 95% mortality in 15 days • Hyperpnea, salivary frothing, hydrothorax, pulmonary edema, hepatic and renal degeneration • 1 mg Se/kg BW—no weight loss in 72 days • 0.5–1 mg Se/kg BW—several deaths between 78–178 days • Oral LD_{50}–1.9 mg Se/kg BW	

OTHER DIAGNOSTIC PROCEDURES
• For most ruminants, normal Se in blood (0.08–0.5 ppm) and liver (0.25–1.0 ppm).
• In acute cases, liver and kidney Se levels are useful for diagnosis. In general, concentrations >1 ppm are suggestive of overexposure, and concentrations >5 ppm are suggestive of toxicosis.
• In chronic cases, liver selenium may range from 2 ppm to 7 ppm and the hair/hoof Se may range from 1.5 ppm up to 45 ppm. Generally, hair Se >5 ppm indicates excessive exposure. Hair samples must be taken from hair that was actually growing at time of intoxication to be diagnostic. Blood Se and blood GPx activity have also been used for diagnostic purposes.

PATHOLOGIC FINDINGS
Acute Selenosis
• Gross lesions include edematous, congested, and/or hemorrhagic lungs. Bloody froth may be present in the trachea, bronchi, and bronchioles. Congestion and hemorrhages are also observed in the liver, kidneys, and GIT. Petechiations of the epicardium may also be seen with or without edema.
• Histologic lesions are minimal if the clinical course is brief. Otherwise, histopathology reveals endocarditis, myocarditis, and myocardial necrosis. Hydropic degeneration of myocardium is seen along with petechial hemorrhages. Focal areas of necrosis are seen in the liver with occasional vacuolation of the hepatocytes. In kidneys, parenchymous and tubular degeneration with casts is a common

finding. Mild hyaline or granular degeneration of skeletal muscle fibers may be present. Variable necrosis of the lymphoid cells may also be present.

Chronic Selenosis
• Gross lesions include edematous and congested lungs, atrophied and cirrhosed liver with discoloration, enlargement of spleen and pancreas, anemia, atrophy of lymphoid tissue, atrophy and dilation of the heart, and erosion of articular surfaces.
• Histopathology indicates congestion and thickening of the alveolar walls in the lungs, hepatic fibrosis, myocardial degeneration, glomerulonephritis, and mild gastroenteritis. Areas primarily affected in the CNS include ventral horns of the cervical and lumbar vertebral segments, with lesser damage in brainstem nuclei. The microscopic appearance of the affected spinal cord includes vacuolation of the neuropils and sometimes within the cytoplasm of the neurons. Neuronal chromatolysis, axonal swelling, multifocal hemorrhage, and endothelial cell swelling and proliferation are also usually present. The white matter has minimal changes.

TREATMENT
THERAPEUTIC APPROACH
No proven therapy for acute selenium toxicity. For chronic selenium toxicity:

• Remove from selenium-containing diet.
• Increase protein and carbohydrate in diet.
• Increase sulfur in the diet.
• 40 ppm arsenic salt or 50–100 ppm arsanilic acid has provided benefit to calves. Arsenic compounds can increase the biliary excretion of selenium.
• Oral administration of 4–5 g naphthalene daily for 5 days, resting for 5 days, and then repeating has been successfully used in the past in mature cattle.

SURGICAL CONSIDERATIONS AND TECHNIQUES
N/A

MEDICATIONS
DRUGS OF CHOICE
• No specific drug/antidote available.
• Analgesics and NSAIDs may be used for pain relief.

CONTRAINDICATIONS
N/A

PRECAUTIONS
Appropriate milk and meat withdrawal times must be followed for all compounds administered to food-producing animals.

POSSIBLE INTERACTIONS
N/A

S

(CONTINUED)

FOLLOW-UP

EXPECTED COURSE AND PROGNOSIS
• Guarded prognosis with acute selenosis
• Prolonged recovery with chronic selenosis

POSSIBLE COMPLICATIONS
N/A

CLIENT EDUCATION
It is important to educate clients on the risks of selenium administration and proper dosing when providing selenium-containing products for on-farm use.

PATIENT CARE
N/A

PREVENTION
• Avoid excess/further selenium exposure.
• Keep the total dietary concentrations within the recommended limits.
• Prevent access to seleniferous plants.
• Monitor selenium status in the blood.
• Avoid selenium supplementation in seleniferous areas.

MISCELLANEOUS

ASSOCIATED CONDITIONS
• Blind staggers (misnomer)
• Polioencephalomalacia

AGE-RELATED FACTORS
Preruminants and young ruminants are considered to be more susceptible to selenosis because the undeveloped rumen is unable to significantly reduce the amount of bioavailable selenium to a non-bioavailable form.

PREGNANCY
• Infertility, abortions, stillbirths, or weak/lethargic calves.
• No teratogenic effects described.
• Hypoplasia of reproductive organs has been observed in lambs from seleniferous areas.

PRODUCTION MANAGEMENT
Analysis of selenium in feed or whole blood for regular monitoring of the overall status

SYNONYMS
• Alkali disease
• Bobtail disease

ABBREVIATIONS
• CNS = central nervous system
• FDA = Food and Drug Administration
• GIT = gastrointestinal tract
• GPx = glutathione peroxidase
• GRAS = generally regarded as safe
• LD_{50} = the estimated dose at which 50% of the population is expected to die
• MLD = minimum lethal dose
• NSAIDs = nonsteroidal anti-inflammatory agents
• ROS = reactive oxygen species

SEE ALSO
• Cardiotoxic Plants
• Selenium/Vitamin E Deficiency

Suggested Reading
Blodgett DJ, Bevill RF. Acute selenium toxicosis in sheep. Vet Hum Toxicol 1987, 29: 233–6.
Osweiler GD, Carson TL, Buck WB, Van Gelder GA. Selenium. In: Clinical and Diagnostic Veterinary Toxicology, 3rd ed. Dubuque, IA: Kendall/Hunt, 1985, pp. 132–42.
O'Toole D, Raisbeck MF. Pathology of experimentally induced chronic selenosis ("alkali disease") in yearling cattle. J Vet Diagn Invest 1985, 7: 364–73.
Raisbeck MF. Selenosis. Vet Clin North Am Food Anim Pract 2000, 16: 465–80.
Authors Adrienne C. Bautista and Birgit Puschner
Consulting Editor Kaitlyn A. Lutz
Acknowledgment The authors and book editors acknowledge the prior contribution of Asheesh K. Tiwary.

S

SELENIUM/VITAMIN E DEFICIENCY

 BASICS

OVERVIEW
• Deficiency of selenium is encountered in many regions of the world, as it is present only in small quantities and is unevenly distributed on the earth's crust. Vitamin E tends to be plentiful in fresh green forages, but can be low in conserved forages and grains.
• The best understood biologic function of selenium involves its role in the antioxidant enzyme glutathione peroxidase (GPx). The consequences of deficiency can thus in part be explained through oxidant damage to cells. Vitamin E also acts as an antioxidant, mainly at the level of the cell membrane. Although selenium and vitamin E requirements are related, the relationship has not been quantified.
• The toxicity of selenium is a recognized clinical problem, while vitamin E is one of the least toxic vitamins.
• Selenium is an essential trace element for animals, whose deficiency has been associated with a range of diseases in ruminants including abortion, infertility, retained placenta, stillborn or weak calves, and calves that fail to thrive. Animals with the greatest growth and production demands will manifest selenium deficiency first.
• An impaired immune response has been associated with selenium and vitamin E deficiencies, with links to mastitis and respiratory diseases.
• Calves and growing heifers are most commonly affected by selenium deficiency. Signs of white muscle disease (WMD) or nutritional myodegeneration (NMD) can be observed in deficient herds.
• Reduction in the activity of selenium-dependent GPx, with an increase in free-radical-induced cellular damage, is associated with muscle damage in the myocardium and skeletal muscle. Immunosuppression around calving leading to mastitis in first-calving heifers is also linked to low selenium intake before calving.
• The reduction in peroxidation is the rationale for feeding increased selenium and vitamin E for cattle in critical periods, such as growing, late gestation, beginning of lactation, and peak of milk yield.

INCIDENCE/PREVALENCE
In regions where selenium deficiency is a concern, the incidence of selenium-responsive disorders in cattle can be higher compared to other regions. Vitamin E deficiency may be common when conserved forages are widely used for feeding cattle.

GEOGRAPHIC DISTRIBUTION
Principally New Zealand, northern Europe, China, the northern part of the United States, eastern Canada, and southern Chile are recognized as having selenium concentrations in soil insufficient to meet livestock requirements.

SYSTEMS AFFECTED
• Musculoskeletal
• Multisystemic

PATHOPHYSIOLOGY
• Selenium exerts its biologic function as a component of selenoproteins. Vitamin E is a lipid-soluble antioxidant essential for protecting cell membranes from oxidative damage by allowing for its own oxidation.
• Several isoenzymes of selenium-dependent GPx have been identified. These reduce hydrogen peroxide and organic hydroperoxides to stop peroxidation of other cytosolic and membrane constituents.
• If peroxidation is uncontrolled, it can initiate chain reactions of reactive oxygen species (ROS) generation, causing tissue damage. WMD is evidenced at slaughter or necropsy by whitish appearance of striated muscle tissue, which is due to bleaching by peroxides and hydroperoxides.
• Selenium deficiency causes an impairment of the phagocytic function of leukocytes, the release of cytokines, and on the response of leukocytes to cytokines. Therefore, infectious diseases (e.g., mastitis) appear as a consequence of the effects of selenium deficiency on the immune response.
• Selenium-dependent iodothyronine deiodinase catalyzes the deiodination of T4 to T3, reverse T3 from T4, and reverse T3 to T2. These enzymes can activate or inactivate the thyroid hormone thyroxine.
• Thioredoxin reductases are dependent upon selenium. Reduced thioredoxin is critical for several redox systems, including those for transcription factors and reductases for DNA synthesis. They have been established as critical for regulating cell growth, prevention of apoptosis, and prevention of embryonic mortality.

SIGNALMENT
• Potentially all ruminant species are affected. Sheep are more susceptible than cattle, and goats are more susceptible than sheep.
• Young, rapidly growing animals are most commonly affected, including newborns, which can be affected prenatally. Older animals are rarely affected by WMD, but are still susceptible to other selenium-responsive diseases such as mastitis, infertility, and retained placenta.
• Both sexes are susceptible to either selenium or vitamin E deficiency.

HISTORICAL FINDINGS
• Rapidly growing animals are most frequently affected with NMD and this can develop either before or after parturition. Older animals have also been reported to be affected by NMD.
• NMD has been reported in goat kids, and suckling and weanling lambs with adequate selenium status but deficient in vitamin E, possibly suggesting inadequate colostrum intake, low colostrum vitamin E concentrations, or inadequate postnatal vitamin E supplementation.
• Other signs that may be associated with deficiency include poor weight gain in young animals, high incidence of retained fetal membranes, high somatic cell counts (SCC) in milk around calving, or a high incidence of clinical cases of mastitis.

PHYSICAL EXAMINATION FINDINGS
• The clinical consequences vary widely within and between species, and likely reflect cellular vulnerability to oxidative stress. A generalized picture of a selenium-deficient herd would include a range of disorders in cows and their calves.
• NMD is characterized by generalized leg weakness and stiffness accompanied by difficulty rising and standing. Impaired suckling ability due to dystrophic tongue muscles, heart failure, and paralysis are also typical.
• In adults, secondary infections such as mastitis and pneumonia are frequently observed. Polypnea may develop in these animals, which can be accompanied by heart disorders.
• An increased incidence of retained placenta, stillborn or weak calves that die soon after birth, and calves that fail to thrive are typical of herds affected by selenium deficiency. Decreased overall calving rates due to subfertility and abortion may be present. Calves will often have diarrhea, and mortality can be high.
• Reduced sperm production and testicular degeneration have been associated with selenium deficiency. Thioredoxin reductase is a testicular selenoprotein that may underlie the defect in spermatogenesis or maturation associated with testicular atrophy in selenium-deficient bulls. This defect is likely due to disruption of ribonucleotide reductase and alteration in the regulation of transcription factors. This may also explain the lower embryo survival noted in selenium-deficient cows.

GENETICS
N/A

CAUSES AND RISK FACTORS
• The general selenium requirement has been established at 0.30 mg/kg ration DM. A dietary selenium concentration less than 0.1 mg/kg DM has been associated with an increased incidence of selenium-responsive disorders.
• The National Research Council recommends about 20 IU of vitamin E/kg DM for lactating cows, and can be as high as 80 IU/kg DM for dry cows and heifers when fed with conserved and stored forages in the last 60 days of gestation. Plasma serum α-tocopherol concentrations >7.0 µmol/L are

S

(CONTINUED) | **SELENIUM/VITAMIN E DEFICIENCY**

considered adequate in adult cattle. Clinical white muscle disease is common when α-tocopherol levels are <4.6 μmol/L.

DIAGNOSIS

DIFFERENTIAL DIAGNOSES
• The diagnosis may present considerable difficulties since the clinical signs are not specific.
• Nutritional deficiency of copper, cobalt, and iodine may confound the diagnosis.
• Other metabolic causes of immunosuppression and thyroid disorders as well as musculoskeletal disorders in young stock.

CBC/BIOCHEMISTRY/URINALYSIS
• Muscle damage may lead to elevated aspartate aminotransferase, creatine kinase, and lactic dehydrogenase.
• Myoglobinuria can be observed in selenium- or vitamin E-deficient cattle.

OTHER LABORATORY TESTS
• Criteria for establishing selenium adequacy are variable among countries. However, responses to selenium supplementation in terms of milk production and reproductive performance are observed when herd blood selenium concentrations are <0.13 μmol/L. Responses in animal performance are less likely to occur when mean herd blood selenium concentrations are >0.25 μmol/L.
• The blood activity of GPx has been used as a biomarker for selenium status; however, supplementation based on marginal GPx levels does not guarantee a clinical or economical response to supplementation.
• Bulk tank milk selenium concentration has been used as an indicator of herd selenium

status, with a concentration >0.28 μmol/L considered adequate. Note that provision of organic forms of Se tends to increase Se concentration in milk when compared to inorganic forms.
• Selenium deficiency affects the thyroid metabolism, causing lowered circulating T3.

IMAGING
N/A

OTHER DIAGNOSTIC PROCEDURES
The best diagnosis is always afforded by a positive response to selenium supplementation.

PATHOLOGIC FINDINGS
• Usually, lesions of NMD are localized in those most actively exercised muscles, suggesting that free radical production is higher in such muscles.
• Postmortem lesions are usually dominated by mineralization of necrotic skeletal and/or cardiac muscles; white foci of calcification and "chicken flesh" appearance with edema are commonly seen in severely affected animals.

TREATMENT

THERAPEUTIC APPROACH
• Selenium and vitamin E injections can dramatically reduce the severity of disease in deficient herds experiencing clinical symptoms; however, lesions are nonreversible when anatomic dysfunction is present.
• Routine supplementation of selenium and vitamin E in the ration, incorporated into salts, meals, grain mixes or total mixed rations, will prevent disease (Table 1).
• Ruminal selenium boluses are also efficacious in prevention of deficiency for at least a year in many cases.

MEDICATIONS

DRUGS OF CHOICE
See Table 1 below

CONTRAINDICATIONS
N/A

PRECAUTIONS
• Oversupplementation of selenium is possible and the margin between the requirement and toxicity is narrow.
• Appropriate milk and meat withdrawal times must be followed for all compounds administered to food-producing animals.

POSSIBLE INTERACTIONS
• Arsenic, mercury, cadmium, and copper, molybdenum, and sulfur have been suggested to alter selenium metabolism.
• Oxalate can decrease selenate transport in sheep and the sulfur amino acids will alter selenium metabolism.
• Dietary protein and sulfur amino acids may limit availability of seleno-amino acid incorporation into proteins. Methionine in the diet will directly influence the proportion of selenomethionine incorporation into proteins; selenomethionine availability for incorporation into GPx can be reduced when methionine is limiting. Increased dietary methionine allows for increased availability of selenomethionine to selenocysteine conversion for incorporation into selenium-specific proteins.
• Other factors influencing retention of selenium are phosphorus and the selenium content of the diet. Multiple factors affect absorption and retention of selenium, with high dietary protein tending to increase absorption while increasing urinary loss.

Table 1

Methods and sources for selenium supplementation in adult cattle.				
Method	*Source*	*Dose rate*		*Duration (months)*
Discontinuous				
Oral drench	Sodium selenate	0.05	mg/kg BW	1
Parenteral injection	Barium selenate	1		12
	Sodium selenate	0.1		1.5
	Sodium selenite	0.05–1.00		2–3
Ruminal pellets	Elemental Se (10%)	6	g	12
Continuous				
Drench	Sodium selenate	1–8	mg/head/d	
Mineral mixes	Sodium selenate/selenite	1–8	mg/head/d or	
	Se yeast*	0.10–0.15	mg/kg of DM	
Indirect				
Fertilizers	Sodium selenate	5–10	g/Ha	12
	Selenium granules	5–10		24[6]

*Used as feed additive, mg/kg of complete feedstuff.

S

SELENIUM/VITAMIN E DEFICIENCY

FOLLOW-UP

EXPECTED COURSE AND PROGNOSIS
Affected animals should have an improvement of gait and growth within weeks of supplementation.

POSSIBLE COMPLICATIONS
• Severely affected recumbent animals will require euthanasia. Animals with intercurrent infectious disease will have a greater likelihood of dying because of their immunosuppression.
• Decreased growth rates.

CLIENT EDUCATION
Taking the time to help your clients better understand nutritional requirements and their effects on growth, reproduction, and health will greatly aid in reducing preventable disease.

PATIENT CARE
• Ensuring adequate nutritional monitoring for all nutrients in the recovery phase is important for repair of muscle damage and prevention of additional damage.
• Ensuring adequate bedding and access to water and feed is critical for recumbent animals.

PREVENTION
• Dietary supplementation when feeds contain <0.3 mg Se/kg DM and 20 IU vitamin E/kg DM.
• Monitoring maternal selenium and vitamin E status is prudent in deficient areas.
• Screening tests for blood GPx activity are relatively simple and cost-effective.

MISCELLANEOUS

ASSOCIATED CONDITIONS
Secondary infectious disease is common in affected herds.

PREGNANCY
Selenium or vitamin E deficient dams will not provide sufficient selenium or vitamin E to the fetus or from colostrum to allow for adequacy in their offspring. It is important that cattle be fed adequately in the last 2 months of gestation to allow offspring to be born without causing nutritional insufficiency.

PRODUCTION MANAGEMENT
Dietary assessment and intervention should be a routine part of management to avoid nutritional disorders related to selenium and vitamin E.

SYNONYMS
• Nutritional myodegeneration (NMD)
• White muscle disease (WMD)

ABBREVIATIONS
DM = dry matter
GPx = glutathione peroxidase
NMD = nutritional myodegeneration
ROS = reactive oxygen species
SCC = somatic cell count
WMD = white muscle disease

SEE ALSO
• Arsenic Toxicosis
• Copper Deficiency and Toxicity
• Iodine Deficiency and Toxicity
• Molybdenum Toxicity
• Sulfur Toxicity

Suggested Reading
Ceballos A. Selenium supplementation in cattle: Transfer to milk and effect on udder health. PhD Thesis. Charlottetown, PEI, Canada: Atlantic Veterinary College, University of Prince Edward Island, 2011.
Ceballos A, Sanchez J, Stryhn H, Montgomery JB, Barkema HW, Wichtel JJ. Meta-analysis of the effect of oral selenium supplementation on milk selenium concentration in cattle. J Dairy Sci 2009, 92: 324–42.
Ceballos-Márquez A, Barkema HW, Stryhn H, Dohoo IR, Keefe GP, Wichtel JJ. Bulk tank milk selenium and its association with milk production parameters in Canadian dairy herds. Can Vet J 2012, 53: 51–6.
Cobo-Angel C, Wichtel J, Ceballos-Marquez A. Selenium in milk and human health. Anim Front 2014, 4: 38–43.
National Research Council. Nutrient Requirements of Dairy Cattle, 7th rev. ed. Washington, DC: National Academy Press, 2001.
Authors Alejandro Ceballos-Márquez and Jeffrey J. Wichtel
Consulting Editor Kaitlyn A. Lutz
Acknowledgment The authors and book editors acknowledge the prior contribution of Thomas W. Graham.

SEMINAL VESICULITIS

BASICS

OVERVIEW
• The paired vesicular glands are the major accessory sex glands in the bull, buck, and ram.
• The vesicular glands are absent in camelids.
• The vesicular glands contribute volume, nutrients, and buffers to the ejaculate but these contributions are not absolutely essential for fertility.
• The vesicular glands have a lobar structure and are found on the floor of the cranial pelvic cavity. Normal glands in the bull are about 2–4 cm wide and 10–15 cm long.
• Seminal vesiculitis is an inflammation of either or both vesicular glands.
• The condition is most commonly described in the bull but this may be due to the accessibility of the pelvic organs in the bull to palpation per rectum as compared to the buck and ram.

INCIDENCE/PREVALENCE
• The prevalence is reported to be between 1% and 10% in bulls.
• The prevalence is significantly higher (10–30%) in young, peripubertal bulls intensively housed and fed high-energy diets.
• The prevalence is also higher in aged bulls (>9 years).
• Clinical diagnostic criteria may significantly underestimate the true disease prevalence, especially in small ruminants where physical examination of the pelvic accessory sex glands is difficult to accomplish and is not routinely performed.

GEOGRAPHICAL DISTRIBUTION
Worldwide

SYSTEMS AFFECTED
Reproductive

PATHOPHYSIOLOGY
• Bacteria are the most commonly incriminated infectious etiologic agents but viral, fungal, and protozoal agents have been isolated. The most commonly isolated organisms include *Trueperella pyogenes, Histophilus somni,* and where not eradicated, *Brucella abortus.*
• The precise mechanism of infection and pathology is not known and ascending, descending, or hematogenous routes of infection are all considered possibilities.
• Primary infections elsewhere in the body, especially chronic ones, may cause seminal vesiculitis by the hematogenous route. Young males on high-energy diets may experience ruminal acidosis, rumenitis, and bacteremia, which potentially explains the higher incidence of seminal vesiculitis in this population.

• Urogenital anomalies may contribute to malfunctioning of the vesicular gland openings on the colliculus seminalis and increase the risk of seminal vesiculitis.
• Retrograde ejaculation or urine reflux into the vesicular gland may predispose to infection or cause a sterile inflammation of the glands.
• Bilateral and unilateral involvement of glands is equally likely.
• In ruminants, seminal vesiculitis is often found as part of a seminal vesiculitis syndrome with concurrent orchitis, epididymitis, ampulitis, bulbourethral adenitis, or prostatitis.

HISTORICAL FINDINGS
• Breeding bulls may have a history of sterility or subfertility but often have acceptable levels of fertility.
• AI sires may have a history of producing semen with poor motility and post-thaw viability along with the presence of white blood cells in the ejaculate.

SIGNALMENT
• Most commonly found in bulls but does affect rams and bucks as well.
• *Bos taurus* and *Bos indicus* bulls are equally affected.
• Most commonly found in peripubertal bulls (10–15 months) and older bulls (>9 years).

PHYSICAL EXAMINATION FINDINGS
• Clinical signs are often completely lacking.
• Unilateral or bilateral enlargement of the glands and loss of lobulations on palpation per rectum are the most common findings.
• In chronic cases, abscess formation and adhesions to adjacent abdominal or pelvic structures may occur.
• Rarely, bulls may show signs of abdominal pain, pain during mounting and thrusting, or pain when semen is collected by electroejaculation.
• Most physical examination findings are normal.
• The finding of infectious or inflammatory lesions anywhere in the genital tract of male ruminants should suggest the possibility of a concurrent seminal vesiculitis.

GENETICS
No known genetic influence or breed distribution

CAUSES AND RISK FACTORS
• Seminal vesiculitis has been attributed to a variety of infectious and noninfectious causes.
• *Mycobacterium tuberculosis, M. avium* subsp. *paratuberculosis, Brucella abortus, B. ovis,* and *B. melitensis* are potential agents of special concern either for their zoonotic potential or local reporting requirements or both.
• In areas free of brucellosis, *Trueperella pyogenes* is the bacterium most commonly isolated from clinical cases.

• *Streptococcus* spp., *Staphylococcus* spp., *Pseudomonas aeruginosa, E. coli, Tritrichomonas foetus, Chlamydophila* spp., *Ureaplasma* spp., *Mycoplasma* spp., and *Haemophilus* spp. have all been reported to cause seminal vesiculitis in bulls.
• A wide variety of bacteria have been isolated from cases of ovine epididymitis and should be considered potential causes of seminal vesiculitis in this species as well.
• Bovine herpesvirus-1 and other viruses have been incriminated as causes of vesiculitis.
• Sperm entering the gland during ejaculation may initiate an autoimmune reaction and subsequent vesiculitis.
• Infections at other body sites (e.g., orchitis, epididymitis, urethritis, rumenitis, pneumonia, omphalophlebitis, or traumatic reticulopericarditis) or congenital anomalies of the urogenital system (e.g., uterus masculinus or malformation of the colliculus seminalis) may predispose to developing seminal vesiculitis.
• High-density housing systems and high-concentrate diets commonly found in bull test stations appear to increase the risk of seminal vesiculitis as well.

DIAGNOSIS

DIFFERENTIAL DIAGNOSES
• Differential diagnoses for enlargement or asymmetry of the vesicular glands are segmental aplasia, hypoplasia, or accessory vesicular glands.
• The presence of a dilated or infected uterus masculinus may mimic seminal vesiculitis.
• Differentials for white blood cells in the semen include infections or inflammation anywhere along the urogenital tract including the prepuce and penis.
• Urinary calculi should be considered, especially in rams and bucks.
• Primary infectious diseases of special concern in cases of seminal vesiculitis include brucellosis, tuberculosis, and paratuberculosis.

CBC/BIOCHEMISTRY/URINALYSIS
• The CBC will usually be normal.
• Certain semen biochemistry values are altered but these have limited clinical relevance.
• Urinalysis may be normal or show an elevated white blood cell count.

OTHER LABORATORY TESTS
• Semen evaluation may reveal an elevated pH, lower sperm motility, increased catalase activity, and lower fructose concentration.
• Leukocytes are not normally seen in ruminant ejaculates but are generally present with seminal vesiculitis. Neutrophils are most commonly seen, but lymphocytes may predominate in some cases.

S

SEMINAL VESICULITIS

• Many bulls with seminal vesiculitis have semen quality problems, typically sperm with poor motility, or morphologic abnormalities are found.

• Changes in sperm morphology may actually be the result of a concurrent orchitis or epididymitis as part of the seminal vesiculitis syndrome, rather than the direct result of seminal vesiculitis.

IMAGING

• Transrectal ultrasonography is useful for imaging the vesicular glands.

• A 5 MHz transrectal probe with a rigid extension can be used for pelvic examination in small ruminants.

• Affected glands are larger and may have a more or less echoic parenchyma with a relatively hyperechoic appearance to the stromal and ductular network.

• Abscessed glands will show a loss of normal lobar architecture with globoid areas of variable echo-density.

OTHER DIAGNOSTIC PROCEDURES

• Culture and antibiotic sensitivity testing are used to confirm cases with a bacterial etiology and to select appropriate treatment.

• Quantitative culture of an ejaculate collected by artificial vagina or electroejaculation may suffice if large numbers of the infectious agent are being secreted in the ejaculate but contamination with urethral, penile, and preputial microflora is unavoidable and may confuse the diagnosis.

• Noncontaminated samples require that the bull be sedated, and the penis be exposed, disinfected, and catheterized followed by transrectal massage of the vesicular glands and collection of fluid.

• Aerobic, anaerobic, and special (e.g., *Mycoplasma, Ureaplasma, T. foetus,* and fungi) cultures should be performed.

• Routine semen evaluation will usually show hypercoagulation of sperm cells and Diff-Quik staining of semen will confirm pyospermia.

PATHOLOGIC FINDINGS

• Gross findings are consistent with the physical examination findings.

• Histologically, the lesions consist of variable leukocytic infiltration of the interstitial and alveolar areas (microabscessation) along with fibrotic and other degenerative changes throughout the glands.

• Spermatozoa are frequently seen in the ductular or alveolar regions of the gland.

TREATMENT

THERAPEUTIC APPROACH

• Medical treatment with antibiotics, local injection of antibiotics or sclerotic agents, have all been attempted but with limited success.

• Medical treatment is usually done on the farm or at the AI center.

• Given the prolonged duration of most medical therapy, the bull will usually be lost for at least the current breeding season.

SURGICAL CONSIDERATIONS AND TECHNIQUES

• Surgical ablation of the vesicular glands (vesiculectomy) may be considered in valuable bulls and usually requires hospitalization.

• Surgery is performed on the standing bull so restraint of the patient is critical.

• Both a perirectal ischiorectal fossa and a ventral pararectal approach to vesiculectomy are described.

• Limited success has been reported following surgery.

MEDICATIONS

DRUGS OF CHOICE

• Antibiotics based on culture and sensitivity for a minimum of 2–4 weeks and potentially for as long as 6–8 weeks.

• Most antibiotics fail to achieve inhibitory concentrations in the seminal vesicles at label dosages. Tulathromycin (2.5 mg/kg IM) and tilmicosin (10 mg/kg SC, q48h for 3 treatments) are reported to more effectively penetrate the seminal vesicles and may offer the potential for more effective and shorter-duration treatment.

• Nonsteroidal anti-inflammatory agents may improve the response to antibiotics in acute cases and reduce the risk of adhesions.

CONTRAINDICATIONS

Appropriate meat withdrawal times must be followed for all compounds administered to food-producing animals.

PRECAUTIONS

No drugs available in the United States are labeled for treatment of seminal vesiculitis, so all therapies represent extra-label drug use and require a determination of appropriate withdrawal times before slaughter.

POSSIBLE INTERACTIONS

N/A

FOLLOW-UP

EXPECTED COURSE AND PROGNOSIS

Guarded to poor prognosis, and recovery may be temporary, so semen from valuable bulls should be collected and frozen as soon as it receives a normal evaluation.

POSSIBLE COMPLICATIONS

Postsurgical abscess formation and peritonitis

CLIENT EDUCATION

It is imperative that clients understand that there is a guarded to poor prognosis for

recovery; therefore, only very valuable bulls should be considered candidates for treatment.

PATIENT CARE

• Sexual rest is recommended during medical therapy and for at least 6 weeks after surgical therapy.

• Repeat a BSE every 6 weeks for up to 6 months.

• Examine the semen carefully for the presence of pyospermia.

PREVENTION

Avoid crowded and unsanitary conditions that may increase the general risk of infectious diseases, especially those caused by *T. pyogenes.*

MISCELLANEOUS

ASSOCIATED CONDITIONS

Seminal vesiculitis can occur in association with primary infections in other organs or as part of the seminal vesiculitis syndrome.

AGE-RELATED FACTORS

• Spontaneous recovery is probably the rule for most young bulls affected with seminal vesiculitis, and treatment of these bulls will often seem to be successful.

• Older bulls are less likely to respond favorably to treatment and have a more guarded prognosis for recovery.

ZOONOTIC POTENTIAL

Brucellosis and tuberculosis can cause seminal vesiculitis in ruminants.

PREGNANCY

N/A

BIOSECURITY

• All males to be used as breeding animals should be subject to the same parasite control and vaccination procedures as the females in the herd or flock except that bulls should not be routinely vaccinated for brucellosis.

• Bulls or bull calves destined for sale to AI centers should be vaccinated only as specifically requested by the AI facility.

• All breeding males entering a herd or flock should undergo a breeding soundness examination and an appropriate period of quarantine followed by reexamination.

PRODUCTION MANAGEMENT

• Animals affected with seminal vesiculitis have the potential to reduce the reproductive efficiency of food and fiber production systems.

• This reduction occurs most often as a result of the decreased fertility of the affected males but may also involve disease transmission to the females.

• Males with evidence of subfertility or infectious or hereditary diseases should be eliminated from the breeding population.

SYNONYMS
- Vesicular adenitis
- Vesiculitis

ABBREVIATIONS
- AI = artificial insemination
- BSE = breeding soundness examination

SEE ALSO
- Beef Bull Management (see www.fiveminutevet.com/ruminant)
- Breeding Soundness Examination: Bovine
- Breeding Soundness Examination: Small Ruminant
- Brucellosis
- Orchitis and Epididymitis

Suggested Reading
Barth A. Vesicular adenitis. In: Hopper RM ed, Bovine Reproduction. Ames: Wiley Blackwell, 2015, p. 109.
Hoover TR. A technique for injecting into the seminal vesicles of the bull. Am J Vet Res 1974, 35: 1135–6.

Jansen BC. The pathology of bacterial infection in the genitalia in rams. Onderstepoort J Vet Res 1980, 47: 263–7.
Parsonson IM, Hall CE, Settergren I. A method for the collection of bovine seminal vesicle secretions for microbiologic examination. J Am Vet Med Assoc 1971, 158: 175–7.

Authors Harry Momont and James Meronek
Consulting Editor Ahmed Tibary

S

SENNA SPECIES

BASICS

OVERVIEW
• Annual or perennial herbs or shrubs that cause musculoskeletal problems in ruminants.
• These plants are members of the Fabaceae (legume) family.
• Between 200–300 different species exist in the Senna genus, primarily located in temperate and tropical regions of the world.
• *Senna occidentalis* (common name coffee senna) and *Senna obtusifolia* (sickle pod) are the two most common species in North America.
• Other less-common species found in the south central United States and Mexico include *S. roemeriana* (twin-leaf senna, two-leaf senna) and *S. lindheimeriana* (Lindheimer senna).
• *S. occidentalis* and *S. obtusifolia* are often found in poorly-maintained pastures, along roadsides, in ditches and fence rows. They may also be found in cultivated fields of corn, sugar cane and other row crops. *S. occidentalis* prefers partial shade and *S. obtusifolia* prefers sandy soil.
• The Sennas are erect, commonly growing up to 8 feet in height.
• They possess alternate, pinnately compound leaves with 4–8 pairs of obovate leaflets.
• Flowers are yellow, 1–2 cm.
• Pods on *S. obtusifolia* are sickle-shaped, almost four-sided, 10–20 cm in length with the ends pointing downward.
• *S. occidentalis* has pods that are more flattened, 10–20 cm in length, and straighter with the tips extending upward.
• Seeds are dark brown.
• The plants may contaminate grains, soybean crops, silage, green chop, and hay.
• Ruminants also become intoxicated by eating the plant in the field.

INCIDENCE/PREVALENCE
• Relative to the availability of the plants.
• The plants are reported to be unpalatable.
• Most intoxication occurs in the fall after a frost damages the plants. The author has seen intoxication after plants were wilted subsequent herbicide treatment. One explanation for this increased consumption of dead or wilting plants may be due to sugars concentrating in the plants as they are dying.
• *S. roemeriana* is more likely a problem in the spring.
• Disease associated with *Senna* spp. is usually limited to a few animals unless plants are inadvertently fed in contaminated silage, hay, etc. This may be due in part to the unpalatable nature of the plants.
• 0.5–3.0% body weight of green plant consumed daily over 5–7 days or overnight fill on *S. occidentalis* will produce toxicity.

GEOGRAPHIC DISTRIBUTION
• Worldwide distribution.
• *S. occidentalis* and *S. obtusifolia* are most common in the Gulf Coast region but are found from Pennsylvania to Texas.
• *S. roemeriana* and *S. lindheimeriana* are found in the south central US and Mexico.

SYSTEMS AFFECTED
• Anthraquinones cause damage to the gastrointestinal tract.
• Other systems affected by *Senna spp.* include skeletal and cardiac muscle and the hepatic system.

PATHOPHYSIOLOGY
• Poorly understood.
• Toxic principles are numerous anthraquinones (obtusin, obtusifolin, emodin, and others). They are known to produce gastrointestinal effects, and are thought to inhibit electron transport of mitochondria, causing myodegeneration, myopathy, and muscular weakness. However, the exact cause of the muscle damage has never been proven.

SIGNALMENT
All ruminants are susceptible, although cattle are most commonly intoxicated.

PHYSICAL EXAMINATION FINDINGS
• Diarrhea (moderate to severe), is seen shortly after consumption and is usually the first observed sign.
• Anthraquinones are known to cause gastrointestinal upset, resulting in depressed appetite and diarrhea.
• Progressive muscular weakness indicated by tremors in rear limbs, ataxia, weakness, and eventual inability to rise occurs later in the course.
• Animals are generally afebrile.
• Cattle are often referred to as "bright-eyed downers" as they will often continue to eat, drink, and remain alert.
• In contrast, some affected animals become lethargic and anorectic.
• The urine is usually dark due to myoglobinuria from muscle degeneration.
• Most animals do not survive once recumbency occurs and death occurs within 1–7 days.

CAUSES AND RISK FACTORS
• Anthraquinones are the toxic principles in *Senna* species. The entire plant is considered toxic when green or dry.
• Mature plants are more toxic than younger specimens.
• Seeds are more toxic than foliage and contain the highest concentration of anthraquinones.
• *Senna* species are not generally very palatable and are more likely consumed in the late summer and fall when other food sources become scarce.
• *S. occidentalis* is more toxic than *S. obtusifolia*.

DIAGNOSIS

DIFFERENTIAL DIAGNOSES
• White muscle disease associated with deficiencies of vitamin E and selenium
• Acute copper poisoning in sheep
• Dallisgrass staggers
• Other causes of "downer" animals

CBC/BIOCHEMISTRY/URINALYSIS
• Marked elevations in serum enzymes AST and CK are commonly noted, reflecting muscle necrosis and degeneration. CK levels may be elevated 10-1000× above normal.
• AST is often elevated 10× above normal levels.
• Myoglobinuria is commonly noted. It may be mistaken for hemoglobinuria (hemoglobin is visible in plasma, whereas myoglobin is not).
• The elevation in AST and CK reflects acute muscle degeneration.

OTHER LABORATORY TESTS
Evidence of plant consumption

PATHOLOGIC FINDINGS
• Signs of toxic myopathy as evidenced by severe muscle necrosis.
• Pale streaking to almost white discoloration of muscle, adjacent to normal muscle may be seen in the shoulder and pelvic limbs, especially in the quadriceps femoris, semimembranosus, and semitendonosus.
• Hyperemia of the mucosa of the stomach and small intestine.
• Mild hepatic necrosis and renal tubular necrosis may be seen microscopically.
• The heart may also contain pale streaking and hemorrhages.

TREATMENT

THERAPEUTIC APPROACH
• Primarily supportive treatment of symptoms as there is no specific therapy available.
• Intravenous fluids to assist maintenance of renal function if myoglobinuria is present.
• Treatment is usually unrewarding after recumbency develops with most animals dying in 1–7 days.

MEDICATIONS

DRUGS OF CHOICE
• Activated charcoal: 2–5 g/kg body weight given orally to control absorption of toxins from the gastrointestinal tract (1 g charcoal per 5 mL water).
• Mineral oil administered orally to more rapidly transport plant materials from gastrointestinal tract.

S

• Generally, it is considered best to use either activated charcoal or mineral oil, but not both at the same time.

CONTRAINDICATIONS
The use of vitamin E and selenium is contraindicated as their use will increase myodegeneration and mortality.

 FOLLOW-UP

EXPECTED COURSE AND PROGNOSIS
• Clinical course may last up to 7–10 days.
• Once recumbency occurs, few animals recover.

PREVENTION
• Prevent animal access to *Senna* spp.
• Maintain appropriate level of nutrition.
• Closely monitor livestock for increased interest in *Senna* species after a frost or herbicide treatment since this may increase plant palatability.

 MISCELLANEOUS

AGE-RELATED FACTORS
The author has noted both calves and adult cattle consuming *Senna* species in sufficient amounts to result in death.

PREGNANCY
Experimentally, fetal deaths have been reported in pregnant animals fed Senna. See Suggested Reading.

ABBREVIATIONS
• AST = aspartate transaminase
• CK = creatine kinase

SEE ALSO
• Grass Tetany/Hypomagnesemia
• Heavy Metal Toxicosis
• Mycotoxins
• Ryegrass Staggers (Perennial, Lolitrem B)
• Selenium/Vitamin E Deficiency

Suggested Reading
Burrows GE, Tyrl RJ. Toxic Plants of North America. Ames: Iowa State University Press, 2001.
Burrows GE, Tyrl RJ eds. Chapter 35. In: Toxic Plants of North America, 2nd ed. Wiley-Blackwell, 2013, pp 598–602. Kindle edition.
Knight AP, Walter RG. A Guide to Plant Poisoning of Animals in North America. Jackson, WY: Teton New Media, 2001.
Poisonous Plants of the Southern United States, Agricultural Extension Services, University of Tennessee, 1980.
Tasaka AC, Sinhorini IL, Dagli MLZ, Haraguchi M, Gorniak SL. Perinatal study of *Senna occidentalis* intoxication in rabbits. In: Acamovic T, Stewart C, Pennycott T eds, Poisonous Plants and Related Toxins, 6th International Symposium on Poisonous Plants. Wallingford, UK: CAB International, 2004, pp. 459–64.

Author Matt G. Welborn
Consulting Editor Christopher C.L. Chase

S

SHEEP AND GOAT POX

 BASICS

OVERVIEW
• Sheep and goat pox caused by separate host-specific capripoxviruses, sheep poxvirus (SPV) and goat poxvirus (GPV). Most strains host-specific for either sheep or goats; some can recombine with other strains causing lesions in one or both species and result in a wide variety of clinical signs.
• Disease is characterized by fever and generalized pox lesions on the skin and mucus membranes. A bronchopneumonia can also be noted in infected animals.
• Transmitted primarily by aerosol from close contact with infected animals. Other methods of viral transmission are abrasions of the skin or mucosa coming into direct contact with dried scabs or contaminated fomites. *Stomoxys calcitrans* is an efficient mechanical vector.
• Disease has not been detected in wild sheep/goat populations.

INCIDENCE/PREVALENCE
• Morbidity and mortality vary with the breed of the animal, its immunity to capripoxviruses, and the strain of the virus.
• Mild infections are common among indigenous breeds in endemic areas, but more severe disease can be seen in young or stressed animals, animals with concurrent infections, or animals from areas where pox has not occurred for some time. Reported morbidity rates in indigenous breeds range from 1% to 75% or higher.
• Although the mortality rate is often <10%, case fatality rates of nearly 100% have been reported in some young animals.
• Imported breeds of sheep and goat usually develop severe disease when they are moved into an endemic area. The morbidity and mortality rates can approach 100% in newly imported, highly susceptible flocks.

GEOGRAPHIC DISTRIBUTION
Endemic in Africa (countries north of the equator), Middle East, India/Pakistan, and most of Asia; recently observed in Southern and Eastern Europe.

SYSTEMS AFFECTED
• Integument
• Ophthalmic
• Respiratory

PATHOPHYSIOLOGY
• The virus enters through the oral, nasal, or respiratory epithelium or via the skin dermis or epidermis. Local viral replication occurs in these affected epithelial tissues.
• Infected macrophage type cells are thought to transport the virus to the regional lymph nodes, where further viral replication takes place. There is a marked proliferative response in the affected lymph nodes, which greatly increase in size.

• A strictly cell-associated viremia then occurs, which introduces infected cells (probably macrophages) throughout the body. The virus then replicates further in the epithelial tissues of the skin, lungs, endothelium, muscle and, more rarely, in nervous tissue.
• The basic lesions in the various affected tissues are due to a vasculitis, thrombosis, and the resulting necrosis. The balloon degeneration of epithelial cells results in the occasional vesicular-type lesions seen with smallpox, but with sheep and goat pox the lesions are necrotic, scabbed epithelium and dermis, with full skin thickness lesions often leaving deep scarring of the hide.

SIGNALMENT
• Severity is influenced by age, sex, breed, and nutritional status of the animal.
• Mortality rate in naïve animals can approach 50–90%. Mortality rate of native sheep from endemic areas can vary from 5% to 10%.
• Young are severely affected with morbidity/mortality approaching 85–95%. Neonates may have a mortality rate of 100%.

PHYSICAL EXAMINATION FINDINGS
• Clinical disease may range from mild to severe.
• Incubation period 4–14 days with the disease lasting up to 6 weeks. Various stages of the pox lesions may be observed at the same time. Complete recovery may take up to 3–4 months.
• Fever, 104–106°F (40–41°C), and depression with conjunctivitis and rhinitis common.
• Pox lesions are soon noted in haired and hairless areas of the body. Swelling of the muzzle, nares, and lips are usually noted first. Macules and papules develop on the muzzle, nares, lips, eyelids, perineum, scrotum, axillary/inguinal regions, and udder.
• Lesions first appear as circular, raised, erythematous areas (macule) that progress to raised blanched regions with a central region of fluid (papule). Papules rupture leaving circular umbilicated lesions that scab over and slowly heal. Associated dermis is thickened, hard, and edematous. Lesions leave deep scars.
• Papules on the eyelid can be very painful and cause blepharitis and mucopurulent discharge.
• Nose, nasal passages, and tracheal lesions cause respiratory distress and mucopurulent discharge. Virus is present in secretions.
• Pneumonia results in severe labored breathing/cough; secondary bacterial infections common. Animals often remain in poor body condition.
• The lesions scab over forming deep slow-healing ulcers in the skin.

CAUSES AND RISK FACTORS
• The poxviruses of sheep and goats (capripoxviruses) are closely related, both antigenically and physicochemically. They are also related to the virus of lumpy skin disease.

• Naïve and young animals are highly susceptible.

 DIAGNOSIS

DIFFERENTIAL DIAGNOSES
• Bacterial pneumonia
• Bluetongue virus
• Contagious ecthyma (orf)
• *Dermatophilus congolensis* (streptothricosis)
• Insect bites
• Photosensitization
• Psoroptic mange

CBC/BIOCHEMISTRY/URINALYSIS
N/A

OTHER LABORATORY FINDINGS
• Virus detected from scabs, vesicle fluid, and oral/nasal secretions.
• Polymerase chain reaction (PCR) assays and sequencing can detect capripoxvirus genomes in tissue samples or cultures, and identify whether the virus is SPV or GPV
• Agar gel immunodiffusion (AGID) test cross reacts with other pox viruses.
• Virus neutralization tests, indirect fluorescent antibody tests and indirect ELISA tests used for antibody measurements for exposure to the viruses.

OTHER DIAGNOSTIC PROCEDURES
Electron microscopy is often used to identify typical large brick-shaped poxvirus particles covered by short tubular elements and measuring 265–295 nm. Viral particles can be difficult to differentiate from orthopoxviruses.

PATHOLOGIC FINDINGS
• Gross lesions include thickened and edematous dermis and epidermis. Lymph nodes draining these areas are often swollen and edematous.
• Pox lesions (circumscribed macules, papules, vesicles, and deep circular ulcerated lesions with scabs in later resolving cases) noted on the muzzle, nares, hairless areas of the axillary and inguinal regions, vulva, prepuce, udder, teats, eyelids, sclera, lips, oral cavity, esophagus, and rumen.
• Lung lesions are randomly distributed throughout the lungs due to hematogenous spread of the virus. Lesions are discrete, hard, gray-white to hemorrhagic nodules that are easily identified in the lungs. The pulmonary parenchyma adjacent to these areas often becomes atelectic due to the affected bronchiole constriction. Secondary bacterial pneumonias are often sequelae to the infection.
• Histologic lesions include acanthosis of epidermis with ballooning degeneration of keratinocytes. Necrosis and microvesiculation of the stratum spinosum occurs as the lesion progresses.
• Eosinophilic intracytoplasmic inclusion bodies are noted in the swollen keratinocytes.

S

• Dermis is edematous with some hemorrhage and neutrophilic infiltrates.
• Macrophages accumulate in the affected dermis with some becoming enlarged and swollen with eosinophilic intracytoplasmic inclusion bodies and large vacuolated nuclei with marginated chromatin (*cellules claveleuses* or sheep pox cells). Fibrocytes and fibroblasts can also become infected and develop intracytoplasmic inclusions.
• Necrosis of the affected dermis and epidermis is due to a severe necrotizing vasculitis that develops in the affected dermis affecting arterioles and venules with thrombosis of affected blood vessels.
• Lung lesions characterized by a proliferative bronchopneumonia with hyperplasia and necrosis of the bronchiolar epithelium. Alveolar septal walls and associated peribronchiolar connective tissue are thickened by edema and hemorrhage. Some type II pneumocyte hyperplasia is noted in alveoli. Variable numbers of macrophages and neutrophils are present in the affected areas with scattered "sheep pox cells" present.
• Eosinophilic intracytoplasmic inclusions can be present in the "sheep pox cells" and type II pneumocytes.
• Mononuclear infiltrates containing "sheep pox cells" can be noted systemically in the heart, kidney, adrenal glands, liver, thyroid, and pancreas.

TREATMENT

THERAPEUTIC APPROACH
• Reportable disease, one should consult with regulatory veterinarians before treatment.
• Treating affected animals is difficult. Supportive treatment should be considered.

MEDICATIONS

DRUGS OF CHOICE
• The administration of antipyretic to make the animal feel better so it will eat and drink are important.
• Antibiotics for secondary bacterial skin or pulmonary disease may be helpful in the survival of the animal.

PRECAUTIONS
If treated for secondary bacterial infections or given antipyretics, appropriate meat and milk withdrawal times must be followed for all compounds administered to food-producing animals.

FOLLOW-UP

EXPECTED COURSE AND PROGNOSIS
Animals living in endemic areas usually have some innate immunity; susceptible adult animals can have a significant mortality.

POSSIBLE COMPLICATIONS
Secondary bacterial infections in the skin and lung are possible.

PATIENT CARE
Animals should be monitored for secondary bacterial infections.

PREVENTION
• Scabs remain infective for months. If reintroducing animals, vaccination would be an appropriate preventive measure.
• Virus shed in body secretions (particularly nasal and ocular). Virus can remain viable in the environment; passage to other sheep by contact with fomites (including contaminated herdsmen) can occur.
• Live attenuated vaccines are available; confer good immunity lasting up to 2 years. New capripoxvirus vector vaccines for sheep/goat pox and lumpy skin disease is currently being developed.
• The ability of the vaccine to protect already exposed /infected animals is questionable. However, good protection can be expected in vaccinated noninfected animals.

MISCELLANEOUS

ASSOCIATED CONDITIONS
Bacterial pneumonia

AGE-RELATED FACTORS
Neonatal lambs and kids can have significant mortality.

ZOONOTIC POTENTIAL
Several suspected human cases of goat pox have been described. However, no virus was isolated from these individuals.

PREGNANCY
• Pregnant animals may abort, probably due to the high fever observed and systemic infection.
• Fetal infections have not been recorded.

BIOSECURITY
• Vaccinate and quarantine new stock entering a flock or herd.
• In an outbreak, vaccinate all animals to develop some immunity to the virus.
• Vector control to decrease insect populations, particularly *Stomoxys calcitrans*, may not help in control.

PRODUCTION MANAGEMENT
• Disease is transmitted by direct contact with virally contaminated dried scabs.
• Respiratory and oral secretions from sick animals and virally contaminated fomites (i.e., clothes, hands and boots of herdsmen, feed, and other equipment) can spread the disease.

ABBREVIATIONS
• AGID = agar gel immunodiffusion
• ELISA = enzyme-labeled immunosorbent assay
• GPV = goat poxvirus
• PCR = polymerase chain reaction
• SPV = sheep poxvirus

SEE ALSO
• Bluetongue Virus
• Dermatophilosis
• Orf (Contagious Ecthyma)
• Parasitic Skin Diseases: Small Ruminant
• Photosensitization
• Respiratory Disease: Small Ruminant

Suggested Reading
Bhanuprakash V, Indrani BK, Hosamani I, Singh RK. The current status of sheep pox disease. Comp Immunol Microbiol Infect Dis 2006, 29: 27–60.
Boshra H, Truong T, Nifon C, et al. Capripoxvirus-vectored vaccine against livestock diseases in Africa. Antiviral Res 2013, 98: 217–27.
Centre for Agriculture and Bioscience International (CABI). Sheep and Goat Pox 2015. http://www.cabi.org/isc/datasheet/81537, accessed August 8, 2016.
Kitching P. Capripoxviruses. In: Brown C, Torres A eds, Foreign Animal Diseases, 7th ed. Committee on Foreign and Emerging Diseases of the United States Animal Health Association. Boca Raton, FL: Boca Publishing Group, 2008, pp. 377–82.
Rao TV, Bandyopadhyay SK. A comprehensive review of goat pox and sheep pox and their diagnosis. Anim Health Res Rev 2000, 1: 127–36.
Rwetemanu M, Paskin R, Benkirane A, Martin V, Roeder P, Wojciechowski K. Emerging diseases of Africa and the Middle East. Ann NY Acad Sci 2000, 916: 61–70.
World Organization for Animal Health. Lumpy skin disease. In: Fernandez PJ, White WR eds, Atlas of Transboundary Diseases. Paris: World Organization for Animal Health, 2010, pp. 150–7.

Author Robert B. Moeller Jr.
Consulting Editor Christopher C.L. Chase

S

SMALL RUMINANT DERMATOLOGY

BASICS

OVERVIEW
• Skin diseases of sheep and goats may be contagious, zoonotic, and/or detrimental to production.
• Common skin diseases of sheep and goats include dermatophytosis, tick and mite infestations, lice, keds and flystrike, contagious ecthyma, and staphylococcal infections.
• Some specific skin diseases of small ruminants, or specific diseases with cutaneous manifestations, may also be reportable to veterinary regulatory authorities.

INCIDENCE/PREVALENCE
Varies with specific conditions, some of which can be endemic in herds or flocks or occur in outbreak fashion.

GEOGRAPHIC DISTRIBUTION
Occur worldwide in areas where sheep and goats are raised; specific diseases will vary in their distributions based on climate, management factors and other influences.

SYSTEMS AFFECTED
Integument

PATHOPHYSIOLOGY
See specific disorders of interest in this text.

HISTORICAL FINDINGS
See specific disorders of interest in this text.

SIGNALMENT
• Skin disease is a common complaint of both sheep and goats.
• Some disorders may have specific signalment associations; for example, contagious ecthyma is more likely to affect juvenile sheep.

GENETICS
N/A

CAUSES AND RISK FACTORS
See specific disorders of interest in this text.

DIAGNOSIS

DIFFERENTIAL DIAGNOSES
• Differential diagnoses can be determined based upon the characteristics of the dermatologic lesions in question, or based upon the area of the body affected by the problem.
• Determination of the primary lesion (pustules, papules, vesicles, wheals, nodules, or presence of a parasite) can be very helpful to establish a differential list. It should also be considered if the observed lesions are secondary to, and a result of, a primary lesion, such as crusts from a concomitant bacterial infection that is secondary to a primary cause.

• Differential diagnoses for small ruminants with specific dermatologic lesions are listed below:

Pustular/Papular/Vesicular Lesions
• Impetigo caused by *Staphylococcus*
• Contagious ecthyma
• Pemphigus foliaceus
• Capripox
• Foot and mouth disease
• Caprine herpesvirus
• Bluetongue
• Peste des petits ruminants

Nodules With or Without Ulcers
• Demodicosis
• Staphylococcal dermatitis
• Mycetoma (fungal tumors)
• Abscesses (caseous lymphadenitis)
• Cutaneous papillomas
• Squamous cell carcinoma
• Melanoma
• Tuberculosis

Pruritus
• Lice
• Sheep keds
• Fleas
• Ticks
• Mites: *Psoroptes* (ear mange), *Sarcoptes*, *Chorioptes*
• Migrating helminths (*Metastrongylus* and *Parelaphostrongylus tenuis*)
• Flies: *Musca* (bush fly), *Stomoxys calcitrans* (stable fly), *Culicoides* (biting midges), *Tabanus* (March flies)
• Scrapie

Crusting and Scaling
• Dermatophytosis
• Dermatophilosis
• *Malassezia* dermatitis
• Protozoa: *Toxoplasma* spp., *Besnoitia* spp.
• Hypothyroidism
• Contagious ecthyma
• Zinc deficiency
• Selenium deficiency and undetermined vitamin E uptake
• Pemphigus foliaceus
• Capripox
• Mites
• *Pelodera* (*Rhabditis*) *strongyloides*

Hair Loss
• Hypothyroidism
• Dermatophytosis
• Contact dermatitis
• Atopic dermatitis
• Mites
• *Pelodera*
• Selenium deficiency and undetermined vitamin E uptake

Erythema
• Sunburn
• Photosensitization

Sloughing of Affected Area
• Frostbite
• Ergotism

• Chemical burns
• Second or third degree burns
• Photosensitization

Differential diagnoses for small ruminants with dermatologic lesions on specific body parts are listed below.

Lips, Face, and Neck
• Contagious ecthyma
• Capripox
• Staphylococcal dermatitis/folliculitis
• Dermatophytosis
• Dermatophilosis
• Demodecosis
• Peste des petits ruminants (morbillivirus)
• Sarcoptic mange
• Pediculosis
• Zinc deficiency
• Selenium deficiency
• Pemphigus foliaceus
• Bluetongue (primarily sheep)
• Urine scald in breeding bucks
• Photosensitization
• Sunburn
• Squamous cell carcinoma
• Contact dermatitis
• Actinobacillosis
• Elaeophoriasis ("sore head")

Ears
• Dermatophytosis
• Dermatophilosis
• Sarcoptic mange
• Ear mites
• Photodermatitis
• Frostbite
• Pemphigus foliaceus
• Squamous cell carcinoma
• Sunburn
• Ergotism
• Fescue toxicosis

Body
• Scrapie
• *Parelaphostrongylus tenuis*
• Dermatophilosis (lumpy wool disease)
• Psoroptic mange
• Goat/sheep pox
• Contagious viral pustular dermatitis
• Vitamin/nutrient deficiency such as:
  ○ Vitamin A
  ○ Vitamin C responsive dermatitis
  ○ Copper deficiency
  ○ Selenium deficiency
  ○ Zinc deficiency
• Anagen defluxion (wool break, sheep)
• Follicular cyst
• Fleece rot
• Contact dermatitis
• Ulcerative dermatosis (sheep)
• Pediculosis

Feet
• Contagious ecthyma
• Foot and mouth disease
• *Staphylococcus* folliculitis
• Interdigital fusiform infection

SMALL RUMINANT DERMATOLOGY

- Dermatophilosis
- Sarcoptic mange
- Chorioptic mange
- Ergotism
- Fescue toxicosis
- *Besnoitia* dermatitis
- Zinc deficiency
- Contact dermatitis
- Pemphigus foliaceus
- Bluetongue

Udder
- Contagious ecthyma
- Staphylococcal dermatitis or folliculitis
- Zinc deficiency
- Hyperpigmentation from exposure to sun
- Cutaneous papillomas in white Saanens

Perineum
- Contagious ecthyma
- Caprine herpesvirus
- Staphylococcal dermatitis
- Ticks
- Neoplasia
- Squamous cell carcinoma
- Urine scald

CBC/BIOCHEMISTRY/URINALYSIS
Usually of limited value unless cutaneous signs relate to a more significant systemic disorder.

OTHER LABORATORY TESTS
N/A

IMAGING
N/A

OTHER DIAGNOSTIC PROCEDURES
- Skin scrapings, particularly useful for diagnosing mite infestations
- Dermatophyte culture
- Potassium hydroxide preparation for the diagnosis of dermatophytosis
- Woods lamp examination
- Cytologic evaluation and impression smears of lesions
- Bacterial culture and sensitivity testing
- Skin biopsy

PATHOLOGIC FINDINGS
See specific disorders of interest in this text.

TREATMENT

THERAPEUTIC APPROACH
- Treatment should always be based on reasonable diagnosis, which can be derived from a thorough historical assessment and physical examination, and from information garnered through selected diagnostic procedures.
- Treatment recommendations vary depending on the disorder in question, but key tenets of therapy include preventing further damage, improving comfort, resolving lesions, and preventing relapses by identifying triggering or influencing factors.

SURGICAL CONSIDERATIONS AND TECHNIQUES
NA

MEDICATIONS

DRUGS OF CHOICE
See specific disorders of interest in this text.

CONTRAINDICATIONS
Corticosteroids should be avoided in pregnant animals.

PRECAUTIONS
Appropriate milk and meat withdrawal times must be followed for all compounds administered to food-producing animals.

POSSIBLE INTERACTIONS
N/A

FOLLOW-UP

EXPECTED COURSE AND PROGNOSIS
See specific disorders of interest in this text. In general, unless associated with significant systemic disease, or refractory to treatment, most dermatologic disorders have a good prognosis for survival and complete recovery.

POSSIBLE COMPLICATIONS
- Secondary bacterial infection of abnormal skin.
- Severe self-trauma with pruritic conditions.
- Opportunistic infection of abnormal skin or wounds with blow flies or screw worm fly.
- Dehydration and protein loss if large areas of skin are inflamed and exudative (such as with extensive burns).

CLIENT EDUCATION
Many dermatologic disorders of small ruminants are infectious or relate to management factors, so targeted client education is often a critical means of decreasing prevalence of skin disorders within groups.

PATIENT CARE
Focus on reducing discomfort and further damage to the skin, and providing appropriate treatment for lesions and monitoring response.

PREVENTION
See specific disorders of interest in this text. Prevention of most skin disorders relies on factors related to management and biosecurity.

MISCELLANEOUS

ASSOCIATED CONDITIONS
N/A

AGE-RELATED FACTORS
See specific disorders of interest in this text.

ZOONOTIC POTENTIAL
Dermatophytosis, orf, and several other skin disorders of small ruminants are caused by zoonotic agents, or can be contracted through similar means in a variety of species. Care should be exercised during handling of animals and during the collection and evaluation of samples.

PREGNANCY
Corticosteroids should be avoided in pregnant animals.

BIOSECURITY
- Quarantine new animal arrivals to prevent disease or parasite transmission to the herd or flock.
- Some disorders with cutaneous manifestations are considered reportable or exotic in specific regions or countries.

PRODUCTION MANAGEMENT
- Dermatologic diseases may have a deleterious effect on production through a variety of mechanisms, including animal comfort, systemic effects, and thriftiness.
- Specific disorders may be managed through vaccination (e.g., contagious ecthyma).

SYNONYMS
See specific disorders in this text.

ABBREVIATIONS
N/A

SEE ALSO
- Dermatophytosis
- Orf (Contagious Ecthyma)
- Parasitic Skin Diseases: Small Ruminant
- Sheep and Goat Pox
- Wool Rot

Suggested Reading
Kahn CM ed. Integumentary system. In: The Merck Veterinary Manual, 10th ed. Merck & Co., 2010.
Pugh DG, Baird AN. Sheep and Goat Medicine, 2nd ed. Maryland Heights, MO: Elsevier, 2012.
Scott DW. Color Atlas of Farm Animal Dermatology. Ames: Blackwell Publishing, 2007.
Smith MC, Sherman DM eds. Skin diseases. In: Goat Medicine. Philadelphia: Lea & Febiger, 1994.
White SD. Diseases of the skin. In: Smith BP ed, Large Animal Internal Medicine, 5th ed. 2015, pp. 1192–222.
Author Cynthia Faux
Consulting Editor Erica C. McKenzie
Acknowledgment The author and book editors acknowledge the prior contribution of Karen A. Moriello and Susan Semrad.

S

SNAKEBITE

BASICS

OVERVIEW
• Pit vipers are responsible for the majority of venomous snakebites in North America.
• The snakes are named for the fossa in the loreal area between the eye and nostril on either side of the head. The loreal pits are external openings to a pair of extremely sensitive infrared-detecting organs which help snakes find prey.
• Pit vipers include rattlesnakes (*Crotalus* spp.), pygmy rattlesnakes, cottonmouths (water moccasins), copperheads (*Agkistrodon* spp.), and massasaugas (*Sistrurus* spp.). These snakes are identifiable by a triangular head, elliptical pupils, keeled scales, and the presence of rattles in adults. Young rattlesnakes have a blunt tip on the tail until it is broken off.
• Pit vipers can be aggressive (depending upon type) and inject a neurotoxic or hemotoxic venom designed to incapacitate or predigest its prey with a small, potent dose.
• Venom is delivered through hinged, hollow, retractable fangs in a rapid stabbing motion. Mature snakes can control the amount of venom injected, while juvenile snakes tend to inject a maximum amount of venom. Older snakes possess more potent venom, and larger snakes are frequently capable of storing larger volumes of venom.
• Coral snakes (*Micruroides euryxanthus* and *Micrurus* spp.) are nocturnal and are rarely responsible for venomous bites to farm animals. They bite with short, fixed fangs and hold on, delivering a neurotoxic venom by chewing.
• Envenomation in all victims is potentially fatal and is a medical emergency.

INCIDENCE/PREVALENCE
Unknown in large animals

GEOGRAPHIC DISTRIBUTION
• Pit vipers are widely distributed throughout North America (United States and parts of Canada), except Alaska, Hawaii, and Maine.
• Pit vipers are also found in Mexico, South America (except Chile), and Australia.
• True vipers are found in Africa, South America, India, and in tropics.
• Coral snakes inhabit the southern US from Arizona to Florida and are found worldwide in the tropics.

SYSTEMS AFFECTED
• Cardiovascular
• Hemolymphatic
• Integument
• Musculoskeletal
• Nervous
• Respiratory

PATHOPHYSIOLOGY
• The composition and mechanism of action of the various components of snake venom continue to be elucidated.
• Venom is classified as hemotoxic or neurotoxic depending upon the predominant physiologic effects.
• Both venoms contain enzymatic proteins that aid in tissue degradation and digestion
  ◦ Metalloproteases
  ◦ Hyaluronidase
  ◦ Collagenase
• Hemotoxic venom affects hemostasis (plasmin-like protease, thrombin-like protease, and kallikrein-like protease); hydrolyze second messengers like cAMP, (phosphodiesterases) and potent, nonenzymatic polypeptides, all of which result in pain, massive swelling, tissue necrosis, and coagulation abnormalities.
• Neurotoxic venom has significantly less local tissue destruction and pain, but has profound effects on both pre- and postsynaptic skeletal and nonskeletal muscle, neuromuscular junction sites including muscarinic and neuronal receptors, and potassium, sodium, and calcium ion channels. Phopholipase A_2 causes membrane disruption and mediates many neurotoxic and cardiotoxic biochemical changes. Numbness, muscle fasciculations, paralysis, and respiratory collapse can be the result.

HISTORICAL FINDINGS
Usually one animal is affected at a time, but several animals may be affected over the course of a season.

SIGNALMENT
All species are susceptible.

PHYSICAL EXAMINATION FINDINGS
• Rapid regional swelling with severe pain, edema, ecchymosis, and petechiation.
• Bleeding and puncture wounds may or may not be apparent.
• Tissue necrosis, inspiratory dyspnea, and epistaxis are common (especially if bite is near or on the muzzle).
• Increased salivation, dysphagia, and anorexia.
• Lethargy, weakness, reluctance to move, muscle fasciculations, paresis, and paralysis.
• Raised temperature, tachycardia, cardiac arrhythmias, shock, numbness, and respiratory collapse.
• Central nervous system signs: Obtundation, seizures, and coma.

CAUSES AND RISK FACTORS
Snakebite with envenomation

Snake
• Size, age, nutritional status, and species of snake (aggressive species such as the Mojave rattlesnake are more likely to strike).
• Amount of venom injected: 25% of bites are "dry" bites with no injection of venom.

• Toxicity of venom, which varies between species: Rattlesnake > water moccasin > copperhead.
• Toxicity of venom will vary within species and within individual snake as it ages or as the size of prey changes.

Victim
• Depends upon the bite and location (tongue, muzzle, face, body wall, or directly into a large vessel pose the greatest risk).
• Age and size of victim (younger animals are more likely to sustain bites resulting in fatality).
• Preexisting conditions that compromise immune response.
• Victim's susceptibility to venom and time to medical treatment.
• Animals often survive the initial bite only to succumb to infection later due to delayed recovery and treatment.
• Activity after the bite also increases the distribution of venom.

Location/Habitat/Time of Year
• Animals that crowd into shaded areas in hot summer months especially adjacent to watering holes, wood piles, rocky outcroppings, overgrazed pastures, and during drought.
• April through October when snakes are most active.

DIAGNOSIS

DIFFERENTIAL DIAGNOSES
• Trauma
• Insect envenomation
• Abscessation
• Lizard bite (Gila monster)

CBC/BIOCHEMISTRY/URINALYSIS
• Hemoconcentration
• Thrombocytopenia
• Hypoalbuminemia
• Leukocytosis
• Echinocytosis
• Elevated creatinine kinase
• Elevated aspartine aminotransferase
• Elevated cardiac troponin I
• Myoglobinuria, hematuria, proteinuria, glucosuria

OTHER LABORATORY TESTS
• Serial coagulation profiles
• Thromboelastography (TEG)
• Fibrinogen
• Serum antibodies to venom
• Detection of venom in serum

IMAGING
• Ultrasound or radiography to rule out traumatic injury or puncture
• Echocardiography: Cardiac function

S

OTHER DIAGNOSTIC PROCEDURES
• Marking leading edge of swelling along with circumferential measurements of limb or muzzle may give an indication of progression.
• Electrocardiograph: Arrhythmias.

PATHOLOGIC FINDINGS
• Gross findings are variable.
• Swelling, serous exudation, tissue necrosis, sloughing.
• Hemorrhage especially at bite site.
• Passive congestion of all organs.
• Hemorrhagic icterus.
• Histopathologic findings are highly variable.

TREATMENT

THERAPEUTIC APPROACH
• Maintenance of airway, preplacement of nasal tubing prior to occlusion or tracheostomy if necessary.
• Intravenous fluid support, polyionic fluids for hypotensive cases.
• Keep animal calm, restrict movement.
• Wash wound to remove topical debris.
• Do not infuse fluid into wound.
• Wound care and debridement as necessary.

SURGICAL CONSIDERATIONS AND TECHNIQUES
Debridement as necessary

MEDICATIONS

DRUGS OF CHOICE
• Antivenin is the treatment of choice. Recommendations for human bite victims are for treatment with multiple vials, but 1–2 vials may be sufficient to improve outcome for animals.
• Administration of antivenin as early as possible after envenomation may preclude the need for treatment with additional vials later.

Antivenin
• Antivenin: CroFab Crotalidae Polyvalent Immune Fab (Ovine) (BTG Specialty Solutions Center, West Conshohocken, PA 19428, USA).
  ◦ Composed of four antivenins: *Crotalus atrox* (Western diamondback rattlesnake), *Crotalus adamenteus* (Eastern diamondback rattlesnake), *Crotalus scutulatus* (Mojave rattlesnake), and *Agkistrodon piscivorus* (cottonmouth or water moccasin). A study in dogs has been conducted with good results utilizing 1–2 vials of antivenin.

• Antivenin (Crotalidae) Polyvalent (ACP) equine origin (Pfizer New York, NY 10017).
  ◦ Composed of four antivenins: *Crotalus adamanteus* (Eastern diamondback rattlesnake), *Crotalus atrox* (Western diamondback rattlesnake), *Crotalus durissus terrificus* (tropical rattlesnake, Cascabel), and *Bothrops atrox* (fer-de-lance).
• Antivenin (*Micrurus fulvius*) equine origin (Pfizer, New York, NY 10017).
  ◦ Will neutralize the venom of *Micrurus fulvius tenere* (Texas coral snake) but will not neutralize venom of *Micruroides euryxanthus* (Arizona or Sonoran coral snake).
• Antivenin (Crotalidae) Polyvalent, equine origin (Boehringer Ingelheim, Saint Joseph, MO 64506). Labeled for use in dogs; studies have shown typical 1–2 vials utilized in dogs.
  ◦ Composed of four antivenins: *Crotalus adamanteus* (Eastern diamondback rattlesnake), *Crotalus atrox* (Western diamondback rattlesnake), *Crotalus durissus terrificus* (Central and South American rattlesnake, Cascabel), and *Bothrops atrox* (fer-de-lance).
• Current use is extra-label in ruminants.
• Be prepared to treat for an allergic reaction.

Other Treatments
• Treatment with broad-spectrum antimicrobials
• Nonsteroidal anti-inflammatory medication for pain
• Revaccinate with tetanus and *Clostridium* toxoids

PRECAUTIONS
• Use caution when and if handling a dead snake. Reflex bites do occur.
• Treatments used previously that have been shown to be detrimental or ineffective are incision, suction, infusion of fluids into wound area in an attempt to dilute toxin, application of hot or cold compress, tourniquets, or electric shock.
• Controversial: Use of corticosteroids in the treatment of venomous snakebites in veterinary medicine.
  ◦ Corticosteroids delay healing and may, although not proven, interfere with effects of antivenin.
  ◦ No studies have shown increased survival rate with use of corticosteroids.
  ◦ Can be used for treatment of allergic reaction associated with antivenin administration.
• Colloid therapy may increase risk of bleeding diathesis, complicate interpretation of coagulation profiles, or cause anaphylaxis. Use with caution.

• Appropriate milk and meat withdrawal times must be followed for all compounds administered to food-producing animals.

POSSIBLE INTERACTIONS
Corticosteroids may interfere with antivenin.

FOLLOW-UP

EXPECTED COURSE AND PROGNOSIS
• Depends on bite location, age and size of victim.
• Depends on size, age, nutritional status, and species of snake, and amount and toxicity of the venom.

PATIENT CARE
• Restrict activity and movement.
• Food and water should be readily accessible and feed should be easy to swallow.
• Serial monitoring of coagulation profiles, complete blood count, biochemistry panel, and urinalysis, and cardiac parameters should be performed as often as warranted by the clinical condition, especially in the first 48 hours.
• Tissue destruction may not peak for several days. Swelling resolves in 3–7 days in most cases that survive.
• Recurrent coagulopathy may occur 1–2 weeks after administration of antivenin due to short persistence of antivenin in the blood compared to venom.

PREVENTION
Crotalus Atrox Toxoid (rattlesnake venom) vaccines are licensed for dogs and horses. There are no vaccines licensed for ruminants and vaccine efficacy is not well established.

MISCELLANEOUS

AGE-RELATED FACTORS
• Young animals are more at risk due to their inquisitive nature.
• A snakebite with envenomation is more likely to result in mortality due to smaller body size.

ZOONOTIC POTENTIAL
• Wear gloves to protect hands with skin abrasions when treating wounds.

PREGNANCY
• Fetal death as a result of venomous snakebite has been reported in humans.
• The safety of antivenin treatment during pregnancy in animals has not been established.

S

SNAKEBITE

ABBREVIATION
• TEG = thromboelastography

SEE ALSO
• Actinobacillosis: Wooden Tongue
• Actinomycosis: Lumpy Jaw
• Anaphylaxis
• Drug Hypersensitivities
• Parasitic Skin Diseases: Bovine
• Parasitic Skin Diseases: Camelid
• Wound Management

Suggested Reading
Banda HS, Brar RS, Chavhan SG, Kammon A. Pathology of snakebite in cow. Toxicol Int 2009, 16: 69–71.
Gawade SP. Snake venom neurotoxins: pharmacological classification. J Toxicol 2004, 23: 37–96. Available at www.dekker.com.
Mackessy SP, Williams K, Ashton KG. Ontogenetic variation in venom composition and diet of *Crotalus oreganus concolor*: a case of venom paedomorphosis? Copeia 2003, 4: 769–82.
Plumlee K. Clinical Veterinary Toxicology. St. Louis: Mosby, 2003.
Sonis JM, Hackett ES, Callan RJ, Holt TN, Hackett TB. Prairie rattlesnake envenomation in 27 New World camelids. J Vet Intern Med 2013, 27: 1238–41.
Stebbins RC. Petersen Field Guide: Western Reptiles and Amphibians, 3rd ed. Boston: Houghton Mifflin Co., 2003.

Author Jenifer Robin Gold
Consulting Editor Christopher C.L. Chase
Acknowledgment The author and book editors acknowledge the prior contribution of Lauren Palmer.

S

SODIUM DISORDERS: HYPERNATREMIA

BASICS

OVERVIEW
Definition—a serum sodium concentration [Na^+] exceeding the upper limit of normal ruminants, usually >152 mmol/L.

INCIDENCE/PREVALENCE
N/A

GEOGRAPHIC DISTRIBUTION
N/A

SYSTEMS AFFECTED
• Cardiovascular • Musculoskeletal • Nervous • Respiratory • Multisystemic

PATHOPHYSIOLOGY
• Hypernatremia—deficit of water in relation to the body's sodium stores. • It can result from a net water loss or a sodium gain. • Sodium is the major extracellular fluid (ECF) cation. Plays a vital role in maintaining the cell membrane potential, ECF volume and osmolality. • Sodium affects water shifts between the ICF and ECF, with hypernatremia and hyperosmolarity leading to a shift of free water from the ICF to the ECF, which results in brain cell shrinkage, vascular rupture, and neurologic deficits in severe cases. • Source of sodium is primary dietary intake. • Renal is the primary route of excretion (~99% reabsorbed in renal tubules). • Cardiovascular effects of hypernatremia—decreased left ventricular contractibility. • Hepatobiliary system—impaired gluconeogenesis and lactate clearance. • Musculoskeletal effects—muscle weakness, cramps, rhabdomyolysis.

SIGNALMENT
All species of ruminant

PHYSICAL EXAMINATION FINDINGS
• Lethargy • Muscle twitching • Hyperreflexia • Spasticity • Coma • Seizures and death

CAUSES AND RISK FACTORS
Sodium Gain
• Salt poisoning. High Na^+ in the diet with inadequate access to water. • Hypertonic fluid. Administration of hypertonic saline or bicarbonate solutions (IV or oral). • Inadequately mixed milk replacer. • High salinity (>1,000 ppm) of water used to prepare milk replacer.

Water Losses
Can be caused by either renal or extrarenal mechanisms.
• Renal—osmotic diuresis (hyperglycemia, mannitol or loop diuretics). • General—pyrexia. • Respiratory—hyperventilation. • Gastrointestinal. Diarrhea, if compensatory water intake has not yet occurred.

Pseudohypernatremia
• Sodium salts of EDTA, fluoride, and heparin. • Decreased plasma protein and/or lipid concentration.

Risk Factors
• Inadequate water intake. • "Salt intoxication" occurs if salt-restricted animals are allowed access to salt (ad libitum consumption).

DIAGNOSIS

DIFFERENTIAL DIAGNOSES
• Meningitis • Polioencephalomalacia • Lead poisoning • Rabies

CBC/BIOCHEMISTRY/URINALYSIS
• Hypernatremia. • Hyposthenuria is associated with diabetes insipidus. • Electrolytes imbalances of K^+, Cl^-, Ca^{2+}, Mg^{2+}.

OTHER LABORATORY TESTS
• Fractional excretion of Na [FE_{Na}]. Suspect extrarenal losses if [FE_{Na}] <1% and dehydration; suspect renal losses if [FE_{Na}] >1% and dehydration. • Plasma osmolality can be elevated. • Urine glucose and osmolality increases with osmotic diuresis.

OTHER DIAGNOSTIC PROCEDURES
• History, physical examination, and laboratory evidence. • Determine the cause of hypernatremia (sodium gain or water losses).

PATHOLOGIC FINDINGS
• Marked congestion and edema of the brain and meninges. Petechiae and ecchymoses within the gray and white matter of the brain.

TREATMENT

THERAPEUTIC APPROACH
• Addressing the underlying cause (e.g., diarrhea; fever, hyperglycemia and correcting the feeding preparation) and correcting the prevailing hypertonicity. • Acute hypernatremia (developed over a period of hours). Reduction of serum [Na^+] by 1 mmol/L/h is appropriate. • Chronic hypernatremia or unknown duration. Reduction of serum [Na^+] at a maximal rate of 0.5 mmol/L/h. It prevents cerebral edema and convulsions during treatment. • The goal of treatment is to reduce the serum [Na^+] to 152 mmol/L.

MEDICATIONS

DRUGS OF CHOICE
Only hypotonic fluids are appropriate.
• Pure water or 5% dextrose (provide 0 mmol/L of [Na^+]) • 0.2 % sodium chloride in 5% dextrose solution (provide 34 mmol/L of [Na^+]) • 0.45 % sodium chloride (provide 77 mmol/L of [Na^+]). • Because the risk of cerebral edema increases with the volume of the infusate, the volume should be restricted to that required to correct hypertonicity.

FOLLOW-UP

EXPECTED COURSE AND PROGNOSIS
Clinical course and prognosis vary and are associated with the underlying disease condition.

POSSIBLE COMPLICATIONS
Neurologic deficits

PATIENT CARE
Monitoring hydration status, acid-base and electrolyte balance.

PREVENTION
• Isotonic saline (0.9%) is unsuitable for correcting hypernatremia. • Salt intake should be gradually increased to salt-deprived animals. • Do not give salt supplementation when cattle are dehydrated or have been starved. • Unlimited access to water can minimize adverse effects of high salt intake.

MISCELLANEOUS

ASSOCIATED CONDITIONS
Renal diseases and diarrhea

PREGNANCY
N/A

ABBREVIATIONS
• ECF = extracellular fluid • FE_{Na} = fractional excretion of Na^+ • ICF = intracellular fluid • IV = intravenous

SEE ALSO
• Sodium Disorders: Hyponatremia

Suggested Reading
Abutarbush SM, Petrie L. Treatment of hypernatremia in neonatal calves with diarrhea. Can Vet J 2007, 48: 184–7.
Senturk S, Huseyin C. Salt poisoning in beef cattle. Vet Hum Toxicol 2004, 46: 26–7.
Cebra CK. Hyperglycemia, hypernatremia, and hyperosmolarity in 6 neonatal llamas and alpacas. J Am Vet Med Assoc 2000, 217: 1701–4.
Author Diego Gomez-Nieto
Consulting Editor Christopher C.L. Chase

S

SODIUM DISORDERS: HYPONATREMIA

 BASICS

OVERVIEW
Definition: A serum sodium concentration ([Na$^+$]) less than the lower limit of normal ruminants, usually <132 mmol/L.

INCIDENCE/PREVALENCE
Unknown.

GEOGRAPHIC DISTRIBUTION
Worldwide

SYSTEMS AFFECTED
• Cardiovascular • Nervous

PATHOPHYSIOLOGY
• Hyponatremia—excess of total body water relative to extracellular sodium. • Sodium is the major extracellular fluid (ECF) cation. Plays a vital role in maintaining the cell membrane potential, ECF volume, and osmolality. • Sodium affects water shifts between the ICF and ECF. • Source of sodium is primary dietary intake. • Renal is the primary route of excretion (~99% reabsorbed in renal tubules). • Effects of hyponatremia include cerebral edema. Noncardiogenic pulmonary edema can occur, resulting in hypoxemia that can worsen the severity of brain edema.

SIGNALMENT
All ruminant species

PHYSICAL EXAMINATION FINDINGS
• Disorientation, weakness, depression, ataxia, blindness, seizures. • If hyperkalemia is present, it increases the risk of cardiac dysrhythmias (i.e., uroabdomen).

CAUSES AND RISK FACTORS
Hypovolemic Hyponatremia
Decreased total body water and serum [Na$^+$], but [Na$^+$] are proportionally lower than body water.
• Diarrhea, third spacing sequestration (i.e., pleuritis, peritonitis, ascites, uroabdomen), intestinal torsion. • Renal disease and/or renal losses (i.e., diuretics including thiazide, furosemide). • Adrenal insufficiency. • Postobstructive diuresis.

Euvolemic or Dilutional Hyponatremia
Total body water volume does not change but serum [Na$^+$] decreases.
• Syndrome of inappropriate antidiuretic hormone (SIADH). • Psychogenic polydipsia. • Iatrogenic—glucose or mannitol administration. • Oral administration of hypotonic fluids. • Diabetes insipidus, if it is compensated with water intake.

Hypervolemic Hyponatremia
Total body water increases but serum [Na$^+$] does not change.

• The hallmark of these conditions is the presence of edema or ascites. • Heart, liver or renal failure. • Severe hypokalemia in which sodium will shift intracellularly.

Pseudohyponatremia
• Hyperlipidemia or hyperglobulinemia. • Mannitol can cause pseudohyponatremia.

Risk Factors
• Diarrhea • Administration of diuretics • Inappropriate fluid therapy • Heart, liver or renal failure

 DIAGNOSIS

DIFFERENTIAL DIAGNOSES
• Severe hypoglycemia • Metabolic acidosis • Meningitis • Polioencephalomalacia

CBC/BIOCHEMISTRY/URINALYSIS
• Hyponatremia. Serum [Na$^+$] <120 mmol/L is considered severe hyponatremia. • Other electrolyte imbalances depend on the underlying causes.

OTHER LABORATORY TEST
• Fractional excretion of Na$^+$ [FE$_{Na}$]: suspect renal losses if [FE$_{Na}$] >1%. • Plasma osmolality is low in hyponatremia.

OTHER DIAGNOSTIC PROCEDURES
• History and physical examination to determine the causes of hyponatremia. • Evaluation of volume status, and analysis of serum and urine sodium levels and osmolality.

PATHOLOGIC FINDINGS
Central pontine myelinolysis can occur after rapid treatment of chronic hypernatremia.

 TREATMENT

THERAPEUTIC APPROACH
• Addressing the underlying cause (i.e., diarrhea, pleuritis, uroabdomen, correcting feeding preparation). • Consider if the animal has signs or symptoms of cerebral edema, time frame for the development of the hyponatremia. • Consider whether the animal has risk factors for developing neurologic complications from hyponatremia or its treatment. • Hyponatremia that has developed <48 hours. Correct rapidly by increasing serum [Na$^+$] to 125 mmol/L over 6 hours. • The amount of [Na$^+$] needed to increase serum [Na$^+$] to 125 mmol/L can be calculated with the following formula: 125 − measured [Na$^+$] (mmol/L) × 0.6 × body weight (kg). Hypertonic saline 3% is the solution recommended for correction of hyponatremia. • Furosemide can be given to

increase excretion of dilute urine. • The serum [Na$^+$] should be checked q2h and the rate of the infusion adjusted accordingly. • Hyponatremia that has developed >48 hours. Correct gradually. Increase serum [Na$^+$] to 125 mmol/L. Correct no more than 8–10 mmol/L/24h initially.

 MEDICATIONS

DRUGS OF CHOICE
Recommended fluid is 3% saline solution with loop diuretic (e.g., furosemide).

PRECAUTIONS
Central pontine myelinolysis can occur after rapid treatment of chronic hypernatremia or may be directly caused by hyponatremia. It has been described in dogs and humans but not in ruminants.

 FOLLOW-UP

EXPECTED COURSE AND PROGNOSIS
Clinical course and prognosis vary and are associated with the underlying disease condition.

POSSIBLE COMPLICATIONS
Neurologic deficits can occur.

PATIENT CARE
Close monitoring of electrolytes and neurologic status during correction of hyponatremia.

PREVENTION
N/A

 MISCELLANEOUS

ASSOCIATED CONDITIONS
• Diarrhea • Heart, liver, or renal failure

PREGNANCY
N/A

ABBREVIATIONS
• ECF = extracellular fluid • FE$_{Na}$ = fractional excretion of Na$^+$ • ICF = intracellular fluid • SIADH = syndrome of inappropriate antidiuretic hormone

SEE ALSO
Sodium Disorders: Hypernatremia

Suggested Reading
Adrogué HJ, Madias NE. Hyponatremia. N Engl J Med 2000, 342: 1581–9.
Author Diego Gomez-Nieto
Consulting Editor Christopher C.L. Chase

S

SOLE LESIONS IN DAIRY CATTLE

BASICS

OVERVIEW
• Lameness is common in dairy cows, with most lesions affecting the sole.
• The most significant lesions of the sole are white line disease and sole ulcers.
• An initial insult to the corium primarily affects the laminar region, and that corium damage increases, with the resulting alteration in the physical forces on the sole.
• The risk of sole lesions is related to stage of lactation, individual cow factors, and farm characteristics.
• Ninety percent or more of lameness in dairy cattle involves the foot. Of that involving the foot, most involves rear feet, particularly the lateral claw.
• Cows most at risk for sole lesions are those with low body condition scores.
• Farms most at risk are those with high stall curbs, long standing times during milking, automatic alley scrapers, and abrasive flooring surfaces or flooring imperfections (e.g., holes in concrete). In pasture based systems, long walking distance to the parlor and rough lane surfaces increase risk.

INCIDENCE/PREVALENCE
• Incidence is influenced by a variety of farm-level factors and varies widely between operations.
• Surveys have suggested that the incidence may be as high as 55 cases per 100 cows per year.
• Another survey estimated an incidence rate of 30 cases per 100 cows per year, a fatality rate of 2%, an increase in days open of 28 days, and costs for treatment and additional labor of $23 per case, estimating an annual cost of $9000 per 100 cows.

GEOGRAPHIC DISTRIBUTION
Worldwide depending on the environment

SYSTEMS AFFECTED
Musculoskeletal

PATHOPHYSIOLOGY
See "Causes and Risk Factors"

HISTORICAL FINDINGS
• Cows with white line disease typically present with severe acute lameness.
• Cows with sole ulcers typically suffer from a low-grade lameness that often progresses to a more severe lameness over time.

SIGNALMENT
Sole ulcers are seen almost exclusively in housed, lactating dairy cattle.

PHYSICAL EXAMINATION FINDINGS
• The site of the lesion can generally be determined by using hoof testers around the periphery of the abaxial wall. Using a hoof knife, the sole should be cleaned and a thin layer of horn removed. The key indicator of a problem is a dark necrotic area within the white line at the site identified with the hoof testers. This is most likely the site at which the lesion is forming.
• Lesions are most commonly seen in the lateral hind claw at the heel-sole junction. The sole of the claw may appear normal on initial examination; however, using hoof testers, an area of pain is typically identified approximately two-thirds of the way back from the toe and toward the axial wall.
• As the sole is trimmed with a knife, it is common to find evidence of an old hemorrhage within the horn of the sole at this site. Eventually, a portion of horn will be removed to reveal a full-thickness defect of the sole with granulation tissue protruding from the underlying corium.
• In complicated cases, a cellulitis develops and spreads to involve articular and soft tissue structures.

GENETICS
N/A

CAUSES AND RISK FACTORS
• The flexible junction between the sole and wall horn, colloquially known as the "white line," is the weakest portion of the sole. Even in a normal animal, it is common to see a small amount of debris impacted into this area.
• Dairy cattle are prone to a subclinical laminitis-like syndrome as a result of being fed diets rich in highly fermentable carbohydrate and low in long-stem fiber. Laminitis is known to make the white line weaker and predispose to white line disease.
• The horn of the white line is formed by the laminar corium which is also the suspensory apparatus of the third phalanx (P3). Conditions such as laminitis which interfere with the vascular supply to the corium are likely to reduce the quality of white line horn produced by the laminar corium, which is believed to increase the potential for white line separation. Areas of hemorrhage may also be visible within the horn in the region of the white line. One thought is that prolonged standing, particularly during the transition period around calving when the suspensory apparatus is weaker and more susceptible to mechanical stresses, may result in inflammation of the suspensory tissues during the time at which it is forming horn of the white line. It is speculated that inflammation of these tissues while they are concurrently forming the horn of the white line would result in hemorrhage and weaker white line horn when it reaches the weight-bearing surface. A weakened white line is more likely to be softer and defective thereby predisposing to the impaction of organic matter within the white line. Should contaminated debris breach the white line and reach the corium, an abscess will form. Such abscesses cause extreme pain as they enlarge due to the great pressures developed between the base of P3 and the hoof capsule, neither of which are flexible.
• Abscesses in both cattle and horses will enlarge and migrate beneath the wall of the hoof and burst out at the coronary band, or they may track caudally below the sole and burst out in the region of the heel.
• The same subclinical laminitis syndrome described above can result in a weakening of the attachments between the laminae of the wall and sinking of P3 within the hoof capsule. This results in the ventral surface of P3 compressing the corium of the sole against the horn of the sole. This compression appears to be most marked in the region of the deep flexor process of P3.
• In addition to changes within the hoof, there are important changes seen in the morphology of the dairy cow's hoof. In the hindlimb, the lateral claw is under asymmetric stress when compared to the medial claw. This overloading of the lateral claw tends to result in hypertrophy of the sole horn, which further overloads the claw.
• In most dairy cows, overgrowth of the claw is characterized by a disproportionate overgrowth of the toe. This, combined with the commonly seen erosion of the heel horn, results in weight bearing by the claw being transferred from the toe back toward the heel region.
• When all these factors are combined, it is apparent that the heel region of the lateral hind claw is under a great deal of stress. As P3 sinks within the hoof capsule, the corium is compressed between the flexor process and the sole. This initially results in a contusion of the corium exhibited as a hemorrhage in the heel-sole junction. The blood is incorporated into the horn and may be seen in the sole as bruising. As the condition progresses, the corium undergoes pressure necrosis and horn formation in the area is halted. This results in a defect in the sole that grows from the inside to the external environment. When the defect is full thickness, a sole ulcer has formed, exposing the underlying corium.

DIAGNOSIS

DIFFERENTIAL DIAGNOSES
• Digital dermatitis
• Lacerations
• Thin soles
• Foreign bodies
• Fractures
• Foot rot—easily distinguished on examination of the foot
• Abscesses secondary to penetrating wound

S

SOLE LESIONS IN DAIRY CATTLE

CBC/BIOCHEMISTRY/URINALYSIS
N/A

OTHER LABORATORY TESTS
N/A

IMAGING
Radiology of the distal limb may be of benefit in cases where there is concern that infection may have spread to either the navicular bursa, distal and/or proximal interphalangeal joints, and the flexor tendon sheaths.

OTHER DIAGNOSTIC PROCEDURES
• Lesions are diagnosed on the basis of the characteristic clinical signs. All that is necessary is close examination of the foot.
• In cases where the infection has spread to the deeper tissues of the foot, it is common to identify that the foot is grossly swollen. The swelling seen in such cases may be distinguished from simple foot rot on the basis that the swelling is asymmetric and centered on one claw.
• The swelling is typically found in either the heel region or around the cranio-lateral aspect of the coronary band.

PATHOLOGIC FINDINGS
See "Causes and Risk Factors"

TREATMENT

THERAPEUTIC APPROACH
• White line abscesses require drainage to provide pain relief and promote healing of the lesion. Having identified the suspected site of the abscess, a hoof knife should be used to resect the wall horn and to follow the lesion to the corium and drain the abscess. Once the abscess is open, the extent of the abscess should be determined using a blunt probe. The entire defect should be opened and all underrun horn removed.
• Care should be taken to avoid leaving any jagged or underrun edges, which would allow foreign material to impact in the lesion.
• When dealing with a sole ulcer, it is important to first trim the foot to normalize weight bearing between the medial and lateral claws as well as adjusting the plane of the sole to prevent excessive weight bearing in the heel region. Next, all undermined sole should be removed from around the ulcer, taking care to not traumatize the corium. The heel of that claw should be lowered (cut deeper than the opposite heel) to prevent any weight bearing in the region of the flexor process. Finally, a wooden or composite block should be placed on the opposite claw to transfer weight bearing away from the affected claw.
• The area of the sole ulcer should be trimmed with great care to remove any underrun horn tissue.

• Bandaging the lesion left by an abscess or sole ulcer is of no value as the dressing simply becomes contaminated with fecal material. The lesions should be left open to heal.

SURGICAL CONSIDERATIONS AND TECHNIQUES
• In chronic cases with severe soft tissue involvement, surgical intervention may be necessary (e.g., lateral wall resection, claw amputation, tenotomy, etc.).
• A number of surgical procedures have been described to salvage the claw, but due to the expense involved, many clinicians opt to amputate the affected digit.

MEDICATIONS

DRUGS OF CHOICE
• Antibiotics are not indicated in the treatment of simple uncomplicated white line disease abscesses or sole ulcers. They are indicated only when infection has spread to the deeper structures of the foot.
• Some clinicians may elect to use NSAIDs to provide analgesia in severe cases.

PRECAUTIONS
Appropriate milk and meat withdrawal times must be followed for all compounds administered to food-producing animals.

CONTRAINDICATIONS
N/A

POSSIBLE INTERACTIONS
N/A

FOLLOW-UP

EXPECTED COURSE AND PROGNOSIS
• Simple uncomplicated white line disease abscesses and sole ulcers typically resolve in 4–6 weeks. On occasion, severe lesions may require additional time.
• The prognosis for infections that involve the deep structures of the hoof is always guarded. Since many of these cases typically present late in the disease course, the infection is well established and there is already significant pathology.
• Aggressive antibiotic therapy is warranted when deep structures of the hoof are involved, but success is limited. Surgery is generally required. Euthanasia may be the only option in some cases where it is not possible to control suffering and the animal is not showing improvement.
• Studies have shown that the life expectancy for a dairy cow following amputation of a digit is <1 year.

POSSIBLE COMPLICATIONS
Spread of infection to soft tissue structures of the distal limb

CLIENT EDUCATION
Prompt attention to lame cattle is not only warranted for welfare purposes but will greatly improve outcomes and minimize losses.

PATIENT CARE
• The majority of animals will show immediate relief after trimming of the lesion and application of an orthopedic block. If the animal fails to have significant improvement after placement of the block, or the lameness is noted to be more severe following treatment, the animal should be reevaluated for another cause of lameness or possible incorrect block placement.
• Animals that remain lame after 3–4 days should be reexamined.
• Orthopedic blocks should always be removed or rechecked within 30 days of application to determine the need for block replacement or permanent removal. Block wear varies according to the distance cows walk and the type of flooring surface. At this time, it is also appropriate to perform a minor hoof trim to encourage complete resolution of the lesion.

PREVENTION
• Attention should be paid to the dairy cow ration to ensure that it always contains sufficient long-stem fiber to prevent ruminal acidosis.
• Since peripartum hormonal changes and metalloproteinase activity are more likely during the transition period (from 2–3 weeks pre-calving to 4 weeks post-calving) it is important to assure the maximum in cow comfort (i.e., no overcrowding, maintain stocking rates at no more than 80%, maximize stall comfort with properly designed and well-maintained stalls, etc.).
• Dairy cows should have their feet trimmed on a regular basis to prevent overloading of the lateral hind claw.

MISCELLANEOUS

ASSOCIATED CONDITIONS
Lameness, decreased milk production, loss of profit

AGE-RELATED FACTORS
Sole ulcer lesions are most common in mid to late lactation multiparous cattle.

PRODUCTION MANAGEMENT
• Body condition scoring should be performed routinely to target high-risk low body condition animals.
• Evaluating barn layout and the cows' time allocation to minimize high steps or stall curbs, long standing times during milking and

abrasive flooring or flooring imperfections (e.g., holes in concrete). Automatic alley scrapers are also a risk that must be managed.
• Attention should be paid to the design of the dairy barn to ensure that cows can always lie down in comfort. Cows at pasture typically lie down for two-thirds of the day. When the animal is recumbent, the feet do not bear weight and therefore the diseases cannot develop.
• In pasture-based herds, cows will ideally walk minimal distances to the parlor during higher risk periods (i.e., very hot or wet conditions) and the need for lane way resurfacing should be assessed annually.

ABBREVIATION
• NSAIDs = nonsteroidal anti-inflammatory drugs

SEE ALSO
• Anesthesia: Local and Regional
• Body Condition Scoring: Dairy Cattle (see www.fiveminutevet.com/ruminant)

• Foot Rot: Bovine
• Lameness: Bovine
• Nonsteroidal Anti-inflammatory Drugs (NSAIDs) (see www.fiveminutevet.com/ruminant)

Suggested Reading
Greenough PA, Collick DW, Weaver AD. Interdigital space and claw. In: Greenough PA ed, Lameness in Cattle, 3rd ed. Philadelphia: Saunders, 1997.
Murray RD, Downham DY, Clarkson MJ, et al. Epidemiology of lameness in dairy cattle: description and analysis of foot lesions. Vet Rec 1996, 138: 586–91.
Shearer JK, Plummer PJ, Schleining JA. Perspectives on the treatment of claw lesions in cattle. Vet Med Res Rep 2015, 6: 273–92.

Smilie RH, Hoblet KH, Eastridge ML, Weiss WP, Schnitkey GL, Moeschberger ML. Subclinical laminitis in dairy cows: use of severity of hoof lesions to rank and evaluate herds. Vet Rec 1999, 144: 17–21.
van Amstel SR, Shearer JK, Palin FL. Moisture content, thickness, and lesions of sole horn associated with thin soles in dairy cattle. J Dairy Sci 2004, 87: 757–63.
Webster AJ. Effects of housing practices on the development of foot lesions in dairy heifers in early lactation. Vet Rec 2002, 151: 9–12.
Westwood CT, Lean IJ. Nutrition and lameness in pasture-fed dairy cattle. Proceedings of the New Zealand Society of Animal Production 2001, 61: 128–34.

Authors Paul J. Plummer and Jan K. Shearer
Consulting Editor Kaitlyn A. Lutz
Acknowledgment The authors and book editors acknowledge the prior contribution of Chris Clark.

S

SQUAMOUS CELL CARCINOMA

BASICS

OVERVIEW
Squamous cell carcinoma (SCC) is a malignant tumor of epidermal cells. In cattle, ocular squamous cell carcinoma (OSCC) is the most common ocular tumor. It can also affect the skin, gastrointestinal tract, and genitourinary tract of ruminants.

INCIDENCE/PREVALENCE
When recording incidence, typically preneoplastic and early neoplastic lesions (plaques, papillomas, and carcinoma in situ) are included in the affected group.

Cattle
• The incidence of OSCC varies between countries. In the United States, estimates of the incidence ranged from 0.8% to 5%, whereas in Australia it is been reported to be as high as 10–20% and in the Netherlands as low as 0.04%. This is consistent with reports that in regions with abundant sunlight the prevalence can be as high as 40%. OSCC is more common in older cattle with a peak around 7–8 years.
• Bladder SCC is very rare except in endemic areas, where the incidence of bladder neoplasia may range from 15% to 25%. Cows with bladder SCC may have more than one type of tumor in their bladder.

Small Ruminants
Most commonly SCC is diagnosed in Merino sheep and older animals (>4 years old) with a reported peak incidence of up to 12% in older animals. Areas that are affected more frequently are the face, ears, and vulva. In goats the perineum appears to be most commonly affected due to their high and short tail which exposes the area to UV light.

Camelids
Overall the second most common malignant tumor in camelids, with half of SCC originating in the skin and the remainder occurring in the GI tract. SCC is the most commonly reported primary neoplasm affecting the GI tract in camelids, usually the first gastric compartment (C1), with potential metastasis seen throughout the abdominal and pleural cavities. In the skin, all regions can be affected with the face, prepuce and perineum most commonly involved.

GEOGRAPHIC DISTRIBUTION
Generally the development of SCC/OSCC is associated with an increase in altitude and mean annual hours of sunlight and with decreases in latitude.

OSCC
• Most OSCC in the United States occurs in the South and Southwest.
• Australia and some regions in Africa also experience a significant number of cattle afflicted with OSCC.

SCC
• SCC of the upper intestinal tract and bladder are most common in regions where bracken fern, containing the cofactor for tumor development, exists along with the presence of infection with bovine papilloma virus 4 (BPV-4). This combination of factors resulting in SCC of the upper intestinal tract was initially reported in Scotland, but additional reports from Europe, Africa, and South America have been published.
• In Australia SCC of the muzzle, ears, and perineal region is a significant problem in sheep.
• In South Africa, lesions on the udder and teats of Saanen and Angora goats have been found.

SYSTEMS AFFECTED
• Integument
• Digestive
• Urinary
• Ophthalmic

PATHOPHYSIOLOGY
The pathogenesis of squamous cell carcinoma is multifactorial and includes extrinsic and intrinsic factors. Factors that have been suggested to play a role in the development of SCC in ruminants include:
• Exposure to solar radiation (ultraviolet light, UV).
• Papillomavirus infection causing precursor lesions that then undergo neoplastic transformation.
• Exposure to carcinogens in bracken fern (*Pteridium aquilinum*) can result in malignant transformation of papillomas of the upper gastrointestinal tract and bladder. In addition, induced immunosuppression can prevent rejection of early neoplastic lesions.
The tumors develop in all species through a series of premalignant stages which progress over time to squamous cell carcinoma. At the same time neoplastic lesions can arise without noticeable precursor stages, and spontaneous regression has been described.

OSCC
Ocular squamous cell carcinomas (OSCC) arise from the epithelial surface of the conjunctiva or cornea. For OSCC the combination of lack of pigmentation in the periocular tissues in the corneoscleral region and exposure to high levels of UV light are linked to an increased prevalence. In addition, it has been found that up to 63.4% of cases with OSCC show an abnormal expression of p53, a tumor suppressor gene that is associated in humans and horses with OSCC development. Abnormal expression is thought to be associated with UV light exposure.

HISTORICAL FINDINGS
Depends on type of SCC. See "Physical Examination Findings" for more details.

SIGNALMENT
• SCC/OSCC of all types is seen primarily in cattle, but has been reported in sheep and less commonly in goats.
• It has also been described as one of the most common tumors in camelids with more reports in llamas than in alpacas.
• In the US, Hereford and Hereford-cross cattle are most likely to be affected with OSCC.
• Other breeds in which OSCC is reported include Simmental, Holstein Friesians, and rarely in other breeds.
• The mean age of cattle with OSCC is 7–8 years, with a decreasing mean age in areas of highest UV light exposure.
• SCC of the upper intestinal tract and bladder is typically found in cattle between 6 and 12 years of age.
• In sheep SCC is most commonly seen in animals >4 years of age.
• The age range in which SCC is seen in camelids is 5–10 years or older, with most camelids that develop SCC of the first gastric compartment >10 years.
• Predominant sex: Although most afflicted cattle are female, that simply reflects the fact that most herds are made up primarily of cows, and bulls are kept in fewer numbers. The same is true of ewes and rams.

PHYSICAL EXAMINATION FINDINGS
OSCC
• Signs depend on the anatomic location, tissues involved, as well as stage of malignancy.
• Precancerous lesions are usually either papilloma-like structures or small, white, elevated, hyperplastic plaques.
• Malignant tumors are more irregular, pink, erosive, and often show signs of necrosis.
• In cattle the most common site is the lateral limbus, followed by the eyelids, nictitating membrane, and medial canthus.
• Invasive OSCC of the palpebrae and medial canthus metastasize more commonly than do OSCC arising from the globe; in advanced stages local invasion of bony structures may be observed.
• Mild to moderate purulent ocular discharge can be present as well as secondary conjunctivitis.

SCC
• Signs depend highly on the location and extent of the lesion.
• SCC of the upper intestinal tract can result in bloat, regurgitation of ruminal contents, loss of condition, painful abdomen, and difficulty swallowing.
• Cutaneous SCC: Horny outgrowths of skin or scales that are painful on manipulation, occurring on unpigmented or lightly pigmented skin in the sacral region, dorsum, and escutcheon as well as mucocutaneus junctions (e.g., vulva).
• SCC of the bladder is typically associated with hematuria.

• Clinical signs associated with distant metastasis are rarely seen.

Camelids
• SCC lesions of the skin (face, prepuce, and perineum): Usually proliferative with some degree of surface ulceration; chains or clumps of nodules may be seen.
• SCC of the GI tract (first gastric compartment, C1): Gradual weight loss with progressive anemia, signs of colic, hypoproteinemia, lethargy and anorexia, abdominal distention or respiratory difficulties due to ascites or pleural effusion, occasionally melena and/or diarrhea.

GENETICS
The high incidence of OSCC seen in Hereford and Hereford-cross cattle was once believed to be associated with a heritable component. Since then, studies have shown that a strong genetic trait for a white face, as well as their use as range animals, predisposes these breeds to the development of OSCC. Selective breeding for more pigmentation around the eyes greatly reduces tumor occurrence.

CAUSES AND RISK FACTORS
Ophthalmic and skin:
• Exposure to ultraviolet light
• Lack of pigmentation
• Infection with bovine papillomavirus
• Correlations with high plane of nutrition
Upper gastrointestinal tract and bladder:
• Infection with BPV-4 and/or BPV-2
• Ingestion of bracken fern or other carcinogenic and immunomodulatory compounds
• Trauma

DIAGNOSIS

DIFFERENTIAL DIAGNOSES
• Papillomas
• Keratoancanthomas
• Carcinoma in situ
• Dermoid cyst
• Fibroma, fibrosarcoma
• Granulation tissue
• Conjunctival follicular hyperplasia

CBC/BIOCHEMISTRY/URINALYSIS
• OSCC and SCC of the upper intestinal tract—results are usually normal.
• SCC of the bladder—anemia, hematuria.

OTHER LABORATORY TESTS
N/A

IMAGING
Radiology:
• Skull radiographs might be indicated if local invasion of bony structures around the orbit can not be ruled out otherwise.
• Thoracic or abdominal radiographs may be used to identify potential metastasis to determine prognosis prior to possible surgical intervention.
Ultrasound:
• Abdominal ultrasound may be helpful to identify additional lesions (metastasis) and for the diagnosis of bladder tumors.
• May also help to determine the extent of locally invasive masses and involvement of underlying structures.

OTHER DIAGNOSTIC PROCEDURES
• Cytologic evaluation of samples obtained by aspiration or scraping followed by Giemsa or Wright's staining may reveal abnormal epithelial cells suggestive of SCC/OSCC.
• A biopsy specimen for histopathology of a suspicious lesion can be used to establish a diagnosis and in 85–90% of cases agrees with the diagnosis made by cytologic examination.
• A biopsy or an aspirate of a local lymph node may help determine presence of metastatic disease (occurrence of metastasis is approximately 10%).

PATHOLOGIC FINDINGS
OSCC
• Invasion into local tissues, including bone and along the optic nerve, may be seen.
• Metastasis to the ipsilateral parotid and lateral retropharyngeal lymph nodes may be seen and on rare occasions they may extent into the thoracic or abdominal organs with approximately 5% of cattle with OSCC having lung metastasis at slaughter.

SCC of the Skin, Upper Gastrointestinal Tract, and Bladder
• Individuals affected with upper GI SCC may have multiple lesions in the oral cavity and throughout the upper and lower GI tract.
• Camelids—usually the first gastric compartment (C1) is involved with potential metastasis throughout the abdominal and pleural cavities. Ascites or pleural effusion can also be present.
• Small ruminants—SCC of the skin can be accompanied by cutaneous papillomas of the udder and teats.
• Findings on histopathology include epidermal hyperplasia, hyperkeratosis, parakeratosis, acanthosis, accentuation of the epidermal rete, and keratinocyte dysplasia.
• Extending into the dermis are cords and islands of neoplastic cells demonstrating a variable degree of epithelial differentiation, sometimes including "keratin pearls."

TREATMENT

THERAPEUTIC APPROACH
• There are currently no treatment options for tumors located in the gastrointestinal tract and bladder.
• OSCC
  ○ Early detection of OSCC is important in order for treatment to be effective. Up to 75% of small lesions (<5 mm in diameter) will regress spontaneously.
  ○ Multiple treatment modalities can be used successfully on early lesions.
• Surgical excision
  ○ *En bloc* resection is best performed for smaller lesions (10–20 mm) for which adequate margins can be obtained. This method is also indicated for lesions of the third eyelid. Nerve blocks are used to facilitate anesthesia of the area (e.g., auriculopalpebral nerve block, retrobulbar or Peterson nerve block) with or without additional infiltration of local anesthetic (e.g., lidocaine 2%).
  ○ Third eyelid removal—The third eyelid is grasped and clamped off using two long tissue forceps in a triangular pattern. The entire third eyelid is then removed using a scalpel blade or scissors and the forceps are left in place for a few minutes to facilitate hemostasis. It is important to ensure that the complete cartilage is removed since a remaining stump can cause chronic irritation and potentially incite further OSCC development. The wound edges can be sutured using a simple interrupted or continuous pattern, or left to heal by second intention.
• Cryosurgery: Can be used alone or in combination with surgical excision. Utilizing two freeze/thaw cycles (freezing to −30°C, a quick freeze and slow thaw cycle appears to result in maximum cryodestruction) has been reported to result in a 97% complete regression rate. The animal again is restrained and local anesthesia is facilitated by nerve blocks and/or local infiltration of local anesthetic (lidocaine 2%). The tissue peripheral to the lesion is protected against freezing by using petroleum jelly. A Styrofoam wedge can be applied to protect the cornea. Frozen tissue sloughs off over the next 7–14 days and is gradually replaced by granulation tissue. A study with more complete follow-up data demonstrated that approximately 71% of lesions treated with cryosurgery had complete regression without recurrence up to 3.5 years.
• Radiofrequency hyperthermia: Raising the temperature in the tumor to 50°C for 30 sec/cm^2 of tumor surface has resulted in complete regression in 90.8% of tumors treated after one or multiple applications. This regression lasted at least for 5.5 months in all animals, and for a year in the cattle available for monitoring at that time in one study. This technique can be used in smaller lesions and after initial debulking. Hyperthermia penetrates 5–10 mm of tissue. Multiple applications may be necessary for larger lesions.
• Radiation therapy: Administered with implants of gamma-emitters such as cobalt-60, gold-198, or cesium-137, this technique has been quite effective at

S

SQUAMOUS CELL CARCINOMA

controlling OSCC; however, these methods are quite costly and are not widely available.
• Immunotherapy: This includes methods to enhance the individual's immune system to induce tumor regression. Different approaches to immunotherapy have been made (e.g., autogenous vaccines made from tumor tissue, infection with Bacillus Calmette Guerin (BCG), and systemic and peri- and intralesional injections of interleukin-2 (IL-2)) with moderate success. Injections of IL-2 for 10 consecutive days resulted in 50–69% regression rates depending on the concentration used and the location of the tumor, with tumors on the third eyelid and limbus being the most responsive.

SURGICAL CONSIDERATIONS AND TECHNIQUES
• See "Therapeutic Approach" for details.
• Surgical removal of OSCC and precursor lesions is only moderately successful in controlling the disease, with recurrence rates of 37–48% reported.
• *En bloc* excision of the tumor (e.g., enucleation, exenteration) and regional lymph nodes can be performed to salvage valuable animals, but is not cost effective in most instances.

MEDICATIONS
DRUGS OF CHOICE
N/A

CONTRAINDICATIONS
The use of intralesional chemotherapeutics (e.g., cisplatin) is not permitted in food-producing animals.

FOLLOW-UP
EXPECTED COURSE AND PROGNOSIS
• Untreated, OSCC will invade normal tissues (potentially including the CNS) and ultimately metastasize to the regional lymph nodes and lungs. Extensive disease can result

in carcass condemnation and thus financial loss.
• With surgical excision (enucleation or mass resection), local recurrence is common (37% in one report), but may allow salvage of the animal for slaughter depending on local regulations.
• Cryosurgery, with a two-freeze cycle, will result in a 77–97% complete response rate. Approximately 71% of responding tumors did not recur in one study following cryosurgery.

POSSIBLE COMPLICATIONS
• Premature loss of breeding cows.
• Carcass condemnation at slaughter due to metastasis or multiple SCC.

CLIENT EDUCATION
• Lesions may recur locally so treated animals should be examined periodically (every 3–4 months) for evidence of recurrence.
• Cryosurgery or hyperthermia can result in hair loss and regrowth of white hairs at the treated site.

PATIENT CARE
All cattle should be examined on a regular basis for OSCC, at least three times a year (including once in the summer months) during routine maintenance health treatments.

PREVENTION
• Breeding cattle for pigmentation in the periocular tissues as well as for pigmentation of the corneoscleral junction will decrease the incidence of OSCC.
• Routine evaluation of all eyes, with cryosurgery or surgical removal of lesions that are enlarging and >5 mm in diameter, greatly decreases the development of lesions that would result in financial loss to the herdsman (through carcass condemnation and premature loss of breeding stock).

MISCELLANEOUS
ASSOCIATED CONDITIONS
Infection with bovine papilloma viruses is thought to cause the initial precancerous lesion.

AGE-RELATED FACTORS
• OSCC are typically diagnosed in animals >4 years of age.
• In camelids, skin and GI lesions are most often diagnosed in older animals (>5 years).

PRODUCTION MANAGEMENT
Routine evaluation of all eyes in a herd allows early detection and treatment of lesions in the epithelium that may be early SCC or premalignant changes.

ABBREVIATIONS
• BPV = bovine papilloma virus
• CNS = central nervous system
• GI = gastrointestinal
• IL-2 = interleukin 2
• OSCC = ocular squamous cell carcinoma
• SCC = squamous cell carcinoma
• UV = ultraviolet

SEE ALSO
• Anesthesia: Local and Regional
• Enucleation/Exenteration (see www.fiveminutevet/com/ruminant)

Suggested Reading
Cebra C. Medical disorders. In: Cebra C, Anderson DE, Tibary A, Van Saun RJ, Johnson LW eds, Llama and Alpaca Care: Medicine, Surgery, Reproduction, Nutrition and Herd Health, 1st ed. St. Louis: Elsevier, 2014, pp. 517–18.
Shaw-Edwards R. Surgical treatment of the eye in farm animals. Vet Clin North Am Food Anim Pract 2010, 26: 459–76.
Sloss V, Smith TJS, Yi GD. Controlling ocular squamous cell carcinoma in Hereford cattle. Aust Vet J 1986, 63: 248–51.
Tsujita H. Bovine ocular squamous cell carcinoma. Vet Clin North Am Food Anim Pract 2010, 26: 511–29.
Author Nora M. Biermann
Consulting Editor Kaitlyn A. Lutz
Acknowledgment The author and book editors acknowledge the prior contribution of Marlene L. Hauck.

S

ST. JOHN'S WORT TOXICITY

BASICS

OVERVIEW
- St. John's wort is an erect perennial herb that stands 1–3 feet tall. Its leaves are opposite, dotted, with many yellow flowers.
- Hypericin is the active ingredient. It is a red florescent pigment found in a semisolid state in the black dots that are scattered over the surface of the leaves, stems, and petals and is present in the plants at all times.
- Hypericin is a naturally occurring naphthodianthrone derivative in the plant species *Hypericum perforatum*. The hypericin concentration in the plant may vary depending on the place of growth, state of plant material, and part of the plant—whole herb concentration 0.00095%–0.466% and flowers up to 0.086%.
- The hypericin concentration in a broadleaf biotype varies from a winter minimum of <100 ppm to a summer maximum approaching 3,000 ppm. In contrast, the narrow-leaf biotype increases from similar winter values to summer maxima approaching 5,000 ppm.
- Consumption causes primary photosensitization, which leads to increased sensitivity of the skin to subsequent light exposure.
- There appears to be an absolute requirement for exposure to bright sunlight before any effects of hypericum will develop.
- St. John's wort is found in dry soil, roadsides, and pasture ranges.

INCIDENCE/PREVALENCE
N/A

GEOGRAPHIC DISTRIBUTION
Potentially worldwide, depending on species and environment

SYSTEMS AFFECTED
- Cardiovascular
- Digestive
- Integument
- Urinary
- Multisystemic

PATHOPHYSIOLOGY
- The mechanism of action is unresolved.
- One study suggested that hypericin was an inhibitor of rat brain mitochondrial monoamine oxidase (MAO).
- Serotonin receptors may be involved in the pharmacologic action of hypericum extracts.
- Another study found that hypericum extract inhibits serotonin uptake by rat synaptosomes derived from rat embryo neurons. Other investigators reported that serotonin receptor expression in neuroblastoma cells was reduced by hypericum extracts.
- When animals ingest the plant, the hypericin is absorbed from the intestinal tract and goes into the circulation. Hypericin is a

photodynamic agent able to cause cellular damage and sunburn.

SIGNALMENT
- Cattle, sheep most commonly affected. Goats are very resistant to toxicity.
- Potentially all ruminant species are affected.

PHYSICAL EXAMINATION FINDINGS
- Extreme hyperesthesia to touch and to contact with cold water.
- Restlessness and discomfort. Animals tend to rub their ears, eyelids, and muzzle.
- Photophobia and/or photosensitization. In sheep with heavy fleece, lesions occur on head and coronary band, but in shorn sheep lesions can occur on the back. Sheep can also have extensive head edema. Onset of lesions may just take hours and initially include erythema and edema followed by blisters, exudation, necrosis, and sloughing of necrotic tissue. In cattle, lesions occur on areas of the body that are nonpigmented and on the teats, udder, perineum, and nose.
- Hyperthermia when exposed to sunlight.
- Diarrhea and tachycardia.
- Seldom lethal. But can markedly affect production of meat, milk or wool and can cause the animal considerable distress.
- Exposure of the tongue to sunlight while licking can cause glossitis with ulceration and deep necrosis.
- Congested mucus membranes and hyperemia of exposed skin on tail and legs. Edema of eyelids and ears, exudation of serum from ears.
- Loss of eyelashes, corneal opacity, and blindness after 5–7 days with high levels of ingestion.
- Animals with pigmented skin and those that remain in subdued light suffer few effects.
- Hemolytic anemia.
- Kidney and liver dysfunction may occur with severe exposure.

CAUSES AND RISK FACTORS
- Hypericum is the toxic principle.
- Severity of effects increases with duration of exposure, but not with dose.
- A single dose of hypericum remains potentially effective for up to 4 days.
- Induces hepatic cytochrome P450 and approximately doubles its metabolic activity.
- Plasma concentration of concomitant medication using cytochrome P450 enzymes will be reduced.
- Rectal temperature rise in affected sheep is a reliable indicator of the early development of an adverse clinical effect.
- There appears to be an absolute requirement for exposure to bright sunlight before any effects of *H. perforatum* will develop.
- A single dose of *H. perforatum* remains potentially effective for up to 4 days.
- In a small group of Merino sheep tested, a tolerance level for *H. perforatum*, eaten at the flowering stage, of <1% (plant wet weight) of body weight and a tolerance level for

hypericin of <2.65 mg per kg live weight were demonstrated.
- Sheep develop restlessness, photophobia, tachycardia, tachypnea, congested mucus membranes, diarrhea, and hyperthermia. Skin lesions include redness of the tail, eyelid edema, and auricular edema. One week later, salivation, perioral and periauricular alopecia, keratoconjunctivitis, corneal opacity, and blindness may be evident.
- Another study found the minimal dose of dried whole hypericum to cause symptoms to be 3 g/kg in calves weighing 100–120 kg. Calves that receive this dose and were exposed to sunlight developed pyrexia and tachypnea 3–4 hours later. The animals became restless, passed soft feces, and developed perinasal and perioral erythema. Calves receiving the same dose but not exposed to sunlight only developed soft feces. Calves receiving 5 g/kg developed similar but more severe symptoms.

DIAGNOSIS

DIFFERENTIAL DIAGNOSES
- Hepatogenous photosensitivity as a result of phylloerythrin accumulating in the blood. Phylloerythrins are formed from the anaerobic breakdown of chlorophyll by microorganisms in the forestomach of ruminants.
- Endogenous photosensitizing agent from aberrant metabolism of hemoglobin.
- Antibiotic-associated photosensitization (sulfonamides and tetracyclines).
- Phenothiazine-induced photosensitization (phenothiazine sulfoxide is the metabolite).
- Plants that can cause sunburn either by contact or ingestion—vetches, various clovers, and buckwheat (*Fagopyrum* spp.)—have caused sunburn and skin scald in animals.

CBC/BIOCHEMISTRY/URINALYSIS
- Elevated serum BUN, Na, K, and bilirubin (total and direct) concentrations.
- Lower than normal serum in Hb, RBC count, PCV, TP, glucose, cholesterol, triglycerides, and serum alkaline phosphatase concentrations.
- Serum sorbitol dehydrogenase, GGT, concentrations within normal limits.
- Transaminases, CPK, sodium, and potassium increase and the BUN may increase up to ninefold. Glucose and hemoglobin decrease, while WBC level does not change.

PATHOLOGIC FINDINGS
- Skin changes typically are limited to the lesser pigmented areas or to the head in sheep. Depending upon the amount of plant material eaten, the changes range from minimal reddening and blister-like effects to extensive areas of sloughing.
- In more severe cases, the skin will be thickened with a gelatinous appearance extending down into the deeper corium.

S

ST. JOHN'S WORT TOXICITY

Crusty and ulcerative or proliferative areas may be present, especially around the face.
• Microscopically, the edema of the skin will be accompanied by necrosis and a polymorphonuclear infiltrate in the deeper corium.

TREATMENT

THERAPEUTIC APPROACH
• Remove animal from source.
• Affected animals should be given full shade or preferably housed and allowed out to graze only during darkness.
• Corticosteroids given parenterally in the early stages may be useful.
• Secondary skin infections and suppuration should be treated with a topical broad-spectrum antibiotic.
• Flystrike should be prevented.
• Emergency evacuation of the gastrointestinal tract is not required since the toxin takes several days to build up in the body and cause signs.

MEDICATIONS

DRUGS OF CHOICE
• 1.1 mg/kg/day prednisone or prednisolone PO for 10 days.
• Depending on the severity of the lesions, antibiotics and anti-inflammatory medications may be indicated.

FOLLOW-UP

EXPECTED COURSE AND PROGNOSIS
• Condition seldom causes death and soon clears once the plant source is removed.

• The prognosis and the eventual productivity of the animal are related to the site and severity of the primary lesion and to the degree of resolution.

PREVENTION
• Weed management—mowing and hand removal.
• Animals will avoid St. John's wort if more palatable forage is available.

MISCELLANEOUS

PREGNANCY
Can cause decreased litter size and reduced body size at birth

PRODUCTION MANAGEMENT
If the pasture contains large stands of St. John's wort, removal is indicated. Mow, spray, and/or reseed to improve the pasture quality.

SYNONYM
Klamath weed

ABBREVIATIONS
• BUN = blood urea nitrogen
• CPK = creatine phosphokinase
• GGT = gamma-glutamyl transferase
• Hb = hemoglobin
• MAO = monoamine oxidase
• PCV = packed cell volume
• PO = per os, by mouth
• RBC = red blood cell
• TP = total protein
• WBC = white blood cell

SEE ALSO
• Drug Toxicities
• Photosensitization

Suggested Reading
Araya OS, Ford EJ. An investigation of the type of photosensitization caused by the ingestion of St. John's wort (*Hypericum*

perforatum) by calves. J Comp Pathol 1981, 91: 135–41.
Burrows GE, Tyrl RJ eds. Toxic Plants of North America, 2nd ed. Ames: Wiley-Blackwell, Kindle edition, 2013, pp. 708–12.
Bourke CA. Sunlight associated hyperthermia as a consistent and rapidly developing clinical sign in sheep intoxicated by St. John's wort (Hypericum perforatum). Aust Vet J 2000, 78: 483–8.
Horn GA Jr, Burrows GE. Primary photosensitization in cattle. Vet Hum Toxicol 1990, 32: 331–2.
Kako MD, al-Sultan II, Saleem AN. Studies of sheep experimentally poisoned with *Hypericum perforatum*. Vet Hum Toxicol 1993, 35: 298–300.
Schey KL, Patat S, Chignell CF, Datillo M, Wang RH, Roberts JE. Photooxidation of lens alpha-crystallin by hypericin (active ingredient in St. John's wort). Photochem Photobiol 2000, 72: 200–3.
Southwell IA, Bourke CA. Seasonal variation in hypericin content of *Hypericum perforatum L*. (St. John's wort). Phytochemistry 2001, 56: 437–41.
Author Troy E.C. Holder
Consulting Editor Christopher C.L. Chase

S

BASICS

OVERVIEW
Starvation is defined as the insufficient intake of energy and nutrients, or the inability to obtain food for an extended period of time.

INCIDENCE/PREVALENCE
N/A

GEOGRAPHIC DISTRIBUTION
N/A

SYSTEMS AFFECTED
Multisystemic

PATHOPHYSIOLOGY
• Many physiologic changes occur as an animal attempts to satisfy its energy requirements in a starvation situation. At the cellular level, catabolism continues to supply the substrates required for anabolism and vital functions. Reserve stores of nutrients are utilized to compensate for the lack of nutritional intake.
• The most readily usable material, glycogen, is utilized first primarily from liver stores and is exhausted in a few hours. Next, stored fat from various subcutaneous deposits (near the kidney, mesentery, and omentum) is utilized. Following this use, fat deposits in the parenchymal organs are utilized, followed by fat deposits in the bone marrow. The final source of energy available to the animal is cell cytoplasm, which is primarily protein. Prolonged catabolism of muscle cells results in muscle atrophy.
• Ketosis is commonly seen.
• Nitrogen excretion rises due to the protein catabolism. The animal eventually reaches a point where it dies because of insufficient blood glucose necessary for brain function and the occurrence of hypoglycemic shock.
• Inadequate food intake, especially in ruminants, results in a rapid decrease in the number of bacteria and protozoa and in the level of volatile fatty acids present in the rumen.
• Nearly 70% of the energy available to ruminants is from fatty acids, thus further impacting on energy availability.
• Decreased microbial populations also diminish the animal's ability to digest fiber.
• Prolonged food deprivation is known to cause a fall in the core body temperature.
• If the animal is subjected to low environmental temperatures with inadequate shelter and/or nutrition then thermoregulation is lost and death by cardiac arrest occurs. This may occur before the loss of significant muscle mass.
• Muscle weakness accompanied by low muscle mass results in prolonged recumbency. This results in lowering of the core body temperature, inability to get up, and eventually asystole, cardiac arrest, and death.

HISTORICAL FINDINGS
• Food unavailability or shortage, wild animals seen by humans more frequently, significant loss in animal body weight.
• Ongoing drought or persistent cold environmental temperatures.

SIGNALMENT
• Thin animals are most susceptible to starvation because of decreased energy stores and environmental tolerance.
• Young and old animals have the highest nutritional demands and the lowest positions in the social environment with respect to food access.
• Young growing animals and pregnant or lactating animals have much higher energy and protein requirements than do dry stock.

PHYSICAL EXAMINATION FINDINGS
• Lethargic, unsteady, listless, unafraid of humans.
• Dehydration, rough hair coat, thin body condition with loss of palpable or visible fat on the ribs or brisket, muscle atrophy, visibility of individual muscle groups especially in the hindquarters.

GENETICS
N/A

CAUSES AND RISK FACTORS
• Inability to ingest, digest, absorb, or utilize food
• Injury, poor teeth, parasitism, chronic disease, foreign bodies, neoplasia
• Inadequate supply of or access to food (competition or overcrowding)
• Insufficient energy and nutrient intake
• Extreme parasitism
• Harsh environmental conditions (drought, deep snow)
• Increased energy demands (pregnancy, lactation, growth)
• Predator stress
• Lack of adequate shelter

DIAGNOSIS

DIFFERENTIAL DIAGNOSES
Malnutrition, parasitism, neoplasia

CBC/CHEMISTRY/URINALYSIS
• Anemia
• Hypoproteinemia, hypoglycemia, hypocalcemia, high anion gap; increased AST, SDH, GGT, and CK
• Proteinuria, ketonuria possible

OTHER LABORATORY TESTS
• Starvation is best diagnosed by gross examination or necropsy (see "Pathologic Findings").
• Femur or mandibular bone marrow fat analysis can be grossly examined in older animals. Some laboratories offer a femur marrow compression method, ether-extract method, kidney fat index, and wet weight-dry weight method.

PATHOLOGIC FINDINGS
• Changes are many and varied. The most striking is the lack of fat in the subcutaneous, visceral, and bone marrow locations.
• Muscle atrophy is generally significant. Serous atrophy of fat is common. The internal organs are generally smaller than normal.
• The digestive tract is generally void of any material and is often shrunken. The gallbladder is generally distended and bile staining may be present. Rumen ulcers may be present and rumen materials are scant and dry. Villous atrophy may be seen in the rumen. Abomasal or duodenal ulcers may be present.
• Femoral bone marrow will be red or yellow in color, transparent and gelatinous.

TREATMENT

THERAPEUTIC APPROACH
• Generally ruminants will not eat large quantities of food when sudden access to unlimited food occurs.
• If food is not provided until late stages of starvation, the animal will likely die. It may take up to 2 weeks for a ruminant to adjust to the new diet and change into a positive energy balance.
• Care must be given to provide a good-quality palatable feed containing readily available carbohydrates, roughage, minerals, and vitamins.
• Moderate quality hay or grass is the safest starting feed along with unlimited access to clean water.
• Treat pre-existing health conditions.
Deficiencies that must be corrected, in order of importance, are:
• Energy.
• Rumen-digestible protein (or alternative nitrogen and sulfur equivalent) required by rumen bacteria to produce energy and protein from low-quality feed.
• High-quality protein required for growth, pregnancy, and lactation.
• Minerals, particularly phosphorus, calcium, and magnesium.
• Vitamins associated with the lack of fresh green feed, particularly vitamins A, D, and E.

MEDICATIONS

DRUGS OF CHOICE
Directed at specific treatments of underlying disease conditions

PRECAUTIONS
N/A

S

STARVATION   (CONTINUED)

CONTRAINDICATIONS

Appropriate milk and meat withdrawal times must be followed for all compounds administered to food-producing animals.

POSSIBLE INTERACTIONS

N/A

 FOLLOW-UP

EXPECTED COURSE AND PROGNOSIS

Will vary greatly depending on chronicity and underlying cause of starvation.

POSSIBLE COMPLICATIONS

The animal is prone to acidosis if a sudden shift of microbial population occurs and the only feed provided is high in carbohydrates, so avoid that practice.

CLIENT EDUCATION

Owners should be educated on appropriate animal husbandry and nutritional requirements.

PATIENT CARE

See "Therapeutic Approach"

PREVENTION

Appropriate animal care and husbandry

 MISCELLANEOUS

ASSOCIATED CONDITIONS

- Malnutrition.
- Metabolic diseases.
- Mineral deficiencies and imbalances.
- Hypocalcemia.
- Hypomagnesemia.
- Reduced fertility in males and females.
- Abortions, stillbirths, birth of underweight offspring, poor growth of neonates due to inadequate lactation in dams.

- Grain toxemia/acidosis:
  ○ Any factor that causes variation in intake (e.g., inclement weather, or palatability of feed) or changes in the availability of the carbohydrate (e.g., a change in grain type, or grain processing) may cause digestive upsets at any time, not just in the period of grain introduction.
- Urea poisoning if excessive amounts of protein supplements are fed during recovery.
- Urinary calculi due to mineral imbalances and dehydration.
- Plant poisoning- hungry animals may consume toxic plants, including shrubs and trees, which they would normally avoid.
- Blue-green algae toxicosis:
  ○ Blooms of blue-green algae are more likely to appear in warmer months during drought.

PREGNANCY

It is common for pregnant animals to abort their fetus during times of starvation. Stillbirths are also common. A fetus that survives will often be small and have an increased chance for mortality. Dams may not allow nursing or may abandon their young.

PRODUCTION MANAGEMENT

- Once pasture is inadequate, cattle should be confined and fed. Confined cattle need significantly less energy for maintenance than do those that are left in the paddock to wander in search of feed.
- Free choice hay, water, and minerals should be available after animals start to eat again.
- Animals should be separated into smaller feeding groups based on age, body condition, and body size.
- The pastures should be left in a condition where they can recover quickly when a drought breaks.
- Any change in feed (especially grain) should be introduced gradually—failure to do this is probably the major cause of illness seen in recovery from drought/starvation.

ABBREVIATIONS

- AST = aspartate aminotransferase
- CK = creatine phosphokinase
- GGT = gamma glutamyl transferase
- SDH = sorbitol dehydrogenase

SEE ALSO

- Animal Welfare (see www.fiveminutevet.com/ruminant)
- Nutritional Assessment (see www.fiveminutevet.com/ruminant)

Suggested Reading

Blum JW, Kunz P, Bachmann C, Colombo JP. Metabolic effects of fasting in steers. Res Vet Sci 1981, 31: 127–9.

Nowak R, Porter RH, Levy F, Orgeur P, Schaal B. Role of mother-young interactions in the survival of offspring in domestic mammals. Rev Reprod 2000, 5: 153–63.

Owens FN, Dubeski P, Hanson CF. Factors that alter the growth and development of ruminants. J Anim Sci 1993, 71: 3138–50.

Poppi DP, McLennan SR. Protein and energy utilization by ruminants at pasture. J Anim Sci 1995, 73: 278–90.

Van Kessel JS, Russell JB. The endogenous polysaccharide utilization rate of mixed ruminal bacteria and the effect of energy starvation on ruminal fermentation rates. J Dairy Sci 1997, 80: 2442–8.

Whiting TL, Postey RC, Chestley ST, Wruck GC. Explanatory model of cattle death by starvation in Manitoba: forensic evaluation. Can Vet J 2012, 53: 1173–80.

Internet Resource

Malnutrition and Starvation. Department of Natural Resources, Michigan. Available at http://www.michigan.gov/dnr/.

Author Stephen R. Purdy

Consulting Editor Kaitlyn A. Lutz

Acknowledgment The author and book editors acknowledge the prior contribution of Angela M. Daniels.

S

BASICS

OVERVIEW

• Strongyloidiasis refers to infection of a variety of mammals, including ruminants, with specific species of *Strongyloides*, a free-living nematode. Other genera of free-living nematodes can also infect mammals, creating a variety of clinical signs depending on the route of infection and organs affected in the host.
• Three genera of the order Rhabditida (free-living soil nematodes) can parasitize ruminants, including *Rhabditis* (*Pelodera*) *strongyloides*, *Halicephalobus gingivalis* (also known as *Micronema deletrix* or *Halicephalobus deletrix*), and *Strongyloides*.
• *R. strongyloides* can create pruritic dermatitis in cattle by penetrating the skin of animals in contaminated environments.
• *H. gingivalis* is a rare and highly pathogenic parasite creating neurologic disease in humans and horses; it has been linked to meningoencephalomyelitis in a small group of dairy calves in Denmark.
• *S. papillosus* affects calves, lambs, and particularly goat kids, with infection occurring via skin penetration and transmammary transmission to nursing neonates. Clinical signs of infection include dermatitis, diarrhea, and coughing.

INCIDENCE/PREVALENCE

Unknown, but increased prevalence with permissive management factors such as confinement, crowding, and poor sanitation are likely.

GEOGRAPHIC DISTRIBUTION

Worldwide

SYSTEMS AFFECTED

• Digestive
• Integument
• Nervous
• Respiratory
• Reproductive

PATHOPHYSIOLOGY

• The life cycle of *Strongyloides* is unique because it has alternate free-living and parasitic generations. The males of this species are not parasitic.
• The parasitic, parthenogenic female is embedded primarily in the mucosa of the proximal small intestine; eggs are laid into the mucosa, develop rapidly, and are embryonated when they are passed in the feces 1–3 weeks after infection.
• On pasture, eggs hatch and develop within 24–48 hours to infective third-stage (filariform) larvae, or alternatively, develop into free-living males or females that can mate to produce infective larvae.
• Grazing hosts ingest infective larvae, or infective larvae penetrate the host skin, typically between the claws of the foot.

• In older animals, larvae accumulate in the subcutaneous tissues and migrate to the mammary gland during impending lactation. Neonates are subsequently infected via ingestion of milk, and egg-laying females may be present in the intestine from about 1 week after birth.
• In young animals, infective larvae penetrate the skin and spread hematogenously to the lungs where they break into the alveoli, migrate up the airways, and/or are coughed up the trachea into the pharynx and swallowed, to develop into mature females 2–3 weeks after ingestion.
• *R. strongyloides* achieves infection by penetrating skin in contact with contaminated surfaces, ground or bedding, particularly the neck, flank, abdomen, and udder, resulting in irritation and inflammation of the skin.
• *H. gingivalis* is thought to penetrate skin and mucus membranes, and appears to display neurotropism in the host, but the life cycle, mode of infection, and risk factors associated with this parasite are poorly understood.

HISTORICAL FINDINGS

Relate to the presence of permissive management factors for *Strongyloides* infection, such as recent births of vulnerable neonates, overcrowding, and confined, poorly sanitized environments.

SIGNALMENT

• Young calves, particularly dairy stock.
• Neonatal and weaned goat kids and lambs.
• Adult ruminants carry a degree of immunity to intestinal infection with this parasite.

PHYSICAL EXAMINATION FINDINGS

• *R. strongyloides*: Dermatitis reflected by marked alopecia of the neck and flank with flaking, thickening and wrinkling of the skin, pruritus, and exudation of serum in severe cases. Pustules may be noted on the ventral abdomen and udder. Cattle in tropical environments can display otitis externa and chronic wasting.
• *H. gingivalis*: Granulomatous encephalomyelitis in calves results in impaired proprioception, central nervous signs, uveitis, and recumbency within the first few weeks of life.
• *Strongyloides* has been studied under natural and experimental conditions, and infection can result in a variety of clinical signs as follows:
   ○ Natural infections can result in clinical signs related to the GI tract (intermittent diarrhea, blood and mucus in feces, anorexia and weight loss); respiratory tract (coughing and tachypnea); and integument of the interdigital space (lameness, stamping, biting at or rubbing feet and legs, increased susceptibility to foot rot) or of the body (pustular, erythematous dermatitis).
   ○ In sheep and lambs, initial skin invasion by *S. papillosus* larvae may not induce any inflammation but subsequent exposures

cause a pustular, erythematous dermatitis. Concurrent enteritis and pulmonary hemorrhage may occur in lambs.
   ○ Adult animals seldom show clinical signs of a *Strongyloides* burden unless stressed, diseased, or exposed to heavy infestation, in which case bulls can show balanoposthitis, and sheep and goats may show unthriftiness, diarrhea, weight loss, and moderate anemia. Tiny white worms may be visible in feces of small ruminants. Reinfection can result in bouts of coughing.
   ○ Experimental infection in kids, lambs and calves has created pallor, coughing, diarrhea, weight loss, neurologic signs and sudden death due to hepatic rupture in some kids, and cardiac arrest in lambs and calves.

GENETICS

N/A

CAUSES AND RISK FACTORS

• Most common when animals are kept confined in a wet, dirty environment.
• Dams that are parasitized at the time of parturition are the major source of *Strongyloides* infection for neonates.

DIAGNOSIS

DIFFERENTIAL DIAGNOSES

• Contact dermatitis or irritation from dirty, wet bedding
• Infectious and noninfectious causes of diarrhea
• Foot rot
• Trombiculidiasis
• Cutaneous larval migrans
• Chorioptic mange
• Dermatophytosis

CBC/BIOCHEMISTRY/URINALYSIS

Anemia in heavily infested animals

OTHER LABORATORY TESTS

N/A

IMAGING

N/A

OTHER DIAGNOSTIC PROCEDURES

• Fecal flotation identifies colorless, small, thin-shelled oval embryonated eggs (40–60 × 20–25 μm). The female is not fecund and therefore a dozen or more eggs in a sample can represent a large load of adults.
• Free-living adults frequently develop from cultures of feces from *Strongyloides* infected animals.
• Skin biopsy identifies pustular dermatitis characterized by edema, inflammatory infiltration (neutrophils, eosinophils, lymphocytes, and giant cells), and destruction of larvae.
• Necropsy: Adults (3–6 mm) may be evident in the small intestine or in scrapings of the intestinal mucosa. Minced tissue can be

placed in a Baermann isolation device to identify immature parasites.
• Serum ELISA may be useful.

PATHOLOGIC FINDINGS
• Catarrhal enteritis with petechiae and ecchymoses may be evident, especially in the duodenum and jejunum.
• Microscopically, larvae establish tunnels in the epithelium of the small intestine at the base of the villi and persist in that location. Villus atrophy can occur, associated with mixed mononuclear inflammatory cell infiltrate into the lamina propria. The epithelium of the crypts of Lieberkuhn is hyperplastic and larvae may be evident in the crypts.
• Embryonated or larvated ova may be retained in the epithelial tunnels and help to distinguish *Strongyloides* from *Trichostrongylus* or other parasitic species.

TREATMENT

THERAPEUTIC APPROACH
• Soiled bedding should be removed and bedding should be kept clean and dry to eliminate moist, warm, habitats for free-living nematodes and larvae.
• Spontaneous recovery may occur if the source of infection is removed and management changes made.
• Anthelmintics can be used which are approved for the ruminant species in question and for the production status of the animal in which it is to be used.

SURGICAL CONSIDERATIONS AND TECHNIQUES
N/A

MEDICATIONS

DRUGS OF CHOICE
• If giving oral medication, reduce feed intake 24 hours before treatment. This has the greatest impact on the benzimidazole class, but can improve other drug classes.
• Albendazole: Goat 10 mg/kg; sheep 7.5 mg/kg body weight PO
• Eprinomectrin: Goat/sheep 0.5 mg/kg PO
• Febantel: Goat/sheep 5 mg/kg PO
• Fenbendazole: Goat/sheep 20 mg/kg PO
• Ivermectin: Goat 0.4 mg/kg; sheep 0.2 mg/kg PO
• Levamisole: Goat 8–12 mg/kg PO
• Morantel: 10 mg/kg PO
• Moxidectin: Goat 0.5 mg/kg PO
• Oxfendazole: Goat 10 mg/kg PO; sheep 5–10 mg/kg PO

CONTRAINDICATIONS
Albendazole should be avoided in pregnant ruminants, particularly within the first 3 months of gestation.

PRECAUTIONS
• Appropriate milk and meat withdrawal times must be followed for all compounds administered to food-producing animals.
• Parasite resistance to anthelmintics is a serious growing danger, so all possible management steps should be favored over anthelmintic use, particularly for parasites such as *Strongyloides* which have relatively limited pathogenicity.

POSSIBLE INTERACTIONS
N/A

FOLLOW-UP

EXPECTED COURSE AND PROGNOSIS
Spontaneous recovery is likely, and rapid response to appropriate anthelmintic treatments is expected.

POSSIBLE COMPLICATIONS
Secondary infection of inflamed skin or secondary bacterial bronchopneumonia.

CLIENT EDUCATION
Focus on management strategies to reduce *Strongyloides* infestation.

PATIENT CARE
Provide clean, dry bedding that is replaced at appropriate intervals.

PREVENTION
• 30–35% of animals carry the majority of nematodes and create pasture contamination.
• To avoid resistance, some of these animals need to remain untreated, so the herd or flock should be managed via targeted selective treatment versus general deworming.
• This ensures a refugia (a population not selected by anthelmintic treatment) of susceptible nematode larvae is maintained on the pasture, to help dilute out resistant genes from resistant nematodes.
• Use of the FAMACHA system can identify clinically anemic animals in need of deworming, leaving healthier animals to host the refugia.
• Similarly, select young animals with poor weight gain for treatment and leave normally growing animals untreated to promote refugia.
• Animals should be kept on "safe pastures"—those where pasture contamination is low and significant reinfection takes longer. This can be a pasture not grazed by the species of interest in 3–6 months, or pastures that have been tilled, burned, or replanted.

MISCELLANEOUS

ASSOCIATED CONDITIONS
Secondary mild bacterial bronchopneumonia

AGE-RELATED FACTORS
Neonates and young animals are more susceptible than adults.

ZOONOTIC POTENTIAL
Cutaneous larval migrans can occur in humans with *S. papillosus*; however, other parasites are more likely to initiate this problem (such as canine hookworms).

PREGNANCY
Routine deworming of dams late in gestation decreases transmammary transmission to neonates.

BIOSECURITY
• In general, to aid parasite control, place all new arrivals in a secure dry lot where they are fed, cleaned, and cared for in order to minimize any contact with herd.
• Perform fecal examination for the presence of nematode eggs.
• Within 2–3 days of arrival, consider treating with three different classes of anthelmintics on the same day, for example, administer a milbemycin (moxidectin), benzimidazole (fenbendazole), and membrane depolarizing agent (levamisole).
• Perform second fecal examination 10–14 days after deworming to check for presence of nematode eggs; if results are negative, repeat the fecal examination in 5–7 days.
• Allow only animals with negative findings on two separate tests to be placed in the herd or flock.

PRODUCTION MANAGEMENT
• Infestation may result in decreased milk production and meat production, pruritic dermatitis may result in damage to the wool and hide, and severe infections in young animals may lead to poor condition, reduced growth, or death.
• Routine deworming of dams in late gestation decreases transmammary transmission of *Strongyloides* to the neonate.
• Early deworming of neonates born to affected untreated dams.
• Provide a clean, dry environment with adequate clean bedding in stalls and rest areas.
• Pasture management to reduce host exposure to parasites by manure removal and rotational grazing.
• Select for parasite resistance by culling animals with chronic, heavy parasite loads.
• Avoid bringing resistant parasites onto properties by isolating new ruminants until fecal egg counts have been performed and deworming performed if needed.

S

SYNONYMS
N/A

ABBREVIATIONS
• ELISA = enzyme linked immunosorbent assay
• PO = per os, by mouth

SEE ALSO
• Dermatophilosis
• Dermatophytosis
• Diarrheal Diseases: Bovine
• Diarrheal Diseases: Small Ruminant
• Parasitic Skin Diseases: Small Ruminant
• Small Ruminant Dermatology

Suggested Reading
Bowman DD, Lunn RC, Eberherd ML eds. Helminths. In: Georgis' Parasitology for Veterinarians, 8th ed. St. Louis: Saunders (Elsevier Science), 2003, pp. 197–201.
Enemark HL, Hansen MS, Jensen TK, Larsen G, Al-Sabi MNS. An outbreak of bovine meningoencephalomyelitis with identification of *Halicephalobus gingivalis*. Vet Parasitol 2016, 218: 82–6.
Miller JE, Kaplan RM, Pugh DG. Internal parasites. In: Sheep and Goat Medicine. Philadelphia: Saunders, 2012, pp. 88–90, 426–28, 435–43.
Nakamura Y, Tsuji N, Taira N, Hirose H. Parasitic females of *Strongyloides papillosus* as a pathogenic stage of sudden cardiac death in infected lambs. J Vet Med Sci 1994, 56: 723–7.
Pienaar JG, Basson PA, du Plessis JL, et al. Experimental studies with *Strongyloides papillosus* in goats. Onderstepoort J Vet Res 1999, 66: 191–235.
Tsuji N, Itabisashi T, Nakamura Y, et al. Sudden cardiac death in calves with experimental heavy infection of *Strongyloides papillosus*. J Vet Med Sci 1992, 54: 1137–43.

Author Jenifer Robin Gold
Consulting Editor Erica C. McKenzie
Acknowledgment The author and book editors acknowledge the prior contribution of Karen A. Moriello and Susan Semrad.

S

STRYCHNINE POISONING

BASICS

OVERVIEW
• Toxin derived from seeds and bark of tree *Strynos nux-vomica* that is native of southeast Asia.
• Strychnine is used in rodenticide baits.

INCIDENCE/PREVALENCE
• Occurs where strychnine grain baits are used. They contain 0.5–1% strychnine alkaloid. Some formulations may contain higher strychnine concentrations. Most baits are used to control rodent populations with below-ground use of these products.
• The lethal oral dose of strychnine for cattle is reported as 0.5 mg/kg body weight. Strychnine is rapidly absorbed from the GIT and metabolized by hepatic enzymes. Strychnine is widely distributed in the body with a small portion excreted unchanged into the urine.

SYSTEMS AFFECTED
Nervous

GEOGRAPHIC DISTRIBUTION
Worldwide

PATHOPHYSIOLOGY
• Strychnine is a selective antagonist in blocking the inhibitory effects of glycine at the glycine receptors of the postsynaptic membrane.
• May also increase levels of glutamic acid.
• End result is neuronal excitation of motor neurons.

HISTORICAL FINDINGS
History of exposure to rodenticide baits that contain strychnine.

SIGNALMENT
All species are susceptible.

PHYSICAL EXAMINATION FINDINGS
Signs can occur within minutes of ingestion.
• Restlessness
• Muscle twitching

• Contracture of skeletal muscles
• Convulsions
• Death

CAUSES AND RISK FACTORS
• Exposure to rodenticide baits that contain strychnine.
• Poor management of rodenticide baits.
• Malicious intent may be cause of exposure.

DIAGNOSIS

DIFFERENTIAL DIAGNOSES
• Botulism
• Metaldehyde or lead toxicosis
• Organophosphorus, carbamate, or chlorinated hydrocarbons
• Sodium ion toxicity
• Tremorgenic mycotoxins
• Tetanus

CBC/BIOCHEMISTRY/URINALYSIS
No characteristic changes

OTHER DIAGNOSTIC PROCEDURES
Detection of toxin in bait, blood, GIT, urine, liver, or kidney using chromatography or mass spectrometry.

PATHOLOGIC FINDINGS
No specific lesions are noted; however, necrosis of the cerebral cortex and brainstem have been reported in humans poisoned with strychnine.

TREATMENT

THERAPEUTIC APPROACH
• Supportive treatment
• Sedation

MEDICATIONS

DRUGS OF CHOICE
None

FOLLOW-UP

EXPECTED COURSE AND PROGNOSIS
Most cases result in death; there have been a few reports of recovery.

PREVENTION
Keep rodenticides away from feedstuffs and livestock.

MISCELLANEOUS

BIOSECURITY
• Monitor all use of rodenticides, particularly around feedstuffs. Keep rodenticides away from livestock.
• Malicious intent may be cause of exposure.

PRODUCTION MANAGEMENT
Keep rodenticides away from livestock and facilities.

ABBREVIATION
GIT = gastrointestinal tract

SEE ALSO
• Carbamate Toxicity
• Clostridial Disease: Nervous System
• Fungal Tremorgens
• Lead Toxicosis
• Metaldehyde Toxicosis
• Organophosphate Toxicity
• Sodium Disorders: Hypernatremia

Suggested Reading
Gupta RC. Non-anticoagulant rodenticides. In: Gupta RC ed, Veterinary Toxicology: Basic and Clinical Principles. London: Academic Press, 2012, pp. 698–700.
Author Jennifer S. Taintor
Consulting Editor Christopher C.L. Chase
Acknowledgment The author and book editors acknowledge the prior contribution of Greg Stoner.

S

SULFUR TOXICITY

BASICS

OVERVIEW
• Sulfur (S) occurs in nature as free S or combined with other elements in sulfides and sulfates. The most common form in water is the sulfate (SO_4^{2-}) ion, although some sulfurous wells may contain relatively high concentrations of dissolved sulfides. The most common naturally occurring forms in feedstuffs are S-containing amino acids (e.g., methionine).
• S is an essential macro element, and, in fact, comprises about 0.15% of the total body in mammals. It is a constituent of the amino acids methionine, cysteine, cystine, homocysteine, cystathionine, taurine, and cysteic acid. It is also a component of biotin, thiamine, estrogens, ergothionine, fibrinogen, heparin, chondroitin, glutathione, coenzyme A, and lipoic acid. Unlike monogastrics, ruminants can synthesize their own organic forms of S from inorganic S.
• S is highly toxic if consumed in excess amounts.
• High doses of S may cause sudden death or polioencephalomalacia (PEM). Somewhat smaller doses can impact productivity (weight gain, reproduction) via its effect upon copper metabolism, and other, poorly understood, chronic effects.

INCIDENCE/PREVALENCE
In 1997, 11.5% of 454 pairs of forage/water samples collected from around the United States yielded dietary S concentrations potentially hazardous for cattle; 37% of these elevated pairs originated from the western United States.

GEOGRAPHIC DISTRIBUTION
S toxicity on western rangelands most commonly results from water-borne SO_4. However, in confinement feeding operations, especially in the mid-west, it is more likely to be associated with feeding ethanol by-products.

SYSTEMS AFFECTED
• Hemolymphatic
• Nervous
• Reproductive
• Respiratory

PATHOPHYSIOLOGY
• The first step in ruminal synthesis of S-amino acids from inorganic S is reduction of the latter to H_2S. Under normal circumstances, the reactive sulfide ion is combined with carbon by rumen microflora to create methionine, homocysteine, cystathionine, cysteine, and other S-amino acids. Under conditions of excessive S intake, however, significant quantities are reduced to H_2S, and the very toxic gas escapes from the

rumen into the systemic circulation, resulting in sudden death or polioencephalomalacia.
• Smaller concentrations of ruminal sulfide react with Cu and/or Mo to form biologically unavailable Cu compounds.
• Chronic exposure to H_2S may impair innate respiratory immunity (phagocytosis and the mucociliary elevator).

HISTORICAL FINDINGS

Acute Toxicity
• Sudden death within 1–2 days of a major change in diet or water supply.
• Cortical neurologic signs within a few days to 2–3 weeks of a major change in diet or water supply.

Chronic Toxicity
• A veterinarian faced with poor conception rates, poor response to vaccine, or increased incidence of respiratory disease should *consider* chronic S toxicity as a possible differential.

SIGNALMENT
• Potentially all ruminant species are susceptible, but cattle seem to be the most sensitive.
• In general, animals need a functional rumen to be affected, thus adults are more likely to be affected than neonates.

PHYSICAL EXAMINATION FINDINGS
• Sudden death with no premonitory signs and no lesions.
• Circling, head-pressing, star-gazing, muscle fasciculations, and convulsions.
• Increased infectious disease with poor response to vaccination and treatment, possibly related to impaired immune function.
• Decreased reproductive efficiency, especially in the first trimester, as a result of Cu deficiency.
• Signs suggestive of cortical neurologic damage, including blindness, tremors, and convulsions.

CAUSES AND RISK FACTORS

Sources
• Naturally occurring S in common forages ranges from 0.17% to 0.48%. This concentration may be drastically altered by human activity.
• Ethanol production by-products, such as DDG, *may* contain S concentrations many times higher than natural feedstuffs.
• The predominate form of S in drinking water is the SO_4^{2-} ion. Concentrations vary widely with the local geosphere. In general, waters from alkaline, arid regions, such as the Great Plains and Intermountain West, tend to contain much higher concentrations of S than other regions of North America.

Toxicity
• Ruminants are more susceptible to S toxicity than nonruminants. All ruminants are susceptible.

• Although there are no experimental side-by-side comparisons of S toxicity in various ruminant species, in the author's experience cattle seem to be more sensitive than sheep and goats. Bison and elk are somewhat intermediate.
• Since S toxicity depends upon generation of the sulfide ion, which may be influenced by a host of other dietary and environmental factors, and because the dose of S received is the sum of the S content of all dietary components including water, it is difficult to settle upon a single number that consistently guarantees safety. The NRC recommends that "the sulfur content of cattle diets be limited to the requirement of the animal, which is 0.2% dietary sulfur for dairy and 0.15% in beef cattle and other ruminants."

DIAGNOSIS

DIFFERENTIAL DIAGNOSES
• Lead poisoning
• Nitrate or cyanide poisoning
• Poor nutrition or trace element deficiencies
• Sodium ion toxicity
• Thiamine deficiency
• Thromboembolic meningoencephalitis

CBC/BIOCHEMISTRY/URINALYSIS
N/A

OTHER LABORATORY TESTS
• Rumen gas cap H_2S concentrations will be higher than background concentrations in some, but not all, acute cases. This is a somewhat exotic test that must be performed on a live or freshly dead animal.
• Analysis of blood or liver for lead and brain for sodium will possibly eliminate two major differentials.
• Hepatic Cu concentration is often depressed in cases of ill-thrift due to chronic S toxicity.

OTHER DIAGNOSTIC PROCEDURES
Analysis of feedstuffs and water for S. All components of the diet must be analyzed and the total dose calculated.

TREATMENT

THERAPEUTIC APPROACH
• Remove animals from source of high dietary S.
• *Massive* doses of parenteral thiamine may provide some improvement in early cases of PEM.
• Dexamethasone may also help with early cases of PEM.
• Switching rations from high carbohydrate (if on them) to high roughage may prevent new cases.

S

MEDICATIONS

DRUGS OF CHOICE

• Thiamine administration at a dosage of 10 mg/kg body weight q6–8h for cattle or small ruminants. The first dose is administered slowly IV; otherwise, the animal may collapse. Subsequent doses are administered IM for 3–5 days.
• Administration of dexamethasone at a dosage of 1–2 mg/kg, IM or SC, to reduce cerebral edema.

CONTRAINDICATIONS

Ionophores increase H_2S production in vitro. The clinical significance of this has not been proven.

FOLLOW-UP

EXPECTED COURSE AND PROGNOSIS

Prognosis is guarded for animals showing signs of PEM.

PREVENTION

Avoid sudden changes in diet or water source, especially during summer months, and allow animals time to adapt to any new combination of feed and water.

MISCELLANEOUS

PRODUCTION MANAGEMENT

• Test each new batch of ethanol by-products before feeding.
• On rangelands with potentially high SO_4 waters, test water before introducing cattle, especially if they are accustomed to low SO_4 waters.

ABBREVIATIONS

• DDG = dry distillers' grains
• IM = intramuscular
• IV = intravenous
• PEM = polioencephalomalacia
• SC = subcutaneous

SEE ALSO

• Cyanide Toxicosis
• *Histophilus somni* Complex
• Lead Toxicosis
• Nitrate and Nitrite Toxicosis
• Sodium Disorders: Hypernatremia
• Vitamin B Deficiency

Suggested Reading

Drewnoski ME, Pogge DJ, Hansen SL. 2014. High-sulfur in beef cattle diets: A review. J Anim Sci 2014, 92: 3763–80.

Gould DH, Dargatz DA, Garry FB, Hamar DW, Ross PF. Potentially hazardous sulfur conditions on beef cattle ranches in the United States. J Am Vet Med Assoc 2002, 221: 673–77.

Levy M. Overview of polioencephalomalacia. In: The Merck Veterinary Manual Online, 2015. http://www.merckvetmanual.com/mvm/nervous_system/polioencephalomalacia/overview_of_polioencephalomalacia.html accessed on August 4, 2016.

McAllister MM, Gould DH, Raisbeck MF, Cummings BA, Loneragan GH. Evaluation of ruminal sulfide concentrations and seasonal outbreaks of polioencephalomalacia in a beef cattle feedlot. J Am Vet Med Assoc 1997, 211: 1275–9.

National Research Council. Sulfur. In: Mineral Tolerance of Animals. Washington DC: National Academies Press, 2005, pp. 372–85.

Raisbeck MF, McAllister MM, Gould DH. Toxic syndromes associated with sulfur. In: Howard J ed, Current Veterinary Therapy: Food Animal Practice. Philadelphia: Saunders, 1997, vol. 4, pp. 280–1.

Author M.F. Raisbeck
Consulting Editor Christopher C.L. Chase

SWEET CLOVER POISONING

BASICS

OVERVIEW
• Three members of *Melilotus* species are a concern within the United States:
  ◦ White sweet clover (*Melilotus alba*) ◦ Sour clover (*Melilotus indica*) ◦ Yellow sweet clover (*Melilotus officinalis*)
• Herb with 3 blade leaflets that are obovate to linear. • Flowers are small and yellow or white. • Coumarin scent (vanilla like) when dried. • Used as hay and silage forage.
• Toxicity occurs when fungi grow in the stems of harvested plants because the plants are not completely dried for hay.

INCIDENCE/PREVALENCE
• Typically, morbidity is low (10–15%) and the case fatality rate high (>50%). • The most devastating episodes occur following surgery, dehorning, and castration. • Disease problems are more likely to appear in winter when animals are fed hay put up in large round bales during a wet summer.

GEOGRAPHIC DISTRIBUTION
This herb is found throughout the US.

SYSTEMS AFFECTED
Hemolymphatic

PATHOPHYSIOLOGY
• Dicoumarol is formed from the interaction of fungal growth in the partially dried or fermented stems with the already present coumarin within the herb. • Coumarin already present in the stems has a relatively low toxicity. • Dicoumarol interferes with vitamin K function, which is needed for activation of coagulation factors II, VII, IX, and X. • Depletion of coagulation factors is seen with dicoumarol concentrations of 10 ppm. • Toxicity effects are seen clinically at 20–30 ppm.

HISTORICAL FINDINGS
• Exposure to sweet clover hay or silage.
• Typically occurs with 4–5 weeks of consumption of toxic hay.

SIGNALMENT
• Although all animals are at some risk, this hemorrhagic disease occurs primarily in cattle.
• Sheep are less susceptible than are cattle.

PHYSICAL EXAMINATION FINDINGS
• Anemia and hemorrhage may be problems in the newborn in the absence of overt signs other than prolonged prothrombin time in the dam. • Subcutaneous hemorrhage. • Body cavity hemorrhage. • Intractable bleeding following surgery or medical procedures. • Spontaneous bleeding. • Tachycardia, tachypnea. • Weakness. • Death.

CAUSES AND RISK FACTORS
• Dicoumarol is the toxic principle.

• Exposure to plant that has been improperly cured for hay or fermented for silage. • These conditions of large bales and moist plants make curing of the tougher stems more difficult and more likely to have fungal growth. • Silage is less often a problem, but it is still a risk, especially in dairy cattle. • There may be no indication prior to surgery of the animal's predisposition for clotting problems, but following surgery, it may be seemingly impossible to stop the bleeding. • Handling animals in squeeze chutes or similar types of facilities also predisposes trauma and subsequent development of subcutaneous hemorrhage.

DIAGNOSIS

DIFFERENTIAL DIAGNOSES
• Blackleg • Warfarin rodenticide toxicity

CBC/BIOCHEMISTRY/URINALYSIS
Anemia

OTHER LABORATORY TESTS
• Coagulation
  ◦ Prolonged prothrombin time ◦ Increased whole blood clotting time

OTHER DIAGNOSTIC PROCEDURES
• History of exposure to the plant • Clinical signs of bleeding or hematomas • Analysis of hay for dicoumarol

TREATMENT

THERAPEUTIC APPROACH
• Severe cases may need blood transfusion.
• Vitamin K_1. • Remove from source and supplement with forage with good quality alfalfa hay.

MEDICATIONS

DRUGS OF CHOICE
• Vitamin K_1 1–5 mg/kg body weight administered IV, IM, or SC depending on severity of the case. • Repeat dose of vitamin K_1 as needed. • Vitamin K_3 has been used at double the dose of vitamin K_1 with some success. • Oral Vitamin K_3 is ineffective.

FOLLOW-UP

EXPECTED COURSE AND PROGNOSIS
• If found and treated, many recover • Death

PATIENT CARE
• PCV • Prothrombin time

PREVENTION
If to be used for forage, must be sown heavily to result in thin stems from dense growth. Cut early while stems are thin, dry thoroughly for hay and pack well for silage.

MISCELLANEOUS

PREGNANCY
• Of special concern is the potential for hemorrhage during parturition or in the newborn calf. • As sheep are more resistant, there is little likelihood of problems at lambing and in newborn lambs.

PRODUCTION MANAGEMENT
• Suspicious sweet clover hay may be fed if it is alternated with good alfalfa hay every 10–14 days. • Pregnant cows should not be fed hay or silage containing *Melilotus* unless these forages have been evaluated for dicoumarol content. • It would be prudent to forgo feeding sweet clover at least 1 month prior to calving. • Cultivars of sweet clover low in coumarin and safe to feed (e.g., Polara) have been developed.

ABBREVIATIONS
• IM = intramuscular • IV = intravenous • PCV = packed cell volume • SC = subcutaneous

SEE ALSO
• Clostridial Disease: Muscular • Rodenticide Toxicity

Suggested Reading
Burrows GE. Fabaceae. In: Burrows GE, Tyrl RJ eds, Toxic Plants of North America. Ames: Iowa State University Press, 2001, pp. 591–4.
Burrows GE, Tyrl RJ. In: Burrows GE, Tyrl RJ eds, Toxic Plants of North America, 2nd ed. Ames: Wiley-Blackwell, Kindle edition, 2013, pp. 579–83.
Casper HH, Alstad AD, Tacke DB, Johnson LJ, Lloyd WE. Evaluation of vitamin K_3 feed additive for prevention of sweet clover disease. J Vet Diag Invest 1989, 1: 116–19.
Puschner B, Galey FD, Holstege DM, Palazoglu M. Sweet clover poisoning in dairy cattle in California. J Am Vet Med Assoc 1998, 212: 857–8.
Author Jennifer S. Taintor
Consulting Editor Christopher C.L. Chase
Acknowledgment The author and book editors acknowledge the prior contribution of Greg Stoner and Larry A. Kerr.

S

SWEET POTATO POISONING

BASICS

OVERVIEW
• Sweet potatoes (*Ipomoea batatas*) produce several toxins in response to injury or mold (*Fusarium solani*) and parasitic infection. • Feeding of sweet potatoes not suitable for human consumption to livestock is the most common exposure.

INCIDENCE/PREVALENCE
• Often seen in the spring when spoiled sweet potatoes are most likely to be fed; however, the disease can occur anytime spoiled sweet potatoes are fed. • Morbidity rates in cattle fed moldy sweet potatoes can be as high as 75% and mortality is usually <10% but can be as high as 30%.

GEOGRAPHIC DISTRIBUTION
Throughout the United States but primarily in the southeast where it is a common practice to feed spoiled sweet potatoes to livestock.

SYSTEMS AFFECTED
Respiratory

PATHOPHYSIOLOGY
• Toxins produced by the sweet potato include 4-ipomeanol, 1-ipomeanol, 1,4-ipomeanol, and ipomeanine • These toxins cause destruction of type 1 pneumocytes and epithelial cells leading to proliferation of type 2 pneumocytes. • Bioactivation of a pneumotoxin, primarily in Clara cells and macrophages of the lung rather than in cells in the liver, results in formation of reactive metabolite intermediates such as 3-methylindole (3-MI). • These reactive metabolites bind to proteins in the lungs and cause tissue destruction, especially of type 1 pneumocytes and epithelial cells. Type 1 pneumocytes are responsible for gas exchange within the alveoli. • Under the stimulus of factors released by macrophages, type 2 pneumocytes proliferate to replace lost type 1 cells and in the process cause formation of foci with massive increase in cellularity. • During this period of proliferation, the ability of type 2 cells to synthesize and secrete functional surface-active phospholipids (surfactants) is decreased. Surfactant produced no longer effectively lowers surface tension. This compromises lung function. • This results in atypical interstitial pneumonia (AIP).

SIGNALMENT
Bovine (most common), ovine, and caprine

HISTORICAL FINDINGS
History of exposure to sweet potatoes

PHYSICAL EXAMINATION FINDINGS
• Labored breathing often open-mouth • Coughing • Salivation • Extended head and neck • Animals may be belligerent

CAUSES AND RISK FACTORS
Consumption of moldy sweet potatoes containing 4-IP

DIAGNOSIS

DIFFERENTIAL DIAGNOSES
• Perilla mint toxicity • DL tryptophan toxicity (fog fever) • Lungworm infection • Irritant gasses inhalation

CBC/BIOCHEMISTRY/URINALYSIS
No characteristic changes

OTHER LABORATORY TESTS
Detection of toxin in rumen samples thru gas chromatography/mass spectrometry

OTHER DIAGNOSTIC PROCEDURES
Sweet potato residue in rumen contents

PATHOLOGIC FINDINGS
• Gross pathology finds distended lungs that fail to collapse with prominent edema and fluid and foam oozes from cut surface. • Histopathologic examination will reveal proliferation of type 2 pneumocytes and alveolar lumens filled with fibrinous exudate.

TREATMENT

THERAPEUTIC APPROACH
• No specific treatment. • Keeping animals as calm as possible is important. • If stressed, animals often become anoxic and die. • Remove animals from etiology (i.e., purple mint, moldy sweet potatoes, or lush pasture).

MEDICATIONS

DRUGS OF CHOICE
• No specific drugs are effective. • Symptomatic treatment such as corticosteroids, atropine, diuretics, antihistamines, and antibiotics. • Supportive treatment: Bronchial dilators. • Weigh the value of therapeutic pharmacology versus the stress involved with handling and treatment.

FOLLOW-UP

EXPECTED COURSE AND PROGNOSIS
• Depending on the amount of lung damage, very guarded early prognosis as death may occur within 12–24 hours. • Clinical course may last 2–3 weeks. • If animals survive 2 or 3 days and are not stressed, prognosis improves. • Even severely affected animals may return to normal in 2–3 weeks when the type 2 pneumocytes resolves to type 1.

CLIENT EDUCATION
Danger associated with feeding moldy sweet potatoes

PREVENTION
Avoid feeding spoiled sweet potatoes

MISCELLANEOUS

ASSOCIATED CONDITIONS
N/A

AGE-RELATED FACTORS
N/A

ZOONOTIC POTENTIAL
N/A

PREGNANCY
N/A

PRODUCTION MANAGEMENT
Avoid spoiled sweet potatoes.

SYNONYMS
• AIP • Atypical interstitial pneumonia • Bovine asthma • Fog fever

ABBREVIATIONS
• AIP = atypical interstitial pneumonia • 3-MI = 3-methylindole • 4-IP = 4 ipomeanol

SEE ALSO
• Aspiration Pneumonia • Atypical Interstitial Pneumonia • Bovine Respiratory Syncytial Virus • *Brassica* spp. Toxicity • Contagious Bovine Pleuropneumonia • Enzootic Pneumonia of Calves • Organophosphate Toxicity • Parasitic Pneumonia • Plants Producing Acute Respiratory Disease Syndrome • Respiratory Disease: Bovine • Toxicology: Herd Outbreaks • Traumatic Reticuloperitonitis

Suggested Reading
Burrows GE. Convolvulaceae. In: Burrows GE, Tyrl RJ eds, Toxic Plants of North America. Ames: Iowa State University Press, 2001, p. 279.
Burrows GE, Tyrl R.J. Toxic Plants of North America. Ames: Wiley. Kindle Edition, 2013.
Doster AR, Mitchell FE, Farrell RL, Wilson BJ. Effects of 4-ipomeanol, a product from mold-damaged sweet potatoes, on bovine lung. Vet Pathol 1978, 15: 367–75.
Peckham JC, Mitchell FE, Jones OH, Doupnik B. Atypical interstitial pneumonia in cattle fed moldy sweet potatoes. J Am Vet Med Assoc 1972, 160: 169–72.
Riet-Correa F, Rivero R, Odriozola, et al. Mycotoxicoses in ruminants and horses. J Vet Diagn Invest 2013, 25: 692–708.
Author Jennifer S. Taintor
Consulting Editor Christopher C.L. Chase
Acknowledgment The author and book editors acknowledge the prior contribution of Kristy Cortright.

S

TEASER PREPARATION

BASICS

OVERVIEW
• Estrus detection is an essential part of any artificial breeding program (AI or ET) in ruminant production systems.
• Heat detection inefficiency is one of the major contributing factors to poor reproductive performance, particularly in dairy animals.
• Teaser animals are used to aid in estrus detection.

INCIDENCE/PREVALENCE
N/A

GEOGRAPHIC DISTRIBUTION
Worldwide

SYSTEMS AFFECTED
Reproductive

PATHOPHYSIOLOGY
• Preparation of teaser aims to increase heat detection efficiency without risk of impregnation.
• Although male sexual behavior may be obtained in females and castrated males through injection of testosterone (i.e., androgenized heifers or steers), this technique is being abandoned to reduce use of hormones in production animals.
• When intact males are used, pregnancy is prevented by eliminating the possibility of full erection, intromission, or ejaculation of viable spermatozoa.
• Vaginal intromission can be prevented mechanically by the use of aprons (small ruminants) or surgically by translocation of the penis and prepuce (penile deviation), penectomy, or penopexy. Erection may also be prevented by injecting an acrylic substance into the corpus cavernosum muscle or creation of a preputial stenosis.
• Ejaculation of viable spermatozoa is eliminated by vasectomy, epididymectomy, or intratesticular injection of a sclerotic agent.
• The combination of vasectomy and penile translocation is the most recommended technique in order to prevent disease transmission and eliminate the risk of pregnancy associated with accidental vaginal intromission.

HISTORICAL FINDINGS
N/A

SIGNALMENT
• Young postpubertal male with good libido.
• Hormone-treated animals can be heifers (usually freemartin), cull cows, or steers.

PHYSICAL EXAMINATION FINDINGS
Animal should be healthy with normal reproductive development.

GENETICS
N/A

CAUSES AND RISK FACTORS
N/A

DIAGNOSIS

DIFFERENTIAL DIAGNOSES
N/A

CBC/BIOCHEMISTRY/URINALYSIS
Total protein and packed cell volume should be determined prior to anesthesia (penile translocation).

OTHER LABORATORY TESTS
Testing for contagious diseases

IMAGING
N/A

OTHER DIAGNOSTIC PROCEDURES
N/A

PATHOLOGIC FINDINGS
N/A

TREATMENT

THERAPEUTIC APPROACH
• Hormone-treated heifers and steers
  ◦ Testosterone enanthate 500 mg IM and 1,500 mg SC, then 1,000 mg every 2 weeks (estrus detection varies 40–60%).
  ◦ Synovex H implants (200 mg testosterone propionate and 20 mg estradiol benzoate, one implant per 100 lb body weight), response rate about 80% and lasts about 6 months.

SURGICAL CONSIDERATIONS AND TECHNIQUES
• Epididymectomy
  ◦ Performed on standing animal in the chute for bulls and in sitting position for sheep and goats.
  ◦ Sedation is not necessary in bulls but is helpful in small ruminants.
  ◦ Local block is applied at the skin incision site. There are two variants of the technique based on the site of skin incision, which can be at the base of the scrotum over the tail of the epididymis or higher with the testis pushed dorsally to expose the tail of the epididymis.
  ◦ A 3 cm incision is made through the scrotal skin and the vaginal tunic to expose the cauda epididymis.
  ◦ The proper ligament of the epididymis is identified and absorbable suture material is passed through in such a way that the tail of the epididymis is ligated at two sites 2 cm apart and the section is transected.
  ◦ The skin incision may be left open.
• Translocation of the penis and penis
  ◦ The technique can be performed in the field under injectable anesthesia. The animal

is placed in slightly tilted dorsal recumbency with the left side slightly extended.
  ◦ The ventral abdomen from the umbilicus to the scrotum and the left lower flank is clipped and prepared for surgery. Care must be taken to thoroughly clean the preputial cavity with dilute iodophor.
  ◦ A catheter is placed as deep as possible within the prepuce and held with towel clamps at the preputial orifice.
  ◦ A 4 cm circular skin incision is made around the preputial orifice and extending caudally on midline to the sigmoid flexure. Mark the proximal part of the preputial orifice with a stay suture to avoid disorientation.
  ◦ The penis within its prepuce is dissected away from the body wall using combined blunt dissection and incision with scissors after ligation of any major blood vessels. It is important to dissect just enough to allow separation of the prepuce and avoid formation of a large dead space.
  ◦ A circular skin incision, slightly smaller than the removed preputial orifice skin, is made just above the flank fold. The site for the incision can be gauged by deviating the dissected prepuce at a 45° angle.
  ◦ The circular flank incision is joined to the midline incision near the base of the penis by tunneling under the skin with a long forceps (Knowles cervical forceps).
  ◦ A sterile sleeve is passed through the formed tunnel and the prepuce is passed through it such that the preputial orifice is brought to the circular skin incision and sutured in place in a simple interrupted pattern.
  ◦ The ventral midline incision is sutured using a Ford interlocking pattern.
• Preputial stenosis
  ◦ This technique is not as common as the previously described techniques and consists of creating a stenosis of the prepuce by placing a purse-string suture circumventing the prepuce and burring it subcutaneously, or by placing a stainless steel ring around an isolated section of the prepuce.
• Penile fixation
  ◦ The surgery is done with the animal sedated, placed in lateral recumbency, and local anesthesia is performed at the surgical site.
  ◦ A 10 cm longitudinal incision through the skin, subcutaneous tissue, and cutaneous trunci muscle is made midway between the preputial opening and the base of the scrotum at the junction of the sheath and the body wall.
  ◦ Blunt dissection is required to locate the dorsal surface of the penis.
  ◦ The penis is exteriorized and its elastic tunics from its dorsal surface are cleared from the preputial reflection to approximately 10 cm caudal.

T

TEASER PREPARATION   (CONTINUED)

○ The linea alba should then be cleared of all loose connective tissue.

○ At least three simple interrupted sutures 1–2 cm apart are then placed through the tunica albuginea on the dorsal surface of the penis and the linea alba using nonabsorbable suture material. Care should be taken to avoid the urethra during suture placement.

○ The skin incision is then closed with nonabsorbable suture material.

MEDICATIONS

DRUGS OF CHOICE
• Sedation and analgesia: Xylazine (0.1 mg/kg body weight IV for bulls; 0.1 mg/kg IM for goats; 0.2 mg/kg for sheep) and ketamine (0.2 mg/kg for bulls; 3–5 mg/kg IM in sheep and goats) and local infiltration of lidocaine or bupivacaine.
• Postsurgical anti-inflammatories: Flunixin meglumine.
• Antibiotic therapy: Procaine penicillin G, 22,000 IU/kg for 5 days) is recommended following penile deviation or fixation.

CONTRAINDICATIONS
Appropriate meat withdrawal times should be followed for all compounds administered to food-producing animals.

PRECAUTIONS
N/A

POSSIBLE INTERACTIONS
N/A

FOLLOW-UP

EXPECTED COURSE AND PROGNOSIS
• Animal should be fasted (small ruminant 24 hours, bulls 24–48 hours) prior to surgery
• Suture are removed 14 days after surgery.
• Vasectomized or epididymectomized males should undergo semen collection and evaluation 2–3 weeks after surgery to make sure that there are no viable spermatozoa in the ejaculate.
• Teasers may be used 4 weeks after penile translocation.

POSSIBLE COMPLICATIONS
• Local infection, adhesions, and formation of sperm granuloma are possible after caudectomy.
• Seroma, abscess, and dehiscence of the surgical site in penile translocation if aseptic technique is not observed.
• Urine accumulation and preputial eversion may occur in penile deviation if preputial swelling is excessive.
• Insufficient retraction or suture breakdown may be experienced after penile fixation technique.

CLIENT EDUCATION
• Welfare issues regarding some techniques.
• Some animals (small ruminants in particular) may still be able to penetrate after penile translocation, particularly if the surgery is performed at young age.
• The duration of service of a teaser animal varies.

PATIENT CARE
• Sexual rest for 3 weeks
• Antibiotic and anti-inflammatory therapy as indicated
• Semen collection and evaluation prior to use for heat detection

PREVENTION
Vaccination against clostridial diseases or administration of tetanus antitoxin and tetanus toxoid at the time of surgery.

MISCELLANEOUS

ASSOCIATED CONDITIONS
N/A

AGE-RELATED FACTORS
N/A

ZOONOTIC POTENTIAL
N/A

PREGNANCY
N/A

BIOSECURITY
• Males to be used as teasers should be free of contagious diseases and selected from known herds or flocks.

• It is preferable to use animals from within the herd.

PRODUCTION MANAGEMENT
• The useful life of the teaser male is longer with vasectomy and penile deviation in the author's experience.
• Performance of the teaser should be monitored as some procedures are associated with loss of libido.
• Bulls used as teasers should not be kept for a long time as they become more and more difficult to handle, particularly in a dairy operation.

SYNONYMS
• Gomer bull, marker
• Estrus detector male

ABBREVIATIONS
• IM = intramuscular
• IV = intravenous
• SC = subcutaneous

SEE ALSO
• Castration/Vasectomy: Bovine
• Castration/Vasectomy: Small Ruminant

Suggested Reading
Aanes WA, Rupp G. Iatrogenic preputial stenosis in preparation of teaser bull. J Am Vet Med Assoc 1984; 184: 1474–6.
Riddell GM. Prevention of intromission by estrus-detector males. In. Wolfe DF, Moll HD eds, Large Animal Urogenital Surgery. Philadelphia: Williams & Wilkins, 1999, pp. 335–44.
Tibary A, Pearson LK, Van Metre DC, et al. Surgery of the sheep and goat reproductive system and urinary tract. In: Fubini S, Ducharme N eds, Farm Animal Surgery, 2nd ed. St. Louis: Elsevier, 2016, pp. 571–9.
Wolfe DF, Powe TA, Push DG. Surgical preparation of estrus detector males. In: Wolfe DF, Moll HD eds, Large Animal Urogenital Surgery. Philadelphia: Williams & Wilkins, 1999, pp. 327–34.

Author Ahmed Tibary
Consulting Editor Ahmed Tibary
Acknowledgment The author and book editors acknowledge the prior contribution of Loren G. Schultz.

T

TEAT LACERATIONS

BASICS

OVERVIEW
• Teat lacerations are most often a result of step-on injury by the animal herself or an adjacent animal.
• The prognosis for laceration repair depends on whether the laceration is partial thickness or full thickness, involving the streak canal, teat sinus, or gland sinus. Prognosis also depends on location, size, and direction of the laceration, degree of tissue loss, age of laceration, and degree of contamination.
• Longitudinal lacerations have a more favorable prognosis because the blood supply flows from the base of the teat towards the apex. Proximal lacerations heal better because perfusion is better closer to the base of the teat.
• Improper healing of teat injuries can result in scar tissue formation, teat obstruction, tcat fistulas, and ultimately loss of the quarter.
• Mastitis is a common sequela of teat laceration especially if it is full thickness.
• The teat is composed of five layers: internal mucosa, submucosa, connective tissue and blood vessels, muscular layer (circular and longitudinal layers), and external squamous epithelium.
• The teat cistern is contained within the teat, the distal opening of which is the rosette of Furstenberg, which leads to the streak canal and teat sphincter. If the streak canal or gland sinus is involved in the laceration, the prognosis for adequate return to function is guarded.
• The teat in general has good blood perfusion so the age of the laceration is not as critical. Lacerations up to 12 hours old are candidates for primary repair. For older lacerations delayed primary closure should be considered.

INCIDENCE/PREVALENCE
N/A

GEOGRAPHIC DISTRIBUTION
N/A

SYSTEMS AFFECTED
• Integument
• Mammary

PATHOPHYSIOLOGY
Wound healing can be divided into three phases: inflammation, proliferation, and maturation/remodeling. The first phase involves influx of white blood cells and inflammatory mediators as well as fibrin clot formation. Proliferation involves granulation tissue formation and epithelialization. Wound remodeling begins after 2 weeks, which is the final stage.

HISTORICAL FINDINGS
History of trauma. Duration is important in determining primary vs. secondary closure.

SIGNALMENT
• Any female ruminant (cattle, sheep, and goats can be affected).
• Dairy cows more likely to be affected than beef cows.
• Animals with large or pendulous udders more commonly affected.

PHYSICAL EXAMINATION FINDINGS
• Teat edema
• Teat hemorrhage
• Milk leakage through teat wall
• Pain
• Bloody milk
• Mastitis

GENETICS
Dairy cattle and goats with poor udder conformation and high milk production will be predisposed to teat lacerations due to their pendulous udder.

CAUSES AND RISK FACTORS
• Self-trauma
• External trauma
• Pendulous or large udders

DIAGNOSIS

DIFFERENTIAL DIAGNOSES
• Mastitis can cause swelling of the teat and/or discoloration, bloody milk without obvious external trauma.
• Teat spiders, webs, and scar tissue can cause swelling and obstruction, but do not have associated bleeding or laceration.
• Teat fistulas cause leaking milk, but without associated traumatized tissue.
• Gangrenous mastitis causes swelling, discoloration, and bleeding, but is progressive and often generalized.

CBC/BIOCHEMISTRY/URINALYSIS
N/A

OTHER LABORATORY TESTS
• California Mastitis Test (CMT) may indicate increased somatic cell count if mastitis is present.
• Milk culture may show bacterial growth if mastitis is present secondary to laceration.

IMAGING
Ultrasound of teat may be helpful to differentiate laceration from other causes.

OTHER DIAGNOSTIC PROCEDURES
Theloscopy can be used to locate and differentiate lesions inside the teat.

PATHOLOGIC FINDINGS
N/A

TREATMENT

THERAPEUTIC APPROACH
• Surgical repair is recommended for a good prognosis.
• Teat must be thoroughly cleaned and evaluated for tissue viability, blood supply, extent of injury.
• Systemic administration of antibiotics is rarely indicated.

SURGICAL CONSIDERATIONS AND TECHNIQUES
• The wound margins should be carefully debrided and rinsed with physiologic saline solution. Any necrotic tissue should be meticulously debrided, but due to the small quantity of the teat tissue, preservation of as much tissue is encouraged to facilitate laceration closure.
• After adequate sedation, an anesthetic ring block with 2% lidocaine around the base of the teat (avoiding the circumferential vein and the teat and gland cistern) should be performed. Alternatively, a caudal epidural can be performed in lieu of the ring block or in addition to it.
• The animal is easiest to work on when restrained in lateral or dorsal recumbency. A tourniquet may be placed around the base of the teat to reduce bleeding and milk flow into the lacerated area during repair. The repair should be performed as aseptically as possible.
• Surgical repair of full thickness lacerations should be in three layers. The submucosa and intermediate layers are closed separately with a continuous horizontal mattress pattern that does not perforate the mucosa. A 3-0 or 4-0 absorbable monofilament suture on a swaged-on tapered needle should be used. The skin should be closed with a 3-0 or 4-0 monofilament suture using a simple interrupted suture pattern.
• Partial thickness lacerations are closed in two layers similar to full thickness repair outlined above, with omission of the first layer in the submucosa.
• Passive drainage using a teat cannula is recommended every other day followed by infusion of intramammary antibiotics every 4 days for 10 days in total. Refer to AMDUCA and FARAD for regulations and withholding times related to off-label use of antimicrobials in food-producing species.
• Tissue adhesives and glue should be avoided in repair due to the inflammatory reaction they can elicit.

T

MEDICATIONS

DRUGS OF CHOICE
• Sedation with acepromazine
 ○ Cattle and goats: 0.05–0.1 mg/kg IV
 ○ Sheep: 0.03–0.05 mg/kg IV
• Xylazine can be used to sedate ruminants at the following doses:
 ○ Goats: 0.05 mg/kg IV or 0.1 mg/kg IM
 ○ Sheep 0.1–0.2 mg/kg IV or 0.2–0.3 mg/kg IM
 ○ Cattle 0.1 mg/kg IV or 0.2 mg/kg IM
 ○ Recumbency will be induced for approximately 1 hour. Low dose xylazine (0.015–0.025 mg/kg IV or IM) will provide sedation without recumbency in ruminants.
• Flunixin meglumine (1.1–2.2 mg/kg IV) can be used at the time of repair, but is rarely necessary after the initial dose.

CONTRAINDICATIONS
• Appropriate milk and meat withdrawal times must be followed for all compounds administered to food-producing animals.
• Acepromazine has been reported to cause sloughing of the tail if inadvertently administered into the coccygeal artery, and therefore care should be taken when administering in the coccygeal vein.

FOLLOW-UP

EXPECTED COURSE AND PROGNOSIS
• Healing should be complete in 10–14 days.
• Prognosis is better with partial thickness lacerations than full thickness lacerations.
• See "Overview" for more details regarding prognostic factors.

POSSIBLE COMPLICATIONS
• Teat fistula formation can occur anywhere along the repair line. Fistulas should be allowed to heal for 3–4 weeks before surgical repair is attempted. Full thickness repair should be performed again in the region of the fistula, following resection of the fistula.
• Mastitis is likely, and should be treated appropriately, avoiding intramammary infusions if possible.

CLIENT EDUCATION
Instill the importance of prompt attention to teat lacerations to dairy workers so that wounds will have a better outcome. Also work with management on culling decisions due to poor udder conformation.

PATIENT CARE
• Laceration should be monitored daily for signs of repair breakdown.
• Suture removal at 7–10 days after surgery.

PREVENTION
• Avoid overcrowding cows or other ruminants.
• Ensure good footing for the animals.
• Animals with pendulous udders may require separate housing or culling.
• Ensure that free stalls are wide enough for easy rising.
• Monitor the length of the medial dew claw(s) as overgrowth can result in teat or udder injury.

MISCELLANEOUS

ASSOCIATED CONDITIONS
None

AGE-RELATED FACTORS
Older cows and does may be more prone due to increased udder size and pendulous nature.

ABBREVIATIONS
• AMDUCA = Animal Medicinal Drug Use Clarification Act
• CMT = California Mastitis Test
• FARAD = Food Animal Residue Avoidance Databank (FARAD) (see www.fiveminutevet.com/ruminant)
• IV = intravenous

SEE ALSO
• Mastitis (multiple chapters)
• Ultrasonography: Mammary
• Wound Management

Suggested Reading
Hull BL. Teat and udder surgery. Vet Clin North Am Food Anim Pract 1995, 11: 1–17.
Steiner A. Teat surgery. In: Fubini SL, Ducharme NG eds, Farm Animal Surgery. St. Louis: Elsevier, 2004.
Turner AS, McIlwraith CW, Hull BL. Repair of teat lacerations. In: Turner AS, McIlwraith CW eds, Techniques in Large Animal Surgery, 2nd ed. Malvern, PA: Lea & Febiger, 1989.
Author Troy E.C. Holder
Consulting Editor Kaitlyn A. Lutz
Acknowledgment The author and book editors acknowledge the prior contribution of Jennifer M. Ivany Ewoldt.

T

BASICS

OVERVIEW
• Teat lesions result from traumatic, milking machine, environmental, infectious, or chemical insults that injure teat skin, dermis, or mucosa resulting in lactation difficulties.
• Mastitis may result if there is penetration and compromise of the teat sinus or external sphincter.

INCIDENCE/PREVALENCE
• More common in animals with the genetic characteristics described under "Genetics."
• Increased incidence can be seen with infectious epidemics, abrupt milking system malfunction, or changes in milking practices.
• Higher prevalence with adverse environmental conditions (close confinement, freezing temperatures, traumatic rough terrain, flies) and higher parity.

GEOGRAPHIC DISTRIBUTION
Worldwide

SYSTEMS AFFECTED
• Integument
• Mammary

PATHOPHYSIOLOGY
• Teat lesions damage the physiologic barriers of the teat skin, wall, and sphincter.
• Loss of barrier integrity can cause the teat and gland sinuses to leak milk and/or allow entry of pathogens into the mammary sinuses resulting in mastitis.
• Teat end lesions usually do not contribute to mastitis unless the lesions are severe.

HISTORICAL FINDINGS
• Reluctance to be nursed or milked.
• Poor milk letdown and reduced production.
• Known trauma, mastitis event, or recent environmental changes may be noted.

SIGNALMENT
Lactating animals

PHYSICAL EXAMINATION FINDINGS
• Teat inflammation (swelling, edema, redness).
• Fever, anorexia, recumbency (secondary mastitis, bacterial sepsis).
• Vesicles, papules, or scabs.
• Bleeding or laceration.
• Teat end hyperkeratosis or sphincter eversion.
• Stamping of feet, brushing udder with hind legs.
• In chronic cases, there is mammary gland atrophy.

GENETICS
• Traits associated with teat lesions include cylindrical teat shape (opposed to funnel-shaped), long teats, disk-shaped external sphincter shape (opposed to round), large and pendulous udders, teat placement and angle of the udder (teats more easily

stepped on), and suspensory ligament breakdown.
• Slow milkers and high-producing animals also have higher incidence of teat lesions.

CAUSES AND RISK FACTORS
Environmental
• Blunt trauma (stepped-on teats)
• Laceration (wire, brambles, other sharp objects)
• Cold (frostbitten and chapped teats)
• Photodermatitis (sunburn)
• Chemicals (defective or inappropriate teat dips or lime from floors and stalls)
• Milking machine trauma (overmilking and excessive vacuum pressure)
• Insects (teat atresia from *Haematobia irritans irritans*—the horn fly)

Infectious Agents
• Pseudocowpox
• Vesicular stomatitis
• Foot and mouth disease virus
• Bovine viral diarrhea
• Bovine malignant catarrhal fever
• Cowpox
• Bovine herpes virus 2
• Vaccinia virus
• Bovine papillomavirus

Mycotoxins
• *Aspergillus* spp.
• *Fusarium* spp.
• *Anacystis* spp.
• *Pithomyces chartarum*

Corpora Amylacea Photosensitization
Plants
• *Ammi majus* (bishop's weed, greater ammi)
• *Cooperia pedunculata* (rain lily)
• *Cymopterus watsonii* (spring parsley)
• *Fagopyrum esculentum* (buckwheat)
• *Heracleum mantegazzianum* (giant hog weed)
• *Hypericum perforatum* (St. John's wort)
• *Thamnosma texana* (Dutchman's breeches)
• *Brassica* spp. (kale)
• *Lantana camara* (lantana)
• *Senecio* spp. (ragwort)
• *Amsinckia* spp. (fiddleneck)
• *Panicum* spp. (millet)

Chemicals
• Phenothiazines
• Thiazides
• Acriflavines
• Rose Bengal
• Methylene blue
• Sulfonamides
• Tetracycline

DIAGNOSIS

DIFFERENTIAL DIAGNOSES
Pseudocowpox, vesicular stomatitis, foot and mouth disease, bovine viral diarrhea, bovine malignant catarrhal fever, cowpox, bovine herpes virus 2, bovine papillomavirus,

environmental causes (see "Causes and Risk Factors/Environmental"), and photosensitization from ingestion of various plants, chemicals, or mycotoxins.

CBC/BIOCHEMISTRY/URINALYSIS
N/A

OTHER LABORATORY TESTS
N/A

IMAGING
Endoscopy and ultrasonography may be useful to assess cause and prognosis of milk flow hindrance.

OTHER DIAGNOSTIC PROCEDURES
• Dependent upon visualization and palpation.
• Milk culture prior to antibiotic treatment may be helpful to combat secondary mastitis.

PATHOLOGIC FINDINGS
• Lacerations, swelling, hemorrhage, sphincter eversion, teat end hyperkeratosis, vesicles, papules, necrotic skin, and/or cracks.
• Scarring with lumen narrowing.

TREATMENT

THERAPEUTIC APPROACH
Milking
• Discontinuing machine milking of affected teat(s) will speed healing by reducing manipulation-associated trauma (milk retrieved with a cannula).
• Culling may be considered in severe cases with refractory mastitis.

Chapped or Sunburned Teats
• Provide shade and apply topical emollients approved for use in lactating cattle (mineral oil, glycerin, or lanolin).
• Teats should be dried after milking.

Frostbite, Virus Infection, and Teat End Trauma
• Preventing mastitis while keeping the teat duct patent may require teat dilators, cannulas, and intramammary or parenteral antimicrobials.
• For teat end lesions caused by the above conditions, using teat dips containing antiseptics such as chlorhexidine, iodophors, and bleach can reduce secondary mastitis.
• Keep teats dry and cows comfortable.

SURGICAL CONSIDERATIONS AND TECHNIQUES
Lacerations
• Surgical correction is appropriate depending on the severity and post-trauma interval.
• Fresh lacerations (<12 hours) with adequate blood supply may be closed with two-layer everting mucosa and skin/muscle sutures.
• Older lacerations warrant cleansing and removal of the skin flap followed by second intention healing with granulation.
• Teats should be bandaged if feasible.

T

TEAT LESIONS   (CONTINUED)

MEDICATIONS

DRUGS OF CHOICE

Antibiotics
• Systemic antibiotics are generally not warranted. Care must be taken in regard to milk contamination if a topical antibiotic is used.
• Refer to specific mastitis pathogen chapters for treatment protocols in the case that mastitis develops secondary to teat lesions.

Teat Dips
• Iodophor solutions: 0.5–1% available iodine
• Hypochlorite solutions: 4% free chlorine
• Chlorhexidine solutions: 0.3%

Emollients
• Glycerin: 15–30%
• Mineral oil
• Lanolin

CONTRAINDICATIONS
N/A

PRECAUTIONS
Appropriate milk and meat withdrawal times must be followed for all compounds administered to food-producing animals.

POSSIBLE INTERACTIONS
N/A

FOLLOW-UP

EXPECTED COURSE AND PROGNOSIS
Common adverse sequelae of severe lesions are teat sphincter scarring and obstruction with integrity loss and resultant mastitis.

POSSIBLE COMPLICATIONS
• Loss of quarter and decreased milk production for permanently damaged teat
• Mastitis
• Reduced milk intake in suckling offspring

CLIENT EDUCATION
• Severe acute teat end lesions are serious injuries with resultant mixed-pathogen mastitis and granulation/canal stenosis.
• Aseptic technique, canal dilation, and appropriate antimicrobial withdrawal times will benefit the patient.

PATIENT CARE
• Aseptic milking techniques will reduce the incidence of mastitis.
• House animals on clean, dry bedding and away from suckling calves and other sources of teat trauma.
• Teat sphincter integrity should be monitored as inflammation subsides and possible granulation ensues.
• Monitoring body temperature, milk consistency, CMT testing, and milk cultures for mastitis.

PREVENTION
• House cows in clean areas with ample space and protection from the elements.
• Practice sound milking hygiene techniques.
• Keep lots, pastures, and fences well maintained and free of debris.
• Use approved fly control.
• Genetically select for desirable udder and teat conformation.

MISCELLANEOUS

ASSOCIATED CONDITIONS
Mastitis, contact dermatitis, loss of productivity

AGE-RELATED FACTORS
Teat lesions increase with parity

ZOONOTIC POTENTIAL
• No zoonotic potential unless caused by cowpox or pseudocowpox virus.
• Gloves should be worn when dealing with suspect or infected animals.

ABBREVIATION
CMT = California Mastitis Test

SEE ALSO
• *Brassica* spp. Toxicity
• Mastitis (specific chapters)
• Photosensitization
• Pseudocowpox
• St. John's Wort Toxicity
• Teat Lacerations

Suggested Reading
Chrystal MA, Seykora AJ, Hansen LB. Heritabilities of teat end shape and teat diameter and their relationship with somatic cell score. J Dairy Sci 1999, 82: 2017–22.
Farnsworth RJ. Observations on teat end lesions. Bov Pract 1995, 29: 89–92.
Osteras O, Ronningen O, Sandvik L, Waage S. Field studies show associations between pulsator characteristics and udder health. J Dairy Res 1995, 62: 1–13.
Rasmussen MD, Madsen NP. Effects of milkline vacuum, pulsator airline vacuum, and cluster weight on milk yield, teat condition, and udder health. J Dairy Sci 2000, 83: 77–84.
Wellenberg GJ, van der Poel WHM, Van Oirschot JT. Viral infections and bovine mastitis: a review. Vet Microbiol 2002, 88: 27–45.
Author Michael Goedken
Consulting Editor Kaitlyn A. Lutz

T

TERATOGENS

 BASICS

OVERVIEW
• A teratogenic is an agent that, on fetal exposure, can alter fetal morphology or subsequent function.
• Teratogens include chemicals, infectious agents, nutritional deficiencies, toxic plants, or physical condition.
• The effects of exposure are not limited to concentration. The timing of exposure during gestation, length of exposure, and concentration of teratogen are all important.
• Teratogenicity depends upon the ability of the agent to cross the placenta.

INCIDENCE/PREVALENCE
• Specific incidence is difficult to determine.
• Occurrence follows seasonal patterns associated with growth characteristics of toxic plants or population dynamics of vectors.

GEOGRAPHIC DISTRIBUTION
Worldwide for some common teratogens. Others are limited to specific regions.

SYSTEMS AFFECTED
• Cardiovascular
• Musculoskeletal
• Nervous
• Ophthalmic
• Reproductive
• Urinary

PATHOPHYSIOLOGY
• The zygote is particularly resilient to the effects of teratogens.
• The embryo is most susceptible to teratogenic agents during periods of rapid differentiation. This susceptibility declines with time, as the embryo becomes more developed. The same trend is seen throughout fetal development (the more developed the fetus, the more resilient it is to the effects of teratogens). While this is generally true, certain structures differentiate relatively late in fetal development. These structures include the cerebellum, palate, and parts of the urinary and reproductive system, which are prone to congenital defects.
• Teratogens affect fetal development by causing abnormal differentiation or specific lesions in developing organs or by limiting fetal development through other mechanisms, such as reduction of motion (e.g., lupine toxicosis).

HISTORICAL FINDINGS
• Increased incidence of pregnancy loss or abortion
• Increased incidence of fetal or neonatal abnormalities
• Stillbirth or neonatal mortality
• History of exposure to teratogen

• Previous occurrence in the herd associated with specific pasture or reproductive management (breeding season).

SIGNALMENT
• Pregnant cows, ewes, and does of any age and breed with a history of exposure to a teratogen.
• Neonates, stillborn or aborted fetuses with developmental abnormalities.

PHYSICAL EXAMINATION FINDINGS
• Physical examination of the dam is often unremarkable.
• Examination of live neonates may show various abnormalities. The most obvious are hydranencephaly, microphthalmia, and arthrogryposis.

GENETICS
Teratogen susceptibility can vary among genotypes within the same species, and possessing certain genes may make the developing animal more susceptible to the effect of a teratogen.

CAUSES AND RISK FACTORS

Nutritional
• Vitamin A deficiency—defects in eye development or harelip.
• Vitamin E/selenium deficiency—white muscle disease in neonates (rarely a cause of abortion), deficiency must be severe to induce white muscle disease in fetus.
• Vitamin D deficiency—neonatal rickets.
• Copper deficiency—dystrophic myelination of spinal cord (enzootic swayback in lambs).
• Iodine deficiency—congenital goiter.

Endocrine
• Polycyclic aromatic hydrocarbons—formed from incomplete combustion of organic material, these compounds have a steric resemblance to steroids. They have been shown to affect serum progesterone (P4), estrogen (E2), prolactin, and luteinizing hormone (LH) and are teratogenic in rats. Livestock are exposed via contaminated water, air, soil, and forages.
• Polychlorinated biphenyls—PCBs are used in hydraulic fluid, plastics, and lubricants. They accumulate in the environment and in fatty tissues and act as synthetic endocrine disruptors with high affinity for estrogen receptors. They may impair normal ovulation and blastocyst implantation. In an experimental rabbit model, PCB exposure induced embryo toxicity and pregnancy loss. Animals may become exposed by ingesting contaminated feed and water.
• Organochlorines (DDT)—chlorinated hydrocarbon used as an insecticide. It can persist for long periods and can be absorbed orally or topically. It is an endocrine disruptor with estrogenic like effects resulting in impaired fertility and pregnancy losses.

• Zearalenone—abnormal fetal development due to estrogenic properties of zearalenone.
• Phytoestrogens—biologically active nonsteroidal plant compounds that are similar in structure to mammalian estrogen and can compete for estrogen receptors. They are found in legumes (alfalfa, soybeans, red clover, subterranean clover, white clover, and alsike clover). Concentrations in plants may increase under cool and wet condition or with stressors such as fungal infection or insect infestation. High concentrations of phytoestrogens can cause cystic ovaries, infertility, and impaired pregnancy maintenance. Also cause decreased lambing rates in ewes due to decreased ovulation rates.
• Bisphenol-A/Bisphenol-S (BPA, BPS)—endocrine disruptor effect results in intrauterine growth restriction, also may negatively affect Leydig cell production of insulin like peptide 3 (INSL3) which is required for testicular descent and therefore may play a role in cryptorchidism.

Drugs
• Acepromazine—fetal CNS depression near term.
• Aminoglycosides—nephrotoxicity in fetus.
• Antifungals—deformation of facial bones, eye, and CNS in cats and rats.
• Atropine—may produce fetal tachycardia.
• Corticosteroids—fetal articular cartilage defects and increased incidence of cleft palate.
• Diazepam—associated with congenital defects in humans, rats, and mice in the first trimester.
• Dimethylsulfoxide (DMSO)—teratogenic in laboratory animals, not advised for use in pregnant animals.
• Sulfonamides—congenital defects reported in rats and mice. Long-acting sulfonamides may antagonize folate (required for neural tube development) and also induce bone marrow suppression.
• Tetracyclines—can induce bone and teeth malformations as well as dental staining in the fetus.

Plants
• *Veratrum californicum* (cyclopamine)—cyclopic malformation in lambs when exposed at day 14 of gestation. Pituitary hypoplasia and prolonged gestation. Embryo death when exposed at days 19–21. Cleft palate when exposed on gestational days 24–30. Metacarpal and metatarsal defects at gestational days 28–31. Ingestion by cows during days 12–30 may cause cleft palate, brachygnathia, syndactyly, decreased number of coccygeal vertebrae.
• *Astragalus* spp. and *Oxytropis* spp. (toxin not identified)—brachygnathia, contracture or overextension of joints, limb rotations, osteoporosis.

T

TERATOGENS

• Lupines (anagyrine and ammodendrine)—maternal ingestion at days 40–70 of gestation results in fetal malformations ("crooked calf syndrome") including arthrogryposis, scoliosis, torticollis, lordosis, kyphosis, or palatoschisis (cleft palate).
• Poison hemlock (*Conium maculatum*; piperidine alkaloids, esp. coniine). Maternal ingestion at days 40–70 of gestation results in fetal malformations including arthrogryposis, scoliosis, torticollis, lordosis, kyphosis, palatoschisis (cleft palate), and excessive flexure of carpal joints.
• Tobacco (*Nicotiana* spp.; piperidine alkaloid, anabasine). Maternal ingestion at 30–60 days of gestation can induce fetal skeletal malformations including arthrogryposis, palatoschisis, torticollis, lordosis, and kyphosis.

Viruses

• Border disease (Pestivirus)—cerebellar hypoplasia, hydrocephalus, hydranencephaly, porencephaly, aberrant hair growth (hair instead of wool) in lambs (may also affect kids).
• Akabane virus (Bunyaviridae)—causes fetal malformations in cattle, sheep, and goats. Arthrogryposis, hydranencephaly, porencephaly, hydrocephalus, cerebellar hypoplasia.
• Schmallenberg virus (Orthobunyavirus)—teratogenic effects in cattle, sheep, and goats include scoliosis, hydrocephalus, arthrogryposis, cerebellar hypoplasia, and an enlarged thymus.
• Bovine viral diarrhea virus—midgestation infections (3–6 months) can cause congenital defects including microophthalmia, microencephaly, brachygnathia, cerebellar hypoplasia, hydranencephaly, hydrocephalus, thymic hypoplasia, cataracts, retinal dysplasia, and optic neuritis.
• Bluetongue virus (Orbivirus)—most severe in sheep but affects many wild and domestic ruminants. Exposure at 40–60 days of gestation usually results in abortion but may see hydranencephaly and retinal dysplasia if fetus survives. Infection at 60–100 days of gestation, exposure results in porencephaly.
• Cache Valley virus (Bunyavirus)—mostly affects sheep. Arthrogryposis, scoliosis, torticollis, hypoplastic musculature, hydranencephaly, hydrocephalus, porencephaly, microencephaly, cerebellar and cerebral hypoplasia.
• Wesselbron virus (Flavivirus)—affects sheep and goats. Neurotropic virus causing necrosis of fetal CNS. Segmental aplasia of spinal cord, hydranencephaly, hydrocephalus, porencephaly, cerebellar hypoplasia, arthrogryposis, brachygnathia.

DIAGNOSIS

DIFFERENTIAL DIAGNOSES
Numerous causes and risk factors (see "Causes and Risk Factors") can result in similar developmental malformations. Differential diagnosis is established by epidemiologic, laboratory investigation.

CBC/BIOCHEMISTRY/URINALYSIS
May be indicated in the dam depending on teratogen exposure.

OTHER LABORATORY TESTS
• Virus isolation (dam), precolostral serology in neonates
• Feed/Water analysis
• Liver biopsy for toxins

IMAGING
N/A

OTHER DIAGNOSTIC PROCEDURES
• Clinical signs, history of exposure/ingestion, finding evidence of exposure/ingestion can be key to diagnosis.
• Epidemiologic data and records analysis.

PATHOLOGIC FINDINGS
Developmental malformations associated with the causes and risk factors can be seen and evaluated on necropsy.

TREATMENT

THERAPEUTIC APPROACH
Live affected neonates with severe abnormalities should be humanely euthanized.

SURGICAL CONSIDERATIONS AND TECHNIQUES
N/A

MEDICATIONS

DRUGS OF CHOICE
N/A

CONTRAINDICATIONS
N/A

POSSIBLE INTERACTIONS
N/A

FOLLOW-UP

EXPECTED COURSE AND PROGNOSIS
• Most cases are discovered after the fact (abortion or birth of fetuses with multiple defects).

• Some infectious causes may require culling of animals that may become potentially shedders.
• If multiple animals are affected, a proper investigation protocol, involving several specialists and laboratory backup, should be set.
• Some infectious diseases are notifiable.

POSSIBLE COMPLICATIONS
• Severe fetal abnormalities may result in abortion or dystocia.
• Developmental malformations/birth defects may result in death or poor quality of life.

CLIENT EDUCATION
• Report abnormalities, stillbirths, and abortions to attending veterinarians.
• Recognize the major regional toxic plants and monitor pastures.

PATIENT CARE
• Remove from source of toxin.
• Neonates with severe developmental abnormalities may need to be euthanized.

PREVENTION
• Limit exposure to teratogens during pregnancy.
• Appropriate adjustment of nutrition to address deficiencies.
• Pasture management or modification of the breeding season to avoid exposure at critical times of pregnancy in cases of toxic plants.
• Biosecurity and preventive measures for infectious causes.

MISCELLANEOUS

ASSOCIATED CONDITIONS
Pregnancy complication

AGE-RELATED FACTORS
N/A

ZOONOTIC POTENTIAL
N/A

PREGNANCY
See "Causes and Risk Factors"

BIOSECURITY
• Mostly applicable to infectious causes. Quarantine, testing, and vaccination when possible.
• Vector control.

PRODUCTION MANAGEMENT
Limit exposure to teratogens during pregnancy.

ABBREVIATIONS
• CNS = central nervous system
• LH = luteinizing hormone

SEE ALSO
• Abortion: Bovine
• Abortion: Small Ruminant
• Abortion: Viral, Fungal, and Nutritional

(CONTINUED) TERATOGENS

- Akabane
- Arthrogryposis
- Bluetongue Virus
- Border Disease
- Bovine Viral Diarrhea Virus
- Cache Valley Virus
- Congenital Defects: Bovine
- Congenital Defects: Camelid
- Congenital Defects: Small Ruminant
- Lupine Toxicity
- Schmallenberg Virus
- Wesselsbron Disease

Suggested Reading

Baughman B. Bovine abortifacient and teratogenic toxins. In: Hopper RM ed, Bovine Reproduction. Ames: Wiley, 2015.

Panter K, Stegelmeier B. Reproductive toxicoses of food animals. Vet Clin North Am Food Anim Pract 2000, 16: 531–44.

Putnam M. Toxicologic problems in food animals affecting reproduction. Vet Clin North Am Food Anim Pract 1989, 5: 325–44.

Roberts SJ. Teratology. In: Veterinary Obstetrics and Genital Diseases. Ithaca, NY: SJ Roberts, 1971.

Author Clare M. Scully
Consulting Editor Ahmed Tibary

T

TESTICULAR DISORDERS: BOVINE

BASICS

OVERVIEW
• Diseases of the bovine testis are often devastating in terms of future reproductive performance but only rarely do they affect the general health of a bull.
• Testicular disorders can be of congenital, inflammatory, or degenerative nature.
• The most common inflammatory disorders are orchitis and epididymitis. These are discussed in detail in a separate chapter, Orchitis and Epididymitis. The focus here is on a more general approach to diagnosis and treatment of testicular disorders in the bull.

INCIDENCE/PREVALENCE
• Studies on the incidence of various testicular disorders are scarce.
• Congenital testicular defects are relatively rare, probably because of the selection pressure through breeding soundness examination (BSE).
• Reported incidence of cryptorchidism is 0.17% with majority (69%) being left-sided.
• Testicular degeneration and small testicular size are common reasons for classification of bulls as unsatisfactory breeders.

GEOGRAPHIC DISTRIBUTION
Worldwide

SYSTEMS AFFECTED
Reproductive

PATHOPHYSIOLOGY
Congenital Disorders
• Cryptorchidism is the most common congenital testicular disorder of domestic animals. Fortunately, it is relatively uncommon in bulls, probably as the result of aggressive selection for normal testicular descent. Although considered hereditary, the mode of inheritance in cattle has not been established adequately.
• Monorchism and polyorchism are rarely seen.
• Hypoplasia of the testis is rare in ruminants and a hereditary predisposition is suspected in most cases.
• While not associated with clinical disease, the appendix epididymis (mesonephric duct remnant) is a vestigial structure present near the head of the epididymis. The appendix epididymis may become cystic and can be detected by ultrasonography or palpation as it enlarges. It is an incidental finding.

Acquired Disorders
• Acquired diseases of the testes can be classified using the traditional DAMNIT system.
• Testicular degeneration is common in bulls. The specific etiology is rarely apparent in clinical cases, likely due to the lag between insult and testis response. Among the conditions known to cause degenerative lesions are heat, toxins, nutritional disorders, obstructive lesions, and ischemia. The initial lesion is a reduction in germ cells number followed by spermiostasis and calcification of the straight tubules near the rete testis. The end stage is characterized by fibrosis and absence of any germinal cells.
• Autoimmune disorders are not commonly reported in ruminants though the bull is capable of producing antisperm antibodies. The true significance of this disorder awaits a reliable commercial test for antisperm antibodies in serum and seminal plasma.
• Neoplastic disorders of the testis are uncommon in bulls. Interstitial cell tumors, seminomas, and sustentacular (Sertoli) cell tumors are the primary testis tumors. Secondary tumors include lymphoma and mesothelioma and are extremely rare.
• Infectious and inflammatory conditions elsewhere (see chapter, Orchitis and Epididymitis).
• Trauma to the testes often results from fighting or crushing injuries from other bulls. Bulls may spontaneously recover from minor trauma but massive trauma can rupture the tunics and result in large hematomas. Bulls seldom recover from this level of insult and the danger exists that scrotal inflammation and antibody production will compromise sperm production in the undamaged testis.
• Inguinal hernia may occur spontaneously or immediately after mating. Congenital inguinal hernia may be hereditary. Excessive fat deposition in the vaginal tunics during puberty has been associated with acquired inguinal hernia. The size of the vaginal ring also seems to be a predisposing factor.

HISTORICAL FINDINGS
• Most testicular abnormalities will be discovered at the time of castration for calves or during BSE.
• Breeding bulls may present with sudden or progressive enlargement of the scrotum or a history of infertility.

SIGNALMENT
• Congenital abnormalities are usually seen in calves at the time of castration or young virgin bulls presenting for BSE.
• Acquired abnormalities are seen in mature breeding bulls.

PHYSICAL EXAMINATION FINDINGS
• Signs vary with the specific disease condition but infertility or subfertility are common findings.
• Most testicular abnormalities are not accompanied by systemic signs of illness except for the case of severe trauma (testicular hemorrhage), inflammatory disorders (epididymitis and orchitis), and possibly incarcerated hernias.

GENETICS
• Sex chromosome aneuploidy and chimerism (degeneration).
• Genetic (hypoplasia).
• Polled Herefords and Shorthorns have reportedly higher incidence of cryptorchidism.

CAUSES AND RISK FACTORS
• Group housing of bulls predisposes them to traumatic injuries.
• Nutrition: Obesity is considered to be one of the leading causes of testicular degeneration in bulls.
• Other systemic diseases.

DIAGNOSIS

DIFFERENTIAL DIAGNOSES
Diagnosis of testicular disorders requires a thorough history and physical examination.

CBC/BIOCHEMISTRY/URINALYSIS
N/A

OTHER LABORATORY TESTS
• Serum hormone concentrations
• Scrotal palpation and measurement
• Microbial culture of the ejaculate
• Testicular biopsy (histopathologic assessment)
• BSE (semen collection and evaluation)

IMAGING
• Ultrasonographic evaluation of the scrotum is an essential diagnostic procedure for assessing testicular disorders in valuable bulls.
• Abnormalities that can be detected by ultrasonography because of variation in echotexture of the parenchyma include calcification, fibrosis, rete testis dilation, and nodules. Cystic dilation of the epididymis may be visualized in cases of segmental aplasia.

OTHER DIAGNOSTIC PROCEDURES
• Transrectal palpation may be helpful in the diagnosis of some pathologies (e.g., inguinal hernia).
• Laparoscopy or laparotomy may be considered for valuable animals.

PATHOLOGIC FINDINGS
• Cryptorchidism: The testis may be retained in the inguinal canal or abdominal cavity. It is generally smaller than the descended testis and has no spermatogenic activity.
• Testicular hypoplasia: Testis is smaller than normal. Histologically, the seminiferous tubules are small, round with no lumen and no spermatogenic activity.
• Testicular degeneration: The testes are usually smaller than normal. Fibrosis and calcification may be evident on the cut surface of the parenchyma. Histologically, the seminiferous tubules present various degrees of vacuolization and collapse.

T

(CONTINUED)

TREATMENT

THERAPEUTIC APPROACH
Treatment for testicular disorders is often unrewarding.

SURGICAL CONSIDERATIONS AND TECHNIQUES
• Hemicastration with parenteral antibiotic and NSAID therapy may improve the prognosis for bulls with severe, unilateral disease.
• Hemicastration should only be considered if the condition is acquired or if the bull is to be used in a terminal cross.

MEDICATIONS

DRUGS OF CHOICE
N/A

CONTRAINDICATIONS
N/A

FOLLOW-UP

EXPECTED COURSE AND PROGNOSIS
Repeated monitoring by BSE and physical examination is necessary for an accurate prognosis.

MISCELLANEOUS

ASSOCIATED CONDITIONS
• Congenital defects
• Infertility and subfertility issues
• Segmental aplasia

AGE-RELATED FACTORS
An age-related degenerative fibrosis occurs in bulls.

ZOONOTIC POTENTIAL
N/A

PREGNANCY
N/A

BIOSECURITY
N/A

PRODUCTION MANAGEMENT
N/A

ABBREVIATIONS
• DAMNIT = (D)egenerative/(D)evelopmental, (A)utoimmune, (M)etabolic, (N)eoplastic, (I)nfectious/(I)atrogenic, (T)raumatic; an organizational system for developing a diagnosis, commonly expanded beyond this initial list
• NSAID = nonsteroidal anti-inflammatory drug

SEE ALSO
• Beef Bull Management (see www.fiveminutevet.com/ruminant)
• Breeding Soundness Examination: Bull
• Congenital Defects: Bovine
• Infertility and Subfertility Issues
• Orchitis and Epididymitis
• Segmental Aplasia of the Reproductive Tract

Suggested Reading

Humphrey JD, Ladds PW. A quantitative histological study of changes in the bovine testis and epididymis associated with age. Res Vet Sci 1975, 19: 135–41.

Kim CA, Parrish JJ, Momont HW, Lunn DP. Effects of experimentally generated bull antisperm antibodies on in vitro fertilization. Biol Reprod 1999, 60: 1285–91.

McEntee K. Reproductive Pathology of Domestic Animals. San Diego: Academic Press, 1990, pp. 224–306.

Steffen D. Genetic causes of bull infertility. Vet Clin North Am Food Anim Pract 1997, 12: 243–52.

Authors Celina Checura and Harry Momont
Consulting Editor Ahmed Tibary

T

TESTICULAR DISORDERS: CAMELID

BASICS

OVERVIEW
• Testicular disorders are the most common cause of subfertility in camelids.
• Testicular disorders can be categorized into congenital and acquired conditions.
• Congenital disorders warrant elimination of the male from breeding due to their possible hereditary nature and association with poor fertility in daughters.
• Breeding males with acquired unilateral testicular disorders are often managed by unilateral castration.
• Testicular degeneration is the most common acquired disorder resulting in reduced or loss of fertility.

INCIDENCE/PREVALENCE
• Examination of 3,015 alpacas showed the following incidence of various congenital abnormalities
   ◦ Testicular hypoplasia: 9.9% (5.9% bilateral)
   ◦ Cryptorchidism: 5.7% (3.5% unilateral left)
   ◦ Ectopic testes: 2.5% (1.7 unilateral left)
• In camels, there are very few clinical observations on incidence of testicular disorders. Orchitis and testicular degeneration seem to be the most common.

GEOGRAPHIC DISTRIBUTION
Worldwide

SYSTEMS AFFECTED
Reproductive

PATHOPHYSIOLOGY
• Congenital testicular disorders in camelids include:
   ◦ Cryptorchidism: Normal testicular descent in camelids occurs late in fetal life. Camelids are born with descended testes in the scrotum. Cryptorchidism is suspected to be hereditary. Unilaterally affected males are fertile if the descended testis is normal. Monorchism is possible but rare. Monorchism has been associated with unilateral renal agenesis in alpacas.
   ◦ Testicular hypoplasia is common in SAC. It is characterized by small, hard testes, poor or lack of development of the seminiferous tubules, and reduced or absent spermatogenesis. Affected males have normal libido but various degrees of infertility due to reduced sperm production and quality.
   ◦ Rete testis cysts are commonly found in SAC. They are believed to be due to tubili recti occlusion. Their effect on fertility depends on their size.
   ◦ Epididymal cysts are due to epididymal segmental aplasia and can result in total sterility if bilateral.
   ◦ Ectopic testicles refers to an abnormal location of the testis. The testis is usually located in the abdominal region lateral to the prepuce or in the medial surface of the hind leg in the femoral canal or crural canal. Because of abnormal thermoregulation, ectopic testes are devoid of any spermatogenic activity.
   ◦ The left testis is more often affected than the right.
• Acquired testicular disorders are suspected due to sudden or progressive change in testicular size or subfertility.
   ◦ Decreased testicular size is generally due to testicular degeneration or atrophy which may be the result of a direct insult to the testis, aging, nutritional deficiencies, or heat stress. Use of testosterone or anabolic steroids (racing camels) downregulates the hypothalamo-pituitary axis resulting in testicular degeneration.
   ◦ Increased scrotal or testicular size may be due to:
      ▪ Hydrocele: The accumulation of fluid in the vaginal cavity and results from heat stress and circulatory disorders. It is rarely a cause of infertility but may contribute over time to testicular degenerative changes.
      ▪ Orchitis and epididymitis: Often result from hematogenous bacteremia. The most common isolates are *Brucella* spp. and *Streptococcus zooepidemicus*. Other bacteria may be introduced directly by puncture wounds or trauma.
      ▪ Testicular hemorrhage: Often the result of biting wounds sustained during a fight with another male.
      ▪ Testicular neoplasia: Seminoma is the most common.
• Infertility is due to poor sperm production, poor motility, and increased sperm abnormalities resulting from loss of seminiferous tubules or epididymal function. The degree of infertility varies depending on whether the condition is unilateral or bilateral and the amount of tissue affected.

HISTORICAL FINDINGS
• Poor libido or infertility.
• Observed increase or decrease in testicular size. In SAC, this is often noticed at the time of shearing.
• Inflammatory or traumatic disorders may be noticed as reluctance to breed or abnormal gait.

SIGNALMENT
• Young animal presented for BSE.
• Adult breeding males with observed external abnormalities or poor fertility.

PHYSICAL EXAMINATION FINDINGS
• Usually normal except for the observed changes in behavior and size of the scrotum.
• Testicular trauma may present as an emergency due to swelling and lameness.

GENETICS
Cryptorchidism and testicular hypoplasia are suspected to be hereditary.

CAUSES AND RISK FACTORS
• Genetics for congenital disorders
• Testicular degeneration: Poor nutrition, heat stress, systemic disease, administration of androgens
• Orchitis, epididymitis: *Brucella abortus*, *Brucella melitensis*

DIAGNOSIS

DIFFERENTIAL DIAGNOSES
• Differential diagnosis between congenital and acquired testicular disorders is very important from legal and ethical perspectives.
• Reproductive history and prior BSE results are important.
• Testicular ultrasonography and biopsy should be considered in order to refine the diagnosis.

CBC/BIOCHEMISTRY/URINALYSIS
• May be indicated in cases of suspected orchitis and epididymitis.
• Indicated before unilateral castration.

OTHER LABORATORY TESTS
• Testing for brucellosis
• Bacteriology of aspirated fluid from the testis
• Semen collection and evaluation

IMAGING
Testicular ultrasonography: Testicular degeneration and fibrosis is characterized by increased echogenicity of the parenchyma. Rete testis cysts are visualized as an anechoic area of variable size in the mediastinum testis. This modality allows differentiation between traumatic lesions, abscesses, and neoplasia.

OTHER DIAGNOSTIC PROCEDURES
Testicular biopsy under heavy sedation using one of the following techniques:
• Wedge incisional or open biopsy: The scrotum is prepared for surgery. A 0.5 cm incision is made through the skin, parietal vaginal tunic, and the exposed tunica albuginea, avoiding vascular areas. Testicular tissue that protrudes from the rent in the tunica albuginea is ablated with a scalpel blade. The tunica albuginea, parietal vaginal tunic, and the scrotal skin are closed with absorbable suture.
• Trucut (self-firing needle): The scrotal skin is blocked with lidocaine. A 4 mm stab incision is made through the skin and vaginal tunic after surgical preparation. A 14–18 gauge self-firing biopsy needle is inserted through the tunica albuginea.
• "Core" biopsy. After surgical preparation of the scrotal skin, a 1 and $\frac{1}{2}$ inch 16 gauge needle is introduced into the testicular parenchyma and redirected by a gentle push-pull movement into two sites. The needle is retracted from the tissue while a finder is placed over the hub to maintain the core sampled. A direct smear is prepared from the sample obtained.

T

(CONTINUED) **TESTICULAR DISORDERS: CAMELID**

• Fine-needle aspirate: Testicular tissue is aspirated with a 20 gauge needle and 12 mL syringe, making sure not to include the epididymis. Cytologic smears stained with DiffQuik® are interpreted based on the different types of spermatogenic cells.

PATHOLOGIC FINDINGS

• Gross and histologic evaluation of the testis after castration confirm the diagnosis.
• Testicular hypoplasia: Small diameter seminiferous tubules without evidence of spermatogenesis.
• Seminiferous tubules are evaluated for spermatogenic activity and presence of degenerative changes (vacuolization, loss of architecture). Inflammatory and neoplastic changes can be evaluated more thoroughly. Atypical spermatogenic cells are associated with testicular neoplasia.

 ## TREATMENT

THERAPEUTIC APPROACH

Males with traumatic or inflammatory injuries should be managed to reduce risk of infection and decrease inflammation.

SURGICAL CONSIDERATIONS AND TECHNIQUES

• Males with congenital and possibly hereditary testicular disorders should be castrated.
• Unilateral castration is recommended for all unilateral acquired conditions, particularly if the interstitial tissue of the affected tests is still functional.

 ## MEDICATIONS

DRUGS OF CHOICE

• Xylazine and ketamine for anesthesia
• Anti-inflammatories: Flunixin meglumine
• Antibiotherapy: Procaine penicillin G, 22,000 IU/kg body weight for 5 days) is recommended postoperatively.

CONTRAINDICATIONS

Appropriate meat withdrawal times should be followed for all compounds administered to food-producing animals.

PRECAUTIONS

N/A

POSSIBLE INTERACTIONS

N/A

 ## FOLLOW-UP

EXPECTED COURSE AND PROGNOSIS

• Semen collection and evaluation should be performed 60 days following unilateral castration.
• Frequency of use of the male should be adjusted based on sperm production ability.

POSSIBLE COMPLICATIONS

• Infection and adhesions are possible after trauma.
• Inflammation may affect spermatogenic activity of the remaining testicle.

CLIENT EDUCATION

• Proper housing and management of breeding males to avoid accidents.
• Maintain proper breeding records.
• Maintain a good herd health preventive program.
• Regular examination of the external genitalia.

PATIENT CARE

• Sexual rest for 4 weeks
• Antibiotic and anti-inflammatory therapy as indicated

PREVENTION

N/A

 ## MISCELLANEOUS

ASSOCIATED CONDITIONS

N/A

AGE-RELATED FACTORS

N/A

ZOONOTIC POTENTIAL

Brucellosis

PREGNANCY

N/A

BIOSECURITY

• Breeding male should be used on healthy females
• Testing for brucellosis

PRODUCTION MANAGEMENT

N/A

SYNONYMS

N/A

ABBREVIATION

BSE = Breeding Soundness Examination

SEE ALSO

• Breeding Soundness Examination: Camelid
• Camelid: Reproduction
• Castration/Vasectomy: Camelid
• Orchitis and Epididymitis

Suggested Reading
Pearson LK, Rodriguez JS, Tibary A. Infertility and subfertility in the male. In: Cebra C, et al. eds, Llama and Alpaca Care: Medicine, Surgery, Reproduction, Nutrition and Herd Health. St. Louis: Elsevier, 2014, pp. 194–216.
Pearson LK, Tibary A. Reproductive disorders of male camelids. Clin Theriogenol 2014, 6: 571–7.
Tibary A; Pearson LK, Anouassi A. Applied andrology in camelids. In: Chenoweth P, Lorton S eds, Animal Andrology: Theories and Applications. Wallingford, UK: CABI, 2014, pp 418–49.
Sumar J. Defectos Congenitos y Hereditarios en la alpaca teratologia. Lima, Peru: Edicion auspiciada por el Consejo Nacional de Cienca y Technologia, 1989.
Author Ahmed Tibary
Consulting Editor Ahmed Tibary

T

TESTICULAR DISORDERS: SMALL RUMINANT

 BASICS

OVERVIEW
Common testicular abnormalities in small ruminants include hypoplasia/testicular degeneration, varicocele, orchitis, epididymitis, sperm granulomas, and cryptorchidism.

INCIDENCE/PREVALENCE
• Cryptorchidism is more common in bucks compared to other ruminants. This condition has an increased incidence in intersex goats.
• The incidence of cryptorchidism depends on selection pressure against the trait. It has been reported as having a 2% incidence in commercial herds, but having a higher incidence in intersex goats.
• Varicocele occurs sporadically in rams.
• Testicular degeneration is associated with other testicular disorders. This can also occur as a result of heat stress and systemic illness (fever).
• Orchitis/epididymitis is more common in rams than in bucks.

GEOGRAPHIC DISTRIBUTION
Worldwide

PATHOPHYSIOLOGY
• Several processes can affect testicular function. Bilateral affection usually results in infertility or sterility.
• Congenital disorders:
  ○ Cryptorchidism is a failure of one or both testicles to descend into the scrotum.
  ○ Testicular hypoplasia is caused as a result of a genetic abnormality. It is commonly seen in intersex goats and with chromosomal abnormalities in rams.
  ○ Sperm granulomas are localized swellings that occur as a result of spermatozoa exposure outside of the immune-privileged tubular duct system of the male reproductive tract. This is caused by misaligned or blind-ended efferent ducts that normally drain into the caput epididymis.
  ○ Inguinal hernia.
• Infectious processes:
  ○ Orchitis is caused by trauma or an extension of infection from the epididymis.
  ○ Epididymitis is a common finding in rams: In older rams, contagious epididymitis due to *Brucella ovis* is common is some regions. In ram lambs several bacterial pathogens (*Histophilus*, *Actinobacillus*, and *Haemophilus*) have been incriminated.
• Degenerative processes:
  ○ Testicular degeneration may be due to nutritional deficiencies, poor health, or age.
  ○ Varicocele is a localized swelling and thrombosis of the pampiniform plexus in the spermatic cord. This condition is more common in rams.

• Neoplastic processes: Testicular neoplasms are rare but seminoma has been reported.
• Trauma and accident: Testicular hemorrhage and scrotal herniation are the most common traumatic injuries.

SYSTEMS AFFECTED
Reproductive

HISTORICAL FINDINGS
• Infertility
• Abnormal appearance of the scrotum
• Sudden increase in scrotal size

GENETICS
Conditions that are considered heritable include cryptorchidism, varicoceles, and granuloma/epididymal aplasia.

SIGNALMENT
• Congenital disorders: Young rams and bucks around the time of puberty or at the first breeding soundness examination.
• Acquired disorders: Incidental findings at BSE or specific complaints in older rams. Testicular degeneration is typically discovered in older animals or following severe systemic disease, poor health and nutrition.
• Sperm granulomas were discovered in males >1 year of age.

PHYSICAL EXAMINATION FINDINGS
• Testicular hypoplasia: Smaller than normal testis. Usually hard on palpation. It can be difficult to assess out of the breeding season.
• Testicular degeneration: Testis is more elongated and the parenchyma can palpate either harder or softer versus the normal. Calcification of testicular parenchyma may be present and affect semen quality.
• Varicocele: The spermatic cord palpates as a fluctuant swelling. It is common for rams to display an abnormal rear limb posture with this condition.
• Orchitis: One or both testicles show significant enlargement and increased temperature. Pain may be elicited on palpation of the affected testicle(s). Systemic illness may result in some severe cases. Libido may be decreased.
• Epididymitis: Characteristic swelling and fibrosis of the epididymis. This condition can lead to the formation of sperm granulomas if the integrity of the epididymis is compromised and haploid cells exit from the immunologically privileged environment.
• Cryptorchidism will be evident on inspection and palpation of the scrotum. It can be unilateral or bilateral. Affected animals have normal masculine characteristics and behaviors. Bilateral cases are azoospermic while unilaterally affected animals are fertile.
• Sperm granulomas: Presence of a localized swelling and inflammation of the epididymis. This condition is most commonly found at the caput epididymis.

CAUSES AND RISK FACTORS
• Testicular hypoplasia is a genetic abnormality that is considered heritable.

• Testicular degeneration can be due to aging or a sequela to many other factors such as extremes in environmental temperatures, scrotal insulation from fat, systemic disease, malnutrition, and parasitism. Blockage of the excurrent duct system can also lead to degeneration.
• Varicocele has an unknown etiology in small ruminants, but some authors suspect a genetic cause.
• Orchitis/epididymitis is an infectious process.
  ○ Virgin ram lamb epididymitis is caused by several organisms such as *Histophilus*, *Actinobacillus*, *Haemophilus* spp. and occasionally *Corynebacterium pseudotuberculosis*. It is common to diagnosis this condition in young rams that are housed together.
  ○ Mature ram epididymitis and orchitis are due to *B. ovis* infection. Other bacterial infections are also possible.
  ○ *B. melitensis* infection in goats.
• Sperm granulomas are caused by a blockage in the excurrent duct system.
• Cryptorchidism is likely a heritable defect.

 DIAGNOSIS

DIFFERENTIAL DIAGNOSES
• An inflamed or enlarged scrotum could be orchitis/epididymitis, hydrocele, hematocele, varicocele, sperm granulomas, inguinal herniation, or neoplasia.
• An abnormally small scrotum or testicle could be testicular hypoplasia or testicular degeneration.
• The absence of one or both testicles in the scrotum could be cryptorchidism or a previous castration.

CBC/BIOCHEMISTRY/URINALYSIS
• An inflammatory leukogram in severe cases of epididymitis/orchitis.
• Leukocytes may be discovered on urinalysis.

OTHER LABORATORY TESTS
• Spermiogram
  ○ Poor motility and morphology due to abnormal thermoregulation (hydrocele, hematocele, varicocele).
  ○ Decreased concentration and increased sperm abnormalities in cases of testicular degeneration or testicular hypoplasia.
  ○ Increased abnormalities and presence of numerous polymorphonuclear neutrophils.
• Culture of semen or urine if ram lamb epididymitis and mature ram epididymitis is suspected.

IMAGING
• Ultrasonography is useful in diagnosing abnormalities in the testicle, epididymis, and spermatic cord.
  ○ Atrophy, inflammatory and degenerative changes results in a heterogeneous

appearance of testicular parenchyma. Comets tails are seen in the parenchyma in case of calcification.
◦ Increased fluid content in the vaginal cavity suggests presence of hydrocele (anechoic), pyocele or hematocele (echogenic). Strands of fibrin and adhesions may also be visualized.
◦ Presence of intestinal loop within the scrotum confirms inguinal/scrotal hernia.
◦ Transabdominal ultrasound may be useful in locating the retained testicle(s).
• Thermography can be useful in diagnosis of problems in the testicle.

OTHER DIAGNOSTIC PROCEDURES
Serologic testing and bacterial culture of semen for infectious causes of epididymitis and orchitis in rams.

PATHOLOGIC FINDINGS
• Testicular hypoplasia and testicular degeneration are characterized histologically by seminiferous tubules lined by one layer of cells with lack of spermatogenic activity. In testicular hypoplasia, the tubules are small, round and often devoid of a lumen.
• Necrosis, edema, and infiltration of inflammatory cells are characteristic of orchitis.
• Varying degrees of fibrosis may be present between seminiferous tubules.

TREATMENT
THERAPETUTIC APPROACH
N/A

SURGICAL CONSIDERATIONS AND TECHNIQUES
Unilateral castration may be considered in unilateral acquired noncontagious conditions for valuable males.

MEDICATIONS
DRUGS OF CHOICE
Culture and sensitivity results from seminal fluid are the basis for antibiotic treatment of infectious causes of testicular disease in small ruminants.

CONTRAINDICATIONS
Meat withdrawal times must be followed.

PRECAUTIONS
N/A

POSSIBLE INTERACTIONS
N/A

FOLLOW-UP
EXPECTED COURSE AND PROGNOSIS
• Antibiotic therapy is often unrewarding in cases of epididymitis/orchitis.
• Hemicastration of affected testicles can result in near normal semen production in the contralateral testicle if there is not damage to the germinal epithelium. Prognosis for return to breeding soundness is guarded.
• Treatment of testicular degeneration is unrewarding and the prognosis is poor.
• All males with congenital abnormalities should be culled.

POSSIBLE COMPLICATIONS
• Infertility
• Death (inguinal herniation)

CLIENT EDUCATION
• All males should undergo BSE.
• Testicular hypoplasia and cryptorchidism are considered heritable conditions. Affected animals should be culled from breeding.
• Valuable males should be submitted for semen cryopreservation.

PATIENT CARE
Animals should be submitted for BSE to determine response to treatment or to monitor the progression of testicular degeneration.

PREVENTION
• Biosecurity measures and serologic testing for *Brucella ovis*.
• Ram/buck management should include an adequate nutritional, parasite control, and vaccination program.

MISCELLANEOUS
ASSOCIATED CONDITIONS
N/A

AGE-RELATED FACTORS
Testicular degeneration is common in old males.

ZOONOTIC POTENTIAL
B. melitensis

PREGNANCY
Brucellosis results in poor pregnancy rates, abortions, stillbirths, and weak lambs.

BIOSECURITY
• Surveillance and strict isolation protocols for new additions to the herd or flock.
• Testing of outside males.
• A diagnosis of brucellosis should be reported to the state veterinary office.

PRODUCTION MANAGEMENT
Regular BSE on all breeding animals

SYNONYMS
N/A

ABBREVIATION
BSE = breeding soundness examination

SEE ALSO
• Breeding Soundness Examination: Small Ruminant
• Brucellosis

Suggested Reading
Edmondson MA, Roberts JF, Baird AN, Bychawski S, Pugh DG. Theriogenology of sheep and goats. In: Baird AN, Pugh DG eds, Sheep and Goat Medicine, 2nd ed. Maryland Heights, MO: Elsevier, 2012.
Kimberling CV, Parson GA. Breeding soundness evaluation and surgical sterilization of the ram. In: Youngquist RS, Threlfall WR eds, Current Therapy in Large Animal Theriogenology. Philadelphia: Saunders, 1997, pp. 620–8.
Mickelsen WD, Memon MA. Infertility and diseaases of the reproductive organs of bucks. In: Youngquist RS, Threlfall WR. Current Therapy in Large Animal Theriogenology. Philadelphia: Saunders, 1997, pp. 519–23.
Memon MA. Male infertility. Vet Clin North Am Large Anim Pract 1983, 5: 619–35.
Author Chance L. Armstrong
Consulting Editor Ahmed Tibary

T

THELAZIASIS

BASICS

OVERVIEW
• Ophthalmic infection by the nematode *Thelazia* spp. eyeworms. • Species include *T. gulosa*, *T. skrjabini*, and *T. rhodesii*. • Additional species can also infect sheep, goats, deer, buffalo, and dromedaries.

INCIDENCE/PREVALENCE
Varies with geographic location and may be decreasing due to extensive use of macrocyclic lactone endectocides in cattle. Prevalence decreased in England from 41.9% in 1978 to 1.5% in 2005.

GEOGRAPHIC DISTRIBUTION
Worldwide

SYSTEMS AFFECTED
Ophthalmic

PATHOPHYSIOLOGY
• *Thelazia* spp. of ruminants requires muscid flies as intermediate hosts; the genus *Musca* is the most important vector in North America. • Adult *Thelazia* live in the lacrimal ducts of the nictitating membrane, in the conjunctival sacs, or under the eyelids and nictitating membranes. Females pass first-stage larvae into ocular secretions where they are ingested by flies during feeding. These develop into infective third-stage larvae in 9–49 days and are deposited on the eye of the host as the fly feeds. • The prepatent period is 2–6 weeks, which is species dependent. • Lesions are caused by the serrated cuticle of the parasite; most lesions are associated with the movement of the active young adults. • Mechanical irritation and inflammation can lead to conjunctivitis, blepharitis, keratitis, and other corneal damage. Inflammation of lacrimal glands/ducts leads to reduced tear production. • Asymptomatic infections may also occur.

HISTORICAL FINDINGS
Asymptomatic to chronic conjunctivitis and keratitis

SIGNALMENT
• *T. rhodesii*: Cattle, buffalo, goats, sheep, and deer in North America, Europe, Africa, Middle East, Asia • *T. gulosa* and *T. skrjabini*: cattle in North America, Europe

PHYSICAL EXAMINATION FINDINGS
• Quite variable, from asymptomatic incidental finding to severe signs. • Conjunctivitis, epiphora, blepharitis, and photophobia. • Keratitis possibly with ulceration, perforation, or scarring. • Visible worms on surface of eye, under eyelids or nictitating membranes.

GENETICS
N/A

CAUSES AND RISK FACTORS
Cause: *Thelazia* spp. infection

Risk factors: Presence of face flies in an endemic area

DIAGNOSIS

DIFFERENTIAL DIAGNOSES
• Chronic bacterial conjunctivitis • Viral conjunctivitis/keratitis • Corneal laceration • Foreign body

CBC/BIOCHEMISTRY/URINALYSIS
N/A

OTHER LABORATORY TESTS
N/A

IMAGING
N/A

OTHER DIAGNOSTIC PROCEDURES
• Gross examination of conjunctival sacs and underlying nictitating membranes. Topical anesthesia may be necessary to aid the manipulation of the third eyelid. • Microscopic examination of lacrimal fluids for larvae.

PATHOLOGIC FINDINGS
May see the parasite emerging from the conjunctival sac or deposited on the skin/hair around the eye of moribund species.

TREATMENT

THERAPEUTIC APPROACH
Administration of an effective anthelmintic has replaced manual removal under local anesthetic.

MEDICATIONS

DRUGS OF CHOICE
• Ivermectin or doramectin at 200 µg/kg body weight given subcutaneously can be 99–100% effective for *T. rhodesii* in cattle. • Levamisole at 5 mg/kg given subcutaneously or administered as a 1% topical aqueous solution is also effective but off-label.

CONTRAINDICATIONS
Do not treat lactating animals producing milk for human consumption with ivermectin or doramectin.

PRECAUTIONS
Appropriate meat and milk withdrawal times must be followed for all compounds administered to food-producing animals.

FOLLOW-UP

EXPECTED COURSE AND PROGNOSIS
Full recovery in about 2 months although long-term persistence of areas of corneal opacity may occur.

POSSIBLE COMPLICATIONS
Scarring of cornea or loss of eye secondary to perforation of cornea is possible in rare severe cases.

CLIENT EDUCATION
N/A

PATIENT CARE
N/A

PREVENTION
• Control of face flies. • Dry, open pastures and less intensely confined conditions help reduce fly numbers.

MISCELLANEOUS

ASSOCIATED CONDITIONS
• Corneal ulceration. • Mechanical irritation and inflammation can lead to lesions involving the lacrimal glands and ducts, conjunctivitis, blepharitis, keratitis, and other corneal damage.

ZOONOTIC POTENTIAL
Reports of other species (*T. californiensis*, *T. callipaeda*) in humans.

PRODUCTION MANAGEMENT
• Control of face flies. • Dry, open pastures and less intensely confined conditions help reduce fly numbers.

SYNONYM
N/A

ABBREVIATIONS
N/A

SEE ALSO
Corneal Disorders

Suggested Reading
Djungu DFL, Retnani EB, Rdwan Y. *Thelazia rhodesii* infection on cattle in Kupang District. Trop Biomed 2014, 31: 844–52.

Otranto D, Traversa D. *Thelazia*: an original endo- and ecto-parasitic nematode. Trends Parasitol 2004, 21: 1–4.

Soll MD, Carmichael IH, Scherer HR, Gross SJ. The efficacy of ivermectin against *T. rhodesii* (Desmaret, 1828) in the eyes of cattle. Vet Parasitol 1992, 42: 67–71.

Tweedle DM, Fox MT, Gibbons LM, Tennant K. Change in the prevalence of *Thelazia* species in bovine eyes in England. Vet Rec 2005, 157: 555–6.

Author Lora R. Ballweber
Consulting Editor Kaitlyn A. Lutz
Acknowledgment The author and book editors acknowledge the prior contribution of Edward L. Powers.

T

TICK PARALYSIS

BASICS

OVERVIEW
• A lower motor neuron (LMN) paralysis resulting from the bite of female ticks of species including *Dermacentor* spp. and *Amblyomma* spp. in the United States and *Ixodes holocyclus* in Australia.
• The potential for inducing paralysis has been suspected in 64 species of tick belonging to the *Ixodid* and *Argasid* genera.
• The tick injects a neurotoxin that causes progressive motor paralysis, respiratory depression, and death in animals that have no immunity to the toxin.

INCIDENCE/PREVALENCE
Unknown

GEOGRAPHIC DISTRIBUTION
• Common in Australia, human and animal cases reported throughout the US (particularly in the Rocky Mountains and Pacific Northwest), and worldwide.
• Distribution patterns reflecting tick populations.
• Exposure to environments favorable to tick infestations such as brushy, woody areas.

SYSTEMS AFFECTED
• Nervous
• Digestive
• Respiratory
• Cardiovascular
• Hemolymphatic
• Musculoskeletal

PATHOPHYSIOLOGY
• Exact pathology is not certain. Signs are caused by a protein neurotoxin possibly produced by the tick itself, by a microbial organism associated with the tick, or by a toxic metabolite resulting from the interaction of tick saliva with host tissue.
• There is a reduction of acetylcholine release and a resulting blockage of neurotransmission at neuromuscular junctions.
• Interference with presynaptic nerve terminal depolarization and acetylcholine release produces a neuromuscular blockade. This manifests primarily as an ascending flaccid paralysis varying from paraparesis to quadriplegia.

HISTORICAL FINDINGS
The owner is not usually aware of the presence of a tick and animals usually present with weakness and ataxia.

SIGNALMENT
• Sheep, goats, cattle.
• Other species such as dogs may be affected.
• All ages potentially are at risk, and both sexes are equally affected.

PHYSICAL EXAMINATION FINDINGS
• Initially, ataxia and weakness in hindlimbs.
• Progression to paralysis of hindlimbs then ascending, symmetrical, flaccid tetraplegia.
• Afebrile.
• Hyporeflexia of the superficial and deep tendons.
• Nystagmus.
• Dyspnea, dysphagia, inability to regurgitate cud normally, weak facial muscles.
• Flaccid tail and anus.
• Disease may progress further and cause respiratory muscle paralysis resulting in death.

GENETICS
N/A

CAUSES AND RISK FACTORS
• Exposure to environments favorable to tick infestations such as brushy, woody areas.
• Seasonal incidence may change in geographic regions where tick populations vary based on ambient temperatures.
• Antitoxic immunity can occur 2 weeks after primary tick exposure and lasts a few weeks. Immunity may be boosted in subsequent infestations.

DIAGNOSIS

DIFFERENTIAL DIAGNOSES
• Botulism
• Acute polyradiculoneuritis
• Spinal cord compression
In early stages:
• Rabies
• Trauma
• Myelopathy
• Metabolic disorders
• *Parelaphostrongylus tenuis* migration

CBC/BIOCHEMISTRY/URINALYSIS
• Results are usually normal.
• Mild metabolic acidosis and dehydration develop. Other changes include increases in blood glucose and cholesterol, and a decrease in blood potassium.
• Increased serum levels of creatine kinase (CK) in tick paralysis caused by *D. andersoni* and *I. holocyclus*.
• Phosphate levels increased in later stages of paralysis caused by *I. holocyclus*.

OTHER LABORATORY TESTS
CSF is normal.

IMAGING
May be useful to rule out other causes of paralysis or to examine degree of lung compromise (e.g., pulmonary edema, aspiration) secondary to respiratory paralysis.

OTHER DIAGNOSTIC PROCEDURES
Examination for the presence of ticks or tick craters on affected animals.

PATHOLOGIC FINDINGS
None specific to the disease, death occurs due to respiratory paralysis.

TREATMENT

THERAPEUTIC APPROACH
• Timely removal of attached ticks, either manually or by using a suitable acaricide. It may be necessary to shave long-haired animals to effectively locate all ticks.
• A canine-derived *Ixodes holocyclus* antivenom (hyperimmune serum) is available in Australia and has been used in lambs and kids. The intravenous route is recommended at a dose of 1 mL/kg body weight. Anaphylactic reactions are possible and treated animals should be monitored closely.
• Supportive therapy—monitor for respiratory paralysis and hypoxia.

SURGICAL CONSIDERATIONS AND TECHNIQUES
N/A

MEDICATIONS

DRUGS OF CHOICE
• Acaricidal dips
• Antivenom

CONTRAINDICATIONS
Steroids should not be used in pregnant animals.

PRECAUTIONS
Appropriate milk and meat withdrawal times must be followed for all compounds administered to food-producing animals.

FOLLOW-UP

EXPECTED COURSE AND PROGNOSIS
• Incubation period is usually 5–7 days.
• Depending on the species of tick involved, prognosis is good to excellent if ticks are removed promptly. Recovery usually occurs within 1–3 days.
• Animals infested with *Ixodes holocyclus* (Australian paralysis tick) may continue to worsen despite removal of all ticks and frequently die within 1–2 days without treatment.

POSSIBLE COMPLICATIONS
N/A

CLIENT EDUCATION
Educate clients on tick prevention strategies and proper removal technique for ticks.

PATIENT CARE
Significant nursing care is required for recumbent animals.

PREVENTION
• Ectoparasite sprays or dips to kill ticks on the animals.

T

TICK PARALYSIS   (CONTINUED)

• Environmental control to reduce tick populations is recommended.
• Cattle and sheep have been shown to develop antibodies to *Dermacentor* and were not susceptible to paralysis after active or passive immunization to tick-specific antigens.

 MISCELLANEOUS

ASSOCIATED CONDITIONS
N/A

AGE-RELATED FACTORS
N/A

ZOONOTIC POTENTIAL
The same ticks can cause tick paralysis in humans. Animals with the disease cannot transmit the disease to humans.

PREGNANCY
N/A

ABBREVIATIONS
• CK = creatine kinase
• CSF = cerebrospinal fluid
• LMN = lower motor neuron

SEE ALSO
• Botulism
• Down Bovine
• Down Camelid
• Down Small Ruminant

Suggested Reading
Aiello SE ed. Tick paralysis. In: Merck Veterinary Manual, 8th ed. Whitehouse Station, NJ: Merck & Co., 1998.
Keirans JE, Hutcheson HJ, Durden LA, Klompen JS. *Ixodes* (Ixodes) *scapularis* (Acari: Ixodidae): redescription of all active stages, distribution, hosts, geographical variation, and medical and veterinary importance. J Med Entomol 1996, 33: 297–318.
Lysyk TJ, Veira DM, Kastelic JP, Majak W. Inducing active and passive immunity in sheep to paralysis caused by *Dermacentor andersoni*. J Med Entomol 2009, 46: 1436–41.
Masina S, Broady KW. Tick paralysis: development of a vaccine. Int J Parasitol 1999, 29: 535–41.
Oliver JE Jr, Lorenz MD, Kornegay JN. Tick paralysis. In: Handbook of Veterinary Neurology, 3rd ed. Philadelphia: Saunders, 1997.
Smith BP ed. Tick paralysis. In: Large Animal Internal Medicine, 5th ed. St. Louis: Mosby, 2015.
Tatchell RJ. Sheep and goat tick management. Parasitologia 1997, 39: 157–60.
Author Kate O'Conor
Consulting Editor Kaitlyn A. Lutz
Acknowledgment The author and book editors acknowledge the prior contribution of Lisa Nashold.

T

BASICS

OVERVIEW
Definition: Intoxication and/or adverse consequences after ingestion of plants of the genus *Nicotiana*. They are members of the nightshade family, Solanaceae.

INCIDENCE/PREVALENCE
• Varies with geographic location • *N. tabacum*—cultivated tobacco • *N. trygonphylla*—wild or desert tobacco in the dry areas of southwest United States • *N. attenuata*—wild or coyote tobacco also in the dry areas of southwest US • *N. glauca*—tree tobacco, an evergreen shrub of low elevation areas of Arizona and California

GEOGRAPHIC DISTRIBUTION
Worldwide; southwestern US and anywhere tobacco is cultivated

SYSTEMS AFFECTED
• Digestive • Musculoskeletal • Nervous • Reproductive

PATHOPHYSIOLOGY
• Two primary toxic compounds are responsible for the adverse effects of tobacco ingestion—nicotine and anabasine. • Nicotine—a potent pyridine alkaloid has poor palatability, but animals will eat it if forage is scarce. It can cause a direct contact irritation to gastrointestinal mucosa. Pharmacologically, it mimics acetylcholine at the autonomic ganglia and myoneural junction acting as a neuromuscular blocking agent. • Anabasine—a piperidine-pyridine alkaloid, a teratogen.

HISTORICAL FINDINGS
Access to *Nicotiana* spp. where forage is poor, pasturing on land where tobacco is cultivated, and ingestion of tobacco products or tobacco-tainted water.

SIGNALMENT
• Potentially any animal can be affected. • Among domestic ruminants, cattle, sheep, and goats have had documented cases.

PHYSICAL EXAMINATION FINDINGS
Neurologic Symptoms
Salivation, vomiting, diarrhea, excitement, increased respiratory rate, twitching, trembling, stiff and uncoordinated gait leading to respiratory paralysis, weakness, bloat, blindness, collapse, and death.

Teratogenic Effects
Calves exhibit arthrogryposis of the forelimbs and spondylosis identical to that seen in lupine toxicity. In sheep, carpal flexure and cleft palate can be seen.

DIAGNOSIS

History of potential exposure to *Nicotiana* spp. and compatible clinical signs.

DIFFERENTIAL DIAGNOSES
• Other toxic plant causes of sudden death—blue-green algae, cyanogenic plants, death camas, larkspur, laurels, lupine, milkweed, oleander, water hemlock. • Other teratogenic causes should be investigated such as bluebonnet, locoweed, and poison hemlock.

CBC/BIOCHEMISTRY/URINALYSIS
No characteristic changes

OTHER LABORATORY TESTS
As an aid to diagnosis, urine or tissues may be analyzed for alkaloid content using GC-MS.

IMAGING
N/A

OTHER DIAGNOSTIC PROCEDURES
N/A

PATHOLOGIC FINDINGS
• In cases of sudden death, no specific lesions may be seen, except the finding of *Nicotiana* spp. in the digestive tract. • Pale mucus membranes, poorly oxygenated blood, myocardial hemorrhage, pulmonary hemorrhages, cerebral congestion, and foam in the trachea are occasionally seen but there are no distinctive pathologic changes. • Teratogenic lesions in calves or lambs as listed above might be seen.

TREATMENT

THERAPEUTIC APPROACH
• No specific treatment except to prevent further ingestion. • Administering activated charcoal and cathartics might be helpful and intravenous fluids may be needed. • Seizures can be treated with diazepam. • Bradycardia can be treated with atropine. • If practical, artificial respiration and supplemental oxygen can be provided in extremely valuable livestock.

MEDICATIONS

DRUGS OF CHOICE
No specific antidote.

CONTRAINDICATIONS
Steroids should not be used in pregnant animals.

PRECAUTIONS
• Appropriate milk and meat withdrawal times must be followed for all compounds administered to food-producing animals.

FOLLOW-UP

EXPECTED COURSE AND PROGNOSIS
If the animal survives acute toxicity, the prognosis is good.

PREVENTION
Prevent access to and consumption of *Nicotiana* spp., especially in forage-scarce areas.

MISCELLANEOUS

PREGNANCY
Teratogenic—prevent access to *Nicotiana* spp. by ruminants.

PRODUCTION MANAGEMENT
Access to *Nicotiana* spp. where forage is poor, pasturing on land where tobacco is cultivated, and ingestion of tobacco products or tobacco-tainted water should be denied to livestock.

ABBREVIATION
• GC-MS = gas chromatography-mass spectrometry

SEE ALSO
• Blue-Green Algae Poisoning • Cyanide Toxicosis • Death Camas • Lupine Toxicity • Milkweed (*Asclepias* spp.) Toxicosis • Oleander and Cardiotoxic Plant Toxicity • Poison Hemlock (*Conium* spp.) Toxicity • Water Hemlock

Suggested Reading
Burrows GE, Tyrl RJ. In Toxic Plants of North America, 2nd ed. Ames: Wiley-Blackwell, Kindle edition, 2013, pp. 1147–51.
Keeler RF, Crowe MW. Teratogenicity and toxicity of wild tree tobacco, *Nicotiana glauca* in sheep. Cornell Vet 1984, 74: 50–9.
Keeler RF, Shupe JL, Crowe MW, Olson A, Balls LD. *Nicotiana glauca*-induced congenital deformities in calves: clinical and pathologic aspects. Am J Vet Res 1981, 42: 1231–4.
Panter KE, James LF, Gardner DR. Lupines, poison-hemlock and *Nicotiana* spp. toxicity and teratogenicity in livestock. J Nat Toxins 1999, 8: 117–34.
Panter KE, Weinzweig J, Gardner DR, Stegelmeier BL, James LF. Comparison of cleft palate induction by *Nicotiana glauca* in goats and sheep. Teratology 2000, 61: 203–10.
Plumlee KH, Holstege DM, Blanchard PC, Fiser KM, Galey FD. *Nicotiana glauca* toxicosis of cattle. J Vet Diagn Invest 1993, 5: 498–9.

Authors Edward L. Powers and Larry Occhipinti
Consulting Editor Christopher C.L. Chase

T

TONGUE TRAUMA

BASICS

OVERVIEW
• Acute or chronic oral ulceration, bruising, and or necrosis may be due to a virus (vesicular stomatitis, bluetongue, epizootic hemorrhagic disease, bovine viral diarrhea virus, malignant catarrhal fever, Seneca valley virus), trauma or irritant (chemical irritants, coarse plants/feed) or oral foreign bodies.
• Abscesses may occur due to actinobacillosis or "woody tongue."
• Because of the tongue's important role in feed prehension and the eating habits of ruminants, tongue trauma is often acutely evident (salivation, blood mixed with saliva, tongue extended from mouth, dysphagia).

SYSTEMS AFFECTED
• Digestive
• Musculoskeletal

PATHOPHYSIOLOGY
• Dependent upon inciting cause.
• *Actinobacillus lignieresii* is a commensal organism of the GI tract and therefore may colonize oral ulcerations.
• Feeding coarse, dry feeds containing goathead (*Tribulus terrestris*) stickers and plant awns (*Hordeum* spp., *Bromus* spp., *Alopecurus* spp., *Setaria* spp.) may result in damage to oral mucosa and colonization of deeper tissues with organisms.
• Oral foreign bodies such as wire may lacerate the tongue or be swallowed such that it is retained by the lingual frenulum leading to salivation, hemorrhage, and eventually infection.

HISTORICAL FINDINGS
Dependent on etiology. History of weight loss may be the first noticeable sign in subtle cases.

SIGNALMENT
• Tongue trauma is more common in younger animals due to their predisposition to suckle on environmental objects (wire, thorns, etc.).
• Vesicular stomatitis in dairy cattle results in large ulcerations of the tongue with lesions evident on teats and coronary bands.
• Bluetongue virus in susceptible sheep results in tongue and dental pad erosions along with other signs compatible with vasculitis.
• Malignant catarrhal fever (cattle) and Rinderpest (cattle sheep and goats) generally manifest as erosive stomatitis not limited to the tongue.

PHYSICAL EXAMINATION FINDINGS
Salivation, blood in saliva, dysphagia, reluctance to allow examination of head,

anorexia, weight loss, dehydration, foul odor to breath, nasal discharge.

CAUSES AND RISK FACTORS
Early weaning, less than optimal housing conditions, salt or water seeking behavior (lack of salt/trace minerals or suitable source of clean water) resulting in consumption of irritant substances (chlorinated naphthalenes). Feeding coarse, dry feeds containing stickers and plant awns may result in damage to oral mucosa and colonization of deeper tissues with organisms. Oral foreign bodies such as wire may lacerate the tongue during prehension leading to hemorrhage and eventually infection.

DIAGNOSIS

DIFFERENTIAL DIAGNOSIS
A complete oral examination should be performed to rule out foreign bodies, abscesses and other disorders. Caution should be practiced during the examination to prevent injury to the examiner (proper animal restraint). Lingual trauma, oral or pharyngeal infection or abscesses should not present with other lesions (coronary bands of feet, teat lesions, generalized vasculitis, CNS signs, disseminated GI disease).

OTHER LABORATORY TESTS
Culture and sensitivity testing is indicated if an infective agent is suspected.

IMAGING
May be helpful with foreign body or fracture.

PATHOLOGIC FINDINGS
Dependent on etiology

TREATMENT

THERAPEUTIC APPROACH
Dependent on underlying management or disease factors

SURGICAL CONSIDERATIONS AND TECHNIQUES
Surgical correction may involve glossectomy or partial glossectomy with consideration of the importance of the tongue to prehension of feed.

MEDICATIONS

DRUGS OF COICE
Will vary depending on etiology.

FOLLOW-UP
Patient outcomes and preventive management plans will vary depending on etiology.

MISCELLANEOUS

ASSOCIATED CONDITIONS
Weight loss and potential culling

PRODUCTION MANAGEMENT
Control of risk factors inlcuding keeping all caustic chemicals away from livestock access.

ABBREVIATION
GI = gastrointestinal

SEE ALSO
• Actinobacillosis: Wooden Tongue
• Agricultural Chemical Toxicities
• Bluetongue Virus
• Calf Diphtheria/Necrotic Stomatitis
• Malignant Catarrhal Fever
• Rinderpest (see www.fiveminutevet.com/ruminant)
• Vesicular Stomatitis

Further Reading
Buttenschon J. The occurrence of lesions in the tongue of adult cattle and their implications for the development of actinobacillosis. Zentralbl Veterinarmed A 1989, 36: 393–400.
Darling R, Dixon R, Honhold N, Taylor N. Oral lesions in cattle and sheep. Vet Rec 2001, 148: 759.
Ducharme NG. Surgical diseases of the oral cavity. In: Fubini SL, Ducharme NG eds, Farm Animal Surgery. Philadelphia: Saunders, 2004, pp. 161–75.
Rebhun WC. Infectious diseases of the gastrointestinal tract. In: Rebhun WC, Diseases of Dairy Cattle, 2nd ed. St. Louis: Saunders Elsevier, 2008.
Roeber DL, Mies PD, Smith CD, et al. National market cow and bull beef quality audit, 1999: A survey of producer-related defects in market cows and bulls. J Anim Sci 2001, 79: 658–65.

Author Jeff Lakritz
Consulting Editor Kaitlyn A. Lutz

T

TOXICOLOGY: HERD OUTBREAKS

BASICS

OVERVIEW
• Food animal practitioners are commonly required to attend toxicologic incidents affecting single or multiple livestock.
• Toxicologic events are usually emergencies occurring day or night, year round.
• Larger herd sizes within certain agriculture sectors (i.e., dairy, calf raisers, and beef feedlots) create the potential for increasingly severe incidents.
• The risk to animals kept on confined feeding operations is more concerning as their sole source of nutrition is the ration and water provided by the farmer.
• Rations can unknowingly become contaminated with toxic weeds included with forage. Ration concentrates can be included at toxic levels due to mixing errors. Components can contain residue contamination from the feed mill as a result of previously produced batches.
• Emotions are strained, whether it is a client's club project or a large operation involving hundreds of animals. One's empathic capabilities can be central to obtaining the owner's cooperation and trust.
• The rapidly deteriorating state of affected livestock requires immediate supportive treatment and care while simultaneously attempting to construct a plan for a diagnosis.
• Smartphones are a very powerful field tool able to provide immediate contact with offsite expertise, internet access, picture documentation and sharing.

INCIDENCE/PREVALENCE
• Toxic events are estimated to be responsible for as much as 3–5% mortality among livestock species (horses, large and small ruminants) in 17 states in the western United States.

SYSTEMS AFFECTED
N/A

PATHOPHYSIOLOGY
N/A

SIGNALMENT
• Poisonings occur in all species, sexes, ages, and production classes of livestock.
• Occasional age-related distinctions may develop such as mature cows being affected by toxic forage while the suckling calves at their side are unaffected.

PHYSICAL EXAMINATION FINDINGS
• Signs associated with a toxicologic event are commonly vague.
• In some instances, signs only become apparent weeks to months following initial exposure.
• Sudden death is commonly the client's only sign in an acute or peracute incident. Poor performance such as slow growth or low milk

production can be associated with chronic toxic exposures.

CAUSES AND RISK FACTORS
• An indepth discussion of the causes and risk factors associated with a toxic event can be found in titles listed under "Suggested Reading."
• Generally speaking, specific toxin sensitivity differences between livestock species have been well documented.
• Some livestock species can adapt to exposure to moderate levels of specific toxins.
• Livestock's level of production or physiologic state (pregnant, ill) can alter an animal's toxin susceptibility.
• Plant stage of maturity as well as growing conditions can alter toxin levels within a given species of plant.
• Certain toxins have a seasonality, as is the case in late summer algal toxicities.
• Inappropriate pesticide or herbicide storage have been the cause of livestock poisonings.

DIAGNOSIS

DIFFERENTIAL DIAGNOSES
• Vague signs commonly associated with poisonings make it important to first rule out other possible causes of illness and death such as nutritional, viral, bacterial, and parasite etiologies.

CBC/BIOCHEMISTRY/URINALYSIS
• The single most important consultation when approaching a toxicologic incident is with the area diagnostic laboratory and specifically with a toxicologist. The laboratory's assistance can prove invaluable when selecting tissues for submission and the tests to request.
• At the bare minimum feed, serum, urine, ruminal contents, brain, liver, kidney, and skeletal muscle should be considered for submission.

OTHER LABORATORY TESTS
Toxins may not be equally distributed throughout the feed or water, therefore submit multiple samples to increase chances of inclusion of offending feed.

OTHER DIAGNOSTIC PROCEDURES
Examination of GIT contents may aid in diagnosis.

PATHOLOGIC FINDINGS
There are few pathognomonic findings for specific toxicologic agents.

TREATMENT

THERAPEUTIC APPROACH
• Largely ineffective as the time elapsed from exposure to diagnosis negates effectiveness of treatment efforts.

• The immediate removal of the toxic source is imperative.
• Many toxic agents require common treatments such as slowing absorption from the GI tract (activated charcoal) or skin (soap and water).
• More specific treatments may include the use of pH modifiers, vegetable oil, or emulsifiers to alter ruminal absorption.
• Palliative treatments such as the use of atropine for parasympatholytic effects or the use of IV fluids for cardiovascular support.
• As with any therapy used in food-producing animals in the USA it is imperative that the treatment falls within AMDUCA. Consultation with FARAD may prove useful for extra-label uses.
• Salvage or euthanasia can be considered under some instances.

MEDICATIONS

DRUGS OF CHOICE
Rarely any specific drug for treatment

FOLLOW-UP

EXPECTED COURSE AND PROGNOSIS
Varies greatly depending on the toxic principle.

POSSIBLE COMPLICATIONS
• Severity of complications are multifactorial and influenced by livestock species, toxin, time exposed, and amount of exposure. Some events result in irreversible, permanent damage to the livestock. Recovery and return to full production can occur in some instances; however, the time required for recovery has to be weighed against the salvage value of the patient and purchase of a replacement animal.
• Carcass disposal issues can be a very important and costly complication depending on local, state, or federal regulations. Improper carcass disposal has resulted in secondary wildlife fatalities.

PATIENT CARE
Dependent on species involved, toxic cause, facilities, and owner capabilities. Large numbers of affected livestock might be economically unfeasible.

PREVENTION
• Sample statistically significant number of feed samples to be analyzed for the commonly occurring toxic weeds growing at the forage origin.
• Regular communication with county agriculture extension service for up-to-date regional information.
• Regular surveillance of pastures (especially roadside fence lines, waterways) to identify

T

TOXICOLOGY: HERD OUTBREAKS   (CONTINUED)

species in pastures as well as removal of noxious volunteers.

MISCELLANEOUS

ASSOCIATED CONDITIONS
Varies greatly depending on the toxic principle.

AGE-RELATED FACTORS
Varies greatly depending on the toxic principle.

ZOONOTIC POTENTIAL
The importance of determining any public health concerns cannot be overemphasized. Primary toxin exposure can occur to animal handlers. Secondary exposure can occur to consumers of the milk, meat, or eggs produced from affected livestock.

PREGNANCY
Many toxic compounds can be abortifacients. As there are many infectious causes of abortion it is important to rule out their involvement beforehand.

BIOSECURITY
• Intentional poisonings have occurred.

• Biosecurity measures described and utilized to counter infectious agents such as foot and mouth disease can also be useful against intentional poisonings.

PRODUCTION MANAGEMENT
• Promote open dialog between nutritionist, veterinarian, hay broker, feeders.
• Document standard operating procedures addressing proper feed sampling and storage, chemical, pesticide and herbicide storage and use, carcass disposal, product (milk, eggs) disposal, biosecurity.
• Work with processors to establish procedures addressing adulterated product handling.

ABBREVIATIONS
• AMDUCA = Animal Medicinal Drug Use Clarification Act
• FARAD = Food Animal Residue Avoidance Databank (FARAD) (see www.fiveminutevet.com/ruminant)
• GIT = gastrointestinal tract
• IV = intravenous

Suggested Reading
Burrows GE, Tyrl RJ. Toxic Plants of North America, 2nd ed. Ames: Wiley-Blackwell, 2013.

Gawande A. The Checklist Manifesto: How to Get Things Right. New York: Picador, 2011.
Gupta RC. Veterinary Toxicology: Basic and Clinical Principles, 2nd ed. London: Academic Press, 2012.
Knight AP, Walter RG. A Guide to Plant Poisoning of Animals in North America. Jackson, WY: Teton NewMedia, 2001.
Osweiler GD. Ruminant toxicology. Vet Clin North Am Food Anim Pract 2011, 27(2).

Internet Resources
• https://www.aphis.usda.gov/publications/animal_health/2014/pub_bioguide_poultry_bird.pdf
• https://www.aphis.usda.gov/animal_health/nahms/beefcowcalf/downloads/beef0708/Beef0708_is_Biosecurity.pdf
• https://www.aphis.usda.gov/animal_health/nahms/feedlot/downloads/feedlot2011/Feed11_is_Biosecurity.pdf
• https://www.aphis.usda.gov/animal_health/nahms/smallscale/downloads/Small_scale_is_Biosecurity.pdf
Author Steven M. Gallego
Consulting Editor Christopher C.L. Chase

T

TRACHEAL EDEMA ("HONKER") SYNDROME

BASICS

OVERVIEW
• Tracheal edema ("honker") syndrome is a potentially life-threatening condition seen sporadically in feedlot cattle.
• Characterized by severe edema and hemorrhage of the dorsal wall of the trachea from the mid-cervical region to the tracheal bifurcation, resulting in partial to complete occlusion of the tracheal lumen.

INCIDENCE/PREVALENCE
Unknown

GEOGRAPHIC DISTRIBUTION
Canada and the United States; potentially worldwide

SYSTEMS AFFECTED
• Respiratory
• Musculoskeletal

PATHOPHYSIOLOGY
• The etiology of the syndrome is unknown.
• Possible causes may include viral or bacterial infection, trauma to the trachea from feed bunks, passive congestion and edema due to fat accumulation at the thoracic inlet, hypersensitivity, and mycotoxicosis.
• Postulated that marked intratracheal pressure changes due to frequent coughing could be the underlying cause of the tracheal lesions.

HISTORICAL FINDINGS
• Seen more often in warm weather. Possible exacerbation due to heat and dust.
• Typically seen during the last half of the feeding period.
• History varies, and can range from subclinically affected animals to those found dead.

SIGNALMENT
• Feedlot beef cattle, similar syndrome reported in pigs
• There appears to be no age or sex predilection.

PHYSICAL EXAMINATION FINDINGS
• Subclinical disease is possible. Tracheal lesions have been demonstrated at slaughter in cattle that did not have clinical signs.
• Typical signs include an acute onset of dyspnea with an increased inspiratory effort, coughing, and a loud, guttural stertor leading to the colloquial term "honker."
• Clinical signs can progress to open-mouth breathing with head and neck extended, cyanosis, belligerence, recumbency, and death.
• Some animals are found acutely dead with no premonitory signs.

GENETICS
N/A

CAUSES AND RISK FACTORS
• Clinical signs are seen predominantly in warm weather and are often brought on by increased movement or exercise.
• The etiology of the syndrome is unknown. Hypothetical causes include viral or bacterial infection, trauma to the trachea from feed bunks, passive congestion and edema due to fat accumulation at the thoracic inlet, hypersensitivity, and mycotoxicosis.

DIAGNOSIS

DIFFERENTIAL DIAGNOSES
• Necrotic laryngitis (calf diphtheria)
• Pharyngeal trauma
• Atypical interstitial pneumonia
• Laryngeal/tracheal foreign body, abscess, granuloma, neoplasia
• Previous severe arytenoid chondritis resulting in permanent narrowing of the rima glottis
• Laryngeal paralysis

CBC/BIOCHEMISTRY/URINALYSIS
N/A

OTHER LABORATORY TESTS
N/A

IMAGING
Tracheal endoscopy may be helpful in making a definitive diagnosis.

OTHER DIAGNOSTIC PROCEDURES
N/A

PATHOLOGIC FINDINGS
• Gross findings include severe submucosal edema and hemorrhage of the dorsal trachea seen from the midcervical trachea to the tracheal bifurcation. On cross section, the lumen of the trachea may be >50% occluded.
• On histopathology, the tracheal mucosa is hyperemic and hyperplastic with focal erosions and loss of cilia. The submucosa is markedly thickened by hemorrhage and edema and infiltrated by white blood cells. The trachealis muscle is separated from the surrounding connective tissue by hemorrhage and edema with swelling and vacuolation of the myocytes.

TREATMENT

THERAPEUTIC APPROACH
• Calm and minimal handling is imperative as asphyxiation and death can ensue if the animal becomes overly excited.
• The provision of shade and cooling with a water spray may be helpful in hot weather.
• Due to the distal location and extent of the typical lesions, temporary or permanent tracheostomy will likely be of no benefit unless an endotracheal tube is placed to the point of the tracheal bifurcation.

• Many cases will relapse, therefore salvage should be considered if the animal can be stabilized and transported comfortably.

SURGICAL CONSIDERATIONS AND TECHNIQUES
N/A

MEDICATIONS

DRUGS OF CHOICE
• Corticosteroids: Dexamethasone 0.05 mg/kg body weight IM or IV or prednisolone 1–2.2 mg/kg IM or IV daily.
• Broad-spectrum antimicrobials may be indicated but results vary.

CONTRAINDICATIONS
If salvage is a better decision from an animal welfare (avoiding chronic or repeated worsening respiratory distress events) and management perspective, then antimicrobials should be withheld.

PRECAUTIONS
Appropriate milk and meat withdrawal times should be followed for all compounds administered to food-producing animals.

POSSIBLE INTERACTIONS
N/A

FOLLOW-UP

EXPECTED COURSE AND PROGNOSIS
Prognosis for full recovery is guarded to poor as relapse often occurs.

POSSIBLE COMPLICATIONS
Poor response to therapy and relapse may require early slaughter or euthanasia.

PATIENT CARE
• Calm and minimal handling is imperative as asphyxiation and death can ensue if the animal becomes overly excited.
• The provision of shade and cooling with a water spray may be helpful in hot weather.

PREVENTION
Movement and exercise of cattle late in the feeding period should be avoided during warmer months and restricted to early morning hours when unavoidable.

MISCELLANEOUS

PRODUCTION MANAGEMENT
• Causes may include viral or bacterial infection, trauma to the trachea from feed bunks, passive congestion and edema due to fat accumulation at the thoracic inlet, hypersensitivity, and mycotoxicosis.
• Calm and minimal handling of affected animals is recommended.

T

TRACHEAL EDEMA ("HONKER") SYNDROME

• Provision of shade and cooling with a water spray may be helpful in hot weather.

SYNONYMS
• Honker
• Bovine honker syndrome
• Tracheal stenosis syndrome
• Tracheal stenosis of feedlot cattle

ABBREVIATIONS
• IM = intramuscular
• IV = intravenous

SEE ALSO
• Atypical Interstitial Pneumonia
• Calf Diphtheria/Necrotic Stomatitis

Suggested Reading
Apley MD, Fajt VR. Feedlot therapeutics. Vet Clin North Am Food Anim Pract 1998, 14: 291–314.

Erickson ED, Doster AR. Tracheal stenosis in feedlot cattle. J Vet Diagn Invest 1993, 5: 449–51.
Fingland RB, Rings DM, Vestweber JG. The etiology and surgical management of tracheal collapse in calves. Vet Surg 1990, 19: 371–9.
Panciera RJ, Williams DE. Tracheal edema (honker) syndrome of feedlot cattle. In: Howard JL ed, Current Veterinary Therapy: Food Animal Practice. Philadelphia: Saunders, 1981.
Rings DM. Tracheal collapse. Vet Clin North Am Food Anim Pract 1995, 11: 171–5.
Szeredi L, Dan A, Makrai L, Takacs N, Biksi I. Acute tracheal oedema and haemorrhage with fibrinonecrotic tracheitis in pigs – a porcine counterpart of bovine honker syndrome? J Comp Pathol 2013, 152: 206–10.

Author Katharine M. Simpson
Consulting Editor Kaitlyn A. Lutz
Acknowledgment The author and book editors acknowledge the prior contribution of William R. DuBois.

T

TRAUMATIC RETICULOPERITONITIS

 BASICS

OVERVIEW
Traumatic reticuloperitonitis (TRP) is a common disease of cattle but rarely seen in small ruminants. The eating habits of cattle predispose them to the accidental swallowing of metal foreign objects that settle in the rumen or reticulum.

INCIDENCE/PREVALENCE
N/A

GEOGRAPHIC DISTRIBUTION
Potentially worldwide, depending on species and environment

SYSTEMS AFFECTED
Digestive

PATHOPHYSIOLOGY
• The foreign object may penetrate the reticulum resulting in localized or generalized peritonitis, or only the wall of the reticulum may be involved and this may result in dysfunction due to interference with chemoreceptors or mechanoreceptors.
• The diaphragm, pericardium, and heart are located cranial to the reticulum and the liver is lateral and dorsal. Any of these organs may be penetrated by the foreign body and become involved in the inflammatory process.

HISTORICAL FINDINGS
In the most severe form of TRP, affected cattle may present with a dramatic change in posture, standing with an arched back, total anorexia, and vocalizing with a grunting noise when forced to move or when urinating. A sudden decrease in milk production is commonly reported.

SIGNALMENT
• This disease is seen primarily in cattle consuming processed forages or concentrates. In at least one study, the risk of TRP decreased with increasing parity and was higher when cattle had feet and leg problems.
• Species affected are dairy and beef cattle; however, potentially all ruminant species can become affected.
• There are no breed or age predilections.
• Females are more likely to have this disease because they are the predominant gender on any farm.

PHYSICAL EXAMINATION FINDINGS
• Physical examination of these cattle is characterized by fever, decreased rumen contractions, and an unwillingness to flex ventrally when pinched over the withers. They may have tachycardia, and auscultation of the heart may reveal increased cardiac intensity or may be muffled due to bacterial contamination and subsequent inflammation of the pericardium.
• Chronic cases present a diagnostic challenge due to signs that are subtle and vague.

Affected cattle in early lactation may have mild ketosis secondary to their anorexia. Mild bloat and changes in fecal consistency are also common signs. Weight loss, roughened hair coat, and diffuse generalized lameness may be the only signs.

GENETICS
N/A

CAUSES AND RISK FACTORS
The indiscriminate eating habits of cattle are the most likely cause of this disease. Construction in and around their environment will also increase the risk. The care and upkeep of the machinery used to process and provide silage to the cattle also plays a role in risk management.

 DIAGNOSIS

DIFFERENTIAL DIAGNOSES
Abomasal ulcers, diaphragmatic hernia, endoparasitism, heart disease, hepatic abscesses, indigestion, laminitis, lymphosarcoma, or other neoplasia may all be confused with TRP. Clinical signs will assist with ruling out laminitis. Further physical examination findings via rectal palpation may assist in ruling out lymphosarcoma or other abdominal neoplasms.

CBC/BIOCHEMISTRY/URINALYSIS
• The white blood cell count and distribution, plasma proteins, and fibrinogen may be normal in the initial stages of TRP. Total plasma proteins of over 10 g/dL have been shown to have a positive predictive value of 76% for TRP in referral populations.
• Biochemical profiles are not of high value in diagnosing TRP, but may be of benefit in ruling out others on the differential diagnosis list.
• Urinalysis would not be of definitive value in this disease, reflecting only the secondary ketosis that accompanies the anorexia commonly observed.

OTHER LABORATORY TESTS
Analysis and cytology of abdominal fluid showing increased protein and leukocyte count and active neutrophils ± bacteria. All normal bovine peritoneal fluid clots upon exposure to air, so samples are placed in small EDTA tubes.

IMAGING
• Abdominal radiographs with the horizontal beam centered over the reticulodiaphragmatic region in an attempt to confirm the presence of metallic foreign bodies can be done with the cow in that standing position or cast into dorsal recumbency.
• One study in which standing radiographs were taken describes the sensitivity of the procedure in detecting TRP as 83%.
• Ultrasound diagnosis has been utilized as well.

OTHER DIAGNOSTIC PROCEDURES
Abdominocentesis is recommended and may be aided by ultrasonography to obtain fluid. Remember that in normal, nonpregnant, adult cattle the amount of abdominal fluid is small.

PATHOLOGIC FINDINGS
• Peritonitis will occur if the reticulum epithelium is breached. This may be walled off by the inflammatory response or it may progress.
• Sudden death has occurred as a result of laceration of a coronary blood vessel or puncture of the heart by the foreign body.

 TREATMENT

THERAPEUTIC APPROACH
• Conservative treatment is most often attempted first and includes administration of a forestomach magnet, antibiotics, and confinement. Many cattle recover after this therapy with resumption of appetite and motility within 3 days.
• Initially affected animals should be stabled with their forequarters higher than their hindquarters.

SURGICAL CONSIDERATIONS AND TECHNIQUES
Those animals that do not recover in 3 days may require a rumenotomy to remove the foreign body in order to allow them to recover. This becomes an economic challenge for the producer and veterinary surgeon.

 MEDICATIONS

DRUGS OF CHOICE
Cattle with diffuse peritonitis have a poor prognosis for return to production or life. Treatment of peritonitis requires systemic antibiotics, possible drainage of the affected area, and surgical correction of the inciting cause.

CONTRAINDICATIONS
Appropriate milk and meat withdrawal times must be followed for all compounds administered to food-producing animals.

PRECAUTIONS
N/A

 FOLLOW-UP

EXPECTED COURSE AND PROGNOSIS
• Cattle with diffuse peritonitis have a poor prognosis for return to production or life.

T

TRAUMATIC RETICULOPERITONITIS

POSSIBLE COMPLICATIONS
• Those cattle that seem to recover in the short term may later develop forestomach outflow problems typical of vagal indigestion.
• It is not uncommon for the foreign body to migrate through the diaphragm and penetrate through the pericardium causing pericarditis and/or pleuritis.

CLIENT EDUCATION
See "Production Management"

PATIENT CARE
Return of rectal temperatures to normal values and increasing appetite and rumen motility are key findings in responding animals.

PREVENTION
Some producers will administer prophylactic magnets to all heifers at 6–8 months of age as another means of prevention of TRP. The implementation of this procedure will depend on the risk or known prevalence within the herd, but in most cases is cost effective.

 MISCELLANEOUS

PREGNANCY
May exacerbate disease symptoms.

PRODUCTION MANAGEMENT
Most producers now have large magnets in place on feed-handling equipment that eliminates the delivery of sharp metal objects to cattle at the time of feeding. Also, many producers have gone away from upright silos for storage of their corn silage in favor of bunkers. This has eliminated another source of metal contamination of feedstuffs by eliminating the mechanical unloader necessary for old upright silos.

SYNONYMS
• Hardware disease
• Wire disease

ABBREVIATION
• TRP = traumatic reticuloperitonitis

SEE ALSO
• Abomasal Ulceration
• Cardiac Failure
• Gastrointestinal Surgeries: Rumenotomy/Rumenostomy (see www.fiveminutevet.com/ruminant)
• Indigestion
• Liver Abscesses
• Lymphosarcoma
• Vagal Indigestion

Suggested Reading
Braun U, Fluckiger M, Gotz M. Comparison of ultrasonographic and radiographic findings in cows with traumatic reticuloperitonitis. Vet Rec 1994, 135: 470–8.
Braun U, Gansohr B, Fluckiger M. Radiographic findings before and after oral administration of a magnet in cows with traumatic reticuloperitonitis. Am. J Vet Res 2003, 64: 115–20.
Farrow CS. Reticular foreign bodies. Causative or coincidence? Vet Clin North Am Food Anim Pract 1999, 15: 397–408.
Fleischer P, Metzner M, Beyerbach M, Hoedemaker M, Klee W. The relationship between milk yield and the incidence of some diseases in dairy cows. J Dairy Sci 2001, 84: 2025–35.
Grohn YT, Bruss ML. Effect of diseases, production, and season on traumatic reticuloperitonitis and ruminal acidosis in dairy cattle. J Dairy Sci 1990, 73: 2355–63.
Rehage J, Kaske M, Stockhofe-Zurwieden N, Yalcin E. Evaluation of the pathogenesis of vagus indigestion in cows with traumatic reticuloperitonitis. J Am Vet Med Assoc 1995, 207: 1607–11.
Ward JL, Ducharme NG. Traumatic reticuloperitonitis in dairy cows. J Am Vet Med Assoc 1994, 204: 874–7.

Author Dennis D. French
Consulting Editor Kaitlyn A. Lutz

T

TREMETOL: WHITE SNAKEROOT AND RAYLESS GOLDENROD

BASICS

OVERVIEW
• White snakeroot is an opposite branching, dark green perennial, which grows 1–4 feet tall in damp, open areas of woods and shaded areas along streams.
• Stems are slender, round, and may be purplish.
• Leaves are 3–5 inches in length and have three distinct veins, coarsely toothed margins, and a sharp tip.
• Flowers are white and clustered in groups of 10–40 at the end of branches and bloom in late summer and fall.
• Roots are shallow and fibrous, and twist and turn, giving the plant its name.
• The plant grows in moist areas bordering streams, woodlands, as well as wooded areas with rich basic soil. It may persist in open areas after clearing.

INCIDENCE/PREVALENCE
• Intoxication requires ingestion of 0.5–1.0% of body weight of green plant over 2–3 weeks.
• Consumption of green plant material equivalent to 5–10% of the animal's body weight is required to produce intoxication.
• Because the toxicant's effects are cumulative, small amounts ingested for several weeks may be almost as toxic as a large amount eaten in a few days.
• There is slow loss of toxicity with heat and/or drying of the plant; however, this is variable, but dried plants in hay and even frost-damaged plants are reported to remain toxic for some time.

GEOGRAPHIC DISTRIBUTION
The geographic distribution is mostly eastern North America and grows from the East Coast including Canada, west to Minnesota, and south to east Texas and the Gulf Coast.

SYSTEMS AFFECTED
• Cardiovascular
• Musculoskeletal
• Multisystemic

PATHOPHYSIOLOGY
• Toxicity is most abundant in the foliage of the mature plant, is resistant to frost, and, although decreased, persists in the dried plant.
• The same toxins found in *Ageratina altissima* (white snakeroot) are also found in *Isocoma wrightii* (rayless goldenrod).
• The specific toxin has not been identified, but the unpurified form has been named tremetol.
• Effect of toxin requires microsomal activation and may explain different effects in different species.
• Intoxication is theorized to inhibit citrate synthase causing ketosis detectable by acetone smell of breath and urine.
• Intoxication in animals is often called trembles.

• Nursing young are clinically affected by high concentration in milk.
• Causes muscle damage and weakness.
• Causes hepatic necrosis.
• May cause photosensitization of small ruminants if animal survives acute disease.
• The toxin is cleared in milk and may cause signs in offspring or humans if ingested.

HISTORICAL FINDINGS
• Disease usually seen in late fall or early winter.
• Animals die soon after becoming recumbent.
• History of weight loss.

SIGNALMENT
• Seen most frequently in sheep, dairy cows, and goats, but all species ingesting the plant are at risk.
• Goats may be at a greater risk.

PHYSICAL EXAMINATION FINDINGS
• Ketosis causes acetone breath
• Afebrile
• Clinical signs different between species

Cattle and Sheep
• Reluctance to move.
• Stiff movements or ataxia.
• Severe trembles after exercise.
• Depression.
• Recumbency.
• Sudden death.
• Dyspnea, salivation, constipation, regurgitation may occasionally occur.
• Clinical signs may appear 3 days to 3 weeks after ingestion.

Goats
• Goats typically show signs of liver failure.
• Depression.
• Weakness.
• Head pressing.
• Icterus.
• Slight tremors with exercise.
• Recumbency.
• Sudden death.
• Photosensitization if animal survives acute disease.
• Clinical signs may appear 1–5 days after ingestion.

CAUSES AND RISK FACTORS
• The specific toxic principle in snakeroot is unknown.
• Moving naïve animals to contaminated pastures when there is inadequate forage (i.e., fall and winter).
• Lactating animals are more resistant due to rapid excretion of toxin in milk, putting nursing animals at high risk for clinical signs.

DIAGNOSIS

DIFFERENTIAL DIAGNOSES
• Selenium/Vitamin E deficiency
• Ionophore toxicosis

• Other causes of liver disease in small ruminants
• Gossypol intoxication
• Botulism in cattle
• Organophosphate intoxication
• CNS trauma
• Other tremorgenic toxicities

CBC/BIOCHEMISTRY/URINALYSIS
• Muscle enzymes (CK, LDH, ALP, AST, troponin) are elevated.
• Animals have ketoacidosis.
• May have myoglobinuria.
• Goats may have elevations in bilirubin.

OTHER DIAGNOSTIC PROCEDURES
• Evidence of plants in rumen
• Evidence of plant exposure

PATHOLOGIC FINDINGS
• Centrolobular hepatic degeneration and necrosis
• Skeletal muscle necrosis
• Cardiac abnormalities reported primarily in horses
• Extreme congestion of liver, kidney, abomasums, brain, and spinal cord
• Extreme fat degeneration of liver and kidney

TREATMENT

THERAPEUTIC APPROACH
• Correct any electrolyte and acid-base abnormalities.
• Ketosis is refractory to treatment.

MEDICATIONS

DRUGS OF CHOICE
• Activated charcoal (AC) (2–5 g/kg PO in a water slurry).
• Evidence in other species of recycling through gastrointestinal system; repeat doses of AC may be beneficial.
• Laxatives.

CONTRAINDICATIONS
• Any drug promoting hepatic microsomal enzymes is contraindicated.
• Any drug inhibiting hepatic microsomal enzymes may be helpful.

PRECAUTIONS
Appropriate milk and meat withdrawal times must be followed for all compounds administered to food-producing animals.

FOLLOW-UP

EXPECTED COURSE AND PROGNOSIS
Animals exhibiting clinical signs have grave prognosis.

T

TREMETOL: WHITE SNAKEROOT AND RAYLESS GOLDENROD   (CONTINUED)

PATIENT CARE
Monitor electrolytes.

PREVENTION
• Prevention of white snakeroot intoxication is possible—monitor pasture and hay for white snakeroot.
• Selective use of herbicides or manual removal of plants may help to diminish problem.

MISCELLANEOUS

AGE-RELATED FACTORS
Nursing animals may show clinical signs before other animals in the herd.

ZOONOTIC POTENTIAL
• During colonial time period hundreds of people were poisoned by milk from affected animals.
• As organic farming becomes more popular, the risk to humans may become more significant. Because the toxin is fat soluble, butter is also toxic.

PREGNANCY
N/A

PRODUCTION MANAGEMENT
Imperative to prevent access to plants during the growing season.

SYNONYMS
• River fever
• Swamp sickness
• Trembles

ABBREVIATIONS
• AC = activated charcoal
• ALP = alkaline phosphatase
• AST = aspartate aminotransferase
• CK = creatine kinase
• LDH = lactate dehydrogenase
• PO = per os, by mouth

SEE ALSO
• Brain Assessment and Dysfunction (see www.fiveminutevet.com/ruminant)
• Clostridial Disease: Gastrointestinal
• Clostridial Disease: Muscular
• Clostridial Disease: Nervous System
• Fungal Tremorgens
• Gossypol Toxicosis
• Liver Abscesses
• Organophosphate Toxicity
• Selenium/Vitamin E Deficiency

Suggested Reading
Beier RC, Norman JO. The toxic factor in white snakeroot: identity, analysis, and prevention. Vet Hum Toxicol 1990, 32 (suppl): 81–8.
Burrows GE, Tyrl RJ eds. In: Toxic Plants of North America, 2nd ed. Ames: Wiley-Blackwell, Kindle edition, 2013, pp. 152–6.
Galey FD. White snakeroot. In: Smith BP ed, Large Animal Internal Medicine. St. Louis: Mosby, 2002.

Author Steve Ensley
Consulting Editor Christopher C.L. Chase
Acknowledgment The author and book editors acknowledge the prior contribution of Benjamin R. Buchanan.

T

BASICS

OVERVIEW

• Trichomoniasis is a bovine venereal disease caused by an extracellular flagellated protozoan, *Tritrichomonas foetus*.
• The disease is asymptomatic in bulls but causes severe economic loss due to early embryonic loss and abortion.
• Trichomoniasis is a reportable disease in many countries. In the United States, some states require all bulls to be tested.
• *T. foetus* has been isolated from camels but its role in infertility and abortion in this species is not yet clear.

INCIDENCE/PREVALENCE

• Prevalence has been studied in several countries including Argentina, Australia, Spain, Switzerland, and the US.
• Prevalence varies from one country to another. In the US herd prevalence varies from 5% to 15% and up to 5% of bulls tested may be positive.
• The disease is more prevalent in beef herds, particularly in the southern and western US.
• Outbreaks have been reported in dairies using natural service.

GEOGRAPHIC DISTRIBUTION

Worldwide, particularly where natural service is the main method of breeding.

SYSTEMS AFFECTED

Reproductive

PATHOPHYSIOLOGY

• Bulls are generally infected if they breed a carrier female.
• The protozoan colonizes the epithelium of the prepuce, penis, and occasionally the urethral orifice of infected bulls.
• Infected bulls are asymptomatic. The parasite is restricted to the mucosal surface and is incapable of invading deeper tissues. The only histologic finding in infected bulls is a lymphocytic and plasmocytic infiltration of the epithelium and subepithelial layer.
• Older bulls (>3 years) become chronically infected whereas younger bulls (<2 years) seem to clear the infection.
• There are no effects on semen quality in infected bulls.
• Cows become infected if they are mated to carrier bulls or inseminated with cryopreserved semen from infected bulls.
• The parasite has cytotoxic and hemolytic activity resulting in an inflammatory response (salpingitis, endometritis, and cervicitis). Pregnant cows experience fetal death in the first trimester and more rarely abortion later in gestation. The pregnancy loss ranges from 5% to 30%. Most abortions occur before 5 months of gestation but later abortions have been observed.
• Pregnancy loss occurs generally 7–9 weeks after infection. Aborting cows show a high number of organisms in the chorioallantois and fetal stomach.
• A high proportion of infected cows may have a pyometra.
• Infected cows develop a local vaginal antigen-specific antibody response (IgG1 and IgA) but this immunity does not always prevent reproductive loss.
• Cows clear the infection within 6–18 weeks.

HISTORICAL FINDINGS

Herds experiencing an outbreak of trichomoniasis share several historical findings including:
• Introduction of open or late calving cows in the herd
• Introduction of nontested bulls
• Use of communal grazing and co-mingling during the breeding season with unknown or untested herds
• Keeping older bulls or open cows from previous season
• Large number of cows returning to estrus
• Low pregnancy rate
• Reduced calving rate or a prolonged calving season

SIGNALMENT

N/A

PHYSICAL EXAMINATION FINDINGS

• Infected bulls do not show any clinical signs.
• Infected aborting cows may show vaginal discharge.
• Clinical suspicion in the herd is made at the time of pregnancy diagnosis. The proportion of open cows varies depending on whether the herd practices early (<90 days) or late (>90 days) pregnancy diagnosis. Overall pregnancy rate may be as low as 70% with a highly variable gestational stage.
• Up to 5% of the open cows may be diagnosed with pyometra (fluid-filled uterus with no positive signs of pregnancy and presence of a corpus luteum).

GENETICS

N/A

CAUSES AND RISK FACTORS

• *Tritrichomonas foetus* is an extracellular flagellated protozoan. The parasite is spindle shaped and measures 8–12 μm by 15–20 μm with three anterior flagellae and a recurrent flagellum (undulating membrane).
• The main risk factor for the disease is the introduction into the herd of carrier bulls.

DIAGNOSIS

DIFFERENTIAL DIAGNOSES

• Other causes of infertility or early pregnancy loss that may present in the same manner as trichomoniasis are nutritional deficiencies and campylobacteriosis.
• Nutritional deficiencies, in particular, poor energy intake, may result in poor reproductive performance due to anestrus, delayed puberty, poor conception rates, and increased early embryo loss. Nutritional deficiencies are suspected based on historical findings, BCS at calving or at breeding, heifer growth performance, and general health of the herd. Ration analysis should provide more information on the nutritional state of the herd.
• Campylobacteriosis due to *Campylobacter fetus* subsp. *venerealis* has the same herd presentation but without the increased rate of pyometra.
• Less commonly, *Histophilus somni* (*Haemophilus somnus*), *Chlamydophila* spp., and *Ureaplasma* spp. may cause outbreaks of venereally transmitted infections resulting in early pregnancy loss. However, these are generally accompanied by clinical genital lesions.
• Use of poor fertility bulls may also results in poor pregnancy rates and a prolonged calving season.

CBC/BIOCHEMISTRY/URINALYSIS

N/A

OTHER LABORATORY TESTS

• In bulls, the most common diagnostic test is culture or culture and PCR from the smegma obtained by preputial scraping.
  ○ The bull is restrained in a chute and the preputial orifice is cleaned. A sterile plastic-covered, 22-inch uterine infusion pipette attached to a 12 mL syringe is introduced deep into the fornix. The plastic cover is pulled back and the pipette is vigorously rubbed against the preputial mucosa while applying a negative pressure with the syringe to allow collection of a good amount of smegma.
  ○ It is important not to contaminate the sample with too much blood or fecal material.
  ○ Other techniques for sampling use preputial scraping devices (Tricamper®, Trichit®) which claim better samples and less blood contamination.
  ○ In the US, several states require training and certification in *T. foetus* sampling before accepting samples from veterinarians.
  ○ The smegma is placed into commercially available special culture media (Diamond's TYM medium or InPouch®; Biomed Diagnostic, San Jose CA, USA).
  ○ Samples are incubated at 37°C (98.6°F) and examined 1, 3, 5, and 7 days after sampling.
  ○ The protozoan is easily identified at 200× to 400× magnification under light microscopy by its wave-like, rapid and irregular rolling and jerky movement.
  ○ Sensitivity of culture for detection of *T. foetus* ranges from 84% to 96% and may be lower under field conditions. Therefore, a culture/PCR test is recommended and improves significantly the sensitivity and specificity. Some states require that the

TRICHOMONIASIS

culture and PCR be performed in an approved or certified laboratory.
• In cows, direct microscopic evaluation of the uterine content from the pyometra reveals the presence of parasite. The fluid may be submitted for culture and PCR.
• The parasite is also isolated from abomasal content of aborted fetuses and can be identified with dark field microscopy.
• Immunohistochemistry using polyclonal and monoclonal antibodies are effective methods for detection of *T. foetus* in fetal and placental tissues.
• In non-autolyzed placentae, the parasite may be identified in the stroma of hematoxylin and eosin stained sections.

IMAGING
Transrectal ultrasonography is not necessary but can confirm palpation diagnosis of pyometra.

OTHER DIAGNOSTIC PROCEDURES
N/A

PATHOLOGIC FINDINGS
• There are no obvious lesions in bulls. Immunohistochemistry may reveal *T. foetus* and/or its surface antigen adhered to the surface of the preputial and penile squamous epithelium.
• In cows, cervicitis and endometritis have been described in cases of *T. foetus* infection. However, these conditions are not common in natural infection. Pyometra is the most commonly found condition. Histologic lesions include mild to moderate infiltration of neutrophils and eosinophils in the stratum compactum and the stratum spongiosum of the endometrium. Many females show aggregations of mononuclear cells in the stratum spongiosum resembling lymphoid follicles, 6–9 weeks after infection.
• There are no gross lesions in the abortus except placental edema in some cases. The fetus may be in a variable state of autolysis. Fetal lung may show bronchopneumonia with neutrophilic and macrophage exudate. On histology, trichomonads may be seen in alveoli and airways along with Langhans and/or foreign body giant cells.

TREATMENT

THERAPEUTIC APPROACH
Treatment is illegal in several countries. Although *T. foetus* may be sensitive to nitro-imidazole drugs, these drugs should not be used.

SURGICAL CONSIDERATIONS AND TECHNIQUES
N/A

MEDICATIONS

DRUGS OF CHOICE
N/A

CONTRAINDICATIONS
N/A

PRECAUTIONS
N/A

POSSIBLE INTERACTIONS
N/A

FOLLOW-UP

EXPECTED COURSE AND PROGNOSIS
• Economic losses vary greatly but are expected to be significant.
• Bulls and open cows should be culled and disposed of according to local/state regulations.
• Trichomoniasis is a reportable disease in several countries. In the US, there are no federal trichomoniasis regulations currently. However, some states have specific regulations. Some states require three consecutive negative tests one week apart before an animal is deemed negative.
• Sample pooling may reduce cost of testing. However, not all states accept results from pooled samples.
• It is important for practitioners to check the protocol for testing with the state veterinarian or other regulating agency.
• The practitioner, producer, and state veterinarian should develop a trichomoniasis elimination program for the herd.
• Positive cows may be maintained in a separate herd and bred by artificial insemination from clean bulls.
• Vaccination of females twice, one month apart, just prior to bull exposure has been suggested as an additional method of control in infected herds.

POSSIBLE COMPLICATIONS
N/A

CLIENT EDUCATION
• Know the risk factors and economic losses for trichomoniasis.
• Understand the limitations of testing protocols.
• Develop a quarantine and testing program, particularly for bulls.
• Develop a prevention and eradication program with their veterinarian.

PATIENT CARE
Positive animals should be culled from breeding.

PREVENTION
• Prevention of trichomoniasis is based primarily on biosecurity measures including testing of all new bulls and avoiding co-mingling with other herds.
• Use of virgin bulls should be part of any preventive measure.
• A commercial killed whole cell vaccine is available. Experimental studies have shown that vaccination of bulls helps prevent or clear infection in bulls. Vaccination of females has been shown to reduce reproductive losses after mating to infected bulls. However, recommendation for widespread use of vaccination as the sole method of control of the disease is controversial.

MISCELLANEOUS

ASSOCIATED CONDITIONS
Abortion, infertility

AGE-RELATED FACTORS
Older bulls (>3 years of age) are more likely to become persistent carriers.

ZOONOTIC POTENTIAL
N/A

PREGNANCY
Early pregnancy loss and abortion

BIOSECURITY
• Test all newly introduced bulls.
• Avoid introduction of open or late calving cows.
• Avoid co-mingling with other herds.

PRODUCTION MANAGEMENT
• Cull all open cows and test all bulls.
• Use artificial insemination with cryopreserved sperm from controlled sources.

SYNONYM
Trichomonosis

ABBREVIATIONS
• BCS = body condition score
• IgA = immunoglobulin A
• IgG1 = immunoglobulin G1
• PCR = polymerase chain reaction

SEE ALSO
• Abortion: Bovine
• Campylobacter
• Pyometra

Suggested Reading
Batzell P, Newton H, O'Connor AM. A critical review and meta-analysis of the efficacy of whole cell killed *Tritrichomonas foetus* vaccines in beef cattle. J Vet Intern Med 2013, 27: 760–70.
Collantes-Fernandez E, Mendoza-Ibarra JA, Pedraza-Diaz S, et al. Efficacy of a control program for bovine trichomonosis based on

testing and culling infected bulls in beef cattle managed under mountain pastoral systems of Northern Spain. Vet J 2014, 200: 140–5.

Garcia Guerra A, Hill JE, Wladner CL, Campbell J, Hendrick S. Sensitivity of a real-time polymerase chain reaction for *Tritrichomonas foetus* in direct individual and pooled preputial samples. Theriogenology 2013, 80:1097–103.

Michi AN, Favetto PH, Kastelic J, Cobo ER. A review of sexually transmitted bovine trichomoniasis and campylobacteriosis affecting cattle reproductive health. Theriogenology 2016, 85: 781–91.

Yao C, Bardsley KD, Litzman E, Davidson MR. *Tritrichomonas foetus* infection in beef bull populations in Wyoming. J Bacteriol Parasitol 2011, 2(5): 117.

Author Ahmed Tibary

Consulting Editor Ahmed Tibary

Acknowledgment The author and book editors acknowledge the prior contribution of Robert H. BonDurant.

T

TRYPANOSOMIASIS

BASICS

OVERVIEW
• Caused by protozoa of the genus *Trypanosoma* that live in the blood and body fluids of their hosts.
• Results in anemia, emaciation of animals, and loss of condition.
• Transmission is by vectors (tsetse flies—*Glossina morsitans, G. palpalis, G. fusca,* and vampire bats) and through mechanical vectors of the genus *Tabanus*. Hematogenous equipment, such as needles and surgical instruments, can also transmit trypanosomes.
• Ruminants are widely known to be active reservoirs.
• Infections with trypanosomes result in diseases such as nagana, surra, Chagas' disease, and African sleeping sickness.

INCIDENCE/PREVALENCE
Unknown

GEOGRAPHIC DISTRIBUTION
Found in the subtropical and tropical areas of Africa, Asia, and South and Central America.

SYSTEMS AFFECTED
• Cardiovascular
• Digestive
• Nervous
• Musculoskeletal
• Hemolymphatic
• Reproductive
• Ophthalmic

PATHOPHYSIOLOGY
• The protozoa multiply in the blood, tissue, or body fluids of the vertebrate host and are transmitted between vertebrate hosts through the saliva of blood-sucking flies as they feed.
• At the site of inoculation, there is a local skin reaction called a chancre.
• From here the trypanosomes reach the bloodstream directly or through the lymphatic system.
• Parasitemia becomes apparent 10–14 days after inoculation.
• Trypanosomes' success lies in their ability to evade the host's immune system by altering the antigenic nature of its surface-coat glycoproteins.

HISTORICAL FINDINGS
Lethargy, depression

SIGNALMENT
• Cattle, sheep, goats, camels, llamas, and buffalo.
• Adult sheep between 1 and 4 years of age with 4 years of age being the norm for susceptibility; lambs are more susceptible to infection if exposed prior to 10 weeks of age.

PHYSICAL EXAMINATION FINDINGS
• There are no pathognomonic signs and the severity of the signs varies depending on the size of the inoculation dose, the species and strain of the trypanosomes, and breed and management of the host.
• Can present as an acute, subclinical, or chronic infection.
• Acute: Anemia, intermittent fever, loss of condition, and abortion may be seen; decrease in milk production; in some cases diarrhea; some become inappetant with a stiff gait and die within a few weeks.
• Chronic: Affected animals are anorexic, apathetic, and emaciated, and have ocular discharge, keratoconjunctivitis, and a dull coat. A marked jugular pulse develops, associated with pale mucus membranes and elevated respiratory and pulse rate. Although the animal continues to eat, it gradually loses weight and death occurs after several months due to heart failure.
• Subclinical: Stress plays a prominent role in the disease process.
• CNS effects include meningoencephalitis, progressive weakness, and ataxia.

GENETICS
Certain breeds of African cattle are considerably more resistant to African trypanosomiasis than others.

CAUSES AND RISK FACTORS
• Nagana or African trypanosomiasis: *Trypanosoma brucei, T. congolense, T. vivax,* and *T. simiae*—variety of animals affected. Transmitted cyclically by tsetse flies and mechanically by other biting flies.
• Surra: *T. evansi*—horses and camels affected; transmitted mechanically by biting flies in Africa, Asia, and South and Central America.
• Found in subtropical and tropical locations; the risk factor is being exposed to vectors, such as tsetse flies, biting flies (tabanids), and vampire bats.

DIAGNOSIS

DIFFERENTIAL DIAGNOSES
• Acute anthrax
• Anaplasmosis
• Babesiosis
• Theileriosis
• Hemorrhagic septicemia
• Gastrointestinal helminths (*Haemonchus*)
• Chronic malnutrition

CBC/BIOCHEMISTRY/URINALYSIS
• Decreased packed cell volume, erythrocyte count, and hemoglobin
• Leukopenia, neutropenia, lymphocytosis, and monocytosis
• Hypoglycemia, hypoalbuminemia, hyperglobinemia
• Thrombocytopenia
• Metabolic acidosis

OTHER LABORATORY TESTS
Serology for other infectious diseases

IMAGING
N/A

OTHER DIAGNOSTIC PROCEDURES
• Microscopic examination (direct)—wet mount of blood slides, thick and thin blood films stained with Giemsa, and stained lymph nodes for visual identification of trypanosomes and exclusion of other blood parasites.
• Indirect method—antigen-detecting ELISA, indirect fluorescent antibody test.
• Molecular test—species-specific DNA probes.
• Subinoculation into experimental animals.

PATHOLOGIC FINDINGS
Most findings are nonspecific but can include serous atrophy of fat, subcutaneous edema, emaciation, petechiation, and enlarged liver, spleen, and lymph nodes. The spleen may also be atrophied or normal in some cases depending on the severity of the disease. Other lesions include necrosis of the kidneys and heart muscle and a sore or chancre at the site of entry.

TREATMENT

THERAPEUTIC APPROACH
• Supportive care
• Blood transfusion from known negative animals

SURGICAL CONSIDERATIONS AND TECHNIQUES
N/A

MEDICATION

DRUGS OF CHOICE
• Treating trypanosomiasis is expensive and not always successful. In some countries, there are prophylactic treatments that have been used with some success.
• Diminazene aceturate (Berenil, 3.5–7 mg/kg body weight, IM) for *T. vivax* and *T. congolense,* well tolerated by ruminants but not by horses.
• Homidium bromide (ethidium B, 1 mg/kg IM) and homidium chloride (novidium or ethidium C, 1 mg/kg IM) for *T. vivax* and *T. congolense*. Cattle and small ruminants.
• Isometamidium chloride is another preferred drug to use against *T. vivax* and *T. congolense* in ruminants as a curative (0.25–0.5 mg/kg, IM) and prophylactic dose (1 mg/kg, IM). Pyrithidium bromide is less widely used against *T. vivax* and *T. congolense* as prophylactic at 2 mg/kg body weight.
• Suramin may also be used against *T. brucei* as a curative and prophylactic drug at 10 mg/kg body weight in horses and camels.
• Melarsomine (0.25–0.5 mg/kg, IM or SC). Registered for use against *T. evansi* in camels. Very widely used in the Middle East.

T

(CONTINUED)

CONTRAINDICATIONS
Appropriate milk and meat withdrawal times must be followed for all compounds administered to food-producing animals.

PRECAUTIONS
Trypanosomiasis is considered a foreign animal disease in several countries including the US, and should be reported immediately to authorities.

POSSIBLE INTERACTIONS
Sudden death can occur.

 FOLLOW-UP

EXPECTED COURSE AND PROGNOSIS
Due to the potential for reinfection, prognosis varies depending on the severity of infection and how rapidly it was detected and treated.

POSSIBLE COMPLICATIONS
Abortion, sudden death can occur after treatment in heavily parasitized animals.

CLIENT EDUCTION
Importance of preventive measures

PATIENT CARE
Because reinfection can occur, monitor weight, appetite, temperature, and PCV.

PREVENTION
• Vector control is recommended.
• Trypano-tolerance—certain breeds of African cattle are considerably more resistant to African trypanosomiasis than others. The mechanisms of trypano-tolerance have been extensively studied and it has been established that it has a genetic basis. Certain small ruminant breeds are also more trypano-tolerant than others. Selective breeding for tolerant animals can reduce the need for medication in endemic areas.

 MISCELLANEOUS

ASSOCIATED CONDITIONS
N/A

AGE-RELATED FACTORS
Sheep aged 1–4 years of age; lambs <10 weeks of age

ZOONOTIC POTENTIAL
• Chagas' disease—*T. cruzi*—occasionally pigs but mainly in dogs and humans susceptible; transmitted by sucking blood vectors in South and Central America and the southern parts of the United States.
• African trypanosomiasis in humans can be caused by *Trypanosoma brucei gambiense* (central and west Africa), which causes a latent chronic infection, and *Trypanosoma brucei rhodesiense* (southern and east Africa), which causes a more virulent acute infection.

PREGNANCY
• African trypanosomiasis can be transmitted in utero from infected mothers resulting in abortion and perinatal death of the fetus; trypanosomiasis can also cause infertility.

BIOSECURITY
Vector control is important although difficult in endemic areas.

PRODUCTION MANAGEMENT
Economic losses can arise from emaciated animals, mortalities, and the cost of vector control programs.

SYNONYMS
• African sleeping sickness
• Chagas' disease
• Nagana
• Surra
• Trypanosomiasis
• Tsetse disease
• Tsetse fly disease

ABBREVIATIONS
• CNS = central nervous system
• ELISA = enzyme-linked immunosorbent assay
• IM = intramuscular
• PCV = packed cell volume
• SC = subcutaneous

SEE ALSO
• Anaplasmosis
• Anemia, Nonregenerative
• Anthrax
• Babesiosis
• Starvation

Suggested Reading
Geerts S, Osaer S, Goossens B, Faye D. Trypanotolerance in small ruminants of sub-Saharan Africa. Trends Parasitol 2009, 25: 132–8.

Gutierrez C, Corbera JA, Morales M, Büscher P. Trypanosomiasis in goats: current status. Ann NY Acad Sci 2006, 1081: 300–10.

Hargrove JW, Ouifki R, Kajunguri D, Vale GA, Torr S. Modeling the control of trypanosomiasis using trypanocides or insecticide-treated Livestock. PLoS Neglected Tropical Diseases, 2012, 6: e1615.

Jaiswal AK, Sudan V, Kumar Verma N, Kumar Verna A. Insight into trypanosomiasis in animals: various approaches for its diagnosis, treatment and control: a review. Asian J Anim Sci 2015, 9: 172–86.

Mare CJ. Trypanosomiasis. In: Foreign Animal Diseases. Richmond, VA: United States Animal Health Association, 1998. http://www.vet.uga.edu/wpp/graybook/FAD.

Ohaeri CC, Eluwa MC. Abnormal biochemical and haematological indices in trypanosomiasis as a threat to herd production. Vet Parasitol 2011, 177: 199–202.

Uilenberg G. A Field Guide for the Diagnosis, Treatment and Prevention of African Animal Trypanosomosis. Rome: Food and Agriculture Organization of the United Nations, 1998.

Van den Bossche P, de La Rocque S, Hendrickx G, Bouyer J. A changing environment and the epidemiology of tsetse-transmitted livestock trypanosomiasis. Trends Parasitol 2010, 26: 236–43.

Wernery U, Kinne J, Schuster RK. Protozoal infections: Trypanosomosis. In: Wernery U, et al. eds, Camelid Infectious Disorders. Paris: OIE (World Organisation for Animal Health), 2014, pp. 359–67.

Author Kate O'Conor
Consulting Editor Ahmed Tibary
Acknowledgment The author and book editors acknowledge the prior contribution of Yessenia Almeida and Danelle Bickett-Weddle.

T

TUBERCULOSIS: BOVINE

BASICS

OVERVIEW
- Bovine tuberculosis (bovine TB) is caused primarily by the bacterium *Mycobacterium bovis*.
- Bovine TB is a reportable disease in many countries, including the United States, and is found in all parts of the world.
- Bovine TB affects primarily the respiratory system and associated lymph nodes. The disseminated form of the disease can be found in other organ systems including the gastrointestinal tract, reproductive tract, mammary glands, and central nervous system.
- *Mycobacterium bovis* infections have been described in numerous domestic and wild animals including sheep, goats, horses, pigs, deer, antelope, dogs, cats, ferrets, camels, foxes, mink, badgers, rats, primates, llamas, kudu, eland, tapir, elk, elephant, sitatunga, oryx, addax, rhinoceros, opossum, ground squirrel, otter, seal, hare, mole, raccoon, coyote, lion, tiger, leopard, and lynx.
- Most species other than cattle are considered to be dead-end hosts; however, some species can serve as reservoir hosts. Known reservoir hosts include brush-tailed opossums in New Zealand, badgers in the United Kingdom and Ireland, deer in the United States, bison in Canada, and greater kudu, common duiker, African buffalo, warthog, and Kafue lechwe in Africa.
- Bovine TB can be transmitted either by the respiratory route or ingestion.
- *Mycobacterium bovis* is a zoonotic agent and is a significant public health concern.

INCIDENCE/PREVALENCE
- In the US where an eradication program has been in place since 1917, the prevalence in cattle is extremely low (0.1 cases per 1 million head). The same is true for many developed countries including New Zealand whose eradication program has been praised.
- In many developing countries prevalence remains high (reports between 3% and 50% in some African countries), with much variability depending on husbandry practices and region.

GEOGRAPHIC DISTRIBUTION
Worldwide

SYSTEMS AFFECTED
- Respiratory
- Reproductive
- Mammary
- Nervous
- Digestive

PATHOPHYSIOLOGY
- Disease is contracted via inhalation of droplets aerosolized from infected reservoirs and less commonly via ingestion of contaminated milk or water.
- If not cleared by alveolar macrophages, the mycobacteria will proliferate and through a cytokine-mediated hypersensitivity reaction a focus of immune cells will form. Eventual formation of a necrotic, caseous, partially calcified center encased by a fibrous capsule is what constitutes the classic tubercle.
- In cases of disseminated TB, these lesions will be found in surrounding lymph nodes and multiple other organs (see "Systems Affected").

HISTORICAL FINDINGS
Bovine tuberculosis is a chronic debilitating disease, but can occasionally be acute and rapidly progressive.

SIGNALMENT
Bovine TB can affect all ages but prevalence is higher in cattle >2 years old.

PHYSICAL EXAMINATION FINDINGS
- Early infections are often asymptomatic; however, in later stages, common symptoms include progressive emaciation, a low-grade fluctuating fever, weakness, and inappetence.
- Animals with pulmonary involvement have a moist cough that is worse in the morning, during cold weather, or during exercise. These animals may also exhibit dyspnea or tachypnea.
- In some animals, the retropharyngeal or other lymph nodes enlarge and may rupture and drain.
- Greatly enlarged lymph nodes can obstruct blood vessels, airways, or the digestive tract.
- If the digestive tract is involved, intermittent diarrhea and constipation may be seen. Lesions are sometimes found on the female genitalia but are rare on the male genitalia.
- Mammary gland involvement typically results in induration and hypertrophy of the affected gland, and enlargement of the supramammary lymph nodes.

GENETICS
N/A

CAUSES AND RISK FACTORS
- Bovine TB is caused primarily by the bacterium Mycobacterium bovis.
- *M. bovis* can survive for several months in the environment, particularly in cold, dark, and moist conditions.
- The major risk factor for infection with bovine TB is exposure to infected reservoirs.

DIAGNOSIS

DIFFERENTIAL DIAGNOSES
- Other causes of chronic respiratory disease—*Mycoplasma bovis*, chronic lung abscesses, aspiration pneumonia.
- Other causes of chronic weight loss and ill thrift—Johne's disease, parasitism, and bovine leukosis.

CBC/BIOCHEMISTRY/URINALYSIS
N/A

OTHER LABORATORY TESTS
N/A

IMAGING
N/A

OTHER DIAGNOSTIC PROCEDURES
- Caudal fold tuberculin test (CFT)—an intradermal skin test that is used as an initial screening test. In the US, an accredited veterinarian must administer this test.
- Comparative cervical test (CCT)—an intradermal skin test used most commonly as a follow-up to the CFT to differentiate immune responses to *Mycobacterium bovis* and *Mycobacterium avium*. In the US, only a state or federal veterinarian can perform this test.
- *Mycobacterium bovis* gamma interferon assay—an assay used most commonly as a follow-up to the CFT test.

PATHOLOGIC FINDINGS
- The characteristic gross lesion seen in an animal infected with bovine TB is the presence of granulomatous tubercles within the body. A tubercle is a white nodule usually 1 mm to 2 cm in diameter.
- Tubercles may be localized to a single organ or disseminated through many organ systems.
- Bovine TB tubercles are most commonly found in the thoracic cavity and associated lymph nodes.
- The lesion most commonly associated with bovine TB is a granuloma.
- On histology, following acid-fast staining of suspect tissue, bacteria that take up stain, including *Mycobacterium bovis*, will appear as short red or pink rods when examined under a microscope.

TREATMENT

Animals diagnosed with the disease are humanely euthanized and those in the herd of contact are quarantined. Specific regulations will vary depending on country.

MEDICATIONS

DRUGS OF CHOICE
N/A

CONTRAINDICATIONS
N/A

PRECAUTIONS
Proper intradermal administration is necessary for accurate test results when performing the CFT and CCT.

POSSIBLE INTERACTIONS
N/A

FOLLOW-UP

EXPECTED COURSE AND PROGNOSIS
Cattle infected with bovine TB are humanely destroyed. Farms where bovine TB positive animals originate are considered infected and subsequently are quarantined. Disposition of these herds is decided upon by the regulatory authorities governing TB control in that area.

POSSIBLE COMPLICATIONS
• Human infections
• Economic implications based on loss of milk sales and herd culling

PATIENT CARE
N/A

PREVENTION
Bovine TB is considered a herd disease; therefore, emphasis is placed on preventing the introduction of the disease onto a farm. Biosecurity procedures should be put in place that prevent the introduction of cattle at high risk of having bovine TB and to prevent potential wildlife reservoirs from having close contact with cattle, cattle feed, or cattle water.

MISCELLANEOUS

ZOONOTIC POTENTIAL
Mycobacterium bovis is a zoonotic agent that historically was spread primarily through the consumption of unpasteurized milk from infected cows. Other potential routes of zoonotic transmission include consumption of undercooked meat and close contact with infected cows.

PREGNANCY
In cattle with advanced bovine TB, fetal infection can occur, resulting in calves being born infected with bovine TB.

BIOSECURITY
Because this is a disease of high consequence both as a zoonosis and as a potential to cause economic disaster for infected herds, employing standard farm biosecurity measures is extremely important. See chapters, Biosecurity: Beef Cow/Calf and Biosecurity: Dairy.

PRODUCTION MANAGEMENT
Routine herd testing may be required depending on government regulations.

ABBREVIATIONS
• CCT = comparative cervical test
• CFT = caudal fold tuberculin test
• TB = tuberculosis

SEE ALSO
• Biosecurity: Beef Cow/Calf (see www.fiveminutevet.com/ruminant)
• Biosecurity: Dairy (see www.fiveminutevet.com/ruminant)
• Cleaning and Disinfection (see www.fiveminutevet.com/ruminant)
• Vaccination Programs: Beef Cattle
• Vaccination Programs: Dairy Cattle
• Vaccinology (see www.fiveminutevet.com/ruminant)

Suggested Reading
de la Rua-Domenech R. Human *Mycobacterium bovis* infection in the United Kingdom: Incidence, risks, control measures and review of the zoonotic aspects of bovine tuberculosis. Tuberculosis (Edinb) 2006, 86: 77–109.
Enticott G, Maye D, Carmody P, et al. Farming on the edge: farmer attitudes to bovine tuberculosis in newly endemic areas. Vet Rec 2015, 177: 439.
Lahuerta-Marin A, Gallagher M, McBride S. Should they stay, or should they go? Relative future risk of bovine tuberculosis for interferon-gamma test-positive cattle left on farms. Vet Res 2015, 46: 90.
Mengistu A, Enguselassi F, Aseffa A, Beyen D. Bovine tuberculosis (BTB) as a risk factor for developing tuberculosis in humans in the rural community of Ethiopia: A case-control study. Ethiop Med J 2015, 53: 1–8.
Morc SJ, Radunz B, Glanville RJ. Lessons learned during the successful eradication of bovine tuberculosis from Australia. Vet Rec 2015, 177: 224–32.
Ramos DF, Silva PE, Dellagostin OA. Diagnosis of bovine tuberculosis: review of main techniques. Braz J Biol 2015, 75: 830–7.

Author Bonnie R. Loghry
Consulting Editor Kaitlyn A. Lutz
Acknowledgment The author and book editors acknowledge the prior contribution of Daniel L. Grooms.

T

ULCERATIVE POSTHITIS AND VULVITIS

BASICS

OVERVIEW
- Ulcerative posthitis is an infectious disease of the external genitalia affecting both male and female small ruminants.
- It is most commonly caused by an aerobic, Gram-positive rod-shaped bacterium, *Corynebacterium renale*.
- This bacterium is a normal inhabitant of the skin and external genitalia of small ruminants and can be spread by venereal transmission.
- The bacteria can survive for 6 months in wool and scabs and can survive freezing in exudates.
- *C. renale* proliferates on the genital mucosa in the presence of urea, which increases in the urine of animals fed high amounts of protein and nonprotein nitrogen (NPN) in rations.
- *C. renale* hydrolyzes urea to ammonia, which results in necrosis of surrounding tissues.

INCIDENCE/PREVALENCE
Sporadic, but a significant proportion of animals in vulnerable groups can be affected, such as pre-sale or pre-breeding rams receiving adjusted rations.

GEOGRAPHIC DISTRIBUTION
Worldwide; distribution influenced by production systems

SYSTEMS AFFECTED
- Reproductive
- Urinary

PATHOPHYSIOLOGY
- *C. renale* is a commensal organism of the skin and external genitalia of small ruminants.
- This organism contains urease and can hydrolyze urea to ammonia.
- Provision of a high-protein ration increases rumen ammonia production, which undergoes hepatic conversion to urea for excretion in the urine.
- High concentrations of urea in the urine allow *C. renale* to proliferate and hydrolyze urea; resulting ammonia creates chemical damage to the skin of the prepuce or vulva.

HISTORICAL FINDINGS
- May include risk factors such as grazing of lush green pastures, or introduction of a high-protein ration to pre-sale, pre-breeding, or finishing animals.
- Signs of disease can commence 2 weeks or later after dietary changes.

SIGNALMENT
- Male and female small ruminants may be affected (males much more commonly).
- Castrated males are predisposed.
- Breeding rams, pet wethers, feedlot lambs, show lambs/kids, and wool and fiber production animals are predisposed.

- Merinos and Angoras are commonly affected due to dense wool and fiber.
- Usually animals >6 months old.

PHYSICAL EXAMINATION FINDINGS
- Moist ulcers at the mucocutaneous junction of the prepuce form, then become covered by a thin, brown, malodorous scab.
- Focal swelling of the prepuce and pain on palpation are evident, with malodorous exudate, necrotic tissue, and urine present in the preputial orifice.
- Infection can ascend to create swelling and ulceration along the internal prepuce, and adhesions can form between the penis and prepuce.
- Stenosis of the preputial orifice may be evident.
- Dysuria may be reflected by vocalization during urination (goats) and may relate to stricture of the vermiform appendage.
- Stilted gait can reflect discomfort and weight loss can occur in chronic disease.
- Bucks which transmit the bacteria may be asymptomatic.
- Does and ewes initially have erythema and swelling of the vulva, which progresses to ulcerative and scabbing lesions of the perineum, vulva, and caudal vagina.
- Dysuria can occur if the urethral orifice is affected, and fibrosis and contracture of the vulva can occur in longstanding cases.

GENETICS
Angora goats and Merino sheep predisposed

CAUSES AND RISK FACTORS
- High-protein rations, generally ≥16%, but disease can occur with as little as 12% protein
- Legume pastures
- Alfalfa hay
- Thick wool or fiber in the preputial region
- Wet grasses
- Venereal spread
- Castration

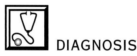

DIAGNOSIS

DIFFERENTIAL DIAGNOSES
- Caprine herpesvirus-1, *Actinobacillus seminis*, *Ureaplasma* spp., and *Trueperella pyogenes* may also cause ulcerative posthitis lesions.
- Obstructive urolithiasis and/or urethral rupture.
- Preputial trauma.
- Ulcerative dermatosis (poxvirus) lesions look similar, but scab removal creates hemorrhage, and lesions are often also present on the legs, lips, and eyes.

- Contagious ecthyma (orf) causes raised, proliferative lesions that are also present on the face, lips, and udder.

CBC/BIOCHEMISTRY/URINALYSIS
Usually unremarkable; rare cases of urinary outflow obstruction may have azotemia and elevated serum potassium.

OTHER LABORATORY TESTS
N/A

IMAGING
N/A

OTHER DIAGNOSTIC PROCEDURES
Diagnosis is generally based on physical examination and lesion characteristics; however, lesions can be cultured or biopsy samples obtained for culture, histopathology, or PCR (herpesvirus).

PATHOLOGIC FINDINGS
- Grossly, there is ulceration and swelling of external genitalia.
- Histologically lesions are consistent with acanthosis, parakeratosis, and hyperkeratosis, or mucosal ulceration, suppurative inflammation, and the presence of bacteria.
- Herpesvirus infection would be reflected by acidophilic intranuclear inclusion bodies, and chromatin margination in epithelial cells adjacent to ulcers.

TREATMENT

THERAPEUTIC APPROACH
- Basic management steps may effect a cure if performed early in disease:
  - Isolate affected individuals from other vulnerable animals.
  - Shear the wool or hair around external genitalia to allow drying.
  - Reduce protein or NPN in the ration, e.g., provide grass hay to animals grazing legume pastures.
- Sheath irrigation with antiseptic solutions and antibiotic administration can be performed for more significant clinical disease.
- Treatment of any kind should continue until lesions are dry and the animal is comfortable.

SURGICAL CONSIDERATIONS AND TECHNIQUES
- Early treatment obviates the need for surgical intervention; however, lesion cleaning and debridement may speed healing.
- Preputial resection may be required to permit urine flow and possible return to breeding after severe infection is cleared.

U

• As a salvage procedure, 2–4 cm incisions can be made through the ventral preputial skin to allow drainage and lavage.
• Strictured vermiform appendages may require resection.

MEDICATIONS

DRUGS OF CHOICE
• Topical antibiotic application can be performed; avoid irritating or caustic solutions.
  ○ Topical mastitis therapy medications and the ointment combination of neomycin, bacitracin, and polymyxin B ("triple antibiotic") have been used but even topical use may require a withdrawal time.
• NSAIDs help decrease pain and inflammation (flunixin, meloxicam).
• Systemic antibiotics are indicated in severe cases (penicillin, ampicillin, tetracycline).

CONTRAINDICATIONS
• Xylazine should not be used in an animal with suspected or known urinary obstruction since it promotes diuresis, which can provoke urinary bladder rupture.
• Avoid iodine-based preparations for sheath lavage as they encourage the formation of adhesions and granulation tissue.

PRECAUTIONS
Appropriate milk and meat withdrawal times must be followed for all compounds administered to food-producing animals.

POSSIBLE INTERACTIONS
N/A

FOLLOW-UP

EXPECTED COURSE AND PROGNOSIS
• If recognized prior to fibrosis/adhesions, animals have a good chance of full recovery with appropriate medical and dietary management.

• Return to breeding soundness is unlikely in severely affected animals, particularly males.

POSSIBLE COMPLICATIONS
• Males:
  ○ Loss of breeding soundness due to adhesion of penis to prepuce
  ○ Scarring of preputial orifice
  ○ Urethral obstruction
  ○ Urethritis
• Females:
  ○ Loss of breeding soundness due to impaired vulvar conformation
  ○ Urine scalding
  ○ Fibrosis of vulva may be severe enough to cause dystocia
  ○ Cystitis/pyelonephritis might occur

CLIENT EDUCATION
Largely a disease of management, so make clients aware of causes, risk factors, and methods of prevention.

PATIENT CARE
Patients must be closely monitored to ensure patency of urinary tract and to monitor discomfort.

PREVENTION
• Maintain protein in feeding regimen below 16% when possible.
• Shear at times of high protein intake.
• Isolate affected animals.
• Increase water availability.
• May include ammonium chloride in feed to reduce urine pH.

MISCELLANEOUS

AGE-RELATED FACTORS
Rare in animals <6 months of age.

PREGNANCY
Fibrosis of vulva may be severe enough to cause dystocia.

BIOSECURITY
• Isolation of affected individuals from herd or flock is indicated.
• Separate males and females.

• Burn any fiber and scabs from treated animals to reduce transmission risk.

PRODUCTION MANAGEMENT
• Limit dietary protein to <16%.
• Shear animals at times of high protein intake.

SYNONYMS
• Pizzle rot
• Enzootic balanoposthitis and vulvitis
• Sheath rot

ABBREVIATIONS
• NPN = nonprotein nitrogen
• NSAIDs = nonsteroidal anti-inflammatory drugs
• PCR = polymerase chain reaction

SEE ALSO
• Orf (Contagious Ecthyma)
• Penile Disorders
• Urolithiasis

Suggested Reading
Byers S. Ulcerative posthitis and vulvitis. In: Smith BP ed, Large Animal Internal Medicine, 5th ed. St. Louis: Elsevier, 2015, pp. 895–7.
Kidanemariam A, Gouws J, van Vuuren M, et al. Ulcerative balanitis and vulvitis of Dorper sheep in South Africa: a study on its aetiology and clinical features. J S Afr Vet Assoc 2005, 76: 197–203.
Loste A, Ramos JJ, Garcia L, et al. High prevalence of ulcerative posthitis in Rasa Aragonesa rams associated with a legume-rich diet. J Vet Med A 2005, 52: 176–9.
Southcott WH. Epidemiology and control of ovine posthitis and vulvitis. Aust Vet J 1965, 41: 225–34.
Uzal FA, Woods L, Stillian M, et al. Abortion and ulcerative posthitis associated with caprine herpesvirus-1 infection in goats in California. J Vet Diagn Invest 2004, 16: 478–84.
Author Meredyth L. Jones
Consulting Editor Erica C. McKenzie

U

ULTRASONOGRAPHY: MAMMARY

BASICS

OVERVIEW
• Ultrasonography is an important evaluation modality of udder conformation and health.
• Ultrasonographic evaluation of mammary gland parenchyma and teat provides information that correlates well with presence of inflammatory changes or abnormality of development.
• Mammary ultrasonography should be used along with clinical evaluation by inspection and palpation of the gland, CMT testing, and gross chemical and bacteriologic evaluation of milk.
• Indications include evaluation of milk flow disorders, isolated abscesses, mammary gland hematoma, neoplasia, and detection of foreign objects.

INCIDENCE/PREVALENCE
N/A

GEOGRAPHIC DISTRIBUTION
Worldwide

SYSTEMS AFFECTED
Mammary

PATHOPHYSIOLOGY
• Anatomy and physiology of the mammary gland
  ◦ The mammary gland originates as primary mammary buds from modified sweat glands of the epidermal epithelium.
  ◦ The primary mammary buds push into the underlying dermis, forming the secondary mammary buds, which protrude and continue to develop into a gland by branching and forming a duct system.
  ◦ From birth to puberty the mammary gland grows at the same rate as other tissues (isometric growth). With the onset of puberty, under the influence of cyclic changes, the gland undergoes allometric growth. Branching and diameter of the ducts increase due to estradiol influence, and alveoli develop under progesterone influence.
  ◦ The final development of the gland occurs during pregnancy under the influence of several hormones (estrogen, progesterone, prolactin, adrenal cortical hormones, and placenta lactogens). The alveoli develop into lobules grouped into lobes that open into a common duct. Milk is synthesized in the secretory cells of the alveoli and delivered to the cistern through intra- and interlobular ducts. The teat consists of a teat canal and the teat cistern surrounded by a well-developed circular muscle forming a teat sphincter that helps retain milk. The junction between the teat canal and the teat cistern has longitudinal mucus membrane folds, the rosette of Fürstenberg. Milk ejection is induced by oxytocin which causes contraction of myoepithelial cells surrounding the alveoli.
  ◦ The external pudendal artery provides the main blood supply to the udder. The lymphatic drainage is provided by the superficial inguinal (supramammary) lymph node. The teat base contains an erectile venous plexus (venous ring of Fürstenberg).
  ◦ Species variation of the anatomy:
    ■ Cow: 4 quarters and 4 teats, one gland, one canal and one cistern per teat
    ■ Sheep and goat: 2 halves and 2 teats, one canal and one cistern per teat
    ■ Camelid: 4 quarters and 4 teats, 2 canals and 2 cisterns per teat
• The udder can be affected by traumatic, inflammatory, neoplastic, and developmental disorders resulting in an alteration of the density of the tissues, which can be revealed by ultrasonographic evaluation.
• Congenital defects include glandular hypoplasia, teat cistern agenesis, partial or complete obstruction due to transverse intraluminal membrane, rudimentary teats, short teats, and supernumerary teats and glands.

HISTORICAL FINDINGS
• Abnormal conformation, size, or sensitivity of the udder
• Poor lactation or milk letdown
• Abnormal milk

SIGNALMENT
Postpubertal or lactating female

PHYSICAL EXAMINATION FINDINGS
• Presence of conformation abnormalities or asymmetry.
• Increase size or sensitivity may be seen in clinical mastitis.
• Bloody or purulent discharge from the teat.
• Enlarged lymph node.
• Abnormal milk.

GENETICS
• Mammary gland conformation and aptitude for milk production.
• Some congenital abnormalities may be hereditary.

CAUSES AND RISK FACTORS
• Genetics
• Infection
• Trauma

DIAGNOSIS

DIFFERENTIAL DIAGNOSES
N/A

CBC/BIOCHEMISTRY/URINALYSIS
N/A

OTHER LABORATORY TESTS
• CMT
• Somatic cell count

IMAGING
• Equipment and technique
  ◦ The glandular parenchyma is scanned with a linear transducer 5–7.5 MHz frequency for small ruminants and SAC and 3.5–5 MHz for the bovine and camel.
  ◦ A higher frequency transducer (7.5–10 MHz) is ideal for the evaluation of the teat and superficial lesions.
  ◦ The gland is cleaned. The hair/fiber is clipped to improve contact. Application of a coupling gel greatly improves the quality of images. For evaluation of the teat, images are improved by placing the teat in a water-filled plastic cup. Alternately a standoff gel pad can be used or the transducer may be placed in a latex condom filled with coupling gel.
• Normal echotexture
  ◦ Skin should appear echogenic and smooth.
  ◦ Glandular parenchyma has a homogeneous echogenicity with visible anechoic areas corresponding to vessels. An echogenic line corresponding to a septum is visible between glands.
  ◦ The teat should be scanned vertically as well as in a transverse manner. The gland cistern is anechoic and demarcated by a hyperechoic line corresponding to the mucosal membrane. Large, round, anechoic structures corresponding to the venous ring of Fürstenberg are seen between the gland cistern and the teat cistern. The teat wall shows, from inside to outside, a thin, bright echoic line (mucus membrane), a thicker hypoechoic homogenous layer with several anechoic vessels (muscle and connective tissue), and a hypoechoic line (skin). In the most ventral aspect, the rosette of Fürstenberg is seen as two parallel echoic lines. Measurement of each component of the teat is helpful if serial evaluations are planned.
• Abnormalities
  ◦ Skin lesions may occasionally be detected. Most of these are abscesses and nodules. Their appearance varies in echogenicity but they should stand out from the rest of the glandular parenchyma.
  ◦ Glandular parenchyma
    ■ Mastitis: Not all types of mastitis produce changes that are visible by ultrasonography. However, acute inflammatory changes may be depicted by increased edema and a more heterogeneous appearance of the parenchyma. The gland may display a comet-tail appearance signaling presence of gas in some Gram-negative bacterial infection. Chronic infection due to *Trueperella pyogenes*, *Klebsiella* spp., and *E. coli* may be detected as round, hypoechoic areas with a hyperechoic center. The milk within the cistern may appear more echogenic.

(CONTINUED) | **ULTRASONOGRAPHY: MAMMARY**

- Hematomas are initially seen as very echogenic masses that progressively show enlarging anechoic or hypoechoic areas with floating fibrin strands and clots as they become more organized.
- Abscesses, due to infection with *Corynebacterium pseudotuberculosis*, are often found in small ruminants and camelids. They usually present as distinct masses with a thick hyperechoic wall and a central cavity with different degrees of echogenicity.
- Foreign bodies are identified as hyperechoic structures casting shadows.
- Neoplasia is rare but has been diagnosed in goats and camelids. Adenocarcinomas present as multiple anechoic cavitary lesions interspaced by hyperechoic tissues.

  ○ Teat
  - Traumatic lesions to the teat canal and rosette of Fürstenberg often produce a heterogeneous appearance with echoic mucosal lesions.
  - Inflammation of the teat cistern produces a thickened, irregular mucosal membrane with increased heterogeneity due to increased blood flow.
  - Lactoliths (milk stones) may be identified as echogenic particles of varying sizes, either free or attached to the mucosal membrane.
  - Polyps and papillomas may be detected as proliferative lesions.
  - Congenital abnormalities should be suspected in primiparous animals with poor milk letdown. Ultrasonographically visible abnormalities include duplication of the teat (conjoined teat), teat agenesis, presence of septum in the cistern, or obstructing intraluminal membranes.
  - Extreme dilation of the teat cistern is a common finding in camels.

OTHER DIAGNOSTIC PROCEDURES
N/A

PATHOLOGIC FINDINGS
N/A

TREATMENT

THERAPEUTIC APPROACH
Depends on diagnosis

SURGICAL CONSIDERATIONS AND TECHNIQUES
Mastectomy should be considered in specific cases.

MEDICATIONS

DRUGS OF CHOICE
N/A

CONTRAINDICATIONS
N/A

PRECAUTIONS
N/A

POSSIBLE INTERACTIONS
N/A

FOLLOW-UP

EXPECTED COURSE AND PROGNOSIS
N/A

POSSIBLE COMPLICATIONS
N/A

CLIENT EDUCATION
- Ultrasonographic udder examination does not replace conventional examination methods.
- Animals with congenital defects should be eliminated from reproduction.

PATIENT CARE
N/A

PREVENTION
See specific condition

MISCELLANEOUS

ASSOCIATED CONDITIONS
N/A

AGE-RELATED FACTORS
N/A

ZOONOTIC POTENTIAL
N/A

PREGNANCY
N/A

BIOSECURITY
N/A

PRODUCTION MANAGEMENT
N/A

SYNONYMS
N/A

ABBREVIATIONS
- CMT = California Milk Test
- SAC = South American camelids

SEE ALSO
- Mastitis: Camelid
- Mastitis: Coliform
- Mastitis: Fungal
- Mastitis: Small Ruminant
- Mastitis: Staphylococcal
- Mastitis: Streptococcal
- Milk Vein Rupture

Suggested Reading
Ashenas J, Vosough D, Massoudifard M, et al. B-mode ultrasonography of the udder and teat in camel (*Camelus dromedarius*). J Vet Res 2007, 62: 27–31.
Bradley KJ, Bradley AJ, Barr FJ. Ultrasonographic appearance of the superficial supramammary lymph nodes in lactating dairy cattle. Vet Rec 2001, 148: 497–501.
Fasulkov I, Karadev M, Vasilev N, et al. Ultrasound and histopathological investigations of experimentally induced *Staphylococcus aureus* mastitis in goats. Small Rumin Res 2015, 129: 114–20.
Fasulkov I, Totov S, Atanasov A, et al. Evaluation of different techniques of teat ultrasonography in goats. J Fac Vet Med Istanbul Univ 2013, 39: 33–9.
Franz S, Floek M, Hofmann-Parisot M. Ultrasonography of the bovine udder and teat. Vet Clin North Am Food Anim Pract 2009, 25: 669–85.
Hussein HA, El Khabaz KAS, Malek S. Is udder ultrasonography a diagnostic tool for subclinical mastitis in sheep? Small Rumin Res 2015, 129: 121–8.
Kotb EZ, Abu-Seida AM, Fadel MS. The correlation between ultrasonographic and laboratory findings of mastitis in buffaloes (*Bubalis bubalis*). Glob Veterinaria 2014, 13: 68–74.
Szencziova I, Strapak P. Ultrasonography of the udder and teat in cattle: Perspective measuring technique. Slovak J Anim Sci 2012, 45: 95–104.
Author Ahmed Tibary
Consulting Editor Ahmed Tibary

U

UMBILICAL DISORDERS

BASICS

OVERVIEW
• Umbilical disorders can occur in all ruminants, usually in newborn and young animals.
• Umbilical masses can be divided into the following categories:
1. Uncomplicated umbilical hernia
2. Umbilical hernia with superficial infection or abscess
3. Umbilical hernia with umbilical remnant infection
4. Umbilical abscess or chronic omphalitis
5. Urachus rupture or cyst
• Umbilical hernias are the most common umbilical disorders in ruminants and camelids.
• The hernia sac has an inner peritoneal membrane and is covered with skin. These hernias have a genetic component but can also result secondary to an umbilical infection.
• Animals with umbilical hernias larger than 4–5 cm should be considered for surgical correction. Unfortunately, umbilical hernias in cattle rarely close spontaneously.
• The hernia usually contains intestines, i.e., abomasum, omentum (most common), or both. If the hernia is reducible there is a decreased incidence of intestinal strangulation. Chronic hernia can result in an abomasal umbilical fistula leading to loss of chloride and resulting in hypochloremic and hypokalemic metabolic acidosis.
• The presence of a patent urachus is not common in ruminants.

INCIDENCE/PREVALENCE
Umbilical disorders are common in veterinary practice.

GEOGRAPHIC DISTRIBUTION
Worldwide

SYSTEMS AFFECTED
• Cardiovascular
• Integument
• Digestive

PATHOPHYSIOLOGY
• At parturition the umbilical cord ruptures and the two umbilical arties retract actively. The urachus is pulled passively by the arteries into the abdomen. The umbilical vein does not retract but collapses due to surrounding smooth muscle contraction. The body wall should close within a few days to a few weeks. Failure of closure of the body wall is referred to as a congenital umbilical hernia.
• Congenital umbilical hernias can have a genetic origin.
• Umbilical hernias may be acquired from infection of the umbilicus in the neonatal period. Bacteria from the environment may seed the umbilical remnants. Less commonly the infection of the umbilical remnants may be hematogenous from a generalized

septicemia or bacteremia. Common bacterial isolates in ruminants include *Trueperella pyogenes, E. coli, Proteus, Enterococcus, Streptococcus,* and *Staphylococcus* species.
• Excessive use of iodine or iodine in high concentrations for dipping of the umbilicus can cause necrosis of the remnants and surrounding tissue, increasing the incidence of infection and subsequent disorders.
• Neonates that develop partial or complete failure of passive transfer have an increased risk for umbilical infection and development of hernia due to compromised immunity.

GENETICS
• Umbilical hernias are the most common bovine congenital defect.
• Increased incidence of umbilical hernias in Holstein-Friesian cattle.
• Beef cattle have a lower risk of developing umbilical hernias in comparison to dairy cattle.

HISTORICAL FINDINGS
• Observation of an umbilical mass.
• Abnormal urination.
• Incidental finding during neonatal examination (camelid).
• Some accidents to the umbilicus may follow dystocia.

SIGNALMENT
• Ruminants and camelids.
• Patent urachus is more common in males.

PHYSICAL EXAMINATION FINDINGS
• Swelling
• Pain
• Presence of hernia sac
• Depressed, lethargic, or anorexic (bacteremia or septicemia or metabolic derangement)
• Purulent discharge or drainage
• Dribbling, scalding urine (patent urachus)
• Colic signs (bowel strangulation)
• Joint distension (septicemia or bacteremia)
• Fever

CAUSES AND RISK FACTORS
• Hereditary.
• Environmental contamination leading to infection of umbilical remnants.
• Excessive use of strong iodine or chlorhexidine for umbilical dipping leads to necrosis.
• Calves derived from SCNT pregnancies are at higher risk because of the abnormally large umbilical cord stump associated with large offspring syndrome and abnormal placentation.

DIAGNOSIS

DIFFERENTIAL DIAGNOSES
• Physical examination, palpation, and ultrasonography of umbilical masses helps differentiate between various conditions of the umbilicus.

• Umbilical hernias have a distinct hernia ring. The hernia may be reducible. Examination of the content by ultrasonography reveals the presence of parts of the gastrointestinal tract.
• Abscesses are usually warm and present typical purulent content which may drain to the surface.
• Patent urachus is diagnosed by observation during urination and by ultrasonographic evaluation of the urachus and bladder.

CBC/BIOCHEMISTRY/URINALYSIS
Hyperfibrinogenemia, hyperproteinemia, neutrophilia, neutrophil-lymphocyte reversal, and mild anemia in cases of infection.

OTHER LABORATORY TESTS
Blood culture: Can be indicated in cases of septicemia.

IMAGING
• Transabdominal ultrasonography of the enlarged umbilical remnants (umbilical arteries, vein, and urachus) may reveal:
  ○ The nature of the content of the hernia sac
  ○ Inflammatory changes and abscess formation with thickening of the umbilical remnants
  ○ Communication between the urachus and the bladder (patent urachus)
  ○ Uroperitoneum in cases of rupture of the urachus.

OTHER DIAGNOSTIC PROCEDURES
Abdominocentesis: If a large amount of fluid is present in the peritoneal cavity, analysis of the fluid can help differentiate between uroperitoneum and peritonitis. Culture of the fluid provides information on the organism in the case of septic peritonitis.

PATHOLOGIC FINDINGS
• Umbilical hernia: The content of the hernia may become strangulated, leading to inflammatory changes and ischemic necrosis. Occasionally, neonates may be born with a complete failure of the skin to close in the umbilical region and eventration of intestines.
• Omphalophlebitis: The umbilical vessels are enlarged and thickened due to inflammation.
• In cases of large offspring syndrome, the umbilical mass may be 4–10 times the size of a normal umbilical stump.

TREATMENT

THERAPEUTIC APPROACH
Umbilical Hernia
Pinning: Clamps or elastrator bands are useful for closing small hernias (<4 cm in length). With the animal sedated, local anesthetic is placed around the hernia sac. The animal is placed in lateral recumbency, the hernia is reduced, and the procedure performed. The elastrator band is placed as close to the body wall as possible and two metal pins are placed in a crossing fashion to retain the band in

place. This will cause necrosis of the tissue distal to the band and an inflammatory reaction that will hopefully cause the hernia ring to close. If this is performed on lambs they should be given tetanus prophylaxis.

Medical Management of Infection of the Umbilicus or Umbilical Remnants
• Some cases of omphalophlebitis and/or omphaloartcritis rcspond to medical treatment.
• Prolonged broad-spectrum antibiotic treatment until infection is resolved.
• If medical treatment is proving ineffective, then surgical excision should be suggested to the owner.

SURGICAL CONSIDERATIONS AND TECHNIQUES
Surgical Resection of Umbilical Hernia
• In cases where the hernia is >4 cm in length, it is advisable to perform surgical closure after resection of the hernia sac. This can be performed under local anesthesia or general anesthesia.
• Large calves should be held off feed for 48 hours.
• The umbilicus is clipped and prepared for surgery. An elliptical incision is made around the hernia sac and dissection performed to expose the hernia ring. The abdominal cavity is opened either just cranial or caudal to the hernia sac on the linea alba to allow introduction of a finger into the abdominal cavity. This allows digital palpation of the hernia ring to ensure no viscera is entrapped.
• The hernia is closed using an absorbable suture of a size determined by the size of the animal. A simple continuous pattern can be used in uncomplicated cases. In larger animals or with larger hernias, the middle of the incision can be closed with a near-far-far-near (tension relieving) suture pattern. The defect both cranial and caudal to this suture is then closed in a simple continuous pattern. This usually provides a secure repair that heals rapidly.
• All animals should receive tetanus prophylaxis.
• Animals should have limited exercise postoperatively and should be monitored for signs of sepsis and dehiscence.

Surgical Management of Infection of the Umbilicus or Umbilical Remnants
• The opening of the umbilicus is oversewn to prevent contamination of the surgical site. The prepuce in male animals can also be oversewn to prevent contamination of the site with urine.
• An elliptical incision is made around the umbilicus. The abdominal cavity is opened either just cranial or caudal to the umbilicus on the linea alba to allow introduction of a finger into the abdominal cavity. This allows digital palpation of the infected umbilical remnants. The incision is continued just lateral to the umbilical remnants on either

side. Care is taken not to transect the umbilical vein, arteries, or urachus. The remnants are inspected for signs of infection.
• The vein and arteries should be ligated to remove as much infection as possible. If the umbilical vein is affected all the way to the liver, then marsupialization of the vein may need to be performed. The urachus is transected at the apex of the bladder within its healthy limits, and closed with a monofilament, absorbable suture in a two-layer closure (simple continuous oversewn with a Cushing or Utrecht suture pattern). The suture should not enter the lumen of the bladder if possible.
• Several suture patterns can be used to close the linea alba. Simple interrupted, interrupted cruciate, or simple continuous patterns are used most commonly. A monofilament absorbable suture material is the best option for closure.
• If marsupialization of the umbilical vein is indicated because of extensive infection, it can be marsupialized at the cranial aspect of the incision. The lumen of the vein is spatulated and sutured to the muscle and skin prior to closure of the incision. The venous stump should be flushed daily with antiseptic solution (1% chlorhexidine or 0.1% providone iodine). Broad-spectrum antibiotics should be administered for a minimum of 14 days post-surgery. The venous stump usually will close within a month. In very rare cases a second surgery may be needed to resect the infected umbilical vein if marsupialization is unsuccessful.

MEDICATIONS
DRUGS OF CHOICE
• Sedation
  ○ Acepromazine: Cattle and goats at 0.05–0.1 mg/kg body weight IV and sheep at 0.03–0.05 mg/kg IV.
  ○ Xylazine: Goats 0.05 mg/kg IV or 0.1 mg/kg IM; sheep 0.1–0.2 mg/kg IV or 0.2–0.3 mg/kg IM; cattle 0.1 mg/kg IV or 0.2 mg/kg IM. Recumbency will be induced for approximately 1 hour. Low dose xylazine 0.015–0.025 mg/kg IV or IM will provide sedation without recumbency in ruminants.
  ○ Anesthesia with xylazine (0.20 mg/kg) followed by ketamine (4 mg/kg IV) has been used in calves.
  ○ Lumbosacral epidural (2% lidocaine, 1 mL/10 lb body weight) after sedation with xylazine can be used in calves with simple hernias.
  ○ In camelids, sedation with butorphanol and gas anesthesia are preferred for umbilical hernia repair or umbilical stump excision.
• Antimicrobials

  ○ Choice of antibiotics and duration of treatment vary depending on the extent of surgery and risk for septicemia.
  ○ Ceftiofur, 2.2 mg/kg q24h
  ○ Oxytertacycline, 20 mg/kg SC q72h
  ○ Procaine Penicillin G, 22,000 IU/kg
  ○ Ampicillin/Amoxicillin 10 mg/kg IM q12h
• Anti-inflammatory drugs
  ○ Flunixin meglumine 1.1–2.2 mg/kg IV can be used at the time of surgery, but is rarely necessary after the initial dose.

CONTRAINDICATIONS
Appropriate milk and meat withdrawal times must be followed for all compounds administered to food-producing animals.

PRECAUTIONS
Acepromazine should not be administered via the coccygeal vein because of the close proximity to the coccygeal artery. Inadvertent infusion into the artery can result in possible loss of the tail.

POSSIBLE INTERACTIONS
N/A

FOLLOW-UP
EXPECTED COURSE AND PROGNOSIS
• Uncomplicated umbilical hernia repair carries a very good prognosis for survival and growth.
• Incarcerated umbilical hernias and post-surgical infection may increase the risk for dehiscence.

POSSIBLE COMPLICATIONS
• Suture abscess.
• Seromas.
• Hematomas.
• Incisional dehiscence which may result in evisceration and incarceration of bowel.
• Tetanus.
• Septic peritonitis especially if there is gross contamination of the abdomen at surgery or severe umbilical vein infection extending far cranially or to the liver.
• Uroabdomen secondary to leakage from closure of the apex of the bladder.
• Urolithiasis in small ruminants due to placement of suture material into the lumen of the bladder.

PATIENT CARE
• Animals should be confined post-surgery and closely monitor for signs of incisional infection or dehiscence.
• Close monitoring for signs of anorexia, fever, depression, or recumbency which may indicate development of bacteremia or sepsis.

PREVENTION
• Ensure adequate ingestion of good quality colostrum. Neonates should be exposed to as little stress as possible, especially in the first

U

UMBILICAL DISORDERS (CONTINUED)

2–3 days of life, to enhance colostrum absorption.
• Judicious care of the umbilicus in neonates. Clean environment and navel dipping with 1% chlorhexidine or 0.1% providone iodine(noncaustic).
• Selective breeding with males who are not genetically predisposed to producing offspring with hernias.

 MISCELLANEOUS

ASSOCIATED CONDITIONS
N/A

AGE-RELATED FACTORS
Most common in neonates

ZOONOTIC POTENTIAL
N/A

PREGNANCY
It is not advisable to breed animals with umbilical hernias. Hernia may increase in size due to intra-abdominal pressure during pregnancy and parturition.

BIOSECURITY
N/A

PRODUCTION MANAGEMENT
• Parturient care: Clean birthing area, monitoring, proper assistance during birth
• Neonatal care: Adequate colostrum intake, umbilical stump care

SYNONYM
Navel ill (omphalophlebitis)

ABBREVIATIONS
• IM = intramuscular
• IV = intravenous
• SCNT = somatic cell nuclear transfer

SEE ALSO
• Neonatology: Beef
• Neonatology: Camelid
• Neonatology: Caprine
• Neonatology: Dairy Cattle (see www.fiveminutevet.com/ruminant)
• Neonatology: Ovine (see www.fiveminutevet.com/ruminant)
• Congenital Defects: Bovine
• Congenital Defects: Camelid
• Congenital Defects: Small Ruminant

Suggested Reading
Marsh P. Umbilical enlargement: disorders and management of the neonate. In: Smith BP ed, Large Animal Internal Medicine, 3rd ed. St. Louis: Mosby, 2002.
Navarre CB, Baird AN, Pugh DG. Pathologic conditions of the umbilicus. In: Pugh DG, Baird N eds, Sheep and Goat Medicine. Philadelphia: Saunders, 2012, pp. 103–5.
Ortved K. Miscellaneous abnormalities of the calf. In: Fubini SL, Ducharme MG eds, Farm Animal Surgery, 2nd ed. Philadelphia: Saunders, 2016, pp. 540–7.
Author Troy E.C. Holder
Consulting Editor Ahmed Tibary

U

BASICS

OVERVIEW
• Urea/nonprotein nitrogen toxicosis is defined as a condition that occurs when large amounts of urea/nonprotein nitrogen are ingested.
• Urea is considered an economical source of crude protein (CP) in ruminant diets. Other nonprotein nitrogen sources will be metabolized in a similar manner.
• Utilization of urea (CH_4N_2O) by the ruminant animal is initiated by its microbial hydrolysis to two ammonia (NH_3) molecules and one carbon dioxide molecule in the rumen environment. This step is accomplished by urease from specific bacterial species such as *Succinivibrio dextrinosolvens*, *Prevotella ruminicola*, and *Ruminococcus bromii*.
• In the rumen, the NH_3 produced from dietary proteins, urea, or other nonprotein nitrogen (NPN) sources is further utilized for synthesis of bacterial amino acids and bacterial proteins. Utilization of NH_3 for bacterial protein synthesis is dependent upon availability of highly fermentable carbohydrate sources such as dietary starch.
• Excess NH_3 is absorbed through the rumen wall and is transferred to the liver for conversion to urea before excretion in the urine.
• Depending on the CP level of the diet, a variable amount of urea is recycled back to the rumen. This is achieved mainly through saliva and to some extent through diffusion across the rumen wall. Urea recycling is intended to increase NH_3 concentrations in the rumen to meet N requirements of the rumen bacteria.
• When the liver's ability to detoxify NH_3 to urea is exceeded, blood NH_3 concentrations are increased to lethal levels (i.e., urea toxicity).

INCIDENCE/PREVALENCE
• The dietary urea levels required to induce toxic symptoms as well as the blood NH_3 concentrations associated with toxicity vary considerably. The conditions that may protect ruminants from urea toxicity are also quite variable. However, urea administration with the diet is less toxic than when administered separately. Younger ruminants are found to be more susceptible to toxicity than older ones.
• In general, urea is used widely in ruminant diets and intakes >0.45 g urea/kg of body weight are known to decrease feed intake and milk production in dairy cows and can induce toxicity.
• Urea toxicity symptoms occur at blood concentrations >1 mg/100 mL and become more severe at higher levels.

• Urea-induced death usually occurs when blood NH_3-N concentrations are in the range 2–4 mg/100 mL.
• Not unusual to find as high as 5–6 mg/100 mL.

GEOGRAPHIC DISTRIBUTION
Worldwide, depending on species and production management

SYSTEMS AFFECTED
• Digestive
• Musculoskeletal
• Nervous
• Respiratory

PATHOPHYSIOLOGY
• Following ingestion of large amounts of urea, a rapid release of NH_3 occurs.
• This increases the rumen pH to reach alkaline levels, which in turn supports high rates of NH_3 absorption through the rumen wall.
• Blood NH_3 is toxic to animal cells at low concentrations and is responsible for cell death. Additionally, NH_3 is carcinogenic.
• Alkaline rumen environments (pH >7.4), therefore, are considered the most important factor in inducing high blood NH_3 concentrations and toxicity.

HISTORICAL FINDINGS
• Elevated concentrations of rumen NH_3 and the subsequent high concentrations of NH_3 in serum are the key characteristics of urea toxicity.
• Complications due to increased serum NH_3 concentrations include alkalosis, rapid uptake of NH_3 by the brain, and central nervous system damage.

SIGNALMENT
• Potentially all ruminant species.
• Younger ruminants are found to be more susceptible to toxicity than adults.

PHYSICAL EXAMINATION FINDINGS
• Clinical signs are apparent within 20–30 min following ingestion of a toxic urea dose.
• Death can occur within hours after exposure.
• The clinical signs include respiratory difficulties (e.g., rapid and/or labored breathing), nervousness, muscular tremors, incoordination, excessive salivation, loss of ability to stand, bloat (due to reduction in rumen motility), and occurrence of tetany. The main cause of death appears to be respiratory arrest.
• Clinical signs can be similar to hypomagnesemia.
• The clinical signs of urea toxicity have been categorized into the following three stages: (1) The stage of depression and fatigue is associated with serum NH_3 concentrations in the range 0.5–1.0 mg/100 mL. (2) The beginning of the stage of convulsion is

associated with serum NH_3 concentrations >2 mg/100 mL. (3) The end of the stage of convulsion is associated with serum NH_3 concentrations in the range 4.0–7.0 mg/100 mL. Damage of the brainstem and paralysis of the respiration center are usually responsible for death.

CAUSES AND RISK FACTORS
• Inadequate mixing of urea or urea-containing supplements with the remaining dietary ingredients may result in consumption of large urea doses at one time and can dispose the animal to urea toxicity.
• Feeding urea to animals that are not adapted to dietary supplementation of NPN such as urea, NH_3, and ammonium salts.
• Allowing free access to palatable sources of high-urea concentrates.
• Feeding poor-quality, forage-based diets.
• Use of urea in low-energy rations.
• Feeding urea-containing diets to cattle that are deprived of feed for extended periods of time (e.g., 24–48 hours).

DIAGNOSIS

Ammonia or NPN poisoning is suggested by signs, lesions, history of acute illness, and dietary exposure.

DIFFERENTIAL DIAGNOSES
• Differential diagnoses include poisonings by nitrate/nitrite, cyanide, organophosphate/carbamate pesticides, raw soybean overload, 4-methylimidazole, lead, chlorinated hydrocarbon pesticides, and toxic gases (carbon monoxide, hydrogen sulfide, nitrogen dioxide).
• Acute infectious diseases; and noninfectious diseases such as encephalopathies (e.g., leukoencephalomalacia, hepatic encephalopathy, polioencephalomalacia), enterotoxemia or rumen autointoxication, protein engorgement, grain engorgement, ruminal tympany, and pulmonary adenomatosis.
• Nutritional and metabolic disorders related to hypocalcemia, hypomagnesemia, and other elemental aberrations should also be considered.

CBC/BIOCHEMISTRY/URINALYSIS
The PCV and serum concentrations of NH_3, glucose, lactate, potassium, phosphorus, AST, ALT, and BUN usually are significantly increased.

OTHER LABORATORY TESTS
• The most accurate indicator of urea toxicity is serum or ocular fluid NH_3 concentrations.
• Specimens for NH_3-N analysis include ruminal-reticular fluid, serum, whole blood, and urine. All specimens should be frozen

UREA TOXICITY

immediately after collection and thawed only for analysis; alternatively, ruminal-reticular fluid may be preserved with a few drops of saturated mercuric chloride solution added to each 100 mL of specimen.
• Animals dead more than a few hours in hot ambient temperatures or 12 hours in moderate climates probably have undergone too much autolysis to be of diagnostic value.
• NH_3-N concentrations of ≥ 2 mg/100 mL in blood, serum, or vitreous humor indicate excess NPN exposure.
• Clinical signs usually appear at ~1 mg/100 mL. The concentration of NH_3-N in ruminal-reticular fluid is >80 mg/100 mL in most cases of NPN poisoning and may be >200 mg/100 mL.
• Acclimated ruminants fed diets high in legume hay, soybean meal, cottonseed meal, linseed meal, fish meal, or milk by-products may have NH_3-N concentrations in rumen fluid approaching 60 mg/100 mL with no apparent toxicity.
• The pH of ruminal-reticular fluid should also be determined; a pH of 7.5–8 (at time of death) is indicative of NPN toxicity.

PATHOLOGIC FINDINGS
• Carcasses of animals dying of NPN poisoning appear to bloat and decompose rapidly, with no specific characteristic lesions.
• Gross brain lesions are not usually reported in NPN-induced ammonia toxicosis, but histopathologic lesions may include neuronal degeneration, spongy degeneration of the neuropil, and congestion and hemorrhage in the pia mater.
• Frequently, pulmonary edema, congestion, and petechial hemorrhages may be seen. Mild bronchitis and catarrhal gastroenteritis are often reported.
• Regurgitated and inhaled rumen contents are commonly found in the trachea and bronchi, especially in sheep.
• The odor of NH_3 may or may not be apparent in ingesta from a freshly opened rumen or cecum.
• A ruminal or cecal pH ≥ 7.5 from a recently dead animal is highly suggestive of NPN poisoning. The ruminal pH remains stable for several hours after death under most circumstances but continues to rise in NPN toxicosis.

TREATMENT

THERAPEUTIC APPROACH

Early Stages
• Oral administration of 5% acetic acid solution to neutralize excess rumen NH_3. This treatment is effective in increasing

potential survival of the animal if it is performed prior to the onset of tetany.
• Oral administration of cold water to slow the rate of urea hydrolysis to NH_3 and to dilute its concentration in the rumen.

Late Stages
Rumen lavage to remove the nonprotein nitrogen.

MEDICATIONS

DRUGS OF CHOICE
• Supportive therapy is indicated and includes IV isotonic saline solutions to correct dehydration, and IV calcium gluconate and magnesium solutions IV to relieve tetanic seizures.
• Convulsions may also be controlled with sodium pentobarbital or other injectable anesthetic agents.

PRECAUTIONS
Appropriate milk and meat withdrawal times must be followed for all compounds administered to food-producing animals.

FOLLOW-UP

EXPECTED COURSE AND PROGNOSIS
Prognosis is grave when severe symptoms are present.

PREVENTION
• Gradual adaptation to urea feeding (e.g., feeding urea to dairy cows at 0.34 g/kg of body weight was achieved after a 6-week adaptation period without inducing negative effects on feed intake, blood composition, milk production, or milk composition).
• Feeding readily fermentable carbohydrate sources (e.g., starch and molasses) in amounts that enable rumen bacteria to capture the released NH_3 for bacterial protein synthesis.
• Uniform mixing of urea with the remaining dietary ingredients.
• Maintaining a regular feeding schedule.
• Feeding urea at rates not exceeding 33% of dietary CP.
• Feeding liquid urea supplements with phosphoric acid to maintain acidic rumen environments and to decrease the rate of NH_3 absorption.
• Coating urea with fat supplements to decrease its rate of hydrolysis to NH_3.
• Extrusion of urea with concentrates such as grains also decreases its rate of hydrolysis.
• Use of urease inhibitors to slow the release of NH_3. These inhibitors include hydroxamic acids, especially caprylhydroxamic acid.

• Urea should not be added to diets that are already meeting the animal's CP requirements.
• The diet should contain sufficient amounts of calcium and phosphorus. The sulfur to N ratio in the diet also should not be less than 1:15. The diet should also contain sufficient amounts of trace minerals, especially cobalt and zinc.
• Feeding low-energy, high-fiber diets, especially poor-quality forages, should be avoided with urea feeding.

MISCELLANEOUS

AGE-RELATED FACTORS
Younger ruminants are found to be more susceptible to toxicity than older ones.

ZOONOTIC POTENTIAL
N/A

PREGNANCY
N/A

PRODUCTION MANAGEMENT
• Urea administration with the diet is less toxic than when administered separately. Younger ruminants are found to be more susceptible to toxicity than older ones.
• In general, urea is used widely in ruminant diets and intakes exceeding 0.45 g urea/kg of body weight are known to decrease feed intake and milk production in dairy cows and can induce toxicity.

SYNONYM
Ammonia toxicosis

ABBREVIATIONS
• AST = aspartate aminotransferase
• BUN = blood urea nitrogen
• CP = crude protein
• IV = intravenous
• NH_3 = ammonia
• NH_3-N = ammonia nitrogen
• NPN = nonprotein nitrogen
• PCV = packed cell volume

SEE ALSO
• Dairy Heifer Nutrition: Basics (see www.fiveminutevet.com/ruminant)
• Dairy Nutrition: Ration Guidelines for Milking and Dry Cows (see www.fiveminutevet.com/ruminant)
• Feeding By-Products to the Beef Cow Herd (see www.fiveminutevet.com/ruminant)
• Milk Cow Nutrition Monitoring (see www.fiveminutevet.com/ruminant)
• Toxicology: Herd Outbreaks

Suggested Reading
Brazil TJ, Naylor JM, Janzen ED. Ammoniated forage toxicosis in nursing calves: a herd outbreak. Can Vet J 1994, 35: 45–7.

Caldow GL, Wain EB. Urea poisoning in suckler cows. Vet Rec 1991, 128: 489–91.

Campagnolo ER, Kasten S, Banerjee M. Accidental ammonia exposure to county fair show livestock due to contaminated drinking water. Vet Hum Toxicol 2002, 44: 282–5.

Haliburton JC, Morgan SE. Nonprotein nitrogen-induced ammonia toxicosis and ammoniated feed toxicity syndrome. Vet

Clin North Am Food Anim Pract 1989, 5: 237–49.

Thompson LJ. Overview of nonprotein nitrogen poisoning. In: The Merck Veterinary Manual Online, 2014. http://www.merckvetmanual.com/mvm/toxicology/nonprotein_nitrogen_poisoning/overview_of_nonprotein_nitrogen_poisoning.html. Accessed August 5, 2016.

Villar D, Schwartz KJ, Carson TL, Kinker JA, Barker J. Acute poisoning of cattle by fertilizer-contaminated water. Vet Hum Toxicol 2003, 45: 88–90.

Author Steve Ensley
Consulting Editor Christopher C.L. Chase
Acknowledgment The author and book editors acknowledge the prior contribution of Hussein S. Hussein.

U

UREAPLASMA

BASICS

OVERVIEW
• Ureaplasmas are cell-wall deficient bacteria of the Mycoplasmataceae family (phylum Terenicutes) which also includes *Mycoplasma*.
• *Ureaplasma diversum* is found only in cattle, where it is a common inhabitant of the respiratory and genital tract.

INCIDENCE/PREVALENCE
• *U. diversum* is commonly isolated or detected by molecular diagnostic techniques in samples from the reproductive tract of apparently normal female cattle (15–70%), particularly from the vulvar and vestibular regions. Heifers with granular vulvitis lesions are reportedly three times as likely to be PCR positive for *U. diversum* as those without vulvovaginal lesions. It is also more frequently detected in uterine flushings from cows with evidence of endometritis.
• Breeding-age beef heifers tend to have the highest prevalence (30–80%) while *U. diversum* has also been isolated from 1-month-old female calves (21%).
• *U. diversum* is also a common inhabitant of the bull reproductive tract (5% to >70%), particularly within the prepuce and distal urethra. While the prevalence is highly variable, there are reports of it being cultured from frozen semen appropriately extended with recommended antibiotics.
• A recent study in Finland detected *U. diversum* in the respiratory tract of 23% of group-housed dairy calves at 1–2 months of age. Calves with clinical respiratory disease were significantly more likely to harbor *U. diversum*.

GEOGRAPHIC DISTRIBUTION
• First isolated from the urogenital tract of cows in western Canada.
• It has been reported in several other countries: Brazil, France, United States, Australia, Finland and may potentially be present worldwide.

PATHOPHYSIOLOGY
• The frequency with which *U. diversum* is isolated from cattle with apparently normal reproductive function has created controversy about its pathogenic significance for over 40 years. It is often considered a commensal bacterium.
• While specific pathologic mechanisms have not been determined, *U. diversum* is associated with a variety of bovine reproductive pathologies including granular vulvitis, endometritis, salpingitis, abortion, weak or stillborn calves, and infertility in female cattle. In bulls it is reported to cause epididymitis, seminal vesiculitis, and balanoposthitis, as well as alterations of sperm morphology and motility.

• Venereal transmission is considered a major source of new infections but transfer of the organism may also result from contaminated obstetric or breeding equipment, use of a common transrectal palpation sleeve, direct contact, congenital transmission, passage through the birth canal during delivery, and via contaminated sperm, oocytes, and embryos used in assisted reproductive programs (i.e., AI, ET, IVF).

HISTORICAL FINDINGS
• Abortion, usually in the last third of pregnancy
• Stillbirths or weak calves
• Infertility
• Lesions of granular vulvovaginitis

SIGNALMENT
U. diversum is found in all breeds of cattle, but more commonly in younger animals of both sexes.

PHYSICAL EXAMINATION FINDINGS
• Most carriers do not present any clinical signs.
• The most common clinical sign is a granular vulvaginitis.

CAUSES AND RISK FACTORS
• It has been suggested that increased blood urea nitrogen predisposes an animal to infection by providing urea substrate for the growth of *Ureaplasma* spp.
• Risk of transmission is increased by high density of cattle in an enclosure and unsanitary breeding techniques.

DIAGNOSIS

DIFFERENTIAL DIAGNOSES
• Granular venereal disease caused by other organisms, including IBR/IPV virus.
• Infertility caused by vibriosis or trichomoniasis.
• Other causes of mid- to late-term abortion.
• Other causes of genital tract inflammation in bulls.
• Calving or breeding trauma.

CBC/BIOCHEMISTRY/URINALYSIS
N/A

OTHER LABORATORY TESTS
• Culture is the gold standard for diagnosis but molecular techniques are becoming more common.
• Samples should be taken carefully to avoid contamination.
• The organism is fastidious so culture samples must be collected, stored, and transported in strict compliance with the recommendations of the diagnostic laboratory that will be processing them. Special transport media is usually required for culture.
• Not all diagnostic facilities offer services for detection of *U. diversum*.

• Diagnosis of *U. diversum* as a cause of abortion should be based on isolation from samples collected aseptically from the placenta, fetal lungs, and fetal stomach content.

IMAGING
N/A

OTHER DIAGNOSTIC PROCEDURES
Fetal necropsy, histopathology

PATHOLOGIC FINDINGS
• *Ureaplasma* infection in female cattle most commonly presents as vestibular hyperemia, usually accompanied by discrete, raised (hence granular) lymphoid cell proliferation with or without mucoid discharge. Granular lesions may progress to a pustular stage. Similar lesions are found on the prepuce and glans penis of affected bulls.
• *U. diversum* is also associated with repeat breeding, abortion, stillbirth, and weak calves.
• Abortion is characterized by a diffuse placentitis and interstitial pneumonia. The amnion is thick and opaque with multifocal areas of hemorrhage, fibrin exudation, necrosis, and fibrosis.

TREATMENT

THERAPEUTIC APPROACH
• Treatment in most cases is considered neither necessary nor practical. Most healthy, well-fed cattle appear to have only brief periods of infertility associated with the organism, so aggressive treatment that would require meat and milk withholding is hard to justify.
• Intrauterine or systemic oxytetracycline has been recommended for granular vulvitis therapy.
• Systemic antibiotic therapy is recommended for salpingitis and seminal vesiculitis when *Ureaplasma* is suspected.
• Eliminating the organism from the vestibulovagina and sheath is difficult.

SURGICAL CONSIDERATIONS AND TECHNIQUES
N/A

MEDICATIONS

DRUGS OF CHOICE
U. diversum is usually sensitive to tetracycline, macrolide, aminoglycoside, and fluoroquinolone antibiotics. In humans, there are concerns about *U. urealyticum* tetracycline resistance but little specific information is available regarding *U. diversum* antibiotic resistance patterns in cattle.

CONTRAINDICATIONS

Appropriate milk and meat withdrawal times must be followed for all compounds administered to food-producing animals.

PRECAUTIONS

N/A

POSSIBLE INTERACTIONS

N/A

 FOLLOW-UP

EXPECTED COURSE AND PROGNOSIS

Most animals that are otherwise healthy appear to be unaffected by the organism or will spontaneously recover from a temporary infertility.

POSSIBLE COMPLICATIONS

• Salpingitis and seminal vesiculitis, while uncommon, represent potentially serious complications of *U. diversum* genital infections.
• Complications are rare but if fertility is significantly affected for a prolonged period of time, affected animals are at an increased risk of being culled.
• Infected calves may have an increased risk of respiratory disease.

CLIENT EDUCATION

Breeding hygiene

PATIENT CARE

• Repeated swabbing for culture or molecular diagnostics is required to confirm elimination of the organism. There seems to be little justification to this approach.
• Monitoring the reproductive performance of individual animals (BSE, pregnancy diagnosis) or the herd on a regular and ongoing basis is a better method for assessing the significance of the disease.

PREVENTION

• No vaccine is currently available.
• Use of a guarded sheath for AI and ET equipment has been suggested as a way to reduce uterine contamination during these procedures.

• Post-breeding intrauterine infusion of tetracycline has been reported to improve fertility in affected animals, but appropriately controlled studies are lacking and the possibility of spontaneous recovery cannot be ruled out.
• Gentamicin, tylosin, lincomycin, and spectinomycin are usually added to extenders for frozen semen.

 MISCELLANEOUS

ASSOCIATED CONDITIONS

• Seminal vesiculitis, balanoposthitis in bulls
• Vaginitis, endometritis, salpingitis, abortion, stillbirth, weak calves in cows

AGE-RELATED FACTORS

Younger cattle seem to be more commonly infected, suggesting the development of immunity over time.

ZOONOTIC POTENTIAL

N/A

PREGNANCY

U. diversum has been implicated in early embryonic loss, mid- to late-term abortion, stillbirth, and birth of low-viability calves.

BIOSECURITY

• The organism appears to be a ubiquitous commensal and there may be no effective way to control exposure. Regardless, routine herd biosecurity protocols should be in place for every farm.
• Semen and embryos should be acquired through reputable, certified sources to minimize the potential for disease introduction.

PRODUCTION MANAGEMENT

• The impact on herd reproductive performance is unclear.
• Routine monitoring of herd reproductive performance should be part of every herd management program.

ABBREVIATIONS

• AI = artificial insemination
• BSE = breeding soundness examination

• ET = embryo transfer
• IBR = infectious bovine rhinotracheitis
• IPV = infectious pustular vulvovaginitis
• IVF = in vitro fertilization

SEE ALSO

• Abortion: Bovine
• Infectious Pustular Vulvovaginitis
• Seminal Vesiculitis
• Vaginitis
• Vulvitis

Suggested Reading

Argue B, Chousalkar KK. Chenoweth P. Presence of *Ureaplasma diversum* in the Australian cattle population. Aust Vet J 2013, 91: 99–101.

Autio T, Pohjanvirta T, Holopainen R, et al. Etiology of respiratory disease in non-vaccinated, non-medicated calves in rearing herds. Vet Microbiol 2007, 119: 256–65.

Doig PA, Ruhnke HL, Palmer N C. Experimental bovine genital ureaplasmosis. I. Granular vulvitis following vulvar inoculation. Can J Comp Med 1979, 44: 242–58.

Machado V., Oikonomou G, Bicalho MLS, Knauer WA., Gilbert R, Bicalho RC. Investigation of postpartum dairy cows' uterine microbial diversity using metagenomic pyrosequencing of the 16S rRNA gene. Vet Microbiol 2012, 159: 460–9.

Marques LM, Buzinhani M, Neto RL, et al. *Ureaplasma diversum* detection in bovine semen straws for artificial insemination. Vet Rec 2009, 165: 572–3.

Rae DO, Chenoweth PJ, Brown MB, Genho PC, Moore SA, Jacobsen K E. Reproductive performance of beef heifers: effects of vulvo-vaginitis, *Ureaplasma diversum* and pre-breeding antibiotic administration. Theriogenology 1993, 40: 497–508.

Authors Harry Momont and Celina Checura
Consulting Editor Ahmed Tibary
Acknowledgment The authors and book editors acknowledge the prior contribution of Peter Chenoweth.

UROLITHIASIS

BASICS

OVERVIEW
• Obstructive urolithiasis is a frequent problem in male small ruminants. It can also occur in bovines to a lesser extent.
• Urinary calculi are concentrations of mucus, protein, and minerals in the urinary tract.
• The composition of uroliths varies depending on diet and geography. The most common uroliths are calcium apatite and phosphatic based calculi. These calculi are usually white or gray, usually smooth, radiopaque, and easily broken. Silicate and calcium carbonate uroliths are occasionally seen.
• Calcium based uroliths are common in ruminants grazing lush, rapidly growing clover pastures or being fed alfalfa hay.
• Urethral obstruction is most commonly seen in show or pet goats and lambs that have a high-concentrate and low-roughage diet.

INCIDENCE/PREVALENCE
• Well recognized in sheep wethers and steers maintained in feedlot conditions and fed high-concentrate, low-forage diets.
• Wethers castrated at an early age are more susceptible due to a lack of testosterone driving development of the urethra and urethral process.

GEOGRAPHIC DISTRIBUTION
Silicate calculi are more commonly diagnosed in animals grazed on sandy soil, high in silica, conditions more frequently seen in the western parts of the United States and Canada.

SYSTEMS AFFECTED
• Urinary
• Cardiovascular
• Integument
• Multisystemic

PATHOPHYSIOLOGY
• Diets that are high in concentrate, phosphorus, and magnesium and low in roughage and calcium will predispose to risk of phosphate urolith formation. Urine is normally highly saturated with mineral solutes. Multiple factors can cause these minerals to leave solution and precipitate in the urine.
• Normally, a ruminant will remove phosphorus from its body by excreting it into saliva and through the manure. Diets high in concentrate and low in roughage decrease the production of saliva so phosphorus has to be excreted from the blood via the urinary system.
• The distal sigmoid flexure is the most common site of obstruction in steers and bulls. In sheep and goats the urethral process and the distal sigmoid flexure are the most common site of obstruction.

• Some breeds of sheep (e.g., Texel and Scottish Blackface) may be predisposed to calculi formation because of excretion of phosphorus via the urinary system in preference to via saliva.

HISTORICAL FINDINGS
• Male castrated animals with history of castration at an early age and diet consisting of high concentrate and low forage.
• History of low water consumption, lethargy, inappetance, and straining ± vocalization.
• In steers, owners may notice preputial swelling as the first sign.

SIGNALMENT
• Males more commonly affected.
• All ages are affected but the incidence is greater in younger ruminants.

PHYSICAL EXAMINATION FINDINGS
• Dysuria, stranguria, hematuria, anuria
• Prolonged urination or urine dribbling
• Tachycardia
• Tachypnea
• Vocalization
• Tail flagging
• Abdominal straining (can lead to rectal prolapse)
• Abdominal pain (stretching, kicking at abdomen, flank watching)
• Abdominal distention
• Preputial/perineal edema ("water belly" in cattle; secondary to urethral rupture)
• Bruxism
• Anorexia, weakness, depression

GENETICS
Texel and Scottish Blackface have a high incidence due to their preferred method of phosphorus excretion.

CAUSES AND RISK FACTORS
• High-grain, low-roughage diets.
• Dietary electrolyte imbalances, decreased water consumption/availability, and abnormal urine pH.

DIAGNOSIS

DIFFERENTIAL DIAGNOSES
A hair ring present around the penis may cause signs of discomfort and dysuria similar to that seen with obstructive urolithiasis.

Hematuria
• Bladder polyps
• Bracken fern toxicity
• Cystitis
• Infarction of kidney
• Papilloma
• Pyelonephritis
• Trauma
• Urethritis

Dysuria
• Actinomyces
• Cystitis

• Mycoplasma
• Orf
• Photosensitivity
• Sacral fracture
• Spinal cord injury
• Trauma
• Ulcerative balantitis and vulvitis

CBC/BIOCHEMISTRY/URINALYSIS
• A complete blood count may reveal a stress leukogram and mild to severe azotemia depending on duration. Mild hemoconcentration, hyperkalemia, hyperglycemia, hyponatremia, hypochloremia, hypocalcemia, and hypophosphatemia can been seen on biochemistry.
• Hematuria and proteinuria are common findings; crystalluria is a variable finding.
• Pyuria can be present with traumatic urethritis, cystitis, or secondary bacterial infection.

OTHER LABORATORY TESTS
If bladder rupture is suspected, an abdominal fluid to serum creatinine ratio can be performed. The ratio should be < 2:1 and if greater suggests urine leakage into the abdomen.

IMAGING
• An enlarged bladder is often visualized on right-sided abdominal or transrectal ultrasound.
• Echogenic material in the bladder or kidneys is occasionally visualized, but lack of this finding does not rule out the diagnosis. A large amount of free fluid (ascites) may also be visualized in the abdomen if the abdominal portion of the urinary tract is ruptured due to unresolved obstruction.
• Abdominal radiography may allow visualization of the calculi depending on composition.
• Calcium oxalate and calcium carbonate crystals are radiopaque while struvite (magnesium ammonium phosphate), apatite, and silicate crystals are radiolucent. Therefore, lack of radiographic visualization does not rule out the presence of obstructive calculi.
• Infusion of contrast media retrograde through a urethral catheter may allow visualization of calculi; however, urethral rupture/fistula formation or bladder rupture can occur.
• Ultrasonographic examination of the kidneys is indicated in chronic (>24 hours) urethral obstruction. The presence of hydronephrosis with loss of cortical tissue warrants a guarded to poor prognosis for restoring normal renal function.

OTHER DIAGNOSTIC PROCEDURES
• Abdominal palpation in small ruminants.
• Urethroscopy has recently been recognized as a modality for diagnosing urethral obstruction in ruminants.

U

• Abdominocentesis yielding urine (be aware of inadvertent cystocentesis with enlarged bladder).

PATHOLOGIC FINDINGS

• Single to multiple calculi lodged along the extent of the urinary tract. The tissues will be hyperemic, hemorrhagic, or necrotic depending on duration of disease.
• Bladder or urethral rupture may be present as well as hydroureter and hydronephrosis.

TREATMENT

THERAPEUTIC APPROACH

• Treatment should be aimed at supportive care and correcting the obstruction.
• In cases of bladder rupture, urine can be drained from the peritoneum to reduce the effects of uremia and correct electrolyte imbalances. Drainage should be performed slowly to reduce the risk of circulatory shock, and IV fluids should be given concurrently.
• IV fluids should be given judiciously in cases of complete obstruction. Choice of fluid therapy should be based on electrolyte imbalances. IV fluids containing potassium should be avoided if hyperkalemia is present.

Cattle

Signs are generally seen after rupture of the urethra once preputial swelling is present. A perineal urethrostomy is the treatment of choice and is used as a salvage procedure to allow animal to survive to slaughter.

Small Ruminants

Although most cases benefit from surgical intervention, partial obstructions may be attempted with medical management along with less-invasive surgical techniques (see *urethral process amputation* and *urethral catheterization and retrograde flushing*). Medical management may include repeated administration of diazepam (0.1–0.5 mg/kg body weight IV) or acepromazine maleate (0.05–0.1 mg/kg IV) to promote urethral relaxation. There are limited reports suggesting the use of acidic solutions (hemiacidrin and Walpole's solution) to dissolve struvite stones through retrograde flushing or ultrasound-guided infusion into the bladder.

SURGICAL CONSIDERATIONS AND TECHNIQUES

Urethral Process Amputation

• If the obstruction is located in the urethral process, amputation may completely alleviate obstruction, as is the case in 37.5–66% of cases.
• Amputation of the urethral process will not affect future breeding ability. This procedure does not prevent future obstruction if

multiple calculi are present in the urinary tract.
• The penis should be exteriorized and urethral process examined in all cases. This may be facilitated by sedation or lumbosacral epidural anesthesia.
• Sedation protocols include diazepam, at a dose range of 0.1–0.5 mg/kg IV, or acepromazine maleate 0.05–0.1 mg/kg IV.
• Acepromazine may promote relaxation of the retractor penis muscle.
• Lumbosacral epidural anesthesia can be performed to provide exteriorization of the penis by eliminating resistance by the retractor penis muscle. Lidocaine (2%) is used at a dose of 1 mL per 5 kg (not to exceed 15 mL). The use of epidural anesthesia may reduce the concentration of inhalant require for surgery.
• Once sedated and/or lumbosacral epidural has been given, the patient can be placed on its rump to allow easier extrusion of the penis. The penis is grasped through the skin at the base of the scrotum and forced cranially. Uroliths may be palpable in the urethra or urethral process and it may be amputated at this time.

Urethral Catheterization and Retrograde Flushing

• Catheterization of the bladder of a ruminant is difficult due to the sigmoid flexure and urethral recess. A catheter can be placed in the distal urethra while occluding the penis. Saline or a lidocaine-saline flush solution (one part lidocaine to three parts saline) is flushed retrograde through the catheter to lavage the calculi into the bladder.
• The disadvantages of this technique are that it is often unsuccessful, can cause trauma to the urethra if catheterization is overly aggressive, and, if successful, the calculus has been returned to the bladder for another chance to cause an obstruction.

Perineal Urethrostomy

• Perineal urethrostomy can be performed in the sedated animal with a lumbosacral epidural.
• Stricture, reduced reproductive ability, and reobstruction are common complications, and this option is best used as a temporary salvage procedure in animals intended for slaughter.

Tube Cystotomy

• Under general anesthesia, a laparotomy is performed, placing an indwelling Foley catheter percutaneously into the bladder wall. The catheter is sutured in place to the abdominal wall enabling voiding of urine through the catheter. The bladder is lavaged to remove remaining calculi. The catheter is left in place to allow the urethra to heal and calculi to be expelled. Periodic challenging of urethral patency is performed until the urethral obstruction is resolved.

• This procedure is the best option for salvage of breeding function in intact males, but it does not prevent recurrence of obstruction.
• Tube cystotomy is the most expensive of the surgical options and is usually performed in pets and breeding animals.

Bladder Marsupialization

• A permanent bladder marsupialization can be performed in which the bladder is sutured to the ventral abdominal wall lateral to the prepuce through a laparotomy incision. This technique requires commitment by the owners as care and cleaning of the stoma are required for the life of the animal.
• Bladder marsupialization has the least chance of reobstruction by calculi but the stoma occasionally strictures and requires surgical modification.
• The breeding capabilities are questionable following this procedure.

MEDICATIONS

DRUGS OF CHOICE

• Sedation can be given for examination and manipulation of the penis and urethral process.
• Diazepam, at a dose range of 0.1–0.5 mg/kg IV (slowly) or acepromazine maleate 0.05–0.1 mg/kg IV or IM. Either as sole agents or in combination with butorphanol 0.05–0.1 mg/kg IV. Alternatively, the use of isoflurane by mask can be used. Acepromazine may promote relaxation of the retractor penis muscle.
• Appropriate antimicrobial therapy should be instituted depending on the specifics of the individual case and route of therapy.
• Preoperative antimicrobials that concentrate in the urine are indicated (e.g., sulfonamides, beta-lactams).

CONTRAINDICATIONS

• Appropriate milk and meat withdrawal times must be followed for all compounds administered to food-producing animals.
• Lidocaine sensitivity is common in goats and should be considered prior to its utilization. (Total dose should never exceed 5 mg/kg or 15 mL of 2% lidocaine in any small ruminant regardless of size.)

PRECAUTIONS

• Alpha-2 agonists (xylazine, detomidine) should not be used in cases of unresolved obstruction due to its diuretic effects.
• Neither diazepam nor acepromazine is approved for use in food animals. The meat withdrawal time for acepromazine maleate is 7 days. There are no withdrawal data for diazepam, therefore consult with FARAD.

U

UROLITHIASIS　(CONTINUED)

POSSIBLE INTERACTIONS
N/A

FOLLOW-UP

EXPECTED COURSE AND PROGNOSIS
Prognosis depends on chronology and severity of obstruction as well as treatment method instituted.

POSSIBLE COMPLICATIONS
Recurrence of obstruction and urethral stricture can be common complications.

CLIENT EDUCATION
• Many small ruminant owners do not know the importance of feeding a low-carbohydrate diet. Small ruminants will preferentially eat grain and owners should feed carbohydrates on a limited basis.
• Mineral supplementation should be done carefully, keeping within recommended ratios.

PATIENT CARE
Animals at risk for obstruction should be monitored closely for signs to enable rapid treatment.

PREVENTION
• A low-carbohydrate, high-roughage diet with a balanced mineral content.
• Free access to water and free-choice salt.
• Urine acidifiers can be used.

MISCELLANEOUS

ASSOCIATED CONDITIONS
Bladder/urethral rupture, uremia, urethral stricture

PRODUCTION MANAGEMENT
• This is a common problem of feedlot lambs fed high-carbohydrate diets.
• Use of ammonium chloride in feed to help reduce the pH of the urine to between 6.0 and 6.5.
• Increasing the quality of long stem ration in the diet.
• Provision of a reliable source of palatable water at all times to encourage water consumption. Heaters should be used to warm the water in winter.

ABBREVIATIONS
• FARAD = Food Animal Residue Avoidance Databank
• IM = intramuscular
• IV = intravenous

SEE ALSO
• Acute Renal Failure
• Bracken Fern Toxicity
• Orf (Contagious Ecthyma)
• Photosensitization
• Pyelonephritis

Suggested Reading
Belknap EB, Pugh DG. Lower urinary tract problems. In: Pugh DG ed, Sheep and Goat Medicine. Philadelphia: Saunders, 2002.
Jones M, Mesner MD, Baird AN, Pugh DG. Obstructive urolithiasis. In: Pugh DG, Baird AN ed, Sheep and Goat Medicine 2nd ed, Maryland Heights: Saunders, 2012.
May KA, Moll HD, Wallace LM, et al. Urinary bladder marsupialization for treatment of obstructive urolithiasis in male goats. Vet Surg 1998, 27: 583–8.
Metre DC, Fecteau G, House JK, et al. Obstructive urolithiasis in ruminants: surgical management and prevention. Comp Cont Educ Pract Vet 1996, 18: S275–S302.
Metre DC, House JK, Smith BP, et al. Obstructive urolithiasis in ruminants: medical treatment and urethral surgery. Comp Cont Ed Pract Vet 1996, 18: 317–28.
Smith MC, Sherman MD. Obstructive urolithiasis. In: Goat Medicine, 2nd ed. Ames: Wiley-Blackwell, 2011.
Tibary A, Pearson LK, Van Metre DC, Ortved K. Surgery of the sheep and goat reproductive and urinary tract. In: Fubini SL, Ducharme NG eds, Farm Animal Surgery. 2nd ed. St. Louis: Elsevier, 2017.
Author Troy E.C. Holder
Consulting Editor Kaitlyn A. Lutz

 Client Education Handout available online

UTERINE ANOMALIES

BASICS

OVERVIEW
• An anomaly is a marked deviation from normal, especially one resulting from a congenital or hereditary defect. • Many of these conditions affecting the uterus are covered individually in other chapters; in this chapter the reader is referred to those chapters for diagnostic and therapeutic information.

INCIDENCE/PREVALENCE
N/A

GEOGRAPHIC DISTRIBUTION
Worldwide

SYSTEMS AFFECTED
Reproductive

PATHOPHYSIOLOGY
The pathophysiology of each condition is highly specific to that condition. This chapter provides a general overview of uterine disease. For specific information about these conditions, the reader is referred to particular chapters.

Congenital Anomalies
This includes arrested development of those structures derived from the embryonic duct systems. Problems caused by either defective or exaggerated fusion of the ducts are reported in most species. It is useful to classify defects on the basis of the underlying anatomic structure. For more information, please consult the following chapters: Segmental Aplasia of the Reproductive Tract; Freemartinism, Congenital Defects (Bovine, Camelid, Small Ruminant).

Acquired Anomalies
• Acquired diseases of the presumptively normal uterus can be classified using the traditional DAMNIT system. • Degenerative, age-associated vascular changes are common in the uterus of the cow and camelid. These usually take the form of a sclerotic lesion and are attributable to previous pregnancies. • Mucometra secondary to chronic ovarian cystic degeneration is associated with uterine atrophy involving both the myometrium and the endometrial glands. • Hydrops allantois can be associated with acquired degenerative uterine changes that impact placental function. • Neoplastic and proliferative disorders of the uterus are uncommon in ruminants, with the exception of lymphosarcoma in cattle. Uterine adenocarcinoma, fibroma, leiomyoma, and leiomyosarcoma are also possible. • Endometrial hyperplasia and cyst formation may occur in association with hyperestrogenism due to toxicity or functional ovarian cysts.

HISTORICAL FINDINGS
• Infertility or subfertility (repeat breeding) • Recurrent pregnancy loss • Abnormal vaginal discharge

SIGNALMENT
• Potentially all ruminant and camelid species. • Congenital anomalies are more common in ruminants.

PHYSICAL EXAMINATION FINDINGS
Signs vary with the specific disease condition but anestrus and repeat breeding are common findings.

GENETICS
• There is evidence for a genetic basis for segmental aplasia of the reproductive tract in female cattle. • Intersex is linked with the gene for polledness in dairy goats.

CAUSES AND RISK FACTORS
• Vary with the specific disease condition. • Degenerative changes of the uterus are often caused by aging and excessive uterine manipulations or chronic infection.

DIAGNOSIS

Diagnosis of uterine anomalies requires a careful history and physical examination.

DIFFERENTIAL DIAGNOSES
Pregnancy should be ruled out in every case of uterine enlargement.

CBC/BIOCHEMISTRY/URINALYSIS
N/A

OTHER LABORATORY TESTS
• Cytogenetic testing or genetic testing (e.g., PCR) • Uterine culture, cytology, and biopsy are useful tools for suspected cases of inflammatory, neoplastic, or degenerative disorders.

IMAGING
• Ultrasonographic evaluation of the uterus is useful for gross pathology such as hydrometra or segmental aplasia. • Radiographs, especially with contrast, may be useful for small ruminants and SAC.

OTHER DIAGNOSTIC PROCEDURES
• Transrectal palpation in cattle and camels. • Exploratory laparotomy or laparoscopy in small ruminants and SAC. • Hysteroscopy is the procedure of choice to investigate intraluminal uterine lesions in SAC.

PATHOLOGIC FINDINGS
The specific findings will vary with the underlying condition.

TREATMENT

Refer to the specific disease conditions.

MEDICATIONS

Refer to the specific disease conditions.

CONTRAINDICATIONS
Appropriate milk and meat withdrawal times must be followed for all compounds administered to food-producing animals.

FOLLOW-UP

N/A

MISCELLANEOUS

ASSOCIATED CONDITIONS
Infertility and subfertility

AGE-RELATED FACTORS
N/A

ZOONOTIC POTENTIAL
N/A

PREGNANCY
N/A

BIOSECURITY
N/A

PRODUCTION MANAGEMENT
N/A

ABBREVIATIONS
• DAMNIT – D)egenerative, (A)utoimmune, (M)etabolic, (N)eoplastic, (I)nfectious/(I)atrogenic, (T)raumatic; an organizational system for developing a diagnosis, commonly expanded beyond this initial list • PCR = polymerase chain reaction • SAC = South American camelid

SEE ALSO
• Congenital Defects: Bovine • Congenital Defects: Camelid • Congenital Defects: Small Ruminant • Endometritis • Freemartinism • Hydrometra • Infertility and Subfertility Issues • Metritis • Pyometra • Segmental Aplasia of the Reproductive Tract

Suggested Reading
McEntee K. Reproductive Pathology of Domestic Animals. San Diego: Academic Press, 1990, pp. 118–90.
Youngquist RS, Braun WF Jr. Abnormalities of the tubular genital organs. Vet Clin North Am Food Anim Pract 1993, 9: 309–22.
Authors Celina Checura and Harry Momont
Consulting Editor Ahmed Tibary
Acknowledgment The authors and book editors acknowledge the prior contribution of Peter Chenoweth.

U

UTERINE ARTERY RUPTURE

BASICS

OVERVIEW
• Uterine artery rupture is a rare, acute, life-threatening hemorrhagic event encountered during the periparturient period. • Rupture is more commonly seen following forced fetal extraction or fetotomy. • Rupture due to arterial wall trauma associated with entrapment and crushing of the uterine artery between the fetus and the maternal pelvis. • May occur subsequent to uterine prolapse as a result of stretching and trauma to the vessels within the broad ligament. • Rarely, it may accompany correction of uterine torsion using the "plank in the flank" technique.

GEOGRAPHIC DISTRIBUTION
N/A

INCIDENCE/PREVALENCE
Unknown

SYSTEMS AFFECTED
• Reproductive • Cardiovascular

PATHOPHYSIOLOGY
• The exact pathophysiology is not known in ruminants and camelids. • May be the result of a combination of traumatic factors associated with dystocia, stretching or sudden drop of the animal and a fragile arterial wall (sclerosis or degenerative changes). • The prolapsed uterus may provide hemostasis by compression of the broad ligament and delay blood loss; death may occur during or soon after repositioning of the uterus.

HISTORICAL FINDINGS
Collapse or sudden death during or soon after parturition.

SIGNALMENT
• More common in dairy cattle • Potentially all ruminant species and camelids

PHYSICAL EXAMINATION FINDINGS
Severe anemia, tachycardia, tachypnea, anxiety, and signs of shock due hypovolemia.

GENETICS
N/A

CAUSES AND RISK FACTORS
• Age • Dystocia

DIAGNOSIS

• Antemortem: History and clinical signs. • Transrectal palpation: Large soft tissue swelling (hematoma) within the broad ligament. • Hemorrhage may be evident at the vulva if the uterine wall is ruptured. • Incidental transrectal findings of a soft tissue mass within the broad ligament and/or a corresponding defect or aneurysm in the uterine artery days or weeks after parturition. • Postmortem: Identification of the rupture within the uterine artery and hemorrhage into the broad ligament or peritoneum.

DIFFERENTIAL DIAGNOSES
• Acute blood loss from other internal sites • Acute septic peritonitis

CBC/BIOCHEMISTRY/URINALYSIS
Evidence of blood loss anemia if the animal survives the first few hours.

OTHER LABORATORY TESTS
Fine-needle aspirate of a soft tissue mass in the broad ligament may allow differentiation of hematoma from an abscess.

IMAGING
Transrectal ultrasonography may help identify a hematoma within the broad ligament and/or a defect in the affected uterine artery.

OTHER DIAGNOSTIC PROCEDURES
N/A

PATHOLOGIC FINDINGS
• Rupture of uterine artery with accompanying massive hemorrhage into the broad ligament. • Hemoabdomen may also be noted. • Extreme pallor of mucus membranes and other tissues noted during postmortem examination.

TREATMENT

THERAPEUTIC APPROACH
• Whole blood transfusion (6–12 liters) • Hypertonic saline (2–4 mL/kg of 7% sodium chloride, IV) may be of acute resuscitative value. • Oxytocin (20–100 IU, IV) to promote uterine contraction and involution—may be given repeatedly. • Aminocaproic acid, a derivative of the amino acid lysine, aids in clot formation by inhibiting fibrinolysis and has been used as a coagulation aid in mares with periparturient hemorrhage (loading dose of 20 g aminocaproic acid diluted in 1 liter of isotonic fluid and given IV followed by 10 g diluted in 1 liter of isotonic fluid q6h).

SURGICAL CONSIDERATIONS AND TECHNIQUES
Vessel ligation may be attempted but will be possible only if a full thickness uterine tear accompanies uterine artery rupture.

MEDICATIONS

DRUGS OF CHOICE
N/A

CONTRAINDICATIONS
Appropriate milk and meat withdrawal times must be followed for all compounds administered to food-producing animals.

PRECAUTIONS
N/A

POSSIBLE INTERACTIONS
N/A

FOLLOW-UP

EXPECTED COURSE AND PROGNOSIS
Prognosis guarded at best

POSSIBLE COMPLICATIONS
Death, infertility, adhesions

CLIENT EDUCATION
Proper observation during parturition

PATIENT CARE
Close confinement with box stall rest to avoid disruption of clot formation and stabilization

MISCELLANEOUS

ASSOCIATED CONDITIONS
N/A

AGE-RELATED FACTORS
More common in multiparous dams

ZOONOTIC POTENTIAL
N/A

PREGNANCY
N/A

BIOSECURITY
N/A

PRODUCTION MANAGEMENT
N/A

ABBREVIATION
IV = intravenous

SEE ALSO
• Anemia, Nonregenerative • Anemia, Regenerative • Down Bovine • Down Camelid • Down Small Ruminant • Dystocia: Bovine • Dystocia: Camelid • Dystocia: Small Ruminant • Postpartum Disorders • Uterine Prolapse • Uterine Torsion

Suggested Reading
Cockroft PD. Diagnosis of a haematoma in the uterine broad ligament associated with a dystocia in a cow using ultrasonography. Vet Rec 1999, 144: 675–6.
Pearson LK, Tibary A. Clinical management of postpartum hemorrhage following failure of cervical dilation in an alpaca. Clin Theriogenol 2014, 6: 111–17.
Roberts SJ. Injuries and diseases of the puerperal period. In: Veterinary Obstetrics and Genital Diseases (Theriogenology), 3rd ed. Woodstock, VT: SJ Roberts, 1986.

Author Jennifer N. Roberts
Consulting Editor Ahmed Tibary
Acknowledgment The author and book editors acknowledge the prior contribution of Simon F. Peek.

U

BASICS

OVERVIEW
• Uterine prolapse is the most dramatic of the reproductive prolapses. It affects all ruminants and camelid species but is most common in multiparous dairy and beef cattle and dromedary camels.
• The protrusion of both uterine horns through the vulva is easily diagnosed and characterizes the uterine prolapse.
• Uterine prolapse usually occurs within a few hours after parturition. In cattle, half occur within 3 hours and >90% occur within a day. More rarely, it can occur up to 5 or 6 days after parturition.
• In camels, uterine prolapse tends to occur immediately after parturition.
• Uterine prolapse is a true emergency and prompt, effective intervention is required to protect the life and reproductive health of the animal.

INCIDENCE/PREVALENCE
The incidence of uterine prolapse is relatively low, ranging from 0.003% to 0.25% but ruminant species are more commonly affected than are other domestic animals.

GEOGRAPHICAL DISTRIBUTION
Worldwide

SYSTEMS AFFECTED
Reproductive

PATHOPHYSIOLOGY
• It is assumed that the loosening and stretching of perineal tissue at parturition creates a laxity that allows the uterus to prolapse.
• Straining, especially after a difficult delivery of a large fetus, along with recumbency and lack of uterine tone are contributing factors. Postpartum uterine inertia may result from excessive distention or hypocalcemia (primary) or dystocia and prolonged effort (secondary).

HISTORICAL FINDINGS
• Recent parturition
• Dystocia

SIGNALMENT
All ruminant species are at risk for the occurrence of uterine prolapse, but cows are at a higher risk. Multiparous cows are at higher risk due to a higher risk for hypocalcemia, a condition that predisposes cows to uterine prolapse.

PHYSICAL EXAMINATION FINDINGS
• Immediately after prolapse occurs, the tissues are normal and there may be fetal membranes still attached to the caruncles (ruminants). Within a few hours after the prolapse, the uterus becomes edematous and is more susceptible to traumatic injury.

• Clinical signs that accompany uterine prolapse are straining, abdominal pain, restlessness, anorexia, and increased pulse and respiratory rate. Uterine prolapse in cows and camels is frequently accompanied by hypocalcemia and, in the more severe cases, milk fever.
• Cows that present with concurrent hypocalcemia may be recumbent and have muscle fasciculation. Although unusual, the condition may progress to shock and death.

GENETICS
The sporadic incidence makes it difficult to confirm a hereditary tendency.

CAUSES AND RISK FACTORS
Dystocia, hypocalcemia

 DIAGNOSIS

The diagnosis is obvious as the uterine horns can be identified protruding from the vulva.

DIFFERENTIAL DIAGNOSES
• Retained fetal membranes
• Vaginal or cervical prolapse

CBC/BIOCHEMISTRY/URINALYSIS
N/A

OTHER LABORATORY TESTS
N/A

IMAGING
N/A

OTHER DIAGNOSTIC PROCEDURES
N/A

PATHOLOGIC FINDINGS
N/A

 TREATMENT

THERAPEUTIC APPROACH
• The correction of uterine prolapse can be performed with the animal standing or in sternum recumbency.
• In camelids, the best approach is to sedate and restrain the animal in a sternal "cush" position with the hindquarter slightly elevated.
• Epidural anesthesia with 2% lidocaine is recommended.
• Administration of clenbuterol is reported to cause uterus relaxation, facilitating replacement of the uterus, reducing the need for epidural anesthesia. Clenbuterol is a prohibited drug in the United States.
• When attempting to reduce uterine prolapse in a recumbent cow, both hindlimbs should be pulled posterior behind the animal so that she is resting on her stifles with the hind legs spread out. This positioning causes the pelvis to be slightly tilted downward and forward, leaving more room in the caudal abdominal cavity, favoring the replacement of the uterus.

The hindquarters of small ruminants should be elevated to assist with replacement.
• It is imperative that when reducing a uterine prolapse the veterinarian and assistant be as clean as possible. Surgical scrub should be used to wash the entire uterine surface and remove fecal material, dirt, bedding material, and fetal membranes. If the membranes are not easily separated from the caruncles, they should be left in place.
• The washed uterus should be supported on a clean surface (e.g., a tray, towel, or sheet) to minimize contamination and assist replacement. For the recumbent cow, the uterus can be supported on the clinician's lap as they kneel between the hind legs. A waterproof obstetric smock provides a clean support surface for both the clinician and the patient.
• Many practitioners attempt to reduce tissue edema to facilitate replacement. This is done by either rinsing the uterus with hypertonic saline or dusting it with sugar.
• The uterus is replaced by alternately pushing on either side of the prolapsed tissue nearest the vulva. Avoid spreading the fingers of the hand while pushing as this may lead to repeated perforation of the organ. Obstetric lubricant should be applied if necessary.
• Once the uterus is replaced, every effort should be made to ensure that the both horns are completely inverted. This simple expedient will prevent recurrence in most cases. If the clinician's arm is too short or too large to accomplish the task, a number of alternatives have been recommended. They include the use of a probang and the infusion of large volumes of sterile fluid. The fluid should be siphoned out after the horns are correctly positioned.
• Oxytocin can be administered after the uterus is successfully replaced to stimulate uterine contraction and involution. Cows that develop uterine prolapse are also at higher risk for hypocalcemia; treatments with calcium intravenous solutions should be considered. Prolonged recumbency after replacement may predispose to recurrence of the prolapse.
• The use of retention sutures after replacement is the subject of some controversy. While there is little evidence that they are necessary if the uterus is correctly replaced, many clinicians (including the author) continue to use them. Options include a Buhner stitch, the shoelace technique, or mattress sutures with stents. These should all be removed within 2–3 days. During this time the animal must be closely monitored for recurrence as the potential for trauma is increased while the sutures are in place.
• Parenteral antibiotic treatment is recommended after uterine prolapse is resolved to avoid the occurrence of metritis. An anti-inflammatory agent should be given for 3–4 days for pain control.

UTERINE PROLAPSE

SURGICAL CONSIDERATIONS AND TECHNIQUES

In cases where replacement of the uterus is impossible or where the tissues are severely damaged, amputation or emergency slaughter may be indicated as salvage options.

MEDICATIONS

DRUGS OF CHOICE

Lidocaine epidural, appropriate parenteral antibiotic, nonsteroidal anti-inflammatory agent

CONTRAINDICATIONS

Appropriate milk and meat withdrawal times must be followed for all compounds administered to food-producing animals.

PRECAUTIONS

N/A

POSSIBLE INTERACTIONS

N/A

FOLLOW-UP

EXPECTED COURSE AND PROGNOSIS

• The prognosis is usually good if the prolapse is recent.
• The prognosis is poor or guarded if there is severe contamination or extensive uterine lesions.

POSSIBLE COMPLICATIONS

• Fatalities are rare but can occur in the event of shock or rupture of a large uterine vessel.
• Cows that develop uterine prolapse are at higher risk for metritis and, consequently, are at higher risk for reproductive problems (e.g., increased calving-to-conception interval and calving interval). Due to reproductive

problems, cows that present with uterine prolapse are at a higher risk for culling than their herd mates.

PATIENT CARE

Animals should be closely observed daily for 5–10 days. Animals showing any signs of straining, fever, anorexia, or depression should be examined and treated appropriately.

CLIENT EDUCATION

Proper handling of animals with prolapse: Keep animal calm, move animal carefully to clean area, protect exposed tissue with clean wet towel or place in a plastic bag.

PREVENTION

• Because hypocalcemic cows are at higher risk of uterine prolapse, the dry cow diet should be formulated to avoid such metabolic imbalance.
• Some studies have shown that cows that have stillborn calves are at higher risk for uterine prolapse, probably due to the longer period between initiation of parturition and assistance provided to the animal. Therefore, it is recommended that the calving area be well monitored at all times and that cows have the proper assistance as they show signs of dystocia or calving difficulties.

MISCELLANEOUS

ASSOCIATED CONDITIONS

Hypocalcemia, dystocia, oversized fetus, retained placenta

AGE-RELATED FACTORS

Because hypocalcemia is more common in multiparous cows, it is expected that multiparous cows are at higher risk for uterine prolapse than primiparous cows.

BIOSECURITY

N/A

PRODUCTION MANAGEMENT

Feeding well-balanced rations in the far-off and close-up periods is important to avoid the occurrence of hypocalcemia, decreasing the risk for uterine prolapse.

ABBREVIATIONS

N/A

SEE ALSO

• Dystocia: Bovine
• Dystocia: Camelid
• Dystocia: Small Ruminant
• Hypocalcemia: Bovine
• Hypocalcemia: Small Ruminant
• Postparturient Paresis (Hypocalcemia)
• Reproductive Prolapse

Suggested Reading

Black B. The Uterine Prolapse.https://youtu.be/Zev6jO6L5N0
Gardner IA, Reynolds JP, Risco CA, Hird DW. Patterns of uterine prolapse in dairy cows and prognosis after treatment. J Am Vet Med Assoc 1990, 197: 1021–4.
Murphy AM, Dobson H. Predisposition, subsequent fertility, and mortality of cows with uterine prolapse. Vet Rec 2002, 151: 733–5.
Peter AT. Vaginal, cervical and uterine prolapse. In: Hopper RM ed, Bovine Reproduction. Ames: Wiley Blackwell, 2015, pp. 383–95.
Tibary A, Pearson LK. Reproductive emergencies in camelids. Clinic Theriogenol 2014, 6: 579–92.

Author Harry Momont
Consulting Editor Ahmed Tibary
Acknowledgment The author and book editors acknowledge the prior contribution of Ricardo Carbonari Chebel.

BASICS

OVERVIEW
• Uterine torsion in cattle involves the rotation of the arc-shaped gravid uterus on its transverse axis. Both uterine horns and broad ligaments are displaced.
• The majority of cases (85–90%) are diagnosed at the time of parturition (late 1st stage or early 2nd stage labor) but some can rarely occur much earlier in gestation.
• Uterine torsion is a relatively common cause of bovine dystocia, accounting for 5–10% of obstetric cases in veterinary practice and up to 20% in referral practices.

INCIDENCE/PREVALENCE
• Uterine torsion represents 5–10% of the dystocia occurring in dairy cattle but in selected populations can represent 20% or more of the dystocias attended by veterinarians.
• Counterclockwise torsion of the uterus is more common than clockwise torsion, probably related to the majority of right horn pregnancies.

GEOGRAPHIC DISTRIBUTION
Worldwide, reportedly less common in *Bos indicus* cattle

SYSTEMS AFFECTED
Reproductive

PATHOPHYSIOLOGY
• The pathophysiology of uterine torsion remains speculative.
• Increased fetal movements in the late 1st and early 2nd stage of labor, uterine instability due to the dorsolateral attachment of the broad ligament, and the fact that cattle rise and lie down with the head lower than the pelvis create the potential for a sudden jarring or fetal movement to rotate the suspended gravid horn. Fetal oversize is another factor that may predispose to uterine torsion.

HISTORICAL FINDINGS
Dystocia

SIGNALMENT
• Gravid females, most often at parturition but has been reported as early as 70 days of gestation in cattle.
• Uterine torsion is more common in pluriparous than primiparous cattle and less common in twin pregnancies.
• Brown Swiss cattle are at greater risk but the condition is common in the Holstein breed.

SIGNS
• Overt clinical signs are often lacking in cows with torsions <270°.
• Cows with uterine torsion may present with signs of anorexia, depression, decreased milk production, and colic/abdominal pain (kicking the abdomen and treading hindlimbs).

• Tenesmus, constipation, and even rectal or vaginal prolapse may be seen in protracted cases.

GENETICS
N/A

CAUSES AND RISK FACTORS
Affected cows are more likely to be carrying a large and/or male fetus.

DIAGNOSIS

The critical aspect of the diagnosis is the correct assessment of the direction of the torsion.

DIFFERENTIAL DIAGNOSES
• Other causes of dystocia, especially fetal malposition
• Other causes of colic

CBC/BIOCHEMISTRY/URINALYSIS
N/A

OTHER LABORATORY TESTS
N/A

IMAGING
N/A

OTHER DIAGNOSTIC PROCEDURES
• Vaginoscopy or manual vaginal examination may show spiral folds in the vaginal walls. However, in one-third of torsions, the vagina is not involved as the torsion is cranial to the cervix.
• Palpation per rectum of the vagina, cervix, uterus, and especially the broad ligaments of the uterus is critical to the correct assessment of the presence and direction of a uterine torsion. The broad ligament on one side is pulled tightly over the top of the genital tract while the ligament on the opposite side is pulled under. In a right/clockwise torsion the right ligament is pulled under. In a left/counterclockwise torsion it is the left ligament that is pulled beneath the tract. The perspective for determining the direction of a torsion is always that of the examiner from behind the cow.
• A fetus in dorso-ileal or dorso-pubic position is a more common finding in cases of uterine torsion than with other causes of dystocia.

PATHOLOGIC FINDINGS
• N/A

TREATMENT

THERAPEUTIC APPROACH
• For intrapartum torsions of 90° or less, it is often possible to rotate the uterus by grasping the calf and swinging it in arc fashion until the torsion is corrected. The calf is rotated in the opposite direction of the torsion.

• If this method is not successful, a detorsion rod can be applied to the calf and again the calf is rotated in the opposite direction of the torsion. A loop on one end of an obstetric chain is placed proximally to the metacarpal/metatarsal joint of the calf. The doubled chain is then passed through the loop of the detorsion rod and the resulting loop is placed proximally to the metacarpal/metatarsal joint of the other limb. A wooden dowel or rod is inserted in the other end of the detorsion rod and the calf is rotated by an assistant while the attending veterinarian monitors the progress and prevents trauma to the birth canal. Detorsion rods should be used with caution and only after adequate training as they may severely injure the cow or calf.
• If access to the calf is prevented by a closed cervix or a severe degree of torsion, then the correction will require rolling the cow. The cow is cast in lateral recumbency (right side for clockwise torsion, left side for counterclockwise). A 2" by 6" and approximately 8–10 feet long plank with a smooth surface is placed over the paralumbar fossa. A 70–100 kg individual stands on the plank, maintaining their position over the cow's abdomen as the cow is rotated by her limbs in the direction of the torsion. The procedure is easier and safer if the fore and hind limbs are tied one to the other.

SURGICAL CONSIDERATIONS AND TECHNIQUES
• Cesarean section should be considered if manipulation fails.
• Either standing flank laparotomy or ventral midline approach have been used.
• Attempt should be made to correct the torsion before incision of the uterus.
• Severe torsions (270° or more) may restrict access to the fetus.
• Vascular compromise makes uterine closure difficult.
• The viability of the calf should be confirmed before this option is selected. It is also possible to correct the torsion through a flank incision and allow the pregnancy to continue if the calf is not at term.

MEDICATIONS

DRUGS OF CHOICE
N/A

CONTRAINDICATIONS
N/A

PRECAUTIONS
N/A

POSSIBLE INTERACTIONS
N/A

UTERINE TORSION: BOVINE

 FOLLOW-UP

EXPECTED COURSE AND PROGNOSIS

The prognosis is usually good; however, it depends on the extent of the torsion and the length of time between occurrence, diagnosis, and treatment.

POSSIBLE COMPLICATIONS

• Complications are rare if the torsion is not severe and manual correction is successful.
• Uterine torsions >270° can cause vascular compromise and potentially uterine rupture.
• Post-surgical complications are similar to those described for cesarean section. Risk of uterine rupture is increased and makes uterine closure more difficult.

CLIENT EDUCATION

Proper calving management procedures

PATIENT CARE

• Patients should be observed for at least 3–5 days after nonsurgical correction to evaluate appetite and to ensure that no fever develops.
• When the uterine torsion is corrected surgically, the patient should be closely observed for 5–10 days. Rectal temperatures should be checked daily, and if signs of fever or loss of appetite appear, the animal should be treated immediately as indicated.

PREVENTION

N/A

 MISCELLANEOUS

ASSOCIATED CONDITIONS

Dystocia and other postpartum complications

AGE-RELATED FACTORS

Multiparous cows may be theoretically at higher risk for uterine torsion due to decreased uterine and mesometrial tone.

ZOONOTIC POTENTIAL

N/A

PREGNANCY

Most uterine torsions in cattle are diagnosed at term. Those that occur earlier may compromise the viability of the fetus. Severe torsions that result in vascular compromise may hasten the death of the calf.

BIOSECURITY

N/A

PRODUCTION MANAGEMENT

Uterine torsion is a relatively uncommon event with limited financial impact on most dairies. For smaller dairy operations it is best managed by timely veterinary intervention.

ABBREVIATIONS

N/A

SEE ALSO

• Cesarean Section: Bovine
• Colic: Bovine
• Dystocia: Bovine

Suggested Reading
Pascale A, Warnick LD, DesCoteaux L, Brouchard E. A study of 55 field cases of uterine torsion in dairy cattle. Can Vet J 2008, 49: 366–72.
Roberts SJ. Veterinary Obstetrics and Genital Diseases (Theriogenology), 3rd ed. Woodstock, VT: SJ Roberts, 1986, pp. 337–43.
Wardrope DD, Boyes GW. Uterine torsion in twin pregnancies in dairy cattle. Vet Rec 2002, 150: 56.

Authors Harry Momont and Celina Checura
Consulting Editor Ahmed Tibary
Acknowledgment The authors and book editors acknowledge the prior contribution of Ricardo Carbonari Chebel.

U

UTERINE TORSION: CAMELID

BASICS

OVERVIEW
• Uterine torsion is diagnosed in gravid females in mid to late gestation, although the torsion event may have occurred earlier.
• The uterus rotates upon its long axis such that tension on the broad ligaments and continued growth of the fetus results in the clinical signs of pain or behavior changes.
• At term, the torsion may result in dystocia.

INCIDENCE/PREVALENCE
Not known but likely higher than reported

GEOGRAPHIC DISTRIBUTION
Worldwide distribution, but incidence seems higher in the United States compared to South America.

PATHOPHYSIOLOGY
• Uterine torsion seems to occur more commonly in SAC than in other species. The exact causes of the torsion are not understood.
• Uterine torsions are characterized by both direction and severity. The direction is either clockwise or counterclockwise, as assessed from standing behind the animal and facing cranially. Severity has been described from 90° to 360°. In one study, 48% of torsions were 360°.
• The overwhelming majority of camelid pregnancies are carried in the left horn (98%) yet both clockwise (81.7%) and counterclockwise (18.3%) torsions were described in a large study of left horn pregnancies.
• 78% of females in one study were multiparous.
• Animals treated by rolling had a cria survival rate of 100%, whereas animals which underwent surgical treatment had a cria survival rate of approximately 70%. Animals were more likely to undergo surgical treatment for more severe torsions, and therefore had increased risk of uterine ischemia and cria compromise.
• Neonatal and dam survival depend on the severity of torsion and the degree of compromise to the uterine vessels and placenta.

SYSTEMS AFFECTED
Reproductive

GENETICS
N/A

HISTORICAL FINDINGS
• The presenting complaint of a female camelid with uterine torsion may be that the producer has observed the animal to be "not quite right," with absence of acute pain.
• Uterine torsion is typically diagnosed in mid to late gestation, or at term, as a cause of dystocia.
• The female may have been observed to have pain or abnormal behavior.

• A few females have had uterine torsions in previous pregnancies, or more than once in the same pregnancy.

SIGNALMENT
• Uterine torsion has been described in alpacas, llamas, and camels.
• In one study of alpacas, the mean ± SD age was 5.9 ± 2.9 years.
• Both primiparous and multiparous animals may be affected.

PHYSICAL EXAMINATION FINDINGS
• The clinical signs may be acute or mild colic signs (rolling, kicking at the belly, increased vocalization) which do not respond to medical therapy.
• Some animals may present with vague clinical signs, such as increased time in lateral recumbency, increased number of trips to the manure pile, or decreased interest in the herd or feeding activities.
• Physical examination may be normal or the female may show signs of systemic debilitation in severe, chronic cases.
• In severe cases, the female may show tachycardia, tachypnea, depression, recumbency, or straining.
• Protracted cases may present as a down animal. Severe profuse diarrhea may be seen in some cases.
• Advanced cases present with lethargy, anorexia, dehydration, and signs of toxemia.

CAUSES AND RISK FACTORS
• The cause of uterine torsion is not known although some risk factors have been suspected.
• Risk factors include shearing on a table, "dusting" or rolling behavior in hot weather, hypocalcemia, fetal sex, fetal size, and maternal body condition score, height, and length.

DIAGNOSIS

• The diagnosis is by transrectal palpation. In alpacas, transrectal palpation may be achieved by clinicians with small hands, and use of lidocaine-infused lubricant. The female is placed in sternal recumbency (the "cush" position) and palpation of the broad ligaments is used to determine the presence of a uterine torsion, and the direction and severity. Palpation of llamas and camels may be more easily performed.
• The fetus is often not easily palpable, particularly when the torsion is severe.
• Diagnosis of the direction of the torsion is based on the position of the broad ligament. The torsion is clockwise (to the right, looking from the back of the animal) if the left broad ligament is stretched diagonally from the left side to the right side of the animal forming a tight band running over the uterine body. The right broad ligament is shorter and

trapped under the uterine body. In the counterclockwise torsion the direction and position of the broad ligaments are reversed.
• Diagnosis of the direction of the torsion can be difficult in small sized animals or if the rectum is swollen.
• Diagnosis of the severity of the torsion remains speculative but can be determined based on the number of rolling actions needed for correction or at surgery.
• The majority of uterine torsions in camelids do not involve the cervix. Therefore, palpation of the cervix will not provide a diagnosis or direction. In addition, vaginal palpation may be extremely difficult and painful for maiden females. Vaginal speculum examination may be performed after correction of a torsion at term, to determine if the cervix is open and labor may ensue.

DIFFERENTIAL DIAGNOSES
• Other causes of colic in camelids.
• Other causes of dystocia, if at term (fetal maldisposition, failure of cervical dilation).

CBC/BIOCHEMISTRY/URINALYSIS
In one study, 65% of blood work was normal. In debilitated animals, the most common abnormalities were toxemia (leukophilia due to neutrophilia, with toxic PMNs evident on a blood smear) (19.9%), toxemia and hypocalcemia (5%), hypocalcemia alone (5%), and hepatic lipidosis (3.4%). Hyperglycemia was a common, nonspecific finding.

OTHER LABORATORY TESTS
N/A

IMAGING
• Transabdominal ultrasonography is used to determine fetal viability, fetal stress, and to examine the health of the uteroplacental unit.
• Persistent fetal tachycardia (>130 bpm) or bradycardia (<50 bpm) suggests fetal compromise.
• Detachment of the fetal membranes or abnormal uterine wall appearance may indicate need for surgical correction.

OTHER DIAGNOSTIC PROCEDURES
N/A

PATHOLOGIC FIDINGS
Postmortem examination may reveal uterine rupture or congestion.

TREATMENT

THERAPEUTIC APPROACH
• Correction of uterine torsion is either by nonsurgical (rolling) or surgical (laparotomy with or without cesarean section) methods.
• To roll, the female is placed in lateral recumbency on the same side as the torsion (i.e., for a clockwise torsion, she is placed in right lateral recumbency). Then one person manually maintains the fetus in position

U

UTERINE TORSION: CAMELID

while two others roll the female from right lateral recumbency, dorsally to left lateral recumbency, then to sternal recumbency. The female is rolled three times, and then transrectal palpation is used to determine if the torsion was corrected.
• Cases diagnosed early and corrected successfully by rolling do not require any further treatment.

SURGICAL CONSIDERATIONS AND TECHNIQUES

• Severely debilitated animals should be stabilized prior to anesthesia.
• Surgical correction is by laparotomy under general anesthesia. In the field, epidural and regional anesthesia may be attempted, with a flank approach. In a clinical setting, ventral midline celiotomy is the approach of choice for SAC. In cases of fetal nonviability, a cesarean section is performed. If possible, viable fetuses are left in situ after correction of the torsion, particularly if not at term. Delivery of a nonviable fetus 3 days postoperatively has occurred.

MEDICATIONS

DRUGS OF CHOICE

To facilitate rolling as a correction method, females may be sedated with butorphanol tartrate IM.

CONTRAINDICATIONS

Appropriate milk and meat withdrawal times must be followed for all compounds administered to food-producing animals.

PRECAUTIONS

• Extreme care should be exercised during the rolling process not to put too much pressure on the uterus.
• Females with a severely compromised uterus should not be rolled.

POSSIBLE INTERACTIONS

N/A

FOLLOW-UP

EXPECTED COURSE AND PROGNOSIS

In one study of SAC, 97% of females survived (fatalities occurred intra- and postoperatively). Cria survival was 100% after correction with rolling and 70% following surgical correction.

POSSIBLE COMPLICATIONS

• Colonic injury during transrectal palpation.
• Expulsion of a nonviable fetus may occur after correction of the torsion.
• Surgical complications (incisional dehiscence, infection, or seroma formation, peritonitis, and adhesion formation).

PATIENT CARE

Perioperative care includes antimicrobials, anti-inflammatories, tetanus toxoid, and may include supportive care including IV fluids, transfaunation, and B vitamins administration.

CLIENT EDUCATION

• Careful monitoring of all pregnant females in the last trimester of pregnancy.
• Refer to a veterinarian any pregnant females exhibiting signs of colic or abnormal behavior.

PREVENTION

N/A

MISCELLANEOUS

ASSOCIATED CONDITIONS

• Dystocia
• Hypocalcemia
• Hepatic lipidosis

AGE-RELATED FACTORS

N/A

ZOONOTIC POTENTIAL

N/A

PREGNANCY

Risk of recurrence in subsequent pregnancies is debatable.

BIOSECURITY

N/A

PRODUCTION MANAGEMENT

Producers should present animals which show vague signs of discomfort in mid to late gestation for veterinary examination.

SYNONYMS

N/A

ABBREVIATIONS

• IM =imtramuscular
• IV = intravenous
• SAC = South American camelids

SEE ALSO

• Cesarean Section: Camelid
• Camelid: Gastrointestinal Disease
• Down Camelid
• Dystocia: Camelid
• Pregnancy Diagnosis: Camelid
• Pregnancy Toxemia: Camelid

Suggested Reading

Anderson DE. Uterine torsion and Cesarean section in llamas and alpacas. Vet Clin North Am Food Anim Pract 2009, 25: 523–38.

Cebra CK, Cebra ML, Garry FB, et al. Surgical and nonsurgical correction of uterine torsion in New World camelids: 20 cases (1990–1996). J Am Vet Med Assoc 1997, 211: 600–2.

Pearson LK, Rodriguez JS, Tibary A. Uterine torsion in late gestation alpacas and llamas: 60 cases (2000–2009). Small Rumin Res 2012, 105: 268–72.

Pearson LK, Rodriguez JS, Tibary A. Disorders and diseases of pregnancy. In: Cebra C, Anderson DE, Tibary A, Van Saun RJ, Johnson LW eds, Llama and Alpaca Care: Medicine, Surgery, Reproduction, Nutrition, and Herd Health. St. Louis: Elsevier, 2014, pp. 256–73.

Author Lisa Pearson
Consulting Editor Ahmed Tibary

U

UTERINE TORSION: SMALL RUMINANT

BASICS

OVERVIEW
• Uterine torsion is a rare cause of dystocia in sheep and goats, accounting for <5% of peripartum complications.
• The condition may be underestimated because it is difficult to diagnose and treat without surgical intervention.
• It can be of mild degree (45–90°) or severe degree (>180°).
• The torsion can be caudal to the cervix, including the vagina, or cranial to the cervix. More often the vagina is included in the torsion.
• It is more common in singleton pregnancies.
• Fetal oversize has seen suggested as a predisposing factor.

INCIDENCE/PREVALENCE
• Uterine torsion represents about 5% of the dystocia occurring in sheep and goats.
• Others have reported up to 10% of all dystocia cases in sheep.

GEOGRAPHIC DISTRIBUTION
Worldwide

PATHOPHYSIOLOGY
The pathophysiology of uterine torsion in small ruminants is not known. In fact this condition is often missed or not diagnosed until surgery (cesarean section).

HISTORICAL FINDINGS
• Down or painful late term female.
• Overdue female that has shown development then regression of the udder.
• No progression beyond first stage of parturition.

SIGNALMENT
• Uterine torsion can occur in sheep and goats.
• Prolific breeds have a lower risk of uterine torsion.
• Multiparous ewes and goats are believed to be at higher risk due to longer and more relaxed broad ligaments of the uterus.

PHYSICAL EXAMINATION FINDINGS
• Dystocia failure to lamb or kid after initial stages of labor preparation
• Sheep and goats with uterine torsion usually present depression, anorexia, elevated respiratory and heart rates. Bruxism (teeth grinding) may be observed in painful animals.
• The perineum can be swollen without appearance of fetal fluid or placenta. However, this may be due to overt manipulation by the owner.
• Development of the mammary gland and colostrum can be present if the animal is in labor.
• Many cases may not present until several days or even weeks after initial signs of parturition.

GENETICS
N/A

CAUSES AND RISK FACTORS
N/A

DIAGNOSIS

DIFFERENTIAL DIAGNOSES
• Clinical diagnosis is often difficult because of impossibility to palpate the uterus. The condition is often suspected after ruling out other causes of dystocia or pregnancy (failure of cervical dilation, fetal maternal disproportion, and twins) or pregnancy toxemia.
• Vaginal speculum examination may be helpful in detecting the presence of vaginal mucosal folds in case of torsion caudal to the cervix. The cervix cannot be visualized.
• Vaginal palpation, if possible, may be helpful.
• Uterine torsion may be suspected by transabdominal ultrasonography based on extensive uterine wall edema and dilated broad ligament vasculature.
• Often the final diagnosis is reached after laparotomy.

CBC/BIOCHEMISTRY/URINALYSIS
• May be performed in ewes or does that are depressed. Usually prior to surgery. The changes are variable depending on the duration of the process.
• Various degrees of dehydration and electrolyte changes, neutrophilia and high fibrinogen are found in cases with severe compromise or rupture of the uterus.
• Severe anemia due to blood loss is present in animals with ruptured uterus and/or if uterine/ovarian blood vessels rupture.

IMAGING
• Transabdominal ultrasonographic evaluation of the entire uterus and cervical area may show several changes including:
  ○ Increased echogenicity and poor definition of fetal fluids
  ○ Loss of fetal fluid if the torsion does completely obliterate the cervical canal
  ○ Increased thickness of the uterine wall with poorly defined placentome
  ○ Thickened/edematous fetal membranes
  ○ Broad ligament edema and severely engorged blood vessels
  ○ In chronic cases, usually presented days to weeks after initiation of parturition, uterine rupture and adhesions to the body wall may already have occurred.
  ○ Fetal viability can be assessed: Fetal death is confirmed by lack of fetal heartbeat. Severely compromised fetuses usually show a very slow and irregular heart beat.

OTHER DIAGNOSTIC PROCEDURES
N/A

PATHOLOGIC FINDINGS
• Death may result from uterine necrosis, uterine rupture, or rupture of the major blood vessels.
• Postmortem examination of ewes shows increased amount of peritoneal fluids, peritonitis, and adhesions to other abdominal organs.

TREATMENT

THERAPEUTIC APPROACH
• Rolling as described in other species has been reported in a few cases in sheep. However, the success rate of this approach depends on accurate diagnosis of the direction of the torsion.
• The rolling technique should only be attempted if the uterine wall is not too compromised.

SURGICAL CONSIDERATIONS AND TECHNIQUES
• Emergency laparotomy and cesarean section should be considered if no diagnosis can be made.
• The best approach for laparotomy is the ventral midline approach in order to better expose the uterus.
• The uterus may already be ruptured or friable, in which case an ovariohysterectomy should be considered.

MEDICATIONS

DRUGS OF CHOICE
• Sedation: Butorphanol and xylazine for rolling.
• General anesthesia (injectable or inhalation) is the preferred approach for surgery.
• NAISDs (flunixin meglumine) and broad-spectrum antibiotics.

CONTRAINDICATIONS
Appropriate milk and meat withdrawal times must be followed for all compounds administered to food-producing animals.

PRECAUTIONS
N/A

POSSIBLE INTERACTIONS
N/A

FOLLOW-UP

EXPECTED COURSE AND PROGNOSIS
• The prognosis depends on the degree and the duration of the torsion. If cesarean section is performed promptly the prognosis for survival in dams is very good. However, the future fertility of the animal can be

compromised depending on the extent of the torsion.
• Severely compromised females should be humanely euthanized.
• Prognosis for fetus or neonate is poor in most cases.

POSSIBLE COMPLICATIONS
• Retained fetal membrane
• Metritis
• Uterine rupture
• Spontaneous vaginal rupture
• Ovarian vein rupture
• Peritonitis

CLIENT EDUCATION
• Lambing and kidding watch and awareness of signs of dystocia.
• Goat and sheep owners often get involved in dystocia management. They should be aware of situations that are beyond their expertise and welfare implications of obstetric manipulations.

PATIENT CARE
• After rolling, parturition may progress normally or may require obstetric assistance. The animal should be monitored is the same manner as for any dystocia. Uterine involution can be verified periodically.
• After cesarean section, the animal should be closely monitored for 7–10 days. Rectal temperature, normal appetite, mentation, urination, and defecation should be recorded. Often evaluation of the skin incision for any signs of infection should be performed.

PREVENTION
N/A

MISCELLANEOUS

ASSOCIATED CONDITIONS
• Dystocia
• Pregnancy toxemia

AGE-RELATED FACTORS
Multiparous ewes and does may be at higher risk for uterine torsion because of decreased broad ligaments tone.

ZOONOTIC POTENTIAL
N/A

PREGNANCY
Depending on the degree of the torsion the pregnancy can be lost spontaneously. Placenta edema, its detachment and subsequent fetal hypoxia of the fetus due to compromised venous return is usually the cause of fetal death.

PRODUCTION MANAGEMENT
• Insufficient cervical dilation and postural abnormalities of the fetus are the most common causes of dystocia in this species. However, recent studies have shown that occurrence of uterine torsion in up to 10% of small ruminant dystocias requiring surgery
• The cost of surgery may be too prohibitive in some production system and humane euthanasia should be considered
• Ewes and does that underwent surgical correction are often culled.

ABBREVIATIONS
• N/A

SEE ALSO
• Cesarean Section: Small Ruminant
• Down Small Ruminant
• Dystocia: Small Ruminant
• Pregnancy Toxemia: Small Ruminant

Suggested Reading
Devi Prasad V. A retrospective study of aetiologies of dystocia in small ruminants. Intas Polivet 2014,15 (II): 284–6.
Ijaz A, Talafha AQ. Torsion of the uterus in an Awassi ewe. Aust Vet J 2002, 77: 652–3.
Kumar A, Bisht S, Nayal SS. Management of uterine torsion in a ewe: A case report. Int J Vet Sci 2014, 3: 222–3.
Mosdol G. Spontaneous vaginal rupture in pregnant ewes. Vet Re 1999, 144: 38–41.
Naidu G. V. A case of uterine torsion in sheep. Indian J Anim Reprod 2012, 33: 102–3.
Scott P. Uterine torsion in the ewe. Livestock 2001, 16: 37–9.
Siddiquee GM, Chaudhary S. Dystocia due to uterine torsion in goats: An analysis of six cases. Intas Polivet 2000, 1: 276–8.
Shwetha KS, Jayakumar C, Chandrashekara Murthy V. Clinical management of uterine torsion in a goat by Schffer's method. Intas Polivet 2014, 15: 250–1.
Wehrand A, Bostedt H, Burkhardt E. The use of trans-abdominal B mode ultrasonography to diagnose intra-partum uterine torsion in the ewe. Vet J 2002, 176: 69–70.
Author Michela Ciccarelli
Consulting Editor Ahmed Tibary

U

VACCINATION PROGRAMS: BEEF CATTLE

BASICS

OVERVIEW
• A strategic vaccination program is part of a total herd health management plan.
• Vaccination is a tool that can help prevent the occurrence of disease or reduce the severity of disease but it is not a substitute for poor management in other areas.
• A successful vaccination program depends on adequate nutrition, proper management and housing, and planning.
• Nutrition must be adequate for the immune system to function properly.
• A vaccine prevents diseases by priming an animal's immune system to fight the disease.
• The animal must be supplied with adequate protein and energy, as well as vitamins A and E, copper, selenium, and zinc for optimum immune system function.
• No vaccine is 100% protective in 100% of the animals. Some animals will have a less than maximal response to a vaccine and some animals may not respond at all.
• Vaccination is simply the act of inoculating an animal with a vaccine. It does not imply immunity.
• Immunization is the development of an immune response in response to a vaccine. It does not imply protection from disease.

INCIDENCE/PREVALENCE
All cattle herds could benefit from a customized vaccination program.

GEOGRAPHIC DISTRIBUTION
• Appropriate vaccination programs must be customized to the specific herd and location for which they are being developed.
• Some vaccines may be appropriate in some areas but unnecessary in others depending on the occurrence of the disease in that area.

SYSTEMS AFFECTED
• Respiratory
• Digestive
• Reproductive
• Musculoskeletal

PATHOPHYSIOLOGY
Passive Immunity
• Antibodies are obtained from a source other than the animal's immune system.
• Passive transfer of colostral antibodies is the most important form of passive immunity.
• Antibodies from passive immunity may interfere with the development of active immunity in response to a vaccination in young animals by "neutralizing" the vaccine.
• Other types of passive immunity include blood or plasma transfusions and antiserum products such as tetanus antitoxin.

Active Immunity
• Humoral, cell mediated, and secretory types.

• With humoral immunity, antibodies are produced by specific lymphocytes in response to exposure to an antigen or in response to a vaccination.
• Cell mediated immunity (CMI) develops when specialized lymphocytes are exposed to a specific organism and develop a "memory" for that organism. When exposed again, these cells attack and kill that organism or cells infected with that organism.
   ○ CMI is not as easily produced as humoral immunity and is rarely produced in response to a killed vaccine.
   ○ In most cases, an infectious organism has to replicate within an animal in order to produce CMI.
• Secretory immunity consists of antibodies produced in response to exposure or vaccination that do not circulate in the bloodstream.
   ○ Antibodies are produced by cells lining the mucosal surfaces of various parts of the body.
   ○ Vaccines that can be administered in the same manner that natural exposure would occur tend to produce the best secretory immune response. An example would be an intranasal vaccine.

Innate Immunity
• Innate immunity consists of natural defense mechanisms such as enzymes, tears, saliva, and gastric acids.
• These mechanisms destroy or mechanically remove infectious organisms before they can cause an infection.
• A failure of any one of these types of immunity predisposes an animal to disease.
• Proper vaccination can improve both passive and active immunity.

HISTORICAL FINDINGS
N/A

SIGNALMENT
• All beef cattle, regardless of age and production status, should be incorporated into a vaccination program.
• Different ages and classes of animals will require different protocols but all animals should be included in the program.

PHYSICAL EXAMINATION FINDINGS
N/A

GENETICS
Genetics play an important role in natural disease resistance including innate immunity and factors such as mothering ability, which affect passive immunity.

CAUSES AND RISK FACTORS
The risk factors associated with vaccine failure are numerous:
• Improper handling of vaccines
• Improper timing of vaccination
• Interference from maternal antibodies
• Improper administration technique
• Improper timing of booster vaccinations

• Animals that are already sick or highly stressed
• Overwhelming disease challenge
• Nutritional deficiencies or other causes of poor health

DIAGNOSIS

DIFFERENTIAL DIAGNOSES
N/A

CBC/BIOCHEMISTRY/URINALYSIS
N/A

OTHER LABORATORY TESTS
N/A

IMAGING
N/A

OTHER DIAGNOSTIC PROCEDURES
Many infectious agents can cause disease and attempts should be made to establish a definitive diagnosis before implementing a vaccination protocol to combat a disease outbreak.

PATHOLOGIC FINDINGS
N/A

TREATMENT

THERAPEUTIC APPROACH
• Ensuring adequate colostral transfer of antibodies is more important and effective than any vaccination program in neonates.
• Animals must be provided a balanced diet that is adequate in vitamins and trace minerals to allow optimum immune system function.
• Vaccines must be used according to the label directions.
• Vaccines should not be mixed in the same syringe unless directed by the label.
• Vaccines should be kept cool and out of direct sunlight. Keep vaccines in an ice chest or some other form of protection while in use.
• Only reconstitute the amount of vaccine that can be used in a 1 hour period. Do not try to store reconstituted MLV products, even if it is just for a few hours.
• Whenever possible, use products that can be administered subcutaneously.
• All injections, both subcutaneous and intramuscular, should be given in the neck, according to BQA guidelines, to avoid damage to the more valuable parts of the carcass.
• Use clean injection equipment to administer vaccines.
   ○ Change needles every 5–10 head.
   ○ Never use chemical disinfectants to disinfect instruments that will be used for MLV products. Residual disinfectant can destroy the effectiveness of MLV products.

VACCINATION PROGRAMS: BEEF CATTLE   (CONTINUED)

MEDICATIONS

DRUGS OF CHOICE

Types of Vaccine

Killed Vaccines
• Require booster dose following initial dose (timing is product dependent). If booster is not properly administered, virtually no protective immunity occurs. Once an animal has received the initial two doses, a single yearly booster may be adequate.
• Provide a shorter duration of immunity.
• Usually do not stimulate CMI.

Modified-Live Vaccines
• Infectious agent is alive but altered so that it does not cause disease in healthy animals.
• Agent replicates within the animal and induces both humoral and cell-mediated immunity.
• Produce long-lasting immunity.
• Usually provide a greater immune response than killed products.
• Some types may cause abortion in pregnant cows or disease in highly stressed animals.
• Some newer MLV products are labeled for use in pregnant cows and calves nursing pregnant cows as long as the vaccines are used according to the label.

Component Vaccines
Vaccines that contain only part of an infectious agent. These products induce immunity to a part of an infectious agent that is necessary for the agent to cause disease.

Toxoids
Vaccines that induce an immune response to certain toxins produced by bacteria.

Recommended Vaccination Programs
A successful vaccination program must be customized to each specific situation.

Branding Vaccines (60–90 days of age)
• Passive immunity to clostridial diseases usually begins to decline around 2–3 months of age. Calves at this age should be given a clostridial bacterin/toxoid.
• Passive immunity to the common respiratory viruses (IBR, BVD, PI-3, and BRSV) usually lasts for 4–5 months so calves at this age should be fairly well protected.
• Respiratory viral vaccines can be administered at this time if the herd has a history of respiratory disease in calves of this age.
• Intranasal vaccines are a good choice in young calves because passive immunity has less effect on these vaccines.

Preweaning Vaccines (2–4 weeks prior to weaning)
• Ideally, calves should be vaccinated 2–4 weeks prior to weaning so that they have had time to develop an immune response and to help reduce the stress of weaning.
• Calves should receive a respiratory virus vaccine and a clostridial booster.
• MLV vaccines are preferable to killed products as long as they can be safely used according to label directions in nursing calves.
• Other vaccines to consider at this time include *Pasteurella* leukotoxoid vaccines and *Histophilus somni*.

Weaning Vaccines
• Calves should receive a respiratory virus booster at this time.
• MLV respiratory virus vaccines can be given at weaning without the risk of abortion in pregnant cows.
• The advantage of giving a second dose at weaning is providing another opportunity for calves that did not respond to previous vaccinations to become immunized.
• Consider calfhood (*Brucella*) vaccination of potential replacement females. Some states require that females be official calfhood vaccinates in order to enter the state.

Replacement Females
• At 1 year of age, replacement heifers should receive MLV respiratory virus vaccine with a five-way leptospirosis.
• *Campylobacter* (vibriosis) can be included if infertility due to vibriosis is a risk.
• Replacement heifers will require two doses of leptospirosis and vibrio vaccines since they will be naïve to these specific vaccines. The first doses can be given 60 days prior to breeding and boosters 30 days prior to breeding, along with the MLV vaccine.

Adult Cows
• Cows should be vaccinated pre-breeding with a respiratory virus vaccine and 5-way leptospirosis annually.
 ○ Adult cows should receive a five-way *Leptospira* bacterin once or twice yearly. Immunity produced by *Leptospira* vaccines is short-lived. This is commonly boostered during routine pregnancy examinations.
 ○ If killed products were used in the replacement heifers, yearly boosters should be given.
• Cows can also be vaccinated with K-99 *E. coli* and rotavirus/coronavirus products to increase the level of passive immunity provided to the calf.
 ○ Pregnant replacements should be given two doses, 3 and 6 weeks prior to calving.
 ○ Previously vaccinated cows only need one dose, 3–4 weeks prior to calving.
 ○ Rotavirus/coronavirus products are available to give to newborn calves prior to the calf's nursing colostrum.
• Campylobacter and trichomoniasis vaccines can be given yearly in at-risk herds.
• Other vaccines such as pinkeye and foot rot vaccines may be considered in problem herds.

Bulls
• Bulls should receive the same pre-breeding vaccinations used in the cow herd with some exceptions.
 ○ Bulls are not vaccinated for brucellosis.
 ○ The currently available trichomoniasis vaccine is not approved for use in bulls.
 ○ IBR virus from MLV products may recrudesce and be shed in semen; therefore, a killed respiratory vaccine is recommended in bulls.
 ○ Bulls should receive leptospirosis and campylobacteriosis vaccines in accordance with the cow herd.
• Other vaccines such as pinkeye and foot rot vaccines may be considered in problem herds.

CONTRAINDICATIONS
• Some MLV viral vaccines can cause abortion if administered to pregnant cows or calves nursing pregnant cows. **Always** follow the label directions.
• Administering vaccines to animals that are already sick or heavily stressed often fails to produce an immune response and may further stress the immune system.
• Administering certain vaccines may complicate international shipment of animals or semen due to positive serologic tests. Consider the ultimate goals of the producer before administering vaccines.

PRECAUTIONS
Appropriate milk and meat withdrawal times must be followed for all compounds administered to food-producing animals.

POSSIBLE INTERACTIONS
Avoid the administration of immunosuppressive drugs such as corticosteroids within 1 week of vaccination.

FOLLOW-UP

EXPECTED COURSE AND PROGNOSIS
• Effective immunity can be expected within 2 weeks after systemic vaccination.
• Mucosal immunity is developed within 48 hours after intranasal administration.

POSSIBLE COMPLICATIONS
Anaphylaxis is possible with some vaccine products. If anaphylaxis occurs, epinephrine is the treatment of choice.

CLIENT EDUCATION
It is important to train workers on proper vaccine handling, administration, and contraindications. See "Treatment."

PATIENT CARE
Patients should be monitored post-vaccination for anaphylactic reactions.

PREVENTION
N/A

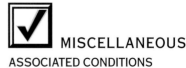

MISCELLANEOUS

ASSOCIATED CONDITIONS
N/A

AGE-RELATED FACTORS

Young calves may not respond to vaccines due to the influence of passive immunity from colostral antibodies. Antibodies to clostridial diseases usually last until the calf is 2–3 months of age and antibodies to the respiratory viruses usually last until 5–6 months of age.

ZOONOTIC POTENTIAL

Brucella vaccine (RB 51) is a live bacterial vaccine that contains zoonotic pathogens.

PREGNANCY

Care must be used when administering MLV products to pregnant cows. Always follow label directions.

BIOSECURITY

Well-designed vaccination programs are an integral part of all biosecurity programs.

PRODUCTION MANAGEMENT

Provision of a well-designed vaccination program is an integral part of any production management system.

ABBREVIATIONS

- BQA = Beef Quality Assurance
- BRSV = bovine respiratory syncytial virus
- BVD = bovine viral diarrhea
- CMI = cell mediated immunity
- GI = gastrointestinal
- IBR = infectious bovine rhinotracheitis
- MLV = modified-live vaccine
- PI-3 = parainfluenza 3

SEE ALSO

- Clostridial Disease (Gastrointestinal, Muscular, Nervous System)
- Neonatal Diarrhea
- Respiratory Disease: Bovine
- Vaccinology (see www.fiveminutevet.com/ruminant)

Suggested Reading

Bagley CV. Vaccination Program for Beef Calves. Utah State University Extension Publication (Electronic). Available at: http://digitalcommons.usu.edu/cgi/viewcontent.cgi?article=1453&context=extension_curall. Accessed April 30, 2017.

Floyd JG. Vaccinations for the Beef Cow Herd. Alabama Cooperative Extension Publication. (Electronic). Available at: http://www.aces.edu/pubs/docs/A/ANR-0968/ANR-0968.pdf. Accessed April 30, 2017.

Thomson DU, White BJ. Backgrounding beef cattle. Vet Clin North Am Food Anim Pract, 2006; 22:373–98.

Author Chelsey R. Ramirez

Consulting Editor Kaitlyn A. Lutz

Acknowledgment The authors and book editors acknowledge the prior contribution of Jim P. Reynolds.

V

VACCINATION PROGRAMS: CAMELID

BASICS

OVERVIEW
• Preventive medicine encompasses all management decisions that affect the health and well-being of camelids (South American camelids, SACs).
• Programs, though unique to camelids, should be based on herd health principles used for other livestock species.
• Vaccinations, parasite control, reproductive management, nutritional consultation, and feet and teeth care should be incorporated into camelid herd health programs.
• Each herd will have different requirements and the program should be developed according to the goals of the producer.
• The following information should be used strictly as a general guideline for vaccinating SACs. It is important to note that protocols for these husbandry practices should be designed according to the particular needs and geographic location of individual farms. The number of animals per group, age of the animals, pasture type, and frequency of animal movement on and off the premises should all be considered.
• There are no vaccines labeled for use in camelids.

INCIDENCE/PREVALENCE
N/A

GEOGRAPHIC DISTRIBUTION
Worldwide, depending on species and environment

PATHOPHYSIOLOGY
Varies according to disease targeted

SYSTEMS AFFECTED
• Digestive
• Respiratory
• Reproductive

GENETICS
N/A

HISTORICAL FINDINGS
Vary according to disease targeted

SIGNALMENT
Camelid species

PHYSICAL EXAMINATION FINDINGS
• Animal should be healthy in order to have a good immune response to vaccination.
• Pregnant females often receive booster vaccines to promote good quality colostrum (high antibodies concentration).

GENETICS
N/A

CAUSES AND RISK FACTORS
• Camelids can be affected by a variety of infectious diseases.
• The most important are clostridial infections, rabies, leptospirosis, West Nile virus, Eastern equine encephalitis, equine herpesvirus, and bovine herpesvirus.
• In some countries, where anthrax is endemic, vaccination is mandatory.
• Camelids can be infected with BVDV but they are not systematically vaccinated against the disease.
• Risk factors for these diseases include co-mingling with other animals (camelids or other species) in pasture, during shows, or in quarantine.
• High stocking density during the birthing period is an important risk factor.

DIAGNOSIS

DIFFERENTIAL DIAGNOSES
N/A

CBC/BIOCHEMISTRY/URINALYSIS
N/A

OTHER LABORATORY TESTS
N/A

IMAGING
N/A

OTHER DIAGNOSTIC PROCEDURES
N/A

PATHOLOGIC FINDINGS
N/A

TREATMENT

THERAPEUTIC APPROACH
• Vaccination programs should be developed with the knowledge that each herd will have different requirements and the program should be developed to the goals of the producer.
• A basic SAC vaccination program should include at least tetanus toxoid and *Clostridium perfringens* type C and D vaccinations on a yearly basis. Intramuscular vaccines may be given in the muscle of the neck in front of the shoulder or in the semimembranosus or tendinosus.
• Vaccine schedules generally include vaccination of dams about 1–2 months before they give birth. Late pregnant animals should be handled cautiously during vaccination due to the risk of stress-induced abortion.
• Tetanus and *C. perfringens* type C and D require two vaccinations given 1 month apart during the first year and one booster vaccination annually.
• Depending on geographic location and herd health history, the following vaccines may be administered in conjunction with those already mentioned:
  ○ *Rabies (IMRAB 3™):* Administer 2 mL IM to crias at 3–4 months of age. Booster annually.

  ○ *Leptospira:* Administer 2 mL dose of a killed bacterin. May need to be repeated 3 or 4 times per year if problematic in the region.
  ○ *West Nile virus:* Research has shown that administration of three doses (1 mL IM) of an equine WNV vaccine (Innovator) at intervals of 3 weeks resulted in an antibody response in nearly all animals tested. Annual boosters should be given 1 month before peak mosquito exposure.
  ○ *Eastern equine encephalitis (EEE):* Research has shown that administration of three doses (1 mL IM) of a killed equine encephalitis vaccine (Encevac) at 4 week intervals resulted in a humoral antibody response.
  ○ *Bovine herpesvirus type 1 (BHV-1), Equine herpesvirus type 1 (EHV-1):* Herpesviruses can infect non-adapted hosts and serious disease or death may result in llamas and alpacas. Blindness in camelids can be caused by EHV-1. The role of BHV-1 in camelids is not well established and the incidence rate is extremely low. Vaccination for BHV-1 is not recommended on a routine basis. EHV-1 vaccination should be considered when camelids are in close contact with equines. Killed virus vaccine has been shown to induce antibodies in llamas when used according to the recommendations for equines. The vaccine has not been tested experimentally to determine the efficacy in preventing disease. Modified-live virus vaccination with EHV-1 should not be attempted. EHV-1 vaccine use is extra-label and has not been tested adequately in camelids.

SURGICAL CONSIDERATIONS AND TECHNIQUES
N/A

MEDICATIONS

DRUGS OF CHOICE
• There are no vaccines labelled for use in camelids.
• Vaccines labelled for use in equine, cattle, or sheep are often used extra-label for SAC.

CONTRAINDICATIONS
Appropriate milk and meat withdrawal times must be followed for all compounds administered to food-producing animals; however, withdrawal times have not been established for camelids.

PRECAUTIONS
• Proper dosing and use of individual needles is important.
• Vaccination of sick animals may not be efficacious.
• Adverse reaction may be seen in some animals, particularly young animals and pregnant females.

(CONTINUED) **VACCINATION PROGRAMS: CAMELID**

• Eight-way vaccines have been associated with abortion, probably due to inflammatory response.

POSSIBLE INTERACTIONS
N/A

 FOLLOW-UP

EXPECTED COURSE AND PROGNOSIS
N/A

POSSIBLE COMPLICATIONS
• Injection site reaction
• Anaphylactic shock is rare but has been reported in some animals.

CLIENT EDUCATION
• Should be aware that most vaccines are used off-label.
• Importance of vaccine handling (refrigeration).
• Injection site and needle requirements.

PATIENT CARE
Response to immunization depends of the health of the animal. Vaccination program should be part of a general herd health program whichs include feeding management, biosecurity, and antiparasite program.

PREVENTION
N/A

 MISCELLANEOUS

ASSOCIATED CONDITIONS
Vaccination against bovine viral diarrhea virus (BVDV) is not recommended for camelids;

rather, increased surveillance and eradication should be the goal.

AGE-RELATED FACTORS
Crias from unvaccinated dams or crias that are orphaned prior to colostrum consumption require special care.

ZOONOTIC POTENTIAL
N/A

PREGNANCY
Some vaccines (8-way clostridial) have been suspected to cause pregnancy loss.

BIOSECURITY
• Isolate and quarantine new stock entering the herd.
• Treat new animals for disease conditions prior to herd introduction; cull if necessary.
• Newly acquired camelids may be started on a vaccine series at any time.
• Crias from unvaccinated dams or crias that are orphaned prior to colostrum consumption require special care.

PRODUCTION MANAGEMENT
N/A

SYNONYMS
N/A

ABBREVIATIONS
• BHV-1 = bovine herpesvirus type 1
• BVDV = bovine viral diarrhea virus
• EHV-1 = equine herpesvirus type 1
• IM = intramuscular

SEE ALSO
• Nutrition and Metabolic Diseases: Camelid (see www.fiveminutevet.com/ruminant)
• Parasite Control Programs: Camelid

Suggested Reading
Bedenice D, Bright A, Pedersen DD, Dibb J. Humoral response to an equine encephalitis vaccine in healthy alpacas. J Am Vet Med Assoc 2009, 234: 530–4.
Cebra CK, Anderson DE, Tibary A, Van Saun RJ, Johnson LW. Llama and Alpaca Care: Medicine, Surgery, Reproduction, Nutrition, and Herd Health. St. Louis: Elsevier, 2014.
Kapil S, Yeary T, Evermann JF. Viral diseases of new world camelids. Vet Clin North Am Food Anim Pract 2009, 25: 323–7.
Kutzler MA, Baker RJ, Mattson DE. Humoral response to West Nile virus vaccination in alpacas and llamas. J Am Vet Med Assoc 2004, 225: 414–16.

Internet Resources
Anderson DE. Camelid Vaccination Protocol. http://www.vet.ohio-state.edu/docs/ ClinSci/camelid/vaccines.html
Purdy SR. Alpaca and Llama Health Information.http://www.purdyvet.com

Author Kate O'Conor
Consulting Editor Ahmed Tibary
Acknowledgment The author and book editors acknowledge the prior contribution of Debbie Terrel.

V

VACCINATION PROGRAMS: CERVIDAE

BASICS

OVERVIEW
• The administration of vaccinations is common in domestic species for the prevention and amelioration of various bacterial and viral diseases.
• Currently, more and more cervids are being raised on a farmed, managed setting, with higher stocking rates and more potential for disease transmission. Due to this, vaccinations are crucial for prevention of different disease processes.
• Preventive health programs should be individualized for each operation, addressing management practices and local disease-related information.

INCIDENCE/PREVALENCE
• Incidence of diseases is variable.
• Prevalence varies according to region and management.

GEOGRAPHIC DISTRIBUTION
Worldwide

SYSTEMS AFFECTED
• Respiratory
• Digestive
• Reproductive

PATHOPHYSIOLOGY
• Cervids are susceptible to common pathogens found in other ruminant species.
• The most common diseases include clostridial diseases which produce a variety of syndromes similar in pathophysiology to other ruminants.
• Response to vaccines is not adequate before 60 days of age because of presence of colostral antibodies.

SIGNALMENT
• There are numerous cervid species currently and commonly being raised for breeding, meat, and hunting. The most common is the white-tailed deer (*Odocoileus virginianus*). Others include mule deer (*Odocoileus hemionus*), fallow deer (*Dama dama*), axis deer or chital (*Axis axis*), sika deer (*Cervus nippon*), elk (*Cervus canadensis*), and red deer (*Cervus elaphus*).

GENETICS
N/A

CAUSES AND RISK FACTORS
Risk factors for disease spread are overstocking, high population density, poor sanitation, poor genetics, and inappropriate vaccination protocols.

 V

DIAGNOSIS

DIFFERENTIAL DIAGNOSES
N/A

CBC/BIOCHEMISTRY/URINALYSIS
N/A

OTHER LABORATORY TESTS
N/A

IMAGING
N/A

OTHER DIAGNOSTIC PROCEDURES
N/A

PATHOLOGIC FINDINGS
N/A

TREATMENT

THERAPEUTIC APPROACH
N/A

SURGICAL CONSIDERATIONS AND TECHNIQUES
N/A

MEDICATIONS

• There is only one vaccine that is routinely recommended for farmed cervid herds: a multivalent clostridial vaccination. There are numerous versions available, most of which are inactivated and consist of bacterins, toxoids, or a mixture of the two. They are developed and manufactured for cattle, but are generally safe to use in cervids.
• Clostridial vaccines can contain as few as 1 and as many as 9 different clostridial strains, including *Clostridium chauvoei*, *C. septicum*, *C. novyi* type B, C, *C. haemolyticum*, *C. sordellii*, *C. tetani*, and *C. perfringens* type C and D.
• Single vaccinations of inactivated clostridial vaccines do not generally provide adequate levels of protection, and most often require a booster dose within 3–6 weeks initially. These vaccinations can be given annually after the initial booster.
• Young fawns generally do not yield adequate protective immunity until around 1–2 months of age, so vaccination strategies against clostridial diseases targeting pregnant dams can allow for maximal immunity transferred to the neonate via the colostrum.
• Gestation times vary between species, and can be 200–280 days; vaccinating pregnant females with killed vaccines within 7 weeks of parturition can help her produce antibodies that will be passed on to the fawn through the colostrum.
• In breeding operations, it may be prudent to vaccinate the pregnant does with a "calf scours" vaccination. These generally include protection against rotavirus, coronavirus, *Clostridium perfringens* type B, C, and D, as well as *Escherichia coli* (using the K99 antigen), all of which are diseases that can kill fawns within days of birth.

• Fawns should be vaccinated at weaning, and given a booster 3–6 weeks later.
• Oral vaccinations, particularly those targeting *E. coli* and *Clostridium* spp. have been used in newborn fawns to provide local immunity and possible passive transfer.

Additional Vaccination Comments
• Antibodies to some cattle respiratory pathogens (PI-3, BVDV, BHV-1) have been found in both white-tailed deer and elk, but no clinical disease has been reported. In heavily managed farm settings, some ranchers vaccinate their cervids using an inactivated cattle respiratory vaccine.
• Depending on the area and the disease prevalence of specific pathogens within the herd (such as leptospirosis, *E. coli*, campylobacteriosis, etc.), specific targeted vaccinations should be considered.
• Autogenous vaccines can be considered and produced if there are problems with atypical strains or pathogens, though none have been published.
• The use of a *Salmonella* vaccine strain that expressed cervid PrP, the main protein that misfolds and is implicated in chronic wasting disease (CWD) has been reported. This vaccine produced mucosal and systemic response to cervid PrP and PrP^{CWD} (the misfolded protein responsible for CWD) in white-tailed deer. The vaccinated deer showed partial protection against CWD. It is currently not commercially available.
• Immunocontraception with porcine zona pellucida (PZP) and gonadotropin-releasing hormone (GnRH) vaccines have been used successfully to control reproduction in deer.
• There are very few published accounts of humoral immune response, safety, and efficacy of vaccinations in cervids, so the decision to vaccinate must be approached cautiously.

DRUGS OF CHOICE
There are no cervid approved vaccines. Vaccines approved for cattle are used extra-label in cervids.

CONTRAINDICATIONS
N/A

PRECAUTIONS
Vaccines should be handled properly to insure a good immunization response.

POSSIBLE INTERACTIONS
N/A

FOLLOW-UP

EXPECTED COURSE AND PROGNOSIS
Animals vaccinated against disease still have the chance of contracting the disease, depending on the strain, host, and situation, but vaccines help reduce the likelihood of this as well as sometimes help ameliorate the disease if it is contracted.

POSSIBLE COMPLICATIONS
Injection site reaction

PATIENT CARE
• Always monitor individuals who have been vaccinated for signs of an immediate or delayed vaccine reaction. This can include sweating, hypersalivation, agitation/restlessness, and anaphylaxis.
• Deer species can also develop abscesses at vaccine injection locations, specifically when the vaccine is administered against the manufacturer's recommendations. Most clostridial vaccinations are recommended to be given subcutaneously.
• In situations where there is not a handling facility available, or anesthesia/capture is not an option, vaccines can be given by darting the individuals, which only allows intramuscular administration and can often cause tissue reactions, swelling, and abscess formation.

PREVENTION
N/A

MISCELLANEOUS

ASSOCIATED CONDITIONS
N/A

AGE-RELATED FACTORS
Vaccination of fawns that are too young is generally useless due to maternal antibody interference.

ZOONOTIC POTENTIAL
N/A

PREGNANCY
Pregnant females should receive a booster with killed vaccine in the last 7 weeks of gestation to improve colostrum quality.

BIOSECURITY
Strict biosecurity measure (testing and quarantine) should be used in conjunction with vaccination.

PRODUCTION MANAGEMENT
N/A

SYNONYMS
N/A

ABBREVIATIONS
• BHV-1 = bovine herpes virus type 1
• BVDV = bovine viral diarrhea virus
• CWD = chronic wasting disease
• GnRH = gonadotropin releasing hormone
• PI-3 = parainfluenza-3
• PrP = prion protein
• PZP = porcine zona pellucida

SEE ALSO
• Abortion: Farmed Cervidae
• Biosecurity: Cervidae (see www.fiveminutevet.com/ruminant)
• Cervidae: Captive Management
• Cervidae Mortality

Suggested Reading
Chirino-Trejo M, Woodbury MR, Huang F. Antibiotic sensitivity and biochemical characterization of *Fusobacterium* spp. and *Arcanobacterium pyogenes* isolated from farmed white-tailed deer (*Odocoileus virginianus*) with necrobacillosis. J Zoo Wildl Med 2003, 34: 262–8.

Gionfriddo JP, Denicola AJ, Miller LA, Fagerstone KA. Efficacy of GnRH Immunocontraception of wild white–tailed deer in New Jersey. Wildl Soc Bull 2011, 35: 142–8.
Goni F, Mathiason CK, Yim L, et al. Mucosal immunization with an attenuated Salmonella vaccine partially protects white-tailed deer from chronic wasting disease. Vaccine 2015, 33: 726–33.
Haigh JC, Mackintosh C, Griffin F. Viral, parasitic and prion diseases of farmed deer and bison. Rev Sci Tech 2002, 21: 219–48.
Mackintosh C, Haigh JC, Griffin F. Bacterial diseases of farmed deer and bison. Rev Sci Tech Off Int Epiz 2002, 21: 249–63.
Smits JEG. Elk disease survey in Western Canada and Northwestern United States. In: Brown RD ed, The Biology of Deer. New York: Springer, 1992, pp. 101–6.
Troxel TR, Burke GL, Wallace WT, et al. Clostridial vaccination efficacy on stimulating and maintaining an immune response in beef cows and calves. J Anim Sci 1997, 75: 19–25.
Wilson PR, Schollum LM. Serological responses of farmed red deer to a vaccine against *Leptospira interrogans* serovars Hardjo and Pomona. N Z Vet J 1984, 32: 117–19.

Author David M. Love
Consulting Editor Ahmed Tibary
Acknowledgment The author and book editors acknowledge the prior contribution of Melissa Weisman.

V

VACCINATION PROGRAMS: DAIRY CATTLE

BASICS

OVERVIEW
• Vaccination is a major part of prevention of infectious diseases on dairy farms.
• There are a few vaccines that are considered basic to the vaccine program on dairies in North America and there are many other vaccines that should be considered for a vaccine program based on the particular disease risks and management of individual farms.
• Vaccines should be chosen carefully because the process can bring both prevention of disease and risk for disease.
• The following principles must be adhered to for a vaccine to work well: The vaccine must be stored and handled properly, the vaccine must be administered to the appropriate animals at the right times using the correct route and dosage, and the animals must be in good health and in positive growth or energy balance.

INCIDENCE/PREVALENCE
N/A

GEOGRAPHIC DISTRIBUTION
Worldwide

SYSTEMS AFFECTED
• Respiratory
• Digestive
• Reproductive
• Musculoskeletal

PATHOPHYSIOLOGY
N/A

SIGNALMENT
Dairy cattle. In particular, the Holstein breed appears to be highly susceptible to the effects of bacterial endotoxin.

HISTORICAL FINDINGS
There should be clinical, laboratory, or other evidence of pathogens in the herd or region for which efficacious vaccines are available to recommend particular vaccines.

PHYSICAL EXAMINATION FINDINGS
N/A

GENETICS
The Holstein breed appears to be highly susceptible to the effects of bacterial endotoxin.

CAUSES AND RISK FACTORS
Typical risks that can be partially managed with vaccines on dairy farms include moving from individual calf hutches to group pens, overcrowding, immunosuppressive periods such as transportation and parturition, and environmental contamination during milking.

DIAGNOSIS

DIFFERENTIAL DIAGNOSES
It is imperative to have knowledge of the infectious diseases the cattle on a farm will be exposed to at different times in the management cycle before recommending vaccine programs.

OTHER DIAGNOSTIC PROCEDURES
Submission of necropsy samples to determine pathogens on the farm is advised.

TREATMENT

THERAPEUTIC APPROACH
Epidemiology
• Vaccines must be given prior to exposure to the pathogen and the animal must have enough time to process the antigens and develop either humoral or cellular immunity.
• Passively acquired immunity from colostrum may interfere with systemic vaccinations for varying periods after colostrum feeding (2–6 months).
• Calves should always receive at least one systemic vaccination for the essential viral vaccines (IBR, BVD, BRSV) after 6 months of age. Intranasal vaccines are not affected by maternal antibody and should be efficacious as soon as the corticosteroids associated with calving have metabolized.
• The concept of herd immunity is important in dairy preventive medicine. Disease prevention and decreased case rate can be expected for most pathogens as long as the majority of animals in the population are effectively immunized.

Dairy Vaccinology
• A basic vaccine program on a dairy should include vaccinations for infectious bovine rhinotracheitis (IBR), bovine virus diarrhea types I and II (BVD), bovine respiratory syncytial virus (BRSV), and *Leptospira hardjo* and *pomona* bacterins.
• Optional vaccines include clostridial (malignant edema, redwater, and blackleg) bacterins, campylobacterosis (vibrio) bacterins, *Moraxella bovis* (pinkeye) bacterins core-antigen J-5 Gram-negative bacterins (coliform mastitis). Rotavirus and coronavirus vaccines may be useful for protecting neonatal calves depending on the dairy.
• Regulations regarding vaccination for *Brucella abortus* vary by country and region.
• The viral pathogens can be administered either as modified-live virus (MLV) or killed vaccines.

• MLV vaccines are generally preferred because of the problem of compliance with boostering killed virus vaccines.
• Killed virus vaccines and bacterins must have a second dose within 2–4 weeks of the primary vaccination to develop an anamnestic response.

Dairy Vaccination Program
• A basic vaccination program for a dairy may include the following vaccines:
  ○ *Birth:* Colostrum (bull and heifer calves). Maternal antibodies are necessary for mucosal and systemic immunity and the white blood cells in colostrum initiate the memory of the calf's immune system.
  ○ *3 days of age:* Temperature-sensitive intranasal IBR.
  ○ *Before weaning or moving to group pens:* Temperature-sensitive intranasal IBR or MLV IBR-BVD-BRSV with Leptospira.
  ○ *6 months of age:* MLV IBR-BVD-BRSV with Leptospira.
  ○ *Before breeding:* MLV IBR-BVD-BRSV with Leptospira.
  ○ *At least 20 days postpartum:* MLV IBR-BVD-BRSV with Leptospira.
  ○ *Or, during the dry period:* MLV IBR-BVD-BRSV with Leptospira.
• Vaccines that may be incorporated based on dairy-specific disease/management include:
  ○ *J-5 Gram-negative vaccines* to reduce the severity of coliform mastitis: 1 or 2 vaccinations prepartum and 1 vaccination 10–20 days in milk. This practice is common on many dairies in the United States and its use has accompanied a significant decline in severity of disease and subsequent mortality from coliform mastitis.
  ○ *Leptospira borgpetersenii* serovar hardjo-bovis (type: *hardjo-bovis*) specific vaccine to prevent early abortions.
  ○ *Rotavirus and coronavirus* vaccine to either dry cows or pre-colostrum calves to prevent diarrhea in calves.
  ○ Clostridial vaccines to control malignant edema (*C. septicum* or *sordelli*), blackleg (*C. chauvoei*) or redwater (*C. hemolyticum*).

MEDICATIONS

DRUGS OF CHOICE
Epinephrine should be on hand in case of anaphylactic reaction after vaccination.

CONTRAINDICATIONS
• Do not administer corticosteroids within 1 week of vaccination.

V

(CONTINUED) **VACCINATION PROGRAMS: DAIRY CATTLE**

• It is commonly recommended to not administer more than two Gram-negative bacterins at the same time because of the risk of endotoxemia.
• Vaccination of animals in negative energy balance may result in decreased efficacy.

PRECAUTIONS
• Only use MLV vaccines in pregnant animals if they are approved and used in accordance with label.
• Do not vaccinate cattle within 1 week after parturition to avoid the immunosuppressive complications of the corticosteroids associated with calving.
• Avoid vaccinating heat-stressed cattle due to the increased risk of endotoxic reaction.

POSSIBLE INTERACTIONS
See "Contraindications" and "Precautions"

 FOLLOW-UP

EXPECTED COURSE AND PROGNOSIS
• Effective immunity can be expected within 2 weeks after systemic vaccinations.
• Mucosal immunity is developed within 48 hours after intranasal vaccination with temperature sensitive IBR vaccines.

POSSIBLE COMPLICATIONS
Abortion, anaphylaxis, or inadequate immunity can result from vaccinating inappropriately.

CLIENT EDUCATION
• Clients must understand the importance of vaccine handling and timing of the vaccinations. All vaccines must be kept cold and out of the sunlight. Modified-live virus vaccines are inactivated quickly by ultraviolet light and should be used within 1 hour of mixing with the diluent.
• Vaccines should not be frozen; MLV vaccines are inactivated and attenuated by freeze-thaw cycles and cells can be ruptured and endotoxin released in bacterins.

• Bacterins must be boostered at the recommended intervals and clients must understand the importance of the booster dose.

PATIENT CARE
• Cattle should be observed for at least 2 hours post-vaccination for signs of anaphylaxis.

PREVENTION
N/A

 MISCELLANEOUS

AGE-RELATED FACTORS
• Calves <1 week of age may not respond well to systemic vaccinations but will respond well to temperature sensitive intranasal vaccines.
• Cellular immunity in the neonatal bovine appears to be decreased between 2 and 5 weeks of age and vaccination with systemic vaccines should be avoided during this period.
• Vaccine programs are generally targeted to bovines based on age. The goal of vaccinating calves is to decrease the case rate and severity of diarrhea and pneumonia while older cattle are vaccinated to protect from abortifacients, mastitis, and pneumonia.

ZOONOTIC POTENTIAL
RB 51 and Strain 19 *Brucella* vaccines are live bacterial vaccines and are zoonotic pathogens.

PREGNANCY
• Bacterins and killed-virus vaccines are generally safe for pregnant cattle, although the endotoxins in bacterins can cause sufficient prostaglandin release during an endotoxic reaction to cause luteolysis and abortion.
• Only MLV vaccines approved for use in pregnant cattle should be used during gestation.
• The first infection with IBR (wild type or vaccine strain) virus can result in infection of the ovary and subsequent luteolysis and abortion. Therefore, cattle should be previously effectively vaccinated with

MLV-IBR prior to MLV-IBR vaccination during pregnancy.

ABBREVIATIONS
• BRSV = bovine respiratory synctial virus
• BVD = bovine viral diarrhea virus
• GI = gastrointestinal
• IBR = infectious bovine rhinotracheitis
• MLV = modified-live virus

SEE ALSO
• Dairy Heifer Management Program (see www.fiveminutevet.com/ruminant)
• Vaccination Programs (by species)
• Vaccinology (see www.fiveminutevet. com/ruminant)

Suggested Reading
Cortese VS. Bovine vaccines and herd vaccination programs. In: Smith BBP ed, Large Animal Internal Medicine, 5th ed. St. Louis: Mosby, 2015, pp. 1465–71.
Ellis JA. The immunology of the bovine respiratory disease complex. Vet Clin North Am Food Anim Pract 2001, 17: 535–50, vi–vii.
Hjerpe CA. Bovine vaccines and herd vaccination programs. Vet Clin North Am Food Anim Pract 1990, 6: 167–260.
Sandvik T. Progress of control and prevention programs for bovine viral diarrhea virus in Europe. Vet Clin North Am Food Anim Pract 2004, 20: 151–69.
van Oirschot JT. Present and future of veterinary viral vaccinology: a review. Vet Q 2001, 23: 100–8.
Zeitlin L, Cone RA, Moench TR, Whaley KJ. Preventing infectious disease with passive immunization. Microbes Infect 2000, 2: 701–8.

Author Jim P. Reynolds
Consulting Editor Kaitlyn A. Lutz

V

VACCINATION PROGRAMS: SMALL RUMINANT

BASICS

OVERVIEW
• A strategic vaccination program is a critical part of herd health management.
• Vaccination can prevent disease or reduce disease severity, but it is not a substitute for poor management in other areas.
• A successful vaccination program depends on adequate nutrition, proper management, and planning.
• Nutrition must be adequate for the immune system to function properly.
  ○ A vaccine prevents disease by priming an animal's immune system to fight the disease.
  ○ The animal must be supplied with adequate protein and energy, as well as vitamins A and E, copper, selenium, and zinc for optimum immune system function.
• No vaccine is 100% protective in 100% of animals. Some animals will have a less than maximal response and some animals may not respond at all.
• Vaccination is the act of inoculating an animal with a vaccine. It does not imply immunity.
• Immunization is the development of an immune response to a vaccine. It does not imply protection from disease.

INCIDENCE/PREVALENCE
N/A

GEOGRAPHIC DISTRIBUTION
• Appropriate vaccination programs must be customized to the specific group and location for which they are being developed.
• Some vaccines may be appropriate in some areas but unnecessary in others depending on the occurrence of the disease in that area.

SYSTEMS AFFECTED
Hemolymphatic

PATHOPHYSIOLOGY
Proper vaccination can improve both passive and active immunity.

Passive Immunity
• Antibodies are obtained from a source other than the animal's immune system.
• Passive transfer of colostral antibodies is the most important form of passive immunity.
• Antibodies from passive immunity may interfere with the development of active immunity in response to vaccination in young animals by "neutralizing" the vaccine.
• Other types of passive immunity include blood or plasma transfusion and antiserum products (e.g., tetanus antitoxin).

Active Immunity
• Humoral and secretory immunity reflect production of antibodies by specific lymphocytes in response to antigen exposure or vaccination.

• Cell mediated immunity (CMI) develops when specialized lymphocytes are exposed to a specific organism and develop a "memory" for that organism. When exposed again, these cells attack and kill that organism or cells infected with that organism.
  ○ CMI is not as easily elicited as humoral immunity and is rarely provoked in response to a killed vaccine.
  ○ In most cases, an infectious organism has to replicate within an animal to produce CMI.

Innate Immunity
• Innate immunity consists of natural defense mechanisms such as enzymes, tears, saliva, and gastric acids.
• These mechanisms destroy or mechanically remove infectious organisms.

HISTORICAL FINDINGS
N/A

SIGNALMENT
Small ruminants of any age or production status can be incorporated into a vaccination program, though protocols may differ for individuals based on age and production role.

PHYSICAL EXAMINATION FINDINGS
Animals with severely abnormal physical examination findings, such as high fever or significant systemic illness, should not be vaccinated until recovered.

GENETICS
Genetics affect natural disease resistance including innate immunity and potentially factors such as mothering ability, which affect passive immunity.

CAUSES AND RISK FACTORS
Vaccine failure can arise from:
• Improper handling of vaccines
• Improper timing of vaccination
• Interference by maternal antibodies
• Improper administration technique
• Improper timing of booster vaccinations
• Vaccinating animals that are already sick or stressed
• Overwhelming disease challenge
• Nutritional deficiencies or other causes of poor health

DIAGNOSIS

DIFFERENTIAL DIAGNOSES
N/A

CBC/BIOCHEMISTRY/URINALYSIS
N/A

OTHER LABORATORY TESTS
N/A

IMAGING
N/A

OTHER DIAGNOSTIC PROCEDURES
N/A

PATHOLOGIC FINDINGS
N/A

TREATMENT

THERAPEUTIC APPROACH
• Ensuring adequate colostral transfer of antibodies is more important and effective than any vaccination program, though appropriate vaccination of the dam boosts this benefit immensely.
• Provide a balanced diet adequate in vitamins and trace minerals to allow optimum immune system function.
• Use vaccines according to label directions.
• Vaccines should not be mixed in the same syringe unless directed by the label.
• Vaccines should be kept cool and out of direct sunlight. Keep vaccines in an ice chest or some other form of protection while in use.
• Only reconstitute the amount of vaccine that can be used in 1 hour. Do not store reconstituted MLV products, even for a few hours.
• Use clean injection equipment to administer vaccines.
• Change needles every 5–10 animals.
• Never disinfect instruments that will be used for MLV products with chemical disinfectants. Residual disinfectant can destroy the effectiveness of MLV products.

SURGICAL CONSIDERATIONS AND TECHNIQUES
N/A

MEDICATIONS

DRUGS OF CHOICE

Killed Vaccines
• Require a booster dose 2–3 weeks after initial dose, otherwise virtually no protective immunity occurs. Once an animal has received two doses, a single yearly booster may be adequate.
• Provide shorter duration of immunity.
• Usually do not stimulate CMI.
• Most approved small ruminant vaccines fall into this category.

Modified-Live Vaccines
• Infectious agent is alive but altered so that it does not cause disease in healthy animals.
• Agent replicates within the animal and induces both humoral and cell-mediated immunity.
• Usually provide a greater immune response than killed products.
• Some types may cause abortion in pregnant animals or disease in stressed animals.

V

Component Vaccines

Vaccines that contain only part of an infectious agent and induce immunity to a component of the infectious agent that is necessary for the agent to cause disease.

Toxoids

Vaccines that induce an immune response to specific toxins produced by bacteria.

CONTRAINDICATIONS

• Only use contagious ecthyma (orf) and caseous lymphadenitis vaccines in herds with a known history of the disease, since these vaccines can produce disease in naïve groups.
• Some MLV vaccines can cause abortion if administered to pregnant animals. Always follow label directions.
• Administering certain vaccines may complicate international shipment of animals or semen due to positive serologic tests. Consider the ultimate goals of the producer before administering vaccines.

PRECAUTIONS

• Administering vaccines to animals that are already sick or heavily stressed often fails to produce an immune response and may induce additional stress.
• Appropriate milk and meat withdrawal times must be followed for all compounds administered to food-producing animals.

POSSIBLE INTERACTIONS

Avoid administration of immunosuppressive drugs such as corticosteroids within 1 week of vaccination.

 FOLLOW-UP

EXPECTED COURSE AND PROGNOSIS

Effective immunity can be expected within 2 weeks of vaccination, and often more rapidly with modified live vaccines.

POSSIBLE COMPLICATIONS

Anaphylaxis can occur with some vaccines.

CLIENT EDUCATION

Focus on educating producers on diseases relevant to their production system, and available vaccines.

PATIENT CARE

Monitor for local or systemic vaccine reactions.

PREVENTION

N/A

☑ MISCELLANEOUS

ASSOCIATED CONDITIONS

Vaccine site reactions or abscesses.

AGE-RELATED FACTORS

Neonates may not respond to vaccines due to the influence of passive immunity from colostral antibodies. Antibodies to clostridial diseases usually persist for the first 2–3 months of age.

ZOONOTIC POTENTIAL

Contagious ecthyma vaccine is a live virus that can cause clinical lesions in humans if handled improperly.

PREGNANCY

MLV products are often unsuitable during pregnancy.

BIOSECURITY

Well-designed vaccination programs are an integral part of herd biosecurity.

PRODUCTION MANAGEMENT

• Clostridial diseases are the only common group of diseases that all sheep and goats should be vaccinated against. Other vaccines that can be used in small ruminants include *Campylobacter, Chlamydia psittaci*, caseous lymphadenitis (CLA), foot rot, rabies, *Leptospira*, and contagious ecthyma. Use of these vaccines should be based on geographic prevalence of disease and the history of disease within each group.
• Previously vaccinated ewes or does should receive an annual booster of clostridial vaccine 4 weeks prior to parturition.
• Previously unvaccinated ewes or does should receive two doses of clostridial vaccine 8 and 4 weeks prior to parturition.
• Rams/bucks should be vaccinated with clostridial vaccine at the same time as pregnant animals.
• Passive immunity to clostridial diseases usually begins to decline around 4–6 weeks of age. Lambs or kids born to previously vaccinated dams can be given a clostridial bacterin/toxoid at this age, with a booster in 3–4 weeks.
• Neonates from dams not vaccinated during late gestation should receive a clostridial vaccination at 1–2 weeks of age, with two boosters given at 3- to 4-week intervals.

• If lambs will be transitioned onto a high energy ration, they should receive an additional vaccination that includes *C. perfringens* type D, 2 weeks prior to a diet change to protect against "enterotoxemia."
• Clostridial vaccines are often manufactured as combination vaccines, ranging from 3-way (C/D/T) to 8-way, and may contain CLA.
• If contagious ecthyma is an issue, lambs should be vaccinated on the inner thigh within the first week of life, and ewes can be vaccinated 2 or more months prior to lambing so that lambs do not come in contact with the scabs.
• *Campylobacter* and *Chlamydia* vaccines can be given 2–3 weeks prior to breeding in at-risk flocks. If a ewe has an unknown history, or has not previously been vaccinated, vaccinate 2–3 weeks prior to breeding and booster mid-pregnancy.
• Other vaccines such as CLA, orf, *Coxiella*, and foot rot vaccines may be considered in problem herds.
• If foot rot is an issue in the herd, vaccinate well in advance of the time of the year when the problem is noted (usually during spring/wet season); it may take several years of vaccinating before beneficial effects are noted.

SYNONYMS

N/A

ABBREVIATIONS

• CLA = caseous lymphadenitis
• CMI = cell mediated immunity
• MLV = modified-live vaccine

SEE ALSO

• Abortion: Small Ruminant
• Campylobacter
• Caseous Lymphadenitis (CLA)
• Clostridial Disease: Gastrointestinal
• Clostridial Disease: Muscular
• Clostridial Disease: Nervous System
• Leptospirosis
• Orf (Contagious Ecthyma)

Suggested Reading

Pugh DG. Sheep and Goat Medicine. Philadelphia: Saunders, 2002, p. 431.

Author Chelsey R. Ramirez
Consulting Editor Erica C. McKenzie

V

VAGAL INDIGESTION

BASICS

OVERVIEW
• Vagal indigestion is a complex syndrome characterized by functional disturbances of the ruminant forestomachs.
• Various causes result in rumen distension with gas and/or fluid.
• Contrary to the name, the most common causes of vagal indigestion are not related to dysfunction of the vagal nerve.
• This syndrome is characterized by and differentiated from other forms of indigestion by its slowly progressive course.

INCIDENCE/PREVALENCE
• No reports list the incidence or prevalence of vagal indigestion.
• It is the most common complication following abomasal volvulus correction.

GEOGRAPHIC DISTRIBUTION
Winter in cold climates may predispose to primary abomasal impaction if water sources freeze, prohibiting drinking.

SYSTEMS AFFECTED
Digestive

PATHOPHYSIOLOGY
The syndrome is composed of four categories of dysfunction.
• Type I: Failure of eructation
  ○ Partial esophageal obstruction by foreign body—feed material, apples, etc.
  ○ Extra-esophageal compression—lymphosarcoma, thyroid tumors, mediastinitis, abscess
  ○ Inflammatory process adjacent to vagal nerve causing neuropraxia—cranial abdominal abscess, peritonitis, chronic pneumonia
• Type II: Omasal transport failure
  ○ Intraluminal reduction in omasal canal—placenta, bags, twine, trichobezoar
  ○ Extramural masses which compress the omasal canal—perireticular adhesions or localized peritonitis related to traumatic reticuloperitonitis (TRP) or perforating abomasal ulcers
  ○ Neoplasia—lymphosarcoma, papilloma, squamous cell carcinoma
  ○ Functional failure of omasal transport (neuropraxia)—abscesses in left lobe of the liver
• Type III: Pyloric outflow failure
  ○ Lymphosarcoma of abomasal wall near pylorus
  ○ Primary abomasal impaction in animals fed dry, coarse roughage or with limited access to water
  ○ Secondary abomasal impaction:
    ■ Functional inability to empty abomasum
    ■ Adhesions from TRP
    ■ Adhesions of right lateral wall of reticulum

■ Poor motility after abomasal volvulus
    ■ Foreign bodies obstructing pylorus (trichobezoars, placenta)
    ■ Misplaced toggle pin fixation for displaced abomasum
• Type IV: Indigestion of late pregnancy
  ○ As fetus enlarges, the abomasum is forced cranially.
  ○ This may interfere with abomasal motility, leading to impaction.
  ○ These animals may have a combination of type II and type III vagal indigestion.

HISTORICAL FINDINGS
• Gradual abdominal enlargement
• Intermittent episodes of indigestion and anorexia
• Reduced milk production
• Weight loss
• Decreased fecal output
• Possible history of abnormal regurgitation
• Animals may be in late pregnancy

SIGNALMENT
• Only reported in bovines; however, abomasal emptying defect of Suffolk sheep is a similar condition to type III vagal indigestion.
• Type IV is more common in late pregnant dairy breeds.
• Lymphoma is most prevalent in cattle 4–8 years of age.

PHYSICAL EXAMINATION FINDINGS
• The hallmark sign of vagal indigestion is gradual abdominal enlargement, with a "papple" or "L-shaped" abdomen (large and round dorsally and ventrally on the left, distended ventrally on the right) due to fluid and/or gas accumulation in the rumen.
• Vagal indigestion is unlikely in acutely sick animals; other diagnoses should be considered first.
• Decreased fecal volume
  ○ Feces may be pasty and have increased fiber length (2–4 cm); the omasum is responsible for reducing feed particle size before delivery to abomasum.
• Melena if abomasal ulceration is involved.
• Abnormal rumen motility
  ○ Often increased with 4–5 contractions per 2 minutes unless there is severe distension, then motility slows.
  ○ Contractions may be nearly silent, but are strong and displace the left paralumbar fossa.
  ○ Absence of rumen motility suggests a very poor prognosis due to likelihood of significant peritonitis and adhesion formation.
• Abdominal percussion may elicit a "ping" from gas-distended rumen and be mistaken for a left displaced abomasum (LDA), but can be differentiated based on size and shape from an LDA.
• Abdominal succussion identifies a "splashy" rumen if there is fluid accumulation.
• Per rectum examination
  ○ L-shaped rumen

○ May palpate a large, distended abomasum, caudally displaced by cranial abdominal pathology.
  ○ May be able to palpate omasum if significant liver pathology, such as abscessation, is present.
• Grunt test and withers pinch to detect cranial abdominal pain can be performed (insensitive).
• Bradycardia is variable and an unusual finding.

GENETICS
No recognized genetic causes or implications for vagal indigestion

CAUSES AND RISK FACTORS
• Type I: Failure of eructation
  ○ Unresolved pneumonia or mediastinal pathology
  ○ Exposure to foreign bodies, particularly spherical objects
• Type II: Omasal transport failure
  ○ Unresolved TRP
  ○ Linear foreign body exposure
• Type III: Pyloric outflow failure
  ○ Grazing on crop residues
  ○ Loss of water access
  ○ Linear foreign body exposure
  ○ Bovine leukemia virus infection
  ○ Toggle repair of LDA
• Type IV: Indigestion of late pregnancy
  ○ Large fetal size

DIAGNOSIS

DIFFERENTIAL DIAGNOSES
• Simple indigestion
• Rumen acidosis
• TRP
• Displaced abomasum
• Frothy bloat
• Hydrops
• Ascites
• Diffuse peritonitis
• Abdominal neoplasia (lymphosarcoma)
• Intestinal obstruction (intussusception, mesenteric volvulus)
• Reticulitis (abnormal regurgitation)
• Ingestion of toxic plants or spoiled feed (abnormal regurgitation; rhododendron and mountain laurel)

CBC/BIOCHEMISTRY/URINALYSIS
• CBC can help differentiate possible etiologies:
  ○ Leukocytosis indicates mild to moderate inflammation, and may occur relatively early in the process.
  ○ Leukopenia occurs with severe inflammation (e.g., diffuse peritonitis).
  ○ Neutrophil : lymphocyte ratio reversal (2:1) suggests inflammation.
  ○ Lymphocytosis suggests lymphosarcoma (if persistent).

○ PCV and total protein may increase due to dehydration, or PCV may be low due to chronic inflammation.
• Biochemistry findings reflect dehydration and electrolyte and acid base anomalies.
  ○ Hypokalemia and hypocalcemia reflect anorexia.
  ○ Hypochloremia indicates abomasal reflux into the rumen from impaction or forestomach stasis decreasing absorption into blood.
    ▪ Occurs in types III and IV
    ▪ Severe hypochloremia (<50 mEq/L) is associated with a grave prognosis.
  ○ Metabolic alkalosis occurs in types II, III, and IV due to HCl sequestration in forestomachs.
  ○ Metabolic acidosis can occur in type I with esophageal obstruction due to loss of salivary bicarbonate.
  ○ Pre-renal azotemia.
  ○ Hypergammaglobulinemia (high total protein) indicates inflammatory process.

OTHER LABORATORY TESTS
• Rumen fluid analysis
  ○ Elevated rumen chloride (>30 mEq/L) indicates HCl reflux into rumen.
  ○ Occurs with abomasal impaction or any abomasal outflow obstruction.

• BLV serology: Positive result indicates viral infection but does not confirm the presence of a tumor, which will arise in only a low percentage of infected cattle.
• Abdominocentesis can identify peritonitis, but may be inconclusive if peritonitis is localized and encapsulated. Increased total protein (>2.5 g/dL) and nucleated cell count (>5,000/μL) suggest peritonitis. Abnormal morphology may suggest lymphoma.
• Fecal occult blood assessment can support presence of GI hemorrhage, including abomasal ulceration, and should be performed prior to per rectum examination.

IMAGING
• Radiography: Visualize cranial abdominal metallic foreign bodies.
• Ultrasonography can assess reticular motility and help identify masses, abscesses, peritonitis or thickening of visceral walls (lymphosarcoma).

OTHER DIAGNOSTIC PROCEDURES
• Exploratory laparotomy can establish diagnosis and possibly treatment.
  ○ Allows localization of masses or abscesses
  ○ Allows needle aspiration or biopsy of masses for evaluation
  ○ Allows removal of masses, drainage of abscesses into the GI tract, or instillation of

fluid into an impacted abomasum and subsequent massage.
• Figure 1 provides a basic plan for differentiating types of vagal indigestion.

PATHOLOGIC FINDINGS
• Type I
  ○ Foreign body, mass obstructing esophagus
  ○ Chronic thoracic pathology (e.g., pneumonia or abscess)
• Type II
  ○ Intraluminal foreign bodies or masses
  ○ Masses impinging upon omasal canal
  ○ Localized peritonitis, adhesions, TRP
  ○ Liver abscesses
• Type III
  ○ Dry, impacted abomasum
  ○ Adhesions, TRP
  ○ Pyloric foreign bodies
  ○ Pyloric stenosis
• Type IV
  ○ Large fetus cranially displacing abomasum
• Histopathology can confirm and define the nature of relevant masses (abscesses, lymphosarcoma, papilloma, squamous cell carcinoma) and can be used to assess other tissues including the vagus nerve, cardia, esophageal groove, reticulo-omasal orifice, omasal canal, and pylorus (often all are normal).

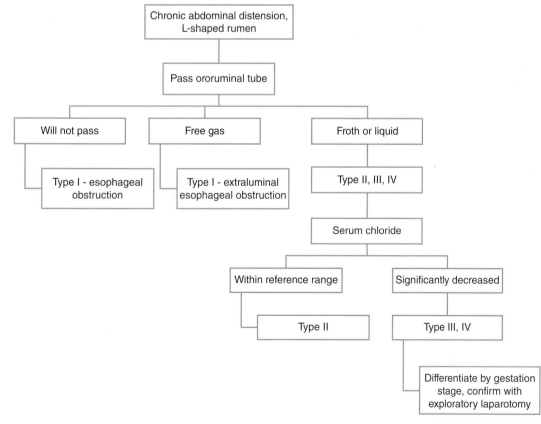

Figure 1.

Algorithm for Distinguishing Different Types of Vagal Indigestion

V

VAGAL INDIGESTION

TREATMENT

THERAPEUTIC APPROACH
• Animals with vagal indigestion generally require hospitalization to be treated for their primary condition and to resolve associated acid-base and electrolyte imbalances
• Type I
  ○ Pending resolution of esophageal obstruction, a rumen fistula can be created to alleviate bloat.
  ○ Self-retaining rumen trocar.
  ○ Rumenostomy can be performed (2–3 cm diameter) by suturing rumen wall to skin. This can granulate over in a few months, allowing time for healing of causative lesion.
  ○ Correct acid-base derangements and electrolyte abnormalities by providing alkalinizing solutions via ororuminal tube or rumenostomy.
  ○ Due to salivary loss of bicarbonate, metabolic acidosis may be severe and require additional IV sodium bicarbonate supplementation.
• Type II
  ○ Supportive therapy based on physical examination and clinicopathologic findings is important, particularly to prepare the animal for additional interventions.
  ○ Parenteral balanced electrolyte solutions high in chloride.
  ○ Potassium supplementation.
  ○ Calcium gluconate.
  ○ Systemic antimicrobials with spectrum to cover mixed gastrointestinal flora, including anaerobes.
  ○ Oral electrolytes (include 20–30 g potassium chloride to improve total body potassium status) and fluids to create mild rumen distension to promote motility.
  ○ Transfaunation with 8–16 L of fresh rumen fluid to reestablish microbial populations and improve to motility and appetite.
  ○ Surgical therapy is required in most animals (see "Surgical Considerations and Techniques").
• Type III
  ○ Generally associated with a poor prognosis.
  ○ Provide balanced electrolyte solutions high in chloride.
  ○ Oral and IV potassium supplementation.
  ○ Limited absorption is expected with limited abomasal outflow.
  ○ Laxatives (mineral oil, magnesium hydroxide) may assist with abomasal impaction.
  ○ Surgical intervention often indicated once hydration, electrolyte and acid-base aberrations addressed.
• Type IV
  ○ Consider value of dam versus calf when determining treatment.

  ○ Also consider stage of gestation and potential viability of calf.
    ▪ If cow is within 4–6 weeks of parturition, it might be possible to provide support until the fetus can be viable after delivery.
    ▪ If there is considerable time to parturition, saving both dam and fetus is less likely, and therapeutic abortion should be considered.
  ○ Provide balanced electrolyte solutions to correct hypokalemia, hypochloremia, alkalosis, and hypocalcemia; however, lack of abomasal outflow will limit utility of orally administered solutions.
  ○ Be prepared to assist delivery in compromised dams if therapeutic abortion is performed.

SURGICAL CONSIDERATIONS AND TECHNIQUES
• In general, left-sided exploration may be selected for suspected type I and II indigestion, or for cesarean section in type IV indigestion.
• Rumenotomy, rumenostomy, and percutaneous abscess drainage may be performed in the standing animal with local anesthesia (using line, paravertebral, or inverted L blocks) to minimize anesthetic risks.
• Left-sided exploration can be paired with rumenotomy to allow investigation of the cardia, reticulum, omasal groove, and abomasum (through rumen wall).
• Right-sided exploration allows enhanced evaluation of the abomasum and pylorus, along with more distal portions of the gastrointestinal tract, and may be selected for type III indigestion.
• Type I: Surgery rarely indicated.
• Type II: Rumenotomy allows diagnostic palpation of cardia, omasal canal, and reticular wall, removal of foreign bodies or masses, and biopsies of masses to aid definitive diagnosis and prognosis.
  ○ Perireticular abscesses, if firmly adherent to the reticular wall, may be incised and drained into the reticulum, or otherwise can be drained percutaneously from the right body wall under ultrasound guidance.
  ○ Paramedian approach may allow attempt at removal *en bloc*.
• Type III: right- or left-sided approaches may be indicated.
  ○ Left-sided approach includes rumenotomy.
    ▪ Palpation for masses or abscesses.
    ▪ Abscesses adhered to the reticulum may be drained into the GI tract.
    ▪ Abomasal contents may be reached through the omasal canal without opening the abomasum.
    ▪ A stomach tube can be passed into the abomasum via the omasal canal with infusion of docusate, magnesium sulfate, and fluids.

    ▪ The abomasum can be massaged though the rumen wall.
  ○ Right-sided approach enhances the ability to examine the abomasum and pylorus, as well as the distal GI tract.
    ▪ Allows for biopsy of infiltrative disease of the abomasum or pylorus.
    ▪ Permits abomasotomy as a last resort to relieve abomasal impactions since it can be associated with adhesion formation, ischemia, and motility disturbances.
• Type IV: Cesarean section with removal of the calf immediately relieves pressure on the forestomachs and generally results in rapid recovery when accompanied by appropriate fluid and electrolyte therapy.

MEDICATIONS

DRUGS OF CHOICE
• Systemic antibiotics are indicated after rumenotomy and GI manipulation.
• Combination analgesia may increase ability to control pain, and improve appetite while assisting preservation of GI motility, and may include NSAIDs and opioids (butorphanol, morphine).
• Therapeutic abortion can be accomplished within 36 hours after concurrent administration of 20 mg dexamethasone and 25 mg dinoprost IM.

CONTRAINDICATIONS
• The use of magnesium oxide/hydroxide is contraindicated in the presence of metabolic alkalosis.
• NSAID use is contraindicated in the presence of abomasal ulcers, increased creatinine, or uncorrected dehydration.

PRECAUTIONS
Appropriate milk and meat withdrawal times must be followed for all compounds administered to food-producing animals.

POSSIBLE INTERACTIONS
N/A

FOLLOW-UP

EXPECTED COURSE AND PROGNOSIS
• In one report, 33/112 (29.5%) of vagal indigestion cases from all causes made a full recovery.
• Type I cases have a good prognosis with rumenostomy, but may not flourish. They have a poorer prognosis if chronic pneumonia was the inciting cause.
• Type II cases have a fair to good prognosis depending on etiology.
• Type III cases have a poor prognosis, particularly if secondary to abomasal volvulus (in one report, 3/26 had a good outcome).

(CONTINUED)

• Type IV cases have improved prognosis with increased proximity to full gestation length. Supporting the dam through several weeks of gestation is intensive and the dam often deteriorates, whereas removal of the fetus at any stage of gestation is likely to improve rumen motility and condition of the cow.
• Neoplasia has a grave prognosis (except papilloma).
• Prognosis with abscesses depends on extent of adhesion formation.
  ◦ Hardware disease (TRP) prognosis:
    ▪ Poor to good outcomes
    ▪ 7/15 (47%) in cases of uncomplicated TRP
    ▪ 6/17 (35%) TRP with obstruction of digesta passage through reticulo-omasal orifice
    ▪ 1/10 (10%) TRP with obstruction of digesta passage though pylorus
  ◦ Peri-omasal or liver abscess—prognosis fair to good:
    ▪ Liver abscess retrospective study
    ▪ 5 of 8 cases made a significant improvement
    ▪ 2 or 3 of 8 recurred at 3 months and 1 year postoperatively
  ◦ Perireticular abscesses involving diaphragm and omasum:
    ▪ 74% (of 29 cases) returned to production for 1–4 years post-operatively.
• Foreign bodies usually have excellent prognosis with removal.

POSSIBLE COMPLICATIONS
• Poor motility despite treatment due to irreversible damage to abomasum.
• Abscess or mass recurrence after drainage or removal (in one report, liver abscess recurrence was 2–3 of 8 cases).
• Postoperative peritonitis.
• Retained fetal membranes and metritis are more common in cattle after artificially induced parturition/abortion.

CLIENT EDUCATION
• Type I
  ◦ Evaluate risk for foreign body exposure in environment.
  ◦ Review evaluation and therapies for pneumonia to prevent chronicity.
• Type II
  ◦ Review risk for hardware disease from environment and feed mixers.
  ◦ Review pasture cleanliness principles regarding twine, bags, etc.
• Type III
  ◦ Evaluate hay and diet quality to reduce risk of impaction.
  ◦ Discuss control strategies for bovine leukemia virus.
• Type IV

  ◦ Review bull selection, nutrition, and other factors associated with fetal size.

PATIENT CARE
• Patients should be monitored for return of appetite and demeanor.
• Abdominal contour must be monitored once animal is eating well to indicate motility and patency.
• Fecal output should be monitored for volume, consistency, and fiber length.
• Supply plenty of fresh water and good quality, highly digestible feed.
• Grains may be added if a laxative effect is desired.

PREVENTION
• Use of magnets in feed mixers and handling equipment to prevent metallic foreign bodies in feed.
• Environmental monitoring and removal of foreign objects.
• BLV control strategies which limit blood transmission of the virus.
• Breeding decisions to control for fetal size.

 MISCELLANEOUS

ASSOCIATED CONDITIONS
• Displaced abomasum
• Abomasal volvulus

AGE-RELATED FACTORS
Older animals are more likely to be affected by neoplastic process.

ZOONOTIC POTENTIAL
N/A

PREGNANCY
Termination of late-term pregnancy, if the dam is considered much more valuable than fetus, may be useful in most types of vagal indigestion, since fetal removal may promote normal abomasal and omasal location and motility.

BIOSECURITY
Consideration for BLV control

PRODUCTION MANAGEMENT
• Animals in dry regions or grazed on crop aftermath should be provided with readily accessible water in order to prevent abomasal impaction.
• Magnets in all feed mixing and handling equipment can reduce metallic foreign body delivery to animals.
• Bale twine and netting should be removed from all bales at feeding.

SYNONYM
Vagus indigestion

ABBREVIATIONS
• BLV = bovine leukemia virus
• GI = gastrointestinal
• IM = intramuscular
• IV = intravenous
• LDA = left displaced abomasum
• NSAIDs = nonsteroidal anti-inflammatory drugs
• TRP = traumatic reticuloperitonitis

SEE ALSO
• Abomasal Impaction
• Bloat
• Bovine Leukemia Virus
• Displaced Abomasum
• Liver Abscesses
• Traumatic Reticuloperitonitis

Suggested Reading
Fubini SL, Ducharme NG, Erb HN, Smith DF, Rebhun WC. Failure of omasal transport attributable to perireticular abscess formation in cattle: 29 cases (1980–1986). J Am Vet Med Assoc 1989, 194: 811–14.
Fubini SL, Ducharme NG, Murphy JP, Smith DF. Vagus indigestion syndrome resulting from a liver abscess in dairy cows. J Am Vet Med Assoc 1985, 186: 1297–300.
Kelton DF, Fubini SL. Pyloric obstruction after toggle-pin fixation of left displaced abomasum in a cow. J Am Vet Med Assoc 1989, 194: 677–8.
Rehbun WC. Vagus indigestion in cattle. J Am Vet Med Assoc 1980, 176: 506–10.
Rehbun WC, Fubini SL, Miller TK, Lesser FR. Vagus indigestion in cattle: Clinical features, causes, treatments and long-term follow-up of 112 cases. Comp Cont Educ Pract Vet 1988, 10: 387–91.
Rehage J, Kaske M, Stockhofe-Zurwieden N, Yalcin E. Evaluation of the pathogenesis of vagus indigestion in cows with traumatic reticuloperitonitis. J Am Vet Med Assoc 1995, 207: 1607–11.
Taguchi K. Relationship between degree of dehydration and serum electrolytes and acid-base status in cows with various abomasal disorders. J Vet Med Sci 1995, 57: 257–60.
VanMetre DC, Fecteau G, House JK, George LW. Indigestion of late pregnancy in a cow. J Am Vet Med Assoc 1995, 205: 625–8.
Wilson AD, Hirsch VM, Osborne AD. Abdominocentesis in cattle: Technique and criteria for diagnosis of peritonitis. Can Vet J 1985, 26: 74.
Author Meredyth L. Jones
Consulting Editor Erica C. McKenzie

V

VAGINITIS

BASICS

OVERVIEW
• Inflammation of the vagina caused by a variety of organisms.
• Transient vaginitis is commonly seen after synchronization of estrus with progesterone intravaginal devices.
• A form of severe necrotic vaginitis may occur following obstetric manipulations.

INCIDENCE/PREVALENCE
• The prevalence of vaginitis was 2.6% in dairy cattle in Austria.
• In herds affected by *Ureaplasma diversum*, clinical signs of vaginitis were reported in 43% of the cows.
• *Ureaplasma diversum* and *Mycoplasma* spp. are commonly isolated from vagina and vestibule of reproductively normal cattle. However, *Ureaplasma diversum* is more commonly isolated from vaginal swabs of cows with vaginitis (40–60%) than cows without vaginitis.
• *Mycoplasma bovigenitalium* was isolated from 55% of cows with vaginitis in one Israeli study.
• The prevalence of *Mycoplasma bovigenitalium* did not differ between cows with and without vaginitis.

GEOGRAPHIC DISTRIBUTION
Potentially worldwide

SYSTEMS AFFECTED
Reproductive

PATHOPHYSIOLOGY
• Infectious granular vulvovaginitis (IGV): Bacteria colonize the vulva and vagina of females, urethra, prepuce, and semen of bulls, and nasal passages in both sexes. Transmission is venereal or by direct contact, environmental contamination, or during passage through the birth canal. Granular vulvovaginitis results 4–10 days after infection, followed by ascending endometritis and salpingitis. Reproductive problems can persist for up to 6 months and nodules can persist for >1 year.
• Infectious pustular vulvovaginitis (IPV): Infection is venereal. Fever, depression, and anorexia may be present during the acute phase 1–3 days post-infection. Small vesicles and 2–3-mm raised pustules are formed in the vaginal mucosa. Pustules may then coalesce forming painful ulcers. Mucopurulent vulvar discharge may develop due to secondary bacterial infection. Lesions heal after 10–14 days. After primary infection, latency is established.
• Caprine herpes virus 1 (CpHV-1): Causes reproductive syndrome in goats similar to that observed in cattle with BHV-1 (IPV).
• Traumatic: Purulent vaginitis is produced by the irritation of the vaginal mucosa after estrus synchronization treatment with CIDR device or sponges.

• The most severe form of bacterial vaginitis is observed following lengthy obstetric manipulation. This form of vaginitis may lead to severe vaginal adhesions. Camelids seem to be more predisposed to this than ruminants.

HISTORICAL FINDINGS
• A herd history of signs described in "Pathophysiology"
• History of dystocia

SIGNALMENT
• Potentially all ruminants: Breeding age females.
• IPV, IGV: Cattle. Heifers are more susceptible to granular vulvovaginitis.
• Caprine herpes virus 1: goats

PHYSICAL EXAMINATION FINDINGS
• Characteristic lesions on vaginal examination.
• Discomfort, arched back, tail twitching or raising, straining, dysuria.
• Mucopurulent vulvar discharge, hyperemia of the vulvar, vestibular, and vaginal mucosa.
• IPV: Vaginal vesicles, raised pustules, painful ulcers.
• IGV: Raised red to gray vaginal nodules, infertility, pregnancy loss.

GENETICS
N/A

CAUSES AND RISK FACTORS
• IPV: Bovine herpes virus 1
• IGV: *Ureaplasma diversum*
• *Mycoplasma bovis*, *Mycoplasma bovigenitalium* (role is controversial)
• Foreign body
• Trauma, most often during calving or breeding
• Urovagina, pneumovagina
• Use of progesterone/progestagen-containing intravaginal devices
• Caprine herpes virus 1 (lesions similar to BHV-1)
• Risk factors include
  ○ Reuse of progesterone-containing intravaginal devices (IGV)
  ○ Vaginal injuries during calving or breeding
  ○ Use of infected semen or bulls

DIAGNOSIS

DIFFERENTIAL DIAGNOSES
• Bovine necrotic vulvovaginitis: Unique to Israel, caused by the anaerobe *Porphyromonas levii*. It is characterized by the development of a necrotic vulvovaginal lesion in the first week postpartum in first calf heifers. Incidence may be 85% initially.
• Vulvar discharge: Metritis, endometritis, pyometra.
• Other causes of infertility and pregnancy loss.

CBC/BIOCHEMISTRY/URINALYSIS
Usually not useful

OTHER LABORATORY TESTS
• Bacterial culture from vulvar and vaginal samples.
• Samples for culture of *Ureaplasma diversum* must be collected with Dacron or polyester-tipped swabs, submersed in appropriate transport medium and frozen.
• Virus isolation, serology, PCR (IPV).

IMAGING
Ultrasonography per rectum may help rule in or out uterine infection.

OTHER DIAGNOSTIC PROCEDURES
Speculum vaginal examination will reveal characteristic lesions, lacerations, urine pooling, or foreign bodies.

PATHOLOGIC FINDINGS
IPV: Necrosis of the vaginal epithelium with intranuclear inclusion bodies.

TREATMENT

THERAPEUTIC APPROACH
• Control infection and inflammation.
• Treat primary cause.
• Vaginal douche with normal saline solution or 0.1% chlorhexidine solution.
• Local antibiotic to prevent secondary bacterial infection.

SURGICAL CONSIDERATIONS AND TECHNIQUES
• Surgical correction of pneumovagina, urovagina, and vaginal lacerations.

MEDICATIONS

DRUGS OF CHOICE
• IGV and Mycoplasma spp.: Tylosin (10 mg/kg) for 5 days.
• Alternative: Tetracycline for *Mycoplasma* spp. infection.

CONTRAINDICATIONS
See "Precautions"

PRECAUTIONS
Appropriate milk and meat withdrawal times must be followed for all compounds administered to food-producing animals.

POSSIBLE INTERACTIONS
N/A

FOLLOW-UP

EXPECTED COURSE AND PROGNOSIS
• IPV is usually self-limiting.
• Cows with IGV usually regain fertility after two or three estrous cycles.

POSSIBLE COMPLICATIONS
• Secondary bacterial infection

V

(CONTINUED)

• Ascending endometritis and salpingitis, infertility

CLIENT EDUCATION
• Work with a veterinarian to design an appropriate biosecurity and vaccination program.
• Work with an experienced insemination technician and veterinarian to insure proper technique during breeding and calving.
• Follow milk and meat withdrawal times if medications are administered.

PATIENT CARE
Supportive as needed

PREVENTION
• Use of sanitary sheath during artificial insemination to prevent introduction of bacteria into the uterus (IGV).
• Tetracycline intrauterine infusion (1 g) 24 h after artificial insemination (IGV).
• Avoid reusing CIDRs and use proper aseptic technique during their application.
• Use proper technique during resolution of dystocia and artificial insemination.
• Optimize the herd's health status by providing appropriate nutritional, stress, and environmental management.

MISCELLANEOUS

ASSOCIATED CONDITIONS
N/A

AGE-RELATED FACTORS
Heifers more susceptible to IGV than cows.

ZOONOTIC POTENTIAL
N/A

PREGNANCY
Ascending infection can cause infertility, embryonic loss, and abortion.

BIOSECURITY
See "Prevention"

PRODUCTION MANAGEMENT
Avoid nutritional, social, and environmental stress by using proper management practices.

SYNONYMS
N/A

ABBREVIATIONS
• BHV-1 = bovine herpesvirus 1
• CIDR = controlled internal drug release
• CpHV-1 = caprine herpesvirus 1
• IGV = infectious granular vulvovaginitis
• IPV = infectious pustular vulvovaginitis
• PCR = polymerase chain reaction

SEE ALSO
• Infectious Bovine Rhinotracheitis
• Infectious Pustular Vulvovaginitis
• *Mycoplasma bovis* Associated Diseases
• Ureaplasma

Suggested Reading
Gaeti JG, Lana MVC, Silva GS, et al. *Ureaplasma diversum* as a cause of pustular vulvovaginitis in bovine females in Vale Guapore, Mato Grosso State, Brazil. Trop Anim Health Prod 2014, 46: 1059–63.
Petit T, Spergser J, Aurich J, Rosengarten R. Prevalence of Chlamydiaceae and Mollicutes on the genital mucosa and serological findings in dairy cattle. Vet Microbiol 2008, 127: 325–33.
Tibary A. Infectious agents: infectious bovine rhinotracheitis. In: Hopper R ed, Bovine Reproduction. Ames: Wiley Blackwell, 2015.
Author Maria Soledad Ferrer
Consulting Editor Ahmed Tibary
Acknowledgment The author and book editors acknowledge the prior contribution of Ramanathan Kasimanickam.

V

VESICULAR STOMATITIS

BASICS

OVERVIEW
- Vesicular stomatitis is a viral disease that causes vesicles, or blisters, in the oral cavity, on the coronary bands, interdigital space, mammary glands, ears, and preputial areas of cattle and horses and occasionally sheep, goats, swine, llamas, and alpacas.
- It cannot be clinically differentiated from foot and mouth disease, and proper identification is imperative to the economics of the United States agriculture industry.
- Vesicular stomatitis virus (VSV) is a reportable disease to state or federal officials in all US states.
- Sheep and goats are fairly resistant and rarely show clinical signs.

INCIDENCE/PREVALENCE
- Incidence varies between geographic locations.
- Morbidity within a herd of naïve animals can reach 90% but typically 5–20% of a herd is symptomatic.
- Mortality is rare.

GEOGRAPHIC DISTRIBUTION
- This disease has been limited to the Americas. It is endemic in some warmer latitudes of North, Central, and South America, and outbreaks occur in more temperate climates sporadically.
- In the southern US and Central America, vesicular stomatitis virus has two domestic strains, New Jersey and Indiana-1, which are found in the southern states.
- Outbreaks in the western US are thought to migrate north out of Mexico and tend to follow waterways and river valleys.

SYSTEMS AFFECTED
- Digestive
- Integument
- Mammary

PATHOPHYSIOLOGY
- Virus enters through an abrasion or mechanical transmission by insects.
- Lesion development is restricted to the site of inoculation.
- However, in some studies, pigs inoculated at the snout via intradermal injection developed vesicles at the coronary band. Short-term viremia was suggested, even though it was not detected in this experiment or in any other in domestic animals to date.
- Vesicles or erosions can be found in the oral cavity, on the feet, and on the mammary gland in cattle.
- Vesicular fluid is very infectious.

HISTORICAL FINDINGS
- Disease can occur at any time of year but cases tend to cluster during the summer and fall, often during or following rainier seasons.
- Cases tend to occur sporadically in endemic areas without large outbreaks.
- Cattle may salivate excessively, have a fever, lose milk production, and develop mastitis.
- The disease is usually self-limiting in approximately 2 weeks.

SIGNALMENT
Cattle, and occasionally sheep and goats.

PHYSICAL EXAMINATION FINDINGS
- Blanched vesicles progressing to erosive ulcers located in one area of the body, such as the oral cavity and muzzle, the feet, or mammary gland.
- Decreased milk production, inappetence and weight loss due to painful oral vesicles, lameness due to vesicles on the coronary band and/or interdigital space, and agitation during milking due to vesicles on the mammary gland.

CAUSES AND RISK FACTORS
- VSV is a member of the genus Vesiculovirus in the family Rhabdoviridae.
- There are two major serotypes of the virus, New Jersey and Indiana. The majority of outbreaks in the US are due to the New Jersey serotype.
- Cases tend to occur sporadically during the warmer months in the southern and western United States and most often near waterways or on pastured animals.
- Introduction route into a herd is not always known but could occur through insect vectors, mechanical transmission, or movement of infected animals.
- Once lesions appear in a herd, direct contact with vesicles and vesicular fluid between animals can spread the virus quite rapidly.
- Transmission can occur through insect vectors, direct contact with infected animals, and indirect contact with contaminated objects.
- Black flies (*Simuliidae*), phlebotomine sand flies (*Lutzomyia shannoni*), and biting midges (*Culicoides*) can transmit the virus to animals and transovarially to their larvae. They have also been shown to overwinter in temperate climates from year to year.
- In the 1982 epizootic of VS in the southwestern US, the New Jersey serotype was isolated from mosquitoes (*Aedes*), house flies (*Musca*), and eye gnats (Chloropidae), but their role in transmission is unknown.
- Moving naïve animals to an endemic area, especially during the late rainy season.

- Increased population of black flies or sand flies.
- Pasture grazing, especially near water sources.

DIAGNOSIS

DIFFERENTIAL DIAGNOSES
- Cattle: Foot and mouth disease, infectious bovine rhinotracheitis, bovine viral diarrhea, rinderpest, malignant catarrhal fever, bluetongue, foot rot, chemical or thermal burns
- Sheep: Bluetongue, contagious ecthyma, lip/leg ulceration, and foot rot

CBC/BIOCHEMISTRY/URINALYSIS
N/A

OTHER LABORATORY TESTS
- Tissue cultures can be used to isolate the virus.
- RT-PCR can be used to detect the virus.
- Viral antibodies (on acute and convalescent sera) and antigen (aseptic vesicular fluid, vesicular epithelium in buffered glycerol or frozen) can be identified using ELISA, CF, and virus neutralization.

OTHER DIAGNOSTIC PROCEDURES
Due to the seriousness of this disease and the inability to clinically differentiate it from FMD, state and federal authorities should be contacted immediately upon suspicion of cases *before* sample collection.

PATHOLOGIC FINDINGS
Vesicles or ulcerative erosions in the oral cavity, on the coronary band, or mammary gland will be seen grossly.

TREATMENT

THERAPEUTIC APPROACH
- Upon confirmatory diagnosis of VSV, animals with lesions should be isolated and given supportive care conducive to the location of the lesions.
- Soft food, or a gruel, and clean water for oral lesions; well-bedded, clean stall for lesions of the feet; milked last if there are mammary lesions.

SURGICAL CONSIDERATIONS AND TECHNIQUES
Local wound debridement may be warranted depending on the extent of the lesion and viable tissue surrounding it, allowing it to heal on its own.

V

MEDICATIONS

DRUGS OF CHOICE
• No treatment for VSV.
• Use of broad-spectrum antimicrobials for prevention and treatment of secondary infections.

FOLLOW-UP

EXPECTED COURSE AND PROGNOSIS
Most recover without complications in 2 weeks. Coronary band lesions and interdigital space lesions can take longer.

POSSIBLE COMPLICATIONS
Secondary bacterial infection of the lesioned area

CLIENT EDUCATION
• Animals with lesions must be isolated to prevent disease spread; no animals can be moved off the property for at least 30 days after the last lesion has healed.
• Equipment and areas of potential exposure at a facility should be cleaned and disinfected before reintroducing any other animals.
• Patients should be monitored for appetite and lesion healing during the course of the disease (approximately 2 weeks).

PATIENT CARE
• Isolated to a pen/stall that has no direct contact with other susceptible animals and no exposure to potential insect vectors.
• Calves should be removed from infected dams.
• Soft forages/gruel for oral lesions, plenty of water.
• Do not feed calves milk or colostrum from infected animals.

PREVENTION
• Do not move animals to an endemic area.
• Insect control and manure management can help prevent disease spread.
• There is no vaccine available in the US.

MISCELLANEOUS

ASSOCIATED CONDITIONS
• Decreased milk production and agitation during milking due to lesions on the mammary gland.
• Inappetence due to oral lesions.
• Lameness due to lesions on the coronary band and/or interdigital space.
• Hypersalivation due to oral lesions.

ZOONOTIC POTENTIAL
• Humans can become infected with VSV New Jersey and Indiana-1 strains; signs include fever, headache, myalgia, and, very rarely, oral vesicles.
• Recovery is usually within 4–7 days.

PREGNANCY
There does not seem to be a concern with pregnant animals unless the lesions impede eating or a severe secondary infection develops.

BIOSECURITY
• Isolation and quarantine of new stock entering the herd or flock.
• Treat or cull new animals for disease conditions prior to herd introduction.
• VSV is a reportable disease.
• Animals with lesions must be isolated to prevent disease spread; no animals can be moved off the property for at least 30 days after the last lesion has healed.
• Equipment and areas of potential exposure at a facility should be cleaned and disinfected before reintroducing any other animals.

ABBREVIATIONS
• CF = complement fixation
• ELISA = enzyme-linked immunosorbent assay
• FMD = foot and mouth disease
• RT-PCR = reverse transcription-polymerase chain reaction
• VSV = vesicular stomatitis virus

SEE ALSO
• Bluetongue Virus
• Bovine Viral Diarrhea Virus
• Burn Management
• Foot and Mouth Disease
• Foot Rot: Bovine
• Foot Rot: Small Ruminant
• Infectious Bovine Rhinotracheitis
• Malignant Catarrhal Fever
• Orf (Contagious Ecthyma)
• Rinderpest (see www.fiveminutevet.com/ruminant)

Suggested Reading
Aiello SE., ed. Merck Veterinary Manual, 8th ed. Whitehouse Station, NJ: Merck & Co., 1998.
Office International des Epizooties. Vesicular stomatitis. http://www.oie.int/fileadmin/Home/eng/Animal_Health_in_the_World/docs/pdf/Disease_cards/VESICULAR_STOMATITIS.pdf. Accessed Feb 9, 2017.
Rebhun WC. Vesicular stomatitis. In: Divers TJ, Peek S eds, Rebhun's Diseases of Dairy Cattle, 2nd ed. St. Louis: Saunders Elsevier, 2007.
United States Animal Health Association. Vesicular stomatitis. http://www.usaha.org/Portals/6/3%202015%20USAHA_IDOHC_VSV%20Modified%20Approach_Pelzel.pdf. Accessed Feb 9, 2017.
USDA APHIS. Vesicular stomatitis. https://www.aphis.usda.gov/aphis/ourfocus/animalhealth/animal-disease-information/horse-disease-information/vesicular-stomatitis/ct_vesicular_stomatitis. Accessed Feb 9, 2017.

Authors Alex K. Turner and Keith A. Roehr
Consulting Editor Christopher C.L. Chase
Acknowledgment The authors and book editors acknowledge the prior contribution of Danelle Bickett Weddle.

V

VITAMIN A DEFICIENCY/TOXICOSIS

 BASICS

OVERVIEW
• Vitamin A occurs as retinol, retinoic acid, and retinal. It is a fat-soluble compound. Together with its precursors, the carotenoids, it is highly labile and rapidly destroyed by light, oxygen, heat, and acid.
• Vitamin A is required by all mammals and is synthesized through the metabolism of carotenoid precursors (carotenes) present in leaves and some grains.
• Of the carotenes, β-carotene has the highest vitamin A activity and is quantitatively the most important for animal nutrition.
• The proximal jejunum is the primary site of vitamin A and carotene absorption. A normal pancreatic, hepatic, and biliary function, together with an adequate dietary fat content and normal fat digestion and absorption, is required for the absorption of β-carotene and its subsequent conversion to retinol.
• Ruminal microbial degradation of biologically active vitamin A is appreciable and varies with diet composition. High-concentrate diets can result in up to 70% pre-intestinal degradation of vitamin A, whereas diets with >75% forage result in <20% degradation, factors to be taken into account for diet formulation and vitamin A or β-carotene supplementation.
• In dairy cows, peripartum decreases in serum concentrations of vitamin A may contribute to impaired immune function.

INCIDENCE/PREVALENCE
N/A

GEOGRAPHIC DISTRIBUTION
N/A

SYSTEMS AFFECTED
Multisystemic

PATHOPHYSIOLOGY
General Functions
Vitamin A is required for cellular differentiation, growth and development, adequate vision, thyroid gland function, protein synthesis, conversion of cholesterol to corticosterone, glycogen synthesis, immune function, regulation of gene expression, and iron metabolism.

Deficiency
• As hepatic stores of vitamin A can last for up to 6 months, deficiency only develops after prolonged periods of inadequate availability.
• Clinical signs occur in young animals more often than adults and include those listed under "Physical Examination Findings."
• Developmental bone abnormalities of the spine may be responsible for some of the neuromuscular deficits in vitamin A–deficient animals.

• Maternal deficiency of vitamin A is associated with congenital ocular abnormalities. In neonatal calves, malformation and closure of the optic foramen resulting in optic nerve compression is described.

Toxicity
• The likelihood of vitamin A toxicity in ruminants is extremely low, because it has a wide safety margin of about 30 times the nutritional requirement (only 4–10 times in monogastrics).
• Experimentally, harmful effects have been reproduced by feeding >100 times the daily requirements for extended periods. Therefore, an accidental dietary excess for short periods of time is unlikely to produce any harmful effects.
• Hypervitaminosis A produces a variety of clinical abnormalities as listed in "Physical Examination Findings."
• Excess intake of vitamin A also impairs absorption and metabolism of the other fat-soluble vitamins, which can result in deficiency of one or more of vitamins D, E, and K in animals fed diets containing marginal levels of these.

HISTORICAL FINDINGS
N/A

SIGNALMENT
• All ruminant species.
• Intestinal absorption of carotene is more efficient in the Jersey and Guernsey breeds.
• Vitamin A deficiency is observed more frequently in young, growing animal than in adults.

PHYSICAL EXAMINATION FINDINGS
Deficiency
• The classic and frequently the first clinical manifestation of vitamin A deficiency in ruminants is nyctalopia, with a gradual reduction of vision in dim light, readily identified as an inability to avoid obstacles in the dark. Characteristic changes in the eye include keratitis, corneal edema, and xerophthalmia characterized by drying of the conjunctiva (not in cattle, where excessive lacrimation occurs).
• Cattle: Reduced feed intake and stunted growth and development rates, abnormal bone and teeth growth, nyctalopia and corneal opacity, epiphora, rough hair coat, diarrhea, joint and brisket edema, seizures, and immunosuppression manifested as increased susceptibility to infectious diseases such as pneumonia, pinkeye, and mastitis.
• Sheep: In addition to the signs observed in cattle, vitamin A deficiency results in xerophthalmia. In lambs, a deficient humoral immune response and abnormal adrenal function have been described.
• Goats: Vitamin A deficiency presents initially as a nonspecific rough, dull hair coat,

followed by the clinical signs described for sheep.
• In females it results in low conception rates and pregnancy losses due to abortions and stillbirths, with offspring born alive being weak and blind. Increased rates of fetal membrane retention have been observed in vitamin A–deficient ewes. Intact males have decreased libido and an increase in sperm abnormalities.
• Advanced hypovitaminosis A most frequently results in characteristic eye changes accompanied by a staggering gait, and convulsive seizures ("fainting" in feedlot cattle) and papilledema of the eye, secondary to elevated cerebrospinal fluid pressure.

Toxicity
• In ruminants fed toxic levels of vitamin A, the most common clinical signs were osteoporosis, reduced feed intake, and decreased cerebrospinal fluid pressure.
• Other signs of hypervitaminosis A include skeletal malformation and osteoporosis leading to spontaneous fractures, anemia, delayed blood clotting and internal hemorrhages, partial or total anorexia, growth retardation and weight loss, alopecia, skin thickening with hyperkeratosis, enteritis with chronic diarrhea, hepatomegaly and splenomegaly with degenerative atrophy and fatty infiltration of liver and kidneys, conjunctivitis, and congenital abnormalities.

GENETICS
N/A

CAUSES AND RISK FACTORS
• Poor dietary formulation with low or excessive vitamin A and/or inadequate fat content.
• Low forage availability.
• Feed exposure to light and heat or the presence of moisture and trace minerals accelerates the loss of vitamin A activity.

 DIAGNOSIS

DIFFERENTIAL DIAGNOSES
Deficiency
Cattle: Polioencephalomalacia, lead poisoning, water deprivation/sodium toxicosis, meningoencephalitis, other causes of increased intracranial pressure and blindness. Small ruminants: Pregnancy toxemia and listeriosis.

Toxicity
All causes of skeletal malformations and spontaneous fractures, hepatic lipidosis, and renal failure.

CBC/BIOCHEMISTRY/URINALYSIS
Nonspecific

V

(CONTINUED) | **VITAMIN A DEFICIENCY/TOXICOSIS**

OTHER LABORATORY TESTS
Plasma and feed vitamin A and carotene concentrations

IMAGING
• Deficiency: Bone deformities
• Toxicity: Decreased bone density and fractures

OTHER DIAGNOSTIC PROCEDURES
Liver biopsy for vitamin A analysis

PATHOLOGIC FINDINGS

Deficiency
Anasarca, corneal opacity and ulceration, papilledema, fundic hemorrhages, retinal degeneration, doming of the head and face, carpal joint enlargement, cerebral and cerebellar compression and tentorial herniation, and focal hyperkeratosis in mucocutaneous junctions and rumen.

Toxicity
Skeletal malformation, decreased bone density, fractures, internal hemorrhages, hyperkeratotic skin, and congenital abnormalities.

TREATMENT

THERAPEUTIC APPROACH
• Deficiency is rapidly corrected with vitamin A supplementation (dietary and injectable).
• Common dietary sources of carotenes are carrots, yellow corn, alfalfa (legumes), green grass (pasture, hay, or silage).
• Advanced clinical signs of both deficiency and toxicity are irreversible.

SURGICAL CONSIDERATIONS AND TECHNIQUES
N/A

MEDICATIONS

DRUGS OF CHOICE
Various formulations for IM or SC injection containing vitamin A usually combined with vitamin D and/or E are available.

PRECAUTIONS
If using products containing vitamin D, hypervitaminosis D, which may result in hypercalcemia, may be induced.

CONTRAINDICATIONS
Vitamins A and D should not be given to meat-producing animals within 2 months of marketing.

POSSIBLE INTERACTIONS
N/A

FOLLOW-UP

EXPECTED COURSE AND PROGNOSIS
• Prognosis is poor for individual animals with advanced clinical signs, and good if treated during the early stages.
• Return to adequate production can be expected at the herd or flock level after correction of dietary vitamin A imbalances.

POSSIBLE COMPLICATIONS
N/A

CLIENT EDUCATION
Awareness of specific nutritional needs is imperative.

PATIENT CARE
Assess for return of vision after a short period of supplementation; animals with loss of vision due to papilledema and not to retinal or optic nerve damage may recover.

PREVENTION
Supplementation in animals with limited access to fresh forage.

MISCELLANEOUS

AGE-RELATED FACTORS
More often observed in young animals

PREGNANCY
Crucial in reproduction and embryogenesis.

ABBREVIATIONS
• IM = intramuscular
• SC = subcutaneous

SEE ALSO
• Selenium/Vitamin E Deficiency
• Vitamin D Deficiency/Toxicosis

Suggested Reading
He X, Li Y, Li M, et al. Hypovitaminosis A coupled to secondary bacterial infection in beef cattle. BMC Vet Res 2012, 8: 222.
LeBlanc SJ, Herdt TH, Seymour WM, Duffield TF, Leslie KE. Peripartum serum vitamin E, retinol, and beta-carotene in dairy cattle and their associations with disease. J Dairy Sci 2004, 87: 609–19.
Mason CS, Buxton D, Gartside JF. Congenital ocular abnormalities in calves associated with maternal hypovitaminosis A. Vet Rec 2003, 153: 213–14.
National Research Council. Nutrient Requirements of Sheep (1985), Nutrient Requirements of Beef Cattle (2016), Nutrient Requirements of Dairy Cattle (2001). Washington DC: National Academy Press.
Solomons NW. Vitamin A and carotenoids. In: Bowman BA, Russell RM eds, Present Knowledge in Nutrition, 8th ed. Washington DC: ILSI Press, 2001.
Waldner CL, Blakley B. Evaluating micronutrient concentrations in liver samples from abortions, stillbirths, and neonatal and postnatal losses in beef calves. J Vet Diagn Invest 2014, 26: 376–89.
Author Carlos E. Medina-Torres
Consulting Editor Kaitlyn A. Lutz
Acknowledgment The author and book editors acknowledge the prior contribution of Daniel C. Rule.

V

VITAMIN B DEFICIENCY

BASICS

OVERVIEW
• Rumen microbes synthesize and meet most B vitamin requirements of the ruminant.
• B vitamins are essential in many critical enzyme systems.
• Thiamine, riboflavin, pantothenic acid, niacin, and biotin are cofactors in the Krebs cycle.
• In ruminants, disease usually relates to B_1 (thiamine) and B_{12} (cobalamin) deficiency.
  ◦ B_1 deficiency has a variety of causes and can result in polioencephalomalacia (PEM).
  ◦ B_{12} deficiency arises from cobalt (Co) deficiency; Co is required for ruminal B_{12} synthesis.

INCIDENCE/PREVALENCE
Usually sporadic; outbreaks of PEM can occur, and subclinical Co deficiency is common.

GEOGRAPHIC DISTRIBUTION
Worldwide; B_1 deficiency influenced by distribution of specific plants (bracken fern) and production systems (feedlots); B_{12} deficiency influenced by Co-deficient soils in large areas of many countries.

SYSTEMS AFFECTED
• Nervous
• Musculoskeletal
• Digestive
• Hemolymphatic

PATHOPHYSIOLOGY
• B_1 is essential for normal Krebs cycle function. Deficiency reduces glucose availability to the brain and can arise from:
  ◦ High starch rations: Ruminal acidosis favors rumen thiaminase.
  ◦ Amprolium: Inhibits thiamine absorption and blocks its phosphorylation.
  ◦ Consumption of plants (bracken) or molds (spoiled feed) that produce thiaminase.
  ◦ Excessive sulfur in feed and water or from hydrogen sulfide gas in the rumen: Sulfur is antagonistic to thiamine enzymes.
• B_{12} is an essential cofactor of methylmalonyl-CoA mutase and methionine synthase. Reductions in these enzymes interfere with folic acid metabolism, utilization of propionate, and immune function, and result in accumulation of methylmalonic acid (MMA) in serum due to incomplete metabolism of absorbed proprionate.
  ◦ Deficiency arises from dietary Co deficiency.
  ◦ Diarrhea results from disturbances of GI flora and reduced resistance to GI parasitism.
  ◦ Anemia is common due to disturbed folic acid metabolism.

HISTORICAL FINDINGS
Young growing ruminants in Co-deficient regions without supplementation, and/or exposed to factors that promote thiamine deficiency: Sudden dietary changes, high dietary concentrate, recent GI disease, recent weaning.

SIGNALMENT
• B_1 deficiency is most common in cattle, sheep, and goats under 18 months; however, adults can be affected. Camelids, camels, and deer occasionally affected.
• B_{12} deficiency typically affects growing animals due to lower liver reserves; sheep are most susceptible.

PHYSICAL EXAMINATION FINDINGS
• B_1 deficiency
  ◦ Weakness, reduced growth, anorexia and diarrhea, with ataxia, apparent blindness, star gazing, separation from the herd, excitability, and circling. Acute disease can bring death within 24 hours, sometimes with diarrhea.
  ◦ In advanced disease the animal becomes recumbent with teeth grinding, absent menace response (often normal bilateral pupillary light reflex), dorsomedial strabismus, horizontal nystagmus, opisthotonos, and seizures. Hyperthermia due to rigidity and seizures can be mistaken for true fever. In sulfur-associated cases, the breath might smell like rotten eggs.
• B_{12} deficiency
  ◦ Failure to grow, ill-thrift, weight loss, diarrhea, pica, emaciation, and lacrimation.
  ◦ Fatty degeneration of the liver ("white liver disease") can produce photosensitization and hepatic encephalopathy.
  ◦ Reduced immunity, anemia, and adverse effects on production variables are common.

GENETICS
N/A

CAUSES AND RISK FACTORS
• B_1 deficiency
  ◦ High soluble carbohydrate, low fiber rations
  ◦ Sudden dietary changes
  ◦ Molasses- and urea-based rations
  ◦ Sulfur in ration and drinking water
  ◦ Amprolium
• B_{12} deficiency
  ◦ Heavily limed pastures and manganese-rich soils decrease Co availability.
  ◦ Heavy rainfall leaches Co from topsoil.
  ◦ Grasses have less Co than legumes, especially if rapidly growing.
  ◦ Coastal soils.

DIAGNOSIS

DIFFERENTIAL DIAGNOSES
• B_1 deficiency
  ◦ Pregnancy toxemia (sheep)
  ◦ Acute coenurosis
  ◦ *C. perfringens* enterotoxemia (sheep)
  ◦ Listerosis
  ◦ Toxicity: Lead, molasses, bracken, salt
  ◦ Rabies
  ◦ Meningitis/Encephalitis
  ◦ Tetanus
  ◦ Vitamin A deficiency (cattle)
  ◦ Hypomagnesemia (cattle)
• B_{12} deficiency
  ◦ Parasitic gastroenteritis
  ◦ Protein-calorie malnutrition
  ◦ Coccidiosis
  ◦ Johne's disease
  ◦ Selenium, copper, and vitamin D deficiencies

CBC/BIOCHEMISTRY/URINALYSIS
• B_1 deficiency: No consistent abnormalities.
• B_{12} deficiency: Macrocytic to normocytic, normochromic anemia; elevated AST and GGT may occur.

OTHER LABORATORY TESTS
• B_1 deficiency is indicated by:
  ◦ Significant percent increase in blood transketolase activity after addition of excess thiamine diphosphate to samples.
  ◦ Low blood thiamine (<50 nmol/L).
  ◦ Increased thiaminase activity in rumen content (submit at least 60 grams, fresh frozen).
• B_{12} deficiency is indicated by:
  ◦ Liver B_{12}: ≤0.3 μg/g WW.
  ◦ Serum B_{12}: <0.1 ng/mL.
  ◦ Low serum (<0.1 ng/mL) or liver (<80 ng/g WW) cobalt.
  ◦ High serum MMA (more reliable than B_{12}): Values >4 μmol/L possibly benefit from supplementation, >13 μmol/L expected to benefit.

IMAGING
N/A

OTHER DIAGNOSTIC PROCEDURES
• Response to B_1 or B_{12} supplementation provides clinical evidence of deficiency.
• B_1 deficiency:
  ◦ Assess ration for sulfur, molasses, salt, urea.
  ◦ Rumen gas hydrogen sulfide concentration: >1,000 ppm suggests excess sulfur consumption (compare to healthy control).
  ◦ Cerebrocortical autofluorescence under ultraviolet lamp.

PATHOLOGIC FINDINGS
• B_1:
  ◦ Gross findings: Focal regions of soft, edematous cortical tissue with gray or yellow discoloration, flattened gyri.
  ◦ Histological findings: Cerebrocortical laminar neuronal necrosis and perineuronal vacuolation with cavitation of endothelial cells in the parietal and occipital lobes.
  ◦ Astrocytic swelling, neuronal shrinkage, and necrosis.

V

(CONTINUED) VITAMIN B DEFICIENCY

○ Lead, sulfur toxicity, and salt poisoning/water deprivation can cause similar lesions.
• B_{12}:
  ○ Cardiovascular lesions resembling arteriosclerosis (sheep).
  ○ Emaciation and hepatic lipidosis.

TREATMENT

THERAPEUTIC APPROACH
Treatment requires supplementation with thiamine or cobalamin, initially by injection in animals with clinical disease.

SURGICAL CONSIDERATIONS AND TECHNIQUES
N/A

MEDICATIONS

DRUGS OF CHOICE
• B_1 deficiency
  ○ Thiamine HCl: 10 mg/kg body weight once IV (slow), then q6–12h SC or IM for 1 day, then q12–24h SC or IM for 3 days.
  ○ Dexamethasone (1–2 mg/kg IM or SC, once) for cerebral edema.
  ○ Seizures may require diazepam (0.5–1.0 mg/kg IV).
  ○ Animals may benefit from IV dextrose during initial therapy.
• B_{12} deficiency
  ○ Cobalamin 100 μg IM (lamb), 300 μg IM (sheep), or 3,000 μg IM (cattle), repeat weekly if needed.
  ○ Drench with cobalt sulfate (1 mg/kg PO).

CONTRAINDICATIONS
Oral medications should be avoided in recumbent, disoriented animals.

PRECAUTIONS
• IV administration of thiamine should be performed slowly and carefully; severe adverse reactions including death are possible.
• Appropriate milk and meat withdrawal times must be followed for all compounds administered to food-producing animals.

POSSIBLE INTERACTIONS
N/A

FOLLOW-UP

EXPECTED COURSE AND PROGNOSIS
• B_1 deficiency
  ○ Treated animals often recover rapidly and stand within 24 hours; vision may take 5–7 days to return.

○ Mild to significant neurologic impairment may remain depending on severity and duration of disease.
  ○ Death is likely in severe cases
• B_{12} deficiency: Rapid improvement with injectable treatment; oral treatment delays improvement for 7–10 days.

POSSIBLE COMPLICATIONS
• Aspiration pneumonia
• Self-trauma

CLIENT EDUCATION
Identify and modify causes and risk factors for these conditions.

PATIENT CARE
Provide a safe warm environment to avoid trauma and distress, accessible food and water; oral or parenteral nutrition may be needed in severely impaired animals.

PREVENTION
• B_1 deficiency
  ○ Avoid exposure to bracken fern and excessive amprolium.
  ○ Avoid feeding excessive concentrate, or moldy or molassed feeds.
  ○ Ensure animals are accustomed to roughage before weaning.
  ○ Supplement grain with brewer's yeast.
  ○ Sulfur intake of cattle should be ≤0.4%.
  ○ Milk replacer containing B vitamins.
• B_{12} deficiency
  ○ Provide 0.1–0.2 mg/kg DM Co in the ration (up to 1 mg/kg).
  ○ Top dressing fields with Co sulfate at 1.5 kg/hectare every 3–4 years.
  ○ Weekly to monthly drenching with Co sulfate.
  ○ Intraruminal soluble glass boluses or pellets release Co over several months.
  ○ Provide salt/mineral mixes with 0.1% Co (1 g Co carbonate per pound of salt).
  ○ Milk replacer containing Co (0.11 mg/kg) for dairy calves.

MISCELLANEOUS

ASSOCIATED CONDITIONS
• Sulfur-induced polioencephalomalacia
• Ovine white liver disease
• Phalaris staggers (Co is protective)

AGE-RELATED FACTORS
Pre-ruminant animals depend on dietary B_1 since the microflora of the forestomach is not developed. Liver reserves of B_{12} are lower in young animals.

ZOONOTIC POTENTIAL
N/A

PREGNANCY
N/A

BIOSECURITY
N/A

PRODUCTION MANAGEMENT
See "Prevention"

SYNONYMS
• B_1 deficiency: Cerebrocortical necrosis or forage poisoning
• B_{12} deficiency: White liver disease

ABBREVIATIONS
• DM = dry matter
• GI = gastrointestinal
• IM = intramuscular
• IV = intravenous
• MMA = methylmalonic acid
• PEM = polioencephalomalacia
• SC = subcutaneous
• WW = wet weight

SEE ALSO
• Brain Assessment and Dysfunction (see www.fiveminutevet.com/ruminant)
• Nutrition and Metabolic Diseases: Beef
• Nutrition and Metabolic Diseases: Small Ruminant
• Sulfur Toxicity

Suggested Reading
Amat S, Olkowski AA, Atila M, O'Neill TJ. A review of polioencephalomalacia in ruminants: Is the development of malacic lesions associated with excess sulphur intake independent of thiamine deficiency? Vet Med Anim Sci 2013, 1:1.
Apley MD. Consideration of evidence for therapeutic interventions in bovine polioencephalomalacia. Vet Clin North Am Food Anim Pract 2015, 31: 151–61, vii.
McDonald P, Edwards RA, Greenhalgh JFD, Morgan CA, Sinclair L, Wilkinson RG. The vitamin B complex. In: Animal Nutrition, 7th ed. Harlow, UK: Pearson Education, 2011, pp. 87–102.
Scott PR. Trace element deficiencies and metabolic disorders. In: Sheep Medicine. Boca Raton FL: CRC Press, 2015, pp. 329–46.
Suttle NF, Jones DG. Micronutrient imbalances: Cobalt deficiency. In: Aitken ID ed, Diseases of Sheep, 4th ed. Oxford, UK: Blackwell, 2007, 377–82.
Author Douglas C. Donovan
Consulting Editor Erica C. McKenzie

V

VITAMIN D DEFICIENCY/TOXICOSIS

BASICS

OVERVIEW
• Vitamin D is a group of compounds of which the most prominent forms are ergocalciferol (vitamin D_2) and cholecalciferol (vitamin D_3), which are supplied through the diet or by irradiation.
• Vitamin D_2 is derived from ergosterol (a plant steroid) and vitamin D_3 from cholecalciferol. The latter is produced from 7-dehydrocholesterol, a precursor exclusively present in animals. This cholesterol-derived provitamin is present in large amounts in the skin, the intestinal wall, and other tissues.
• Vitamin D precursors require ultraviolet (UV) irradiation (exposure to sunlight) to be activated. In ruminants, sufficient exposure to UV radiation results in adequate amounts of vitamin D and the lack of an absolute requirement of dietary intake.
• Vitamin D toxicity is the result of oversupplementation of enteral or parenteral formulations of vitamin D_3 or from ingestion of plants with vitamin D_2 activity.
• Risk of vitamin D deficiency is higher in the winter months and in animals kept in confinement systems.

INCIDENCE/PREVALENCE
N/A

GEOGRAPHIC DISTRIBUTION
• Higher risk for deficiency in northern latitudes during winter months.
• Non-iatrogenic toxicity is more likely where plants with high vitamin D_2 activity are present (*Cestrum diurnum, Solanum* spp., *Trisetum flavescens*).

SYSTEMS AFFECTED
Multisystemic

PATHOPHYSIOLOGY
• The main role of vitamin D is linked to calcium and phosphorus homeostasis through metabolic changes in the intestine, bone, and kidney.
• It also participates in various other processes through a hormonal action, with receptors being present in a variety of tissues.

Deficiency
The most common disease associated with hypovitaminosis D is the skeletal disorder of growing animals known as rickets, which is characterized by low levels of calcium and phosphorus in cartilage and bone matrices. In adults, the resultant condition is osteomalacia due to bone demineralization caused by decreased calcium and phosphorus in the bone matrix.

Toxicity
The deleterious effects of hypervitaminosis D are associated with hypercalcemia secondary to increased bone resorption and intestinal absorption, leading to generalized soft tissue calcification. In addition to calcification, inflammation, tissue necrosis, and pain are observed. Bone resorption results in skeletal demineralization and weakness.

HISTORICAL FINDINGS
• Hypovitaminosis D: Prolonged confinement with no vitamin D supplementation.
• Hypervitaminosis D: Parenteral administration of vitamin D or the presence of plants with high vitamin D_2 content, together with clinical signs.
• Use of vitamin D-containing rodenticides can result in accidental consumption and toxicity.

SIGNALMENT
The Jersey breed is suggested to be more susceptible to toxicosis.

PHYSICAL EXAMINATION FINDINGS
Deficiency
• Clinical signs of rickets include weak, curved, deformed long bones seen as bowing of the extremities, enlarged, painful carpal and tarsal joints with erosion of joint surfaces and difficult ambulation, thoracic deformation with rib beading, stiff gait and hindlimb dragging, deviation of the spine, and arching of the back.
• In adults, osteomalacia will eventually result in pathologic fractures, but earlier signs include decreased milk yields and reduced weight gain, reproductive failure, and an increased incidence of diseases associated with hypocalcemia.
• The skull, vertebrae, and epiphyses of long bones suffer the most severe demineralization, followed by the scapula, sternum and ribs, with diaphysis of long bones of the limbs being the most resistant.
• Additionally: Anorexia, stunted growth, gastrointestinal dysfunction, labored breathing, and sometimes seizures and tetany, which in some cases occur before skeletal abnormalities become apparent.
• An increase in stillbirths, congenital defects, and weak or deformed calves, lambs and kids may be recorded.

Toxicity
• Early on, affected animals show anorexia and dullness, weight loss, drop in production, and formation of a thick ocular discharge. This is followed by muscle stiffness leading to recumbency, respiratory distress, polyuric and subsequently anuric renal failure, in some cases accompanied by cutaneous emphysema. Cardiac arrhythmias may be present.
• Immediately preceding death, a rapid pounding pulse has been noted.
• Soft tissue mineralization results in the observed clinical signs (e.g., tendon and muscle calcification leads to stiffness and recumbency; renal calcification leads to polyuria, hypercalciuria, and renal failure).

GENETICS
N/A

CAUSES AND RISK FACTORS
Deficiency
The main cause and highest risk is lack of exposure to UV radiation.

Toxicity
• The main causes are iatrogenic due to overdosing of vitamin D supplements and consumption of plants with high vitamin D_2 content.
• For iatrogenic cases, injectable presentations pose a higher risk.
• High dietary calcium, which allows more calcium to be absorbed, and hypovitaminosis A exacerbate the likelihood of vitamin D toxicity.
• Pregnant cattle are more prone to toxicity.

DIAGNOSIS

DIFFERENTIAL DIAGNOSES
Deficiency
In rare cases, severe calcium deficiency in growing animals can lead to similar clinical manifestations.

Toxicity
All causes of hypercalcemia: Iatrogenic, hyperparathyroidism and neoplastic processes leading to hypercalcemia of malignancy.

CBC/BIOCHEMISTRY/URINALYSIS
Deficiency
Nonspecific

Toxicity
• Hypercalcemia is the hallmark of vitamin D toxicity. However, if the source of vitamin D has been removed, calcium levels may be normal.
• Hyperphosphatemia, hypercalciuria, isosthenuria, azotemia will be present depending on the stage and severity of disease.

OTHER LABORATORY TESTS
N/A

IMAGING
• Deficiency: Bone deformities, decreased bone density, and fractures can be confirmed radiographically.
• Toxicity: Calcification of fibroelastic layers in the periphery of blood vessels in all soft tissues and organs throughout the body can be radiographically identified.

OTHER DIAGNOSTIC PROCEDURES
• Deficiency: Low serum vitamin D concentrations with compatible history and clinical signs.
• Toxicity: Serum vitamin D concentrations >80 ng/mL along with biochemistry and urinalysis findings (see "CBC/Biochemistry/Urinalysis") and compatible history and clinical signs.

PATHOLOGIC FINDINGS

Deficiency
• Grossly, bone deformity and laxity are observed.
• Microscopically, a lack of mineralization of the cartilage and bone matrices, especially in cancellous bone, is present.

Toxicity
• Grossly, the lungs may fail to collapse because of dystrophic calcification, and soft tissue mineralization of the heart, aorta, kidney, stomach, lungs, tendons, and muscles can be readily identified.
• Histopathologically a high degree of osteoclastic activity may be seen. If dietary calcium is low, this will progress to demineralization and rarefaction of bone. Adequate or excessive dietary calcium will result in osteosclerosis and increased bone mineralization.
• Osteoblasts will produce a pattern of abundant basophilic matrix, characteristic for vitamin D toxicity.

TREATMENT

THERAPEUTIC APPROACH
• Deficiency is rapidly corrected with vitamin D supplementation. Provision of UV radiation with lamps or by limiting confinement.
• Toxicity is managed by prompt removal of the source of vitamin D. In addition, dietary calcium should be limited to reduce tissue calcium deposition.
• Adequate supportive care for weak and recumbent animals is essential and severe cases may require euthanasia.

MEDICATION

DRUGS OF CHOICE
• In deficiency, injectable vitamin D formulations are most effective.

• In toxicity, vitamin A can have some sparing effects on soft tissue mineralization, as can thyroxin, glucagon, and estrogen.

PRECAUTIONS
Oversupplementation with vitamin D is detrimental (see "Pathologic Findings").

CONTRAINDICATIONS
Vitamins D and A should not be given to meat-producing animals within 2 months of marketing.

POSSIBLE INTERACTIONS
N/A

FOLLOW-UP

EXPECTED COURSE AND PROGNOSIS
• Prognosis and duration of disease is dependent on severity and duration of exposure.
• Vitamin D supplementation rapidly correct deficits, but bone deformity and cartilage loss are irreversible.
• In toxicosis, withdrawal of the source of vitamin D stops disease progression after tissue storage depots are depleted.

POSSIBLE COMPLICATIONS
Overdosing of vitamin D is the primary complication of treating hypovitaminosis.

CLIENT EDUCATION
See "Prevention"

PATIENT CARE
Severely affected animals should be sold if suitable for human consumption, or euthanized.

PREVENTION
• Vitamin D deficiency and toxicity are prevented through adequate supplementation.
• Deficiency can be avoided by limiting animal confinement and increasing exposure to sunlight or supplementing when exposure is limited.

MISCELLANEOUS

ASSOCIATED CONDITIONS
• Hypercalcemia; stunted growth; bone deformities; myopathy; renal failure; reproductive failure; pathologic fractures.
• Enteque seco or Manchester wasting disease is caused by ingestion of 1,25-OH-cholecalciferol glycoside-containing plants, which induces hypervitaminosis D in grazing animals.

PREGNANCY
• Pregnant animals are at higher risk.
• Crucial for reproduction, embryogenesis, and fetal development.

ABBREVIATION
• UV= ultraviolet

SEE ALSO
• Acute Renal Failure
• Hypocalcemia: Bovine
• Hypocalcemia: Small Ruminant
• Postparturient Paresis (Hypocalcemia)

Suggested Reading
Dittmer KE, Thompson KG. Vitamin D metabolism and rickets in domestic animals: a review. Vet Pathol 2011, 48: 389–407.
Horst RL. Regulation of calcium and phosphorus homeostasis in the dairy cow. J Dairy Sci 1986, 69: 604–16.
National Research Council, Subcommittee on Vitamin Tolerance, Committee on Animal Nutrition, Board of Agriculture, National Research Council. Vitamin Tolerance of Animals. Washington DC: National Academy Press, 1987, pp. 11–30.
Mearns R, Scholes SF, Wessels M, Whitaker K, Strugnell B. Rickets in sheep flocks in northern England. Vet Rec 2008, 162: 98–9.

Author Carlos E. Medina-Torres
Consulting Editor Kaitlyn A. Lutz
Acknowledgment The author and book editors acknowledge the prior contribution of Daniel C. Rule.

V

VOMITOXIN

BASICS

OVERVIEW
• Vomitoxin or deoxynivalenol (DON) is a sesquiterpenoid compound with an epoxy group at C12–13 in the trichothecene structure, which is essential for toxicity.
• Vomitoxin is a type B trichothecene that is a common field contaminant of grains and forages produced by *Fusarium graminearum* (*Gibberella zeae*), *F. culmorum*, and other closely related fungi under wet, warm conditions at flowering and during plant growth.
• In addition to vomitoxin, the interaction of plant and fungi can generate other derivatives of DON, including acetyl-DON (3 and 15 ADON), glucoside-DON (D3G) and animal derived glucuronide metabolite (D3 and D15GA) that can be more or less toxic than DON.
• The majority of trichothecene exposures are subchronic to chronic in nature with low dietary DON concentrations in the feed and are associated with nutritional impairment, reduced production, and possible lowered immune responses, but DON is not associated with fatal disease.

INCIDENCE/PREVALENCE
• Vomitoxin is produced as a secondary metabolite by *Fusarium* fungi primarily in the field, with mold growth in equilibrium with relative humidity >90–95%.
• *Fusarium graminearum* and *F. culmorum* growth in cereal grains and corn are favored by warm, wet weather at anthesis and shortly after.
• Wet weather and warm days/cool evenings after pollination, delayed harvest, and hail damage can enhance fungal growth and mycotoxin production.

GEOGRAPHIC DISTRIBUTION
Worldwide in crops and forages

SYSTEMS AFFECTED
• Digestive
• Hemolymphatic

PATHOPHYSIOLOGY
Vomitoxin can cause cellular effects by targeting ribosomes and causing ribotoxic stress. The suggested mechanism of ribosome binding is by chemical reactivity of the vomitoxin epoxide moiety with nucleotides forming nucleic acids (RNA and DNA). However, the precise nature of the chemical reaction of DON binding to rRNA is not known. It is known that binding of vomitoxin to rRNA can cause their cleavage and activation of several cellular signaling pathways affecting cell functions and possibly initiate cell apoptosis. DON can affect the function of intestinal, immune, and brain cells.

SIGNALMENT
• Potential effects can occur in ruminants ingesting moldy grains, forages, and other feedstuffs.
• Dairy cows are more sensitive to adverse effects, which may be due to the higher stress levels that dairy cows undergo. Dairy have higher levels of dry matter intake that can result in faster rumen turnover rate and perhaps less rumen microbial degradation of vomitoxin.

PHYSICAL EXAMINATION FINDINGS
• Vomitoxin has been associated with reduced feed intake and feed efficiency, and perhaps diarrhea and lowered milk production. However, definite cause and effect relationships have not been established in ruminants for loss in milk production.
• Beef cattle and sheep appear to tolerate a higher concentration of DON in feed without measurable effects.

CAUSES AND RISK FACTORS
• The toxic principle is DON.
• Ingestion of moldy feedstuffs containing significant concentrations of vomitoxin can lead to clinical effects. Pre-ruminants, which lack rumen microbial metabolism, and dairy cows, which are more highly stressed, are more at risk.

DIAGNOSIS

DIFFERENTIAL DIAGNOSES
Inadequate nutrition, inadequate rumen microbial population, other causes of mild gastroenteritis and diarrhea (e.g., endotoxins, poisonous plants, petroleum hydrocarbons).

CBC/BIOCHEMISTRY/URINALYSIS
Possible hypoproteinemia, mild anemia, leukopenia

OTHER LABORATORY TESTS
Detection of vomitoxin in feed by liquid or gas chromatography-mass spectrometry, gas chromatography, and other reliable methods validated for the feed matrix.

OTHER DIAGNOSTIC PROCEDURES
Laboratory analysis of feed for mycotoxins

PATHOLOGIC FINDINGS
Very high, acute concentrations of vomitoxin could result in enteritis, perhaps hemorrhagic.

TREATMENT

THERAPEUTIC APPROACH
• Stop feeding vomitoxin-contaminated feed or reduce exposure to vomitoxin concentrations associated with no clinical signs in ruminants (see regulatory guidelines).
• Provide clean feed and supportive fluids if necessary.

• Animals generally recover quickly and residues in milk and tissues are of minimal concern because of rapid metabolism and excretion.

MEDICATIONS

DRUGS OF CHOICE
N/A

FOLLOW-UP

EXPECTED COURSE AND PROGNOSIS
Recovery is anticipated with a good prognosis.

PREVENTION
• Follow regulatory or guidance levels for vomitoxin in animal feed.
• In the United States, the Food and Drug Administration issued advisory levels for DON in feed for cattle that "would not appear to present an animal or public health hazard." Advisory levels of 10 ppm DON on grains and grain by-products (88% DM) and 30 ppm in distiller's grains and brewer's grains (88% DM) destined for ruminating beef and feedlot cattle >4 months and ruminating dairy cattle older than 4 months, with the added recommendations that the TOTAL RATION for ruminating beef and feedlot cattle >4 months NOT exceed 10 ppm DON, and the total ration for ruminating dairy cattle >4 months NOT exceed 5 ppm DON.
• The advisory level for ruminants <4 months and sheep, goats (and other ruminants) is 5 ppm DON on grains and grain by-products with the added recommendation that these ingredients NOT exceed 40% of the diet. Hence the DON concentrations should be <2 ppm in the final ration.
• In the US, mycotoxin binders have not been approved by the Food and Drug Administration. The use of agents to "bind" vomitoxin in ruminants is equivocal.

MISCELLANEOUS

ASSOCIATED CONDITIONS
• The interaction of plant and fungi can generate other derivatives of DON, including acetyl-DON (3 and 15 ADON), glucoside-DON (D3G), and animal derived glucuronide metabolite (D3 and D15GA) that can be more or less toxic than DON.
• Little research has been done in ruminants with these DON derivatives.

AGE-RELATED FACTORS
Older animals with a functioning rumen capable of metabolizing vomitoxin to the

(CONTINUED)

relatively nontoxic DOM-1 are less affected than pre-ruminants.

PREGNANCY
N/A

BIOSECURITY
Avoid feeding moldy feedstuffs. Analyze suspect feed for vomitoxin prior to use and utilize appropriate guidelines.

PRODUCTION MANAGEMENT
• Stop feeding mycotoxin-contaminated feed or reduce exposure to concentrations associated with no clinical signs in ruminants when regulatory guidelines are available.
• Dilution with noncontaminated feedstuffs is one possibility, but this may not be acceptable on a regulatory basis.

ABBREVIATIONS
• DOM-1 = de-epoxydeoxynivalenol
• DON = deoxynivalenol

SEE ALSO
• Abomasal Ulceration
• Emesis
• Indigestion
• Mycotoxins

Suggested Reading
Food & Drug Administration. Guidance for Industry and FDA: Advisory levels for deoxynivalenol (DON) in finished wheat products for human consumption and grains and grain by-products used for Animal Feed. June 29, 2010.
Gallo A, Giubert G, Frisvad J, Bertuzzi T, Nielsen KF. Review on mycotoxin issues in ruminants: Occurrence in forages, effects of mycotoxin ingestion on health status and animal performance and practical strategies to counteract their negative effects. Toxins 2014, 7: 3057–111.

Jouany J-P, Diaz DE. Effects of mycotoxins in ruminants. In: Diaz DE ed, The Mycotoxin Blue Book. Nottingham, UK: Nottingham University Press, 2005, pp. 295–322.
Maresca M. From the gut to the brain: Journey and pathophysiological effects of the food-associated trichothecene mycotoxin deoxynivalenol. Toxins 2013, 5: 784–820.
Mostrom MS, Jacobsen BJ. Ruminant mycotoxicosis. Vet Clin North Am Food Anim Pract 2011, 27: 315–44.

Internet Resources
http://www.fda.gov/downloads/Food/ GuidanceRegulation/UCM217558.pdf
Author Michelle Mostrom
Consulting Editor Christopher C.L. Chase
Acknowledgment The author and book editors acknowledge the prior contribution of Heidi Coker.

V

VULVITIS

BASICS

• Vulvitis is relatively common in ruminants where it is often associated with vaginitis (vulvovaginitis). • It should be noted that many of the disorders classified as vulvitis are more correctly an inflammation of the vestibule. • Ruminants and camelidae have a very simple vulvar anatomy, and trauma associated with coitus or parturition along with poor perineal conformation are the most common disorders of the vulva proper. Other lesions specific to the vulva are associated with chemical irritation, trauma, and microbial agents.

INCIDENCE/PREVALENCE
Common in all ruminants but most cases have little long-term clinical significance.

GEOGRAPHIC DISTRIBUTION
Worldwide

SYSTEMS AFFECTED
Reproductive

PATHOPHYSIOLOGY
• The vestibule contains subepithelial foci of inflammatory cells, activated more or less constantly by local flora (commensal and pathogenic). It is not unusual to see evidence of hyperemia and lymphoid proliferation, which defines granular vulvitis (granular venereal disease or vestibulitis). • Necrotic vulvitis associated with severe edema and tissue sloughing may result from chemical irritation, allergic reactions, or local infection with anaerobic bacteria. • A variety of infectious agents have been associated with the caudal reproductive tract including *Ureaplasma diversum*, *Mycoplasma* spp., *Trueperella pyogenes*, *Streptococcus* spp., *Staphylococcus* spp., *E. coli*, *H. somni* as well as the IBR/IPV and contagious ecthyma viruses. • Enzootic ovine vulvitis is the female analog of pizzle rot in the ram. It is associated with high protein diets and local infection with *Corynebacterium renale*. • Ulcerative vulvitis and balanoposthitis in sheep has been attributed to local infection with a variety of bacterial agents (*Mycoplasma* spp., *Histophilus* spp., *T. pyogenes*).

GENETICS
N/A

HISTORICAL FINDINGS
N/A

SIGNALMENT
Potentially all ruminant and camelid species

PHYSICAL EXAMINATION FINDINGS
• Systemic signs of disease are usually absent. • Edema, ulceration, vestibular lymphoid hyperplasia, and mucopurulent discharge are most frequently seen. • Vestibular and vulvar hyperemia and edema. • Mucoid or mucopurulent discharge. • Ulceration of vulvar and/or perineal skin. • Pneumovagina.

CAUSES AND RISK FACTORS
• Presence of pathogenic microorganisms • High protein diet in sheep and goats • Parturient or coital trauma • Poor perineal conformation and perivulvar tissue folds in ewes

DIAGNOSIS

DIFFERENTIAL DIAGNOSES
• Transmissible fibropapillomas (cattle) • Neoplasia (e.g., fibroma, squamous cell carcinoma) • Trauma (coital, parturient, predation) • Ectopic mammary tissue (doe) • External parasites (mange in sheep and tick infestation in camels) • Contagious ecthyma (sheep and goats) • Cystic vestibular (Bartholin's) glands • Tubercular Gartner's ducts

CBC/BIOCHEMISTRY/URINALYSIS
N/A

OTHER LABORATORY TESTS
Culture and sensitivity, viral isolation, or molecular diagnostics may be indicated if infective agents are suspected of causing an economically significant problem.

IMAGING
N/A

OTHER DIAGNOSTIC PROCEDURES
Speculum examination and visual observation of vulva is essential.

TREATMENT

THERAPEUTIC APPROACH
• Treatment is often unnecessary, especially with milder cases of granular venereal disease. • Treatment for suspected clostridial infections when indicated.

SURGICAL CONSIDERATIONS AND TECHNIQUES
Surgery for wounds or conformational defects may be indicated.

MEDICATIONS

DRUGS OF CHOICE
N/A

CONTRAINDICATIONS
Appropriate milk and meat withdrawal times must be followed for all compounds administered to food-producing animals.

PRECAUTIONS
N/A

POSSIBLE INTERACTIONS
N/A

FOLLOW-UP

EXPECTED COURSE AND PROGNOSIS
Usually good

POSSIBLE COMPLICATIONS
• Occasionally, severe necrotic vulvovaginitis may lead to vaginal stenosis. • In sheep, fly strike may lead to complications.

CLIENT EDUCATION
N/A

PATIENT CARE
N/A

PREVENTION
• Avoid feeding of excess protein. • Minimize dystocia prevalence and provide appropriate, gentle and sanitary obstetric assistance.

MISCELLANEOUS

ASSOCIATED CONDITIONS
Retained placenta, puerperal metritis, or physical injury to the vulva

AGE-RELATED FACTORS
GVD is seen most commonly in heifers in their first or second natural breeding season.

ZOONOTIC POTENTIAL
Care must be taken in the collection of laboratory samples and the diagnosis/treatment of affected animals, especially if TB or contagious ecthyma (orf) are suspected.

PREGNANCY
N/A

BIOSECURITY
• Isolation and quarantine of new stock entering the herd or flock. • Treat and or cull new animals for disease conditions prior to herd introduction. • GVD appears to be easily and rapidly spread, and it varies considerably in severity.

PRODUCTION MANAGEMENT
N/A

ABBREVIATIONS
• GVD = granular venereal disease • IBR = infectious bovine rhinotracheitis • IPV = infectious pustular vulvovaginitis • TB = tuberculosis

SEE ALSO
• Infectious Pustular Vulvovaginitis • Ureaplasma • Vaginitis

Suggested Reading
McEntee K. Reproductive Pathology of Domestic Animals. San Diego: Academic Press, 1990, p. 201.
Authors Harry Momont and Celina Checura
Consulting Editor Ahmed Tibary
Acknowledgment The authors and book editors acknowledge the prior contribution of Peter Chenoweth.

WATER BUFFALO DISEASES

BASICS

OVERVIEW
• Water buffalo are hardier than cattle to resist disease and also can thrive in a hot and humid environment.
• Their weak thermoregulatory mechanism means they need to wallow and be sprayed with water in hot weather.
• Water buffalo are susceptible to most diseases and parasites affecting cattle. Treatment and vaccination protocols are generally similar between the two species.
• High yielding buffalo are more prone to reproductive and metabolic diseases than low yielders.
• Mortality among buffalo calves is higher than cow calves because they are more susceptible to ascariasis and calf scour due to colibacillosis and salmonellosis.
• The wallowing habit of water buffalo also helps transmission of waterborne diseases.
• Tail necrosis is a common medical condition in water buffalo.
• Reproductive problems such as infertility, repeat breeding, dystocia, retained placenta, prolapse of uterus and vagina, and metabolic diseases are more common in stall-fed animals than in free range systems.
• Mange mites, dermatophyte infection, Degnala disease, alopecia, and ulceration are common skin disease conditions.

INCIDENCE/PREVALENCE
• Neoscariasis: Very common problem with an incidence of >30% in humid conditions.
• Tapeworms: Reported at an incidence of 15% in some tropical environments (*Moniezia* spp.).

GEOGRAPHIC DISTRIBUTION
• Some 42 countries; 97% of water buffalo are in Asian countries.
• There are two general types of water buffalo: the swamp buffalo (*Bubalus carabanesis*) which is found from the Philippines to as far west as India; and the river buffalo or domestic Asian buffalo (*Bubalus bubalis*) which is found farther west from India to Egypt and Europe.

PATHOPHYSIOLOGY
See specific diseases

SYSTEMS AFFECTED
All systems, depending on the disease process

HISTORICAL FINDINGS
Vary depending on the disease process. Some disease may present as an outbreak; others may affect individual animals.

SIGNALMENT
The swamp buffalo (*Bubalus carabanesis*) and the river buffalo (*Bubalus bubalis*)

PHYSICAL EXAMINATION FINDINGS
Vary depending on the complaint and the disease (see "Differential Diagnoses").

GENETICS
N/A

CAUSES AND RISK FACTORS
See "Differential diagnoses"

DIAGNOSIS

DIFFERENTIAL DIAGNOSES

Skin Diseases
• Yoke gall—chronic injury to the ligamentum nuchae caused by the continuous pressure of a yoke (collar) on the buffalo's neck
• Cutaneous filariasis (*Parafilaria bovicola*)
• Cutaneous onchocerciasis—cutaneous lesions in the dermis, most apparent in the xiphoid region (*Onchocerca* spp.)
• Cowpox as well as the buffalo poxvirus
• Mange—three types—psoroptic (*Psoroptes natalensis*), sarcoptic (*Sarcoptes scabiei* var. *bubalus*), and demodectic (*Demodex bovis*)
• Dermatomycosis
• Tail necrosis—several causes have been postulated—*Corynebacterium bovis*, fatty acid deficiency, and microfilaria
• Lumpy skin disease
• Warts

Bacterial, Viral, and Protozoal Diseases
• Hemorrhagic septicemia/pasteurellosis—outbreak occurs in summer season
• Anaplasmosis
• BVD/mucosal disease
• Anthrax—sporadic in nature
• Tuberculosis
• Rabies—a very danger zoonotic disease
• Blackquarter
• Foreign body syndrome (similar to TRP)
• Brucellosis—cause late abortion
• Foot and mouth disease
• Johne's disease
• Rinderpest—eradicated from most countries of the world
• Bovine ephemeral fever—seen in hot summer and rainy season
• Malignant catarrhal fever
• Toxoplasmosis
• Nephritis, hydronephrosis, and renal calcification
• Piroplasmosis—transmitted by tick
• Pleuropneumonia (mycoplasmal)
• Hypophosphatemia
• Peste des petits ruminants—very common in small ruminants

Parasitic Diseases
• Ascarid infection—heavy losses of young buffalo calves caused by *Toxocara vitulorum*.
• Strongyles—adult buffalo are resistant.
• Echinococcosis/hydatid cyst disease (*Echinococcus granulosum*).
• Coccidiosis (*Eimeria* spp.).
• Filarial nematodiasis.
• Trypanosomiasis—buffalo more susceptible to *Trypanosoma evansi* than cattle.

• Pediculosis—caused by the sucking louse (*Hematopinus tuberculatus*).
• Babesia (*Babesia argentina* and *B. bigemini*)—secondary to infection by ticks *Boophilus microplus* and *Hyalomma anatolicum*.
• Lungworm—infestation of the respiratory tract by *Dictyocaulus viviparous*.
• Cutaneous filariasis (*Parafilaria bovicola*).
• Cutaneous onchocerciasis—cutaneous lesions in the dermis, most apparent in the xiphoid region (*Onchocerca* spp.).
• Leeches.
• Ticks—buffalo are resistant to ticks.
• Tapeworms—reported at an incidence of 15% in some tropical environments (*Moniezia* spp.).
• Ectoparasitism—a primary ectoparasite in Australia and Southeast Asia is the buffalo fly (*Siphona* spp.). Lice and mites may infest buffalo all year, but primarily during the winter season. Mosquitoes and flies affect buffalo during hot/humid weather.
• Mange—psoroptic (*Psoroptes natalensis*), sarcoptic (*Sarcoptes scabiei var. bubalus*), and demodectic (*Demodax bovis*).
• Ophthalmic parasites—conjunctivitis caused by *Thelazia* spp. is common.
• Several moth species feed nocturnally on buffalo lacrimal secretions in Asia.
• Syngamosis (*Syngamus laryngeus*).
• Hepatic flukes—*Fasciola hepatica* and/or *F. gigantica* are very common worldwide. Snails of *Lymnaea* spp. are common vectors.
• Intestinal flukes—common flukes are *Cotylophoron cotylophorum*, *Calicophoron* spp., *Paramphistomum* spp., *Olveria* spp., and *Ceylonocotyle* spp. Fluke infestations (intestinal and hepatic) are the most common cause of mortality in adult water buffalo maintained in tropical Asian climates.
• Biliary leach—*Gigantocotyle explanatum* causes calf loss.
• Sarcosporidosis.
• Schistosomiasis—can cause enteritis in young buffalo calves <2 years of age.
• Theileriosis.

Reproductive Diseases
• Anestrus—nutritional, anatomic, hereditary, and functional. Anestrus has its highest incidence during the hot season. Small, hard, and inactive ovaries generally are present.
• Subactive/inactive ovaries—secondary to nutritional deficiency.
• Excessive follicular atresia with a failure of maturation and ovulation.
• Cystic ovaries.
• Small, inactive ovaries—often related to a low-phosphorus diet.
• Persistent CL.
• Encapsulation of ovaries.
• Salpingitis.
• Cervicitis.
• Metritis.
• Pyometra.
• Endometritis.

W

• Vaginitis.
• Iatrogenic reproductive problems commonly occur when artificial insemination programs reflect poor technical abilities and rough handling.
• The incidence of dystocia, abortions, and retained placenta is similar to that in cattle.

Management-Related Issues
• Respiratory infections—primarily due to poor management
• Diarrhea—found mainly in calves
• Decreased milk production
• Lameness
• Iatrogenic infertility
• Bloat/tympany
• Mastitis

CBC/BIOCHEMSTRY/URINALYSIS
Similar changes as in other ruminants for specific disease processes.

OTHER LABORATORY TESTS
Serology, bacteriology, virology, and parasitology tests have been established for some diseases as in other ruminants.

IMAGING
Varies according to diseases process. Ultrasonography is important in reproductive medicine (similar to bovine reproductive ultrasonography).

TREATMENT
THERAPEUTIC APPROACH
See specific disorders in the bovine

SURGICAL CONSIDERATIONS AND TECHNIQUES
See specific disorders in the bovine

MEDICATIONS
DRUGS OF CHOICE
See specific disorders in the bovine

CONTRAINDICATIONS
Appropriate milk and meat withdrawal times must be followed for all compounds administered to food-producing animals.

PRECAUTIONS
N/A

POSSIBLE INTERACTIONS
N/A

FOLLOW-UP
EXPECTED COURSE AND PROGNOSIS
See specific disorders in the bovine

POSSIBLE COMPLICATIONS
See specific disorders in the bovine

CLIENT EDUCATION
See specific disorders

PATIENT CARE
See specific disorders

PREVENTION
See specific disorders

MISCELLANEOUS
ASSOCIATED CONDITIONS
See specific disorders

AGE-RELATED FACTORS
• Buffalo calf deaths are a significant problem and impact profitability.
• Diarrhea found mainly in calves.
• Adult buffalo are resistant to Strongyles.
• Schistosomiasis can cause enteritis in young buffalo calves <2 years of age.

ZOONOTIC POTENTIAL
Zoonotic diseases are similar to those described for cattle.

PREGNANCY
Abortion-causing diseases are similar to those described for cattle.

BIOSECURITY
• See specific disease.
• Isolation and quarantine of new stock entering the herd.
• Treat and or cull new animals for disease conditions prior to herd introduction.

PRODUCTION MANAGEMENT
Water buffalo are susceptible to most diseases and parasites affecting cattle. Poor ventilation, insufficient sanitation, inappropriate reproductive management, and poor quality nutrition programs all impact production of water buffalo.

ABBREVIATIONS
• BVD = bovine viral diarrhea
• CL = corpus luteum
• TRP = traumatic reticuloperitonitis

SEE ALSO
• Biosecurity: Beef Cow/Calf (see www.fiveminutevet.com/ruminant)
• Biosecurity: Dairy (see www.fiveminutevet.com/ruminant)
• Parasite Control Programs: Beef
• Parasite Control Programs: Dairy
• Vaccination Programs: Beef Cattle
• Vaccination Programs: Dairy Cattle
• Water Buffalo Parasite Issues

Suggested Reading
Govindarajan R, Koteeswaran A, Venugopalan AT, et al. Isolation of pestes des petits ruminants virus from an outbreak in Indian buffalo (*Bubalus bubalis*). Vet Rec 1997, 141: 573–4.
Gundran RS, More SJ. Health and growth of water-buffalo calves in Nueva Ecija, the Philippines. Prev Vet Med 1999, 40: 87–100.
Nanda AS, Brar PS, Prabhakar S. Enhancing reproductive performance in dairy buffalo: major constraints and achievements. Reprod Suppl 2003, 61: 27–36.
Oswin Perera BM. Reproduction in water buffalo: comparative aspects and implications for management. J Reprod Fertil Suppl 1999, 54: 157–68.
Selim SA. Oedematous skin disease of buffalo in Egypt. J Vet Med B Infect Dis Vet Public Health 2001, 48: 241–58.
Author Egendra Kumar Shrestha
Consulting Editor Ahmed Tibary
Acknowledgment The author and book editors acknowledge the prior contribution of Ravi Kumar Putluru.

WATER BUFFALO MANAGEMENT

BASICS

OVERVIEW
• Buffalo is one of major livestock species of some Asian countries such as India, Nepal, Pakistan, and China generally kept for milk, meat, manure, hide, and draft purposes. Dairy buffalo production is very popular in the Caucasian countries, Asia, and Egypt.
• In recent years mozzarella cheese made from buffalo milk has become very popular in Italy, in other European countries, and also in the United States.
• Besides milk and meat purposes, buffalo are extensively used to plough fields, cultivate crops, pump water, and haul carts and draft boats. They are also used to carry people, thresh grain, press sugar cane, haul logs, and so on.
• World buffalo population in 2008 has been estimated at 185.29 million spread over some 42 countries; 97% of water buffalo are in Asian countries.
• India has the largest population of buffalo, approx.105.1 million (56.7 % of the world population), followed by Pakistan 29.0 million (15.65 %), and China 23.27 million (12.55%). Bangladesh and Nepal have positive growth with annual growth of 5.7 1% and 2.1% respectively.

INCIDENCE/PREVALENCE
N/A

GEOGRAPHIC DISTRIBUTION
Asian countries such as India, Nepal, Pakistan, and China, and also in the Caucasian countries and Egypt.

SYSTEMS AFFECTED
N/A

PATHOPHYSIOLOGY
N/A

HISTORICAL FINDINGS
N/A

SIGNALMENT
• *Bubalus carabanensis* (swamp buffalo) and *Bubalus bubalis* (river buffalo).
• Body size of buffalo varies from small breeds of approx. 250 kg to heavy breeds up to 1,000 kg.
• They have black and dark gray body coat color with little hair. Therefore, the skin absorbs heat easily and has few sweat glands.
• The horns spread outward and upward, measuring up to 7 ft (2 m) across.
• First calves are usually produced at about 24–36 months of age, but recent studies show that with adequate nutrition and good management, buffalo can reach puberty at about the same age as cattle (18 months).
• They generally produce two calves every 3 years.

• The gestation period for buffalo is about the same as for cattle, 287 days.
• Peak calving season is mid-June to mid-September in Northern India and Nepal while in southern parts it is January and February.
• Birthweight of buffalo calves is generally 20–25 kg.

PHYSICAL EXAMINATION FINDINGS
N/A

GENETICS
• Buffalo are classified into two groups: swamp buffalo (*Bubalus carabanesis*) and river buffalo (*Bubalus bubalis*).
• Chromosome number of river buffalo is 50 (25 pairs) and swamp buffalo is 48 (24 pairs).
• The swamp buffalo are most common in Southeast Asian countries and generally kept for draft power for rice cultivation. They have very low milk yield. Recently they have been employed for meat production.
• The river buffalo are the most common type of buffalo in India, Pakistan, Nepal, Bulgaria, Hungary, Turkey, Italy, and Egypt. They are also found in Brazil and Caucasia.
• River buffalo have been used for milk production and some breeds such as Murrah, Nili-Ravi and Surti are used for dairy production only.

CAUSES AND RISK FACTORS
N/A

DIAGNOSIS
N/A

TREATMENT
N/A

MEDICATIONS
N/A

FOLLOW-UP
N/A

MISCELLANEOUS

ASSOCIATED CONDITIONS
N/A

AGE RELATED FACTORS
N/A

ZOONOTIC POTENTIAL
N/A

PREGNANCY
N/A

BIOSECURITY
N/A

PRODUCTION MANAGEMENT

Economic Considerations
• For thousands of years, this animal species has provided draft power, milk, meat, and hide to millions of people, mainly small-scale farmers.
• Buffalo are used for a variety of agricultural operations such as plowing paddy fields, lifting water from wells, and transporting farm produce to nearby markets.
• More than 5% of world milk comes from buffalo and 95% of it comes from Asia.
• India is the world's largest buffalo milk producer with about 35% of milk animals producing almost 70% of the total Indian milk.
• Buffalo feeding and management is cheaper than cattle feeding and management, and buffalo farmers also get a 30–50% higher price for their milk.
• Buffalo milk contains more total solids (16%) compared with the solids (12–14%) found in cow's milk. Buffalo milk butterfat content is usually 6–8% compared with domestic dairy cow butterfat levels of 3–5%.
• Buffalo farming is one of the substantial secondary income sources for small farmers in Asia. Usually women take care of buffalo feeding, milking, and selling of milk.
• Water buffalo offer a major source of meat in Asia. The buffalo meat industry is expanding.
• Asia produces 91–92% of the world's total buffalo meat, with India being the world's largest buffalo meat producer followed by Pakistan, China, Nepal, and Thailand.
• Carcass characteristics of buffalo are similar to domestic cattle with the average dressing percentage of 53%.
• In Nepal and some Indian states, slaughtering of cows is prohibited because of Hinduism. So the salvage value of buffalo is higher than cattle.
• Water buffalo also provide a major work force in Asia, and it is probably the most adaptable and versatile of all work animals.

Specific Considerations
• Buffalo require more drinking water, more grazing field area, and more standing space than cows.
• Because of their poorly developed thermoregulatory mechanisms, buffalo need to wallow or need to be sprayed during hot weather in order to keep their bodies cool.
• Their housing generally requires higher roofing to improve ventilation and to protect from direct heat during summer months.

W

• Buffalo need stronger barriers than those used for cattle, and the wires should be closer together and lower to the ground to avoid having them lift fences up with their horns.
• They must be handled quietly and calmly because of their timid nature.

Management
• The classic buffalo in Asia belongs to a small farm, and millions of water buffalo are managed in intensive "backyard" systems. Herds of 2–50 animals are owned by small or marginal farmers; close to urban centers herds of 20–50 are common.
• In the United States, Brazil, Venezuela, and Australia, water buffalo are managed on rangelands.
• They require more drinking water and more standing space than cows.
• Because of their poorly developed thermoregulatory mechanisms, buffalo need to wallow or need sprinklers during hot weather in order to keep their bodies cool.
• Their housing generally requires higher roofing to improve ventilation.
• Buffalo need stronger barriers than those used for cattle, and the wires should be closer together and lower to the ground to avoid having them lift the fences up with their horns.

SYNONYMS
N/A

ABBREVIATIONS
N/A

SEE ALSO
• Biosecurity: Beef Cow/Calf (see www.fiveminutevet.com/ruminant)
• Biosecurity: Dairy (see www.fiveminutevet.com/ruminant)
• Nutrition and Metabolic Diseases: Water Buffalo
• Parasite Control Programs: Beef
• Parasite Control Programs: Dairy
• Vaccination Programs: Beef Cattle
• Vaccination Programs: Dairy Cattle
• Water Buffalo Diseases
• Water Buffalo Parasite Issues
• Water Buffalo: Reproduction

Suggested Reading
Cassiano LAP, Mariante A da S, McManus C, Marques JRF, da Costa NA. Phenotypic characterization of national Brazilian buffalo breeds and Baio type. Pesq Agropec Bras 2003, 38: 1337–42.
Chandra BS, Das N. Behaviour of Indian river buffaloes (*Bubalus bubalis*) during short-haul road transportation. Vet Rec 2001, 148: 314–15.
McCool C. Buffalo and Bali cattle—exploiting their reproductive behaviour and physiology. Trop Anim Health Prod 1992, 24: 165–72.
Nanda AS, Brar PS, Prabhakar S. Enhancing reproductive performance in dairy buffalo: major constraints and achievements. Reprod Suppl 2003, 61: 27–36.
Oswin Perera BM. Reproduction in water buffalo: comparative aspects and implications for management. J Reprod Fertil Suppl 1999, 54: 157–68.
Thomas CS, Svennersten-Sjaunja K, Bhosrekar MR, Bruckmaier RM. Mammary cisternal size, cisternal milk and milk ejection in Murrah buffaloes. J Dairy Res 2004, 71: 162–8.
Author Egendra Kumar Shrestha
Consulting Editor Ahmed Tibary
Acknowledgment The author and book editors acknowledge the prior contribution of Ravi Kumar Putluru and Scott R.R. Haskell.

W

WATER BUFFALO PARASITE ISSUES

BASICS

OVERVIEW
• Water buffalo belong to the family Bovidae, Subfamily Bovinae, and the genus *Bubalus*.
• Buffalo are important multipurpose farm animals in the Indian subcontinent, contributing significantly to meat and milk production.
• The total population of buffalo in the world is 151.5 million, of which 96.6 million are found in Asia.
• Parasites including both ectoparasites and endoparasites are a major cause for decreased health and productivity as well as mortality.

INCIDENCE/PREVALENCE
Variable by region. Generally higher in Asia.

GEOGRAPHIC DISTRIBUTION
Potentially worldwide depending on favourable environment

SYSTEMS AFFECTED
Multisystemic

PATHOPHYSIOLOGY
Dependent on parasite species involved

HISTORICAL FINDINGS
Important history to determine includes age of affected animals, duration of onset of symptoms, past infections, feed quality, animal movement, grazing pattern, and treatment history.

SIGNALMENT
Young buffalo are more susceptible to parasitic infection than calves and adult buffalo.

PHYSICAL EXAMINATION FINDINGS
• Internal parasites cause weakness and debility, decrease in production, unthriftiness, decreased immune function, dry skin, brittle and coarse hair, diarrhea, and loss of body condition.
• External parasites cause annoyance, uneasiness, weakness, loss of production, hair loss, skin wounds, and dry skin.

GENETICS
N/A

CAUSES AND RISK FACTORS
Ectoparasites
• Louse (*Haematopinus tuberculatus*)
• Leech (*Hirudinaria manillensis*)
• Flies (*Siphona* spp.)
• Mange (psoroptic, *Psoroptes natalensis*; sarcoptic, *Sarcoptes scabiei* var. *bubalus*; and demodectic, *Demodex bovis*)

Endoparasites
Nematodes
• *Haemonchus* spp. (abomasum)
• *Strongyloides* spp. (small intestine)
• *Capillaria* spp. (small intestine)
• *Oesophagostomum* spp. (large intestine)
• *Trichostrongylus* spp. (small intestine)
• *Toxocara vitulorum* (small intestine)

• *Nematodirus* spp. (small intestine)
• *Dictyocaulus viviparus* (respiratory system)
• *Thelazia rhodesii* (eye)
• *Cooperia* spp. (small intestine)
• *Setaria digitata* (peritoneal cavity)
• *Ostertagia circumcincta* (abomasum)
• *Gongylonema pulchrum* (esophageal/buccal mucosa)
• *Onchocera gibsoni* (aorta)
• *Dicrocoelium dendriticum* (bile duct)
Trematodes
• *Fasciola* spp. (liver)
• *Paramphistomum* spp. (rumen)
• *Schistosoma* spp. (blood flukes)
• *Cotylophoron* spp. (small intestine)
Cestodes
• *Moniezia expansa* (small intestine)
• *Echinococcus* spp. (cysts in muscles and organs)
Protozoans
• *Toxoplasma gondii* (intestine)
• *Trypanosoma* spp. (bloodstream)
• *Sarcocystis* spp. (muscles)
• *Theileria* spp. (RBC, lymphocytes)
• *Babesia* spp. (RBC)
• *Anaplasma* spp. (RBC)
• *Eimeria zuernii* (intestine)
• *Cryptosporidium* (intestinal epithelium)
• *Neospora caninum* (tachyzoites are found intracellularly in neural cells, macrophages, fibroblasts, vascular endothelial cells, hepatocytes and muscular cells of myocardium and placenta. Bradyzoites are found in tissue cysts in the brain, spinal cord, and retina).

Risk Factors
• Cattle, deer, pigs, sheep
• Feces of dogs, wolves, or coyotes
• Feeding on infested pasture, usually early in the grazing period
• Inadequate or inappropriate use of anthelmintics and preventive pasturing practices

DIAGNOSIS

DIFFERENTIAL DIAGNOSES
Metabolic diseases, dermatologic diseases

CBC/BIOCHEMISTRY/URINALYSIS
Diagnosis of all those parasites found in the liver can be aided by examining the hepatic enzymes GLDH, GGT, and AST.

OTHER LABORATORY TESTS
• Endoparasites:
   ○ Fecal sample examination and ELISA are mainly used for diagnosing nematodes.
   ○ Muscle biopsy, ELISA, PCR (copro-DNA assay), indirect immunofluorescence, indirect hemagglutination, immunoblotting, latex agglutination and, rarely, complement fixation tests are used for cestode diagnosis.

   ○ Fecal sample examination, ELISA, and PCR techniques are used for trematodes.
• Protozoans: Microhematocrit centrifugation technique (MHCT), ELISA.

IMAGING
Imaging techniques such as X-ray, magnetic resonance imaging (MRI) scan, computed tomography (CT) scan, ultrasonographic imaging, positron emission tomography (PET) combined with CT, and single photon emission computed tomography can also be used to diagnose the presence of parasites.

OTHER DIAGNOSTIC PROCEDURES
Ectoparasites: Skin scraping followed by microscopic examination

PATHOLOGIC FINDINGS
N/A

TREATMENT

THERAPEUTIC APPROACH
Therapeutic treatments with anthelmintics, antiprotozoals and ectoparasiticides are effective.

SURGICAL CONSIDERATIONS AND TECHNIQUES
Surgical removal of cysts could be done but this is complicated and is not practiced.

MEDICATIONS

DRUGS OF CHOICE
For Protozoans
Metronidazole (25–30 mg/kg body weight/day in divided doses, PO, at 20 mg/kg BW/day in divided doses, IV).

For Hemoprotozoans
Diminazine aceturate (0.8–1.6 g/100 kg BW, IM), quinapyramine—anti-trypanosomiasis (quinapyramine sulfate 1.5 g + quinapyramine chloride 1 g at 4.4 mg/kg BW, IM), buparvaquone—anti-theilerial (2.5 mg/kg BW, IM), oxytetracycline—anti-theilerial and anti-anaplasma (10–20 mg/kg BW, IV).

For Helminths
Albendazole (5–10 mg/kg BW, single dose, PO), fenbendazole (5–7.5 mg/kg BW, single dose, PO), levamisole (7.5 mg/kg BW, single dose, PO/SC), mebendazole (10–15 mg/kg BW, PO), niclosamide (50–100 mg/kg BW, PO), oxfendazole (5 mg/kg BW, PO), oxyclozanide (10–15 mg/kg BW, PO), piperazine (200–300 mg/kg BW, PO), tetramisole (15 mg/kg BW, PO).

For Ectoparasites
Amitraz, carbaryl, coumaphos, cypermethrin, deltamethrin, fenvalerate, fipronil, flumethrin, lindane, permethrin as per label instructions.

W

WATER BUFFALO PARASITE ISSUES

CONTRAINDICATIONS
Some of the above listed compounds are illegal for use in food-producing animals in certain countries (i.e. metronidazole in the United States).

PRECAUTIONS
• Avoid administration of albendazole during first trimester of pregnancy.
• Parenteral overdose of levamisole may be lethal and oral overdose may produce nervous symptoms.
• Overdose of oxyclozanide may cause toxicity.
• Piperazine may produce neurologic signs when given in overdose.
• Overdose of tetramisole may produce clinical signs similar to phosphorus poisoning.
• Anti-protozoal drugs should be avoided during pregnancy.
• Diminazine aceturate dose should not exceed 9 g/animal/day.
• Avoid direct contact of ectoparasiticides with eyes and skin and prevent licking.
• Appropriate milk and meat withdrawal times must be followed for all compounds administered to food-producing animals.

POSSIBLE INTERACTIONS
N/A

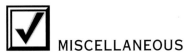 MISCELLANEOUS

ASSOCIATED CONDITIONS
Water buffalo are generally more resistant than cattle to diseases.

AGE-RELATED FACTORS
Young buffalo are more susceptible to parasitic infection than calves and adult buffalo.

ZOONOTIC POTENTIAL
Several of the parasitic disease conditions are zoonotic. Special precautions should be followed while collecting and handling laboratory samples.

PREGNANCY
Several of the parasitic disease conditions cause infertility, sterility, reproductive disorders, and abortion in water buffalo.

BIOSECURITY
• Avoid keeping different species together in a shed.
• Isolation and quarantine of new stock entering the herd.
• Treat and or cull new animals for disease conditions prior to herd introduction.

PRODUCTION MANAGEMENT
See "Biosecurity"

ABBREVIATIONS
• ALT = alanine aminotransferase
• AST = aspartate aminotransferase
• CT = computed tomography
• ELISA = enzyme-linked immunosorbent assay
• GGT = Gamma-glutamyl transferase
• GLDH = Glutamate dehydrogenase
• IM = intramuscular
• IV = intravenous
• MHCT = microhematocrit centrifugation technique
• MRI = magnetic resonance imaging
• PCR = polymerase chain reaction
• PET = positron emission tomography
• PO = per os, by mouth

• RBC = red blood cell
• SC = subcutaneous

SEE ALSO
• Water Buffalo Diseases
• Water Buffalo Management

Suggested Reading
Bastianetto E, Cerqueira LR. Epidemiological aspects and parasitic disease control of water buffaloes. Eighth World Water Buffalo Congress. The Turkey Creek Corporation, 2015.
Current Indian Veterinary Index (CINVEX), 2009–10.
Fagiolo A, Roncoroni C, Lai O, Borghese A. Buffalo Pathologies. ftp://ftp.fao.org/docrep/fao/010/ah847e/ah847e04.pdf. Accessed Jan 26, 2016.
Islam FMS, Rahman MH, Chowdhury SMZH. Prevalence of parasites of water buffaloes in Bangladesh. Asian-Australas J Anim Sci 1992, 5: 601–4.
Mamun MAA, Mondal MMH. A coprological survey of gastro-intestinal parasites of water buffaloes (*Bubalus bubalis*) in Kurigram District of Bangladesh. J Bangladesh Agric Univ 2011, 9: 103–9.
Patel HC, Hasnani JJ, Patel PV, Solanki JB, Jadav SJ. A study on helminth parasites of buffaloes brought to Ahmedabad Slaughter House, Gujarat, India. Int J Life Sci Pharma Res 2015, 5: 20–7.
Authors Saluna Pokhrel and Egendra Kumar Shrestha
Consulting Editor Kaitlyn A. Lutz

WATER BUFFALO: REPRODUCTION

BASICS

OVERVIEW
• The water buffalo, *Bubalus bubalis*, is a major dairy, draft, and meat animal especially in South Asia.
• There are two main types—river buffalo and swamp buffalo—based on wallowing in running water or stagnant pools, respectively.

INCIDENCE/PREVALENCE
N/A

GEOGRAPHIC DISTRIBUTION
• The total world buffalo population is about 199 million. About 96% of it is found in Asia, with minor numbers in the Mediterranean region, Australia, and parts of Central and South America.
• The river type is mainly found in the India-Pakistan region and the swamp type in China and Southeast Asia.

SYSTEM AFFECTED
Reproductive

PATHOPHYSIOLOGY
Male Reproduction
• The anatomy of the male reproductive system is very similar to the reproductive anatomy of male cattle; however, testes are comparatively smaller and prepuce is less pendulous.
• Testes grow in size until about 3 years of age with the fastest growth rate during the second year of age.
• Spermatogenesis starts from about 12–15 months of age; however, motile spermatozoa in the ejaculate are not seen before puberty, i.e., at about 24 months of age.
• The duration of spermatogenesis is 38 days and the cycle of seminiferous epithelium is 8.6 days.
• The spermatozoa of a buffalo bull are longer than those of a cattle bull and have a specific rectangular shape.

Female Reproduction
Female Reproductive Anatomy
• The female reproductive anatomy and physiology of the buffalo are very similar to that of cattle, with few differences. The cervix is less conspicuous, cervical canal is narrower and more tortuous, number of caruncles is about 60–90, uterine horns are smaller but more coiled. Ovaries are smaller and contain much fewer primordial follicles (10,000–20,000) in a cyclic buffalo heifer.
Female Reproductive Physiology
• The buffalo is a polyestrous animal. The swamp type is generally nonseasonal; however, the river buffalo has a seasonal tendency (short day breeder) governed by photoperiod and summer heat.
• The minimum size of an ovulatory follicle is about 10–12 mm, a mature CL is about 10–15 mm, and CL is more deeply embedded in the ovarian tissue as compared to CL of cattle. Mostly, the CL is not crowned.
• The mean age at puberty under optimum condition is 15–18 months for the river buffalo and 21–24 months for the swamp buffalo; however, under field conditions it rises to 30 (16–46) months, after attaining 55–60% of adult body weight, i.e., 275 (200–350) kg.
• The majority of buffalo have two follicular waves per estrous cycle, with some having three and few having one per cycle.
• The buffalo does not show overt estrus sign and is known as a silent estrus or subestrus animal. Homosexual behavior during estrus is uncommon. The estrus usually occurs late at night and in the early morning, making estrus detection more difficult and giving further weight to the description of silent estrus animals.
• The length of the estrous cycle is 21 (17–26) days; duration of estrus is 10 (5–27) hours, an LH surge lasts about 9 hours, and ovulation happens 15 (6–21) hours after the end of estrus.

Reproductive Disorders
• The buffalo has inherently poor reproductive efficiency, especially when compared to cattle, mainly due to the lesser number of primordial follicles in the ovaries, delayed age at puberty and maturity, reproductive seasonality, silent estrus, lower conception rate, longer calving intervals, summer anestrus, and longer postpartum anestrus.
• Genital prolapse, retention of fetal membranes, and abortions are more common in buffalo than in cattle, and more common in the river buffalo than the swamp buffalo.
• Uterine torsion is common in the buffalo due to more length and lower number of smooth muscles in the broad ligament.
• Endometritis is more prevalent in the buffalo than in cattle, while dystocia is less common. The most common cause of dystocia is fetopelvic disproportion, leading to different fetal disposition.
• Abortions and reproductive losses by nonspecific infectious agents are more prevalent than those caused by specific infections such as brucellosis, leptospirosis, listeriosis, campylobacteriosis, bubaline herpes virus-1 infection, bovine viral diarrhea, chlamydophilosis, Q fever, and neosporosis.
• Summer anestrus is a very prevalent problem in the river buffalo.

Artificial Breeding
Embryo Biotechnology
• All the reproductive biotechnologies used in cattle work for the buffalo but with lower success.
• Offspring have been produced from embryo transfer, from in vitro matured oocytes, and vitrified embryos.
• Ovum pickup (OPU) oocytes have significantly better embryo development capacity, embryo transferable quality, and blastocyst hatching than those from abattoir-derived ovaries. Oocyte recovery with OPU from 2–8 mm follicles ranges from 0.7 to 2.4 oocytes per ovary.
• Transgenic and cloned buffalo calves have been produced.
Hormonal Control of Ovarian Activity and Ovulation
• A combination of PRID for 10–12 days followed by 750–1,000 IU of eCG is the method of choice to induce estrus in noncycling heifers, resulting in >50% conception rate.
• For superovulation, FSH yields a better response than eCG. Overall, poor superovulatory response is due to the lower follicular reservoir in the ovaries.
• Estrus synchronization is achievable with the protocols used for cattle. Seemingly, PRID for 10–12 days followed by PGF2$_\alpha$ and 750–1,000 international units eCG at day 7, or ovulation synchronization protocol (GnRH, PGF2$_\alpha$ after 7 days, GnRH after 36–48 hours), are reported to achieve a better conception rate than other estrus synchronization protocols.
• Two fixed-time inseminations, at 48 hours and 72 hours during peak breeding season and at 72 hours and 96 hours during low breeding season, offer an acceptable conception rate.
Semen Collection and Artificial Insemination
• Semen can be collected by massage method, with a cattle electro-ejaculator and with an artificial vagina maintained at about 40–42°C.
• The sperm concentration in the ejaculate ranges from 1 billion to 4 billion sperm per mL of ejaculate.
• The sperm motility and sperm freezability are lower than for cattle.
• The egg yolk in semen extender must be <20%.
• Optimum time of insemination is 8–42 hours after onset of estrus. So the AM, PM rule of insemination is valid for the buffalo.
• The success rate and adoption of AI is lower than in cattle due to poor heat detection efficiency and poor conception rate with freeze-thawed semen.
• Semen sexing in the buffalo has resulted in birth of calves of pre-selected sex.

Water Buffalo Hybrid
• The fertile hybrid of the river buffalo with the swamp buffalo has been produced to combine dairy capacity of the water buffalo with meat and draft capacity of the swamp buffalo.
• Though fertilization takes place, a hybrid of water buffalo with domestic cattle could not be produced because embryos do not develop well beyond the eight-cell stage, few embryos develop to blastocyst stage, and no pregnancy is established after embryo transfer.

HISTORICAL FINDINGS
Depends on complaint

W

WATER BUFFALO: REPRODUCTION

SIGNALMENT
• Species: Water buffalo (*Bubalus bubalis*)
• Nili-ravi and Murrah are two top milk breeds of the river buffalo.

PHYSICAL EXAMINATION FINDINGS
N/A

GENETICS
The river buffalo has 50 chromosomes and the swamp buffalo has 48 chromosomes.

CAUSES AND RISK FACTORS
Causes and risk factors for reproductive disorders are similar to those described in cattle.

DIAGNOSIS

DIFFERENTIAL DIAGNOSES
Differential diagnosis approach for abortion and reproductive failure is similar to that used in cattle.

CBC/BIOCHEMISTRY/URINALYSIS
N/A

OTHER LABORATORY TESTS
Serum progesterone assay may be used to monitor cyclicity, as in cattle.

IMAGING
Transrectal ultrasonography for follicular dynamics, cyclicity, and pregnancy diagnosis.

OTHER DIAGNOSTIC PROCEDURES
N/A

PATHOLOGIC FINDINGS
N/A

TREATMENT

THERAPEUTIC APPROACH
• Therapeutic approach for reproductive disorders is similar to that described for cattle.
• Estrus synchronization programs used in cattle have been adapted with moderate success in buffalo and yak.

SURGICAL CONSIDERATIONS AND TECHNIQUES
N/A

MEDICATIONS

DRUGS OF CHOICE
Drugs used for hormonal therapy are similar to those used in cattle.

CONTRAINDICATIONS
Appropriate milk and meat withdrawal times must be followed for all compounds administered to food-producing animals.

PRECAUTIONS
N/A

POSSIBLE INTERACTIONS
N/A

FOLLOW-UP

EXPECTED COURSE AND PROGNOSIS
N/A

POSSIBLE COMPLICATIONS
N/A

PATIENT CARE
N/A

PREVENTION
N/A

MISCELLANEOUS

ASSOCIATED CONDITIONS
N/A

AGE-RELATED FACTORS
• Age at maturity for the buffalo is delayed compared to cattle. However, overall reproductive lifespan is longer than for cattle.

ZOONOTIC POTENTIAL
The abortigenic diseases: Brucellosis and leptospirosis.

PREGNANCY
• The physiology of gestation and parturition are very similar to that of cattle.
• The length of gestation is 310 (300–320) days for the river buffalo and 330 (320–340) days for the swamp buffalo.
• The placenta is epitheliochorial cotyledonary.
• The CL persists through the entire gestation.
• Pregnancy rate to first service is 50–75% with natural mating and 30–50% with AI, in the river buffalo.
• An accurate pregnancy diagnosis using per rectum ultrasonography is recommended from 30th day of insemination.
• Pregnancy can be diagnosed by transrectal palpation from day 30–45 post-insemination depending upon expertise of the clinician.

• The incidence of twinning is <0.1%. The buffalo usually produces two calves within three years.
• The involution of uterus completes within 30 (25–30) days after parturition.
• First postpartum ovulation occurs at about 96 days in the swamp buffalo and 60 days in the river buffalo.

BIOSECURITY
N/A

PRODUCTION MANAGEMENT
• Some buffalo breeds can yield 4,000 L of milk per 305 days.
• In general, the buffalo is kept under harsh field conditions by poor farmers in developing countries. It survives in harsh environment better, consumes dry roughages better, and copes with specific tropical diseases better than do cattle.
• In the females calving during winter or spring, postpartum estrus and conception are delayed till the next fall and winter, leading to increased calving interval compared with females calving during summer or fall and conceiving during fall or the following winter.

SYNONYMS
N/A

ABBREVIATIONS
• AI = artificial insemination
• CL = corpus luteum
• eCG = equine chorionic gonadotropin
• FSH = follicle stimulating hormone
• GnRH = gonadotropin releasing hormone
• LH = luteinizing hormone
• OPU = ovum pickup
• PGF2$_\alpha$ = prostaglandin F2$_\alpha$
• PRID = progesterone releasing intravaginal device

SEE ALSO
• Nutrition and Metabolic Diseases: Water Buffalo
• Water Buffalo Diseases
• Water Buffalo Management

Suggested Reading
Drost M. Bubaline versus bovine reproduction. Theriogenology 2007, 68: 447–9.
Perera B. Reproduction in domestic buffalo. Reprod Domest Anim 2008, Suppl 2: 200–6.
Author Muhammad Salman Waqas
Consulting Editor Ahmed Tibary

W

WATER HEMLOCK

BASICS

OVERVIEW
• Water hemlock or *Cicuta* species of which all members are toxic.
• Perennials that grow within wet habitats such as swamps, marshes, streams, and water banks.
• Thickened tuber at the base of a stem that is chambered and exudes a yellow oily substance that has a parsnip odor.
• Leaves are pinnately covered with veins extending to notches between teeth.
• Flowers are tiny and white and grow in umbrella-like fashion.
• Seeds may be present.
• New growth is readily eaten; however, unless tubers, excessive vegetation or flowers consumed, toxic signs are not seen.
• Tubers are reported to be palatable.

INCIDENCE/PREVALENCE
• Typically, few animals will be involved, although on occasion, circumstances will prevail that result in larger losses.
• There is a report of illness in 17 bull calves in a group of 62; 10 of the 17 eventually died.

GEOGRAPHIC DISTRIBUTION
Throughout Northwest, Midwest and Northeast United States and all of Canada

SYSTEMS AFFECTED
Nervous

PATHOPHYSIOLOGY
• Cicutoxin is a potent neurotoxin believed to block gamma-aminobutryric acid (GABA) leading to neuronal depolarization.
• Tubers and flowers contain toxin, with tubers being the most common source.
• Lethal dose has been reported in sheep as 1.0 mg of tuber (wet weight) per kg body weight.

HISTORICAL FINDINGS
History of exposure to plants

SIGNALMENT
Bovine, ovine, caprine

PHYSICAL EXAMINATION FINDINGS
• Develop within few hours of exposure
• Initially uneasiness and muscle twitching of head
• Seizures
• Death

CAUSES AND RISK FACTORS
• Cicutoxin is the toxic principle.
• Plants are said to be most toxic when dormant and least toxic when actively growing.
• The first new leaves and stems in early spring are particularly dangerous because they may be avidly eaten.
• The tuberous roots are apparently not too distasteful—cattle will sometimes eat them

readily. The concentration of toxin in roots is sufficient to pose a serious hazard throughout the year. This presents a particular problem if plants are pulled up and allowed to remain lying on the ground where livestock can eat the roots or when the ground becomes wet enough to allow entire plants to be easily pulled up and the roots eaten.
• Toxin levels, which are lowest in the upper leafy parts, decline as the leaves mature and dry.

DIAGNOSIS

DIFFERENTIAL DIAGNOSES
Acute grass tetany

CBC/BIOCHEMISTRY/URINALYSIS
In those animals who survive, there may be significant increases in serum LDH, AST, and CK enzymes 1–2 days after ingestion.

OTHER LABORATORY TESTS
Detection of toxin in rumen samples thru gas chromatography/mass spectrometry.

IMAGING
N/A

OTHER DIAGNOSTIC PROCEDURES
• History of exposure to the plants
• Clinical signs
• Identification of plant in oral cavity or GI contents

TREATMENT

THERAPEUTIC APPROACH
Supportive treatment:
• Sedation
• Administration of fluids and electrolytes and possibly respiratory support are appropriate as needed.

SURGICAL CONSIDERATIONS AND TECHNIQUES
In some instances, rumenotomy and flushing with water to remove the root fragments may be appropriate.

MEDICATIONS

DRUGS OF CHOICE
• No antidote
• Treatment with 30 mg/kg BW of pentobarbital and 75 mg of atropine prevented development of signs, lesions, and death in sheep experimentally fed water hemlock.

FOLLOW-UP

EXPECTED COURSE AND PROGNOSIS
• Most cases result in death; there have been reports of recovery.
• Death may occur within 1–8 hours of ingestion due to anoxia and cardiopulmonary arrest. Survival beyond 8 hours is a good indicator for eventual recovery if no complications from the convulsions ensue.

PREVENTION
Avoid grazing animals in areas where the plants are pulled up and allowed to remain lying on the ground where livestock can eat the roots or when the ground becomes wet enough to allow entire plants to be easily pulled up and the roots eaten.

MISCELLANEOUS

PRODUCTION MANAGEMENT
Plant is easily killed by broad leaf herbicides but caution in spraying around water source.

ABBREVIATIONS
• AST = aspartate aminotransferase
• CK = creatine kinase
• GI = gastrointestinal
• LDH = lactate dehydrogenase

SEE ALSO
Grass Tetany/Hypomagnesemia

Suggested Reading
Burrows GE. Apiaceae. In: Burrows GE, Tyrl RJ eds, Toxic Plants of North America. Ames: Iowa State University Press, 2001, pp. 49–53.
Burrows GE, Tyrl RJ. In: Toxic Plants of North America, 2nd ed. Iowa: Wiley-Blackwell, Kindle edition, 2013, pp. 58–62.
Panter KE, Gardner DR, Stegelmeier BL, et al. Water hemlock poisoning in cattle: Ingestion of immature *Cicuta maculate* seed as possible cause. Toxicon 2011, 57: 157–61.
Panter KE, Baker DC, Kechele PO. Water hemlock (*Cicuta douglasii*) toxicoses in sheep: pathologic description and prevention of lesions and death. J Vet Diagn Invest 1996, 8: 474–80.
Author Jennifer S. Taintor
Consulting Editor Christopher C.L. Chase
Acknowledgment The author and book editors acknowledge the prior contribution of Patricia Talcott.

W

WATER QUALITY ISSUES

 BASICS

OVERVIEW

• Water is the single most important nutrient for all livestock species. Water is involved either directly or indirectly in virtually every physiologic process essential to life. While animals can survive for a week or more without food, death is likely in a matter of days without adequate water intake. Poor water quality (or inadequate quantity) may result in decreased productivity, and adverse effects on animals' health, including death.

• Physical, chemical, and microbial constituents determine water quality. Physical components can range from gross contamination of water by fecal, organic materials and biofilms to stray voltage and the depth and condition of containers used to hold drinking water.

• Some chemical attributes of water can be detrimental to animal health at excessive concentrations. These include pH, soluble salts, various organic and inorganic compounds, and sulfates, nitrates, and nitrites.

• Ruminants are unique in that they are more sensitive to the toxic effects of both nitrates and sulfates than monogastrics. This is due to ruminal conversion/reduction to toxic nitrites and sulfides.

• Rate of consumption and adaptation influence the potential toxicity of many contaminants. Concentrations of (e.g.) sulfate which have no effect in winter, when water consumption is low, may be acutely lethal in summer, when consumption is several fold greater. Ruminants can adapt to moderately high concentrations of some toxicants, if introduced to them gradually.

• The microbiologic quality of water may also be important. Standing and running water may contain pathogens such as *Escherichia coli*, *Salmonella* spp., or *Leptospira* spp., and toxigenic cyanobacteria (blue-green algae).

• Drinking-water quality and availability should be included in a practitioner's differential diagnosis for poor performance or nonspecific disease conditions in livestock.

• Diagnosing water quality problems involves obtaining a thorough history, evaluating chemical and physical properties of water samples, and asking questions relevant to the water supply, such as "Where does it come from?," "How long have they been on it?," and "how much are they drinking?"

INCIDENCE/PREVALENCE

N/A

GEOGRAPHIC DISTRIBUTION

Worldwide depending on environment

SYSTEMS AFFECTED

Multisystemic

SIGNALMENT

All ruminant species

PHYSICAL EXAMINATION FINDINGS

• Ill-thrift (poor gain, infertility, etc.) is often associated with poor water quality or inadequate intake. In many cases, the problem is not any particular contaminant per se, but the fact that contaminants have rendered the water unpalatable, and animals are not drinking enough.

• Nitrates in excess of 500 mg/L (measured as the NO_3 ion) *may* cause abortion and/or sudden death. Although there are numerous anecdotal reports of lower nitrate concentrations causing a variety of chronic maladies, there is no experimental evidence to support such claims, and, in fact, several large, well-designed studies in cattle have failed to demonstrate any effects at substantially higher concentrations.

• Sulfate contamination (measured as the SO_4 ion) in excess of 1800 mg/L has caused polioencephalomalacia and acute death in a small percentage (~1%) of exposed cattle under field conditions, although higher concentrations were reportedly tolerated in small (n~10), experimental studies. Concentrations as low as 500 ppm have interfered with productivity in large, controlled, experiments.

• *Salmonella* spp.: Diarrhea, fever, loss of production, abortions.

• *E. coli*: Gastrointestinal signs, coliform mastitis, septic meningitis/arthritis in younger animals.

• *Leptospira* spp.: Infertility, low or diminished milk production, widespread late-term abortion.

• Three species of cyanobacteria (blue-green algae) are associated with most field cases of poisoning in North America. Each produces a characteristic syndrome, involving either convulsions, hypersalivation and other parasympathetic signs, or liver necrosis. The feature common to all three is rapid onset and high mortality.

CAUSES AND RISK FACTORS

• Sudden changes in water supply.

• Natural or anthropogenic contamination of surface runoff and wells.

• Damaged casings in old wells.

• Poor sanitation practices in confinement operations.

 DIAGNOSIS

Diagnosis is based upon the traditional triad of clinical presentation, pathology, and "testing." Merely because a water quality parameter exceeds some published "standard" does not necessarily prove that water is the problem. The clinical signs and history must match what is known about the contaminant.

CBC/BIOCHEMISTRY/URINALYSIS

Blood and urine analysis may indicate dehydration or hypernatremia if palatability is poor or some physical problem has interfered with consumption.

OTHER LABORATORY TESTS

Some water-borne toxicants may be directly or indirectly detectable in tissues and body fluids.

OTHER DIAGNOSTIC PROCEDURES

• Basic laboratory evaluation of water quality for livestock should include measurement of sulfate, nitrate-nitrite, and bacteria. Supplementary water tests may include pH, TDS, sodium, magnesium, chloride, calcium, potassium, manganese, and area-specific contaminants such as selenium, arsenic, or fluoride.

• It is important to use a laboratory that specializes in water quality for livestock, or else have a thorough understanding of the methodologies and reporting format used by the laboratory. For example, nitrate may be reported as "NO_3-N" or the NO_3 ion. The difference is more than two-fold.

• Many water quality laboratories offer "rural health" panels which, while inexpensive, are tailored to human residences and include tests (e.g., "hardness") and cite standards which are either inappropriate or irrelevant to animal health. It pays to know what you're asking for and understand how to interpret results.

PATHOLOGIC FINDINGS

N/A

 TREATMENT

See under specific toxicants, e.g., blue-green algae, *E. coli*, leptospirosis, nitrates, *Salmonella*, sulfur.

 MEDICATIONS

N/A

 FOLLOW-UP

PREVENTION

Regular tests of livestock water supplies for specific contaminants should be conducted if there has been a water-related problem, or the local environment is known to be prone to certain kinds of contamination.

 MISCELLANEOUS

PREGNANCY

Nitrate is known to cause abortion in ruminants.

BIOSECURITY

While there are no scientifically established safety standards for microbial contamination of livestock drinking water, common sense dictates that water supplies be kept as clean and free from microbial contamination as possible.

PRODUCTION MANAGEMENT

N/A

SYNONYMS

N/A

ABBREVIATION

• TDS = total dissolved solids

SEE ALSO

• Blue-Green Algae Poisoning
• Copper Deficiency and Toxicity
• Molybdenum Toxicity
• Nitrate and Nitrite Toxicosis
• Selenium Toxicity

• Sodium Disorders: Hypernatremia
• Sodium Disorders: Hyponatremia
• Sulfur Toxicity

Suggested Reading

Carson TL. Current knowledge of water quality and safety for livestock. Vet Clin North Am Food Anim Pract 2000, 16: 455–64.

Canadian Council of Ministers of the Environment. Canadian Water Quality Guidelines for the Protection of Agricultural Water Uses, 1999. http://ceqg-rcqe.ccme.ca/en/index.html#void. Accessed Jan 16, 2016.

Food and Agriculture Organization of the United Nations. Water Quality for Livestock and Poultry, 1985. Accessed Jan 10, 2016.

LeJeune JT, Besser TE, Merrill NL, Rice DH, Hancock DD. Livestock drinking water microbiology and the factors influencing the quality of drinking water offered to cattle. J Dairy Sci 2001, 84: 1856–62.

Pfost DL, Casteel S. Water quality for livestock drinking. University of Missouri Extension, EQ381, 2001. http://muextension.missouri.edu/explore/envqual/eq0381.htm. Accessed Aug 1, 2004.

Raisbeck MF, Riker SL, Tate CM, et al. Water Quality for Wyoming Livestock and Wildlife. University of Wyoming Agricultural Experiment Station, Bulletin B1183, 2007.

Author Merl F. Raisbeck
Consulting Editor Christopher C.L. Chase
Acknowledgment The author and book editors acknowledge the prior contribution of Dipa Pushkar Brahmbhatt.

W

WEIGHT LOSS: BOVINE

BASICS

OVERVIEW
Weight loss is defined as a decrease in body weight. The loss may be acute, chronic, physiologic, or pathologic. Although it is not considered a specific type of weight loss, decrease in daily weight gain is an abnormal physiologic condition as well.

INCIDENCE/PREVALENCE
Incidence of weight loss will depend directly or indirectly on the occurrence of disease related to a decrease in feed intake or the increase of nutritional requirements. All lactating animals, especially during the first trimester of lactation, mobilize body reserves, potentially causing a decline in weight and body condition.

GEOGRAPHIC DISTRIBUTION
Worldwide, weight loss commonly occurs in locations where drought is common or the feed supply is compromised.

SYSTEMS AFFECTED
• Multisystemic
• Musculoskeletal

PATHOPHYSIOLOGY
• Weight loss may occur as a result of anorexia, an increase in nutritional requirements, unbalanced diets, or a combination of these factors.
• Anorexia may be pathologic or physiologic.
• Pathologic anorexia occurs secondary to any systemic disease or local condition affecting the digestive system or oral cavity.
• Physiologic anorexia may occur during the last month of gestation and the first weeks of lactation. This decrease in feed intake is markedly evident at calving and during the peripartum period. Heat stress is another physiologic condition that noticeably affects dry matter intake.
• Increases in nutritional requirements occur under normal and pathologic conditions.
• Fever or any inflammatory process including tissue damage increases nutritional requirements, specifically the need for protein. Parasitism is an additional cause of pathologic weight loss.
• Examples of physiologic increases in nutritional requirements include lactation, last trimester of gestation, and overall animal growth. Unbalanced diets, especially diets deficient in microminerals and vitamins, and diets reduced in energy and protein, may promote poor growth rates or weight loss.
• Weight loss may be acute or chronic.
• Acute weight loss is typical with pathologic conditions that markedly affect dry matter intake, such as lameness, rumen acidosis, and displaced abomasum; or physiologic conditions, such as early lactation.
• Chronic weight loss is typical with pathologic conditions such as parasitism, chronic diarrhea (e.g., Johne's disease); or physiologic conditions that occur in aging animals.

HISTORICAL FINDINGS
Vary depending on underlying condition

SIGNALMENT
All breeds, ages, sex, and production stage may be affected.

PHYSICAL EXAMINATION FINDINGS
Anatomically depressed left paralumbar fossa, decrease in body condition score, visibility of skeletal prominences, and emaciation.

GENETICS
Several genetic or congenital conditions might affect growth and performance. Examples include dwarfism, cleft lip/palate (palatoschisis), and ventricular septal defect.

CAUSES AND RISK FACTORS
Any factor that decreases the animal's appetite, increases nutritional requirements, or inconsistent feed management (e.g., unbalanced diets, poor feed quality, macro/micro-nutrient deficiency, etc.). Risk factors include diseased animals, poor environmental management (e.g., heat stress, mud, insect control, etc.), inadequate feed management, low nutritional quality, drought, age, gender, physiologic stage, season, location.

DIAGNOSIS

DIFFERENTIAL DIAGNOSES
• Weight loss may be difficult to diagnose.
• May be secondary to other pathologic conditions (see Table 1).

CBC/BIOCHEMISTRY/URINALYSIS
Anemia, altered white cell profile, altered albumin to globulin ratio, elevated nonesterified fatty acids, increased creatinine and blood urea nitrogen, increase of specific enzymes related to tissue damage (AST, alkaline phosphatase, GGT, creatine kinase), elevated ketone bodies, low micromineral levels.

OTHER LABORATORY TESTS
Dependent upon specific disease condition(s) and differential diagnoses.

IMAGING
May be helpful to rule out a foreign body (traumatic reticuloperitonitis) in individual animals.

OTHER DIAGNOSTIC PROCEDURES
• Visual observation, body condition scoring, weight of animals, record analysis.
• Assessment of management.
• Complete dietary/nutritional analysis may be indicated.

PATHOLOGIC FINDINGS
Emaciation, decrease or absence of adipose tissue, especially in abdominal organs, and

Table 1

Major Differential Diagnosis of Weight Loss in the Bovine
Actinobacillosis
Actinomycosis
Bovine leucosis
Cryptosporidiosis
Deficiencies
• Copper
• Selenium
Dental abnormalities
Diarrhea
• Enterotoxigenic *E. coli*
• Salmonellosis
• Undifferentiated Enterotoxigenic *E. coli*
Failure of passive transfer (neonates)
Fescue toxicity
Gastrointestinal problems
• Abomasal ulcer
• Displaced abomasum
• Fat necrosis
• Hepatic abscess
• Johne's disease
• Pharyngeal, retropharyngeal abscess
• Salmonellosis
• Traumatic reticuloperitonitis (hardware)
• Vagal indigestion
• Winter dysentery
Intussusception/Torsions
Lameness
• Footrot
• Septic arthritis
• Sole abscess
Malnutrition
Mastitis
Metabolic diseases
• Ketosis
• Lactic acidosis
• Hypomagnesemia
• Hypocalcemia
Parasites
• Anaplasmosis
• Coccidiosis
• Flukes
• Gastrointestinal worms
• Lice
• Lungworm
• Ostertagiasis
• Sarcoptic mange
Pasteurellosis
Peritonitis
Pneumonia
Urinary problems
• Pyelonephritis/cystitis
• Urolithiasis
Viruses
• Bluetongue
• Bovine viral diarrhea virus (BVDV)
• Coronavirus
• Infectious bovine rhinotracheitis (IBR)
• Rotavirus

W

(CONTINUED) WEIGHT LOSS: BOVINE

decreased or stunted growth. Evaluate body condition scores. Mature animals break down fat reserves, initially utilizing peripheral fat, followed by abdominal and perirenal fat. After fat utilization, animals catabolize muscle proteins.

 TREATMENT

THERAPEUTIC APPROACH
Dependent upon whether the weight loss is secondary to a pathologic or physiologic condition.

SURGICAL CONSIDERATIONS AND TECHNIQUES
N/A

 MEDICATIONS

DRUGS OF CHOICE
• Vitamins (A, D, E, B complex), minerals (mostly microminerals), feed additives (monensin, probios, propionate, propylene glycol), and growth stimulants may be indicated dependent upon the type of weight loss.
• Treatment should be predicated based upon disease condition.
• If lameness is evident, hoof care should be established.

CONTRAINDICATIONS
Appropriate milk and meat withdrawal times must be followed for all compounds administered to food-producing animals.

POSSIBLE INTERACTIONS
N/A

 FOLLOW-UP

EXPECTED COURSE AND PROGNOSIS
Dependent upon the primary cause of weight loss

POSSIBLE COMPLICATIONS
Down cow syndrome, weakness

CLIENT EDUCATION
Institute programs where body condition scoring, or weighing if possible, and feed evaluation are routinely performed. Behavior surrounding feeding or grazing is important to observe also as less obvious factors such as limited feed space, social dominance, and palatability/sorting behavior may play a role in weight loss.

PREVENTION
Based on the primary cause of weight loss

 MISCELLANEOUS

ASSOCIATED CONDITIONS
Decrease in productivity

AGE-RELATED FACTORS
Older animals are more likely to lose weight inherently due to aging; young stock are particularly susceptible to diarrheal diseases.

ZOONOTIC POTENTIAL
Some infectious conditions (e.g., salmonellosis, leptospirosis) are zoonoses.

PREGNANCY
Can negatively affect growth and weight gain.

BIOSECURITY
Considered in the case of infectious disease associated with weight loss, (e.g., Johne's disease, salmonellosis, etc.).

PRODUCTION MANAGEMENT
Adequate feed intake, general management, and cow comfort. Specific management recommendations will follow diagnosis of underlying disease or underlying management/facilities issues.

SYNONYMS
N/A

ABBREVIATIONS
• AST = aspartate aminotransferase
• BVDV = bovine viral diarrhea virus
• GGT = gamma glutamyltransferase
• IBR = infectious bovine rhinotracheitis

SEE ALSO
• Body Condition Scoring (by species) (see www.fiveminutevet.com/ruminant)
• Weight Loss: Small Ruminant

Suggested Reading
Allen MS, Piantoni P. Carbohydrate nutrition: managing energy intake and partitioning through lactation. Vet Clin North Am Food Anim Pract 2014, 30: 577–97.
Connor EE. Invited review: improving feed efficiency in dairy production: challenges and possibilities. Animal 2015, 9: 395–408.
Gifford CA, Holland BP, Mills RL, et al. Growth and Development Symposium: Impacts of inflammation on cattle growth and carcass merit. J Anim Sci 2012, 90: 1438–51.
Sweeney RW. Pathogenesis of paratuberculosis. Vet Clin North Am Food Anim Pract 2011, 27: 537–46.

Author Pedro Melendez
Consulting Editor Kaitlyn A. Lutz
Acknowledgment The author and book editors acknowledge the prior contribution of Jeff W. Tyler.

W

WEIGHT LOSS: CAMELID

BASICS

OVERVIEW
• Weight loss is a common presenting complaint in camelids and the cause can be difficult to diagnose.
• Thorough examination and appropriate diagnostic tests frequently result in diagnosis.

INCIDENCE/PREVALENCE
Common

GEOGRAPHIC DISTRIBUTION
Worldwide

SYSTEMS AFFECTED
• Musculoskeletal
• Digestive

PATHOPHYSIOLOGY
• Camelids have a highly efficient compartment system of rumination, so even moderate quality forages are usually sufficient to maintain adult animals; true starvation is rare.
• Growing animals and late pregnant or lactating females are typically the first to display weight loss.
• Extremes of environmental temperature can increase energy requirements.
• Any disease process can increase energy requirements, and many also suppress appetite, which can cause rapid weight loss.

HISTORICAL FINDINGS
• Depend upon the etiology.
• Early detection of weight loss can be difficult for clients with animals in heavy fiber; reports of acute weight loss should be viewed cautiously unless clients are regularly performing body condition scoring.
• History should include age, number of animals affected, stage of pregnancy or lactation, appetite, and duration over which weight loss occurred.
• Investigate deworming and supplementary feeding practices, vitamin D supplementation strategy, and housing.
• Determine if this is a herd versus individual animal problem to refine the differential list.
• Inspection of the premises may help identify relevant management issues.

SIGNALMENT
• Camelids of any age, gender, and breed can be affected.
• Vitamin D deficiency is most prevalent in crias 3–6 months of age, darkly pigmented, and born in late fall/winter.
• Young animals are also more prone to vitamin E/selenium deficiency.

PHYSICAL EXAMINATION FINDINGS
• Vary with cause. Particular attention should be paid to mucus membrane color (conjunctival more reliable than oral) to evaluate potential anemia. Detection of

edema is difficult and it is most reliably found in the axillary, mammary, and scrotal regions.
• Observation from a distance can detect subtle changes such as increased time in cush, mild colic (shifting or abnormal limb position in cush), and increased separation from the herd.
• Assessment of the dung pile can detect diarrhea and tapeworm infestations in the herd. Diarrhea should be suspected if fecal consistency is anything softer than individual pellets, which disperse on hitting the ground.
• Pneumonia is difficult to detect by auscultation in camelids; thoracic ultrasound or radiography are more reliable.
• Cardiac murmurs are abnormal in camelids and generally require further investigation.
• Palpation of the mandibles and maxillae should be performed to evaluate dental disease.
• Reluctance to move, arched stance, shifting limb lameness, joint enlargement, and angular limb deformities (carpal valgus) occur with vitamin D deficiency.
• Camelids with head-shaking, pruritis, shade seeking, and weight loss might be exposed to sporidesmin toxin, produced by the fungus *Pithomyces chartarum*. Jaundice can occur in severe cases.
• Weakness and reluctance to move can indicate nutritional myodegeneration due to selenium deficiency.
• Bruxism, frothing at the mouth, or mild colic can occur with third compartment ulcers; however, in many cases signs may be restricted to lethargy, weight loss, and reduced appetite.

GENETICS
N/A

CAUSES AND RISK FACTORS
• Causes vary (listed under "Differential Diagnoses").
• Inadequate nutrition should be suspected in animals with weight loss, despite a good appetite, and no other abnormal findings.
• Risk factors include intensive management systems with high stocking densities.
• Anthelmintic resistance can result in high parasite burdens even in treated animals.

DIAGNOSIS

DIFFERENTIAL DIAGNOSES
• Inadequate nutrition
• Hepatic lipidosis
• Endoparasitism
• Vitamin D deficiency
• Dental disease
• Selenium deficiency
• Facial eczema (sporidesmin toxicity)
• Perennial ryegrass staggers
• Blood parasites: *Candidatus Mycoplasma haemolamae, Theileria orientalis*

• Third compartment ulcers
• Chronic infections: Pneumonia, endocarditis, Johne's disease, bovine viral diarrhea virus, *Yersinia enterocolitica*, tuberculosis, caseous lymphadenitis
• Congenital abnormalities: Cardiac abnormalities, portosystemic shunts, vascular ring anomalies
• Neoplasia: Malignant round cell tumor, intestinal adenocarcinoma
• Megaesophagus
• Chronic renal failure

CBC/BIOCHEMISTRY/URINALYSIS
• CBC and serum chemistry analysis help diagnose vitamin D deficiency (phosphorus <3 mg/dL), selenium deficiency, blood parasites, chronic infections, and hepatic and renal disorders.
• Measurements of triglycerides, β-hydroxybutyrate, and nonesterified fatty acids are often relevant.
• Hypoproteinemia due to hypoalbuminemia (often severe) is a common finding with *Eimeria macusaniensis* infection.

OTHER LABORATORY TESTS
• Fecal examination should comprise part of the investigation. *E. macusaniensis* is rarely detected using the McMasters technique; the Modified Wisconsin Sugar Flotation Method is recommended. The prepatent period is 32–43 days, with clinical signs occurring from 21 days, so clinical signs can occur before detectable fecal shedding.
• BVDV and mycoplasma PCR (on blood).
• Assessment of blood selenium or glutathione peroxidase activity (selenium deficiency).

IMAGING
• Ultrasonography is useful to assess GI, cardiac, urogenital, and respiratory disease.
• Thoracic and abdominal radiographs are useful for specific disorders.
• Computed tomography can be performed with IV contrast; orogastric contrast is useful to specifically investigate GI disorders 3 hours after administration.

OTHER DIAGNOSTIC PROCEDURES
• Liver biopsy: Hepatic lipidosis, fibrosis, neoplasia.
• Exploratory laparotomy is an option in valuable animals unable to be diagnosed by less extreme measures.

PATHOLOGIC FINDINGS
Vary with etiology

TREATMENT

THERAPEUTIC APPROACH
• Depends upon the cause of weight loss; however, reinstituting appropriate caloric intake is critical in avoiding, or treating, hepatic lipidosis. Appetite is best stimulated by transfaunation with bovine rumen fluid obtained from a freshly slaughtered or

(CONTINUED)

WEIGHT LOSS: CAMELID

fistulated cow. Otherwise reconstituted feces from a healthy herd mate can be used. Fluid can be administered via orogastric tube, or if repetition is expected, a small bore indwelling naso-esophageal tube can be left in place for transfaunation to be performed once or twice daily for 3–5 days.
• Anemia is common and extremely well tolerated in camelids, and clinical signs of pallor, tachycardia, and lethargy may not be recognized until the PCV is critically low. Blood transfusion is well tolerated and can be performed by acquiring blood from either a healthy alpaca or llama. Cross-matching is not required unless subsequent transfusions are performed more than 48 hours later.

SURGICAL CONSIDERATIONS AND TECHNIQUES
N/A

MEDICATIONS

DRUGS OF CHOICE
• Anthelmintics are indicated when GI parasites are confirmed in relationship to clinical disease. Resistance is common, particularly in areas where camelids are treated prophylactically for *Parelaphostrongylus tenuis* with avermectins. Moxidectin likely has the best efficacy but a narrow margin of safety so individual animals should be weighed prior to administration of the drug (0.4 mg/kg body weight PO).
• Coccidiostats: Toltrazuril 15 mg/kg PO once; ponazuril 20 mg/kg PO q24h for 3 days.
• Vitamin D: 1500 IU/kg SC q12 weeks for young and all darkly pigmented animals. 1,500 IU/kg q6 months for lightly pigmented animals.
• Selenium should only be given to animals with known deficiency to avoid toxicity (50 µg/kg once SC or IM).
• Antibiotics are commonly preferred over surgical intervention for dental abscesses: Florfenicol (20 mg/kg IM q48h for 3 weeks); penicillin, long-acting ceftiofur and other drugs have been used.
• Ulcer medications are largely ineffective due to poor absorption. Reestablishing appetite is the best treatment for ulcers; pantoprazole can be administered SC (2 mg/kg IV, q24h) or IV (1 mg/kg IV, q24h) with efficacy if medication is indicated.

• Thiamine (10 mg/kg SC) is indicated in animals with prolonged inappetance.

CONTRAINDICATIONS
N/A

PRECAUTIONS
Appropriate milk and meat withdrawal times must be followed for all compounds administered to food-producing animals.

POSSIBLE INTERACTIONS
N/A

FOLLOW-UP

EXPECTED COURSE AND PROGNOSIS
Varies with etiology. Chronic weight loss is more likely to carry a poor prognosis if a reversible cause cannot be established and addressed.

POSSIBLE COMPLICATIONS
Hepatic lipidosis can occur in any camelid (particularly crias) with prolonged periods of reduced caloric intake and/or high metabolic demands.

CLIENT EDUCATION
See "Prevention"

PATIENT CARE
Ensure provision of high quality, adequate volume, readily accessible feed.

PREVENTION
• Appropriate vaccination and parasite control methods help prevent common diseases.
• Fecal parasite examination should be repeated 10 days after anthelmintic therapy to ensure efficacy of the selected drug.
• Educated assessment of rations and pasture conditions is important.
• Periodic body condition scoring, regular weighing, and fecal egg counts are valuable tools for maintaining animal condition and for early identification of disease.

POSSIBLE COMPLICATIONS
• Hepatic lipidosis
• Refeeding syndrome

MISCELLANEOUS

ASSOCIATED CONDITIONS
N/A

AGE-RELATED FACTORS
N/A

ZOONOTIC POTENTIAL
N/A

PREGNANCY
N/A

BIOSECURITY
N/A

PRODUCTION MANAGEMENT
N/A

SYNONYMS
N/A

ABBREVIATIONS
• BVDV = bovine viral diarrhea virus
• GI = gastrointestinal
• IM = intramuscular
• IV = intravenous
• PCR = polymerase chain reaction
• PCV = packed cell volume
• PO = per os, by mouth
• SC = subcutaneous

SEE ALSO
• Body Condition Scoring: Alpacas and Llamas (see www.fiveminutevet.com/ruminant)
• Camelid: Dentistry
• Camelid: Gastrointestinal Disease
• Camelid: Parasitology
• Nutrition and Metabolic Diseases: Camelid (see www.fiveminutevet.com/ruminant)
• Parasite Control Programs: Camelid
• Respiratory Disease: Camelid

Suggested Reading
Cebra CK, Valentine BA, Schlipf JW, et al. *Eimeria macusaniensis* infection in 15 llamas and 34 alpacas. J Am Vet Med Assoc 2007, 230: 94–100.
Niehaus A. Dental disease in llamas and alpacas. Vet Clin North Am Food Anim Pract 2009, 25: 281–93.
Van Saun RJ. Nutritional diseases of South American camelids. Small Rumin Res 2006, 61: 153–64.
Author Laura Y. Hardefeldt
Consulting Editor Erica C. McKenzie

W

WEIGHT LOSS: SMALL RUMINANT

BASICS

OVERVIEW
• Weight loss is a common and nonspecific sign which can be an indicator of poor management or true medical disease.
• It may be the focus of case assessment or the consequence of more specific conditions to be assessed.
• Weight loss should be defined into the following categories to help with differential diagnosis construction:
  ◦ Weight loss with increased appetite
    ▪ Malassimilation—maldigestion or malabsorption of nutrients
    ▪ Malutilization—nutrients are digested and absorbed normally but utilized abnormally by tissues
  ◦ Weight loss with normal appetite and intake
  ◦ Weight loss with reduced appetite

INCIDENCE/PREVALENCE
Varies with specific conditions

GEOGRAPHIC DISTRIBUTION
Worldwide

SYSTEMS AFFECTED
Multisystemic

PATHOPHYSIOLOGY
• Weight loss can arise from
  ◦ Undersupply of nutrition
  ◦ Conditions preventing adequate ingestion of food and/or water
  ◦ Conditions causing malabsorption
  ◦ Disturbed metabolic processes

HISTORICAL FINDINGS
• Vary with specific conditions.
• Weight loss can be acute or chronic.
• Weight loss may or may not be accompanied by more overt clinical indicators of disease.
• Assess management features, particularly feed supply and housing characteristics.
• Determine herd versus individual animal problem to refine the differential list.
• If possible, inspection of the premises may help identify relevant management issues.

SIGNALMENT
All small ruminant species of any age or gender can be afflicted.

PHYSICAL EXAMINATION FINDINGS
• Vary with specific conditions.
• Critical to define a body condition score for the animal, using a scoring system appropriate for the species and breed in question.
• Differentiate muscle loss from fat loss.
• Identify any other anomalies that may relate to weight loss and disease.
• Include a thorough inspection of the oral cavity.

GENETICS
N/A

CAUSES AND RISK FACTORS
Vary with specific conditions

DIAGNOSIS

DIFFERENTIAL DIAGNOSES
• Management and nutrition inadequacies:
  ◦ Inadequate energy density of ration
  ◦ Inadequate supply or palatability of water (reduces DM intake)
  ◦ Poor forage quality (late autumn and undergrazed pasture) or inadequate quantity (grass length of 4–6 cm optimal)
  ◦ Competitive exclusion from food: Different age groups housed together or inadequate feed trough space
  ◦ Vitamin deficiencies: E, B_{12}
  ◦ Mineral deficiencies: Sodium, potassium, sulfur, cobalt, copper, selenium
  ◦ Toxic plant ingestion (particularly sheep): Acorns, fiddleneck, groundsel, locoweed, phalaris, yellow star thistle
• Disease conditions creating weight loss due to impaired prehension/ingestion:
  ◦ Dental disease
  ◦ Oral cavity infections: orf, *Fusobacterium necrophorum, Actinobacillus lignieresii*
  ◦ Pharyngeal or retropharyngeal trauma and/or abscessation
  ◦ Esophageal diseases
• Other GI disorders:
  ◦ Impaction of the rumen or abomasum
  ◦ Rumen acidosis
  ◦ Abomasal emptying defect (Suffolk sheep)
  ◦ Parasitism: Cestodes, nematodes, *Coccidia, Cryptosporidium*
  ◦ Johne's disease
  ◦ Intestinal neoplasia
• Other disorders:
  ◦ Severe lameness inhibiting mobility to food
    ▪ Foot rot
    ▪ Contagious ovine digital dermatitis
    ▪ White line abscesses
    ▪ Infectious arthritis: *Streptococcus* (lambs), *Erysipelothrix, Chlamydia,* maedi-visna virus (MVV), caprine arthritis encephalitis virus (CAEV)
    ▪ Limb fractures/trauma
  ◦ Hepatobiliary disease
    ▪ Cobalt deficiency
    ▪ Fasciolosis
    ▪ Pyrrolizidine alkaloid ingestion
  ◦ Cardiovascular disease
    ▪ Vegetative endocarditis
    ▪ Congestive heart failure
  ◦ Respiratory disease
    ▪ Pasteurellosis and/or chronic viral infection
    ▪ Enzootic nasal adenocarcinoma
    ▪ *Oestrus ovis*
    ▪ Laryngeal chondritis
    ▪ *Dictyocaulus filaria*
    ▪ Chronic bacterial pneumonia (*F. necrophorum, Trueperella pyogenes*)
    ▪ Sheep pulmonary adenomatosis
    ▪ MVV
    ▪ Caseous lymphadenitis (CLA): Pulmonary abscesses
  ◦ Central nervous system
    ▪ Scrapie
    ▪ Polioencephalomalacia
    ▪ Louping ill
    ▪ Listeriosis
  ◦ Reproductive
    ▪ Pregnancy toxemia
    ▪ Postpartum peritonitis
  ◦ Integument
    ▪ Pruritic disorders: Mange (*Sarcoptes scabiei* var. *ovis, Sarcoptes scabiei* var. *caprae*), mites (sheep scab, *Psoroptes ovis*), lice (*Mallophaga* and *Anoplura*) and biting flies (*Melophagus ovinus*)
    ▪ Parapox virus
    ▪ Contagious pustular dermatitis (orf)
  ◦ Ophthalmic
    ▪ Vitamin A deficiency
  ◦ Urinary
    ▪ Enterotoxemia (pulpy kidney)
    ▪ Pyelonephritis
    ▪ Urolithiasis
    ▪ Renal amyloidosis (sheep with CLA)
    ▪ Chronic renal failure

CBC/BIOCHEMISTRY/URINALYSIS
• CBC and serum chemistry are indicated to assess inflammation and abnormalities of liver enzymes and function (AST, GGT, SDH, bilirubin), renal function (BUN and creatinine), electrolyte and mineral status, and blood protein profile (total protein, albumin, globulin).
• Measurement of triglycerides, β-hydroxybutyrate, and nonesterified fatty acids may be relevant.
• Urinalysis is indicated when urinary tract disorders are suspected, or to evaluate glucose and ketone content.

OTHER LABORATORY TESTS
• Fecal egg counts
• Serum bile acids (hepatic disease)
• Vitamin and trace mineral assessments

IMAGING
• Ultrasound of the thoracic and abdominal organs may confirm specific diagnoses.
• Ultrasound in early pregnancy (fetal counting) assists prevention of pregnancy toxemia.
• Radiographs and computed tomography are also useful methods of imaging small ruminants.

OTHER DIAGNOSTIC PROCEDURES
Depend on suspected diagnosis

PATHOLOGIC FINDINGS
Depend on system affected

W

TREATMENT

THERAPEUTIC APPROACH
Identify underlying cause of weight loss to determine if and how it can be resolved. This is particularly critical for herd issues.

SURGICAL CONSIDERATIONS AND TECHNIQUES
N/A

MEDICATIONS

DRUGS OF CHOICE
Antibiotics and anthelmintics may be relevant to specific bacterial or parasitic disorders causing weight loss.

CONTRAINDICATIONS
N/A

PRECAUTIONS
N/A

POSSIBLE INTERACTIONS
N/A

FOLLOW-UP

EXPECTED COURSE AND PROGNOSIS
Depends on the specific causative condition

POSSIBLE COMPLICATIONS
Depends on the specific causative condition

CLIENT EDUCATION
Depends on the specific causative condition

PATIENT CARE
Depends on the specific causative condition

PREVENTION
• Appropriate vaccination and parasite control methods are valuable for preventing common causes of weight loss.
• Assessment of rations and pasture conditions is also important.
• Periodic body condition scoring, regular weighing, and fecal egg counts are valuable tools for maintaining the condition of flocks and herds and for early identification of disease.

MISCELLANEOUS

ASSOCIATED CONDITIONS
N/A

AGE-RELATED FACTORS
N/A

ZOONOTIC POTENTIAL
• *Cryptosporidium parvum*
• Contagious pustular dermatitis

PREGNANCY
Pregnancy toxemia can cause weight loss in advanced gestation.

BIOSECURITY
• Pathogens can spread readily via animal contact within a herd, particularly in intensive management conditions.
• Control contact with wild animals and other domesticated species.
• Ensure security of feed and water sources to avoid contamination.
• Minimize vehicles or visitors on farm.
• Avoid substantial mixing of different age groups or animals from different sources.

PRODUCTION MANAGEMENT
Ration assessment, periodic body condition scoring or regular weighing, and solid vaccination and parasite control protocols are paramount to maintaining healthy production animals.

SYNONYMS
N/A

ABBREVIATIONS
• AST = aspartate aminotransferase
• BUN = blood urea nitrogen
• CAEV = caprine arthritis encephalitis virus
• CLA = caseous lymphadenitis
• DM = dry matter
• GGT = gamma glutamyltransferase
• GI = gastrointestinal
• MVV = maedi-visna virus
• SDH = sorbitol dehydrogenase

SEE ALSO
• Blood Chemistry (see www.fiveminutevet.com/ruminant)
• Body Condition Scoring: Goats (see www.fiveminutevet.com/ruminant)
• Body Condition Scoring: Sheep (see www.fiveminutevet.com/ruminant)
• Ewe Flock Nutrition (see www.fiveminutevet.com/ruminant)
• Nutrition and Metabolic Diseases: Small Ruminant
• Parasite Control Programs: Small Ruminant

Suggested Reading
Forero L, Nader G, Craigmill A, Ditomaso JM, Puschner B, Maas J. Livestock-Poisoning Plants of California. University of California Agriculture and Natural Resources. Publication 8398. January 2011.

Hindson J. Differential diagnosis of weight loss in the ewes. In Practice 1994, 16: 204–8.

Hindson JC, Winter AC. Adult weight loss. In: Outline of Clinical Diagnosis in Sheep, 2nd ed. Oxford, UK: Blackwell Science, 1996, pp. 108–14.

Hindson JC, Winter AC. Respiratory diseases. In: Manual of Sheep Diseases. Oxford, UK: Blackwell Science, 2002.

Maas J, Stratton-Phelps M. Alterations in body weight or size. In: Smith BP ed, Large Animal Internal Medicine, 4th ed. St. Louis: Elsevier, 2009, p. 159.

Maddison J. Weight loss. In: Maddison JE, Volk HA, Church DB eds, Clinical Reasoning in Small Animal Practice. Chichester, UK: Wiley Blackwell, 2015, pp. 55–64.

National Research Council. Nutrient Requirements of Small Ruminants. Washington, DC: National Academies Press, 2007.

Sager R, Maas J. Diseases of the Alimentary Tract: Cobalt deficiency in ruminants. In: Smith BP ed, Large Animal Internal Medicine, 5th ed. St. Louis: Elsevier Mosby, 2015, pp. 840–1.

Sherman DM. Unexplained weight loss in sheep and goats. A guide to differential diagnosis, therapy, and management. Vet Clin North Am Large Anim Pract 1983, 5: 571–90.

Smith MC, Sherman DM. Goat Medicine. Philadelphia: Lea & Febiger, 1994.

Author Douglas C. Donovan
Consulting Editor Erica C. McKenzie

W

WESSELSBRON DISEASE

BASICS

OVERVIEW
• Acute arthropod-borne viral infection of the genus Flavivirus.
• Predominantly affects sheep, cattle, and goats in sub-Saharan Africa.

INCIDENCE/PREVALENCE
• Seroprevalence in endemic regions is approximately 50%.
• Mortality rates up to 30% in infected lambs.
• Infections are seen to occur year round in most endemic regions; some regions observe increased incidence following periods of heavy rainfall.

GEOGRAPHIC DISTRIBUTION
• Africa, including Madagascar.
• Serologic evidence of presence in other countries (especially those with warm and moist climates).

SYSTEMS AFFECTED
• Digestive
• Nervous
• Musculoskeletal
• Reproductive

PATHOPHYSIOLOGY
• No evidence to support animal-to-animal transmission.
• *Aedes* mosquitoes are responsible for virus transmission.
• Reservoir host is unknown (suspected to be rodents).
• 1–3 day incubation period.

HISTORICAL FINDINGS
Location within an endemic region and periods of heightened vector activity are pertinent.

SIGNALMENT
• Neonatal lambs and kids (<7 days of age) are most susceptible to clinical disease.
• Adult infection is usually subclinical, unless preexisting liver disease is present.
• Cattle, goats, and sheep are the predominant species affected.
• There are reports of Wesselsbron disease in horses, pigs, ostriches, guinea pigs, rabbits, a gerbil, a dog, and a camel; serologic evidence exists in other wild ruminants.

PHYSICAL EXAMINATION FINDINGS
• Lambs, kids, and calves: Nonspecific signs including fever, anorexia, weakness, listlessness, tachypnea, and icterus. Infected lambs are usually 1–3 days of age, and may progress to death within 72 hours of clinical signs.
• Calves and mature sheep, goats, and cattle typically develop subclinical infection, or occasionally nonfatal febrile illness.
• Abortion with congenital malformations of the CNS and arthrogryposis of the fetus can be observed in some pregnant ewes.

• Hydrops amnii can occur in ewes.

GENETICS
N/A

CAUSES AND RISK FACTORS
• Enveloped, positive-sense RNA Flavivirus with properties of a hemagglutinating flavivirus.
• Mosquitoes from the *Aedes* genus, including *A. caballus* and *A. circumluteolus*, are responsible for transmission.
• Neonatal lambs and pregnant ewes are at increased risk of clinical disease.
• Infection can occur in conjunction with Rift Valley fever, especially during heavy rainfall periods.

DIAGNOSIS

DIFFERENTIAL DIAGNOSES
• Rift Valley fever (RVF): Similar geographic distribution, but Wesselsbron disease is usually milder with lower mortality rates, reduced abortion rate, and less severe liver pathology. Wesselsbron disease is more neurotropic than RVF and can cause severe teratology of the fetal CNS.
• Other abortive diseases including toxic plant ingestion and other viral diseases that can result in teratogenesis.

CBC/BIOCHEMISTRY/URINALYSIS
N/A

OTHER LABORATORY TESTS
• Virus isolation via intracerebral inoculation of newborn mice with samples from virtually any organ from RVF affected neonates.
• Can be differentiated from RVF by intraperitoneal inoculation of weaned mice which results in death (RVF) versus survival (Wesselsbron disease virus).
• Serodiagnosis can be achieved via hemagglutination-inhibition, complement fixation, or virus neutralization tests, with virus neutralization used to confirm virus identity.
• There is a high degree of cross-reactivity with other flaviviruses on hemagglutination-inhibition assays.

IMAGING
N/A

OTHER DIAGNOSTIC PROCEDURES
N/A

PATHOLOGIC FINDINGS
• Diffuse icterus and hepatomegaly of neonates, with hepatic discoloration (yellow–orange brown), and focal to extensive necrosis of parenchyma.
• Hepatocytes may contain eosinophilic inclusion bodies and Kupffer cell proliferation is present.
• Petechiae and ecchymoses are found in the abomasal mucosa, and the abomasal contents

contain evidence of hemorrhage (brown discoloration).
• Diffuse lymphadenopathy.
• Lesions in adult animals are usually very mild.
• Congenital malformations of the CNS can occur in ovine and bovine fetuses, including porencephaly, hydranencephaly, and cerebellar hypoplasia, with arthrogryposis often also evident.

TREATMENT

THERAPEUTIC APPROACH
N/A

SURGICAL CONSIDERATIONS AND TECHNIQUES
N/A

MEDICATIONS

DRUGS OF CHOICE
N/A

CONTRAINDICATIONS
N/A

PRECAUTIONS
N/A

POSSIBLE INTERACTIONS
N/A

FOLLOW-UP

EXPECTED COURSE AND PROGNOSIS
• Up to 30% mortality rate in neonatal lambs.
• Prognosis for survival and reproductive future is good for ewes following abortion.

POSSIBLE COMPLICATIONS
N/A

CLIENT EDUCATION
N/A

PATIENT CARE
N/A

PREVENTION
• Utilization of the previously available attenuated vaccine should be avoided in pregnant ewes because it can cause early embryonic death, CNS teratogenesis, arthrogryposis of the fetus, hydrops amnii, abortion, or fetal mummification. The attenuated vaccine was discontinued in 2000 due to the high prevalence of these adverse side effects.
• Attempts to control mosquito vectors is helpful but challenging.
• Immunity is life-long.
• Confine valuable animals to avoid exposure.
• Reduce sources of standing, stagnant water.

W

☑ **MISCELLANEOUS**

ASSOCIATED CONDITIONS
• Abortion: primarily due to malformation of the CNS with arthrogryposis in cattle and sheep.
• Hydrops amnii in pregnant ewes.

AGE-RELATED FACTORS
Newborn animals suffer high mortality rates.

ZOONOTIC POTENTIAL
• The virus has been associated with influenza-like disease in humans with signs including fever, headache, arthralgia, and myalgia.
• Infection can be transmitted to humans by *Aedes* mosquitoes or by handling virus-contaminated organs or materials; therefore, precautions should be taken while performing necropsy of suspected Wesselsbron disease cases.

PREGNANCY
Abortion with CNS malformation and arthrogryposis.

BIOSECURITY
No studies performed specifically into the sensitivity of Wesselsbron virus to disinfectants; however, due to similarities of this virus with other hemagglutinating flaviviruses, it is likely sensitive to temperatures over 104°F (40°C), detergents, and lipid solvents.

PRODUCTION MANAGEMENT
N/A

SYNONYMS
N/A

ABBREVIATIONS
• CNS = central nervous system
• RVF = Rift Valley Fever

SEE ALSO
• Arthrogryposis
• Rift Valley Fever

Suggested Reading
Barnard BJH. Wesselsbron disease. In: Howard JL ed, Current Veterinary Therapy, Food Animal Practice, 2nd ed. Philadelphia: Saunders, 1986.
Coetzer JAW, Theodoridis A. Clinical and pathological studies in adult sheep and goats experimentally infected with Wesselsbron disease virus. Onderstepoort J Vet Res 1982, 49: 19–22.
Coetzer JAW, Theodoridis A, Herr S, Kritzinger L. Wesselsbron disease: a cause of congenital porencephaly and cerebellar hypoplasia in calves. Onderstepoort J Vet Res 1979, 46: 165–9.
Jupp PG, Kemp A. Studies on an outbreak of Wesselsbron virus in the Free State Province, South Africa. J Am Mosq Control Assoc 1998, 14: 40–5.
Smith MC, Sherman DM eds. Goat Medicine. Philadelphia: Lea & Febiger, 1994.
Theodoridis A, Coetzer JAW. Wesselsbron disease: virological and serological studies in experimentally infected sheep and goats. Onderstepoort J Vet Res 1980, 47: 221–9.
Weyer J, Thomas J, Leman PA, Grobbelaar AA, Kemp A, Paweska JT. Human cases of Wesselsbron disease, South Africa 2010–2011. Vector Borne Zoonotic Dis 2013, 13: 330–6.
Author Sian A. Durward-Akhurst
Consulting Editor Erica C. McKenzie
Acknowledgment The author and book editors acknowledge the prior contribution of Kent M. Jackson.

W

WINTER DYSENTERY

BASICS

OVERVIEW
• Acute, contagious diarrheal disease of cattle with worldwide distribution, occurring in closely confined cattle during winter months (November to March).
• The feces are usually recognized as dark and fluid, often containing frank blood, and may have bubbles present and a foul odor. The odor from feces is unusual.
• In lactating cows there is a significant drop in milk production associated with anorexia and depression. Milk production decreases and clinical disease in individual animals is usually short (<1 week); however, outbreaks within a herd can persist for 2–8 weeks, depending upon herd size and housing. Lactating cows are most commonly affected.
• Calves may also demonstrate similar clinical signs and attack rates.
• Mortality is low, but morbidity can be quite significant (40–50%).
• Herds not experiencing outbreaks of winter dysentery (WD) for several years are at risk for subsequent outbreaks.

INCIDENCE/PREVALENCE
Acute, contagious diarrhea in cattle that occurs sporadically in epizootic form during the colder months of the year (November to March). Morbidity is generally high, with low mortality.

GEOGRAPHIC DISTRIBUTION
Disease occurs more commonly in northern states of the United States and Canada, but also has been documented to occur in Australia, northern United Kingdom, Europe, Israel, and Japan.

SYSTEMS AFFECTED
• Digestive
• Respiratory

PATHOPHYSIOLOGY
To date the exact cause is unknown. However, increasing evidence suggests that bovine coronavirus may be causal when appropriate animal and environmental conditions are present. Viral particles invade the colonic mucosae resulting in death and necrosis of the colonic epithelial cells. The loss of epithelial barrier function results in transudation of proteinaceous fluid and blood. The increased volume of fluid presumably results in loose, dark and sometimes bloody stool.

HISTORICAL FINDINGS
N/A

SIGNALMENT
Primarily adult dairy cows, either soon after calving or within the first 100 days in milk. Pregnant cows appear to be at reduced risk. Winter dysentery may also cause diarrhea and respiratory signs in calves, as shown

experimentally. Some outbreaks have been reported in beef cattle and feedlot calves.

PHYSICAL EXAMINATION FINDINGS
• Acute onset of voluminous, tan to dark diarrhea with clots of blood interspersed within liquid occurring in anorexic, depressed cows with reduced milk production. Reduced rumen fill and dehydration result in weight loss. Blood in feces may be mixed evenly in feces or may be present in clots.
• Rectal examination may reveal mildly distended loops of bowel and the manure generally has a fetid odor. Affected animals may develop diarrhea and respiratory signs (dyspnea, coughing, nasal and lacrimal discharge) but these are not consistent.
• Usually epizootic in nature with 10–100% morbidity.
• Excluding other causes of contagious diarrhea (coccidiosis, parasitism, salmonellosis) leads one to suspect WD.

GENETICS
No breed predilection. More common in dairy animals.

CAUSES AND RISK FACTORS
• Cattle in herds with recent exposure and immunologic response to BVDV or BCV (>4 fold increase in serum titer), cattle housed in tie stalls or stanchion barns and facilities using the same equipment to manage manure as well as feed are at increased risk for development of WD.
• Cows with high fecal BCV ELISA antigen and high acute serum BCV IgG antibody titers that seroconvert (> 4-fold increase) are at greater risk for development of WD. Pregnant cows are at reduced risk for WD.

DIAGNOSIS

DIFFERENTIAL DIAGNOSES
Diarrheic diseases caused by BVDV, coccidia, gastrointestinal parasites, *Salmonella* spp., *Campylobacter* spp., *Mycobacterium avium* ssp. *paratuberculosis* (Johne's disease), heavy metal intoxications (As, Cd), organophosphate toxicity, and dietary induced gut disturbances. *Mycobacterium avium* ssp. *paratuberculosis* is not often a problem in outbreak form. *Campylobacter* spp. has not been isolated from cattle with WD. Coccidiosis is not generally a problem in adult cattle, fecal evaluation may rule out coccidia and gastrointestinal nematodiasis. Heavy metal intoxication is often accompanied by high mortality in groups of cattle. Organophosphate intoxication includes acute death, neurologic animals, salivation, lacrimation, urination, defecation. Dietary induced diarrhea is often accompanied by lameness, reduced milk fat or protein/fat inversion. Bloody stool, or diarrheic feces with blood clots may indicate

clostridial enteritis (jejunal hemorrhage syndrome).

CBC/BIOCHEMISTRY/URINALYSIS
Not generally helpful in diagnostics. If persistent, dysentery may result in anemia.

OTHER LABORATORY TESTS
• BCV, the suspected etiologic agent, is diagnosed via fecal evaluation (electron microscopy, PCR, or ELISA).
• Differential diagnoses can be ruled out via fecal culture (*Salmonella* spp., *Campylobacter*, *Mycobacterium avium* subspecies *paratuberculosis*), serology (BVDV, IBR, Johne's, rotavirus, campylobacter, BRSV, BAV3, and BLV), fecal flotation and smear (coccidiosis, cryptosporidium).

IMAGING
N/A

OTHER DIAGNOSTIC PROCEDURES
N/A

PATHOLOGIC FINDINGS
In acute cases, BCV can be found in colonic tissue via immunohistochemical staining.

TREATMENT

THERAPEUTIC APPROACH
• Provision of adequate feed and fresh water is important. Access to salt and trace minerals is also advisable.
• Most cases will recover with supportive treatment with anti-diarrheal agents.
• More severe cases may require parenteral calcium, oral fluids, and propylene glycol for secondary hypocalcemia, dehydration, and ketosis respectively.
• Very rarely, animals will become severely dehydrated or anemic due to colonic blood loss and require IV fluids and whole blood transfusion.

MEDICATIONS

DRUGS OF CHOICE
• Oral anti-diarrheal agents (e.g., bismuth subsalicylate, kaolin/pectin)
• Oral isotonic fluid preparations (5–10 gallons q12–24h)
• IV hypertonic saline with fresh water available

CONTRAINDICATIONS
N/A

PRECAUTIONS
Appropriate milk and meat withdrawal times must be followed for all compounds administered to food-producing animals.

POSSIBLE INTERACTIONS
N/A

W

FOLLOW-UP

EXPECTED COURSE AND PROGNOSIS
• Morbidity is generally high with low mortality.
• Cows with high fecal BCV ELISA antigen and high acute serum BCV IgG antibody titers that seroconvert (>4-fold increase) are at greater risk for development of WD.

POSSIBLE COMPLICATIONS
N/A

CLIENT EDUCATION
Educate clients on risk factors associated with WD.

PATIENT CARE
Supportive care

PREVENTION
Management practices that prevent cross-contamination of feed with manure appear to be important.

MISCELLANEOUS

AGE-RELATED FACTORS
More common in adults but calves can be affected

ZOONOTIC POTENTIAL
Salmonella spp., *Campylobacter* spp., and possibly Johne's disease may be zoonotic.

PREGNANCY
Pregnant cows appear to be at reduced risk.

BIOSECURITY
Management practices that prevent cross-contamination of feed with manure appear to be important.

PRODUCTION MANAGEMENT
Cattle in herds with recent exposure and immunologic response to BVDV or BCV (>4-fold increase in serum titer), cattle housed in tie stalls or stanchion barns, and facilities using the same equipment to manage manure as well as feed are at increased risk for development of WD.

SYNONYM
Winter scours

ABBREVIATIONS
• BAV3 = bovine adenovirus type 3
• BCV = bovine corona virus
• BLV = bovine leukosis virus
• BRSV = bovine respiratory syncytial virus
• BVDV = bovine viral diarrhea virus
• ELISA = enzyme-linked immunosorbent assay
• IBR = infectious bovine rhinotracheitis
• IgG = immunoglobulin G
• PCV = packed cell volume
• WD = winter dysentery

SEE ALSO
• Biosecurity: Beef/Cow Calf (see www.fiveminutevet.com/ruminant)
• Biosecurity: Dairy (see www.fiveminutevet.com/ruminant)
• Bovine Viral Diarrhea Virus
• Coccidiosis
• Coronavirus
• Diarrheal Diseases: Bovine
• Epidemiology: Diagnostic Test Use (see www.fiveminutevet.com/ruminant)
• Salmonellosis

Suggested Reading
Boileau MJ, Kapil S. Bovine coronavirus associated syndromes. Vet Clin North Am Food Animal Pract 2010, 26: 123–46.

Cho K-O, Halbur PG, Bruna JD, et al. Detection and isolation of coronavirus from feces of three herds of feedlot cattle during outbreaks of winter dysentery-like disease. J Am Vet Med Assoc 2000, 217: 1191–4.

Cho K-O, Hoet AE, Loerch SC. Evaluation of concurrent shedding of bovine coronavirus via the respiratory tract and enteric route in feedlot cattle. Am J Vet Res 2001, 62: 1436–41.

Fecteau G, Guard CL. Winter dysentery in cattle (bovine coronavirus). In: Smith BP ed, Large Animal Internal Medicine. St. Louis: Mosby, 2015, p. 829.

Saif LJ. A review of evidence implicating bovine coronavirus in the etiology of winter dysentery in cows: an enigma resolved? Cornell Vet 1990, 80: 303–11.

Smith DR, Fedorka-Cray PJ, Mohan R, et al. Epidemiologic herd-level assessment of causative agents and risk factors for winter dysentery in dairy cattle. Am J Vet Res 1998, 59: 994–1001.

Smith DR, Fedorka-Cray PJ, Mohan R, et al. Evaluation of cow-level risk factors for the development of winter dysentery in dairy cattle. Am J Vet Res 1998, 59: 986–93.

Traven M, Naslung K, Linde N, et al. Experimental reproduction of winter dysentery in lactating cows using BCV: comparison with BCV infection in milk fed calves. Vet Microbiol 2001, 81: 127–51.

Tsunemitsu H, Smith DR, Saif LJ. Experimental inoculation of adult dairy cows with bovine coronavirus and detection of coronavirus in feces by RT-PCR. Arch Virol 1999, 144: 167–75.

Author Jeff Lakritz
Consulting Editor Kaitlyn A. Lutz

W

WOOL ROT

BASICS

OVERVIEW
• Wool rot (fleece rot) is a skin disease caused by prolonged and excessive wetting of the skin resulting in exudation and discoloration of the wool.
• The primary etiologic agent is *Pseudomonas aeruginosa*, although other bacteria may also be significant.
• Wool rot is characterized by superficial inflammation, seropurulent exudation, and putrefaction that attracts blowflies (*Lucilia cuprina*) to oviposition.
• Wool rot causes severe financial loss through downgrading of wool and promoting cutaneous myiasis by blowflies.

INCIDENCE/PREVALENCE
• Common problem in sheep.
• Incidence varies from 15% to 90%.
• It is most problematic in Australia, where reported prevalence can exceed 20%.

GEOGRAPHIC DISTRIBUTION
• Worldwide but most commonly occurs in Australia and New Zealand during wet season.
• Also of concern in South Africa and United Kingdom.
• Occasionally reported in the United States, where it is far less economically or clinically significant.

SYSTEMS AFFECTED
Integument

PATHOPHYSIOLOGY
• The main inciting factor is prolonged wetting of the skin and matting of the wool, arising from rain or dipping procedures.
• Continued wetting of the skin for at least 8 days or 100 mm of rain will provoke the disease.
• Temperature is not a factor in disease development.
• The primary factor for susceptibility is the sensitivity of the skin to prolonged wetting.
• Chronic wetting of the skin results in acanthosis, hyperkeratosis, and edema of the lower layers of the epidermis and subsequent infiltration of the area by neutrophils and other inflammatory cells.
• Microabscesses form and exudate is discharged into the lower layers of the epidermis.
• Prolonged wetting of the skin, high humidity in the fleece environment, and the availability of nutrients from serous exudates allow for indigenous skin flora, opportunistic flora, and bacteria such as *P. aeruginosa* to proliferate.
• Chromogenic bacteria (*Pseudomonas* spp.) cause discoloration of the fleece. *P. indigofera* produces a blue color, *P. aeruginosa* produces a green color, and *P. maltophilia* can cause yellow discoloration. Other bacteria may

produce brown, greenish-brown, or red discoloration.

HISTORICAL FINDINGS
Recent relevant weather conditions or management activities (dipping).

SIGNALMENT
• Can occur in any age, gender, or breed of sheep.
• Most common in younger sheep after succession of wet days from either rain or repeated dipping.

PHYSICAL EXAMINATION FINDINGS
• Except for the fleece, sheep are otherwise normal.
• Some sheep may show evidence of pain, rubbing, and/or biting at affected skin sites.
• Lesions are most common on the dorsum with the skin becoming red-purple in the early stages followed by exudation and matting of the wool.
• Affected areas are wet and the wool easily epilates.
• Parting of wool in affected areas reveals exudation and commonly diffuse discoloration or bands of discoloration.
• Fleece rot is characterized by a greenish discoloration of the wool fibers with a seropurulent crust. Most commonly discoloration is greenish but it may be yellow, yellow-brown, blue, or red-brown. Greenish coloration is due to bacterial production of the pigment pyocyanin.
• The virulence of this disease is determined by the presence of the enzyme phospholipase C in *P. aeruginosa*.
• Affected areas emanate a putrid odor and attract blowflies.
• General health is unaffected, but in cases with severe ulceration, death can occur due to sepsis.
• A chronic ulcerative necrotic dermatitis on the tail, udder, and legs associated with a greenish discoloration of fleece following excessive rain has been seen in the Mediterranean.

GENETICS
• There is a genetic predisposition to fleece rot with some sheep breeds being more susceptible than others, and some individuals within a breed being more vulnerable.
• Breeds with lower wax content, irregular fiber size, and thicker wool fibers are more susceptible.

CAUSES AND RISK FACTORS
• Major cause is prolonged wetting coupled with a "less waterproof" fleece.
• Fleece staple is a major factor in wool rot. A long fleece reduces skin wettability but, once wet, the skin and fleece dry more slowly. Short staple fleece is rapidly penetrated by water but dries more quickly.
• Compact fleeces with high wax contents are most resistant. This is probably due to the effect of the wax on waterproofing the fleece.

• Breeds with open fleece and poor staple structure are more prone.
• Susceptible sheep have smaller follicle groups and higher densities of follicle populations with more primary follicles; sheep with more secondary to primary hair follicle ratios are more resistant.
• Susceptible sheep have thicker wool fibers growing from primary follicles.
• Susceptible sheep have irregular wool fibers that retain water in the fleece for longer, making the fleece more susceptible to rot.
• Resistant sheep have better fleece closure and higher wax content allowing water to run off the wool; sheep that are more "waterproof" are more resistant.
• Yellowish fleece color (high suint content) is found in more susceptible sheep.

DIAGNOSIS

DIFFERENTIAL DIAGNOSES
• Major differential diagnosis is dermatophilosis.
• Scab formation and skin ulceration are absent in fleece rot, but present in dermatophilosis.

CBC/BIOCHEMISTRY/URINALYSIS
Affected sheep may have leukocytosis and neutrophilia.

OTHER LABORATORY TESTS
• If needed, bacterial isolation of causative agents by culture can be performed.
• Impression smears of exudate reveal Gram-negative rods.

IMAGING
N/A

OTHER DIAGNOSTIC PROCEDURES
Skin biopsy

PATHOLOGIC FINDINGS
Skin biopsy reveals suppurative intraepidermal pustular dermatitis and superficial folliculitis.

TREATMENT

THERAPEUTIC APPROACH
• Affected sheep are typically not treated, and treatment is usually of limited benefit.
• Chemical drying of fleece may decrease wetness and incidence of fleece rot.
• A mixture of zinc and aluminum oxides with sterols and fatty acids applied as a mist may be protective. This mixture has been shown to reduce fleece moisture for 10–12 weeks, reducing fleece rot by 60%.
• Prevention through selection of sheep with fleece resistant to wool rot is the most practical approach.

(CONTINUED) **WOOL ROT**

SURGICAL CONSIDERATIONS AND TECHNIQUES
N/A

MEDICATIONS

DRUGS OF CHOICE
Antibiotic treatment is of limited value due to the nature of *P. aeruginosa* to be resistant to many antibiotics.

CONTRAINDICATIONS
N/A

PRECAUTIONS
• Chemical drying agents should be compatible with other dipping chemicals (e.g., insecticides).
• Appropriate milk and meat withdrawal times must be followed for all compounds administered to food-producing animals.

POSSIBLE INTERACTIONS
N/A

FOLLOW-UP

EXPECTED COURSE AND PROGNOSIS
N/A

POSSIBLE COMPLICATIONS
• Affected animals are susceptible to blowfly strike.
• Affected sheep may develop secondary *P. aeruginosa* infections of the skin characterized by granulomatous scabs on the wool-free areas of the legs and scrotum.

CLIENT EDUCATION
Knowledge of risk factors and methods of prevention of fleece rot will help reduce prevalence in flocks.

PATIENT CARE
N/A

PREVENTION
• Shearing sheep before wet season may minimize wool rot, along with selection of breeds that are resistant to fleece rot.

• Heritability of resistance is estimated to be between 0.35 and 0.4 and selective breeding programs are recommended for high-risk areas.
• In the Merino breed the FBLN1 (fibulin) and FABP4 (fatty acid binding protein 4) genetic markers have been identified as key factors in the ability to resist fleece rot. Future efforts to select for these markers could allow for selection of a more resistant population of sheep.
• A killed *P. aeruginosa* vaccine has been found to be protective against severe exudation and may become a viable option in the future.

MISCELLANEOUS

ASSOCIATED CONDITIONS
• Affected sheep are at risk for blowfly strike.
• Prolonged wetting of the skin may predispose sheep to "pink rot," which is caused by a bacterial infection of the skin with *Bacillus* spp. Affected fibers are found at shearing and appear as a mat of wool in creamy pink exudate.

AGE-RELATED FACTORS
Wool rot is more common in young sheep.

ZOONOTIC POTENTIAL
N/A

PREGNANCY
N/A

BIOSECURITY
N/A

PRODUCTION MANAGEMENT
• Fleece rot is of major economic concern.
• Fleece wettability can be determined by taking a sample of staple and placing it in a wet plastic cylinder with one end in water. The mass of water taken up in a given time is measured. Results are consistent and capable of distinguishing resistant sheep from susceptible sheep.
• Susceptible fleeces are identified as having thin staples of unevenly crimped wool.

SYNONYMS
• Canary stain
• Fleece rot
• Water rot
• Wool rot
• Yolk rot

ABBREVIATIONS
N/A

SEE ALSO
• Dermatophilosis
• Lumpy Skin Disease
• Sheep Genetics and Selection (see www.fiveminutevet.com/ruminant)

Suggested Reading
Kimberling C. Diseases of the skin. In: Jensen R ed, Jensen and Swift's Diseases of Sheep, 3rd ed. Philadelphia: Lea & Febiger, 1988.
Plant, J. Bacterial and fungal infections of the skin and wool. In: Martin WB, Aitken ID eds, Diseases of Sheep, 3rd ed. Edinburgh: Blackwell Science, 2000.
Pugh DG, Baird AN. Diseases of the integumentary system. In: Pugh DG ed, Sheep and Goat Medicine, 2nd ed. Maryland Heights MO: Elsevier Health Sciences, 2012.
Radostits OM. Diseases caused by bacteria. In: Radostits OM, Gay CC, Hinchcliff KW, Constable PD eds, Veterinary Medicine: A Textbook of the Diseases of Cattle, Horses, Sheep, Pigs, and Goats, 10th ed. Edinburgh: Saunders Elsevier, 2007.
Scott DW. Ovine fleece rot. In: Howard JL, Smith RA eds, Current Veterinary Therapy 4: Food Animal Practice. Philadelphia: Saunders, 1999.
Smith WJM, Li Y, Ingham A, Reverter A. A genomics-informed, SNP association study reveals FBLN1 and FABP4 as contributing to resistance to fleece rot in Australian Merino sheep. BMC Vet Res 2010, 6: 1.

Author Joe S. Smith
Consulting Editor Erica C. McKenzie
Acknowledgment The author and book editors acknowledge the prior contribution of Susan Semrad and Karen A. Moriello.

W

WOUND MANAGEMENT

BASICS

OVERVIEW
Wound: An interruption in the continuity of the external surface of the body. Wounds may be restricted to the skin but often involve underlying and adjacent tissues.
Wound healing: A host's attempt to restore tissue continuity.
Proper understanding of the mechanism of wound healing allows the practitioner to select appropriate wound management techniques to decrease mortality and improve outcome.

SYSTEMS AFFECTED
• Musculoskeletal
• Integument

PATHOPHYSIOLOGY
Wound healing: A dynamic process which involves complex interactions between cellular and biochemical events. For simplicity it is divided into three phases.
1. Inflammation (1–6 days)—after initial vasoconstriction this phase is dominated by increased vascular permeability and subsequent edema with resulting influx of white blood cells and inflammatory mediators. Fibrin clot formation and debridement of contamination and necrotic tissue by white blood cells occurs.
2. Proliferation (3–14 days)—epithelialization, fibroplasia and angiogenesis result in granulation tissue formation and ingrowth of epithelium from the wound edges.
3. Maturation/Remodeling (14 days onwards)—wound contraction and remodeling, with fibroblast degradation and a balance between collagen synthesis and catabolic activity.

PHYSICAL EXAMINATION FINDINGS
Variable depending on location, severity, and involved structures. See "Therapeutic Approach" for details on patient and wound evaluation.

CAUSES AND RISK FACTORS
• Common causes—mechanical trauma.
• Other causes—neoplasia, burns, hypothermia, chemical-induced trauma, and infection.
• Generally:
  ◦ Penetrating or puncture wounds—deceptive in nature and can appear minor, but should always be considered serious. Bacteria, dirt, and foreign material can be translocated into the deep tissue by the penetrating object.
  ◦ Incised wound—injury created by a sharp object that leaves clean-edged wounds.
  ◦ Lacerated wounds—unlike incised wounds, these have rough and irregular edges and are more prone to infection.

  ◦ Abrasion—a scrape, friction burn, or excessive rubbing are common causes. They are a minor problem compared to the others and involve only the top layer of the skin.

DIAGNOSIS

DIFFERENTIAL DIAGNOSES
N/A

CBC/BIOCHEMISTRY/URINALYSIS
CBC—unremarkable in minor cases, but might be warranted in complicated wounds with involvement of deeper structures (e.g., osteomyelitis) or body cavities.

OTHER LABORATORY TESTS
• Cytology—evaluation of synovial, peritoneal, or pleural fluid is indicated when involvement of synovial structures or body cavities is suspected.
• Bacterial culture—evaluation of deep and chronically infected wounds as well as synovial, peritoneal, or pleural fluid when indicated.

IMAGING
• Ultrasonography—assessment of degree and severity of soft tissue involvement (e.g., ligaments, tendons), joint abnormalities, and presence of foreign bodies.
• Radiography—assessment of bony involvement (e.g., fractures, sequestrum formation) and radiodense foreign bodies.
• Contrast radiography—to evaluate the extent of wound tracts (puncture wounds).

OTHER DIAGNOSTIC PROCEDURES
• Palpation—using digital palpation or a probe to explore the wound and surrounding tissue to assess the extent of the wound and soft tissue damage. Perform after initial preparation and removal of gross contamination.
• See also "Imaging."

TREATMENT

THERAPEUTIC APPROACH
• Physical examination—vital parameters to assess systemic involvement (e.g., shock, blood loss, generalized or localized sepsis).
• Evaluation of the wound and involved structures
  ◦ Chemical restraint (use of sedation)
  ◦ Local anesthesia—regional anesthesia or a local block (e.g., lidocaine 2%). General anesthesia may be necessary for extensive injuries or for cast application.
  ◦ Preparation of the wound—clipping of hair and scrubbing of wound surroundings (povidone-iodine or chlorhexidine scrub). Wound lavage with lactated Ringer's

solution or isotonic saline. A 60 mL syringe with an 18-gauge needle can be used. It applies a pressure between 8–15 psi, preventing further damage and deeper translocation of bacteria into the wound.
  ◦ Povidone-iodine 0.1% solution or chlorhexidine 0.05% solution—recommended at this concentration to minimize cytotoxic effects on the tissue. Further debridement—sharp resection of devitalized tissue (scalpel blade, scissors).
  ◦ Exploration of the wound—digital palpation or use of a probe. Evaluation of soft tissue structures, extent of the wound, potential involvement of synovial structures or body cavities.
• Suspected synovial structure involvement—synoviocentesis (cytology and culture), infusion of sterile saline, and observation for fluid leakage from the wound.

SURGICAL CONSIDERATIONS AND TECHNIQUES

Primary Wound Closure
• Provides the greatest rate of healing and faster return to normal function. Indicated for recent wounds with minimal contamination.
• Closure—simple continuous or interrupted sutures. Tension relieving sutures (e.g., horizontal or vertical mattress, far-near-near-far) may also be required.
• Drain placement—when dead space is present (first 48–72 hours).
Suture removal: 10–14 days.

Delayed Primary Closure
• Indicated for older wounds, presence of intermediate contamination, and/or history of topical application of irritants.
• Closure—perform after initial treatment (debridement and lavage) when healthy granulation tissue has developed and no signs of infection are present.

Second Intention Wound Healing
• Indicated for heavy contamination, excessive soft tissue damage or dead space, or extensive tissue loss. Requires greatest time to heal and functionality might be impaired due to scar formation.
• Treat with topical medication and bandage application; highly mobile areas (e.g., joint surfaces on distal limbs) may require application of a splint bandage or cast for immobilization.

MEDICATIONS

DRUGS OF CHOICE

Systemic Medications
• Anti-inflammatory drugs—NSAIDs (e.g., flunixin meglumine 1.1 mg/kg body weight, IV, q24h; ketoprofen 3 mg/kg, IV/IM, q24h)

W

can have some negative effects on wound healing but are indicated for patient comfort and control of swelling.

• Antimicrobial drugs—depending on severity of the wound. With involvement of synovial structures and/or body cavities, broad-spectrum antimicrobial therapy might be indicated based on common contaminants. A more targeted approach can be instituted after receiving culture results. Beta-lactam antimicrobials (penicillin, ceftiofur, amoxicillin, ampicillin) or potentiated sulfonamides (where permitted) are most commonly used.

• Tetanus toxoid—animals with significant tissue damage, penetrating wounds, and risk of anaerobic infection. Administer as per manufacturer's instructions.

• Regional medications
  ◦ Regional limb perfusion—distal limb wounds. Delivery of high antimicrobial concentrations (broad spectrum, concentration dependent antibiotic) to the affected area.
  ◦ The addition of a local anesthetic (e.g., lidocaine 2%) can facilitate patient management and manipulation of the wound (e.g., debridement).

Topical Medications

A variety of different wound dressings and wound care products are available, with little research performed on their effects on wound healing in ruminants. Extrapolation from other species (human, small animal, and horse) may guide the practitioner in their choice. Restrictions for food-producing animals must be considered. Note: all products containing nitrofurazone are prohibited from use in food-producing species.

Wound Dressings

• Inflammatory phase—adherent dressings aid in debridement (e.g., mesh gauze can be used to create a wet-to-dry bandage).

• Proliferative phase/Maturation and remodeling—semi-occlusive and nonadherent bandages can be used when bed of granulation tissue has developed (e.g., coated gauze, amnion).

CONTRAINDICATIONS

Glucocorticosteriods—can cause inhibition of the normal inflammatory response, leading to delayed wound healing. Contraindicated in pregnant animals.

PRECAUTIONS

Appropriate milk and meat withdrawal times must be followed for all compounds administered to food-producing animals.

 FOLLOW-UP

EXPECTED COURSE AND PROGNOSIS

Variable, depending on type of wound, structures involved, and severity of the lesion.

POSSIBLE COMPLICATIONS

• Septicemia
• Localized spread of infection—synovial sepsis (joints, tendon sheath, bursae), osteomyelitis, myositis
• Tissue necrosis
• Loss of function (severe scar formation, degenerative joint disease)

PATIENT CARE

• Monitor for progression of wounds through the different phases and insure that applied treatments are not detrimental to progress.
• Monitor for signs of infection (color, size, and discharge), systemic sepsis, localized septic processes, and primary dehiscence, or tissue necrosis.

 MISCELLANEOUS

ASSOCIATED CONDITIONS

Generalized or localized sepsis, loss of function, degenerative joint disease can all be associated depending on location and severity of the wound.

AGE-RELATED FACTORS

Wounds can be acquired throughout all life stages but the ability to heal has been shown to be best in young animals.

ZOONOTIC POTENTIAL

Certain secondary wound diseases are zoonotic.

ABBREVIATION

NSAID = nonsteroidal anti-inflammatory drug

SEE ALSO

• Anesthesia: Local and Regional
• Burn Management
• Food Animal Residue Avoidance Databank (FARAD) (see www.fiveminutevet.com/ruminant)
• Pain Management (see www.fiveminutevet.com/ruminant)

Suggested Reading

Hackett CH, Hackett RP, Nydam CW, Nydam DV, Gilbert RO. Surgery of the bovine (adult) integumentary system. In: Fubini SL, Ducharme NG eds, Farm Animal Surgery, 2nd ed. St. Louis: Elsevier, 2017.

Jones M, Gibbons P, Hartnack A. Surgery of the sheep and goat integumentary system. In: Fubini SL, Ducherme NG eds, Farm Animal Surgery 2nd ed. St. Louis: Elsevier, 2017.

Miesner MD. Bovine surgery of the skin. Vet Clin North Am Food Anim Pract 2008, 24: 517–26.

Stashak TS, Farstvedt E. Update on wound dressings: Indications and best use. In: Stashak TS, Theroret CL eds, Equine Wound Management, 2nd ed. Ames: Blackwell, 2009.

Author Nora M. Biermann
Consulting Editor Kaitlyn A. Lutz
Acknowledgment The author and book editors acknowledge the prior contribution of Yessenia Almedia.

W

YAK MANAGEMENT AND DISEASE

BASICS

OVERVIEW
• Yak (*Poephagus grunniens* or *Bos grunniens*) is a long-haired, flat-headed, bushy-tailed domesticated bovine found in the mountain regions of Northern India, Nepal, Bhutan, Mongolia, Russia and predominately in the Qinghai-Tibetan Plateau.
• Yak can survive in very low temperatures (down to −55°C) and are found at an altitude of 3,000–5,000 meters above sea level and generally not below 2,000 m. They thrive well in the extreme harshness of cold mountain climates.
• Yak are raised for milk, cheese, butter, ghee (clarified butter), churpee (dry cheese), wool, draft power, manure, and pack purposes; they are closely linked with the social, cultural, and ritual activity and livelihood of Himalayan people such as the Sherpa community of Nepal.
• Population of yak and chauri (yak/hill cow hybrid) is estimated at 13 million in China, 6 million in Mongolia, and 26,288 in Nepal.
• In general, the male is called a yak and the female is called a nak.
• Crossing between male yak and local hill cow (*Bos indicus*) is very popular and the offspring are called Urang Jhopkyo (male) and Urang Chauri (female). Males are sterile and females are popular for milk production.

INCIDENCE/PREVALENCE
Data on incidence of disease in yak is scarce.

GEOGRAPHIC DISTRIBUTION
Himalayan region of Northern India, Nepal and Bhutan, Mongolia, Russia, and predominately on the Qinghai-Tibetan Plateau of China.

SYSTEMS AFFECTED
Depends on the disease.

PATHOPHYSIOLOGY
Depends on the disease but generally similar to other ruminants.

HISTORICAL FINDINGS
Depends on the disease but generally similar to other ruminants.

SIGNALMENT
Depends on the disease but generally similar to other ruminants.

PHYSICAL EXAMINATION FINDINGS
Depends on the disease but generally similar to other ruminants.

GENETICS
• Yak and cattle have same number of chromosome (2n = 60).

• Crossing of yak with local hill cattle is popular to increase meat and milk production and for better reproductive performance.
• The hybrids are found at lower altitudes and less harsh conditions than the highland environment of the yak.
• In Nepal, Brown Swiss bovine semen was used for cross-breeding with yak, with satisfactory results.
• F2, F3, and F4 generations and back-crossing are practiced in the yak mating system; however, farmers prefer F1 generation.
• F1 males are sterile.
• F1 hybrids grow faster and the milk yield is higher than with the purebred nak.
• The fat percentage in the milk of hybrids is lower than that of purebred nak.

CAUSES AND RISK FACTORS
Bacterial Diseases
• Anthrax—common in many regions of Asia
• Blackquarter— common in Nepal and perhaps other places
• Brucellosis—common throughout Asia
• Botulism—*Clostridium botulinum* type C has been identified in Tibet
• Hemorrhagic septicemia (HS)
• Johne's disease
• Mastitis—very common
• Tuberculosis—researchers tested 1,749 yaks in Tibet, found 12.7% positive reactors
• Calf scour—mostly due to *E. coli*
• Leptospirosis—causes abortion
• Contagious bovine pleuropneumonia
• Salmonellosis—common among yak in China
• Tetanus
• *Coxiella burnetii*
• Campylobacteriosis

Viral Diseases
• Foot and mouth disease—common in yak producing areas of Asia
• Rinderpest—yak are highly susceptible to rinderpest but now outbreaks not reported
• Bovine viral diarrhea/mucosal disease—detected in several provinces of Tibet
• Other—rabies, calf diphtheria

Parasitic Diseases
• Lice, tick, flea, mites—Psoroptidae and Sarcoptidae family of mites are commonly found in yak
• Babesiosis
• Hypodermiasis
• Gid (coenurosis)—reported in Bhutan
• Liver fluke disease—*Fasciola hepatica* and *F. gigantica*
• *Strongyles* spp.*, Trichuris*, coccidia, *Dicrocoelim* and *Ascaris* are other common endoparasites of yak reported throughout Asia.

DIAGNOSIS

DIFFERENTIAL DIAGNOSES
Depends on the disease but generally similar to other ruminants.

CBC/BIOCHEMISTRY/URINALYSIS
Depends on the disease but generally similar to other ruminants.

OTHER LABORATORY TESTS
Depends on the disease but generally similar to other ruminants.

IMAGING
Depends on the disease but generally similar to other ruminants.

OTHER DIAGNOSTIC PROCEDURES
Depends on the disease but generally similar to other ruminants.

PATHOLOGIC FINDINGS
Depends on the disease but generally similar to other ruminants.

TREATMENT

THERAPEUTIC APPROACH
Depends on the disease but generally similar to other ruminants.

SURGICAL CONSIDERATIONS AND TECHNIQUES
Depends on the disease but generally similar to other ruminants.

MEDICATIONS

DRUGS OF CHOICE
Yak farmers use local medicines to treat diseases, such as locally brewed alcohol (Chhyang), Tibetan tea leaves, and the excreta of insects collected from trees in the case of red water disease, mustard oil and garlic in the case of bloat, Nirmasi (aconite roots) in poisoning, and Timur (prickly wood seed) for digestive problems.

CONTRAINDICATIONS
Appropriate milk and meat withdrawal times must be followed for all compounds administered to food-producing animals.

PRECAUTIONS
N/A

POSSIBLE INTERACTIONS
N/A

YAK MANAGEMENT AND DISEASE

FOLLOW-UP

EXPECTED COURSE AND PROGNOSIS
Depends on the disease but generally similar to other ruminants.

POSSIBLE COMPLICATIONS
Depends on the disease but generally similar to other ruminants.

CLIENT EDUCATION
Depends on the disease but generally similar to other ruminants.

PATIENT CARE
Depends on the disease but generally similar to other ruminants.

PREVENTION
Depends on the disease but generally similar to other ruminants.

MISCELLANEOUS

ASSOCIATED CONDITIONS
Depends on the disease but generally similar to other ruminants.

AGE-RELATED FACTORS
• Young calves are more susceptible to ascariasis and adults are susceptible to *Fasciola*.
• By 3–3.5 years Chauri and Jiulong males have reached nearly 58% of their adult weight.

ZOONOTIC POTENTIAL
Similar to cattle: Anthrax, tuberculosis, brucellosis, Q fever, rabies, salmonellosis.

PREGNANCY
• 90% of mating takes place during August to November
• Most calves born from April to July when they reach upper pasture area.

BIOSECURITY
• Quarantine and testing
• Isolate sick animal, especially if the disease is contagious, e.g., HS, rinderpest, FMD

PRODUCTION MANAGEMENT
• Yak are open grazers.
• The transhumance system of moving animals to upper pastures in summer and autumn and to lower pastures in winter and spring months is practiced for yaks and chauri.
• Due to the nomadic system of animal husbandry, yak are housed in a temporary type of shed for a short period (2–3 weeks) at one place and then moved on to the next stopping point in a similar way.
• During the winter months the yak are kept outside in a fenced open area close to the herder's house. During periods of heavy snowfall the young and productive yak are kept indoors on the ground floor of the permanent house.
• Average age of first calving of purebred nak is 4.23 years while for Dimjo and Urang Chauri it is 3.33 years and 3.87 years respectively.
• Average milk yield of nak is 720 L per lactation and for Dimjo and Urang Chauri it is 1,690 L and 1,300 L respectively.

Nutrition
• Yak consume less feed as compared to cattle due to their smaller rumen relative to body weight.
• Dry matter intake in kg per day for growing yak is calculated as $DMI = 0.0165W + 0.04869$ (W = body weight in kg).
• Dry matter intake in kg per day for lactating yak is calculated as $DMI = 0.008W^{0.52} + 1.369Y$ ($W^{0.52}$ = metabolic body weight and Y = milk yield in kg per day)
• Voluntary intake (VI) ranges from 18–25 kg fresh forage in summer season to 6–8 kg per day under cold grazing conditions.
• Rumen volume ranges from 32.3 to 66.8 L in mature adult yak.

Energy
• The thermoneutral zone for the growing yak is estimated as 8°C–14°C.
• The fasting heat production (FHP) of the growing yak can be estimated as $FHP = 916$ kJ per kg $W^{0.52}$ per day.
• The metabolizable energy requirement for maintenance (ME_m) in growing yak is around 460 kJ per kg $W^{0.75}$ per day.
• The daily metabolizable energy requirement of growing yak has been estimated as ME $(MJ/d) = 0.45W^{0.75} + (8.73 + 0.091W)$ DG, where W is the body weight and DG is daily gain (kg), and the efficiency of utilization of metabolizable energy for growth (k_g) in yak is 0.49.
• Researchers observed that lactating yak have better utilization of dietary energy than dry yak cows. Another study with lactating yak indicated that yak cows have a lower efficiency of metabolizable energy utilization for milk production (averaging 0.46) than dairy cattle (*Bos taurus*).

Protein
• There is no difference in the digestibility of dietary nitrogen between lactating and dry yak cows.
• Yak can use nonprotein nitrogen as efficiently as domestic cattle.
• Rumen degradable crude protein requirements for maintenance ($RDCP_m$; g per day) in the growing yak are around $6.09W^{0.52}$ g per day.
• Crude protein requirements for daily gain (DG $RDCP_g$; g per day) in growing yak can be estimated as $RDCP_g = (1.16/DG + 0.05/W^{0.52})^{-1}$.
• Total crude protein requirements for growing yak can be calculated as RDCP (g per day) = $6.09W^{0.52} + (1.16/DG + 0.05/W^{0.52})^{-1}$.
• Yak may have evolved a mechanism to recycle more nitrogen to the rumen than cattle.

Minerals
• Mineral nutrition is poorly understood in the yak.
• Researchers have found that inorganic phosphate (P) is sufficient for various categories of yak (calves, heifers, dry cows, and lactating cows) during the warm season when grazing was on alpine meadows with good-quality pasture. But in the spring and early summer, dietary phosphate failed to meet yak requirements.
• Chinese researchers suggest that yak living in the Qinghai Lake area are suffering sodium (Na) and copper (Cu) deficiency and there may be a shortage of molybdenum on Tianzhu alpine rangelands.

SYNONYMS
N/A

ABBREVIATIONS
• DG = daily gain
• DMI = dry matter intake
• FHP = fasting heat production
• FMD = foot and mouth disease
• HS= hemorrhagic septicemia
• ME = metabolizable energy
• RDCP = rumen degradable crude protein
• W = body weight

SEE ALSO
• Biosecurity: Beef Cow/Calf (see www.fiveminutevet.com/ruminant)
• Biosecurity: Dairy (see www.fiveminutevet.com/ruminant)
• Diarrheal Diseases: Bovine
• Foot and Mouth Disease
• Johne's Disease
• Parasite Control Programs: Beef
• Parasite Control Programs: Dairy
• Respiratory Disease: Bovine
• Weight Loss: Bovine
• Yak Reproduction

Suggested Reading
Claus M, Dierenfeld ES. Susceptibility of yak (*Bos grunniens*) to copper deficiency. Vet Rec 1999, 145: 436–7.

Guo S, Chen W. The situation of yaks in China. In: Miller DG, Craig SR, Rana GM eds, Proceedings of a Workshop on Conservation and Management of Yak Genetic Diversity. Kathmandu: ICIMOD (International Centre for Integrated Mountain Development), 1996.

Y

YAK MANAGEMENT AND DISEASE (CONTINUED)

Kharel M, Shrestha BS, Shrestha R. The Nepali Yak. Bhaktapur, Nepal: Himalayan College of Agricultural Sciences and Technology (HICAST), 2010.

Lensch JH, Geilhausen HE. Infectious and parasitic diseases in the yak. Proceedings of the Second International Congress on Yak. Xining, China: Qinghai People's Publishing House, 1997.

Long RJ, Apori SO, Castro FB, Ørskov ER. Feed value of native forages of the Tibetan Plateau of China. Anim Feed Sci Technol 1999, 80: 101–13.

Long RJ, Zhang DG, Wang X, Hu ZZ, Dong SK. Effect of strategic feed supplementation on productive and reproductive performance in yak cows. Prev Vet Med 1999, 38: 195–206.

Pal RN. Domestic yak (*Poephagus grunniens* L.): A research review. Indian J Anim Sci 1993, 63: 743–53.

Wiener G, Jianlin H, Ruijun L. The Yak. Bangkok, Thailand: Food and Agriculture Organization of the United Nations, 2003.

Xu G, Wang Z. Present situation and proposal for future development of yak industry in China. Forage and Livestock, 1998, Supplement: 6–8.

Author Egendra Kumar Shrestha
Consulting Editor Ahmed Tibary
Acknowledgment The author and book editors acknowledge the prior contribution of Scott R.R. Haskell.

BASICS

OVERVIEW
• The yak (*Poephagus grunniens* or *Bos grunniens*) is a unique species that thrives well in the extremely harsh conditions of mountain regions and is nomadic in nature.
• The crosses of yak (*Bos grunniens*) and local hill cattle (*Bos indicus*) are called chauri. The chauri are more productive than the female yak (nak) and can adapt to lower altitudes.
• Chauri farming is a main source of livelihood in the Himalayan regions.

INCIDENCE/PREVALENCE
N/A

GEOGRAPHIC DISTRIBUTION
Yak are found in the Himalayan regions of Nepal, Northern India, Bhutan, Mongolia, Russia, and on the Qinghai-Tibetan Plateau of China.

SYSTEMS AFFECTED
Reproductive

PATHOPHYSIOLOGY
• There is little information on the pathophysiology of reproductive disorders in the yak.
• Reproductive physiology in this species presents several characteristics.

Male Reproduction
• Male yak may display sexual behavior as early as 6 months of age but are not able to ejaculate spermatozoa until 18–24 months of age.
• Bulls tends to graze separately in winter and early spring and join the herd during the breeding season. They can detect estrous females from a long distance.
• Bulls have smaller testicular size compared to *Bos taurus* or *Bos indicus* cattle. Sperm production is similar to cattle but total sperm production is about 60% that of cattle.
• The yak scrotum is small with abundant hair, apparently an adaptation to the cold environment.
• The reproductive life varies from 3.5 to 14 years of age and may be breed-dependent. In general, bulls are used starting at 4 years of age and reach peak reproductive efficiency at 7 years.

Female Reproduction
Reproductive Anatomy
• The reproductive organs of the female yak are similar to those of the bovine, with several differences. The cervix is long (5–6 cm), the uterine body is short (1.5–3 cm), the ovaries are smaller than those of cattle and present fewer primordial oocytes.
Reproductive Physiology
• Puberty occurs between 13 and 30 months of age and is determined mainly by the body condition at the beginning of the breeding season. Age at first calving varies from 3 to 4 years.
• Follicular activity is seasonal.
• The breeding season starts in late spring and early summer, between May and July, depending on the geographic location. Peak activity is observed in the height of summer (July and August), when temperatures are at their highest and grass growth is at its best. Estrus frequency decreases and stops around November.
• Estrus cycle length varies between 18 and 22 days. A greater variation in the length of the estrus cycle has been reported but may be due to factors such as silent or nondetected estrus, delayed ovulation, or pregnancy loss.
• Estrus in the yak is greatly affected by the environment. Signs of estrus are similar but not as strongly displayed as in *B. taurus*. Physical changes of the reproductive organs during estrus are more obvious and include reddening and swelling of the vulva and mucus vaginal discharge.
• Signs of estrus are more intense in the early morning and evening. The duration of estrus is estimated at 12–16 hours. Ovulation generally occurs 12–24 hours after the end of estrus.
• Conception rates are very high in females with good body condition scores and approach 70% per cycle for both natural cover and artificial insemination. Under extensive management, pregnancy rates may vary from 40% to 80%.
• The average gestation period of the yak is 258 days, range 228–280 days. Almost all births take place during the day and only very few at night.
• Premonitory signs of parturition include isolation from the herd by the female that seeks a sheltered area. The first stage of labor is characterized by alternating body position between lateral recumbence and standing. Calves may be delivered in the standing position. Complete cervical dilation lasts up to 4 hours. The second stage of labor, fetal expulsion, lasts 20–30 minutes, and the third stage of labor, expulsion of the placenta, lasts 2–6 hours. The dam generally licks the newborn calf for about 10 minutes, after which the calf attempts to stand up and suck.
• Dystocia is a rare event in purebred yaks. Twinning incidence is about 0.5% of all births, but may be higher in some breeds.
Postpartum
• Postpartum anestrus duration varies from 70 to 125 days and seems to be influenced by body condition and month of calving.
• Most yak females are managed to calve twice in 3 years.

Artificial Breeding
Hormonal Control of Ovarian Activity and Ovulation
• Several techniques in cattle for estrus synchronization and induction of ovulation have been attempted in yaks. Induction of follicular activity and ovulation in anestrous yaks has been done using eCG or FSH.
• Treatment with eCG (100 IU) induces estrus 1–10 days later. GnRH injection is reported to induce estrus in >80% of anestrous females within 7 days, with conception rates >70%. Estrus synchronization in cycling yaks is possible using two injections of PGF2$_\alpha$ or analogs 10 days apart. Fertility at the induced estrus is excellent.
Artificial Insemination
Artificial insemination is used in some breeding projects both for purebred yaks and in cross-breeding schemes with *Bos taurus*.
Semen Collection and Evaluation
Yak bulls can readily be trained to serve an artificial vagina. Semen can be collected twice weekly. Ejaculates of adult yak bulls have a volume of 2–5 mL and a concentration of 7.5–16 million/mL. The proportion of normal spermatozoa is generally >70%. Motility varies between 70% and 85%.
Semen Processing
• Techniques for extending and freezing yak semen are similar to those used for the bovine. Many authors use yak milk as the milk extender. Extenders frequently used are sucrose based or lactose-citrate with 20% egg yolk and 3–7% glycerol. Glycerolated semen is equilibrated for 2–3 hours before freezing. Semen is frozen in various packages including ampules, pellets, and straws.
• Semen frozen in pellets is thawed out by agitation for 3–5 seconds in 2.9% sodium citrate solution, glucose-sodium citrate solution, or fresh skim milk solution at 38–42°C.
Insemination
• Technique of insemination is similar to that used for cattle. The cervix of estrous yaks is reportedly easier to penetrate than that of cattle. Females are inseminated twice, 12 hours apart, with 10 million progressively motile spermatozoa. The first insemination is generally performed 24 hours after the beginning of estrus and repeated 12 hours later.
• Conception rates of >80% are reported with two inseminations, the first at the end of estrus and the second 12 hours later. For optimum fertility, semen should be deposited in the uterine body.

Cross-breeding Between Yak and Bos taurus
• Cross-breeding between yak and species of cattle is often practiced to improve milk and meat yield in Asia. Pregnancy rates are generally lower in cross-breeding programs.
• Pregnancy loss (abortion or premature birth) are more frequent in females carrying hybrids. Pregnancy length is increased in female yaks carrying crossbred fetuses.
• Yak cows carrying hybrid calves are at higher risks for dystocia and may require more obstetric assistance.

YAK REPRODUCTION

Reproductive Failure
• Abortion, anestrus, and repeat breeding are common reproductive disorders.
• Reported abortion causes include brucellosis and chlamydiosis.

HISTORICAL FINDINGS
Depends on complaint

SIGNALMENT
Breeding age male and female yak

PHYSICAL EXAMINATION FINDINGS
N/A

CAUSES AND RISK FACTORS
Causes and risk factors for reproductive disorders are similar to those described in cattle.

DIAGNOSIS

DIFFERENTIAL DIAGNOSES
Differential diagnosis approach to abortion and reproductive failure is similar to that used in cattle.

CBC/BIOCHEMISTRY/URINALYSIS
N/A

OTHER LABORATORY TESTS
Serum progesterone assay may be used to monitor cyclicity as in cattle.

IMAGING
Transrectal ultrasonography for follicular dynamics, cyclicity, and pregnancy diagnoses.

OTHER DIAGNOSTIC PROCEDURES
N/A

PATHOLOGIC FINDINGS
N/A

TREATMENT

THERAPEUTIC APPROACH
• Therapeutic approach for reproductive disorders in similar to that described for cattle.
• Estrus synchronization programs used in cattle have been adapted with moderate success in yaks.

SURGICAL CONSIDERATIONS AND TECHNIQUES
N/A

MEDICATIONS

DRUGS OF CHOICE
Drugs used for hormonal therapy are similar to those used for cattle.

CONTRAINDICATIONS
Appropriate milk and meat withdrawal times must be followed for all compounds administered to food-producing animals.

PRECAUTIONS
N/A

POSSIBLE INTERACTIONS
N/A

FOLLOW-UP
N/A

MISCELLANEOUS

ASSOCIATED CONDITIONS
N/A

AGE-RELATED FACTORS
• Male yaks may display sexual behavior as early as 6 months of age but are not able to ejaculate spermatozoa until 18–24 months of age.
• In general, bulls are used starting at 4 years of age and reach peak reproductive efficiency at 7 years.
• Puberty in yaks occurs between 13 and 30 months of age and is determined mainly by the body condition at the beginning of the breeding season. Age at first calving varies from 3 to 4 years.

ZOONOTIC POTENTIAL
Brucellosis

PREGNANCY
• Dystocia is a rare event in purebred yaks. Twinning incidence is about 0.5% of all births, but may be higher in some breeds.
• Conception rates are very high in females with good body condition scores and approach 70% per cycle for both natural cover and artificial insemination. Under extensive management pregnancy rates may vary from 40% to 80%.
• The average gestation length of yaks is 258 days, range 228–280 days according to some observations. Almost all births take place during the day and only very few at night.

BIOSECURITY
N/A

PRODUCTION MANAGEMENT
The Performance of the Yak (Nak)
• The age of first calving is 48 months
• The milk yield is 470 liters per lactation
• The calving interval is 687 days
• The lactation length is about 174 days

The Performance of the Chauri
• The age of first calving is 36 months
• The milk yield is 1,960 liters per lactation
• The calving interval is 425 days
• The lactation length is 254–400 days

SYNONYMS
N/A

ABBREVIATIONS
• eCG = equine chorionic gonadotropin
• FSH = follicle stimulating hormone
• GnRH = gonadotropin releasing hormone
• $PGF2_\alpha$ = prostaglandin $F2_\alpha$

SEE ALSO
Yak Management and Disease

Suggested Reading
Aryal S, Paudel K. Reproductive disorders and seroprevalence of brucellosis in Yak. Nepal Agric Res J 2007, 8: P130–3.
Kharel M, Shrestha BS, Shrestha R. The Nepali Yak. Bhaktapur, Nepal: Himalayan College of Agricultural Sciences and Technology (HICAST), 2010.
Li Z, Cao X, Fu B, et al. Identification and characterization of *Chlamydia abortus* isolated from yaks in Quighai, China. Biomed Res Int 2015, 2015: 658519. doi: 10.1155/2015/658519. Epub 2015 Apr 28.
Long RJ, Zhang DG, Wang X, Hu ZZ, Dong SK. Effect of strategic feed supplementation on productive and reproductive performance in yak cows. Prev Vet Med 1999, 38: 195–206.
Wiener G, Jianlin H, Ruijun L. The Yak. Bangkok, Thailand: Food and Agriculture Organization of the United Nations, 2003.
Xiang-Dong Zi. Reproduction in female yaks (*Bos grunniens*) and opportunities for improvement. Theriogenology 2003, 59: 1303–12.
Zhao XX, Zhang RC. Recent Advances in Yak Reproduction. Ithaca NY: International Veterinary Information Service (www.ivis.org), 2001.
Author Egendra Kumar Shrestha
Consulting Editor Ahmed Tibary
Acknowledgment The author and book editors acknowledge the prior contribution of Ahmed Tibary.

YEW TOXICITY

BASICS

OVERVIEW
• Yew or *Taxus* family of which all members are toxic.
• Evergreen shrubs or trees commonly used for landscaping.
• Leaves are simple, alternate needle-like that often appear as 2-ranked.
• Flexible seed cones that contain seeds that are nutlike and partially or wholly enclosed by a fleshy cup-like aril that varies from green to red orange to brilliant scarlet.
• Relatively palatable.

INCIDENCE/PREVALENCE
Mortality rate is high

SYSTEMS AFFECTED
• Cardiovascular
• Digestive

GEOGRAPHIC DISTRIBUTION
Worldwide

PATHOPHYSIOLOGY
• Toxicity is result of toxic alkaloids of which taxine A and B are the most toxic.
• Antagonism of myocardial calcium channels thus interferes with cardiac conduction leading to depression of atrioventricular conduction and heart block.
• Taxine at low dose also affects smooth muscle tone, thus manifests as decreased intestinal motility and uterine contractions.
• Volatile irritant oils are also present within the plant and in subacute cases will result in gastrointestinal inflammation.
• All parts, except for the avril, are toxic.
• Lethal dose in cattle is 2.0 g/kg body weight while goats are more resistant with lethal dose of 12 g/kg.

HISTORICAL FINDINGS
History of exposure to plants

SIGNALMENT
• Bovine, ovine, caprine
• Wild ruminants seem to be resistant to some species of *Taxus*.

PHYSICAL EXAMINATION FINDINGS
• Develop within minutes of exposure
• Acute collapse and death
• Dyspnea
• Tremors
• Subacute exposure: gastroenteritis

CAUSES AND RISK FACTORS
• Toxic principles are taxines A and B.
• Both fresh and dried leaves toxic; seeds toxic.
• Clippings are highly toxic.

DIAGNOSIS

• History of exposure to the plants
• Clinical signs
• Identification of plant in oral cavity or GI contents

DIFFERENTIAL DIAGNOSES
• Oleander
• Foxglove
• Rhododendron

CBC/BIOCHEMISTRY/URINALYSIS
No characteristic changes

PATHOLOGIC FINDINGS
• There are few lesions other than nonspecific organ congestion, including moderate pulmonary congestion and edema, and perhaps a few scattered ecchymotic hemorrhages which are changes typical of circulatory disturbances.
• Evidence of myocardial fibrosis on necropsy although this is not specific to this toxicity.

TREATMENT

THERAPEUTIC APPROACH
Supportive treatment

MEDICATIONS

DRUGS OF CHOICE
No antidote

FOLLOW-UP

EXPECTED COURSE AND PROGNOSIS
Extremely grave, most animals die.

PREVENTION
Do not allow access to *Taxus* spp. or clippings

MISCELLANEOUS

PRODUCTION MANAGEMENT
• Remove *Taxus* spp. from pastures.
• Do not allow access to yew clippings.

SEE ALSO
• Cardiotoxic Plants
• Oleander and Cardiotoxic Plant Toxicity

Suggested Reading
Burrows GE. Taxaceae. In: Burrows GE, Tyrl RJ eds, Toxic Plants of North America. Ames: Iowa State University Press, 2001, pp. 1149–55.
Burrows GE, Tyrl RJ. In: Toxic Plants of North America, 2nd ed. Ames: Wiley-Blackwell, Kindle edition, 2013, pp. 1179–83.
Sula MJM, Morgan S, Bailey KL, et al. Characterization of cardiac lesions in calves after ingestion of Japanese yew (*Taxus cuspidata*). J Vet Diagn Invest 2015, 25: 522–6.
Author Jennifer S. Taintor
Consulting Editor Christopher C.L. Chase
Acknowledgment The author and book editors acknowledge the prior contribution of Jerry R. Roberson.

ZINC DEFICIENCY AND TOXICITY

OVERVIEW

Zinc (Zn) is an essential trace element that is a component of several enzymes, serves catalytic, structural and regulatory functions, and is essential for keratinization.

INCIDENCE/PREVALENCE
• Zn deficiency: Low
• Zn toxicity: Rare

GEOGRAPHIC DISTRIBUTION
Western United States and Canada: Forages with low concentrations of Zn; does not coincide with widespread clinical Zn deficiency.

SYSTEMS AFFECTED
Zinc Deficiency
• Dermatologic
  ◦ Parakeratosis
• Digestive
  ◦ Decrease in microvillus length → maldigestive, malabsorptive diarrhea
• Endocrine system
  ◦ Decreased production of thyroid hormone, growth hormone, insulin, and testosterone
• Reproductive
  ◦ Degeneration of the seminiferous tubules
  ◦ Abnormal Leydig cell numbers and morphology
  ◦ Reduced circulating testosterone
  ◦ Abnormal sperm development and function
  ◦ Abortion, fetal mummification, low birthweights, teratogenic defects, and reduced neonatal survival
  ◦ Altered myometrial contractility and increased risk of hemorrhage postpartum
• Ophthalmology
  ◦ Zn is needed for multiple steps in the metabolism of vitamin A to rhodopsin, and in its absence night blindness is seen.
• Immunology
  ◦ Decreased response to hypersensitivity, decreased CD4 positive T-lymphocytes and B-lymphocytes, and neutropenia
• Musculoskeletal
  ◦ Weakness
  ◦ Poor suckle reflex
  ◦ Reduced bone density and growth
• Neurologic
  ◦ Altered concentration of hypothalamic neurotransmitters → altered sense of taste and smell → decreased appetite
  ◦ Required for normal brain development and function
• Hematology
  ◦ Decreased erythrocyte precursors in the bone marrow and increased erythrocyte osmotic fragility

  ◦ Impaired platelet aggregation and increased bleeding time

Zinc Toxicity
• Digestive: Hepatic dysfunction, pancreatitis
• Urogenital: Glomerular damage and renal tubular epithelial necrosis (protein losing nephropathy)
• Hematology: Interference with glutathione reductase → oxidative damage → intravascular hemolysis

PATHOPHYSIOLOGY
• Plasma: ~0.1% total body Zn (99% protein-bound)
• No storage system → homeostasis primarily controlled at the level of intestinal absorption → largely dependent on the Zn status of the animal
• *Zn deficiency* affects multiple systems
  ◦ Systems that have a high cellular turnover are most affected.
  ◦ Alteration in prostaglandin metabolism affects the arachidonic acid cascade, luteal function, and myometrial contractions.
• *Zn toxicity:* Soluble Zn salts form in acidic abomasum → direct mucosal irritation and ulceration → absorbed into circulation and rapidly distributed to the liver, kidneys, prostate, muscles, bones, and pancreas. Zn salts interfere with the metabolism of other ions (Cu, Ca, and Fe) and inhibit erythrocyte production and function.
  ◦ Mechanisms of toxicity are not completely understood.
  ◦ Acute toxicity LD50 of Zn salts ~100 mg/kg.
  ◦ Chronic Zn toxicosis in large animals caused by diets containing Zn >2,000 ppm.

HISTORICAL FINDINGS
Variable. See "Physical Examination Findings."

SIGNALMENT
Young pre-ruminants more susceptible to Zn deficiency because rumen microbes digest phytate, increasing Zn bioavailability.

PHYSICAL EXAMINATION FINDINGS
Zinc Deficiency
• Anorexia
• Reduced weight gain
• Diarrhea
• Lesions of the integument
  ◦ Alopecia, rough hair coat
  ◦ Deep fissures
  ◦ Serum crusts
  ◦ ± Pruritis
  ◦ Distribution: face, neck and distal extremities and mucocutaneous junctions
• Poliosis: Reduced pigmentation of the hair around the orbits
• Loss of crimping in wool

• Deformed hooves
• Excessive lacrimation, nasal discharge, salivation
• Testicular atrophy, poor reproductive performance
• Reduced milk production, increased incidence of mastitis
• Immunodeficiency, delayed wound healing
• Poor suckle reflex in calves
• Night blindness

Zinc Toxicity
• Diarrhea
• Anorexia
• Lethargy
• Decrease in weight gain and milk production
• Intravascular hemolysis—icterus, hemoglobinuria
• Cardiac arrhythmia
• Seizures
• Ulcers in the oral cavity and esophagus
• Signs of copper deficiency

GENETICS
• Bovine hereditary zinc deficiency (lethal trait A46, Adema disease, hereditary parakeratosis, hereditary thymus hypoplasia)
  ◦ Autosomal recessive
  ◦ Reduced ability to absorb Zn
  ◦ Friesian cattle
  ◦ Signs seen 4–8 months after birth → fatal around 4 months if untreated
  ◦ Prompt treatment of calves with oral zinc → recovery and normal development. Continued poor immune function.
• Inherited parakeratosis in Shorthorn beef cattle
  ◦ Autosomal recessive
  ◦ Reduced ability to absorb Zn

CAUSES AND RISK FACTORS
Zinc Deficiency
• Consuming a Zn-deficient diet
  ◦ Diets high in phytates (seeds, nuts, legumes, cereals, and soy-based products), oxalates, or minerals (Cu, Ca, P, Mg, Fe) reduce Zn bioavailability
  ◦ Successive cuttings of hay crops within a season
  ◦ Highly mature forages
  ◦ Cow's milk in diet
• Failure to absorb Zn from the gastrointestinal tract
  ◦ Hereditary zinc deficiency
  ◦ Hypothyroidism
  ◦ Intestinal parasitism
  ◦ Malabsorptive syndromes
  ◦ Competes with Cu, Fe, and Ca for absorption

Zinc Toxicity
• Sources: Paint, old car batteries, automotive parts, galvanized material, Zn oxide creams
• Over-supplementation

ZINC DEFICIENCY AND TOXICITY

DIAGNOSIS

DIFFERENTIAL DIAGNOSES

Zinc Deficiency
- Endo- or ectoparasitism
- Other mineral deficiency
- Primary vitamin A deficiency
- Inherited epidermal dysplasia (Baldy calf syndrome)

Zinc Toxicity
- Primary Cu deficiency
- Immune mediated hemolytic anemia
- BVDV

CBC/BIOCHEMISTRY/URINALYSIS

Zinc Deficiency
- Lymphopenia
- ⇓ ALP (Zn-dependent enzyme), lacks specificity
- ⇓ free T4

Zinc Toxicity
- Regenerative hemolytic anemia
- ⇑ bilirubin
- ⇑ ALP
- ± ⇑ BUN and ⇑ creatinine
- Hemoglobinemia, bilirubinemia
- Hemoglobinuria, proteinuria
- Urinary casts

OTHER LABORATORY TESTS
- Serum [Zn]
  ○ Normal values: 0.8–1.2 µg/mL
  ○ Low sensitivity
  ○ Decreased with hypoalbuminemia, 60% bound to albumin
  ○ Inflammation → Zn sequestered
  ○ Spurious
    ■ Leach from RBC—serum should be separated within 4–6 hours
    ■ Rubber stoppers in many blood collection tubes are lubricated with a Zn-containing substance—use tubes with royal blue top
- Preferred samples for postmortem analysis—pancreas, bone, liver, and reproductive organs
- Erythrocyte [MT] (ELISA): Decrease in Zn deficiency. Levels are unaffected by transient plasma [Zn], but are affected by other metallo-ions.
- Feed trace mineral analysis

IMAGING
N/A

OTHER DIAGNOSTIC PROCEDURES
Skin biopsy: Hyperplastic superficial perivascular dermatitis with marked diffuse and follicular parakeratotic hyperkeratosis.

PATHOLOGIC FINDINGS

Zinc Deficiency
- Irregular epidermal hyperplasia, marked neutrophilic exocytosis, and extensive confluent parakeratosis
- Oral and esophageal ulcers
- Thymic atrophy
- Depletion of lymphoid tissue
- Inflamed gastrointestinal mucosa
- Decreased accessory sex gland size and Leydig cell number
- Degeneration of the seminiferous tubules
- Abnormal sperm morphology

Zinc Toxicity
- Hepatocellular centrilobular necrosis
- Renal tubular necrosis
- Pancreatic duct necrosis with fibrosis of interlobular fat
- Inflamed gastrointestinal mucosa

TREATMENT

THERAPEUTIC APPROACH

Zinc Deficiency
- Oral Zn supplementation (Zn oxide and Zn sulfate).
- Treat soil and forages with Zn-rich fertilizers.
- Antibiotics if secondary bacterial infections are present.
- Nutritional support: Total parenteral nutrition if diarrhea persists.

Zinc Toxicity
- Removal of the source of the Zn (rumenotomy) normally results in rapid decrease in plasma [Zn].
- Diuresis.
- Chelators (calcium disodium EDTA, D-penicillamine, or dimercaprol); No studies published to support beneficial effect or optimal therapeutic regimen.

SURGICAL CONSIDERATIONS AND TECHNIQUES
N/A

MEDICATIONS

DRUGS OF CHOICE

Zinc Deficiency
- Pre-ruminants: 0.5–1 g elemental Zn q24h mixed into milk replacer
- Adult: 20–40 mg elemental Zn/kg q24h orally
- Oral boluses of Zn in gel capsules can be used q48h.

- Zn complexed with amino acids or other low-M_r organic ligands (citrate, ascorbate, picolinate, proprionate) appear to be more bioavailable.
- Low-dose corticosteroids might enhance Zn absorption through induction of MT in some nonresponsive cases.

Zinc Toxicity
- Calcium disodium (EDTA) 100 mg/kg body weight, q24h, IV or SC for 3 days (diluted and divided into four doses)
- D-penicillamine: 110 mg/kg q24h for 7–14 days
- Dimercaprol: 3–6 mg/kg q8h for 3–5 days

CONTRAINDICATIONS
Zn competes with Cu, Cd, and Mn for binding site on MT. Excess Zn administered → deficiency of these metallo-ions.

PRECAUTIONS
Appropriate milk and meat withdrawal times must be observed for all compounds administered to food-producing animals.

POSSIBLE INTERACTIONS
Chelators might increase systemic absorption of Zn from GIT and nonspecifically bind and promote elimination of Fe, Cu, and Ca.
- Ca-EDTA may exacerbate Zn-induced nephrotoxicity.
- Requires monitoring of serum [Zn].

FOLLOW-UP

EXPECTED COURSE AND PROGNOSIS
- *Zn deficiency*: Good with treatment. Response to treatment should occur within days:
  ○ Adults—resolution of hypersalivation and diarrhea
  ○ Calves—improved suckle
- *Zn toxicity*: May have long-term effects on the animal's health and productivity.

POSSIBLE COMPLICATIONS
Zn deficiency during periods of long bone growth → stunted indefinitely.

CLIENT EDUCATION
Proper trace mineral supplementation

PATIENT CARE
Serum [Zn] should be monitored to ensure correct dosing.

PREVENTION
- Supplementation in geologically Zn-deficient areas.
- Remove stray sources of Zn in pastures.

Z

ZINC DEFICIENCY AND TOXICITY   (CONTINUED)

MISCELLANEOUS

ABBREVIATIONS
- ALP = alkaline phosphatase
- BVDV = bovine viral diarrhea virus
- EDTA = ethylene diamine tetraacetic acid
- ELISA = enzyme-linked immunosorbent assay
- GIT = gastrointestinal tract
- M_r = relative molecular weight
- MT = metallothionein
- T4 = thyroxine

SEE ALSO
- Copper Deficiency and Toxicity
- Vitamin A Deficiency/Toxicosis

Suggested Reading
Christian P, West KP. Interactions between zinc and vitamin A: an update. Am J Clin Nutr 1998, 68(suppl): 435–441S.
Cummings JE, Kovacic JP. The ubiquitous role of zinc in health and disease. J Vet Emerg Crit Care 2009, 19: 215–40.
Herdt TH, Hoff B. The use of blood analysis to evaluate trace mineral status in ruminant livestock. Vet Clin North Am Food Anim Pract 2011, 27: 255–83.

Machen MR, Montgomery T, Holland R, et al. Bovine hereditary zinc deficiency: lethal trait A 46. J Vet Diagn Invest 1996, 8: 219–27.
Smith JC. The vitamin A–zinc connection: a review. Ann N Y Acad Sci 1980, 355: 62–75.
Vogt DW, Carlton CG, Miller RB. Hereditary parakeratosis in Shorthorn beef calves. Am J Vet Res 1988, 49: 120–1.

Author Laura Johnstone
Consulting Editor Kaitlyn A. Lutz
Acknowledgment The author and book editors acknowledge the prior contribution of Margo R. Machen.

APPENDIX 1: CLIENT COMMUNICATION

BASICS

OVERVIEW

• Good communication is the foundation of a good veterinarian-client relationship. It is among the most important factors determining the volume of future caseload from your clients.

• Client communication can be the most difficult yet the most important skill we must master to be successful. Many veterinarians have changed careers because of their frustrations in dealing with clients and coworkers. With so much riding on the quality of your communication, you should be compelled to be the best communicator possible. This requires that you take 100% responsibility for all communication in which you are involved. That means having good command of both ends of the communication process.

• Most financially successful veterinarians are not only skilled in a specialized area, but are very good at client communication.

• Clients frustrated by automatic bank tellers, electronic supermarket checkout stations, and similar depersonalizing machines will place ever-increasing value on their scarcer human contacts.

• Seek first to understand, and then be understood; be empathetic. Ask questions and let the client talk. If we start by finding out what clients think is urgent and important, they are more likely to be receptive to what we think they need to improve or manage better.

Effective Listening Skills

The most significant of all veterinarian-client rapport builders is good listening skills. It is extremely important to become a good listener. It will benefit your practice in the following ways:

• Accurate history—good listening skills allow for an accurate exchange of information, which is critical for serving the client and patient properly.

• Reduced misunderstandings—good listening skills help eliminate misunderstandings, thereby increasing client satisfaction with your services and enhancing their perception of your professional competence.

• Increased client rapport—when clients feel you understand them and have listened effectively, it creates greater client trust. Good listening improves trust and maximizes the probability of maintaining a professional relationship in the future.

• Differentiation—since most people are poor listeners, good listening skills will improve your practice competence.

• The initial interview—(1) shapes client perception of the veterinarian and staff; (2) defines the service to be provided in terms of both problem and goal, and (3) is an important opportunity for client education (e.g., production management, herd health improvements, possible increased client/producer profits). In many cases, the initial interview may in fact be the most significant communication before outcome determinative events.

Self-Evaluation Skills

• How good are you at communicating with your clients? Let us examine ourselves. Self-critical thinking involves our ability to evaluate objectively one's own thought processes and beliefs, with reflective skepticism.

• Francis Bacon stated, "Man prefers to believe what he prefers to be true." This is reinforced by a survey of one million high school seniors (Gilovich, 1991). Seventy percent thought they were above average in leadership ability, and only 2% thought they were below average. *All* students thought they were above average in ability to get along with others, 60% thought they were in the top 10%, and 25% thought they were in the top 1%. A survey of college professors showed that 94% thought they were better at their jobs than their colleagues (ibid).

Effective Communication with Your Clients

• Valuing client feedback.

• Seven canons of client communications (adapted from Collins 2004, *Effective Communication with your Clients*).
  ○ Ignorance is folly.
  ○ Speed of reply to messages.
  ○ Awareness of feedback.
  ○ Treat all clients with courtesy.
  ○ Respect your client's confidentiality.
  ○ Correlating information between you and your clients.
  ○ Securing client information.

Being an Effective Listener

• There are two tests of effective listening:
  ○ Is the information being received and understood by the listener?
  ○ Does the speaker perceive that he/she is being understood?

• By necessity, most veterinarians are reasonably proficient as listeners. Since they rely heavily on information the client provides, they listen carefully to get the facts straight.

• However, many veterinarians are not as good at creating the perception that they are receiving the information.

Obstacles to Good Communication

• Most people are not very good listeners. It is estimated that only about 60% of spoken information is accurately received.

• There are several reasons the information doesn't get through (adapted from J.A. Kline, *Listening Effectively*):
  ○ The veterinarian/speaker is unclear or not specific enough, causing the listener to make assumptions.
  ○ The listener is not paying attention due to lack of interest in the subject matter.
  ○ The listener is preoccupied with other matters.
  ○ The veterinarian/speaker is not saying what the listener wants to hear.
  ○ The listener is busy formulating a rebuttal to something the speaker said previously.
  ○ Most miscommunications are the result of poor listening, not poor articulation. Most people are passive listeners. Even when information is received and understood, the listener fails to acknowledge it.
  ○ Passive listening also allows misunderstandings to go undetected.

Active Listening Skills

• The communication process consists of speaking and listening.

• Passive listeners take an active role in communication only when it is their turn to speak, leaving the process beyond their control at least half the time. Taking 100% responsibility for communication requires you to be specific and articulate in your own speech, and to actively facilitate the quality of the other party's communication when you are listening.

The Power of Questions

• Used properly, questions can give you great power in facilitating excellent communication with your clients as well as everyone else.

• Questions are the key to taking control of a conversation. The person asking the question is in control.

• Ineffective communicators don't ask enough questions. They tend to make statements and then stop, allowing the other person to make a statement. When you do that you relinquish control to the other party.

• The purpose of communication is the effective exchange of information.

Asking Relevant Questions (adapted from Italo, 1996)

The first rule of good communication is to ask frequent relevant questions. This is a very simple process where you listen carefully to the content and then ask questions that seek clarification, verification, motivation, or specificity.

• Clarification—Clarifying questions are those you ask when there seem to be inconsistencies or when you are not sure you understand what the person is trying to say. These questions are very important in avoiding misunderstandings.

• Verification—Verifying questions are questions you ask to verify that the information has been correctly received. It is particularly important to ask verifying questions when you have drawn a conclusion based on what has been said.

• Motivation—Motivational questions help you understand the reasons why people act and they give you insight into how they are likely to behave in the future.

- Specificity—People tend to speak in generalities. It is particularly important to ask specifying questions if the speaker is in an emotionally charged state. The more emotional we are, the more we tend to generalize. This is because our thought patterns become much more reactive and less analytic when we are upset.
- Relevant questions—Show interest in what the speaker is saying. When the speaker perceives you are interested, it creates a feeling of mutual respect.
- Acknowledging the speaker—There is little that is more frustrating than the feeling that someone you are talking to isn't listening. Speakers look for certain cues that acknowledge the message is being received. When speakers don't notice the cues they are looking for, they get the impression you aren't listening.
- Auditory and visual cues—When the speaker is speaking you should give both auditory and visual signs that you are listening.
- Listening check—This is a powerful tool that is extremely effective in creating rapport and improving the quality of your communication. A listening check is a statement that summarizes your understanding of what was just said. For instance: "So, what I hear you saying is that you are unhappy with your workers' heat detection ability." There are two types of listening checks: Listening checks for content and listening checks for feelings. Use listening checks frequently with your clients. It will improve your professional relationships.
- Don't get defensive—Defensiveness in communication only causes each party to become more entrenched in their position.
- Don't make the client wrong—No one likes to be wrong. If you make your clients feel wrong, it will surely embarrass them.
- Don't use absolutes—There are very few absolutes in life. Phrases using always, never, impossible, every, none, are seldom true and only serve to supercharge and polarize the conversation.
- Encourage interruptions—Interruptions are vital to good communication. They allow immediate feedback and prevent frustration and preoccupation. Encourage interruptions. You should also interrupt when appropriate. An appropriate interruption should be immediate, making a comment or asking a question that is directly relevant to the speaker's latest idea.
- Use an open body language—Your body language communicates how you are feeling. You should be very aware of maintaining a friendly and open body language with clients. Lean forward and listen with interest. Don't cross your arms or legs. This makes you look uneasy and defensive.

Client-Veterinarian Communications
- Help staff members streamline, personalize, and customize their communications to individual clients.
- Help associates and staff effectively manage their services to their existing client base. Effective communications help:
  ○ Deliver more revenue, a higher degree of client satisfaction, and higher client retention.
  ○ Reduce the frequency and length of calls to the veterinarian.
  ○ Eliminate misunderstandings and poor communications.
  ○ Increase professional integrity.
  ○ Allow staff and associates to track the results of the management implementation.
- Empower client communications through:
  ○ A consultative approach to develop an effective solution to clients' agriculture- and management-based problems.
  ○ A full array of integrated services that would enable clients to use one veterinary provider.
  ○ Superior customer service, utilizing new technologies, while ensuring confidentiality and integrity.

Client's Expectations, Objectives, and Options
With effective communication, veterinarians should discuss the following with their clients.
Client Objectives and Expectations
- Specific veterinary services the client will receive from the veterinarian.
- Specific results the veterinarian is likely to achieve for the client.
- Costs associated with achieving those objectives.
- Time required to complete the veterinary services and achieve the results.
Client's Instructions
- Choice of options or strategies the client instructs the veterinarian to pursue.
- Impact of choosing particular options or strategies.
- Estimated fees and disbursements relative to those instructions.
Advice Given to the Client
- Options of treatments and procedures recommended by the veterinarian.
- Explanation of the drug withdrawal times.
- Importance of a valid veterinarian-client-patient-relationship (VCPR).
- Referral to other veterinary, animal science, university, or consulting professionals.
Course of Action
- Strategy to be undertaken by the veterinarian.
- Estimated length of time required to complete the plan of action.
Risk Analyses
- The client's potential liability
- The veterinarian's potential liability
- Risks or benefits associated with the services

- Veterinarian's and, if different from the veterinarian, the client's assessment of whether or not the likely outcome is justified by the expense or risk involved.

Fees and Disbursement Communications
The veterinarian should provide the client with a timely estimate of the fees or disbursements involved so that the client is able to make an informed decision. The estimate should reasonably include the following.
Basis for Charging Professional Fees
- Hourly rate
- Flat fee (i.e., per head basis)
- Other method of charging
Amount and Payment Date Agreements
- Initial monetary retainer
- Ongoing monetary retainers
- Accounts
Billing Details
- Facts or circumstances that form the basis of the cost estimate.
- Possible facts or circumstances that may result in an increase or decrease in the estimate.

SUMMARY
- In your clinic, client communication starts with the receptionist who answers the phone. Is he or she warm, friendly, and helpful? If not, the clients will already be insistent and defensive when you talk to them.
- The words "no" or "we can't" have harsh implications. You can always find a way around using it by saying, "we'll try, but . . . ." After all, we are always trying.
- If we recognize and have the desire to improve our communication skills, we need to take a critical look at our approach and how the client reacts to our suggestions.
- If your attitude is positive, there is always a better or improved way to deal with people.
- Communication is a life-long learning experience.

ABBREVIATION
VCPR = veterinarian-client-patient-relationship

SEE ALSO
- Employee Management (see www.fiveminutevet.com/ruminant)
- Veterinary Legal Liability (see www.fiveminutevet.com/ruminant)

Suggested Reading
Blayney N. Communicating with clients. Vet Rec 2001, 149: 531.
Collins J. Effective communication with your clients, 2004. http://www.akamarketing.com/communicating-with-clients.html. Accessed May 2, 2008.
Covey S. The Seven Habits of Highly Effective People. New York: Simon & Schuster, 1998.

Fudin CE. Basic skills for successful client relations. Probl Vet Med 1991, 3: 7–19.

Gilovich T. How we know what isn't so: the fallibility of human reason in everyday life. New York: Free Press, 1991.

Italo A. Effective Communication with Clients, 1996. http://www.mindspring.com/~italco/com.html. Accessed May 2, 2008.

Kline JA. Listening Effectively. Air University Press Maxwell Air Force Base, Alabama, 1996.

Kogan LR, Butler CL, Lagoni LK, Brannan JK, McConnell SM, Harvey AM. Training in client relations and communication skills in veterinary medical curricula and usage after graduation. J Am Vet Med Assoc 2004, 224: 504–7.

Mendel E. Friendly communication is key to effective client interactions. J Am Vet Med Assoc 1991, 198: 1707–8.

Milani M. Practitioner-client communication: when goals conflict. Can Vet J 2003, 44: 675–8.

Osborne CA. Client confidence in veterinarians: how can it be sustained? J Am Vet Med Assoc 2002, 221: 936–8.

Shaw JR, Adams CL, Bonnett BN. What can veterinarians learn from studies of physician-patient communication about veterinarian-client-patient communication? J Am Vet Med Assoc 2004, 224: 676–84.

Shilling V, Jenkins V, Fallowfield, L. Factors affecting patient and clinician satisfaction with the clinical consultation: can communication skills training for clinicians improve satisfaction? Psychooncology 2003, 12: 599–611.

Authors Dennis Hermesch, Sergio Gonzales, Scott R.R. Haskell, and Bonnie R. Loghry
Consulting Editor Kaitlyn A. Lutz

APPENDIX 2: EUTHANASIA AND DISPOSAL

BASICS

OVERVIEW

• Humane procedures should be used to ensure that death is rapid, painless, and as distress free as possible. It is important to remember that not all methods used on a worldwide basis are humane and many cannot be classified as euthanasia.

• Animal handling prior to humane euthanasia is a key element of ethical euthanasia and should be carried out in a calm and respectful manner in appropriate facilities or areas.

• Humane euthanasia results in the rapid, complete, and irreversible loss of consciousness followed by cardiac and/or respiratory arrest.

• Death must be confirmed prior to animal disposal. Absence of a heartbeat or pulse is the best confirmation method but others include no movement over a prolonged period of time, continued absence of respiratory sounds with a stethoscope, lack of corneal reflex, and development of blue to gray mucus membranes and rigor mortis.

• Carcass disposal is considered a standard part of euthanasia and, if possible, planned prior to euthanasia.

SYSTEMS AFFECTED

• Cardiovascular
• Respiratory
• Nervous

GEOGRAPHIC DISTRIBUTION

Worldwide

SIGNALMENT

All ruminants

EUTHANASIA

METHODOLOGY

• Modified from 2013 AVMA *Guidelines on Euthanasia*

• May involve sedation or anesthesia prior to euthanasia

  ○ Useful in an isolated case; often not performed in ruminant medicine

  ○ Not practical in herd conditions where humans may be endangered by an injured animal

• Carcass disposal is the responsibility of both the veterinarian and owner/producer.

  ○ Poisoning of wildlife from poorly disposed carcasses is the responsibility of the veterinarian.

ACCEPTABLE METHODS OF EUTHANASIA

• Sole means of euthanasia, no other agents used

• Humane death consistently occurs

Systemic Agents (Noninhaled)

• Barbiturates (e.g., pentobarbital, others)

  ○ Advantages

    ▪ Good for single, restrained animal.

    ▪ Generally safe for veterinarian, handler, and animal.

    ▪ Rapid and pain-free onset of death.

  ○ Disadvantages

    ▪ Not useful for herds or poorly restrained animal.

    ▪ Costly, depending on size of animal.

    ▪ DEA schedule II or III drugs require accurate accounting and paperwork and necessitate a secured, locked compartment in practice vehicle.

    ▪ Carcass disposal problematic due to drug residues.

ACCEPTABLE METHODS WITH CONDITIONS

• Specific conditions need to be met to ensure consistent humane death.

• May require an adjunctive method.

• Possibility of human error or injury to humans may occur with this method.

Physical Methods

• Gunshot—most common method for euthanasia on the farm; death from brain tissue destruction.

  ○ Handguns

    ▪ Short barreled

    ▪ Fired with one hand within close range (1–2 feet)

    ▪ From .32 to .45 caliber for cattle (.22 caliber NOT recommended for adult cattle)

    ▪ Solid, lead bullets recommended over hollow point bullets.

  ○ Rifles

    ▪ Long barrel

    ▪ Fired from shoulder

    ▪ Distance shooting

    ▪ 0.22 magnum, .223, .243, .270, .308, others for cattle

    ▪ 0.22 LR for sheep and goats

  ○ Shotguns

    ▪ Close range (1–2 yards)

    ▪ Birdshot or slugs

    ▪ 20, 16, or 12 gauge preferred for adult cattle

• Penetrating captive bolt

  ○ Mature cattle that can be restrained

  ○ Various styles available

  ○ Use doesn't always result in death and an adjunct method such as a second shot or IV potassium chloride may be needed.

ADJUNCTIVE METHODS

• Not acceptable as the solitary means of euthanasia.

• Used to ensure death after an acceptable means of causing unconsciousness.

Systemic Agents (Noninhaled)

• IV potassium chloride or magnesium sulfate; **after** captive bolt or administration of alpha 2 adrenergic receptor agonists that render the animal unconscious

• Lower residue risk (except alpha 2 receptor agonist medications)

Physical Methods (Unconscious Animals)

• Second shot or third shot, in event first was unsuccessful

• Exsanguination

  ○ Controversial use

  ○ Ventral portion of neck, used to ensure death

• Pithing—use entry site of bullet or captive bolt

UNACCEPTABLE METHODS

Considered inhumane under any circumstances.

Systemic Methods (Noninhaled)

• Use of IV or IM chemical agents such as disinfectants and high doses of salts (potassium chloride or magnesium sulfate) in a conscious animal

• Use of alpha 2 adrenergic receptor agonists alone or followed by large doses of IV salts in a conscious animal

• Air embolism

• Strychnine

• Sole use of neuromuscular blocking agents

Physical Methods

• Blunt trauma to the head or neck

• Electrocution with 120-volt electrical cord

• Drowning of a conscious or unconscious animal

• Exsanguination in a conscious animal

SPECIAL CONSIDERATIONS

• Neonates: Skulls are smaller so accurate placement is required for gunshot or captive bolt.

• Dams and fetuses

  ○ Barbiturate overdose

    ▪ Fetus remains in a "sleep-like" state of unconsciousness

    ▪ Death in dam precedes fetus by 20–25 minutes

    ▪ If not rescued, do not remove from uterus or remove only after >25 minutes have passed; check closely to be sure fetus is not alive.

  ○ Physical method recommended if fetus is to be rescued; follow with adjunctive method after fetus is removed.

FUTURE CONSIDERATIONS

• Carbon dioxide either alone or in combination has been used successfully in swine as an appropriate (with conditions) euthanasia agent.

• Recently studied in kid goats as an alternative to current methods.

• More work needs to be done but may provide an alternative for other ruminant species.

CARCASS DISPOSAL

LEGALITIES

• Must be legal and safe.

• Regional laws regarding disposal methods vary considerably; species to species variation as well

• Particularly important in large outbreaks of infectious diseases (e.g., anthrax) and reportable diseases.

- Barbiturate contamination of soil and water should be considered.

METHODS

Rendering
- Common and easy method; not a good choice for carcasses with known infectious agents and barbiturate-induced euthanasia.
- Carcass is cooked and separated into animal fat and protein which are used for animal foodstuffs and other industrial products.
- Most rendering facilities will not accept sheep carcasses due to scrapie and subsequent BSE concerns.
- Use of barbiturates must be disclosed.
- Vehicle should be sealed and not allow any drainage during transportation.

Closed Pit Burial
- Open pit no longer recommended due to groundwater contamination and access by scavengers.
- Good if permitted and owner/producer able to do under local laws.
- Preferred for many infectious diseases (except prions).
- Commonly used in natural disasters.
- Depth of burial, height of water table, soil composition, surface slope, and other factors must be considered.
- USDA READEO burial site recommendations: 4–6 feet depth, 150 feet from water wells and 100 feet from dwellings.
- Deep burial needed for anthrax-contaminated carcasses.

Composting
- Carcass goes through a two-stage slow "cooking" process. Stage 1 takes 2–3 months and stage 2 another 2–3 months. Core temperature must reach 130–160°F (55–71°C) for pathogen destruction.
- End result is water, carbon dioxide, and organic material.
- Bin composting generally involves a concrete floor below and roof above.

Organic matter (e.g., manure) must cover carcass.
- Must be scavenger and predator free.

Incineration
- Good option if available.
- Burning carcasses successfully yields bone and ash free of pathogens (except prions).
- Recommended disposal for anthrax suspect carcasses in some states. Anthrax carcasses must be burned only to ash and the contaminated ash disinfected in sodium hydroxide (lye) and buried deeply.
- Open air burning banned in some regions.
- Biologic incineration by some laboratories and veterinary schools.
  ○ Good for their specific needs but not a large-scale disaster.
  ○ Requires transportation of carcass to the facility.
  ○ Good for infectious diseases with prion agents (e.g., BSE).
- Controlled burning in an air-curtain incinerator or trench burner.
  ○ Portable and environmentally friendly
  ○ Useful in large-scale disasters
  ○ Can also be used to burn contaminated vegetation.

Alkaline Hydrolysis (Tissue Digestion)
- Carcass is cooked with alkalis at high temperatures to produce a sterile solution composed of amino acids, sugar, and soap.
- Generally good for smaller animals (<200 pounds).
- Utilized for deer and elk contaminated with CWD.

Landfills
No longer an option in many areas.

ABBREVIATIONS
- AVMA = American Veterinary Medical Association
- BSE = bovine spongiform encephalitis
- CWD = chronic wasting disease
- DEA = Drug Enforcement Administration
- IM = intramuscular
- IV = intravenous

- LR = long rifle
- READEO = Regional Emergency Animal Disease Eradication Organization
- USDA = United States Department of Agriculture

Suggested Reading

Anthrax in Humans and Animals. 4th edition. World Health Organization, Geneva; 2008. Available from http://www.ncbi.nlm.nih.gov/books/NBK310492/. Accessed February 20, 2016.

AVMA Guidelines for the Euthanasia of Animals: 2013 edition. Available from https://www.avma.org/KB/Policies/Documents/euthanasia.pdf. Accessed February 5, 2016.

Ellis DB. Carcass Disposal Issues in Recent Disasters, Accepted Methods, and Suggested Plan to Mitigate Future Events. 2001. Available from https://digital.library.txstate.edu/bitstream/handle/10877/3502/fulltext.pdf. Accessed February 7, 2016.

Gilliam JN, Shearer JK, Woods J, et al. Captive-bolt euthanasia of cattle: determination of optimal-shot placement and evaluation of the Cash Special Euthanizer Kit® for euthanasia of cattle. Anim Welfare 2012, 21(S2): 99–102.

Passler T. Euthanasia of farm animals. In: Lin H, Walz P eds, Farm Animal Anesthesia: Cattle, Small Ruminants, Camelids, and Pigs. Chichester, UK: Wiley, 2014, pp. 248–62.

Withrock IS. The use of carbon dioxide (CO_2) as an alternative euthanasia method for goat kids. Graduate thesis and dissertations, Paper 14718. Ames, Iowa State University, 2015. Available from http://lib.dr.iastate.edu. Accessed February 18, 2016.

Author Lynn Rolland Hovda
Consulting Editor Kaitlyn A. Lutz
Acknowledgment The author and book editors acknowledge the prior contribution of Scott R.R. Haskell and Sergio Gonzales.

APPENDIX 3: MEDICAL WASTE MANAGEMENT: EXPIRED DRUGS

BASICS

OVERVIEW

Note: Although the specific government agencies and acts mentioned below are specific to the US, the information is relevant globally.

- The therapeutic use of expired medications, medical devices or intravenous (IV) fluids is unacceptable in veterinary medicine, does not represent appropriate standard of care, and violates the FD&C Act.
- The proper disposal of these products and all other medical waste is the responsibility of each clinic, which should have routine policies and procedures in place to ensure appropriate disposal.
- Improper disposal of medical waste, including expired drugs, represents a significant burden on the environment, clean water, and impacts human and animal health. Detectable levels of some prescription and nonprescription drugs have been found in water supplies.
- Action should be taken to ensure proper disposal of medical waste, including expired drugs, wherever the source. Proper policies and procedures for medications either used in-clinic or dispensed to animal owners will prevent improper discharge of medications into the environment.
- Due to periodic changes in statutes, clinics should coordinate efforts with local and state hazardous waste agencies as well as state public health agencies to ensure proper collection, storage, and disposal of all waste from the clinic, including expired drugs.
- The AVMA provides directions and links to applicable agencies involved in medical waste management through their website (refer to "Internet Resources" section).

OVERVIEW OF MEDICAL WASTE

- Medical waste (which includes pharmaceuticals) in the United States is regulated, broadly, under the Medical Waste Tracking Act (MWTA) of 1988. Other Federal Acts including the FD&C Act, TSCA, FIFRA, RCRA, the Clean Air Act, and the Safe Drinking Water Act are also involved with medical and hazardous waste disposal.
- Medical waste is broadly defined under the MWTA as "any solid waste that is generated in the diagnosis, treatment, or immunization of human beings or animals … "
- Clinics produce medical waste from multiple sources including therapeutic agents (e.g., drugs, vaccines, pesticides), diagnostic materials (e.g., laboratory reagents, radiographic agents), sharps and medical or surgical products (e.g., intravenous supplies), blood or body fluids, and animal tissues or carcasses.
- Additional hazardous waste is generated from cleaning and disinfecting supplies and office and facility management supplies (e.g., batteries, light bulbs, paint).

OVERVIEW OF THE DISPOSAL OF MEDICAL WASTE

- The MWTA established a "Cradle-to-the-Grave" tracking system for parties that generate medical waste, standards for segregation, labeling and storage of medical waste, and penalties for organizations that fail to comply.
- Medical waste is often segregated at the site of generation by color-coded bins based on source of the waste or pathogenicity potential. These systems often lack consistency.
- Medical waste generated in the clinic should be segregated and secured away from usual trash until it can be properly collected and disposed of.
- Following site collection, most medical waste is incinerated down to ash or autoclaved to eliminate microbes before ultimate disposal at a landfill.
- No perfect system exists from the various disposal methods due to concerns over potential release of toxic agents into the air. Improvements in air scrubbers have dramatically reduced the amount of air pollution generated in the process.

Health Risks from Improper Disposal of Pharmaceuticals

- The stability or effectiveness of medications beyond their expiration date cannot be assured. Bacterial overgrowth in liquid formulations or problems with dissolution of solid dosage formulations of drugs poses a risk to the animal receiving an expired drug.
- Pharmaceuticals pose a risk to the environment, aquatic life, and the safe drinking water supply if improperly disposed.
- Measurable levels of some drugs have been identified in lakes, rivers, and streams sourced for potable water. Potential sources may include illegal or improper disposal into these bodies or leachate from landfills.
- Long-term health consequences from exposure to small amounts of drugs from potable water among humans or animals have not been well established; some have raised concerns that antibiotic resistance may be related to their presence in water supplies.

DISPOSAL OF CLINIC MEDICATIONS

- Clinics should develop policies and procedures to manage the inventory of prescription drugs.
- Limit storage areas for all drugs to prevent them from becoming "lost" in the clinic.
- Staff should be assigned to review expiration dates for all medications on hand at least every four weeks to identify medications approaching their date of expiration to ensure that they are disposed of before they are dispensed.
- Clinics should work with their supply chain to identify medication return or buy-back programs.

- Disposal of medications (even in small quantities) into the water supply via sinks and toilets is no longer acceptable practice in many jurisdictions.
- Safety Data Sheets (SDS) can identify special handling and disposal requirements for any medical waste including drugs, and cytotoxic or biologic agents including vaccines; however, in all cases, clinics should work closely with local and state hazardous waste disposal agencies to ensure appropriate measures are taken to segregate and dispose of all clinic waste.
- Special restrictions and requirements are in place for retrieval and disposal of federally controlled substances. Contact your local DEA office to discuss these requirements.
- Maintain records identifying specific medications, amounts, and the lot number and expiration date for each item removed from stock and the manner in which it was disposed of.

DISPOSAL OF CHEMOTHERAPEUTIC AGENTS

- Chemotherapeutic agents are occasionally used in ruminant animal practice.
- Policies and procedures should be developed to manage these unique agents from the time of intake and storage of the medication through the administration and disposal.
- In addition to the drug vials, all medical equipment used in their administration (e.g., IV bags, gloves, sharps) requires special handling and disposal as well.
- Professional organizations have established guidelines for handling antineoplastic agents to limit exposure risk from time of administration to disposal.

DISPOSAL OF DISPENSED MEDICATIONS

- Policies and procedures should be developed to address disposal of medications that have been dispensed to animal owners.
- To prevent wastage, only sufficient doses to cover treatment should be dispensed or prescribed and should be dispensed in appropriate containers to prevent loss or spillage.
- Veterinarians should be familiar with local and state statutes governing disposal of medications they have dispensed from the clinic to direct animal owners accordingly.
- Anti-parasitic agents (e.g., ivermectin, fenbendazole) used in ruminants are regulated as pesticides under FIFRA by the EPA and should be disposed of appropriately.
- Many towns and cities host "Medication Take Back" programs together with state and federal agencies such as the DEA to ensure that unused medication is disposed of correctly. These events can be highlighted to animal owners to increase safe disposal. (Refer to "Internet Resources.")

ABBREVIATIONS
- AVMA = American Veterinary Medical Association
- DEA = Drug Enforcement Administration
- EPA = Environmental Protection Agency
- FD&C = Federal Food, Drug and Cosmetic Act
- FIFRA = Federal Insecticide, Fungicide and Rodenticide Act
- IV = intravenous
- MWTA = Medical Waste Tracking Act
- RCRA = Resource Conservation and Recovery Act
- SDS = Safety Data Sheets (previously named Material Safety Data Sheets)
- TSCA = Toxic Substance Control Act

Internet Resources
- AVMA Waste Disposal Guidelines: https://www.avma.org/PracticeManagement/Administration/Pages/Federal-Regulation-of-Waste-Disposal.aspx
- Safe Disposal of Medications at Home: http://www.fda.gov/Drugs/ResourcesForYou/Consumers/BuyingUsingMedicineSafely/EnsuringSafeUseofMedicine/SafeDisposalofMedicines/ucm186187.htm

Suggested Reading
Connor TH, Cordes B. Safe handling of hazardous drugs for veterinary healthcare workers. DHHS Pub No. 2010-150. Washington DC: Department of Health and Human Services, 2010. Available from: www.cdc.gov/niosh/docs/wp-solutions/2010-150/pdfs/2010-150.pdf

Easty AC, Coakley N, Cheng R, Cividino M, Savage P, Tozer R, White RE. Safe handling of cytotoxics: guideline recommendations. Current Oncol 2015, 22: e27–37.

Hayes A. Safe use of anticancer chemotherapy in small animal practice. Comp Anim Pract 2005, 27: 118–27.

Kwon JW, Rodriguez JM. Occurrence and removal of selected pharmaceuticals and personal care products in three wastewater-treatment plants. Arch Environ Contam Toxicol 2014, 66: 538–48.

Wick JY. Getting the upper hand on expired drugs. Consult Pharm 2010, 25: 122–4.

Windfeld ES, Brooks MS. Medical waste management: A review. J Environ Manage 2015, 163: 98–108.

Authors Stephen H. LeMaster and Lynn Rolland Hovda

Consulting Editor Kaitlyn A. Lutz

Acknowledgment The authors and editors acknowledge the prior contribution of Scott R.R. Haskell, Larry P. Occhipinti, and Ed. L. Powers.

APPENDIX 4: PHYSICAL EXAMINATION: BOVINE

BASICS

OVERVIEW
• Gather information by asking appropriate questions and use interpersonal skills to clarify concerns and expectations; methodically evaluate body systems, and identify possible health problems. Obtain history, perform physical examination, and evaluate the herd environment. The overall goal of examination is to establish an accurate diagnosis or conclusion and to establish a plan of action.
• Formulate a complete problem list, define appropriate differential diagnoses, and determine the need for additional diagnostic tests.
• There are four major parts to a thorough health evaluation: History collection, physical examination, diagnostic testing, and data analysis.
• Physical examination on a herd basis requires a detailed history of the problem, number of animals affected, duration, factors that may have contributed to development or exacerbation of the problem, and how the problem has been managed to date.

INCIDENCE/PREVALENCE
N/A

GEOGRAPHIC DISTRIBUTION
N/A

SYSTEMS AFFECTED
All systems must be examined in a thorough physical examination.

PATHOPHYSIOLOGY
N/A

GENETICS
N/A

HISTORICAL FINDINGS
Prior to beginning the clinical examination ask the owner for the presenting problem(s), the signalment (age, sex, production group), history of the animal(s) affected, and other relevant information. The history should encompass the type, onset, and duration of clinical signs, and epidemiologic data such as the number of affected animals and the distribution of disease in the herd.

SIGNALMENT
Bovine

PHYSICAL EXAMINATION FINDINGS
• Observe the animal(s) at a distance for abnormalities of behavior, posture, gait, body condition, symmetry, and abdominal distention.
• If the animal is lame, identify the affected leg by observing the animal walk, or via abnormal weight bearing at rest. For more subtle lameness, examine carriage of the head and hips when the animal walks. Lameness often affects the front feet and the animal will raise its head while bearing weight on the affected front leg and lower its head while bearing weight on the non-affected front leg. The animal will hike its hip when bearing

weight on an affected hind leg. Once the affected leg is identified, the animal should be restrained and the foot and leg examined. The most common causes of foot lameness are sole ulcer, sole abscess, "strawberry foot rot" (digital dermatitis), and "foot rot" (interdigital necrobacillosis). Palpate joints and tendon sheaths for size, effusion and pain. Septic joints are generally enlarged, distended with fluid, and very painful.
• Use a geographic approach to perform a detailed examination. Commence at the rear of the animal and proceed to examine the left and right sides of the animal. Perform a per rectum examination and examine the head last. Follow the same sequence of steps (steps 1–7 [Figure 1] and steps 8–12 [Figure 8]) each time an examination is performed to avoid missing abnormal findings.

Step 1. Rear of the Animal
• Obtain a urine sample. Normal passage of urine that is clear and amber suggests a normal urinary tract. A urine sample may be obtained from a cow or heifer by stroking the vulva or perineum. Straining and/or difficult urination suggest an abnormality of the urinary tract and requires further examination. Observe the vulva for blood, fetal membranes, discharge, or pus. In the male, observe the prepuce for blood, pus, or ventral swelling. Examine the preputial hairs of male animals for crystals/uroliths.
• Urine, blood, or milk should be examined for ketone bodies using a cow-side test. The presence of ketone bodies indicates the cow is mobilizing body fat faster than the liver can metabolize it. The circulating ketones are acetone, acetoacetate, and beta-hydroxybutyrate (BHBA). Cow-side

tests measure both acetone and acetoacetate or BHBA. The gold standard for ketone testing is measurement of BHBA. Routine monitoring of BHBA in early lactation cows on a herd level using >1.4 mmol/L BHBA as positive, is often used as a diagnostic tool to monitor the transition period from dry to lactating cow.
• Insert a lubricated thermometer into the rectum. Normal temperature is 38.5°C (101.3°F; range 38.0–39.0°C [100.4–102.2°F]) for adults, and for calves is 39.0°C (38.5–39.5°C [101.3–103.1°F]). Temperatures of pen mates can be used to assess seasonal influences.
• Obtain a pulse from the coccygeal artery on the ventral midline of the tail. The normal pulse is 60–80 beats per minute (bpm). Examine the vulvar mucus membranes of cows and heifers, which should be moist and pink.

Step 2. Left Side: Heart
• Observe the jugular and mammary veins for distention or pulsation. Examine the jugular vein for filling and emptying and check the brisket and submandibular area for edema. Distended jugular veins are abnormal and suggest right-sided heart failure or pericardial effusion. Normal animals should not have significant jugular pulses when the head is elevated. Occlude the jugular vein with a finger. The jugular vein will fail to empty after releasing the occlusion if cardiac disease is present. Pinch the skin of the neck to assess hydration status.
• The stethoscope should be placed deep into the left axilla to find the pulmonic (3rd intercostal space), aortic (4th intercostal space), and mitral (5th intercostal space)

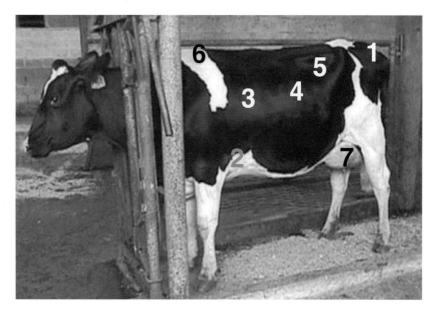

Figure 1.

Examination steps on the left side of the cow. (Also availalbe in color at www.fiveminutevet.com/ruminant)

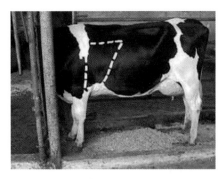

Figure 2.

Normal lung field on the left side of the cow. (Also availalbe in color at www.fiveminutevet.com/ruminant)

valves. Carefully evaluate the rate, rhythm, and heart sounds. The heart should be clearly audible on the left side. S1 and S2 heart sounds are expected and S3 and S4 heart sounds occasionally heard. Muffled heart sounds can be caused by pericardial or pleural effusion. Normal heart rate is 60–80 bpm in adults, and 80–120 bpm in calves. Most animals with cardiac disease have tachycardia, but fever or toxemia also cause tachycardia. Bradycardia (<60 bpm) is most often associated with vagal indigestion. Occasionally bacterial endocarditis of the mitral valve will cause a left systolic murmur. Traumatic reticuloperitonitis typically presents with muffled hearts sounds and a "washing machine murmur." Atrial fibrillation is a common rhythm abnormality, reflected by an irregularly irregular heart rhythm. It is most often associated with GI problems such as a left displaced abomasum (LDA).

Step 3. Left Side: Lungs and Skin
• Observe the rate and effort of respiration. Respiratory disease is common in cattle and is often first diagnosed by observation from a distance. Signs of respiratory disease include coughing, respiratory distress, open-mouth breathing, and mucopurulent nasal discharge. Most cattle with respiratory disease will initially have a fever. The normal respiratory rate in adult cattle is 15–35 breaths per minute and in calves 20–40 breaths per minute.
• Auscult the lungs, moving the stethoscope systematically over the entire lung field. The lung field in the bovine is small and the caudal border extends from the 11th rib to the elbow (Figure 2). Normal lung sounds are quiet during auscultation and louder on inspiration than expiration, and in the ventral lung fields compared to the dorsal lung fields. Upper airway abnormalities can create referred abnormal inspiratory sounds. Breath sounds of increased or decreased intensity can be abnormal. Lung consolidation (pneumonia) often results in louder than normal large airway breath sounds in the ventral lung

fields. Crackles, wheezes, and pleural friction rubs are abnormal sounds. The animal can be induced to take deeper breaths by either holding off the nostrils or placing a plastic bag over the animal's muzzle for 30–60 seconds.
• Palpate the trachea. A cough can generally be elicited in animals with pneumonia.
• Palpate the skin on the left side and ventral abdomen. Feel dorsally for subcutaneous emphysema. Examine the prescapular (superficial cervical) lymph node cranial to the point of the shoulder and the prefemoral (subiliac) lymph node cranial to the stifle. Lymph nodes are enlarged in lymphosarcoma.

Step 4. Left Side: Pings
• "Ping" the left side of the animal by simultaneously percussing and ausculting the whole left abdomen by firmly flicking a finger against the body wall. A "ping" represents a fluid-gas interface or gas accumulation. On the left side of the animal, gas may be present in the abomasum (LDA), rumen, or peritoneal cavity (Figure 3). Classically, an LDA ping occurs in the mid-thoracic area on a line between the elbow and the tuber coxa (Figure 4), and may extend to the cranial edge of the left paralumbar fossa. LDA pings and rumen pings often occur concurrently and are usually distinguished by location and different tones during auscultation and percussion (Figure 3). A rumen void ping occasionally occurs when the rumen is small on per rectum palpation and extends over both the rumen and LDA area. The monotone nature of the rumen void ping helps to distinguish it from a concurrent LDA and rumen ping.
• Observe the abdomen from a distance. The left caudal rib can have a "sprung" appearance with an LDA. Animals with rumen bloat or vagal indigestion will have distention over the rumen and right ventral abdominal quadrant.

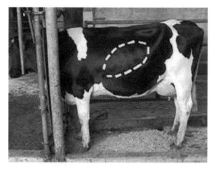

Figure 4.

Dashed line is typical location of ping for LDA. (Also availalbe in color at www.fiveminutevet.com/ruminant)

Step 5. Left Side: Rumen
• Listen to the rumen by placing the stethoscope over the left paralumbar fossa. Normal rumen contractions (1–3 per minute) are strong. Palpate, auscult, and ballot the rumen to assess consistency. The dorsal sac of the rumen has a gas cap. The rumen becomes doughier towards the ventral fluid-filled sac.

Step 6. Left Side: Withers Pinch Test
• Pinch the withers (Figure 5). A normal animal will flex ventrally when its withers are pinched, and an animal with thoracic or abdominal pain will not, although false negatives are common. Animals with GI pain will often stand hunched with their elbows abducted. They may tread their hind feet, but overt signs of "colic" are rare. Common reasons for abdominal pain are traumatic reticuloperitonitis (hardware disease) and abomasal ulceration.
• Perform a "grunt test" by either using a fist pushed up with a knee (Figure 6), or a board with one person on each side lifting the board

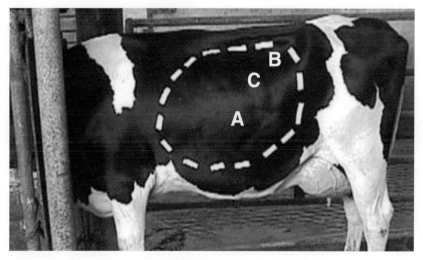

Figure 3.

Dashed line is area to percuss for a "ping" on the left side. A = location of left displaced abomasum (LDA) ping; B = location of rumen ping; C = location of both rumen and LDA ping. (Also availalbe in color at www.fiveminutevet.com/ruminant)

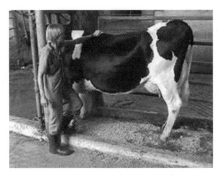

Figure 5.

Withers pinch test. (Also availalbe in color at www. fiveminutevet.com/ruminant)

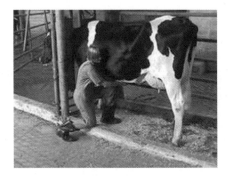

Figure 6.

Grunt test. (Also availalbe in color at www. fiveminutevet.com/ruminant)

to apply pressure to the xiphoid area. Grunting or kicking indicates pain. Often a grunt is only heard while simultaneously applying pressure to the xiphoid area at the peak of inspiration and ausculting over the trachea. As with the "withers pinch test" false negatives are common.

Step 7. Left Side: Udder
• Strip milk from each quarter into a strip cup (Figure 7) or onto a mastitis plate. It is possible to compare quarters by stripping each quarter's secretion onto the last quarter's secretion, then repeat in reverse order.

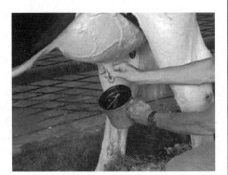

Figure 7.

Obtaining milk from each quarter. (Also availalbe in color at www.fiveminutevet.com/ruminant)

Subtle abnormalities in secretions from quarter to quarter will be detected by this method.
• Palpate each quarter for edema, hardening, and swelling to detect clinical mastitis.
• Palpate the mammary lymph nodes in the proximal caudal aspect of the udder.
• Integrate findings with the rest of the physical examination; e.g., a cow with clots in the milk and a normal examination is not likely to be sick from the mastitis; whereas a cow with a watery secretion, acute swelling of the udder, and an elevated heart rate and temperature is likely sick from the mastitis.
• Bacterial culture of the milk can identify specific bacterial agents causing mastitis.
• Many cow-side tests are available to determine degree of inflammation in the udder. The California Mastitis Test gives a semi-quantitative estimate of the somatic cell count (SCC) in milk.
• Electronic SCC counters are commonly used to assess inflammation in the udder and to determine udder infection status on a herd level. The SCC data can be used to identify cows with high SCC, the percentage of SCC each cow contributes to the bulk tank, and overall SCC trends in the herd. Ideally a composite milk sample should have SCC <200,000 cells/mL.

Step 8. Right Side: Heart
• Examine the right jugular vein for filling. Distended jugular veins are abnormal and suggest cardiac disease (Figure 9) or thrombosis. Jugular pulses should be minimal when the head is elevated. Occlude the jugular vein; failure to empty after releasing occlusion suggests cardiac disease is present.
• The heart is ausculted similarly on the right side as the left (Figure 8), but cardiac sounds

are usually quieter than from the left side. The tricuspid valve is located at the third intercostal space halfway between the elbow and shoulder, and is the most common site for bacterial endocarditis in cows. Early signs of bacterial endocarditis are fever, pain, and tachycardia. Advanced signs include murmur, distended jugular veins, and submandibular (Figure 10) and brisket edema (Figure 11), resulting from right-sided heart failure.

Step 9. Right Side: Lungs and Skin
• Auscult the lungs by moving the stethoscope systematically over the entire right lung field. It is comparable in size to the left lung field and the caudal border extends from the 11th rib to the right elbow.
• Palpate the skin of the right side and ventral abdomen. Examine the prescapular and prefemoral lymph nodes.

Step 10. Right Side: Pings
• "Ping" the right abdomen and carefully delineate the borders of any pings (Figure 12). Right side pings can arise from gas and fluid accumulation in the cecum, spiral colon, small intestine, duodenum, uterus (post-calving), peritoneum, rectum, or abomasum (from right displaced abomasum [RDA] or right displacement with torsion [RTA]). It is not uncommon to find a ping in the right paralumbar fossa of sick cows. A distended cecum will produce a large ping and is palpable per rectum. Pings from RDA or RTA are usually cranial to the 8th rib, and more cranial in location compared to LDA pings. The severity and degree of torsion of a right displaced abomasum is associated with the heart rate and degree of dehydration of the cow.

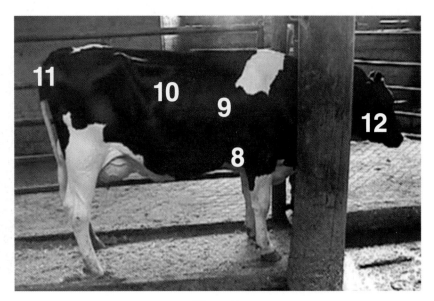

Figure 8.

Examination steps on the right side of the cow. (Also availalbe in color at www.fiveminutevet.com/ruminant)

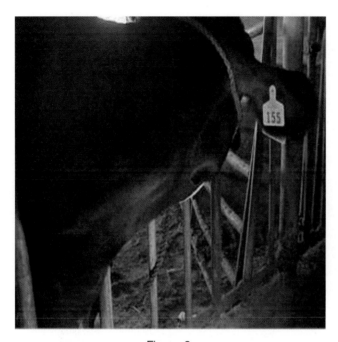

Figure 9.

Jugular venous distension. (Also availalbe in color at
www.fiveminutevet.com/ruminant)

The dorsal contents may have some gas and are generally doughy or will "pit" compared to the ventral more fluid contents. Absence of a readily palpable rumen often results in a "rumen void" ping which can be confused with an LDA. Then palpate the left kidney located to the right of the rumen on the midline. The palpator's arm is normally inserted beyond the elbow to find the left kidney unless it is enlarged, which most commonly occurs in pyelonephritis. Continue to palpate towards the right abdominal wall. The right abdomen should feel empty in normal animals. There should be no discernible distention of the cecum or small intestine in this region. An RTA can occasionally be palpated in the far cranial right abdominal region. Palpate the deep inguinal (iliofemoral) lymph nodes cranially along each shaft of the ileum.
• In female animals the cervix lies on the floor of the pelvis. Examine the reproductive tract and determine the reproductive stage of the cow. The bladder is occasionally palpated cranial to the brim of the pelvis if it is full.
• In intact male animals used for breeding purposes a detailed examination of both the internal and external genital organs should be performed. Per rectum, examine the pelvic urethra, ampullae of the vas deferens, prostate gland, seminal vesicles, and bulbourethral glands. Examine all the external genital organs including the scrotum, testes, epididymis, spermatic cord, and penis.

Step 12. Head
• Examine the head last, since cattle often resent manipulation. Palpate the ears;

• Ballot the right abdomen for detection of a fetus (≥7 months) or infrequently a mass (abscess, tumor, etc.).

Step 11. Rear: Per Rectum Examination
• Examine the perineum and tail for blood, mucus, and feces. Normal cows have a clean perineal area. Fresh blood on the tail indicates recent estrus; clear mucus suggests a cow's proximity to estrus or parturition. Postpartum metritis can cause watery, brown-red malodorous uterine discharge. Examine quantity, color, and consistency of feces in the rectum. Lack of feces suggests reduced fecal output. Large quantities of liquid feces suggest an intestinal problem such as Johne's disease, winter dysentery, or salmonellosis. Black feces (melena) suggests bleeding from

the small intestine or abomasum (ulcer). Fresh blood indicates bleeding from the distal large intestine (e.g., coccidiosis). Cows with hemorrhagic bowel syndrome often have large quantities of fresh blood in the feces.
• Perform per rectum examination in a consistent sequence. Palpate the rumen left of midline for size and consistency. The rumen should be palpable in the cranial abdomen.

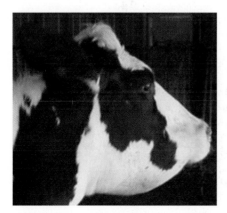

Figure 10.

Submandibular edema. (Also availalbe in color at
www.fiveminutevet.com/ruminant)

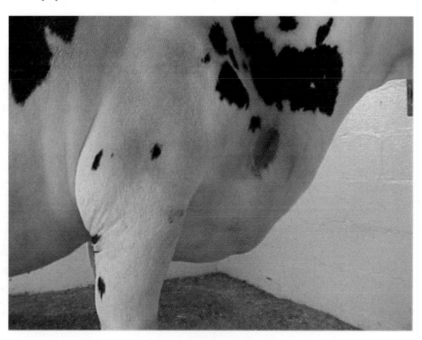

Figure 11.

Brisket edema. (Also availalbe in color at www.fiveminutevet.com/ruminant)

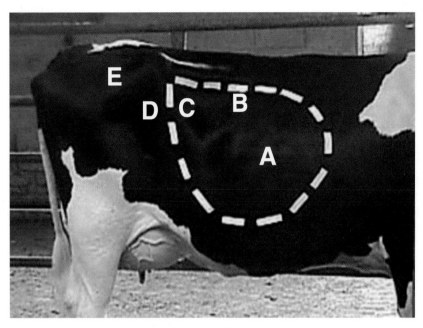

Figure 12.

Dashed line represents area to percuss ("ping") on the right side. A = Location of RDA or RTA; B = location of spiral colon ping; C = location of cecal ping; D = location of uterine ping; E = location of rectal ping. (Also availalbe in color at www.fiveminutevet.com/ruminant)

coolness indicates poor perfusion (shock, milk fever). Evaluate symmetry and ocular and nasal discharge. Although nasal discharge commonly occurs with respiratory conditions, a dry dirty nose usually indicates the cow is sick. Neurologic signs such as a head tilt, droopy ear, and eyelid paresis are commonly associated with listeriosis. Cows with listeriosis may have asymmetry of the muzzle with uneven flaring of the nostrils. Failure to swallow suggests botulism or listeriosis. Tent the eyelid to assess hydration. Assess the eyes for vision, position, and pupillary reflexes. Blindness is associated with polioencephalomalacia, and constricted pupils with organophosphate toxicity. Check the sclera for color and injection of the scleral vessels. Pale sclera indicate anemia often due to blood loss (abomasal ulceration in adults, parasites in younger animals). Icterus is almost always due to hemolytic disease. Large prominent scleral vessels and hypopyon are associated with septic conditions.

• Examine the mouth by pressing the fingers against the hard palate to induce the animal to open its mouth. Examine the gums and palate for ulcers and vesicles which can occur with bovine virus diarrhea (BVD) and other viral disorders. Check the mucosal papillae for blunting (BVD), and the nasal passages for vesicles commonly seen in viral infections such as infectious bovine rhinotracheitis. The pharynx can be examined by pushing the tongue between the molars with the back of the hand. Retropharyngeal abscesses and "wooden tongue" are palpable conditions. "Lumpy jaw" causes osteomyelitis of the mandible. Palpate the mandibular lymph nodes in the intermandibular space.

MISCELLANEOUS

ASSOCIATED CONDITIONS
N/A

AGE-RELATED FACTORS
N/A

ZOONOTIC POTENTIAL
N/A

PREGNANCY
N/A

BIOSECURITY
N/A

PRODUCTION MANAGEMENT
N/A

SYNONYMS
N/A

ABBREVIATIONS
• BHBA = beta-hydroxybutyrate
• BVD = bovine viral diarrhea
• LDA = left displaced abomasum
• RDA = right displaced abomasum
• RTA = right displaced torsion of the abomasum
• SCC = somatic cell count

SEE ALSO
• Abomasal Ulceration
• Actinobacillosis: Wooden Tongue
• Actinomycosis: Lumpy Jaw
• Bacterial Endocarditis
• Cardiac Failure
• Diarrheal Diseases: Bovine
• Displaced Abomasum
• Lameness: Bovine
• Physical Examination: Small Ruminant (Appendix 6)
• Pregnancy Diagnosis: Bovine
• Pyelonephritis

Suggested Reading

Fowkes FG, Dobson AJ, Hensley MJ, Leeder SR. The role of clinical epidemiology in medical practice. Eff Health Care 1984, 1: 259–65.

Fox FH. Diagnostic techniques for diseases of cattle. J Am Vet Med Assoc 1972, 161: 1251–5.

Jackson, P, Cockcroft, P. Clinical Examination of Farm Animals. Oxford UK: Blackwell Publishing, 2002.

Lees GE. History-taking and development of the examination record. Vet Clin North Am Small Anim Pract 1981, 11: 441–52.

Stauffer VD. Health examinations. J Am Vet Med Assoc 1968, 153: 234–5.

Wilson JH. Physical examination. The Veterinary Clinics of North America. Philadelphia: Saunders, 1992.

Author Michaela Kristula
Consulting Editor Erica C. McKenzie

APPENDIX 5: PHYSICAL EXAMINATION: CAMELID

BASICS

OVERVIEW
• Physical examination should be performed in a methodic and thorough manner.
• Proper physical restraint in the form of a chute or halter is important.
• Because camelids are covered with fiber, a thorough hands-on examination should always be performed.

INCIDENCE/PREVALENCE
N/A

GEOGRAPHIC DISTRIBUTION
Worldwide

SYSTEMS AFFECTED
All systems

PATHOPHYSIOLOGY
• Pathologic processes produce specific or nonspecific changes in the physical examination parameters.
• Change in BCS (particularly weight loss) is a reflection of poor nutrition or of poor absorption of nutrients due to gastrointestinal disorder. Other disorders such as genetic defect or overall poor health may result in ill thrift and loss of condition.
• The general demeanor of the animal is often affected by chronic diseases.
• Rectal temperature outside of the norm may reflect an acute inflammatory/infectious process (fever) or a severe depression of the animal's health (hypothermia) or exposure to the elements (hypothermia in debilitated animals and high temperature in the case of heat stress).
• The pulse and respiratory rates are often increased in a stressful or painful situation.
• Deviations from normal auscultation characteristics of the heart, lungs, and gastrointestinal system warrant detailed examination of each.

HISTORICAL FINDINGS
• A detailed history should be obtained including present and past problems, routine health, nutritional and environmental management, and exposure to other animals.
• History should be obtained at an individual and herd level.

SIGNALMENT
• New World camelids. Reproductive examination differs with sex of the animal.
• Age-specific reference ranges should be considered for interpretation of findings.

PHYSICAL EXAMINATION FINDINGS
Behavioral Observation
• Camelids are normally bright, alert, and responsive to stimuli and their surrounding environment.
• In general, camelids show reluctance to being approached and examined, especially by strangers or in a strange environment.
• In the face of stress or fear, camelids may adopt sternal recumbency or "cush."

• Muscle strength, gait, posture, and proprioception are evaluated while the animal is being led or is spontaneously moving in the pasture to identify lameness and neurologic deficits.

Body Condition Scoring
• Palpation and observation of the midback (T8 to L2), fiberless area of the chest behind the elbows, dorsal pelvis, brisket, and perineal region allows estimation of body condition score.
• A scale from 1 (thin) to 9 (obese) is used. Ideal body condition score is 5.

Conformation of the Animal
• Conformation should be evaluated from a distance looking at the animal from the front, rear, and both sides.
• Common conformation problems in camelids include various angular limb deformities and dropped pasterns.

PHYSICAL EXAMINATION
Physical examination is performed in a methodical manner (Figure 1). Accurate information is best obtained via a specific pattern performed on a properly restrained animal that is calm. Figure 1 outlines a number pattern to follow while performing a camelid physical examination. Begin at number 1 and continue sequentially until information from all of the numbered sites has been obtained.

1: Rectal Temperature
Resting rectal temperature is 99.5–102°F (37.5–38.9°C).

Peripheral Pulse
• Pulse is best evaluated in the medial saphenous artery.
• Reference range is 60–90 beats/minute.

2: Respiratory Rate and Character
• Respiratory rate is best evaluated by observation of nostril flaring or auscultation of the trachea in the lower neck. Reference range is 10–30 breaths/minute.
• There is normally a combined thoracic and abdominal effort. However, excessive abdominal effort should be considered a sign of respiratory distress, as is increased nostril flaring and open-mouthed breathing.

3: Examination of the Head
• Oral mucosa and conjunctiva are normally pink and moist. Capillary refill time is <2 seconds.
• The facial skin and ears are normally free of hyperkeratosis, crusting, erythema, or dermatitis. Attention should also be paid to the mucocutaneous junctions.
• Alignment of the jaw is examined by inspection. Maxillary jaw distortion known as wry face is thought to have a genetic origin.
• On oral inspection, the lower incisors should be in contact with the anterior margin of the dental pad. Superior and inferior

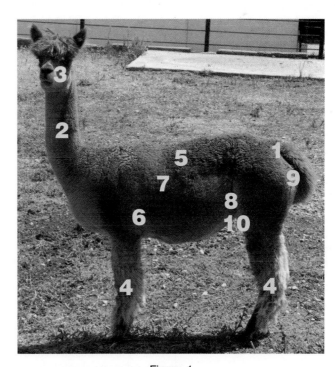

Figure 1.

Camelid. With animal restrained, follow numbers for methodical order of examination. (Also availalbe in color at www.fiveminutevet.com/ruminant)

brachygnathism with an under- or overshot, respectively, of more than 3 mm leads to uneven wear of teeth and the need for dental care treatment.
• The mouth is inspected for missing or broken teeth. Palpation and inspection of the jaws and retropharyngeal space may help identify bony masses, abscesses, or enlarged salivary glands or lymph nodes.
• Nares have clear moistness and uniform bilateral air flow. Presence of dryness, mucus purulent or bloody discharge, as well as alterations in air flow are abnormal.
• External evaluation of ears may reveal lacerations, frostbite injury, and alopecia. Animals with ear problems may show head tilt, ear droop, or neurologic signs.
• Otoscopic examination is difficult due to the anatomy of camelid ears. Abnormal findings include foreign bodies and ticks. Observation of the tympanic membrane is not always possible.
• Eyelids are usually pigmented and are inspected for abnormalities such as entropion or ectropion. Tearing may be associated with blocked tear ducts.
• The cornea is inspected for presence of opacity, scarring, or ulcers. Vision can be determined by observing obstacle avoidance on the lead, menace response, and the animal's ability to track moving objects.
• Direct and consensual pupillary light reflexes are normally sluggish. Eye position is evaluated in a neutral position and a few abnormal positions of the head.
• Facial sensation and motor function are evaluated by probing the face, assessing the palpebral reflex, and observing the position and symmetry of lips, nostrils and ears.
• Food can be offered to evaluate mastication and deglutition.
• The neck should be palpated and passively flexed to evaluate mobility, pain, and palpable abnormalities.

4: Examination of the Limbs
• The nails are non-weight-bearing and wear with exercise on rough surfaces. Excessively long or curled toenails can lead to permanent alteration in growth or damage to tendons and ligaments, and require trimming.
• The interdigital skin is inspected for signs of mange or dermatitis.
• Foot pads are normally free of cracks, ulcers, or lesions.

5: Examination of the Skin and Fiber
• In general, there is a coverage with long, dense fiber over the back and flanks, dorsum of the tail, neck and proximolateral limbs. Alpacas also have long fleece over the crown of the head.
• Fiber needs to be parted for evaluation of skin in fleece-covered areas of the body. Presence of scaling, crustiness, and ectoparasites should be noted.

• Fiber normally does not come out with pulling. Matted fiber that comes out in clumps is abnormal.
• Lumpy lesions on the back and neck may be due to abscesses (*Corynebacterium pseudotuberculosis*) or furunculosis.

6: Examination of the Heart
• Cardiac auscultation can be done in the short-fleeced axillary area. On the left side, the pulmonic valve can be best heard over the third intercostal space under the triceps brachii. The aortic valve is found more dorsally at the fourth intercostal space, and the mitral valve more ventrally at the chondrocostal junction at the fourth or fifth intercostal space. On the right, the tricuspid valve is best heard over the fourth intercostal space caudal to the triceps brachii (see Figure 1, No. 6).
• The valve areas are palpated for presence of thrill.
• Normal heart rate is 60–90 bpm in adults and 90–120 bpm in neonates.
• First and second heart sounds are normally heard, as well as physiologic murmurs. Loud third and fourth sounds or systolic murmurs are abnormal.

7: Examination of the Lungs
The lung field is delimited by the caudal border of the triceps muscle, a line extending 20–25 cm caudally, and triangling back to the olecranon. Fiber must be parted to allow proper auscultation of the entire lung field.

8: Examination of the Abdomen
• Gastric motility can be auscultated in the fiberless area in front of the left stifle. Normal motility is 3–5 movements/minute.
• Intestinal borborygmus can be evaluated in the fiberless area in front of the right stifle.
• Abdominal contour is inspected for signs of distension or ventral edema.
• Normal feces are well-formed pellets. Loose stools may be temporarily present because of anxiety, change in diet or green pastures, but persistently loose or watery stools are abnormal.

9: Examination of the Reproductive Tract
• The nonpendulous scrotum is located in the perineal area (Figure 1, No. 9). Inspection may reveal skin lesions, lacerations, dermatitis, enlargement, or asymmetry. Heat or pain are abnormal.
• Two testicles are present within the scrotum. Testicles are ovoid in shape, symmetric, painless, freely movable within the scrotum, and resilient and painless on palpation.
• The epididymis is palpated. The head is normally bigger than the tail in camelids.
• The tip of the prepuce is directed caudally in nonaroused camelids. The skin and prepucial orifice should be free of lesions.
• A sigmoid flexure is present cranial to the scrotum. The penis and sigmoid flexure can be palpated transcutaneously for presence of

masses or abnormalities. Exteriorization of the penis by manual manipulation requires general anesthesia or heavy sedation.
• In the female, the vulva is observed for conformation, size, lesions, lacerations, swelling, or discharge. Vulvar discharge may be seen during the first week postpartum but it is otherwise considered abnormal in camelids.
• Digital vaginal examination and vaginoscopic examination are performed using aseptic technique to identify vaginal or cervical lacerations, inflammation, or adhesions.

10: Examination of the Mammary Glands
The mammary gland possesses four teats. Camelids are reluctant to allow palpation of the mammary glands, but they should be nonpainful, symmetric, and free of lesions.

GENETICS
N/A

CAUSES AND RISK FACTORS
N/A

DIAGNOSIS
DIFFERENTIAL DIAGNOSES
N/A

CBC/BIOCHEMISTRY/URINALYSIS
N/A

OTHER LABORATORY TESTS
N/A

IMAGING
N/A

OTHER DIAGNOSTIC PROCEDURES
Additional diagnostic tests and imaging may be indicated depending on the findings of the physical examination.

PATHOLOGIC FINDINGS
N/A

TREATMENT
THERAPEUTIC APPROACH
N/A

SURGICAL CONSIDERATIONS AND TECHNIQUES
N/A

MEDICATIONS
DRUG(S) OF CHOICE
• Chemical restraint may be necessary to complete the physical examination.
• Butorphanol 0.5–0.1 mg/kg IV or IM
• Xylazine 0.1–0.2 mg/kg IV or IM

CONTRAINDICATIONS
Appropriate milk and meat withdrawal times must be followed for all compounds administered to food-producing animals.

PRECAUTIONS
Use of chemical restraint will affect evaluation of cardiovascular status and other physical parameters.

POSSIBLE INTERACTIONS
N/A

FOLLOW-UP
EXPECTED COURSE AND PROGNOSIS
N/A
POSSIBLE COMPLICATIONS
N/A
CLIENT EDUCATION
• Clients should be instructed to conduct BCS periodically.
• Client should be observant of any changes in demeanor or behavior which often are the first warning signs of sickness.
PATIENT MONITORING
N/A
PREVENTION
N/A

MISCELLANEOUS
ASSOCIATED CONDITIONS
N/A
AGE-RELATED FACTORS
Age-specific reference ranges should be used for interpretation of findings.

ZOONOTIC POTENTIAL
N/A
PREGNANCY
N/A
BIOSECURITY
N/A
PRODUCTION MANAGEMENT
N/A
SYNONYMS
N/A
ABBREVIATIONS
• BCS = body condition scoring
• IM = intramuscular
• IV = intravenous
SEE ALSO
• Body Condition Scoring: Alpacas and Llamas (see www.fiveminutevet.com/ruminant)
• Breeding Soundness Examination: Camelid
• Camelid: Dentistry
• Camelid: Dermatology
• Camelid: Gastrointestinal Disease
• Camelid: Heat Stress
• Camelid Parasitology
• Camelid: Reproduction
• Colic: Camelid
• Congenital Defects: Camelid
• Down Camelid
• Lameness: Camelid
• Mastitis: Camelid
• Neonatology: Camelid
• Nutrition and Metabolic Diseases: Camelid (see www.fiveminutevet.com/ruminant)
• Parasitic Skin Diseases: Camelid
• Respiratory Disease: Camelid
• Weight Loss: Camelid

Suggested Reading
Bedenice D. Approach to the critically ill camelid. Vet Clin North Am Food Anim Pract 2009, 25: 407–21.
Johnson LW. Physical examination and conformation. In: Cebra C, Anderson DE, Tibary A, Van Saun RJ, Johnson LW eds, Llama and Alpaca Care: Medicine, Surgery, Reproduction, Nutrition, and Herd Health, 1st ed. St. Louis: Elsevier, 2014.
Author Maria Soledad Ferrer
Consulting Editor Ahmed Tibary

APPENDIX 6: PHYSICAL EXAMINATION: SMALL RUMINANT

BASICS

OVERVIEW

• Physical examination entails systematic evaluation of an animal's body. In small ruminants the procedure is generally performed from anterior to posterior and dorsal to ventral and includes auscultation of the heart and lungs. Additionally, activity/behavior (e.g., lethargy, seizures), anatomy (e.g., body condition score, tumors, lacerations, fractures), and indicators of systemic physiology (e.g., increased respiration, heart rate, temperature) are assessed.

• The physical examination identifies abnormalities that, along with the history, allow formulation of appropriate differential diagnoses. Diagnostic tests may then be selected and performed to gain more information and to refine the list of possible differential diagnoses.

• The development of a problem list, differential diagnosis list, and working or final diagnosis is intimately linked with successful physical examination. Prevention, treatment, and management options can then be methodically developed.

• The detection of disease, and the organ systems affected, occurs during the examination procedure. There are three types of examination: comprehensive, screening, and emergency or limited examination.

• A complete, thorough examination is not time-consuming or expensive, and is essential to formulate a complete and accurate diagnosis.

INCIDENCE/PREVALENCE
N/A

GEOGRAPHIC DISTRIBUTION
Worldwide

SYSTEMS AFFECTED
Multisystemic

PATHOPHYSIOLOGY
N/A

HISTORICAL FINDINGS
N/A

SIGNALMENT
Sheep and goats of all ages and genders

GENETICS
N/A

HISTORICAL FINDINGS

Prior to beginning the clinical examination, retrieve information regarding the presenting problem(s), the signalment (age, sex, production group), history of the animal(s) affected, and other relevant information. The history should encompass the type, onset, and duration of clinical signs, and epidemiologic data such as the number of affected animals and the distribution of disease in the flock or herd.

PHYSICAL EXAMINATION FINDINGS

• Sheep and goats are generally alert and somewhat flighty, with a strong desire to run away from the observer. This normal behavior allows one to compare sick animals with healthy ones. Sick animals will closely follow the flock or herd movements to the best of their ability but may lag or be completely unable to keep up.

• Observe the patient to evaluate locomotion, mentation, breathing, urination, and defecation behavior. For a successful assessment of the patient's health, it is vital to use information from both the history and physical examination.

• Accurate information is best obtained via a specific pattern performed on a properly restrained animal that is calm. Figures 1 and 2 outline a number pattern to follow while performing a small ruminant physical examination. Begin at number 1 and continue sequentially until information from all of the numbered sites has been obtained.

Number 1: Rectal Temperature

• Normal range 101.5–104°F (38.6–40°C), and can be as high as 104.5°F (40.3°C) in fully fleeced animals on hot days.

• Neonates suffering from hypothermia/hypoglycemia will often have a rectal temperature below 90°F (32.2°C).

• Temperatures can be compared to normal flock or herd mates to determine the impact of ambient conditions.

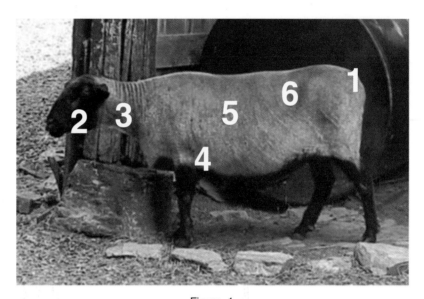

Figure 1.

Left side. (Also availalbe in color at www.fiveminutevet.com/ruminant)

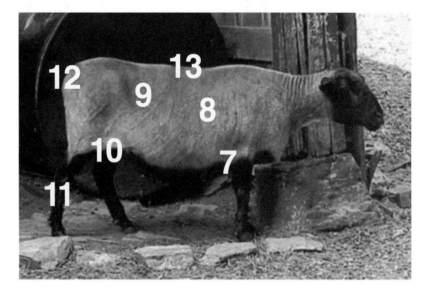

Figure 2.

Right side. (Also availalbe in color at www.fiveminutevet.com/ruminant)

Number 2: Examination of the Head

• Mucus membrane color can be assessed from the conjunctiva, gums, or vulva. In animals with pigmented oral mucosa, the bulbar or palpebral conjunctiva is often superior. Applying pressure to the dorsal globe to expose the third eyelid allows for good visualization.

• Pale to white coloration is suggestive of anemia which in small ruminants is often compatible with haemonchosis. A yellow to light brown color is suggestive of hemolysis which can occur in sheep with copper toxicosis or other toxicities. Large, congested vessels in the bulbar conjunctiva can indicate toxemia.

• Ulcerative or proliferative lesions of the gums, lips, or skin near the mucus membrane junction is often associated with contagious ecthyma (orf) or bluetongue virus infection.

• The eyes are normally centrally positioned in the orbit with a strong pupillary light reflex and menace response. The lids should be examined for symmetry, position, and size. The bulbar and palpebral conjunctiva should be evaluated for color and secretions. The lack of a menace response with an intact pupillary light reflex is common with polioencephalomalacia, and is often accompanied by characteristic dorsomedial strabismus of the eye. The presence of a watery or mucopurulent ocular discharge may indicate conjunctivitis, which could be due to trauma or infection.

• Asymmetry of the face, with flaccid paralysis of the ear, eyelid, muzzle, cheek, and/or nostrils on one side of the head represents unilateral cranial nerve damage. When combined with excessive drooling and/or tongue protrusion, listeriosis is suspected. Trauma can also cause various degrees of asymmetry.

• It is normal for small ruminants to have bilateral clear-to-serous nasal discharge. Animals suffering from respiratory disease may have mucopurulent discharge or a buildup of crusty material due to failure to clean their nose. In sheep, a unilateral discharge could indicate infection with *Oestrus ovis* (nasal bot).

• Abscesses, salivary gland mucoceles, or impacted cud can produce swelling in the cheek area. A firm swelling involving the mandible can indicate actinobacillosis in sheep.

• Teeth should be thoroughly evaluated with a good oral cavity examination, which may require a mouth gag and light source for the posterior oral cavity. Broken and worn teeth are commonly seen in older, thin ewes (broken mouth).

• Severe gastrointestinal parasitism may cause an accumulation of fluid in the submandibular space ("bottle jaw") as well as pale mucus membranes.

• Caseous lymphadenitis caused by *Corynebacterium pseudotuberculosis* often infects lymph nodes and produces focal, firm, round nodules caudal to the ramus of the mandible or ventral to the mandible.

• Breath can smell foul with necrotic stomatitis, pharyngitis, or pneumonia; acetone odor or a chemical smell to the breath is typical of ketoacidosis (ketosis), which is associated with pregnancy toxemia in sheep. The presence of a rumen smell to the breath or visualization of vomitus at the mouth is often associated with toxic plant ingestion. Rhododendrons and azaleas are common plants in the United States and ingestion of these plants by small ruminants causes vomiting as a prominent clinical sign.

Number 3: Examination of the Neck

• Abnormalities such as goiter or abscesses can produce swellings of the neck.

• Also, the thymus gland appears as a soft, distinct swelling in the upper neck region of young goats.

• Nonpainful, round, fluctuant swellings that form at the base of a wattle are cysts. They are benign and can be surgically removed.

• Large, round, firm swellings in the upper neck and along the jugular furrow may indicate lymph node abscessation, most commonly associated with caseous lymphadenitis.

Number 4: Examination of the Heart

• Normal heart rate is 70–90 beats/minute. The heart is easily ausculted on the left side over the 4th to 5th intercostal spaces. The heart rate is most likely to elevate during times of stress, excitement, pain, and toxemia.

• Congenital heart disease, endocarditis, or intrathoracic masses such as abscesses or thymomas can result in murmurs. Anemia can also cause cardiac murmurs associated with reduced blood viscosity.

• Muffled heart sounds are also associated with intrathoracic masses and pericardial effusion. Congestive heart failure is very rare in the small ruminant.

Number 5: Examination of the Lungs

• Normal respiration rate is 12–20 breaths/minute, and can elevate to as high as 60 breaths/minute on hot days. Respiratory rate and effort should be determined at rest and after exertion when signs of lower respiratory tract disease (coughing and open-mouth breathing) may become evident.

• Auscultation of the lungs of small ruminants is difficult due to their small lung field and normally harsh bronchovesicular sounds. It is important to listen cranially and ventrally to the lungs because involvement of this region with lower respiratory disease is common.

• Short, shallow breathing is often overlooked but may indicate pleural pain, even in the presence of normal lung sounds.

• Tracheal palpation that elicits a cough may indicate tracheitis, bronchitis, or a combination of the two.

• Other diagnostic procedures including thoracic radiography, ultrasonography, computed tomography and transtracheal wash are easily performed in the small ruminant.

• Elevated rectal temperature, high respiratory rate, nasal discharge, and the presence of a cough often accompany respiratory disease.

Number 6: Examination of the Left Abdomen

• The normal rate of rumen contraction is 1–2 contractions/minute, which can be ausculted over the left paralumbar area. It is important to also determine the strength of contraction during auscultation. A strong, healthy contraction will push outward against the hand when ausculting.

• Ballotment of the normal rumen will reveal a soft, gas-filled indentible area dorsally with a more firm, ingesta-filled doughy area ventrally.

• Small ruminants spend several hours a day ruminating (chewing cud).

• A distended abdomen may indicate bloat, advanced pregnancy, or peritonitis, but some breeds such as the pygmy goat always appear very round.

• Evaluate the hair or wool near the perineum for fecal material, which could indicate a digestive disturbance such as diarrhea.

Number 7: Examination of the Heart (Right Side)

• The heart should be ausculted on the right side over the 4th to 5th intercostal spaces as described above in No. 4.

Number 8: Examination of the Lungs (Right Side)

The lungs should be ausculted on the right side as described in No. 5.

Number 9: Examination of the Right Abdomen

• Auscultation of the right abdomen is mainly done in neonates to assess borborygmi (gut sounds).

• The absence of gut sounds in an anorexic animal with a distended abdomen warrants further diagnostics.

Number 10: Examination of the Udder or Testes

• Udder
  ◦ Visual examination should note shape, color, symmetry, and contour. Blue discoloration is often indicative of gangrenous mastitis due to *Staphylococcus aureus*. Red discoloration is often indicative of toxic mastitis due to coliform bacteria or trauma. These diseases of the mammary gland also cause swelling and therefore create asymmetry.
  ◦ Manual examination should note firmness, tenderness, and fibrosis. Most cases of mastitis will produce these findings. However, in sheep, a diffusely firm udder with minimal milk secretion and no pain noted immediately after lambing could be due to ovine progressive pneumonia (OPP).

In goats, a similar finding of the udder may be due to caprine arthritis encephalitis (CAE).

° Milk examination using a strip plate should note discoloration, consistency, and the presence of clots or clumps. The use of the California Mastitis Test (CMT) will help identify animals with subclinical mastitis. Small ruminants normally have higher cellular contents in their milk secretions than cattle; therefore, careful interpretation of this test is necessary. A trace to plus 1 is considered normal. A milk culture is indicated when mastitis is identified.

° Ulcerated lesions with scabs may be seen near the teat orifice in animals suffering from contagious ecthyma (orf).

° An enlarged mammary gland in a nonlactating small ruminant is known as a precocious udder and can be considered common in high-producing small ruminants.

° Male goats (bucks) may have overdeveloped mammary glands. This abnormality is referred to as gynecomastia.

• Testes

° A breeding soundness examination (BSE) should be performed on all rams or bucks that will be used for breeding stock.

° The testes and epididymis should be palpated, taking note of size, shape, freedom of movement, and consistency. An abnormal size and shape could indicate epididymitis, orchitis, or hypoplasia. A lack of movement within the scrotum could indicate adhesions and a soft consistency to the testes could indicate poor sperm production.

Number 11: Examination of the Feet and Legs

• Care must be taken to differentiate primary musculoskeletal problems from secondary problems that include neurologic, metabolic, or infectious disease. Small ruminants with pain associated with a mammary gland infection may present as lame due to limb contact with the enlarged gland. Also, excited animals may appear sound, so care should be taken as to when the animals are examined.

• Overgrown toes, a common problem in small ruminants, are easily corrected by regular trimming.

• Interdigital infection with *Dichelobacter nodosus* causes a characteristic foul odor and symmetric swelling that may lead to severe necrosis and underrunning of the hoof horn, i.e., "foot rot." These animals are very painful and because multiple feet are involved, they are often seen walking on their knees.

• Hoof testers can be used to identify foot abscesses. Affected animals are typically lame in only one foot.

• Joints should be palpated for swelling, pain, and decreased range of motion, which is indicative of septic arthritis. Septic joints are generally very painful.

• In goats, enlarged, painful joints, specifically the carpal joints, are indicative of caprine arthritis encephalitis (CAE).

• Lambs and kids that have stiff limbs and that are unwilling to rise and walk may be suffering from white muscle disease (nutritional myodegeneration).

• Injury to the spinal cord via trauma or parasitic migration of *Parelaphostrongylus tenuis* can result in paresis or paralysis.

Number 12: Examination of the Urogenital Tract

• Occluding the nostrils for a brief period of time induces urination in sheep. This should not be performed in extremely sick animals. In goats, there is no specific trick to induce urination. However, most small ruminants will urinate at some point during physical examination so a container should be kept in close proximity.

• The presence of ketone bodies in the urine is indicative of a negative energy balance often seen in sheep with pregnancy toxemia.

• Straining to urinate with vocalization is commonly seen in male small ruminants suffering from obstructive urolithiasis.

Number 13: Examination of the Integument

• Initially observe the patient from a distance to gain an impression of skin, hair, or wool abnormalities and their distribution. Next, examine the coat for alopecia or color change. The skin should also be examined for color, elasticity, and lesions.

• Ectoparasites such as biting and sucking lice are common in small ruminants and their presence may result in pruritus with skin excoriation.

• Goats with demodectic mange present with nodules that exude a thick, white material. These nodules are typically present over the neck and back.

• Patches of loose or missing wool in sheep, known as "wool break," are often associated with systemic illness or nutritional stress.

MISCELLANEOUS

ASSOCIATED CONDITIONS
N/A

AGE-RELATED FACTORS
N/A

ZOONOTIC POTENTIAL
N/A

PREGNANCY
N/A

BIOSECURITY
N/A

PRODUCTION MANAGEMENT
N/A

SYNONYMS
N/A

SEE ALSO
• Body Condition Scoring: Goats (see www.fiveminutevet.com/ruminant)
• Body Condition Scoring: Sheep (see www.fiveminutevet.com/ruminant)
• Caprine Arthritis Encephalitis
• Maedi-Visna (Ovine Progressive Pneumonia)
• Nutrition and Metabolic Diseases: Small Ruminant

ABBREVIATIONS
• BCS = body condition score
• BSE = breeding soundness examination
• CAE = caprine arthritis-encephalitis
• CMT = California Mastitis Test
• OPP = ovine progressive pneumonia

Suggested Reading

Anderson DE, Whitehead CE. Alpaca and llama health management. Vet Clin North Am Food Anim Pract 2009, 25(2).

Ballweber LR. Ruminant parasitology. Vet Clin North Am Food Anim Pract 2006, 22(3).

Coetzee J, Smith RA. Pain management. Vet Clin North Am Food Anim Pract 2013, 29(1).

Constable PD. Ruminant neurologic diseases. Vet Clin North Am Food Anim Pract 2004, 20(2).

Fagan DA. Diagnosis and treatment planning. Vet Clin North Am Small Anim Pract 1986, 16: 785–99.

Fthenakis GC, Menzies PI. Therapeutics and control of sheep and goat diseases. Vet Clin North Am Food Anim Pract 2011, 27(1).

Jackson P, Cockcroft P. Clinical Examination of Farm Animals. Oxford, UK: Blackwell Publishing, 2002.

Ketner G, Van Camp SD. Assessment of the reproductive system of the female ruminant. Vet Clin North Am Food Anim Pract 1992, 8: 317–30.

Pringle JK. Assessment of the Ruminant respiratory system. Vet Clin North Am Food Anim Pract 1992, 8: 233–42.

Pugh DG. Sheep and Goat Medicine. Philadelphia: Saunders, 2002.

Roussel AJ, Smith GW, Smith RA. Fluid and electrolyte therapy. Vet Clin North Am Food Anim Pract 2014, 30(2).

Sherman DM, Robinson RA. Clinical examination of sheep and goats. Vet Clin North Am Large Anim Pract 1983, 5: 409–26.

Wilson JH. Physical examination. The Veterinary Clinics of North America. Philadelphia: Saunders, 1992.

Van Metre DC. Update on small ruminant medicine. Vet Clin North Am Food Anim Pract 2001, 17(2).

Author Billy I. Smith
Consulting Editor Erica C. McKenzie

INDEX

Notes: Text in **boldface** denotes topic discussions. Topics marked as "*website*" can be found on the companion website at www.fiveminutevet.com/ruminant rather than in the printed book.